W9-AGK-376

for Instructors

INSTRUCTOR'S ELECTRONIC RESOURCE

Available in CD and online formats, this useful instructor's package provides all of the tools needed to quickly and consistently develop lectures and student assignments and evaluate student comprehension. The Instructor's Manual includes chapter outlines and teaching strategies, activities for students, case studies, and curriculum guides for courses of various lengths. The ExamView Test Bank contains questions in NCLEX® format, including new alternate format questions, and an answer key with page references to the text, rationales, and NCLEX® coding. Also included are a full-color Image Collection, PowerPoint Lecture Slides for building presentations and developing lectures, and answer guidelines for the Critical Thinking Exercises included in the text.

EVOLVE COURSE MANAGEMENT SYSTEM

http://evolve.elsevier.com/Lowdermilk/MWHC/

Evolve is an interactive teaching and learning environment that works in coordination with *Maternity & Women's Health Care, 9th edition,* providing Internet-based course content that reinforces and expands on the concepts that instructors deliver in class. In addition to the resources available to students, instructors are able to access all of the components of the Instructor's Electronic Resource, including the computerized test bank and PowerPoint slides. Instructors can also use Evolve to: publish class syllabi, outline, and lecture notes; set up "virtual office hours" and email communication; share important dates and information through the online class calendar; and encourage student participation through chat rooms and discussion boards. Instructors are encouraged to contact their sales representative for more information about integrating Evolve into their curriculum.

EVOLVE SELECT

http://evolveselect.elsevier.com

Evolve Select is a unique and innovative new learning tool that revolutionizes the way instructors teach and students study and learn. It provides electronic access to leading Elsevier nursing books, including *Maternity & Women's Health Care, 9th edition,* together in one resource. Students can electronically search, highlight, and notate within an individual book or across multiple books, providing a fully electronic nursing curriculum. With Evolve Select, your students spend less time searching and more time learning!

Contents

Companion CD Contents

From patient preparation through documentation, learn maternity nursing skills from the inside out!

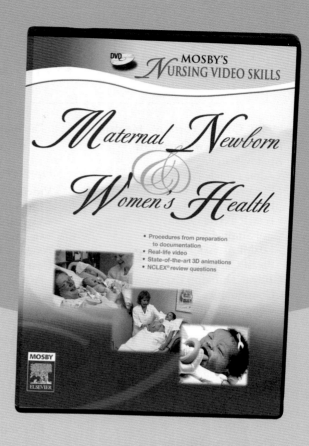

Mosby's Nursing Video Skills DVD: Maternal-Newborn & Women's Health

See how easy and convenient it can be to learn essential maternity nursing skills! This interactive DVD presents 23 of the most common procedures used to care for today's maternity, neonatal and women's health patients. Coverage includes essential procedures such as gestational assessment, fundal height, fetal heart tones, Leopold's maneuvers, postpartum assessment, newborn reflexes, and more.

November 2006 • ISBN: 0-323-04569-3
ISBN-13: 978-0-323-04569-8

Watch and learn essential maternity nursing skills — each procedure includes:

- ✔ **A step-by-step skills video** that shows you exactly how to perform key maternity, neonatal, and women's health procedures.
- ✔ **Dynamic 3-D animations** that simplify difficult concepts by helping you visualize what's happening inside the body.
- ✔ **Preparation steps** that outline essential equipment and patient instructions.
- ✔ **Step-by-step checklists** that can be printed to use as portable quick-reference sheets.
- ✔ **Follow-up care** coverage that includes essential nursing interventions and patient education.
- ✔ **Documentation guidelines** that highlight information needed to accurately, safely, and legally complete procedures.
- ✔ **NCLEX® examination-style review questions** that reinforce your understanding of key concepts.

Get your copy today!

Order securely at **www.elsevierhealth.com** | Call toll-free **1-800-545-2522** | Visit your **local bookstore**

NM-06205

edition **9**

Maternity & Women's Health Care

Deitra Leonard Lowdermilk
RNC, PhD, FAAN

Clinical Professor Emerita, School of Nursing
University of North Carolina at Chapel Hill
Chapel Hill, North Carolina

Shannon E. Perry
RN, CNS, PhD, FAAN

Professor Emerita, School of Nursing
San Francisco State University
San Francisco, California

MOSBY
ELSEVIER

MOSBY
ELSEVIER

11830 Westline Industrial Drive
St. Louis, Missouri 63146

MATERNITY & WOMEN'S HEALTH CARE, NINTH EDITION   ISBN: 978-0-323-04367-0
Copyright © 2007, 2004, 2000, 1997, 1993, 1989, 1985, 1981, 1977 by Mosby, Inc., an affiliate of Elsevier Inc.

All rights reserved. No part of this publication may be reproduced or transmitted in any form or by any means, electronic or mechanical, including photocopying, recording, or any information storage and retrieval system, without permission in writing from the publisher. Permissions may be sought directly from Elsevier's Health Sciences Rights Department in Philadelphia, PA, USA: Phone: (+1) 215 239 3804, fax: (+1) 215 239 3805, e-mail: healthpermissions@elsevier.com. You may also complete your request online via the Elsevier homepage (http://www.elsevier.com), by selecting "Customer Support" and then "Obtaining Permissions."

Notice

Knowledge and best practice in this field are constantly changing. As new research and experience broaden our knowledge, changes in practice, treatment, and drug therapy may become necessary or appropriate. Readers are advised to check the most current information provided (i) on procedures featured or (ii) by the manufacturer of each product to be administered, to verify the recommended dose or formula, the method and duration of administration, and contraindications. It is the responsibility of the practitioner, relying on his or her own experience and knowledge of the patient, to make diagnoses, to determine dosages and the best treatment for each individual patient, and to take all appropriate safety precautions. To the fullest extent of the law, neither the Publisher nor the Authors assume any liability for any injury and/or damage to persons or property arising from or related to any use of the material contained in this book.

Library of Congress Cataloging-in-Publication Data
Maternity & women's health care / [edited by] Deitra Leonard Lowdermilk, Shannon E.
Perry. — 9th ed.
    p. cm.
  Includes bibliographical references and index.
  ISBN-13: 978-0-323-04367-0
  ISBN-10: 0-323-04367-4
  1. Maternity nursing. 2. Gynecologic nursing. 3. Women's health services. I.
Lowdermilk, Deitra Leonard. II. Perry, Shannon E. III. Title: Maternity and women's
health care.

RG951.M318 2007
618.2'0231—dc22

2006046937

Acquisitions Editor: Catherine Jackson
Senior Developmental Editor: Laurie K. Gower
Publishing Services Manager: Jeff Patterson
Senior Project Manager: Anne Konopka
Design Direction: Amy Buxton

Printed in China
Last digit is the print number: 9 8 7 6 5 4 3 2

**Working together to grow
libraries in developing countries**

www.elsevier.com | www.bookaid.org | www.sabre.org

ELSEVIER | BOOK AID International | Sabre Foundation

About the Authors

Deitra Lowdermilk is Clinical Professor Emerita, School of Nursing, University of North Carolina at Chapel Hill (UNC CH). She received her BSN from East Carolina University and her MEd (and minor in Obstetric Nursing) and PhD in Education from UNC CH. She is certified in In-Patient Obstetrics by the National Certification Corporation (NCC). She is a Fellow in the American Academy of Nursing. In addition to being a nurse educator for over 34 years, Dr. Lowdermilk has clinical experience as a public health nurse and as a staff nurse in labor and delivery, postpartum, and newborn units, and has worked in gynecologic surgery and cancer care units. Dr. Lowdermilk continues to teach undergraduate maternal-newborn theory and clinical experiences for the 24- and 14-month BSN program options at UNC CH.

Dr. Lowdermilk has been recognized for her expertise in nursing education. She has repeatedly been selected as Classroom and Clinical Teacher of the Year by graduating seniors. She was a recipient of the Educator of the Year Award from both the District IV Association of Women's Health, Obstetric and Neonatal Nurses (AWHONN) and the North Carolina Nurses Association. She also received the 2005 AWHONN Excellence in Education Award.

She is active in AWHONN, having served as Chair of the North Carolina Section of AWHONN and has served as chair and member of various committees in AWHONN at the national, district, state, and local levels. She has served as guest editor for the *Journal of Obstetric, Gynecologic, and Neonatal Nursing (JOGNN)* and served on editorial boards for other publications. She has been a board member and officer for other nursing organizations in North Carolina.

Dr. Lowdermilk's most significant contribution to nursing has been to promote excellence in nursing practice and education in women's health through integration of knowledge into practice. She has published extensively in nursing texts, served as associate editor for two texts, including *Maternal Child Nursing Care,* third edition, and is co-author of *Maternity Nursing,* seventh edition. She has published articles in refereed journals and made invited presentations nationally and internationally. She has published computer-assisted instruction programs, one of which received a Media Award for Excellence in Nursing Journalism from Sigma Theta Tau International, as well as presented continuing education programs. She has also served as a consultant to nursing schools in the United States, Australia, Thailand, and Taiwan. In 2005 she received the first Distinguished Alumni Award from East Carolina University School of Nursing for her exemplary contributions to the nursing profession in the area of maternal-child care and the community.

Shannon Perry is Professor Emerita, School of Nursing, San Francisco State University. She received her diploma in nursing from St. Joseph Hospital School of Nursing, Bloomington, Illinois; a Baccalaureate in Nursing from Marquette University, Milwaukee, Wisconsin; an MSN in Maternal-Child Nursing from the University of Colorado Medical Center, Denver, Colorado; and a PhD in Educational Psychology with a specialization in child development from Arizona State University, Tempe, Arizona. She completed a 2-year postdoctoral fellowship in perinatal nursing at the University of California, San Francisco, as a Robert Wood Johnson Clinical Nurse Scholar.

Dr. Perry has had clinical experience as a staff nurse, head nurse, and supervisor in surgical nursing, obstetrics, pediatrics, gynecology, and neonatal nursing. She has taught nursing in schools of nursing in several states. She is a Fellow in the American Academy of Nursing, has been an officer or board member in a number of professional organizations, recently completed a 2-year term on the National League for Nursing Board of Governors, and is nursing consultant to the International Education Research Foundation. She is interested in international nursing and has traveled extensively, learning about nursing and health care in various countries, and she has taught international nursing courses for which she traveled with nursing students to the United Kingdom, Italy, Thailand, Ghana, and China.

Her current research interests include the history of nursing and evidence-based practice. She has published widely on perinatal topics and on the nurse as an expert witness. Dr. Perry is also co-author of two other successful Elsevier titles: *Maternity Nursing,* seventh edition, and *Maternal Child Nursing Care,* third edition.

Contributors

Kathryn R. Alden, RN, MSN, IBCLC
Clinical Assistant Professor, School of Nursing
University of North Carolina at Chapel Hill
Chapel Hill, North Carolina

Debbie Fraser Askin, MN, RNC
Associate Professor, Neonatal Nurse Practitioner
University of Manitoba
Winnipeg, Manitoba, Canada

Bonnie Callen, PhD, RN
Assistant Professor, College of Nursing
University of Tennessee, Knoxville
Knoxville, Tennessee

Kitty Cashion, RN, BC, MSN
Clinical Nurse Specialist
Department of Obstetrics and Gynecology
Division of Maternal-Fetal Medicine
University of Tennessee Health Science Center
Memphis, Tennessee

Robin Webb Corbett, PhD, RN, C
Associate Professor, School of Nursing
East Carolina University
Greenville, North Carolina

Gayle Tart Davis, BSN, MSN, EdD, CPNP
Associate Professor, School of Nursing
University of North Carolina at Chapel Hill
Chapel Hill, North Carolina

Dusty Dix, RN, MSN
Clinical Instructor, School of Nursing
University of North Carolina at Chapel Hill
Chapel Hill, North Carolina

Karen Dorman, RN, MS
Research Instructor, School of Medicine
University of North Carolina at Chapel Hill
Chapel Hill, North Carolina

Susan M. Ellerbee, RNC, PhD, IBCLC
Associate Professor, College of Nursing
University of Oklahoma
Oklahoma City, Oklahoma

Anne H. Fishel, BSN, MSN, PhD
Professor, School of Nursing
University of North Carolina at Chapel Hill
Chapel Hill, North Carolina

Catherine Ingram Fogel, PhD, RNC (WHCNP), FAAN
Professor, School of Nursing
University of North Carolina at Chapel Hill
Chapel Hill, North Carolina

Cynthia Garrett, MSN, RN, BC
Clinical Systems Analyst
University of North Carolina Health Care
Chapel Hill, North Carolina

S. Kim Genovese, RNC, MSN, MSA
Executive Director
Nursing 2000, Northern Indiana Region
Valparaiso, Indiana

Margaret Wagoner Gilliam, RNC, MSN, CCE
Education Coordinator
Alamance Regional Medical Center
Burlington, North Carolina

Pat Mahaffee Gingrich, RN-C, MSN, WHNP
Clinical Assistant Professor, School of Nursing
University of North Carolina at Chapel Hill
Chapel Hill, North Carolina

†Sharron Humenick, PhD, FAAN
Professor, School of Nursing
Virginia Commonwealth University
Richmond, Virginia

Carole Kenner, DNS, RNC, FAAN
Dean and Professor, College of Nursing
University of Oklahoma Health Sciences Center
Oklahoma City, Oklahoma

Sharon E. Lock, PhD, ARNP
Associate Professor, College of Nursing
University of Kentucky
Lexington, Kentucky

†Deceased

Jane McAteer, RN, BSN, MN
Director of Nursing
San Mateo Community College District
San Mateo, California

Margaret Shandor Miles, BSN, MSN, PhD, FAAN
Professor, School of Nursing
University of North Carolina at Chapel Hill
Chapel Hill, North Carolina

Mary Courtney Moore, MSN, PhD
Research Associate Professor, School of Medicine
Vanderbilt University
Nashville, Tennessee

Maureen A. Nalle, PhD, RN
Assistant Professor, College of Nursing
University of Tennessee, Knoxville
Knoxville, Tennessee

Karen A. Piotrowski, RNC, MSN
Associate Professor of Nursing
D'Youville College
Buffalo, New York

Barbara Rynerson, APRN, BC
Associate Professor Emerita, School of Nursing
University of North Carolina at Chapel Hill
Chapel Hill, North Carolina

Angela Sammarco, PhD, RN
Assistant Professor, Department of Nursing
College of Staten Island
Staten Island, New York

Linda Fowler Shahzad, BSN, MSN, RNC
Clinical Nurse II, Women's Services
University of North Carolina Health Care
Chapel Hill, North Carolina

Susan Speraw, PhD, RN
Associate Professor, College of Nursing
University of Tennessee, Knoxville
Knoxville, Tennessee

Marcia Van Riper, RN, PhD
Associate Professor, School of Nursing
University of North Carolina at Chapel Hill
Chapel Hill, North Carolina

Wendy Wetzel, RN, MSN, FNP, AHN-BC, SANE
Nurse Practitioner, A Woman's Place
Medical Director, Northern Arizona Center Against
    Sexual Assault
Flagstaff, Arizona

Jan Lamarche Zdanuk, MSN, RN, CWS, FNP-BC
Certified Family Nurse Practitioner
Private Practice
Fort Worth, Texas

Reviewers

Johnett Benson-Soros, RN, MSN, CNP
Assistant Professor of Nursing
Kent State University
Ashtabula, Ohio

Carrie L. Davis, RNC, MSN, WHNP
Instructor, School of Nursing
Norfolk State University
Norfolk, Virginia

Marian L. Farrell, PhD, CRNP, CNS, CS
Professor of Nursing
University of Scranton
Scranton, Pennsylvania

Jo Garner, RN, BSN
Clinical Nurse II
UNC Hospitals
Chapel Hill, North Carolina

Jennifer G. Hensley, EdD, RN, MSN, CNM
Assistant Professor, School of Nursing
Director, Midwifery Program
University of Colorado at Denver and Health
   Sciences Center
Denver, Colorado

Helen W. Jones, RN, BSN, MN, PhD
Professor, Nurse Education
Raritan Valley Community College
Somerville, New Jersey

Edward L. Lowdermilk, BS, RPh
Clinical Pharmacist
Piedmont Health Services
Siler City, North Carolina

Deborah A. Redd-Terrell, BSN, MS, CFNP, CS
Associate Professor and Chair, Department of Nursing
Harry S Truman College
Chicago, Illinois

Kathleen Sebrey Schafer, BSN, MSN, RNC, NP
Clinical Associate Professor, Nursing
Purdue University
West Lafayette, Indiana

M. Terese Verklan, PhD, RNC, CCNS
Associate Professor, Neonatal Clinical Nurse Specialist
University of Texas Health Science Center at Houston
Houston, Texas

Gail L. Withers, RN, MSN, ARNP-CNS
Dean of Nursing and Allied Health
Pratt Community College
Pratt Regional Medical Center
Pratt, Kansas

Preface

WOMEN'S health care encompasses reproductive health care and the unique physical, psychologic, and social needs of women throughout their life span. The specialty of women's health and maternity nursing offers both challenges and opportunities. Nurses are challenged to assimilate knowledge and develop the technical and critical thinking skills needed to apply that knowledge to practice. Each woman, with her individual needs that must be identified and met, presents a challenge. However, the opportunities are sufficiently extraordinary to make this one of the most fulfilling specialties of nursing practice.

The goal of nursing education is to prepare today's students to meet the challenges of tomorrow. This preparation must extend beyond mastery of facts and skills. Nurses must be able to combine clinical competence with caring and critical thinking. They must address both the physiologic and the psychosocial needs of their clients. They must look beyond the condition and see the woman as an individual with distinctive needs. Above all, they must strive to improve nursing practice on the basis of sound, evidence-based information. In a time of a nursing shortage and shrinking financial resources for health care, nurses can use evidence-based practice to produce measurable outcomes that can validate their unique and necessary role in the health care delivery system.

Maternity & Women's Health Care was developed to provide students with the knowledge and skills they need to become clinically competent, think critically, and attain the necessary sensitivity to become caring nurses. *Maternity & Women's Health Care* has been a leading maternity nursing text since it was first published in 1977, 30 years ago. We are proud of the continued support this text has received. With this ninth edition, we have a responsibility to continue this leading tradition.

This ninth edition has been revised and refined in response to comments and suggestions from educators, clinicians, and students. It includes the most accurate, current, and clinically relevant information available. We have had the assistance of expert faculty, nurse clinicians, and specialists from other health disciplines who authored, reviewed, and revised the text. Many exciting updates and new additions will be noted throughout the book; they demonstrate the various dimensions of women's health care and areas of rapid and complex changes such as genetics, fetal assessment, and alternative therapies. However, we have retained the underlying philosophy that has been the strength of previous editions: our belief that pregnancy and childbirth and developmental changes in a woman's life are natural processes. We have also retained a strong, integrated focus on the family and on evidence-based practice.

The text is also used as a reference for the practicing nurse. The most recent recommendations based on evidence from research and clinical experts have been included from professional organizations such as the Association for Women's Health, Obstetric, and Neonatal Nurses; the National Association of Neonatal Nurses; the American College of Obstetricians and Gynecologists; the American Academy of Pediatrics; the American Diabetes Association; the Centers for Disease Control and Prevention; and the United States Preventive Health Services Task Force.

Approach

Professional nursing practice continues to evolve and adapt to society's changing health priorities. The ever-changing health care delivery system offers new opportunities for nurses to alter the practice of maternity and women's health nursing and to improve the way care is given. Consumers of maternity and women's health care vary in age, ethnicity, culture, language, social status, marital status, and sexual preference. They seek care with obstetricians, gynecologists, family practice physicians, nurse-midwives, nurse practitioners, and other health care providers in a variety of health care settings, including the home. Increasingly, many are self-treating, using a variety of alternative and complementary therapies.

Nursing education must reflect these changes. Clinical education must be planned to offer students a variety of maternity and women's health care experiences in settings that include hospitals and birth centers, the home health setting, clinics and private physician offices, shelters for the homeless or women in need of protection, prisons, and other community-based settings. The changing needs of nursing students also must be addressed. Today's nursing students are challenged to learn more than ever before and often in less time than their predecessors. Students are diverse. They may be new high school graduates, college students, or older adults with families. They may be male or female. They may have college degrees in other fields and be interested in changing careers. They may represent various cultures; English may not be their primary language.

This ninth edition of *Maternity & Women's Health Care* is designed to provide the most current information for nurses to meet the needs of women during their reproductive years and beyond, as well as to meet the needs of students in all types of nursing programs, including accelerated ones. This edition presents focused content in a clearly written and easily read manner while retaining the comprehensiveness of previous editions.

Health care today emphasizes *wellness*. This focus is an integral part of our philosophy. Likewise, the developmental changes a woman experiences throughout her life are considered natural and normal. In women's health care, the goal is promotion of wellness for the woman through knowledge of her body and its normal functioning throughout her life span, while developing an awareness of conditions that require professional intervention. The unit on women's health care emphasizes the wellness aspect of care but also includes information about common gynecologic problems as well as gynecologic cancers. This unit has been placed before the units on pregnancy because many of the aspects of assessment and care can be applied to later chapters. Pregnancy and childbirth are also part of a natural developmental process. We believe that students need to thoroughly understand and recognize the normal processes before they can identify complications and comprehend their implications for care. We present the entire normal childbearing cycle before discussing potential complications.

Features

The ninth edition features a contemporary design and spacious presentation. Students will find that the logical, easy-to-follow headings and attractive full-color design highlight important content and increase visual appeal. More than 750 color photographs (many of them new) and drawings throughout the text illustrate important concepts and techniques to further enhance comprehension. Each chapter begins with a list of *Learning Objectives* designed to focus students' attention on the important content to be mastered. *Electronic Resources* that can be found on the companion website and/or the interactive companion CD are listed at the beginning of each chapter to provide the student with additional information. *Key Terms* that alert students to new vocabulary are in blue, defined within the chapter, and included in a glossary at the end of the book. Each chapter consistently ends with a **NEW** *Community Activity* and *Key Points*, which summarize important content. All **NEW** *Critical Thinking Exercises* are integrated in each chapter to guide students

in applying their knowledge and increasing their ability to think critically about maternity and women's health care issues. *References* have been updated significantly, with most citations being less than 5 years old and all chapters having citations within 1 year of publication. More of the additional outstanding features follow:

- *Care Management* is used as the consistent framework throughout to discuss collaborative care and specifically nursing care incorporating the five steps of the *Nursing Process*.
- *Plans of Care* help students apply the nursing process in the clinical setting and use NANDA-approved nursing diagnoses, describe expected outcomes for client care, provide rationales for interventions, and include evaluation of care.
- *Care Paths, Protocols, and Procedures* provide students with examples of various approaches to implementation of care.
- *Teaching for Self-Care* boxes emphasize guidelines for the client to practice self-care and provide information to help students transfer learning from the hospital to the home setting.
- *Emergency* boxes alert students to the signs and symptoms of various emergency situations and provide interventions for immediate implementation.
- *Signs of Potential Complications* boxes alert students to signs and symptoms of potential problems and are included in chapters that cover uncomplicated pregnancy and childbirth.
- *Nurse Alerts* highlight critical information for the student.
- *Evidence-Based Practice* is incorporated throughout in **NEW** boxes that integrate findings from several studies on selected clinical practices and changing practice. In addition, research findings summarized in the ***Cochrane Pregnancy and Childbirth Database*** and other resources for evidence-based practices that confirm effective practices or identify practices that have unknown, ineffective, or harmful effects are integrated throughout the text and identified by this icon in the margin.
- *Alternative and Complementary Therapies* are discussed for many women's health and pregnancy-related problems and are identified in the text by this icon in the margin.
- *Cultural Considerations* boxes describe beliefs and practices about pregnancy, childbirth, parenting, and women's health concerns and the importance of understanding cultural variations when providing care.
- *Legal Tips* are integrated throughout to provide students with relevant information to deal with these important areas in the context of maternity and women's health nursing.
- *Medication Guide* boxes include key information about medications used in maternity and women's health care, including their indications, adverse effects, and nursing considerations.

Organization

The ninth edition of *Maternity & Women's Heath Care* comprises eight units organized to enhance understanding and learning and to facilitate easy retrieval of information.

Unit One, Introduction to Maternity & Women's Health Care, begins with an overview of contemporary issues in maternity and women's health nursing practice. Chapter 1 includes a new section on historic milestones in maternity care. It then addresses the community as a unit of care, incorporating family theory, cultural aspects of care, and home care in relation to maternity and women's health nursing. The unit continues with a chapter on genetics that provides essential discussion about genetics in relation to maternity and women's health care. The last chapter in the unit describes alternative and complementary therapies, providing an overview of the important therapies that can be used instead of or in addition to traditional techniques used in maternity and women's health care.

Unit Two, Women's Health, is a significantly revised unit on women's health. Eight chapters discuss health promotion, screening, and physical assessment, and then present common reproductive concerns. The chapter on assessment and health promotion incorporates normal anatomy and physiology of the female reproductive system and integrates health promotion for common women's health problems. There are separate chapters on reproductive problems and concerns, sexually transmitted infections and other infections, contraception and abortion, infertility, violence, problems of the breast, and structural disorders and neoplasms of the female reproductive system.

Unit Three, Pregnancy, describes nursing care of the woman and her family from conception through preparation for childbirth. Nursing care during pregnancy includes both physiologic and psychologic aspects of care. A separate chapter on maternal and fetal nutrition emphasizes the important aspects of care, highlights cultural variations on diet, and stresses the importance of early recognition and management of nutritional problems. The preparation for childbirth chapter includes information on incorporating doula care during pregnancy and labor and birth.

Unit Four, Childbirth, focuses on collaborative care among physicians, nurse-midwives, nurses, and women and their families during the processes of labor and birth. Separate chapters deal with the nurse's role in management of discomfort during labor and childbirth, and fetal monitoring, both of which have been updated significantly. All four chapters familiarize students with current childbirth practices and focus on evidence-based interventions to support and educate the woman and her family.

Unit Five, Postpartum, deals with a time of significant change for the entire family. The mother requires both physical and emotional support as she adjusts to her new role. The chapter on transition to parenthood discusses family dynamics in response to the birth of a child and describes ways nurses can facilitate parent-infant adjustment.

Unit Six, The Newborn, has been updated and addresses physiologic adaptations of the newborn and assessment and care of the newborn. Information on the nutritional needs of the newborn and nursing care associated with breastfeeding and formula feeding are highlighted in a separate chapter. A chapter on care of the newborn at home includes anticipatory guidance for the first few weeks at home and home follow-up care.

Unit Seven, Complications of Pregnancy, discusses the conditions that place the woman, fetus, infant, and family at risk. This unit has been revised and updated and includes a chapter on high risk assessment of pregnancy complications and eight other chapters on hypertensive disorders, antepartal hemorrhagic disorders, endocrine and metabolic problems, medical-surgical problems, obstetric critical care, mental health problems and substance abuse, labor and birth complications, and postpartum complications. Care management focuses on achieving the best possible outcomes, as well as supporting the woman and family when expectations are not met.

Unit Eight, Newborn Complications, addresses the most common acquired conditions of the neonate and hematologic disorders and congenital anomalies. It then describes the nursing care for high risk newborns, emphasizing the care of the preterm infant. All chapters have been revised and updated. This unit addresses the continuing trend of providing care to moderately compromised newborns including near-term and late preterm infants in the newborn nursery. A separate chapter on loss and grief discusses care management of the family experiencing a fetal or neonatal maternal loss.

Teaching and Learning Package

Several ancillaries to this text have been developed to assist instructors and students in the teaching and learning process.

The *Instructor's Resource Manual and Test Bank* are keyed chapter by chapter to the text to help coordinate course objectives to chapter content. Each chapter includes an outline of content with course guidelines, suggested learning activities, and a summary of key concepts. The test bank portion includes more than 975 questions that parallel the NCLEX format. The answer key provides page references and coding of questions according to the NCLEX test plan category of cognitive level.

A *Curriculum Guide* that includes a proposed class schedule and reading assignments for courses of varying lengths is provided. This gives educators suggestions for using the text in the most essential manner or in a more comprehensive way. Also, answers are provided for the Critical Thinking Exercises found in the text.

An *Electronic Image Collection*, another valuable tool for instructors, provides easy access to electronic images from the main textbook. Each image can easily be imported to a slide, transparency, or PowerPoint presentation to enhance lecture materials. *PowerPoint Lecture Slides* for building presentations and developing lectures are also included.

A separate *Student Study Guide* includes chapter review activities and critical thinking exercises to reinforce learning and evaluate comprehension. The Study Guide can be used for homework assignments or for remedial practice. The exercises in the guide were developed to assist students in synthesizing knowledge of maternity and women's health care and to foster critical thinking.

A new *Clinical Companion* provides students with an accessible, quick reference to the information needed in the clinical setting.

The *Companion CD* packaged with the text provides the student with case studies; critical thinking questions with categories and rationales; video segments, including births and assessments; a care plan constructor; illustrated skills; anatomy reviews; resources; animations; English/Spanish guidelines; review questions; and an English/Spanish audio glossary.

The *Evolve website* includes case studies, review questions, and WebLinks.

Acknowledgments

THE ninth edition of *Maternity & Women's Health Care* would not have been possible without the contributions of many people. First, we want to thank the many nurse educators, clinicians, and nursing students in the United States, Canada, Australia, and Taiwan whose comments and suggestions about the manuscript led to this collaborative effort by an outstanding group of contributors. A special thanks goes to these contributors, many of whom are new to this edition, whose names are listed in the list of Contributors. Their expertise and knowledge of current clinical practice and research have added to the relevancy and accuracy of the materials presented. Kitty Cashion, Kathy Alden, and Karen Piotrowski deserve special recognition for their continuing extra efforts. We acknowledge the contributions to the chapter on Alternative and Complementary Therapies from The American Holistic Nurses' Association, and Phillip Fenske, LAc. We also thank Pat Gringrich for contributing to the Evidence-Based Practice boxes; Jane McAteer for developing Plans of Care; Jo Garner, Marilyn Selkirk, and Laurie Gower for assisting with Spanish translations; and Ed Lowdermilk for his assistance with Medication Guides and verification of other medication information.

We remember especially our contributor, Sharron Humenick, who died September 9, 2006, after a long illness. Sharron was a friend, breastfeeding advocate, editor of the *Journal of Perinatal Education*, researcher, and professor at Virginia Commonwealth University at the time of her death. She will be sorely missed.

We are also appreciative of the critiques given by the reviewers, especially their attention to validating the accuracy of content and their challenge to present content differently and to include new ideas. These combined efforts have resulted in a revision that incorporates the most recent research and current information about the practice of maternity and women's health care.

We offer thanks for shared expertise and photographs to the staffs of University of North Carolina Women's Hospital; University of North Carolina School of Nursing; Nurses Certificate program in Interactive Imagery; Jane Stansbury, SRS Medical Systems, Inc.; Phil Wilson, Momentum, Inc.; Leonard Nihan, Sea-Band International; Gayle Kipnis, RNC, CHTP, HNC; Tina Whitehorn; Polly Perez, Cutting Edge Press; and Barbara Harper, Global Maternal/Child Health Association.

We also would like to thank the following photographers: Cheryl Briggs, RN, Annapolis, MD; Michael S. Clement, MD, Mesa, AZ; Julie Perry Nelson, Gilbert, AZ; and Marjorie Pyle, RNC, Lifecircle, Costa Mesa, CA.

Thanks to the following individuals who allowed us to use their beautiful photos: Jodi Brackett, Phoenix, AZ; David A. Clarke, Philadelphia, PA; Thomas and Christie Coghill, Clayton, NC; Shelley Conroy, Ogden, UT; Bernadine Cunningham, Phoenix, AZ; Skip Davis, San Francisco, CA; Eugene Doerr, Litchfield, KY; Kara George, Phoenix, AZ; Sara Kossuth, Los Angeles, CA; Mahesh Kotwal, MD, Phoenix, AZ; Paul Vincent Kuntz, Houston, TX; Nicole Larson, Eden Prairie, MN; Wendy and Marwood Larson-Harris, Roanoke, VA; Ed Lowdermilk, Chapel Hill, NC; Jonas N. McCoy, Raleigh, NC; Judy Meyr, St. Louis, MO; Kim Molloy, Knoxville, IA; Bill and Tricia Olson, North Ogden, UT; Chris Rozales, San Francisco, CA; H. Gil Rushton, MD, Washington, DC; Brian and Mayannyn Sallee, Las Vegas, NV; Edward S. Tank, MD, Portland, OR; and Amy and Ken Turner, Cary, NC.

Special words of gratitude are extended to Catherine Jackson, Acquisitions Editor; Laurie Gower, Senior Developmental Editor; Jeff Patterson, Publishing Services Manager; Anne Konopka, Senior Project Manager; and Amy Buxton, Senior Designer, for their encouragement, inspiration, and assistance in the preparation and production of this text. These talented and hardworking people helped change our manuscript into a beautiful book by editing the manuscript, designing an attractive format for our special features, and overseeing the production of the book from start to finish. We are especially thankful to Laurie Gower, who always had time to answer our questions, kept track of innumerable details, found just the right photo or resource, obtained that elusive permission, and always reassured us that we were doing a great job.

Deitra Leonard Lowdermilk
Shannon E. Perry

Special Features

Learning Objectives begin each chapter to focus attention on the important content to be mastered.

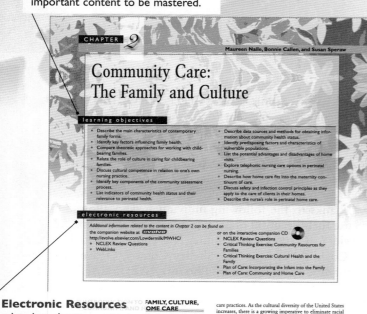

CHAPTER 2

Maureen Nalle, Bonnie Callen, and Susan Speraw

Community Care: The Family and Culture

learning objectives

- Describe the main characteristics of contemporary family forms.
- Identify key factors influencing family health.
- Compare theoretic approaches for working with childbearing families.
- Relate the role of culture in caring for childbearing families.
- Discuss cultural competence in relation to one's own nursing practice.
- Identify key components of the community assessment process.
- List indicators of community health status and their relevance to perinatal health.

- Describe data sources and methods for obtaining information about community health status.
- Identify predisposing factors and characteristics of vulnerable populations.
- List the potential advantages and disadvantages of home visits.
- Explore telephonic nursing care options in perinatal nursing.
- Describe how home care fits into the maternity continuum of care.
- Discuss safety and infection control principles as they apply to the care of clients in their homes.
- Describe the nurse's role in perinatal home care.

electronic resources

Additional information related to the content in Chapter 2 can be found on the companion website at **evolve**
http://evolve.elsevier.com/Lowdermilk/MWHC/
- NCLEX Review Questions
- WebLinks

or on the interactive companion CD
- NCLEX Review Questions
- Critical Thinking Exercise: Community Resources for Families
- Critical Thinking Exercise: Cultural Health and the Family
- Plan of Care: Incorporating the Infant into the Family
- Plan of Care: Community and Home Care

Electronic Resources related to chapter content are included at the beginning of each chapter and highlighted throughout the text.

FAMILY, CULTURE,
ND H... OME CARE

... function of the American
...lly in recent years, largely
...graphic, sociocultural, and
...ce family life and health
...2003). Despite great im-
...lth of the nation, there is
...ly health and well-being as
...unity, and national health
...003) observed that the cur-
...t provide adequate services
... areas of prenatal care, be-
havioral health, nutrition, and chronic illness, or for special
care needs. Families face significant barriers in accessing
needed services and overcoming discrimination in health

care practices. As the cultural diversity of the United States
increases, there is a growing imperative to eliminate racial
and ethnic health disparities by providing access to quality
care for diverse populations (Weissman et al., 2005).
Healthy People 2010 established national health priorities that focus on two major goals: (1) increased quality
and years of healthy life, and (2) elimination of health disparities. The 28 diverse focus areas and 467 objectives provide a systematic approach to health improvement for all
people (USDHHS, 2000a) (www.healthypeople.gov) (see
Chapter 1). Maternal-child focus areas address the most
significa...
includin...
women-...
care—an...
mortalit...

18

examination (including pelvic examination), and laboratory tests are usually completed.

Informed consent is a vital component in the education
of the client concerning contraception or sterilization. The
nurse often has the responsibility of documenting information provided and the understanding of that information by the client. Use of the acronym *BRAIDED* may be
useful (see Legal Tip).

▬ LEGAL TIP   Informed Consent
B—Benefits: information about advantages and success rates
R—Risks: information about disadvantages and failure rates
A—Alternatives: information about other available methods
I— Inquiries: opportunity to ask questions
D—Decisions: opportunity to decide or to change mind
E—Explanations: information about method and how it is
    used
D—Documentation: information given and client's understanding

Nursing diagnoses reflect analysis of the assessment
findings. Examples of nursing diagnoses that may emerge
regarding contraception include those listed.

- *Decisional conflict related to*
  -contraceptive alternatives
  -partner's willingness to agree on contraceptive
   method
- *Fear related to*
  -contraceptive method side effects
- *Risk for infection related to*
  -unprotected sexual intercourse
  -type of contraceptive method used
  -broken skin or mucous membrane after surgery or
   intrauterine device (IUD) insertion
- *Ineffective sexuality patterns related to*
  -fear of pregnancy
- *Acute pain related to*
  -postoperative recovery after sterilization
- *Risk for spiritual distress related to*
  -discrepancy between religious or cultural beliefs and
   choice of contraception

▬ Expected Outcomes of Care

Planning is a collaborative effort among the woman, her
sexual partner (when appropriate), the primary health care
provider, and the nurse. The expected outcomes are determined and stated in client-centered terms and may include
that the woman or couple will do the following:
- Verbalize understanding about contraceptive methods
- Verbalize understanding of all information necessary to
  give informed consent
- State comfort and satisfaction with the chosen method
- Use the contraceptive method correctly and
  consistently
- Experience no adverse sequelae as a result of the chosen
  method of contraception
- Prevent unplanned pregnancy or plan a pregnancy

Legal Tips provide students with relevant information regarding legal aspects in the context of maternity and women's health nursing.

▬ Plan of Care and Interventions
Unbiased client teaching is fundamental to initiating and
maintaining any form of contraception. A care provider
relationship based on trust is important for adherence by
the client. To foster a safe environment for consultation, a
private setting should be provided in which the client can
feel free to be open. Distractions should be minimized,
and samples of birth control devices for interactive teaching should be available. The nurse counters myths with
facts, clarifies misinformation, and fills in gaps of knowledge. The ideal contraceptive should be safe, easily available, economical, acceptable, simple to use, and promptly
reversible. Although no method may ever achieve all these
objectives, significant advances in the development of new
contraceptive technologies have occurred over the past 30
years (World Health Organization [WHO], 2004).

Contraceptive failure rate refers to the percentage of contraceptive users expected to have an unplanned pregnancy
during the first year, even when they use a method consistently and correctly. Contraceptive effectiveness varies
from couple to couple (Box 9-1) and depends on both the
properties of the method and the characteristics of the user
(Trussell, 2004). Failure rates decrease over time, either because a user gains experience and uses a method more appropriately or because the less effective users stop using the
method.

CRITICAL THINKING EXERCISE

Choosing a Contraceptive

Joyce is a 45-year-old woman who has an appointment in the
local health department family planning clinic. She is seeking
information about which type of contraception would be best
for her at this time in her life. She smokes a pack of cigarettes
a day and has been having irregular periods.
1. Evidence—Is there sufficient evidence to draw conclusions about what response the nurse should give?
2. Assumptions—Describe underlying assumptions about
   the following issues:
   a. Personal considerations for choosing a birth control
      method
   b. Appropriate methods for perimenopausal women
3. What implications and priorities for nursing care can be
   made at this time?
4. Does the evidence objectively support your conclusion?
5. Are there alternative perspectives to your conclusion?

Box 9-1   **Factors Affecting Method Contraceptive Effectiveness**
- Frequency of intercourse
- Motivation to prevent pregnancy
- Understanding of how to use the method
- Adherence to method
- Provision of short-term or long-term protection
- Likelihood of pregnancy for the individual woman
- Consistent use of method

Critical Thinking Exercises depict real-life situations that challenge students to choose the best interventions and make good clinical judgments.

EVIDENCE-BASED PRACTICE

Uterine-Conserving Treatments Versus Hysterectomy for Uterine Fibroids

BACKGROUND
- Benign tumors of the uterine smooth muscle, or leiomyomata,
  are thought to occur in nearly one third of women aged 25
  to 45 years. The risk of uterine fibroids is almost three times
  higher for African-American women than the general population. Although frequently present without symptoms, fibroids
  can cause abnormal bleeding and pain, as well as urinary frequency and constipation due to pelvic mass. Fibroids are also
  associated with pregnancy complications and infertility.
- Treatments vary considerably. Medical therapies include nonsteroidal antiinflammatory drugs and hormonal therapies.
  Uterine-sparing surgical procedures include uterine artery
  embolization, coagulation using cautery or laser, and myomectomy. Uterine fibroids are the most common reason for
  hysterectomy.

OBJECTIVES
- The reviewers set out to compare the efficacy, the risks for
  complications, and the benefits of treatments for uterine fibroids. Outcomes were to include physiologic, symptomatic,
  pregnancy rates and complications, quality of life, adverse outcomes, and need for additional treatment.

METHODS
Search Strategy
- After a comprehensive search of health databases and reference lists, the authors identified few randomized controlled
  trials or prospective cohort studies, the two highest quality
  studies. Therefore, they also accepted large cohort studies,
  retrospective reviews, and large case studies, which had to
  meet certain internal and external validity criteria. The dates,
  countries, and numbers of studies or subjects were not
  noted.

Statistical Analyses
- Data also came from a survey of 1,000 hospitals (or 20% of all
  U.S. hospitals), and from the hospital administration of Duke
  University Medical Center, for statistics on client trends and
  costs. Similar data were pooled. Differences between groups
  that exceeded the 95% confidence interval were accepted as
  significant.

FINDINGS
- African-American women were more likely than caucasian
  women to receive hysterectomy or myomectomy. Hyster-

ectomies led to favorable outcomes and symptomatic relief,
even two years out. Complications of myomectomy increased
with additional fibroids, while a single fibroid lowered the risk
of recurrence. Use of GnRH agonists, (e.g., Lupron) before
surgery led to decreased blood loss. In pregnancy, fibroids
were associated with increased preterm labor, placental abruption, cesarean birth, and breech presentation. Ovarian hormone levels may have been altered by removal of the uterus,
even when the ovaries were spared. Hysterectomy did not
adversely affect sexual functioning, and may have improved it,
in severely symptomatic women.
- The lowest cost treatment for symptomatic fibroids was
  nonsteroidal antiinflammatory drugs, at around $60 a month,
  followed by oral contraceptives at $90 a month, and GnRH
  inhibitors at $500 for a standard 3-month course. Myomecto-
  mies cost less than hysterectomies.

LIMITATIONS
- There are insufficient data to compare the risks and benefits of myomectomy versus hysterectomy, or to recommend
  the most appropriate treatment for symptomatic clients.
  Randomized controlled data were sparse.

IMPLICATIONS FOR PRACTICE
- Although hysterectomy is the second most common major
  surgical procedure performed in the United States, there is
  little evidence upon which to base recommendations for interventions and alternatives for management of leiomyomata.
  Hysterectomy had the best record of long-term symptom
  relief. Nurses can question clients about their history of fibroids, and alert them to the increased concerns for pregnancy. Uterus-preserving interventions may be cost effective
  and preserve fertility.

IMPLICATIONS FOR FURTHER RESEARCH
- There is a need for research on the genetics and long-term
  natural history of fibroids. Randomized controlled trials with
  standardized measures comparing medical versus surgical interventions would facilitate metaanalysis and therefore the
  power of research to allow comparison of outcomes and recommendations for management. Researchers need to address
  costs, quality of life, and racial disparities of health care access
  of fibroid management.

Reference: Management of uterine fibroids: Summary, evidence report/technology assessment: Number 34. (2001). AHRQ Publication No. 01-E051. Rockville,
MD: Agency for Healthcare Research and Quality.

Hysteroscopic uterine *ablation* (vaporization of tissues) can
be performed under local or general anesthesia, usually as
an outpatient procedure. Medical therapy using GnRH
agonists to control bleeding temporarily and to suppress
endometrial tissue may be given for 8 to 12 weeks before
surgery. Although the uterus remains in place, the vaporization process can cause scarring and adhesions in the
uterine cavity, affecting future fertility. Thus this procedure
is for women who wish to retain their uterus but no longer
desire childbearing potential (Lefebvre et al., 2003). Risks

of the procedure include uterine perforation, cervical injury, and fluid overload (caused by the leaking into blood
vessels of fluid used to expand the uterus during surgery).
The woman may experience postoperative cramping and
a slight vaginal discharge for a few days. Before discharge,
the following information is given:
- Analgesics or NSAIDs may be used for pain relief as
  needed.
- Normal activities may be resumed within several days.
- Vaginal discharge is to be expected for 4 to 6 weeks.

Evidence-Based Practice boxes highlight both research and critical thought processes that support and guide the outcomes of nursing care.

Medication Guide boxes provide students with key information about medications and their effects on the woman and her newborn.

Signs of Potential Complications boxes alert students to signs and symptoms of potential problems.

Teaching for Self-Care boxes promote client wellness and encourage preventive care.

Full-color photos and illustrations help clarify information.

Community Activity boxes focus on maternal, newborn, and women's health activities that can be pursued in local community settings.

---

medication guide

Opioid Agonist Analgesics for Intrathecal and Epidural Use

Fentanyl citrate (Sublimaze)
Sufentanil citrate (Sufenta)

ACTION ■ Opioid agonist analgesics that stimulate both mu and kappa opioid receptors to decrease the transmission of pain impulses; rapid action with short duration (0.5-1 hr IV; 1-2 hr epidural); sufentanil citrate has a more potent analgesic action than fentanyl citrate with less passage across the placenta to the fetus

INDICATION
■ Because of their short duration of action when given intravenously, they are most commonly administered epidurally or intrathecally, alone or in combination with a local anesthetic agent, to relieve moderate to severe labor pain and postoperative pain after cesarean birth.

DOSAGE AND ROUTE
■ Fentanyl citrate: 25 to 50 mg IV; 1 to 2 mg with 0.125% bupivacaine at rate of 8 to 10 ml/hr epidurally
■ Sufentanil citrate: 1 mg with 0.125% bupivacaine at rate of 10 ml/hr.

ADVERSE EFFECTS
■ Dizziness, drowsiness, allergic reactions, rash, pruritus, maternal and fetal/neonatal respiratory depression, nausea and vomiting, urinary retention

NURSING CONSIDERATIONS
■ Assess for respiratory depression; naloxone should be available as antidote

IV, Intravenous.

medication guide

Opioid Agonist-Antagonist Analgesics

Butorphanol tartrate (Stadol)
Nalbuphine hydrochloride (Nubain)

ACTION
■ Mixed agonist-antagonist analgesics; stimulate kappa opioid receptors and blocks or weakly stimulates mu opioid receptors, resulting in good analgesia but with less respiratory depression and nausea and vomiting when compared with opioid agonist analgesics

INDICATION
■ Moderate to severe labor pain and postoperative pain after cesarean birth

DOSAGE AND ROUTE
■ Butorphanol tartrate: 1 mg (range 0.5 to 2 mg) IV every 3-4 hr as needed; 2 mg (range 1 to 4 mg) IM every 3-4 hr as needed
■ Nalbuphine hydrochloride: 10 mg IV; 10 to 20 mg IM every 3-4 hours as needed

ADVERSE EFFECTS
■ Confusion, sedation, drowsiness, headache, dizziness, nervousness, sweating; maternal palpitations/tachycardia or bradycardia; transient nonpathologic sinusoidal-like FHR rhythm; respiratory depression; nausea and vomiting; difficulty with urination (retention, urgency)

NURSING CONSIDERATIONS
■ See opioid agonist analgesics; may precipitate withdrawal symptoms in opioid-dependent women and their newborns

IM, Intramuscular; IV, intravenous.

signs of potential complications

Maternal Opioid Abstinence Syndrome (Opioid Withdrawal)

- Yawning, rhinorrhea (runny nose), sweating, lacrimation (tearing), mydriasis (dilation of pupils)
- Anorexia
- Irritability, restlessness, generalized anxiety
- Tremor
- Chills and hot flashes
- Piloerection ("gooseflesh")
- Violent sneezing
- Weakness, fatigue, and drowsiness
- Nausea and vomiting
- Diarrhea, abdominal cramps
- Bone and muscle pain, muscle spasm, kicking movements

respiratory depression in the mother or neonate. They are less likely to cause nausea and vomiting, but sedation may be as great or greater when compared with pure opioid agonists. As a result of these effects, parenteral opioid agonist-antagonist analgesics are used more commonly during labor than the opioid agonist analgesics. Both IM and IV routes of administration can be used, but the IV route is preferred. This classification of opioid analgesics, especially nalbuphine, is not suitable for women with an opioid dependence because the antagonist activity could precipitate withdrawal symptoms (abstinence syndrome) in both the mother and her newborn (Florence & Palmer, 2003; Hawkins et al., 2002; Lehne, 2004) (see Medication Guide and Signs of Potential Complications box).

Opioid Antagonists. Opioids such as hydromorphone, meperidine, and fentanyl can cause excessive CNS depres-

tramuscularly (see Medication Guide). The woman should be told that the pain that was relieved with the use of the opioid analgesic will return with the administration of the opioid antagonist. Some authorities believe that unless maternal CNS depression is severe enough to affect her well-being and that of her fetus, the woman should not receive naloxone just before birth in an attempt to prevent neonatal CNS depression. Placental transfer of naloxone is unpredictable; the newborn may not require treatment with an opioid antagonist; and the sudden return of severe pain could have adverse physiologic and psychologic effects on the mother (Hawkins et al., 2002; Lehne, 2004).

---

the primary health care provider. Occasionally the reaction is one of anger or indifference; the woman turns away from the baby, concentrates on her own pain, and sometimes makes hostile comments. These varied reactions can arise from pleasure, exhaustion, or deep disappointment. When evaluating parent-newborn interactions after birth, the nurse also should consider the cultural characteristics of the woman and her family and the expected behaviors of that culture. In some cultures, the birth of a male child is preferred, and women may grieve when a female child is born (D'Avanzo & Geissler, 2003).

Whatever the reaction and its cause may be, the woman needs continuing acceptance and support from all staff. Notation regarding the parents' reaction to the newborn can be made in the recovery record. Nurses can assess this reaction by asking themselves such questions as, "How do the parents look?" "What do they say?" "What do they do?" Further assessment of the parent-newborn relationship can be conducted as care is given during the period of recovery. This is especially important if warning signs (e.g., passive or hostile reactions to the newborn, disappointment with gender or appearance of the newborn, absence of eye contact, or limited interaction of parents with each other) were noted immediately after birth. The nurse may find it helpful to discuss any warning signs that may have been noted with the woman's primary health care provider.

Siblings, who may have appeared only remotely interested in the final phases of the second stage, tend to experience renewed interest and excitement when the newborn appears. They can be encouraged to hold the baby (Fig. 21-28).

Parents usually respond to praise of their newborn. Many need to be reassured that the dusky appearance of their baby's extremities immediately after birth is normal until circulation is well established. If appropriate, the nurse should explain the reason for the molding of the newborn's head. Information about hospital routine can

be communicated. It is important, however, for nurses to recognize that the cultural background of the parents may influence their expectations regarding the care and handling of their newborn immediately after birth. For example, some traditional Southeast Asians believe that the head should not be touched because it is the most sacred part of a person's body. They also believe that praise of the baby is dangerous because jealous spirits may then cause the baby harm or take it away (D'Avanzo & Geissler, 2003). Hospital staff members, by their interest and concern, can provide the environment for making this a satisfying experience for parents, family, and significant others.

■ **Evaluation**

Determining a woman's satisfaction with and impressions of her childbirth experience is a critical component in the provision of high-quality maternal-newborn health care that meets the individual needs of women and families using these services. The woman may find it helpful to review her childbirth experience with a caring nurse who will listen, support, and provide explanations for events that occurred. This review process can help the woman to express her feelings about this significant event that will change her life forever (Semenic et al., 2004).

FIG. 21-28 Big brother becomes acquainted with new baby sister. (Courtesy Marjorie Pyle, RNC, Lifecircle, Costa Mesa, CA.)

community activity

1. Survey your community for doulas and complete the following activities:
   a. Create a list of the doulas that includes the following information:
      - Name of the doula and her credentials (e.g. education, certification)
      - Contact information: address, phone number, email
      - Cost and payment method
   b. Contact one of the doulas on your list and arrange to interview her. Write a description of this doula and her practice that includes the following information:
      - Her beliefs regarding the process of labor and her role in facilitating its progress
      - When she begins her contact with the women she will care for; what does she do to assist these women before the onset of their labor
      - How she supports women in labor including physical comfort measures, emotional support, information giving, and advocacy
      - How she supports the woman's partner and support system
      - How she interacts with members of the labor and birth staff; how does she see her role different from theirs; has she encountered any difficulties and if so how did she handle the situation
      - Number of births she attends each year
      - Persons involved in the care of women and their families during labor
      - Length of stay including follow-up after discharge

TEACHING FOR SELF-CARE

Breast Self-Examination

1. The best time to do breast self-examination is about a week after your period, when breasts are not tender or swollen. If you do not have regular periods or sometimes skip a month, do it on the same day every month. If you are breastfeeding or no longer menstruating, choose a date and examine your breasts at the same time each month.
2. Lie down and put a pillow under your right shoulder. Place your right arm behind your head (Fig. 1).
3. Use the finger pads of your three middle fingers on your left hand to feel for lumps or thickening. Your finger pads are the top third of each finger.
4. Press firmly enough to know how your breast feels. If you're not sure how hard to press, ask your health care provider or try to copy the way your health care provider does the finger pads during a breast examination. Learn what your breast feels like most of the time. A firm ridge in the lower curve of each breast is normal.
5. Move around the breast in a set way. You can choose either circles (Fig. 2, A), vertical lines (Fig. 2, B), or wedges (Fig. 2, C). Do it the same way every time. It will help you to make sure that you've gone over the entire breast area and to remember how your breast feels.
6. Gently compress the nipple between your thumb and forefinger and look for discharge.
7. Now examine your left breast using the finger pads of your right hand.
8. If you find any changes, see your health care provider right away.
9. You may want to check your breasts while standing in front of a mirror right after you do your breast self-examination each month. See if there are any changes in the way your breasts look: dimpling of the skin, changes in the nipple, or redness or swelling.
10. You may also want to do an extra breast self-examination while you're in the shower (Fig. 3). Your soapy hands will glide over the wet skin, making it easy to check how your breasts feel.
11. It is important to check the area between the breast and the underarm and the underarm itself. Also examine the area above the breast to the collarbone and to the shoulder.

Fig. 2

Fig. 1

Fig. 3

transitional stage between childhood and sexual maturity. Increasing amounts and variations in gonadotropin and estrogen secretion develop into a cyclic pattern at least a year before menarche. In North America, this occurs in most girls at about age 13 years.

Initially, periods are irregular, unpredictable, painless, and *anovulatory* (no ovum released from the ovary). After 1 or more years, a hypothalamic-pituitary rhythm develops, and the ovary produces adequate cyclic estrogen to make a mature ovum. *Ovulatory* (ovum released from ovary) periods tend to be regular, monitored by progesterone.

Although pregnancy can occur in exceptional cases of true precocious puberty, most pregnancies in young girls occur after the normally timed menarche. All young adolescents of both sexes would benefit from knowing that pregnancy can occur at any time after the onset of menses.

Menstrual Cycle

Menstruation is the periodic uterine bleeding that begins approximately 14 days after ovulation. It is controlled by a feedback system of three cycles: hypothalamic-pituitary, ovarian, and endometrial. The average length of a menstrual

Contents

■ UNIT EIGHT
NEWBORN COMPLICATIONS

Contemporary Maternity Nursing and Women's Health Care

learning objectives

- Describe the scope of maternity nursing and women's health care.
- Evaluate contemporary issues and trends in maternity nursing and women's health care.
- Describe sociopolitical issues affecting the care of women and infants.
- Compare selected biostatistical data among races and countries.

- Examine social concerns in maternity nursing and women's health care.
- Explain quality management and standards of practice in the delivery of nursing care.
- Debate ethical issues in perinatal nursing.
- Examine the *Healthy People 2010* goals related to maternal and infant care.

electronic resources

Additional information related to the content in Chapter 1 can be found on

the companion website at **evolve**
http://evolve.elsevier.com/Lowdermilk/MWHC/
- NCLEX Review Questions
- WebLinks

or on the interactive companion CD
- NCLEX Review Questions

Maternity nursing focuses on the care of childbearing women and their families through all stages of pregnancy and childbirth, as well as the first 4 weeks after birth. Throughout the prenatal period, nurses, nurse practitioners, and nurse-midwives provide care for women in clinics and physicians' offices and teach classes to help families prepare for childbirth. Nurses care for childbearing families during labor and birth in hospitals, in birthing centers (e.g., www.birthcenters.org), and in the home. Nurses with special training may provide intensive care for high risk neonates in special care units and for high risk mothers in antepartum units, in critical care obstetric units, or in the home. Maternity nurses teach about pregnancy; the process of labor, birth, and recovery; and parenting skills; and they provide continuity of care throughout the childbearing cycle.

Women's health care focuses on the physical, psychologic, and social needs of women throughout their lives. In caring for women, their overall experience is emphasized: general physical and psychologic well-being, childbearing functions, and diseases. Women's health nurses specialize in and investigate conditions unique to women (such as reproductive malignancies and menopause) and sociocultural and occupational factors that may be related to women's health problems (such as poverty, rape, incest, and family violence). They may also provide care for women and their families during the childbearing cycle. An excellent model for nurses who care for women and children is the International Confederation of Midwives' Vision for Women and Their Health (Box 1-1).

Nurses caring for women have helped make the health care system more responsive to women's needs. Nurses have been critically important in developing strategies to improve the well-being of women and their infants and have led the efforts to implement clinical practice guidelines and to practice using an evidence-based approach. Through professional associations, nurses can have a voice in setting standards and in influencing health policy by actively participating in the education of the public and of state and federal legislators (e.g., www.ana.org; www.can-nurses.ca). Some nurses hold elective office and influence policy directly.

box 1-1 **The Vision for Women and Their Health**

International Confederation of Midwives envisions a world where

- Women are respected and treated as persons in their own right in all societies.
- Women stand as equal partners with men in the world order.
- Women are recognized as crucial to the health of any nation.
- Women and their families are part of a health care system with high-quality care and easy access when needed.
- Women have the right to choose among safe options for care throughout their lives including high-quality, state-of-the-art

care from competent providers who truly care about the woman and her health.

- Women are educated and empowered to delight in a strong sense of self, to trust their bodies, to plan their pregnancies, and to make wise choices in their health care.
- Women experience a reasonable standard of living, including a clean and safe environment, healthy food, and a reasonable place to live.
- Women need have no fear for their lives or the lives of their babies when they are pregnant.
- Women believe that birth is normal and prefer to avoid unnecessary intervention.

From International Confederation of Midwives. Accessed http://www.internationalmidwives.org/May 19, 2006.

box 1-2 **Historic Overview of Milestones in the Care of Mothers and Infants**

1847—James Young Simpson in Edinburgh, Scotland, used ether for an internal podalic version and birth; the first reported use of obstetric anesthesia

1861—Ignaz Semmelweis wrote *The Cause, Concept and Prophylaxis of Childbed Fever*

1906—First U.S. program for prenatal nursing care established

1908—Childbirth classes started by the American Red Cross

1909—First White House Conference on Children convened

1911—First milk bank in the United States established in Boston

1912—U.S. Children's Bureau established

1916—Margaret Sanger established first American birth control clinic in Brooklyn, NY

1923—First U.S. hospital center for premature infant care established at Sarah Morris Hospital in Chicago

1933—*Natural Childbirth* published by Grantly Dick-Read

1941—Penicillin used as a treatment for infection

1953—Virginia Apgar, an anesthesiologist, published Apgar scoring system of neonatal assessment

1958—Edward Hon reported on the recording of the fetal electrocardiogram (ECG) from the maternal abdomen (first commercial electronic fetal monitor produced in the late 1960s)

1958—Ian Donald, a Glasgow physician, was the first to report clinical use of ultrasound to examine the fetus

1959—*Thank You, Dr. Lamaze* published by Marjorie Karmel

1960—American Society for Psychoprophylaxis in Obstetrics (ASPO/Lamaze) formed

1960—International Childbirth Education Association founded

1960—Birth control pill introduced in the United States

1962—Thalidomide found to cause birth defects

1963—Title V of the Social Security Act amended to include comprehensive maternity and infant care for women who were low income and high risk

1965—Supreme Court ruled that married people have the right to use birth control

1967—$Rh_o(D)$ immune globulin produced

1967—Reva Rubin published article on Maternal Role Attainment

1968—Rubella vaccine became available

1969—Nurses Association of the American College of Obstetricians and Gynecologists (NAACOG) founded; renamed AWHONN (Association of Women's Health, Obstetric and Neonatal Nurses) and incorporated as a 501 (c)3 organization in 1993

1972—WIC (Special Supplemental Food Program for Women, Infants, and Children) started

1973—Abortion legalized in the United States

1974—First standards for obstetric, gynecologic, and neonatal nursing published by NAACOG

1975—The Pregnant Patient's Bill of Rights published by the International Childbirth Education Association

1978—Louise Brown, first test-tube baby, born

1991—Society for Advancement of Women's Health Research founded

1992—Office of Research on Women's Health authorized by U.S. Congress

1993—Human embryos cloned at George Washington University

1993—Family and Medical Leave Act enacted

1998—Newborns' and Mothers' Health Act went into effect

2000—Working draft of sequence and analysis of human genome completed

Tremendous advances have taken place in the care of mothers and their infants during the past 150 years (Box 1-2). However, in the United States, serious problems exist related to the health and health care of mothers and infants. Lack of access to prepregnancy and pregnancy-related care for all women and the lack of reproductive health services for adolescents are major concerns. Sexually transmitted infections, including acquired immunodeficiency syndrome (AIDS), continue to adversely affect reproduction.

Racial and ethnic diversity is increasing within North America. It is estimated that by the year 2050, 50% of the population will be European-American, 15% will be African-American, 24% will be Hispanic, and 8% will be Asian-American (U.S. Census Bureau, 2004). This presents a challenge for health care providers to provide culturally sensitive health care.

Despite the great strides in public health that the United States has made, significant disparity exists in health outcomes among people of various racial and ethnic groups. In addition, people may have lifestyles, health needs, and health care preferences related to their ethnic or cultural backgrounds. They may have dietary preferences and health practices that are not understood by caregivers. To meet the health care needs of a culturally diverse society, the nursing workforce must reflect the diversity of its clients.

This chapter presents a general overview of issues and trends related to the health and health care of women and infants.

▬ CONTEMPORARY ISSUES AND TRENDS

Problems with the U.S. Health Care System

The U. S. health care system is fragmented and is, in many respects, inefficient and wasteful. The United States spends twice as much on health care per capita on average as do other industrialized nations. In spite of this expenditure, there are significant disparities in access to care related to income, insurance status, race, and ethnicity. Consumer-driven health coverage is designed to make people more cost-conscious. Critics are concerned that combining a medical savings account with a high-deductible health plan will result in high out-of-pocket expenses and thus discourage the use of health services that are needed (Hollander, 2006).

Medical errors result in as many as 98,000 deaths per year (Gauthier & Serber, 2005). Of the medical errors, approximately 60% occurred in ambulatory settings (Schoen et al., 2005), suggesting that efforts to reduce errors must be directed to outpatient as well as inpatient settings.

High Cost of Health Care

Health care is one of the fastest-growing sectors of the U.S. economy. Even though the United States spends proportionately more on health care than any of the other 190 countries that make up the World Health Organization, it ranks thirty-seventh in quality (Rubin, 2000). A shift in demographics, an increased emphasis on high-cost technology, and the liability costs of a litigious society contribute to the high cost of care. Most researchers agree that caring for the increased number of low-birth-weight (LBW) infants in neonatal intensive care units contributes significantly to the overall health care costs.

Midwifery care has helped contain some health care costs. However, not all insurance carriers reimburse nurse practitioners and clinical nurse specialists as direct care providers. Nor do they reimburse for all services provided by nurse-midwives, a situation that continues to be a problem. Nurses must become involved in the politics of cost containment because they, as knowledgeable experts, can provide solutions to many health care problems at a relatively low cost.

Early postpartum discharge programs also are used to reduce costs. The American Academy of Pediatrics

CRITICAL THINKING EXERCISE

Safety and Efficacy of Midwifery Care

A group of nurse-midwives is setting up practice in your home town. They are to collaborate with one of the groups of obstetricians in the city. A letter to the editor appeared in the local newspaper stating that the presence of midwives will jeopardize care of pregnant women in the community because midwives usually care for the poor and indigent, deliver babies at home, and therefore don't have the skills to work in hospitals and care for middle-class women who have insurance. The letter-writer urged the community to boycott the midwives to ensure safe deliveries for women in the community.

1. Evidence—Is there sufficient evidence to document the qualifications of nurse-midwives and their safety record to write a response to this letter?
2. Assumptions—What assumptions can be made about midwifery care and the knowledge base of the public regarding that care?
3. What implications and priorities for nursing can be made at this time?
4. Does the evidence objectively support your conclusion?
5. Are there alternative perspectives to your conclusion?

(www.apa.org) has published minimal criteria for early discharge of a newborn (American Academy of Pediatrics Committee on Fetus and Newborn, 2004) (see Box 23-2).

Limited Access to Care

Barriers to access must be removed so pregnancy outcomes can be improved. The most significant barrier to access is the inability to pay. Lack of transportation and dependent child care are other barriers. In addition to a lack of insurance and high costs, a lack of providers for low-income women exists because many physicians either refuse to take Medicaid clients or take only a few such clients. This presents a serious problem because a significant proportion of births are to mothers who receive Medicaid.

Status of Nursing

A national nursing shortage exists, including a shortage of nursing faculty. The workforce is aging; the average age of registered nurses is 46.8 years, with 25.5% over 54 years of age. The employment rate of nurses is high (83.2% of nurses are employed in nursing, and 56.2% work in hospitals), and clients are sicker and require a higher level of nursing care (The registered nurses population: National Sample Survey of Registered Nurses, 2004). Nurses are working longer hours, which jeopardizes client safety (Rogers, Hwang, Scott, Aiken, & Dinges, 2004). A minimum nurse-client ratio has been legislated to protect nurses and their clients.

Advanced practice nurses comprise 8.3% of RN population; of these, 13,684 are midwives. The educational level of nurses is increasing with a 37% increase in the numbers of nurses earning the master's or doctoral degree (U.S. Department of Health and Human Services Health

Resources and Services Administration, 2004). The role of the nurse is evolving from primary caregiver to leader of the interdisciplinary care team. Documentation of client outcomes has become essential (see later discussion). Advanced practice roles have increased as nurses assume more responsibility for client care.

Integrative Health Care

Integrative health care encompasses complementary and alternative therapies in combination with conventional Western modalities of treatment. Many popular alternative healing modalities offer human-centered care based on philosophies that recognize the value of the client's input and honor the individual's beliefs, values, and desires. The focus of these modalities is on the whole person, not just on a disease complex. Clients often find that alternative modalities are more consistent with their own belief systems and also allow for more client autonomy in health care decisions (see Chapter 4). Complementary and alternative therapy will be identified throughout the text with an icon ✐.

Approximately 40% of the general population uses complementary and alternative therapies (Barrett, 2003), and most of these users do not tell their physicians. Throughout the world the use of traditional medicine presents unique challenges in terms of health care policy, efficacy, accessibility, and utilization (World Health Organization, 2002).

In 1992 the National Institutes of Health (NIH) developed the Office of Alternative Medicine (OAM) in the United States to support research and evaluation of various alternative and complementary modalities and to provide information to health care consumers about such modalities. In 1998, Congress instituted the National Center for Complementary and Alternative Medicine (NCCAM), which incorporates the work of the OAM in its mission and function.

Childbirth Practices

Prenatal care may promote better pregnancy outcomes by allowing early risk assessment and promoting healthy behaviors such as improved nutrition and smoking cessation. In 2004, 83.9% of all women received care in the first trimester and 3.5% had only late or no prenatal care. There is disparity in use of prenatal care in the first trimester by race and ethnicity: 89% of non-Hispanic whites, 76% of non-Hispanic blacks, and 78% of Hispanic women receive care in the first trimester (Hoyert, Mathews, Menacker, Strobino, & Guyer, 2006) (see Chapter 16).

Women can choose physicians or nurse-midwives as primary care providers. In 2003, physicians attended 91% and nurse-midwives attended 8% of all births (Martin, Hamilton, Sutton, Ventura, Menacker, & Munson, 2005). Women who choose nurse-midwives as their primary providers participate actively in childbirth decisions and receive fewer interventions during labor (Jackson et al., 2003). Women can give birth in a hospital labor room (rather than a delivery

room), in a birthing room, in a freestanding birthing center, or at home. In 2003, 99% of births in the United States occurred in the hospital. Of the out-of-hospital births, 65% were in the home and 27% in freestanding birthing centers (Martin et al., 2005). Cesarean births increased to 29.1% of live births in the United States in 2004, making it unlikely that the *Healthy People 2010* goal of 15% can be accomplished. The rate of vaginal births after cesarean (VBACs) declined to 9.2% (Hoyert et al., 2006).

Changes are occurring in the conduct of the second stage of labor (from 10-cm dilation to birth of the baby); positions are varied, with more emphasis on upright posture. The arbitrary limit of 2 hours for the second stage is less rigid as delayed pushing (waiting until the forces of labor propel the fetus down in the birth canal instead of encouraging pushing as soon as the cervix is 10 cm dilated) is instituted. Delayed pushing conserves the energy of the mother, results in fewer instrumental births, and is less costly. The rates of episiotomy are declining, resulting in fewer severe perineal lacerations; midwives perform fewer episiotomies than do physicians (see Chapter 21).

The method of analgesia varies, depending on the condition and choice of the mother and preferences of the providers. Mothers typically are awake and aware during labor and birth. Contrasting philosophies exist regarding analgesia during labor. Some women prefer to experience the sensations of birth with little or no analgesia; others opt for epidural analgesia to provide comfort and control over their behavior during the experience (see Chapter 19).

Increasing numbers of infants are born after the use of assisted reproductive technology. In 2003, 112,872 procedures were performed. These procedures resulted in 35,785 live births and 48,756 infants (Centers for Disease Control and Prevention, 2006).

With family-centered care, fathers, partners, grandparents, siblings, and friends may be present for labor and birth. Fathers or partners may be present for cesarean births. Father participation may include cutting the umbilical cord (Fig. 1-1). Doulas—trained and experienced female labor attendants—provide a continuous, one-on-one, caring

FIG. 1-1 Father cutting cord of his newborn daughter. (Courtesy Bill Olson, North Ogden, UT.)

presence throughout the labor and birth. Newborn infants remain with the mother and may breastfeed immediately after birth. Parents participate in the care of their infants in nurseries and neonatal intensive care units. Kangaroo care—skin-to-skin holding—is supported for preterm infants.

Childbirth education and parenting classes encourage the participation of a support person, teach breathing and relaxation techniques, and give general information about birth, infant development, and parenting. Other classes or parent support groups may be organized for the weeks and months after birth (see Chapter 17).

In some cases, a woman labors, gives birth, and recovers in the same room (labor-delivery-recovery); she may stay in the same room for the entire birth experience (labor-delivery-recovery-postpartum). Instead of having one nurse care for the baby and another nurse care for the mother, some hospitals have one nurse care for both the mother and baby (couplet or mother-baby care). In some hospitals, central nurseries have been eliminated, and babies "room-in" with their mothers. Many hospitals use lactation consultants to assist mothers with breastfeeding.

Discharge of a mother and baby within 24 hours of birth has created a growing need for follow-up or home care. In some settings, discharge may occur as early as 6 hours after birth. Legislation has been enacted to ensure that mothers and babies are permitted to stay in the hospital for at least 48 hours after vaginal birth and 96 hours after cesarean birth. Focused and efficient teaching is necessary to enable the parents and infant to make the transition safely from the hospital to the home. Nurses may use follow-up telephone calls or home visits to assist families needing information and reassurance.

Neonatal security in the hospital setting is of concern. Cases of "baby-napping" and of sending parents home with the wrong baby have been reported. Security systems are placed in nurseries (Fig. 1-2), and nurses are required to wear photo identification or some other security badge.

FIG. 1-2 Infant security system. (Courtesy Shannon Perry, Phoenix, AZ.)

Certified Nurse-Midwives

Certified nurse-midwives (CNMs) are registered nurses with education in the two disciplines of nursing and midwifery. Certified midwives (direct-entry midwives) are educated only in the discipline of midwifery. In the United States, certification of midwives is through the American College of Nurse-Midwives (ACNM), the professional association for midwives in the United States (www.midwife. org). The Royal College of Midwives is the professional association for midwives in the United Kingdom (www. rcm.org.uk). In Canada, the Association of Ontario Midwives is the professional association (www.aom.on.ca), and the College of Midwives of Ontario is the regulatory body for midwives in Ontario (www.cmo.on.ca); the other provinces of Canada have similar regulatory bodies (e.g., College of Midwives of British Columbia, www.cmbc. bc.ca). Many national associations belong to the International Confederation of Midwives, which comprises 85 member associations from 75 countries in the Americas and Europe, Africa, and the Asia-Pacific region (www. internationalmidwives.org).

Family Leave

The Family and Medical Leave Act of 1993 provides for up to 12 weeks' unpaid leave to eligible employees for birth, adoption, or foster placement; for care of a child, spouse, or parent who is seriously ill; or for the employee's own illness. This is of great benefit to women because they are usually the primary caretakers of family members.

International Concerns

Female genital mutilation, infibulation, and circumcision are terms used to describe procedures in which part or all of the female external genitalia are removed for cultural reasons (Ahmed & Abushama, 2005; Momoh, 2004). Worldwide, many women undergo such procedures. With the growing number of immigrants from African and other countries where female genital mutilation is practiced, nurses will increasingly encounter women who have undergone the procedure. Ethical dilemmas arise when the woman requests that after birth the perineum be repaired as it was after infibulation and the health care provider believes that such repair is unethical. The International Council of Nurses and other health professionals have spoken out against the procedures as harmful to women's health.

Health of Women

Various factors and conditions affect the health of women. Race is a major factor: Caucasian women have a life expectancy at birth of 80.5 years, in contrast with 76.1 years for African-American women (Hoyert et al., 2006). In 2006, there will be an estimated 212,920 new cases of invasive breast cancer in women in the United States, and 40,970 women are expected to die of the disease (American Cancer Society, 2006). Early detection of breast cancer through breast self-examination and mammography can reduce the mortality rate resulting from this type of cancer. However, because of lack of information or lack of insurance and access, many women never have mammograms. Wide disparity exists between Caucasian women and women of other races and between older and younger women in their rates of mammography, detection, and treatment of breast cancer, and in their survival rates (see Chapter 11).

The population has grown older: approximately 50 million women are older than 50 years of age; 51 is the median age for menopause. Hormone replacement therapy for menopausal women has been used for many years and has both benefits and risks (see Chapter 7).

Violence is a major factor affecting women (see Chapter 6). Violence includes battery, rape or other sexual assaults, and attacks with various weapons. Rates of reported intimate partner violence have increased, possibly because of better assessment and reporting mechanisms. Approximately 8% of pregnant women are battered; the incidence of battering increases during pregnancy. Violence is associated with complications of pregnancy such as bleeding. Alcoholism and substance abuse by the woman and her abuser are associated with violence and homelessness, which affect a growing number of women and children and place them at risk for a variety of health problems.

The rates of pregnancy and elective abortion among adolescents have declined (Hoyert et al., 2006) but are still higher in the United States than in any other industrialized country. Single mothers gave birth to 35.7% of the babies born in the United States in 2004 (Hoyert et al., 2006). Births to unmarried women are frequently related to less favorable outcomes, such as LBW infants or preterm birth, because a large number of these mothers are teenagers.

Cases of perinatally acquired immunodeficiency virus (HIV) infection and AIDS peaked in 1992; since then the rate of AIDS among infants has continued to decline. Treatment with antiretroviral prophylaxis of mothers who tested positive for HIV before giving birth has resulted in a dramatic decrease in the number of infants infected with the virus; highly active antiretroviral therapy (HAART–3 or more anti-HIV drugs) and elective cesarean birth reduce the rate of mother-to-child transmission of HIV (European Collaborative Study, 2005). Universal HIV testing in pregnancy and access to quality prenatal care will contribute to reducing the transmission of HIV and prolonging survival. For women in labor who have had no prenatal care, rapid HIV testing is available (European Collaborative Study, 2005).

Healthy People 2010 Goals

Healthy People 2010 is the United States' agenda for improving health. It has two overarching goals: to increase the quality and years of healthy life and to eliminate health disparities. In *Healthy People 2010,* the 467 objectives to improve health are organized into 28 specific focus areas, including one related to maternal, infant, and child health (Box 1-3). Current information about the goals of *Healthy People 2010* is available on the Internet at www.health. gov/healthypeople.

Trends in Fertility and Birth Rate

Fertility trends and birth rates reflect women's needs for health care. Box 1-4 defines biostatistical terminology useful in analyzing maternity health care. In 2004 the fertility rate, births per 1000 women from 15 to 44 years of age, was 66.3 (Hoyert et al., 2006). The highest birth rates occurred among women between 20 and 29 years of age (Table 1-1). The birth rate, number of live births in 1 year per 1000 population, was 14 in 2004; the teen birth rate was 41.2 (Hoyert et al., 2006). In 2004 the proportion of births by unmarried women varied widely among racial groups in the United States: African-American, 69.2%; Native-American, 62.3%; Hispanic, 46.4%; Caucasian, 24.5%; and Asian or Pacific Islander, 15.5% (Hoyert et al., 2006).

Low-Birth-Weight and Preterm Birth

The risks of morbidity and mortality increase for newborns weighing less than 2500 g (5 lb, 8 oz)–low-birth-weight

---

box 1-3 *Healthy People 2010,* Focus Area 16, Maternal, Infant, and Child Health

Goal: Improve the health and well-being of women, infants, children, and families
- Fetal, infant, child, and adolescent deaths
- Maternal deaths and illnesses
- Prenatal care
- Obstetric care
- Risk factors
- Developmental disabilities and neural tube defects
- Prenatal substance exposure
- Breastfeeding, newborn screening, and service systems

From U.S. Department of Health and Human Services. (2000). *Healthy People 2010* (conference edition, in two volumes). Washington, DC: Author.

---

box 1-4 **Maternal-Infant Biostatistical Terminology**

Abortus: An embryo or fetus that is removed or expelled from the uterus at 20 weeks of gestation or less, weighs 500 g or less, or measures 25 cm or less

Birthrate: Number of live births in 1 year per 1000 population

Fertility rate: Number of births per 1000 women between the ages of 15 and 44 years (inclusive), calculated on a yearly basis

Infant mortality rate: Number of deaths of infants under 1 year of age per 1000 live births

Maternal mortality rate: Number of maternal deaths from births and complications of pregnancy, childbirth, and puerperium (the first 42 days after termination of the pregnancy) per 100,000 live births

Neonatal mortality rate: Number of deaths of infants under 28 days of age per 1000 live births

Perinatal mortality rate: Number of stillbirths and the number of neonatal deaths per 1000 live births

Stillbirth: An infant who, at birth, demonstrates no signs of life, such as breathing, heartbeat, or voluntary muscle movements

table 1-1	Birth Rate According to Age—2004
AGE (YR)	**100 WOMEN**
15-17	22.1
18-19	70.0
20-24	101.8
25-29	115.5
30-34	95.5
35-39	45.4
40-44	9.0

Data from Hoyert, D., et al. (2006). Annual summary of vital statistics: 2004. *Pediatrics, 117*(1), 168-183.

(LBW) infants. Multiple births contribute to the incidence of LBW. In 2003, 58% of all multiple births were LBW. In 2004 the incidence of LBW infants increased to 8.1% (Hoyert et al., 2006). African-American infants are more than twice as likely as non-Hispanic white infants to be of LBW and to die in the first year of life. For African-American births, the incidence of LBW was 13.7%, whereas the rate was 7.2% for non-Hispanic white births and 6.8% for Hispanic births (Hoyert et al., 2006). Cigarette smoking is associated with LBW, prematurity, and intrauterine growth restriction. In 2004, 10.2% of pregnant women smoked, a proportion that has declined from 19.5% in 1989 (Hoyert et al., 2006).

The percentage of infants born preterm (i.e., born before 38 weeks of gestation) was 12.5% in 2004. There was variation in the percentage according to race and Hispanic origin: 17.9% for non-Hispanic black births, 12.0% for Hispanic births, and 11.5% for non-Hispanic white births (Hoyert et al., 2006). Multiple births accounted for 3.2% of births in 2003, with most of the increase associated with increased use of fertility drugs and older age at childbearing (Hoyert et al., 2006) (see Chapter 40).

Infant Mortality in the United States

A common indicator of the adequacy of prenatal care and the health of a nation as a whole is the infant mortality rate, the number of deaths of infants younger than 1 year of age per 1000 live births. The U.S. infant mortality rate for 2003 was 6.9 (Hoyert et al., 2006). The disparity in infant mortality rate between African-American infants and Caucasian infants has increased over time. The infant mortality rate continues to be higher for non-Hispanic black babies (14.1 per 1000) than for non-Hispanic whites (5.8 per 1000) and Hispanic (5.6 per 1000) babies (Martin et al., 2005). Limited maternal education, young maternal age, unmarried status, poverty, lack of prenatal care, and smoking appear to be associated with higher infant mortality rates. Poor nutrition, smoking and alcohol use, and maternal conditions such as poor health or hypertension also are important contributors to infant mortality. A shift from the current emphasis on high-technology medical interventions to a focus on improving access to preventive care for low-income families is necessary.

International Infant Mortality Trends

In 2002, the infant mortality rate of Canada (5.4/1000) ranked twenty-fourth, and that of the United States (7.0/1000) ranked twenty-seventh, when compared with those of other industrialized nations (Hoyert et al., 2006). Decreases in the infant mortality rate in the United States do not keep pace with the rates of other industrialized countries. One reason for this is the high rate of LBW infants in the United States in contrast with the rates in other countries.

Maternal Mortality Trends

Worldwide, approximately 1600 women die each day of problems related to pregnancy or childbirth; many of these deaths are preventable. In the United States in 2003, the annual maternal mortality rate (number of maternal deaths per 100,000 live births) was 8.2 (Hamilton, Martin, Ventura, Sutton, & Menacker, 2005; Hoyert, Kung, & Smith, 2005). The rates have significant racial differences: "African-American women are four times more likely and Hispanic women are 1.3 times more likely than Caucasian women to die of pregnancy-related complications" (National Center for Health Statistics, 2005). The predominant causes of these deaths are embolism, hemorrhage, gestational hypertension, and infection. The *Healthy People 2010* goal of 3.3 maternal deaths per 100,000 poses a significant challenge. To achieve this goal, early diagnosis and appropriate intervention must occur. Worldwide strategies to reduce maternal mortality rates include improving access to skilled attendants at birth, providing postabortion care, improving family planning services, and providing adolescents with better reproductive health services (Millennium Development Goals, 2004).

Involving Consumers and Promoting Self-Care

Self-care is appealing to both clients and the health care system because of its potential to reduce health care costs. Maternity care is especially suited to self-care because childbearing is essentially health focused, women are usually well when they enter the system, and visits to health care providers can present the opportunity for health and illness interventions. Measures to improve health and reduce risks associated with poor pregnancy outcomes and illness can be addressed. Topics such as nutrition education, stress management, smoking cessation, alcohol and drug treatment, improvement of social supports, and parenting education are appropriate for such encounters.

Efforts to Reduce Health Disparities

Significant disparities in morbidity and mortality rates are experienced by African-Americans, Native Americans, Hispanics, Alaska natives, and Asians/Pacific Islanders. Shorter life expectancy, higher infant and maternal mortality rates, more birth defects, and more sexually transmitted infections are found among these groups. The disparities are thought to result from a complex interaction among biologic factors, environment, and health behaviors. Disparities in education and income are associated with differences in occurrence of morbidity and mortality. The cause-specific mortality ratio was three to four times higher for black women when compared with white women for each cause of death (Chang et al., 2003). The National Institutes of Health has a commitment to improve the health of minorities and provides funding for research and training of minority researchers. The National Institute of Nursing Research has included the goal of reducing disparities in its strategic plan and supports research for that purpose (www.nih.gov/ninr). The nation must make a concerted effort to eliminate health disparities.

Health Literacy

Almost half of all American adults have difficulty in understanding and using health information (Nielsen-Bohlman, Panzer, & Kindig, 2004). Health literacy involves a spectrum of abilities, ranging from reading an appointment slip to interpreting medication instructions. These skills must be assessed routinely to recognize a problem and accommodate clients with limited literacy skills. An excellent resource is *Teaching Patients with Low Literacy Skills* (Doak, Doak, & Root, 1996).

As a result of the increasingly multicultural U.S. population, there is a more urgent need to address health literacy as a component of culturally and linguistically competent care. Health care providers contribute to health literacy by using simple, common words, avoiding jargon, and assessing whether the client is understanding the discussion. Speaking slowly and clearly and focusing on what is important will increase understanding (Roberts, 2004).

Emphasis on High-Technology Care

Advances in scientific knowledge and the large number of high risk pregnancies have contributed to a health care system that emphasizes high-technology care. Maternity care has branched out to include preconception counseling, more and better scientific techniques to monitor the mother and fetus, more definitive tests for hypoxia and acidosis, and neonatal intensive care units. Point-of-care testing is available. Personal data assistants are used to enhance comprehensive care (Lewis & Sommers, 2003); the medical record is often in an electronic form. Virtually all women are monitored electronically during labor despite the lack of evidence of efficacy of such monitoring.

Telemedicine is an umbrella term for the use of communication technologies and electronic information between participants—those providing and those needing care—who are separated by distance. Telemedicine permits specialists, including nurses, to provide health care and consultation at a distance. For example, Baby CareLink (Gray et al., 2000) is an Internet-based program that incorporates teleconferencing and the World Wide Web to enhance interactions among health care providers, families, and community providers. It includes distance learning, virtual home visits, and remote monitoring of the infant after discharge. This technology will save billions of dollars annually for health care.

Strides are being made in identifying genetic codes, and genetic engineering is taking place. Women's health has expanded to emphasize care of older women, new cancer-screening techniques, advances in the diagnosis and treatment of breast cancer, and work on an AIDS vaccine. In general, high-technology care has flourished, whereas "health" care has become relatively neglected. These technologic advances also have contributed to higher health care costs. Nurses must use caution and prospective planning and assess the effect of the emerging technology.

Community-Based Care

A shift in settings, from acute care institutions to ambulatory settings including the home, has been occurring (see Chapter 2). Even childbearing women at high risk are cared for on an outpatient basis or in the home. Technology previously available only in the hospital is now found in the home. This has affected the organizational structure of care, the skills required in providing such care, and the costs to consumers.

Home health care also has a community focus. Nurses are involved in providing care for women and infants in homeless shelters, in caring for adolescents in school-based clinics, and in promoting health at community sites, churches, and shopping malls. Nursing education curricula are increasingly community based.

Increase in High Risk Pregnancies

The number of high risk pregnancies has increased, which means that a greater number of pregnant women are at risk for poor pregnancy outcomes. Escalating drug use and abuse (ranging from 11% to 27% of pregnant women, depending on the geographic location) has contributed to higher incidences of prematurity, LBW, congenital defects, learning disabilities, and withdrawal symptoms in infants. Alcohol use in pregnancy has been associated with miscarriages, mental retardation, LBW, and alcohol-related birth defects. Hypertension associated with pregnancy and diabetes, and the increasing number of multiple pregnancies associated with reproductive technology, contribute to the increasing number of pregnancies at risk.

▬ TRENDS IN NURSING PRACTICE

The increasing complexity of care for maternity and women's health clients has contributed to specialization of nurses working with these clients. This specialized knowledge is gained through experience, advanced degrees, and certification programs. Nurses in advanced practice (e.g., nurse practitioners and nurse-midwives) may provide primary care throughout a woman's life, including during the pregnancy cycle. In some settings, the clinical nurse specialist and nurse practitioner roles are blended, and nurses deliver high-quality, comprehensive, and cost-effective care in a variety of settings. Lactation consultants provide services in the postpartum unit or on an outpatient basis, including during home visits.

box 1-5 **Childbearing Care Interventions**

LEVEL I DOMAIN: FAMILY
- Care that supports the family

LEVEL 2 CLASS: CHILDBEARING CARE
- Interventions to assist in the preparation for childbirth and management of the psychologic and physiologic changes before, during, and immediately after childbirth

LEVEL 3: INTERVENTIONS
- Amnioinfusion
- Birthing
- Bleeding reduction: antepartum uterus
- Bleeding reduction: postpartum uterus
- Breastfeeding assistance
- Cesarean section care
- Childbirth preparation
- Circumcision care
- Electronic fetal monitoring: antepartum
- Electronic fetal monitoring: intrapartum
- Environmental management: attachment process
- Family integrity promotion: childbearing family
- Family planning: contraception
- Family planning: infertility
- Family planning: unplanned pregnancy
- Fertility preservation
- Genetic counseling
- Grief work facilitation: perinatal death
- High risk pregnancy care
- Intrapartal care
- Intrapartal care: high risk delivery
- Kangaroo care
- Labor induction
- Labor suppression
- Lactation suppression
- Newborn care
- Newborn monitoring
- Nonnutritive sucking
- Phototherapy: neonate
- Postpartal care
- Preconception counseling
- Pregnancy termination care
- Prenatal care
- Reproductive technology management
- Resuscitation: fetus
- Resuscitation: neonate
- Risk identification: childbearing family
- Surveillance: late pregnancy
- Tube care: umbilical line
- Ultrasonography: limited obstetric

From Dochterman, J., & Bulechek, G. (2004). *Nursing interventions classification (NIC)* (4th ed.). St. Louis: Mosby.

Nursing Interventions Classification

When the National Institute of Medicine proposed that all client records be computerized by the year 2000, a need for a common language to describe the contributions of nurses to client care became evident. Nurses from the University of Iowa developed a comprehensive standardized language that describes interventions that are performed by generalist or specialist nurses. This language is included in the *Nursing Interventions Classification (NIC)* (Dochterman & Bulechek, 2004). Interventions commonly used by maternal-child nurses include those in Box 1-5.

Evidence-Based Practice

Evidence-based practice—providing care based on evidence gained through research and clinical trials—is increasingly emphasized. Although not all practice can be evidence based, practitioners must use the best available information on which to base their interventions. The Association of Women's Health, Obstetric and Neonatal Nurses (AWHONN) (www.awhonn.org) *Standards and Guidelines for Professional Nursing Practice in the Care of Women and Newborns* (2003) and the *Standards for Professional Perinatal Nursing Practice and Certification in Canada* (2002) include an evidence-based approach to practice. Discussion of nursing care and evidence-based practice boxes throughout this text provide examples of evidence-based practice in perinatal and women's health nursing.

box 1-6 **AWHONN Research-Based Practice Programs**

- Transition of the Preterm Infant to an Open Crib
- Management of Women in Second-Stage Labor
- Continence for Women
- Neonatal Skin Care
- Cyclic Pelvic Pain and Discomfort Management
- Setting Universal Cessation Counseling, Education, and Screening Standards: Nursing Care for Pregnant Women Who Smoke (SUCCESS)

Accessed http://www.awhonn.org/awhonn/?pg=0-874 May 19, 2006

AWHONN has conducted six research-based practice projects (Box 1-6). These projects were conducted in several states, and staff nurses were involved in their implementation and in data collection. The AWHONN practice guidelines incorporate evidence-based practices for second-stage labor management, continence for women, breastfeeding support, midlife well-being, perianesthesia care, neonatal skin care, and cardiac health. By using such guidelines and published reports, nurses can develop protocols and procedures based on published research and incorporate an evidence base into their own practice. AWHONN research priorities include the aforementioned topics as well as family violence, fetal surveillance, genetics, infertility, and early parenting (Box 1-7).

box 1-7 **AWHONN Research Priorities for Women's and Neonatal Health**

WOMEN ACROSS THE LIFE SPAN
- Disparities in care
- Weight management
- Exercise
- Cardiovascular health, including smoking cessation
- Mental health and stress management
- Cancer screening and risk reduction
- Access to reproductive services
- Menopause adjustment and symptom management
- Chronic illness
- Alternative therapies

PROFESSIONAL PRACTICE AND NURSING ISSUES
- Staff and student education
- Nursing shortage
- Client safety
- Cultural/linguistic competency
- Staffing
- Diverse workforce
- Ethics
- Quality of care
- Interdisciplinary collaboration
- Organizational culture
- Health promotion

CHILDBEARING/NEWBORN
- Near-term infant
- Breastfeeding
- Diabetes evidence-based guidelines (EBG)
- Cardiovascular risk in pregnancy
- Social risks: domestic violence
- Mental health (selective serotonin reuptake inhibitors [SSRIs] in pregnancy, breastfeeding)
- Reduce disparities in low-birth-weight births
- Prematurity
- Genetics
- Reproductive technology
  —Management of information acquired through technology in perinatal care
  —Use of technology
  —Impact of technology (anticipatory guidance)
  —Parent education
- Complementary therapies

Recommended by AWHONN Research Review and Advisory Panel, April 2005. Approved by AWHONN Board of Directors, June, 2005.

Introduction to Evidence-Based Practice Reviews

Evidence-based practice review groups systematically examine all relevant research studies on a certain topic and communicate their findings to the professionals who make clinical decisions and write protocols for clinical practice. Many studies are too small to be generalizable to the general population. With the studies combined, several smaller studies together achieve more "power," or predictive value. The review by Gupta, Hofmeyr, and Smyth (2006), for example, combined eight smaller trials to include a total of 3600 women.

A review group searches large databases, such as Cochrane, MEDLINE, CINAHL, PsycINFO, or PubMed, using combinations of words related to the topic. They also hand search the reference lists of relevant citation and ask experts in that field. The authors may choose to review only randomized trials, because these are the most generalizable to the larger population. In addition, they may choose only controlled trials (one group gets the intervention and one group, the control, does not), which makes a stronger case that any difference between the groups is actually a result of the intervention rather than some other influence. In the study of "Positions Beneficial for Birth" in the Evidence-Based Practice box, the studies ranged from the years 1963 to 1999 and were from five continents. The reviewers examined research on a variety of maternal outcomes, such as pain, blood loss, perineal trauma (episiotomies or perineal

tears), and duration of labor. They also looked at fetal outcomes, such as trauma, neonatal intensive care unit (NICU) admission, and death. The trials included a variety of birthing positions and protocols. In this case, the reviewers combined studies with similar definitions, and reported overall findings, as well as significant variations.

Conclusions are the review committee's best recommendations for clinical practice, based on the best available evidence. Reviewers may find that some of our long-standing assumptions about clinical care are not beneficial, or may even be harmful for mother or baby. In the Gupta, Hofmeyr, and Smyth review, the upright birth position was found to be a safe alternative for mother or baby, except for the caution about increased blood loss. Although this review found upright position superior on many outcomes, the authors stop short of recommending upright position over supine until better-quality and larger studies can confirm their findings.

Cochrane Pregnancy and Childbirth Database

The Cochrane Pregnancy and Childbirth Database was first planned in 1976 with a small grant from the World Health Organization to Dr. Iain Chalmers and colleagues at Oxford. In 1993, the Cochrane Collaboration was formed, and the Oxford Database of Perinatal Trials became known as The Cochrane Pregnancy and Childbirth Database. The Cochrane Collaboration oversees up-to-date, systematic reviews of randomized controlled trials of

EVIDENCE-BASED PRACTICE

Positions Beneficial for Birth

BACKGROUND

- Historically, women have tended to assume upright positions for birth, such as squatting, supported by a birth stool, crouching, or kneeling. The dorsal position is a more recent cultural norm within Western hospital settings, where the semi-recumbent or lithotomy position is thought to be favorable for monitoring the fetus, as well more convenient for the health care provider doing medical procedures. Advantages of an upright birth position include augmentation of progress from gravity, increased uteroplacental perfusion and less fetal acidosis, improved pelvic alignment and roomier outlet, and stronger and more efficient contractions. While the squatting position may be the most natural position in cultures where women squat to defecate and to rest, Western women may not have the necessary muscle stretch or tone to tolerate the position for long without support.

OBJECTIVE

- The reviewers sought to compare the different positions assumed for birth. Possibly affected outcomes included maternal pain, blood pressure, duration and trauma of labor, blood loss, long-term perineal changes, and satisfaction. The authors also hoped to compare fetal outcomes of heart rate patterns, occipitoposterior position, and neonatal conditions leading to neonatal intensive care or death.

METHOD

Search Strategy

- From the research literature, the authors chose 19 randomized controlled trials involving 5764 women, dated 1963-1999. They represented trials in Australia, Canada, England, Finland, France, Hong Kong, India, Ireland, New Zealand, Scotland, South Africa, Sweden, and Kuwait. No U.S. studies met the criteria.

Statistical Analyses

- Similar data were pooled. Reviewers calculated relative risk for dichotomous (categoric) data, such as episiotomy, and weighted mean difference for continuous data, such as pain scale. Differences between groups outside the 95% confidence interval were accepted as significant. Most were analyzed in their original, randomly assigned "intention to treat" categories, even if they changed their minds.

FINDINGS

- The upright position was significantly superior to supine or lithotomy positions in reducing duration and severity of pain in second-stage labor, and was associated with fewer worrisome fetal heart rate patterns and assisted births. There were fewer episiotomies, offset partially by an increase in second-degree perineal tears. Increased estimated blood loss of greater than 500 ml was reported in the upright position. Use of birth or squatting stools and birth chairs resulted in significantly fewer episiotomies, increased blood loss, and less pain; use of birth cushions also contributed to a considerably shorter second stage of labor and fewer perineal tears. Lateral positions were similar to supine positions in duration of the second stage, assisted births, and episiotomies.

LIMITATIONS

- Since it was not possible to allow blinding, observer bias may have affected results. Some subjects were excluded after randomization or had some difficulty assuming their assigned position. Abnormal skewing of results and sample size caused the reviewers to label the overall quality of the studies as poor and report their results with caution.

IMPLICATIONS FOR PRACTICE

- Most women in the non-Western world expect to use the upright position for birth. The upright position for birth can use gravity and mechanics to augment the progress of the second stage of labor. Nurses must advocate for upright positions as an alternative for their clients during birth. The reviewers recommend any position that is comfortable for the woman.

IMPLICATIONS FOR FURTHER RESEARCH

- This review was transcultural, which greatly strengthens its generalizability. Randomized controlled trials with excellent data analysis are needed to determine more fetal and infant outcomes. More positions need comparison, such as hands and knees (which is not upright). Research should explore whether the upright position can decrease operative or instrumental births. There may be differences in outcomes between health care providers (physicians and certified nurse-midwives), related to provider familiarity with the birth position. Blood loss, an important parameter, should be explored with continuous data, and it should be accurately measured, rather than estimated.

Reference: Gupta, J., Hofmeyr, G., & Smyth, R. (2006). Position of second stage of labour for women without epidural anaesthesia. In *The Cochrane Database of Systematic Reviews,* 2006, Issue 3. Chichester, UK: John Wiley & Sons.

health care and disseminates these reviews. The premise of the project is that these types of studies provide the most reliable evidence about the effects of care.

The evidence from these studies should encourage practitioners to implement useful measures and to abandon those that are useless or harmless. Studies are ranked in six categories:

1. Beneficial forms of care
2. Forms of care that are likely to be beneficial
3. Forms of care with a trade-off between beneficial and adverse effects
4. Forms of care with unknown effectiveness
5. Forms of care that are unlikely to be beneficial
6. Forms of care that are likely to be ineffective or harmful

Practices that have been reviewed by the Collaboration as well as other evidence for practice will be identified with a symbol ❋ throughout this text.

Joanna Briggs Institute

Founded in 1995 as an initiative of the Royal Adelaide Hospital and the University of Adelaide in Australia, the Joanna Briggs Institute (JBI) uses a collaborative approach for evaluating evidence from a range of sources (www. joannabriggs.edu.au). The JBI has formed collaborations with a variety of universities and hospitals around the world including in the United States and Canada.

In its reviews, the JBI categorizes studies by strength of evidence according to the following classification:

I: Evidence obtained from a systematic review of all relevant randomized controlled trials.

II: Evidence obtained from at least one properly designed randomized controlled trial.

III.1: Evidence obtained from well-designed pseudo-randomised controlled trials (alternate allocation or some other method).

III.2: Evidence obtained from comparative studies with concurrent controls and allocation not randomized (cohort studies), case control studies or interrupted time series with a control group.

III.3: Evidence obtained from comparative studies with historical control, two or more single arm studies, or interrupted time series without a parallel control group.

IV: Evidence obtained from case series, either post-test or pre-test and post-test (the Joanna Briggs Institute Approach to "Evidence," 2006).

The JBI provides another source for perinatal nurses to access information to support evidence-based practice.

Outcomes-Oriented Practice

Outcomes of care (that is, the effectiveness of interventions and quality of care) are receiving increased emphasis. Outcomes-oriented care measures effectiveness of care against benchmarks or standards. It is a measure of the value of nursing using quality indicators and answers the question, "Did the client benefit or not benefit from the care provided?" (Moorhead, Johnson, & Maas, 2004). The Outcome Assessment Information Set (OASIS) is an example of an outcome system important for nursing. Its use is required by the Centers for Medicare and Medicaid Services, formerly the Health Care Financing Administration (HCFA), in all home health organizations that are Medicare accredited. The Nursing Outcomes Classification (NOC) is an effort to identify outcomes and related measures that can be used for evaluation of care of individuals, families, and communities across the care continuum (Moorhead et al., 2004). An example of outcomes classification is provided in Table 1-2.

A Global Perspective

Advances in medicine and nursing have resulted in increased knowledge and understanding in the care of mothers and infants and reduced perinatal morbidity and mortality rates. However, these advances have affected predominantly the industrialized nations. For example, the majority of the 3.2 million children living with HIV or AIDS acquired the infection through perinatal transmission and live in sub-Saharan Africa. This illustrates the inequities that exist between industrialized and resource-poor parts of the world (Cohan, 2003).

As the world becomes smaller because of travel and communication technologies, nurses and other health care providers are gaining a global perspective and participating in activities to improve the health and health care of people worldwide. Nurses participate in medical outreach, providing obstetric, surgical, ophthalmologic, orthopedic, or other services; attend international meetings; conduct research; and provide international consultation. International student and faculty exchanges occur (Fig. 1-3) (Perry & Mander, 2005). More articles about health and health care in various countries are appearing in nursing journals. Several schools of nursing in the United States are World Health Organization Collaborating Centers.

Millennium Development Goals

The member states of the United Nations adopted the Millennium Declaration in September 2000. The Millennium Development Goals are a guide to implementing the Millennium Declaration. The goals are to (1) eradicate extreme poverty and hunger, (2) achieve universal primary education, (3) promote gender equality and empower women, (4) reduce child mortality, (5) improve maternal health, (6) combat HIV and AIDS, malaria, and other diseases, (7) ensure environmental sustainability, and (8) develop a global partnership for development. The target date for achievement of the goals is 2015. The goals help to define a yardstick with which to measure results. With the rich resources of many developed countries, poorer countries can be provided with additional resources and assistance (Millennium Development Goals, 2004).

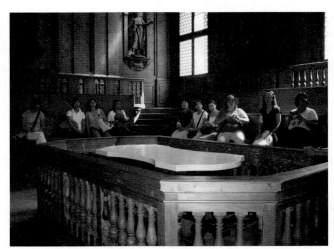

FIG. 1-3 Nursing students visiting an anatomy museum in Bologna, Italy, as part of a course on international perspectives in nursing. (Courtesy Shannon Perry, Phoenix, AZ.)

table I-2 **Nursing Outcomes Classification**

BREASTFEEDING ESTABLISHMENT: INFANT (1000)

Domain—Physiologic Health (II)
Class—Nutrition (K)
Scale—Not adequate to Totally adequate (f)
Definition: Infant attachment to and sucking from the mother's breast for nourishment during the first 3 weeks of breastfeeding

BREASTFEEDING ESTABLISHMENT: INFANT	NOT ADEQUATE 1	SLIGHTLY ADEQUATE 2	MODERATELY ADEQUATE 3	SUBSTANTIALLY ADEQUATE 4	TOTALLY ADEQUATE 5
Indicators					
100001 Proper alignment and latch on	1	2	3	4	5
100002 Proper areolar grasp	1	2	3	4	5
100003 Proper areolar compression	1	2	3	4	5
100004 Correct suck and tongue placement	1	2	3	4	5
100005 Audible swallow	1	2	3	4	5
100006 Swallowing a minimum of 5 to 10 minutes per breast	1	2	3	4	5
100007 Minimum 8 feedings per day	1	2	3	4	5
100008 Urinations per day appropriate for age	1	2	3	4	5
100009 Loose, yellow, seedy stools per day appropriate for age	1	2	3	4	5
100010 Appropriate weight gain for age	1	2	3	4	5
100011 Infant contentment after feeding	1	2	3	4	5

Outcome Content References:

Biancuzzo, M. (2003). *Breastfeeding the newborn* (2nd ed.). St. Louis: Mosby.

Henderson, A., Pincombe, J., & Stamp, G. (2000). Assisting women to establish breastfeeding: Exploring midwives practices. *Breastfeeding Review, 8*(3), 11-17.

Lang, S. (2002). *Breastfeeding special care babies* (2nd ed.). London: Bailliere Tindall.

Lawrence, R. A., & Lawrence, R. M. (1999). *Breastfeeding: A guide for the medical professional* (5th ed.). St. Louis: Mosby.

Minchin, M. (1989). Positioning for breastfeeding. *Birth: Issues in Perinatal Care and Education, 16*(2), 67-80.

Mulford, C. (1992). The mother-baby assessment (MBA): an "Apgar Score" for breastfeeding. *Journal of Human Lactation, 8*(2), 79-82.

Neifert, M., & Seacat, J. (1986). A guide to successful breastfeeding. *Contemporary Pediatrics, 3,* 1-14.

Page-Goertz, S. (1989). Discharge planning for the breastfeeding dyad. *Pediatric Nursing, 15*(5), 543-544.

Righard, L., & Alade, M. (1992). Sucking technique and its effect on success of breastfeeding. *Birth: Issues in Perinatal Care and Education, 19*(4), 185-189.

Riordan, J., & Auerbach, K. (1999). *Breastfeeding and human lactation* (2nd ed.) . Boston: Jones and Bartlett.

Shrago, L., & Bocar, D. (1990). The infant's contribution to breastfeeding. *Journal of Obstetric, Gynecologic, and Neonatal Nursing, 19*(3), 209-215.

Walker, M. (1989). Functional assessment of infant breastfeeding patterns. *Birth: Issues in Perinatal Care and Education, 16*(3), 140-147.

From Moorhead, S., Johnson, M., & Maas, M. (Eds.). (2000). *Nursing outcomes classification (NOC)* (3rd ed.). St. Louis: Mosby.

▀ STANDARDS OF PRACTICE AND
▀ LEGAL ISSUES IN DELIVERY OF CARE

Nursing standards of practice in perinatal and women's health nursing have been described by several organizations, including the American Nurses Association (ANA), which publishes standards for maternal-child health nursing; AWHONN, which publishes standards of practice and education for perinatal nurses (Box 1-8); ACNM, which publishes standards of practice for midwives; and the National Association of Neonatal Nurses (NANN), which publishes standards of practice for neonatal nurses (www.nann.org). These standards reflect current knowledge, represent levels of practice agreed on by leaders in the specialty, and can be used for clinical benchmarking.

In addition to these more formalized standards, agencies have their own policy and procedure books that outline standards to be followed in that setting. In legal terms, the standard of care is that level of practice that a reasonably prudent nurse would provide. In determining legal negligence, the care given is compared with the standard of care. If the standard was not met and harm resulted, negligence is concluded to have occurred. The number of legal suits in the perinatal area has typically been high. As a consequence, malpractice insurance costs are high for physicians, nurse-midwives, and nurses who work in labor and delivery.

▀ LEGAL TIP Standard of Care

When you are uncertain about how to perform a procedure, consult the agency procedure book and follow the guidelines printed therein. These guidelines are the standard of care for that agency.

box 1-8 **Standards of Care for Women and Newborns**

STANDARDS THAT DEFINE THE NURSE'S RESPONSIBILITY TO THE CLIENT

Assessment
- Collection of health data of the woman or newborn

Diagnosis
- Analysis of data to determine nursing diagnosis

Outcome Identification
- Identification of expected outcomes that are individualized

Planning
- Development of a plan of care

Implementation
- Performance of interventions for the plan of care

Evaluation
- Evaluation of the effectiveness of interventions in relation to expected outcomes

STANDARDS OF PROFESSIONAL PERFORMANCE THAT DELINEATE ROLES AND BEHAVIORS FOR WHICH THE PROFESSIONAL NURSE IS ACCOUNTABLE

Quality of Care
- Systemic evaluation of nursing practice

Performance Appraisal
- Self-evaluation in relation to professional practice standards and other regulations

Education
- Participation in ongoing educational activities to maintain knowledge for practice

Collegiality
- Contribution to the development of peers, students, and others

Ethics
- Use of Code for Nurses to guide practice

Collaboration
- Involvement of patient, significant others, and other health care providers in the provision of client care

Research
- Use of research findings in practice

Resource Utilization
- Consideration of factors related to safety, effectiveness, and costs in planning and delivering client care

Practice Environment
- Contribution to the environment of care delivery

Accountability
- Legal and professional responsibility for practice

Source: Association of Women's Health, Obstetric and Neonatal Nurses (AWHONN). (2003). *Standards and guidelines for professional nursing practice in the care of women and newborns* (6th ed.). Washington, DC: Author.

Risk Management

Risk management is an evolving process that identifies risks, establishes preventive practices, develops reporting mechanisms, and delineates procedures for managing lawsuits. Nurses should be familiar with concepts of risk management and their implications for nursing practice. These concepts can be viewed as systems of checks and balances that ensure high-quality client care from preconception until after birth. Effective risk management minimizes the risk of injury to clients and the number of lawsuits against nurses, doctors, and hospitals. Each facility or site develops site-specific risk management procedures based on accepted standards and guidelines. The procedures and guidelines must be reviewed periodically.

To decrease risk of errors in the administration of medications, the Joint Commission on Accreditation of Healthcare Organizations (JCAHO) developed a list of abbreviations, acronyms, and symbols *not* to use (Table 1-3). In addition, each agency must develop its own list.

Sentinel Events

JCAHO describes a sentinel event as "an unexpected occurrence involving death or serious physical or psychologic injury, or the risk thereof. Serious injury specifically includes loss of limb or function." These events are called "sentinel" because they signal a need for an immediate investigation and response (JCAHO, 2002). Reportable sentinel events in perinatal nursing include any maternal death related to the process of birth and any perinatal death that is not related to a congenital condition in an infant with a birth weight greater than 2500 g.

Failure to Rescue

Failure to rescue is used to "evaluate the quality and quantity of nursing care by comparing the number of surgical clients who develop common complications who survive versus those who do not" (Simpson, 2005). As mothers and babies are generally healthy, complications leading to death in obstetrics are comparatively rare. Simpson (2005) proposes evaluating the perinatal team's ability to decrease risk of adverse outcomes by measuring processes involved in common complications and emergencies in obstetrics. Key components of failure to rescue are (1) careful surveillance and identification of complications, and (2) acting quickly to initiate appropriate interventions and activating a team response. For the perinatal nurse, this involves timely

table 1-3 JCAHO "Do Not Use" List

ABBREVIATION	POTENTIAL PROBLEM	PREFERRED TERM
U (for unit)	Mistaken for ")" (zero), the number "4" (four), or "cc".	Write "unit."
IU (for international unit)	Mistaken for IV (intravenous) or the number 10 (ten).	Write "International Unit."
Q.D., QD, q.d., qd (daily)	Mistaken for each other.	Write "daily"
Q.O.D., QOD, q.o.d., qod (every other day)	Period after the Q mistaken for an "I" and the "O" for "I."	Write "every other day."
Trailing zero (X.0 mg)	Decimal point is missed.	Write X mg
Lack of leading zero (.X mg)		Write 0.X mg
MS	Can mean morphine sulfate or magnesium sulfate.	Write "morphine sulfate"
MSO_4 and $MgSO_4$	Confused for one another.	Write "magnesium sulfate."

Source: Official "Do not use" List. Accessed http://www.jointcommission.org/PatientSafety/DoNotUseList/May 19, 2006.

identification of complications, appropriate interventions, and efforts of the team to minimize client harm. Maternal complications that are appropriate for process measurement are placental abruption, postpartum hemorrhage, uterine rupture, eclampsia, and amniotic fluid embolism (Simpson, 2005). Fetal complications include nonreassuring fetal heart rate and pattern, prolapsed umbilical cord, shoulder dystocia, and uterine hyperstimulation (Simpson, 2005). Perinatal nurses can use these complications to develop a list of expectations for monitoring, timely identification, interventions, and roles of team members. The list can be used to evaluate the perinatal team's response.

■ ETHICAL ISSUES IN PERINATAL
■ NURSING AND WOMEN'S HEALTH CARE

Ethical concerns and debates have multiplied with the increased use of technology and with scientific advances. For example, with reproductive technology, pregnancy is now possible in women who thought they would never bear children, including some who are menopausal or postmenopausal. Should scarce resources be devoted to achieving pregnancies in older women? Is giving birth to a child at an older age worth the risks involved? Should older parents be encouraged to conceive a baby when they may not live to see the child reach adulthood? Should a woman who is HIV positive have access to assisted reproduction services? Should third-party payers assume the costs of reproductive technology? With induced ovulation and in vitro fertilization, multiple pregnancies occur, and multifetal pregnancy reduction (selectively terminating one or more fetuses) may be considered. Innovations such as intrauterine fetal surgery, fetoscopy, therapeutic insemination, genetic engineering, stem cell research, surrogate childbearing, surgery for infertility, "test tube" babies, fetal research, and treatment of very LBW (VLBW) babies have resulted in questions about informed consent and allocation of resources. The introduction of long-acting contraceptives has created moral choices and policy dilemmas for health care providers and legislators; that is, should some women (substance abusers, women with low incomes, or women who are HIV positive) be required to take the contraceptives? With the potential for great good that can come from fetal tissue transplantation, what research is ethical? What are the rights of the embryo? Should cloning of humans be permitted? Discussion and debate about these issues will continue for many years. Nurses and clients, as well as scientists, physicians, attorneys, lawmakers, ethicists, and clergy, must be involved in the discussions.

■ RESEARCH IN PERINATAL NURSING
■ AND WOMEN'S HEALTH CARE

Research plays a vital role in the establishment of maternity and women's health science. Nurses can promote research funding and conduct research on maternity and women's health, especially concerning the effectiveness of nursing strategies for these clients. Research can validate that nursing care makes a difference. For example, although prenatal care is clearly associated with healthier infants, no one knows exactly which nursing interventions produce this outcome. The research into women's health must increase. In the past, medical researchers rarely included women in their studies, so more research in this area is crucial. Many possible areas of research exist in maternity and women's health care. The clinician can identify problems in the health and health care of women and infants. Through research, nurses can make a difference for these clients.

Ethical Guidelines for Nursing Research

Nurses must protect the rights of human subjects (that is, clients) in all of their research. For example, nurses may collect data on or care for clients who are participating in clinical trials. The nurse ensures that the subjects are fully informed and aware of their rights as subjects. Research with perinatal clients may create ethical dilemmas for the nurse. For example, participating in research may cause additional stress to a woman concerned about outcomes of genetic testing or one who is waiting for an invasive procedure. Obtaining amniotic fluid samples or performing cordocentesis poses risks to the fetus. The nurse may be involved in determining whether the benefits of research outweigh the risks to the mother and the fetus. Following the ANA ethical guidelines in the conduct, dissemination, and implementation of nursing research helps nurses ensure that research is conducted ethically.

community activity

Obtain statistics from your state and local health departments on racial and ethnic makeup of the state and your community, and the number of deaths from breast cancer and the infant mortality rate according to racial and ethnic categories. Then do a short search of the World Wide Web by using your preferred search engine to access information on research addressing access to mammography and prevention of infant mortality. Describe one research project that deals with (1) prevention or treatment of breast cancer or (2) prevention of infant mortality. Is the principal investigator a nurse? Are nurses involved in the research? What is the ethnic and racial composition of the participants in the study? Where were the findings published? Do consumers have access to this information? Have the results appeared in the popular press?

key points

- Maternity nursing focuses on women and their infants and families during the childbearing cycle.
- Women's health nursing focuses on the special physical, psychologic, and social needs of women throughout their life spans.
- Nurses caring for women can play an active role in shaping health care systems to be responsive to the needs of contemporary women.
- Childbirth practices have changed to become more focused on the family and to allow alternatives in care.
- Home care is a cost-effective alternative site for providing health care.
- A variety of factors, including race, age, and violence, affect women's health.
- Canada ranks twenty-fourth and the United States ranks twenty-seventh among industrialized nations in infant mortality rates.
- Integrative medicine combines modern technology with ancient healing practices and encompasses the whole of body, mind, and spirit.
- Evidence-based practice and outcomes orientation are emphasized in current practice.
- Risk management and learning from sentinel events can improve quality of care.
- *Healthy People 2010* provides goals for maternal and infant health.
- Research plays a vital role in establishing a scientific base for the care of women and infants.
- Ethical concerns have multiplied with the increasing use of technology and scientific advances.

REFERENCES

Ahmed, B., & Abushama, M. (2005). Female genital mutilation and childbirth. *Saudi Medical Journal, 26*(3), 376-378.

American Academy of Pediatrics Committee on Fetus and Newborn. (2004). Policy Statement. Hospital stay for healthy term newborns. *Pediatrics, 113*(5), 1434-1436.

American Cancer Society. (2006). *Cancer facts and figures 2006. Estimated new cancer cases and deaths by sex for all sites, US, 2006.* Accessed www.cancer.org, February 19, 2006.

Association of Women's Health, Obstetric and Neonatal Nurses (AWHONN). (2003). *Standards and guidelines for professional nursing practice in the care of women and newborns* (6th ed.). Washington, DC: Author.

Association of Women's Health, Obstetric and Neonatal Nurses (AWHONN). (2002). *Standards for professional perinatal nursing practice and certification in Canada,* Washington, DC: Author.

Barrett, B. (2003). Alternative, complementary, and conventional medicine: Is integration upon us? *Journal of Alternative and Complementary Medicine, 9*(3), 417-427.

The Joanna Briggs Institute Approach to "Evidence." (2006). Accessed www.joannabriggs.edu.au/about/history_approach.php, May 19, 2006.

Centers for Disease Control and Prevention. (2006). 2003 Assisted reproductive technology (ART) report. Accessed www.cdc.gov/Art/ART2003, May 19, 2006.

Chang, J., Elam-Evans, L., Berg, C., Herndon, J., Flowers, L., Seed, K., et al. (2003). Pregnancy-related mortality surveillance–United States, 1991-1999. *Morbidity and Mortality Weekly Report Surveillance Summary, 52*(SS02), 1-8.

Cohan, D. (2003). Perinatal HIV: Special considerations. *Topics in HIV Medicine, 11*(6), 200-213.

Doak, C., Doak, L., & Root, J. (1996). *Teaching patients with low literacy skills* (2nd ed.). Philadelphia: JB Lippincott.

Dochterman, J., & Bulechek, G. (2004). *Nursing interventions classification (NIC)* (4th ed.). St. Louis: Mosby.

European Collaborative Study. (2005). Mother-to-child transmission of HIV infection in the era of highly active antiretroviral therapy. *Clinical Infectious Diseases, 40*(3), 458-465.

Gauthier, M., & Serber, M. (2005). *A need to transform the U.S. health care system: Improving access, quality, and efficiency.* The Commonwealth Fund. Accessed www.cmwf.org/publications/publications_show.htm?doc_id=302833, February 10, 2006.

Gray, J., Safran, C., Davis, R., Pompilio-Weitzner, G., Stewart, J., Zaccagnini, L., et al. (2000). Baby CareLinks: Using the Internet and telemedicine to improve care for high-risk infants. *Pediatrics, 106*(6), 1318-1324.

Gupta, J., Hofmeyr, G., & Smyth, R. (2006). Position of second stage of labour for women without epidural anaesthesia (Cochrane Review). In *The Cochrane Database of Systematic Reviews,* 2006, Issue 3. Chichester, UK: John Wiley & Sons.

Hamilton, B., Martin, J., Ventura, S., Sutton, P., & Menacker, F. (2005). Births: Preliminary data for 2004. *National Vital Statistics Reports, 54*(8), 1-17.

Hollander, C. (Digest Ed.). (2006). *"Consumer-driven" plans not so consumer-friendly. The Commonwealth Fund Digest,* January/February. Accessed www.cmwf.org/funddigest/funddigest_list.htm?issue_id=2289&doc_id=342311, February 16, 2006.

Hoyert, D., Mathews, T., Menacker, F., Strobino, D., & Guyer, B. (2006). Annual summary of vital statistics: 2004. *Pediatrics, 117*(1), 168-183.

Hoyert, D., Kung, H-C., & Smith, B. (2005). Deaths: Preliminary data for 2003. *National Vital Statistics Reports, 53*(15), 1-48.

Jackson, D., Lang, J., Swartz, W., Ganats, T., Fullerton, J., Ecker, J., et al. (2003). Outcomes, safety and resource utilization in a collaborative care birth center program compared with traditional physician-based perinatal care. *American Journal of Public Health, 93*(6), 999-1006.

Joint Commission on Accreditation of Healthcare Organizations (JCAHO). *"Do not use" list required in 2004:* LTC Update, Issue e. Accessed http://www.jcaho.org/accredited+organizations/patient+safety/dnu.htm, February 19, 2006.

Joint Commission on Accreditation of Healthcare Organizations (JCAHO). (2002). *Sentinel event policy and procedures. Revised: July 2002.* Accessed www.jcaho.org, February 19, 2006.

Lewis, J., & Sommers, C. (2003). Personal data assistants: Using new technology to enhance nursing practice. *MCN American Journal of Maternal/Child Nursing, 28*(2), 66-73.

Martin, J., Hamilton, B., Sutton, P., Ventura, S., Menacker, F., & Munson, M. (2005). Births: Final data for 2003. *National Vital Statistics Report, 54*(2), 1-116.

Millennium Development Goals. (September, 2004). Accessed www.developmentgoals.org, February 17, 2006.

Momoh, C. (2004). Female genital mutilation. *Current Opinion in Obstetrics and Gynecology, 16*(6), 477-480.

Moorhead, S., Johnson, M., & Maas, M. (2004). *Nursing outcomes classification (NOC)* (3rd ed.). St. Louis: Mosby.

National Center for Health Statistics (2005). *Health, United States, 2005. Table 43. Maternal mortality for complications of pregnancy, childbirth, and the puerperium, according to race, Hispanic origin, and age: United States, selected years 1950-2002.* Accessed www.cdc.gov/nchs/hus.htm, February 19, 2006.

Nielsen-Bohlman, L., Panzer, A., & Kindig, D. (Eds.). (2004). *Health literacy: A prescription to end confusion.* Washington, DC: Institute of Medicine.

Perry, S., & Mander, R. (2005). A global frame of reference: Learning from everyone, everywhere. *Nursing Education Perspectives, 26*(3), 148-151.

Roberts, K. (2004). Simplify, simplify: Tackling health literacy by addressing reading literacy. *American Journal of Nursing, 104*(3), 118-119.

Rogers, A., Hwang, W., Scott, L., Aiken, L., & Dinges, D. (2004). The working hours of hospital staff nurses and patient safety. *Health Affairs (Millwood), 23*(4), 202-232.

Rubin, R. (2000, June 21). U.S. ranks 37th in health care. *USA Today,* p. 1.

Schoen, C., Osborn, R., Huynh, P., Doty, M., Zapert, K., Peugh, J., et al. (2005). Taking the pulse of health care systems: Experiences of patients with health problems in six countries. *Health Affairs* Web Exclusive November 3, 2005 W5-509-W5-525. Accessed www.cmwf.org/publications/publications_show.htm?doc_id=303012, August 16, 2006.

Simpson, K. (2005). Failure to rescue in obstetrics. *MCN American Journal of Maternal/Child Nursing, 30*(1), 76.

U.S. Department of Health and Human Services. (2000). *Healthy People 2010* (Conference edition, in two volumes). Washington, DC: Author.

U.S. Department of Health and Human Services Health Resources and Services Administration. (2004). *The registered nurse population: National Sample Survey of Registered Nurses March 2004.* Accessed http://bhpr.hrsa.gov/healthworkforce/reports/rnpopulation/preliminaryfindings.htm, February 14, 2006.

U.S. Census Bureau. (2004). *U.S. interim projections by age, sex, race, and Hispanic origin.* Accessed www.census.gov/ipc/www/usinterimproj/, February 19, 2006.

World Health Organization. (May 2, 2002). *Traditional medicine: Growing needs and potential, WHO Policy Perspectives on Medicine.* Geneva: Author. Accessed http://www.who.int/medicines/publications/policyperspectives/en/index.html, February 19, 2006.

CHAPTER 2

Maureen Nalle, Bonnie Callen, and Susan Speraw

Community Care: The Family and Culture

learning objectives

- Describe the main characteristics of contemporary family forms.
- Identify key factors influencing family health.
- Compare theoretic approaches for working with childbearing families.
- Relate the role of culture in caring for childbearing families.
- Discuss cultural competence in relation to one's own nursing practice.
- Identify key components of the community assessment process.
- List indicators of community health status and their relevance to perinatal health.

- Describe data sources and methods for obtaining information about community health status.
- Identify predisposing factors and characteristics of vulnerable populations.
- List the potential advantages and disadvantages of home visits.
- Explore telephonic nursing care options in perinatal nursing.
- Describe how home care fits into the maternity continuum of care.
- Discuss safety and infection control principles as they apply to the care of clients in their homes.
- Describe the nurse's role in perinatal home care.

electronic resources

Additional information related to the content in Chapter 2 can be found on

the companion website at **evolve**
http://evolve.elsevier.com/Lowdermilk/MWHC/
- NCLEX Review Questions
- WebLinks

or on the interactive companion CD
- NCLEX Review Questions
- Critical Thinking Exercise: Community Resources for Families
- Critical Thinking Exercise: Cultural Health and the Family
- Plan of Care: Incorporating the Infant into the Family
- Plan of Care: Community and Home Care

▪ INTRODUCTION TO FAMILY, CULTURE, COMMUNITY, AND HOME CARE

The composition, structure and function of the American family have changed dramatically in recent years, largely in response to economic, demographic, sociocultural, and technologic trends that influence family life and health (Friedman, Bowden, & Jones, 2003). Despite great improvements in the overall health of the nation, there is widespread concern about family health and well-being as a reflection of individual, community, and national health status. Pincus and colleagues (2003) observed that the current health care system does not provide adequate services for mothers and children in the areas of prenatal care, behavioral health, nutrition, and chronic illness, or for special care needs. Families face significant barriers in accessing needed services and overcoming discrimination in health

care practices. As the cultural diversity of the United States increases, there is a growing imperative to eliminate racial and ethnic health disparities by providing access to quality care for diverse populations (Weissman et al., 2005).

Healthy People 2010 established national health priorities that focus on two major goals: (1) increased quality and years of healthy life, and (2) elimination of health disparities. The 28 diverse focus areas and 467 objectives provide a systematic approach to health improvement for all people (USDHHS, 2000a) (www.healthypeople.gov) (see Chapter 1). Maternal-child focus areas address the most significant health issues for mothers, infants, and children, including those related to pregnant and postpartum women—maternal illness and death rates, access to prenatal care—and those affecting infant health and survival—infant mortality, birth outcomes, and prevention of birth defects

(USDHHS, 2000b). National objectives for each maternal-child health indicator are used to track progress, highlight achievement, and identify areas for further action.

Trends in maternal and infant health in the United States reveal that progress has been made in relation to reduced infant and fetal deaths, and use of prenatal care (see Chapter 1), but notable gaps remain in as the rates of low birth weight, preterm birth, and infant mortality that continue to fall short of *Healthy People 2010* target goals, with persistent disparities between non-Hispanic whites and African-Americans (March of Dimes, 2003). That many of these outcomes are preventable through access to prenatal care and use of preventive health practices clearly demonstrates the need for comprehensive, community-based care for mothers, infants, and families. As perinatal health trends emerge, nurses are assuming greater roles in assessing family health status and providing care across the perinatal continuum. This continuum begins with family planning and continues with the following categories of care: preconception, prenatal, intrapartum, postpartum, newborn, interconception, and the child from infancy to 1 year of age. In the community, health care ranges from individual care to group and community services, and from primary prevention to tertiary care experiences and home visiting. Depending on the needs of the individual family unit, independent self-care, ambulatory care, home care, low risk hospitalization, or specialized intensive care may be appropriate at different points along this continuum.

In community-based health care, both the aggregate (group of people who have shared characteristics) and the population become the focus of intervention. Health professionals are required not only to determine health priorities but also to develop successful plans of care to be delivered in the health clinic, the community health center, or the client's home. This home- and community-based delivery system presents unique challenges for perinatal and maternity nurses.

This chapter discusses the integration of home, community, and family-focused nursing in relation to culture, *Healthy People 2010,* and perinatal health outcomes.

■ THE FAMILY IN CULTURAL AND ■ COMMUNITY CONTEXT

The perinatal experience must be viewed within the context of the family, group, and community, including cultural, economic, work environment, provider access, and other factors that influence health and health care. By far, the most important of these influences is the family and its cultural context, which define the work of maternity nurses in a significant way. Family structure and function, care-seeking behavior, and relationships with providers are all influenced by culturally related health beliefs and values. Ultimately all of these factors have the power to affect maternal and child health outcomes. It therefore is important to recognize these influences, discuss current trends in families, and explore nursing implications.

Defining Family

The family has traditionally been viewed as the primary unit of socialization, the basic structural unit within a community. However, Chen and Rankin (2002) expanded on this definition, describing family as "the primary institution in society that preserves and transmits culture." Although a family is the primary cultural and socialization unit within a community, it also plays a pivotal role in health care, representing the primary target of health care delivery for maternal and newborn nurses. Most models of health behavior view family as a "system" within the larger social framework of a community. These definitions and understandings affect our approaches to health and health care of individuals within the family unit.

As one of society's most important institutions, the family represents a primary social group that influences and is influenced by other people and institutions. Most people have more continuous contact with this social group than with any other. A family is considered a fundamental social unit because it assumes most of the responsibility for affection, socialization, and health care functions of its members (Friedman et al., 2003) and transmits its cultural background and core values in this context. This unique social network provides a powerful support system for each family member.

Family Organization and Structure

Census data clearly indicate significant alterations in the definition and social configuration of families over the past several decades. The Urban Institute (newfederalism.urban.org/nsaf) recognizes five categories of families: married parents, married-blended family, cohabiting parents, the single-parent family, and no-parent families (Wherry & Finegold, 2004). A broader view of the contemporary family is offered by Brooks (2002), who defines a family as "a group of two or more persons related by blood, marriage, adoption, or emotional commitment who have a permanent relationship and who work together to meet life goals and needs." Beyond these basic characteristics, family trends are difficult to monitor, since current national data systems do not provide extensive information on family structure or caregiving patterns (Federal Interagency Forum on Children and Family Statistics, 2005).

The nuclear family has long represented the traditional American family in which male and female partners and their children live as an independent unit, sharing roles, responsibilities, and economic resources (Fig. 2-1). In contemporary society, this "idealized" family structure actually represents only a relatively small number of families. Married-parent families (biologic or adoptive parents) account for approximately 64% of American families, representing 69% of Caucasian, 55% of Hispanic, and 26.6% of African-American families (Wherry & Finegold, 2004).

Many nuclear families have other relatives living in the same household. These extended family members, called *kin,* are grandparents, aunts or uncles, or other people related by blood (McEwen, 2002) (Fig. 2-2). For some

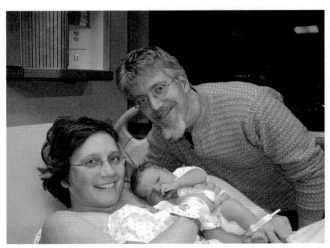

FIG. 2-1 Nuclear family. (Courtesy Wendy and Marwood Larson-Harris, Roanoke, VA.)

groups, such as African-American and Latin-American women, the family kin network is an important resource in terms of preventive health behavior. The extended family is becoming more common as American society ages. The need to care for elderly parents within the same household often creates a "sandwich generation" where parents of the nuclear family provide care for their children as well as for elderly grandparents or other relatives.

Married-blended families, those formed as a result of divorce and remarriage, consist of unrelated family members (stepparents, stepchildren, and stepsiblings) who join together to create a new household. These family groups frequently involve a biologic or adoptive parent whose spouse has not adopted the child.

Cohabiting-parent families are those in which children live with two unmarried biologic parents or two adoptive parents. Hispanic children are more than twice as likely as African-American children to live in cohabiting-parent

FIG. 2-2 Extended family. (Courtesy Shannon Perry, Phoenix, AZ.)

families and about four times as likely as Caucasian children to live in this kind of family arrangement (Wherry & Finegold, 2004).

Single-parent families comprise an unmarried biologic or adoptive parent who may or may not be living with other adults. The single-parent family may result from the loss of a spouse by death, divorce, separation, or desertion; from either an unplanned or planned pregnancy; or from the adoption of a child by an unmarried woman or man. This family structure is becoming more prevalent, with estimates at less than one fifth (18.2%) of Caucasian families, less than one third (27.3%) of Hispanics, and more than half (53.4%) of African-American families in the United States (Wherry & Finegold, 2004). Although the share of single-mother families has decreased significantly, the share of children living in cohabiting families has increased (Acs & Nelson, 2003).

The single-parent family tends to be vulnerable economically and socially, creating an unstable and deprived environment for the growth of children. Research demonstrates the impact of single-parenthood not only in economic instability but also in relation to health status, school achievement, and high risk behaviors for these children. Single mothers are more likely to live in poverty and have poor perinatal outcomes (Schor, 2004; Spencer, 2005; Weitoft, Hjern, Haglund, & Rosen, 2003).

Another family configuration that is less well documented is the increasing number of homosexual families (lesbian and gay), who may live together with or without children. It is estimated that between 800,000 and 7 million homosexual parents are raising between 1 and 9 million children (Cameron, 2004). Although there is no consensus as to what constitutes a gay and lesbian family, these families are rich and diverse in their form and composition. Usually formed by same-sex couples, they can also consist of single gay or lesbian parents or multiple parenting figures (Friedman et al., 2003).

Children in lesbian and gay families may be the offspring of previous heterosexual unions, conceived by one member of a lesbian couple through therapeutic insemination, or adopted. These trends reflect the increased opportunities for alternative forms of parenthood within our society, owing both to more liberal social mores and to technologic and medical advances that offer the possibility of parenthood to single men and women (Greenfield, 2005).

No-parent families are those in which children live independently in foster or kinship care such as living with a grandparent. An estimated 2 million grandparents are primary caretakers for their grandchildren; nearly half of these have assumed this responsibility for more than 5 years (U.S. Census, 2002).

The Family in Society

The social context for the family can be viewed in relation to social and demographic trends that define the population as a whole. U.S. Census data indicate that the racial and ethnic diversity of the population has grown dramatically in the last three decades: 29.5% of all U.S. citizens belong to racial or ethnic minority groups (USDHHS, 2005). Current statistics reflect a population that is 75% Caucasian, 12% African-American, and 13% Hispanic (U.S. Census Bureau, 2002). In 2002, the Hispanic population in the United States for the first time became larger than the African American population (U.S. Census Bureau, 2003).

■ THEORETIC APPROACHES TO ■ UNDERSTANDING FAMILIES

A family theory can be used to describe families and how the family unit responds to events both within and outside the family. Each family theory makes certain assumptions about the family and has inherent strengths and limitations. Most nurses use a combination of theories in their work with families. A brief discussion of a theory commonly used with families, systems theory, and the implications of this theory for maternal-child nursing is presented. A brief synopsis of several other theories useful in working with families is included in Table 2-1.

Family Systems Theory

Among the caring disciplines, a systems approach to understanding the family is almost universally applied. Many systems concepts are central to the delivery of holistic nursing care. These include recognition that changes occurring in one member affect the entire family, and an appreciation that nurses who work with families also enter into a systemic relationship with them. This is especially true for nurses who provide perinatal nursing care through community- or home-based agencies. Understanding how family members influence and interact with each other can help the nurse develop empathy with and respect for different ways of functioning.

When applied to families, the systems theory allows nurses to "view the family as a unit and thus focus on observing the interaction among family members rather than studying family members individually" (Wright & Leahey, 2005). Key characteristics of the family systems theory as identified by Wright and Leahey are:

- A family system is part of a larger suprasystem and in turn is composed of many subsystems.
- The family as a whole is greater than the sum of its individual members.
- A change in one family member affects all family members.
- The family is able to create a balance between change and stability.
- Family members' behaviors are best understood from a view of circular rather than linear causality.

---

table 2-1 **Theories and Models Relevant to Family Nursing Practice**

THEORY	SYNOPSIS OF THEORY
Family Life Cycle (Developmental) Theory (Carter & McGoldrick, 1999)	Families move through stages. The family life cycle is the context in which to examine the identity and development of the individual. Relationships among family members go through transitions. Although families have roles and functions, a family's main value is in relationships that are irreplaceable. The family involves different structures and cultures organized in various ways. Developmental stresses may disrupt the life cycle process.
Family Stress Theory (Boss, 2002)	Ways families react to stressful events is the focus. Family stress can be studied within the internal and external contexts in which the family is living. The internal context involves elements that a family can change or control, such as family structure, psychologic defenses, and philosophic values and beliefs. The external context consists of the time and place in which a particular family finds itself and over which the family has no control, such as the culture of the larger society, the time in history, the economic state of society, maturity of the individuals involved, success of the family in coping with stressors, and genetic inheritance.
McGill Model of Nursing (Allen, 1997)	Strength-based approach in clinical practice with families, as opposed to a deficit approach is the focus. Identification of family strengths and resources; provision of feedback about strengths; assistance given to family to develop and elicit strengths and use resources.
Health Belief Model (Becker, 1974; Janz & Becker, 1984)	The goal of the model is to reduce cultural and environmental barriers that interfere with access to health care. Key elements of the Health Belief Model include the following: perceived susceptibility, perceived severity, perceived benefits, perceived barriers, cues to action, and confidence.
Human Developmental Ecology (Bronfenbrenner, 1979; Bronfenbrenner, 1989)	Behavior is a function of interaction of traits and abilities with the environment. Major concepts include ecosystem, niches (social roles), adaptive range, and ontogenetic development. Individuals are "embedded in a microsystem (role and relations), a mesosystem (interrelations between two or more settings), an exosystem (external settings that do not include the person), and a macrosystem (culture)" (Klein & White, 1996). Change over time is incorporated in the chronosystem.

Using Theories to Guide Practice

People interact with each other in many ways. The nurse must understand that countless factors influence ways in which family members relate among themselves and with the health care community. Some of these factors include the natural history of the family, culture, roles, values, beliefs, and traditional customs. Because so many variables affect ways of relating, the nurse must be aware that most family members will interact and communicate with each other in ways that are very different from those of the nurse's own family of origin. Most families will hold at least some beliefs about health that are very different from those of the nurse; in some instances, their beliefs will conflict with principles of health care management predominant in the Western health care system. Therefore to be effective in working with families, the nurse must possess a degree of personal openness and acceptance and be willing to work with families in a way that is respectful and adapts to their ways of learning and communicating.

Because family relationships are always complex, viewing the interaction of the whole family helps nurses to understand more fully the functioning of individual family members. Family systems theory encourages nurses to view individual family members as part of a larger family system influenced by and influencing others. The extent to which this suprasystem influences the family in matters such as prenatal care, childbirth education, and infant care depends on the family's boundary permeability. A family that has recently immigrated to this country may want to receive health information only from others within the family or the immediate cultural community, whereas a family that has more experience in dealing with the American health care system may be more receptive to nurses who are culturally different. When interacting with a family, the nurse becomes part of a system with them. The behaviors and interaction style of the nurse not only affect the individual who is identified as the "client" but also contribute to family members' responses to each other. Finally, the quality of the nurse-family system strongly influences how the family will interact with the greater health care community in the future.

Knowing about the phases of the life cycle can assist nurses in providing anticipatory guidance for families. For example, helping childbearing families prepare for the birth of a newborn may minimize the development of crises. By using developmental theory, a nurse can anticipate that a family who has a child with a serious anomaly might experience a crisis or state of disequilibrium because the birth of an ill child is not a normative event. Because such a family may revert to a state of dependence, the nurse will realize that their need for extra support and nurturing from the nurse is a natural response to stress (see Plan of Care, "Incorporating the Infant into the Family").

Because today's families experience a great deal of pressure, they must develop effective stress-management strategies. Maternity nurses working in community settings may care for a full range of family situations including healthy but highly stressed families, families coping with the extraordinary stress of ill infants, and mothers who have recently had major surgical procedures such as cesarean births. Nurses can assist families in changing their stress levels by helping families control internal and external context factors. The nurse can intervene through educational strategies to correct misconceptions and reduce stress. Explaining normal infant growth and development (maturation) may reduce the stress of parenting.

A family assessment tool such as the one outlined by Friedman (1998) (Fig. 2-3) can be used as a guide for assessing aspects of the family discussed in this chapter. A family genogram, a family tree format depicting relationships of family members over at least three generations (Fig. 2-4) provides valuable information about a family and can be placed in the nursing care plan for easy access by care providers.

By using the Health Belief Model as a guide to assessment, nurses can better address concerns specific to an individual from a different cultural group and motivate the individual to take action on her own behalf. Understanding a woman's concerns from her own point of view can help the nurse to provide interventions that will place women at ease in the health care setting. For example, the nurse can modify or adjust her care in assessing uterine involution as part of postpartum care for a woman who holds traditional Mexican beliefs and fears of having cold enter her uterus during a normal examination. The culturally competent nurse can close the door to the room, pull curtains to minimize air flow around the woman, position the woman so that the perineum is facing away from the door or air vents, and keep the perineum draped so that the examination takes place with a minimum of exposure.

Within the larger society, individuals and families have a variety of stressors that affect their ability to function and to engage consistently in behaviors that will promote health and wellness. These individuals and families fall into high risk or vulnerable populations. Their stresses relate to many aspects of life: ethnic and cultural minority status, immigration status, poverty, challenges with English language fluency and literacy, malnutrition, and limited access to housing.

Some families have multiple stressors, placing them at especially high risk for poor health outcomes. However, it should be noted that not only low-income or minority groups are at risk for high morbidity and mortality. Some stressors affect families at all strata of society. These antecedents to vulnerability include mental illness, substance use, domestic violence, and reduced access to medical care due to unemployment, loss of medical insurance, or inadequate insurance coverage. Nurses cannot make the assumption that a family is invulnerable because its members live in an exclusive neighborhood, are well educated, and are fully employed. The concepts of high risk and vulnerability apply to everyone.

The Friedman Family Assessment Model (Short Form)

Identifying Data

1. Family name
2. Address and phone
3. Family composition
4. Type of family form
5. Cultural (ethnic) background
6. Religious identification
7. Social class status
8. Family's recreational or leisure-time activities

Developmental Stage and History of Family

9. Family's present developmental stage
10. Extent of family developmental tasks fulfillment
11. Nuclear family history
12. History of family of origin of both parents

Environmental Data

13. Characteristics of home
14. Characteristics of neighborhood and larger community
15. Family's geographic mobility
16. Family's associations and transactions with community
17. Family's social support system or network

Family Structure

18. Communication patterns
    Extent of functional and dysfunctional communication (types of recurring patterns)
    Extent of emotional (affective) messages and how expressed
    Characteristics of communication within family subsystems
    Extent of congruent and incongruent messages
    Types of dysfunctional communication processes seen in family
    Areas of open and closed communication
    Familial and contextual variables affecting communication
19. Power structure
    Power outcomes
    Decision-making process
    Power bases
    Variables affecting family power
    Overall family system and subsystem power (Family power continuum placement)
20. Role structure
    Formal role structure
    Informal role structure
    Analysis of role models (optional)
    Variables affecting role structure
21. Family values
    Compare the family to American or family's reference group values and/or identify important family values and their importance (priority) in family.
    Congruence between the family's values and the family's reference group or wider community

Congruence between the family's values and family member's values
Variables influencing family values
Values consciously or unconsciously held
Presence of value conflicts in family
Effect of the above values and value conflicts on health status of family

Family Functions

22. Affective function
    Family's need–response patterns
    Mutual nurturance, closeness, and identification
    Separateness and connectedness
23. Socialization function
    Family child-rearing practices
    Adaptability of child-rearing practices for family form and family's situation
    Who is (are) socializing agent(s) for child(ren)?
    Value of children in family
    Cultural beliefs that influence family's child-rearing patterns
    Social class influence on child-rearing patterns
    Estimation about whether family is at risk for child-rearing problems and if so, indication of high risk factors
    Adequacy of home environment for children's need to play
24. Health care function
    Family's health beliefs, values, and behavior
    Family's definitions of health–illness and their level of knowledge
    Family's perceived health status and illness susceptibility
    Family's dietary practices
    Adequacy of family diet (recommended 3-day food history record)
    Function of mealtimes and attitudes toward food and mealtimes
    Shopping (and its planning) practices
    Person(s) responsible for planning, shopping, and preparation of meals
    Sleep and rest habits
    Physical activity and recreation practices (not covered earlier)
    Family's drug habits
    Family's role in self-care practices
    Medically based preventive measures (physicals, eye and hearing tests, and immunizations)
    Dental health practices
    Family health history (both general and specific diseases—environmentally and genetically related)
    Health care services received
    Feelings and perceptions regarding health services
    Emergency health services
    Source of payments for health and other services
    Logistics of receiving care

Family Stress and Coping

25. Short- and long-term familial stressors and strengths
26. Extent of family's ability to respond, based on objective appraisal of stress-producing situations
27. Coping strategies utilized (present/past)
    Differences in family members' ways of coping
    Family's inner coping strategies
    Family's external coping strategies
28. Dysfunctional adaptive strategies utilized (present/past; extent of usage)

Family Composition Form

Name (last, first)	Gender	Relationship	Date/place of birth	Occupation	Education
1. (Father)					
2. (Mother)					
3. (Oldest child)					
4.					
5.					
6.					
7.					
8.					

FIG. 2-3 The Friedman Family Assessment Model (short form). (From Friedman, M. [1998]. *Family nursing theory and assessment* [4th ed.]. New York: Appleton & Lange.)

plan of care ❯ **Incorporating the Infant into the Family**

NURSING DIAGNOSIS Readiness for enhanced family coping related to adaptation of family to new infant

Expected Outcome *Family members will verbalize that individual and family goals are met during a smooth transition of new family member into the home.*

Nursing Interventions/*Rationales*
- Assess type and amount of support available to family on a daily basis during the postpartum period *to facilitate adaptation of the family to situation of a new member.*
- Encourage family to use past successful coping mechanisms *to enhance ability to cope with new situation and promote self-esteem.*
- Encourage mother to use family and other support or services *to carry out daily household tasks to permit her to focus on herself and infant.*
- Suggest that woman take time to rest when infant sleeps *to conserve energy for healing and limit responsibility to herself and infant.*
- Assess family structure and relationships, including culture, *to evaluate if longer period of adjustment may be expected.*
- Teach family about sensory needs and capabilities of infant *to motivate family to meet infant's needs and set realistic expectations for infant's capabilities.*
- Refer to parent support group or community agencies, as needed, *to facilitate and validate ongoing positive adjustment of family to new family member.*

NURSING DIAGNOSIS Ineffective role performance related to developmental challenge of addition of new family member

Expected Outcomes *Each family member will verbalize realistic expectations regarding his or her role in the family and formulate a plan to incorporate role into overall family goals.*

Nursing Interventions/*Rationales*
- Assess family structure, roles, and each member's perception of his or her role in the family *to evaluate the impact of the new member on the structure and roles of the family as perceived by the members.*
- Evaluate individual's perception of goals and new roles during this transition *to promote early intervention and correct any misinterpretation.*
- Encourage discussion of family members' thoughts and feelings regarding this transition *to promote open communication and trust.*
- Provide positive reinforcement for family members' actions that promote a positive environment for the infant *to increase self-esteem and provide encouragement.*
- Refer to community support groups *to provide group reinforcement and further assistance.*
- Give information about sibling and grandparent classes and support groups as available *to promote empowerment and self-esteem for significant others in the family.*

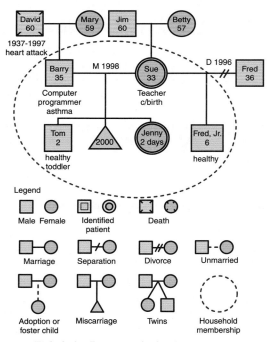

FIG. 2-4 Example of a family genogram.

■ THE FAMILY IN A CULTURAL CONTEXT
Cultural Factors Related to Family Health

Culture has many definitions. According to the classic definition by Fejos (1959), culture is "the sum total of socially inherited characteristics of a human group that comprises everything which one generation can tell, convey, or hand down to the next; in other words, the nonphysically inherited traits we possess." Leininger, a world-renowned nurse anthropologist, says that culture is the values, beliefs, norms, and practices of a group of people that are learned and shared and guide thinking, decisions, and actions in a patterned way (Leininger & McFarland, 2002). Giger and Davidhizar (2004) add that "culture is a patterned behavioral response that develops over time as a result of imprinting the mind through social and religious structures and intellectual and artistic manifestations."

All of these definitions include the recognition that culture helps shape a person's interpretation of every life experience. Cultural knowledge includes beliefs and values about each facet of life and is passed from one generation to the next. Cultural beliefs and traditions relate to food, language, religion, art, health and healing practices, kinship relationships, and all other aspects of community, family, and individual life. Culture has also been shown to have a direct effect on health behaviors. Values, attitudes, and beliefs that are culturally acquired may influence perceptions of illness, as well as health care–seeking behavior and response to treatment (National Academy Press [NAP], 2002). The political, social, and economic context of people's lives is also part of the cultural experience.

Culture plays a powerful role in an individual's behavior, particularly when the individual is sick. Understanding of a culture can provide insight into how a person reacts to illness, pain, and invasive medical procedures, as well as patterns of human interaction and expressions of emotion (Munoz & Luckmann, 2005). The impact of these influences must be assessed by health professionals in providing health care and developing effective intervention strategies (Taylor, 2005). Culture is not static; it is an ongoing process that influences a woman throughout her entire life, from birth to death. Culture is an essential element of what defines us as people.

Many subcultures may be found within each culture. Subculture refers to a group existing within a larger cultural system that retains its own characteristics. A subculture may be an ethnic group or a group organized in other ways. For example, in the United States and Canada, many ethnic subcultures such as African-Americans, Asian-Americans, Hispanic-Americans, and Native Americans exist, as do subcultures within these groups. In addition, the Caucasian population in America has multiple subcultures of its own. Because every identified cultural group has subcultures, and because it is impossible to study every subculture in depth, greater differences may exist among and between groups than is generally acknowledged.

In a multicultural society, many groups can influence traditions and practices. As cultural groups come in contact with each other, acculturation and assimilation may occur.

Acculturation refers to the changes in one's cultural pattern to those of the host society (Spector, 2004). These changes take place within one group or among several groups when people from different cultures come in contact with one another. People may retain some of their own culture while adopting some of the cultural practices of the dominant society. This familiarization among cultural groups results in some overt behavioral similarity, especially in mannerisms and dress. Language patterns, food choices, and health practices are often much slower to adapt to the influence of acculturation. Furthermore, during times of family transitions such as childbearing, or during crisis or illness, a person may rely on old cultural patterns even after she has become acculturated in many ways. This is consistent with family developmental theory that states that during times of stress, people revert to practices and behaviors that are most comfortable and familiar.

Assimilation means becoming in all ways like the members of the dominant culture (Spector, 2004). This process involves the complete loss of cultural identity while acquiring a new cultural identity. Assimilation is the process by which groups "melt" into the mainstream, thus accounting for the notion of a "melting pot," a phenomenon that has been said to occur in the United States. This is illustrated by individuals who identify themselves as being of "Irish" or "German" descent, without having any remaining cultural practices or values linked specifically to that culture such as food preparation techniques, style of dress, or proficiency in the language associated with their reported cultural heritage. Spector (2004) asserts that in the United States the melting pot, with its dream of a common culture, is a myth. Instead, a mosaic phenomenon exists in which we must both accept and appreciate the differences among people.

Implications for Nursing

Nurses must be aware that some factors may prevent some health care practitioners from providing optimal care, whereas others can enhance nursing practice. Understanding the concepts of ethnocentrism and cultural relativism may help nurses care for families in a multicultural society.

Ethnocentrism refers to the view that one's own culture's way of doing things is best (Giger & Davidhizar, 2004). Although the United States is a culturally diverse nation, the prevailing practice of health care is based on the beliefs and practices held by members of the dominant culture, primarily Caucasians of European descent. This practice is based on the biomedical model that focuses on curing disease states. From this biomedical perspective, pregnancy and childbirth are viewed as processes with inherent risks that are most appropriately managed by using scientific knowledge and advanced technology.

The medical perspective stands in direct contrast with the belief systems of many cultures. Among many women, birth is traditionally viewed as a completely normal process that can be managed with a minimum of involvement from health practitioners. When encountering behavior in women unfamiliar with the biomedical model, the nurse may become frustrated and impatient. The nurse may label the women's behavior inappropriate and believe that it conflicts with "good" health practices. If the Western health care system provides the nurse's only standard for judgment, the behavior of the nurse is called ethnocentric.

Childbearing Beliefs and Practices

Nurses working with childbearing families care for families from many different cultures and ethnic groups. To provide culturally competent care, the nurse should be aware of the spectrum of cultural beliefs and practices important to individual families. When working with childbearing families, a nurse should consider all aspects of culture including communication, space, time orientation, and family roles.

Communication often creates the most challenging obstacle for nurses working with clients from diverse cultural groups. This is because communication is not merely the exchange of words. Instead it involves (1) understanding the individual's language, including subtle variations in meaning and distinctive dialects; (2) appreciation of individual differences in interpersonal style; and (3) accurate interpretation of the volume of speech as well as the meanings of touch and gestures. For example, members of some cultural groups tend to speak more loudly when they are excited, with great emotion and with vigorous and animated gestures; this is true whether their excitement is related to positive or negative events or emotions. It is important, therefore, for the nurse to avoid rushing to judgment regarding a client's intent when the client is speaking, especially in a language not understood by the nurse. Instead, the nurse should withhold an interpretation of what has been expressed until it is possible to clarify the client's intent. The nurse must quickly enlist the assistance of a person who can help, and seek to verify with the client the true intent and meaning of the communication.

Inconsistencies between the language of clients and the language of providers present a significant barrier to effective health care. Because of the diversity of cultures and languages within the U.S. and Canadian populations, health care agencies are increasingly seeking the services of interpreters (of oral communication from one language to another) or translators (of written words from one language to another) to bridge these gaps and fulfill their obligation for culturally and linguistically appropriate health care (Box 2-1). Finding the best possible interpreter in the circumstance is critically important as well. However, ideal interpretive services sometimes are impossible to find when they are needed, because the nature of nursing care is not always predictable and because nursing care that is provided in a home or community setting does not always allow expert, experienced, or mature adult interpreters. In crisis or emergency situations, or when family members are having extreme stress or emotional upset, it may be necessary to use relatives, neighbors, or children as interpreters. If this situation occurs, the nurse must ensure that the client is in agreement and comfortable with using the available interpreter to assist.

When using an interpreter, the nurse respects the family by creating an atmosphere of consideration and privacy. Questions should be addressed to the woman and not to the interpreter. Even though an interpreter will of necessity be exposed to sensitive and privileged information about the family, the nurse should take care to ensure that confidentiality is maintained. A quiet location free from interruptions is the ideal place for interpretive services to take place. In addition, culturally and linguistically appropriate educational materials that are easy to read, with appropriate text and graphics, should be available to assist the woman and her family in understanding health care information (Simmons, Bennett, Schwartz, Sharifyz, & Short, 2002).

Cultural traditions define the appropriate personal space for various social interactions. Although the need for personal space varies from person to person and with the situation, the actual physical dimensions of comfort zones differ from culture to culture. Actions such as touching, placing the woman in proximity to others, taking away personal possessions, and making decisions for the woman

---

box 2-1 **Working with an Interpreter**

STEP 1: BEFORE THE INTERVIEW
A. Outline your statements and questions. List the key pieces of information you want/need to know.
B. Learn something about the culture so that you can converse informally with the interpreter.

STEP 2: MEETING WITH THE INTERPRETER
A. Introduce yourself to the interpreter and converse informally. This is the time to find out how well he or she speaks English. No matter how proficient or what age the interpreter is, be respectful. Some ways to show respect are to ask a cultural question to acknowledge that you can learn from the interpreter, or you could learn one word or phrase from the interpreter.
B. Emphasize that you do want the client to ask questions, because some cultures consider this inappropriate behavior.
C. Make sure the interpreter is comfortable with the technical terms you need to use. If not, take some time to explain them.

STEP 3: DURING THE INTERVIEW
A. Ask your questions and explain your statements (see Step 1).
B. Make sure that the interpreter understands which parts of the interview are most important. You usually have limited time with the interpreter, and you want to have adequate time at the end for client questions.
C. Try to get a "feel" for how much is "getting through." No matter what the language is, if in relating information to the client, the interpreter uses far fewer or far more words than you do, "something else" is going on.
D. Stop every now and then and ask the interpreter, "How is it going?" You may not get a totally accurate answer, but you will have emphasized to the interpreter your strong desire

to focus on the task at hand. If there are language problems: (1) speak slowly; (2) use gestures (e.g., fingers to count or point to body parts); and (3) use pictures.
E. Ask the interpreter to elicit questions. This may be difficult, but it is worth the effort.
F. Identify cultural issues that may conflict with your requests or instructions.
G. Use the interpreter to help problem solve or at least give insight into possibilities for solutions.

STEP 4: AFTER THE INTERVIEW
A. Speak to the interpreter and try to get an idea of what went well and what could be improved. This will help you to be more effective in the future with this or another interpreter.
B. Make notes on what you learned for your future reference or to help a colleague.

Remember:
Your interview is a *collaboration* between you and the interpreter. *Listen* as well as speak.

Notes:
1. The interpreter may be a child, grandchild, or sibling of the client. Be sensitive to the fact that the child is playing an adult role.
2. Be sensitive to cultural and situational differences (e.g., an interview with someone from urban Germany will likely be different from an interview with someone from a transitional refugee camp).
3. Younger females telling older males what to do may be a problem for both a female nurse and a female interpreter. This is not the time to pioneer new gender relations. Be aware that in some cultures it is difficult for a woman to talk about some topics with a husband or a father present.

Courtesy Elizabeth Whalley, PhD, San Francisco State University.

can decrease personal security and heighten anxiety. Conversely, if nurses respect the need for distance, they allow the woman to maintain control over personal space and support the woman's autonomy, thereby increasing her sense of security. For example, many Asian groups have reserved attitudes about physical contact, and this may at times create anxiety when health care is delivered.

Nurses often use touch, and frequently do so without any awareness of the emotional distress they may be causing to clients from some cultures. In the home care setting, a nurse who must provide physical care to a woman with a disease may cause the woman great anxiety, as she fears that her disease will be spread to the nurse. Fears about spreading the disease also may interfere with her acceptance of physical comfort and care from family members.

Time orientation also is a fundamental way in which culture affects health behaviors. People in cultural groups may be relatively more oriented to past, present, or future. Those who focus on the past strive to maintain tradition or the status quo and have little motivation for formulating future goals. In contrast, individuals who focus primarily on the present neither plan for the future nor consider the experiences of the past. These individuals do not necessarily adhere to strict schedules and are often described as "living for the moment," or "marching to their own drummer." Individuals oriented to the future maintain a focus on achieving long-term goals.

The time orientation of the childbearing family may affect nursing care. For example, talking to a family about bringing the infant to the clinic for follow-up examinations (events in the future) may be difficult for the family that is focused on the present concerns of day-to-day survival. Because a family with a future-oriented sense of time plans far in advance, thinking about the long-term consequences of present actions, they may be more likely to return as scheduled for follow-up visits. Despite the differences in time orientation, each family may be equally concerned for the well-being of its newborn.

Family roles involve the expectations and behaviors associated with a member's position in the larger family system (e.g., mother, father, or grandparent). Social class and cultural norms also affect these roles, with distinct expectations for men and women clearly determined by social norms. For example, culture may influence whether a man actively participates in the pregnancy and childbirth, yet maternity care practitioners working in the Western health care system expect fathers to be involved. This can create a significant conflict between the nurse and the role expectations of very traditional Mexican or Arab families, who usually view the birthing experience as a female affair (see Cultural Considerations box). The way that health care practitioners manage such a family's care molds its experience and perception of the Western health care system.

In maternity nursing and women's health care, the nurse supports and nurtures the beliefs that promote physical or emotional adaptation to childbearing. However, if certain beliefs might be harmful, the nurse should

cultural considerations

Questions to Ask to Elicit Cultural Expectations About Childbearing

1. What do you and your family think you should do to remain healthy during pregnancy?
2. What can you do or not do to improve your health and the health of your baby?
3. Who do you want with you during your labor?
4. What can he or she do to help you be most comfortable during labor?
5. What actions are important for you and your family after the baby's birth?
6. What do you and your family expect from the nurse(s) caring for you?
7. How will family members participate in your pregnancy, childbirth, and parenting?

carefully explore them with the woman and use them in the reeducation and modification process. Strategies for care delivery and providing appropriate care are presented in Box 2-2.

Few families are exclusively "Asian" or "Caucasian." Instead they are often blended composites, with one partner bringing to the relationship the traditions of one culture or family of origin, whereas the other partner brings a slightly differing perspective. Even when partners are both of Asian ancestry, for example, their families of origin may come from different regions of the same country and follow completely different health practices. Table 2-2 provides examples of some cultural beliefs and childbearing practices frequently encountered by the nurse who works with women who identify themselves as European-American (Caucasian), Latin-American, Asian-American, African-American (black), or Native American. The cultural beliefs

box 2-2 Strategies for Care Delivery and Providing Appropriate Care

STRATEGIES FOR CARE DELIVERY
- Break down the language barriers
- Explain your rationale and reasons for suggestions
- Integrate folk and Western treatments
- Enlist the family caretaker and others
- Get consent from the right person
- Provide language-appropriate materials

PROVIDING APPROPRIATE CARE
- Ask about traditional beliefs, such as the role of hot and cold
- Be sensitive regarding interpreters and language barriers
- Ask about important dietary practices, particularly those related to events such as childbirth
- Ask about group practices and beliefs
- Ask about a woman's fears, and those of her family, regarding an unfamiliar care setting

From Mattson, S. (2000). Providing culturally competent care: Strategies and approaches for perinatal clients. *AWHONN Lifelines, 4*(5), 37-39.

table 2-2   Traditional* Cultural Beliefs and Practices: Childbearing and Parenting

PREGNANCY	CHILDBIRTH	PARENTING

HISPANIC

(Based primarily on knowledge of Mexican-Americans; members of the Hispanic community have their origins in Spain, Cuba, Central and South America, Mexico, Puerto Rico, and other Spanish-speaking countries.)

Pregnancy	*Labor*	*Newborn*
Pregnancy desired soon after marriage	Use of *"partera"* or lay midwife preferred in some places; may prefer presence of mother rather than husband	Breastfeeding begun after third day; colostrum may be considered "filthy" or "spoiled" or just not enough nourishment
Late prenatal care		
Expectant mother influenced strongly by mother or mother-in-law	After birth of baby, mother's legs brought together to prevent air from entering uterus	Olive oil or castor oil given to stimulate passage of meconium
Cool air in motion considered dangerous during pregnancy	Loud behavior in labor	Male infant not circumcised
Unsatisfied food cravings thought to cause a birthmark		Female infant's ears pierced
Some pica observed in the eating of ashes or dirt (not common)	*Postpartum*	Belly band used to prevent umbilical hernia
Milk avoided because it causes large babies and difficult births	Diet may be restricted after birth; for first 2 days only boiled milk and toasted tortillas permitted (special foods to restore warmth to body)	Religious medal worn by mother during pregnancy; placed around infant's neck.
Many predictions about sex of baby	Bed rest for 3 days after birth	Infant protected from "evil eye"
May be unacceptable and frightening to have pelvic examination by male health care provider	Keep warm	Various remedies used to treat *mal ojo* (evil eye) and fallen fontanel (depressed fontanel)
	Delay bathing	
Use of herbs to treat common complaints of pregnancy	Mother's head and feet protected from cold air; bathing permitted after 14 days	
Drinking chamomile tea thought to ensure effective labor	Mother often cared for by her own mother	
May wear ribbon or band around pregnant belly in belief that baby will be born healthy	Forty-day restriction on sexual intercourse	
	Mother may want baby's first wet diaper to wipe her face in belief that it aids in making "mask of pregnancy" go away.	

AFRICAN-AMERICAN

(Members of the African-American community, many of whom are descendants of slaves, have different origins. Today a number of black Americans have emigrated from Africa, the West Indies, the Dominican Republic, Haiti, and Jamaica.)

Pregnancy	*Labor*	*Newborn*
Acceptance of pregnancy depends on economic status	Use of "Granny midwife" in certain parts of United States	Feeding very important: "Good" baby thought to eat well
Pregnancy thought to be state of "wellness," which is often the reason for delay in seeking prenatal care, especially by lower-income African-Americans	Varied emotional responses: some cry out, some display stoic behavior to avoid calling attention to selves	Early introduction of solid foods
		May breastfeed or bottle-feed; breastfeeding may be considered embarrassing
"Old wives' tales" include beliefs that having a picture taken during pregnancy will cause stillbirth and reaching up will cause cord to strangle baby	Woman may arrive at hospital in far-advanced labor	Parents fearful of spoiling baby
	Emotional support often provided by other women, especially the woman's own mother	Commonly call baby by nicknames
		May use excessive clothing to keep baby warm
Craving for certain foods, including chicken, greens, clay, starch, and dirt	*Postpartum*	Belly band used to prevent umbilical hernia
Pregnancy may be viewed by African-American men as a sign of their virility	Vaginal bleeding seen as sign of sickness; tub baths and shampooing of hair prohibited	Abundant use of oil on baby's scalp and skin
		Strong feeling of family, community, and religion

Data from Amaro, H. (1994). Women in the Mexican-American community: Religion, culture, and reproductive attitudes and experiences. *Journal of Comparative Psychology, 16*(1), 6-19; Bar-Yam, N. (1994). Learning about culture: A guide for birth practitioners. *International Journal of Childbirth Education, 9*(2), 8-10; Galanti, G. (1997). *Caring for patients from different cultures: Case studies from American hospitals.* (2nd ed.). Philadelphia: University of Pennsylvania Press; D'Avanzo, C., & Geissler, E. (2003). *Pocket guide to cultural health assessment* (3rd ed.). St. Louis: Mosby; Mattson, S. (1995). Culturally sensitive prenatal care for Southeastern Asians. *Journal of Obstetric, Gynecologic, and Neonatal Nursing, 24*(4), 335-341; Spector, R. (2004). *Cultural diversity in health and illness* (6th ed.). Upper Saddle River, NJ: Prentice Hall and Williams, R. (1989). Issues in women's health care. In B. Johnson (Ed.), *Psychiatric mental health nursing: Adaptation and growth.* Philadelphia: JB Lippincott.

NOTE: Most of these cultural beliefs and customs reflect the traditional culture and are not universally practiced. These lists are not intended to stereotype patients but rather to serve as guidelines while discussing meaningful cultural beliefs with a patient and her family. Examples of other cultural beliefs and practices are found throughout this text.

*Variations in some beliefs and practices exist within subcultures of each group.

table 2-2 **Traditional* Cultural Beliefs and Practices: Childbearing and Parenting—cont'd**

PREGNANCY	CHILDBIRTH	PARENTING
AFRICAN-AMERICAN—cont'd		
Pregnancy—cont'd	***Postpartum—cont'd***	
Self-treatment for various discomforts of pregnancy, including constipation, nausea, vomiting, headache, and heartburn	Sassafras tea thought to have healing power Eating liver thought to cause heavier vaginal bleeding because of its high "blood" content	
ASIAN-AMERICANS		
(Typically refers to groups from China, Korea, the Philippines, Japan, Southeast Asia [particularly Thailand], Indochina, and Vietnam.)		
Pregnancy	***Labor***	***Newborn***

Pregnancy considered time when mother "has happiness in her body"
Pregnancy seen as natural process
Strong preference for female health care provider
Belief in theory of hot and cold
May omit soy sauce in diet to prevent dark-skinned baby
Prefer soup made with ginseng root as general strength tonic
Milk usually excluded from diet because it causes stomach distress
Inactivity or sleeping late may cause difficult delivery
	Mother attended by other women, especially her own mother
	Father does not actively participate
	Labor in silence
	Cesarean birth not desired
	
	Postpartum
	Must protect self from *yin* (cold forces) for 30 days
	Ambulation limited
	Shower and bathing prohibited
	Warm room
	Diet:
	  Warm fluids
	  Some women are vegetarians
	  Korean mother served seaweed soup with rice
	  Chinese diet high in hot foods
	  Chinese mother avoids fruits and vegetables
		Concept of family important and valued
		Father is head of household; wife plays a subordinate role
		Birth of boy preferred
		May delay naming child
		Some groups (e.g., Vietnamese) believe colostrum is dirty; therefore they may delay breastfeeding until milk comes in

EUROPEAN-AMERICAN		
(Members of the European-American [Caucasian] community have their origins in countries such as Ireland, Great Britain, Germany, Italy, and France.)		
Pregnancy	***Labor***	***Newborn***
Pregnancy viewed as a condition that requires medical attention to ensure health Emphasis on early prenatal care Variety of childbirth education programs available, and participation encouraged Technology-driven Emphasis on nutritional science Involvement of the father valued Written sources of information valued	Birth is a public concern Technology-dominated Birthing process in institutional setting valued Involvement of father expected Physician seen as head of team ***Postpartum*** Emphasis or focus on early bonding Medical interventions for dealing with discomfort Early ambulation and activity emphasized Self-care valued	Increased popularity of breastfeeding Breastfeeding begins as soon as possible after childbirth ***Parenting*** Motherhood and transition to parenting seen as stressful time Nuclear family valued, although single-parenting and other forms of parenting more acceptable than in the past Women often deal with multiple roles Early return to prenatal activities
NATIVE AMERICAN		
(Many different tribes exist within the Native American culture; viewpoints vary according to tribal customs and beliefs.)		
Pregnancy	***Labor***	***Newborn***
Pregnancy considered a normal, natural process Late prenatal care Avoid heavy lifting Herb teas encouraged	Prefers female attendant, although husband, mother, or father may assist with birth Birth may be attended by whole family Herbs may be used to promote uterine activity Birth may occur in squatting position ***Postpartum*** Herb teas to stop bleeding	Infant not fed colostrum Use of herbs to increase flow of milk Use of cradle boards for infant Babies not handled often

and customs in Table 2-2 are categorized based on distinct cultural traditions and are not practiced by all members of the cultural group in every part of the country. Women from these cultural and ethnic groups may adhere to some, all, or none of the practices listed. In using this table as a guide, the nurse should use caution to avoid making stereotypic assumptions about any person based on sociocultural-spiritual affiliations. Nurses should exercise sensitivity in working with every family, being careful to assess the ways in which they apply their own mixture of cultural traditions.

■ DEVELOPING CULTURAL COMPETENCE

In today's society, with its ever-expanding diversity, it is of critical importance that nurses develop more than technical skills. They need to develop cultural competence. There are as many varying definitions of cultural competence as there are for culture. According to Giger and Davidhizar (2004), cultural competence is the adaptation of care in a manner that is congruent with the client's culture. It refers to learning about and applying the standards of another person's culture to activities within that culture. It is, therefore, the opposite of ethnocentrism (www.cecp.air.org/cultural/default.htm).

A number of authors have discussed the key components of culturally competent care:

- Personal insight into the reality that there is disparity between one's own culture and that of the client
- The ability of the nurse to understand the behaviors of clients from her own unique cultural background, and educate and promote healthy behaviors in a cultural context that has meaning for the clients (Bushy, 2002)
- The ability to take abstract knowledge about other cultures and apply it in a practical way, so that the quality of service improves and policies are enacted that meet the needs of all clients
- The ability to communicate respectfulness for a wide range of differences, including client use of nontraditional healing practices and alternative therapies
- Recognition of the importance of culturally different communication styles, problem-solving techniques, concepts of space and time, and desires to be involved with care decisions
- Anticipating the need to address varying degrees of language ability and literacy, as well as barriers to care and compliance with treatment, is key to the ability to plan effective care

Cultural competence affirms the uniqueness and value of every culture in nursing practice (www.bphc.hrsa.gov/cultural competence). For over a decade, the American Academy of Nursing has pledged to promote transcultural nursing and to foster nursing expertise in culturally competent care, defined as a complex integration of knowledge, attitudes, and skills that enhance cross-cultural communications and lead to appropriate and effective interaction with others (American Academy of Nursing, 1992) (see Critical Thinking Exercise). It has always been vital that nurses develop the ability to relate to others, but the challenges of meeting the broad scope of these needs have never been so great.

Cultural competence proceeds along a continuum. It is a process, not an end point (Andrews & Boyle, 2003). Nurses at every level of preparation, and throughout their professional lives, must engage in a continual process of developing and refining attitudes and behaviors that will promote culturally competent care (Taylor, 2005).

The development of cultural competence is of equal importance in terms of health outcomes as it is to issues of preserving and promoting human dignity. Nurses who relate effectively with clients are able to motivate them in the direction of health-promoting behaviors. Provider competence to address language barriers facilitates appropriate tailoring of health messages and preventive health teaching (Brown, Villarruel, Oakley, & Eribes, 2003). Cross-cultural experiences also present an opportunity for the health care professional to expand cultural sensitivity, awareness, and skills.

Implications for Nursing

When nurses develop plans of care for clients who are culturally different from themselves or from the dominant culture of the community, they should be certain to include an assessment that addresses psychosocial issues

---

CRITICAL THINKING EXERCISE

Transcultural Communication

The home care nurse receives a referral for home care visits to Maria, a 21-year-old Hispanic mother who has just been discharged from the hospital following cesarean birth of a healthy baby boy. Maria lives with her husband and a 1-year-old daughter. Several members of her extended family live in nearby apartments. Maria speaks only a few words of English. The nurse wants to provide culturally competent care for Maria.

1. Evidence—Is there sufficient evidence to determine what culturally competent care for Maria consists of?
2. Assumptions—What assumptions can be made about culturally competent care and the role language plays in providing that care?
   a. How the nurse, who speaks no Spanish, might effectively communicate with Maria
   b. How the nurse can provide culturally competent postpartum teaching
   c. Factors the nurse should keep in mind before discussing birth control with this young mother
   d. Appropriate teaching materials and resources; appropriate questions to gain information about current birth control beliefs and practices
3. What implications and priorities for nursing can be made at this time?
4. Does the evidence objectively support your conclusion?
5. Are there alternative perspectives to your conclusion?

related to that diversity. No nursing care plan is complete without attention to nursing diagnoses that address cultural diversity issues.

- *Compromised family coping related to*
  - –immigration or refugee status
- *Impaired verbal communication related to*
  - –inability to speak or understand English
- *Risk for loneliness related to*
  - –separation from family and country of origin
- *Post-trauma syndrome related to*
  - –impact of war, persecution, or civil and political unrest
- *Social isolation related to*
  - –separation from family and friends due to immigration status
- *Chronic sorrow related to*
  - –refugee status, separation from family, and death of family members.

■ COMMUNITY HEALTH PROMOTION

Health promotion in the community moves beyond individual health behavior to address population health issues that impact on families, groups, or whole communities. Pender, Murdaugh, and Parsons (2002) noted that community-based, coordinated health promotion programs have the potential to bring about widespread change in community health status. Population health initiatives vary in scope and focus, from local group efforts to solve a single health problem to multiorganizational or coalition efforts to address a broader public health agenda (Chrisman, Senturia, Tang, & Gheisar, 2002).

Best practices in community-based health initiatives involve understanding of community relationships and resources as well as participation of community leaders. As Averill (2003) suggests, a fundamental principle of nursing is empowering the community through creative, collaborative practices. This empowerment of people, organizations, and communities working together is necessary for lasting change (Cottrell, Girvan, & McKenzie, 2006; Jackson & Phillips, 2003). A community-based framework helps to bring together multiple perspectives and diverse community resources to address a specific health priority. Such approaches promote engagement of those most affected by social and health concerns within the community (Schulz, Kreiger, & Galea, 2002; Schultz, Parker, Israel, Allen, Decarlo, & Lockett, 2002).

The emphasis on community-based health promotion has grown in recent years, with recognition that many health issues require the collaborative efforts of a diverse community network to achieve public health goals (Cottrell et al., 2006). These efforts are particularly relevant in relation to maternal-newborn health, which is affected by multiple public health issues: lack of health insurance, teen pregnancy, substance abuse, and the consequences of inadequate prenatal care.

Levels of Preventive Care

Population-based care involves prevention activities focused on target needs identified in the community assessment process. These levels of prevention provide a framework for nursing interventions. Primary prevention involves health promotion and disease prevention activities to decrease the occurrence of illness and enhance general health and quality of life. Sometimes referred to as "true prevention," primary prevention precedes disease or dysfunction and encourages individuals to achieve the optimal level of health possible (Allender & Spradley, 2005). Examples of primary prevention include health education and counseling about healthy lifestyle behaviors including nutrition and exercise. Other examples are immunizations, injury prevention through the use of seat belts and safety helmets, and environmental modifications to improve air quality. Educational programs that teach safer-sex practices or the dangers of smoking and drug use are also examples of primary prevention.

Secondary prevention is aimed at early detection of a disease and prompt treatment to either cure a disease or to slow its progression and prevent subsequent disability (Maurer & Smith, 2005). Screening programs to detect disease while persons are asymptomatic are the most frequent forms of secondary prevention. Examples of this level of prevention are community blood pressure and cholesterol screenings that identify persons at high risk for heart attack and stroke and facilitate early treatment. The goal is to shorten disease duration and severity, thus enabling an individual to return to normal function as quickly as possible.

Tertiary prevention follows the occurrence of a defect or disability and is aimed at preventing disability through restoration of optimal functioning (Porche, 2004). Persons who have developed disease are provided with treatment and rehabilitation to prevent complications and further deterioration. Examples of tertiary prevention are early treatment and management of diabetes to reduce problems, and rehabilitation of persons after a stroke.

Because most women are healthy during pregnancy, maternal-newborn nursing emphasizes primary and secondary prevention activities regardless of where care is provided. Tertiary prevention is frequently the focus for the ill pregnant woman at home or in the hospital.

Promoting Family Health

Functioning within the social, cultural, environmental, and economic context of the community, the family becomes an integral component of community health promotion efforts (Friedman et al., 2003). For childbearing families, health promotion is primarily focused on early intervention through prenatal care and prevention of complications during the perinatal period. Often this early exposure to health information sets the stage for a successful birth and positive outcomes for mother and baby. Family systems and developmental theories provide a framework for the appropriate timing and content of health promotion activities. The nurse's role in this process is focused on collaboration with the family, identifying risk factors, and providing health information to facilitate positive health behaviors (Best, Stokols, Green, Leischow, Holmes, & Bucholz, 2003). Involving expectant mothers and fathers in identification of their learning needs is an essential first step to securing their participation in the health promotion process.

A wide variety of strategies have been used to engage families and groups in health-promoting activities or community health programs. Some are more successful than others. Generally, participant engagement in the planning process and empowerment to create internal solutions are considered key factors in effective interventions. Many communities have organized coalitions to address specific health promotion agendas related to sharing information, educating community members, or advocating for health policies around maternal and child health issues. An example of this is the National Friendly Access Program (2003), a community-based initiative to improve access to maternal and child care by changing provider behaviors. In recent years, the benefits of partnership with faith-based organizations for community health improvement have been demonstrated in health promotion efforts aimed at lifestyle choices, health education, and maternal-child health outcomes (Zahner & Corrado, 2004). Another community-based partnership demonstrated the potential for policy and practice improvements in maternal child health systems around the issues of provider access, transportation, and discrimination in health care practices (Pincus et al., 2003).

Prenatal classes are a well-established mechanism for increasing awareness of healthy behaviors during pregnancy and preparing parents for the care of themselves and their newborn during the postpartum period. Mass media efforts such as those presented by the March of Dimes "Baby Your Baby" advertisements are clear, consumer-friendly messages designed to reach a large target audience. Other venues include public health education in newspapers and magazines, and health department programs such as the Special Supplemental Program for Women, Infants, and Children (WIC), which offers a variety of health education and written information to mothers.

▬ ASSESSING THE COMMUNITY

Community, in its broadest definition, refers to a geographically defined area; its residents; their cultural, religious, and ethnic characteristics; and the activities or functions through which the needs of the residents are met. Community may also refer to groupings of people with common characteristics or interests (Smith, Hamilton, Sheats, Mensah, Apantaku, & Sullivan, 2003).

Community assessment is a complex, yet well-defined, process through which the unique characteristics of the populations and their special needs are identified to plan and evaluate health services for the community as a whole. The desired outcome of this process is identification of

direct service as well as advocacy needs of the targeted aggregate or group, and improved health for the community as a whole (Kuehnert, 2002).

A community assessment framework or model provides criteria for conducting a community assessment, identifies types and methods of data collection, and organizes the data of a community assessment (Ervin, 2002). Many models and frameworks are available, but the actual process often depends on the extent and nature of the assessment to be performed, the time and resources available, and the way the information is to be used.

The community *asset mapping* approach provides an overview of community attributes and strengths that may facilitate long-term change and improved quality of life for community residents (Averill, 2003). Community *capacity* looks at a community's ability to address social and health problems, or the development of knowledge, systems and resources that contribute to a community health status (Freudenberg, 2004). Both of these approaches help to direct the health promotion process by identifying community priorities and areas of needed change.

Data Collection and Sources of Community Health Data

Data collection is often the most time-consuming phase of the community assessment process, but it provides an important definition and description of the community (Ervin, 2002). Important measures of community health include access to care, level of provider services available, as well as other social and economic factors. Consideration of individual, interpersonal, community, organizational, and policy-level data, as well as the interaction of these factors, is important in providing a comprehensive framework for community health promotion (Brennan, Baker, Haire-Joshu, & Brownson, 2003). A community assessment model (Fig. 2-5) is often used to provide a comprehensive guide to data collection.

The most critical community indicators of perinatal health relate to access to care; maternal mortality; infant mortality; low birth weight; first trimester prenatal care; and rates for mammography, Papanicolau smears, and other similar screening tests (AHRQ, 2005; USDHHS, 2005). Nurses may use these indicators as a reflection of access, quality, and continuity of health care in a community. For women and infants, access to a consistent source of care is critical. Those with a regular source of care are more likely to use preventive services and receive timely treatment for illness and injury (USDHHS, 2005), but current statistics indicate that many women lack access to a usual source of care or rely primarily on emergency services.

Access to health care is also an important measure of community health. This indicator relates not only to the *availability* of health department services, hospitals, public clinics, or other sources of care, but also to *accessibility* of care. In many areas where facilities and providers are available, geographic and transportation barriers render the care inaccessible for certain populations. This is particularly

CD Critical Thinking Exercise: Cultural Health and the Family

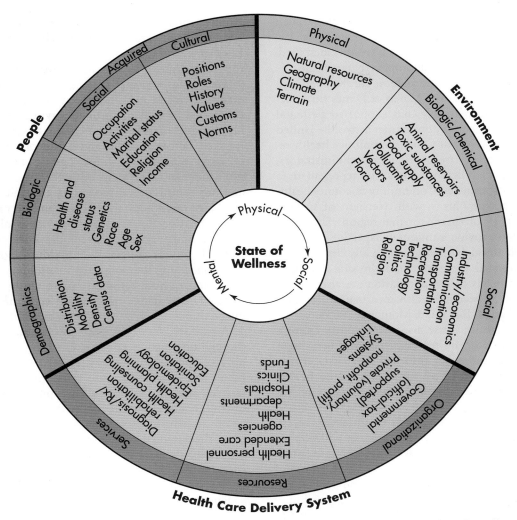

FIG. 2-5 Community health assessment wheel. (From Clemen-Stone, S., McGuire, S., & Eigsti, D. [2002]. *Comprehensive community health nursing: Family, aggregate, & community practice* [6th ed]. St. Louis: Mosby.)

true in rural areas or other remote locations (Huttlinger, Schaller-Ayers, & Lawson, 2004). Other barriers to care should also be evaluated including cultural and language barriers, and lack of providers or specialty care. An analysis by Mete, Cioffi, and Lichtveld (2003) shows that local health departments provide varied levels and types of services, which may or may not meet the needs of the populations they serve. For example, primary care services are limited in many areas, although health education is offered by most health departments. There is a growing trend in the U.S. to have walk-in clinics in grocery stores, an easily accessible location.

Health departments at the city, county, and state level are a valuable resource for annual reports of births and deaths. Maternal and infant death rates are particularly important, since they reflect health outcomes that may be preventable (McDevitt & Wilbur, 2002). Local health departments also compile extensive statistics about the birth complications, causes of death, and leading causes

of morbidity and mortality for each age group. Local and state health data are compiled and reported through the Centers for Disease Control and Prevention (CDC) (www.cdc.gov) to the National Center for Health Statistics (NCHS). The National Health Survey published annually from this source describes national health trends (Stanhope & Lancaster, 2004). However, national data are only as accurate and reliable as the local data on which they are based, so caution is needed in interpreting the data and applying it to specific population groups.

The U.S. government census provides data on population size, age ranges, sex, racial and ethnic distribution, socioeconomic status, educational level, employment, and housing characteristics. Summary data are available for most large metropolitan areas, arranged by zip code and census tract, which usually corresponds to a neighborhood comprising approximately 3000 to 6000 people. Looking at individual census tracts within a community helps to identify subpopulations or aggregates whose needs may differ

CD Critical Thinking Exercise: Community Resources for Families

from those of the larger community. For example, women at high risk for inadequate prenatal care according to age, race, and ethnic or cultural group may be readily identified, and outreach activities may be appropriately targeted.

Other sources of useful information are hospitals and voluntary health agencies. The March of Dimes Birth Defects Foundation, for example, has supported perinatal needs assessments in many communities across the United States (www.modimes.org). Other community health resources include health care providers or administrators, government officials, religious leaders, and representatives of voluntary health agencies. Community or county health councils exist in many areas, with oversight of specific health initiatives or programs for that region. These key informants often provide a unique perspective that may not be accessible through other sources. Community gate-keepers who are at the forefront of addressing the social and health care needs of the population are also critical links to population-specific health information (Surani, Baezconde-Garbanati, Bastani, & Montano, 2003).

The perinatal health nurse also may explore existing community health program reports, records of preventive health screenings, and other informal data. Established programs often provide good indicators of the health promotion and disease prevention characteristics of the population.

Professional publications are a rich and readily accessible source of information for all nurses. In addition to nursing and public health journals, behavioral and social science literature offers diverse perspectives on community health status for specific populations and subgroups. The Internet has increased the availability and accessibility of national, state, and local health data as well. However, the use of Internet-based resources for health information requires some caution, since data reliability and validity are difficult to verify. (Some guidelines for evaluation of Internet health resources can be found at the Health on the Net website, www.hon.org).

Data collection methods may be either qualitative or quantitative and may include visual surveys that can be completed by walking through a community, participant observation, interviews, focus groups, and analysis of existing data. Potential clients and health care consumers may be asked to participate in focus groups or community forums to present their views on needed community services and programs. Formal surveys, conducted by mail, telephone, or face-to-face interviews, can be a valuable source of information not available from national databases or other secondary sources. Several drawbacks exist with this method: surveys are generally expensive to develop and time-consuming to administer. In addition to the cost of such surveys, poor response rates often preclude a sufficiently representative response on which to base nursing interventions.

A walking survey is generally conducted by a walk-through observation of the community (Box 2-3), taking note of specific characteristics of the population, economic and social environment, transportation, health care services, and other resources. This method allows the nurse to collect subjective data and may facilitate other aspects of the assessment (Ervin, 2002). Participant observation is another useful assessment method in which the nurse actively participates in the community to understand the community more fully and to validate observations (Stanhope & Lancaster, 2004).

Finally, as part of the assessment process, nurses working in multiethnic and multicultural groups need an in-depth assessment of culturally based health behaviors.

---

box 2-3 **Community Walk-Through**

As you observe the community, take note of the following:
- **Physical environment**—Older neighborhood or newer subdivision? Sidewalks, streets, and buildings in good or poor repair? Billboards and signs? What are they advertising? Are lawns kept up? Is there trash in the streets? Parks or playgrounds? Parking lots? Empty lots? Industries?
- **People in the area**—Old, young, homeless, children, predominant ethnicity, language? Is the population homogeneous? What signs do you see of different cultural groups?
- **Stores and services available**—Restaurants: chain, local, ethnic? Grocery stores: neighborhood or chain? Department stores, gas stations, real estate or insurance offices, travel agencies, pawn shops, liquor stores, discount or thrift stores, newspaper stands?
- **Social**—Clubs, bars, fraternal organizations (e.g., Elks, American Legion), museums?
- **Religious**—Churches, synagogues, mosques? What denominations? Do you see evidence of their use other than on religious/holy days?
- **Health services**—Drug stores, doctors' offices, clinics, dentists, mental health services, veterinarians, urgent care

facilities, hospitals, shelters, nursing homes, home health agencies, public health services, traditional healers (e.g. herbalists, palmists)?
- **Transportation**—Cars, bus, taxi, light rail, sidewalks, bicycle paths, access for disabled persons?
- **Education**—Schools, before- and after-school programs, child care, libraries, bookstores? What is the reputation of the schools?
- **Government**—What is the governance structure? Is there a mayor? City council? Are meetings open to the public? Are there signs of political activity (e.g. posters, campaign signs)?
- **Safety**—How safe is the community? What is the crime rate? What types of crimes are committed? Are police visible? Is there a fire station?

Evaluation of the community based on your observations—What is your impression of the community? Is the environment pleasing? Are services and transportation adequate? How difficult is it for residents to obtain needed services—i.e., how far do they have to travel? Would you want to live in this community? Why or why not?

Analysis and synthesis of data obtained during the assessment process help to generate a comprehensive picture of the community's health status, needs, and problem areas, as well as its strengths and resources for addressing these concerns. The goal of this process is to assign priorities to community health needs and to develop a plan of action for correcting them. A comparison of community health data with state and national statistics may be useful in identification of appropriate target populations as well as interventions to improve health outcomes.

Vulnerable Populations in the Community

Assessment of population health includes indicators related to diverse groups and cultures, particularly disenfranchised or "vulnerable" community members (www.crosshealth.com). Vulnerability in terms of health status and health outcomes may take many forms–including sociocultural, economic, and environmental risk factors that contribute to disparities in health. Health disparities are conditions that disproportionately affect certain racial, ethnic, or other groups. African-Americans, Hispanics or Latinos, Native Americans, Pacific Islanders, and Asian-Americans are all considered vulnerable populations because they are more likely to have poor health and die prematurely (CDC, 2005a).

The Institute of Medicine report, *Unequal Treatment: Confronting Racial and Ethnic Disparities in Care* (2002), provided evidence of racial and ethnic disparities for a number of health conditions and services. According to the National Health Care Disparities Report (AHRQ, 2004), disparities are pervasive and improvement is possible, but there are still gaps in information for many groups. Although health disparities have been evident across all domains of health care for several decades, the etiology of these differences is still unclear (Jacobs, Karavolos, Rathouz, Ferris, & Powell, 2005). Smith and colleagues (2003) suggest that poverty, poor access to care, lack of preventive services, and inadequate health knowledge and skills all contribute to excess disease burden for some groups, particularly African-American, Hispanic, and Asian populations.

Women

Women compromise 51% of the U.S. population, representing a very diverse, and largely "at risk," group in relation to health (USDHHS, 2005). Although women assume leadership for health care decision making in most families, they also face significant challenges in accessing the health care system and meeting their own health needs and those of family members (Kaiser Family Foundation, 2003) (www.kff.org/womenshealth). What is the source of women's vulnerability? Although there is no single contributing factor, the primary sources of health disparities for women fall into the areas of gender, socioeconomic status, and race/ethnicity. Significant gaps exist in the quality of care for women when compared to men (www.hispanichealth.org).

The *National Report Card on Women's Health* describes significant deficiencies in women's health (National Women's Law Center [NWLC], 2004). Assessing states' performance in relation to 27 key areas, most were rated as *unsatisfactory* in relation to women's health status and policies influencing women's health. Key indicators focused on access to services, use of preventive health care and health promotion activities, the occurrence of certain health conditions, and an assessment of the community's impact on women's health. This report suggested that one of the primary factors compromising women's health is lack of access to acceptable-quality health care, which may manifest itself in many forms: lack of health insurance, living in a medically underserved area, or an inability to obtain needed services, particularly basic services such as prenatal care. Federal and state policies and programs also fail to safeguard women's interests in relation to reproductive health and health care coverage (NWLC, 2004).

Although many women report that they are in good to excellent health, statistics reveal significant disparities in health status of women from all age groups and racial and ethnic backgrounds (USDHHS, 2005). Low levels of educational attainment (high school or lower) are also associated with lack of resources, and difficulty navigating the health care system. This is particularly true of women of ethnic and racial minorities, whose limited English proficiency may compromise provider access and quality of care (Kaiser Family Foundation, 2003). Access to primary health care and use of preventive services by women is often dictated by costs and insurance availability. In 2003, nearly 15% of all women were uninsured, with minority women disproportionately affected by lack of health care coverage (USDHHS, 2005).

Within the larger group of vulnerable women, a number of subgroups present challenges to the community-based perinatal nurse.

Racial and Ethnic Minorities

In addition to social, economic, and cultural barriers to optimal health, women who are in racial and ethnic minorities (29.3% of all U.S. women), experience a disproportionate burden of disease, disability, and premature death. Whereas 63% of non-Hispanic white females reported that they are in excellent or good health, only 53% of Hispanic and 51% of non-Hispanic black women reported this level of health (USDHHS, 2005).

Significant health disparities continue to exist in terms of adult women's health and the health of their infants. Although some positive trends are evident, there are persistent disparities among racial and ethnic groups in early prenatal care, an important factor in achieving healthy pregnancy outcomes (USDHHS, 2005). Infant mortality rates reveal the depth of health disparities with significant differences in three major perinatal indicators: low birth weight, preterm birth, and infant mortality (March of Dimes [MOD], 2003). Infant mortality rates are highest among Native American, Alaska Native, and Puerto Rican women (CDC, 2005b).

Minority women, many of whom live in poverty, also have higher rates of chronic disease including heart disease, cancer, hepatitis, and acquired immunodeficiency syndrome (AIDS), and mental health issues (USDHHS, 2005). Women with underlying health conditions are at especially high risk for poor obstetric outcomes for both themselves and their infants. They have high rates of preterm labor and gestational hypertension, and often have intrauterine growth restriction resulting in the birth of infants who are small for gestational age. These are the clients for whom the community-based perinatal nurse will be providing care, and their needs are complex, demanding high levels of expertise and skill.

Adolescent Girls

The adolescent population in the United States is generally considered healthy. Yet this group of women is often vulnerable due to high risk behaviors (NWLC, 2004). Blum, McNeely, and Nonnemaker (2002) reveal that 75% of adolescent mortality can be attributed to social factors, (disadvantaged environments) and high risk behaviors (substance abuse, diet and exercise, injury and violence, and sexuality). Adolescent girls, especially those from minorities and low-income or disrupted families, are more likely to engage in early sexual activity and other high risk behaviors (Doswell, Kouyate, & Taylor, 2003), with both immediate and long-term health consequences.

Female adolescents in the United States also experience a high rate of teen pregnancy, with 4 out of 10 becoming pregnant before the age of 20 years (Crosby et al., 2002).

Although teen pregnancy rates among all racial and ethnic groups have declined in recent years, the highest rates are still seen in non-Hispanic blacks (100.7/1000), and Hispanics (83.1/1000). Sexually transmitted infection (STI) rates, primarily chlamydia and gonorrhea, are highest among adolescent and young adult females (USDHHS, 2005).

Adolescent health is another broad target area for community health promotion efforts, including both health education and policy initiatives. Because adolescents fail to perceive their own vulnerability, they need help navigating a complex environment and dealing with risk behaviors through preventive strategies that enhance decision making and increase protective factors (Blum et al., 2002; Nightingale & Fischoff, 2002).

A report (Kaiser Family Foundation, 2003) revealed that although adolescents are concerned about becoming pregnant, they still engage in unprotected sex. Adolescents also use a variety of sources for health information—the media, friends, and sex education—yet they are very misinformed, particularly about STIs and HIV transmission. These findings have significant implications for perinatal outcomes and emphasize the importance of aggressive prevention programs and community outreach related to sexuality, teen pregnancy, and substance abuse (Montgomery, 2003).

Older Women

In 2003, the U.S. population comprised 19.5 million women over the age of 65 years. This represents almost 58% of the population ages 65 and older. Although women have a greater life expectancy than men, they are more likely to have chronic illnesses, less likely to use preventive services, and ultimately spend more on health care (USDHHS, 2005).

However, there is a great deal of emphasis on preventive interventions that are effective in delaying or controlling age-related changes. Improving self-care activities such as diet and exercise are important health promotion elements for this population (Miller & Iris, 2002).

Low Literacy

Individuals and groups for whom English is a second language often lack the skills necessary to seek medical care and function adequately in the health care setting. Communication barriers may affect access to care, particularly in such areas as making appointments, applying for services, and obtaining transportation (NAP, 2002).

Health literacy involves a spectrum of abilities, ranging from reading an appointment slip to interpreting medication instructions. There is growing evidence of the effects of low health literacy on adult health status (Rosal, Goins, Carbone, & Cortes, 2004) (www.hsph.harvard.edu/healthliteracy). Low health literacy may also be an independent contributor to a disproportionate disease burden among disadvantaged populations (Schillinger et al., 2002). Disparities in preventive care, early screening for cancer, and utilization of health care services, particularly among minority women, have also been linked to language barriers (Jacobs, Karavalos, Rathous, Ferris, & Powell, 2005) (www.prenataled.com/healthlit).

As the United States becomes increasingly multicultural, nurses will be required to interact with non–English–speaking groups or those with limited health literacy. Consequently, health literacy must be viewed as a component of culturally and linguistically competent care. These skills must be assessed routinely to recognize a problem and accommodate clients with limited literacy skills.

Incarcerated Women

The number of incarcerated women in the United States has continued to climb in recent years, increasing at a significantly greater rate than for men. In 2003, nearly 182,000 were in prison, with the highest number of these being black, non-Hispanic women (Harrison & Karlberg, 2004). Many of these women report a history of sexual and physical abuse.

Because their relationship histories are often unstable, and because they often lack the support of family, incarcerated women or those with a history of repeated incarceration frequently have difficulty providing emotional stability, secure housing, and health promotion role modeling for their children.

EVIDENCE-BASED PRACTICE

Coronary Heart Disease: The Leading Cause of Death in Women

BACKGROUND

- A quarter of a million women die every year as a result of coronary heart disease (CHD), defined as impaired circulation to the heart muscle, causing hypoxia. Major studies have greatly increased the identification of risk factors, diagnostic tools, and treatment options for CHD, but most of their subjects were male. In order to determine the generalizability of the research on CHD to women, the Agency for Healthcare Research and Quality and the National Institutes of Health commissioned a preliminary review of evidence. The reviewers found the following:

  1. Risk factors for CHD in women include hyperlipidemia, diabetes, and hyperhomocysteinemia. Other risk factors for women have not been well researched.
  2. For women, ceasing smoking after myocardial infarction (MI) and decreasing blood pressure and lipids all lower the risk for CHD events. Other interventions to mitigate risk factors in women have not been investigated.
  3. Women are more likely than men to be treated for hypertension, but less likely to undergo diagnostic testing.
  4. Women with CHD benefit from administration of beta-blockers, aspirin, and ACE inhibitors, but not nitrates. The efficacy of other medical and surgical treatments to women with heart disease is not well researched.

- From that preliminary study, four promising topics were selected for systematic review and metaanalysis.

OBJECTIVES

- The reviewers explored the evidence specific to women on echocardiography and myocardial perfusion imaging (MPI), diabetes, lipid management, and prognostic value of troponin.

METHOD

Search Strategy

- The reviewers searched available research diligently. Eligible research included cross-sectional studies (which analyze a population at a given point in time), prospective cohort studies (which begin the study before any treatment effect), and randomized controlled trials.
- The findings include the number of studies, publication dates, total number of subjects, and results of the study. Countries were not all noted, but included Finland, Fiji, Scotland, and the United States.

Statistical Analyses

- Each topic was calculated separately. Similar data were pooled. In some cases, the reviewers contacted the authors of the individual studies to extract the information about women.
- Reviewers calculated relative risk for dichotomous data, and weighted mean difference for continuous data. Results outside the 95% confidence interval were accepted as significant differences.

FINDINGS

- Echocardiography and MPI: Results from 14 studies (893 women), dated 1990-1998, found low diagnostic accuracy for MPI and echocardiography detecting CHD in women.
- Diabetes: Seventeen studies, published 1971-2002, of 43,944 women (4,522 with diabetes and 39,422 without diabetes) show a nonsignificant trend for women to have higher CHD mortality and nonfatal MI due to diabetes than men. Men, however, had a trend toward higher all-cause mortality.
- Lipid Management: Eleven trials (15,917 women), dated 1986-1999, confirmed that for women with CHD, lowering lipids led to significantly fewer major CHD events and nonfatal MI's, and less CHD mortality. However, there was no decrease in total mortality. There was not enough evidence to draw conclusions about the benefits of lowering lipids for women without CHD.
- Prognostic Value for Troponin: The findings in eight studies (3,169 women and 4,070 men), published 1996-1999, found that elevated troponin in women marks a greater risk for nonfatal MI than in men. Women are typically older and more likely to have diabetes and hypertension than men when they first exhibit symptoms of myocardial ischemia. The mortality risk for men and women with elevated troponin was similar.

LIMITATIONS

- More well-designed studies are needed to distinguish the role that gender plays in the prevention, diagnosis, and treatment of CHD. Evidence about efficacy for women is weak or nonexistent for many mainstream treatments, such as stents, heparin, coronary bypass surgery, angioplasty, and commonly used medications,

IMPLICATIONS FOR PRACTICE

- Women often fear cancer, but are often unaware that they are more likely to suffer and die from CHD, which is generally perceived as a "man's disease." Nurses can identify known risk factors for CHD in women; they can work with patients to improve lifestyle choices to lower blood pressure and lipids, decrease stress, stop smoking, improve rest and diet, and exercise regularly. The nurse can also advocate for his or her female patients to be diagnosed and treated using evidence-based, gender-specific guidelines.

IMPLICATIONS FOR FURTHER RESEARCH

- Comparing the results of healthy subjects prospectively can identify the efficacy of MPI and echocardiography as screening tools. Well-designed studies can identify which CHD risk factors in diabetes are specific for women. Adequate numbers are needed to identify the preventive benefits of lipid-lowering interventions in healthy women. The gender differences in troponin necessitate research to increase understanding of its prognostic value. More accurate, noninvasive forms of diagnostic testing can benefit men and women.

Grady, D., Chapur, L., & Kristof, M. (2003). *Results of systematic review of research on diagnosis and treatment of coronary heart disease in women* (AHRQ Publication No. 03-E035). Rockville, MD: Agency for Healthcare Research and Quality.
Grady, D., Chapur, L., & Kristof, M. (2003). *Diagnosis and treatment of coronary heart disease in women: Systematic reviews of evidence on selected topics* (AHRQ Publication No. 03-E036). Rockville, MD: Agency for Healthcare Research and Quality.

The lifestyle choices of this group, including risky sexual relationships, illicit drug use, and smoking, place them at high risk for sexually transmitted infections, HIV and AIDS, other chronic and communicable diseases, and complicated pregnancies (USDHHS, 2005).

Migrant Women

There are an estimated 3 million migrant and seasonal farmworkers in the United States, 21% of whom are women. Diverse ethnic and cultural groups are represented among migrant workers; however, 75% of these workers were born in Mexico. The majority (81%) speak Spanish, their average age is 33, and seventh grade was the highest completed on average (U.S. Department of Labor National Agricultural Workers Survey, 2005).

Migrant workers in the United States are primarily in regions associated with agriculture, tobacco production, and fishing and mining industries. The three primary migrant streams are East Coast states, midwestern and western states, and West Coast states (Bushy, 2002).

Migrant laborers and their families face many problems, including financial instability, child labor, poor housing, lack of education, language and cultural barriers, and limited access to health and social services (Clemen-Stone, 2002). Poor dental health, diabetes, hypertension, malnutrition, tuberculosis, and parasitic infections are common health issues among migrant populations. Primary health care services are largely provided by a number of migrant health centers, of which there are over 400 throughout the United States. Routine prenatal care, as well as screening and treatment for hypertension and diabetes, are provided. Community health nurses frequently encounter the challenges of providing culturally and linguistically appropriate care while facing numerous health issues (Lausch, Heuer, Guasasco, & Bengiamin, 2003).

Numerous reproductive health issues exist for migrant women, including less consistent use of contraception and increased rates of STIs. Migrants are less likely to receive early prenatal care and have a greater incidence of inadequate weight gain during pregnancy than do other poor women.

Rural Versus Urban Community Settings

In the United States, approximately 20% of the population lives in a rural area. Characteristically, rural residents are older, less educated, and generally in poorer health than their urban counterparts. Rural communities are disproportionately affected by poverty and poor access to health care services (APHA, 2004; Kaiser Commission, 2003b). Lack of insurance presents an additional factor for poor health in rural areas. Of the 41 million uninsured residents of the United States, one in five lives in rural communities. In some states, up to 70% of rural residents lack insurance or rely on Medicaid (Kaiser Commission, 2003a).

Rural women are especially vulnerable to financial and transportation barriers to health care. While women in rural counties report only *fair* to *poor* health, they pay considerably more for their health care (USDHHS, 2004). In rural communities, women have less access to prenatal care, which contributes to higher rates of adverse pregnancy outcomes including higher rates of preterm birth, low birth weight, and infant mortality. Peck and Alexander (2003) suggest that this disproportionate distribution of poverty and of variations in race/ethnicity, age, education, and availability and access to medical resources may be the link to infant mortality in rural areas.

Homeless Women

Homelessness among women is an increasing social and health issue in the United States. Although exact numbers are unknown, it is estimated that women make up one third of America's 2 to 3 million homeless people. The Bureau of Primary Health Care (BPHC, 2001) identifies poverty, acute and chronic health problems, substance abuse, and domestic violence as major factors for homelessness. As women are increasingly affected by poverty, homelessness is becoming more prevalent for families and children, particularly among rural populations.

Health issues among the homeless are numerous and result primarily from a lack of preventive care and a lack of resources in general. Health problems including chronic illness, asthma, circulatory problems, and diabetes are rampant. Homeless women face a number of health issues, related both to lifestyle factors and the vulnerability resulting from being homeless. In addition to extreme poverty, women are at increased risk for illness and injury; many have been victims of domestic abuse, assault, and rape (American College of Obstetricians and Gynecologists [ACOG], 2005).

Although little is known about pregnancy in this population, about 20% of women do become pregnant while homeless. Conversely, pregnancy and recent birth are highly correlated with becoming homeless (ACOG, 2005). In addition to risk factors related to inadequate nutrition, inadequate weight gain, anemia, bleeding problems, and preterm delivery, homeless women face multiple barriers to prenatal care: transportation, distance, and wait times. Most women also underutilize available prenatal services (Bloom, Bednarzyk, Devitt, Renault, Teaman, & VanLoock, 2004). The unsafe environment and high risk lifestyles often result in adverse perinatal outcomes (Lewis, Andersen, & Gelberg, 2003).

Refugees and Immigrants

Along with their profound resilience and determination, refugees and immigrants have brought rich diversity to the United States in several important dimensions including cultural heritage and customs, economic productivity, and enhanced national vitality. At the same time, multiple challenges accompany the dramatic influx of individuals and families from other countries.

Immigrants also differ from U.S.-born persons in demographics: overall they are younger, with lower incomes and educational attainments. While 73% of immigrants are legal citizens (Kaiser Commission, 2003b), this population is disproportionately affected by health disparities related to cultural and language barriers, having no usual source of care, and lack of insurance (Mohanty, Woolhandler, Himmelstein, Pati, Carrasquillo, & Bor, 2005). Current (2006) legislative efforts may address some of these inequities.

Women without U.S. citizenship are less likely to have a usual source of care (26.1%) and more likely to be without health insurance coverage (45.5%). Nearly 25% of these women have not seen a health care provider in the past year (USDHHS, 2005).

Access to care is further limited by health care policies that restrict Medicaid eligibility for these groups (Kaiser Commission, 2003a). Mohanty and coworkers (2005) compared the health care costs of immigrants to those of U.S. citizens. Refuting the assumption that immigrants place an extra burden on the health care system, the study revealed that total health care expenditures for immigrant adults and children were significantly lower than those of U.S.-born citizens.

Refugee status imposes a particular type of vulnerability on affected individuals and groups. Of primary significance are the precipitating factors by which people are displaced suddenly or forced to leave their country of origin: persecution, civil unrest, or war. Families are thus forced from their own homes to seek residence and employment elsewhere (Murray, Zentner, & Samiezade-Yazd, 2001). Often these groups are extremely impoverished and face extreme physical and emotional stress when they arrive in the United States.

In general, refugees are more likely to live in poverty than are immigrants (Murray et al., 2001). Over time, measures of health and well-being actually decline for the immigrant population as they become part of American society (NAP, 2002). Many of the conditions or illnesses that they acquire contribute to the persistence of disparities in maternal and neonatal health outcomes for both immigrants and refugees.

Implications for Nursing

Although the long-term consequences of contemporary immigration for American society are unclear, the successful incorporation of immigrant families depends on the resources, benefits, and policies that ensure their healthy development and successful social adjustment. Culturally competent health care and involvement of the immigrant community in health care programs are recommended strategies for improving the access to and effectiveness of health care for this population (NAP, 2002).

The use of camp volunteers has been effective in assisting families living in migrant worker camps to obtain prenatal, postpartum, and infant care. Working in partnership with health professionals such as nurses, lay camp aides have been used effectively for outreach and health education; however, more strategies are needed to link traditional practices with the formal health care system. Guidance and information about other health resources are available to health care providers through the National Migrant Resource Program and the Migrant Clinicians Network.

Nurses working with homeless women and families are challenged to treat them with dignity and respect to establish a therapeutic relationship. Case management is recommended to coordinate the services and disciplines that may be involved in meeting the complex needs of these families. Whenever possible, general screening and preventive health services must be provided when the woman seeks treatment, as this may be the only opportunity to provide health information and intervention. Building on existing coping strategies and strengths, the health care provider helps the woman and her family to reconnect with a social support system. Nurses also have an important role in advocating for funding to support homeless health services and to improve access to preventive care for all homeless populations.

■ HOME CARE IN THE COMMUNITY

Modern home care nursing has its foundation in public health nursing, which provided comprehensive care to sick and well clients in their own homes. Specialized maternity home care nursing services began in the 1980s when public health maternity nursing services were limited and services had not kept pace with the changing practices of high risk obstetrics and emerging technology. Lengthy antepartal hospitalizations for such conditions as preterm labor and gestational hypertension created nursing care challenges for staff members of inpatient units.

Many women expressed their concern for the negative effect of antepartal hospitalizations on the family. Although clinical indications showed that a new nursing care approach was needed, home health care did not become a viable alternative until third-party payers (i.e., public or private organizations or employer groups that pay for health care) pushed for cost containment in maternity services.

In the current health care system, home care is an important component of health care delivery along the perinatal continuum of care (Fig. 2-6). The growing demand for home care is based on several factors:
- Interest in family birthing alternatives
- Shortened hospital stays
- New technologies that facilitate home-based assessments and treatments
- Reimbursement by third-party payers

As health care costs continue to rise, and because millions of American families lack health insurance, there is greater demand for innovative, cost-effective methods of health care delivery in the community. Large health care systems are developing clinically integrated health care delivery networks whose goals are (1) improved coordination of care and care outcomes; (2) better communication among health care providers; (3) increased client, payer, and provider satisfaction; and (4) reduced cost. The integration of clinical services changes the focus of care to a continuum of services that are increasingly community-based.

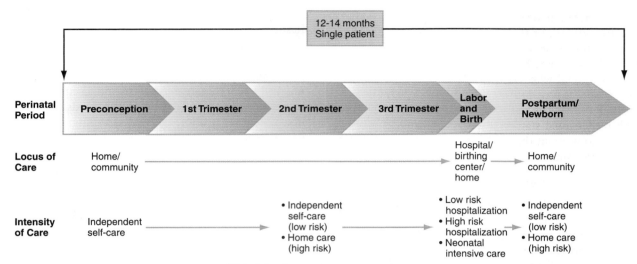

FIG. 2-6 Perinatal continuum of care.

Communication and Technology Applications

As maternity care continues to consist of frequent and brief contacts with health care providers throughout the prenatal and postpartum periods, services that link maternity clients throughout the perinatal continuum of care have assumed increasing importance; these include critical pathways, telephonic nursing assessments, discharge planning, specialized education programs, parent support groups, home visiting programs, nurse advice lines, and perinatal home care. Some hospitals provide cross-training for hospital-based nurses to make postpartum home visits or to staff outpatient centers for postpartum follow-up.

Telephonic nursing care through services such as "warm lines," nurse advice lines, and telephonic nursing assessments is a valuable means of managing health care problems and bridging the gaps among acute, outpatient, and home care services. Some providers are using the Internet to communicate with clients who have an Internet service provider (ISP). Nursing care that occurs by telephone is interactive and responsive to immediate health care questions about particular health care needs. Warm lines are telephone lines that are offered as a community service to provide new parents with support, encouragement, and basic parenting education. Nurse advice lines, or toll-free nurse consultation services, often are supported by third-party payers or health management organization/managed care organization (HMO/MCO) nurse case managers and are designed to provide answers to medical questions. These nurses are prepared to guide callers through urgent health care situations, suggest treatment options, and provide health education. Telephonic nursing assessments, or nurse consultation, assessment, and health education that take place during a telephone conversation, can be added to the plan of care in conjunction with skilled nursing visits, or they may comprise a separate nursing contact for the woman. Telephonic nursing assessments are commonly used after a postpartum home care visit to reassess a woman's knowledge about the signs and symptoms of adequate hydration in breast-feeding, or, after initiating home phototherapy, to assess the caregiver's knowledge regarding problems with equipment.

Guidelines for Nursing Practice

The Association of Women's Health, Obstetric, and Neonatal Nurses (AWHONN, 2003) defines home care as the provision of technical, psychologic, and other therapeutic support in the client's home rather than in an institution. The scope of nursing care delivered in the home is necessarily limited to practices deemed safe and appropriate to be carried out in an environment that is physically separated from a health care institution and its resources. Nursing practice at home is consistent with federal and state regulations that direct home care practice. The nurse demonstrates practice competence through formalized orientation and ongoing clinical education and performance evaluation in the respective home care agency. Standards for practice from key specialty organizations such as AWHONN, the American College of Obstetricians and Gynecologists (ACOG), the American Academy of Pediatrics (AAP), and the Intravenous Nursing Society (INS) provide the basis for clinical protocols and pathways and organizational programs in home care practice. The Joint Commission on Accreditation of Healthcare Organizations (JCAHO) (www.jcaho.org) provides criteria for home care operations based on Centers for Medicare and Medicaid Services (formerly Health Care Financing Administration, or HCFA) regulations (cms.hhs.gov).

A wide range of professional health care services and products can be delivered or used in the home by means of technology and telecommunication. For example, telehealth and telemedicine make it possible for clients in the home to be interviewed and assessed by a specialist located hundreds of miles away. Some view home health care as an extension of in-hospital care. Essentially, the primary difference between health care in a hospital and home care is the absence of the continuous presence of professional health care providers in a client's home. Generally, but not always, home health care entails intermittent care by a professional who visits the client's home for a particular reason and/or provides care on site for fewer than 4 hours at a time. The home health care agency maintains on-call professional staff to assist home care clients who have questions about their care and for emergencies, such as equipment failure.

Perinatal Services

Home care perinatal services may be provided by hospital-based programs, independent proprietary (for-profit) agencies, or nonprofit home care agencies, and official or tax-supported agencies. Innovative programs may be supported by research grants for a period of years, but ultimately they must be sponsored by an agency with long-term funding. Home visits have both advantages and disadvantages. The pregnant woman is able to maintain bed rest if indicated, and vulnerable neonates are not exposed to the weather or external sources of infection. The nurse can observe and interact with family members in their most natural and secure environment. Adequacy of resources and safety factors can be assessed. Teaching can be tailored to the actual home conditions, and other family members can be included. A home visit is less expensive than a day's hospitalization, but a 60- to 90-minute visit requires 2.5 to 3 hours of nursing time, including travel and documentation. Travel time may be even greater when a client resides in a rural area because of distance and travel- and weather-related factors (Bosch & Bushy, 1997). It is more cost-effective for the health care provider to see clients in an office, since professional time is not spent in travel. Availability of nurses with expertise in maternity care may be limited, and concerns about the nurse's physical safety in some communities may limit visits.

Visits for outreach and health promotion are an integral part of community (or public) health nursing. In countries with national health systems, a nurse or midwife may see all women during pregnancy and after birth. In the United States, visits of this sort have been provided mainly to low-income families without health insurance and Medicaid recipients who use the clinics provided by local health departments. Until recently, private insurers did not reimburse for health promotion visits. Managed care organizations (MCOs) now recognize that anticipatory guidance can be cost-effective, but home visitation programs for the most part still target specific, high risk populations, such as adolescents and women at risk for preterm labor.

Home care agencies are subject to regulation by governmental and professional organizations and provide interdisciplinary services including social work, nutrition, and occupational and physical therapy. Increasingly, their case loads are made up of clients who require high-technology care, such as infusions or home monitoring. Although the home health nurse develops the care plan, all care must be ordered by a physician. In addition, interventions must meet the insurer's criteria for reimbursement, and services are limited to registered clients. Preconception care and low risk antepartum care can usually be provided more efficiently in offices and are not currently reimbursable. High risk antepartum care can be provided by home care agencies; for example, women with hyperemesis gravidarum who require parenteral nutrition may be treated at home. Conditions requiring bed rest, such as preterm labor and hypertension, are other common indications for home care. Other conditions often managed with home care may include cardiac disease, substance abuse, and diabetes in pregnancy.

Some insurers reimburse for at least one postpartum visit to families after early discharge or in the presence of high risk factors. Home phototherapy is used for treatment of neonatal hyperbilirubinemia and to avoid separation of mother and infant. Many other neonates who require long-term high-technology care are also managed with home care. The AAP (1998) recommends home visits as an effective early intervention strategy to improve child health in families at risk.

Client Selection and Referral

The office- or hospital-based nurse is often the key person in making effective referrals to home care. When considering a referral to home care, the following factors are evaluated:

- Health status of mother and fetus or infant: Is the condition serious enough to warrant home care, and is it stable enough for intermittent observation to be sufficient?
- Availability of professionals to provide the needed services within the client's community
- Family resources, including psychosocial, social, and economic resources: Will the family be able to provide care between nursing visits? Are relationships supportive? Is third-party reimbursement available, or can it be negotiated with the insurer? Could a voluntary or tax-supported community agency provide needed care without payment?
- Cost-effectiveness: Is it more reasonable for the client to receive these services at home or to go to a local outpatient facility to receive them?

Community referrals should not be limited to women with physiologic complications of pregnancy that require medical treatment. Clients at risk (e.g., young adolescents, families with a history of abuse, members of vulnerable population groups, developmentally disabled individuals) may need follow-up care at home. In consultation with the social worker, the hospital-based nurse should become familiar with agencies in the community that accept such referrals. When the client lives in a rural area, hospital-based nurses should familiarize themselves with available formal and informal resources in that community, since these may be different from those in a more populated setting (Bushy, 2000).

Standardized referral forms simplify the referral process and ensure that all needed information will be forwarded to the home health agency. The nursing assessment should include the woman's physical and psychologic status, her level of knowledge about self-care activities, her willingness to learn, the availability of caregivers and social support in the home, and her level of comfort with home care. If the referral is for a mother-and-infant home care visit, the nursing assessment should include newborn data.

High-technology home care requires additional information to be collected from the chart, and consultation with the referring physician and other members of the health care team, before a home care referral is made. These additional data include the medical diagnosis, medical prognosis, prescribed therapies, medication history, drug-dosing information, potential ancillary supplies, type of infusion and access device, and the available systems of social support for the client and family. The nursing assessment and therapy data provide baseline information for the home care nurse and other health care providers involved in the care plan.

Whenever a referral is called in to a home health care agency, a member of the nursing or admissions staff determines the agency's ability to accept the client for service. The use of telecommunication modalities such as fax machines, cellular phones, and the Internet to transmit information has eliminated delays in initiating home care services, even in more remote rural areas.

▬ CARE MANAGEMENT

▬ Preparing for the Home Visit

The home care nurse reviews the available clinical data, demographic information, and completed plan of care form and consults with the home care pharmacist or other health care team members who have previously contacted the woman to determine the goals of the visit. At this point, the nurse uses the medical diagnosis and the place where the case falls on the perinatal continuum as a starting point to organize the woman's care. The nurse reviews agency policies and procedures, professional literature about diagnosis, and community resources as part of the previsit preparation work (Box 2-4).

Before going on a home visit, the nurse contacts the woman. Contact by telephone before the visit has several goals besides establishing a convenient time to visit and exact directions; it also sets the stage for the first home care visit.

The nurse identifies himself or herself by name, title, and agency. He or she then explains who referred the woman to the agency for home care and the purpose of the home care visits. The nurse briefly explains what will occur during the visit and approximately how long the visit will last. The woman should be asked to restrain any pets during the visit. Last, the nurse asks about health supplies that may be needed for the woman's care.

▬ First Home Care Visit

Making the first home care visit can be stressful for the nurse and the client. The home care nurse is faced with an unknown environment controlled by the woman and her family. The woman and her family also experience feelings about the unknown, such as anxiety about the way the nurse will treat them or what the nurse will do during the visit. The challenge for the home care nurse is to establish a positive nurse-client relationship and provide the prescribed home care services within the time provided for the initial home visit. One of the most important roles of the home care nurse is modeling health-related behaviors for the woman and others who are in the home during the visit.

Introductions generally begin the visit; the nurse identifies himself or herself and the home care agency. The woman introduces herself and the other family members who are present. Sometimes the woman may feel uncertain of her role or be uncomfortable in taking the lead in introductions, so other people in the home may not be introduced to the nurse. In these situations, the nurse can politely ask about other people in the home and their relationship to the woman.

In the first visit to the home, the home care nurse completes extensive documentation with the client. Before performing any services, the nurse must obtain written agreement and consent for the home health care services. This consent-for-care serves two major purposes: agreement for care and authorization to release medical information. Many third-party payers require written documentation of the services provided; therefore the agency obtains authorization from the woman to give information to her physician and any individual or company involved in payment for the services. Agencies that bill third-party payers for the rendered services will include agreement language for assignment of benefits and

FIG. 2-7 Home care nurse visits with a woman in preterm labor at home on bed rest. (Courtesy Shannon Perry, Phoenix, AZ.)

| box 2-4 | **Protocol for Perinatal Home Visits** |

PREVISIT INTERVENTIONS

1. Contact the family to arrange details for home visit.
   a. Identify self, credentials, and agency role
   b. Review purpose of home visit follow-up
   c. Schedule convenient time for visit
   d. Confirm address and route to family home
2. Review and clarify appropriate data.
   a. All available assessment data for mother and fetus or infant (i.e., referral forms, hospital discharge summaries, identified learning needs of the family)
   b. Review records of any previous nursing contacts
   c. Contact other professional caregivers as necessary to clarify data (i.e., obstetrician, nurse- midwife, pediatrician, referring nurse)
3. Identify community resources and teaching materials appropriate to meet those needs already identified.
4. Plan the visit, and prepare a bag with equipment, supplies, and materials necessary for assessments of mother and fetus or infant, actual care anticipated, and teaching.

IN-HOME INTERVENTIONS: ESTABLISHING A RELATIONSHIP

1. Reintroduce yourself and establish the purpose of the visit for mother, infant, and family; offer the family the opportunity to clarify their expectations of the contact.
2. Spend a brief time socially interacting with the family to become acquainted and establish trusting relationship.

IN-HOME INTERVENTIONS: WORKING WITH FAMILY

1. Conduct a systematic assessment of the mother and the fetus or newborn to determine their physiologic adjustment and any existing complications (Fig. 2-7).
2. Throughout visit, collect data to assess the emotional adjustment of individual family members to the pregnancy or birth and lifestyle changes. Note any evidence of family-newborn bonding and sibling rivalry; note relationships among mother, father, children, and grandparents.
3. Determine the adequacy of support system.
   a. To what extent does someone help with cooking, cleaning, and other home management tasks?
   b. To what extent is help being provided in caring for the newborn and any other children?
   c. Are support persons encouraging the new mother to care for herself and get adequate rest?
   d. Who is providing helpful information? Emotional support?
4. Throughout the visit, observe the home environment for adequacy of resources:
   a. Space: privacy, safe play of children, sleeping
   b. Overall cleanliness and state of repair

   c. Number of steps pregnant woman/new mother must climb
   d. Adequacy of cooking arrangements
   e. Adequacy of refrigeration and other food storage areas
   f. Adequacy of bathing, toilet, and laundry facilities
   g. Arrangements in home for newborn: sleeping, bathing, formula preparation (if needed), layette items, and diapers
5. Throughout the visit, observe the home environment for overall state of repair and existence of safety hazards:
   a. Storage of medications, household cleaners, and other substances hazardous to children
   b. Presence of peeling paint on furniture, walls, or pipes
   c. Factors that contribute to falls, such as dim lighting, broken steps, scatter rugs
   d. Presence of vermin
   e. Use of crib or playpen that fails to meet safety guidelines
   f. Existence of emergency plan in case of fire; fire alarm or extinguisher
6. Provide care to the mother, the newborn, or both as prescribed by their respective primary care provider or in accord with agency protocol.
7. Provide teaching on the basis of previously identified needs.
8. Refer the family to appropriate community agencies or resources, such as warm lines and support groups.
9. Ascertain that the woman knows potential problems to watch for and who to call if they occur.
10. Ensure that used disposable items have been handled appropriately and that reusable items are cleaned and repacked appropriately in the nurse's bag.

IN-HOME INTERVENTIONS: ENDING THE VISIT

1. Summarize the activities and main points of the visit.
2. Clarify future expectations, including the schedule of the next visit.
3. Review the teaching plan and provide major points in writing.
4. Provide information about reaching the nurse or agency if needed before the next scheduled visit.

POSTVISIT INTERVENTIONS

1. Document the visit thoroughly, using the necessary agency forms to serve as a legal record of the visit and to allow third-party reimbursement, as possible.
2. Initiate the plan of care on which the next encounter with the woman and/or family will be based.
3. Communicate appropriately (by telephone, letter, progress notes, or referral form) with the primary care provider, other health professionals, or referral agencies on behalf of the woman and family.

---

financial remuneration. By agreeing to assign insurance benefits to the agency, the woman allows her insurance company to pay the home health care agency directly.

All clients have the right to participate actively in their plan of care. These client rights and responsibilities should begin the discussion about the nurse and client roles during this initial visit.

▬ Assessment and Nursing Diagnoses

The primary goals of the assessment phase are to develop a trusting relationship and collect data by various methods to obtain a comprehensive client profile. It may not be feasible or appropriate to collect in-depth information about all areas of assessment during the first visit. However, in many instances, the nurse may be limited to one visit and must obtain information pertinent to the current situation in that hour.

The establishment of a trusting relationship begins with the previsit telephone call. Several techniques facilitate the development of that trusting relationship: an interview style that reflects sensitivity; a nonjudgmental, accepting attitude; and respect for the woman's rights. A skillful interviewer avoids barriers to communication such as false reassurance, advice giving, excessive talking, and the showing of approval or disapproval. This nurse-client relationship continues to develop over the course of home visits.

The nurse is a guest in the woman's home and should show respect for her and her belongings. Some adaptation of the home visit schedule may be made if numerous distractions interrupt a visit, such as caring for the needs of small children. The nurse may ask to have the volume of the television reduced or suggest moving to another room where it is more quiet and private.

The major areas of the assessment are demographics, medical history, general health history, medication history, sociocultural assessment, home and community environment, and physical assessment. Some of this information can be obtained from client records sent to the home care agency at the time of referral or from the previsit interview. These data will be used to develop the nursing care plan and complete the plan of care, which is required for many licensed home health care agencies (Box 2-5).

Each plan of care has a different emphasis in the home environment. For example, women receiving infusion therapy for hyperemesis gravidarum need a safe place to store medications and infusion supplies that is out of reach of small children living in the home. The home care nurse should incorporate the agency policies and procedures for the storage and handling of infusion supplies into her walk-through inspection. During the walk-through, the home care nurse looks at the potential storage areas that are dry and clean, and where the temperature can be maintained. The home care nurse should include an inspection of the work areas such as countertops, tabletops, sinks, and trash areas that the woman or caregiver may use for mixing medications, changing infusion tubing, handling supplies, or disposing of used equipment and supplies.

The homes of clients using electronic home health care equipment, such as phototherapy equipment or infusion pumps, require physical inspection of any electrical outlets, electrical cords, and extension cords that will be used. Homes with faulty electrical wiring may place the client at risk for being involved in an electrical fire; faulty wiring may require inspection and repair by a professional electrician before electronic devices are used. Findings from the assessment are incorporated into the plan of care.

Nursing diagnoses are derived from the data collected at the first home visit. Nursing diagnoses for perinatal home health care clients include the following:

- *Deficient knowledge related to*
  - management of therapeutic regimen (e.g., nausea and vomiting, preterm labor, gestational diabetes)
  - newborn care and feeding
- *Compromised family coping related to*
  - lack of child care while mother is on bed rest
  - care of newborn receiving oxygen therapy
- *Impaired parenting related to*
  - maternal immaturity and lack of family support
- *Deficient diversional activity related to*
  - prolonged bed rest

▬ Expected Outcomes of Care

Examples of expected outcomes for perinatal clients include that the woman/family will do the following:
- Verbalize understanding of treatments.

---

box 2-5 Psychosocial Assessment

LANGUAGE
- Identify the primary language spoken in the home
- Assess whether there are any language barriers to receiving support

COMMUNITY RESOURCES/ACCESS TO CARE
- Identify primary and secondary means of transportation
- Identify community agencies family currently uses for health care and support
- Assess cultural and psychosocial barriers to receiving care

SOCIAL SUPPORT
- Determine the people living with the pregnant woman
- Identify who assists with household chores
- Identify who assists with child care and parenting activities
- Identify who the pregnant woman turns to for problems or during a crisis

INTERPERSONAL RELATIONSHIPS
- Identify the way decisions are made in the family
- Identify the family's perception of the need for home care
- Identify roles of adults in caring for family members

CAREGIVER
- Identify the primary caregiver for home care treatments
- Identify other caregivers and their roles
- Assess the caregiver's knowledge of treatments and the care process
- Identify potential strain from the caregiver role
- Identify the level of satisfaction with the caregiver role

STRESS AND COPING
- Identify what the woman perceives as lifestyle changes and their impact on her and her family
- Identify the changes she and her family have made to adjust to her health condition and home health care treatments

- Report decreased anxiety about performing procedures (e.g., blood glucose monitoring).
- Use support systems to cope effectively with problems (e.g., pregnancy complications, newborn complications or treatments).
- Perform procedures accurately, as evidenced by return demonstration.
- Verbalize decreased role strain.

■ Plan of Care and Interventions

The nursing plan of care is developed in collaboration with the client, based on the health care needs of the individual. Home care nurses working in home health care agencies regulated by the Centers for Medicare and Medicaid Services use a plan of care that includes client demographics, the health care provider's orders, home care goals, and the client's level of functioning. This document is initiated at the time of referral to the home care agency and must be updated every 60 days or as specified by state regulations. The frequency of the skilled nursing visit may vary with the individual plan of care and reimbursement criteria established by the third-party payers.

■ *Nursing Considerations*

In home care, the woman or family members are responsible for administration of medications in the absence of the nurse. A careful medication history should be obtained to see if the woman is taking her medications correctly and understands their desired action and potential side effects. Sometimes when orders are changed, women continue to take both the old and new prescriptions, which can lead to dangerous overdoses or medication interactions. The culturally competent nurse ensures that there is an adequate supply and a safe place for proper storage of medications to prevent deterioration or accidental ingestion by children or pets. The nurse inquires about any other medications that the woman might be taking concurrently. Over-the-counter drugs or herbal supplements may not be considered medications by the women and not mentioned unless such information is specifically asked for. Even more important is ensuring that the woman and her caregivers fully understand the information that they are exposed to by health care providers.

High-technology home care involves many diagnostic and therapeutic procedures. A focused physical assessment is always part of the visit. Nurses involved in perinatal home care must be skilled in prenatal, postpartal, and newborn assessment. Many women require additional diagnostic tests. The nurse may need to collect blood or other specimens. Portable fetal monitoring equipment or even ultrasound can be used in the home for fetal assessment. Home infusion for women with hyperemesis gravidarum often replaces hospitalization. Women with preterm labor may receive parenteral tocolytic therapy. Phototherapy devices or apnea monitors can be provided in the home for newborns. Family members may need to be taught to monitor equipment between nurse visits and to prevent accidental damage.

Medical emergencies may occur during or between the nurse's visits to the home. Prior planning and education can reduce the risk of problems. All parents of newborns should know how to perform infant cardiopulmonary resuscitation (CPR). There should be immediate telephone access to call for emergency medical assistance. Women and their families should be taught to recognize danger signs related to their condition. For example, women at risk for preterm labor should learn to palpate the uterus and recognize contractions in the absence of pain; women with diabetes must learn the signs of hypoglycemia and what to do if it occurs; women with preeclampsia must know the danger signs that indicate worsening of their condition and to notify the health care provider immediately. In a more remote rural community that does not have an obstetrician in the region, the nurse may have to assist the client's family to arrange for "boarding" somewhere that is closer to a medical specialist.

Client and family education in home care includes information about the specific high risk condition(s) involved, implications for pregnancy outcome, and measures for self-monitoring. Verbal explanations should be supplemented with clearly written instructions. General information to promote well-being, such as about nutrition and common discomforts of pregnancy, should also be included. The need for preparation for childbirth can be addressed by using books or videos and supplemented by individual teaching at home. Coping with bed rest or other limitation of activity is a problem for many women with high risk pregnancies. The nurse may share strategies that others have used, help with time management, and provide information about support services. Teaching about infant care or the special needs of the preterm infant may be appropriate during the prenatal period.

Clear documentation of assessments, problems identified, treatments and interventions performed, and the client's response is essential. Third-party payers base reimbursement on the nurse's written record of providing skilled nursing care and assessments that support the woman's continuing need for those services. The nurse must promptly inform the health care provider by telephone or facsimile of any significant changes. When new orders are transmitted by telephone, a written copy must be sent for the physician's signature.

Nursing documentation should reflect an objective description of the nursing assessment data collected at each visit. Statements such as "no change" or "same as last visit" do not accurately reflect the monitoring of the woman's condition that occurred during the skilled nursing visit. Once the home care outcomes are achieved and the client is discharged from the home care agency, documentation should include information about the client's status at the time of discharge, progress made toward attaining health care goals, and plans for follow-up care (see Plan of Care, "Community and Home Care").

The role of the clinical record in home care has been affected by social, economic, and legal health care changes.

plan of care ▶	**Community and Home Care**

NURSING DIAGNOSIS Readiness for enhanced family coping related to family growth and development in new community

Expected Outcome *Family will identify at least three community groups that can serve as appropriate resources for an expectant family with small children.*

Nursing Interventions/Rationales

• Assess family structure and availability of significant others, friends, or family members to assist family with new baby and siblings *to provide database for further interventions.*

• Encourage family to enlist assistance of individuals who are available to help family at birth of new baby *to provide physical and emotional support.*

• Using therapeutic communication, assist the family to assess coping strategies used in the past for new situations *to provide clarification and promote empowerment of family in new situations.*

• Suggest strategies to find resources available in the community *to assist family during pregnancy, with new baby, and with small siblings.*

• Give information regarding community workshops, classes, or support groups *to promote networking, community bonding, and support.*

NURSING DIAGNOSIS Ineffective community management of therapeutic regimen

Expected Outcome *The community will develop programs to meet the needs of new members of the community.*

Nursing Interventions/Rationales

• Conduct a needs assessment of the community *to identify priority needs for new members of the community.*

• Initiate health education programs based on topics identified in the needs assessment *to meet the needs of members of the community.*

• Prepare client education materials in a variety of languages *to enhance understanding of community members.*

• Identify risks in the community (e.g., environmental hazards, drug sales) *to provide a target for community improvement.*

• With community leaders, develop a plan to cope with and reduce environmental hazards *to improve public health and safety.*

• Develop a monitoring or surveillance system *to ensure that progress will continue and new problems will be identified.*

NURSING DIAGNOSIS Ineffective community coping

Expected Outcome *Health status of the community will improve.*

Nursing Interventions/Rationales

• Initiate health screening programs for community members *to identify effects of environmental hazards in the community.*

• Work with politicians and policy makers to develop the community *to provide a safe environment with means of economic survival for community members.*

• Initiate programs such as Block Watch, Safe Houses, and Neighborhood Watch *to enhance the safety of the environment.*

• Work with community leaders to develop or clean up playgrounds *to provide a safe place for children to play.*

• With community leaders, develop community grass roots initiatives *to enable community members to take ownership in the community.*

• Identify sites of lead exposure *to decrease the potential for lead poisoning in children.*

• Participate in immunization or vaccination clinics *to reduce the risk in the community of infectious diseases.*

Appropriate care should be taken to complete the necessary home health care records accurately and in a timely manner. Documentation guidelines include writing or dictating notes or using a laptop computer at the client's home or shortly after the visit.

■ Evaluation

Evaluation is a continuous process through which the nurse must reassess the woman's and family condition and any response to the interventions in relation to expected outcomes of care. The nurse, in collaboration with the woman and family, then revises the nursing diagnoses and plan of care as necessary to meet mutually determined goals.

■ SAFETY ISSUES FOR THE ■ HOME CARE NURSE

Nurse safety and infection control are two important aspects specific to home care. The nurse should be fully aware of the home environment and the neighborhood in which the home care is being provided. Unlike hospitals, in which the environment is more predictable and controlled,

the client's neighborhood and home have the potential for uncertainty. Home care nurses should take necessary safety precautions and avoid dangerous areas.

Agencies that serve clients in high crime areas may conduct a violence potential assessment by telephone before the visit and enlist the client's cooperation in minimizing risk. Others have hired full-time security personnel to accompany nurses on their visits. Personal strategies recommended for nurses visiting families with a history of violence or substance abuse include (1) self-awareness; (2) environmental assessment; (3) using listening and observation skills with clients to be aware of behavioral changes indicating aggression or lack of impulse control; (4) planning for dealing with aggressive behavior (i.e., allowing personal space and taking a nonaggressive stance); (5) making visits in pairs; and (6) having access to a cellular phone at all times.

Personal Safety

The home care nurse must be aware of personal safety behaviors before going on a home visit. Dress should be casual but professional in appearance, with a name identification tag. Limited jewelry should be worn. Valuable personal items, such as an expensive purse or coat, should not be worn on a visit. Carrying an extra set of car keys in the nursing home care bag saves time and frustration if the nurse becomes locked out of the automobile. Automobile keys spread between the fingers with sharp ends outward can be used as a weapon if necessary. The same commonsense behaviors and precautions that guide a person's behavior when alone in any setting should be followed by home care nurses.

The agency should have a copy of the nurse's home care itinerary, including contact telephone numbers if a client does not have a telephone and information on the nurse's car (make, model, color, and license plate number). Many home care nurses carry agency-provided pagers or cellular telephones that allow the agency to contact the nurse throughout the day to give information about client updates, changes in orders or services, schedule changes, and new clients who require an initial visit. The telephone also is useful to notify clients when the nurse is delayed.

The automobile used for the home care visits, whether a personal or an agency-owned vehicle, should have regular preventive maintenance checks, an adequate fuel level, and road safety items stored in the trunk. Items to carry in the vehicle include change for telephone calls and tolls, maps, emergency telephone numbers, a flashlight, a first aid kit, flares, a blanket, and equipment for inclement weather conditions. When making a visit to a client in a more remote rural setting, other travel considerations may be needed, as well as taking additional supplies or medication to the client (Bosch & Bushy, 1997).

Home care nurses should park and lock their cars in a safe place that is visible from the street and the client's home and away from hidden alleys. While driving to the client's home, the nurse should assess the neighborhood for safety, especially if the neighborhood is unfamiliar. All valuable items should be stored out of sight before leaving the office. While walking to the client's home, nurses should not walk near groups of strangers hanging out in doorways or alleys, enter into vacant buildings, or enter a yard that has an unrestrained dog. The home or building should not be entered if the nurse has any safety concerns. All home care agencies should have policies to follow for such situations.

Client's Home

Once inside the woman's home, the nurse may encounter unsafe situations such as the presence of weapons, abusive behavior, or health hazards. Each potentially hazardous situation must be dealt with according to agency policies and procedures. If abuse or neglect is reasonably suspected, the home care nurse should follow home care agency and state and federal regulations for reporting and documenting the situation. Nurses should maintain their own safety first and act accordingly throughout the visit.

Infection Control

The nurse carries the necessary supplies and equipment to provide nursing care to the woman. Home care bags should contain infection control supplies, such as personal protection equipment; disposable nonsterile, sterile, and utility gloves; disinfectants; disposable CPR masks; gowns; shoe covers; caps; leak-proof and puncture-resistant specimen containers; sharps container; dry hand disinfectants; and leak-proof barriers. Proper infection control techniques should be used in stocking, storing, handling, and transporting this bag. When a procedure is to be performed, the nurse should set up a clean area for necessary supplies. A "dirty" area is designated with a trash bag for the collection of soiled equipment and supplies. Hands are washed before all supplies and equipment for the visit are removed from the bag and placed in a clean area.

The importance of infection control does not diminish because nursing care is provided in the client's home rather than in a hospital. Clients are not likely to become infected because of their home environment, but the nurse may become exposed to an infectious disease.

The CDC has recommended Standard Precautions guidelines for the protection of health care workers from blood-borne pathogens. These guidelines recommend that Standard Precautions be used whenever a treatment is performed because it is difficult to determine which clients have a communicable disease (see Box 8-4).

Handwashing remains the single most important infection-control procedure, and the caregiver is in a position to educate about the importance of this practice in preventing disease. Hands should be washed before and after each client contact. Wearing gloves does not eliminate the necessity of handwashing. If running water or clean facilities are unavailable, the hands can be cleaned with a self-drying antiseptic solution.

Using gloves reduces the incidence of exposure to blood-borne pathogens. Gloves should be selected according to the nursing activity to be performed. Nonsterile latex or vinyl gloves should be worn with each procedure that incurs potential contact with bodily substances (e.g., performing venipunctures, heel sticks on the newborn, and perineal care). Sterile gloves should be worn for clinical procedures requiring sterile technique, such as insertion of peripherally inserted central lines and certain dressing changes. General-purpose utility gloves should be used for housekeeping activities, such as cleaning equipment or spills. Nonsterile and sterile gloves should be discarded after each use in a leak-resistant waste receptacle. Utility gloves may be disinfected and reused.

Disposable personal protection equipment should be removed after each use and discarded in a plastic trash container. Safety glasses and goggles can be cleaned with soap and water after each use.

Whenever specimens are collected, Standard Precautions should be used. Any specimen of bodily fluids should be placed in a leak-proof bag and secured in a puncture-proof container. The outside of the container is washed off, if it was soiled, before transporting it. Specimens should be labeled with the woman's name and additional identifying information according to the home health care agency or laboratory policies. If specimens are being transported, they should be placed in a container on a flat surface in the vehicle. An insulated container may be used to keep specimens cool in transit. The nurse should be aware of the time sensitivity for certain types of specimens and laboratory procedures.

Sharps containers are puncture-proof and leak-proof containers labeled with a biohazard sign on the outside and should be used to collect needles and sharp objects. Clients are instructed to fill containers between two-thirds and three-fourths full to prevent spillage of their contents. As part of the client teaching process, information about storage and handling is covered by the home care nurse. When the container reaches its maximal capacity, it should be returned to the home health care agency and replaced. Medical waste such as urine and secretions can be discarded through the sewer or septic system.

Contaminated dressings and disposable supplies should be placed in a leak-proof plastic bag and securely fastened for disposal at the client's home. The client should be instructed regarding the proper disposal of medical waste in the home. Agency policies and procedures and local waste management ordinances should be consulted before the client is instructed.

community activity

Select a *Healthy People 2010* priority area related to maternal, newborn, or women's health (such as obesity or cancer). Identify an "at risk" target population in your community for a health promotion program.
- Outline the main steps in developing a health promotion program for this target population.
- Identify key sources of data that might be used for assessing health status of this group.
- Discuss the cultural beliefs, values, and health behaviors that are characteristic of your target population.
- Describe real or potential barriers to health promotion with the target population.
- Identify community assets and resources to facilitate the health promotion effort.
- Recommend health promotion strategies for effective intervention with the target population.

key points

- Contemporary American society recognizes and accepts a variety of family forms.
- The family is a social network that acts as an important support system for its members.
- Family theories provide nurses with useful guidelines for understanding family function.
- Family socioeconomics, response to stress, and culture are key factors influencing family health.
- The reproductive beliefs and practices of a culture are embedded in its economic, religious, kinship, and political structures.
- To provide quality care to women in their childbearing years and beyond, nurses should be aware of the cultural beliefs and practices important to individual families.
- A community is defined as a locality-based entity composed of systems of societal institutions, informal groups, and aggregates that are interdependent and whose function is to meet a wide variety of collective needs.
- Of necessity, most changes aimed at improving community health involve partnerships among community residents and health workers.

- Methods of collecting data useful to the nurse working in the community include walking surveys, analysis of existing data, informant interviews, and participant observation.
- Vulnerable populations are groups who are at higher risk for developing physical, mental, or social health problems.
- Perinatal home care is a unique nursing practice that incorporates knowledge from community health nursing, acute care nursing, family therapy, health promotion, and client education.
- Perinatal home care can be provided for women and infants throughout the perinatal period, beginning before conception and ending in the postpartum period.
- Telephonic nurse advice lines, telephonic nursing assessments, and warm lines are low-cost health care services that facilitate continuous client education, support, and health care decision making, even though health care is delivered in multiple sites.
- Communication protocols among members of the home health care team are critical to diminish fragmentation and duplication of health care services.

REFERENCES

Acs, G., & Nelson, S. (2003). *Changes in family structure and child well-being: Evidence from the 2002 National Survey of American Families.* Accessed www.urban.org/url.cfm?ID=311025, August 4, 2005.

Agency for Health Care Research and Quality (AHRQ). (2004). *National Health Care Disparities Report, 2004.* Accessed http://www.qualitytools.ahrq.gov/disparitiesreport/browse/browse.aspx?id=3223, September 5, 2005.

Agency for Healthcare Research and Quality (AHRQ). (May, 2005). *Women's Health Care in the United States: Selected Findings From the*

2004 National Healthcare Quality and Disparities Reports. Fact Sheet. AHRQ Publication No. 05-P021. Rockville, MD. Accessed http://www.ahrq.gov/qual/nhqrwomen/nhqrwomen.htm, September 5, 2005.

Allen, F. (1997). Comparative theories of the expanded role in nursing and implications for nursing practice. *Nursing Papers, 9*(2), 38-45.

Allender, J., & Spradley, B. (2005). *Community health nursing; Promoting and protecting the public's health* (6th ed.). Philadelphia: Lippincott Williams & Wilkins.

American Academy of Nursing. (1992). AAN expert panel report: Culturally competent health care. *Nursing Outlook, 40*(6), 277-283.

American Academy of Pediatrics Council on Child and Adolescent Health. (1998). The role of home-visitation programs in improving health outcomes for children and families. *Pediatrics, 101*, 486-489.

American College of Obstetricians and Gynecologists (ACOG). (2005). Health Care for Homeless Women. ACOG Committee Opinion No. 312. *Obstetrics and Gynecology, 106*, 429-434.

American Public Health Association. (April 15, 2004). *Rural Health Disparities Fact Sheet.* Accessed http://www.apha.org/NPHW/facts/Rural-PHW04_Facts.pdf, September 15, 2005.

Andrews, M., & Boyle, J. (2003). *Transcultural concepts in nursing care.* (4th ed.). Philadelphia, PA: Lippincott Williams & Wilkins.

Association of Women's Health, Obstetric, and Neonatal Nurses (AWHONN). (2003). *Standards and guidelines for professional nursing practice in the care of women and newborns* (6th ed.). Washington, DC: Author.

Averill, J. (2003). Keys to the puzzle: Recognizing strengths in a rural community. *Public Health Nursing, 20*(6), 449-455.

Becker, M. (1974). The Health Belief Model and sick role behavior. *Health Education Monographs, 2*, 409-419.

Best, A., Stokols, D., Green, W., Leischow, S., Holmes, B., & Bucholz, K. (2003). An integrative framework for community partnering to translate theory into effective health promotion strategy. *American Journal of Health Promotion, 18*(2), 168-76.

Bloom, K., Bednarzyk, M., Devitt, D., Renault, R., Teaman, V., & VanLoock, D. (2004). Barriers to prenatal care for homeless pregnant women. *Journal of Obstetric, Gynecologic and Neonatal Nursing, 33*(4), 428-435.

Blum, R., McNeely, C., & Nonnemaker, J. (2002). Vulnerability, risk, and protection. *Journal of Adolescent Health, 31*(1 Suppl.), 28-39.

Bosch, D., & Bushy, A. (1997). Case management: Implementing home care in rural areas. *Home Healthcare Consultant, 4*(7), 19-42.

Boss, P. (1996). *Family stress management* (2nd ed.). Newbury Park, CA: Sage.

Brennan, L., Baker, E., Haire-Joshu, D., & Brownson, R. (2003). Linking perceptions of the community to behavior: Are protective social factors associated with physical activity? *Health Education & Behavior, 30*(6), 740-755.

Bronfenbrenner, U. (1979). *The ecology of human development.* Cambridge, MA: Harvard University Press.

Bronfenbrenner, U. (1989). Ecological systems theory. In R. Vasta (Ed.), *Annals of child development* (Vol. 6). Greenwich, CT: JAI.

Brooks, E. (2002). Family assessment and cultural diversity. In S. Clemen-Stone, S. McGuire, & D. Eigsti (Eds.), *Comprehensive community health nursing: Family, aggregate, and community practice* (6th ed.). St. Louis: Mosby.

Brown, J., Villarruel, A., Oakley, D., & Eribes, C. (2003). Exploring contraceptive pill taking among Hispanic women in the United States. *Health Education & Behavior, 30*(6), 663-682.

Bureau of Primary Health Care (BPHC). (2001). *Homeless population statistics.* Accessed www.bphc.hrsa.gov/hchirc/about/face_homelessness.htm, September 29, 2005.

Bushy, A. (2002). *Resource manual: Rural minorities, their health issues and resources.* Kansas City, MO: National Rural Health Association.

Cameron, P. (2004). Number of homosexual parents living with their children. *Psychological Reports, 94*(1), 179-88.

Carter, B., & McGoldrick, M. (1999). *The expanded family life cycle: Individual, family, and social perspectives* (3rd ed.). Boston: Allyn & Bacon.

Centers for Disease Control and Prevention (CDC), Office of Minority Health. (2005a). *Disease burden and risk factors.* Accessed www.cdc.gov/omh/AboutUS/disparities.htm, September 5, 2005.

Centers for Disease Control and Prevention (CDC), Office of Minority Health. (2005b). *Infant Mortality Fact Sheet.* Accessed www.cdc.gov/omh/AMH/factsheets/infant.htm, September 5, 2005.

Chen, J., & Rankin, S. (2002). Using the resiliency model to deliver culturally sensitive care to Chinese families. *Journal of Pediatric Nursing, 17*(3), 157-166.

Chrisman, N., Senturia, K., Tang, G., & Gheisar, B. (2002). Qualitative process evaluation of urban community work: A preliminary view. *Health Education & Behavior, 29*(2), 232-248.

Clemen-Stone, S. (2002). Community assessment and diagnosis. In S. Clemen-Stone, S. McGuire, & D. Eigsti (Eds.), *Comprehensive community health nursing: Family, aggregate, and community practice* (6th ed.). St. Louis: Mosby.

Cottrell, R., Girvan, J., & McKenzie, J. (2006). *Health promotion and education* (3rd ed.). San Francisco: Pearson Benjamin Cummings.

Crosby, R., DiClemente, R., Wingood, G., Cobb, B., Harrington, K., Davies, S., et al. (2002). Condom use and correlates of African American adolescent females' infrequent communication with sex partners about preventing sexually transmitted diseases and pregnancy. *Health Education & Behavior, 29*(2), 219-231.

Doswell, W., Kouyate, M., & Taylor, J. (2003). The role of spirituality in preventing early sexual behavior. *American Journal of Health Studies, 18*(4), 195-202.

Ervin, N. (2002). *Advanced community health nursing practice: Population-focused care.* Upper Saddle River, NJ: Prentice Hall.

Federal Interagency Forum on Children and Family Statistics. (2005). *Population and family characteristics.* Accessed www.childstats.gov, August 3, 2005.

Fejos, P. (1959). Man, magic, and medicine. In L. Goldston, (Ed.), *Medicine and anthropology.* New York: International University Press.

Friedman, M. (1998). *Family nursing theory and assessment* (4th ed.). New York: Appleton & Lange.

Friedman, M., Bowden, V., & Jones, E. (2003). *Family nursing: Research, theory, and practice.* Upper Saddle River, New Jersey: Prentice-Hall.

Freudenberg, N. (2004). Community capacity for environmental health promotion: Determinants and implications for practice. *Health Education & Behavior, 31*(4), 472-490.

Giger, J., & Davidhizar, R. (2004). *Transcultural nursing: Assessment and intervention* (4th ed.). St. Louis: Mosby.

Greenfeld, D. (2005). Reproduction in same sex couples: Quality of parenting and child development. *Current Opinion in Obstetrics and Gynecology, 17*(3), 309-12.

Harrison, P., & Karlberg, J. (May, 2004). *Prison and jail inmates at Midyear 2003.* Washington, DC: U.S. Department of Justice. Bureau of Justice Statistics Bulletin.

Huttlinger, K., Schaller-Ayers, J., & Lawson, T. (2004). Health care in Appalachia: A population-based approach. *Public Health Nursing, 21*(2), 103-110.

Institute of Medicine (IOM). (2002). *Unequal treatment: Confronting racial and ethnic disparities in health care.* Washington, DC: National Academies Press.

Jackson, F., & Phillips, M. (2003). Collaborative research and reproductive health outcomes among African American women. *American Journal of Health Studies, 18*(4), 178-187.

Jacobs, E., Karavalos, K., Rathous, P., Ferris, T., & Powell, L. (2005). Limited English proficiency and cervical cancer screening in a multiethnic population. *American Journal of Public Health, 95*(8), 1420-1416.

Janz, N., & Becker, M. (1984). The Health Belief Model: A decade later. *Health Education Quarterly, 11*(1), 1-47.

Kaiser Commission on Medicaid and the Uninsured. (2003a). *The uninsured in rural America.* Accessed www.kff.org/uninsured/up-load/The-Uninsured-in-Rural-America-Update-PDF.pdf, September 15, 2005.

Kaiser Commission on Medicaid and the Uninsured. (August, 2003b*). Immigrants' health care coverage and access.* Accessed www.kff.org/uninsured/upload/Immigrants-Health-Care-Coverage-and-Access-fact-sheet.pdf, September 15, 2005.

Kaiser Family Foundation. (2003). *National survey of adolescents and young adults: Sexual health, knowledge, attitudes and experiences.* Accessed www.kff.org/youthhivstds/upload/National-Survey-of-Adolescents-and-Young-Adults-Sexual-Health-Knowledge-Attitudes-and-Experiences-Summary-of-Findings.pdf, September 30, 2005.

Klein, D., & White, J. (1996). *Family theories: An introduction.* Newberry Park, CA: Sage.

Kuehnert, P. (2002). Overview of program planning. In N. Ervin (Ed.), *Advanced community health nursing practice.* Upper Saddle River, NJ: Prentice Hall.

Lausch, C., Heuer, L., Guasasco, C., & Bengiamin, M. (2003). The experiences of migrant health nurses employed in seasonal satellite nurse-managed centers: A qualitative study. *Journal of Community Health Nursing, 20*(2), 67-80.

Leininger, M., & McFarland, M. (2002). *Transcultural nursing concepts, theory, research, and practice.* New York: McGraw-Hill Professional.

Lewis, J., Andersen, R., & Gelberg, L. (2003). Health care for homeless women: Unmet needs and barriers to care. (AHRQ grant HS08323). *Journal of General Internal Medicine, 18*(11), 921-928.

Lowe, J. (2002). Balance and harmony through connectedness: The intentionality of Native American nurses. *Holistic Nursing Practice, 16*(4), 4-11.

March of Dimes (MOD). (2003). *Perinatal Profiles, 2003*: U.S. Accessed www.marchofdimes.com/peristats/alldata.aspx?reg=16, September 10, 2005.

Maurer, F., & Smith, C. (2005). *Community/public health nursing practice: Health for families and populations* (3rd ed.). St. Louis: Saunders.

McDevitt, J., & Wilbur, J. (2002). Locating sources of data. In N. Ervin (Ed.), *Advanced community health nursing practice: Population-focused care.* Upper Saddle River, NJ: Prentice Hall.

McEwen, M. (2003). *Community-based nursing: An introduction* (2nd ed). St. Louis: Saunders.

Mete, C., Cioffi, J., & Lichtveld, M. (2003). Are public health services available where they are needed most? An examination of local health department services. *Journal of Public Health Management and Practice, 9*(3), 214-233.

Miller, A., & Iris, M. (2002). Health promotion attitudes and strategies in older adults. *Health Education & Behavior, 29*(2), 249-267.

Mohanty, S., Woolhandler, S., Himmelstein, D., Pati, S., Carrasquillo, O., & Bor, D. (2005). Health care expenditures of immigrants in the United States: A nationally representative analysis. *American Journal of Public Health, 95*(8), 1431-1438.

Montgomery, K. (2003). Health promotion for pregnant adolescents. *AWHONN Lifelines, 7*(5), 432-444.

Munoz, C., & Luckmann, J. (2005). *Transcultural communication in nursing* (2nd ed.). Clinton Park, NY: Thompson.

Murray, R., Zentner, J., & Samiezade-Yazd, C. (2001). Sociocultural influejnces on the person and family. In R. Murray & J. Zentner (Eds.), *Health promotion strategies through the lifespan* (7th ed.). Upper Saddle River, NJ: Prentice Hall.

National Academy Press (NAP). (2002). *From generation to generation: The health and well-being of children in immigrant families.* Accessed www.search.nap.edu/html/generation/summary.html, September 29, 2005.

National Alliance for Hispanic Health. (2001). *A primer for cultural proficiency: Towards quality health services for Hispanics.* Washington, DC: Author.

National Friendly Access Program. (2003). *The Lawton and Rhea Chiles Center for Healthy Mothers and Babies.* Accessed www.chilescenter.org/programs4.htm, September 25, 2005.

National Women's Law Center (NWLC). (2004). *Making the grade on women's health: A national and state-by-state report card.* Accessed www.nwlc.org/details.cfm?id=1861&section=health, Sept. 25, 2005.

Nightingale, E., & Fischoff, B. (2002). Adolescent risk and vulnerability: An overview. *Journal of Adolescent Behavior, 31*(1 Suppl.), 3-9.

Peck, J., & Alexander, K. (2003). Maternal, infant, and child health in rural areas. *Rural Healthy People 2010: A companion document to Healthy People 2010.* Volume 1. College Station, TX: The Texas A&M University System Health Science Center, School of Rural Public Health, Southwest Rural Health Research Center. Accessed www.srph.tamhsc.edu/centers/rhp2010/07Volume1MIC.htm, September 25, 2005.

Pender, N., Murdaugh, C., & Parsons, M. (2002). *Health promotion in nursing practice.* Upper Saddle River, NJ: Prentice Hall.

Pincus, H., Thomas, S., Keyser D., Castle, N., Dembosky, J., Firth, R., et al. (2003). *Improving maternal and child health care.* Santa Monica, CA: Rand Health.

Porche, D. (2004). *Public & community health nursing practice: A population-based approach.* Thousand Oaks, CA: Sage.

Purnell, L., & Paulanka, B. (2003). *Transcultural health care: A culturally competent approach* (2nd ed.). Philadelphia: F.A. Davis.

Rosal, M., Goins, K., Carbone, E., & Cortes, D. (2004). Views and preferences of low-literate Hispanics regarding diabetes education: Results of formative research. *Health Education & Behavior, 31*(3), 388-405.

Schillinger, D., Grumbach, K., Piette, J., Wang, F., Osmond, D., Daher, C., et al. (2002). Association of health literacy with diabetic outcomes. *Journal of the American Medical Association, 288*(4), 475-482.

Schor, E. (2003). Family pediatrics: Report of the Task Force on the Family. *Pediatrics, 111*(6 Pt 2), 1542-71.

Schulz, A., Kreiger, J., & Galea, S. (2002). Addressing social determinants of health: Community-based participatory approaches to research and practice. *Health Education & Behavior, 29*(3), 287-295.

Schultz, A., Parker, E., Israel, B., Allen, A., Decarlo, M., & Lockett, M. (2002). Addressing social determinants of health through community-based participatory research: The East Side Village Health Worker Partnership. *Health Education & Behavior, 29*(3), 326-341.

Simmons, R., Bennett, E., Schwartz, M., Sharifyz, D., & Short, E. (2002). Health education and cultural diversity in the health care setting: Tips for the practitioner. *Health Promotion Practice, 3*(1), 8-11.

Smith, S., Hamilton, S., Sheats, J., Mensah, E., Apantaku, F., & Sullivan, L. (2003). Stay beautiful, stay alive: A successful approach to community-based participatory research. *American Journal of Health Studies, 18*(4), 219-224.

Spector, R. (2004). *Cultural diversity in health and illness* (6th ed.). Upper Saddle River, NJ: Prentice Hall.

Spencer, N. (2005). Does material disadvantage explain the increased risk of adverse health, educational, and behavioral outcomes among children in lone parent households in Britain? A cross-sectional study. *Journal of Epidemiology and Health, 59*(2), 152-157.

Stanhope, M., & Lancaster, J. (2004). *Community and public health nursing* (6th ed.). St. Louis: Mosby.

Surani, Z., Baezconde-Garbanati, L., Bastani, R., & Montano, B. (2003). Improving community capacity to develop cancer awareness programs. *American Journal of Health Studies, 18*(4), 203-210.

Taylor, R. ((2005). Addressing barriers to cultural competence. *Journal for Nurses in Staff Development, 21*(4), 135-142.

U.S. Census Bureau. (2002). *The population profile of the United States: 2000.* Accessed www.census.gov/population/www/pop-profile/profile2000.html, September 15, 2005.

U.S. Census Bureau. (2003). *U.S. Census Bureau guidance on the presentation and comparison of race and Hispanic origin data.* Accessed http://www.census.gov/population/www/socdemo/compraceho.html, September 15, 2005.

U.S. Department of Health and Human Services (USDHHS). (2000a). *Healthy people 2010: Understanding and improving health.* Washington, DC: Author, Government Printing Office.

U.S. Department of Health and Human Services (USDHHS). (2000b). *Healthy People 2010: Chapter 16: Maternal, infant, and child health.* Accessed www.health.gov/healthypeople/Document/HTML/ Volume2/16MICH.htm, September 15, 2005.

U.S. Department of Health and Human Services (USDHHS). Health Resources and Services Administration. (2003). *Minority Women Health Report.* Accessed www.hrsa.govv/womenshealth, September 5, 2005.

U.S. Department of Health and Human Services (USDHHS). (2005). Health Resources and Services Administration. *Women's Health USA 2005.* Accessed www.hrsa.gov/womenshealth, September 5, 2005.

U.S. Department of Health and Human Services (USDHHS). Centers for Disease Control and Prevention Office of Minority Health. *Disease burden and risk factors.* Accessed www.cdc.gov/omh/Populations/populations.htm, September 25, 2005.

U.S. Department of Labor, Office of the Assistant Secretary for Policy, Office of Programmatic Policy. (2005). *Findings from the National Agricultural Workers Survey (NAWS) 2001-2002. A demographic and employment profile of United States farm workers.* Washington, DC: Author, Office of the Assistant Secretary for Policy, Office of Programmatic Policy, Research Report No. 9. March 2005. Accessed www.doleta.gov/agworker/naws.cfm, March 24, 2006.

Weissman, J., Betancourt, J., Campbell, E., Park, E., Kim, M., Clarridge, B., et al. (2005). Resident physician's preparedness to provide cross-cultural care. *Journal of the American Medical Association, 294*(9), 1058-1067.

Weitoft, G., Hjern, A., Haglund, B., & Rosen, M. (2003). Mortality, severe morbidity, and injury in children living with single parents in Sweden: A population based study. *Lancet, 361*(9354), 289-295.

Wherry, L., & Finegold, K. (2004). *Marriage promotion and the living arrangements of black, Hispanic and white children.* The Urban Institute. Accessed www.urban.org/url.cfm?ID=311064, August 4, 2005.

Wright, L., & Leahey, M. (2005). *Nurse and families* (4th ed.). Philadelphia: F.A. Davis.

Zahner, S., & Corrado, S. (2004). Local health department partnerships with faith-based organizations. *Journal of Public Health Management and Practice, 10*(3), 259-265.

Genetics

Marcia Van Riper

learning objectives

- Explore how recent advances in genetics have changed the field of health care.
- List the five main genetics-related competencies that all nurses should be prepared to acquire and put into practice.
- Identify ongoing initiatives designed to improve the genetics expertise of nurses.
- Explore challenges and opportunities related to integrating genetics into nursing practice.
- Describe expanded roles for nurses in genetics and genetic counseling.
- Explore the possible benefits and risks of pharmacogenomics.
- Discuss the purpose and key findings of the Human Genome Project.

- Examine the ethical, legal, and social implications of the Human Genome Project.
- Discuss the current status of gene therapy (gene transfer).
- Explain the key concepts of basic human genetics.
- Discuss the different types of genetic testing.
- Identify genetic disorders commonly tested for in maternity and women's health nursing.
- Discuss the education and counseling needs of individuals and families who undergo genetic testing.
- Explore the availability of genetic testing to individuals and families from diverse backgrounds.
- Describe the role of genetics in cancer.
- Identify genetics resources for nurses and other health care professionals.

electronic resources

Additional information related to the content in Chapter 3 can be found on

the companion website at **evolve**
http://evolve.elsevier.com/Lowdermilk/MWHC/
- NCLEX Review Questions
- WebLinks

or on the interactive companion CD
- NCLEX Review Questions
- Critical Thinking Exercise: Genetic Counseling
- Plan of Care: The Family Living with Down Syndrome

ECENT advances in molecular biology and genomics have revolutionized the field of health care by providing the tools needed to determine the hereditary component of many diseases, as well as improve our ability to predict susceptibility to disease, onset and progression of disease, and response to medications (Guttmacher & Collins, 2005; Loescher & Merkle, 2005; Seo & Ginsburg, 2005). With this increase in genetic knowledge there has been a gradual shift from genetics to genomics (Khoury, 2003). According to Guttmacher and Collins (2002), genetics is the "study of single genes and their effects," whereas genomics is the "study not just of single genes, but the functions and interactions of all the genes in the genome." Khoury (2003) described the shift from genetics to genomics as a continuum ranging from the concept of disease in genetics to the concept of genetic information in genomics.

The demand for genetic services, especially genetic testing, has never been greater. In addition, the convergence of genetics, genomics, biotechnology, and informatics has dramatically changed how these services are accessed and delivered (Lea, 2000). With growing public interest in genetics and genomics, increasing commercial pressures, and web-based opportunities for individuals, families, and communities to participate in the direction and design of their genomic health care, genetic services are rapidly becoming an integral part of routine health care (Collins & Guttmacher, 2001; Collins & McKusick, 2001; Rubinstein & Roy, 2005).

Health care professionals in all settings and roles are caring for individuals and families who want, and deserve, high-quality genomic health care. Nowhere is this more apparent than in the area of maternity and women's health care. A growing number of health care professionals working in this area are offering and interpreting genetic tests to individuals and families. Although most of these tests are being used to determine a client's risk of having a child affected by a genetic condition such as Down syndrome or cystic fibrosis (CF), the number of tests being used to determine the presence of, or susceptibility to, adult-onset disorders (e.g., hereditary breast and ovarian cancer, Huntington's disease [HD], Alzheimer's disease) is increasing at a rapid rate. Health care professionals working in maternity and women's health care are caring for individuals and families who are dealing with complex ethical, legal, and social issues associated with genetic testing and the experience of living with someone who has a genetic condition (Hamilton, Bowers, & Williams, 2005; Jones & Fallon, 2002; Klipstein, 2005; Lewis, 2002; Van Riper, 2004; Van Riper, 2005).

■ NURSING AND GENETICS EXPERTISE

Historically, few nurses had formal education in genetics (Burke & Kirk, 2006; Lea, Feetham, & Monsen, 2002; Prows, Glass, Nicol, Shirton, & Williams, 2005). It was considered relatively unusual for a nurse to be caring for a client with a genetic condition. Nurses could choose whether they wanted to learn genetics and become involved in the delivery of genetics health care. Today, with genetics rapidly moving into the mainstream of health care, understanding genetics is not an option for nurses (Lea & Williams, 2001).

The pace and significance of recent genetics discoveries has made it virtually impossible for nurses not to be involved in some aspect of genomic health care. Because of their frontline position in the health care system and their long-standing history of providing holistic, family-centered care, nurses are likely to be the first health care professional to whom individuals and families turn with questions about genetic risk and susceptibility (Lea & Williams, 2001; Tinkle & Cheek, 2002), and to seek guidance regarding the complexities of genetic testing and interpretation.

Expanded or New Roles

Expanded or new roles for nurses with expertise in genetics and genomics are developing in many areas of maternity and women's health nursing. These areas include but are not limited to preconception counseling and preimplantation diagnosis for clients at risk for the transmission of a genetic disorder (Jones & Fallon, 2002; Klipstein, 2005); prenatal screening and testing (Gates, 2004; Grant, 2000; Jones, 2000; Lewis, 2002); prenatal care for women with psychiatric disorders that have a genetic component, such as bipolar disorder and schizophrenia (Carlson-Sabelli & Lessick, 2001; Lamberg, 2005); newborn screening and testing (Kenner & Moran, 2005; Lloyd-Puryear & Forsman, 2002); the care of families who have lost a fetus or a child affected by a genetic condition (Korenromp, 2005); the identification and care of children with genetic conditions and their families (Gallo, Angst, Knafl, Hadley, & Smith, 2005; Kenner, Gallo, & Bryant, 2005; Lessick & Anderson, 2000; Tinkle, 2002; Van Riper & Cohen, 2001), and the

care of women with genetic conditions who require specialized care during pregnancy, such as women with congenital heart disease (Khairy, Ouyang, Fernandes, Lee-Parritz, Economy, & Landzberg, 2006), cystic fibrosis (McMullen et al., 2006), Marfan syndrome (Rahman, 2003, www.marfan.org), and Factor V Leiden (Horne & McKloskey, 2006). Oncology nurses are beginning to integrate genomics into all phases of care for individuals and families affected by cancer (Loud, Peters, Fraser, & Jenkins, 2002).

Initiatives to Improve Expertise in Genetics and Genomics

A number of ongoing initiatives are designed to help nurses in all stages of their careers gain the knowledge, skills, and confidence they need to provide high-quality genomic health care in a wide variety of settings (Cragun, Couch, Prows, Warren, & Christianson, 2005; Diekelmann & Diekelmann, 2000; Lea et al., 2002). Many of these can be found on websites for the International Society for Nurses in Genetics (ISONG), the National Coalition for Health Professional Education in Genetics (NCHPEG), and the Genetics Education Program for Nurses (http://gepn.cchmc.org).

ISONG, a nursing specialty organization dedicated to fostering the scientific and professional growth of nurses in human genetics, was founded in 1981 and incorporated in 1988. Through annual education conferences, newsletter communication, and credentialing efforts, ISONG strives to ensure that practicing nurses around the world are adequately prepared to provide genetics health care. ISONG members have worked collaboratively with other professionals on interdisciplinary initiatives, such as NCHPEG, to promote genetics education.

NCHPEG, established in 1996, is a national effort to promote health professional education and access to information about advances in human genetics (www.nchpeg.org). Nursing, represented by ANA and 15 other nursing organizations, plays a key role in this initiative. Leaders from two nursing organizations (American Nurses Association and Sigma Theta Tau International) now serve on NCHPEG's board of directors.

NCHPEG members have developed a list of core competencies in genetics that all health professionals should possess (Engstrom, Sefton, Matheson, & Healy, 2005). Minimally, each health care professional should be able to appreciate limitations of his or her genetics expertise; understand the social and psychologic implications of genetics services; and know how and when to make referrals to genetics professionals.

Importance of Family History

Recently there has been a resurgence of interest in family history. Although it is easy to be impressed by the over 1000 genetic tests currently available, the single most cost-effective piece of genetic information continues to be the family history (Bennett, 2004). Rich and colleagues (2004) described the family history as the most important tool for diagnosis and risk assessment in health care genetics and a critical tool in the use of predictive testing in primary care. In 2004, the U.S. Department of Health and Human Services launched a Family History Initiative by designating Thanksgiving Day as the first annual National Family History Day. The U.S. Surgeon General encouraged families to use their family gatherings as a time to talk about and collect important family health history. A newly developed computerized tool called *My Family Health Portrait* was made available free of charge (www.hhs.gov/familyhistory/download.html). Additional family history tools were made available for the second annual National Family History Day in 2005. Nurses are ideally suited to take the lead in ongoing efforts to recognize the significance of the family history as an important source of genetic information.

Genetics-Related Nursing Activities

In 2005, a panel of over 50 nursing leaders from clinical, research, and academic settings developed and came to consensus on a document, *Essential Nursing Competencies and Curricula Guidelines for Genetics and Genomics*. The competencies in the document reflect the minimal amount of genetic and genomic competency expected of all nurses. The competencies are not intended to replace or recreate current standards of practice. The document is currently available for review and consideration at www.nursingworld. org/ethics/genetics. To date, it has been endorsed by 36 nursing organizations. Five examples of competencies included in the document are the following:

* Constructs pedigree from collected family history information using standardized symbols and terminology
* Develops plan of care that incorporates genetic and genomic assessment information
* Identifies credible, accurate, appropriate, and current genetic and genomic information, resources, services, and/or technologies specific to given clients
* Identifies ethical, ethnic/ancestral, cultural, religious, legal, fiscal, and societal issues related to genetic and genomic information and technologies
* Facilitates referrals for specialized genetic and genomic services for clients as needed.

Genetics-related activities that all nurses should be able to provide are further delineated in the *Statement on the Scope and Standards of Genetics Clinical Nursing Practice* (ISONG, 1998), which is in the process of being revised. This document includes standards and levels of practice for genetics nursing that were established cooperatively by ISONG and ANA. Efforts are under way to strengthen genetics knowledge and skills requirements for nursing licensure and certification examinations (Lea et al., 2002). ISONG has developed two credentials: one to recognize advanced practice nurses in genetics for their advanced knowledge, skills, and abilities, and another to recognize the special knowledge base and skills of genetics nurses who have a bachelor's degree. In addition, ISONG is working cooperatively with the American Nurses Credentialing Center to develop recognition of nurses in genetics.

▬ HUMAN GENOME PROJECT

The Human Genome Project was a publicly funded international effort coordinated by the NIH and the U.S. Department of Energy (www.doegenomes.org). Not only was the Human Genome Project responsible for a long list of amazing genetics discoveries, but it also stimulated and facilitated the work of thousands of scientists worldwide. Within 24 hours after a piece of deoxyribonucleic acid (DNA) had been sequenced by Human Genome Project scientists, the results were posted on a public database (www.ncbi.nlm.nih.gov/genome/guide/human/) and there are no restrictions on its use or redistribution. "The argument for doing this was simple: the sequence would only benefit the public fully if it could be understood, and that required making it immediately available so that all the creative minds of the planet would work on it" (Collins, 2001).

When the Human Genome Project was initiated in 1990, the ultimate goal of the project was to map the human genome (complete set of genetic instructions in the nucleus of each human cell) by 2005. Considering that the human genome consists of approximately 3 billion base pairs of DNA, many people considered this to be an impossible task. By February 1999, less than 15% of the human genome had been sequenced. Then a turning point occurred: a decision was made to aim for working draft coverage of the human genome, rather than complete coverage, by the spring of 2000 (Collins, 2001). This decision was based on findings from an earlier study in which draft sequences of DNA were compared with finished sequences of DNA, and they were found to be very useful.

On June 26, 2000, an announcement was made at the White House that a working draft of the Human Genome Project had been completed by two groups: scientists working on the Human Genome Project and scientists from Celera Genomics, a privately funded effort. Simultaneous publications describing the initial draft sequence and analysis of the human genome appeared in *Nature* (International Human Genome Sequencing Consortium, 2001) and *Science* (Venter et al., 2001) on February 12, 2001. A substantially complete version of the human genome was announced in April, 2003 (www.genome.gov/11006929).

Current Outcomes

Two key findings from initial efforts to sequence and analyze the human genome are that (1) all human beings are 99.9% identical at the DNA level, and (2) approximately 20,000 to 25,000 genes (pieces or sequences of DNA that contain information needed to make proteins) make up the human genome (International Human Genome Sequencing Consortium, 2001). The finding that human beings are 99.9% identical at the DNA level should help to discourage the use of science as a justification for drawing biologically precise racial boundaries around certain groups of people (Collins & Mansoura, 2001). Originally, scientists had estimated that there were 80,000 to 150,000 genes in the human genome. It had been assumed that the main reason that humans are more evolved and more highly sophisticated than other species is that they have more genes. A new explanation for human complexity, given the relatively small number of genes, is that humans are more efficient with their genes. Humans are able to do much more with their genes than are other species. Instead of producing only one protein per gene, most human genes produce at least three proteins.

Gene Identification and Testing

Initial efforts to sequence and analyze the human genome have proven invaluable in the identification of genes involved in disease and in the development of genetic tests. Hundreds of genes involved in diseases such as HD, breast cancer, colon cancer, Alzheimer's disease, achondroplasia, and CF have been identified. The number of commercially available genetic tests continues to increase and can be found at GeneTests (www.genetests.org).

Genetic testing involves the analysis of human DNA, ribonucleic acid (RNA), chromosomes (threadlike packages of genes and other DNA in the nucleus of a cell), or proteins to detect abnormalities related to an inherited condition. Genetic tests can be used to examine directly the DNA and RNA that make up a gene (direct or molecular testing), look at markers that are coinherited with a gene that causes a genetic condition (linkage analysis), examine the protein products of genes (biochemical testing), or examine chromosomes (cytogenetic testing). Cytogenetic analysis of malignant tissue has become a mainstay of oncology.

Most of the genetic tests now offered in clinical practice are tests for single-gene disorders in clients with clinical symptoms or who have a family history of a genetic disease (Yoon et al., 2001; [http://iml.dartmouth.edu/education/cme/Genetics; http://webct.isu.edu/public/GENETICS]). Some of these genetic tests are prenatal tests or tests used to identify the genetic status of a pregnancy at risk for a genetic condition. Current prenatal testing options include maternal serum screening (a blood test used to see if a pregnant woman is at increased risk for carrying a fetus with a neural tube defect or a chromosomal abnormality such as Down syndrome) and invasive procedures (amniocentesis and chorionic villus sampling). Other tests are carrier screening tests, which are used to identify individuals who have a gene mutation for a genetic condition but do not show symptoms of the condition, because it is a condition that is inherited in an autosomal recessive form (e.g., CF, sickle cell disease, and Tay-Sachs disease). Another type of genetic testing is predictive testing, which is used to clarify the genetic status of asymptomatic family members. The two types of predictive testing are presymptomatic and predispositional. Mutation analysis for Huntington's disease, a neurodegenerative disorder, is an example of presymptomatic testing. If the gene mutation for HD is present, symptoms of HD are certain to appear if the individual lives long enough. Testing for a BRCA1 gene mutation to determine breast cancer susceptibility is an example of predispositional testing. Predispositional testing differs from presymptomatic testing in that a positive result (indicating that a BRCA1 mutation is present) does not indicate a 100% risk of developing the condition (breast cancer).

In addition to using genetic tests to test for single-gene disorders, genetic tests are being used for population-based screening, for example state-mandated newborn screening for phenylketonuria (PKU) and other inborn errors of metabolism (IEMs), and to test for common complex diseases such as cancer and cardiovascular conditions. Genetic tests also are being used to determine paternity, identify victims of war and other tragedies, and profile criminals (www.genetests.org).

Pharmacogenomics

One of the most immediate clinical applications of the Human Genome Project may be pharmacogenomics, or the use of genetic information to individualize drug therapy (Phillips, Veenstra, Oren, Lee, & Sadee, 2001). There has been speculation that pharmacogenomics may become part of standard practice for a large number of disorders and drugs by 2020 (Collins & McKusick, 2001). The expectation is that by identifying common variants in genes that are associated with the likelihood of a good or bad response to a specific drug, drug prescriptions can be individualized, based on the individual's unique genetic make-up (Prows & Prows, 2004; Roses, 2000). A primary benefit of pharmacogenomics is the potential to reduce adverse drug reactions. Considering that adverse drug reactions result in significant morbidity, mortality, and excess medical costs, pharmacogenomics could prove to be very important.

Gene Therapy (Gene Transfer)

In the early 1990s, a great deal of optimism was felt about the possibility of using genetic information to provide quick solutions to a long list of health problems (Collins & McKusick, 2001). Although the early optimism about gene therapy was probably never fully justified, it is likely that the development of safer and more effective methods for gene delivery will ensure a significant role for gene therapy in the treatment of some diseases (Collins & McKusick, 2001). Major challenges include targeting the right gene to the right location in the right cells, expressing the transferred gene at the right time, and minimizing adverse reactions (Brower, 2001). There have been reports of exciting possibilities regarding the application of gene therapy for hemophilia B (Kay et al., 2000) and severe combined immunodeficiency (Anderson, 2000; Cavazzana-Calvo et al., 2000). However, gene therapy for individuals with severe combined immunodeficiency was suspended in 2003 because four of the clients had developed leukemia as a result of where the gene was inserted (Marwick, 2003). "Gene therapy will succeed with time. And it is important that it does, because no other area of medicine holds as much promise for providing cures for the many devastating diseases that ravage humankind" (Anderson, 2000).

Ethical, Legal, and Social Implications

Before the beginning of the Human Genome Project, widespread concern about misuse of the information gained through genetics research resulted in 5% of the Human Genome Project budget being designated for the study of the ethical, legal, and social implications (ELSIs) of human genome research. Two large ELSI programs were created to identify, analyze, and address the ELSIs of human genome research at the same time that the basic science issues were being studied. The two ELSI programs are separate but complementary. During the past decade, issues of high priority for these programs have been privacy and fairness in the use and interpretation of genetic information; clinical integration of new genetics technologies; issues surrounding genetics research, such as possible discrimination and stigmatization; and education for professionals and the general public about genetics, genetics health care, and ELSI of human genome research. Both ELSI programs have excellent websites that include vast amounts of educational information, as well as links to other informative sites (www.genome.gov/10001618; www.ornl.gov/sci/techresources/Human_Genome/elsi/elsi.shtml).

The major risk associated with genetic testing concerns what happens with the information gained: it may result in increased anxiety and altered family relationships; it may be difficult to keep confidential, especially if the test results are shared with the individual; and it may result in discrimination and stigmatization; and about which little, if anything, can be done (Thomson, 1997). Thomson noted that informed consent is very difficult to ensure when some of the outcomes, benefits, and risks of genetic testing remain unknown. In addition, many of the tests being used are as yet imperfect. That is, few have a 100% detection rate. Individuals and families who receive false-positive results (the test results indicate that a person or fetus is affected by a genetic condition when they are not) may terminate an unaffected pregnancy or undergo unwarranted extreme measures such as bilateral prophylactic mastectomy. Individuals and families who receive false-negative results (the test results indicate that a person or fetus is not affected by genetic condition when they are) may fail to follow surveillance strategies designed to improve their health outcomes because they have been falsely reassured that they are not at increased risk for a specific condition (Critical Thinking Exercise).

Factors Influencing the Decision to Undergo Genetic Testing

The decision to undergo genetic testing is seldom an autonomous decision based solely on the needs and preferences of the individual being tested. Instead, it is often a decision based on feelings of responsibility and commitment to others (Burgess & d'Agincourt-Canning, 2002; Van Riper, 2005; Van Riper & McKinnon, 2004). For example, a woman who is receiving treatment for breast cancer may undergo BRCA1/BRCA2 mutation testing not because she wants to find out if she carries a BRCA1 or

---

CRITICAL THINKING EXERCISE

Counseling About Genetic Risk

Sylvia confides in you that several infants have been born into her family with serious anomalies. From previous conversations, you know that she is opposed to abortion and would never consider having one. Sylvia is currently 6 weeks pregnant, and her physician has urged her to have chorionic villus sampling (CVS). Sylvia asks you for information about CVS and the implications of a finding that her fetus has serious anomalies.

1. Evidence—Is there sufficient evidence to provide Sylvia with answers to her questions about CVS?
2. Assumptions—What assumptions can be made about CVS and what can be discovered using this technology?
   a. The risks of this technology
   b. The benefits of this technology
   c. The fit between Sylvia's beliefs and the implications of a positive diagnosis
   d. Sylvia's acceptance of the birth of a child with an anomaly
3. What implications and priorities for nursing can be made at this time?
4. Does the evidence objectively support your conclusion?
5. Are there alternative perspectives to your conclusion?

BRCA2 mutation, but because her two unaffected sisters have asked her to be tested, and she feels a sense of responsibility and commitment to them. A female airline pilot with a family history of HD, who has no desire to find out if she has the gene mutation associated with HD, may undergo mutation analysis for HD because she feels she has an obligation to her family, her employer, and the people who fly with her.

Decisions about genetic testing are shaped, and in many instances constrained, by factors such as social norms, where care is received, and socioeconomic status. Most pregnant women in the United States now have at least one ultrasound examination, many undergo some type of multiple-marker screening, and a growing number undergo other types of prenatal testing (Grant, 2000). The range of prenatal testing options available to a pregnant woman and her family may vary significantly, based on where the pregnant woman receives prenatal care and her socioeconomic status. Certain types of prenatal testing may not be available in smaller communities and rural settings (e.g., chorionic villus sampling and FISH analysis [fluorescent in situ hybridization]). In addition, certain types of genetic testing may not be offered in conservative medical communities (e.g., preimplantation diagnosis). Some types of genetic testing are expensive and typically not covered by health insurance. Because of this, these tests may be available only to a relatively small number of individuals and families: those who can afford to pay for them.

Cultural and ethnic differences also have a significant impact on decisions about genetic testing. When prenatal diagnosis was first introduced, the principal constituency was a self-selected group of Caucasian, well-informed, middle- to upper-class women. Today the widespread use of genetic testing has introduced prenatal testing to new groups of women, women who had not previously considered genetics services. The fact that many of the women currently undergoing prenatal testing may not share mainstream U.S. views about the role of medicine and prenatal care, the meaning of disability, or how to respond to scientific risks and uncertainties further amplifies the complexity of ethical issues associated with prenatal testing.

The genetic testing experience raises fundamental questions about the mutual obligations of kin (Burgess & d'Agincourt-Canning, 2002). Are individuals morally obligated to alert extended family members about inherited health risks? Conversely, do extended family members have a moral obligation to participate in research designed to determine genetic risk when unwanted information about them may be generated in the process? In a case presentation involving familial conflict over genetic testing for breast cancer, Green and Thomas (1997) raised another important question that must be considered: "Whose gene is it?" This question is likely to stimulate a great deal of debate, especially in the area of preimplantation genetic testing.

■ CLINICAL GENETICS

Genetic Transmission

Human development is a complicated process that depends on the systematic unraveling of instructions found in the genetic material of the egg and the sperm. Development from conception to birth of a normal, healthy baby occurs without incident in most cases; occasionally, however, some anomaly in the genetic code of the embryo creates a birth defect or disorder. The science of genetics seeks to explain the underlying causes of congenital disorders (disorders present at birth) and the patterns in which inherited disorders are passed from generation to generation.

Genes and Chromosomes

The hereditary material carried in the nucleus of each of the somatic (body) cells determines an individual's physical characteristics. This material, called DNA, forms threadlike strands known as chromosomes. Each chromosome is composed of the many smaller segments of DNA referred to as genes. Genes, or combinations of genes, contain coded information that determines an individual's unique characteristics. The "code" is found in the specific linear order of the molecules that combine to form the strands of DNA. Genes control both the types of proteins that are made and the rate at which they are produced. Genes never act in isolation; they always interact with other genes and the environment.

All normal human somatic cells contain 46 chromosomes arranged as 23 pairs of homologous (matched) chromosomes; one chromosome of each pair is inherited from each parent. There are 22 pairs of autosomes that control most traits in the body, and one pair of sex chromosomes.

Whereas the Y chromosome is primarily concerned with sex determination, the X chromosome contains genes that are involved in much more than sex determination. The larger female chromosome is called the X; the smaller male chromosome is the Y. Generally the presence of a Y chromosome causes an embryo to develop as a male; in the absence of a Y chromosome, the individual develops as a female. Thus in a normal female, the homologous pair of sex chromosomes are XX, and in a normal male, the homologous pair are XY.

Homologous chromosomes (except the X and Y chromosomes in males) have the same number and arrangement of genes. In other words, if one chromosome has a gene for hair color, its partner chromosome also will have a gene for hair color, and these hair-color genes will have the same loci or be located in the same place on the two chromosomes. Although both genes code for hair color, they may not code for the *same* hair color. Genes at corresponding loci on homologous chromosomes that code for different forms or variations of the same trait are called alleles. An individual having two copies of the same allele for a given trait is said to be homozygous for that trait; with two different alleles, the person is heterozygous for the trait.

The term genotype typically is used to refer to the genetic makeup of an individual when discussing a specific gene pair, but at times, genotype is used to refer to an individual's entire genetic makeup or all the genes that the individual can pass on to future generations. Phenotype refers to the observable expression of an individual's genotype, such as physical features, a biochemical or molecular trait, and even a psychologic trait. A trait or disorder is considered dominant if it is expressed or phenotypically apparent when only one copy of an allele associated with the trait is present. It is considered recessive if it is expressed only when two copies of the alleles associated with the trait are present.

As more is learned about genetics, the concepts of dominance and recessivity have become more complex, especially in X-linked disorders (Lashley, 2005). For example, traits considered to be recessive may be expressed even when only one copy of a gene located on the X chromosome is present. This occurs frequently in males because males have only one X chromosome; thus they have only one copy of the genes located on the X chromosome. Whichever gene is present on the one X chromosome determines which trait is expressed. Females, conversely, have two X chromosomes, so they have two copies of the genes located on the X chromosome. However, in any female somatic cell, only one X chromosome is functioning (otherwise, there would be inequality in gene dosage between males and females). This process, known as X-inactivation or the Lyon hypothesis, is generally a random occurrence. That is, there is a 50:50 chance as to whether the maternal X or the paternal X is inactivated. Occasionally the percentage of cells that have the X with an abnormal or mutant gene is very high. This helps explain why hemophilia, an X-linked recessive disorder, can clinically manifest itself in a female known to be a heterozygous carrier (a female who has only one copy of the gene mutation). It also helps explain why traditional methods of carrier detection are less effective for X-linked recessive disorders; the possible range for enzyme activity values can vary greatly, depending on which X chromosome is inactivated.

Chromosomal Abnormalities

Chromosomal abnormalities are a major cause of reproductive loss, congenital problems, and gynecologic disorders (Simpson & Elias, 2003), accounting for approximately 4% to 7% of perinatal deaths and 0.5% to 1% of infants born with multiple anomalies (Jones, 2006). Errors resulting in chromosomal abnormalities can occur during mitosis (cell division occurring in somatic cells that results in two identical daughter cells containing a diploid number of chromosomes) or meiosis (division of a sex cell into two and four haploid cells). These errors can occur in either the autosomes or the sex chromosomes. Even without the presence of obvious structural malformations, small deviations in chromosomes can cause problems in fetal development.

The pictorial analysis of the number, form, and size of an individual's chromosomes is known as a karyotype. Cells from any nucleated, replicating body tissue (not red blood cells, nerves, or muscles) can be used (Scheuerle, 2001). The most commonly used tissues are white blood cells and fetal cells in amniotic fluid. The cells are grown in a culture and arrested when they are in metaphase (during metaphase, the chromosomes are condensed and visible with a light microscope), and then the cells are dropped onto a slide. This breaks the cell membranes and spreads the chromosomes, making them easier to visualize. Next the cells are stained with special stains (e.g., Giemsa stain) that create striping or "banding" patterns. These patterns

aid in the analysis because they are consistent from person to person. Once the chromosome spreads are photographed or scanned by a computer, they are cut out and arranged in a specific numeric order according to their length and shape. The chromosomes are numbered from largest to smallest, 1 to 22, and the sex chromosomes are designated by the letter X or Y. Each chromosome is divided into two "arms" designated by p (short arm) and q (long arm). A female karyotype is designated as 46, XX and a male karyotype is designated as 46, XY. Figure 3-1 illustrates the chromosomes in a body cell.

Autosomal Abnormalities

Autosomal abnormalities involve differences in the number or structure of autosome chromosomes (pairs 1–22). They result from unequal distribution of genetic material during gamete (egg and sperm) formation.

Abnormalities of Chromosome Number. Euploidy is the term used to denote the correct number of chromosomes. Deviations from the correct number of chromosomes or the diploid number (2N, 46 chromosomes) can be one of two types: (1) polyploidy, in which the deviation is an exact multiple of the haploid number of chromosomes or one chromosome set (23 chromosomes); or (2) aneuploidy, in which the numerical deviation is not an exact multiple of the haploid set (Lashley, 2005). A triploid (3N) cell is an example of a polyploidy. It has 69 chromosomes. A tetraploid (4N) cell, also an example of a polyploidy, has 92 chromosomes.

Aneuploidy is the most commonly identified chromosome abnormality in humans. Aneuploidy occurs in at least 5% of all clinically recognized pregnancies, and it is the leading known cause of pregnancy loss (Hassold & Hunt, 2001). Aneuploidy also is the leading genetic cause of mental retardation. A monosomy is the product of the union between a normal gamete and a gamete

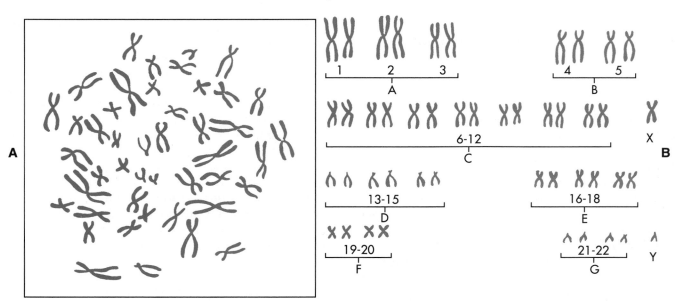

FIG. 3-1 Chromosomes during cell division. **A,** Example of photomicrograph. **B,** Chromosomes arranged in karyotype; female and male sex-determining chromosomes.

that is missing a chromosome. Monosomic individuals only have 45 chromosomes in each of their cells. The product of the union of a normal gamete with a gamete containing an extra chromosome is a trisomy. The most common autosomal aneuploid conditions involve trisomies. Trisomic individuals have 47 chromosomes in each of their cells.

During the past decade, DNA polymorphisms have been used to determine the origin of different aneuploid conditions (Hassold & Hunt, 2001). Limited data are available concerning the origin of monosomies because when an embryo is missing an autosomal chromosome, the embryo never survives. Although a great deal of variation exists among trisomies with regard to the parent and stage of origin of the extra chromosome, most trisomies are maternal meiosis I (MI) errors. This means that most trisomies are caused by nondisjunction during the first meiotic division. The first meiotic division involves the segregation of homologous or similar chromosomes. One pair of chromosomes fails to separate. One resulting cell contains both chromosomes, and the other contains none. The fact that most trisomies are maternal MI errors is not that surprising, because maternal MI occurs over a long time span. It is initiated in precursor cells during fetal development, but it is not completed until the time those cells undergo ovulation after menarche.

The most common trisomal abnormality is Down syndrome, or trisomy 21 (47, XX +21, female with Down syndrome; or 47, XY +21, male with Down syndrome). The incidence of Down syndrome is approximately one in approximately every 733 live births (National Down Syndrome Society, 2006). Ninety-five percent of individuals with Down syndrome have trisomy 21 or an extra chromosome 21. Individuals with Down syndrome have various degrees of mental retardation, but most fall within the mild to moderate range. Common characteristics seen in individuals with Down syndrome are as follows:

- Oblique palpebral fissures or an upward slant to the eyes
- Epicanthal folds or small skin folds on the inner corners of the eyes
- Small, white, crescent-shaped spots on the irises called Brushfield spots
- A flat facial profile that usually includes a somewhat depressed nasal bridge and a small nose
- Enlargement of the tongue in relationship to size of the mouth
- Small, low-set ears, which may be abnormally shaped
- Short, broad hands with a fifth finger that has one flexion crease instead of two
- A single deep crease across the center of the palm, often referred to as a simian crease
- Excessive space between large and second toe
- Hyperflexibility, an excessive ability to extend the joints
- Muscle hypotonia or low muscle tone

Some individuals with Down syndrome have all of these characteristics, but others have only a few. Figure 3-2

FIG. 3-2 Infant with Down syndrome. Note upward slant to eyes, flat nasal bridge, slightly protruding tongue, and mottled skin. (Courtesy Thomas and Christie Coghill, Clayton, NC.)

is a picture of an infant with Down syndrome who has some of the characteristics commonly associated with that syndrome (see Plan of Care).

Congenital abnormalities and diseases found in individuals with Down syndrome are the same as those that occur in the general population, but individuals with Down syndrome are affected more often and more severely by specific abnormalities and diseases than are normally developing individuals (Van Riper & Cohen, 2001). For example, congenital heart disease occurs in 40% to 60% of individuals with Down syndrome, but only 8 of every 1000 individuals in the general population have congenital heart disease (Freeman et al., 1998). Children with Down syndrome are 10 to 30 times more likely to acquire leukemia than are normally developing children. Individuals with Down syndrome have increased susceptibility to infections and a higher mortality rate from infectious disease than do individuals who do not have Down syndrome. Detailed guidelines have been developed for the care of individuals with Down syndrome (www.ds-health.com/ds_sites.htm; www.ndsccenter.org; www.ndss.org).

Although the risk of having a child with Down syndrome increases with maternal age (incidence is approximately 1 in 1350 for a 25-year-old woman; 1 in 400 for a 35-year-old woman; and 1 in 30 for a 45-year-old woman), children with Down syndrome can be born to mothers of any age. Eighty percent of children with Down syndrome are born to mothers younger than 35 years (National Down Syndrome Society, 2006). The average age of mothers when they give birth to children with Down syndrome is about 27 years. The risk of a mother having a second child with Down syndrome is about 1% when the cause of the Down syndrome is trisomy 21.

During the past 30 years, fundamental changes have occurred in the care of individuals with Down syndrome (Van Riper & Cohen, 2001). These changes, which underscore the importance of the family and emphasize the need for health promotion and health protection activities, have

CD Plan of Care: The Family Living with Down Syndrome

plan of care ▶ **The Family Living with Down Syndrome**

NURSING DIAGNOSIS Interrupted family processes related to birth of a neonate with Down syndrome

Expected Outcome *The couple will verbalize accurate information about Down syndrome, including implications for future pregnancies.*

Nursing Interventions/Rationales
- Assess knowledge base of couple regarding the clinical signs and symptoms of Down syndrome *to correct any misconceptions and establish basis for teaching plan.*
- Provide information throughout the genetic evaluation regarding risk status and clinical signs and symptoms of Down syndrome *to give couple a realistic picture of neonate's defects and assist with decision making for future pregnancies.*
- Use therapeutic communication during discussions with the couple *to provide opportunity for expression of concern.*
- Refer to support groups, social services, or counseling *to assist family with cohesive actions and decision making.*
- Refer to child development specialist *to provide family with realistic expectations regarding cognitive and behavioral differences of child with Down syndrome.*

NURSING DIAGNOSIS Situational low self-esteem related to diagnosis of Down syndrome as evidenced by parents' statements of guilt and shame

Expected Outcome *The parents will express an increased number of positive statements regarding the birth of a neonate with Down syndrome.*

Nursing Interventions/Rationales
- Assist parents to list strengths and coping strategies that have been helpful in past situations *to use appropriate strategies during this situational crisis.*
- Encourage expression of feelings using therapeutic communication *to provide clarification and emotional support.*
- Clarify and provide information regarding Down syndrome *to decrease feelings of guilt and gradually increase feelings of positive self-esteem.*
- Refer for further counseling as needed *to provide more in-depth and ongoing support.*

NURSING DIAGNOSIS Risk for impaired parenting related to birth of neonate with Down syndrome

Expected Outcomes *Parents will bond with and provide appropriate care for the infant*

Nursing Interventions/Rationales
- Assist parents to see and describe normal aspects of infant *to promote bonding.*

- Encourage and assist with breastfeeding if that is parents' choice of feeding method *to facilitate closeness with infant and provide benefits of breast milk.*
- Assure parents that information regarding the neonate will remain confidential *to assist the parents to maintain some situational control and allow for time to work through their feelings.*
- Discuss and role play with parents ways of informing family and friends of infant's diagnosis and prognosis *to promote positive aspects of infant and decrease potential isolation from social interactions.*
- Provide anticipatory guidance about what to expect as infant develops *to assist family to be prepared for behavior problems or mental deficits.*

NURSING DIAGNOSIS Spiritual distress related to situational crisis of child born with Down syndrome

Expected Outcome *Parents will seek appropriate support persons (family members, priest, minister, rabbi) for assistance.*

Nursing Interventions/Rationales
- Listen for cues indicative of parents' feelings ("Why did God do this to us?") *to identify messages indicating spiritual distress.*
- Acknowledge parents' spiritual concerns and encourage expression of feelings *to help build a therapeutic relationship.*
- Facilitate visits from clergy and provide privacy during visits *to demonstrate respect for parents' relationship with clergy.*
- Encourage parents to discuss concerns with clergy *to use expert spiritual care resources to help the parents.*
- Facilitate interaction with family members and other support persons *to encourage expressions of concern and seek comfort.*

NURSING DIAGNOSIS Social isolation related to full-time caretaking responsibilities for a neonate with Down syndrome

Expected Outcome *Parents will describe a plan to utilize resources to prevent social isolation.*

Nursing Interventions/Rationales
- Provide opportunity for parents to express feelings about caring for a neonate with Down syndrome *to facilitate effective communication and trust.*
- Discuss with parents their expectations about caring for the neonate *to identify potential areas of concern.*
- Assist parents to identify potential caregiving resources *to permit parents to return to a routine at home.*
- Identify appropriate referrals for home care *to provide continuity of care.*

---

resulted in individuals with Down syndrome living longer and enjoying an improved quality of life. The median age at the time of death has increased from 25 years in 1987 to 49 years in 1997 (Yang, Rasmussen, & Friedman, 2002). Some individuals with Down syndrome are living beyond the age of 70 years. For decades, it was assumed that the experience of living in a family that includes a child with Down syndrome was a negative experience. Findings from three large programs of research concerning families of

children with Down syndrome do not provide support for this notion (Van Riper, 1999). Many families living with a child with Down syndrome have described the experience as positive and growth producing (see also Chapter 37).

Other identified autosomal trisomies are trisomy 18 and trisomy 13. Trisomy 18 (Edward syndrome) is more common than trisomy 13 (Patau syndrome). Infants with trisomy 18 may exhibit more than 130 different anomalies, but some of the major phenotypic features and medical complications are small-for-gestational-age or low-birth-weight infants; small mouth; feeding difficulties; weak cry; central nervous system manifestations including hypertonia, seizures, and apnea; craniofacial abnormalities; cardiac malformations; unusual or absent fingerprints; and extremity malformations such as clenched hands with overlapping fingers and rocker-bottom feet (Lewis, 2001).

As with trisomy 18, infants with trisomy 13 have numerous abnormalities, the most common of which are central nervous system anomalies, holoprosencephaly (one large eyelike structure in the center of the face due to fusion of the developing eyes), craniofacial malformations such as microcephaly (small head), capillary hemangiomas, cardiac defects, extremity deformities including polydactyly (extra fingers or toes), renal abnormalities, and genital abnormalities.

Infants with trisomy 18 and trisomy 13 are usually severely to profoundly retarded. Although both conditions have a very poor prognosis, with the vast majority of affected infants dying within the first few days of life, a significant percentage of these infants will survive the first 6 months to 1 year of life; some children with trisomy 18 and trisomy 13 have lived beyond age 10 years.

Nondisjunction also can occur during mitosis. If this occurs early in development when cell lines are forming, the individual has a mixture of cells, some with a normal number of chromosomes and others either missing a chromosome or containing an extra chromosome. This condition is known as mosaicism. Mosaicism in autosomes is most commonly seen as another form of Down syndrome. Approximately 1% to 2% of individuals with Down syndrome have mosaic Down syndrome.

Depending on when the nondisjunction occurs during development, different body tissues will have different numbers of chromosomes. The clinical characteristics of Down syndrome may be mild or with varying degrees of severity, depending on the number and location of the abnormal cells. An individual with mosaic Down syndrome may have normal intelligence. Mosaicism of both trisomy 18 and trisomy 13 has been reported. Both situations usually lead to a partial clinical expression of the phenotype. Infants who have mosaic trisomy 18 or trisomy 13 usually have a longer life span than infants with these disorders who are not mosaic.

Abnormalities of Chromosome Structure. Structural abnormalities can occur in any chromosome (Simpson & Elias, 2003). Types of structural abnormalities include translocation, duplication, deletion, microdeletion, and inversion. Translocation results when there is an exchange of chromosomal material between two chromosomes. Exposure to certain drugs, viruses, and radiation can cause translocations, but often they arise for no apparent reason (Lewis, 2001). The two major types of translocation are reciprocal and robertsonian. Reciprocal translocations are the most common. In a *reciprocal translocation,* either the parts of the two chromosomes are exchanged equally (balanced translocation) or a part of a chromosome is transferred to a

different chromosome, creating an unbalanced translocation because there is extra chromosomal material—extra of one chromosome but correct amount or deficient amount of other chromosome. In a balanced translocation, the individual is phenotypically normal because there is no extra chromosome material; it is just rearranged. In an unbalanced translocation, the individual will be both genotypically and phenotypically abnormal.

In a *robertsonian translocation,* the short arms (p arms) of two different acrocentric chromosomes (chromosomes with very short p arms) break, leaving sticky ends that then cause the two long arms (q arms) to stick together. This forms a new, large chromosome that is made of the two long arms. The individual with a balanced robertsonian translocation will have 45 chromosomes. Because the short arm of acrocentric chromosomes contains genes for ribosomal RNA and these genes are represented elsewhere, the individual usually does not show any symptoms. The individual may produce an unbalanced gamete (sperm or egg with too many or two few genes). This can lead to reproductive difficulties such as miscarriages or birth defects. Of all cases of Down syndrome, 3% to 4% occur because one parent has a balanced robertsonian translocation, a translocation between chromosomes 21 and 14. The child with this type of Down syndrome has an unbalanced translocation because there is an extra part of chromosome 21. The second most common robertsonian translocation occurs between chromosomes 13 and 14.

Deletions result in the loss of chromosomal material and partial monosomy for the chromosome involved (Simpson & Elias, 2003). Loss of chromosomal material at the end of a chromosome is referred to as a terminal deletion. In contrast, loss of chromosomal material anywhere else in the chromosome is called an interstitial deletion. The resulting clinical phenotype of either a terminal or an interstitial deletion will depend on how much of the chromosome has been lost and the number and function of the genes contained in the missing segment. Microdeletions are deletions too small to be detected by standard cytogenetic techniques. These deletions can be identified with FISH analysis. FISH technology uses a single-stranded piece of DNA with a florescent label that will adhere to its complementary piece of DNA in the chromosome being investigated.

Whenever a portion of a chromosome is deleted from one chromosome and added to another, the gamete produced may have either extra copies of genes or too few copies. The clinical effects produced may be mild or severe, depending on the amount of genetic material involved. Two of the more common conditions are the deletion of the short arm of chromosome 5 (*cri du chat* syndrome) and the deletion of the long arm of chromosome 18. *Cri du chat* syndrome, so named after the typical mewing cry of the affected infant, causes severe mental retardation with microcephaly and unusual facial appearance. Deletion of the long arm of chromosome 18 causes severe psychomotor retardation with multiple organ malformations. *Velocardiofacial syndrome,* characterized by cardiac and craniofacial abnormalities, is an example of a microdeletion. In this syndrome, a very small piece of the long arm of chromosome 22 is missing. Microdeletions in the Y chromosome have been found in men with infertility problems.

Inversions are deviations in which a portion of the chromosome has been rearranged in reverse order. Few birth defects have been attributed to the presence of inversions, but it is suspected that inversions may be responsible for problems with infertility and miscarriages. Some inversions can be detected prenatally. Inversions do not appear to occur randomly; more than 40% of all inversions involve chromosome 9 (Lashley, 2005).

Sex Chromosome Abnormalities

Several sex chromosome abnormalities are caused by nondisjunction during gametogenesis in either parent. The most common deviation in females is *Turner syndrome* or monosomy X (45, X). The affected female is missing an X chromosome. She usually exhibits juvenile external genitalia with undeveloped ovaries. She is short and often has webbing of the neck and lymphedema of her hands and feet. Intelligence may be impaired. Most affected embryos miscarry spontaneously. DNA polymorphism studies suggest that in most cases of Turner syndrome, it is the paternal X or Y that is lost (Hassold & Hunt, 2001)

The most common deviation in males is *Klinefelter syndrome,* or trisomy XXY. The affected male has an extra X chromosome and exhibits poorly developed secondary sexual characteristics and small testes. He is infertile, usually tall, effeminate, and may be slow to learn. Males who have mosaic Klinefelter syndrome may be fertile.

Patterns of Genetic Transmission

Heritable characteristics are those that can be passed on to offspring. The patterns by which genetic material is transmitted to the next generation are affected by the number of genes involved in the expression of the trait. Many phenotypic characteristics result from two or more genes on different chromosomes acting together (referred to as multifactorial inheritance); others are controlled by a single gene (referred to as unifactorial inheritance). Specialists in genetics (e.g., geneticists, genetic counselors, and nurses

with advanced expertise in genetics) predict the probability of the presence of an abnormal gene from the known occurrence of the trait in the individual's family and the known patterns by which the trait is inherited.

Multifactorial Inheritance

Most common congenital malformations result from multifactorial inheritance, a combination of genetic and environmental factors. Examples are cleft lip, cleft palate, congenital heart disease, neural tube defects, and pyloric stenosis. Each malformation may range from mild to severe, depending on the number of genes for the defect present or the amount of environmental influence. A neural tube defect may range from spina bifida, a bony defect in the lumbar region of the vertebrae with little or no neurologic impairment, to anencephaly, absence of brain development, which is always fatal. Some malformations occur more often in one sex. For example, pyloric stenosis and cleft lip are more common in males, and cleft palate is more common in females.

Unifactorial Inheritance

If a single gene controls a particular trait or disorder, its pattern of inheritance is referred to as *unifactorial mendelian,* or single-gene inheritance. The number of single-gene disorders far exceeds the number of chromosomal abnormalities. Potential patterns of inheritance for single-gene disorders include autosomal dominant, autosomal recessive, and X-linked dominant and recessive modes of inheritance.

Autosomal Dominant Inheritance. Autosomal dominant inheritance disorders are those in which only one copy of a variant allele is needed for phenotypic expression. The variant allele may be a result of a mutation, a spontaneous and permanent change in the normal gene structure, in which case the disorder occurs for the first time in the family. Usually an affected individual comes from multiple generations having the disorder. An affected parent who is heterozygous for the trait has a 50% chance of passing the variant allele to each offspring (Fig. 3-3, *B* and *C*). There is a vertical pattern of inheritance (there is no skipping of generations; if an individual has an autosomal dominant disorder such as HD, so must one of his or her parents). Males and females are equally affected.

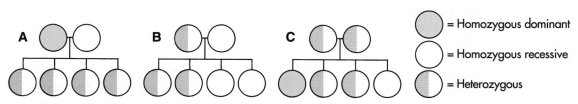

FIG. 3-3 Possible offspring in three types of matings. **A,** Homozygous-dominant parent and homozygous-recessive parent. Children all heterozygous, displaying dominant trait. **B,** Heterozygous parent and homozygous-recessive parent. Children 50% heterozygous, displaying dominant trait; 50% homozygous, displaying recessive trait. **C,** Both parents heterozygous. Children 25% homozygous, displaying dominant trait; 25% homozygous, displaying recessive trait; 50% heterozygous, displaying dominant trait.

Autosomal dominant disorders are not always expressed with the same severity of symptoms. For example, a woman who has an autosomal dominant disorder may show few symptoms and may not become aware of her diagnosis until after she gives birth to a severely affected child. Predicting whether an offspring will have a minor or severe abnormality is not possible. Examples of autosomal dominant disorders are HD, Marfan syndrome, neurofibromatosis, myotonic dystrophy, Stickler syndrome, Treacher Collins syndrome, and achondroplasia (dwarfism).

Neurofibromatosis (NF) is a progressive disorder of the nervous system that causes tumors to form on nerves anywhere in the body. NF affects all races, all ethnic groups, and both sexes equally. Half of the cases of NF result from spontaneous genetic mutation, whereas the other half of cases are inherited in an autosomal dominant manner. Individuals with NF due to a spontaneous mutation have a 50% chance of transmitting the variant allele to the next generation with each pregnancy. Two genetically distinct forms of NF include NF1, the most common type, with an incidence of 1 in 3000 (Mueller & Young, 2001), and NF2, with an incidence of 1 in 35,000. Individuals with NF1 generally are able to live a normal, healthy life.

NF1 is inherited in an autosomal dominant manner with almost complete penetrance by age 5 years (Mueller & Young, 2001). Penetrance is defined as the proportion of heterozygotes for a dominant trait who express a trait, even mildly. Expression of NF1 is very variable. Affected members of the same family can look strikingly different as far as disease severity is concerned. The NF2 gene has been mapped to chromosome 22. The gene product, merlin, is thought to be a cytoskeleton protein that acts as a tumor suppressor. No treatment for NF is available, other than the surgical removal of the tumors. Once removed, the tumors may grow back.

Factor V Leiden (FVL) is the most common inherited risk factor for primary and recurrent venous thromboembolisms (Moll, 2006). It is an autosomal dominant disorder that markedly increases an individual's risk for deep venous thrombosis (blood clots in the large veins of the legs) and pulmonary emboli (blood clots that travel through the bloodstream and become embedded in the lungs), especially if the individual is a woman who (a) uses oral contraceptives, (b) is pregnant, or (c) is on hormone replacement therapy during menopause. FVL is due to a mutation in the Factor V gene, which leads to activated protein C (APC) resistance. According to Kujovich (2004), if a woman is heterozygous (has inherited one copy of the FVL mutation), she has a fourfold to eightfold increase in her chance of developing venous blood clots, but her risk increases by a factor as high as 75 if she is homozygous (has inherited two copies of the FVL mutation). Women who carry the FVL mutation should not take oral contraceptives (Ament, 2004). In addition, if they become pregnant and they have a history of blood clots, it is recommended that they receive prophylactic anticoagulation (with low-dose heparin) during their pregnancy and for 6 weeks postpartum (Kujovich, 2004).

FVL can be accurately detected with genetic testing, but the most cost-effective way to screen for FVL is taking a careful individual and family history. Women with a personal or close family history of venous blood clots, pulmonary emboli, early onset and recurrent preeclampsia, recurrent fetal growth restriction, recurrent pregnancy loss and stillbirth, or placental abruption should be screened for FVL (Ament, 2003).

Autosomal Recessive Inheritance. Autosomal recessive inheritance disorders are those in which both genes of a pair are forms associated with the disorder to be expressed. Heterozygous individuals have only one variant allele and are unaffected clinically because their normal gene (wild-type allele) overshadows the variant allele. They are known as carriers of the recessive trait. Because these recessive traits are inherited by generations of the same family, an increased incidence of the disorder occurs in consanguineous matings (closely related parents). For the trait to be expressed, two carriers must each contribute a variant allele to the offspring (see Fig. 3-3, *C*). The chance of the trait occurring in each child is 25%. A clinically normal offspring may be a carrier of the gene. Autosomal recessive disorders have a horizontal pattern of inheritance, rather than the vertical pattern seen with autosomal dominant disorders. That is, autosomal recessive disorders are usually observed in one or more siblings, but not in earlier generations (Jorde, Carey, Bamshad, & White, 2003). Males and females are equally affected. Most recessive disorders tend to have severe clinical manifestations, and affected offspring may not reproduce. If they do, all their offspring will at least be carriers for the disorder. Most IEMs, such as PKU, galactosemia, maple syrup urine disease, Tay-Sachs disease, sickle cell anemia, and CF, are autosomal recessive inherited disorders.

Inborn Errors of Metabolism. More than 350 inborn errors of metabolism have been recognized (Jorde et al., 2003). Individually, IEMs are relatively rare, but collectively, they are common (1 in 5000 live births). Archibald Garrod first used the term "inborn errors of metabolism" in 1908 when he described variants of metabolism. Garrod recognized that IEMs illustrate our "chemical individualities." As noted previously, most IEMs are inherited in an autosomal recessive pattern. IEMs occur when a gene mutation reduces the efficiency of encoded enzymes to a level at which normal metabolism cannot occur. Defective enzyme action interrupts the normal series of chemical reactions from the affected point onward. The result may be an accumulation of a damaging product, such as phenylalanine in PKU, or the absence of a necessary product, such as the lack of melanin in albinism caused by lack of tyrosinase. Diagnostic and carrier testing is available for a growing number of IEMs. In addition, many states in the United States have started screening for specific IEMs as part of their expanded newborn screening programs using tandem mass spectrometry. Unfortunately, many of the deaths caused by IEMs are due to enzyme variants not currently screened for in many of the newborn screening programs (Jorde et al., 2003).

Phenylketonuria is a relatively uncommon autosomal recessive disorder. A deficiency in the liver enzyme phenylalanine hydroxylase results in failure to metabolize the amino acid phenylalanine, allowing its metabolites to accumulate in the blood. The incidence of this disorder is 1 in every 10,000 to 20,000 births. The highest incidence is found in Caucasians (from northern Europe and the United States). It is rarely seen in Jewish, African, or Japanese populations. Screening for PKU is routinely performed on all newborns through a blood test.

Tay-Sachs disease is a lipid-storage disease that occurs more commonly in Ashkenazi Jews and French-Canadians from Quebec (Lashley, 2005). It results from a deficiency in hexosaminidase. Until age 4 to 6 months, infants with Tay-Sachs disease appear normal; their facial features are considered very beautiful. Then the clinical symptoms appear: apathy and regression in motor and social development and decreased vision. Death occurs between ages 3 and 4 years. No treatment exists for Tay-Sachs disease.

Infantile Krabbe's disease or *globoid-cell leukodystrophy* is a lysosomal storage disorder characterized by failure of the process of myelination in the central and peripheral nervous systems, rapidly progressive neurologic deterioration, and death (often before the age of 2 years). Findings from a study by Escolar and colleagues (2005) suggest that transplantation of umbilical-cord blood from unrelated donors in newborns with infantile Krabbe's disease favorably altered the natural history of this disease. Infants who underwent transplantation before the development of symptoms demonstrated continued gains in developmental skills and progressive central myelination, and most had age-appropriate cognitive function and receptive language skills. However, if transplantation occurred after the onset of symptoms, there was minimal neurologic improvement. These findings have implications for decisions regarding the addition of screening for lysosomal storage disorders to existing newborn screening programs.

X-linked Dominant Inheritance. X-linked dominant inheritance mimics autosomal dominant inheritance, except that male-to-male transmission cannot occur unless the father has Klinefelter syndrome due to XY disomy (Simpson & Elias, 2003). X-linked dominant inheritance disorders occur in males and heterozygous females, but because of X inactivation, affected females are usually less severely affected than affected males and they are more likely to transmit the abnormal gene (variant allele) to their offspring (Lashley, 2005). Heterozygous females (females who have one wild-type allele and one variant allele) have a 50% chance of transmitting the abnormal gene (variant allele) to each offspring. The variant allele is often lethal in affected males since, unlike affected females, they have no normal gene (wild-type allele). Mating of an affected male and an unaffected female is uncommon as a result of the tendency for the variant allele to be lethal in affected males. Relatively few X-linked dominant disorders have

been identified. Two examples are vitamin D–resistant rickets and fragile X syndrome (FXS).

FXS is the most common inherited form of mental retardation. Unlike Down syndrome, FXS is not generally detectable through behavioral observation or physical examination at birth. Delays and behavioral abnormalities gradually become apparent during the first 2 years of life, but ultimately its presence can be verified only through DNA testing (Sherman, Pletcher, & Driscoll, 2005). Males with FXS usually have some degree of mental retardation (typically in the moderate range) and often have characteristic physical features (large ears, long face, hypermobile joints, and macroorchidism or increased testicular volume in postpubertal males) and behavior (repetitive speech, avoids eye contact, self-injurious behavior, hyperarousal). Since the mutation is X-linked, males are more severely affected than females. Thus the degree of mental retardation tends to be milder and more variable in females than in males (Jorde et al., 2003). FXS is caused by a trinucleotide repeat expansion (CGG) at a "fragile site" (Xq27.3) on the long arm of the X chromosome in the FMR1 (fragile X mental retardation) gene (Lashley, 2005). Individuals who do not have FXS have 29-30 CGG repeats, with a range of 7 to 54 CGG repeats. Individuals with more than 55 but fewer than 200 CGG repeats are said to be permutation carriers. These individuals were originally thought to be unaffected, but recent research has shown that about 20% of adult carrier females may develop premature ovarian failure (cessation of menses before 40 years of age). Elderly male permutation carriers may manifest the fragile X–associated tremor/ataxia syndrome (FXTAS), which consists of parkinsonism, intention tremors, autonomic dysfunction, peripheral neuropathy, weakness in the legs, cognitive decline, and cerebellar ataxia (www.nfx.org).

X-linked Recessive Inheritance. Abnormal genes for X-linked recessive inheritance disorders are carried on the X chromosome. Females may be heterozygous or homozygous for traits carried on the X chromosome, because they have two X chromosomes. Males are hemizygous because they have only one X chromosome, which carries genes with no alleles on the Y chromosome. Therefore X-linked recessive disorders are most commonly manifested in the male, with the abnormal gene on his single X chromosome. Hemophilia, color blindness, and Duchenne muscular dystrophy are X-linked recessive disorders.

The male receives the disease-associated allele from his carrier mother on her affected X chromosome. Female carriers (those heterozygous for the trait) have a 50% probability of transmitting the disease-associated allele to each offspring. An affected male can pass the disease-associated allele to his daughters, but not to his sons. The daughters will be carriers of the trait if they receive a normal gene on the X chromosome from their mother. They will be affected only if they receive a disease-associated allele on the X chromosome from both their mother and their father.

▬ CANCER GENETICS

Genes That Cause Cancer When Mutated

Cancer is genetic in origin (Vogelstein & Kinzler, 2002; Zawacki & Phillips, 2002). It begins with one or more genetic mutations that make cells unstable. Three classes of genes lead to cancer if they are mutated: (1) protooncogenes, (2) tumor suppressor genes, and (3) DNA damage-recognition-and-repair genes including DNA mismatch genes (Lashley, 2005). Mutations that go unchecked start a cascade of further genetic events that lead to uncontrolled growth and tumor formation.

Oncogenes are mutated forms of protooncogenes. The main functions of protooncogenes are to encourage and promote normal growth and development. When protooncogenes mutate to become carcinogenic oncogenes, the result is excessive cell multiplication. The activation of oncogenes has been compared to a jammed accelerator in a car. Two examples of oncogenes are ERBB2, located on chromosome 13, and KRAS2, located on chromosome 12. ERBB2 is involved in breast, ovarian, lung, gastric, and salivary gland cancers. KRAS2 is involved in breast, pancreatic, thyroid, colorectal, bladder, and lung cancers, as well as acute myeloid leukemia.

Tumor suppressor genes normally function to inhibit or "put the brakes on" the cell growth and division cycle. They function to prevent the development of tumors. Mutations in tumor suppressor genes cause the cell to ignore one or more of the components of the network of inhibitory signals, removing the brakes from the cell cycle. This results in a higher rate of uncontrolled growth: cancer. Examples of tumor suppressor genes include APC, located on chromosome 5 and involved with familial adenomatous polyposis of the colon (FAP); BRCA1, located on chromosome 17 and associated with hereditary breast cancer and ovarian cancer; and RB1, found on chromosome 13 and involved with familial retinoblastoma.

DNA damage-recognition-and-repair genes hunt down and excise mistakes in copying (mutations) to ensure an accurate DNA strand. Mutations in DNA repair genes limit the efficiency of their identification and repair functions, leading to an increase in the frequency of mutations in replicated DNA strands. Disorders associated with faulty DNA damage-recognition-and-repair genes include Bloom syndrome, ataxia telangiectasia, Fanconi anemia, and hereditary nonpolyposis colon cancer (HNPCC).

People acquire mutations in genes in three main ways. The first is from the environment. Known factors in the environment that cause cancer are ultraviolet (UV) light (skin cancer) and tobacco smoke (lung cancer). The second way that people acquire mutations is by chance. Normal metabolic processes can generate chemicals that damage DNA. Third, people acquire mutations through heredity. Sometimes people are born with specific mutations in critical genes. For example, people in whom HNPCC develops were born with a mutation in a DNA repair gene.

Hereditary Breast and Ovarian Cancer (HBOC)

Breast cancer is a common disease and a central concern in women's health. In the United States, breast cancer is the most common form of cancer for women and the second most common cause of death. According to the American Cancer Society (2006), it is estimated that 212,920 women will be diagnosed with breast cancer in 2006 and over 40,970 will die from it. It is estimated that 5% to 10% of all breast and ovarian cancers are hereditary cancers that can be attributed to a mutation in a gene strongly associated with breast and ovarian cancer susceptibility (Blackwood & Weber, 1998). Another 15% to 20% of female breast cancers occur in women who have a family history of breast and ovarian cancer but do not carry a mutation in one of the genes that are known to be strongly associated with breast and ovarian cancer susceptibility. BRCA1 and BRCA2 mutations account for approximately 70% to 85% of hereditary breast and ovarian cancer (HBOC). These mutations are inherited in an autosomal dominant pattern; thus each offspring of an individual found to carry a BRCA mutation has a 50% chance of inheriting the same mutation. Ashkenazi Jews are 10 times more likely to have BRCA1 and/or BRCA2 mutations than are the general population. Even though only about 6% of the men who carry a BRCA mutation develop breast cancer, men who carry a BRCA mutation have a 50% chance of passing the mutation on to their offspring (www.nci.nih.gov).

BRCA1, the first major breast cancer gene, was identified and isolated in 1994. A second breast cancer gene, designated BRCA2, was mapped to chromosome 13 in 1994 and cloned in 1995. Although it is clear that BRCA1 and BRCA2 mutations confer high risks of breast and ovarian cancer, the magnitude of the risk remains unclear. A metaanalysis of data from 22 studies found that the average cumulative risks in BRCA1-mutation carriers by age 70 years were 65% for breast cancer and 39% for ovarian cancer (Antoniou et al., 2003). Corresponding estimates for BRCA2-mutation carriers were 45% for breast cancer and 11% for ovarian cancer. The risk of developing a second breast cancer in carriers who have undergone breast conserving therapy is as high as 70% at 10 years. Carriers of BRCA1 mutations may also be at increased risk for colon cancer, though this has been disputed. Carriers of BRCA2 mutations may be at increased risk for pancreatic, prostate, gallbladder and bile duct, and stomach cancers, hematologic malignancies, and malignant melanoma.

Genetic testing for HBOC has been commercially available in the United States since 1995. The cost for testing (current in 2006) ranges from $3,000 to $3,311 for full-sequence BRCA1 and BRCA2 testing, and $350 to $585 for an analysis of relatives of an individual with an identified mutation. Women newly diagnosed with breast cancer are increasingly being asked to consider undergoing

CD Critical Thinking Exercise: Genetic Counseling

BRCA1 and BRCA2 testing before they make decisions about their treatment options (Daly, 2004), however, the cost may be prohibitive. This request for testing is occurring because a number of studies have shown that a woman's short-term risk of developing a second breast cancer is substantially affected by whether she carries a BRCA1 or BRCA2 mutation, and prophylactic surgery has been found to decrease the risk of breast and ovarian cancer by more than 90% (Hartmann, Degnim, & Schaid, 2004; McDonnell et al., 2001; Rebbeck et al., 2004). The main advantage to offering BRCA1 and BRCA2 testing before the onset of treatment is that it gives women who are found to carry a deleterious mutation the option of choosing risk-reduction surgery concurrent with therapeutic surgical treatment.

Colon Cancer

Colon cancer is the third leading cause of cancer-related death in women. According to the American Cancer Society (2006), it is estimated that 106,680 new cases of colon cancer will be diagnosed in 2006, and there will be 55,170 deaths due to colon and rectal cancer. Of colon cancer cases, 10% are likely to involve a mutation in one of several predisposing genes. Two examples of predisposing genes are mutations in the APC tumor suppressor gene and mutations in a mismatch repair gene. Mutations in the APC tumor suppressor gene, which is located on chromosome 5, have been associated with FAP, a rare, autosomal dominant syndrome that accounts for about 1% of all colon cancer (Vogelstein & Kinzler, 2002). It is typically diagnosed clinically. Affected individuals have 100 to 1000 polyps in their colon by the time they are 20 to 30 years old. Genetic testing is greater than 80% sensitive. Identification of high risk individuals guides surveillance strategies and the timing of a prophylactic colectomy. Low risk individuals can stop the increased surveillance.

HNPCC results from mutations in one of many mismatch repair (MMR) genes. Mutations in MSH2 and MLH1 account for 50% to 60% of HNPCC. Families at high risk for HNPCC often have three or more relatives with colorectal cancer; colorectal cancer present in at least two generations; and a diagnosis of colorectal cancer before age 50 years in at least one case. HNPCC is characterized by an increased risk of colon cancer and other cancers that include cancers of the ovary, endometrium, stomach, small intestine, upper urinary tract, hepatobiliary tract, brain, and skin. The lifetime risk of colon cancer for individuals with HNPCC is approximately 80%. The majority of these cancers occur in the proximal colon. Genetic tests are available to test for MSH2 and MLH1. Testing should be done first on the affected family member. At-risk clients should be offered a prophylactic colectomy. Women may be offered a total abdominal hysterectomy with a salpingo-oophorectomy to decrease cancer risk. If colon cancer develops, a total colectomy is recommended.

▬ GENETIC COUNSELING

Genetic counseling is a service that grew out of a need for professionals who could provide genetics information, education, and support to individuals and families with ongoing or potential genetic health concerns (www.genome. bov/glossary.cfm). As of 2006, there are 27 master's-level genetic counseling programs in the United States, and international genetic counseling programs in 15 different countries. The number of graduate nursing programs with an advanced practice course in genetics is growing rapidly (see Box 3-1 for examples). The National Society of Genetic Counselors, formed in 1979, now has more than 2000 members (www.nsgc.org, www.faseb.org/genetics/mainmenu.htm).

Definition of Genetic Counseling

In 1975, an ad hoc committee of the American Society of Human Genetics developed a formal definition of genetic counseling. According to this definition,

> Genetic counseling is a communication process that deals with the human problems associated with the occurrence or risk of occurrence of a genetic disorder in a family. This process involves an attempt by one or more appropriately trained person to help the individual or family to (1) comprehend the medical facts including the diagnosis, probable course of the disorder, and the available management; (2) appreciate the way heredity contributes to the disorder and the risk of recurrence in specified relatives; (3) understand the alternatives for dealing with the risk of recurrence; (4) choose a course of action that seems to them appropriate in view of their risk, their family goals, and their ethical and religious standards and act in accordance with that decision; and (5) make the best possible adjustment to the disorder in an affected family member and/or to the risk of recurrence of that disorder.

Access and Referral to Genetic Counseling

Genetic counseling is typically provided by a team of genetics specialists that includes clinical geneticists (physicians with an MD or DO), medical geneticists with a PhD, genetics fellows, genetics counselors, and, in a growing number of cases, advanced practice genetics nurse specialists. Cytogeneticists, biochemical geneticists, and molecular geneticists support the clinical genetics team by providing laboratory expertise that helps with the diagnosis and management of individuals and families affected by genetic conditions.

Until recently, most individuals and families interested in receiving genetic counseling went to regional genetics centers or major medical centers. Genetic counseling also was provided in outreach or satellite genetics clinics, public health clinics, and some community hospitals. Now that genetics is entering the mainstream of health care, genetic counseling is being offered in a wide variety of other settings. These include, but are not limited to, managed health care organizations, commercial facilities, and private practices. A number of specialized groups provide genetics

box 3-1 **Initiatives to Improve Genetics Expertise**

GENETICS INITIATIVES FOR NURSES AND OTHER HEALTH CARE PROVIDERS

- National Coalition of Health Professional Education in Genetics (NCHPEG); www.nchpeg.org/
- International Society of Nurses in Genetics (ISONG); www.nursing.creighton.edu/isong/

SUMMER INSTITUTES

- Genetics Interdisciplinary Faculty Training Program, Duke University Genetics Program for Nursing Faculty; www.gift.duke.edu/index.html
- Cincinnati Children's Hospital Medical Center; www.cincinnatichildrens.org/Professional_Education/programs/Genetics_Program_for_Nursing_Faculty/GPNF/About_GPNF/default.htm
- Summer Genetics Institute, Intensive Research Training, NINR; www.fmp.cit.nih.gov/ninr/

ADVANCED DEGREE PROGRAMS

- Rush University, Chicago, IL; www.rushu.rush.edu./nursing/
- University of California, San Francisco, CA; http://nurseweb.ucsf.edu/
- University of Cincinnati, OH; www.nursing.uc.edu/
- University of Iowa, Ames, IA; http://coninfo.nursing.uiowa.edu/
- University of Washington, Seattle, WA; www.son.washington.edu/
- Teacher's College at Columbia University, New York, NY; www.tc.edu/hbs/NurseEd/

education and counseling for individuals and families affected by specific genetic disorders, such as Down syndrome, CF, diabetes, muscular dystrophy, HD, and cancer. Genetic counseling also is offered over the Internet.

Individuals and families seek out, or are referred for, genetic counseling for a wide variety of reasons and at all stages of their lives. Some seek preconception or prenatal information; others are referred after the birth of a child with a birth defect or a suspected genetic condition; still others seek information because they have a family history of a genetic condition. Regardless of the setting or the individual and family's stage of life, genetic counseling should be offered and available to all individuals and families who have questions about genetics and their health. However, there is currently a shortage of appropriately trained genetics professionals who can provide genetic counseling (Begleiter, 2002; Greendale & Pyeritz, 2001). This means that many individuals and families will not be offered genetic counseling when they undergo genetic testing. Moreover, some of the genetics education and counseling that is provided will be less than adequate.

At present, more individuals who can provide genetic counseling are needed urgently. It has been suggested that primary care providers will have to assume prominent roles in the provision of genetic counseling and other genetics services (Collins, 1997; Touchette, Holzman, Davis, & Feetham, 1997). This suggestion has not met with overwhelming support (Begleiter, 2002; Greendale & Pyeritz, 2001). The main criticism of this suggestion is that most primary care providers (physicians and nurses) lack an adequate understanding of genetics. This deficit reflects both rapid advances in the field of genetics and historical limitations in genetics education in medical and nursing curricula (Burke & Emery, 2002). As noted previously, a number of initiatives are under way to help nurses and other health care professionals gain the knowledge, skills, and confidence they need to provide high quality genetics health care in a wide variety of settings.

It may take years before a sufficient number of health care professionals feel comfortable and are proficient in providing genetic counseling. Until then, it is imperative that all health care professionals become familiar with existing genetics resources (www.hsl.unc.edu/Services/Guides/focusonclingen.cfm, www.cdc.gov/genetics/activities/ogdp.htm). Some of these resources may be in their own communities, but others will be regional, national, and international resources (e.g., www.genome.gov/glossary.cfm). As noted earlier in this chapter, at a minimum, each health care professional should be able to appreciate limitations of his or her genetics expertise; understand the social and psychologic implications of genetics services; and know how and when to make referrals to genetics professionals.

Estimation of Risk

Most families with a history of genetic disease want an answer to the following question: What is the chance that our future children will have this disease? Because the answer to this question may have profound implications for individual family members and the family as a whole, health care professionals must be able to answer this question as accurately as they can in a timely manner. In some cases, estimation of risk is rather straightforward; in other cases, it becomes rather complicated. Because of this, health care professionals should be prepared to refer families with a history of genetic disease to genetics professionals if they are at all unsure. Again, the answer to this question can have profound implications for individual family members and the family as a whole, so health care professionals must do their best to ensure that the question is answered accurately.

If a couple has not yet had children, but they are known to be at risk for having children with a genetic disease, they will be given an occurrence risk. Once the mating of a couple has produced one or more children with a genetic disease, the couple will be given a recurrence risk. Both occurrence and recurrence risks are determined by the mode of inheritance for the genetic disease in question. For genetic diseases caused by a factor that segregates during cell division (genes and chromosomes), risk can be estimated with a high degree of accuracy by application of the mendelian principles (http://www3.ncbi.nlm.nih.gov/entrez/query.fcgi?db=OMIM).

In an autosomal dominant disorder, both the occurrence and recurrence risk is 50%, or one in two, when one parent is affected and the other is not. The recurrence risk for autosomal recessive disorders is 25%, or one in four, if both parents are carriers (they each have one recessive disease gene and one normal gene). Occasionally an individual homozygous for a recessive disease gene mates with an individual who is a carrier of the same recessive gene. In this case, the recurrence risk is 50%, or one in two. If two individuals affected by an autosomal recessive disorder mate, all of their children will be affected. For X-linked disorders, recurrence risk is related to the sex of the child. Translocation disorders have a high risk of recurrence.

A number of autosomal disorders display fairly complex patterns of inheritance, making estimation of risk somewhat difficult. For example, if a child is born with a genetic disease and there has been no history of the disease in the family, the disease may have been caused by a new mutation (this is more likely if the disease in question is an autosomal dominant disorder, such as achondroplasia). If the child's genetic disease has been caused by a new mutation, the recurrence risk for the parents' subsequent children is low (1% to 2%), but it is not as low as that for the general population. Offspring of the affected child may have a substantially elevated occurrence risk.

The risk of recurrence for multifactorial conditions can be estimated empirically. An empiric risk is based not on genetics theory but rather on experience and observation of the disorder in other families. Recurrence risks are determined by applying the frequency of a similar disorder in other families to the case under consideration.

An important concept to be emphasized to individuals and families during a genetic counseling session is that *each pregnancy is an independent event.* For example, in monogenic disorders in which the risk factor is one in four that the child will be affected, the risk remains the same no matter how many affected children are already in the family. Families may maintain the erroneous assumption that the presence of one affected child ensures that the next three will be free of the disorder. However, "chance has no memory." The risk is one in four for each pregnancy. Conversely, in a family with a child who has a disorder with multifactorial causes, the risk increases with each subsequent child born with the disorder.

Interpretation of Risk

The guiding principle for genetics counselors has traditionally been the principle of nondirectiveness. According to the principle of nondirectiveness, the individual who is providing genetic counseling respects the right of the individual or family being counseled to make autonomous decisions. Counselors using a nondirective approach avoid making recommendations, and they try to communicate genetics information in an unbiased manner. The first step in providing nondirective counseling is becoming aware of one's own values and beliefs. Another important step is recognizing how one's values and beliefs can influence or interfere with the communication of genetics information.

If the individual who is providing genetic counseling has difficulty being nonjudgmental and objective, he or she may either intentionally or unintentionally influence the decision-making process. Individuals and families also may pressure the counselor to make decisions for them with questions such as, "What would you do if you were me?" Families and individuals need education, guidance, and support throughout the counseling process. They should be given the facts and possible consequences, as well as all of the assistance they need in problem solving, but the final decision regarding a course of action must be their own.

Role of Nurses in Genetic Counseling

The role of nurses in genetic counseling continues to expand (www.cincinattichildrens.org/ed/clinical/gpnf/resources/curriculum/multiple-roles.htm). Some nurses play a key role in the identification of families in need of genetic counseling, and they collaborate with other health care professionals to make referrals to specialists in genetics. Other nurses take a more active role in genetic counseling. For example, these nurses might provide appropriate genetics information before, during, and after the initial genetic counseling session; construct family pedigrees of three or more generations; clarify the genetics information that family members receive during counseling sessions or from other sources such as the public library, the Internet, or support groups (www.geneticalliance.org); help families manage the ongoing challenges associated with living with a genetic disorder; make referrals to support groups and national organizations; and provide long-term follow-up of families affected by genetic conditions.

Probably the most important of all nursing functions is to provide emotional support during all aspects of the counseling process. Feelings that are generated under the real or imagined threat posed by a genetic disorder are as varied as the people being counseled. Responses may include a variety of stress reactions, such as apathy, denial, anger, hostility, fear, embarrassment, grief, and loss of self-esteem. Guilt and self-blame are universal reactions. Many look on the disorder as a stigma, especially if the disorder is visible to others. Old wives' tales, superstitions, and long-held misconceptions may influence a family's reaction to a genetic disorder.

▪ FUTURE PROMISE OF GENETICS

Overall, the Human Genome Project and other sequencing efforts have been a huge success. Our understanding of the human genome, as well as other genomes, has grown exponentially during the past decade. The increased availability of genetic testing and other genetics services gives individuals and families unprecedented opportunities to learn whether they have heightened risk for certain diseases or the potential to transmit gene mutations to their offspring. Awareness of genetic risk also can facilitate informed health care decisions and, in some cases, can

EVIDENCE-BASED PRACTICE

The Paradoxes of Abnormal Prenatal Diagnosis

BACKGROUND

- Until the last generation or so, parents had to wait until after the birth to discover whether their child had an impairment. As prenatal diagnostic technology has improved the ability to diagnose an abnormality in the second trimester or sooner, parents are faced with decisions for which they have no precedents. Qualitative researchers have interviewed parents about their experiences with prenatal diagnostic tests.

OBJECTIVE

- The authors wished to analyze and synthesize the body of research on parental experiences with abnormal prenatal diagnosis. Since this research is qualitative, there are neither intervention trials nor numerical data to metaanalyze. Instead, the authors sought to systematically discover the major topics and themes that emerged in the studies.

METHOD

Search Strategy

- The authors searched nursing, social sciences, humanities and women's resources literature. All 17 qualitative studies of U.S. parents receiving abnormal prenatal diagnosis were included, regardless of the population studied or when during the pregnancy the results were known. The studies were published from 1984 to 2001.

Statistical Analyses

- Each study was analyzed using a 14-item reading guide, so that similar data could be extracted and compared. Those items included the research problem, the literature review, theoretical orientation, methods, data collection, validity, and findings, among others. The reviewers used qualitative metasummary and metasynthesis to show thematic patterns recurring in the parent interviews.

FINDINGS

- Parents who received abnormal prenatal diagnoses had four dominant types of experiences and issues: (1) time-sensitive decision-making; (2) selective management about what information they would allow in (so as not to be overwhelmed or feel their decision to be undermined) and what information they could allow out (to friends and family, so as not be judged); (3) devastation, particularly for the mothers; and (4) the traumatic sequelae to the relationships, personal growth, subsequent pregnancies, and chronic feelings of loss.
- Topics in the studies focused on the prenatal diagnosis, sometimes ambiguous prognosis, and pregnancy termination, if available and timely. The themes were primarily about decision making. Couples could not look to their family history for guidance, nor could they share with their usual community. The loss of the fantasy child is the same whether the diagnosis occurs prenatally or after birth, but prenatal diagnosis puts the onus on the parents to paradoxically love and terminate a pregnancy. The unbounded possibilities of the virtual baby became limited choices of life with an impaired (or dead) infant or a pregnancy termination, and the stigma of impairment and abortion. The intensity of their attachment (the "wantedness" of this baby) paradoxically relieved their grief.

LIMITATIONS

- Qualitative research is dependent upon interpretation by the researcher in defining the problem, obtaining the data, and reporting the themes. This injects human bias, but can also allow intuitive leaps of insight. The quandary of parents who receive abnormal results will change as the technology evolves.

IMPLICATIONS FOR PRACTICE

- No two people grieve the same way, but the nurse can be sensitive to the particular information management style of a couple, especially timing information to their readiness. Particularly useful is helping them develop narrative strategies, such as how they will remember the experience and what they will tell their friends and family. The nurse can select language that supports the couple's strategy. Acknowledging their grief as profound and real is the most important issue to parents.

IMPLICATIONS FOR FURTHER RESEARCH

- Future research can explore families' experiences with the differences between other types of pregnancy loss. There is little research following up on couples who choose to continue an impaired pregnancy. More information about the stigma of impairment and termination would be illuminating.

Reference: Sandelowski, M., & Barroso, J. (2005). The travesty of choosing after positive prenatal diagnosis. *Journal of Obstetric, Gynecologic, and Neonatal Nursing,* 34(3), 307-318.

promote risk reduction behaviors that have the potential to reduce morbidity and mortality. Ultimately it is hoped that advances in molecular biology and genomics will make it possible to offer diagnostic, preventive, and treatment options not only for genetic diseases but also for common diseases such as cancer, atherosclerosis, diabetes, and Alzheimer's disease.

Recent advances made possible through the Human Genome Project have been remarkable, but our ability to offer treatment options, even for single-gene disorders, remains very limited. Progress in the acquisition of genetics information and the development of genetics technology continues to outpace the development of therapeutic interventions. For most genetic conditions, therapeutic interventions are nonexistent or disappointingly limited. Consequently the most useful means of reducing the incidence of genetic disorders now is preventing transmission. Only three reproductive options exist for individuals at risk for transmitting a genetic disorder: the avoidance of pregnancy; genetic diagnosis during an ongoing pregnancy; and prevention of transmission of an altered gene or genes through preimplantation genetics (Jones &

Fallon, 2002). For many families, none of these options is viewed as acceptable.

Dialogue among pregnant women, expectant families, health care professionals, and disability advocates concerning prenatal testing for Down syndrome and other genetic disorders is urgently needed. Clinical and technical information must be complemented by social understanding of the experience of disability in contemporary society. The picture of life with a disability should be more balanced than that currently portrayed (Marteau & Dormandy, 2001). It is critical that the voices of individuals and families living with disabilities be heard.

Nurses are in an ideal position to help individuals and families maximize the benefits of the genetics revolution, but first, nurses need (1) a working knowledge of human genetics, (2) an awareness of recent advances in genetics and genomics, and (3) an understanding of the potential effects of genomic discoveries on individual and family well-being. More research is needed concerning the family experience of genetic testing (Van Riper, 2005; Van Riper & Gallo, 2006). Nurses must understand why individuals and families decide to undergo genetic testing. Nurses also need to be aware of how individuals and families define and manage ethical, legal, and social issues that emerge during the genetic testing experience. The following quote by Juengst (1998) underscores why this knowledge is needed:

> The promise of accessible genetic information lies in its ability to allow individuals and families to identify, understand, and sometimes control their inherited health risks. This promise puts the individual and families that receive genetic services at the moral center of the enterprise: if genetic assessment is to be judged a success, it must be from the recipients' point of view, in terms of their ability to use the information to enrich their lives.

community activity

Select two web addresses for resources on genetics for parents. Access the sites.
- Compare and contrast the appearance, readability, and information contained in the sites.
- Is the information available for parents who do not read English?
- Do you agree that these sites are appropriate for parents?
- Is the information contained culturally relevant?
- How could you, as a nurse, use this information?
- Role play with a classmate reviewing the information with a parent undergoing genetic testing.

key points

- Recent advances in molecular biology and genomics have revolutionized the field of health care by providing the tools needed to determine the hereditary component of many diseases.
- Increasingly, nurses from all specialty areas, as well as all practice settings, are expected to have competencies in genetics and genomics.
- The major force behind the genetics revolution has been the Human Genome Project.
- All humans are 99.9% identical at the DNA level.
- Approximately 20,000 to 25,000 genes are found in the human genome.
- Most of the genetic tests being offered in clinical practice are tests for single-gene disorders.

- Pharmacogenomics will probably be the most immediate clinical application of the Human Genome Project.
- The decision to undergo genetic testing is often based on feelings of responsibility and commitment to others.
- Genes are the basic units of heredity responsible for all human characteristics. They comprise 23 pairs of chromosomes: 22 pairs of autosomes and 1 pair of sex chromosomes.
- Chromosomal abnormalities occur in both autosomes and sex chromosomes.
- Multifactorial inheritance includes genetic and environmental contributions.
- Advances in genetics have complex ethical, legal, and social implications.

REFERENCES

Ad Hoc Committee on Genetic Counseling, American Society of Human Genetics. (1975). Genetic counseling. *American Journal of Human Genetics, 27*(2), 240-242.

Ament, L. (2003). Factor V Leiden: A review of the literature. *Journal of Perinatal and Neonatal Nursing, 17*(3), 190-195.

Ament, L. (2004). Factor V Leiden and contraception. *Journal of Midwifery & Women's Health, 49*(1), 51-52.

American Cancer Society. (2006) *Breast cancer facts & figures 2005-2006.* Accessed http://www.cancer.org/docroot/STT/stt_0.asp, June 16, 2006.

Anderson, W. (2000). Gene therapy: The best of times, the worst of times. *Science, 288*(5466), 627-629.

Antoniou, A., Pharoah, P., Narod, S., Risch, H., Eyfjord, J., Hopper, J., et al. (2003). Average risks of breast and ovarian cancer associated with BRCA1 or BRCA2 mutations detected in case series unselected for family history: A combined analysis of 22 studies. *American Journal of Human Genetics, 72*(5), 1117-1130.

Begleiter, M. (2002). Training for genetic counselors. *National Review of Genetics, 3,* 557-561.

Bennett, R. (2004). The family medical history. *Primary Care, 31*(3), 479-495.

Blackwood, M., & Weber, B. (1998). BRCA1 and BRCA2: From molecular genetics to clinical medicine. *Journal of Clinical Oncology, 16*(5), 1969-1977.

Brower, V. (2001). Gene therapy revisited: In spite of problems and drawbacks, gene therapy moves forward. *EMBO Reports, 2*(12), 1064-1065.

Burgess, M., & d'Agincourt-Canning, L. (2002). Genetic testing for hereditary disease: Attending to relational responsibility. *Journal of Clinical Ethics, 12*(4), 361-372.

Burke, S., & Kirk, M. (2006). Genetics education in the nursing profession: Literature review. *Advances in Nursing Science, 54*(2), 228-237.

Burke, W., & Emery, J. (2002). Genetics education for primary-care providers. *Nature Review Genetics, 3*(7), 561-566.

Carlson-Sabelli, L., & Lessick, M. (2001). Genetic advances in bipolar disorder. *AWHONN Lifelines, 5*(3), 34-41.

Cavazzana-Calvo, M., Hacein-Bey, S., de Saint Basile, G., Gross, F., Yvon, E., Nusbaum, P., et al. (2000). Gene therapy of human severe combined immunodeficiency (SCID)-XI disease. *Science, 288*(5466), 669-672.

Collins, F. (1997). Preparing health care professionals for the genetic revolution. *Journal of the American Medical Association, 278*(15), 1285-1286.

Collins, F. (2001). Contemplating the end of the beginning. *Genome Research, 11*(5), 641-643.

Collins, F., & Guttmacher, A. (2001). Genetics moves into the medical mainstream. *Journal of the American Medical Association, 286*(18), 2322-2324.

Collins, F., & Mansoura, M. (2001). The human genome project: Revealing the shared inheritance of all humankind. *Cancer Supplement, 91*(1 Suppl), 221-225.

Collins, F., & McKusick, V. (2001). Implications of the Human Genome Project for medical science. *Journal of the American Medical Association, 285*(5), 540-544.

Cragun, D., Couch, S., Prows, C., Warren, N., & Christianson, C. (2005). A success of a genetics educational intervention for nursing and dietetic students: A model for incorporating genetics into nursing and allied health curricula. *Journal of Allied Health, 34*(2), 90-96.

Daly, M. (2004). Tailoring breast cancer treatment to genetic status: The challenges ahead. *Journal of Clinical Oncology, 22*(10), 1776-1777.

Demsey, S. (2000). Carrier screening for cystic fibrosis: A perinatal perspective. *Nursing Clinics of North America, 35,* 14-26.

Diekelmann, N., & Diekelmann, J. (2000). Learning ethics in nursing and genetics: Narrative pedagogy and the grounding of values. *Journal of Pediatric Nursing, 15*(4), 226-231.

Engstrom, J., Sefton, M., Matheson, J., & Healy, K. (2005). Genetic competencies essential for health care professionals in primary practice. *Journal of Midwifery & Women's Health, 5*(3), 177-183.

Escolar, M., Poe, M., Provenzale, J., Richards, K., Allison, J., Wood, S., et al. (2005). Transplantation of umbilical-cord blood in babies with Infantile Krabbe's disease. *New England Journal of Medicine, 352*(20), 2069-2081.

Freeman, S., Taft, L., Dooley, K., Allran, K., Sherman, S., Hassold, T., et al. (1998). Population-based study of congenital heart defects in Down syndrome. *American Journal of Medical Genetics, 80*(3), 213-217.

Gallo, A., Angst, D., Knafl, K., Hadley, E., & Smith, C. (2005). Parents sharing information with their children about genetic conditions. *Journal of Pediatric Health Care, 19*(5), 267-275.

Gates, E. (2004). Communicating risk in prenatal genetic testing. *Journal of Midwifery & Women's Health, 49*(3), 220-227.

Grant, S. (2000). Prenatal genetic screening, *Online Journal of Issues in Nursing, 5,* 2. Accessed www.nursingworld.org/ojin/topic13/tpc13_3.htm, August 20, 2006.

Green, R., & Thomas, A. (1997). Whose gene is it? A case discussion about familial conflict over genetic testing for breast cancer. *Journal of Genetic Counseling, 6*(2), 245-253.

Greendale, K., & Pyeritz, R. (2001). Empowering primary care health professionals: How soon? How fast? How far? *American Journal of Medical Genetics, 106*(3), 223-232.

Guttmacher, A., & Collins, F. (2002). Genomic medicine: A primer. *New England Journal of Medicine, 347*(19), 1512-1520.

Guttmacher, A., & Collins, F. (2005). Realizing the promise of genomics in biomedical research. *Journal of the American Medical Association, 294*(11), 1399-1402.

Hamilton, R., Bowers, B., & Williams, J. (2005). Disclosing genetic test results to family members. *Journal of Nursing Scholarship, 37*(1), 18-24.

Hartmann, L., Degnim, A., & Schaid, D. (2004). Prophylactic mastectomy for BRCA 1/2 carriers: Progress and more questions. *Journal of Clinical Oncology, 22*(6), 981-983.

Hassold, T., & Hunt, P. (2001). Too err (meiotically) is human: The genesis of human aneuploidy. *National Review of Genetics, 2*(4), 280-291.

Horne, M., & McCloskey, D. (2006). Factor V Leiden as a common genetic risk factor for venous thromboembolism. *Journal of Nursing Scholarship, 38*(1), 19-25.

International Human Genome Sequencing Consortium. (2001). Initial sequencing and analysis of the human genome. *Nature, 409*(6822), 860-921.

International Society for Nurses in Genetics (ISONG). (1998). *Statement on the scope and standards of genetics clinical nursing.* Washington, DC: American Nurses Association.

Jones, K. (2006). *Smith's recognizable patterns of human malformation* (6th ed.). Philadelphia: Saunders.

Jones, S. (2000). Reproductive genetic technologies: Exploring ethical and policy implications. *AWHONN Lifelines, 4*(5), 33-36.

Jones, S., & Fallon, L. (2002). Reproductive options for individuals at risk for transmission of a genetic disorder. *Journal of Obstetric, Gynecologic, and Neonatal Nursing, 31*(2), 193-199.

Jorde, L., Carey, J., Bamshad, M., & White, R. (2003). *Medical genetics* (3rd ed.). St. Louis: Mosby.

Juengst, E. (1998). Caught in the middle again: Professional ethical considerations in genetic testing for health risks. *Genetic Testing, 1*(3), 189-200.

Kay, M., Manno, C., Ragni, M., Larson, P., Couto, L., McClelland, A., et al. (2000). Evidence for gene transfer and expression of factor IX in haemophilia B patients treated with an AAV vector. *Nature Genetics, 24*(3), 257-261.

Kenner, C., Gallo, A., & Bryant, K. (2005). Promoting children's health through understanding of genetic and genomics. *Journal of Nursing Scholarship, 37*(4), 308-314.

Kenner, C., & Moran, M. (2005). Newborn screening and genetic testing, *Journal of Midwifery & Women's Health, 50*(3), 219-226.

Khairy P., Ouyang, D., Fernandes, S., Lee-Parritz, A., Economy, K., & Landzberg, M. (2006). Pregnancy outcomes in women with congenital heart disease. *Circulation, 113*(4), 517-524.

Khoury, M. (2003). Genetics and genomics in practice: The continuum from genetic disease to genetic information in health and disease. *Genetics in Medicine, 5*(4), 261-268.

Klipstein, S. (2005). Preimplantation genetic diagnosis: Technological promise and ethical perils. *Fertility and Sterility, 83*(5), 1347-1353.

Korenromp, M. (2005). Long-term psychological consequences of pregnancy termination for fetal abnormality: A cross-sectional study. *Prenatal Diagnosis, 25*(3), 253-260.

Kujovich, J. (2004). Thrombophilia and pregnancy complications. *American Journal of Obstetrics and Gynecology, 191*(2), 412-424.

Lamberg, L. (2005). Risks and benefits key to psychotropic use during pregnancy and postpartum period. *Journal of the American Medical Association, 294*(13), 1604-1608.

Lashley, F. (2005). *Clinical genetics in nursing practice* (3rd ed.) New York: Springer.

Lea, D. (2000). A new world view of genetics service models. *Online Journal of Issues in Nursing, 5.* Accessed www.nursingworld.org/ojin/ topic13/tpc13_6.htm, November 8, 2006.

Lea, D., Feetham, S., & Monsen, R. (2002). Genomic-based health care in nursing: A bi-directional approach to bringing genetics into nursing's body of knowledge. *Journal of Professional Nursing, 18*(3), 120-129.

Lea, D., & Williams, J. (2001). Are you ready for the genetics revolution? *American Journal of Nursing, 101*(8), 11.

Lessick, M., & Anderson, L. (2000). Genetic discoveries: Challenges for nurses who care for children and their families. *Journal of the Society of Pediatric Nursing, 5*(1), 47-51.

Lewis, J. (2002). Genetics in perinatal nursing: Clinical applications and policy considerations. *Journal of Obstetric, Gynecologic, and Neonatal Nursing, 31*(2), 188-192.

Lewis, R. (2001). *Human genetics: Concepts and applications.* Boston: McGraw-Hill.

Lloyd-Puryear, M., & Forsman, I. (2002). Newborn screening and genetic testing. *Journal of Obstetric, Gynecologic, and Neonatal Nursing, 31*(2), 200-207.

Loescher, L., & Merkle, C. (2005). The interface of genomic technologies and nursing. *Journal of Nursing Scholarship, 37*(2), 111-119.

Loud, J., Peters, J., Fraser, M., & Jenkins, J. (2002). Applications of advances in molecular biology and genomics to clinical cancer care. *Cancer Nursing, 25*(2), 110-122.

Marwick, C. (2003). FDA halts gene therapy trials after leukaemia case in France. *BMJ, 326*(7382), 181.

Marteau, T., & Dormandy, E. (2001). Facilitating informed choice in prenatal testing: How well are we doing? *American Journal of Medical Genetics, 106*(3), 185-190.

McDonnell, S., Schaid, D., Myers, J., Grant, C., Donohue, J., Woods, J., et al. (2001). Efficacy of contralateral prophylactic mastectomy in women with a personal and family history of breast cancer. *Journal of Clinical Oncology, 19*(19), 3938-3943.

McMullen, A., Pasta, D., Frederick, P., Konstan, M., Morgan, W., Schechter, M., et al. (2006). Impact of pregnancy on women with cystic fibrosis. *Chest, 129*(3), 706-711.

Moll, S. (2006). Thrombophilias–practical implications and testing caveats. *Journal of Thrombosis and Thrombolysis, 21*(1), 7-15.

Mueller, R., & Young, I. (2001). *Emery's elements of medical genetics* (11th ed.). New York: Churchill Livingstone.

National Down Syndrome Society. (2006). *NDSS Statement on the CDC's new study on the prevalence of Down Syndrome.* Accessed www.ndss.org/content.cfm?fuseaction_InfoResGeneralArticle& article_29, November 8, 2006.

Phillips, K., Veenstra, D., Oren, E., Lee, J., & Sadee, W. (2001). Potential role of pharmacogenomics in reducing adverse drug reactions. *Journal of the American Medical Association, 286*(18), 2270-2279.

Prows, C., Glass, M., Nicol, M., Shirton, H., & Williams, J. (2005). Genomics in nursing education. *Journal of Nursing Scholarship, 37*(3), 196-202.

Prows, C., & Prows, D. (2004). Medication selection by genotype: How genetics is changing drug prescribing and efficacy. *American Journal of Nursing, 104*(5), 60-70.

Rahman, J. (2003). Obstetric and gynecologic complications in women with Marfan syndrome. *Journal of Reproductive Medicine, 48*(9), 723-728.

Rebbeck, T., Friebel, T., Lynch, H., Neuhausen, S., van't Veer, L., Garber, J., et al. (2004). Bilateral prophylactic mastectomy reduces breast cancer risk in BRCA1 and BRCA2 mutation carriers: The PROSE study group. *Journal of Clinical Oncology, 22*(6), 1055-1062

Rich, E., Burke, W., Heaton, C., Haga, S., Pinsky, L., Short, M., et al. (2004). Reconsidering the family history in primary care. *Journal of General Internal Medicine, 19*(3), 273-280.

Roses, A. (2000). Pharmacogenetics and the practice of medicine. *Nature, 405*(6788), 857-865.

Rubinstein, W., & Roy, H. (2005). Practicing medicine at the front lines of the genomic revolution. *Archives of Internal Medicine, 165*(16), 1815-1817.

Scheuerle, A. (2001). Diagnosis of genetic disease. In M. Mahowald, A. Scheuerle, V. McKusick, & T. Aspinwall (Eds.), *Genetics in the clinic: Clinical, ethical, and social implications for primary care.* St. Louis: Mosby.

Seo, D., & Ginsburg, G. (2005). Genomic medicine: Bringing biomarkers to clinical medicine. *Current Opinion in Chemical Biology, 9*(4), 381-386.

Sherman, S., Pletcher, B., & Driscoll, D. (2005). Fragile X syndrome: Diagnostic and carrier testing. *Genetics in Medicine, 7*(8), 584-587.

Simpson, J., & Elias, S. (2003). *Genetics in obstetrics and gynecology.* Philadelphia: Saunders.

Thomson, E. (1997). Ethical, legal, social, and policy issues in genetics. In F. Lashley (Ed.), *The genetics revolution: Implications for nursing.* Washington, DC: American Academy of Nursing.

Tinkle, M. (2002). Cystic fibrosis carrier screening: Are nurses ready to be on the front line? *AWHONN Lifelines, 6*(2), 134-139.

Tinkle, M., & Cheek, D. (2002). Human genomics: Challenges and opportunities. *Journal of Obstetric, Gynecologic, and Neonatal Nursing, 31*(2), 178-187.

Touchette, N., Holtzman, N., Davis, J., & Feetham, S. (Eds.). (1997). *Toward the 21st century: Incorporating genetics into primary health care.* Cold Spring Harbor, NY: Cold Spring Harbor Laboratory Press.

Van Riper, M. (1999). Living with Down syndrome: The family experience. *Down Syndrome Quarterly, 4*(1), 1-11.

Van Riper, M. (2003). A change of plans: The birth of a child with Down syndrome. *American Journal of Nursing, 103*(6), 71-74.

Van Riper, M. (2004). What families need to thrive. *Down Syndrome News, 27*, 18-22.

Van Riper, M. (2005). Genetic testing and the family. *Journal of Midwifery & Women's Health, 50*(3), 227-233.

Van Riper, M., & Cohen, W. (2001). Caring for children with Down syndrome and their families. *Journal of Pediatric Health Care, 15*(3), 123-131.

Van Riper, M., & Gallo, A. (2006). Family, health, and genomics. In D. Crane & E. Marshall (Eds.), *Handbook of families and health: Interdisciplinary perspectives.* Thousand Oaks, CA: Sage.

Van Riper, M., & McKinnon, W. (2004). Genetic testing for breast and ovarian cancer susceptibility: A family experience. *Journal of Midwifery & Women's Health, 43*(3), 210-219.

Venter, J., Adams, M., Myers, E., Li, P., Mural, R., Sutton, G., et al. (2001). The sequence of the human genome. *Science 291*(5507), 1304-1351.

Vogelstein, B., & Kinzler, K. (2002). *The genetic basis of human cancer* (2nd ed.). New York: McGraw-Hill.

Yang, Q., Rasmussen, S., & Friedman, J. (2002). Mortality associated with Down's syndrome in the USA from 1983 to 1997: A population-based study. *Lancet, 359*(9311), 1019-1025.

Yoon, P., Chen, B., Faucett, A., Clyne, M., Gwinn, M., Lubin, I., et al. (2001). Public health impact of genetic tests at the end of the 20th century. *Genetic Medicine, 3*(6), 405-410.

Zawacki, K., & Phillips, M. (2002). Cancer genetics and women's health. *Journal of Obstetric, Gynecologic, and Neonatal Nursing, 31*(2), 208-216.

Alternative and Complementary Therapies

learning objectives

- Describe the differences between standard (allopathic or Western) and holistic health care.
- Define the biopsychosocial and spiritual implications of holistic health care.
- Outline the advantages of a holistic philosophy.

- Compare and contrast touch, energetic, mind-body, and alternative pharmacologic healing modalities.
- Discuss the limitations of research in holistic healing.
- Identify the appropriate modalities for integrative women's health care.

electronic resources

Additional information related to the content in Chapter 4 can be found on

the companion website at *evolve*
http://evolve.elsevier.com/Lowdermilk/MWHC/
- NCLEX Review Questions
- WebLinks

or on the interactive companion CD
- NCLEX Review Questions

IT began as a quiet revolution. Consumers, feeling dismayed with the depersonalization of health care and the increasing reliance on high technology and specialization, began investigating alternatives to standard (allopathic or Western) medicine. Voicing dissatisfaction with hurried providers, decisions being made by insurance companies, and increasing health care costs, some consumers turned to folk healers, spiritual healers, massage therapists, or herbalists.

It has long been argued that the current U.S. health care system is disease focused. For example, insurance companies may offer reimbursement for the treatment of various illnesses but not for health maintenance activities; new drugs for chronic illnesses appear in large numbers, but little attention is paid to the role of diet in health and in disease. Stress has been identified as a major health problem, but the treatment of choice has often been pharmaceutical agents rather than lifestyle change and stress management techniques at a fraction of the cost.

In an emerging paradigm, health is valued, and a new appreciation for the connection of body, mind, and spirit is honored and nurtured. Human values, including spirituality (that which brings values, meaning, and purpose to

life, blending with the sense of the divine, the natural environment, other individuals, and the inner self), ethics, and partnership within health care, are coming together with the finest in technology and research. In her classic work, Ferguson (1980) suggested that holistic healing, including alternative and complementary therapies, focuses on the correction of underlying disharmony in the interaction of body, mind, and spirit and demonstrates concern and compassion for the whole client, not just the client's symptoms (Box 4-1). Holism (a philosophy that an integrated whole has an independent reality that is greater than the sum of its parts, that patterns and processes combine to form the whole, and that evaluation, acceptance, and modulation of those patterns can lead to profound personal healing) encompasses attitude, acceptance, perception, and purpose.

Many of the popular alternative healing modalities offer human-centered care, with philosophies that recognize the value of the client's input and honor the individual's beliefs, values, and desires. The focus of these modalities is the whole person, not just a disease complex. Clients often find that alternative modalities are more consistent with their own belief systems and allow more client autonomy in health care decisions (Gordon, 2004).

---

box 4-1 **Definitions**

An understanding of the following terms used to describe alternative therapies is essential:

- **Acupressure** Massage techniques applied to specific points along certain energy pathways of the body called meridians. A form of treatment based in the theories of traditional Chinese medicine.
- **Acupuncture** A form of treatment using slender needles to stimulate points along energy pathways to correct, enhance, and rebalance the flow of body energy.
- **Alternative and complementary therapies** Nontraditional approaches to health care and healing, often philosophically different from Western medicine. Often involve interventions that are said to induce healing from within the client or improve the internal environment so that the body, mind, or spirit can heal. Often referred to as "natural healing." Can be used in place of or in conjunction with standard health care practices. Also defined as therapeutic modalities not commonly taught by U.S. medical schools or available in U.S. hospitals. Alternative healing often refers to those modalities used *in place of* conventional (or other) health care. Complementary healing refers to those modalities used *in conjunction with* conventional (or other) health care. Many therapies can be either alternative or complementary.
- **Biofeedback** Techniques that teach the client to consciously control certain body functions usually thought of as unconscious (breathing, heart rate, etc.). Often involves electronic instrumentation that provides immediate visual and auditory feedback to assist the learning process.
- **Energy healing** A variety of techniques and disciplines that are said to augment, modulate, stimulate, or remedy certain deficiencies or blocks in the human energy system.
- **Guided imagery** The use of imagination and thought processes in a purposeful way to change certain physiologic and emotional conditions.
- **Healing** The integrating and balancing of the body, mind, and spirit. May or may not effect physical healing from illness. Often perceived as improved sense of well-being, acceptance, and inner peace and harmony.
- **Healing touch** A combination of energetic healing techniques used by nurses and other health care professionals.
- **Holism** Philosophy that states that the whole is greater than the sum of its parts. In healing, refers to consideration and treatment of the whole client as a unified being. May

include alternative and complementary modalities but is more a philosophic base than a modality in and of itself.
- **Holistic medicine** Health care treatment with techniques not commonly taught in U.S. medical schools or widely available in U.S. hospitals. May include a variety of disciplines involving diet, exercise, vitamin and nutritional supplements, body work, or alternative pharmacologic agents. Philosophy of medicine that encompasses holism.
- **Holistic nursing** Nursing practice that stems from the philosophy of holism, one that views the client as an integrated whole and as influenced by a variety of internal and external factors, including the biopsychosocial and spiritual dimensions of the person, an integrated whole.
- **Meditation** Any activity that focuses the attention in the present moment and, in the process, quiets and relaxes the mind and body.
- **Reflection** Looking within for solutions and answers to certain dilemmas, using intuition and inner wisdom as guides for attainment of healing.
- **Relaxation** The absence or alleviation of mental, physical, and emotional tension through purposeful activities that quiet the mind and body.
- **Spirituality** The individual's connection to one's own values, purpose, and meaning of life. May encompass organized religion or belief in higher power or authority. Recognition of wisdom, imagination, spirit, and intuition. A perception of the unity of nature and the interconnectedness of all beings; inner strength.
- **Standard (Western or allopathic) medicine** Interchangeable terms used to describe the current American health care system. With foundations in germ theory and reductionism, standard medical practice often focuses on one body system or disease complex. Treatments are often pharmaceutical or surgical and produce effects that are different from those of the disease complex.
- **Therapeutic touch** A modern interpretation of the laying on of hands for healing, as interpreted by Dolores Krieger, PhD, RN, and Dora Kunz, a noted healer. Originally taught within nursing programs.
- **Traditional Chinese medicine** Ancient methods of healing that combine herbs, energy healing, and movement as a pathway to health. Seeks to heal on deeper levels rather than just deal with symptoms.

Sources: Dossey, B. (Ed.). (1997). *Core curriculum for holistic nursing.* Gaithersburg, MD: Aspen; Dossey, B., Keegan, L., & Guzzetta, C. (2005). *Holistic nursing: A handbook for practice* (4th ed.). Sudbury, MA: Jones and Bartlett; Ferguson, M. (1980). *The Aquarian conspiracy.* Los Angeles: J. P. Tarcher; and Goldberg, B., Anderson, J., & Trivieri, L. (Eds.). (2002). *Alternative medicine: The definitive guide* (2nd ed.). Berkeley, CA: Ten Speed Press.

Although standard medical practice excels in many areas, alternative methods are often cited as being more beneficial for the treatment of chronic illness, as well as being more cost-effective because of the emphasis on preventive care and health maintenance (Weil, 2004).

Consumerism has driven the need for scholarly investigation of these therapies. Increasing numbers of American adults have sought alternative care, in spite of the fact that these services are not generally covered by health care insurance. These clients want a more active role in their health care decision making, more choices, and fewer

interventional procedures. Those with chronic or debilitating diseases often search for alternatives that will improve the quality of their lives, rather than effect a total cure (Barnes, Powell-Griner, McFann, & Nahin, 2004; Gordon, 2004; Kessler et al., 2001; Ni, Simile, & Hardy, 2002).

Although skeptical at first, physicians, nurses, and other providers began to see the value in integrating some of these alternative methods into health care. The research and knowledge base for alternative and complementary therapies has grown and will continue to expand as the interest in and quest for healing continues.

This chapter presents an overview of alternative and complementary therapies, their place in current health care practices, current research endeavors, the role of the nurse in holistic health care, and possibilities for use in women's health care.

OVERVIEW OF ALTERNATIVE AND COMPLEMENTARY MODALITIES

Alternative health care options are many and diverse. Some modalities focus on the body structure and balance, and some on the biochemical environment. Various treatment forms address emotional and psychologic health, and others work with the human energy field. It is beyond the scope of this chapter to address all the philosophic and procedural specifics of current alternative and complementary therapies; many texts and reference volumes provide detailed information (Goldberg, Anderson, & Trivieri, 2002).

Regardless of modality, several concepts are shared by many of these systems. First, there is an emphasis on the client as a whole being, capable of decision making and an integral part of the health care team. Clients are encouraged to take responsibility for their health and healing. Equal consideration is provided for all the biopsychosocial and spiritual needs of the client. Each client is seen as a unique individual, and treatment is tailored to that specific person (Dossey, Keegan, & Guzzetta, 2005).

Second, proper nutrition, adequate rest, relaxation, exercise, and emotional health are cornerstones of good health and are thought to promote healing. Although various philosophies advocate a variety of dietary regimens, there is agreement that nutrition is often overlooked by mainstream medicine and must be emphasized for healing to occur. Our fast-paced culture often seems to deny individuals the chance to make time for rest, relaxation, exercise, and spiritual renewal (Dossey et al., 2005; Weil, 2004).

Third, signs and symptoms of disease states are seen as reflective of deeper processes, including those on the emotional and spiritual levels. Alternative healing modalities attempt to treat those deeper levels and the underlying causes, rather than just the symptoms. Physical symptoms are seen as signals from the mind and the spirit that change is in order (Ferguson, 1980; Gerber, Tiller, & Cousens, 2001; Weil, 2004). The road to healing therefore becomes an individual journey, encompassing the client's entire being while addressing specific physical, mental, emotional, spiritual, and social needs.

Integrative Health Care

The health care community exists as a fluid and dynamic environment. With a variety of clinicians, from physicians and nurses, physical therapists, and mental health counselors to acupuncturists and massage therapists, energy healers, and herbalists, a variety of philosophies and treatment options exist.

Western medicine excels in the treatment of acute diseases, bacterial diseases, surgical emergencies, and trauma. It has also, by necessity, become highly specialized and systematic. With the vast amount of information and research available, it is virtually impossible for one practitioner to know and absorb all of the current data. With increasing specialization in health care, providers often focus on one body system or disease, and other symptoms may be overlooked or not evaluated. Clients who seek alternative health care often do so in an attempt to find a practitioner who will address the client as a whole person and who shares the client's own philosophy, convictions, and values (Gordon, 2004; Weil, 2004).

Western medicine has been less successful in the treatment of chronic disease states, such as diabetes, heart disease, immune disorders, and environmental illnesses. Over time, the role of the mind in the health of the body has been forgotten or neglected. Chronic disease states have been treated with an increasing number of pharmaceutical agents or invasive surgery, but the root causes of such ailments have not been considered. The avenues to continued and improved health have not been fully explored (Dossey et al., 2005; Weil, 2004).

It is imperative that health care become an integrative and cooperative venture, one in which both mainstream and alternative medicine can be accessed and used. Fortunately, an environment is being created in which healing forms are used for what they do best and work side by side in harmony. Medical schools, hospitals, and health care institutions are devising integrative health care models, and these programs are expected to proliferate as the health care system responds to increased consumer demand. Barriers still exist to complete integration, including a lack of research; opposing or competing philosophies and paradigms; health care cost concerns; lack of consistency in state licensing laws; and lasting biases, attitudes, and prejudices (Adams, Cohen, Eisenberg, & Jonsen, 2002; Wetzel, Kaptchuk, Haramatil, & Eisenberg, 2003).

Research Efforts

In 1992 the National Institutes of Health (NIH) developed the Office of Alternative Medicine (OAM). Mandated by Congress, the OAM was designed to support research and evaluation of various alternative and complementary modalities and to provide information to health care consumers about such modalities. Funding has provided research grants; development and maintenance of a research database; dissemination of information to both health care providers and consumers; funds to support, evaluate, and coordinate domestic and worldwide research; and help to train researchers. In 1998, Congress instituted the National Center for Complementary and Alternative Medicine (NCCAM), which incorporates the work of the OAM in its mission and function (altmed.od.nih.gov/nccam). Funding has been granted to researchers investigating guided imagery, biofeedback, prayer, movement (dance, yoga, qi gong, and tai chi), music, acupuncture, chiropractic, massage, homeopathy, herbs, and other therapies for a variety of disease processes and health concerns (NCCAM, 2005).

To facilitate definitions and research, the NIH established seven categories of alternative and complementary healing (Table 4-1). Although many therapies belong in more than one category, this system provides a starting point for research and data collection.

table 4-1 **National Institutes of Health Categories of Alternative Healing Modalities**

CATEGORY	EXAMPLES
Alternative systems of medical practice	Acupuncture
	Ayurveda
	Environmental medicine
	Homeopathy
	Native American healing
	Naturopathic medicine
	Shamanism
	Traditional Chinese medicine
Bioelectromagnetic applications	Electroacupuncture
	Neuromagnetic stimulation devices
Diet, nutrition, lifestyle changes	Changes in lifestyle
	Diet
	Macrobiotics
	Megavitamins and other nutritional supplements
Herbal medicine	Herbal approaches from a variety of cultures including the Americas, Europe, and the Far East
Manual healing	Acupressure
	Chiropractic
	Massage therapy
	Osteopathy
	Reflexology
	Therapeutic touch/healing touch
	Trager method
Mind-body control	Art therapy
	Biofeedback
	Counseling
	Dance therapy
	Guided imagery and hypnosis
	Humor therapy
	Meditation
	Music therapy
	Prayer
	Psychotherapy
	Relaxation
	Support and self-help groups
	Yoga
Pharmacologic and biologic treatments	Antioxidizing agents
	Chelation therapy
	Oxidizing agents
	Vaccines (not currently accepted by mainstream medicine)

Source: National Center for Complementary and Alternative Medicine (NCCAM)/Office of Alternative Medicine (OAM). (2005). Accessed http://nccam.nih.gov, August 21, 2006.

▬ THE NURSE'S ROLE: HOLISTIC NURSING

Nursing is coming full circle. As consumers seek medical treatment that is more caring and personal, nurses are playing a key role in the rehumanization of health care. Although it was originally grounded in the holistic theories of Nightingale (Dossey, 2000), nursing has moved into highly technical areas, often losing some of the human-centered caring that was once its hallmark. Many nurses now are rediscovering the value of client-centered care that addresses the whole person, not just a diagnosis or condition. With that realization, these nurses often self-identify as holistic nurses.

Holistic nurses can be found in every area of nursing practice. Being holistic refers more to one's underlying philosophy than to the tasks assigned to a specific nurse. Holistic nurses provide care that is relationship centered rather than disease or task oriented. By seeing the client as a whole individual, nurses can then provide care that encompasses all of the needs of the individual: physical, emotional, spiritual, or social. Seeking to blend technology with healing, holistic nurses are striving to create models of health care that embrace the whole person while enhancing healing and the interconnectedness of all beings (Dossey et al., 2005). Holistic nurses recognize the need

box 4-2 **What is Holistic Nursing?**

- Holistic nursing embraces all nursing that has as its goal the enhancement of healing the whole person from birth to death. Holistic nursing recognizes that there are two views regarding holism: (1) that holism involves identifying the interrelationships of the bio-psycho-social-spiritual dimensions of the person, recognizing that the whole is greater than the sum of its parts; and (2) that holism involves understanding the individual as a unitary whole in mutual process with the environment. Holistic nursing responds to both views, believing that the goals of nursing can be achieved within either framework.
- The holistic nurse is an instrument of healing and a facilitator in the healing process. Holistic nurses honor the individual's subjective experience about health, health beliefs, and values. To become therapeutic partners with individuals, families, and communities, holistic nursing practice draws on nursing knowledge, theories, research, expertise, intuition, and creativity. Holistic nursing practice encourages peer review of professional practice in various clinical settings and integrates knowledge of current professional standards, laws, and regulations governing nursing practice.
- Practicing holistic nursing requires nurses to integrate self-care, self-responsibility, spirituality, and reflection in their lives. This may lead the nurse to greater awareness of the interconnectedness with self, others, nature, and God/Life-Force/Absolute/Transcendent. This awareness may further enhance the nurses' understanding of all individuals and their relationships to the human and global community, and permits nurses to use this awareness to facilitate the healing process.

Source: American Holistic Nurses' Association. (2005). Flagstaff, AZ: Author.

for health care to be based on the interrelated relationships between client and provider, provider and provider, and community and provider.

Although many holistic nurses incorporate and integrate alternative and complementary healing modalities into their practices, these techniques are not prerequisites for holistic nursing practice. Holistic nursing practice reflects the attitudes and philosophy brought to the nursing situation, rather than the techniques or modalities used during the course of nursing care. Holistic nurses also involve themselves in self-care activities, striving to attain their own levels of wellness and integration (Box 4-2) (Dossey et al., 2005; Frisch, Dossey, Guzzetta, & Quinn, 2000).

As the body of knowledge grows, more methods will be integrated into nursing practice. Many modalities require intensive training, additional certification, or both. As with basic nursing practice, certain competencies must be established before using the skill with clients. With the introduction of dozens of various modalities into health care, nurses are cautioned to examine carefully the reputation, research, and educational criteria of any program of study.

The North American Nursing Diagnosis Association (NANDA) also has acknowledged the emergence of holism with several nursing diagnoses. These include "imbalanced," "risk for," and "readiness for enhanced" spiritual well-being, spiritual distress, and energy field disturbance. The Nursing Interventions Classification (NIC) lists several alternative modalities as nursing interventions. These include but are not limited to therapeutic touch (TT), simple massage, touch, relaxation, meditation, imagery, and hypnosis (Dossey et al., 2005; Frisch et al., 2000).

■ **LEGAL TIP** Scope of Practice
for Healing Modalities

Although a vast array of alternative healing modalities are available, not all of them are within the scope of nursing practice, as defined by licensing bodies (Box 4-3). Nurses are advised to consult their own state's nurse practice act for details on the additional training required to integrate complementary healing into their nursing practice.

Support and Education for Holistic Nursing

In 1980 a group of nurses and supporters formed the American Holistic Nurses' Association (AHNA) to assist and support nurses in their journeys to holism (www.ahna. org). A vital force in nursing today, AHNA has established basic and advanced certification in holistic nursing and published a core curriculum of holistic nursing practice (Dossey, 1997). It is the mission of AHNA "to unite nurses in healing" (AHNA, 2005). This is to be accomplished through the development, implementation, and evaluation of the standards, education, and research for holistic nursing. This mission is accomplished through various educational offerings, certification, and support of holistic nursing research. AHNA also supports the individual

---

box 4-3 **Holistic Therapies and Modalities Most Commonly Used in Nursing**

- *Body therapies,* including acupressure, healing touch, massage, therapeutic touch, reflexology
- *Mind-body healing,* including art therapy, biofeedback, cognitive therapy, counseling (in cases of addiction, grief, environmental concerns, relationships, spiritual crisis, violence and sexual abuse, and wellness issues), exercise and movement, goal setting and contracts, holistic self-assessment, journaling and self-reflection, meditation, prayer, humor and laughter, imagery, music and sound therapy, play therapy, rituals of healing (combining several modalities)
- *Lifestyle modifications,* including smoking cessation, weight management

Sources: Dossey, B. (Ed.). (1997). *Core curriculum for holistic nursing.* Gaithersburg, MD: Aspen; Dossey, B., Keegan, L., & Guzzetta, C. (2005). *Holistic nursing: A handbook for practice* (4th ed.). Sudbury, MA: Jones and Bartlett.

---

journey toward wholeness and healing by encouraging self-care and personal growth for nurses (AHNA, 2005; Frisch et al., 2000).

Across the country, more and more schools of nursing are offering and integrating classes that reflect the holistic perspective. Examples of offered coursework include holistic nursing concepts, herbal healing, energetic modalities, environmental concerns, and body work. These classes increase critical thinking, self-care, and leadership skills, as well as cultural awareness. Several major universities now offer graduate-level degrees with a focus in holistic nursing (Richardson, 2004).

■ ALTERNATIVE AND COMPLEMENTARY
■ THERAPIES IN WOMEN'S HEALTH CARE

Women's health care is an emerging specialty. There is increased realization that the human female body is biochemically different from the male body. The long-standing gender biases of Western medicine are giving way to a broader view of women's health care. In the realm of holistic medicine, too, an increasing number of modalities are seen as appropriate and are being integrated into care. Thousands of articles and books exist on these topics; this section addresses only an overview of a representative sample of those most often used in women's health care and specific to nursing practice (Box 4-4).

Touch and Energetic Healing

One of the most primitive yet effective healing gestures is that of touch. First recorded more than 5000 years ago by ancient Asian healers, touch has been a key element of healing through the ages. It is a natural instinct to touch that which hurts or needs comfort. The touch of a mother's hand to her child's feverish head and the touch of one friend to another in a time of crisis are clear images of this intuitive healing method.

---

box 4-4 **Representative Alternative Therapies**

TOUCH AND ENERGETIC THERAPIES
- Massage
- Acupressure
- Therapeutic touch
- Healing touch

MIND-BODY HEALING
- Imagery
- Meditation, prayer, reflection
- Biofeedback
- Other modalities that may fall outside of nurse practice guidelines unless the nurse has completed additional training or certification:
  Herbs
  Homeopathy
  Traditional Chinese medicine

The use of touch for healing has many forms. Most people are familiar with massage therapy and its various methods. Massage involves rubbing, stroking, and manipulating the muscle groups and other connective tissue to relieve tension and pain and increase blood flow to the area, thus promoting healing. Various claims are made for the different modes of massage therapy, including increasing circulation, promoting lymphatic drainage, relieving muscle tension, aiding in recovery from certain musculoskeletal injuries, decreasing edema, and improving the functioning of certain body systems. Although simple massage is listed in the nursing intervention categories, therapeutic massage requires additional formal training, and national certification is available. Massage therapists are subject to individual state laws and regulations (Goldberg et al., 2002; Reilly, 2005).

Other forms of touch in healing combine physical touch and energetic theory. A variety of alternative and complementary therapies use an energy-based philosophy that essentially states that the human body has an energy field around and in it. That energy field not only is detectable, but also can be modulated and changed. Energy-based healing seeks to improve the health of the energy field, balance it, and restore it, so that the body then can heal. Any physical, emotional, or spiritual illness is said to be detectable in the field, as well as healed with the field (Hover-Kramer, Mentgen, & Scandrett-Hibdon, 2001; Oschman, 2000). In many respects, this is congruent with the nursing theory of Martha Rogers (1970), who spoke of the person as a four-dimensional being.

Energy healing (www.healingtouch.net) has its roots in the writings of the ancient Hindus (who spoke of *prana*), Asians (who referred to it as *chi,* or *qi*), and Greeks and early Christians. The healing ability of Jesus is interpreted by some as an energetic healing form. Healing as part of a spiritual path was routinely practiced by clergy and lay persons alike within the context of their religious practices until Pope Alexander mandated a halt to the healing

mission of the church in the twelfth century. Although this took healing out of the hands of the church, history records many talented healers who continued to use energetic techniques (Dossey et al., 2005; Gerber et al., 2001; Hover-Kramer et al., 2001).

Acupressure is a variation on massage and touch that has its origins in traditional Chinese medicine (TCM). TCM states that *qi,* or *chi,* is the vital force of life, the energy of the body. If the energy is blocked or stagnated in any way, illness, pain, or other dysfunction can result. Energy travels on defined pathways throughout the body, called meridians, and on each meridian, a series of points corresponds to body function and various organs. Practitioners of TCM believe that by massaging or compressing a given point, the body energy to that corresponding organ or system can be restored or changed. When the energy flow is restored, healing can occur (Flaws, 2004; Gerber et al., 2001; Goldberg et al., 2002; Oschman, 2000). Although nurses can learn a few select points to use with their clients, a comprehensive education program is desirable for the treatment of more complex health problems.

In nursing circles, one of the best-known methods of touch healing is therapeutic touch (TT) (www.therapeutic-touch.org). TT was designed by Dolores Krieger, PhD, RN, a professor of nursing at New York University. She documented a reproducible manner of touch, one in which the practitioner begins in a calm and centered state (called "centering") and holds thoughts of desiring to help or heal (called "intention"). TT has several steps in which the practitioner perceives the client's energy field and notes any areas of uneven activity, deficit, or increase. After observing and feeling the client's energy field, the practitioner can use techniques to modulate the energy and correct the deficiencies or abnormal areas. Krieger's seminal work in the field of human energy is well described in her many publications (Krieger, 1979, 1987, 1993, 2002; Kunz & Krieger, 2004). TT has been widely researched in the nursing field. Early studies documented pain relief, anxiety reduction, and wound healing; later work focused more on physiologic data (Quinn, 1994; Snyder & Lindquist, 2002, Ventegodt, Morad, & Merrick, 2004).

Healing Touch (HT) is another energy-based touch healing modality. Whereas Krieger's work emphasizes a single sequence of energy modulation, HT combines a variety of techniques from a series of disciplines. This gives the practitioner an array of "tools" to use with clients. Practitioners are taught energetic diagnosis and treatment forms and the means for documenting the client's response and progress. These techniques are said to align and balance the human energy field, thereby enhancing the body's ability to heal itself. Proponents assert that HT can be useful for a variety of physical, mental, emotional, and spiritual disorders (Hover-Kramer et al., 2001).

Nursing research on HT is expanding rapidly. Studies focusing on its use by nurses with clients experiencing chronic and acute pain, wound infections, cancer, human immunodeficiency virus infection, depression, fatigue, anxiety, and other health problems are being conducted or have been completed. Nurses also are investigating the phenomenologic implications of this modality, from both the client's and the provider's perspective. Of special note to nurses involved in women's health care are studies on HT with stress disorders, chronic and acute pain, surgical recovery, and cancer (Healing Touch, 2005; Hover-Kramer et al., 2001) (www.therapeutictouch.org).

TT and HT have been integrated in many health care facilities and institutions, and policies have been written and accepted to make these modalities part of inpatient care. As independent nursing interventions, they do not require a physician's order for the nurse to provide this service.

Mind-Body Healing

Use of the mind as a healing tool also is rooted in ancient teachings. The use of imagination, prayer, and meditation is found in numerous spiritual traditions dating back to the beginning of recorded history.

Guided imagery, the purposeful development of mental images while in a deep state of relaxation (Heinschel, 2005), is used for relaxation, stress management, and enhancing immune function (www.academyforguidedimagery.com). Imagery allows or guides the normal flow of thoughts within the imagination. It can be likened to the sense of being worried, when mental pictures and thoughts of a dreaded event occur. Although there may not be a direct threat to the person at the time, the mind can induce feelings of fear with associated body symptoms such as tightening the chest or stomach or the onset of sweating. These symptoms are in response to a perception or a thought, but not always to a concurrent event. Imagery uses the power of the mind to induce positive images of healing, improve performance, and reduce anxiety. The mind will then influence the body to meet the image (Dossey et al., 2000; Heinschel, 2005; LeMaire, 2002; Snyder & Lindquist, 2002).

Proponents also state that a relaxed body and focused mind can bring about changes in perception and solutions to problems, and heal emotional trauma. Imagery also has been used with clients with allergies, musculoskeletal pain, and acute injuries, and in preoperative and postoperative situations. Cancer clients have used imagery to decrease the side effects of treatment. Nurses use guided imagery in private practice as well as in health care settings (Fig. 4-1). Imagery can assist relaxation, reduce anxiety, minimize the need for pain medications, and increase the client's ability to focus, while enhancing creativity. By using recall to enhance change, imagery also may alter emotional and biochemical processes (Dossey et al., 2005; Heinschel, 2005) (www.integrativeimagery.com).

Meditation, prayer, reflection, and relaxation are similar modalities, all creating an environment of inner quiet. These are ways of looking inside the self and connecting with inner wisdom and intuition. Although some religious traditions define prayer as a communication with God, others simply define it in terms of connecting with a divine or absolute power found within all beings. Prayer is said to

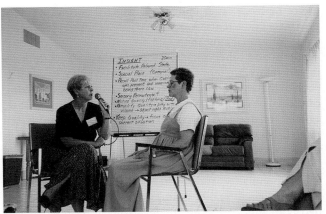

FIG. 4-1 Nurse and client during guided imagery session. (Courtesy Nurses Certificate Program in Interactive Imagery, Foster City, CA.)

be a speaking out, whereas meditation is a quiet listening. Reflection, then, is the evaluation and synthesis of the experience (Dossey et al., 2005; Henry & Henry, 2004).

These techniques can aid in the relaxation response and decrease heart rate and blood pressure, thereby reducing stress, decreasing pain perception, and increasing self-understanding. This is thought to allow insight, cognitive awareness of body functioning, and an intuitive comprehension of what is needed for the individual healing process (Dossey et al., 2005; Goldberg et al., 2002; Snyder & Lindquist, 2002).

Biofeedback combines relaxation with consciously learning to regulate those body functions normally seen as automatic to improve health and decrease pain, blood pressure, and pulse rate. With specially designed equipment that can monitor heart rate, muscle tension, and skin temperature, moisture, and electrical conductivity, clients are taught the means to reduce tension, induce relaxation, and isolate and exercise certain muscle groups. Biofeedback instruments provide immediate information to the client and show the progress made, thus reinforcing the client behaviors that brought about the desired change. For example, if a certain breathing technique induces a significant and desired change in heart rate and blood pressure, the client can immediately see the effects on the biofeedback instrumentation and feel the change within the body (Goldberg et al., 2002; Snyder & Lindquist, 2002).

Biofeedback also can assist with muscle training. By enabling the client to focus on specific muscle groups, correct exercises can be learned with the help of biofeedback. After several sessions, the client is usually able to isolate and exercise the same muscle groups, even without the biofeedback equipment. Applications for women's health include continence training, pain control, and stress reduction.

Alternative Pharmacologic Modalities

Some of the complementary therapies most frequently used by American consumers today are those involving alternatives to drug therapy. These modalities involve the use of herbs or other remedies outside the usual scope of pharmaceutic agents. Proper use of these therapies mandates additional education.

Herbs and other botanic substances were used for healing in many ancient civilizations. Although it is often considered a folk remedy, herbal medicine plays a significant role even today. Many of our current pharmacologic agents are derived from or originated in a plant-based model. Digitalis, for example, is a derivative of plants in the foxglove family, and atropine was first derived from the deadly nightshade. Recently herbal preparations have gained popularity, and several have been investigated for their medicinal qualities. St. John's wort has been identified as an antidepressant, and feverfew has been researched for its role in preventing migraines.

By definition, one is practicing herbal medicine if one uses a cup of mint tea to soothe an upset stomach. However, the science of herbal medicine is complex and precise. Herbs can vary in potency from day to day and season to season; whereas a small dose may be beneficial, a larger one can be hazardous. Herbal preparations are readily available to the public in a variety of settings, including health food stores and supermarkets. However, they can vary in concentration, and consumers should be advised to read all labels carefully for information about the actual herbal component of the selected preparation (Skidmore-Roth, 2004; Weed, 2001).

Herbs are classified according to their properties and effects (Fig. 4-2). Most herbal medicine texts list the desired effect and the properties of the herb itself. Herbs can be delivered in whole form (dried and powdered), as a tea (steeped in water), as extracts and tinctures (small amounts dissolved in an alcohol base), in capsules or tablets, as concentrated "essential" oil, and in creams and salves.

Herbs are medicine. They can have side effects and contraindications. Clients should be asked about their use of herbs in conjunction with standard pharmaceuticals. Herbs can counteract or intensify pharmaceutical effects, and they

can be dangerous if taken in higher than recommended doses (Simpkins, Thurston, Colyer, & Talbot, 2005).

Homeopathy is a system of healing founded by Samuel Hahnemann, a German physician, in the late 1700s. Hahnemann, also known for his work in pharmacology and toxicology, sought to find a more sensible and compassionate alternative to the medical practices of his day (for example, bloodletting with leeches and use of toxic laxatives). By experimenting with certain botanic agents, he confirmed Hippocrates' observation that small doses of the same agent that caused a disease would cure it. This also is the basis for modern immunologic medicine, wherein a small amount of a toxin, allergen, or virus stimulates the body to create immunity (Goldberg et al., 2002; Lansky, 2003).

Homeopathic practitioners believe that each client is a unique individual, and care is directed to create and prescribe a remedy specific to that person. Although many standard remedies exist, practitioners often blend individual remedies based on the client's specific needs. Homeopathy also dictates that illness, as perceived on the physical level, is evidence of disturbances on other, deeper levels; the remedies are thought to work through those other levels, from the most recent through the oldest, until full healing is achieved (Goldberg et al., 2002; Lansky, 2003).

Combining herbal and energy medicine, Traditional Chinese Medicine (TCM) is experiencing a resurgence of popularity. It has been practiced for more than 3000 years and was one of the first methods of healing to be documented. TCM incorporates theories of energetic healing, often describing the energy flow as an excess or a deficiency. The goal of TCM is to restore total harmony on all levels: emotional, spiritual, and physical. Although acupressure is a discipline within TCM, traditional methods include acupuncture (the stimulation of specific points on the body with needles, herbs, or heat) and herbal treatments. Various movement forms such as *tai chi* and *qi gong* may be integrated into a program of TCM (Flaws, 2004; Goldberg et al., 2002).

Acupuncture is widely practiced in the United States for a variety of conditions and is showing promise in the areas of pain management (postoperative states, dental procedures, fibromyalgia, and myofascial pain) and nausea caused by pregnancy or chemotherapy. Research is continuing to determine its efficacy in other areas (NCCAM, 2006).

Nutrition and Exercise

The current North American diet is changing; we have become a nation of "fast-food" eaters, quickly consuming meals that are high in fat and calories and often lacking in essential nutrients. Stress, lifestyle choices, and time constraints are most often cited as reasons for the lack of balanced food intake. Although there is no consistent agreement regarding actual intake and dietary structure, most will agree that reduction of saturated fats and calories and proportionate consumption of high-quality protein and complex carbohydrates are the keys to a balanced diet. Scores of weight-loss and food-management programs are

FIG. 4-2 Traditional Chinese medicine pharmacy in a Hong Kong hospital. (Courtesy Shelley Conroy, Ogden, UT.)

available to the consumer, but not all provide the essential balance of nutrients (Martin & Jung, 2002; Northrup, 2002; Padden, 2002; Weil, 2004).

Adequate nutrition benefits the human system on all levels. These include but are not limited to normal organ development and functioning, appropriate metabolism, immune system response, optimal energy, reproductive function, functional repair of injury or tissue damage, appropriate emotional responses, and behavior (Dossey, 1997). Women seem especially sensitive to the lack of micronutrients and macronutrients in their diets, and deficiencies can manifest as hormonal changes or irregular menstrual periods, as well as affecting other endocrine functions (Martin & Jung, 2002; Northrup, 2002, 2003). Nurses should be aware that a diet history should be part of any care plan.

Citizens of our nation also lack the motivation for consistent exercise. Our lifestyle has become more sedentary, with hours spent in front of computers or television sets. Our children spend countless hours with video games. Current guidelines promote 60 minutes of some form of physical exercise daily to achieve the known benefits of improved cardiovascular health, decreased body fat, disease prevention, and increased sense of well-being. Exercise programs should be less outcome oriented and should focus more on daily progress. Weight-bearing exercise (especially walking) is extremely beneficial for women to prevent osteoporosis. Nursing interventions for the promotion of adequate physical exercise include providing motivation and support, working with the client to find an exercise form that suits the client's needs and ability, facilitating education regarding the numerous health benefits, and monitoring of the client's progress (Martin & Jung, 2002; Padden, 2002). Unlimited forms of exercise can be beneficial on a multitude of levels, including yoga, martial arts, aerobics, and weight and endurance training (Box 4-5, Fig. 4-3).

Applications in Women's Health Care

Many women seek "natural" alternatives to invasive health care practices. Whether looking for natural childbirth or alternatives for menopause, women have been more open to complementary modalities and have more actively sought care from practitioners of holistic medicine. Research is ongoing, and significant strides are being made to open the doors to health care that encompasses the whole person while providing comprehensive health care (Collins, 2002; Northrup, 2002, 2003) (Critical Thinking Exercise).

Pregnancy and Maternity Care

Pregnancy is usually seen as a naturally occurring event, but highly technical medical practices have shifted the

---

box 4-5 | Yoga: An Example of Lifestyle Choice

With the increasing emphasis on diet and exercise programs, the practice of yoga can be used as an example of a lifestyle choice that meets a variety of needs, envisioning the client from a bio-psycho-social-spiritual perspective.

BIOLOGY

- Yoga provides structured exercise that can increase strength, flexibility, and endurance. Postures, or *asanas,* focus on various body systems, are seen as corrective for certain disease states, and increase endorphin release. Although some definitions may be regionally different, yoga is practiced in a variety of forms, each presenting its own challenge and focus. *Hatha yoga* focuses on slowly and deliberately stretching within the asanas, lengthening and strengthening the various muscle groups. *Astanga yoga* promotes endurance with more difficult and athletic poses and stretches. *Vinyasa yoga* adds an aerobic component with more rapid progression with athletic postures. The postures are said to affect a variety of body functions, including balance, muscle tone, and coordination.
- Yoga also incorporates controlled deep breathing, or *pranayama,* to energize and stimulate the body. This also is said to enhance cardiovascular functioning, stimulate blood flow, and reduce the effects of stress. Reduction in blood pressure has been noted.
- Many practitioners adopt a vegetarian lifestyle, although that is not required. Practitioners state that the yoga lifestyle helps them to make healthier lifestyle choices, which may include goals of weight management and improved diet.

PSYCHOLOGY

- Yoga seeks to relieve stress through the quieting of the mind and focused concentration. This meditative state is said to raise the level of consciousness beyond the daily mundane thought processes and bring inner peace. This, then, is a path to increased awareness.
- Exercise has been shown to increase the release of endorphins, neurochemicals that can positively affect mood and mental state. This provides an increased sense of well-being, enhanced energy, and mental focus for other tasks.

SOCIAL

- Yoga provides a community structure of other practitioners, offering common goals and experiences. Yoga comes for the Sanskrit word for "union," thus seeking to bring the practitioner from a fragmented state to one of unity of body, mind, and spirit. Yoga promotes a lifestyle of balance, harmony, unity, ethics, morals, and personal conduct.

SPIRITUALITY

- Yoga promotes a form of meditation, focuses the flow of body energy, and connects the practitioner to the divine. This is said to promote inner peace and harmony. Yoga is congruent with a variety of spiritual practices and is not promoted as a religion.

Sources: Iyengar, B. (2001). *Yoga: The path to holistic health.* London: Dorling Kindersley; Martin, L., & Jung, P. (2002). *Taking charge of the change.* Albany, NY: Delmar; Mehta, M. (2001). *How to use yoga.* London: Anness; Mehta, S., Mehta, M., & Mehta, S. (2001). *Yoga: The Iyengar way.* New York: Alfred A. Knopf.

FIG. 4-3 Pregnant women participating in a Yoga for Pregnancy class. (Courtesy Julie Perry Nelson, Gilbert, AZ.)

CRITICAL THINKING EXERCISE

Natural Treatments for Menopausal Symptoms

Sandra is a new client in your facility. She is 52 years old and had a hysterectomy (removal of uterus) for fibroids 5 years ago. She is now complaining of frequent hot flashes and night sweats that interrupt her sleep. She states that intercourse is painful for her, and that lubricants are no longer helpful. She wants only natural treatments for what she considers to be menopause.

1. Evidence—Is there sufficient evidence to draw conclusions about her diagnosis and preferred treatment?
2. Assumptions—What assumptions can be made for the following items?
   a. Possible diagnosis for Sandra
   b. Physical assessment, laboratory tests, and/or diagnostic procedures that will be done to make a diagnosis
   c. Treatment options available
   d. Methods to assess efficacy of treatment
3. What implications and priorities for nursing care can be made at this time?
4. Does the evidence support your conclusion?
5. Are there alternative perspectives to your conclusion?

emphasis from a condition of health to one of potential disease. Although there is no disputing the advances in care of high risk obstetrics clients, most normal pregnancies can proceed safely with little or no intervention. Several commonly used alternative therapies can assist the expectant mother through gestation.

The nausea and vomiting of pregnancy can be a difficult problem. Although women with hyperemesis gravidarum must receive prompt and comprehensive care, the lesser nausea of the first trimester can be effectively treated with herbal teas. Herbs such as peppermint, spearmint, chamomile, and ginger can be used in teas and have been cited as possible remedies for "morning sickness." Other herbs, including fennel, hops, and wild yam, also have been named but are less accessible. Women may need to try several different herbal teas or alternate their use to achieve efficacy (Goldberg et al., 2002; Skidmore-Roth, 2004; Strong, 2001).

Certain homeopathic remedies also are noted to be effective for nausea. Many are available as over-the-counter products; or a skilled homeopath can construct an appropriate mixture based on the severity of the woman's symptoms (Goldberg et al., 2002; Lansky, 2003).

TCM also offers some alternatives in its herbal pharmacy, administered under the direction of a skilled practitioner. Certain acupressure or acupuncture points assist with the relief of nausea. One of these, pericardium 6 (P6), is a point that women can use for self-treatment. P6 is located two to three finger widths below the flexion crease of the wrist on the palmar side and between the flexor tendons (Fig. 4-4). By stimulating this point (with a fingertip or other blunt object), nausea can be relieved. Certain elasticized wristbands (Sea-Bands, for example) use a bead or other firm object to stimulate the P6 point and can be worn continuously (Fig. 4-5). Several studies have shown that clients report a decrease in nausea when using the wrist bands on the appropriate point. This acupressure technique also has been studied in cases of nausea occurring with chemotherapy and after anesthesia (Carlsson et al., 2000; Flaws, 2004; Norheim, Pedersen, & Fonnebo, 2001; Smith, Crowther, & Beilby, 2002).

When appropriate acupressure alone does not relieve nausea or vomiting, acupuncture treatments may be more effective. By using slender needles gently inserted into the specific points, licensed acupuncturists can treat not only the P6 point, but also various other points that govern the digestive process. Daily treatments often are required until the nausea subsides (Strong, 2001).

Musculoskeletal discomforts of pregnancy can be addressed with a variety of alternatives. Massage, physical therapy, chiropractic, and TCM all offer treatments to maintain flexibility and ease pain (Lie, 2005).

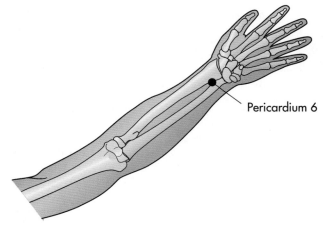

Pericardium 6

FIG. 4-4 Pericardium 6 (P6) acupressure/acupuncture point for nausea.

FIG. 4-5   Sea-Bands used for stimulation of acupressure point P6. (Courtesy Sea-Band International, Newport, RI.)

The management of labor pain long has been a nursing function. The Lamaze method encourages parents to take an active role in their pregnancy and obstetric care, to make informed choices, and to be guided by their inner wisdom. Techniques for stress reduction and pain management are taught in classes as life skills. Modalities such as imagery and progressive relaxation are emphasized along with communication skills and comfort measures (heat and cold, pressure points). The Lamaze method encourages realistic decision making and active participation on the part of the expectant parents (Lamaze International, 2005). Other methods, including the Bradley and the Read methods, also are taught nationwide, although Lamaze still enjoys the greatest popularity and widest appeal (see also Chapter 18).

Energetic healing modalities also are being used for labor management. Nurses practicing HT and TT have brought these modalities into the hospital setting. Krieger (1987) reported a study conducted with pregnant women and their partners and the use of TT in labor as an adjunct to the Lamaze method. Although pain control was not measured, couples using TT in addition to the Lamaze method reported a greater marital (relationship) satisfaction for their childbirth experience than did the control group. This small study points to the need for further research into pain management in laboring women. Healing touch (Fig. 4-6) also is used for labor care, but no studies have been published (Healing Touch, 2005; Hover-Kramer et al., 2001).

Massage techniques also are integrated into labor care. Studies have shown that therapeutic massage decreased labor time, hospital stay, and postpartum depression. Women receiving massage during pregnancy and labor had an increased positive outlook, reported less discomfort, and were less agitated than were those who did not receive massage (Caton et al., 2002; Simpkin & Bolding, 2004).

FIG. 4-6   Healing Touch session with pregnant client. (Courtesy Wendy Wetzel, Flagstaff, AZ.)

EVIDENCE-BASED PRACTICE

Labor Pain Management with Complementary and Alternative Medicine

BACKGROUND

- Pain in labor is caused by uterine contractions, cervical dilation, and perineal stretching, and is heightened by the fear-tension-pain cycle. Pain relief options now include some complementary and alternative medicine (CAM), defined as therapies neither typically taught in medical school nor used in conventional medicine. Many women prefer alternative, nonpharmacologic pain relief. Complementary therapies can potentiate conventional medication, improving pain relief with less sedation.

- The most common complementary practices involve mind-body interventions that can be taught in prenatal classes or even early labor, such as breathing, relaxation, and visualization, which apply the gate control theory of blocking pain impulses by providing other stimulation. More advanced concentration is required for yoga, meditation, and self-hypnosis, where discipline serves to relax and distract from the pain. Acupuncture and acupressure may stimulate the nervous system to produce endorphins, providing a blocking mechanism for pain. Aromatherapy uses essential oils to improve mood and may provide stimulation or sedation. Homeopathy uses very dilute substances that mimic the symptoms to paradoxically extinguish them. Selection of the substance is based on the type of pain and the women's emotions. Massage and reflexology use pressure points to interrupt pain and improve blood flow.

OBJECTIVE

- The authors wished to compare labor pain relief using CAM with conventional pharmacologic management of labor, placebo, or no treatment. Outcome measures included maternal satisfaction, use of pharmacologic labor pain relief, duration of labor, blood loss, perineal trauma, need for augmentation with oxytocin, bonding, breastfeeding, neonatal Apgar score and admission to a neonatal intensive care unit (NICU).

METHOD

Search Strategy

- From an extensive search and evaluation of the literature, seven randomized controlled trials met the criteria. They were published from 1965 to 2002, representing 336 laboring women in the United States, England, Sweden, and New Zealand.

Statistical Analyses

- Each therapy was examined separately, and similar data were pooled. The reviewers calculated relative risk for dichotomous (categorical) data, such as perineal trauma, and weighted mean differences for continuous data, such as pain scale. Results outside the 95% confidence interval were accepted as significant.

FINDINGS

- *Acupuncture*: Significantly more laboring women receiving acupuncture required no additional pain relief, including epidurals. They were also more relaxed. Interestingly, this made no difference to maternal satisfaction or pain scores. *Aromatherapy*: There was no difference found between ginger and lemongrass baths for laboring women. There were no controls in this trial. *Audio-Analgesia* (sea noise): No differences between groups were found. *Music*: There was a trend to less analgesia use among the treatment group, but it did not reach the level of significance. *Hypnosis*: Women using hypnosis were more likely to give birth vaginally, and less likely to need augmentation by oxytocin than the control group. However, the duration of labor in the hypnosis group was longer (mean 12.4 hours) than the control group (mean 9.7 hours). There were no differences in neonatal outcomes.

LIMITATIONS

- There is a lack of systematic and well-designed randomized controlled trials for all CAM therapies, including applications for labor pain relief. The number of women studied was small. Only one topic, hypnosis, had more than one study to combine data. Results from a study of audio-analgesia were reported, but there was no prior discussion of this as a CAM therapy. The aromatherapy group had no control group, and therefore no way to know what difference aromatherapy makes.

IMPLICATIONS FOR PRACTICE

- Hypnosis may be helpful at safely relieving the pain of laboring women and improving their satisfaction, but it also may increase labor duration. Although there appears to be no harm to mother or baby with any of these CAM therapies, there is insufficient evidence to endorse aromatherapy, audio-analgesia, biofeedback, or music as effective against labor pain.

IMPLICATIONS FOR FURTHER RESEARCH

- The authors recommend more trials where women choose which therapies they will use. This could increase satisfaction. Studies should include the training of the CAM practitioners, which varies markedly. Researchers can continue to look for the most effective timing and intensity and dosing of the therapies, and the additive effects of combinations of acupuncture and hypnosis. Characteristics of the individual women, such as parity, might give some insight into pain relief.

Reference: Smith, C., Collins, C., Cyna, A., & Crowther, C. (2003). Complementary and alternative therapies for pain management in labour. In *The Cochrane Library*, 2006, Issue 3. Chichester, UK: John Wiley & Sons.

Alternative care can extend beyond the immediate pregnancy period. Lactation can be enhanced and supported through the judicious use of herbs (Skidmore-Roth, 2004). Investigational studies are examining the value of herbs, vitamins and supplements, bodywork (especially massage), aromatherapy, and acupuncture in the support and treatment of postpartum depression (Weier & Beal, 2004).

Gynecology

Gynecologic complaints generate a large number of visits to health care practitioners. Menstrual cramps, irregular periods, pelvic pain, fibroids, and menopausal concerns make up the majority of episodic visits. Women in increasing numbers are seeking alternatives to standard surgical and pharmacologic treatments.

Menstrual cramping, or dysmenorrhea, affects a large number of women in all age groups. Various drug therapies, including nonsteroidal antiinflammatory agents, have been proposed over time with a measure of success; however, a vast number of alternatives can provide relief. Dietary changes, such as eliminating milk and dairy products and reducing the intake of complex carbohydrates and red meat, have been shown to decrease the incidence and severity of cramping. Dietary supplements, especially vitamin B_6 (100 mg per day), vitamin E (400 international units per day), calcium (1200 mg per day), and magnesium (up to 600 mg per day), are recommended. Certain herbal preparations, especially those containing cramp bark, white willow, red raspberry, and black cohosh, also may provide relief. Moderate aerobic exercise will stimulate blood flow and prevent congestion in the pelvic region. Visualization of healthy pelvic organs with guided imagery also can reduce pain and discomfort. Acupuncture has been shown to be useful as a complementary modality (Goldberg et al., 2002; Northrup, 2002, 2003) (see Chapter 7).

Irregular menstrual cycles and heavy menstrual flow are common problems. Often a result of hormonal imbalances, dysfunctional uterine bleeding may respond to synthetic hormone treatment. However, a significant number of women experience adverse effects that cause them to stop therapy. After other physiologic problems (thyroid dysfunction, bleeding disorders, diabetes, and other metabolic diseases) have been ruled out, treatment with human-identical hormones, especially progesterone, may be useful. Herbal therapy with black cohosh, red raspberry, and yarrow also is recommended. Increased soy in the diet also may provide some additional support (Martin & Jung, 2002; Northrup, 2002, 2003).

Premenstrual syndrome (PMS), or premenstrual dysphoria, is a common complaint. Some women experience a variety of disturbing symptoms during the postovulatory period. These symptoms often are alleviated with the onset of menses but cause significant disability and discomfort while they exist. Various theories, including hormonal, emotional, and behavioral, have been proposed. Northrup (2003) suggested that PMS is a social condition brought about by years of shame regarding menstrual functioning; other authors proposed that environmental stressors and dietary habits are contributing factors. Suggested remedies include dietary changes; herbal treatments with chaste tree, evening primrose oil, dandelion, cramp bark, and valerian root; homeopathic remedies to treat the underlying imbalances; bodywork such as massage and energy healing; and acupuncture. Increasing attention has been paid to the role of hormones in PMS. Supplementation with "natural" or human-identical progesterone has been reported to provide some relief (see Chapter 8) (Lee & Hopkins, 2004; Mancho, & Edwards, 2005; Northrup, 2003).

As the number of menopausal women increases, so do the requests for "natural" hormone therapy. For almost 50 years, women have been offered only estrogens derived from the urine of pregnant horses (conjugated equine estrogens) and synthetic progestins. With the introduction of other botanically based formulas, there are more options than ever before. Although truly natural hormones may be difficult to obtain, certain plants (soy and yam, for example) have been found to have molecular components that are identical in structure and function to human hormones and can be used in these preparations. These offer a new horizon for menopausal treatment, often without the side effects of standard agents, but with similar benefits and actions (Boothby, Doering, & Kipersztok, 2004; Conrad, 2005; Malat, 2005; Northrup, 2002, 2003; Reiss & Zucker, 2002).

For women who cannot or choose not to take hormonal treatment for menopausal complaints, herbs and homeopathy offer some alternatives. With the increasing awareness and diagnosis of breast cancer, there is consensus that women with a history of breast cancer should not take hormone replacement until they have been in remission for several years. However, these women often need some support and treatment for their symptoms. Herbs such as black cohosh, chasteberry, motherwort, burdock, yam, valerian, and St John's wort can provide symptomatic relief of hot flashes, night sweats, irritability, depression, and insomnia. A skilled herbalist can combine the ingredients into a mixture suited to the individual woman. Vitamin E oil can soothe atrophic vaginal tissues, and certain homeopathic remedies also can ease this time of transition. Chinese herbs such as dong quai and ginseng also may provide some essential relief (Boothby et al., 2004; Kronenberg & Fugh-Bermen, 2002; Lansky, 2003; Martin & Jung, 2002; Newton, Buist, Keenan, Anderson, & LaCroix, 2002; Northrup, 2003; Skidmore-Roth, 2004; Weed, 2001) (see Chapter 8).

Bone health and osteoporosis prevention must be addressed with any menopausal woman. Diet, calcium, vitamin D and micronutrient supplementation, and weight-bearing exercise are paramount to maintaining bone integrity during the premenopausal and postmenopausal periods. Dietary restrictions of foods known to deplete calcium stores should be outlined. Excessive intake of protein, salt, and caffeine may leach calcium from the bones. Some medications interfere with calcium absorption. Exercise programs such as tai chi, yoga, and Pilates help by strengthening the supporting muscles, improve balance and mobility, and reduce stress. Fall prevention should be outlined with all clients (Horowitz, 2004).

■ IMPLICATIONS FOR NURSING PRACTICE

With increased client awareness of health care models that are different from standard medical practice, the nurse is often the first to be consulted for her professional opinion and advice. Nurses can assist by being knowledgeable about current research, certification or licensure requirements, and professional organizations, and by fostering local networks of resources and practitioners. By maintaining an open and compassionate atmosphere, the nurse can determine the woman's level of knowledge about a given healing modality, as well as serve as a resource for concise and factual information.

At the intake interview, women should be asked if they are using any alternative or complementary modalities in their health plan. This also includes asking about the use of vitamins and over-the-counter remedies.

▬ NURSE ALERT

Women should inform their health care providers that they are using herbal remedies; as part of their history taking, health care providers should inquire if women are using herbal remedies.

Beliefs and values can be explored by the nurse and the woman to determine her desires and value system. A congruent plan of care can then be formulated to integrate the woman's biopsychosocial and spiritual needs. By approaching the woman with a nonjudgmental attitude, the nurse can gain her trust and assist her in incorporating her desires for alternative and complementary healing into the overall plan of care.

Holistic nurses often are called on to guide clients through the healing process and may themselves be the care providers with certain modalities. In ever-increasing numbers, nurses are gaining the knowledge and skills to maintain independent practices in various modalities. In this role, they can provide nursing support and guidance along with their chosen modality, thus creating a more comprehensive program of wellness and healing.

community activity

Visit a local health food store and observe the various types of vitamins, herbs, and supplements. Pay particular attention to those products marketed for women's health concerns. What claims are made? What are the main ingredients? If possible, interview the store owner or the person in charge of the supplement department. What specialized training does he or she possess? How does he or she counsel customers who are seeking these supplements? What books does he or she recommend? Does he or she make referrals to health care providers?

key points

- Integrative medicine combines modern technology with ancient healing practices and encompasses the whole of body, mind, and spirit.
- Alternative and complementary modalities address the whole client and seek to treat on a variety of levels.
- Although holistic research has been limited in the past, increasing efforts and governmental support are paving the way for more inquiries.
- Holistic nursing refers to a philosophic understanding and may integrate alternative and complementary therapies into nursing care.

- Holistic nurses recognize the importance of relationships within healing, as well as the necessity of self-care.
- A variety of alternative and complementary therapies are currently integrated into maternity and women's health care.
- Nurses are continuing to identify research opportunities to document the efficacy of integrative women's health care.

REFERENCES

Adams, K., Cohen, M., Eisenberg, D., & Jonsen, A. (2002). Ethical considerations of complementary and alternative medical therapies in conventional medical settings. *Annals of Internal Medicine, 137*(8), 660-664.

American Holistic Nurses' Association (AHNA). (2005). *About AHNA.* Flagstaff, AZ: Author. Accessed www.ahna.org/about/about.html, March 25, 2006.

Barnes, P., Powell-Griner, E., McFann, K., & Nahin, R. (2004). Complementary and alternative medicine use among adults: United States, 2002. *Advance Data, 343.* Accessed www.cdc.gov/nchs/data/ad/ad343.pdf, March 25, 2006.

Benson, H., & Proctor, W. (1984). *Beyond the relaxation response.* New York: Putman/Berkley.

Boothby, L., Doering, P., & Kipersztok, S. (2004). Bioidentical hormone therapy: A review. *Menopause: The Journal of the North American Menopause Society, 11*(3), 356-367.

Carlsson, C., Axemo, P., Bodin, A., Corstensen, H., Ehrenroth, B., Modegard-Lind, I., et al. (2000). Manual acupuncture reduces hyperemesis gravidarum: A placebo-controlled, randomized, single-blind, crossover study. *Journal of Pain Symptom Management, 20*(4), 273-279.

Caton, D., Corry, M., Frigoletto, F., Hopkins, D., Lieberman, E., Mayberry, L., et al. (2002). The nature and management of labor pain: Executive summary. *American Journal of Obstetrics and Gynecology, 186*(5 Suppl Nature), S1-S15.

Collins, J. (2002). *Discover your menopause type.* Roseville, CA: Three Rivers Press.

Conrad, C. (2005). *A woman's guide to natural hormones.* New York: Perigree Trade.

Dossey, B. (Ed.). (1997). *Core curriculum for holistic nursing.* Gaithersburg, MD: Aspen.

Dossey, B. (2000). *Florence Nightingale: Mystic, visionary, healer.* Springhouse, PA: Springhouse.

Dossey, B., Keegan, L., & Guzzetta, C. (2005). *Holistic nursing: A handbook for practice* (4th ed.). Sudbury, MA: Jones and Bartlett.

Ferguson, M. (1980). *The Aquarian conspiracy.* Los Angeles: J.P. Tarcher.

Flaws, R. (2004). *Chinese medical obstetrics.* Boulder, CO: Blue Poppy.

Frisch, N., Dossey, B., Guzzetta, C., & Quinn, J. (2000). *AHNA standards of holistic nursing practice: Guides for caring and healing.* Gaithersburg, MD: Aspen.

Gerber, R., Tiller, W., & Cousens, G. (2001). *Vibrational medicine.* Rochester, VT: Inner Traditions.

Goldberg, B., Anderson, J., & Trivieri, L. (Eds.). (2002). *Alternative medicine: The definitive guide* (2nd ed.) Berkeley, CA: Ten Speed Press.

Gordon, R. (2004). Why more patients are seeking alternative therapies. *Advance for Nurse Practitioners, 12*(5), 45-47.

Healing Touch International. (2005). *The healing touch research survey.* Lakewood, CO: Author.

Heinschel, J. (2005). A descriptive study of the interactive guided imagery experience. *Journal of Holistic Nursing, 20*(5), 325-346.

Henry, L., & Henry J. (2004). *The soul of the caring nurse: Stories and resources for revitalizing professional passion.* Washington, DC: American Nurses Association.

Horowitz, S. (2004). Natural, active approaches to osteoporosis prevention and treatment. *Alternative and Complementary Therapies, 10*(3), 125-130.

Hover-Kramer, D., Mentgen, J., & Scandrett-Hibdon, S. (2001). *Healing touch: A resource for health care professionals.* Albany, NY: Delmar.

Kessler, R., Davis, R., Foster, D., Van Rompay, M., Walters, E., Wilkey, S., et al. (2001). Long term trends in the use of complementary and alternative medical therapies in the United States. *Annals of Internal Medicine, 135*(4), 262-8.

Krieger, D. (1979). *The therapeutic touch: How to use your hands to help or to heal.* Englewood Cliffs, NJ: Prentice Hall.

Krieger, D. (1987). *Living the therapeutic touch: Healing as a lifestyle.* New York: Dodd, Mead.

Krieger, D. (1993). *Accepting your power to heal: The personal practice of therapeutic touch.* Santa Fe, NM: Bear.

Krieger, D. (2002). *Therapeutic touch as transpersonal healing.* New York: Lantern Books.

Kronenberg, F., & Fugh-Bermen, A. (2002). Complementary and alternative medicine for menopausal symptoms. *Annals of Internal Medicine, 137*(10), 805-813.

Kunz, D. & Krieger, D. (2004). *The spiritual dimension of therapeutic touch.* Santa Fe, NM: Bear.

Lamaze International. (2005). *About Lamaze.* Accessed www.lamaze.org, March 25, 2006.

Lansky, A. (2003). *The impossible cure: The promise of homeopathy.* Portola Valley, CA: R.L. Ranch Press.

Lee, J., & Hopkins, V. (2004). *What your doctor may not tell you about pre-menopause.* New York: Warner Books.

LeMaire, B. (2002). Something extra. *Nurseweek, 3*(7), 10-12.

Lie, D. (2005). Acupuncture may be helpful for pelvic girdle pain during pregnancy. *Medscape CME.* Accessed www.medscape.com/viewarticle/50170, March 25, 2006.

Malat, B. (2005). *Exploring alternative care for menopausal symptoms.* Presented at The American Academy of Physican Assistants Conference. Accessed www.medscape.com/viewarticle/510527, March 25, 2006.

Mancho, P., & Edwards, Q. (2005). Chaste tree for premenstrual syndrome. An evolving therapy in the United States. *Advance for Nurse Practitioners, 13*(5), 43-46.

Martin, A. (2002). It's never too late: Seven steps toward good health. *Topics in Advanced Practice Nursing E-journal, 2*(1). Accessed www.medscape.com/viewarticle/421471, March 25, 2006.

Martin, L., & Jung, P. (2002). *Taking charge of the change.* Albany, NY: Delmar.

National Center for Complementary and Alternative Medicine (NCCAM)/Office of Alternative Medicine (OAM). (2005). *Get the facts. What is complementary and alternative medicine.* Accessed nccam.nih.gov/health/whatiscam, March 25, 2006.

National Center for Complementary and Alternative Medicine (NCCAM) /Office of Alternative Medicine (OAM). (2006). *Get the facts. Acupuncture.* Accessed nccam.nih.gov/health/acupuncture/, June 17, 2006.

Newton, K., Buist, D., Keenan, N., Anderson, L., & LaCroix, A. (2002). Use of alternative therapies for menopause symptoms: Results of a population-based survey. *Obstetrics and Gynecology, 100*(1), 18-25.

Ni, H., Simile, C., & Hardy, A. (2002). Utilization of complementary and alternative medicine by United States adults. *Medical Care, 40*(4), 353-358.

Norheim, A., Pedersen, E., Fonnebo, V., & Berge, L. (2001). Acupressure treatment of morning sickness in pregnancy: A randomized, double-blind, placebo-controlled study. *Scandinavian Journal of Primary Health Care, 19*(1), 43-47.

Northrup, C. (2002). *Women's bodies, women's wisdom.* New York: Bantam.

Northrup, C. (2003). *The wisdom of menopause.* New York: Bantam.

Oschman, J. (2000). *Energy medicine.* New York: Churchill Livingstone.

Padden, D. (2002). The role of the advanced practice nurse in the promotion of exercise and physical activity. *Topics in Advanced Practice Nursing E-journal, 2*(1). Accessed www.medscape.com/viewarticle/421475, March 25, 2006.

Quinn, J. (1994). *Therapeutic touch: Healing through human energy fields, theory and research* [videotapes and study guide]. New York: National League for Nursing.

Reilly, A. (2005). Massage therapy. *Advance for Nurse Practitioners, 13*(5), 37-42.

Reiss, U., & Zucker, M. (2002). *Natural hormone balance for women: Look younger, feel stronger, and live life with exuberance.* New York: Pocket Books.

Richardson, S. (2004). Complementary health and healing in nursing education. *Journal of Holistic Nursing, 21*(1), 20-35.

Rogers, M. (1970). *The theoretical basis of nursing.* Philadelphia: F.A. Davis.

Simpkin, P., & Bolding, A. (2004). Update on nonpharmacologic approaches to relieve labor pain and prevent suffering. *Journal of Midwifery & Women's Health, 49*(6), 489-504.

Simpkins, A., Thurston, D., Colyer, M., & Talbot, S. (2005). Nature's wrath? A closer look at complications with five popular herbs. *Advance for Nurse Practitioners, 13*(6), 55-58.

Skidmore-Roth, L. (2004). *Mosby's handbook of herbs and natural supplements* (2nd ed.). St. Louis: Mosby.

Smith, C., Crowther, C., & Beilby, J. (2002). Acupuncture to treat nausea and vomiting in early pregnancy: A randomized controlled trial. *Birth, 29*(1), 1-9.

Snyder, M., & Lindquist, R. (Eds.). (2002). *Complementary/alternative therapies in nursing* (4th ed.). New York: Springer.

Strong, T. (2001). Alternative therapies of morning sickness. *Clinical Obstetrics and Gynecology, 44*(4), 653-660.

Ventegodt, S., Morad, M., & Merrick, J. (2004). Clinical holistic medicine: Classic art of healing or the therapeutic touch. *Scientific WorldJournal, 4*(4), 134–147.

Weed, S. (2001). *The new menopausal years: The wise woman way.* Woodstock, NY: Ash Tree.

Weier, K., & Beal, M. (2004). Complementary therapies as adjuncts in the treatment postpartum depression. *Journal of Midwifery & Women's Health, 49*(2), 96-104.

Weil, A. (2004). *Natural health, natural medicine: A comprehensive manual for wellness and self-care.* Boston: Houghton Mifflin.

Wetzel, M., Kaptchuk, T., Haramatil A., & Eisenberg, D. (2003). Complementary and alternative medical therapies: Implications for medical education. *Annals of Internal Medicine, 138*(3), 191-196.

CHAPTER 5

Jan Lamarche Zdanuk

Assessment and Health Promotion

learning objectives

- Identify the structures and functions of the female reproductive system.
- Compare the menstrual cycle in relation to hormonal, ovarian, and endometrial response.
- Identify the four phases of the sexual response cycle.
- Analyze financial, cultural, and communication barriers that may affect a woman's decision to seek and follow through with health care.
- Investigate how the history and physical examination can be adapted for women with special needs.
- Compare the strategies for teaching safety and injury prevention during routine health examinations.
- Examine indications of abuse, appropriate screening, and referral to community agencies.

- Describe the components of taking a woman's history and performing a physical examination.
- Identify the correct procedure for assisting with and collecting specimens for Papanicolaou testing.
- Review client teaching of breast self-examination.
- Analyze conditions and characteristics that increase health risks for women across the life span.
- Evaluate programs of anticipatory guidance that promote health and prevention of disease.
- Outline health-screening schedules for women in the childbearing years.

electronic resources

Additional information related to the content in Chapter 5 can be found on

the companion website at **evolve**
http://evolve.elsevier.com/Lowdermilk/MWHC/
- NCLEX Review Questions
- Case Study: Health Assessment
- WebLinks

or on the interactive companion CD
- NCLEX Review Questions
- Anatomy Review: Adult Female Pelvis, External Female Genitalia, Female Breast, Female Pelvic Organs
- Animations: Ovarian Torsion, Ovulation
- Case Study: Health Assessment
- Skill: Breast Self-Examination

CD: Anatomy Review: External Female Genitalia

MANY women initially enter the health care system because of a gender-related concern such as vaginal infection, irregular menses, pregnancy, a desire for contraception, or an episodic illness such as a sinus infection. Once women are in the system, it is important for health care providers to recognize the need for health promotion and health maintenance and to offer these services across the life span of women.

This chapter reviews female anatomy and physiology including the menstrual cycle. Physical assessment and screening for disease prevention for women are presented. Barriers to seeking health care and an overview of conditions and circumstances that increase health risks across the life span are discussed. Anticipatory guidance suggestions including nutrition and stress management also are included.

■ FEMALE REPRODUCTIVE SYSTEM

The female reproductive system consists of external structures visible from the pubis to the perineum and internal structures located in the pelvic cavity. The external and internal female reproductive structures develop and mature in response to estrogen and progesterone, starting in fetal life and continuing through puberty and the childbearing years. Reproductive structures atrophy with age or in response to a decrease in ovarian hormone production. A complex nerve and blood supply supports the functions of these structures. The appearance of the external genitals varies greatly among women. Heredity, age, race, and the number of children a woman has borne determine the size, shape, and color of her external organs.

External Structures

The external genital organs, or *vulva,* include all structures visible externally from the pubis to the perineum: the mons pubis, the labia majora, the labia minora, the clitoris, the vestibular glands, the vaginal vestibule, the vaginal orifice, and the urethral opening. The external genital organs are illustrated in Figure 5-1. The *mons pubis* is a fatty pad that lies over the anterior surface of the symphysis pubis. In the postpubertal female, the mons is covered with coarse, curly hair. The *labia majora* are two rounded folds of fatty tissue covered with skin that extend downward and backward from the mons pubis. The labia are highly vascular structures whose outer surfaces develop hair after puberty. They protect the inner vulvar structures. The *labia minora* are two flat, reddish folds of tissue visible when the labia majora are separated. No hair follicles are in the labia minora, but many sebaceous follicles and a few sweat glands are present. The interior of the labia minora is composed of connective tissue and smooth muscle and supplied with extremely sensitive nerve endings. Anteriorly, the labia minora fuse to form the *prepuce* (hoodlike covering of the clitoris) and the *frenulum* (fold of tissue under the clitoris). The labia minora join to form a thin flat tissue called the *fourchette* underneath the vaginal opening at midline. The *clitoris* is located underneath the prepuce. It is a small structure composed of erectile tissue with numerous sensory nerve endings. During sexual arousal, the clitoris increases in size.

The vaginal *vestibule* is an almond-shaped area enclosed by the labia minora that contains openings to the urethra, Skene glands, vagina, and Bartholin glands. The urethra is not a reproductive organ but is considered here because of its location. It usually is found about 2.5 cm below the clitoris. Skene glands are located on each side of the urethra and produce mucus, which aids in lubrication of the vagina. The vaginal opening is in the lower portion of the vestibule and varies in shape and size. The hymen, a connective tissue membrane, surrounds the vaginal opening.

It can be perforated during strenuous exercise, insertion of tampons, masturbation, and vaginal intercourse. Bartholin glands (see Fig. 5-1) lie under the constrictor muscles of the vagina and are located posteriorly on the sides of the vaginal opening, although the ductal openings are usually not visible. During sexual arousal, the glands secrete a clear mucus to lubricate the vaginal introitus.

The area between the fourchette and the anus is the perineum, a skin-covered muscular area that covers the pelvic structures. The perineum forms the base of the perineal body, a wedge-shaped mass that serves as an anchor for the muscles, fascia, and ligaments of the pelvis. The pelvic organs are supported by muscles and ligaments that form a sling.

Internal Structures

The internal structures include the vagina, the uterus, the uterine tubes, and the ovaries. The vagina is a fibromuscular, collapsible, tubular structure that extends from the vulva to the uterus and lies between the bladder and rectum. During the reproductive years, the mucosal lining is arranged in transverse folds called rugae. These rugae allow the vagina to expand during childbirth. Estrogen deprivation that occurs after childbirth, during lactation, and at menopause causes dryness and thinning of the vaginal walls and smoothing of the rugae. The vagina, particularly the lower segment, has few sensory nerve endings. Vaginal secretions are slightly acidic (pH 4 to 5) so that vaginal susceptibility to infections is reduced. The vagina serves as a passageway for menstrual flow, as a female organ of copulation, and as a part of the birth canal for vaginal childbirth. The uterine cervix projects into a blind vault at the upper end of the vagina. There are anterior, posterior, and lateral pockets called fornices that surround the cervix. The internal pelvic organs can be palpated through the thin walls of these fornices.

The *uterus* is a muscular organ shaped like an upside-down pear that sits midline in the pelvic cavity between

CD: Anatomy Review: Adult Female Pelvis, Female Pelvic Organs

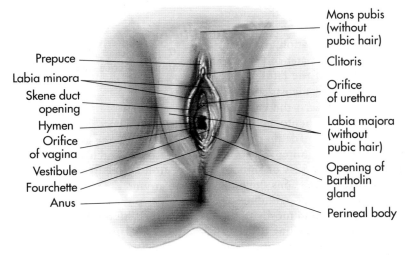

Prepuce
Labia minora
Skene duct opening
Hymen
Orifice of vagina
Vestibule
Fourchette
Anus

Mons pubis (without pubic hair)
Clitoris
Orifice of urethra
Labia majora (without pubic hair)
Opening of Bartholin gland
Perineal body

FIG. 5-1   External female genitalia.

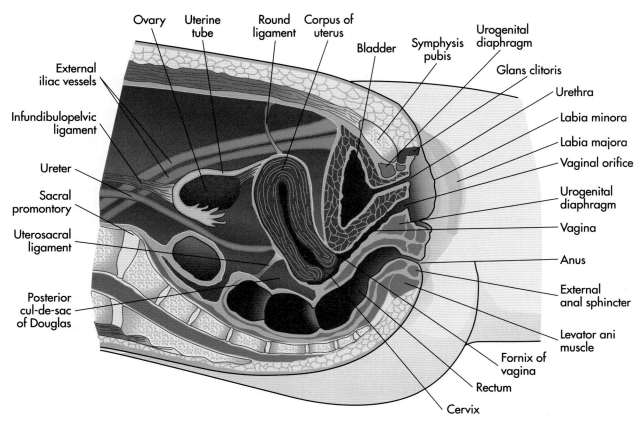

FIG. 5-2   Midsagittal view of female pelvic organs with woman lying supine.

the bladder and rectum and above the vagina. Four pairs of ligaments support the uterus: the cardinal, the uterosacral, the round, and the broad. Single anterior and posterior ligaments also support the uterus. The cul-de-sac of Douglas is a deep pouch, or recess, posterior to the cervix formed by the posterior ligament.

The uterus is divided into two major parts, an upper triangular portion called the corpus and a lower cylindric portion called the *cervix* (Fig. 5-2). The *fundus* is the dome-shaped top of the uterus and is the site at which the uterine tubes enter the uterus. The isthmus (lower uterine segment) is a short, constricted portion that separates the corpus from the cervix.

The uterus serves for reception, implantation, retention, and nutrition of the fertilized ovum and later of the fetus during pregnancy, and for expulsion of the fetus during childbirth. It also is responsible for cyclic menstruation.

The uterine wall comprises three layers: the endometrium, the myometrium, and part of the peritoneum. The endometrium is a highly vascular lining made up of three layers, the outer two of which are shed during menstruation. The myometrium is made up of layers of smooth muscles that extend in three different directions (longitudinal, transverse, and oblique) (Fig. 5-3). Longitudinal fibers of the outer myometrial layer are found mostly in the fundus, and this arrangement assists in expelling the fetus during the birth process. The middle layer contains fibers from all three directions, which form a figure-eight pattern

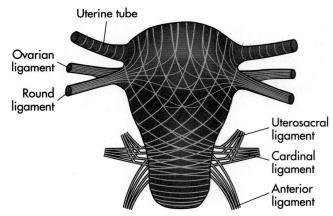

FIG. 5-3   Schematic arrangement of directions of muscle fibers. Note that uterine muscle fibers are continuous with supportive ligaments of uterus.

encircling large blood vessels. These fibers assist in ligating blood vessels after childbirth and control blood loss. Most of the circular fibers of the inner myometrial layer are around the site where the uterine tubes enter the uterus and around the internal cervical os (opening). These fibers help keep the cervix closed during pregnancy and prevent menstrual blood from flowing back into the uterine tubes during menstruation.

The cervix is made up of mostly fibrous connective tissues and elastic tissue, making it possible for the cervix to stretch during vaginal childbirth. The opening between the uterine cavity and the canal that connects the uterine cavity to the vagina (endocervical canal) is the internal os. The narrowed opening between the endocervix and the vagina is the external os, a small circular opening in women who have never been pregnant. The cervix feels firm (like the end of a nose) with a dimple in the center, which marks the external os.

The outer cervix is covered with a layer of squamous epithelium. The mucosa of the cervical canal is covered with columnar epithelium and contains numerous glands that secrete mucus in response to ovarian hormones. The squamocolumnar junction, where the two types of cells meet, is usually located just inside the cervical os. This junction also is called the *transformation zone,* the most common site for neoplastic changes (see Fig. 12-12); cells from this site are scraped for the Papanicolaou (Pap) test (see later discussion).

The *uterine tubes* (fallopian tubes) attach to the uterine fundus. The tubes are supported by the broad ligaments and range from 8 to 14 cm in length. The tubes are divided into four sections: the interstitial portion is closest to the uterus; the isthmus and the ampulla are the middle portions; and the infundibulum is closest to the ovary. The uterine tubes form passages between the ovaries and the uterus for the passage of the ovum. The infundibulum has fimbriated ends, which pull the ovum into the tube. The ovum is pushed along the tubes to the uterus by rhythmic contractions of the muscles of the tubes and by the current that is produced by the movement of the cilia that line the tubes. The ovum is usually fertilized by the sperm in the ampulla portion of one of the tubes.

The *ovaries* are almond-shaped organs located on each side of the uterus below and behind the uterine tubes. During the reproductive years, they are approximately 3 cm long, 2 cm wide, and 1 cm thick; they diminish in size after menopause. Before menarche, each ovary has a smooth surface; after menarche, they become nodular because of repeated ruptures of follicles at ovulation. The two functions of the ovaries are ovulation and hormone production. Ovulation is the release of a mature ovum from the ovary at intervals (usually monthly). Estrogen, progesterone, and androgen are the hormones produced by the ovaries.

The Bony Pelvis

The bony pelvis serves three primary purposes: protection of the pelvic structures, accommodation of the growing fetus during pregnancy, and anchorage of the pelvic support structures. Two innominate (hip) bones (consisting of ilium, ischium, and pubis), the sacrum, and the coccyx make up the four bones of the pelvis (Fig. 5-4). Cartilage and ligaments form the symphysis pubis, the sacrococcygeal joint, and two sacroiliac joints that separate the pelvic bones. The pelvis is divided into two parts: the false pelvis and the true pelvis (Fig. 5-5). The false pelvis is the upper portion above the pelvic brim or inlet. The true pelvis is the lower, curved bony canal, which includes the inlet, the cavity, and the outlet through which the fetus passes during vaginal birth. The upper portion of the outlet is at the level of the ischial spines, and the lower portion is at the level of the ischial tuberosities and the pubic arch (see Fig. 5-4). Variations that occur in the size and shape of the pelvis are usually due to age, race, and sex. Pelvic ossification is complete at about age 20 years.

Breasts

The breasts are paired mammary glands located between the second and sixth ribs (Fig. 5-6). About two thirds of the breast overlies the pectoralis major muscle, between the

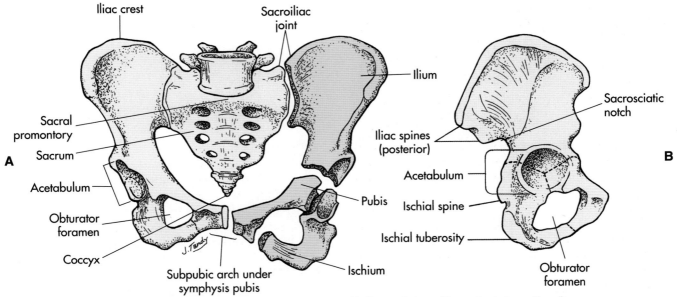
FIG. 5-4 Adult female pelvis. **A,** Anterior view. **B,** External view of innominate bone (fused).

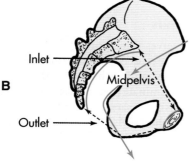

FIG. 5-5 Female pelvis. **A,** Cavity of false pelvis is shallow. **B,** Cavity of true pelvis is an irregularly curved canal (*arrows*).

sternum and midaxillary line, with an extension to the axilla referred to as the tail of Spence. The lower one third of the breast overlies the serratus anterior muscle. The breasts are attached to the muscles by connective tissue or fascia.

The breasts of healthy mature women are approximately equal in size and shape, but often are not absolutely symmetric. The size and shape vary depending on the woman's age, heredity, and nutrition. However, the contour should be smooth, with no retractions, dimpling, or masses. Estrogen stimulates growth of the breast by inducing fat deposition in the breasts, development of stromal tissue

(i.e., increase in its amount and elasticity), and growth of the extensive ductile system. Estrogen also increases the vascularity of breast tissue.

Once ovulation begins in puberty, progesterone levels increase. The increase in progesterone causes maturation of mammary gland tissue, specifically the lobules and acinar structures. During adolescence, fat deposition and growth of fibrous tissue contribute to the increase in the gland's size. Full development of the breasts is not achieved until after the end of the first pregnancy or in the early period of lactation.

Each mammary gland comprises 15 to 20 lobes, which are divided into lobules. Lobules are clusters of acini. An *acinus* is a saclike terminal part of a compound gland emptying through a narrow lumen or duct. In discussions of mammary glands, the correct anatomic term (acinus) often is used interchangeably with the term alveolus. The acini are lined with epithelial cells that secrete colostrum and milk. Just below the epithelium is the myoepithelium (*myo,* or muscle), which contracts to expel milk from the acini.

The ducts from the clusters of acini that form the lobules merge to form larger ducts draining the lobes. Ducts from the lobes converge in a single nipple (mammary papilla) surrounded by an areola. Just as the ducts converge, they dilate to form common lactiferous sinuses, which also are called ampullae. The lactiferous sinuses serve as milk reservoirs. Many tiny lactiferous ducts drain the ampullae and exit in the nipple.

The glandular structures and ducts are surrounded by protective fatty tissue and are separated and supported by fibrous suspensory *Cooper's ligaments.* Cooper's ligaments provide support to the mammary glands while permitting their mobility on the chest wall (see Fig. 5-6). The round

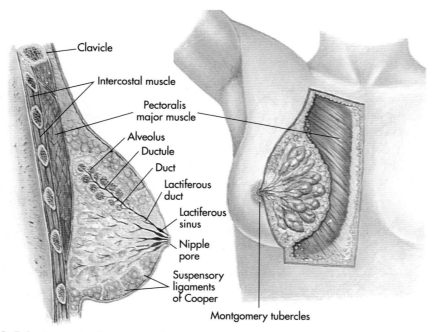

FIG. 5-6 Anatomy of the breast, showing position and major structures. (From Seidel, H., Ball, J., Dains, J., & Benedict, G. [2006]. *Mosby's guide to physical examination* [6th ed.]. St. Louis: Mosby.)

table 5-1 Female Reproductive Physical Assessment Across the Life Cycle

	ADOLESCENT	ADULT	POSTMENOPAUSAL
Breasts	Tender when developing; buds appear; small, firm; one side may grow faster; areola diameter increases; nipples more erect	Grow to full shape in early adulthood; nipples and areola become pinker and darker	Become stringy, irregular, pendulous, and nodular; borders less well delineated; may shrink, become flatter, elongated, and less elastic; ligaments weaken; nipples are positioned lower
Vagina	Vagina lengthens; epithelial layers thicken; secretions become acidic	Growth complete by age 20	Introitus constricts; vagina narrows, shortens, loses rugation; mucosa is pale, thin, and dry; walls may lose structural integrity
Uterus	Musculature and vasculature increase; lining thickens	Growth complete by age 20	Size decreases; endometrial lining thins
Ovaries	Increase in size and weight; menarche occurs between 8 and 16 years of age; ovulation occurs monthly	Growth complete by age 20	Size decreases to 1 to 2 cm; follicles disappear; surface convolutes; ovarian function ceases between 40 and 55 years of age
Labia majora	Become more prominent; hair develops	Growth complete by age 20	Labia become smaller and flatter; pubic hair sparse and gray
Labia minora	Become more vascular	Growth complete by age 20	Become shinier and drier
Uterine tubes	Increase in size	Growth complete by age 20	Decrease in size

nipple is usually slightly elevated above the breast. On each breast, the nipple projects slightly upward and laterally. It contains 15 to 20 openings from lactiferous ducts. The nipple is surrounded by fibromuscular tissue and covered by wrinkled skin. Except during pregnancy and lactation, there is usually no discharge from the nipple.

The nipple and surrounding areola are usually more deeply pigmented than the skin of the breast. The rough appearance of the areola is caused by sebaceous glands, *Montgomery tubercles,* directly beneath the skin. These glands secrete a fatty substance, thought to lubricate the nipple. Smooth muscle fibers in the areola contract to stiffen the nipple to make it easier for the breastfeeding infant to grasp.

The vascular supply to the mammary gland is abundant. In the nonpregnant state, the skin does not have an obvious vascular pattern. The normal skin is smooth without tightness or shininess. The skin covering the breasts contains an extensive superficial lymphatic network that serves the entire chest wall and is continuous with the superficial lymphatics of the neck and abdomen. In the deeper portions of the breasts, the lymphatics form a rich network as well. The primary deep lymphatic pathway drains laterally toward the axillae.

Besides their function of lactation, breasts function as organs for sexual arousal in the mature adult.

The breasts change in size and nodularity in response to cyclic ovarian changes throughout reproductive life. Increasing levels of both estrogen and progesterone in the 3 to 4 days before menstruation increase the vascularity of the breasts, induce growth of the ducts and acini, and promote water retention. The epithelial cells lining the ducts proliferate in number, the ducts dilate, and the lobules distend. The acini become enlarged and secretory, and lipid (fat) is deposited within their epithelial cell lining. As a result, breast swelling, tenderness, and discomfort are common symptoms just before the onset of menstruation. After menstruation, cellular proliferation begins to regress; the acini begin to decrease in size; and retained water is lost. After breasts have undergone changes numerous times in response to the ovarian cycle, the proliferation and involution (regression) are not uniform throughout the breast. In time, after repeated hormonal stimulation, small persistent areas of nodulations may develop. This normal physiologic change must be remembered when breast tissue is examined. Nodules may develop just before and during menstruation, when the breast is most active. The physiologic alterations in breast size and activity reach their minimal level about 5 to 7 days after menstruation stops. Therefore, breast self-examination (BSE) (systematic palpation of breasts to detect signs of breast cancer or other changes) is best carried out during this phase of the menstrual cycle (see Teaching for Self-Care). Table 5-1 compares the variations in physical assessment related to age differences in women.

■ MENSTRUATION AND MENOPAUSE

Nurses should be knowledgeable about menarche, the hypothalamic-pituitary cycle, the ovarian cycle, the endometrial cycle, and other cyclic changes, and the climacteric since they provide care for women across the life span.

Menarche and Puberty

Although young girls secrete small, rather constant amounts of estrogen, a marked increase occurs between ages 8 and 11 years. The term menarche denotes first menstruation. Puberty is a broader term that denotes the entire

Skill: Breast Self-Examination

TEACHING FOR SELF-CARE

Breast Self-Examination

1. The best time to do breast self-examination is about a week after your period, when breasts are not tender or swollen. If you do not have regular periods or sometimes skip a month, do it on the same day every month. If you are breastfeeding or no longer menstruating, choose a date and examine your breasts at the same time each month.

2. Lie down and put a pillow under your right shoulder. Place your right arm behind your head (Fig. 1).

3. Use the finger pads of your three middle fingers on your left hand to feel for lumps or thickening. Your finger pads are the top third of each finger.

4. Press firmly enough to know how your breast feels. If you're not sure how hard to press, ask your health care provider or try to copy the way your health care provider uses the finger pads during a breast examination. Learn what your breast feels like most of the time. A firm ridge in the lower curve of each breast is normal.

5. Move around the breast in a set way. You can choose either circles (Fig. 2, A), vertical lines (Fig. 2, B), or wedges (Fig. 2, C). Do it the same way every time. It will help you to make sure that you've gone over the entire breast area and to remember how your breast feels.

6. Gently compress the nipple between your thumb and forefinger and look for discharge.

7. Now examine your left breast using the finger pads of your right hand.

8. If you find any changes, see your health care provider right away.

9. You may want to check your breasts while standing in front of a mirror right after you do your breast self-examination each month. See if there are any changes in the way your breasts look: dimpling of the skin, changes in the nipple, or redness or swelling.

10. You may also want to do an extra breast self-examination while you're in the shower (Fig. 3). Your soapy hands will glide over the wet skin, making it easy to check how your breasts feel.

11. It is important to check the area between the breast and the underarm and the underarm itself. Also examine the area above the breast to the collarbone and to the shoulder.

Fig. 2

Fig. 1

Fig. 3

transitional stage between childhood and sexual maturity. Increasing amounts and variations in gonadotropin and estrogen secretion develop into a cyclic pattern at least a year before menarche. In North America, this occurs in most girls at about age 13 years.

Initially, periods are irregular, unpredictable, painless, and *anovulatory* (no ovum released from the ovary). After 1 or more years, a hypothalamic-pituitary rhythm develops, and the ovary produces adequate cyclic estrogen to make a mature ovum. *Ovulatory* (ovum released from ovary) periods tend to be regular, monitored by progesterone.

Although pregnancy can occur in exceptional cases of true precocious puberty, most pregnancies in young girls occur after the normally timed menarche. All young adolescents of both sexes would benefit from knowing that pregnancy can occur at any time after the onset of menses.

Menstrual Cycle

Menstruation is the periodic uterine bleeding that begins approximately 14 days after ovulation. It is controlled by a feedback system of three cycles: hypothalamic-pituitary, ovarian, and endometrial. The average length of a menstrual cycle is 28 days, but variations are normal. The first day of bleeding is designated day 1 of the menstrual cycle, or menses (Fig. 5-7). The average duration of menstrual flow is 5 days (range, 3 to 6 days), and the average blood loss is 50 ml (range, 20 to 80 ml), but these vary greatly.

For about 50% of women, menstrual blood does not appear to clot. The menstrual blood clots within the uterus, but the clot usually liquefies before being discharged from the uterus. Uterine discharge includes mucus and epithelial cells in addition to blood.

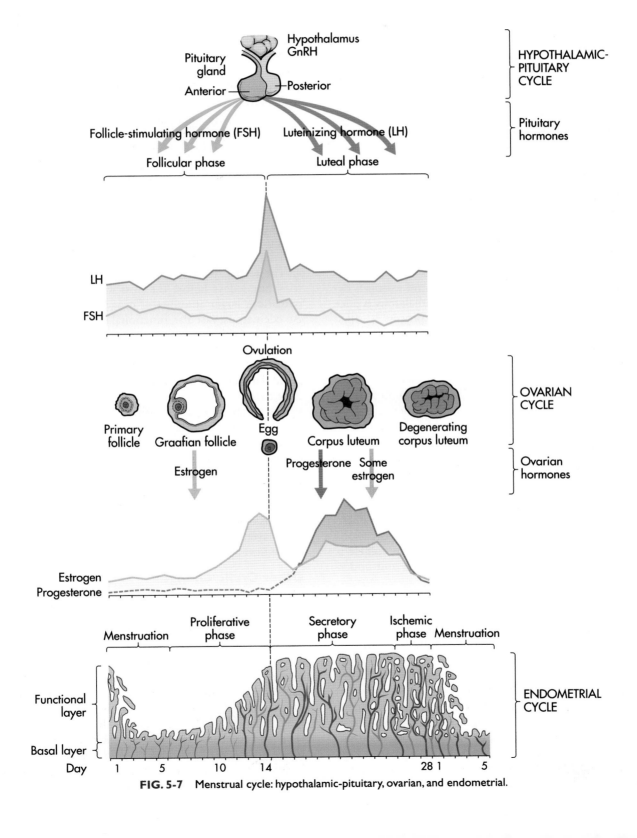

FIG. 5-7   Menstrual cycle: hypothalamic-pituitary, ovarian, and endometrial.

The menstrual cycle is a complex interplay of events that occur simultaneously in the endometrium, the hypothalamus, the pituitary glands, and the ovaries. The menstrual cycle prepares the uterus for pregnancy. When pregnancy does not occur, menstruation follows. The woman's age, physical and emotional status, and environment influence the regularity of her menstrual cycles.

Hypothalamic-Pituitary Cycle

Toward the end of the normal menstrual cycle, blood levels of estrogen and progesterone decrease. Low blood levels of these ovarian hormones stimulate the hypothalamus to secrete gonadotropin-releasing hormone (GnRH). In turn, GnRH stimulates anterior pituitary secretion of follicle-stimulating hormone (FSH). FSH stimulates development of ovarian graafian follicles and their production of estrogen. Estrogen levels begin to decrease, and hypothalamic GnRH triggers the anterior pituitary to release luteinizing hormone (LH). A marked surge of LH and a smaller peak of estrogen (day 12; see Fig. 5-7) precede the expulsion of the ovum from the graafian follicle by about 24 to 36 hours. LH peaks at about day 13 or 14 of a 28-day cycle. If fertilization and implantation of the ovum have not occurred by this time, regression of the corpus luteum follows. Levels of progesterone and estrogen decline, menstruation occurs, and the hypothalamus is once again stimulated to secrete GnRH. This process is called the hypothalamic-pituitary cycle.

Ovarian Cycle

The primitive graafian follicles contain immature oocytes (primordial ova). Before ovulation, from 1 to 30 follicles begin to mature in each ovary under the influence of FSH and estrogen. The preovulatory surge of LH affects a selected follicle. The oocyte matures, ovulation occurs, and the empty follicle begins its transformation to the corpus luteum. This follicular phase (preovulatory phase; see Fig. 5-7) of the ovarian cycle varies in length from woman to woman. Almost all variations in ovarian cycle length are the result of variations in the length of the follicular phase (Fehring, Schneider, & Raviele, 2006). On rare occasions (i.e., 1 in 100 menstrual cycles), more than one follicle is selected, and more than one oocyte matures and undergoes ovulation.

After ovulation, estrogen levels decrease. For 90% of women, only a small amount of withdrawal bleeding occurs, so that it goes unnoticed. In 10% of women, there is sufficient bleeding for it to be visible, resulting in what is termed *midcycle bleeding.*

The luteal phase begins immediately after ovulation and ends with the start of menstruation. This postovulatory phase of the ovarian cycle usually requires 14 days (range, 13 to 15 days). The corpus luteum reaches its peak of functional activity 8 days after ovulation, secreting the steroids estrogen and progesterone. Simultaneously with peak luteal functioning, the fertilized ovum is implanted in the endometrium.

If implantation does not occur, the corpus luteum regresses, steroid levels decrease, and the functional layer of the uterine endometrium is shed through menstruation.

Endometrial Cycle

The four phases of the endometrial cycle are (1) the menstrual phase, (2) the proliferative phase, (3) the secretory phase, and (4) the ischemic phase (see Fig. 5-7). During the menstrual phase, shedding of the functional two thirds of the endometrium (the compact and spongy layers) is initiated by periodic vasoconstriction in the upper layers of the endometrium. The basal layer is always retained, and regeneration begins near the end of the cycle from cells derived from the remaining glandular remnants or stromal cells in this layer.

The proliferative phase is a period of rapid growth lasting from about the fifth day to the time of ovulation. The endometrial surface is completely restored in approximately 4 days, or slightly before bleeding ceases. From this point on, an eightfold to tenfold thickening occurs, with a leveling off of growth at ovulation. The proliferative phase depends on estrogen stimulation derived from ovarian follicles.

The secretory phase extends from the day of ovulation to about 3 days before the next menstrual period. After ovulation, larger amounts of progesterone are produced. An edematous, vascular, functional endometrium becomes apparent. At the end of the secretory phase, the fully matured secretory endometrium reaches the thickness of heavy, soft velvet. It becomes luxuriant with blood and glandular secretions, a suitable protective and nutritive bed for a fertilized ovum.

Implantation of the fertilized ovum generally occurs about 7 to 10 days after ovulation. If fertilization and implantation do not occur, the corpus luteum, which secretes estrogen and progesterone, regresses. With the rapid decrease in progesterone and estrogen levels, the spiral arteries go into spasm. During the ischemic phase, the blood supply to the functional endometrium is blocked, and necrosis develops. The functional layer separates from the basal layer, and menstrual bleeding begins, marking day 1 of the next cycle (see Fig. 5-7).

Other Cyclic Changes

When the hypothalamic-pituitary-ovarian axis functions properly, other tissues undergo predictable responses. Before ovulation, the woman's basal body temperature (BBT) is often less than 37° C; after ovulation, with increasing progesterone levels, her BBT increases. Changes in the cervix and cervical mucus follow a generally predictable pattern. Preovulatory and postovulatory mucus is viscous (thick), so that sperm penetration is discouraged. At the time of ovulation, cervical mucus is thin and clear. It looks, feels, and stretches like egg white. This stretchable quality is termed *spinnbarkeit.* Some women have localized lower abdominal pain called *mittelschmerz* that coincides with ovulation. Some spotting may occur.

CD:Animations: Ovarian Torsion, Ovulation

Prostaglandins

Prostaglandins (PGs) are oxygenated fatty acids classified as hormones. The different kinds of PGs are distinguished by letters (PGE, PGF), numbers (PGE$_2$), and letters of the Greek alphabet (PGF$_{2\alpha}$).

Prostaglandins are produced in most organs of the body, including the uterus. Menstrual blood is a potent prostaglandin source. PGs are metabolized quickly by most tissues. They are biologically active in minute amounts in the cardiovascular, gastrointestinal, respiratory, urogenital, and nervous systems. They also exert a marked effect on metabolism, particularly on glycolysis. Prostaglandins play an important role in many physiologic, pathologic, and pharmacologic reactions. PGF$_{2\alpha}$, PGE$_4$, and PGE$_2$ are most commonly used in reproductive medicine.

Prostaglandins affect smooth muscle contractility and modulation of hormonal activity. Indirect evidence suggests that PGs have an effect on ovulation, fertility, changes in the cervix, and cervical mucus that affect receptivity to sperm, tubal and uterine motility, sloughing of endometrium (menstruation), onset of abortion (spontaneous and induced), and onset of labor (term and preterm).

After exerting their biologic actions, newly synthesized PGs are rapidly metabolized by tissues in such organs as the lungs, the kidneys, and the liver.

Prostaglandins may play a key role in ovulation. If PG levels do not increase along with the surge of LH, the ovum remains trapped within the graafian follicle. After ovulation, PGs may influence production of estrogen and progesterone by the corpus luteum.

The introduction of PGs into the vagina or into the uterine cavity (from ejaculated semen) increases the motility of uterine musculature, which may assist the transport of sperm through the uterus and into the oviduct.

Prostaglandins produced by the woman cause regression of the corpus luteum, regression of the endometrium, and sloughing of the endometrium, resulting in menstruation. PGs increase myometrial response to oxytocic stimulation, enhance uterine contractions, and cause cervical dilation. They may be a factor in the initiation of labor, the maintenance of labor, or both. They also may be involved in dysmenorrhea (see Chapter 7) and preeclampsia-eclampsia (see Chapter 30).

Climacteric and Menopause

The climacteric is a transitional phase during which ovarian function and hormone production decline. This phase spans the years from the onset of premenopausal ovarian decline to the postmenopausal time when symptoms stop. Menopause (from the Latin *mensis,* month, and Greek *pausis,* to cease) refers only to the last menstrual period. Unlike menarche, however, menopause can be dated with certainty only 1 year after menstruation ceases. The average age at natural menopause is 51.4 years, with an age range of 35 to 60 years. Perimenopause is a period preceding menopause that lasts about 4 years. During this time, ovarian function declines. Ova slowly diminish, and menstrual cycles may be anovulatory, resulting in irregular bleeding. The ovary stops producing estrogen, and eventually menses no longer occurs (Stenchever, Droegemueller, Herbst, & Mishell, 2001).

■ SEXUAL RESPONSE

The hypothalamus and anterior pituitary gland in females regulate the production of FSH and LH. The target tissue for these hormones is the ovary, which produces ova and secretes estrogen and progesterone. A feedback mechanism between hormone secretion from the ovaries, the hypothalamus, and the anterior pituitary aids in the control of the production of sex cells and steroid sex hormone secretion.

Although the first outward appearance of maturing sexual development occurs at an earlier age in females, both females and males achieve physical maturity at approximately age 17 years; however, individual development varies greatly. Anatomic and reproductive differences notwithstanding, women and men are more alike than different in their physiologic response to sexual excitement and orgasm. For example, the glans clitoris and the glans penis are embryonic homologues. Little difference exists between female and male sexual response; the physical response is essentially the same whether stimulated by coitus, fantasy, or masturbation. Physiologically, according to Masters (1992), sexual response can be analyzed in terms of two processes: vasocongestion and myotonia.

Sexual stimulation results in an increase in circulation to circumvaginal blood vessels (lubrication in the female), causing engorgement and distention of the genitals. Venous congestion is localized primarily in the genitals, but it also occurs to a lesser degree in the breasts and other parts of the body. Arousal is characterized by myotonia (increased muscular tension), resulting in voluntary and involuntary rhythmic contractions. Examples of sexually stimulated myotonia are pelvic thrusting, facial grimacing, and spasms of the hands and feet (carpopedal spasms).

The sexual response cycle is divided into four phases: excitement phase, plateau phase, orgasmic phase, and resolution phase. The four phases occur progressively, with no sharp dividing line between any two phases. Specific body changes take place in sequence. The time, intensity, and duration for cyclic completion also vary for individuals and situations. Table 5-2 compares male and female body changes during each of the four phases of the sexual response cycle.

■ REASONS FOR ENTERING THE ■ HEALTH CARE SYSTEM

Women's health assessment and screening focus on a systems evaluation, beginning with a careful history and physical examination. During the assessment and evaluation, the responsibilities for self-care, health promotion, and enhancement of wellness are emphasized. Nursing care

table 5-2 Four Phases of Sexual Response

REACTIONS COMMON TO BOTH SEXES	FEMALE REACTIONS	MALE REACTIONS
EXCITEMENT PHASE		
Heart rate and blood pressure increase. Nipples become erect. Myotonia begins.	Clitoris increases in diameter and swells. External genitals become congested and darken. Vaginal lubrication occurs; upper two thirds of vagina lengthen and extend. Cervix and uterus pull upward. Breast size increases.	Erection of the penis begins; penis increases in length and diameter. Scrotal skin becomes congested and thickens. Testes begin to increase in size and elevate toward the body.
PLATEAU PHASE		
Heart rate and blood pressure continue to increase. Respirations increase. Myotonia becomes pronounced; grimacing occurs.	Clitoral head retracts under the clitoral hood. Lower one third of vagina becomes engorged. Skin color changes occur—red flush may be observed across breasts, abdomen, or other surfaces.	Head of penis may enlarge slightly. Scrotum continues to grow tense and thicken. Testes continue to elevate and enlarge. Preorgasmic emission of 2 or 3 drops of fluid appears on the head of the penis.
ORGASMIC PHASE		
Heart rate, blood pressure, and respirations increase to maximum levels. Involuntary muscle spasms occur. External rectal sphincter contracts.	Strong rhythmic contractions are felt in the clitoris, vagina, and uterus. Sensations of warmth spread through the pelvic area.	Testes elevate to maximum level. Point of "inevitability" occurs just before ejaculation and an awareness of fluid in the urethra. Rhythmic contractions occur in the penis. Ejaculation of semen occurs.
RESOLUTION PHASE		
Heart rate, blood pressure, and respirations return to normal. Nipple erection subsides. Myotonia subsides.	Engorgement in external genitalia and vagina resolves. Uterus descends to normal position. Cervix dips into seminal pool. Breast size decreases. Skin flush disappears.	Fifty percent of erection is lost immediately with ejaculation; penis gradually returns to normal size. Testes and scrotum return to normal size. Refractory period (time needed for erection to occur again) varies according to age and general physical condition.

includes assessment, planning, education, counseling, and referral as needed, as well as commendations for good self-care that the woman has practiced. This enables women to make informed decisions about their own health care.

Preconception Counseling and Care

Preconception health promotion provides women and their partners with information that is needed to make decisions about their reproductive future. Preconception counseling and care can be provided as part of routine health examinations such as premarital, employment, school, and family planning. Preconception counseling guides couples on how to avoid unintended pregnancies, how to identify and manage risk factors in their lives and their environment, and how to identify healthy behaviors that promote the well-being of the woman and her potential fetus (Moos, 2003). The components of preconception care, such as health promotion, risk assessment, and interventions, are discussed in Chapter 17.

Pregnancy

A woman's entry into health care is often associated with pregnancy, either for diagnosis or for actual care. The possibility of pregnancy is realized most commonly when a woman is late with her menses. If she is pregnant, it is desirable for a woman to enter prenatal care within the first 12 weeks. This allows early pregnancy counseling, especially for the woman who has had no preconception care. Major goals of prenatal care are found in Box 5-1 and should be initiated at the first visit. Extensive discussion of pregnancy is found in Chapter 16.

Well-Woman Care

Current trends in the health care of women have expanded beyond a reproductive focus. A holistic approach to women's health care includes a woman's health needs

box 5-1 Major Goals of Prenatal Care

- Define health status of mother and fetus.
- Determine the gestational age of the fetus, and monitor fetal development.
- Identify the woman at risk for complications, and minimize the risk whenever possible.
- Provide appropriate education and counseling.

throughout her lifetime. This view goes beyond simply her reproductive needs. This restructuring places women's health within the primary health care delivery system. Women's health assessment and screening focus on a multisystem evaluation emphasizing the maintenance and enhancement of wellness (Moos, 2003).

Many women first enter the health care delivery system for a Pap test or contraception. Visits to the nurse may be their only contact with the system unless they become ill. Some women postpone examination until a specific need arises, such as pregnancy, pain, abnormal bleeding, or vaginal discharge.

Health care needs vary with culture, religion, age, and personal differences. The changing responsibilities and roles of women, their socioeconomic status, and their personal lifestyles also contribute to differences in the health and behavior of women. Employment outside of the home, physical disability, inadequate or no health insurance, divorce, single parenthood, and sexual orientation also can affect women's ability to seek and receive health care in clinical settings. As women age, many continue to address their primary health care needs within their established gynecologic care setting; therefore, well-women's health care should include a complete history, physical examination, and age-appropriate screening, and health promotion.

Fertility Control and Infertility

As women become more informed about themselves and their health care, they are more willing to seek counseling and contraception appropriate to their varied and specific needs. Some women first enter the health care system to obtain such advice. More than half of the pregnancies in the United States each year are unintended, and the majority of these occur in the 10% of women who do not use birth control (Kowal, 2004). Education is the key to encouraging women to make family planning choices based on preference and actual benefit-to-risk ratios. Providers can influence the user's motivation and ability to use the method correctly (see Chapter 9 for further discussion of contraception).

The concept of health promotion applies to contraception, as can be seen in Box 5-2. The nurse is in an ideal situation to influence women positively regarding the need for child spacing, methods of family planning that are consistent with religious and personal preferences, noncontraceptive benefits of certain methods, the appropriate use of methods selected, and the protection of future fertility when so desired.

Women also enter the health care system because of their desire to achieve a pregnancy. Approximately 15% of couples in the United States have some degree of infertility. Many couples have delayed starting their families until they are in their 30s or 40s, which allows more time to be exposed to situations negatively affecting fertility (including age-related infertility for the woman). In addition, sexually transmitted infections (STIs), which can

---

> **box 5-2** **Contraceptive Health Promotion**
>
> - Child spacing and quality maternity care improve perinatal outcomes and health in general of mother and children.
> - Achieving desired family size enables a better sharing of all resources, with attendant increases in education, health care, and other positive societal parameters.
> - Contraceptives themselves may positively affect future health. For example, use of condoms may prevent acquisition of HIV infection; combined OCs may provide some protection against later development of cancer of ovary and endometrium; barrier methods decrease transmission of STIs, which can develop into pelvic inflammatory disease with resultant infertility or sterility and thus affect future childbearing capacity.

HIV, Human immunodeficiency virus; *OCs,* oral contraceptives; *STIs,* sexually transmitted infections.

---

predispose to decreased fertility, are becoming more common, and many women and men are in workplaces and home settings where they may be exposed to reproductive environmental hazards.

Steps toward prevention of infertility should be undertaken as part of ongoing routine health care, and such information is especially appropriate in preconception counseling. Primary care providers can undertake initial evaluation and counseling before couples are referred to specialists. For additional information about infertility, see Chapter 10.

Menstrual Problems

Irregularities or problems with the menstrual period are among the most common concerns of women and often cause them to seek help from the health care system. Common menstrual disorders include amenorrhea, dysmenorrhea, premenstrual syndrome, endometriosis, and menorrhagia or metrorrhagia. Simple explanation and counseling may handle the concern; however, history and examination must be completed, as well as laboratory or diagnostic tests, if indicated. Questions should never be considered inconsequential, and age-specific reading materials are recommended, especially for teenagers. See Chapter 7 for an in-depth discussion of menstrual problems.

Perimenopause

The body responds to this natural transition in a number of ways, most of which are due to the decrease in estrogen. Most women seeking health care during the perimenopausal period do so because of irregular bleeding. Others are concerned about vasomotor symptoms (hot flashes and flushes). Although fertility is greatly reduced during this period, women are urged to maintain some method of birth control because pregnancies still can occur. All women need to have factual information, the dispelling of myths, a thorough examination, and periodic health screenings thereafter. See Chapter 7 for discussion of perimenopause and menopause.

▬ BARRIERS TO SEEKING HEALTH CARE

Financial Issues

Parts of the health care delivery system remain in a state of flux. Great variation occurs depending on type and size of the system, source of payment for services, private versus public programs, availability of and accessibility to providers, individual preferences, and insurance coverage or ability to pay. The existing system continues to be oriented to treatment of acute or episodic conditions rather than the promotion of health and comprehensive care.

In the United States, disparity among races and socioeconomic classes affects many facets of life, including health. With limited money and awareness, there is a lack of access to care, delay in seeking care, few prevention activities, and little accurate information about health and the health care system. Women use health services more often than do men but are more likely than men to have difficulty in financing the services; they are twice as often underinsured (i.e., have limited coverage with high-cost copayments or deductibles). Women make up the majority of Medicaid recipients; however, only 42% of poor women are eligible. Medicaid includes special benefits for pregnant women, but they are limited to treatment of pregnancy-related conditions and terminate 60 days after birth. More states are requiring their Medicaid recipients to enroll in managed care programs; whether this improves access and outcomes is yet to be determined.

Insurance coverage varies significantly by age, marital status, race, and ethnicity. Caucasians of all ages are more likely than African-Americans and other racial or ethnic groups to have private insurance. Caucasians possess insurance 2.5 times more often than Hispanics and 1.8 times more often than African-Americans. Single, separated, or divorced individuals are less likely to have insurance. Often unmarried teenagers, who are usually covered by their parents' medical insurance, do not have maternity coverage because policies have inclusion statements that cover only the employee or spouse.

Midwifery care has helped contain some health care costs, but reimbursement issues still exist in some areas. Nurses should be involved with the politics concerning cost-containment health care policies, because they, as knowledgeable experts, can provide solutions to many of the health care problems at a relatively low cost.

Cultural Issues

As our nation becomes more racially, ethnically and culturally diverse, the health of minority groups becomes a major issue. A variety of reasons are given to explain some of the differences in accessing care when financial barriers are adjusted. Unfair treatment was described by women who experienced racial discrimination or disrespectful, disillusioning, or discouraging encounters with community service providers such as social services and health care providers. A lack of training in cross-cultural communication may present problems. Desired health outcomes are best

cultural considerations

Female Genital Mutilation

Female circumcision occurs in women of many different ethnic, cultural, and religious backgrounds. Although circumcision is usually performed during childhood, some communities circumcise infants or older females.

The procedure involves the removal of a portion of the clitoris but may extend to the removal of the entire clitoris and labia minora. Additionally, the labia majora, which are often stitched together over the urethral and vaginal openings, may be affected.

The extent of the circumcision site affects the seriousness of complications. Common complications include bleeding, pain, local scarring, keloid or cyst formation, and infection. Impaired drainage of urine and menstrual blood may lead to chronic pelvic infections, pelvic and back pain, and chronic urinary tract infections. Some women may require surgery before vaginal examination, intercourse, or childbirth if the vaginal opening is obstructed.

Nurses are providing care to a growing number of women who have emigrated from the Middle East, Asia, and Africa, where female circumcision is more common. Nurses must be sensitive to the unique needs of these clients, especially if these women have concerns about maintaining or restoring the intactness of the circumcision after childbirth.

Reference: Kelly, E., & Hillard, P. (2005). Female genital mutilation. *Current Opinion in Obstetrics and Gynecology, 17*(5), 490-494; Sala R., & Manara, D. (2001). Nurses and requests for female genital mutilation: Cultural rights versus human rights. *Nursing Ethics, 8*(3), 247-258.

achieved when the health care providers have a knowledge and understanding about the culture, language, values, priorities, and health beliefs of minority groups. Conversely, members of the group should understand the health goals to be achieved and the methods proposed to do so. Language differences can produce profound barriers between women and health care providers. Even with an interpreter, information may be skewed in either direction.

Providers must consider culturally based differences that could affect the treatment of diverse groups of women, and the women themselves should share their practices and beliefs that could influence their management, responses, or willingness to comply (see Cultural Considerations box). Religious beliefs may dictate a specified plan of care, such as limiting assisted reproductive technology, birth control measures, blood transfusions, cardiopulmonary resuscitation, or assisted ventilation. Some cultural groups prefer folk medicine, homeopathy, or prayer to traditional Western medicine, and others attempt combinations of various practices (see Chapter 2).

Gender Issues

Gender influences provider-client communication and may influence access to health care in general. The most obvious gender consideration is that between men and women. Researchers have reported significant male-female differences in receipt of major diagnostic and therapeutic interventions, especially with cardiac and kidney problems.

Women tend to use primary care services more often than men and, some believe, more effectively. The sex of the provider plays a role; studies have shown that female clients have Pap tests and mammograms more consistently if they are seen by female providers.

Sexual orientation may produce another barrier. Lesbian women have primary erotic attractions and relations with other women. Some lesbians may not disclose their orientation to health care providers because they feel they may be at risk for hostility, inadequate health care, or breach of confidentiality. In many health care settings, heterosexuality is assumed, and the setting may be one in which the woman does not feel welcome (magazines, brochures, and environment reflect heterosexual couples, or the health care provider shows discomfort interacting with the woman). Another problem is that lesbians themselves may hold beliefs that are incorrect, such as that they have immunity to human immunodeficiency virus (HIV), STIs, and certain cancers (e.g., cervical). The perceived lack of risk can result in lesbians avoiding medical care as well as in health care providers giving incorrect advice or not doing appropriate cancer screening for these women. Not all gynecologic cancers are related to sexual activity; lesbians who have never had children may be more at risk for breast, ovarian, and endometrial cancer. Their risk for heart disease, cancer of the lung, and colon cancer is not different from that of the heterosexual woman. To offset stereotypes, it is necessary for providers to develop an approach that does not assume that all women are heterosexual (Bonvicini & Perlin, 2003).

■ HEALTH RISKS IN THE
■ CHILDBEARING YEARS

Maintaining optimal health is a goal for all women. Essential components of health maintenance are identification of unrecognized problems and potential risks and the education and the health promotion needed to reduce them. This is especially important for women in their childbearing years, because conditions that increase a woman's health risks are not only of concern for her well-being but also are potentially associated with negative outcomes for both mother and baby in the event of a pregnancy. Prenatal care is an example of prevention that is practiced after conception; however, prevention and health maintenance are needed before pregnancy because many of the mother's risks can be identified and then eliminated or at least modified. An overview of conditions and circumstances that increase health risks in the childbearing years follows.

Age
Adolescence

As a girl progresses through development, she may be at risk for conditions that are age related. All teens undergo progressive growth of sexual characteristics and also undertake developmental tasks of adolescence, such as establishing identity, developing sexual preference, emancipating from family, and establishing career goals. Some of these

situations can produce great stress for the adolescent, and the health care provider should treat her carefully. Female teenagers who enter the health care system usually do so for screening (Pap tests start at age 21 or 3 years after the girl becomes sexually active) or because of a problem such as episodic illness or accidents. Gynecologic problems are often associated with menses (either bleeding irregularities or dysmenorrhea), vaginitis or leukorrhea, STIs, contraception, or pregnancy. The adolescent also is at risk for a major depressive disorder (Hauenstein, 2003).

Teenage Pregnancy. Pregnancy in the teenager who is 16 years old or younger often introduces additional stress into an already stressful developmental period. The emotional level of such teens is commonly characterized by impulsiveness and self-centered behavior, and they often place primary importance on the beliefs and actions of their peers. In attempts to establish a personal and independent identity, many teens do not realize the consequences of their behavior, and planning for the future is not part of their thinking processes.

Teenagers usually lack the financial resources to support a pregnancy and may not have the maturity to avoid teratogens or to have prenatal care and instruction or follow-up care. Children of teen mothers may be at risk for abuse or neglect because of the teen's inadequate knowledge of growth, development, and parenting. Implementation of specialized adolescent programs in schools, communities, and health care systems is demonstrating continued success in reducing the birth rate in teens.

Young and Middle Adulthood

Because women aged 20 to 40 years have need for contraception, pelvic and breast screening, and pregnancy care, they may prefer to use their gynecologic or obstetric provider as their primary care provider also. During these years, the woman may be "juggling" family, home, and career responsibilities, with resulting increases in stress-related conditions. Health maintenance includes not only pelvic and breast screening but also promotion of a healthy lifestyle, that is, good nutrition, regular exercise, no smoking, little or no alcohol consumption, sufficient rest, stress reduction, and referral for medical conditions and other specific problems. Common conditions requiring well-woman care include vaginitis, urinary tract infections, menstrual variations, obesity, sexual and relationship issues, and pregnancy.

Parenthood after Age 35 Years. The woman older than 35 years does not have a different physical response to a pregnancy, per se, but rather has had health status changes as a result of time and the aging process. These changes may be responsible for age-related pregnancy conditions. For example, a woman with type 2 diabetes may not have had expression of her diabetes at age 22 years, but may have full-blown disease at age 38 years. Other chronic or debilitating diseases or conditions increase in severity with time, and these, in turn, may predispose to increased risks during pregnancy. Of significance to women in this age group is the risk for certain genetic anomalies (e.g., Down syndrome), and the opportunity for genetic counseling should be available to all (Viau, Padua, & Eddy, 2002).

Late Reproductive Age

Women of later reproductive age are often experiencing change and reordering of their personal priorities. Generally, the goals of education, career, marriage, and family have been achieved, and now the woman has increased time and opportunity for new interests and activities. Conversely, divorce rates are high at this age, and children leaving home may produce an "empty nest syndrome," resulting in increased levels of depression. Chronic diseases also become more apparent. Most problems for the well woman are associated with perimenopause (e.g., bleeding irregularities and vasomotor symptoms). Health maintenance screening continues to be of importance because some conditions such as breast disease or ovarian cancer occur more often during this stage.

Socioeconomic

Socioeconomic status affects birth outcomes. The rates of perinatal and maternal deaths, preterm births, and low-birth-weight babies are considerably higher in disadvantaged populations (Hoyert, Mathews, Menacker, Strobino, & Guyer, 2006). Social consequences for poor women as single parents are great, because many mothers with few skills are caught in the bind of having income that is insufficient to afford child care. These families generate fewer and fewer resources and increase their risks for health problems. Multiple roles for women in general produce overload, conflict, and stress, resulting in higher risks for psychologic illness.

Substance Use and Abuse

Use of illicit drugs and inappropriate use of prescription drugs continue to increase and are found in all ages, races, ethnic groups, and socioeconomic strata. Addiction to substances is seen as a biopsychosocial disease, with several factors leading to risk. These include biogenetic predisposition, lack of resilience to stressful life experiences, and poor social support. Women are less likely than men to abuse drugs, but the rate in women is increasing significantly. Substance-abusing pregnant women create severe problems for themselves and their offspring, including interference with optimal growth and development and addiction. In many instances, the use of substances is identified through screening programs in prenatal clinics and obstetric units (see Chapter 35).

Smoking

Cigarette smoking is a major preventable cause of death and illness. Smoking is linked to cardiovascular heart disease, various types of cancers (especially lung and cervical), chronic lung disease, and negative pregnancy outcomes. Tobacco contains nicotine, which is an addictive substance

---

CRITICAL THINKING EXERCISE

Smoking Cessation During Pregnancy

Sally is a 22-year-old who is 8 weeks pregnant. At her first prenatal visit, a history is taken and she reports that she smokes about half a pack of cigarettes a day. She says she knows that she should probably try to cut down, but she has tried before and not been successful. How would you respond to her statement?

1. Evidence: Is there sufficient evidence to draw conclusions about what the nurse should say?
2. Assumptions: What assumptions can be made about the following issues?
   a. Effects of smoking on pregnancy
   b. Cessation interventions for pregnant women
3. What implications and priorities for nursing care can be made at this time?
4. Does the evidence objectively support your conclusion?
5. Are there alternative perspectives to your conclusion?

---

that creates a physical and a psychologic dependence. Among adolescents and young adults, more women than men smoke (American Cancer Society [ACS], 2006). Cigarette smoking impairs fertility in both women and men, may reduce the age for menopause, and increases the risk for osteoporosis after menopause. Smoking during pregnancy is known to cause a decrease in placental perfusion and is a cause of low birth weight (Bernstein, Mongeon, Badger, Solomon, Heil, & Higgins, 2005; Kliegman, 2006). (see Critical Thinking Exercise).

Alcohol

Women aged 35 to 49 years have the highest rates of chronic alcoholism, but women aged 21 to 34 have the highest rates of specific alcohol-related problems. About one third of alcoholics are women, and many relate onset of their drinking problem to stressful events. Women who are problem drinkers are often depressed, have more motor vehicle injuries, and have a higher incidence of attempted suicide than women in the general population. They also are at risk for alcohol-related liver damage. Early case finding and treatment are important in alcoholism for both the ill individual and for family members. See Chapter 35 for further discussion about alcohol use in women.

Prescription Drugs

Psychotherapeutic medications such as stimulants, sleeping pills, tranquilizers, and pain relievers are used by an estimated 2% of American women. Such medications can bring relief from undesirable conditions such as insomnia, anxiety, and pain, but because the medications have mind-altering capacity, misuse can produce psychologic and physical dependency in the same manner as illicit drugs. Risk-to-benefit ratios should be considered when such medications are used for more than short periods.

Depression is the most common mental health problem in women. Many kinds of medications are used to treat depression. All of these psychotherapeutic drugs can have some effect on the fetus when taken during pregnancy and must be very carefully monitored (see Chapter 35).

Illicit Drugs

Illicit drugs are taken for unlawful purposes. When they are unprescribed, they are usually obtained on the street for the purpose of getting high or for their body-mind–altering characteristics. Almost any drug can be abused or even illegal if taken in excess, including alcohol and prescription medication. Some examples of illicit drugs are listed in Box 5-3 (see Chapter 35 for further discussion of substance abuse).

Nutrition

Good nutrition is essential for optimal health. A well-balanced diet helps prevent illness and also is used to treat certain health problems. Conversely, poor eating habits, eating disorders, and obesity are linked to disease and debility. *Dietary Guidelines for Americans 2005* provides evidenced-based recommendations to promote health and reduce risks for chronic diseases through diet and physical activity. This guide contains resources for health professionals and consumers on dietary guidelines, the food guide pyramid (see Fig. 15-4), food composition, dietary supplements, and resource lists (U.S. Department of Health and Human Services [USDHHS] & U.S. Department of Agriculture [USDA], 2005) (http://www.nal.usda.gov/fnic/).

Nutritional Deficiencies

Overt disease caused by lack of certain nutrients is rarely seen in the United States; however, insufficient amounts or imbalances of nutrients do pose problems for individuals

and families. Overweight or underweight status, malabsorption, listlessness, fatigue, frequent colds and other minor infections, constipation, dull hair and thin nails, and dental caries are examples of problems that can be related to nutrition and indicate the need for further nutritional assessment. Poor nutrition, especially related to obesity and high fat and cholesterol intake, may lead to more serious conditions and is said to contribute to 4 of the 10 leading causes of death in the United States: diseases of the heart, malignant neoplasms, cerebrovascular diseases, and diabetes.

Obesity

During the past 20 years, the prevalence of obesity has doubled in the United States. It is estimated that 25% of the women older than 20 years are obese (body mass index [BMI], 30 or higher), and 51% of the women older than 20 years are overweight (BMI, 25 to 25.9) (Kealy, 2003; National Center for Chronic Disease Prevention and Health Promotion, 2000). In the United States the prevalence of obesity is highest among non-Hispanic black women, followed by Hispanic women and non-Hispanic white women (Flegal, Carroll, Ogden, & Johnson, 2002).

The BMI is defined as a measure of an adult's weight in relation to his or her height, specifically the adult's weight in kilograms divided by the square of his or her height in meters (Box 5-4 and Table 15-2).

Overweight and obesity are known risk factors for premature death, diabetes, heart disease, dyslipidemia, stroke, hypertension, gallbladder disease, diverticular disease, some anemias, oral disease, constipation, osteoarthritis, gout, osteoporosis, respiratory dysfunction and sleep apnea, and some types of cancer (uterine, breast, colorectal, kidney, and gallbladder) (American Cancer Society, 2006). In addition, obesity is associated with high cholesterol, menstrual irregularities, hirsutism (excess body/facial hair), stress incontinence, depression, complications of pregnancy, increased surgical risk, and shortened life span (USDHHS & USDA, 2005). Pregnant women who are morbidly obese are at increased risk for hypertension, diabetes, gallbladder disease, postterm pregnancy, and musculoskeletal problems (Cesario, 2003).

Other Considerations

Other dietary extremes also can produce risk. For example, insufficient amounts of calcium can lead to osteoporosis, too much sodium can aggravate hypertension, and

---

box 5-3 | Drugs of Abuse

- Acid/lysergic acid diethylamide (LSD)
- Alcohol
- Club drugs
   Gamma-hydroxybutyrate (GHB)
   Methylenedioxymethamphetamine (MDMA or ecstasy)
   Flunitrazepam (Rohypnol)
   Ketamine
   Methamphetamines
- Cocaine/crack
- Hallucinogens
- Heroin
- Inhalants (e.g., paint thinners)
- Marijuana
- Phencyclidine (PCP)
- Prescription drugs
   Depressants
   Opioids—morphine derivatives
   Stimulants—amphetamines
- Smoking/nicotine

Source: Community Epidemiology Work Group. (2005). *Epidemiologic trends in drug abuse—advance report.* Washington, DC: National Institute on Drug Abuse.

---

box 5-4 | Ideal Body Weight with Body Mass Index (BMI)

- BMI ≤18.5, underweight
- BMI 18.5 to 24.9, normal weight
- BMI 25.0 to 29.9, overweight
- BMI 30.0 to 34.5, obese
- BMI 35.0 to 40, very obese

Source: Weiss, J., & Scott, L. (2001). Stalking the no. 1 killer of women: Detecting diabetes and heart diseases. *AWHONN Lifelines, 5*(5), 26-34.

mega-doses of vitamins can cause adverse effects in several body systems. Fad weight-loss programs and yo-yo dieting (repeated weight gain and weight loss) result in nutritional imbalances and, in some instances, medical problems. Such diets and programs are not appropriate for weight maintenance. Adolescent pregnancy produces special nutritional requirements because the metabolic needs of pregnancy are superimposed on the teen's own needs for growth and maturation at a time when eating habits are less than ideal.

Anorexia Nervosa. Some women have a distorted view of their bodies and, no matter what their weight, perceive themselves to be much too heavy. As a result, they undertake strict and severe diets and rigorous extreme exercise. This chronic eating disorder is known as anorexia nervosa. Women can carry this condition to the point of starvation, with resulting endocrine and metabolic abnormalities. If not corrected, significant complications of arrhythmias, amenorrhea, cardiomyopathy, and congestive heart failure occur and, in the extreme, can lead to death. The condition commonly begins during adolescence in young women who have some degree of personality disorder. They gradually lose weight over several months, have amenorrhea, and are abnormally concerned with body image. Diagnosis can be difficult, especially if the person tries to hide the problem. Denial of a problem and secrecy around eating are common features of anorexia. Depression usually accompanies anorexia. There are no specific tests to diagnose anorexia nervosa. A medical history, physical examination, and screening tests help identify women at risk for eating disorders. Several tools are available to use in primary care settings. The SCOFF questionnaire is easy to administer and can help the nurse decide whether an eating disorder is likely and if the woman needs further assessment and possibly psychiatric and medical intervention (Parker, Lyons, & Bonner, 2005; Perry, Morgan, Reid, Brunton, O'Brien, Luck, et al., 2002) (Box 5-5).

Bulimia Nervosa. Bulimia refers to secret, uncontrolled binge eating alternating with methods to prevent weight gain: self-induced vomiting, use of laxatives or diuretics, strict diets, fasting, and rigorous exercise. During a binge episode, large numbers of calories are consumed, usually consisting of sweets and "junk foods." Binges occur at least twice per week. Bulimia usually begins in early adulthood (ages 18 to 25 years) and is found primarily in women. Complications can include dehydration and electrolyte imbalance, gastrointestinal abnormalities, and cardiac arrhythmias. Bulimia is somewhat similar to anorexia in that it is an eating disorder and usually involves some degree of depression. Unlike those with anorexia, individuals with bulimia may feel shame or disgust about their disorder and tend to seek help earlier. The SCOFF screening assessment also can be used (see Box 5-5).

Binge Eating Disorder. The hallmark of binge eating disorder is eating large amounts of food in a short period (a couple of hours) and not being able to stop eating. The woman may eat when she's not hungry or until uncomfortably full. She may choose to eat alone because she is embarrassed about how much she eats. Binge eating disorder involves binging that alternates with a restricted dietary intake. An associated syndrome called night eating syndrome is when limited food is eaten early in the day and most of the day's food intake is consumed after the evening meal. Over time, obesity and related complications of being overweight can develop. Common personality traits found in those with binge eating disorder include excessive concern about body size and shape and low self-esteem. Depression and anxiety commonly occur along with binge eating, which makes treatment and recovery more difficult. Binge eating is not associated with anorexia nervosa or bulimia nervosa.

Physical Fitness and Exercise

Exercise contributes to good health by reducing risks for a variety of conditions that are influenced by obesity and a sedentary lifestyle. It is effective in the prevention of cardiovascular disease and in the management of chronic conditions such as hypertension, arthritis, diabetes, respiratory disorders, and osteoporosis. Exercise also contributes to stress reduction and weight maintenance. Women report that engaging in regular exercise improves their body image and self-esteem and acts as a mood enhancer. Aerobic exercise produces cardiovascular involvement because increasing amounts of oxygen are delivered to working muscles. Anaerobic exercise, such as weight training, improves individual muscle mass without stress on the cardiovascular system. Because women are concerned about both cardiovascular and bone health, weight-bearing aerobic exercises such as walking, running, racket sports, and dancing are preferred. However, excessive or strenuous exercise can lead to hormonal imbalances, resulting in amenorrhea and its consequences. Physical injury also is a potential risk.

Stress

The modern woman faces increasing levels of stress and as a result is prone to a variety of stress-induced complaints and illness. Stress often occurs because of multiple roles, such as when coping with job and financial responsibilities conflicts with parenting and duties at home. To add to this

---

box 5-5 | **Screening for Eating Disorders**

SCOFF QUESTIONS

Each questions score 1 point. A score of 2 or more indicates the person may have anorexia nervosa or bulimia.

1. Do you make yourself **S**ick (i.e., induce vomiting) because you feel too full?
2. Do you worry about loss of **C**ontrol over the amount you eat?
3. Have you recently lost more than **O**ne stone (6.4 kg [14 lbs]) in a 3-month period?
4. Do you think you are too **F**at even if others think you are too thin?
5. Does **F**ood dominate your life?

Reference: Morgan, J., Reid, F., & Lacey, J. (1999). The SCOFF questionnaire: Assessment of a new screening tool for eating disorders. *BMJ, 319*(7223), 1467-1468.

burden, women are socialized to be caretakers, which is an emotionally draining role in itself. They also may find themselves in positions of minimal power that do not allow them to have control over their everyday environments. Some stress is normal and contributes to positive outcomes. Many women thrive in busy surroundings. However, excessive or high levels of ongoing stress trigger physical reactions in the body, such as rapid heart rate, elevated blood pressure, slowed digestion, release of additional neurotransmitters and hormones, muscle tenseness, and a weakened immune system. Consequently, constant stress can contribute to clinical illnesses such as flare-ups of arthritis or asthma, frequent colds or infections, gastrointestinal upsets, cardiovascular problems, and infertility. Box 5-6 lists symptoms that may be related to chronic or extreme stress. Psychologic signs such as anxiety, irritability, eating disorders, depression, insomnia, and substance abuse also have been associated with stress.

Sexual Practices

Potential risks related to sexual activity are undesired pregnancy and STIs. The risks are particularly high for adolescents and young adults who engage in sexual intercourse at earlier and earlier ages. Adolescents report many reasons for wanting to be sexually active, among which are peer pressure, desire to love and be loved, experimentation, enhancing self-esteem, and having fun. However, many teens do not have the decision-making or values-clarification skills needed to take this important step at a young age, and they lack the knowledge base regarding contraception and STIs. They also do not believe that becoming pregnant or getting an STI will happen to them.

Although some STIs can be cured with antibiotics, many can cause significant problems. Possible sequelae include infertility, ectopic pregnancy, neonatal morbidity and mortality, genital cancers, acquired immunodeficiency syndrome (AIDS), and even death (Centers for Disease Control and Prevention [CDC], Workowski, & Berman, [2006]). The incidence of STIs is increasing rapidly and reaching epidemic proportions. Choice of contraception has an impact on the risk of contracting an STI; however, no method of contraception offers complete protection. (See Chapter 8 for discussion of STIs and Chapter 9 for contraception.)

▬ NURSE ALERT

A comprehensive sexual assessment should be integrated into all health histories.

Medical Conditions

Most women of reproductive age are relatively healthy. Heart disease, lung, breast, colon, and gynecologic cancers, stroke, chronic lung disease, and diabetes are all concerns for adult women, since they are among the leading causes of death in women (Box 5-7). Certain medical conditions present during pregnancy can have deleterious effects on both the woman and the fetus. Of particular concern are risks from all forms of diabetes, urinary tract disorders,

| box 5-6 | **Stress Symptoms** |

PHYSICAL
- Perspiration/sweaty hands
- Increased heart rate
- Trembling
- Nervous tics
- Dryness of throat and mouth
- Tiring easily
- Urinating frequently
- Sleeping problems
- Diarrhea, indigestion, vomiting
- Butterflies in stomach
- Headaches
- Premenstrual tension
- Pain in the neck and lower back
- Loss of appetite or overeating
- Susceptibility to illness

BEHAVIOR
- Stuttering and other speech difficulties
- Crying for no apparent reason
- Acting impulsively
- Startling easily
- Laughing in a high-pitched and nervous tone of voice
- Grinding teeth
- Increasing smoking
- Increasing use of drugs and alcohol
- Being accident-prone
- Losing appetite or overeating

PSYCHOLOGIC
- Feeling anxious
- Feeling scared
- Feeling irritable
- Feeling moody
- Low self-esteem
- Fear of failure
- Inability to concentrate
- Embarrassing easily
- Worrying about the future
- Preoccupation with thoughts or tasks
- Forgetfulness

Modified from The State University of New York Counseling Center. (2002). *Stress management.* Buffalo: University of Buffalo, The State University of New York.

thyroid disease, hypertensive disorders of pregnancy, cardiac disease, and seizure disorders. Effects on the fetus vary and include intrauterine growth restriction, macrosomia, anemia, prematurity, immaturity, and stillbirth. Effects on the woman also can be severe. These conditions are discussed in later chapters.

Gynecologic Conditions

Women are at risk throughout their reproductive years for pelvic inflammatory disease, endometriosis, STIs and other vaginal infections, uterine fibroids, uterine deformities such as bicornuate uterus, ovarian cysts, interstitial cystitis, and urinary incontinence related to pelvic relaxation. These gynecologic conditions may contribute negatively

Evolve/CD: Case Study: Health Assessment

box 5-7 Top Ten Leading Causes of Death in the United States*

1. Diseases of the heart (1)
2. Malignant neoplasms (cancer) (2)
3. Cerebrovascular diseases (stroke) (3)
4. Chronic lower respiratory disease (chronic obstructive pulmonary disease [COPD]) (4)
5. Accidents (7)
6. Diabetes mellitus (6)
7. Influenza and pneumonia (8)
8. Alzheimer's disease (5)
9. Nephritis, nephritic syndrome, and nephrosis (9)
10. Septicemia (10)

* NOTE: Top 10 ranking for general population is on the left. Rank of top ten leading causes of death for women in parentheses.
Reference: Centers for Disease Control and Prevention. Office of Women's Health. (2006). *Leading causes of deaths Females-United States, 2002.* Accessed www.cdc.gov, February 27, 2006; Hoyert, D., Mathews, T., Menacker, F., Strobino, D., & Guyer, B. (2006). Annual summary of vital statistics-2004. *Pediatrics, 117*(1), 168-183.

to pregnancy by causing infertility, miscarriage, preterm labor, and fetal and neonatal problems. Gynecologic cancers also affect women's health, although the risk for most cancers is low in pregnancy. Risk factors depend on the type of cancer. The impact of developing a gynecologic problem or cancer in women and their families is shaped by a number of factors including the specific type of problem or cancer, the implications of the diagnosis for the woman and her family, and the timing of the occurrence in the woman's and the family's lives. These conditions are discussed in Chapters 7, 8, and 12.

Environmental and Workplace Hazards

Environmental hazards in the home, the workplace, and the community can contribute to poor health at all ages. Categories and examples of health-damaging hazards include the following: (1) pathogenic agents (viruses, bacteria, fungi, parasites); (2) natural and synthetic chemicals (natural toxins from animals, insects, and plants; consumer and industrial products such as pesticides and hydrocarbon gases; medical and diagnostic devices; tobacco; fuels; and drug and alcohol abuse); (3) radiation (radon, heat waves, sound waves); (4) food substances (added components that are not necessary for nutrition); and (5) physical objects (moving vehicles, machinery, weapons, water, and building materials).

Environmental hazards can affect fertility, fetal development, live birth, and the child's future mental and physical development. Environmental hazards are discussed throughout other chapters as they are identified as specific risks to women's and infants' health.

Violence Against Women

Violence against women is a major health care problem in the United States, affecting millions of women each year and costing millions of dollars in annual medical costs. Women of all races and of all ethnic, educational, religious, and socioeconomic backgrounds are affected. Pregnancy is often a time when violence begins or escalates. The

magnitude of the problem is far greater than the statistics indicate, because violent crimes against women are the most underreported data as a result of fear, lack of understanding, and stigma surrounding violent situations. Maternity and women's health nurses, by the very nature of their practice, are in a unique position to conduct case finding, provide sensitive care to women experiencing abusive situations, engage in prevention activities, and influence health care and public policy toward decreasing the violence. For further discussion of violence against women, see Chapter 6.

▬ HEALTH ASSESSMENT

Women's health trends have expanded beyond a reproductive focus to include a holistic approach to health care across the life span and places women's health within the scope of primary care. Women's health assessment and screening focuses on a systems evaluation beginning with a careful history and physical examination. During the assessment and evaluation, the responsibility for self-care, health promotion, and enhancement of wellness is emphasized.

In a market-driven system such as managed care, specific guidelines may be provided for health screening by the insurer or the managed care organization. A nurse often takes the history, orders diagnostic tests, interprets test results, makes referrals, coordinates care, and directs attention to problems requiring medical intervention. Advanced practice nurses who have specialized in women's health, such as nurse practitioners, clinical nurse specialists, and nurse-midwives, perform complete physical examinations, including gynecologic examinations.

Interview

The contact with the woman usually begins with an interview. This interview should be conducted in a private, comfortable, and relaxed setting (Fig. 5-8). The woman is addressed by her title and name (e.g., Mrs. Gonzalez), and the nurse introduces herself or himself by using name and

FIG. 5-8 Nurse interviews client as part of annual physical examination. (Courtesy Skip Davis, San Francisco, CA.)

title. It is important to phrase questions in a sensitive and nonjudgmental manner. Body language should match verbal communication. The nurse is cognizant of a woman's vulnerability and assures her of strict confidentiality. For many women, fear, anxiety, and modesty make the examination a dreaded and stressful experience. Many women are uninformed, misguided by myths, or afraid they will appear ignorant by asking questions about sexual or reproductive functioning. The woman is assured that no question is irrelevant. The history begins with an open-ended question such as, "What brings you in to the office/clinic/hospital today? Anything else? Tell me about it."

Additional ways to get women to share information include the following:

- **Facilitation:** Using a word or posture that communicates interest; leaning forward; making eye contact; or saying "Mm-hmmm" or "Go on"
- **Reflection:** Repeating a word or phrase that a woman has used
- **Clarification:** Asking the woman what is meant by a word or phrase
- **Empathic responses:** Acknowledging the feelings of a woman by statements such as "That must have been frightening"
- **Confrontation:** Identifying something about the woman's behavior or feelings not expressed verbally or apparently inconsistent with her history
- **Interpretation:** Putting into words what you infer about the woman's feelings or about the meaning of her symptoms, events, or other matters

Direct questions may be necessary to elicit specific details. These should be worded in language that is understandable to the woman and expressed neutrally, so that the woman will not be led into a specific response. The nurse asks about one item at a time and proceeds from the general to the specific (Seidel, Ball, Dains, & Benedict, 2006).

Cultural Considerations and Communication Variations

Recognizing signs and symptoms of disease and deciding when to seek treatment is influenced by cultural perceptions. It is essential that a nurse have respect for the rich and unique qualities that cultural diversity brings to individuals. In recognizing the value of these differences, the nurse can modify the plan of care to meet the needs of each woman. Trust that the woman is the expert on her life, culture, and experiences. If the nurse asks with respect and a genuine desire to learn, the woman will tell the nurse how to care for her. Modifications may be necessary for the physical examination. In some cultures, it may be considered inappropriate for the woman to disrobe completely for the physical examination. In many cultures, a woman examiner is preferred (Mattson, 2003).

Communication may be hindered by different beliefs even when the nurse and woman speak the same language. Examples of communication variations are listed in the Cultural Considerations Box.

---

cultural considerations

Communication Variations

- **Conversational style and pacing:** Silence may show respect or acknowledgment that the listener has heard. In cultures in which a direct "no" is considered rude, silence may mean no. Repetition or loudness may mean emphasis or anger.
- **Personal space:** Cultural conceptions of personal space differ. Based on one's culture, for example, someone may be perceived as distant for backing off when approached, or aggressive for standing too close.
- **Eye contact:** Eye contact varies among cultures from intense to fleeting. Consistent with the effort to refrain from invading personal space, avoiding direct eye contact may be a sign of respect.
- **Touch:** The norms about how people should touch each other vary among cultures. In some cultures, physical contact with the same sex (embracing, walking hand in hand) is more appropriate than that with an unrelated person of the opposite sex.
- **Time orientation:** In some cultures, involvement with people is more valued than being "on time." In other cultures, life is scheduled and paced according to clock time, which is valued over personal time.

Reference: Mattson, S. (2000). Striving for cultural competence: Providing care for the changing face of the U.S. *AWHONN Lifelines, 4*(3), 48-52.

Women with Special Needs
Women with Disabilities

Women with emotional or physical disorders have special needs. Women who have vision, hearing, emotional, or physical disabilities should be respected and involved in the assessment and physical examination to the full extent of their abilities. The nurse should communicate openly and directly with sensitivity. It is often helpful to learn about the disability directly from the woman while maintaining eye contact. Family and significant others should be relied on only when absolutely necessary. The assessment and physical examination can be adapted to each woman's individual needs.

Communication with a woman who is hearing impaired can be accomplished without difficulty. Most of these women read lips, write, or both; thus an interviewer who speaks and enunciates each word slowly and in full view may be easily understood. If a woman is not comfortable with lip reading, she may use an interpreter. In this case, it is important to continue to address the woman directly, avoiding the temptation to speak directly with the interpreter.

The visually impaired woman needs to be oriented to the examination room and may have her guide dog with her. As with all women, the visually impaired woman needs a full explanation of what the examination entails before proceeding. Before touching her, the nurse explains, "Now I am going to take your blood pressure. I am going to place the cuff on your right arm." The woman can be asked if she would like to touch each of the items that will be used in the examination to reduce her anxiety.

Many women with physical disabilities cannot comfortably lie in the lithotomy position for the pelvic examination. Several alternative positions may be used, including a lateral (side-lying) position, a V-shaped position, a diamond-shaped position, and an M-shaped position (Fig. 5-9). The woman can be asked what has worked best for her previously. If she has never had a pelvic examination, or has never had a comfortable pelvic examination, the nurse proceeds by showing her a picture of various positions and asking her which one she prefers. The nurse's support and reassurance can help the woman to relax, which will make the examination go more smoothly.

Abused Women

Nurses should screen all women entering the health care system for potential abuse. Help for the woman may depend on the sensitivity with which the nurse screens for abuse, the discovery of abuse, and subsequent intervention. The nurse must be familiar with the laws governing abuse in the state in which she or he practices.

Pocket cards listing emergency numbers (abuse counseling, legal protection, and emergency shelter) may be available from the local police department, a women's shelter, or an emergency department. It is helpful to have these on hand in the setting where screening is done. An abuse-assessment screen (Fig. 5-10) can be used as part of the interview or written history. If a male partner is present, he should be asked to leave the room because the woman may not disclose experiences of abuse in his presence, or he may try to answer questions for her to protect himself. The same procedure would apply for partners of lesbians, parents of teens, or adult children of older women.

Fear, guilt, and embarrassment may keep many women from giving information about family violence. Clues in the history and evidence of injuries on physical examination should give a high index of suspicion. The areas most commonly injured in women are the head, the neck, the chest, the abdomen, the breasts, and the upper extremities. Burns and bruises in patterns resembling hands, belts, cords, or other weapons may be seen as well as multiple traumatic injuries. Attention should be given to women who repeatedly seek treatment for somatic complaints such as headaches, insomnia, choking sensation, hyperventilation, gastrointestinal symptoms, and pain in the chest, back, and pelvis. During pregnancy, the nurse should assess for injuries to the breasts, the abdomen, and the genitals. See Chapter 6 for further discussion of violence.

Adolescents (Aged 13 to 19 Years)

As a young woman matures, she should be asked the same questions that are included in any history. Particular attention should be paid to hints about risky behaviors, eating disorders, and depression. Do not assume that a teenager is not sexually active. After rapport has been established, it is best to talk to a teen with the parent (partner or friend) out of the room. Questions should be asked with sensitivity and in a gentle and nonjudgmental manner (Seidel et al., 2006).

A teen's first speculum examination is the most important because she will develop perceptions that will remain with her for future examinations. What the examination entails should be discussed with the teen while she is

FIG. 5-9 Lithotomy and variable positions for women who have a disability.

ABUSE ASSESSMENT SCREEN

1. Have you ever been emotionally or physically abused by your partner or someone important to you?

YES ☐   NO ☐

2. Within the last year, have you been hit, slapped, kicked, or otherwise physically hurt by someone?

YES ☐   NO ☐

If YES, by whom _____

Number of times _____

Mark the area of injury on body map.

3. Within the last year, has anyone forced you to have sexual activities?

YES ☐   NO ☐

If YES, by whom _____

Number of times _____

4. Are you afraid of your partner or anyone you listed above?

YES ☐   NO ☐

FIG. 5-10 Abuse assessment screen. (Modified from the Nursing Research Consortium on Violence and Abuse. [1991].)

---

dressed. Models or illustrations can be used to show exactly what will happen. All of the necessary equipment should be assembled so that there are no interruptions. Pediatric specula that are 1 to 1.5 cm wide can be inserted with minimal discomfort. If the teen is sexually active, a small adult speculum may be used.

Injury prevention should be a part of the counseling at routine health examinations, with special attention to seat belts, helmets, firearms, recreational hazards, and sports involvement. The use of drugs and alcohol and the nonuse of seat belts contribute to motor vehicle injuries, accounting for the greatest proportion of accidental deaths in women. Contraceptive/STI prevention information may be needed for teens who are sexually active.

To provide developmentally appropriate care, it is important to review the major tasks for women in this stage of life. Major tasks for teens include values assessment; education and work goal setting; formation of peer relationships that focus on love, commitment, and becoming comfortable with sexuality; and separation from parents. Individuality may be reflected in areas such as sexuality, politics, and career choices. Conflict exists between making and keeping commitments to keep options open. The teen is egocentric as she progresses rapidly through emotional and physical change. Her feelings of invulnerability may lead to serious misconceptions, such as that unprotected sexual intercourse will not lead to pregnancy.

Midlife and Older Women (Aged 50 Years and Older)

The assessment of women aged 50 and older presents unique challenges. Women may be experiencing major lifestyle changes, such as children leaving home, care for their aging parents, job change, retirement, separation, divorce or death of a partner, and aging-related changes and health problems. The nurse has an opportunity to use reflection and empathy while listening and ensuring open and caring communication. It may be necessary to schedule a longer appointment time because older women have longer histories or have a need to talk. Some women may fail to report symptoms because they fear their complaints will be attributed to old age, or they feel that they have lived with a chronic condition (e.g., incontinence, dyspareunia, interstitial cystitis, decreased libido, depression) for so long that nothing can be done. Women may choose to ignore a problem if they have symptoms that are life threatening (e.g., chest pain or a breast lump) because they traditionally put the needs of others first. As a result, the nurse should encourage the woman to express her concerns and fears and reassure her that her problems are important and will be addressed. Hormone therapy, diet, vitamin and calcium supplementation, daily aspirin, breast self-examination, mammogram, sigmoidoscopy, colonoscopy, updating immunizations, and need for exercise and sun protection should be discussed.

Functional assessment is included as part of the history in women older than 70 years and those with disabilities. In the review of systems, the nurse should ask about self-care activities such as walking, getting to the bathroom, bathing, hair combing, dressing, and eating. Questions about driving, using public transportation, the telephone or the Internet, hanging up clothes, buying groceries, taking medications, and meal preparation should be included.

Sexual assessment continues to be important in women aged 50 and older. Unless directly asked, women may omit mention of sexual concerns. Questions asked with sensitivity may invite responses regarding changes in sexual desire or response or physical issues that challenge her sexual enjoyment. Open and reflective questions also affirm a woman's right to sexual enjoyment throughout the life span.

Women older than 50 years commonly experience menopause and have physical changes associated with decreased estrogen. A decrease in estrogen causes thinning of the mucosal tissue layers, resulting in a narrowing and a decrease in lubrication of the vagina. Estrogen also plays a role in the formation of bone matrix, and a decrease may lead to osteoporosis. The risk for heart disease increases because of changes in lipid metabolism related to declining estrogen levels. Decreases in estrogen also can cause a relaxation of the ligaments and connective tissue, which affects the support of the bladder and uterus. Decreases in estrogen also affect the hypothalamus, causing hot flashes, which are disturbing to most women (see Chapter 7).

Physical changes can result in increased discomfort during the pelvic examination. It is important to be both gentle and thorough during the examination. A small adult speculum may be used to view the cervix. The uterus in a menopausal woman is small and firm, and the ovaries are non-palpable. In postmenopausal women, the specimen from the vaginal pool may be useful to detect endometrial cells. A woman with palpable adnexal masses or vaginal bleeding after menopause needs immediate gynecologic referral.

A respectful and reassuring approach toward caring for women aged 50 and older will ensure their continued participation in seeking health care. Because the risk of breast, ovarian, uterine, cervical, and colon cancer increases with age, the nurse has the opportunity to educate women about the importance of preventive screening. It is the nurse's responsibility to ensure a positive health care experience that encourages future visits for prevention and chronic and acute care.

Advance directives can be introduced on any entry into a health care system. It is a good idea to have a formal statement in the medical record regarding a woman's wishes in the event of accident or illness regarding life-maintenance measures or organ donation. Most states have laws formalizing such statements in writing. The Durable Power of Attorney for Health Care can be used by a woman to delegate decision-making authority to a trusted relative or friend.

Many studies done on religion and health suggest that religious people are healthier and generally live longer than nonreligious people. Religious people have lower rates of

---

box 5-8 | **Spiritual Wellness Self-Assessment**

The more questions for which you have an answer other than "I don't know," the higher the level of spiritual wellness.
1. What is your purpose in life?
2. What activities do you do regularly that bring you joy?
3. Do you believe in a higher power?
4. Who can you count on for encouragement and/or support?
5. To whom do you give encouragement and/or support?
6. Who loves you?
7. Who do you love or care about?
8. In what areas are you growing?
9. What activities nurture you?
10. Is there something that you do just for yourself every day?
11. How do you go about forgiving yourself?
12. How do you go about forgiving others?
13. To whom do you confide your hopes, dreams, and pain?
14. What do you hope for in the future?
15. What do you do regularly just for fun?
16. When do you reach out to people?
17. What goals do you have for 6 months from now?
18. What goals do you have for 2 years from now?
19. Do you look forward to getting up in the morning?
20. Would you like to live to be 100?

Reference: Condon, M. (2004). *Women's health: Body, mind, spirit: An integrated approach to wellness and illness.* New Jersey: Prentice Hall.

---

uterine, cervical, and intestinal cancer, ulcer disease, coronary artery disease, and high blood pressure. Those who attend church once a week are less likely to become ill than those who do not. The studies did not control for rates of smoking and drinking, so no inference can be made as to whether the improved health status was from better health habits or religion. In general, it is known that religious people do tend to have healthier lifestyles overall than people who are not religious (Condon, 2004). Spiritual wellness can be estimated by answering questions such as those suggested in Box 5-8.

Healthy Aging. Women in the United States can expect on average to live to be 80 years old and may spend one third of their lives as postmenopausal women. With a healthy lifestyle, many women are living to be 100 years old or older. Proper nutrition, exercise, and mental and social stimulation are critical to keeping the body healthy and the mind active and alert into old age. Menopause is a time to evaluate, take stock, and prepare for many healthy years to come (Minikin & Wright, 2005).

History

At a woman's first visit, she is often expected to fill out a form with biographic and historic data before meeting with the examiner. This form aids the health care provider in completing the history during the interview. Most forms include information about the following categories:
- Biographic data
- Reason for seeking care
- Present health or history of present illness

- Past health
- Family history
- Review of systems
- Functional assessment (activities of daily living)

The following section describes a complete health history based on the above categories.

- **Identifying data:** Name, age, race, sex, marital status, occupation, religion, and ethnicity
- **Reason for seeking care:** A response to the question, "What problem or symptom brought you here today?" If the woman lists more than one reason, focus on the one she thinks is most important.
- **Present health:** Current health status is described with attention to the following:
  - Use of safety measures: seat belts, bicycle helmets, designated driver
  - Exercise and leisure activities: regularity
  - Sleep patterns: length and quality
  - Sexuality: Is she sexually active? With men, women, or both? Safer-sex practices?
  - Diet, including beverages: 24-hour dietary recall; caffeine: coffee, tea, cola, or chocolate intake
  - Nicotine, alcohol, illicit or recreational drug use: type, amount, frequency, duration, and reactions
  - Environmental and chemical hazards: home, school, work, and leisure setting; exposure to extreme heat or cold, noise, industrial toxins such as asbestos or lead, pesticides, diethylstilbestrol (DES), radiation, cat feces, or cigarette smoke
- **History of present illness:** A chronologic narrative that includes onset of the problem, the setting in which it developed, its manifestations, and any treatments received are noted. The woman's state of health before the onset of the present problem is determined. If the problem is of long standing, the reason for seeking attention at this time is elicited. The principal symptoms should be described with respect to the following:
  - Location
  - Quality or character
  - Quantity or severity
  - Timing (onset, duration, frequency)
  - Setting
  - Factors that aggravate or relieve
  - Associated factors
  - Woman's perception of the meaning of the symptom
- Past health:
  - Infectious diseases: For example, measles, mumps, rubella, whooping cough, chickenpox, rheumatic fever, scarlet fever, diphtheria, polio, tuberculosis (TB), hepatitis
  - Chronic disease and system disorders: arthritis, cancer, diabetes, heart, lung, kidney, seizures, thyroid, stroke, ulcers, sickle cell anemia
  - Adult injuries, accidents
  - Hospitalizations, operations, blood transfusions
  - Obstetric history

  - Allergies: medications, previous transfusion reactions, environmental allergies
  - Immunizations: diphtheria; pertussis; tetanus; polio; measles; mumps; rubella (MMR); hepatitis B; varicella; influenza; pneumococcal vaccine; last TB skin test
  - Last date of screening tests: Pap test, mammogram, stool for occult blood, sigmoidoscopy/colonoscopy, hematocrit, hemoglobin, rubella titer, urinalysis, cholesterol test; electrocardiogram, last vision, dental, hearing examination
  - Current medications: name, dose, frequency, duration, reason for taking, and compliance with prescription medications; home remedies, over-the-counter drugs, vitamin and mineral or herbal supplements used over a 24-hour period
- **Family history:** Information about age and health of family members may be presented in narrative form or as a family tree or genogram: age, health/death of parents, siblings, spouse, children. Check for history of diabetes; heart disease; hypertension; stroke; respiratory, renal, or thyroid problems; cancer; bleeding disorders; hepatitis; allergies; asthma; arthritis; TB; epilepsy; mental illness; HIV; or other disorders.
  - **Screen for abuse:** Has she ever been hit, kicked, slapped, or forced to have sex against her wishes? Has she been verbally or emotionally abused? Does she have a history of childhood sexual abuse? If yes, has she received counseling or does she need referral?
- **Review of systems:** It is probable that all questions in each system will not be included every time a history is taken. Some questions regarding each system should be included in every history. The essential areas to be explored are listed in the following head-to-toe sequence. If a woman gives a positive response to a question about an essential area, more detailed questions should be asked.
  - General: weight change, fatigue, weakness, fever, chills, or night sweats
  - Skin: skin, hair, and nail changes; itching, bruising, bleeding, rashes, sores, lumps, or moles
  - Lymph nodes: enlargement, inflammation, pain, suppuration (pus), or drainage
  - Head: trauma, vertigo (dizziness), convulsive disorder, syncope (fainting); headache: location, frequency, pain type, nausea/vomiting, or visual symptoms present
  - Eyes: glasses, contact lenses, blurriness, tearing, itching, photophobia, diplopia, inflammation, trauma, cataracts, glaucoma, or acute visual loss
  - Ears: hearing loss, tinnitus (ringing), vertigo, discharge, pain, fullness, recurrent infections, or mastoiditis
  - Nose/sinuses: trauma, rhinitis, nasal discharge, epistaxis, obstruction, sneezing, itching, allergy, or smelling impairment

–Mouth/throat/neck: hoarseness, voice changes, soreness, ulcers, bleeding gums, goiter, swelling, or enlarged nodes

–Breasts: masses, pain, lumps, dimpling, nipple discharge, fibrocystic changes, or implants; BSE practice

–Respiratory: shortness of breath, wheezing, cough, sputum, hemoptysis, pneumonia, pleurisy, asthma, bronchitis, emphysema, or TB; date of last chest X-ray

–Cardiovascular: hypertension, rheumatic fever, murmurs, angina, palpitations, dyspnea, tachycardia, orthopnea, edema, chest pain, cough, cyanosis, cold extremities, ascites, intermittent claudication (leg pain caused by poor circulation to the leg muscles), phlebitis, or skin-color changes

–Gastrointestinal: appetite, nausea, vomiting, indigestion, dysphagia, abdominal pain, ulcers, hematochezia (bleeding with stools), melena (black, tarry stools), bowel-habit changes, diarrhea, constipation, bowel-movement frequency, food intolerance, hemorrhoids, jaundice, or hepatitis; sigmoidoscopy, colonoscopy, barium enema, ultrasound

–Genitourinary: frequency, hesitancy, urgency, polyuria, dysuria, hematuria, nocturia, incontinence, stones, infection, or urethral discharge; menstrual history (e.g., age at menarche, length/flow of menses, last menstrual period [LMP], dysmenorrhea, intermenstrual bleeding, age at menopause or signs of menopause), dyspareunia, discharge, sores, itching

–Sexual health–sexual activity: with men, women, or both; contraceptive use; sexually transmitted infections

–Peripheral vascular: coldness, numbness and tingling, leg edema, claudication, varicose veins, thromboses, or emboli

–Endocrine: heat/cold intolerance, dry skin, excessive sweating, polyuria, polydipsia, polyphagia, thyroid problems, diabetes, or secondary sex characteristic changes

–Hematologic: anemia, easy bruising, bleeding, petechiae, purpura, or transfusions

–Musculoskeletal: muscle weakness, pain, joint stiffness, scoliosis, lordosis, kyphosis, range-of-motion instability, redness, swelling, arthritis, or gout

–Neurologic: loss of sensation, numbness, tingling, tremors, weakness, vertigo, paralysis, fainting, twitching, blackouts, seizures, convulsions, loss of consciousness or memory

–Mental status: moodiness, depression, anxiety, obsessions, delusions, illusions, or hallucinations

• Functional assessment: ability to care for self

Physical Examination

In preparation for the physical examination, the woman is instructed on undressing and given a gown to wear during the examination. She is usually given the opportunity to undress privately. Objective data are recorded by system or location. A general statement of overall health status is a good way to start. Findings are described in detail.

• General appearance: age, race, sex, state of health, posture, height, weight, development, dress, hygiene, affect, alertness, orientation, cooperativeness, and communication skills

• Vital signs: temperature, pulse, respiration, blood pressure

• Skin: color; integrity; texture; hydration; temperature; edema; excessive perspiration; unusual odor; presence and description of lesions; hair texture and distribution; nail configuration, color, texture, condition, or presence of nail clubbing

• Head: size, shape, trauma, masses, scars, rashes, or scaling; facial symmetry; presence of edema or puffiness

• Eyes: pupil size, shape, reactivity, conjunctival injection, scleral icterus, fundal papilledema, hemorrhage, lids, extraocular movements, visual fields and acuity

• Ears: shape and symmetry, tenderness, discharge, external canal, and tympanic membranes; hearing—Weber should be midline (loudness of sound equal in both ears) and Rinne negative (no conductive or sensorineural hearing loss); should be able to hear whisper at 3 feet

• Nose: symmetry, tenderness, discharge, mucosa, turbinate inflammation, frontal or maxillary sinus tenderness; discrimination of odors

• Mouth and throat: hygiene, condition of teeth, dentures, appearance of lips, tongue, buccal and oral mucosa, erythema, edema, exudate, tonsillar enlargement, palate, uvula, gag reflex, ulcers

• Neck: mobility, masses, range of motion, trachea deviation, thyroid size, carotid bruits

• Lymphatic: cervical, intraclavicular, axillary, trochlear, or inguinal adenopathy; size, shape, tenderness, and consistency

• Breasts: skin changes, dimpling, symmetry, scars, tenderness, discharge or masses; characteristics of nipples and areolae

• Heart: rate, rhythm, murmurs, rubs, gallops, clicks, heaves, or precordial movements

• Peripheral vascular: jugular vein distention, bruits, edema, swelling, vein distention, Homans sign, or tenderness of extremities

• Lungs: chest symmetry with respirations, wheezes, crackles, rhonchi, vocal fremitus, whispered pectoriloquy, percussion, and diaphragmatic excursion; breath sounds equal and clear bilaterally

• Abdomen: shape, scars, bowel sounds, consistency, tenderness, rebound, masses, guarding, organomegaly, liver span, percussion (tympany, shifting, dullness), costovertebral angle tenderness

• Extremities: edema, ulceration, tenderness, varicosities, erythema, tremor, or deformity

- Genitourinary: external genitalia, perineum, vaginal mucosa, cervix, inflammation, tenderness, discharge, bleeding, ulcers, nodules, masses, internal vaginal support; bimanual and rectovaginal palpation of cervix, uterus, and adnexae
- Rectal: sphincter tone, masses, hemorrhoids, rectal wall contour, tenderness, and stool for occult blood
- Musculoskeletal: posture, symmetry of muscle mass, muscle atrophy, weakness, appearance of joints, tenderness or crepitus, joint range of motion, instability, redness, swelling, or spine deviation
- Neurologic: mental status, orientation, memory, mood, speech clarity and comprehension, cranial nerves II to XII, sensation, strength, deep tendon and superficial reflexes, gait, balance, and coordination with rapid alternating motions

Pelvic Examination

Many women are intimidated by the gynecologic portion of the physical examination. The nurse in this instance can take an advocacy approach that supports a partnership relationship between the woman and the care provider.

The woman is assisted into the lithotomy position (see Fig. 5-9, *A*) for the pelvic examination. When she is in the lithotomy position, the woman's hips and knees are flexed, with the buttocks at the edge of the table, and her feet are supported by heel or knee stirrups.

Some women prefer to keep their shoes or socks on, especially if the stirrups are not padded. Many women express feelings of vulnerability and strangeness when in the lithotomy position. During the procedure, the nurse assists the woman with relaxation techniques.

One method of helping the woman relax is to have her place her hands on her chest at about the level of the diaphragm, breathe deeply and slowly (in through her nose and out through her O-shaped mouth), concentrate on the rhythm of breathing, and relax all body muscles with each exhalation (Barkauskas, Baumann, & Darling-Fisher, 2002). This breathing technique is particularly helpful for the adolescent or the woman whose introitus may be especially tight or for whom the experience may be new or may provoke tension. Some women relax when they are encouraged to become involved with the examination with a mirror placed so that they can view the area being examined. This type of participation helps with health teaching as well. Distraction is another technique that can be used effectively (e.g., placement of interesting pictures on the ceiling over the head of the table).

Many women find it distressing to attempt to converse in the lithotomy position. Most women appreciate an explanation of the procedure as it unfolds, as well as coaching for the types of sensations they may expect. Generally, however, women prefer not to have to respond to questions until they are again upright and at eye level with the examiner. Questioning during the procedure, especially if they cannot see their questioner's eyes, may make women tense.

External Inspection. The examiner sits at the foot of the table for the inspection of the external genitals and for the speculum examination. In good lighting, external genitals are inspected for sexual maturity: clitoris, labia, and perineum. After childbirth or other trauma, there may be healed scars.

External Palpation. The examiner proceeds with the examination by using palpation and inspection. The examiner wears gloves for this portion of the assessment. Before touching the woman, the examiner explains what is going to be done and what the woman should expect to feel (e.g., pressure). The examiner may touch the woman in a less sensitive area such as the inner thigh to alert her that the genital examination is beginning. This gesture may put the woman more at ease. The labia are spread apart to expose the structures in the vestibule: urinary meatus, Skene glands, vaginal orifice, and Bartholin glands (Fig. 5-11). To assess the Skene glands, the examiner inserts one finger into the vagina and "milks" the area of the urethra. Any exudate from the urethra or the Skene glands is cultured. Masses and erythema of either structure are assessed further. Ordinarily the openings to the Skene glands are not visible; prominent openings may be seen if the glands are infected (e.g., with gonorrhea). During the examination, the examiner keeps in mind the data from the review of systems, such as history of burning on urination.

The vaginal orifice is examined. Hymenal tags are normal findings. With one finger still in the vagina, the examiner repositions the index finger near the posterior part of the orifice. With the thumb outside the posterior part of the labia majora, the examiner compresses the area of Bartholin glands located at the 8 o'clock and 4 o'clock positions and looks for swelling, discharge, and pain.

The support of the anterior and posterior vaginal wall is assessed. The examiner spreads the labia with the index and middle fingers and asks the woman to strain down. Any bulge from the anterior wall (urethrocele or cystocele) or posterior wall (rectocele) is noted and compared with the history, such as difficulty to start the stream of urine or constipation.

FIG. 5-11 External examination. Separation of the labia. (From Edge, V., & Miller, M. [1994]. *Women's health care.* St. Louis: Mosby.)

The perineum (area between the vagina and anus) is assessed for scars from old lacerations or episiotomies, thinning, fistulas, masses, lesions, and inflammation. The anus is assessed for hemorrhoids, hemorrhoidal tags, and integrity of the anal sphincter. The anal area also is assessed for lesions, masses, abscesses, and tumors. If there is a history of STI, the examiner may want to obtain a culture specimen from the anal canal at this time. Throughout the genital examination, the examiner notes the odor. Odor may indicate infection or poor hygiene.

Vulvar Self-Examination. The pelvic examination provides a good opportunity for the practitioner to emphasize the need for regular vulvar self-examination (VSE) and to teach this procedure. Because there has been a dramatic increase in cancerous and precancerous conditions of the vulva in recent years, a VSE should be performed as an integral part of preventive health care by all women who are sexually active or aged 18 years or older, monthly between menses, or more frequently if there are symptoms or a history of serious vulvar disease. Most lesions, including malignancy, condyloma acuminatum (wartlike growth), and Bartholin cysts, can be seen or palpated and are easily treated if diagnosed early.

The VSE can be performed by the practitioner and woman together, by using a mirror. A simple diagram of the anatomy of the vulva can be given to the woman, with instructions to perform the examination herself that evening to reinforce what she has learned. She does the examination in a sitting position with adequate lighting, holding a mirror in one hand and using the other hand to expose the tissues surrounding the vaginal introitus. She then systematically examines the mons pubis, the clitoris, the urethra, the labia majora, the perineum, and the perianal area and palpates the vulva, noting any changes in appearance or abnormalities, such as ulcers, lumps, warts, and changes in pigmentation.

Internal Examination. A vaginal speculum consists of two blades and a handle. Speculums come in a variety of types and styles. A vaginal speculum is used to view the vaginal vault and cervix (see Procedure box). The speculum is gently placed into the vagina and inserted to the back of the vaginal vault. The blades are opened to reveal the cervix and are locked into the open position. The cervix is inspected for position and appearance of the os: color, lesions, bleeding, and discharge (Fig. 5-12). Cervical findings that are not within normal limits include ulcerations, masses, inflammation, and excessive protrusion into the vaginal vault. Anomalies, such as a cockscomb (a protrusion over the cervix that looks like a rooster's comb), a hooded or collared cervix (seen in DES daughters), or polyps, are noted.

Collection of Specimens. The collection of specimens for cytologic examination is an important part of the gynecologic examination. Infection can be diagnosed through examination of specimens collected during the pelvic examination. These infections include candidiasis, trichomoniasis, bacterial vaginosis, group B streptococcus, gonorrhea, chlamydia, and herpes simplex virus. Once the diagnoses have been made, treatment can be instituted.

Papanicolaou (Pap) Test. Carcinogenic conditions, potential or actual, can be determined by examination of cells from the cervix collected during the pelvic examination (see Procedure box). This is termed a Pap test (see Evidence-based Practice box).

Vaginal Examination. After the specimens are obtained, the vagina is viewed when the speculum is rotated. The speculum blades are unlocked and partially closed. As the speculum is withdrawn, it is rotated, and the vaginal walls are inspected for color, lesions, rugae, fistulas, and bulging.

procedure

Assisting with Pelvic Examination

- Wash hands. Assemble equipment (see Fig.).
- Ask woman to empty her bladder before the examination (obtain clean-catch urine specimen as needed).
- Assist with relaxation techniques. Have the woman place her hands on her chest at about the level of the diaphragm, breathe deeply and slowly (in through her nose and out through an O-shaped mouth), concentrate on the rhythm of breathing, and relax all body muscles with each exhalation.*
- Encourage the woman to become involved with the examination if she shows interest. For example, a mirror can be placed so that she can see the area being examined.
- Assess for and treat signs of problems such as supine hypotension.
- Warm the speculum in warm water if a prewarmed one is not available.
- Instruct the woman to bear down when the speculum is being inserted.
- Apply gloves and assist the examiner with collection of specimens for cytologic examination, such as a Pap test. After handling specimens, remove gloves and wash hands.
- Lubricate the examiner's fingers with water or water-soluble lubricant before bimanual examination.
- Assist the woman at completion of the examination to a sitting position and then a standing position.
- Provide tissues to wipe lubricant from perineum.
- Provide privacy for the woman while she is dressing.

Equipment used for pelvic examination. (Courtesy Michael S. Clement, MD, Mesa, AZ.)

* From Barkauskas, V., Baumann, L., & Darling-Fisher, C. (2002). *Health and physical assessment* (3rd ed.). St Louis: Mosby.

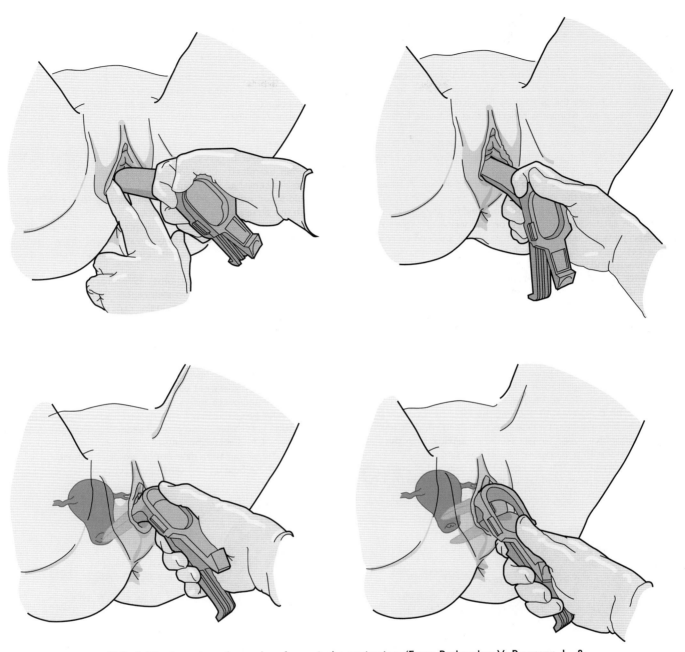

FIG. 5-12 Insertion of speculum for vaginal examination. (From Barkauskas, V., Baumann, L., & Darling-Fisher, C. [2002]. *Health and physical assessment* [3rd ed.]. St Louis: Mosby.)

Bimanual Palpation. The examiner stands for this part of the examination. A small amount of lubricant is placed on the first and second fingers of the gloved hand for the internal examination. To avoid tissue trauma and contamination, the thumb is abducted and the ring and little fingers are flexed into the palm (Fig. 5-13 on p. 118).

The vagina is palpated for distensibility, lesions, and tenderness. The cervix is examined for position, shape, consistency, motility, and lesions. The fornix around the cervix is palpated.

The other hand is placed on the abdomen halfway between the umbilicus and the symphysis pubis and exerts pressure downward toward the pelvic hand. Upward pressure from the pelvic hand traps reproductive structures for assessment by palpation. The uterus is assessed for position, size, shape, consistency, regularity, motility, masses, and tenderness.

With the abdominal hand moving to the right lower quadrant and the fingers of the pelvic hand in the right lateral fornix, the adnexa is assessed for position, size, tenderness, and masses. The examination is repeated on the woman's left side.

Just before the intravaginal fingers are withdrawn, the woman is asked to tighten her vagina around the fingers as much as she can. If the muscle response is weak, the woman is assessed for her knowledge about Kegel exercises.

Papanicolaou (Pap) Test

- In preparation, make sure the woman has not douched, used vaginal medications, or had sexual intercourse for 24 to 48 hours before the procedure (Gingrich, 2004). Reschedule the test if the woman is menstruating. Midcycle is the best time for the test.
- Explain to the woman the purpose of the test and what sensations she will feel as the specimen is obtained (e.g., pressure but not pain).
- The woman is assisted into a lithotomy position. A speculum is inserted into the vagina.
- The cytologic specimen is obtained before any digital examination of the vagina is made or endocervical bacteriologic specimens are taken. A cotton swab may be used to remove excess cervical discharge before the specimen is collected.
- The specimen is obtained by using an endocervical sampling device (cytobrush, cervex-brush, spatula, or broom) (see Figs., A and B). If the two-sample method of obtaining cells is used, the cytobrush is inserted into the canal and rotated 90 to 180 degrees, followed by a gentle smear of the entire transformation zone by using a spatula. Broom devices are inserted and rotated 360 degrees five times. They obtain endocervical and ectocervical samples at the same time. If the client has had a hysterectomy, the vaginal cuff is sampled. Areas that appear abnormal on visualization will require colposcopy and biopsy. If using a one-slide technique, the spatula sample is smeared first. This is followed by applying the cytobrush sample (rolling the brush in the opposite direction from which it was obtained), which is less subject to drying artifact; then the slide is sprayed with preservative within 5 seconds.
- The ThinPrep Pap Test is a liquid-based method of preserving cells that reduces blood, mucus, and inflammation. The Pap specimen is obtained in the manner described above except that the cervix is not swabbed before collection of the sample. The collection device (brush, spatula, or broom) is rinsed in a vial of preserving solution that is provided by the laboratory. The sealed vial with solution is sent off to the appropriate laboratory. A special processing device filters the contents, and a thin layer of cervical cells is deposited on a slide, which is then examined microscopically. The AutoPap and Papnet tests are similar to the ThinPrep test. If cytology is abnormal, liquid-based methods allow follow-up testing for HPV DNA with the same sample (Gingrich, 2004).
- Label the slides or vial with the woman's name and site. Include on the form to accompany the specimens the woman's name, age, parity, and chief complaint or reason for taking the cytologic specimens.
- Send specimens to the pathology laboratory promptly for staining, evaluation, and a written report, with special reference to abnormal elements, including cancer cells.
- Advise the woman that repeated tests may be necessary if the specimen is not adequate.
- Instruct the woman concerning routine checkups for cervical and vaginal cancer. The American Cancer Society (2006) advises women who have been sexually active for 3 years or who are 21 years old to have yearly Pap tests (or every 2 years if liquid-based test is used). At age 30, after 3 normal Pap results, screening may be every 2 to 3 years. A pelvic examination is recommended every 3 years from ages 20 to 40 and every 1 to 3 years thereafter.

Record the examination date on the woman's record.
Communicate findings to woman per agency protocol.

Pap test. **A,** Collecting cells from endocervix using a cytobrush. **B,** Obtaining cells from the transformation zone using a wooden spatula. (From Stenchever, M., et al. [2001]. *Comprehensive gynecology* [4th ed.]. St. Louis: Mosby.)

Sources: Gingrich, P. (2004). Management and follow-up of abnormal Papanicolaou tests. *Journal of the American Medical Women's Association, 59*(1), 54-60; American Cancer Society (ACS). (2006). *Cancer facts and figures 2006*. New York: ACS.

Rectovaginal Palpation. To prevent contamination of the rectum from organisms in the vagina (such as *Neisseria gonorrhoeae*), it is necessary to change gloves, add fresh lubricant, and then reinsert the index finger into the vagina and the middle finger into the rectum (Fig. 5-14). Insertion is facilitated if the woman strains down. The maneuvers of the abdominovaginal examination are repeated. The rectovaginal examination permits assessment of the rectovaginal septum, the posterior surface of the uterus, and the region behind the cervix and the adnexa. The vaginal finger is removed and folded into the palm, leaving the middle finger free to rotate 360 degrees. The rectum is palpated for rectal tenderness and masses.

After the rectal examination, the woman is assisted into a sitting position, given tissues or wipes to cleanse herself, and given privacy to dress. The examiner returns after the woman is dressed to discuss findings and the plan of care.

EVIDENCE-BASED PRACTICE

Cervical Cancer Screening Devices

BACKGROUND

- The Papanicolaou test has shown itself to be an effective screening test for cervical cancer, when followed up with treatment to prevent invasive disease. To decrease false negative results, it was believed that the best samples include both ectocervical (squamous) cells and endocervical (columnar, or glandular) cells. The presence of endocervical cells (ECC) in the sample is accepted as an indication of adequate sampling of the transformation zone (squamocolumnar junction), the site of most premalignant changes. Anatomically, the endocervical canal can be challenging to access. Samples that are inadequate due to inadequate cellularity or cells obscured by blood or inflammation lead to the cost and inconvenience of retesting, or missed opportunities for treatment. To potentiate collection of endocervical cells, several sampling devices are in use.

OBJECTIVES

- The reviewers had two goals: to investigate if the presence of endocervical cells correlates with quality of cervical screening's ability to detect disease, and to examine if well-designed sampling devices may increase the presence of endocervical cells detected.

METHODS

Search Strategy

- The authors identified six spatulas, two endocervical testing devices, and three brushes ("brooms") intended to sample endocervix and ectocervix simultaneously. They searched the literature extensively and found 36 randomized controlled trials and 6 nonrandomized controlled trials, dated 1976 through 1996, from Australia, Denmark, Italy, the Netherlands, the United Kingdom, and the United States, representing 1,626,000 cervical smears.

Statistical Analyses

- Cytologic results span a period across four successive classification systems, and some trials did not distinguish atypia, dysplasia severity, or invasive carcinoma. None of the trials specified glandular atypia, now thought to be suspicious for higher-grade lesions. Therefore, in order to compare rates of detection (sensitivity), the authors pooled all abnormal cervical results.

FINDINGS

- The cytobrush was the best for ECC collection, followed in order by the cotton swab, extended tip spatulas, and classic round spatulas. Order of use affected outcomes. One study showed the cytobrush followed by the spatula was the gold standard at collecting endocervical cells. The cytobrush/spatula combination consistently collected more ECCs than the cotton swab/spatula, the combined cervical brush, and the spatula plus bulb aspirator. The main problem with the cytobrushes was bleeding, but it wasn't enough to obscure the cells on the smear. Cytobrushes were generally avoided during pregnancy, for fear of nicking the amniotic membrane. The extended tip spatula and the cytobrush were also correlated with higher capture of cervical abnormalities. The presence of ECC improved detection of abnormality, especially with higher-grade lesions.

LIMITATIONS

- Practices changed during the years of this metareview: the introduction of the cytobrush and liquid cytologic collection system greatly increased the uptake of endocervical cells, and the criterion for adequacy of cervical sample was changed to require identification of at least 10 endocervical cells.

IMPLICATIONS FOR PRACTICE

- Good cervical sampling increases the capture of endocervical cells, and therefore the sensitivity for abnormalities. Regardless of the collection medium of slide or liquid, the best collection devices are the cytobrush followed by the extended-tip spatula, especially if the transformation zone is not visible. Clinicians should be trained to improve their technique at ECC collection to decrease the incidence of collecting inadequate samples and having to schedule retesting, both of which are costly to the woman in terms of time, money, and stress.

IMPLICATIONS FOR FURTHER RESEARCH

- More research comparing devices used to collect endocervical cells are needed. Information about cost-effectiveness would be helpful.

Reference: Martin-Hirsch, P., Jarvis, G., Kitchener, H., & Lilford, R. (2005). Collection devices for obtaining cervical cytology samples. In *The Cochrane Library*, Database of Systematic Reviews, 2006, Issue 3. Chichester, UK: John Wiley & Sons.

Pelvic Examination during Pregnancy

The pelvic examination is done in the same way as it is during a routine examination on a nonpregnant woman. Pelvic measurements are completed, and uterine size is estimated. A Pap test may be done initially, as well as collection of cytologic specimens to test for gonorrhea, chlamydia, human papillomavirus, herpes simplex virus, and group B streptococcus. As the pregnancy progresses, the nurse will inspect the woman's abdomen, palpate fetal size and position, auscultate fetal heart tones, and measure fundal height at each visit.

While the pregnant woman is in lithotomy position, the nurse must watch for supine hypotension, caused by the weight of the abdomen pressing on the vena cava and aorta and triggering a decrease in blood pressure (see Fig 21-5). Symptoms of supine hypotension include pallor, dizziness, faintness, breathlessness, tachycardia, nausea, clammy skin, and sweating. The woman should be positioned on her side until symptoms resolve and vital signs stabilize. The vaginal examination can be done with the woman in the lateral position.

FIG. 5-13   Bimanual palpation of the uterus.

FIG. 5-14   Rectovaginal examination. (From Seidel, H., et al. [2006]. *Mosby's guide to physical examination* [6th ed.]. St. Louis: Mosby.)

Pelvic Examination after Hysterectomy

The pelvic examination is done much as it is done on a woman with a uterus. Vaginal screening using the Pap test is not recommended in women who have had a hysterectomy for benign disease (ACS, 2006; National Comprehensive Cancer Network [NCCN], 2004). Because of the epidemic of human papillomavirus, which causes vaginal intraepithelial neoplasia, sampling of the vaginal cuff and vaginal walls after hysterectomy may still be practiced, with schedules varying from every year to every 2 to 3 years (DiSaia & Creasman, 2002).

Laboratory and Diagnostic Procedures

The following laboratory and diagnostic procedures are ordered at the discretion of the clinician, considering the woman and her family history: hemoglobin, fasting plasma glucose, total blood cholesterol, lipid profile, urinalysis, syphilis serology (Venereal Disease Research Laboratory [VDRL] or rapid plasma reagin [RPR]) and other screening tests for sexually transmitted infections, mammogram, tuberculosis skin testing, hearing, visual acuity, electrocardiogram, chest X-ray, pulmonary function, fecal occult blood, flexible sigmoidoscopy, and bone mineral density scan). Results of these tests may be reported in person, by phone call, or by letter. Tests for HIV and drug screening may be offered with informed consent in high risk populations. These test results usually are reported in person.

▬ ANTICIPATORY GUIDANCE FOR HEALTH PROMOTION AND ILLNESS PREVENTION

Over the last several decades, women have made tremendous strides in education, careers, policy making, and overall participation in today's complex society. There have been costs for these advances, and although women are living longer, they may not be living better. As a result, the health care system must pay greater attention to the health consequences for women. In addition, women must be active participants in their own health promotion and illness prevention. Health promotion is the motivation to increase well-being and actualize health potential. Illness prevention is the desire to avoid illness, detect it early, or maintain optimal functioning when illness is present.

Nurses have a major opportunity and responsibility to help women understand risk factors and to motivate them to adopt healthy lifestyles that prevent disease. Lifestyle factors that affect health over which the woman has some control include diet; tobacco, alcohol, and substance use; exercise; sunlight exposure; stress management; and sexual practices. Other influences, such as genetic and environmental factors, may be beyond the woman's control, although some opportunities for prevention exist (e.g., through environmental legislation activism or genetic counseling services).

Knowledge alone is not enough to bring about healthy behaviors. The woman must be convinced that she has some control over her life and that healthy life habits, including periodic health examinations, are a sound investment. She must believe in the efficacy of prevention, early detection, and therapy and in her ability to perform self-care practices, such as BSE. Many people believe that they have little control over their health, or they become immobilized by fear and anxiety in the face of life-threatening illnesses, such as cancer, so they delay seeking treatment. The nurse must explore the reality of each woman's perceptions about health behaviors and individualize teaching if it is to be effective.

Nutrition

To maintain good nutrition, women should be counseled to include recommended servings from the major food categories of the food pyramid (see Fig. 15-4). Recommended servings from the food groups also provide adequate vitamins, minerals, iron, and fiber. Fluid intake is not included in the food pyramid, but individuals should be encouraged to drink at least six to eight glasses of water every day in addition to other fluids such as juices. Coffee, tea, soft drinks, and alcoholic beverages should be used in moderation.

Folic acid helps to reduce high levels of homocysteine, an amino acid that damages the heart and blood vessels and increases the risk of heart disease, stroke, and dementia (Corrada & Kawas, 2005). Folic acid is present in citrus fruits, broccoli, spinach, asparagus, peas, lettuce, beans, whole grains, and orange juice. It is in many fortified grains and pasta or can be taken as a daily vitamin supplement (USDHHS and USDA, 2005).

Antioxidants are thought to be effective in helping to prevent oxidative damage in the body such as cancer, heart disease, and stroke; however, more research is needed in this area. Vitamins C and E; selenium (a mineral); and a group known as beta-carotenes (carotenoids) can be found in a diet containing fruits, vegetables, and whole grains.

Most women do not recognize the importance of calcium to health, and their diets are insufficient in calcium. Women who are unlikely to get enough calcium in the diet may need calcium supplements in the form of calcium carbonate, which contains more elemental calcium than do other preparations.

The diet can be assessed by using a standard assessment form—a 24-hour recall is adequate and quick—and then food likes and dislikes, including cultural variations and typical food portions and dietary habits should be discussed and incorporated into counseling (see Chapter 15).

Exercise

Physical activity and exercise counseling for women of all ages should be undertaken at schools, work sites, and primary care settings. American Heart Association (AHA) (2006) recommendations include 30 to 60 minutes of moderate to vigorous activity on most days of the week at 50% to 75% of maximum heart rate. Activities do not need to be strenuous to bring health benefits. What is important is to include activities as part of a regular health routine. Activities that are especially beneficial when performed regularly include brisk walking, hiking, stair climbing, aerobic exercise, jogging, running, bicycling, rowing, swimming, soccer, and basketball. Few Americans exercise as often as they should, and physical activity is known to decrease with age, especially during adolescence and early adulthood.

The nurse should stress the importance of daily exercise throughout life for weight management and health promotion, suggesting exercises that are enjoyable to the individual (Fig. 5-15). Physical activity builds healthy bones, muscles, and joints and reduces the risk of colon and breast cancer.

FIG. 5-15 Weight-bearing exercise such as dancing may delay bone loss and increase bone mass. (Courtesy Shannon Perry, Phoenix, AZ.)

It also reduces feelings of depression and anxiety and improves mood and promotes a feeling of well-being. Many women who are sedentary during leisure time can benefit from gradually increasing their physical activity. They may be encouraged to exercise with their children or in groups with friends. Programs such as Curves for women, worksite fitness programs, or community-based programs such as the American Heart Association's Choose To Move are increasingly available. Young women can be involved in fitness centers, cheerleading, gymnastics, sports teams, or individual competitive sports.

For women who are sedentary or are not able to exercise vigorously, even moderate and low intensity activities, when performed daily, can have long-term health benefits such as lowering the risk of cardiovascular disease. Regular physical activity can reduce or eliminate some of these risk factors by lowering blood pressure, maintaining a reasonable weight or facilitating weight loss, and lowering cholesterol levels to below 200 mg/dl.

Home maintenance, yard work, and gardening are other activities that promote health and a sense of well-being, especially for older adults. Attention to safety factors and wearing clothing and shoes appropriate to each activity are advised. Care should be taken not to aggravate existing conditions or create muscle and joint discomfort by an overly aggressive approach to exercise.

Kegel Exercises

Kegel exercises, or pelvic muscle exercises, were developed to strengthen the supportive pelvic floor muscles to control or reduce incontinent urine loss. These exercises also are beneficial during pregnancy and postpartum. They strengthen the muscles of the pelvic floor, providing support for the pelvic organs and control of the muscles surrounding the vagina and urethra. Educational strategies for teaching women how to perform Kegel exercises were compiled by nurse researchers who conducted a research

TEACHING FOR SELF-CARE

Kegel Exercises

DESCRIPTION AND RATIONALE

Kegel exercise, or pelvic muscle exercise, is a technique used to strengthen the muscles that support the pelvic floor. This exercise involves regularly tightening (contracting) and relaxing the muscles that support the bladder and urethra. By strengthening these pelvic muscles, a woman can prevent or reduce accidental urine loss.

TECHNIQUE

The woman needs to learn how to target the muscles for training and how to contract them correctly. One suggestion for teaching is to have the woman pretend she is trying to prevent the passage of intestinal gas. Have her use this tightening motion on the muscles around her vagina and the upper pelvis. She should feel these muscles drawing inward and upward. Other suggested techniques are to have the woman pretend she is trying to stop the flow of urine in midstream or to have her think about how her vagina is able to contract around and move up the length of the penis during intercourse.

The woman should avoid straining or bearing-down motions while performing the exercise. She should be taught how bearing down feels by having her take a breath, hold it, and push down with her abdominal muscles as though she were trying to have a bowel movement. Then the woman can be taught how to avoid straining down by exhaling gently and keeping her mouth open each time she contracts her pelvic muscles.

SPECIFIC INSTRUCTIONS

1. Each contraction should be as intense as possible without contracting the abdomen, thighs, or buttocks.
2. Contractions should be held for at least 10 seconds. The woman may have to start with as little as 2 seconds per contraction until her muscles get stronger.
3. The woman should rest for 10 seconds or more between contractions, so that the muscles have time to recover and each contraction can be as strong as the woman can make it.
4. The woman should feel the pulling up over the three muscle layers so that the contraction reaches the highest level of her pelvis.

OTHER SUGGESTIONS FOR IMPLEMENTATION

1. At first the woman should set aside about 15 minutes a day to do the Kegel exercises.
2. The woman may want to put up reminders to do the exercises, such as notes on her bathroom mirror, her refrigerator, her television, or her calendar.
3. Guidelines for practicing Kegel exercises suggest performing between 24 and 100 contractions a day; however, positive results can be achieved with only 24 to 45 a day.
4. The best position for learning how to do Kegel exercises is to lie supine with the knees bent. Another position to use is on the hands and knees. Once the woman learns the proper technique, she can perform the exercises in other positions such as standing or sitting.

Sources: Sampselle, C. (2003). Behavior interventions in young and middle-aged women: Simple interventions to combat a complex problem. *American Journal of Nursing, 103*(Suppl), 9-19; Sampselle, C. (2000). Behavioral interventions for urinary incontinence in women: Evidence for practice. *Journal of Midwifery & Women's Health, 45*(2), 94-103; Sampselle, C. Wyman, J., Thomas, K., Newman, D., Gray, M., Dougherty, M., Burns, P., et al. (2000). Continence for women: A test of AWHONN's evidence-based protocol. *Journal of Obstetric, Gynecologic, and Neonatal Nursing, 29*(1), 312-317.

utilization project for the Association of Women's Health, Obstetric, and Neonatal Nurses (AWHONN) are described in the Teaching for Self-Care box.

Stress Management

Because it is neither possible nor desirable to avoid all stress, women must learn how to manage stress. The nurse should assess each woman for signs of stress by using therapeutic communication skills to determine risk factors and the woman's ability to function. See Box 5-6 for identifying symptoms of stress.

Women are twice as likely as men to have depression, anxiety, or panic attacks (National Women's Health Resource Center, 2003). Nurses must be alert to the symptoms of serious mental disorders, such as depression and anxiety. Women having major life changes such as divorce and separation, bereavement, serious illness, and unemployment also need special attention.

For many women, the nurse is able to provide comfort, reassurance, and advice concerning helping resources, such as support groups. Many centers offer support groups to help women prevent or manage stress. The nurse can help women become more aware of the relationship between good nutrition, rest, relaxation, and exercise, and

diversion, and their ability to deal with stress. In the case of role overload, determining what needs immediate attention and what can wait is important. Practical advice includes having regular breaks, taking time for friends, developing interests outside of work or the home, setting realistic goals, and learning self-acceptance. Discussing how women can maintain meaningful relationships is important. Social support and good coping skills can improve a woman's self-esteem and give her a sense of mastery. Anticipatory guidance for developmental or expected situational crises can help her plan strategies for dealing with potentially stressful events.

The abundant literature on stress management interventions includes role-playing, relaxation techniques, biofeedback, meditation, desensitization, imagery, assertiveness training, yoga, diet, exercise, and weight control, techniques nurses can include in their repertoire of helping skills. Insufficient time prevents one-on-one assistance in many situations, but the more nurses know about these interventions, the better able they are to intervene, counsel, and direct women to appropriate resources.

Some women must be referred for counseling or other mental health therapy. Careful follow-up of all women experiencing difficulty in dealing with stress is important.

Substance Use Cessation

Women of all ages will receive substantial and immediate benefits from smoking cessation. This is not easy, however, and most people stop temporarily several times before they accomplish their goal. Many are never able to do so.

New approaches to increase cessation among smokers and to discourage smoking among young women—especially in adolescence and during pregnancy—are needed. Health care providers can have an impact on smoking behavior and should attempt to motivate smokers to stop.

Women who are not pregnant and wish to stop smoking can be referred to a smoking-cessation program in which individualized methods can be implemented. A five-step intervention program is recommended to help pregnant women stop smoking (American College of Obstetricians and Gynecologists [ACOG], 2005) (Box 5-9). AWHONN

box 5-9 Interventions for Smoking Cessation: The Five A's

ASK
- What was her age when she started smoking?
- How many cigarettes does she smoke a day? When was her last cigarette?
- Has she tried to quit?
- Does she want to quit?

ASSESS
- What were her reasons for not being able to quit before, or what made her start again?
- Does she have anyone who can help her?
- Does anyone else smoke at home?
- Does she have friends or family who have quit successfully?

ADVISE
- Give her information about the effects of smoking on pregnancy and her fetus, on her own future health, and on the members of her household.

ASSIST
- Provide support; give self-help materials.
- Encourage her to set a quit date.
- Refer to a smoking cessation program, or provide information about nicotine replacement products (not recommended during pregnancy) if she is interested.
- Teach and encourage use of stress-reduction activities.
- Provide for follow-up with a phone call, letter, or clinic visit.

ARRANGE FOLLOW-UP
- Arrange to follow the woman to find out about smoking-cessation status.
- Make a phone call around the time of her quit date. Assess her status at every prenatal visit.
- Congratulate her on her success, or provide support for her if she relapses.
- Referral to intensive treatment may be necessary.

Source: American College of Obstetricians and Gynecologists Committee on Health Care for Underserved Women; ACOG Committee on Obstetric Practice. (2005). ACOG Committee Opinion No. 316, October, 2005. Smoking cessation during pregnancy. *Obstetrics and Gynecology, 106*(4), 883-888.

also has a smoking cessation counseling program for pregnant women (Albrecht, Maloni, Thomas, Jones, Halleran, & Osborne, 2004). At the very least, individuals should be guided to self-help materials available from the March of Dimes Birth Defects Foundation, the American Lung Association, and the American Cancer Society (www.cancer.org). During pregnancy, women seem to be highly motivated to stop or at least to limit smoking to 10 or fewer cigarettes a day. Insult to the fetus can be reduced or even avoided if this is done by the end of the first trimester (Bernstein, Mongeon, Badger, Soloman, Heil, & Higgins, 2005).

Counseling women who appear to be drinking alcohol excessively or using drugs may include promoting strategies to increase self-esteem and teaching new coping skills to resist and maintain resistance to alcohol abuse and drug use. Appropriate referrals should be made, with the health care provider arranging the contact and then following up to be sure that appointments are kept. General referral to sources of support also should be provided. National groups that provide information and support for those who are chemically dependent have local branches or contacts that are listed in the local telephone book.

Anticipatory guidance includes teaching about the health and safety risks of alcohol and mind-altering substances and discouraging drug experimentation among preteen and high school students, because the use of drugs at an early age tends to be a predictor of greater involvement later.

Safer Sexual Practices

Prevention of STIs is predicated on the reduction of high risk behaviors by educating toward a behavioral change. Behaviors of concern include multiple and casual sexual partners and unsafe sexual practices. Specific self-care measures for "safer sex" can be reviewed in Box 5-10. The abuse of alcohol and drugs also is a high risk behavior and results in impaired judgment and thoughtless acts.

box 5-10 Safer Sex

- Safer sex is possible only if there is no oral, genital, or rectal exchange of body fluids or if a person is in a long-term mutually monogamous relationship with an uninfected partner.
- Correct use of latex condoms, although greatly reducing risk, is not 100% protective.
- Sexual partners should be selected with great care.
- Partners should be asked about any history of STIs.
- A new condom should be used for each act of sexual intercourse (e.g., oral, vaginal, and anal).
- Abstinence from sexual intercourse is encouraged for persons who are being treated for an STI or whose partners are being treated.

Source: Centers for Disease Control and Prevention, Workowski, K; & Berman, S. (2006). Sexually transmitted diseases treatment guidelines, 2006. *MMWR Morbidity and Mortality Weekly Report, 55*(RR11), 1-94.
HIV, Human immunodeficiency virus; *STIs*, sexually transmitted infections.

table 5-3 Health Screening Recommendations for Women Aged 18 Years and Older

INTERVENTION	RECOMMENDATION*
PHYSICAL EXAMINATION	
Blood pressure	Every visit, but at least every 2 years
Height and weight	Every visit, but at least every 2 years
Pelvic examination	Annually until age 70; recommended for any woman who has ever been sexually active
Breast examination	
Self-examination	Initiated or taught at time of first pelvic examination; done monthly at end of menses
Clinical examination†	Every 3 years, ages 20 to 39; annually after age 40
High risk	Annually after age 18 with history of premenopausal breast cancer in first-degree relative
Risk groups	At least annually:
Skin examination	Family history of skin cancer or increased exposure to sunlight after age 40; every 3 years between ages 20 to 40; monthly self-examinations also recommended
Oral cavity examination	Mouth lesion or exposure to tobacco or excessive alcohol
LABORATORY AND DIAGNOSTIC TESTS	
Blood cholesterol (fasting lipoprotein analysis)	Every 5 years
High risk	More often per clinical judgment with potential for cardiac or lipid abnormalities
Papanicolaou test†	Initially, 3 years after becoming sexually active but no later than age 21; yearly with conventional Pap test or every 2 years with liquid-based Pap tests. After age 30 and after three normal test results in a row, every 2 to 3 years; after age 70 and no abnormal test results in 10 years, screening may be stopped
Mammography‡	Annually over age 50
	Annually over age 40
	Every 1 to 2 years between ages 40 and 49 and annually thereafter
Colon cancer screening	Fecal occult blood test annually and flexible sigmoidoscopy every 5 years or colonoscopy every 10 years after age 50; more often if family history of colon cancer or polyps
Risk groups	
Fasting blood sugar	Annually with family history of diabetes or gestational diabetes or if significantly obese; every 3 to 5 years for all women older than 45 years of age
Hearing screen	Annually with exposure to excessive noise or when loss is suspected
Sexually transmitted infection screen	As needed with multiple sexual partners
Tuberculin skin test	Annually with exposure to persons with tuberculosis or in risk categories for close contact with the disease
Endometrial biopsy	At menopause for women at risk for endometrial cancer
Vision	Every 2 years between ages 40 and 64; annually after age 65
Bone mineral density testing	All women age 65 and older; younger women with risk for osteoporosis may need periodic screenings
IMMUNIZATIONS	
Tetanus-diphtheria	Booster is given every 10 years after primary series
Measles, mumps, rubella	Once if born after 1956 and no evidence of immunity
Hepatitis A	Primary series of 2 injections for all who are in risk categories
Hepatitis B	Primary series of 3 injections for all who are in risk categories
Influenza	Annually after age 65 or in risk categories, such as chronic diseases, immunosuppression, renal dysfunction
Human papillomavirus (HPV) vaccine	Primary series of 3 injections for young girls ages 9 to women 26 years old. Intended for those not previously exposed to HPV.

Sources: American Cancer Society (ACS). (2006). *Cancer facts and figures 2006.* New York: ACS; Centers for Disease Control and Prevention (CDC), Workowski, K. & Berman, S. (2006). Sexually transmitted diseases treatment guidelines, 2006. *Morbidity and Mortality Weekly Report, 55*(RR11) 1-94. Expert Panel on Detection, Evaluation, and Treatment of High Blood Cholesterol in Adults. (2001). Executive summary of the third report of the national education program (NCEP) expert panel on detection, evaluation, and treatment of high blood cholesterol in adults (Adult Treatment Panel III). *Journal of the American Medical Association, 285*(19), 2486-2497; National Women's Health Information Center. (2005). *Recommended screenings and immunizations for women at average risk for most diseases.* Accessed www.4woman.gov, February 28, 2006; United States Preventive Services Task Force (USPSTF). (2005). *Guide to clinical preventive services.* U.S. Department of Health and Human Services, Agency for Healthcare Research and Quality, AHRQ Pub. No. 05-0570, Baltimore: Williams & Wilkins. Centers for Disease Control and Prevention (2006). CDC Advisory Committee on Immunization Practices recommends human papillomavirus vaccination. Accessed www.cdc.gov/od/oc/media/pressrel/R060629.htm. August 21, 2006.
* Unless otherwise noted, the recommended intervention should be performed routinely every 1 to 3 years.
† American Cancer Society (ACS). (2006).
‡ NOTE: There is no consensus regarding mammograms for women between 40 and 49 years of age; therefore various recommendations are listed. Women are urged to discuss circumstances with their health care providers.

In addition to the prevention of STIs, women of child-bearing years need information regarding contraception and family planning (see Chapter 9).

Health Screening Schedule

Periodic health screening includes history, physical examination, education, counseling, and selected diagnostic and laboratory tests. This regimen provides the basis for overall health promotion, prevention of illness, early diagnosis of problems, and referral for appropriate management. Such screening should be customized according to a woman's age and risk factors. In most instances, it is completed in health care offices, clinics, or hospitals; however, portions of the screening are now being carried out at events such as community health fairs. An overview of health screening recommendations for women older than 18 years is provided in Table 5-3.

Health Risk Prevention

Simple safety factors often are forgotten or perceived not to be important, yet injuries continue to have a major impact on the health status of all age groups. Being aware of hazards and implementing safety guidelines will reduce risks. The nurse should frequently reinforce the following common sense concepts that will protect the individual:

- Wear seat belts at all times in a moving vehicle.
- Wear safety helmets when riding a motorcycle, bicycle, or inline skates.
- Follow driving "rules of the road."
- Place smoke alarms throughout the home and workplace.
- Avoid secondhand smoke.
- Reduce noise pollution or safeguard against hearing loss.
- Protect skin and eyes from ultraviolet light with the use of sunscreen, protective clothing, sunglasses, and hats.
- Handle and store firearms appropriately.
- Practice water safety.

Taking necessary precautions and avoiding dangerous situations is imperative.

Health Protection

Nurses can make a difference in stopping violence against women and preventing further injury. Educating women that abuse is a violation of their rights and facilitating their access to protective and legal services constitutes a first step. Encouraging health care institutions to implement appropriate domestic violence screening programs also is of great value (see Chapter 6). Other helpful measures for women to discourage their entry into abusive relationships include promoting assertiveness and self-defense courses; suggesting support and self-help groups that encourage positive self-regard, confidence, and empowerment; and recommending educational and skills development classes that will enhance independence and self-care.

Numerous national and local organizations provide information and assistance for women in abusive situations. All nurses who work in women's health care should become familiar with local services and legal options.

---

community activity

Visit the nearest office of the American Heart Association to assess resources for promoting cardiovascular health in women. If there is not an office in the community to do this, visit the website (www.americanheart.org). What recommendations are given for maintaining cardiovascular health? Design an exhibit on Women's Cardiovascular Health for a health fair targeting women in your community who may not have regular access to health care to educate about heart disease being the number one killer of all women.

---

key points

- Culture, religion, socioeconomic status, personal circumstances, the uniqueness of the individual, and stage of development are among the factors that influence a person's recognition of a need for care and response to the health care system.
- The changing status and roles of women affect their health, needs, and ability to cope with problems.
- Assessment is more comprehensive and learning is enhanced in a safe environment in which the atmosphere is nonjudgmental and sensitive and the interaction is strictly confidential.
- Every woman is entitled to be respected and fully involved in the assessment and educational process.
- Preconception counseling allows identification and possible remediation of potentially harmful personal and social conditions, medical and psychologic conditions, environmental conditions, and barriers to care before conception.

- Conditions that increase a woman's health risks also increase risks for her offspring.
- Periodic health screening, including history, physical examination, immunizations, and diagnostic and lab tests, provide the basis for overall health promotion, prevention of illness, early diagnosis of problems, and referral for management.
- AHA recommendations include 30 to 60 minutes of moderate to vigorous activity on most days of the week at 50% to 70% of maximum heart rate to lower the risk of cardiovascular disease, the leading cause of death in women.
- Health promotion and prevention of illness assists women in actualizing health potential by increasing motivation, providing information, and incorporating recommendations for accessing specific resources.

REFERENCES

Albrecht, S., Maloni, J., Thomas, K., Jones, R., Halleran, J., & Osborne, J. (2004). Smoking cessation counseling for pregnant women who smoke: Scientific basis for AWHONN's SUCCESS project. *Journal of Obstetric, Gynecologic, and Neonatal Nursing, 33*(3), 298-305.

American Cancer Society (ACS). (2006). *Cancer facts and figures 2006.* New York: Author.

American College of Obstetricians and Gynecologists (ACOG) Committee on Health Care for Underserved Women; ACOG Committee on Obstetric Practice. (2005). ACOG Committee Opinion No. 316, October, 2005. Smoking cessation during pregnancy. *Obstetrics and Gynecology, 106*(4), 883-888.

American Heart Association. (2006). *Physical activity and cardiovascular health: Questions and answers.* Accessed www.americanheart.org, June 6, 2006.

Barkauskas, V., Baumann, L., & Darling-Fisher, C. (2002). *Health and physical assessment* (3rd ed.). St. Louis: Mosby.

Bernstein, I., Mongeon, J., Badger, G., Solomon, L., Heil, S., & Higgins, S. (2005). Maternal smoking and its association with birth weight. *Obstetrics and Gynecology, 106*(5 Part 1), 986-991.

Bonvicini, K., & Perlin, M. (2003).The same but different: Clinician-patient communication with gay and lesbian patients. *Patient Education and Counseling, 51*(2), 115-122.

Centers for Disease Control and Prevention (CDC), Workowski, K., & Berman, S. (2006). Sexually transmitted diseases treatment guidelines 2006. *MMWR Morbidity and Mortality Weekly Report, 55*(RR11), 1-94.

Cesario, S. (2003). Obesity in pregnancy. What every nurse needs to know. *AWHONN Lifelines, 7*(2), 118-125.

Community Epidemiology Work Group. (2005). *Epidemiologic trends in drug abuse—advance report.* Washington, DC: National Institute on Drug Abuse.

Condon, M. (2004). *Women's health: Body, mind, spirit: An integrated approach to wellness and illness.* New Jersey: Prentice Hall.

Corrada, M., Kawas, C. (2005). Reduced risk of Alzheimer's disease with high folate intake: The Baltimore longitudinal study on aging. *Alzheimer's & Dementia: The Journal of the Alzheimer's Association, 1*(1) p. 11-18.

DiSaia, P., & Creasman, W. (2002). *Clinical gynecologic oncology* (6th ed.). St. Louis: Mosby.

Edge, V., & Miller, M. (1994). *Women's health care.* St. Louis: Mosby.

Fehring, R., Schneider, M., & Raviele, K. (2006). Variability in the phases of the menstrual cycle. *Journal of Obstetric, Gynegologic, and Neonatal Nursing, 35*(3), 376-384.

Flegal, K., Carroll, M., Ogden, C., & Johnson, C. (2002). Prevalence and trends in obesity among U.S. adults, 1999-2000. *Journal of the American Medical Association, 288*(14), 1723-1727.

Hauenstein, E. (2003). Depression in adolescence. *Journal of Obstetric, Gynecologic, and Neonatal Nursing, 32*(2), 239-248.

Hoyert, D., Mathews, T., Menacker, F., Strobino, D., & Guyer, B. (2006). Annual summary of vital statistics-2004. *Pediatrics, 117*(1), 168-183.

Kealy, M. (2003). Preventing obesity. *AWHONN Lifelines, 7*(1), 24-27.

Kliegman, R. (2006). Intrauterine growth restriction. In R. Martin, A. Fanaroff, & M. Walsh (Eds). *Fanaroff and Martins's neonatal-perinatal medicine: Diseases of the fetus and infant.* St Louis: Philadelphia: Mosby.

Kowal, D. (2004). Expanding perspectives on reproductive health. In R. Hatcher, J. Trussell, & F. Stewart, *Contraceptive technology* (18th ed.). New York: Ardent Media.

Masters, W. (1992). *Human sexuality* (4th ed.). New York: HarperCollins.

Mattson, S. (2003). Caring for Latino women. *AWHONN Lifelines, 7*(3), 258-260.

Minikin, M., & Wright, C. (2005). *A woman's guide to menopause and perimenopause.* New Haven: Yale University Press.

Moos, M. (2003). Preconceptional wellness as a routine objective for women's health: An integrated strategy. *Journal of Obstetric, Gynecologic, and Neonatal Nursing, 32*(4), 550-556.

National Center for Chronic Disease Prevention and Health Promotion. (2000). *U.S. obesity trends 1985 to 2000.* Atlanta: Centers for Disease Control and Prevention.

National Comprehensive Cancer Network, Inc. (2004). *NCCN practice guidelines in oncology. Cervical screening. Version 1. 2005.* Accessed www.nccn.org, January 12, 2006.

National Women's Health Resource Center. (2003). Depression and women. *National Women's Health Report, 25*(4), 1-4.

Parker, S., Lyons, J., & Bonner, J. (2005). Eating disorders in graduate students: Exploring the SCOFF questionnaire as a simple screening tool. *Journal of American College Health, 52*(2), 103-107.

Perry, L., Morgan, J., Reid, F., Brunton, J., O'Brien, A., Luck, A. et al. (2002). Screening for symptoms of eating disorders: Reliability of the SCOFF screening tool with written compared to oral delivery. *International Journal of Eating Disorders, 32*(4), 466-472.

Seidel, H., Ball, J., Dains, J., & Benedict, G. (2006). *Mosby's guide to physical examination* (6th ed.). St. Louis: Mosby.

Stenchever, M., Droegemueller, W., Herbst, A., & Mishell, D. (2001). *Comprehensive gynecology* (4th ed.). St. Louis: Mosby.

United States Department of Health and Human Services (USD-HHS), & United States Department of Agriculture (USDA). (2005). *Dietary Guidelines for Americans.* Hyattsville, MD: US Department of Agriculture.

Viau, P., Padua, C., & Eddy, B. (2002). An exploration of health concerns and health-promotion behaviors in pregnant women over age 35. *MCN American Journal of Maternal/Child Nursing, 27*(6), 328-334.

Violence Against Women

learning objectives

- Describe the beliefs and practices that historically have perpetuated violence against women.
- Examine the prevalence and effects of intimate partner violence.
- Contrast the theoretic premises underlying the victimization of women.
- Explain the cycle of violence and its use in assessment and intervention for battered women.

- Develop a plan of care for a battered woman.
- Review the dynamics of rape.
- Describe the rape-trauma syndrome.
- Develop a nursing plan of care for a woman in the acute phase of rape-trauma syndrome.
- Evaluate resources available to women experiencing abuse.

electronic resources

Additional information related to the content in Chapter 6 can be found on

the companion website at **evolve**
http://evolve.elsevier.com/Lowdermilk/MWHC/
- NCLEX Review Questions
- WebLinks

or on the interactive companion CD
- NCLEX Review Questions
- Critical Thinking Exercise: Women's Health and Safety
- Plan of Care: The Battered Woman

*I*ntimate partner violence (IPV) is the most common form of violence experienced by women worldwide, with a reported incidence of one out of every six women having been a victim of domestic violence (World Health Organization [WHO], 2005). Although there is no consensus on the definition of IPV, the National Violence Against Women survey definition will be used here: the actual or threatened physical, sexual, psychologic, or emotional abuse by a spouse, ex-spouse, boyfriend, girlfriend, ex-boyfriend, ex-girlfriend, date, or cohabiting partner. IPV also may include rape and stalking (Tjaden & Thoennes, 2000). The term often implies female victims and male perpetrators, since only 7.4% of IPV is committed against men (Tjaden & Thoennes).

IPV is a significant social problem and a major health and health care problem around the world. A study of 9938 women in India found a 13% prevalence rate of moderate to severe violence, including slapping, beating, kicking, and use of a weapon, during pregnancy (Peedicayil et al., 2005). The WHO (2005) study reported an incidence of IPV ranging from of 15% to 71% in a sample of 24,000

women in 10 countries not including the United States. An estimated 1.3 million women in the United States are assaulted by an intimate partner annually (Tjaden & Thoennes, 2000). Many abused women also report being forced into sexual activities. An average of three women a day are murdered by their intimate partners (Walton-Moss & Campbell, 2002). Women who are abused during pregnancy have a threefold increase in risk of being murdered (McFarlane, Campbell, Sharps, & Watson, 2002).

In spite of all the publicity and available information, violence against women continues to be an unabating epidemic and, given the extensive violence in the United States in general, may even be increasing. In the United States, violence is the second leading cause of injuries to women in the 15- to 44-year-old age group (National Women's Health Information Center [NWHIC], 2002). In one study, women who had experienced abuse had a 50% to 70% increase in central nervous system (CNS), gynecologic, and anxiety-related problems (Campbell, J. et al., 2002). In a study of 82 women with diagnoses of depression, the researchers found that 61% of them had experienced IPV in their lifetimes and that the severity of

CRITICAL THINKING EXERCISE

Intimate Partner Violence

Angela, a 21-year-old college student, is screened for abuse in student health as she stated that her cohabiting partner is very caring and handsome, but he is very jealous and occasionally gets "tough." When he goes out with his male friends, he insists that she stay at home and study, rather than spending time with her girlfriends, and frequently calls to check up on her. She asks the nurse if this behavior is "fair" and how might she "keep peace" and yet have a life of her own.

1. Evidence—Is there sufficient evidence to label her as an "abused" woman?
2. Assumptions—What assumptions can be made about the following?
   a. Characteristic behaviors of abuse
   b. Gender equality
   c. Blame and self-doubt
   d. Relationship expectations
3. What implications and priorities for nursing care can be made at this time?
4. Does the evidence objectively support your conclusion?
5. Are there alternative perspectives to your conclusion?

violence was significantly correlated with the severity of depression (Dienemann, Boyle, Baker, Resnick, Wiederhorn, & Campbell, 2000). Annual costs of interpersonal violence are estimated to be $7.6 billion in medical expenses, police and court costs, shelters, foster care, sick leave, absenteeism, and nonproductivity (Centers for Disease Control and Prevention [CDC], 2003). A *Healthy People 2010* objective is to decrease the rate of IPV to 4 per 1000 women older than 12 years, as well as development of protocols by health care facilities for abuse intervention and prevention (U.S. Department of Health and Human Services [USDHHS], 2000).

Statistical data on IPV are limited. The numerous and complex factors related to IPV research, and the lack of reporting in many instances of violence, often result in inconsistent information. However, they do reflect the extent and complexity of IPV problems. Maternity and women's health nurses are in unique positions to identify and assist in the treatment of women experiencing any type of violence or sexual assault; to help prevent further harm through identification, treatment and education; and to influence public policy aimed at decreasing violence.

▰ HISTORICAL PERSPECTIVE

Women have been treated inhumanely throughout history and often still are. For example, a television news broadcast reported that a woman was doused with gasoline and set on fire by her intimate partner, resulting in third-degree burns over 50% of her body (October, 2005). In 2002, a woman from a middle-Eastern country was stoned to death, a punishment that was socially acceptable in her

culture. Her crime was having been raped by a family member. Another woman was ordered to be raped by four men as punishment for a male cousin of hers who had been seeing a woman above his social class. Her relatives were prevented, by armed officials, from rescuing her, and she was ordered by the tribal jury to walk home naked after the group assault (Fisher, 2002).

In ancient Roman times, wives were divorced or killed by husbands for adultery, public drunkenness, or attending public games, whereas men could engage in these activities daily. In the 1700s, under English Common Law, the "rule of thumb" gave men permission to chastise their wives physically as long as the implement they used was no wider than their thumbs. This legacy carried over to the United States and into the nineteenth century, when wife abuse became illegal in the United States. Even so, it did not cease to occur. Misogyny, patriarchy, devaluation of women, power imbalance, viewing women as property, sex-role stereotyping, and acceptance of aggressive male behavior as appropriate all contributed and continue to contribute to the subordinate status of women in many of the world's societies.

The power imbalance and the concept that family problems are private often kept women from disclosing abuse. There was little awareness and even less response from both medical professionals and the legal and justice systems to the plight of women in intimate relationships. As late as the 1960s, it was believed that violence in the family was rare and committed only by mentally ill or otherwise disturbed people. The women's movement of the 1970s first called attention to the inequality of women in all forms of interpersonal relationships; intolerance of violence then was manifested, and public sanctions against such behavior were initiated. Recognition of the extent of both female and male injustices, including incest, rape, and elder abuse, also increased at this time.

▰ CONCEPTUAL PERSPECTIVES

Many attempts have been made to apply theoretic explanations to the causes and understanding of violence, none of which is conclusive. A brief summary of these is provided to assist in analyzing the persistent acts of violence against women.

Psychologic Perspective

Psychology, the study of individual behavior, places responsibility for all behavior, including aggression, on the individual. Early psychoanalytic theory postulated aggression as a basic instinctual drive leading to mastery and accomplishment and, particularly in men, as a positive force that connotes boldness, forcefulness, energy, and enterprise. From psychoanalytic theory, the gender-stereotypic expectations for women are to be caring and nurturing; thus, aggression is viewed negatively. Aggressive women are labeled hostile and belligerent.

Another psychologic myth is that abuse is committed by people who are mentally ill or deranged in some way. This misconception perpetuates the notion that violence occurs among people who are not "normal." Mental illness accounts for very little interpersonal violence; however, borderline and antisocial personality disorders may be more prevalent in men who batter. A mental health diagnosis of alcohol abuse is frequently found in abusers but should not be misconstrued as the cause of violence. There is evidence that alcohol may increase the risk of violent behavior, since survivors of violence often report abuser substance abuse (Torres & Han, 2003). There is no diagnostic profile of an abuser, but Box 6-1 provides some characteristics of men who batter that nurses can use to assess clients' relationships.

Women with severe and persistent mental illness are likely to be more vulnerable to being involved in controlling and violent relationships. However, numerous mental health problems (such as depression, psychophysiologic illnesses, substance abuse, eating disorders, posttraumatic stress disorder [PTSD], and anxiety reactions) experienced by women with abusive partners are more likely to be consequences of long-term abuse rather than causes (Moracco et al., 2004).

Biologic Factors

A complete biologic perspective is beyond the scope of this chapter, but evidence indicates that neurobiologic and hormonal factors influence aggression in men. Areas in the brain believed to play a role in aggressive behavior are the limbic system, the frontal lobes, and the hypothalamus. Changes in structural functioning of the limbic system, such as occur with brain lesions, substance use, epilepsy, and head injuries, affect both emotional experience and behavior of the individual and thus may increase or decrease the potential for aggressive behavior (Hamolia, 2005).

Neurochemical factors also may play a role in aggressive behavior so that dysfunction or disregulation of certain neurotransmitters may result in aggression. Increased levels of both norepinephrine and L-dopa foster aggressive behavior. Reducing the levels of serotonin in animals causes aggressive behavior. The amino acid gamma-aminobutyric acid (GABA) inhibits aggressive behavior. The occurrence of violence in neurologic disorders also is reported, especially when violent reactions are out of proportion to the provoking events (Hamolia, 2005).

In studies of animals, aggression is associated with abnormally high levels of testosterone. Soler, Vinayak, and Quadagno (2000) reported higher testosterone levels in abusive male subjects and suggested that heritability is an issue that warrants the inclusion of this variable in future studies of violent behavior. There is no conclusive evidence in biologic theory, except perhaps in instances of neurologic damage, that it is impossible to control aggressive behavior.

Sociologic Perspective

The social structure and conditions in Western society provide the basis for the prevailing attitudes toward violent behavior. The United States has a long history of using violence for social control reasons, as in wars and riots. Approval of violence in men is promoted in the double standard dictating that women are expected to be nonviolent, whereas men are expected to be aggressive; therefore, men's violence is treated with more leniency and less stigma, particularly in the justice system. The more a culture uses physical force for socially approved ends, the more the violence becomes generalized to other areas of social life (Fishwick, Parker, & Campbell, 2005).

The structure and dynamics of the family often set the stage for violent behaviors: ascribed roles of family members, the amount of time spent together, the private nature of the family, the intensity of emotional involvement, and stress and conflict inherent in families (Fishwick et al., 2005). Power and violence, or even the threat of physical force, serve to maintain the patriarchal view of woman's place in the home and in the rest of society. Gender inequality, in both economic opportunities and physical strength, serves to perpetuate the power imbalance in relationships.

Another family issue is the multigenerational transmission of violence; both perpetrators of violence and victims learn about violence in families of origin by either witnessing or experiencing violence while growing up (Fishwick et al., 2005). In violent families, both the lack of emotional support experienced by children and the awareness that people who love each other can be violent are prominent factors. The authors caution that abuse as a child does

---

box 6-1 Characteristics of a Potential Batterer

- Low self-esteem
- Problems with abandonment, loss, helplessness, dependency, insecurity, and intimacy
- Inadequate verbal skills, especially difficulty expressing feelings
- Deficits in assertiveness
- Personality disorders frequently diagnosed
- Low frustration tolerance (loses temper easily)
- Higher incidence of growing up in an abusive or violent home
- Denies, minimizes, blames, and lies about own actions
- Violence is consistent with his view of himself and the world; it is an acceptable way of dealing with everyday life
- Inability to empathize with others
- Rigidity in male and female behaviors (sex-role stereotypes)
- Perception of self as "special" and deserving special attention for being the provider, protector
- Substance abuse problems are common
- Display of an unusual amount of jealousy (e.g., expects partner to spend all of her time with him or to keep him informed of her whereabouts)

not completely determine later violent behavior since many children who were abused grow up to avoid violent behavior.

Other significant social factors in violent behavior include the following (Hamolia, 2005):

- Poverty and oppression
- Low income, with its subsequent stress, and limited resources making it difficult to meet basic needs
- Unemployment
- Difficulty in maintaining interpersonal ties
- Disruption in marriages
- Single-parent families

Feminist Perspective

The contemporary social view of violence is derived from feminist theory. This view, with the primary theme of male dominance and coercive control, enhances our understanding of all forms of violence against women, including wife battering, stranger and acquaintance rape, incest, and sexual harassment in the workplace. This gender and power perspective evolved from women's descriptions of their abusive experiences and from activists attempting to understand the victimization that occurred. In numerous cases, power and control tactics were central events leading to the violence (Renzetti, Edleson, & Bergen, 2001). The power and control wheel developed by the Duluth, Minnesota Domestic Abuse Intervention Project identifies the ways in which men exercise the power and control that underlie all types of intimate partner violence (Fig. 6-1).

Campbell and Fishwick (1993) discussed the concept of machismo, or compulsive masculinity, associated particularly with wife abuse. Machismo encompasses the traditional male values of "toughness" and aggression and the characterization of the male identity as a preoccupation with physical strength, athletic prowess, demonstrations of daring and valor through aggression and violence, an inability to verbalize emotions, treatment of women as commodities and conquest objects, and inability to be gentle toward and to cooperate with women. Men may say, "I only hit her because I needed to keep her in line." This machismo framework is consistent with the feminist perspective on abuse.

Most research indicates that a combination of environmental, physical, and social factors results in violence; in essence, aggressive behavior is an individual's response to

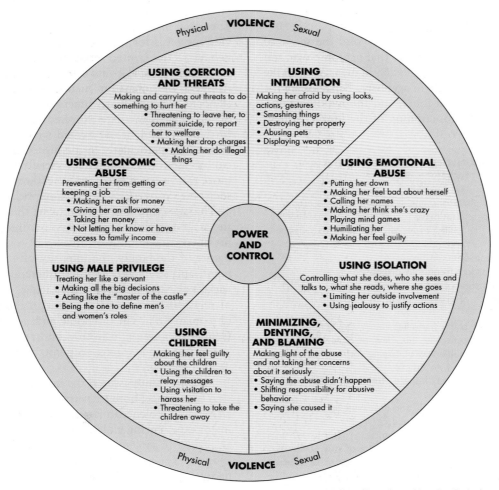

FIG. 6-1 Model of how power and control issues perpetuate battering. (Developed by the Duluth Domestic Abuse Intervention Project, Duluth, MN.).

his or her perception of the situation. This model suggests that trauma experienced by an individual, such as child abuse and/or neglect as well as the experience of multiple lifetime traumas, may contribute to the cycle of violence (Neller, Denney, Pietz, & Thomlinson, 2005). Thus, trauma is another factor which should be considered in the feminist perspective.

Implications for Nursing

Theoretic frameworks assist the nurse to understand the dynamics and the many variables in the victimization of women. This knowledge is vital in dispelling myths that prevail among professionals and their clients. The more cognizant nurses become, the more information they can share with women, who ultimately make their own decisions about the quality of their lives and relationships.

■ CULTURAL CONSIDERATIONS

Women of all races, ethnicity, religions, and socioeconomic backgrounds are abused or at risk (NWHIC, 2002). In the United States, Caucasian women report less IPV than do non-Caucasians. Native American and Alaska Native women report significantly more instances of IPV than do women of any other racial background; Asian women report significantly less IPV than do other racial groups (Tjaden & Thoennes, 2000). Reporting rates may not reflect the magnitude of the problem, since many women do not disclose violence because of fear, embarrassment, or not having been asked by those from whom they seek help.

Culturally, women differ on their perceptions of violence and options for treatment depending on the women's sense of self as a member of a family and community. The most salient mechanism of cultural influence is the worldview—that is, collectivism or individualism—to which a woman subscribes (Yoshioka & Choi, 2005). According to the authors, collectivism emphasizes obedience to and harmony within the group; thus in conflict, collectivists tend to use collaborative strategies in the face of personal cost to maintain relationships and save face with others. In contrast, individualist cultural emphases are personal pleasure, achievement and autonomy; thus one tends to use confrontation and adversarial strategies to save face; in essence, a high personal cost justifies breaking an intimate relationship (Yoshioka & Choi).

Another cultural consideration relates to refugees and immigrants. The nurse must be cognizant of the extent to which these women and/or their intimate partners become acculturated or not, in a new society, since care should be delivered as much as possible, according to the cultural norms to which people subscribe (Shiu-Thornton, Senturia, & Sullivan, 2005).

The objectification of women and power inequalities in human social arrangements support the abuse of women. These are especially apparent in any social or cultural system of oppression. The cross-cultural meaning of violence is difficult to ascertain because cultures also differ in their perceptions and definitions of abuse. Accurate data about the incidence and prevalence of violence in ethnic groups are lacking because they are infrequently represented in research studies; violence may be underreported as a result of cultural norms. For example, groups that distrust police or immigration officials may not report abuse, since they fear the repercussions.

Nurses must consider all forces that shape the client's identity: ethnicity, race, class, language, citizenship, religion, and culture, while recognizing that abuse is against the law and injurious to the health and well-being of women and children. More than basic awareness of cultural influences on violence toward women is helpful to the nurse who seeks to be more sensitive to the needs of women whose cultural experiences differ from the nurse's own. Becoming familiar with the client's cultural influences and increasing the numbers of nurses from various ethnic groups will increase the opportunity to provide culturally appropriate care.

African-American Culture

The African-American culture supports unity among humans, nature, and the spiritual world, and social connectedness and relatedness as important norms. African-American men are more likely to be psychologically, socially, and economically oppressed and discriminated against. Violence may occur more frequently as a result of anger generated by environmental stresses and limited resources (Campbell, D., Sharps, Gary, Campbell, & Lopez, 2002).

No valid evidence of greater violence seems to exist in this population although African-American women tend to report violence at a slightly higher rate than Caucasian women (McFarlane, Groff, O'Brien, & Watson, 2005). The devalued status of the female survivor and racial stereotypes may be barriers to African-American women seeking and receiving help.

Hispanic Culture

Hispanics in general are family oriented and have a strong family network in which unity, cooperation, respect, and loyalty are important. However, traditional families are very hierarchic, with authority often given to elderly people, parents, and men. Sex roles are clearly delineated. Hispanics typically seek health care from their families first, and thus women sometimes are less likely to disclose abuse. "Latinas are known to under-use traditional intervention services such as domestic violence shelters, health care, and law enforcement agencies because they lack health insurance, face language and cultural barriers, and distrust formal systems" (Glass, 2005).

Native American Culture

Empiric evidence about abuse in the Native American culture is lacking, but many believe that incest, sexual abuse, and domestic abuse may be the cultural norm rather than the exception, although this sounds offensive. Native American and Alaska Native women report the highest rates of IPV in the United States; however, research is needed to determine whether the rate is higher in these women, or the rate of reporting is higher (Tjaden & Thoennes, 2000).

Asian Women

A study from a community of Vietnamese women provides some perspective on domestic violence among Asian women and is an example of collectivism. The needs of the family take precedence over individual needs, and the woman's role is to maintain harmony in the family. Conflict means failure to be a good wife. Also the woman's role is to be subordinate to men in social and family life. Conflict is perceived as ordinary, personal, and a private matter (Shiu-Thornton et al, 2005).

■ BATTERED WOMEN

Although IPV is the preferred term, *wife battering*, spouse abuse, and *domestic* or *family violence* are all terms that may be applied to a pattern of assaultive and coercive behaviors inflicted by a male partner in a marriage or other heterosexual, significant, intimate relationships. It is probable that partners engage in occasional pushing and poking as they work out the myriad of conflicts that arise in any intimate relationship. Common elements of battering are economic deprivation, sexual abuse, intimidation, isolation, and stalking and terrorizing victims and their children (NWHIC, 2002).

Characteristics of Women in Abusive Relationships

Every segment of society is represented among abused women. Race, religion, social background, age, and educational level are not significant factors in differentiating women at risk. Poor and uneducated women tend to be disproportionately represented because they are seen in emergency departments (EDs), they are financially more dependent, they have fewer resources and support systems, and they may have fewer problem-solving skills.

Battered women may believe they are to blame for their situations because they are "not good enough, not efficient enough, not pretty enough." The woman may also blame herself for bringing on the violent behavior in her relationship because she believes she must "try harder" to please the abuser. In many cases, a traumatic bonding with the man hinges on loyalty, fear, terror, and learned helplessness. Some women have low self-esteem and may have histories of domestic violence in their families of origin.

The value women place on their social roles may have some influence in intimate partner violence. Traditional feminine characteristics such as compassion, sympathy, and yielding often result in a positive attitude toward male dominance and more acceptance of partner violence. In contrast the traits of assertiveness, independence, and willingness to take a stand are more characteristic in

women who are in nonviolent relationships (Faramarzi, Esmailzadeh, & Mosavi, 2005.) Social isolation seems to be another characteristic of battered women, which may result from stigma, fear, or restrictions placed on them by their partners.

Battered women may be formally diagnosed as having *posttraumatic stress disorder (PTSD)*, provided that the symptoms meet the criteria in the Diagnostic and Statistical Manual of Mental Disorders (American Psychiatric Association, 2000). Table 6-1 compares the characteristics of PTSD sufferers with characteristics of battered women and those of rape-trauma victims (discussed later in this chapter). Professionals making the diagnosis must guard against implying that the woman's problems are her issues alone.

Myths About Battered Women

Many people have difficulty believing the tragedies inflicted on women and have even more trouble accepting that women stay in harmful relationships. IPV often entraps a woman in a relationship with conflicting realities. One reality consists of the good aspects of the partner relationship and is supported by the partner and others. The second is the reality of the abuse, which the woman may not recognize or may minimize or deny (McCosker, Barnard, & Gerber, 2003). Both realities may elicit the woman's hopefulness that things will change.

Health professionals often become frustrated by women they see repeatedly who have numerous signs of abuse but seem unable to liberate themselves from the battering relationships. As with other human dynamics that are not easily explained, people tend to rationalize the woman's behaviors and justify their own noninvolvement. A number of misconceptions have emerged to account for this perceived self-destructive behavior. If nurses believe these misconceptions, making judgments (such as blaming the victim) or unhelpful responses may be the result, rather than empathy and empowering women to take control over their lives. Empowering includes providing supportive empathy and information that can be lifesaving. Table 6-2 lists some myths and facts about abuse and battering.

Cycle of Violence: The Dynamics of Battering

Lenore Walker pioneered the cause of women as victims of violence in the United States when she published her research in her book, *The Battered Woman* (1979). By using the qualitative research method, she recorded results from interviews with 120 battered women.

Their accounts of the progress of the abuse were remarkably similar; the resulting pattern is now recognized as the cycle of violence. According to this concept, battering is neither random nor constant; rather, it occurs in repeated cycles (Fig. 6-2). A three-phase cyclic pattern in the battering behavior has been described as a period of increasing tension leading to the battery, which is then followed by a period of calm and remorse in which the male partner

table 6-1 Comparison of Characteristics of Posttraumatic Stress Syndrome, Battered Woman's Syndrome, and Rape-Trauma Syndrome

POSTTRAUMATIC STRESS SYNDROME*	BATTERED WOMAN'S SYNDROME	RAPE-TRAUMA SYNDROME
The person experienced an event that involved or threatened death, a serious injury, or a threat to physical integrity of self or others.	Deliberate and repeated physical or sexual assault experienced by a woman at the hands of an intimate partner.	A violent, aggressive sexual assault on a woman without her consent from a stranger or someone she knows.
The person's response involved intense fear, helplessness, or horror.	The woman responds with terror, entrapment, and helplessness.	The woman responds with shock, terror, and humiliation.
The traumatic event is persistently reexperienced, such as through distressing recollections or dreams.	If the woman remains in the relationship, the repeated experience may be real rather than recalled.	The woman relives the scene and considers what she "should have done"; she experiences a range of emotions and may feel guilty.
Psychologic reactivity occurs on exposure to internal or external cues symbolic of the traumatic event.	The woman feels anxious and isolated (or alone) and reacts to any expression of anger or threat by cowering or attempting to placate the abuser.	Physical symptoms such as muscle tension, hyperventilation, and flushing may occur in response to reexperiencing the rape or when approached by men, especially strangers.
The person persistently avoids stimuli associated with the trauma; responses are numbed.	The woman attempts to avoid arousing the anger of the abuser and tries to please him; she exerts effort to control situations to avoid abuse.	The woman avoids situations in which she feels vulnerable; if in an intimate relationship, she may avoid intercourse.
The person has persistent symptoms of increased arousal, such as difficulty sleeping, hypervigilance, and exaggerated startle response.	The woman is alert to signs of increasing tension in the abuser during the tension-building stages; she withdraws from interaction.	The woman is afraid of being alone or in a crowd and of being attacked from behind; she takes extra precautions when going out and is suspicious.

*Modified from American Psychiatric Association. (2000). *Diagnostic and statistical manual of mental disorders* (4th ed. rev.). Washington, DC: American Psychiatric Association.

table 6-2 Myths and Facts About Intimate Partner Violence

MYTHS	FACTS
Battering occurs in a small percentage of the population.	One fourth of all women experience battering by an intimate partner.
Being pregnant protects the woman from battering.	From 4% to 8% of all women who are battered are battered during pregnancy.
	Battering frequently begins or escalates in frequency and intensity during pregnancy. Pregnancy may be the result of forced sex or of the man's control of contraception.
Battering occurs only in "problem" or lower class families.	Intimate partner violence can occur in any family. Although lower class families have a higher reported incidence of battering, it also occurs in middle- and upper-income families. Incidence is not really known because of the tendency of middle- and upper-income families to hide their battering.
Battered women like to be beaten and deliberately provoke the attack. They are masochistic.	Women are terrified of their assailants and go to great lengths to avoid a confrontation. In some cases, the woman may provoke her partner to release tension that, if left unchecked, might lead to a more severe beating and possible death.
Only men with psychologic problems abuse women.	Many batterers are successful professionals, including politicians, ministers, physicians, and lawyers. Research indicates that only a small number of abusers have psychologic problems.
Only people who come from abusive families end up in abusive relationships.	Most battered women report that their partners were the first person to beat them.
Alcohol and drug abuse cause battering.	Although alcohol may be involved in abusive incidents, it is not the cause. Many batterers use alcohol as an excuse to batter, and shift the blame to the alcohol.
Women would leave the relationship if the abuse were really that bad.	Those women who stay in the relationship do so out of fear and financial dependence. Shelters have long waiting lists.
Batterers and battered women cannot change.	Counseling may effectively help both batterers and battered women.

From Gelles, R. (1997). *Intimate violence in families* (3rd ed.). Thousand Oaks, CA: Sage; National Institute on Alcohol and Alcoholism. (1997). Alcohol, violence, and aggression. *Alcohol Alert, 38,* 1-6; National Women's Health Information Center. (2002). *Violence against women.* Accessed http://www.4woman.gov/violence/index.cfm, March 2, 2006.

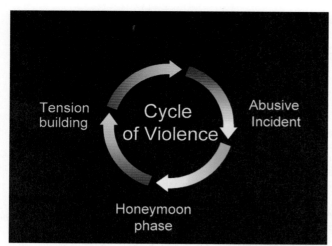

FIG. 6-2 Cycle of violence. (Courtesy Barbara Rynerson, Chapel Hill, NC.)

displays kind, loving behavior and pleas for forgiveness. This "honeymoon" phase lasts until stress or other factors cause conflict and tension to mount again toward another episode of battering. Over time, the tension and battering phases last longer, and the calm phase becomes shorter, until there is no honeymoon phase (Walker, 1984).

Phase I: The Tension-Building State

Tension gradually escalates. The batterer expresses dissatisfaction and hostility without violent outbursts. He may be angered because the food is too cold, he cannot find his socks, or the children are unruly. The woman senses the danger and anxiously tries to placate him. These tactics work for a time but only reinforce the woman's unrealistic belief that she can control his violent behavior. Eventually, she can no longer control his anger, and she withdraws to cope. He senses this withdrawal and becomes angrier until the violent outburst occurs. The woman suppresses the knowledge of her mate's impending abuse.

Phase II: The Acute Battering Incident

The acute battering phase is characterized by the man's uncontrollable discharge of the tension that has been building for the purpose of "teaching her a lesson." The phase can last for hours to several days. The types of behaviors are slaps, punches to face and head, kicking, stomping, punching, choking, pushing, breaking of bones, burns from irons, and mutilation from knives and guns. The woman's injuries are usually to her face, buttocks, and hands and forearms, as she tries to protect herself. The woman denies to herself and others the severity of the damage and may not seek medical assistance even when it is needed.

Phase III: Kindness and Contrite, Loving Behavior

This "honeymoon" phase is characterized by the batterer feeling remorseful and apologizing profusely. He may try to help her, take her to the hospital, or shower her with gifts they may not be able to afford. He promises it will

never happen again, and he may believe at that time that it will not. She desperately wants to believe him, and this behavior restores her hope that he will change. This stage is the positive reinforcement for remaining in the relationship. The woman denies the inevitable recurrence of the abuse. Not all abusive relationships follow this cycle, but many women recognize this pattern. See Box 6-2 for a poem by an unknown author that graphically illustrates the cycle of violence.

Battering During Pregnancy

Estimates of prevalence of battering in pregnancy vary, ranging from 4% to 8% (Martin, Mackie, Kupper, Buescher, & Moracco, 2001). Most women abused before pregnancy will be abused during the pregnancy, and the incidence may escalate. Abuse also may happen for the first time during pregnancy. Huth-Brooks, Levendosky, and Bogart (2002) found that maternal complications of depression, suicide, low weight gain, infections, and substance abuse were related to being in an abusive relationship.

Pregnancy is often a time of initial or increased battering episodes in violent relationships for a variety of reasons: (1) the biopsychosocial stresses of pregnancy may strain the relationship beyond the couple's ability to cope, and frustration is followed by violence; (2) the man may be jealous of the fetus, resenting the intrusion into the couple's relationship and the woman's displacement of attention; (3) the man may be angry at the unborn child or the woman; and (4) the beating may be the man's conscious or

---

box 6-2 I Got Flowers Today

I got flowers today. It wasn't my birthday or any other special day.

We had our first argument last night, and he said a lot of cruel things that really hurt me.

I know he is sorry and didn't mean the things he said because he sent me flowers today.

I got flowers today. It wasn't our anniversary or any other special day.

Last night he threw me into a wall and started to choke me. It seemed like a nightmare. I couldn't believe it was real. I woke up this morning sore and bruised all over.

I know he must be sorry because he sent me flowers today, and it wasn't Mother's Day or any other special day.

Last night he beat me up again, and it was much worse than all the other times. If I leave him, what will I do? How will I take care of my kids? What about money? I'm afraid of him and scared to leave.

But I know he must be sorry. Because he sent me flowers today.

I got flowers today. Today was a very special day.
It was the day of my funeral.
Last night he finally killed me. He beat me to death.
If only I had gathered enough courage and strength to leave him,
I would not have gotten flowers today.
—Author unknown

subconscious attempt to end the pregnancy. After birth, the mother may be so physically and emotionally drained that she may have difficulty bonding with her infant (Lindgren, 2001). She may be at risk of becoming an abusive mother whether or not she remains in the abusive relationship.

Physical and sexual abuse may predict poor health during pregnancy and the postpartum period. Studies indicate that women who are abused report as many medical symptoms, especially headaches, pain, and high levels of depression, as nonpregnant women (Plichta, 2004). Gastrointestinal symptoms may occur from chronic stress, as may hypertension and chest pain. Other conditions are gynecologic problems such as sexually transmitted infections (STIs), bleeding, urinary tract infections, chronic pelvic pain, and genital trauma. Use of contraception may be hindered. Depression and PTSD are the most prevalent mental health sequelae, but substance abuse is common as a method of coping (Campbell, J., et al., 2002).

During pregnancy, the target body parts change during abusive episodes. Women report physical blows directed to the head, breasts, abdomen, and genitalia. Sexual assault is common.

If the pregnant woman remains with her partner, she is at additional risk for repeated physical and psychologic trauma and even death (McFarlane et al., 2002). The potential for child abuse is great, especially if the batterer's anger is directed at the unborn child or if he is jealous of the fetus. If battering begins in pregnancy, it is likely to continue after the birth. This information is vital to share with the woman and other nurses involved in her care. Another factor in the health of both the mother and the newborn child is that the woman may expend energy on coping with the battering rather than on caring for the newborn child.

Pregnant women's difficulties may assist the nurse in identifying battering during pregnancy. These include consumption of an inadequate diet including too little milk and milk products, lack of sleep, and minimal forms of self-relaxation; in short, the battered pregnant woman may not take proper care of herself.

Physical abuse is harmful not only to the mother; the risk of fetal injury is very high. Studies have demonstrated that battery during pregnancy also results in a higher rate of low-birth-weight newborns, preterm birth, placental abruptions, and even neonatal death (Yost, Bloom, McIntire, & Leveno, 2005). In addition some woman may engage in smoking or using alcohol or other drugs as means of coping with IPV, which activities are significantly related to low-birth-weight infants (Huth-Brooks et al., 2002).

Pregnant adolescents are abused at higher rates than are adult women, so they should be considered at high risk. There is a greater likelihood of unintended pregnancy in adolescents who often delay prenatal care (Plichta, 2004). Battering and pregnancy in teenagers constitutes a particularly difficult situation. Adolescents may be more trapped in the abusive relationship than adult women because of their inexperience. They may ignore the violence because the jealous and controlling behavior is interpreted as love and devotion. Because pregnancy in young adolescent girls is frequently the result of sexual abuse, feelings about the pregnancy should be assessed. Teens report abuse from partners, former partners, and family members (Renker, 2002). Many who had been abused through the pregnancy also were abused afterward, and others who were not abused during pregnancy reported initial abuse after giving birth (Harrykissoon, Rickert, & Wiemann, 2002). Adolescents have been found to be at very high risk for abuse in the postpartum period. Quinlivan and Evans (2005) found that both intimate partner violence and drug abuse in adolescents affected both maternal attachment and infant temperament.

Nurses must remember that although pregnancy is a time of risk for women owing to preeclampsia, diabetes, sepsis, coagulopathy, and other pregnancy-related disorders, IPV-related homicide may be the biggest risk facing pregnant women (McFarlane et al., 2002).

■ CARE MANAGEMENT

Care of the battered woman must begin with the nurse's self-assessment. An exploration of attitudes toward women in abusive situations, awareness of feelings that may result in judgmental communication, and knowledge about the many aspects of IPV are preparations for care. Dienemann, Glass, and Hyman (2005) found that women desired health care providers to take an active role; that is, to provide documentation, protection, immediate response, to give options, and to be there for the survivor later. They also wanted to be treated with respect and concern.

Exactly what drives a woman to seek assistance is not clear. Women who belong to any of the following three groups are more likely to seek assistance: (1) women who are beaten frequently and severely; (2) those who have not experienced or witnessed family violence in their family of origin; and (3) those who see an alternative to life in an abusive relationship, specifically women with jobs. Sometimes women seek help after their children have been hurt or when their children start imitating the abuser's behavior.

Battered women may be reluctant to seek help for various reasons, including the need to avoid the stigma associated with the nature of the family violence; the fear that they will not be believed; the fear of reprisal from their husbands or partners; and in some states in which battering is a reportable crime, the desire to avoid involvement with police (see Legal Tip).

■ LEGAL TIP Mandatory Reporting of Domestic Violence

Domestic violence is considered a crime in all states, but it varies between being categorized a misdemeanor and a felony, the majority calling it a misdemeanor. Forty states and the District of Columbia have laws that mandate reporting by health care providers in situations in which the woman has an injury that may be caused by a deadly weapon. Some states also require reports when there is a reason to believe that the woman's injury may have resulted from an illegal act or an act of violence.

California has the strongest reporting law. Colorado, New Mexico, and Kentucky mandate health provider reporting of injuries resulting from IPV to law enforcement or public welfare. Ohio mandates that IPV be documented in the medical record. Rhode Island requires that domestic violence injuries be reported for statistical purposes only. Texas mandates that IPV be documented and that clients be informed that IPV is against the law and be offered shelter referral.

Because of the wide variation from state to state in mandatory reporting, nurses *must* be knowledgeable about the reporting requirements of the state in which they practice (Family Violence Prevention Fund [FVPF], 2004). Nurses can check the FVPF website—**www.endabuse.org**—for a current listing and evaluation of reporting laws.

■ Assessment and Nursing Diagnoses

Clients in women's health care settings are all at risk for abuse; nurses should assess all women entering the health care system for potential abuse (McFarlane et al., 2002). Health care providers are often the first and only contact that a severely isolated woman will make with someone outside the relationship. Failure to identify spousal abuse and to recognize the risk of serious injury or even death further endangers the lives of women and their children.

A woman suspected of having been assaulted should be examined and interviewed in private, and she may feel safer and more comfortable with a female health care provider.

EVIDENCE-BASED PRACTICE

Preventing Intimate Partner Violence

BACKGROUND
- By some definitions, intimate partner violence (IPV) affects one quarter to one third of all women during their lifetimes. Significant psychologic and physical damage can result from IPV, not the least of which is the perpetuation of violent behavior from one generation to another. Violence during pregnancy jeopardizes mother and baby, leading to increased risk for preterm birth, low birth weight, injury, and no prenatal care. Battered women typically experience markedly increased gynecologic, central nervous system, and stress-related symptoms, including serious mental health problems. Many health care providers are encouraged to screen and refer for IPV, but without real evidence of beneficial outcomes.

OBJECTIVE
- Although IPV can be perpetrated by women against men, or in same sex relationships, women experience the preponderance of serious injuries from abuse by men. The reviewers' goal was to systematically review the evidence on primary care interventions that might prevent abuse of women by men. The authors focused on the outcomes for women of primary care screening and intervention, which is usually referral to a safe place and/or community resource for women, and batterer treatment for men.

METHOD
Search Strategy
- After an extensive literature search, the authors found 11 articles which met the inclusion criteria. Nine randomized controlled trials and 1 quasi-randomized noncontrolled trial, dated 1991-1999, represented a total of 2416 participants, from the United States and New Zealand. The systematic review synthesized four quasi-experimental and two randomized controlled trials dated 1986-1997; number of participants and countries of origin were not addressed.

Statistical Analyses
- Similar data were pooled and metaanalyzed. Differences among groups outside the 95% confidence interval were accepted as significant.

FINDINGS
- Women who received weekly counseling for 10 weeks experienced less violence, less reabuse at 2 years, more social support, more skill at obtaining resources, and a greater quality of life than women in the shelter stay–only group. This counseling included information on safety planning, accessing community services, housing, and employment. Personal and vocational counseling alone increased self-esteem, but no other differences were noted. Prenatal counseling sessions, printed material with resource phone numbers, and outreach resulted in less reported violence than in the control group. Interventions with the batterer or with the couple in a military setting were not effective at reducing reabuse.

LIMITATIONS
- Outcomes would ideally include disease morbidity and mortality, social support, safety behaviors, safety planning, and use of community resources (counseling, shelters, legal assistance), but most literature just reports incidence of reabuse. Much evidence suggests that women underreport abuse and reabuse. Some studies may have had selection bias and may not have had a lengthy enough follow-up to detect reabuse.

IMPLICATIONS FOR PRACTICE
- Nurses are often the first to suspect abuse, and are a primary resource for relief. This review provides evidence that a stay in shelter plus ongoing counseling on practical issues offer some better outcomes for women. The authors do not yet recommend universal screening, since the potential harms from screening have not been evaluated. However, for certain psychologic or medical symptoms, IPV screening is very appropriate and necessary.

IMPLICATIONS FOR FURTHER RESEARCH
- Health outcomes have not been examined. Some studies have targeted education of young people as a primary prevention strategy. Protective societal changes, such as legislation and enforcement, must be informed and reformed by research. Well-designed studies will also have to measure long-term benefits of interventions. The potential harms of IPV screening have not been investigated. It has been suggested that women should choose their own outcomes.

Reference: Wathen, C., & MacMillan, H. (2003). Interventions for violence against women. *Journal of the American Medical Association, 289*(5), 589-599.

Nurses should *never* ask about abuse with a partner present, since this may place the woman in danger. When one is taking a psychosocial history, the following information provides clues to violence or potential for violence: how the woman and her partner resolve conflict; what happens when the woman's partner becomes angry; whether fighting occurs during disagreements; and when such fighting occurs, if it ever escalates to restraining or physical means. It may help the woman to disclose information if these events are normalized by the nurse stating, "Many people (families) have difficulty in expressing anger or dealing with conflict. What is that like for you and your partner?" The nurse listens for any evidence of power and control in the relationship. While inquiring about past trauma or injuries, the nurse also should ask directly if the woman has been injured by her husband or intimate partner. At least the following questions should be asked:

- Are you with a spouse or partner who threatens or physically hurts you?
- Within the past year or in this pregnancy has anyone hit, slapped, kicked, or otherwise hurt you?
- Has anyone forced you to have sexual activities that made you uncomfortable? (American College of Obstetricians and Gynecologists [ACOG], 2006). These questions give a woman permission to disclose sensitive information.

Assessment tools can be a part of the interview (see Fig. 5-10) that give the nurse useful information. Reports show an increase in the identification of victims of domestic violence when the nurse inquires at each visit whether a woman has been hit or threatened since her last visit (Walton-Moss & Campbell, 2002). Other cues to abuse are delay in seeking medical assistance (hours or days), missed appointments, vague explanation of injuries, nonspecific somatic complaints, social isolation, lack of eye contact, a husband or partner who does not want to leave the woman alone with the primary health care provider, and substance abuse.

In the United States a pregnant woman is often accompanied by her husband to the antepartum appointment if the woman does not speak English and the husband does. The use of an interpreter is preferred; the interpreter needs to be a woman who can communicate the nurse's sensitivity and concern accurately.

Because of the cycle of violence and the loving respite phase, abused women may cope by denying the probabilities of impending abuse, severity of injury, future recurrence, and death. Women may be embarrassed about their abusive relationships and believe the abuse is caused by their inadequacies. By asking a woman directly about abuse, telling her that similar injuries are common in women who have been abused, and pointing out that she is not responsible for another's violent behavior, the nurse may help her disclose the violence she is experiencing. During pregnancy, the nurse should assess for abuse at each prenatal visit and on admission to labor, although it is not appropriate to ask questions during active labor.

Assessment for abuse continues after birth, since abuse may begin or escalate then; well-baby clinics may be important settings for screening women for abuse (Martin et al., 2001).

During the physical examination, the nurse should observe for injuries to the face, breasts, abdomen, and buttocks. These injuries may be old or new and may range from minor bruising to serious injuries. Psychosocial assessment findings may include anxiety, insomnia, self-directed abuse, depression, smoking, and drug or alcohol abuse (Downs & Rindels, 2004; Gerber, Gantz, Lichter, Williams, & McCloskey, 2005). Other physical signs include fractures that required significant force or that would rarely occur by accident; multiple injuries at various stages of healing; and patterns left by whatever might inflict injury, such as teeth, utensils, fists, or hot objects.

Examples of potential nursing diagnoses for battered women include the following:

- *Hopelessness related to*
  - –prolonged exposure to physical, mental, psychologic, and sexual abuse
- *Powerlessness related to*
  - –phenomenon of being battered and isolated
  - –cycle of violence
- *Ineffective and family coping related to*
  - –persistence of victim-abuser relationship
- *Injury related to*
  - –battering episode
- *Situational low self-esteem related to*
  - –continuing victim-abuser relationship
- *Deficient knowledge about*
  - –the cycle of violence
  - –available resources

▬ Expected Outcomes of Care

Expected outcomes for care should be formulated in collaboration with the woman. An overall outcome is to have the woman recognize the abuse she has experienced, to recognize that it is not her fault and is against the law, and to state all her options in making decisions about what actions to take. Specific expected outcomes are that the woman will do the following:

- Identify her areas of strength and develop goals for herself
- State her knowledge of alternatives, options, and choices; community resources (shelters, financial aid, child care, education, job or financial assistance); counseling for the partner
- Express a feeling of empowerment and control as a survivor
- Perceive herself as deserving of respect and not as "deserving" to be victimized
- Express measures to protect her children or, if she is pregnant, the fetus from abuse
- Formulate a plan for safety

CD: Spanish Guidelines

CD: Critical Thinking Exercise: Women's Health and Safety

▬ Plan of Care and Interventions

A therapeutic relationship and skillful interviewing help women disclose and describe their abuse. Language is important when talking with women. A major factor in addressing abuse is to identify the woman as a survivor, not a victim. Victim connotes someone who is harmed, is made to suffer, and has no control. Survivor is an empowering term that connotes coping and decision making in relation to taking control of one's life. Women who have identified their abuse may appear passive, hostile, anxious, depressed, or hysterical because they may think they are at the mercy of the man's temper. In addition, they may be embarrassed, afraid, angry, sad, and shocked. A tool that provides a framework for sensitive nursing interventions is the *ABCDEs* of caring for the abused woman (Campbell & Furniss, 2002):

- *A* is reassuring the woman that she is not *alone.* The isolation and denigration by the abuser keep her from knowing that others are in the same situation and that health care providers can help.
- *B* is expressing the *belief* that violence against the woman is not acceptable in any situation and that it is not her fault; no one deserves to be hurt or mistreated. This may be the first step in empowering her to think about self-protection and acceptable boundaries.
- *C* is *confidentiality* of the information being shared, particularly because the woman may believe that if the abuse is reported, the perpetrator will retaliate (and in reality, this may happen). Explain the mandatory reporting laws, where applicable.
- *D* is for descriptive *documentation* and includes the following: (1) the woman's quoted statement, "My husband punched me," a clear statement by the client about the abuse. It should not include her subjective opinion, such as "I provoked the abusive behavior"; (2) accurate descriptions of injuries and a history of the first, worst, and most recent incident of violence may be included; and (3) with the woman's consent, evidence or photographs (Box 6-3).
- *E* is for *education,* especially about the cycle of violence, which is likely to recur and escalate, and about options. Also, educate about community resources such as where a woman can be referred for help and information about local shelters: for example, National Domestic Violence/Abuse Hotline—800-799-SAFE. Ask if she knows how to obtain a restraining order.
- *S* is for *safety,* the most significant part of the intervention, since one of the most dangerous times for a woman is when she decides to leave. Tell the woman to call 911 if she is in imminent danger, and to consider alerting neighbors to call the police if they hear or see signs of conflict. The woman can be offered a telephone to call the shelter if this is an option she chooses. If she chooses to go back to the abuser, a safety plan includes necessities for a quick escape: a

---

box 6-3 **Documenting Abuse**

Documentation can be useful to women later in court should they choose to press charges or obtain child support, custody, or alimony. Write legibly. Medical records are most helpful if they do the following:

- Take photographs of the injuries known or believed to have been caused by domestic violence.
- Write clearly.
- Set off the woman's words in quotation marks and use such phrases as "client states" to indicate the information recorded reflected the woman's words. Describe the offender and the event in the words of the woman, for example, the client said, "My husband kicked me in the stomach."
- Avoid such legalistic phrases as "woman claims" or "woman alleges" that cast doubt about the truth of the statements. Avoid terms such as "alleged perpetrator." If the health care provider's observations differ from the woman's account of the victimization, state the reason for the difference.
- Do not summarize a client's report in conclusive terms that lack the supporting factual information, for example, "the client is a battered woman," because it will render the report inadmissible. In the same theme, do not place the term "domestic violence" in the diagnosis section of the medical record, because it does not convey factual information and is not medical terminology.
- Describe the woman's demeanor, whether she is crying, shaking, angry, calm, laughing, or sad, even if it belies the evidence of abuse.
- Record the time of day of the examination and indicate whenever possible how much time has passed since the abuse.

Source: Meuer, T., Seymour, A., & Wallace, H. (2002). Domestic violence. *National Victim Assistance Academy 2003.* Accessed www.nvaa.org/assist/chapter9sup.html, March 2, 2006.

---

bag packed with personal items for an overnight stay (can be hidden or left with a neighbor), money or a checkbook, an extra set of car keys, and any legal documents to use for identification. Legal options, such as those for restraining orders or arrest of the perpetrator, also are important aspects of the safety plan. A restraining order can be obtained 24 hours a day from the county court or police department. Many communities have battered women's hotlines where they can get counseling. Pennell and Francis (2005) discuss safety conferencing as a means of building the individual and collective strength to assist women to reshape connections, make sound choices, and promote their safety.

If the woman is pregnant, collaboration with maternity nurses who will be involved in her care during the pregnancy may be helpful. Each nurse can plan care that will point out the woman's strengths and increase her self-esteem. The husband or partner may attend prenatal visits and classes and is included in other ways if the woman chooses to stay with him. The first days after birth are particularly crucial because the mother is physically and emotionally vulnerable and usually tired, and the baby's crying may be intolerable to both the father and the mother. The danger of abuse to mother and child is acute during this time. Facilitating the woman's establishment of a support network of maternity and pediatric staff, community health nurses, and shelter and parental crisis center personnel is important during this crucial period. Referral to resources and provision for follow-up examination by health care providers also should be part of the nursing intervention.

Many nurses become frustrated when a battered woman returns to a previously abusive situation (Davis, Park, Kaups, Bennink, & Bilello, 2003). It is important to remember that many victims have been abused for a long time, which may make it difficult for them to seek and accept help. Women in repeatedly abusive situations may have lost their ability to perceive the possibility of success and may have become very passive. In addition to understanding the many reasons women stay in abusive relationships, recognizing that the most dangerous period for a battered woman is when she is in the process of leaving may help nurses to be less judgmental about the woman's dilemma.

A woman may indicate her readiness to leave the relationship when she believes that she is capable of planning for herself, investing in herself, and recognizing that the abuse is part of a continuing pattern. She also needs to believe that she will have economic and other resources to "make it" on her own. Going to a shelter may be an option; however, shelter stays are typically limited to 30 to 90 days, and therefore a long-term plan must be in place. Also, her being in a shelter may make the batterer more angry. Shelter staff assist women with this planning. Nurses can be helpful in directing women to sources of information, continuing to be expert listeners, and offering encouragement as women struggle in their decision-making process toward freedom and control in their lives.

▬ *Prevention*

Nurses can make a difference in stopping the violence and preventing further injury. Educating women that abuse is a violation of their rights and facilitating their access to protective and legal services constitute a first step. Other helpful measures for women to discourage the risk of abusive relationships are promoting assertiveness and self-defense courses; suggesting support and self-help groups that encourage positive self-regard, confidence, and empowerment; and recommending educational and skills-development classes that will enhance independence or at least the ability to take care of oneself (Pennell & Francis, 2005). Classes for English language learning may be particularly helpful to immigrant women. Nurses can offer information on local classes.

Preventive education with children encourages and teaches them androgynous gender roles: both male and female persons are equal; both can be nurturing; and neither needs to dominate the other or to engage in violent behavior to have needs met. Helping children to gain problem solving and conflict management skills may eliminate the need for violent solutions to life stresses. Encouraging schoolchildren to form and participate in Students Against Violence Everywhere (SAVE) groups, which is a nationwide pro-peace effort that promotes justice, respect, and love, gives them an appreciation for these qualities in all facets of life. Adolescents benefit from discussion about sex roles, their relationships, and the consequences of the "macho" concept. School nurses can be instrumental in developing and implementing informational activities for adolescents (Walton-Moss & Campbell, 2002). Other means of prevention are to advocate against violence in all arenas and to participate actively in promoting legislation and policies toward stopping violent acts.

▬ Evaluation

Evaluation of the care of the abused woman must be based on expected outcomes and must be in harmony with the choices the woman has made (see Plan of Care).

▬ SEXUAL ASSAULT AND RAPE

Sexual assault is a broad term that encompasses a wide range of sexual victimization including rape, unwanted or uncomfortable touches, kisses, hugs, petting, intercourse, or other sexual acts. Rape is an act of violence. It is not a sexual act, but is intended to humiliate, defile, and dominate the victim (Fishwick et al., 2005). The term is a legal and not a medical one and, in its strictest sense, comprises forced sexual intercourse or the penile penetration of the female sex organ or labia without consent; it may or may not include the use of a weapon. Molestation consists of noncoital sexual activity between a child and an adolescent or adult. Statutory rape involves penetration by a person who is 18 years or older of a person under the age of consent, which varies from state to state.

The key feature to establish rape is the absence of consent: bribery, threat, or coercion implies the lack of consent. The victim who is mentally retarded, who is unconscious or otherwise physically unable to move, who has been drugged without her knowledge, or who is a minor (statutory rape) is not capable of giving consent. The court must prove absence of consent; thus the term alleged rape or alleged sexual assault is used in medical records.

More than 300,000 women are raped each year in the United States. Adolescents have the highest rates of rape and sexual assault. More than half of all rape victims are females younger than 18 (National Center for Injury Prevention and Control [NCIPC], 2005). Drugs often are involved in date rapes, and alcohol potentiates the effects. Date rape drugs such as flunitrazepam (Rohypnol, or "ruffies" [not a legal drug in the United States]) and gamma-hydroxybutyrate (GHB) are often available at bars and clubs (Poirier, 2002). Signs indicating that a woman may have been drugged include having no recall after taking a drink laced with the drug, feeling as if sex has occurred but not having any memory of the incident, feeling more intoxicated than what would be a usual response to the

CD: Plan of Care: The Battered Woman

---

plan of care | The Battered Woman

NURSING DIAGNOSIS Risk for self-directed violence related to history of battering by partner as evidenced by physical injuries

Expected Outcomes *Woman will identify factors leading to cycle of violence and develop plan for safety.*

Nursing Interventions/*Rationales*
- Provide opportunity to verbalize feelings in a nonthreatening atmosphere *to give emotional support.*
- Be alert for cues indicative of battering *to provide database for interventions.*
- Provide information on options available to battered women (e.g., shelters, legal assistance) *to provide information in developing a future plan for safety for herself and any children.*
- Refer to social services and support groups *to give further information and share experiences.*

NURSING DIAGNOSIS Social isolation related to stigma of battering as evidenced by behaviors of withdrawal

Expected Outcome *Woman will demonstrate an increase in social contacts.*

Nursing Interventions/*Rationales*
- Provide private opportunity to express feelings of aloneness *to initiate and maintain a therapeutic relationship.*
- Support opportunities for social interaction *to increase feelings of self-worth and self-confidence.*
- Encourage interaction with groups for socialization and support *to increase number of social contacts.*

NURSING DIAGNOSIS Ineffective family coping related to situational crisis

Expected Outcome *Family will identify feelings and the need for support during this situational crisis.*

Nursing Interventions/*Rationales*
- Provide appropriate time and place for therapeutic communication *to promote trust and allow expression of feelings.*
- Identify effective coping mechanisms *to provide the family with a foundation of familiar interventions.*
- List support systems available *to assist the family to use outside resources.*
- Refer the woman and family to counseling and social services *to provide ongoing support.*

---

amount of alcohol consumed, or feeling fuzzy on awakening (Kilpatrick, Whalley, & Edmunds, 2002).

Many factors deter a woman from reporting the crime, so accurate statistics concerning psychosocial and demographic variables relating to rape are not available. One in every six women report experiencing an attempted or completed rape at some time in their lives. Data regarding sexual assaults greatly underestimate the magnitude of the problem; rape is one of the most underreported crimes (NCIPC, 2005). Women do not report rape because of the associated stigma; embarrassment; guilt that in some way they provoked the assault; fear of retribution from the rapist or his friends; dread of being humiliated and figuratively "raped" again by the criminal justice system publicity; and discouragement generated by the dismally small number of convictions. Rape survivors often fear the reactions of husbands, lovers, friends, family, and children and prefer to suffer alone.

The types of rape are date or acquaintance rape, marital rape, gang rape, stranger rape, and psychic rape. *Acquaintance rape* involves persons who know one another, such as a classmate, neighbor, family member, or date; it is sexual assault that occurs when the trust of a relationship is violated, and one person is forced by another into sexual activity. Victims of date and acquaintance rape are most often between ages 15 and 19 years.

Marital rape occurs partly because some men believe it is their right to engage in sex whenever they desire, regardless of the partner's desire or condition. Marital rape is particularly devastating to the woman because she is in a committed relationship and living with the partner. Most states now recognize marital rape as a legitimate, reportable crime.

Gang rape occurs when one woman is raped by two or more men. *Stranger rape* describes an unknown attacker actively seeking a woman who is vulnerable and is the most feared by women. *Psychic rape* occurs when one's personal dignity and self-respect are assaulted. *Sexual harassment,* although not classified as rape, is another form of using power and control tactics to victimize women sexually, particularly in workplaces.

Dynamics of Rape

Rape is not an act of lust or overzealous passion. Rape is a legal term and involves the use of power and control tactics in a violent, aggressive assault on the victim's body and integrity. As one victim said, "No matter how terrible people think rape is, it's worse than they know. It's like a bomb going off at the center of your soul." The rapist has no regard for his victim's age, race, sexual attraction, or physical condition: 10-day-old infants as well as handicapped elderly women confined to wheelchairs have been sexually assaulted. Most rapes occur intraracially rather than interracially.

Victims of date and acquaintance rape may be less prone to recognize what is happening to them; the dynamics are different from those of stranger rape and may begin rather subtly. The rapist may begin contact by asking personal questions, invading personal space, and proceed to touching that is unwanted and uncomfortable. The woman may not be too alarmed by the perpetrator's actions, believing them to be normal and usual behavior. As she becomes less mindful of the uncomfortable behavior, she may find herself isolated, taken to an apartment, an isolated area in a car, or any place where the two are alone, which is where the forced act of sex frequently occurs (Fishwick et al., 2005).

Rape-Trauma Syndrome

To assess and provide care to a woman who experiences rape, the nurse must first understand the rape-trauma syndrome. This syndrome is characterized by extreme anxiety and stress, resulting in emotional and psychologic reactions and often somatic complaints in the woman. Burgess and Holmstrom, in their classic work (1986), defined three phases of the syndrome.

Acute Phase: Disorganization

The assault itself marks the beginning of this phase of rape-trauma syndrome, which can last for several days or up to 3 weeks. Reactions such as shock, denial, and disbelief are similar to those described by Kübler-Ross in the process of grief and dying. In addition, the rape survivor feels embarrassed, degraded, fearful, angry, and vengeful, and she usually blames herself. She feels unclean and wants to bathe and douche, although that may destroy evidence. Her affect may change rapidly from crying to being calm and controlled. She relives the scene over and over in her mind and considers things she "should have done." Physiologically she may be uncomfortable, experiencing skeletal muscle pain or tension, gastrointestinal irritability, sighing respirations, hyperventilation, flushing, or a sense of feeling too hot or too cold.

Outward Adjustment Phase

During the adjustment phase, the survivor may appear to have resolved her crisis. She may return to a job or to maintaining a household, or both, but she is denying and suppressing her thoughts and feelings. She needs this time to regain some control in her life. She may move, change jobs, buy a weapon to protect herself, or install an alarm system in her home. She becomes less interested in discussing the rape. She may develop specific or generalized fears that restrict her activities.

Long-Term Process: Reorganization Phase

The third phase is reorganization. Denial and suppression cannot be maintained forever. Disclosing personal thoughts and feelings has a profound effect on improving health and reducing stress. As a rape survivor's suppression of feelings and emotions starts to deteriorate, she becomes depressed and anxious. Her own healthy spirit pressures her to discuss the rape with someone. Because she is losing her control of denial, her fears start to surface; she may be afraid to be alone or in a crowd or may fear being attacked from behind. Nightmares and eating disorders are common in these last two phases.

The recovery process may take years and can be difficult and painful. The victim has progressed through recovery when the physical distress and the constant memories of the rape have diminished. She no longer blames herself for what happened and can truly call herself a survivor.

Rape trauma syndrome may meet the criteria for PTSD and be formally diagnosed (see Table 6-1).

Collaborative Care

Nurses in women's health care and EDs are most likely to see rape victims in the acute phase. However, all women who manifest any of the signs of other phases should be assessed for posttraumatic experiences.

Facilities that treat rape victims vary in protocols and resources. In its 1992 guidelines, the Joint Commission on Accreditation of Healthcare Organizations (JCAHO) required EDs and ambulatory care departments to have protocols on physical assault; rape or sexual assault; and domestic abuse of elders, spouses, partners, and children. These protocols must address client consent, examination, and treatment guidelines and the health care facility's responsibility for collecting evidence, photographing injuries, and releasing evidence to law enforcement officials. In addition, the EDs and ambulatory care departments must provide to victims a referral list of community-based and private service agencies dealing with family violence. The nurse interacting with the sexual assault client should be guided by the particular treatment center's protocol (Box 6-4).

Many treatment centers have initiated the use of Sexual Assault Nurse Examiners (SANEs). A SANE is educated in the specialty of forensic nursing and is prepared to examine clients; recognize, collect, and preserve evidence; counsel the client; link the client with vital community resources; follow up cases; and, if necessary, testify in court (Stermac & Stirpe, 2002). If a SANE is not available in a particular facility, JCAHO member organizations must implement a plan for educating an appropriate staff member about identifying, treating, and referring abuse victims. Additional resources may include a social worker who is called when a woman who has been raped is admitted. A local rape crisis center may have volunteers on call who may help by providing emotional support; providing transportation; helping the woman interact with her family, friends, and various authorities; informing her of rape-trauma syndrome; and finding other resources for her as needed. Male volunteers may counsel male members of the victim's family and her male friends.

History

History taking is an important first step in care, and the client should be informed of all the steps involved in the rape examination and follow-up examination. Because rape is a crime, the first nurse to see the sexually assaulted client must consider the need to preserve evidence (see Legal Tip). However, the preservation of evidence should not overshadow a survivor's rights to be treated as a human being with respect, courtesy, and dignity.

▬ **LEGAL TIP** Collector of Evidence

Consent forms must be signed before evidence can be collected and released to the police and before photographs can be taken. If the victim is under 16 years of age, a pediatrician is notified. A parent or guardian is required to sign the consent forms. A children's protective service may need to be called to facilitate consent.

---

box 6-4 **Adult Sexual Assault Protocol: Emergency Department**

PURPOSE

To outline nursing care of sexual assault (rape and/or sexual offense) clients, which includes participation in the collection of forensic evidence and in the referral of clients for follow-up treatment.

Whenever possible, the sexual assault client will be cared for by a SANE (Sexual Assault Nurse Examiner) RN. These nurses have successfully completed a continuing education course in forensic and sexual assault evidence collection. This course provides those nurses with the information and skills to care properly for clients after sexual assault by recognizing, collecting, and preserving evidence; interviewing the client; and linking the client to vital community resources for follow-up.

ASSESSMENT

- Assess the client for any life-threatening injuries.
- Assess the client's level of coping, coherence, and ability to control behavior.
- Assess the client's priorities:
  - –Is client seeking care for prevention of pregnancy or disease only?
  - –Is client seeking forensic evidence collection?
  - –Does the client want both?
- **NOTE:** Notify a SANE nurse to perform the examination if the client is seeking evidence collection for filing of police charges either at this time or in the future.
- Assess the client's entire body for bruises, lacerations, and/or other skeletal or soft tissue injuries.
- Initiate the collection of evidence using the sexual assault collection kit if client consents.
  If SANE nurse is available:
  –SANE: Complete collection.

–SANE: Examine the vagina and rectum to include the speculum examination.
NOTE: Toluidine blue dye and a colposcope may be used to collect evidence.
  –Physician performs the bimanual examination.
  If SANE nurse is not available:
  –Primary nurse initiates collection with the exception of vaginal, rectal, and bimanual examinations.
  –Physician performs vaginal, rectal, and bimanual examinations.
  –Ask client whether or not those who are with the client know that the client has been sexually assaulted.
NOTE: This information cannot be given to secondary victims without the client's permission.

SAFETY

- Notify hospital police when a sexual assault client enters the emergency department.
NOTE: Hospital police will complete a risk assessment of client safety.

CARE

- Provide care for any physical injuries.
- Provide for client privacy and nonjudgmental support.
- Protect client confidentiality by identifying the client as "7273" rather than by name or chief complaint.
- Assign one nurse to the client for the duration of his or her stay and disposition of evidence collection.
- Notify the sexual assault advocate office.
NOTE: The client has the right to refuse an advocate. It is the policy of the emergency department to allow the advocate to offer services directly to the client unless the client expressly forbids it. Notify the advocate of any secondary victims who may

---

History includes a statement of the traumatic event. Box 6-5 lists information to be collected. The woman needs privacy but should not be left alone. She also needs assurance of confidentiality and may need a great deal of support and assistance in verbalizing the offender's acts. For example, giving the woman permission to describe the situation however she chooses and restating what the client has said (without minimizing) will show empathy. It is important to tell the woman that she is safe, that the incident is not her fault, and that she is not alone in what she has experienced. It also is important to obtain sexual, gynecologic, and obstetric histories (see Chapter 5). Because determination of rape is made in court, the wording of the history should reflect the woman's report, and her exact words should be used as often as possible (Poirier, 2002).

Physical Examination and Laboratory Tests

The nurse may assist with or, if trained, may perform the physical examination, which is conducted after the procedure is explained to the woman and consent is obtained. Preservation of the woman's dignity is of utmost importance during the examination. She remains clothed while her vital signs and blood pressure are determined, and her clothing is inspected for stains, tears, and foreign material. Clothing is handled only by the woman and may be

collected and sealed in a bag to be checked for evidence. She is assisted to undress and is draped for the physical examination. A female attendant, rape counselor, or other person of her choice may remain with her during the examination. The physician or nurse practitioner informs her of every step of the procedure. Her body is inspected for bruises, swelling, scratches, lacerations, stab wounds, and body lice. A head-to-toe examination is performed. Many victims have injuries to other parts of their body, mostly involving head, face, and neck (Poirier, 2002). Special attention is given to the area assaulted, that is, pelvic structures and genitalia. External genitals, thighs, buttocks, and lower abdomen are assessed, and if there are injuries, photographs may be taken or drawings made. Pubic and scalp hair is combed for collection. Perianal, oral, and vaginal swabs are collected. If the victim scratched her attacker, her nails are scraped to obtain material that may aid in identification. Necessary equipment for the examination is usually packaged in standard rape kits, which should be available in most EDs.

A speculum examination is performed gently to detect tears or bruises and to collect appropriate specimens. Most victims have some type of genital injury, even if it is asymptomatic. The cervix is cultured for *Neisseria gonorrhoeae, Chlamydia* organisms, and herpes simplex virus, and

box 6-4 | **Adult Sexual Assault Protocol: Emergency Department—cont'd**

have accompanied the client and if the secondary victim is aware that the client has been sexually assaulted.

- Reassure the client that he or she is safe.
- Reassure the client that the incident is not his or her fault.
- Prepare the client for the possibility that some questions asked may be embarrassing.
- Obtain informed consent for the physical examination, to include photographs of injuries.

NOTE: If the client permits the release of information to law enforcement agencies, explain to the victim that the evidence will be turned over to the appropriate jurisdiction for processing. If the client is unwilling to have law enforcement notified at this time, the client should mark "do not" on the release form. The client may later change this if he or she chooses to file charges or have law enforcement involved.

- Collect the evidence as directed and in accordance with client consent.

NOTE: All evidence should be marked with the client's identification. Any photographs taken should be labeled with the client's information and described in the nursing notes. These photographs should then be sealed in an envelope and secured per Department of Emergency Medicine policy. The evidence *must* remain in the possession of *one nurse* throughout the entire assessment procedure and treatment period, until it is released to a police agency.

- Perform a urine test for pregnancy; the urine can also be tested for drugs if the client suspects that he or she was drugged.
- Provide the opportunity for bathing and clean clothing after the examination.
- Discuss and provide emergency contraception and prophylaxis against sexually transmitted infections (STIs), including human immunodeficiency virus (HIV) if desired.

- Arrange for follow-up care per client preference for any medical and/or psychologic problems and/or injury.

CLIENT/SIGNIFICANT OTHER (SO) TEACHING

- Explain to the client/SO:
  - All procedures and rationale for them
  - That feelings of anger, anxiety, and fear are normal
  - That options for medical, legal, and emotional counseling are available to both primary and secondary victims

NOTE: Do not assume that a friend or SO is aware of the assault.

- Inform client/SO of resources available:
  - Judicial system options (e.g., official police report, "blind" report)
  - Financial assistance
  - Other available resources:
  - Local rape crisis center
  - Mental health agency
  - Sites and phone numbers for HIV counseling and testing
  - Resource list of phone numbers (e.g., law enforcement)

DOCUMENTATION

- Complete the forms for sexual assault evidence collection.
- Attach forms to appropriate documents.
- Seal the evidence kit as directed, and deliver it to a sworn law enforcement officer.
- Seal all photographs in an envelope marked with client identification, and secure per Department of Emergency Medicine policy.
- Document care rendered, teaching done, and client response and level of understanding on emergency department nursing record.

box 6-5 | **Sexual Assault History Taking and Assessment**

- Assess the woman for life-threatening injuries.
- Assess the woman's level of coping, coherency, and ability to control behavior.
- Assess the woman's priorities:
  Is the woman seeking care for prevention of disease or pregnancy only?
  Is the woman seeking forensic evidence collection?
  Does the woman want both?
- Ask the woman to describe the event:
  - Time and place of the event
  - Her relationship to the assailant, if any
  - Nature of suspected physical and sexual acts
  - Time lapse between assault and current examination.
- Did the woman bathe, douche, or shower? Did she urinate or defecate?
- Ask woman whether those who are with her know that she has been sexually assaulted.
- Ask the woman if she can think of any other information that would help in her care, and inform her that it is safe to say whatever she needs to and that her disclosures are confidential.
- Inspect the entire body for bruises, lacerations, and other injuries.
- Initiate collection of evidence using the sexual assault collection kit (or notify the Sexual Assault Nurse Examiner).

vaginal fluid is aspirated for analysis. One slide is fixed and dried to be stained and examined for sperm. Fluid is evaluated for seminal contents, including acid phosphatase (an enzyme found in high concentrations in seminal fluid), p30 protein (specific to the prostate and indicates ejaculation), and seminal vesicle specific antigen and ABO antigens (McGregor, Mont, & Myhr, 2002). Cultures for gonorrhea and chlamydia may be obtained from any other sites of penetration or contact such as vagina, anus, and pharynx. Standard wet-mount slides and cultures also may be obtained to test for trichomoniasis. Colposcopy may be used to visualize small abrasions. Some care providers use a hand-held magnifying glass. A bimanual pelvic examination is performed carefully to determine the size and position of the uterus and adnexa. A pelvic mass, caused by bleeding into the broad ligament, may be palpated. Internal pelvic assessment ends with a rectovaginal examination if the woman has given consent, and it is deemed necessary.

Sexual assault kits are intended to facilitate collection of specimens, particularly if they are to be used as evidence should the woman decide to report the rape; they give specific instructions on what specimens to collect from what body parts or articles of clothing, and ways to preserve the evidence.

Laboratory tests may include a urine or serum pregnancy test and serum tests for syphilis, hepatitis B virus, and human immunodeficiency virus (HIV) (CDC, Workowski, & Berman, 2006).

During the examination, the woman's emotional status is assessed, and findings are recorded: what reactions she exhibits to the assault; her orientation to time and place; and her attention span, affect, and verbal description and feelings about the assault. The availability of family or peer-support systems is assessed. She is asked about her plans to report or not to report the crime to the police.

After the physical examination, the woman should be allowed to shower and be offered fresh clothes or a gown. She may be offered time to rest and to talk with the nurse, rape crisis counselor, family, or friends.

Nursing diagnoses for the rape victim during the immediate and later posttrauma periods include the following:

IMMEDIATE POSTTRAUMA PERIOD
- *Anxiety/fear related to*
  - –rape-trauma experience
  - –interactions with police and caregivers
  - –physical examination to assess injury and collect evidence
- *Acute pain related to*
  - –physical injury from rape
  - –examination
- *Disturbed body image related to*
  - –the rape
- *Rape-trauma syndrome related to*
  - –aftermath of being sexually assaulted
  - –feelings of being unclean and humiliated
  - –silent reaction of being unable to discuss the rape
- *Decisional conflict related to*
  - –discussing rape with family
  - –possible pregnancy

LATER POSTTRAUMA PERIOD
- *Risk for infection related to*
  - –sexually transmitted infections
  - –sexual assault by an assailant of unknown sexual history
- *Impaired social interaction related to*
  - –the rape
  - –strained relationships with family, friends, intimate partners

---

Immediate Care

Medical management includes (1) treating the physical injuries, including tetanus toxoid booster if indicated; (2) providing prophylactic antibiotic therapy for STIs (e.g., gonorrhea, syphilis); and (3) providing prophylaxis for pregnancy if the woman is not pregnant. If physical trauma is life threatening, appropriate intervention takes precedence over collecting evidence.

If the victim is at risk for pregnancy, emergency contraception should be discussed with her. Over 32,000 pregnancies result from rape every year (NCIPC, 2005). Emergency contraception with progestin-only or combined estrogen and progestin pills must be used within 72 hours of the sexual assault (ACOG, 2005) (see Table 9-2). She should be advised that emergency contraception does not guarantee pregnancy prevention, and that she should repeat the pregnancy test if she has not had a menstrual period within 3 to 4 weeks. The woman is apprised of the availability of abortion or menstrual extraction as a backup measure. If the woman is pregnant at the time of the assault, she should be observed for several hours for uterine contractility.

The woman may be provided with prophylactic antibiotic therapy to prevent STIs, hepatitis B immunization if needed, and human immunodeficiency virus (HIV) postexposure prophylaxis (PEP) (CDC, Workowski, & Berman, 2006).

Discharge

The woman is discharged with medications and printed instructions about their use, printed instructions for self-care, and names and telephone numbers of resource people if she requires assistance. Money as needed and transportation to wherever she is staying (an alternative place may be found for her) add to the woman's comfort and perception of being in control. A medical follow-up examination in the gynecology or pediatric clinic is scheduled in 1 to 2 weeks for repeated cultures for gonorrhea and other STIs; at 6 weeks for assessment of healing injuries; and at 6, 12, and 24 weeks for repeated serology tests for syphilis and HIV infection if initial test results were negative. The woman and her counselor determine whether there is a need for an additional medical or psychologic follow-up examination between the scheduled visits. The woman has a choice of site for follow-up testing. Some women choose to continue with the health care provider who first performed the examination; others prefer their primary health care provider; and still others need referral to a clinic in the area (city, state) in which they live.

Nurses must be aware that responses to rape are variable. Self-blame and humiliation may alternate with anger and fear. The client needs to be reassured again before she leaves that her feelings are normal and that she is not alone. The initial care of a woman will affect her recovery and her decision to return for follow-up care. Nurses can assist clients through an examination that is as nontraumatic as possible, with kindness, skill, and empathy.

After Discharge

Because of the phases of recovery, telephone contact by the health care provider to whomever the woman is referred is continued until the woman has no further need for such help. Education in prevention strategies is often offered by community agencies or rape-awareness groups. The focus of the classes is usually on increasing women's awareness of situations that put them at high risk for rape or sexual assault. Other courses may teach self-defense methods or how to change personal behaviors to reduce the risk of being victimized, such as avoiding being alone in isolated places and being alert to unusual activities or persons in one's environment. Still other courses may focus on changing societal attitudes about rape. Nurses can play a role in preventive education by offering courses or participating in courses offered by community or health care groups. Nurses must be knowledgeable about the epidemiology of sexual assault, reporting requirements, and services available in their community for victims, and should screen all women for a history of assault and any sequelae.

community activity

October is National Intimate Partner Awareness Month. Negotiate with the manager of a local mall or superstore to display a poster and pamphlets that provide accurate information about the extent and costs of violence as well as what preventive measures the public might take. There may be a local violence against women coalition that can be consulted; alternatively, you can use Internet resources to design your display.

key points

- Violence against women is a major social and health care problem in the United States, costing thousands of lives and billions of dollars in direct and indirect health care costs.
- Intimate partner violence includes physical, sexual, emotional, psychologic, and economic abuse.
- To provide effective care, nurses must increase awareness of their own beliefs and values regarding victimization of women.
- Theoretic frameworks—psychologic, sociologic, biologic, and feminist perspectives—provide the foundation for understanding the complexity of the victimization of women.
- Cultural influences regarding violent behaviors and relationships sensitize the nurse to the special needs of women from various ethnic groups.
- Battering affects young, middle-aged, and older women of all races; all socioeconomic, educational, and religious groups; and pregnant women.

- All states have mandatory reporting of the abuse of children and elderly people; some states have initiated mandatory reporting of wife abuse. Mandatory reporting may be helpful to some women who just are not comfortable making the call, whereas other women would prefer to have control over their own reporting choices.
- Rape is a legal term meaning a violent, aggressive sexual assault carried out against one's will.
- Nurses in all professional areas should respond with sensitivity and caring to women who experience abuse and victimization.
- Follow-up and collaborative care are important in all instances of abuse.
- Nurses should be knowledgeable about reporting requirements and available community service for women who have been sexually assaulted.

REFERENCES

American College of Obstetricians and Gynecologists (ACOG). (2005). Emergency contraception. ACOG Practice Bulletin No. 69. *Obstetrics and Gynecology, 106*(6), 1443-1451.

American College of Obstetricians and Gynecologists (ACOG). (2006). *Screening tools for domestic violence.* Accessed www.acog.org, March 2, 2006.

American Psychiatric Association. (2000). *Diagnostic and statistic manual of mental disorders* (4th rev. ed.). Washington, DC: American Psychiatric Association Press.

Burgess, A., & Holmstrom, L. (1986). *Rape, crisis, and recovery.* West Newton, MA: Awab.

Campbell, D., Sharps, P., Gary, F., Campbell, J., & Lopez, L. (2002). Intimate partner violence in African American women. *Online Journal of Issues in Nursing, 7*(1), 5.

Campbell, J., & Fishwick, N. (1993). Abuse of female partners. In J. Campbell & J. Humphreys (Eds.), *Nursing care of survivors of family violence.* St. Louis: Mosby.

Campbell, J., & Furniss, K. (2002). Violence against women: Identification, screening and management of intimate partner violence. Washington, DC: Association of Women's Health, Obstetric, and Neonatal Nurses.

Campbell, J., Jones, A., Dienemann, J., Kub, J, Schollenberger, J, O'Campo, P., et al. (2002). Intimate partner violence and physical health consequences. *Archives of Internal Medicine, 162*(10), 1157-1163.

Centers for Disease Control and Prevention (CDC). (2003). Costs of intimate partner violence against women in the United States. Atlanta, GA: *US Department of Health and Human Services.* Accessed http://www.cdc.gov/ncipc/pub-res/ipv_cost/00_preface.htm, March 2, 2006.

Centers for Disease Control and Prevention (CDC), Workowski, K., & Berman, S. (2006). Sexually transmitted diseases treatment guidelines 2006. *MMWR Morbidity and Mortality Weekly Report, 55*(RR11), 1-94.

Davis, J., Park, S., Kaups, K., Bennink, L., & Bilello, J. (2003). Victims of domestic violence on the trauma service: Unrecognized and underreported. *Journal of Trauma, 54*(2), 352-355.

Dienemann, J., Boyle, E., Baker, D., Resnick, W., Wiederhorn, N., & Campbell, J. (2000). Intimate partner abuse among women diagnosed with depression. *Issues in Mental Health Nursing, 21*(5), 499-513.

Dienemann, J., Glass, N., & Hyman, R. (2005). Survivor preferences for response to IPV disclosure. *Clinical Nursing Research, 14*(3), 215-233.

Downs, W., & Rindels, B. (2004). Adulthood depression, anxiety, and trauma symptoms: A comparison of women with nonabusive, abusive, and absent father figures in childhood. *Violence and Victims, 19*(6), 659-671.

Family Violence Prevention Fund (FVPF). (2004). Mandatory reporting of domestic violence by health care providers. Accessed www.endabuse.org/health/mandatoryreporting, March 2, 2006.

Faramarzi, M., Esmailzadeh, S., & Mosavi, S. (2005). A comparison of abused and non-abused women's definitions of domestic violence and attitudes to acceptance of male dominance. *European Journal of Obstetrics, Gynecology, and Reproductive Biology, 122*(2), 225-231.

Fisher, I. (2002, July 12). Doubt cast on charges that led to Pakistan rape. *New York Times*, Section A, p 8.

Fishwick, N., Parker, B., & Campbell, J. (2005). Care of survivors of abuse and violence. In G. Stuart & M. Laraia (Eds.), *Principles and practice of psychiatric nursing* (8th ed.). St. Louis: Mosby.

Gerber, M., Gantz, M., Lichter, E., Williams, C., & McCloskey, K. (2005). Adverse health behaviors and the detection of partner violence by clinicians. *Archives of Internal Medicine, 165*(9), 1016-1021.

Glass, N. (2005). *Discovery, Oregon Health Sciences University School of Nursing, Annual Research Publication*. Portland, OR: Oregon Health Sciences University School of Nursing.

Hamolia, C. (2005) Preventing and managing aggressive behavior. In G. Stuart, & M. Laraia, (Eds.), *Principles and practice of psychiatric nursing* (8th ed.). St. Louis: Mosby.

Harrykissoon, S., Rickert, V., & Wiemann, C. (2002). Prevalence and patterns of intimate partner violence among adolescent mothers during the postpartum period. *Archives of Pediatric and Adolescent Medicine, 156*(4), 325-330.

Huth-Brooks, A., Levendosky, Q., & Bogart, G. (2002). The effects of domestic violence during pregnancy on maternal and infant health. *Violence and Victims, 17*(2), 169-185.

Kilpatrick, D., Whalley, A., & Edmunds, C. (2002). Sexual assault. *National Victim Assistance Academy 2002*. Accessed www.nvaa.org/assist/chapter10sup.html, March 2, 2006.

Lindgren, K. (2001). Relationships among maternal fetal attachment, prenatal depression and health practices in pregnancy. *Research in Nursing and Health, 24*(3), 203-217.

Martin, S., Mackie, L., Kupper, L., Buescher, P., & Moracco, K. (2001). Physical abuse of women before, during, and after pregnancy. *Journal of the American Medical Association, 285*(12), 1581-1584.

McCosker, H., Barnard, A., & Gerber, R. (2003). Phenomenographic study of women's experiences of domestic violence during the childbearing years. *Online Journal of Issues in Nursing, 9*(1), 12.

McFarlane, L., Campbell, J., Sharps, P., & Watson, K. (2002). Abuse during pregnancy and femicide: Urgent implications for women's health. *Obstetrics and Gynecology, 100*(1), 27-35.

McFarlane, J., Groff, J., O'Brien, A.. & Watson, K. (2005). Populations at risk: empirical studies of prevalence of partner violence against 7,443 African American, White, and Hispanic women receiving care at urban public primary care clinics. *Public Health Nursing, 22*(2), 98-107.

McGregor, M., Mont, J., & Myhr, T. (2002). Sexual assault forensic medical examination: Is evidence related to successful prosecution? *Annals of Emergency Medicine, 39*(6), 639-647.

Moracco, K., Brown, C., Martin, S., Chang, J. Dulli, L., Loucks-Sorrell, M., et al.. (2004). Mental health issues among female clients of domestic violence programs in North Carolina. *Psychiatric Services, 55*(9), 1036-1040.

National Center for Injury Prevention and Control (NCIPC). (2005). *Sexual violence: fact sheet*. Accessed http://www.cic.gov/ncipc/factsheets/svfacts.htm, March 2, 2006.

National Women's Health Information Center (NWHIC). (2002). *Violence against women*. Accessed http://www.4woman.gov/violence/index.cfm, March 2, 2006.

Neller, J., Denney, R., Pietz, C., & Thomlinson, R. (2005). Testing the trauma model of violence. *Journal of Family Violence, 20*(3), 151-159.

Peedicayil, A., Sadowski, L., Lakshman, J., Shankar, V., Jain, D., Suresh, S., et al. (2005). Spousal physical violence against women during pregnancy. *British Journal of Obstetrics and Gynaecology, 111*(7), 682-687.

Pennell, J., & Francis, S. (2005). Safety conferencing: toward a coordinated and inclusive response to safeguard women and children. *Violence Against Women, 11*(5), 666-692.

Plichta, S., (2004). Intimate partner violence and physical health consequences. *Journal of Interpersonal Violence, 19*(11), 1296-1323.

Poirier, M. (2002). Care of the female adolescent rape victim. *Pediatric Emergency Care, 18*(1), 53-59.

Quinlivan, J., & Evans, S. (2005). Impact of domestic violence and drug abuse in pregnancy on maternal attachment and infant temperament in teenage mothers in the setting of best clinical practice. *Archives of Women's Mental Health, 8*(3), 191-199.

Renker, P. (2002). "Keep a blank face. I need to tell you what has been happening to me." Teens' stories of abuse and violence before and during pregnancy. *MCN American Journal of Maternal/Child Nursing, 27*(2), 109-116.

Renzetti, C., Edleson, J., & Bergen, R. (2001). *The sourcebook on violence against women*. Thousand Oaks, CA: Sage.

Shiu-Thornton, S., Senturia, K., & Sullivan, M. (2005). "Like a bird in a cage": Vietnamese women survivors talk about domestic violence. *Journal of Interpersonal Violence, 20*(8), 959-976.

Soler, H., Vinayak, P., & Quadagno, D. (2000). Biosocial aspects of domestic violence. *Psychoneuroendocrinology, 25*(7), 721-739.

Stermac, L., & Stirpe, T. (2002). Efficacy of a 2-year-old sexual assault nurse examiner program in a Canadian hospital. *Journal of Emergency Nursing, 28*(1), 18-23.

Tjaden, P., & Thoennes, N. (2000). *Extent, nature and consequences of intimate partner violence: Findings from the national violence against women survey*. Washington, DC: U.S. Department of Justice.

Torres, S., & Han, H. (2003). Women's perceptions of their male batterers' characteristics and level of violence. *Issues in Mental Health Nursing, 24*(6), 667-673.

U.S. Department of Health and Human Services (USDHHS). (2000). *Healthy people 2010: National health promotion and disease prevention objectives*. Washington, DC: Author.

Walker, L. (1979). *The battered woman*. New York: Harper & Row.

Walker, L. (1984). *The battered woman syndrome* (Vol. 6). New York: Springer.

Walton-Moss, B., & Campbell, J. (2002). Intimate partner violence: Implications for nursing. *Online Journal of Issues in Nursing, 7*(1), 6.

World Health Organization (WHO). (2005). *WHO multi-country study on women's health and domestic violence against women. Summary report of initial results on prevalence, health outcomes, and women's responses*. Geneva: Author.

Yoshioka, M., & Choi, D. (2005). Culture and interpersonal violence research. *Journal of Interpersonal Violence, 20*(4), 513-519.

Yost, N., Bloom, S., McIntire, G., & Leveno, K. (2005). A prospective observational study of domestic violence during pregnancy. *Obstetrics and Gynecology, 106*(1), 61-65.

CHAPTER 7

Catherine Ingram Fogel

Reproductive System Concerns

learning objectives

- Differentiate signs and symptoms of common menstrual disorders.
- Develop a nursing plan of care for the woman with primary dysmenorrhea.
- Outline client teaching about premenstrual syndrome (PMS).
- Relate the pathophysiology of endometriosis to associated symptoms.
- Identify the health risks of perimenopausal women.

- Develop an assessment guide for perimenopausal women.
- Develop a nursing plan of care for the postmenopausal woman.
- Examine the risks and benefits of menopausal hormone therapy.
- Summarize client teaching strategies for prevention of osteoporosis.
- Evaluate the use of alternative therapies for menstrual disorders and menopausal symptoms.

electronic resources

Additional information related to the content in Chapter 7 can be found on

the companion website at *evolve*
http://evolve.elsevier.com/Lowdermilk/MWHC/
- NCLEX Review Questions
- WebLinks

 or on the interactive companion CD
- NCLEX Review Questions
- Plan of Care: Endometriosis
- Plan of Care: Premenstrual Syndrome

---

*P*ROBLEMS may occur at any point in the menstrual cycle. In addition, many factors, including anatomic abnormalities, physiologic imbalances, and lifestyle, can affect the menstrual cycle. Many women seek out nurses as advisors, counselors, and health care providers for information about menstrual cycle experiences, concerns, or disorders. If they are to meet their clients' needs, nurses must have accurate, up-to-date information. This chapter provides information on menstrual cycle experiences, including menarche and menopause, common menstrual disorders, and problems associated with menopause.

Knowledge of the normal parameters of menstruation is essential to the assessment of menstrual cycle experiences and disorders. The menstrual cycle is a result of a complex interplay among the reproductive, neurologic, and endocrine systems (Blackburn, 2003). The hypothalamus produces gonadotropin-releasing hormone (GnRH), which stimulates the pituitary gland to produce follicle-stimulating

hormone (FSH) and luteinizing hormone (LH). In turn, FSH and LH stimulate the ovaries to produce first estrogen and then progesterone. In response to the hormones, the endometrium, or lining of the uterus, proliferates and then sheds. Chapter 5 provides additional information on the menstrual cycle and endocrine physiology.

Normal menstrual patterns are averages based on observations and reports from large groups of healthy women. When counseling an individual woman, remember that these values are averages only. Generally a woman's menstrual frequency stabilizes at 28 days within 1 to 2 years after puberty, with a range from 26 to 34 days (Blackburn, 2003). Although no woman's cycle is exactly the same length every month, the typical month-to-month variation in an individual's cycle is usually plus or minus 2 days. However, greater but still normal variations are noted frequently.

During her reproductive years, a woman may have more than one physiologic variation in her menstrual cycle. An understanding of the physiologic variations that occur in several age groups is essential knowledge for nurses. Menstrual cycle length is most irregular at the extremes of the reproductive years including the 2 years after menarche and the 5 years before menopause, when anovulatory cycles are most common. Irregular bleeding, both in length of cycle and amount, is the rule, rather than the exception, in early adolescence. It takes approximately 15 months for completion of the first 10 cycles and an average of 20 cycles before ovulation occurs regularly. Cycle lengths of 15 to 45 days are not unusual, and during the first 2 years after menarche, intervals of 3 to 6 months between menses can be normal.

Women's knowledge and understanding of the menstrual cycle may be limited and is often influenced by myths and misunderstandings. Women typically have menstrual cycles for about 40 years. Once the irregular nature of menses in the first 1 to 2 years after menarche subsides and a cyclic, predictable pattern of monthly bleeding is established, women may worry about any deviation from that pattern, or from what they have been told is normal for all menstruating women. A woman may be concerned about her ability to conceive and bear children, or she may believe that she is not really a woman without monthly evidence. A sign such as amenorrhea or excess menstrual bleeding can be a source of severe distress and concern for women.

■ COMMON MENSTRUAL DISORDERS

Amenorrhea

Amenorrhea, the absence of menstrual flow, is a clinical symptom of a variety of disorders. Although these criteria for a clinical problem of amenorrhea are not universal, these circumstances should generally be evaluated: (1) the absence of both menarche and secondary sexual characteristics by age 14 years; (2) absence of menses by age 16 years, regardless of presence of normal growth and development (primary amenorrhea); or (3) a 3- to 6-month absence of menses after a period of menstruation (secondary amenorrhea) (Harlow, 2000; Speroff & Fritz, 2005).

Although amenorrhea is not a disease, it is often the sign of one. Still, most commonly and most benignly, amenorrhea is a result of pregnancy. It also may result from anatomic abnormalities such as outflow tract obstruction, anterior pituitary disorders, other endocrine disorders such as polycystic ovarian syndrome, hypothyroidism or hyperthyroidism, chronic diseases such as type 1 diabetes, medications such as phenytoin (Dilantin), illicit drug abuse (alcohol, tranquilizers, opiates, marijuana, cocaine), or oral contraceptive use.

In addition, it may occur from any defect or interruption in the hypothalamic-pituitary-ovarian-uterine axis. In rare instances, a pituitary lesion or genetic inability to produce FSH and LH is at fault. Hypogonadotropic amenorrhea often results from hypothalamic suppression as a result of stress (in the home, school, or workplace) or a sudden and severe weight loss, eating disorders, strenuous exercise, or mental illness (Parent-Stevens & Burns, 2000). Research

on the interaction between nervous system or neurotransmitter functions and hormonal regulation throughout the body has demonstrated a biologic basis for the relation of stress to physiologic processes. Women who are more than 20% underweight for height or who have had rapid weight loss may report amenorrhea, as may women with eating disorders such as anorexia nervosa (Alexander, Shimp, & Smith, 2000; Parent-Stevens & Burns, 2000). Amenorrhea is one of the classic signs of anorexia nervosa, and the interrelatedness of disordered eating, amenorrhea, and premature osteoporosis has been described as the female athlete triad (Kleposki, 2002; Sabatini, 2001). A loss of calcium from the bone, comparable to that seen in postmenopausal women, may occur with this type of amenorrhea.

Exercise-associated amenorrhea can occur in women undergoing vigorous physical and athletic training (Sanborn, Horea, Siemers, & Dieringer, 2000). The pathophysiology is complex and is thought to be associated with many factors, including body composition (height, weight, and percentage of body fat); type, intensity, and frequency of exercise; nutritional status; and presence of emotional or physical stressors (Kleposki, 2002; Speroff & Fritz, 2005). In addition, it is probably due to diminished secretion of GnRH. Women who participate in sports emphasizing low body weight are at greatest risk, including the following (Sabatini, 2001):

- Sports in which performance is subjectively scored (e.g., dance, gymnastics)
- Endurance sports favoring participants with low body weight (e.g., distance running, cycling)
- Sports in which body contour–revealing clothing is worn for competition (e.g., swimming, diving, volleyball)
- Sports with weight categories for participation (e.g., rowing, martial arts)
- Sports in which prepubertal body shape favors success (e.g., gymnastics, figure skating)

Assessment of amenorrhea begins with a thorough history and physical examination. An important initial step, often overlooked, is to be sure that the woman is not pregnant. Specific components of the assessment process depend on a client's age—adolescent, young adult, or perimenopausal—and whether she has previously menstruated.

Once pregnancy has been ruled out by a β-human chorionic gonadotropin (β-hCG) pregnancy test, diagnostic tests may include FSH level, thyroid-stimulating hormone (TSH) and prolactin levels, radiographic or computed tomography scan of the sella turcica, and a progestational challenge (Hall, 2002).

Management. When amenorrhea is due to hypothalamic disturbances, the nurse is an ideal health professional to assist women because many of the causes are potentially reversible (e.g., stress, weight loss for nonorganic reasons). Counseling and education are primary interventions and appropriate nursing roles. When a stressor known to predispose a client to hypothalamic amenorrhea is identified, initial management involves addressing the stressor.

Together the woman and the nurse plan how the woman can decrease or discontinue medications known to affect menstruation, correct weight loss, deal more effectively with psychologic stress, address emotional distress, and alter exercise routine.

The nurse works with the woman to help her identify, cope with, and possibly resolve sources of stress in her life. Deep-breathing exercises and relaxation techniques are simple yet effective stress reduction measures. Referral for biofeedback or massage therapy also may be useful. In some instances, referrals for psychotherapy may be indicated.

If a woman's exercise program is thought to contribute to her amenorrhea, several options exist for management. She may decide to decrease the intensity or duration of her training if possible or to gain 2% to 3% in body weight. Coming to accept this alternative may be difficult for one who is committed to a strenuous exercise regimen, and the nurse and the client may have several sessions before the woman elects to try exercise reduction. Many young female athletes may not understand the consequences of low bone density or osteoporosis; nurses can point out the connection between low bone density and stress fractures. The nurse and the woman also should investigate other factors that may be contributing to the amenorrhea and develop plans for altering lifestyle and decreasing stress.

A daily calcium intake of 1200 to 1500 mg/day, accomplished by drinking 3 glasses of skim milk or taking a calcium supplement, is recommended for women with amenorrhea associated with the female athlete triad (Kleposki, 2002). Some researchers have found that oral contraceptives have a positive effect on bone density in amenorrhoeic premenopausal women (Liu & Lebrun, 2006).

Cyclic Perimenstrual Pain and Discomfort

Cyclic perimenstrual pain and discomfort (CPPD) is a concept developed by a nurse science team for a research project for the Association of Women's Health, Obstetric and Neonatal Nurses (Collins Sharp, Taylor, Thomas, Killeen, & Dawood, 2002). This concept includes dysmenorrhea, premenstrual syndrome (PMS), and premenstrual dysphoric disorder (PMDD) as well as symptom clusters that occur before and after the menstrual flow starts. CPPD is a health problem that can have a significant impact on the quality of life for a woman. The following discussion focuses on the three main conditions of CPPD. See the Evidence-Based Practice box for further discussion of the clinical guidelines for nursing practice for CPPD.

Dysmenorrhea

Dysmenorrhea, pain during or shortly before menstruation, is one of the most common gynecologic problems in women of all ages. Many adolescents have dysmenorrhea in the first 3 years after menarche. Young adult women ages 17 to 24 years are most likely to report painful menses. Dysmenorrhea decreases in most women after a full-term pregnancy (Speroff & Fritz, 2005). Between 30% and 40% of women report some level of discomfort associated with menses, and 7% to 15% report severe dysmenorrhea (Parent-Stevens & Burns, 2000); however, the amount of disruption in women's lives is difficult to determine. It has been estimated that up to 10% of women with dysmenorrhea have severe enough pain to interfere with their functioning for 1 to 3 days a month. Menstrual problems, including dysmenorrhea, are more common in women who smoke and those who are obese. Severe dysmenorrhea is also associated with early menarche, nulliparity, and stress (Stenchever, Droegemueller, Herbst, & Mishell, 2001). Traditionally, dysmenorrhea is differentiated as primary or secondary. Symptoms usually begin with menstruation, although some women have discomfort several hours before onset of flow. The range and severity of symptoms are different from woman to woman and from cycle to cycle in the same woman. Symptoms of dysmenorrhea may last several hours or several days.

Pain is usually located in the suprapubic area or lower abdomen. Women describe the pain as sharp, cramping, or gripping or as a steady dull ache; pain may radiate to the lower back or upper thighs.

Primary Dysmenorrhea

Primary dysmenorrhea, a condition associated with abnormally increased uterine activity, is due to myometrial contractions induced by prostaglandins in the second half of the menstrual cycle. During the luteal phase and subsequent menstrual flow, prostaglandin $F_{2\alpha}$ ($PGF_{2\alpha}$) is secreted. The uterine muscle of both normal and dysmenorrhoeic women is sensitive to prostaglandins; however, the amount of prostaglandin produced is the major differentiating factor (Speroff & Fritz, 2005). Excessive release of $PGF_{2\alpha}$ increases the amplitude and frequency of uterine contractions and causes vasospasm of the uterine arterioles, resulting in ischemia and cyclic lower abdominal cramps. Systemic responses to $PGF_{2\alpha}$ include backache, weakness, sweating, gastrointestinal symptoms (anorexia, nausea, vomiting, and diarrhea), and central nervous system symptoms (dizziness, syncope, headache, and poor concentration). Pain begins at the onset of menstrual flow and lasts from 8 to 48 hours. The release of most prostaglandins during menstruation occurs in the first 48 hours, which coincides with the greatest intensity of symptoms (Stenchever et al., 2001).

Primary dysmenorrhea is not caused by underlying pathology; rather it is the occurrence of a physiologic alteration in some women. Primary dysmenorrhea usually appears within 6 to 12 months after menarche when ovulation is established. Anovulatory bleeding, common in the few months or years after menarche, is painless. Because both estrogen and progesterone are necessary for primary dysmenorrhea to occur, it is experienced only with ovulatory cycles. This problem is most common in women in their late teens and early twenties; the incidence declines with age.

AWHONN Research-Based Practice Guidelines for Cyclic Perimenstrual Pain and Discomfort

BACKGROUND

- Most women experience some perimenstrual symptoms, which can cause loss of work or school and extra medical visits and costs. Conventionally, research has focused on discrete aspects of menstrual changes, such as pain or negative affect. However, most women experience several symptoms simultaneously. A more comprehensive and functional concept of cyclic perimenstrual pain and discomfort (CPPD) includes the symptom clusters that occur throughout the luteal phase and menstruation. Up to 100 perimenstrual symptoms have been identified.

OBJECTIVES

- Many women do not seek medical advice about CPPD, and many health care providers are poorly informed about CPPD management. Women often use over-the-counter treatments ineffectively. Nurses are ideally positioned to offer first-line screening and advice about management of CPPD. The Association of Women's Health, Obstetric and Neonatal Nurses (AWHONN) selected CPPD as a focus for its research-based practice project, with the goal of providing guidelines for nursing practice.

METHODS

Search Strategy

- The AWHONN science team researched CINAHL, MEDLINE, and the Cochrane databases, as well as references. Search keywords included *cyclic pain, pelvic pain, comfort, pain guidelines,* and *dysmenorrhea.* Thirty-three relevant research articles, dated 1992-1999, were selected, ranging from case studies to clinical trials.

Statistical Analyses

- Because the studies were so varied, the research team analyzed the data holistically. Three nursing diagnoses emerged: perimenstrual cyclic pain, perimenstrual discomfort, and perimenstrual negative affect.

FINDINGS

- Research-based nursing interventions fell into six categories:
  1. Fundamental symptom management: Principles of general pain management and assisting with coping enhancement and mutual goal setting are appropriate for CPPD.
  2. Self-monitoring: Instruction on daily tracking of symptoms and stressors increases self-esteem and efficacy.
  3. Self-regulation:
     a. Pharmacologic agents had the strongest research. Nonsteroidal antiinflammatory drugs (NSAIDs) and low-dose, combined oral contraceptives were very effective.
     b. Nutritional supplements were supported by moderately good evidence.
        i. Calcium, 1200 mg/day, may significantly decrease premenstrual syndrome symptoms by the third cycle.
        ii. Magnesium helps stabilize blood sugar and decreases constipation and bloating.
     iii. Vitamin B_6 (pyridoxine) may relieve negative affect symptoms but can be toxic in overdose.
     iv. Essential fatty acids, such as evening primrose oil, borage, and black currant oil, may decrease dysmenorrhea, breast tenderness, and fluid retention.
     c. Topical—cutaneous: The strongest research supported the use of transcutaneous electrical nerve stimulation (TENS), which may disrupt the sensory perception of pain, combined with NSAIDs. Moderately strong research backed the use of abdominal heat and massage, which may increase blood flow. Weaker evidence showed some pain relief using acupressure points at the abdomen, back, and inner ankle.
     d. Behavioral—cognitive: There was some evidence of symptom relief with daily practice of relaxation, breathing, stretching, meditation, or guided imagery.
  4. Self-Modification:
     a. Nutritional: Eliminating smoking, alcohol, salt, caffeine, and sugars, eating frequent small meals, and drinking six to eight glasses of fluids a day resulted in some improvement in symptoms. Moderate evidence supported a program of multivitamins and minerals, which may be individualized to include vitamin E, essential fatty acids, B-complex vitamins, calcium, and amino acids L-tyrosine and L-tryptophan.
     b. Research was equivocal that exercise may increase blood flow, metabolism, and endorphins.
  5. Environmental: Time management and communication skills helped somewhat to modify the stressors that compound CPPD.
  6. Referral: Chinese herbals, chiropractic treatment, acupuncture, and homeopathy have shown some promise anecdotally, but lack strong evidence.

LIMITATIONS

- The complexity of CPPD, combined with the range of qualitative and quantitative studies, made synthesis of the literature a Herculean task. Each woman has her own cluster of discomforts each cycle, and the treatment must be as dynamic as the symptoms. No critical pathway or decision tree can be established yet. Treatment is still an art, with some science.

IMPLICATIONS FOR PRACTICE

- CPPD is a quality-of-life issue for women. The authors recommended routine screening for CPPD, specifically pelvic pain and other discomforts, and efficacy of self-treatment. Individualized, multimodal management should produce treatment options based on the strongest evidence.

IMPLICATIONS FOR FURTHER RESEARCH

- Further research, especially randomized controlled complementary and alternative medicine research, is needed to yield more generalizability to the studies. Possible combinations of therapies may show promise for symptom relief.

Reference: Collins Sharp, B., Taylor, D., Thomas, K., Killeen, M., & Dawood, M. (2002). Cyclic perimenstrual pain and discomfort: The scientific basis for practice. *Journal of Obstetric, Gynecologic, and Neonatal Nursing, 31*(6), 637-649.

CRITICAL THINKING EXERCISE

Cyclic Perimenstrual Pain and Discomfort

Marianne, 34, has come to Women's Clinic for her annual gynecologic checkup. She reports perimenstrual symptoms of pain, breast tenderness, bloating, edema, and feeling irritable and depressed. She says she takes ibuprofen for the pain with fairly good relief, but so far it does not relieve the other symptoms. How should the nurse respond?

1. Evidence—Is there sufficient evidence to draw conclusions about what advice the nurse should give to Marianne?
2. Assumptions—Describe underlying assumptions about the following issues:
   a. Cyclic perimenstrual pain and discomfort
   b. Self-help strategies (e.g., symptom management, monitoring symptoms, modification)
   c. Quality of life issues for women experiencing perimenstrual pain and discomfort
   d. Coping enhancement as a nursing strategy
3. What implications and priorities for nursing care can be made at this time?
4. Does the evidence objectively support your conclusion?
5. Are there alternative perspectives to your conclusion?

Management. Management of primary dysmenorrhea depends on the severity of the problem and an individual woman's response to various treatments. Important components of nursing care are information and support. Because menstruation is so closely linked to reproduction and sexuality, menstrual problems such as dysmenorrhea can have a negative influence on sexuality and self-worth. Nurses can correct myths and misinformation about menstruation and dysmenorrhea by providing facts about what is normal. Nurses must support their clients' feelings of positive sexuality and self-worth.

Often more than one alternative for alleviating menstrual discomfort and dysmenorrhea can be offered. Women can then try options and decide which ones work best for them. Heat (heating pad or hot bath) minimizes cramping by increasing vasodilation and muscle relaxation and minimizing uterine ischemia. Massaging the lower back can reduce pain by relaxing paravertebral muscles and increasing pelvic blood supply. Soft rhythmic rubbing of the abdomen (effleurage) may be useful because it provides distraction and an alternative focal point. Guided imagery, progressive relaxation, hatha yoga, and meditation also have been used successfully to decrease menstrual discomfort.

Exercise has been found to help in relieving menstrual discomfort through increased vasodilation and subsequently decreased ischemia; release of endogenous opiates, specifically β-endorphins; suppression of prostaglandins; and shunting of blood flow away from the viscera, resulting in less pelvic congestion. A specific exercise that nurses can suggest to their clients is pelvic rocking.

In addition to maintaining good nutrition at all times, specific dietary changes may be helpful in decreasing some of the systemic symptoms associated with dysmenorrhea. Decreased salt and refined sugar intake 7 to 10 days before expected menses may reduce fluid retention. Increasing water intake may serve as a natural diuretic. Including natural diuretics such as asparagus, cranberry juice, peaches, parsley, and watermelon in the diet may help reduce edema and related discomforts. Decreasing red meat intake also may help minimize dysmenorrheal symptoms. Some women with primary dysmenorrhea reported a decrease in symptoms when they switched from a high-fat to a low-fat diet.

Medications used to treat primary dysmenorrhea in women not desiring contraception include prostaglandin synthesis inhibitors, primarily nonsteroidal antiinflammatory drugs (NSAIDs) (American College of Obstetricians and Gynecologists [ACOG], 2004b) (Table 7-1). NSAIDs are effective if begun 2 to 3 days before menses or with the sign of first bleeding; this regimen decreases the possibility of a woman taking these drugs early in pregnancy (Speroff & Fritz, 2005). Often if one NSAID is ineffective, a different one will be effective. All NSAIDs have potential gastrointestinal side effects, including nausea, vomiting, and indigestion. All women taking NSAIDs should be warned to report dark-colored stools, because this may be an indication of gastrointestinal bleeding. Women with a history of aspirin sensitivity or allergy should avoid all NSAIDs. Approximately 80% of dysmenorrheic women obtain relief with prostaglandin inhibitors.

Oral contraceptive pills (OCPs) are a reasonable choice for women who want a contraceptive agent. The benefits of OCP use are attributed to decreased prostaglandin synthesis associated with an atrophic decidualized endometrium (ACOG, 2004b; Speroff & Fritz, 2005). No single OCP has been shown to be superior to another for the relief of primary dysmenorrhea. OCPs are a particularly good choice for therapy because they combine contraception with a positive impact on dysmenorrhea, menstrual flow, and menstrual irregularities. It should be remembered that OCPs have side effects, and that women who do not need or want them may not wish to use them for dysmenorrhea. OCPs also may be contraindicated for some women. (See Chapter 9 for a complete discussion of OCPs.)

Over-the-counter (OTC) preparations that are indicated for primary dysmenorrhea include the same active ingredients (e.g., ibuprofen, naproxen sodium) as prescription preparations; however, the labeled recommended dose may be subtherapeutic. Preparations containing acetaminophen are even less effective because acetaminophen does not have the antiprostaglandin properties of NSAIDs.

If dysmenorrhea is not relieved by one of the NSAIDs, further investigation into the cause of the symptoms is necessary. Conditions associated with dysmenorrhea include müllerian duct anomalies, endometriosis, and pelvic inflammatory disease.

Alternative and complementary therapies are increasingly popular and used in developed countries. Therapies

table 7-1 Medications Used to Treat Dysmenorrhea*

DRUG	BRAND NAME AND STATUS	RECOMMENDED DOSAGE†	COMMON SIDE EFFECTS‡
Diclofenac	Cataflam Rx Votaren-XR-Rx Votaren-Rx	50 mg tid or 100 mg initially, then 50 mg tid to 150 mg/day	Nausea, diarrhea, constipation, abdominal distress, dyspepsia, flatulence
Ibuprofen	Motrin Rx Advil OTC, Nuprin OTC, Motrin IB OTC	400 mg every 4-6h 200 mg every 4-6h to 1200 mg/day	Nausea, dyspepsia, rash, pruritus
Ketoprofen	Orudis Rx Orudis KT OTC Actron OTC	25-50 mg every 6-8h to 300 mg/day 12.5 mg every 6-8h to 75 mg/day	Nausea, diarrhea, constipation, abdominal distress, dyspepsia, flatulence
Meclofenamate	Meclomen Rx	100 mg tid to 300 mg	See ketoprofen
Mefenamic acid	Ponstel Rx	50 mg initially, then 250 mg every 6-8h to 1000 mg/day	See ketoprofen
Naproxen	Naprosyn Rx	500 mg initially, then 250 mg every 6-8h to 1250 mg/day	See ibuprofen
Naproxen sodium	Anaprox Rx	550 mg initially, then 275 mg every 6-8h to 1375 mg/day	See ibuprofen
	Aleve OTC	440 mg initially, then 220 mg every 6-8h to 660 mg/day	

Sources: Clinical Pharmacology. (2004). *Drugs used to treat dysmenorrhea.* Gold Standard Multimedia. Accessed http://cp.gsm.com, August 22, 2006. Facts and Comparisons. (2006). *Drug Facts and Comparison* (60th ed). St. Louis: Facts and Comparisons; Parent-Stevens, L., & Burns, E. (2000). Menstrual disorders. In M. Smith & L. Shimp (Eds.), *20 Common problems in women's health care.* New York: McGraw-Hill.
GI, Gastrointestinal; *h,* hours; *NSAIDs,* nonsteroidal antiinflammatory drugs; *OTC,* over the counter; *Rx,* prescription; *qid,* 4 times a day; *tid,* 3 times a day.
*Nonsteroidal antiinflammatory drugs.
†Dosages are current recommendations and should be verified before use. Recommended dosages for over-the-counter preparations are generally less than recommendations for therapeutic dosages. As-needed dosing is recommended by manufacturer; scheduled dosing may be more effective.
‡Risk with all NSAIDs is gastrointestinal ulceration, possible bleeding, and prolonged bleeding time. Incidence of side effects is dose related. Reported incidence, 3% to 9%.

such as acupuncture, acupressure, biofeedback, desensitization, hypnosis, massage, reiki, relaxation exercises, and therapeutic touch have been used to treat pelvic pain (Dehlin & Schuiling, 2006; Proctor & Farquhar, 2004). Herbal preparations have long been used for management of menstrual problems including dysmenorrhea (Table 7-2). Herbal medicines may be valuable in treating dysmenorrhea; however, it is essential that women understand that these therapies are not without potential toxicity and may cause drug interactions. It is important that women use herbal preparations from well-established companies.

■ **NURSE ALERT**
Nurses must routinely ask women about use of herbal and other alternative therapies and document their use.

Secondary Dysmenorrhea

Secondary dysmenorrhea is acquired menstrual pain that develops later in life than primary dysmenorrhea, typically after age 25 years. This condition is associated with pelvic pathology, such as adenomyosis, endometriosis, pelvic inflammatory disease, endometrial polyps, or submucous or interstitial myomas (fibroids). Women with secondary dysmenorrhea often have other symptoms that may suggest an underlying cause. For example, heavy menstrual flow with dysmenorrhea suggests a diagnosis of leiomyomata, adenomyosis, or endometrial polyps. Pain associated with endometriosis often begins a few days before menses, but can be present at ovulation and continue through the first days of menses or start after menstrual flow has begun. In contrast to primary dysmenorrhea, the pain of secondary

COMMENTS	CONTRAINDICATIONS
Enteric coated: immediate release Take with food and 6-8 oz water Do not lie down for 30 min after taking drug	For all NSAIDs: Do not give if client has hemophilia or bleeding ulcers; do not give if client has had an allergic or anaphylactic reaction to aspirin or another NSAID; do not give if client is taking anticoagulant medication
If GI upset occurs, take with food, milk, or antacids; avoid alcoholic beverages; do not take with aspirin See ibuprofen	
See ibuprofen Very potent and effective prostaglandin-synthesis inhibitor Antagonizes already formed prostaglandins Increased incidence of adverse GI side effects See ibuprofen	
See ibuprofen	

dysmenorrhea is often characterized by dull, lower abdominal aching radiating to the back or thighs. Often women experience feelings of bloating or pelvic fullness. In addition to a physical examination with a careful pelvic examination, diagnosis may be assisted by ultrasound examination, dilation and curettage, endometrial biopsy, or laparoscopy. Treatment is directed toward removal of the underlying pathology. Many of the measures described for pain relief of primary dysmenorrhea also are helpful for women with secondary dysmenorrhea.

Premenstrual Syndrome

Premenstrual syndrome (PMS) is a complex, poorly understood condition that includes a number of cyclic symptoms occurring in the luteal phase of the menstrual cycle. About 85% of women experience mood and/or somatic symptoms that coincide with their menstrual cycles (ACOG, 2000b). Between 5% to 14% of women report symptoms severe enough to be disabling (Angst, Sellaro, Merikangas, & Endicott, 2001). All age-groups are affected, with women in their twenties and thirties most frequently reporting symptoms. Ovarian function is necessary for the condition to occur, since it does not occur before puberty, after menopause, or during pregnancy. The condition is not dependent on the presence of monthly menses: women who have had a hysterectomy without bilateral salpingo-oophorectomy still can have cyclic symptoms.

It is difficult to establish a universal definition of PMS, since so many symptoms have been associated with the condition. However, Speroff and Fritz (2005) suggest that the simplest definition is a commonsense one: "The cyclic appearance of one or more of a large constellation of symptoms just prior to menses, occurring to such a degree that lifestyle or work is affected, followed by a period of time entirely free of symptoms." PMS symptoms include distressing physical, mood, and behavioral experiences.

Premenstrual Dysphoric Disorder (PMDD) is a diagnostic term for a smaller percentage of women who suffer from severe PMS with an emphasis on mood symptoms

table 7-2 Herbal Therapies for Menstrual Disorders

SYMPTOMS OR INDICATIONS	HERBAL THERAPY	ACTION
Menstrual cramping	Black haw Ginger	Uterine antispasmodic Antiinflammatory
Premenstrual discomfort	Black cohosh root Chaste tree fruit	Estrogen-like LH suppressant; binds to estrogen receptors Decreases prolactin levels
Tension, breast pain	Bugleweed	Antigonadotropic; decreases prolactin levels
Dysmenorrhea	Potentilla Dong quai	Uterotonic Antiinflammatory; possibly analgesic activity
Menorrhea, metrorrhagia	Shepherd's purse	Uterotonic

Sources: Bascom, A. (2002). *Incorporating herbal medicine into clinical practice.* Philadelphia: F.A. Davis; Dog, L. (2001). Conventional and alternative treatments for endometriosis. *Alternative Therapies, 7*(6), 50-56; Fugh-Berman, A., & Awang, D. (2001). Black cohosh. *Alternative Therapies in Women's Health, 39*(11), 81-85; Stevinson, C., & Ernst, E. (2001). Complementary/alternative therapies for premenstrual syndrome: A systemic review of random controlled trials. *American Journal of Obstetrics and Gynecology, 185*(1), 227-235.
LH, Luteinizing hormone.

(American Psychiatric Association [APA], 2000). Commonly, symptoms occur in the final 7 to 10 days of the menstrual cycle. Symptoms commonly reported include abdominal bloating, anxiety, tension, breast tenderness, crying episodes, depression, fatigue and lack of energy, irritability, difficulty concentrating, appetite changes, thirst, and swelling of the extremities (Speroff & Fritz, 2005). The most common symptoms are those associated with mood disturbances.

A diagnosis of PMS is made when the following criteria are met (ACOG, 2000b; Association of Women's Health, Obstetrical and Neonatal Nurses [AWHONN], 2003; Taylor, Schuiling, & Sharp, 2006):

- Symptoms consistent with PMS occur in the luteal phase and resolve within a few days of menses onset.
- Symptom-free period occurs in the follicular phase.
- Symptoms are recurrent.
- Symptoms have a negative impact on some aspect of a woman's life
- Other diagnoses that better explain the symptoms have been excluded.

For a diagnosis of PMDD, the following criteria must be met (APA, 2000):

- Five or more affective and physical symptoms are present in the week before menses and are absent in the follicular phase of the menstrual cycle.
- At least one of the symptoms is irritability, depressed mood, anxiety, or emotional lability.
- Symptoms interfere markedly with work or interpersonal relationships.
- Symptoms are not due to an exacerbation of another condition or disorder.

These criteria must be confirmed by prospective daily ratings for at least two menstrual cycles (APA, 2000).

The etiology of PMS and PMDD is not clear, but there is general agreement that they are distinct psychiatric and medical syndromes rather than an exacerbation of an underlying psychiatric disorder. They do not occur if there is no ovarian function. A number of biologic and neuroendocrine etiologies have been suggested; however, none have been conclusively substantiated as the causative factor. It is likely that biologic, psychosocial, and sociocultural factors contribute to PMS and PMDD (Speroff & Fritz, 2005; Taylor, Schuiling, & Sharp, 2006). Readers are encouraged to explore current feminist, medical, and social science literature for more information on PMS.

Management. There is little agreement on management. A careful, detailed history and daily log of symptoms and mood fluctuations spanning several cycles may give direction to a plan of management. Any changes that assist a woman with PMS to exert control over her life have a positive impact. Education is an important component of the management of PMS. Nurses can advise women that self-help modalities often result in significant symptom improvement. Women have found a number of complementary and alternative therapies to be useful in managing the symptoms of PMS. Diet and exercise changes are a useful way to begin and provide symptom relief for some women. Nurses can suggest that women not smoke and limit their consumption of refined sugar (less than 5 tbsp/day), salt (less than 3 g/day), red meat (up to 3 oz/day), alcohol (less than 1 oz/day), and caffeinated beverages. Women can be encouraged to include whole grains, legumes, seeds, nuts, vegetables, fruits, and vegetable oils in their diet. Three small-to-moderate-sized meals and three small snacks a day that are rich in complex carbohydrates and fiber have been reported to improve symptoms (Jones, 2001). Use of natural diuretics (see section on dysmenorrhea management on p. 149) may help reduce fluid retention as well. Nutritional supplements may assist in symptom relief. Calcium (1200 mg daily), magnesium (300 to 400 mg daily), and vitamin B_6 (100 to 150 mg daily) have been shown to be moderately effective in relieving symptoms, to have few side effects, and to be safe. Although research findings regarding the benefits of evening primrose oil have been mixed, consumption of evening primrose oil was found to decrease premenstrual mood symptoms, breast pain, and fluid retention (Budeiri, Li Wan Po, & Dornan, 1996). The safety of this herb is well-established; however, approximately 2% of those taking evening primrose oil may have stomach distress, nausea, or headaches. Other herbal therapies have long been used to treat PMS; specific suggestions are found in Table 7-2.

Regular exercise (aerobic exercise 3 to 4 times a week), especially in the luteal phase, is widely recommended for relief of PMS symptoms. A monthly program that varies in intensity and type of exercise according to PMS symptoms is best. Women who exercise regularly seem to have less premenstrual anxiety than do nonathletic women. It is thought that aerobic exercise increases β-endorphin levels to offset symptoms of depression and elevate mood.

Yoga, acupuncture, hypnosis, chiropractic therapy, and massage therapy have all been reported to have a beneficial effect on PMS.

Nurses can explain the relation between cyclic estrogen fluctuation and changes in serotonin levels, that serotonin is one of the brain chemicals that assist in coping with normal life stresses, and the ways in which the different management strategies recommended help maintain serotonin levels. Counseling, in the form of support groups or individual or couples counseling, may be helpful. Stress reduction techniques also may assist with symptom management (Collins Sharp et al., 2002; Rapkin, 2003).

If these strategies do not provide significant symptom relief in 1 to 2 months, medication is often begun. Many medications have been used in treatment of PMS, but no single medication alleviates all PMS symptoms. Medications often used in the treatment of PMS include diuretics, prostaglandin inhibitors (NSAIDs), progesterone, and OCPs. Serotonergic-activating agents including the selective serotonin reuptake inhibitors (SSRIs) fluoxetine (Prozac or Sarafem), sertraline (Zoloft), paroxetine (Paxil), and citalopram (Celexa) have been shown to decrease severe

CD: Plan of Care: Premenstrual Syndrome

plan of care **Premenstrual Syndrome**

NURSING DIAGNOSIS Acute pain related to cyclic breast changes as evidenced by woman's report

Expected Outcome *Woman will report a decrease in the intensity of pain or discomfort after interventions.*

Nursing Interventions/Rationales
- Assess timing and intensity of pain or discomfort *to validate relation to cyclic changes.*
- Counsel woman to take medications if prescribed *to minimize breast tenderness.*
- Suggest that woman wear a supportive bra *to minimize breast tenderness.*

NURSING DIAGNOSIS Situational low self-esteem related to cyclic hormonal changes as evidenced by woman's verbal report

Expected Outcome *Woman will report increased number of feelings of self-worth.*

Nursing Interventions/Rationales
- Provide therapeutic communication *to validate feelings of depression and mood swings.*
- Encourage woman to limit caffeine and eat small, frequent meals *to lessen irritability aggravated by caffeine and hypoglycemia.*
- Refer woman to support groups *to encourage the sharing of experiences, feelings, and self-help tips.*

NURSING DIAGNOSIS Excess fluid volume related to cyclic hormonal influences as evidenced by weight gain before start of menstrual period

Expected Outcome *Woman will report no significant changes in body weight before start of menstrual period.*

Nursing Interventions/Rationales
- Encourage woman to limit intake of salt- and sodium-containing foods *to decrease fluid retention.*
- Counsel woman to take diuretics as prescribed *to facilitate fluid excretion.*
- Encourage consumption of natural diuretic foods *to encourage fluid excretion.*

NURSING DIAGNOSIS Anxiety related to anticipation of cyclical pain

Expected Outcome *Woman will report a decrease in anxiety level.*

Nursing Interventions/Rationales
- Teach woman to recognize anxiety *to prompt early preventive interventions.*
- Identify relaxation techniques *to decrease anxiety to promote self-care.*
- Encourage woman to attend support groups *to encourage expression of feelings and self-help interventions.*

premenstrual symptoms including depression (Jones, 2001; Lin & Thompson, 2001). Common side effects are headaches, sleep disturbances, dizziness, weight gain, dry mouth, and decreased libido (see Plan of Care).

Endometriosis

Endometriosis is characterized by the presence and growth of endometrial glands and stroma outside of the uterus. The tissue may be implanted on the ovaries, the anterior and posterior cul-de-sac, the broad, uterosacral, and round ligaments, the uterine tubes, the rectovaginal septum, the sigmoid colon, the appendix, the pelvic peritoneum, the cervix, and the inguinal area (Fig. 7-1). Endometrial lesions have been found in the vagina and surgical scars, as well as on the vulva, the perineum, and the bladder, and sites far from the pelvic area such as the thoracic cavity, the gallbladder, and the heart. A cystic lesion of endometriosis found in the ovary is sometimes described as a chocolate cyst because of the dark coloring of the contents of the cyst caused by the presence of old blood.

Endometrial tissue contains glands and stoma and responds to cyclic hormonal stimulation in the same way that the uterine endometrium does. During the proliferative and secretory phases of the cycle, the endometrial tissue grows. During or immediately after menstruation, the tissue bleeds, resulting in an inflammatory response with subsequent fibrosis and adhesion to adjacent organs.

An accurate incidence of endometriosis is unknown; however, current estimates are 5% to 20% for women with

FIG. 7-1 Common sites of endometriosis. (From Stenchever, M. et al. [2001]. *Comprehensive gynecology* [4th ed.]. St. Louis: Mosby.)

pelvic pain, 20% to 40% in women with infertility, and 3% to 10% among the general population of reproductive-age women (Speroff & Fritz, 2005). Endometriosis is diagnosed in 50% to 70% of adolescents having a laparoscopy for pelvic pain unrelieved by medical treatment

(Laufer, Sanfilippo, & Rose, 2003). Further, endometriosis has been found in adolescents with abnormal vaginal bleeding (Motta, 2004). In addition, endometriosis has been reported to occur in about 5% of postmenopausal women receiving menopausal hormone therapy (Nakad & Isaacson, 2002). At one time, endometriosis was believed to be more prevalent in Caucasian middle-class women; however, the condition appears equally in Caucasian, African-American, and Asian women (Nakad & Isaacson). Furthermore, endometriosis occurs across all socioeconomic levels. There appears to be a familial tendency to develop endometriosis; the condition is six to seven times more prevalent in women who have a first-degree relative with endometriosis as compared to the general population (Speroff & Fritz). Endometriosis may worsen with repeated cycles, or it may remain asymptomatic and undiagnosed, eventually disappearing after menopause. Endometriosis can occur in women who have been pregnant and may be a cause of secondary infertility (Speroff & Fritz).

Several theories to account for the cause of endometriosis have been suggested, yet the etiology and pathology of this condition continue to be poorly understood. One of the most widely accepted, long-debated theories is transplantation or retrograde menstruation. According to this theory, endometrial tissue is refluxed through the uterine tubes during menstruation into the peritoneal cavity, where it implants on the ovaries and other organs. Retrograde menstruation has been documented in a number of surgical studies and is estimated to occur in 90% of menstruating women. For most women, endometrial tissue outside the uterus is destroyed before it can implant or seed in the peritoneal cavity or elsewhere. Perhaps endometriosis develops in only 10% to 15% of women because of differences in the functioning of an individual's immune system. It also may reflect differences in genetic makeup or environmental challenges (Speroff & Fritz, 2005).

Symptoms vary among women, from nonexistent to incapacitating. Severity of symptoms can change over time and may be disconnected from the extent of the disease. The major symptoms of endometriosis are pelvic pain, dysmenorrhea, dyspareunia (painful intercourse), abnormal menstrual bleeding, and infertility. Women also may experience chronic noncyclic pelvic pain, pelvic heaviness, or pain radiating into the thighs. Many women report bowel symptoms such as diarrhea, pain with defecation, and constipation caused by avoiding defecation because of the pain. Less common symptoms include abnormal bleeding (hypermenorrhea, menorrhagia, or premenstrual staining) and pain during exercise as a result of adhesions (Lemaire, 2004). Women who have endometriosis may also have other conditions such as chronic fatigue syndrome, fibromyalgia, endocrine disorders, and autoimmune disorders (Conversations with Colleagues, 2002-2003).

Impaired fertility may result from adhesions around the uterus that pull the uterus into a fixed, retroverted position. Adhesions around the uterine tubes may block the fimbriated ends or prevent the spontaneous movement that carries the ovum to the uterus.

Management. Treatment is based on the severity of symptoms and the goals of the woman or couple. Women without pain who do not want to become pregnant need no treatment. In women with mild pain who may desire a future pregnancy, treatment may be limited to use of NSAIDs during menstruation (see earlier discussion of these medications).

Suppression of endogenous estrogen production and subsequent endometrial lesion growth is the cornerstone of management of the disease in adult women. Two main classes of drugs are used to suppress endogenous estrogen levels: GnRH agonists and androgen derivatives. GnRH-agonist therapy (leuprolide [Lupron], nafarelin [Synarel]) acts by suppressing pituitary gonadotropin secretion. FSH and LH stimulation of the ovary declines markedly, and ovarian function decreases significantly. A medically induced temporary menopause develops, resulting in anovulation and amenorrhea. Shrinkage of already established endometrial tissue, significant pain relief, and an interruption in further lesion development follow. The hypoestrogenism results in hot flashes in almost all women. Trabecular bone loss is common, although most loss is reversible within 12 to 18 months after the medication is stopped. Leuprolide (3.75 mg intramuscular injection given once a month) or nafarelin (200 mg administered twice daily by nasal spray) are both effective and well tolerated. Both medications reduce endometrial lesions and pelvic pain associated with endometriosis and have posttreatment pregnancy rates similar to those of danazol therapy (Speroff & Fritz, 2005). Common side effects of these drugs are those of natural menopause—hot flashes and vaginal dryness. Occasionally women report headaches and muscle aches. Treatment is usually limited to 6 months to minimize bone loss. Although unlikely, it is possible for a woman to become pregnant while taking a GnRH agonist. Because the potential teratogenicity of this drug is unclear, women should use a barrier contraceptive during treatment.

Danazol (Danocrine), a mildly androgenic synthetic steroid, suppresses FSH and LH secretion, thus producing anovulation and hypogonadotropinism, with consequently decreased secretion of estrogen and progesterone and regression of endometrial tissue. This medication was widely used to treat endometriosis in the 1970s and 1980s. Danazol side effects can cause a woman to discontinue the drug. Side effects include masculinizing traits in the woman (weight gain, edema, decreased breast size, oily skin, hirsutism, and deepening of the voice), all of which often disappear when treatment is discontinued. Other side effects are amenorrhea, hot flashes, vaginal dryness, insomnia, and decreased libido. Migraine headaches, dizziness, fatigue, and depression also are reported. Danazol treatment has been reported to affect lipids adversely, with a decrease in high-density lipoprotein (HDL) levels and an increase in low-density lipoprotein (LDL) levels. Danazol should never be prescribed when pregnancy is suspected, and contraception (e.g., barrier) should be used with it because ovulation may not be suppressed. Danazol can produce pseudohermaphroditism in female fetuses. The medication is contraindicated in women with liver disease and should be used with caution in women with cardiac and renal disease. The recommended dosage is 200 to 400 mg/day for 3 to 6 months.

Women who have early symptomatic disease and can postpone pregnancy may be treated with continuous oral contraceptives that have a low estrogen-to-progestin ratio to shrink endometrial tissue. Any low-dose OCPs can be used if taken for 15 weeks followed by 1 week of withdrawal. This therapy is associated with minimal side effects and can be taken for extended periods (Nakad & Isaacson, 2002).

Continuous combined hormonal therapy (oral contraceptive pills, estrogen/progestin patch, estrogen/progestin vaginal ring) for menstrual suppression and administration of NSAIDs are the usual treatment of adolescents under the age of 16 who have endometriosis. Gonadotropin-releasing hormone (GnRH) agonists are not usually used since the resultant hypoestrogenic state can affect bone mineralization (ACOG Committee on Adolescent Health Care, 2005).

Surgical intervention is often needed for severe, acute, or incapacitating symptoms. Decisions regarding the extent and type of surgery are influenced by a woman's age, desire for children, and location of the disease. For women who do not want to preserve their ability to have children, the only definitive cure is total abdominal hysterectomy with bilateral salpingo-oophorectomy (TAH with BSO). In women who are in their childbearing years and want children and in whom the disease does not prevent it, reproductive capacity should be retained through careful removal by surgery or laser therapy of all endometrial tissue possible and with retention of ovarian function (Nakad & Isaacson, 2002).

Regardless of the type of treatment, short of TAH with BSO, endometriosis reoccurs in approximately 40% of women; thus for many women, endometriosis is a chronic disease with conditions such as chronic pain or infertility. Counseling and education are critical components of nursing care for women with endometriosis. Women need an honest discussion of treatment options, with potential risks and benefits of each option reviewed. Because pelvic pain is a subjective, personal experience that can be frightening, support is important. Sexual dysfunction resulting from painful intercourse (dyspareunia) is common and may necessitate referral for counseling. Support groups for women with endometriosis may be found in some locations; Resolve (www.resolve.org), an organization for infertile couples, or the Endometriosis Association (www.ivf.com/endohtml.html) also may be helpful. The nursing care discussed in the earlier section on dysmenorrhea is appropriate for managing chronic pelvic pain and dysmenorrhea in the woman with endometriosis (see Plan of Care).

Alterations in Cyclic Bleeding

Women often have changes in amount, duration, interval, or regularity of menstrual cycle bleeding. Often women worry about menstruation that is short, that is small in amount, or that occurs too frequently.

Oligomenorrhea/Hypomenorrhea

The term oligomenorrhea often is used to describe decreased menstruation, either in amount, time, or both. However, oligomenorrhea more correctly refers to infrequent menstrual periods characterized by intervals of 40 to 45 days or longer, and hypomenorrhea to scanty bleeding at normal intervals. The causes of oligomenorrhea are often abnormalities of hypothalamic, pituitary, or ovarian function. Oligomenorrhea also can be physiologic, or part of a woman's normal pattern for the first few years after menarche or for several years before menopause.

Treatment is aimed at reversing the underlying cause, if possible. Hormonal therapy using progestins, with or without estrogens, also may be used to prevent complications of unopposed estrogen production (endometrial hyperplasia or carcinoma) or of absent estrogen (vaginal dryness, hot flashes or flushes, or osteoporosis).

Women with menstruation characterized by prolonged intervals between cycles need education and counseling. The cause of the condition and the rationale for a specific treatment should be discussed, as should advantages and disadvantages of hormonal therapy. If a woman chooses medical intervention, she should be provided with written instructions, taught how to take the medications, and made aware of side effects of any medications. Teaching and counseling should emphasize the importance of the woman keeping careful records of her vaginal bleeding.

One of the most common causes of scanty menstrual flow is OCPs. If a woman is considering OCPs for contraception, it is important that the nurse explain in advance that the use of OCPs can decrease menstrual flow by as much as two thirds. This effect is caused by the continuous action of the progestin component, which produces a decidualized endometrium with atrophic glands.

Hypomenorrhea also may be caused by structural abnormalities of the endometrium or the uterus that result in partial destruction of the endometrium. These conditions include Asherman syndrome, in which adhesions resulting from curettage or infection obliterate the endometrial cavity, and congenital partial obstruction of the vagina.

Metrorrhagia

Metrorrhagia, or intermenstrual bleeding, refers to any episode of bleeding, whether spotting, menses, or hemorrhage, that occurs at a time other than the normal menses. *Mittlestaining,* a small amount of bleeding or spotting that occurs at the time of ovulation (14 days before onset of the next menses), is considered normal. The cause of mittlestaining is not known; however, its common occurrence can be documented by its repetition in the menstrual cycle.

CD: Plan of Care: Endometriosis

plan of care ▶ Endometriosis

NURSING DIAGNOSIS Acute pain related to menstruation secondary to endometriosis

Expected Outcome *Woman will verbalize a decrease in intensity and frequency of pain during each menstrual cycle.*

Nursing Interventions/*Rationales*
- Assess location, type, and duration of pain and history of discomfort *to determine severity of dysmenorrhea.*
- Administer analgesics *to assist with pain relief.*
- Administer hormone-altering medications if ordered *to suppress ovulation.*
- Provide nonpharmacologic methods such as heat *to increase blood flow to the pelvic region.*

NURSING DIAGNOSIS Deficient knowledge related to unfamiliarity with treatment, as evidenced by woman's statements

Expected Outcome *Woman will verbalize correct understanding of the use of self-care methods and prescribed therapies.*

Nursing Interventions/*Rationales*
- Assess woman's current understanding of the disorder and related therapies *to validate the accuracy of knowledge base.*
- Give information to woman regarding the disorder and treatment regimen *to empower the client to become a partner in her own care.*

NURSING DIAGNOSIS Situational low self-esteem related to infertility as evidenced by woman's statements of decreased self-worth

Expected Outcome *Woman will verbalize positive feelings of self-worth.*

Nursing Interventions/*Rationales*
- Provide therapeutic communication *to validate feelings and provide support.*
- Refer to support group *to enhance feelings of self-worth through group communication.*

NURSING DIAGNOSIS Anxiety related to possible invasive surgical procedure as evidenced by woman's verbal report

Expected Outcome *Woman will report a decreased number of anxious feelings.*

Nursing Interventions/*Rationales*
- Provide opportunity to discuss feelings *to identify source of anxiety.*
- Reinforce information provided *to keep expectations realistic and dispel myths or inaccuracies.*
- Provide emotional support *to encourage verbalization of feelings.*

NURSING DIAGNOSIS Risk for injury related to disease progression

Expected Outcome *Woman will report any changes in health status to health care provider.*

Nursing Interventions/*Rationales*
- Teach woman to report any changes in health status *to initiate prompt treatment.*
- Review side effects of medications *to recognize possible causes for changes in health status.*
- Encourage ongoing communication with health care provider *to promote trust and comfort.*

Women taking OCPs may have midcycle bleeding or spotting. (See Chapter 9 for a discussion of the side effects of OCPs.) If the OCP does not maintain a sufficiently hypoplastic endometrium, the endometrium will begin to shed, usually in small amounts at a time, a process termed *breakthrough bleeding.* Breakthrough bleeding is most common in the first three cycles of OCPs. The reduced potency of OCPs (resulting in increased safety) has decreased the amount of available hormones, making it more important that blood levels be kept constant. Taking the pill at exactly the same time each day may alleviate the woman's problem. If the spotting continues, a different formulation of the OCP that increases either the estrogen or progestin component of the pill can be tried.

Progestin-only contraceptive methods (oral and injectable) also may cause midcycle bleeding, especially in the first several cycles. Women should be advised of this and counseled to report continuation of breakthrough bleeding after the first three to six cycles to their health care provider.

Women with an intrauterine device (IUD) may have spotting between their periods and possibly heavier menstrual flow.

The causes of intermenstrual bleeding are varied (Table 7-3). It is important that the nurse always consider the possibility that any woman who has not undergone menopause and who seeks care for intermenstrual bleeding is or recently has been pregnant.

table 7-3 Causes of Intermenstrual Bleeding

REPRODUCTIVE DISORDER	PREGNANCY PROBLEMS	INFECTIONS
Functional ovarian cyst	Pregnancy: implantation	Endometritis
Cervical erosion infection	Miscarriage	Sexually transmitted infections
Leiomyoma	Ectopic pregnancy	
Polyps, uterine or endocervical	Molar pregnancy	
Trauma	Retained placenta, miscarriage or induced abortion	
Foreign body	Retained placenta, birth	
Malignancy of reproductive tract		

Treatment of intermenstrual bleeding depends on the cause and may include reassurance and education concerning mittlestaining, observation of three menstrual cycles for suspected functional ovarian cyst, adjustment of an OCP, removal of foreign bodies, and treatment for vaginal infections. More complex treatment may consist of removal of polyps; evaluation and treatment of an abnormal Papanicolaou (Pap) smear, including colposcopy, biopsy, cautery, cryosurgery, or conization; and surgery, chemotherapy, or radiation treatment for malignancy. Important nursing roles include reassurance, counseling, education, and support.

Menorrhagia

Menorrhagia (hypermenorrhea) is defined as excessive menstrual bleeding, in either duration or amount. The causes of heavy menstrual bleeding are many, including hormonal disturbances, systemic disease, benign and malignant neoplasms, infection, and contraception (IUDs). A single episode of heavy bleeding may occur, or a woman may have regular flooding as a pattern in which she changes tampons or pads every few hours for several days.

■ NURSE ALERT

If the woman herself considers the amount or duration of bleeding to be excessive, the problem should be investigated.

Hemoglobin and hematocrit provide objective indicators to actual blood loss and should always be assessed.

A single episode of heavy bleeding may signal an early pregnancy loss. This type of bleeding is often thought to be a period that is heavier than usual, perhaps delayed, and is associated with abdominal pain or pelvic discomfort. When early pregnancy loss is suspected, a hematocrit and serum β-hCG pregnancy test should be done.

Infectious and inflammatory processes such as acute or chronic endometritis and salpingitis may cause heavy menstrual bleeding. Although rare, systemic diseases of nonreproductive origin such as blood dyscrasias, hypothyroidism, and lupus erythematosus also can cause hypermenorrhea. In obese women, anovulation caused by increased peripheral conversion of androstenedione to estrogen may develop and manifest as menorrhagia. Medications also may cause abnormal bleeding. Chemotherapy, anticoagulants, neuroleptics, and steroid hormone therapy all have been associated with excessive flow.

Uterine *leiomyoma* (fibroids or myomas) are a common cause of menorrhagia. Fibroids are benign tumors of the smooth muscle of the uterus, the etiology of which is unknown. Fibroids are estrogen sensitive and commonly develop during the reproductive years and shrink after menopause. Other uterine growths ranging from endometrial polyps to adenocarcinoma and endometrial cancer are other common causes of heavy menstrual bleeding, as well as of intermenstrual bleeding.

Treatment for menorrhagia depends on the cause of the bleeding. If the bleeding is related to contraceptive method, the nurse provides factual information and reassurance and discusses other contraceptive options. If bleeding is related to presence of fibroids, the degree of disability and discomfort associated with the fibroids and the woman's plans for childbearing will influence treatment decisions. Treatment options include medical and surgical management. Most fibroids can be monitored by frequent examinations to judge growth, if any, and correction of anemia, if present. Women with menorrhagia should be warned not to use aspirin because of its tendency to increase bleeding. Medical treatment is directed toward temporarily reducing symptoms, shrinking the myoma, and reducing its blood supply (Stenchever et al., 2001). This reduction is often accomplished with the use of a GnRH agonist. If the woman wishes to retain childbearing potential, a myomectomy may be done. Myomectomy, or removal of the tumors only, is particularly difficult if multiple myomas must be removed. If the woman does not want to preserve her childbearing function, or if she has severe symptoms (severe anemia, severe pain, considerable disruption of lifestyle), hysterectomy or endometrial ablation (laser surgery or electrocoagulation) may be done (see Chapter 12). Uterine artery embolization, based on the assumption that control of arterial blood flow to the fibroid will control symptoms, has been reported to result in reduced menorrhagia, less dysmenorrhea, and reduced pelvic pressure and urinary symptoms. This method of treatment is used for women who have completed their childbearing since there is a risk for loss of fertility (see Chapter 12).

Dysfunctional Uterine Bleeding

Abnormal uterine bleeding (AUB) is any form of uterine bleeding that is irregular in amount, duration, or timing and not related to regular menstrual bleeding. Box 7-1 lists possible causes of AUB. Although often used interchangeably, the terms AUB and dysfunctional uterine bleeding (DUB) are not synonymous. Dysfunctional uterine bleeding is a subset of AUB defined as "excessive uterine bleeding with no demonstrable organic cause, genital or extragenital" (Stenchever et al., 2001). DUB is most frequently caused by anovulation. When there is no LH surge, or if there is not sufficient progesterone produced by the corpus luteum to support the endometrium, it will begin to involute and shed. This most often occurs at the extremes of a woman's reproductive years—when the menstrual cycle is just becoming established at menarche or when it draws to a close at menopause. DUB also can be found with any condition that gives rise to chronic anovulation associated with continuous estrogen production. Such conditions include obesity, hyperthyroidism and hypothyroidism, polycystic ovarian syndrome, and any of the endocrine conditions discussed in the sections on amenorrhea and oligomenorrhea.

Women also may unknowingly use medications with an impact on the endometrium; for example, ginseng, an herbal root, has been associated with estrogen activity and abnormal bleeding. A diagnosis of DUB is made only after all other causes of abnormal menstrual bleeding have been

box 7-1	**Possible Causes of Abnormal Uterine Bleeding**

ANOVULATION
- Hypothalamic dysfunction
- Polycystic ovary syndrome

PREGNANCY-RELATED CONDITIONS
- Threatened or spontaneous miscarriage
- Retained products of conception after elective abortion
- Ectopic pregnancy

LOWER REPRODUCTIVE TRACT INFECTIONS
- Chlamydial cervicitis
- Pelvic inflammatory disease

NEOPLASMS
- Endometrial hyperplasia
- Cancer of cervix and endometrium
- Endometrial polyps
- Hormonally active tumors (rare)
- Leiomyomata (fibroids)
- Vaginal tumors (rare)

TRAUMA
- Genital injury (accidental, coital trauma, sexual abuse)
- Foreign body
- Primary coagulation disorders

SYSTEMIC DISEASES
- Diabetes mellitus
- Thyroid dysfunction (hypothyroidism, hyperthyroidism)
- Severe organ disease (renal or liver failure)

IATROGENIC CAUSES
- Exogenous hormone use (oral contraceptives, menopausal hormone therapy)
- Medications with estrogenic activity
- Herbal preparation (ginseng)

Sources: American College of Nurse-Midwives (ACNM). (2002). Abnormal and dysfunctional uterine bleeding. ACNM Clinical Bulletin No. 6. *Journal of Midwifery and Women's Health, 47*(3), 207-213; Stenchever, M., Droegemueller, W., Herbst, A., & Mishell, D. (2001). *Comprehensive gynecology* (4th ed.). St. Louis: Mosby.

ruled out (American College of Nurse-Midwives [ACNM], 2002).

When uterine bleeding is profuse and a woman's hemoglobin level is less than 8 g/dl (hematocrit of 23% or 24%), the woman may be hospitalized and given conjugated estrogens (e.g., Premarin), 25 mg intravenously. The dose may be repeated until bleeding stops or slows significantly (usually within 1 to 5 hours) (Dodd & Sinert, 2006). If the bleeding has not stopped in 12 to 24 hours, dilation and curettage (D&C) may be done to control severe bleeding and hemorrhage. An endometrial biopsy may be collected at the same time to evaluate endometrial tissue or rule out endometrial cancer. After this treatment, oral conjugated estrogen, 2.5 mg, is given daily followed by the addition of progesterone (e.g., medroxyprogesterone [Provera], 10 mg by mouth), given in the final 10 days of therapy to initiate withdrawal bleeding. Alternatively, a combined OCP is given for 21 days after intravenous therapy. Once the acute phase has passed, the woman is maintained on cyclic, low-dose OCPs for 3 to 6 months. Such long-term treatment will help prevent recurrence of the pattern of dysfunctional uterine bleeding and hemorrhage. If she wants contraception, she should continue to take OCPs. If the woman has no need for contraception, the treatment may be stopped to assess her bleeding pattern. If menstruation does not resume, a progestin regimen (e.g., medroxyprogesterone, 10 mg/day for 10 days before the expected date of her menstrual period) may be prescribed after ruling out pregnancy. This is done to prevent persistent anovulation with chronic unopposed endogenous estrogen hyperstimulation of the endometrium, which can result in eventual atypical tissue changes.

If the recurrent, heavy bleeding is not controlled by hormonal therapy or D&C, ablation of the endometrium through laser treatment may be performed. Nursing roles include informing clients of their options, counseling and education as indicated, and referring to the appropriate specialists and health care services.

▬ CARE MANAGEMENT

▬ Assessment and Nursing Diagnoses

In addition to taking a careful menstrual, obstetric, sexual, and contraceptive history, the nurse should explore the woman's perceptions of her condition, cultural or ethnic influences, experiences with other caregivers, lifestyle, and patterns of coping. The amount of pain or bleeding and its effect on daily activities should be evaluated. Home remedies and prescriptions to relieve discomfort are noted. A symptom diary, in which the woman records emotions, behaviors, physical symptoms, diet, and exercise and rest patterns, is a useful diagnostic tool.

Nursing diagnoses for women with menstrual disorders may include the following:

- *Ineffective coping related to*
  - insufficient knowledge of the cause of the disorder
  - emotional and physiologic effects of the disorder
- *Deficient knowledge related to*
  - self-care
  - available therapy for the disorder
- *Disturbed body image related to*
  - menstrual disorder
  - sexual dysfunction
- *Risk for situational low self-esteem related to*
  - others' perception of her discomfort
  - inability to conceive
- *Acute pain related to*
  - menstrual disorder

■ Expected Outcomes of Care

After data collection and review, mutual expected outcomes are established, and a plan of care is developed. The expected outcomes for the woman are that she will do the following:

- Verbalize understanding of reproductive anatomy, etiology of her disorder, medication regimen, and diary use.
- Verbalize her understanding and acceptance of her emotional and physical responses to her menstrual cycle.
- Develop personal goals that benefit her emotionally and physically.
- Choose appropriate therapeutic measures for her menstrual problems.
- Adapt successfully to the condition if cure is not possible.

■ Plan of Care and Interventions

During the history and diagnostic workup, the clinician's concern and acceptance of the woman's symptoms as valid are in themselves therapeutic. Data from the daily diary of emotional status, subjective feelings, and physical state are correlated with physiologic changes. If the woman has a partner, she and her partner should keep separate diaries that include how each perceives the other's responses day by day. Through the diaries, feelings are vented, problems are identified and clarified, insights occur, and possible solutions begin to develop. The clinician facilitates insights and suggests therapeutic options. The woman (couple) makes choices considered best for her (them).

Nurses should discuss the options available to women with menstrual disorders. Women must understand basic information about the anatomy and physiology, pathophysiology, psychologic impact, and treatment for the condition, including alternative therapies.

Support groups are an important resource. Nurses can use a local women's center or clinic to bring together women who want to learn more about their condition and support each other.

■ Evaluation

The nurse can be assured that care has been effective when the woman reports improvement in the quality of her life, skill in self-care, and a positive self-concept and body image.

■ MENOPAUSE

With the increasing life span of American women, most women can expect to live one third of their lives after their reproductive years. As women age, many experience transitions that present challenges and require adaptation such as changing health, work, or marital status. Nowhere is this more true than with the changes associated with menopause. In the United States, most women have menopause during their late forties and early fifties, with the median age being 51 to 52 years (Speroff & Fritz,

2005). The average age for the onset of the perimenopausal transition is 46 years; 95% of women experience the onset between ages 39 and 51. The average duration of the perimenopause is 5 years, with a range of 2 to 8 years for 95% of women (Speroff & Fritz). Cigarette smoking and a history of short intermenstrual intervals seem to decrease the age at onset of menopause. However, the popular belief that an early menarche predisposes to a late menopause is not substantiated. Unlike menarche, the average age of menopause has remained about the same since the Middle Ages.

Perimenopause is the period that encompasses the transition from normal ovulatory cycles to cessation of menses and is marked by irregular menstrual cycles. Another term used to signal the period when a woman moves from the reproductive stage of life through the perimenopausal transition and menopause to the postmenopausal years is the climacteric. Menopause refers to the complete cessation of menses and is a single physiologic event said to occur when women have not had menstrual flow or spotting for 1 year, and it can be identified only in retrospect. Surgical menopause occurs with hysterectomy and bilateral oophorectomy. Postmenopause is the time after menopause.

Although all women have similar hormonal changes with menopause, the experience of each woman is influenced by her age, cultural background, health, type of menopause (spontaneous or surgical), childbearing desires, and relationships. Women may view menopause as a major change in their lives—either positive, such as freedom from troublesome dysmenorrhea or the need for contraception, or negative, such as feeling "old" or losing childbearing possibilities.

Physiologic Characteristics

Knowledge of the normal changes that occur during the perimenopause is essential to the assessment of menopausal experiences and problems. Natural menopause is a gradual process with progressive increases in anovulatory cycles and eventual cessation of menses. In the 2 to 8 years preceding menopause, subtle hormonal changes eventually lead to altered menstrual function and later to amenorrhea. When women are in their forties, anovulation occurs more often, menstrual cycles increase in length, and ovarian follicles become less sensitive to hormonal stimulation from FSH and LH. Because of these changes, a follicle is stimulated to the point that an ovum grows to maturity and is released in some months, and in other months, no ovulation takes place. Without ovulation and release of an ovum, progesterone is not produced by the corpus luteum. The lining continues to grow until it lacks a sufficient blood supply, at which point it will bleed. During this time, a woman's cycle will become more irregular. She may skip or miss periods; have shorter or lighter periods or longer, heavier periods; and have clotting. FSH levels become elevated, reflecting an attempt to stimulate a follicle to produce estrogen.

Physical Changes During the Perimenopausal Period
Bleeding

During the perimenopausal years, women may have longer menstrual periods that differ in the type of bleeding. They may have 2 to 3 days of spotting followed by 1 to 2 days of heavy bleeding, or they may have regular menses followed by 2 to 3 days of spotting. Such symptoms are characteristic of degenerating corpus luteum function. After menopause, women continue to have small amounts of circulating estrogen. Although the ovaries do not produce estrogen, androgens (androstenedione and testosterone) are produced for some time after menopause. Androgens produced by the adrenal glands are converted to estrone, a form of estrogen, in the liver and fat cells. With advanced age, the ovaries stop producing androstenedione, which further limits the amount of estrone in the body. Obese women are more likely to have dysfunctional uterine bleeding and endometrial hyperplasia because women with more body fat have higher estrone levels.

Genital Changes

The vagina and urethra are estrogen-sensitive tissues, and low levels of estrogen can cause atrophy of both. Age-related vaginal changes not affected by estrogen also occur. Through both processes, the vaginal membranes thin, hold less moisture, and lubricate more slowly. However, not all women have symptoms of genital atrophy. Women who are sexually active have less vaginal atrophy and fewer problems related to intercourse. Thin women are more likely to have more symptoms related to reduced estrogen levels such as vaginal dryness because of lack of adipose tissue and thus stored estrogen. Additionally, vaginal pH increases, lactobacilli growth can be depressed, and other bacteria tend to multiply. This combination of factors can lead to vaginitis.

Dyspareunia (painful intercourse) can occur because the vagina becomes smaller, the vaginal walls become thinner and dryer, and lubrication during sexual stimulation takes longer. Intercourse becomes painful and may result in postcoital bleeding. Some women may decide to forego intercourse altogether.

In some women, the shrinking of the uterus, the vulva, and the distal portion of the urethra associated with aging leads to disturbing symptoms, including urinary frequency, dysuria, uterine prolapse, and stress incontinence. Vaginal relaxation with cystocele, rectocele, and uterine prolapse is not caused by reduced estrogen levels but may be a delayed result of childbearing or other cause of weakness of pelvic support structures. Urinary frequency sometimes occurs after menopause because the distal portion of the urethra, which has the same embryologic origin as the reproductive organs, shortens and shrinks. Irritants have easier access to the urinary tract with its shorter urethra and may cause frequency and urinary tract infections.

Urinary incontinence and uterine displacement are two other common age-related rather than menopause-related findings in the postmenopausal period. These conditions are discussed in Chapter 12.

Vasomotor Instability

During the past three decades, investigators have devoted significant attention to identifying ovarian, hypothalamic, and pituitary hormonal mechanisms that produce symptoms related to menopause. Two symptoms appear to increase in incidence as women progress through menopause: hot flashes and night sweats. Many of the other changes commonly associated with menopause, such as decrease in size of genital structures, skin changes, and changes in breast size, are more correctly attributed to aging.

Vasomotor instability in the form of hot flashes or flushes is a result of fluctuating estrogen levels and is the most common disturbance of the perimenopausal years, occurring in up to 75% of women having natural menopause and 90% of women who have a surgical menopause. Vasomotor instability occurs most frequently in the first 2 postmenopausal years; the number of episodes decreases over time. However, some women have hot flashes before menopause and continue to have them for 10 to 20 years afterward. During this time, women experience changeable vasodilation and vasoconstriction as a hot flush (visible red flush of skin and perspiration) or hot flash (sudden warm sensation in neck, head, and chest) and night sweats. These disturbances vary widely in severity, and only a minority of women seek health care for them. Hot flushes and flashes can occur often throughout the day and may continue for several months or years. For some women, hot flashes may be an infrequent, possibly pleasant, sensation of warmth; for others, they may be an intensely unpleasant sensation of heat or warmth that may occur 20 to 50 times a day, create intense anxiety, and significantly decrease quality of life. Surveys of midlife women have found that, in the absence of menopausal hormonal therapy, most affected women will have disturbances for 1 to 2 years, and 25%, up to 5 years (Speroff & Fritz, 2005). Several factors can precipitate or aggravate an episode, including crowded or warm rooms, alcohol, hot drinks, spicy foods, proximity to a heat source, and stress.

Night sweats, characterized by profuse perspiration and heat radiating from the body during the night, are another form of vasomotor instability experienced by many women. Sleep may be interrupted nightly because nightclothes and bed linens may be soaked. Women may find that they are not able to go back to sleep. Other problems that may be associated with perimenopausal fluctuations of vasoconstriction or vascular spasms include dizziness, numbness and tingling in fingers and toes, and headaches.

Mood and Behavioral Responses

The tendency to associate hormonal changes with psychologic symptoms in midlife that has been prevalent in medical literature for decades and continues today was fueled by a belief that postmenopausal women have "estrogen deficiency." Contrary to this common belief, there is no concrete evidence that menopause has a deleterious effect on mental health of midlife women. Reviews of epidemiologic studies on menopause and depression found no causal association between menopause and depression (Sowers, 2000). Women with hot flashes and night sweats do report insomnia, fatigue from loss of sleep, and depressed mood. Women complain of feeling more emotionally labile, nervous, or agitated, with less control of their emotions. However, the interaction of psychologic, biologic, and sociocultural factors is so complex that it is difficult to determine whether a woman's reported mood shifts are the result of hormonal changes, normal aging, or cultural conditioning. Most likely a woman's psychologic makeup, cultural background, intercurrent stresses, and changing life roles and circumstances are more important than estrogen levels. Dealing with teenage children; having teenagers leave home; helping aging parents; becoming widowed or divorced; the onset of a major illness or disability (even death) in a spouse, relative, or friend; grieving for friends and family who are ill or dying; retirement; and financial insecurity are among the many stresses of women in their forties and fifties.

Cultural messages also influence individual women's perception of menopause. Women's experiences with menopause are not universal and vary among cultural groups. Most North American women do not believe that menopause interferes with their quality of life (National Institutes of Health [NIH], 2005). Women do not find symptoms to be a cause for concern; however, they do report that symptoms are bothersome. Many women have accepted childbearing and child rearing as their major role in life, and the inability to bear children is a significant loss. Others see menopause as the first step to old age and associate it with a loss of attractiveness, physical ability, and energy. Western culture values youth and physical attractiveness; the wisdom gained from life experience is not valued, and the elderly have a loss of status, function, and role. No rituals give older women a special place and function. In cultures where postmenopausal women gain status, such as India, the Far East, and the South Pacific Islands, depression among menopausal women is not observed. Western women, however, may have little to compensate for their losses.

For other women, menopause is not a loss or a symbol of losses, but a relief. For some, menopause is a relief from the fear of pregnancy, the discomfort and bother of menstruation, and the inconveniences of contraception.

The ability to cope with any stress involves three factors: the person's perception or understanding of the event, the support system, and coping mechanisms. Nurses counseling women in their perimenopausal years must therefore assess their understanding of perimenopausal changes, their perceptions of stressful experiences, their support systems, and their repertoire of coping skills.

Health Risks of Perimenopausal Women

Osteoporosis and coronary heart disease are the major health risks of perimenopausal women and are the focus of the following discussion.

Osteoporosis

Aging is associated with a progressive decrease in bone density in both men and women. Osteoporosis is a generalized, metabolic disease characterized by decreased bone mass and increased incidence of bone fractures. Normally there is a dynamic balance between bone formation (osteoblastic activity) and bone resorption (osteoclastic activity). Because one of the functions of estrogen is to stimulate the osteoblasts, the postmenopausal decrease in estrogen levels causes an imbalance between bone formation and resorption. Old bone deteriorates faster than new bone is formed, resulting in a slow thinning of the bones. Estrogen also is required for the conversion of vitamin D into calcitonin, which is essential in the absorption of calcium by the intestine. Reduced calcium absorption from the gut, in addition to the thinning of the bones, places postmenopausal women at risk for problems associated with osteoporosis.

Osteoporosis is a major health problem in the United States, affecting more than 10 million women older than 45 years (Speroff & Fritz, 2005). Approximately 50% of women in the United States have some degree of osteoporosis. One in two will have changes severe enough to predispose them to fractures. In the United States, the incidence of osteoporosis-related fractures has increased in the past 20 years. Postmenopausal women with a hip or symptomatic vertebral fracture have a six- to eightfold increased risk of death in the year following their fracture (Zizic, 2004). During the first 5 to 6 years after menopause, women lose bone 6 times more rapidly than men. By age 65 years, one third of women have had a vertebral fracture; by age 81 years, one third have had a hip fracture. By the time women reach age 80 years, they have lost 47% of their trabecular bone, concentrated in the vertebrae, the pelvis and other flat bones, and the epiphyses. The most well-defined risk factor for osteoporosis is the loss of the protective effect of estrogen associated with cessation of ovarian function, particularly at menopause. Women at risk are likely to be Caucasian or Asian, small boned, and thin. Obese women have higher estrogen levels resulting from the conversion of androgens in adipose tissue; mechanical stress from extra weight also helps preserve bone mass. A family history of the disease is common. The influences of heredity, race, and sex may result in differences in peak bone mass.

Inadequate calcium intake is a risk factor, particularly during adolescence and into the third and fourth decade, when peak bone mass is attained (Speroff & Fritz, 2005). An excessive caffeine intake increases calcium excretion, causing a systemic acidosis that stimulates bone resorption. Smoking is associated with earlier and greater bone loss and decreases estrogen production. Excessive alcohol intake interferes with calcium absorption and depresses bone formation. A greater phosphorus than calcium intake, which occurs with soft drink consumption, may be a risk factor. Other risk factors include steroid therapy and disorders such as hypogonadism and hyperthyroidism.

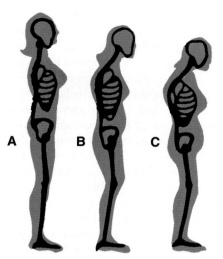

FIG. 7-2 Skeletal changes secondary to osteoporosis assessed by height and body shape at **A,** age 55 years; **B,** age 65 years; and **C,** age 75 years.

The first sign of osteoporosis is often loss of height resulting from vertebral fracture and collapse (Fig. 7-2). Back pain, especially in the lower back, may or may not be present. Later signs include "dowager's hump," in which the vertebrae can no longer support the upper body in an upright position, and fractured hip, in which the fracture often precedes a fall. Damage to the vertebrae usually precedes bone loss in the hip by an average of 10 years. Osteoporosis cannot be detected by radiographic examination until 30% to 50% of the bone mass has been lost; thus routine screening is not warranted in women under age 65. However, bone density testing is recommended for women at high risk for osteoporosis at age 60 and for all women older than 65 years to assess fracture risk (National Osteoporosis Foundation [NOF], 2003; United States Public Health Services Task Force, 2005). Medicare will pay for tests for high risk women once every 2 years. Insurance reimbursement varies for the tests, which cost about $700.

Coronary Heart Disease

A woman's risk of developing and dying of cardiovascular disease increases after menopause. Diseases of the heart are the leading cause of death for women in the United States. Known risk factors for coronary heart disease include obesity, cigarette smoking, elevated cholesterol and blood pressure levels, diabetes mellitus, family history of cardiac disease, alcohol abuse, and the effects of aging on the cardiovascular system (Alexander & Andrist, 2006; Speroff & Fritz, 2005). Estrogen has a favorable effect on circulating lipids, decreasing LDL and total cholesterol and increasing HDL, and has a direct antiatherosclerotic effect on arteries. Postmenopausal women are at risk for coronary artery disease because of changes in lipid metabolism: a decline in serum levels of HDL cholesterol and an increase in LDL levels. These changes can be favorably reduced by diet and exercise.

Menopausal Hormonal Therapy

Until 2002, menopausal hormonal therapy (MHT)—either as estrogen replacement therapy (ERT) or estrogen therapy (ET), in which a woman takes only estrogen, or hormonal replacement therapy (HRT) or hormonal therapy (HT), in which she takes both estrogen and progestins—was widely prescribed for discomforts associated with the perimenopausal years, including hot flashes and vaginal and urinary tract atrophy. Further, MHT was aggressively used for both therapeutic and preventive management. At the same time, its use remained a highly controversial issue in women's health. Some authorities recommended HT or ET for all women; these proponents viewed the perimenopause as a disease or deficiency state. Others insisted that the use of hormones was never indicated for menopausal symptoms. The middle-ground approach advocated the use of MRT for women who have specific discomforts (therapeutic management) and for women in certain high risk groups (preventive management). Research studies challenged these beliefs in the preventive and beneficial effects of HT (Kaunitz, 2002; Rossouw et al., 2002) and documented increased risks for blood clots, heart attack, stroke, and invasive breast cancer in older women with a uterus (mean age 63, range 50-79 years) with long-term use of continuous combined estrogen plus progestin.

These findings changed the way MHT is used. Many women stopped taking MHT and sought alternative therapies to treat their menopausal symptoms. Others chose to continue with the MHT but had questions about the available regimens and associated risks. Although the absolute risk for these adverse outcomes in an individual woman is very low, menopausal women should be aware of the most current research to make an informed decision regarding if, when, and for how long they use MHT.

Decision to Use Hormone Therapy

All women considering ET or HT must understand that studies on MHT are ongoing, and there is still much to be learned. Nurses can provide information and counseling to assist women to make decisions regarding MHT use (Wilhelm, 2002) Important teaching points include the following (ACOG, 2004a & b; American Health Consultants, 2002; Berg, 2002; Jaffe & Santen, 2006; Klaiber, Vogel, & Rako, 2005; National Women's Health Information Center, 2006 [www.4women.gov]).

- For women taking MHT for short-term (1 to 3 years) relief of menopausal discomforts and who do not have increased risks for cardiovascular disease, the benefits may outweigh the risks. The decision to use MRT should be made between a woman and her health care provider.
- Older women who are taking or considering MHT only for the prevention of cardiovascular disease should be counseled on other methods to reduce their risks of cardiovascular disease.

Menopause

BACKGROUND

- Menopause, the cessation of menses, is typically a natural process lasting several years around age 51 years, but can span ages 40-58 years. As the ovaries age, they produce less estrogen and become less sensitive to follicle-stimulating hormone. Decreased estrogen results in the hot flashes of vasomotor instability and thinning and drying of the vagina. Other symptoms may also include sleep disturbance (alone or from night sweats), mood symptoms, somatic complaints, loss of libido, cognitive disturbances, uterine bleeding, and decreased quality of life.

OBJECTIVES

- Although there are many studies on the symptoms and management of menopause, the definitions and measurements lack validity and reliability. The authors sought to systematically review the literature for meaningful, usable research on menopausal symptoms and timing, management, and impact of complicating health issues.

METHODS

Search Strategy

- Regarding menopause symptoms and timing: After searching the literature, the authors selected 48 randomized controlled trials from 14 cohorts and 22 cross-sectional studies from other populations. The studies originated in Australia, Canada, Denmark, Netherlands, the United Kingdom, and the United States, and were dated 1993 to 2003.
- Regarding treatment for menopausal symptoms, 192 randomized controlled trials met the authors' criteria. The citations dated 1977 to 2002, and included participants from Denmark, Israel, South Africa, Sweden, the United Kingdom, and the United States.
- There were 15 randomized controlled trials addressing management of perimenopausal symptoms complicated by breast cancer. The dates and countries of those trials were not noted in the review.

Statistical Analyses

- All similar data were pooled. Reviewers calculated relative risks for dichotomous (categoric) data, such as night sweats, and weighted mean differences for continuous data, such as age. Differences between groups outside the 95% confidence interval were accepted as significant.

FINDINGS

- Half of all perimenopausal women experience vasomotor symptoms lasting several years, which may include night sweats and sleep disturbances. Vaginal dryness is an increasing problem for one out of three perimenopausal and postmenopausal women. There were no strong associations of menopause with somatic symptoms, mood symptoms, or cognitive disturbances. Findings equating menopause to urinary leakage, declining sexual function, and reduced quality of life were equivocal. No studies of uterine bleeding problems in menopause met the criteria to be reviewed. Data on the timing of menopause were inconclusive, except to differentiate the symptoms experienced by women with surgical or sudden menopause from those undergoing natural menopause.

- Estrogen remains the most effective therapy for vasomotor, sleep and mood disturbances, sexual function, and quality of life. Adverse effects include cardiovascular and thromboembolic events, nausea and vomiting, breast soreness, weight gain, headache, rash, and liver or gallbladder dysfunction. Data on benefits of progestin were mixed. Testosterone improved sexual function, but at risk of acne or hirsutism. Tibolone showed benefits for vasomotor, sleep, and somatic complaints similar to estrogen, and also some similar side effects of weight gain and headache. Vasomotor effects showed mixed improvements with paroxetine, veralipride, gabapentin, and phytoestrogens, including soy.

- Vasomotor symptoms in women with breast cancer were reduced with clonidine, venlafaxine, and megestrol acetate, but not with black cohosh, isoflavones, vitamin E, magnets, or fluoxetine.

LIMITATIONS

- Dissimilar definitions and methods made comparisons difficult. Volunteer participants may not have been representative of the population. Adjustments were lacking for relevant variables such as body mass index (BMI), age, race, or history of depression. Few studies reported adverse treatment effects. Some trials were of limited duration, had small sample size, were lost to follow-up, and used measures lacking validation or standardization. Industry sponsorship may have affected interpretation.

IMPLICATIONS FOR PRACTICE

- Nurses can recognize vasomotor and sleep disturbances and vaginal dryness as expected perimenopausal symptoms. Other symptoms have weaker associations with menopause, and may be causally related or concurrent. Most women must tailor their treatment through trial and error.

IMPLICATIONS FOR FURTHER RESEARCH

- Much basic information remains unclear—the timing and definitions of menopause, the optimum treatments and dosing, placebo effects, adverse effects, and nonpharmacologic therapies. Factors such as race, age, BMI, premature ovarian failure, lifestyle, surgical or sudden menopause, and medications all may affect timing, symptoms, and treatment of menopausal symptoms. Uniform definitions and measures and large, longitudinal, population-based studies are needed to improve generalizability and power of findings about the advisability, dosing, and tapering of estrogen and alternatives.

Reference: Nelson, H., Haney, E., Humphrey, L., Miller, J., Nedrow, A., Nicolaidis, C., et al. (2005). *Management of menopause-related symptoms*. (AHRQ Publication No. 05-E016-1). Rockville, MD: Agency for Healthcare Research and Quality.

- Alternatively, there may be beneficial cardiovascular effects associated with MHT for younger, more recently menopausal women, but research is needed.
- Women who are taking MHT only for prevention of osteoporosis should be counseled regarding their personal risks and benefits for continuing the therapy and reassured that there are effective alternatives for long-term prevention. Bone density studies also may be indicated to determine the degree of risk in an individual woman.
- Women with a high risk for breast cancer or who have had breast cancer should be counseled against using MHT.
- MHT may worsen myomas of the uterus and porphyria.
- Conjugated estrogens are associated with an increased incidence of gallbladder disease, and women with a known history of gallbladder disease should not use MHT.
- If used, MHT should be taken at the lowest effective dose for the shortest possible duration.
- When a woman decides to stop MHT, gradual withdrawal to prevent return of symptoms by rapid withdrawal of estrogen is advised.

Nurses are encouraged to stay current with ongoing MHT research findings. As other Women's Health Initiative (WHI) data on MHT are analyzed, further clarification of the issues will be published. One easily accessible resource is the American College of Obstetricians and Gynecologists; this organization regularly produces national guidelines and standards of practice with midlife and menopausal women and will update recommendations as new information becomes available (see www. ACOG.org).

Side Effects

Side effects associated with estrogen use include headaches, nausea and vomiting, bloating, ankle and feet swelling, weight gain, breast soreness, brown spots on the skin, eye irritation with contact lenses, and depression. The type of estrogen used for postmenopausal hormonal therapy is much less potent than ethinyl estradiol used in OCPs and has fewer serious side effects. Side effects that occur with MHT may disappear with a change in estrogen preparation or a decrease in the dose prescribed.

Treatment Guidelines

Although many women will discontinue use of MHT based on the current research findings, others will continue because they believe the benefits of the therapy in relieving their symptoms or preventing osteoporosis to outweigh the risks. Research in this important area continues; however, nurses who must counsel women about MHT must understand what is available and teach women who choose to continue MHT how to take the medications correctly. Thus the following discussion about the different regimens of MHT is included.

Many different estrogen preparations, natural and synthetic, and ways of administering them—oral tablets, topical creams, transdermal preparations, injectables, suppositories, and vaginal rings—exist (Table 7-4). However, most women today use either tablets or the transdermal patch.

Previous regimens of sequential HT prescribed estrogen in combination with progesterone to simulate the normal menstrual cycle. This created a 5- to 6-day period at the end of the month when no hormones were taken and breakthrough bleeding occurred. This regimen was cumbersome to explain and difficult for women to follow; therefore a more convenient regimen of a continuous dose of estrogen (0.625 mg) on days 1 to 28 and intermittent progestins (2.5 mg medroxyprogesterone) on days 14 to 28 is the most commonly prescribed. Women usually do not have cyclical bleeding with this regimen and are less likely to have progestin side effects. An alternative regimen is continuous combined HT with estrogen and progestin taken daily, but this regimen is no longer recommended.

The transdermal estrogen patch is applied once a week to a hairless area of skin. Any site on the trunk or upper arms provides adequate absorption. Sites should be rotated. The patches should not be placed on the breasts because of their sensitivity. Some women report minor skin irritation and reddening at the patch site. Generally transdermal estrogen offers the same relief of menopausal symptoms as the oral preparation. The transdermal method of delivery of estrogen does not have the same side effects such as breast tenderness and fluid retention. Oral progestin therapy can be used with transdermal ET. Combined estrogen-progestin transdermal patches also are available.

Alternative Therapies

Many complementary and alternative therapies are useful for relieving some of the changes associated with altered estrogen levels. Homeopathy, acupuncture, and herbs have been used successfully for menopausal problems such as heavy bleeding, hot flashes, irritability, and headaches (Box 7-2).

Homeopathy views menopausal symptoms as the body's efforts to heal itself from the hormonal changes it is experiencing. Examples of remedies commonly prescribed during menopause by homeopaths are sepia, made from the inky juice of the cuttlefish, to relieve symptoms such as dry mouth, eyes, and vagina; nux vomica, derived from the poison nut, to relieve backaches, constipation, and frequent awakenings; and pulsatilla, made from the windflower, to relieve severe menstrual symptoms and hot flashes. Homeopathic remedies are subject to regulation by the U.S. Food and Drug Administration (FDA), although the FDA does not require proof of effectiveness.

Acupuncturists also treat hot flashes, but it is important that women evaluate their acupuncturists carefully. The American Association of Acupuncturists and Oriental Medicine will supply a list of acupuncturists in a given state. Questions to ask are, "Is the acupuncturist certified by the National Commission for the Certification of

table 7-4 Estrogen, Progestin, and Combination Estrogen/Progestin Medications for Menopausal Symptoms

TRADE NAME	CHEMICAL NAME	DOSAGES	METHOD
ESTROGEN EQUIVALENCES			
Premarin	Conjugated estrogens	0.3 mg; 0.45 mg; 0.625 mg; 0.9 mg; 1.25 mg; 2.5 mg	Oral
Estrace	Micronized estradiol	0.5 mg; 1.0 mg; 2.0 mg	Oral
Estratab Menest	Esterified estrogens	0.3 mg; 0.625 mg; 1.25 mg; 2.5 mg	Oral
Estratest	Esterified estrogens with methyltestosterone	0.635 mg esterified estrogen +1.25 mg methyltestosterone 1.25 mg esterified estrogens +1.25 mg methyltestosterone	Oral
Ortho-Est Ogen	Estropipate	0.625 mg; 1.25 mg; 2.5 mg	Oral
Estraderm	Transdermal estradiol	0.05 mg; 0.1 mg	Transdermal patch
Climera		0.05 mg; 0.1 mg	Release rates mg/24 hr for all
FemPatch		0.025 mg	
Esclim		0.025 mg; 0.0375 mg; 0.075 mg; 0.1 mg	
Vivelle		0.0375 mg; 0.05 mg; 0.075 mg; 0.1 mg	Transdermal patch
Vivelle-Dot		0.025 mg	Transdermal patch
Alora		0.05 mg; 0.075 mg; 0.1 mg	Transdermal patch
VAGINAL ESTROGEN CREAMS, RINGS, AND TABLETS			
Premarin	Conjugated estrogens	0.625 mg/g	Vaginal cream
Estrace	Estradiol	0.1 mg/g	Vaginal cream
Ogen	Estropipate	1.5 mg/g	Vaginal cream
Estring	Estradiol	2 mg	Vaginal ring
Vagifem	Estradiol	25 mcg	Vaginal tablet
PROGESTIN EQUIVALENCIES			
Provera	Medroxyprogesterone acetate	2.5 mg; 5.0 mg; 10 mg	Oral
Curretabs	Medroxyprogesterone	10 mg	Oral
Aygestin	Norethindrone acetate	5 mg	Oral
Micronor	Norethindrone	0.35 mg	Oral
Prometrium	Progesterone USP	200 mg	Oral
COMBINATION ESTROGEN-PROGESTIN			
Prempro	Conjugated estrogens Medroxyprogesterone acetate	0.3 mg; 0.45 mg; 0.625 mg 1.5 mg; 1.5 mg; 2.5 mg; 5 mg	Oral (1 combination tablet/day for 28 days)
Premphase	Conjugated estrogens Medroxyprogesterone acetate	0.625 mg 5 mg	Oral (14 days of estrogen only, then 14 days of both)
CombiPatch	Estradiol/norethindrone acetate (NETA)	0.05 mg estradiol/0.14 mg NETA or 0.05 mg estradiol/0.25 mg NETA	Transdermal (release rates mg/24 hr)
Activella	Estradiol and (NETA)	1 mg/0.5 mg	Transdermal
Climera Pro	Estradiol and Levonorgestrel	0.045 mg/0.015 mg	Transdermal
FemHRT 1/5	NETA and ethinyl estradiol	1 mg/0.5 mcg 0.5 mg/2.5 mcg	Transdermal

Source: *Activella*. (2006). Accessed www.activella.com, April 16, 2006; American Society of Health-System Pharmacists. (2006). MedlinePlus drug information: *Estradiol transdermal system*. Accessed www.nlm.nih.gov/medlineplus, April 13, 2006; *Climera Pro*. (2006). Accessed www.climerapro.com, April 16, 2006; Facts and Comparisons. (2002). *Loose-leaf drug information service*. St. Louis: Facts and Comparisons; *FemHRT*. (2006). Accessed www.femhrt.com, April 16, 2006; Healthwise. (2005). *Low-dose vaginal estrogen for dryness and atrophy*. Accessed www.questdiagnostics.com, April 13, 2006; *Vagifem*. (2006). Accessed www.vagifem.com, April 16, 2006.

Acupuncture? Is the acupuncturist certified in the state in which he or she practices? Does the acupuncturist carry malpractice insurance?"

Herbal therapy also has been used to treat menopausal discomforts (Table 7-5). Herbs can be ingested as teas or tinctures. Many herbal preparations also are available in capsule form. It is important that women understand mechanisms of action, contraindications, and potential side effects of each herb.

▬ NURSE ALERT

Most herbal preparations have not undergone long-term testing for safety and efficacy. Benefits and risks are not completely known. Women should always consult with their health care provider before beginning herbal therapy. Questions regarding the use of herbal therapy and other supplements must be a component of a client history.

In addition to resolving physical symptoms, herbs also are used to combat mood swings and depression. Ginseng

---

box 7-2 | **Alternatives to Hormonal Therapy for Menopausal Symptoms**

HOT FLASH/FLUSH

- Vitamin E: 100-800 international units daily (≤100 international units in the presence of high blood pressure, diabetes, or rheumatic heart disease). Start with a low dose and increase over 6 to 8 weeks to 800 international units or less if symptoms improve.
- Bioflavonoids (500 mg to 1 g) combined with vitamin C. Dietary sources include wheat germ, whole grains, vegetable oils, soybeans, peanuts, spinach and other dark-green leafy vegetables, and cold pressed oils.
- Herbal therapy: see Table 7-5
- Soy: 40 to 100 mg isoflavones or approximately 30 to 50 g soy protein
- Vitamin B complex: 1 to 2 daily. Dietary sources include whole grains, wheat germ, yogurt, brewer's yeast, and milk.
- Vitamin C
- Acupuncture
- Medications other than hormone replacement:
  Bellergal (can increase high blood pressure)
  Belladonna (side effects: dry mouth, rapid pulse, constipation)
  Clonidine (side effects: sleepiness, dry mouth, decreased blood pressure)

INSOMNIA

- Herbal therapy:
  Valerian (natural tranquilizer)
  Peppermint, catnip, hops, passionflower
  Chamomile

HEADACHES

- Herbal therapy:
  Natural diuretics (parsley)
  Chasteberry, peppermint oil, feverfew, royal jelly products

UROGENITAL SYMPTOMS

- For vaginal dryness and itching:
  Vitamin E: 400 to 800 international units daily or vitamin E oil on the skin
  Evening primrose oil, aloe vera, slippery elm paste
  Witch hazel and glycerin (dip pads in mixture and apply to skin for itching)

NERVOUSNESS/IRRITABILITY

- Vitamin B₆: 5 to 25 mg daily. Dietary sources include brewer's yeast, bran, wheat germ, organ meats, molasses, walnuts, peanuts, and brown rice.

Sources: ACOG Committee on Practice. (2001). Use of botanicals for management of menopausal symptoms. ACOG Practice Bulletin No. 28. *Obstetrics and Gynecology, 97*(6), Suppl 1-11; Blumenthal, M. (Ed.). (1998). *The complete German Commission E monographs: Therapeutic guide to herbal medicines.* Austin, TX: The American Botanical Council; Lowdermilk, D., & Fogel, C. (1996). *Health care issues of midlife women.* Edwardsville, KS: Educational Software.

---

has been claimed to be helpful in alleviating hot flashes, although research studies have not supported this assertion. Women should be advised against prolonged use of ginseng in high doses because it can increase blood pressure. Oriental herbal teas composed of licorice, ginseng, coptis, red raspberry leaf, and Chinese rhubarb may be of some help in relieving hot flashes.

Dong quai and black cohosh have been used to treat menopausal discomforts; both have been investigated for effectiveness, with varying results (ACOG, 2003). Black cohosh has been used by Native Americans for a variety of problems, including gynecologic ones, and it was a major ingredient in Lydia Pinkham's Vegetable Compound, a well-known nineteenth-century patent medicine.

Some plant foods contain phytoestrogens (isoflavones) and are capable of interacting with estrogen receptors in the body. These foods include wild yams, dandelion greens, cherries, alfalfa sprouts, black beans, and soybeans. Use of soy-rich foods as an alternative to traditional hormonal therapy for menopause has been studied, and beneficial effects on menopausal symptoms and on reducing cholesterol have been documented (Albertazzi, 2005; Faure, Chante, & Mares, 2002; Han, Soares, Haidar, de Lima, & Baracat, 2002; Upmalis, Lobo, Bradley, Warren, Cone, & Lamia, 2000). However, more research is needed to better understand the potential effects of soy intake on prevention of osteoporosis and reducing risks of coronary heart disease (Stokes, 2004). For women who want to add soy to their diets, tofu, roasted soy nuts, and soy milk are good sources. Foods should be added gradually because some women have gastrointestinal discomfort from the high fiber content of these foods. Spreading out the daily intake over several meals may be the best way to include soy products into the diet. The consumption of 100 mg or less per day of isoflavones is likely to be safe (Stokes).

Vitamin E is a popular alternative among women who do not take MHT. Women who take vitamin E regularly report relief from hot flushes, leg cramps, and loss of energy. Vitamin E is found in a variety of foods, including spinach, peanuts, wheat germ, vegetable oils, and soybeans, or may be taken as a supplement. Dosage varies widely, from 400 to 800 international units/day.

Layered clothing, ice packs, iced water, and fans may offer symptomatic relief from hot flashes (see Teaching for Self-Care box). Women can be counseled to avoid hot curries and other spicy foods. Reassurance that hot flashes will not last forever may be of comfort even if duration of the problem cannot be predicted accurately. Most women find that hot flashes disappear within 4 to 6 years after menopause.

Nurses should be aware of the availability of natural remedies for menopausal symptoms and be knowledgeable about the indications for complementary and alternative therapies so clients can be counseled appropriately.

▬ CARE MANAGEMENT

▬ Assessment and Nursing Diagnoses

A thorough health history, physical examination, and laboratory tests are essential to distinguish pathologic conditions from the normal perimenopausal experiences.

table 7-5 Herbals for Menopausal Symptoms

SYMPTOM/INDICATION	HERB	ACTIONS	CONSIDERATIONS/ SIDE EFFECTS	CONTRAINDICATIONS
Menopausal symptoms "hot flashes"	Black cohosh*	Binds estrogen receptor; inhibits LH secretion and non-receptor– mediated actions	Additive hypotensive effects with antihypertensive agents GI side effects, headaches, dizziness, and bradycardia with high doses	Pregnancy, lactation
	Sage	Estrogenic, uterotonic	NK	NK
	Licorice	Adrenal stimulant	Excess amounts can deplete potassium and elevate blood pressure	Avoid if hypertensive
	Red clover	Ovarian stimulant	NK	NK
Sleep disturbances, GI complaints, nervousness	Lemon balm	Tranquilizer/sedative	No known side effects, no known drug interactions	NK
Memory deficits, impaired concentration	Ginkgo	Stimulates circulation and oxygen flow	Side effects: allergic reactions, mild GI upset	Inhibits platelet-activating factor; not to be used with antithrombotic therapy
Fatigue, loss of concentration	Ginseng	Stimulant	Side effects: insomnia, tachycardia, palpitations, hypertension, ginseng abuse syndrome reported with overuse	Do not take with vitamin C; avoid if diabetic; do not use if have cardiac problems May be associated with postmenopausal bleeding
Anxiety, insomnia, nervousness	Passionflower	Tranquilizer/sedative	NK side effects NK drug interactions	NK
Depression, anxiety	St. John's wort	Antidepressive	Photosensitivity can occur	Contraindicated with MAO inhibitors or SSRIs
	Chaste tree fruit*	Alters FSH and LH levels; increases progesterone levels	May inhibit prolactin secretion; may interfere with dopamine antagonist Pruritic rash, GI side effects	Pregnancy and lactation
Nervousness, insomnia	Valerian	Tranquilizer/sedative	Allergic and GI side effects rare NK drug interactions with long-term use Headaches, restlessness, insomnia, cardiac dysfunction possible	NK
"Women's discomforts"	Dong quai	Stimulate/relax uterus; antiinflammatory; possibly analgesic activity	Phototoxicity Liver and renal damage in animal studies; abortifacient	Pregnancy; Coumarin components may increase risk of bleeding

Sources: ACOG. (2003). *Herbal products for menopause.* Accessed www.medem.com, April 11, 2006; ACOG Committee on Practice. (2001). Use of botanicals for management of menopausal symptoms. ACOG Practice Bulletin No. 28. *Obstetrics and Gynecology, 97(6),* Suppl. 1-11; Blumenthal, M. (Ed.). (1998). *The complete German Commission E monographs: Therapeutic guide to herbal medicines.* Austin, TX: The American Botanical Council; Huntley, A. (2002). Complementary therapies for the relief of menopausal symptoms. *Focus on Alternative and Complementary Therapies, 7(2),* 121-125; No author. (2006). *Alternative medicine for menopause: Herbal medicine.* Accessed www.holistic-online.com, April 11, 2006.
FSH, Follicle-stimulating hormone; *GI,* gastrointestinal; *LH,* luteinizing hormone; *MAO,* monoamine oxidase; *NK,* not known; *SSRIs,* selective serotonin reuptake inhibitors.
*Approved by Commission E specifically for treatment of menopausal symptoms.

TEACHING FOR SELF-CARE

Comfort Measures

HOT FLASHES/FLUSHES

During the Day
- Wear layered clothing so you can take things off if you get warm.
- Avoid "triggers" that bring on a flash/flush; these include vigorous exercise on hot days, eating spicy foods, caffeine, hot beverages, and alcohol.
- Splash your face with cool water, drink iced water, or take a cool shower if you get warm.
- Try slow, deep breathing.

At Night
- Sleep in cotton clothes, use cotton sheets, and keep room cool.
- Avoid heavy blankets that make you too warm at night.
- Keep a thermos of water by the bed.

INSOMNIA
- Avoid caffeine, alcohol, or tobacco in the evening.
- Avoid liquids after dinner.
- Exercise regularly but limit exercise to the daytime and early evening.
- Develop a bedtime routine.
- Establish a regular time to go to bed.
- Try drinking warm milk or having a hot bath.
- Use your bed only for sleeping or sexual activity; don't watch TV, read, etc.
- Encourage your body's circadian rhythm.
- If you can't sleep, get up and do something until you feel tired.
- Avoid naps during the day.
- Sprinkle lavender oil on the pillow.
- Drink chamomile tea (do not use if allergic to ragweed or chrysanthemums).

HEADACHES
- Try to avoid stress and get plenty of rest.
- Eat or drink foods that contain natural diuretics (parsley).

UROGENITAL SYMPTOMS
- Drink lots of water (i.e., at least 8 glasses a day), and empty bladder frequently.
- Practice Kegel exercises daily.
- Wear cotton underwear and avoid wet bathing suits for a prolonged time.
- Use water-soluble lubricants for vaginal dryness.

NERVOUSNESS, IRRITABILITY
- Practice yoga or other meditation.
- Do relaxation or deep-breathing exercises.
- Practice guided imagery.

Source: Lowdermilk, D., & Fogel, C. (1996). *Health care issues of midlife women.* Edwardsville, KS: Educational Software.

Personal or family history of breast or uterine cancer, hypertension, thrombophlebitis, liver or gallbladder disease, undiagnosed uterine bleeding, and other acute or chronic diseases are noted, as are hysterectomy and bilateral oophorectomy. Recent changes in menstrual history help identify the phase of the perimenopausal period the woman is experiencing, and risk factors for osteoporosis are identified. The woman's perception of this stage of life, ethnic and cultural factors, and knowledge and concerns about sexuality and care available are all recorded. The practices and remedies the woman has used for menopausal symptoms are assessed, including pharmacologic and alternative therapies.

Nursing diagnoses for perimenopausal women may include the following:

- *Deficient knowledge related to*
  –menopause and its management
- *Readiness for enhanced family coping related to*
  –receiving information about the condition, its management, and prognosis
  –emotional support
- *Risk for injury related to*
  –osteoporosis
  –heart disease

- *Sexual dysfunction related to*
  –changes associated with decreasing estrogen levels
- *Risk for situational low self-esteem related to*
  –physical and emotional changes during the perimenopausal period

▬ Expected Outcomes of Care

Planning requires knowledge of the perimenopausal period and great sensitivity. Informed consent regarding MHT, weight-bearing exercise, and calcium supplements is a major concern because treatment may involve expense, inconvenience, and side effects. Expected outcomes are stated in terms of client behaviors. The woman will do the following:

- Explain the physical changes associated with menopause.
- View the perimenopausal period as a normal developmental phase instead of a deficiency disease.
- Have no discomforts that interfere with daily activities.
- Develop no symptoms or signs of osteoporosis or experience only minimal effect.
- Experience a healthy perimenopausal transition.
- Report concerns about changes associated with menopause and treatment.

▬ Plan of Care and Interventions

Most women know little about menopause, and old wives' tales and misinformation can cause anxiety. They need to know what to expect, why it happens, and what measures will help make them more comfortable. Women appreciate the opportunity to discuss what they are experiencing. They need to know that their discomforts have a normal physiologic basis and that other women experience similar discomforts.

Treatment must be individualized for the specific woman. Menopause clinics are needed where research on the effects of various treatments can be developed and evaluated and where care by the various specialty groups involved, such as endocrinology, radiology, psychosocial resources, exercise physiology, and nutrition, can be effectively coordinated. Women's support groups also are needed. Areas that need further discussion include sexuality, nutrition, exercise, and support.

▬ *Sexual Counseling*

Sexuality is a lifelong behavior, and contrary to common stereotypes, sex does not end with menopause. Many women remain sexually active throughout their entire lives. However, women and their partners may change their expression of sexuality during and after menopause, depending on physical changes, changes in the partner, and cultural myths and messages. Some women report decreases in interest and desire. These decreases in sexuality with aging are influenced more by culture and attitudes than by nature and physiology (hormones). Although some women report that it takes longer to reach orgasm and that the orgasm is not so intense, the capacity for orgasm is not decreased. There is no way to prevent the inevitable aging process that the body undergoes. For people who see aging as loss, sexuality may become difficult to incorporate into what they perceive to be a less attractive identity. The fear of rejection may be present.

Changes in a male partner may influence whether he continues to want to engage in sexual activity. As men age, they, too, take longer to reach orgasm; erections take longer to occur and are less firm. Men may believe they are becoming impotent or ill and give up sexual activity, viewing it as too frustrating. Women may believe their partners are losing interest in them. Couples may need counseling to understand these changes.

The two most important influences on older women's sexual activity are the strength of a relationship and the physical condition of each partner. The lack of available male partners can have a negative effect on sexual expression for many midlife and older women. Women outlive men, and older widowed and divorced women frequently have fewer opportunities to develop relationships because they are less sought after. In counseling older women who do engage in intercourse, the nurse cannot assume that new or nonmonogamous partners are free of sexually transmitted infections (STIs) and should inform clients of their risk for human immunodeficiency virus infection and other STIs and the need to use condoms.

As long as women are able to bear children, some accept intercourse as part of their responsibility as wives. When menopause frees them from this duty, they may choose to forego intercourse. For other women, libido may increase without the fuss of contraception, fear of pregnancy, or interruption from menses.

Older lesbian women largely have been a silent group whose sexual needs and special social circumstances have not been acknowledged or recognized. Although lesbian women in midlife and in later years do not face the problem of a lack of available male partners, they are faced with negative attitudes accompanying being old, female, and lesbian—all of which can adversely affect sexuality and sexual expression.

Nurses must give accurate information on matters such as appropriate contraception, sexuality, and the physiology of menopause and should offer support and nonjudgmental guidance. Women need advice about contraception, because ovulation may not cease for a year after the last menstrual cycle, and menopausal women can still become pregnant. The nurse's attitude toward sex and the older woman is important. Negative attitudes can reinforce the client's misgivings about maintaining an active and satisfying sex life. The nurse can reassure the woman grieving over lost youth and attractiveness that the desire for sex into old age is a natural one and that the body has the capacity for sexual satisfaction. Only minor adjustments may be required.

Muscle tone around the reproductive organs decreases after menopause. Kegel exercises strengthen these muscles, improve tone, and, if practiced regularly, help prevent prolapsed uterus and stress incontinence. This is a low-cost, effective, noninvasive intervention to control symptoms. However, symptoms return if exercises are discontinued.

Lubricating jelly (e.g., K-Y, Femglide, Aqualube), are water-soluble lubricants that provide relief from painful intercourse. They may be applied directly to the vulva and the penis. Vaginal moisturizers may be water based but also contain other products such as vitamin E and aloe (e.g., K-Y Longlasting, Replens, Astroglide). They are inserted into the vagina using a prefilled applicator. Oil-based lubricants such as petroleum jelly (Vaseline) should not be used because they clog vaginal glands, which can then be sites for bacterial infection.

The nurse can refer couples to a counselor or physician for problems beyond the scope of nursing practice.

Prolonged hospitalization of an elderly partner may have a significant impact on the couple's sexual relationship. They may have difficulty renewing sexual activity when the separation is over and may need counseling or referral. In the event that a couple is admitted to a nursing home, the nurse should encourage placement of the couple together. With the aging of the American population and changing attitudes about the appropriateness of lifelong sexual expression, long-term care, extended care, and full-term care facilities are more receptive to providing opportunities for sexual activity between marital partners.

■ Nutrition

Obesity and osteoporosis are common health problems of midlife and older women. As women move out of their childbearing years, they may need to change their diets. Because metabolic rates decrease with age and many women exercise less, fewer calories are needed for weight maintenance as women age. In general, foods chosen should be high in nutrients, fiber, and calcium but moderate in calories and low in fat to allow adequate nutritional intake while maintaining body weight. Nurses can suggest that women substitute skim for whole milk or chicken without skin for steak. Foods high in calcium and low in phosphorus are recommended. Excessive protein should be avoided. Fat-free milk and yogurt are good sources of calcium and vitamin D. Women should avoid excessive intake of alcohol, soft drinks, and caffeinated coffee.

Calcium is an essential part of any therapeutic regimen for women with osteoporosis and those who want to prevent osteoporosis. The best source of calcium is food; however, it is difficult to eat other foods that contain calcium (sesame seeds, spinach, greens, broccoli, and seaweed) in quantities sufficient to meet daily requirements. Calcium supplements are recommended when a woman's diet does not supply recommended amounts of calcium. Although calcium cannot reverse loss of bone mass or prevent fractures, calcium supplementation may retard the development of osteoporosis after menopause. Menopausal women without contraindications to calcium supplementation (history of kidney stones, kidney failure, hypercalcemia) should be encouraged to consume a diet that has 1200 to 1500 mg of calcium a day or to add an amount of calcium supplementation that will increase their daily intake to this level. Calcium supplements are best taken in divided doses and with meals because of the increase in acid secretions and extended time in the stomach. At least 8 ounces of water to increase solubility is recommended. Calcium supplements should not be taken with caffeinated beverages. Calcium is most commonly available as calcium carbonate, calcium lactate, and calcium phosphate. Some of the calcium preparations (e.g., some generic brands) on the market are useless because they do not dissolve; Tums are most soluble. A combination of vitamin D and calcium (1200 mg) may be recommended as a supplement because vitamin D aids in calcium absorption. Mineral supplements are not classified as drugs by the FDA and are therefore not regulated, making it difficult for consumers to know which product is best.

■ Exercise

All too often, midlife women are sedentary—the demands of family and work constraints increase, and energy levels decrease. Unfortunately little or no exercise predisposes women to weight gain and does not help prevent cardiac disease or osteoporosis. Exercise alone cannot prevent or reverse osteoporosis, but data indicate that weight-bearing exercise, such as walking and stair climbing for 30 to 60 minutes a day, may delay bone loss and increase bone mass at any age.

Water aerobics is excellent for cardiovascular fitness and is a good choice for older women who may be unable to engage in weight-bearing exercises. The nurse can help women plan an exercise program. Examples of exercises are available from the National Osteoporosis Foundation (Fig. 7-3).

■ Medications for Osteoporosis

In addition to calcium and exercise, there are a number of FDA-approved medications for the prevention and treatment of osteoporosis (Box 7-3). The medications assist in delaying bone loss, increasing bone mass, and preventing fractures. These include salmon calcitonin (Miacalcin), bisphosphonates (alendronate sodium [Fosamax], risedronate sodium [Actonel]), selective estrogen receptor modulators (SERMs) such as raloxifene (Evista), parathyroid hormone (teriparatide [Forteo]), and estrogen or hormone therapy (NOF, 2006; Zizic, 2004).

Calcitonin reduces the rate of bone turnover and stabilizes bone mass in women with osteoporosis and may have some analgesic effects. Although calcitonin can reduce the incidence of spinal fractures, no data are available

---

box 7-3 | **Prevention of Osteoporosis**

- Significant bone loss can be prevented by a well-balanced diet, including 200 to 400 international units of vitamin D and 1200 to 1500 mg of calcium a day, and regular weight-bearing exercise. Good sources of calcium are dairy products, fish, oysters, tofu, dark-green leafy vegetables, and whole wheat bread.
- Supplements of vitamin D and calcium can be taken, but the body cannot use them without the right balance of other vitamins and minerals.
- Eliminating environmental hazards in the home can decrease the risk of falls.
- Weight-bearing exercise 30 to 60 min/day may delay bone loss and increase bone mass.
- Raloxifene may be prescribed for prevention of osteoporosis in postmenopausal women.
- Alendronate sodium may be prescribed for women who already have osteoporosis to delay bone loss and increase bone mass.
- Estrogen therapy (ET) can be prescribed to prevent fractures from osteoporosis. The risks and benefits of ET used solely for osteoporosis prevention must be weighed on an individual basis with the health care provider.

FIG. 7-3 A, Wall standing and pelvic tilt. **B,** Isometric posture correction. **C,** Standing back bend. **D,** The bridge. **E,** The elbow prop. **F,** Prone press-ups with deep breathing. (From *Boning Up On Osteoporosis,* courtesy the National Osteoporosis Foundation.)

about the use of calcitonin to protect against hip fractures. Calcitonin may be used with women in whom estrogen is contraindicated or not tolerated. The drug is administered intranasally or subcutaneously on a daily basis. The medication is considered safe; however, side effects of nausea, vomiting, anorexia, and rhinitis (if used intranasally) have been reported (NOF, 2006).

Bisphosphonates are approved for prevention and treatment of osteoporosis, especially in reducing the incidence of spinal fractures. Side effects include gastrointestinal problems such as difficulty swallowing, inflammation of the esophagus, and gastric ulcer. Depending on the medication used, this oral drug may be taken daily or monthly. Some formulations contain vitamin D (NOF, 2006).

■ NURSE ALERT

Because food and certain minerals reduce the absorption of bisphosphonates, women must take alendronate sodium and risedronate sodium on an empty stomach with 6 to 8 ounces of plain water only, at least 30 minutes before eating or drinking to improve absorption (Zizic, 2004); remaining upright for these 30 minutes also is recommended.

Raloxifene is approved by the FDA for osteoporosis prevention and treatment in postmenopausal women only. This medication seemingly preserves the beneficial effects of estrogen, including protection against cardiovascular diseases and osteoporosis, without stimulating breast and uterine tissues. However, the effects of raloxifene and the risks of breast cancer and heart disease are still under study (NOF, 2006). The medication modestly increases bone density. Calcium supplements up to 1500 mg should be taken if dietary intake is inadequate.

Parathyroid hormone is approved for the treatment of osteoporosis in postmenopausal women at high risk for fractures. It is administered by daily subcutaneous injection. Safety and efficacy have not been demonstrated beyond 2 years of use (NOF, 2006).

Estrogen therapy is approved for the prevention of osteoporosis, but the FDA recommends that it should not be used solely for this purpose until after approved nonestrogen treatments are tried (NOF, 2006).

■ *Midlife Support Groups*

Nurses should be familiar with local resources and direct women to classes that supply appropriate information and

FIG. 7-4 Midlife women can develop a supportive network. (Courtesy Ed Lowdermilk, Chapel Hill, NC.)

support. They can encourage women to develop a supportive network with other women with whom they can share their concerns (Fig. 7-4).

Women's centers and clinics may have support groups and classes for women who want to discuss menopause and other midlife events. If no group or class is available in the community, nurses should consider starting one.

▬ Evaluation

The nurse can be reasonably assured that care was effective to the degree that the expected outcomes of care have been met.

---

key points

- Menstrual disorders diminish the quality of life for affected women and their families.
- PMS, no longer considered a purely psychologic problem, is a disorder with symptoms that begin in the luteal phase of the menstrual cycle and end with the onset of menses.
- Endometriosis is characterized by secondary amenorrhea, dyspareunia, abnormal uterine bleeding, and infertility.
- The perimenopause is a normal developmental phase during which a woman passes from the reproductive to the nonreproductive stage.
- During the perimenopause, women seek care for symptoms that arise from bleeding irregularities, vasomotor instability, fatigue, genital changes, and changes related to sexuality.
- Alternative therapies are beneficial in relieving discomforts associated with menstrual disorders and menopause.
- Osteoporosis, a progressive loss of bone mass that results from decreasing levels of estrogen after menopause, can be prevented or minimized with lifestyle changes and medication.
- Estrogen increases calcitonin levels to prevent bone resorption and maintain bone density.
- Postmenopausal women are at increased risk for coronary artery disease because of changes in lipid metabolism.
- Sexuality and the capacity for sexual expression continue after menopause.

---

community activity

- Locate resources in your community for women who have menstrual and menopausal problems. Make a list of these resources complete with contact information, accessibility, costs, and a brief description of service(s) provided.
- Alternately, if there are limited resources in your community, locate resources on the Internet for women who are looking for symptom management of menstrual problems or menopause.

REFERENCES

Albertazzi, P. (2005). Alternatives to estrogen to manage hot flushes. *Gynecological Endocrinology, 20*(1), 13-21.

Alexander, E., Shimp, L. & Smith, M. (2000). Obesity and eating disorders. In M. Smith & L. Shimp (Eds.), *20 common problems in women's health care.* New York: McGraw-Hill. Alexander, I. & Andrist, L. (2006). Menopause. In K. Schuiling & F. Liskis (Eds.), *Women's Gynecologic Health.* Sudbury, MA: Jones & Bartlett.

American College of Nurse-Midwives (ACNM). (2002). Abnormal and dysfunctional uterine bleeding. ACNM Clinical Bulletin No. 6. *Journal of Midwifery & Women's Health, 47*(3), 207-213.

American College of Obstetricians and Gynecologists (ACOG). (2000a). Management of anovulatory bleeding. *ACOG Practice Bulletin No. 14.* Washington DC: Author.

American College of Obstetricians and Gynecologists. (2000b). Premenstrual syndrome. *ACOG Practice Bulletin, No. 15.* Washington, DC: Author.

American College of Obstetricians and Gynecologists (ACOG). (2003). *Herbal products for menopause.* Accessed www.medem.com, April 11, 2006.

American College of Obstetricians and Gynecologists (ACOG). (2004a). ACOG statement on the NIH announcement to halt estrogen-only arm of the WHI study. *ACOG News Release,* March 2, 2004. Accessed www.acog.org, April 11, 2006.

American College of Obstetricians and Gynecologists (ACOG). (2004b). Chronic pelvic pain. ACOG Practice Bulletin No. 51. *Obstetrics and Gynecology, 103*(3), 589-605.

American College of Obstetricians and Gynecologists Committee on Adolescent Health Care. (2005). Endometriosis in adolescents. ACOG Committee Opinion No. 310. *Obstetrics and Gynecology, 105*(4), 921-927.

American Health Consultants. (2002). Hormone replacement therapy: Review choices in light of new data. *Contraceptive Technology Update, 23*(9), 97-103.

American Psychiatric Association (APA). (2000). *Diagnostic and statistical manual of mental disorders* (4th ed., text revision). Washington, DC: American Psychiatric Association Press.

Angst, J., Sellaro, R., Merikangas, K., & Endicott, J. (2001). The epidemiology of perimenstrual psychological symptoms. *Acta Psychiatrica Scandinaciva, 104*(2), 110-116.

Association of Women's Health, Obstetric and Neonatal Nurses (AWHONN). (2003). *Evidence-based clinical practice guideline: Nursing management for cyclic perimenstrual pain and discomfort.* Washington, DC: Author.

Berg, E. (2002). When should HT be discontinued? *Journal Watch Women's Health, 7*(9), 71.

Blackburn, S. (2003). *Maternal, fetal, & neonatal physiology: A clinical perspective* (2nd ed.). St. Louis: Saunders.

Budeiri, D., Li Wan Po, A., & Dornan, J. (1996). Is evening primrose oil of value in the treatment of premenstrual syndrome? *Controlled Clinical Trials, 17*(1), 60-68.

Collins Sharp, B., Taylor, D., Thomas, K., Killeen, M., & Dawood, M. (2002). Cyclic perimenstrual pain and discomfort: The scientific basis for practice. *Journal of Obstetric, Gynecologic, and Neonatal Nursing, 31*(6), 637-649.

Conversations with Colleagues. (2002-2003). Endometriosis sufferers risk other diseases. *AWHONN Lifelines, 6*(6), 502-504.

Dehlin, L., & Schuiling, K. (2006). Chronic pelvic pain. In K. Schuiling & F. Lokis (Eds.) *Women's gynecologic health*. Boston: Jones & Bartlett.

Dodd, N., & Sinert, R. (2006). *Dysfunctional uterine bleeding*. Accessed www.emedicine.com, April 11, 2006.

Faure, E., Chante, P., & Mares, P. (2002). Effects of a standardized soy extract on hot flushes: A multicenter, double-blind, randomized, placebo-controlled clinical trial. *Menopause, 9*(5), 329-334.

Hall, J. (2002). Amenorrhea. In K. Carlson et al. (Eds.), *Primary care of women* (2nd ed.). St. Louis: Mosby.

Han, K., Soares, J., Haidar, M., de Lima, G., & Baracat, E. (2002). Benefits of soy isoflavone therapeutic regimen on menopausal symptoms. *Obstetrics and Gynecology, 99*(3), 389-394.

Harlow, S. (2000). Menstruation and menstrual disorders. In M. Goldman & M. Hatch (Eds.), *Women and health*. San Diego: Academic Press.

Jaffe, R., & Santen, R. (2006). *Hormone therapy for menopausal symptoms: The first few years*. Accessed www.hormone.org, April 11, 2006.

Jones, C. (2001). Premenstrual dysphoric disorder. *Advance for Nurse Practitioners, (March, 2001),* 87-90.

Kaunitz, A. (2002). Menopausal hormone therapy: Where do we go now? *Breast Journal, 8*(6), 329-337.

Klaiber, E., Vogel, W., & Rako, S. (2005). A critique of the WHI hormone therapy study. *Fertility and Sterility, 84*(6), 1589-1601.

Kleposki, R. (2002). The female athlete triad: A terrible trio implications for primary care. *Journal of the American Academy of Nurse Practitioners, 14*(10), 26-31.

Laufer, M., Sanfilippo, J., & Rose, G. (2003). Adolescent endometriosis: Diagnosis and treatment approaches. *Journal of Pediatric and Adolescent Gynecology, 16*(Suppl 3), S3-S11.

Lemaire, G. (2004). More than just menstrual cramps: Symptoms and uncertainty among women with endometriosis. *Journal of Obstetric, Gynecologic, and Neonatal Nursing, 33*(10), 71-79.

Lin, J., & Thompson, D. (2001). Treating premenstrual dysphoric disorder using serotonin agents. *Journal of Women's Health & Gender-Based Medicine, 10*(6), 745-750.

Liu, S., & Lebrun, C. (2006). Effect of oral contraceptives and hormone replacement therapy on bone mineral density in premenopausal and perimenopausal women: A systematic review. *British Journal of Sports Medicine, 40*(1), 11-24.

Motta, G. (2004). Teenage endometriosis. *Advance for Nurses Southwestern States, 6*(9), 32-34.

Nakad, T., & Isaacson, K. (2002). Endometriosis. In K. Carlson, et al. (Eds.), *Primary care of women* (2nd ed.). St. Louis: Mosby.

National Institutes of Health (NIH). (2005). National Institutes of Health state-of-the-science conference statement: Management of menopause-related symptoms. *Annals of Medicine, 142*(12 Part 1), 1003-1013.

National Osteoporosis Foundation (NOF). (2003). *Physician's guide for the prevention and treatment of osteoporosis*. Washington, DC: Author.

National Osteoporosis Foundation (NOF). (2006). *Medication to prevent and treat osteoporosis*. Accessed www.nof.org/patientinfo/medications.htm, April 9, 2006.

National Women's Health Information Center. (2006). *Menopause and hormone therapy*. Accessed www.4women.gov/menopause, April 11, 2006.

Parent-Stevens, L., & Burns, E. (2000). Menstrual disorders. In M. Smith & L. Shimp (Eds.), *20 Common problems in women's health care*. New York: McGraw-Hill.

Proctor, M., & Farquhar, C. (2004). Dysmenorrhoea. *Clinical Evidence, Dec*(12), 2524-2547.

Rapkin, Q. (2003). A review of treatment of premenstrual syndrome and premenstrual dysphoric disorder. *Psychoneuroendocrinology, 28*(Suppl 3), 39-53.

Rossouw, J., Anderson, G., Prentice, R., LaCroix, A., Kooperberg, C., Stefanick, M. et al. (2002). Risks and benefits of estrogen plus progestin in healthy postmenopausal women: Principal results from the Women's Health Initiative randomized control trial. *Journal of the American Medical Association, 288*(3), 321-333.

Sabatini, S. (2001). The female athlete triad. *American Journal of the Medical Sciences, 322*(4), 193-195.

Sanborn, C., Horea, M., Siemens, B., Derringer, B. (2000). Disordered eating and the female athlete triod. *Clinics in Sports Medicine, 19*(2), 199-213.

Sowers, M. (2000). Menopause: Its epidemiology. In M. Goldman & M. Hatch, (Eds.), *Women & health*. San Diego: Academic Press.

Speroff, L., & Fritz, M. (2005). *Clinical gynecologic endocrinology and infertility* (7th ed.). Philadelphia: Lippincott Williams & Wilkins.

Stenchever, M., Droegemueller, W., Herbst, A., & Mishell, D. (2001). *Comprehensive gynecology* (4th ed.). St. Louis: Mosby.

Stokes, M. (2004). Soy and menopausal symptoms. Accessed www.ahcpub.com/hot_topics, April 10, 2006.

Taylor, D., Schuiling, K., & Sharp, B. (2006). Menstrual pain and discomforts. In K. Schuiling & F. Liskis (Eds.), *Women's gynecologic health*. Sudbury, MA: Jones & Bartlett.

United States Public Health Services Task Force. (2005). Screening for osteoporosis in postmenopausal women. In *The Guide to Clinical Preventive Health Services, 2005*. Rockville, MD: Agency for Healthcare Research and Quality.

Upmalis, D., Lobo, R., Bradley, L., Warren, M., Cone, F., & Lamia, C. (2000). Vasomotor symptoms relief by soy isoflavone extract tablets in postmenopausal women: A multicenter, double-blind, randomized, placebo-controlled study. *Menopause, 7(4)*, 236-242.

Wilhelm, S. (2002). Factors affecting a woman's intent to adopt hormone replacement therapy for menopause. *Journal of Obstetric, Gynecologic, and Neonatal Nursing, 31*(6), 698-707.

Zizic, T. (2004). Pharmacologic prevention of osteoporosis. *American Family Physician, 70*(7), 1293-1300.

Catherine Ingram Fogel

Sexually Transmitted and Other Infections

learning objectives

- Describe prevention of sexually transmitted infections in women.
- Differentiate signs, symptoms, diagnosis, and management of nonpregnant and pregnant women with bacterial sexually transmitted infections.
- Examine the care of nonpregnant and pregnant women with selected viral infections (human immunodeficiency virus; hepatitis A, B, and C; human papillomavirus).
- Discuss the effect of group B streptococcus (GBS) on pregnancy and management of pregnant clients with GBS.

- Compare and contrast signs, symptoms, and management of selected vaginal infections in nonpregnant and pregnant women.
- Review principles of infection control for human immunodeficiency virus (HIV) and blood-borne pathogens.
- Describe the health consequences for women who are infected with reproductive tract infections (e.g., sexually transmitted infections and vaginal infections).

electronic resources

Additional information related to the content in Chapter 8 can be found on

the companion website at **evolve**
http://evolve.elsevier.com/Lowdermilk/MWHC/
- NCLEX Review Questions
- WebLinks

or on the interactive companion CD
- NCLEX Review Questions
- Animation: Pelvic Inflammatory Disease
- Plan of Care: Sexually Transmitted Infections

---

*R*eproductive tract infection is a term that encompasses both sexually transmitted infections and other common genital tract infections (Cates, 2004). Sexually transmitted diseases (STDs), or sexually transmitted infections (STIs), include more than 25 infectious organisms that cause infections or infectious disease syndromes primarily transmitted by close, intimate contact (Box 8-1). These terms, used interchangeably in this text, have replaced the older designation, *venereal disease,* which described primarily gonorrhea and syphilis. Caused by a wide spectrum of bacteria, viruses, protozoa, and ectoparasites (organisms that live on the outside of the body, such as a louse), STIs are a direct cause of tremendous human suffering, place heavy demands on health care services, and cost society hundreds of millions of dollars to treat. Despite the U.S. Surgeon General's targeting STIs as a priority for prevention and control efforts, STIs are among the most common health problems in the United States. The Centers for Disease Control and Prevention (CDC) estimates that more than 19 million Americans are infected with

STIs every year (CDC, 2006b). The most common STDs or STIs in women are chlamydia, human papillomavirus, gonorrhea, herpes simplex virus type 2, syphilis, and human immunodeficiency virus (HIV) infection; these are discussed in this chapter. Common vaginal infections are also discussed. Neonatal effects of STIs are discussed in Chapter 38.

■ PREVENTION

Preventing infection (primary prevention) is the most effective way of reducing the adverse consequences of STIs for women and for society. With the advent of serious and potentially lethal STIs that are not readily cured or are incurable, primary prevention becomes critical. Prompt diagnosis and treatment of current infections (secondary prevention) also can prevent personal complications and transmission to others.

Preventing the spread of STIs requires that women at risk for transmitting or acquiring infections change their behavior. A critical first step is for the nurse to include questions about a woman's sexual history, risky sexual behaviors, and drug-related risky behaviors as a part of her assessment (Box 8-2). Techniques that are effective in providing prevention counseling include using open-ended questions, using understandable language, and reassuring the woman that treatment will be provided regardless of consideration such as ability to pay, language spoken, or lifestyle (CDC, Workowski, & Berman, 2006). Prevention messages should include descriptions of specific actions to be taken to avoid acquiring or transmitting STIs (e.g., refrain from sexual activity if you have STI-related symptoms) and should be tailored to the individual woman, with attention given to her specific risk factors.

To be motivated to take preventive actions, a woman must believe that getting a disease will be serious for her and that she is at risk for infection. Unfortunately most individuals tend to underestimate their personal risk of infection in a given situation; thus many women may not perceive themselves as being at risk for contracting an STI, and telling them that they should carry condoms may not be well received. Although levels of awareness of STIs are generally high, widespread misconceptions or specific gaps in knowledge also exist. Therefore nurses have a responsibility to ensure that their clients have accurate, complete knowledge about transmission and symptoms of STIs and risky behaviors that place them at risk for contracting an infection.

Primary preventive measures are individual activities aimed at deterring infection. Risk-free options include complete abstinence from sexual activities that transmit semen, blood, or other body fluids or that allow skin-to-skin contact (CDC et al., 2006). Alternatively, involvement in a mutually monogamous relationship with an uninfected partner also eliminates risk of contracting STIs. When neither of these options is realistic for a woman, however, the nurse must focus on other, more feasible measures.

Safer Sex Practices

An essential component of primary prevention is counseling women regarding safer sex practices, including knowledge of her partner, reduction of number of partners, low risk sex, and avoiding the exchange of body fluids.

---

box 8-1 Sexually Transmitted Infections

BACTERIA
- Chlamydia
- Gonorrhea
- Syphilis
- Chancroid
- Lymphogranuloma venereum
- Genital mycoplasmas
- Group B streptococcus

VIRUSES
- Human immunodeficiency virus
- Herpes simplex virus, types 1 and 2
- Cytomegalovirus
- Viral hepatitis A and viral hepatitis B
- Human papillomavirus

PROTOZOA
- Trichomoniasis

PARASITES
- Pediculosis (may or may not be sexually transmitted)
- Scabies (may or may not be sexually transmitted)

---

box 8-2 Assessing STI and HIV Risk Behaviors

SEXUAL RISK
- Are you sexually active now?
- If no, have you had sex in the past?
- Ever had an oral, vaginal, or anal sexual experience with another person?
- With how many different people? 1? 2 or 3? 4 to 10? More than 10?
- Have your partners been men, women, both?
- Ever thought that a sex partner put you at risk for AIDS or an STI (IV drug user, bisexual)?
- Ever had an STI (herpes, gonorrhea, genital warts, chlamydia)?
- Ever had sex against your will?
- What do you do to protect yourself from AIDS and STIs?
- Do you use male condoms? Female condoms? Other barriers?

DRUG USE–RELATED RISK
- Ever injected drugs using shared equipment, including street drugs, steroids?
- Ever had sex with a person who uses and shares?
- Ever had sex while stoned, high, or drunk, so that you can't remember the details?
- Ever exchanged sex for drugs, money, shelter?

BLOOD-RELATED RISKS
- Ever had a blood transfusion?
- Ever had sex with a person who had a blood transfusion?
- Ever had sex with a person with hemophilia?
- Ever received donor semen, egg, transplanted organ or tissue?
- Ever shared equipment for tattoo, body piercing?

OTHER
- Ever had a test for HIV?
- Ever worried about AIDS and would like to talk with someone about it?

Adapted from Guest, F. (2004). HIV/AIDS and reproductive health. In R. Hatcher, J. Trussell, F. Stewart, A. Nelson, W. Cates, F. Guest, et al. (Eds). *Contraceptive technology* (18th ed.). New York: Ardent Media.
AIDS, Acquired immunodeficiency virus; *HIV,* human immunodeficiency virus; *IV,* intravenous; *STIs,* sexually transmitted infections.

No aspect of prevention is more important than knowing one's partner. Reducing the number of partners and avoiding partners who have had many previous sexual partners decreases a woman's chance of contracting an STI. Deciding not to have sexual contact with casual acquaintances also may be helpful. Discussing each new partner's previous sexual history and exposure to STIs will augment other efforts to reduce risk; however, sexual partners are not always truthful about their sexual history. Women must be cautioned that safer sex measures are always advisable, even when partners insist otherwise. Critically important is whether male partners resist or accept wearing condoms. This is crucial when women are not sure about their partners' history. Women should be cautioned against making decisions about a partner's sexual and other behaviors based on appearances and unfounded assumptions such as the following (Guest, 2004):

- Single people have many partners and risky practices.
- Older people have few partners and infrequent sexual encounters.
- Sexually experienced people know how to practice safer sex.
- Married people are heterosexual, low risk, and monogamous.
- People who look healthy are healthy.
- People with good jobs do not use drugs.

Sexually active persons also may benefit from carefully examining a partner for lesions, sores, ulcerations, rashes, redness, discharge, swelling, and odor before initiating sexual activity.

Women should be taught low risk sexual practices and which sexual practices to avoid (Table 8-1). Sexual fantasizing is safe, as are caressing, hugging, body rubbing, and massage. Mutual masturbation is low risk as long as there is no contact with a partner's semen or vaginal secretions. All sexual activities when both partners are monogamous, trustworthy, and known to be free of disease (by testing) are safe.

The physical barrier promoted for the prevention of sexual transmission of HIV and other STIs is the condom (male and female). Nurses can help motivate clients to use condoms by iniating a discussion of the subject with them. This gives women permission to discuss any concerns, misconceptions, or hesitations they may have about using condoms. Information to be discussed includes the importance of using latex or plastic male condoms rather than natural skin condoms for STI protection. The nurse should remind women to use a condom with every sexual encounter, to use each one only once, to use a condom with a current expiration date, and to handle it carefully to avoid damaging it with fingernails, teeth, or other sharp objects. Condoms should be stored away from high heat. Although it is not ideal, women may choose to safely carry condoms in wallets, shoes, or inside a bra. Women can be taught the differences among condoms: price ranges, sizes, and where they can be purchased. Explicit instructions for how to apply a male condom are included in Box 9-3.

The female condom—a lubricated polyurethane sheath with a ring on each end that is inserted into the vagina—has been shown in laboratory studies to be an effective mechanical barrier to viruses, including HIV. Although no clinical studies have been completed to evaluate the efficacy of female condoms in protecting against STIs, laboratory studies have demonstrated that polyurethane can block smaller viruses such as the herpes virus and HIV (Murphy, Morgan, & Likis, 2006). Further, studies suggest that the female condom is at least as effective as male condoms in preventing transmission of STIs (Hoffman, Mantell, Exner, & Stein, 2004), and the CDC et al., 2006 states that, when used correctly and consistently, the female condom may substantially reduce STI risk and recommends its use when a male condom cannot be used properly. What is important and should be stressed by nurses is the consistent use of condoms for every act of sexual intimacy where there is the possibility of transmission of disease.

Despite recent concern about the potential for cervicovaginal epithelial disruption with nonoxynol-9 (N-9)–based spermicides (Wilkinson, Ramjee, Tholandi, & Rutherford, 2002), interest in vaginally applied chemical barriers that provide dual contraceptive and protection against bacterial STIs remains. Recent evidence has shown that vaginal spermicides do not protect against certain STIs, although more than 60 potential microbicides are in development and 18 are in clinical trials (Murphy et al., 2006). Condoms lubricated with N-9 are not recommended (CDC et al., 2006).

A key issue in condom use as a preventive strategy is to stress to women that in sexual encounters, men must comply with a woman's suggestion or request that they use a condom. Moreover, condom use must be renegotiated with every sexual contact, and women must address the issue of control of sexual decision making every time they request a male partner to use a condom. Women may fear that their partner would be offended if a condom were introduced. Some women may fear rejection and abandonment, conflict, potential violence, or loss of economic support if they suggest the use of condoms to prevent STI transmission. For many individuals, condoms are symbols of extrarelationship activity. Introduction of a condom into a long-term relationship where one has not been used previously threatens the trust assumed in most long-term relationships.

Nurses must suggest strategies to enhance a woman's condom negotiation and communication skills. It can be suggested that she talk with her partner about condom use at a time removed from sexual activity, which may make it easier to bring up the subject. Role playing possible partner reactions with a woman and her alternative responses can be helpful. Asking a woman who appears particularly uncomfortable to rehearse how she might approach the topic is useful, particularly when a woman fears her partner may be resistant. The nurse might suggest her client begin by saying, "I need to talk with you about something that is important to both of us. It's hard for me, and I feel embarrassed, but I think we need to talk about safer sex." If

table 8-1 Safer Sex Guidelines

SAFEST	LOW RISK	POSSIBLY RISKY (POSSIBLE EXPOSURE)	HIGH RISK (UNSAFE)
BEHAVIOR			
Abstinence	Wet kissing*	Cunnilingus†	Unprotected anal intercourse
Self-masturbation	Vaginal intercourse with	Fellatio‡	Unprotected vaginal
Monogamous (both partners	condom	Mutual masturbation with skin	intercourse
and no high risk activities)	Anal intercourse with	breaks	Oral-anal contact
Hugging,* massage,* touching*	condom	Vaginal intercourse after	Any sex (fisting, rough vaginal
Dry kissing	Urine contact with intact skin	anal contact without new	or anal intercourse, rape)
Mutual masturbation§		condom	that causes tissue damage
Drug abstinence			or bleeding
Sexual fantasy			Multiple sexual partners
Erotic conversation, books,			Sharing sex toys, douche
movies, video			equipment
Erotic bathing, showering			Sharing needles
Eroticizing feet, fingers,			Blood contact, including
buttocks, abdomen, ears			menstrual blood
PREVENTION			
Avoid high risk behaviors	Avoid exposure to potentially	Use dental dam or female	Avoid exposure to potentially
	infected body fluids	condom with cunnilingus	infected body fluids
	Consistent use of condom	Use condom with fellatio	Use condom and spermicide
	and spermicide	Use latex gloves	consistently
	Avoid anal intercourse		Avoid anal penetration
			If anal penetration occurs, use
			condom with intercourse,
			latex glove with hand
			penetration
			Avoid oral-anal contact
			Do not share sex toys,
			needles, douching
			equipment
			If sharing needles, clean with
			bleach before and after use

Adapted from Centers for Disease Control and Prevention, Workowski, K., & Berman, S. (2006). Sexually transmitted diseases treatment guidelines, 2006. *MMWR Morbidity and Mortality Weekly Report, 55*(RR11), 1-94; Fogel, C. (2003). Female sexuality. In E. Breslin & V. Lucas (Eds.), *AWHONN women's health nursing: Toward evidence-based practice.* Philadelphia: Saunders.
*Assumes no breaks in skin.
†Cunnilingus: oral stimulation of the female genitalia.
‡Fellatio: oral stimulation of the male genitalia.
§Assumes no contact with semen or vaginal secretions.

women are able to sort out their feelings and fears before talking with their partners, they may feel more comfortable and in control of the situation. Women can be reassured that it is natural to be uncomfortable and that the hardest part is getting started. Nurses should help their clients clarify what they will and will not do sexually because it will be easier to discuss their concerns with their partners if they have thought about what to say. Women can be reminded that their partner may need time to think about what they have said and that they must pay attention to their partner's response. If the partner seems to be having difficulty with the discussion, a woman may slow down and wait a while. She can be reminded that if her partner resists safer sex, she may wish to reconsider the relationship.

Many women do not anticipate or prepare for sexual activity in advance; embarrassment or discomfort in purchasing condoms may prevent some women from using them. Cultural barriers also may impede the use of condoms; for example, Latino gender roles make it difficult for Latina women to suggest using condoms to a partner. In general, suggesting condom use implies that a woman is sexually active, that she is "available" for sex, and that she is "seeking" sex; these are messages that many women are uncomfortable conveying, given the prevailing mores of our country. In a society that commonly views a woman who carries a condom as overprepared, possibly oversexed, and willing to have sex with any man, expecting her to insist on the use of condoms in a sexual encounter is somewhat optimistc at best and unrealistic at worst.

Finally, women should be counseled to watch out for situations that make it hard to talk about and to practice safer sex. These include romantic times when condoms are not available and when alcohol or drugs make it impossible to make wise decisions about safer sex.

Certain sexual practices should be avoided to reduce one's risk of infection. Abstinence from any sexual activities that could result in exchange of infective body fluids will help decrease risk. Anal-genital intercourse, anal-oral contact, and anal-digital activity are high risk sexual behaviors and should be avoided. Sexual transmission occurs through direct skin or mucous membrane contact with infectious lesions or body fluids. Because mucosal linings are delicate and subject to considerable mechanical trauma during intercourse, small abrasions often may occur, facilitating entry of infectious agents into the bloodstream. The rectal epithelium is especially easy to traumatize with penetration. Sexual practices that increase the likelihood of tissue damage or bleeding, such as fisting (inserting a fist into the rectum), should be avoided. Deep kissing when lips, gums, or other tissues are raw or broken also should be avoided (Guest, 2004). Because enteric infections are transmitted by oral-fecal contact, avoiding oral-anal activities, "rimming" (licking the anal area), and anal-digital activities should reduce the likelihood of infection. Vaginal intercourse should never follow anal contact unless a condom has been used and then removed and replaced with a new condom.

BACTERIAL SEXUALLY TRANSMITTED INFECTIONS

Chlamydia

Chlamydia trachomatis is the most common and fastest spreading STI in American women (CDC et al., 2006). These infections are often silent and highly destructive; their sequelae and complications can be very serious. In women, chlamydial infections are difficult to diagnose; the symptoms, if present, are nonspecific, and the organism is expensive to culture.

Early identification of *C. trachomatis* is important because untreated infection often leads to acute salpingitis or pelvic inflammatory disease. Pelvic inflammatory disease is the most serious complication of chlamydial infections, and past chlamydial infections are associated with an increased risk of ectopic pregnancy and tubal factor infertility. Furthermore, chlamydial infection of the cervix causes inflammation, resulting in microscopic cervical ulcerations, and thus may increase the risk of acquiring HIV infection. More than half of infants born to mothers with chlamydia will develop conjunctivitis or pneumonia after perinatal exposure to the mother's infected cervix. *C. trachomatis* is the most common infectious cause of ophthalmia neonatorum. Neonatal ocular prophylaxis with silver nitrate solution or antibiotic ointment does not prevent perinatal transmission from mother to infant, nor does it adequately treat chlamydial infection (see Chapter 38). Sexually active women younger than 20 years are 2 to 3 times as likely to become infected with chlamydia as are women between 20 and 29 years. Women older than 30 years have the lowest rate of infection. Risky behaviors, including multiple partners and nonuse of barrier methods of birth control, increase a woman's risk of chlamydial infection. Lower socioeconomic status may be a risk factor, especially with respect to treatment-seeking behaviors.

Screening and Diagnosis

In addition to obtaining information regarding the presence of risk factors, the nurse should inquire about the presence of any symptoms. The CDC and others (2006) and U.S. Preventive Services Task Force (USPSTF, 2005b) strongly recommends screening of asymptomatic women at high risk in whom infection would otherwise go undetected (see websites CDC, www.cdc.org, and USPSTF, www.ahrq.gov). CDC guidelines recommend screening of all sexually active adolescents, women between ages 20 and 25 years, and women older than 25 years who are at high risk (e.g., those with new or multiple partners). In addition, whenever possible, all women with two or more of the risk factors for chlamydia should be cultured. All pregnant women should have cervical cultures for chlamydia at the first prenatal visit. Screening late in the third trimester (36 weeks) may be carried out if the woman was positive previously, or if she is younger than 25 years, has a new sex partner, or has multiple sex partners.

Although chlamydial infections are usually asymptomatic, some women may experience spotting or postcoital bleeding, mucoid or purulent cervical discharge, or dysuria. Bleeding results from inflammation and erosion of the cervical columnar epithelium. Women taking oral contraceptives also may have breakthrough bleeding.

Diagnosis of chlamydia is by culture (expensive and labor intensive), deoxyribonucleic acid (DNA) probe (less expensive but less sensitivity), enzyme immunoassay (less expensive but less sensitivity), and nucleic acid amplification (expensive but about 90% sensitivity) (Rawlins, 2001). The chlamydial culture procedure requires collection of a sample that contains many epithelial cells. Endocervical (columnar) cells are required; cell scrapings provide better specimens, so the cervix should be swabbed with cotton or rayon swabs before collecting the specimen to remove mucus and discharge from the cervical os. Special culture media and proper handling of specimens are important, so the nurse should always know what is required in her individual practice site. Chlamydial culture testing is not always available, primarily because of expense.

Management

The CDC recommendations for treatment of urethral, cervical, and rectal chlamydial infections, which are summarized in Table 8-2, are doxycycline (100 mg orally twice a day for 7 days) or azithromycin (1 g orally in a single dose) (CDC et al., 2006). Azithromycin is often prescribed when compliance may be a problem, because only one dose is needed; however, expense is a concern with this medication. If the woman is pregnant, erythromycin (500 mg orally 4 times a day for 7 days) or amoxicillin (500 mg orally 3 times a day for 7 days) is used. Women who have a chlamydial infection and also are infected with

HIV should be treated with the same regimen as those who are not infected with HIV.

Because chlamydia is often asymptomatic, the woman should be cautioned to take all medication prescribed. All exposed sexual partners should be treated. Woman treated with recommended or alternative regimens do not need to be retested unless symptoms continue. It is recommended that pregnant women be retested 3 weeks after completing the medication, although the validity of this practice has not been established (CDC, et al., 2006).

table 8-2 Sexually Transmitted Infections and Drug Therapies for Women*

DISEASE	NONPREGNANT WOMEN (13-17 YR)	NONPREGNANT WOMEN (>18 YR)	PREGNANT WOMEN	LACTATING WOMEN‡
Chlamydia	*Recommended:* Azithromycin, 1 g orally once or Doxycycline, 100 mg orally bid for 7 days *Alternatives:* Erythromycin base, 500 mg orally qid 7 days or Erythromycin ethylsuccinate, 800 mg orally qid for 7 days or Ofloxacin, 300 mg orally bid for 7 days or Levofloxacin, 500 mg orally for 7 days	*Recommended:* Azithromycin, 1 g orally once or Doxycycline, 100 mg orally bid for 7 days *Alternatives:* Erythromycin base, 500 mg orally qid 7 days or Erythromycin ethylsuccinate, 800 mg orally qid for 7 days or Ofloxacin, 300 mg orally bid for 7 days or Levofloxacin, 500 mg orally for 7 days	*Recommended:* Azithromycin, 1 g orally once or Amoxicillin, 500 mg orally tid for 7 days *Alternatives:* Erythromycin base, 500 mg orally qid for 7 days or Erythromycin base, 250 mg orally qid for 14 days or Erythromycin ethylsuccinate, 800 mg orally qid for 14 days or Erythromycin ethylsuccinate, 400 mg orally qid for 14 days	*Recommended:* Azithromycin, 1 g orally once or Amoxicillin, 500 mg orally tid for 7 days *Alternatives:* Erythromycin base, 500 mg orally qid for 7 days or Erythromycin base, 250 mg orally qid for 14 days or Erythromycin ethylsuccinate, 800 mg orally qid for 7 days or Erythromycin ethylsuccinate, 400 mg orally qid for 14 days
Gonorrhea	*Recommended:* Ceftriaxone, 125 mg IM once (Adolescents who weigh >45 kg can be treated with any regimen recommended for adults)	*Recommended:* Ceftriaxone, 125 mg IM once or Cefiximine 400 mg orally once or Ciprofloxacin, 500 mg orally once or Ofloxacin, 400 mg orally once or Levofloxacin, 250 mg orally once PLUS† Azithromycin, 1 g orally once or other treatment for chlamydia *Alternatives:* Spectinomycin, 2 g IM once	*Recommended:* Ceftriaxone, 125 mg IM once If cephalosporin-allergic, spectinomycin, 2 g IM once PLUS† Azithromycin, 1 g orally once or other treatment for chlamydia	*Recommended:* Ceftriaxone, 125 mg IM once If cephalosporin-allergic, spectinomycin, 2 g IM once PLUS† Azithromycin, 1 g orally once or other treatment for chlamydia
Syphilis	Primary, secondary, early latent disease:	Primary, secondary, early latent disease:	Primary, secondary, early latent disease:	Primary, secondary, early latent disease:

Source: American Academy of Pediatrics Committee on Drugs. (2002). The transfer of drugs and other chemicals into human milk. *Pediatrics, 108*(3), 776-789; Centers for Disease Control and Prevention et al.,2006. Sexually transmitted diseases treatment guidelines, 2006. *MMWR Morbidity and Mortality Weekly Report, 55*(RR11), 1-94.
*List may not be inclusive of all drugs that may be used as alternatives.
†If chlamydial infection not ruled out, treatment is recommended.
bid, Twice daily; *IM,* intramuscularly; *qid,* four times daily.
‡These medications are usually compatible with breastfeeding.

Continued

table 8-2 Sexually Transmitted Infections and Drug Therapies for Women*—cont'd				
DISEASE	NONPREGNANT WOMEN (13-17 YR)	NONPREGNANT WOMEN (>18 YR)	PREGNANT WOMEN	LACTATING WOMEN‡
Syphilis—cont'd	*Recommended:* Benzathine penicillin G, 2.4 million units IM once Late latent or unknown duration disease: *Recommended:* Benzathine penicillin G, 7.2 million units total, administered as three doses, 2.4 million units each, at 1-wk intervals Penicillin allergy: Doxycycline, 100 mg orally bid for 14 days *or* Tetracycline, 500 mg orally qid for 14 days	*Recommended:* Benzathine penicillin G, 2.4 million units IM once Late latent or unknown duration disease: *Recommended:* Benzathine penicillin G, 7.2 million units total, administered as three doses, 2.4 million units each, at 1-wk intervals Penicillin allergy: Doxycycline, 100 mg orally qid for 14 days *or* Tetracycline, 500 mg orally qid for 14 days	*Recommended:* Benzathine penicillin G, 2.4 million units IM once (some experts recommend a second dose of benzathine penicillin, 2.4 million units, 1 wk later) Late latent or unknown duration disease: *Recommended:* Benzathine penicillin G, 7.2 million units total, administered as three doses, 2.4 million units each, at 1-wk intervals No proven alternatives to penicillin in pregnancy. Pregnant women who have a history of allergy to penicillin should be desensitized and treated with penicillin	*Recommended:* Benzathine penicillin G, 2.4 million units IM once
Human papillomavirus	Recommended for external genital warts: Client-applied Podofilox, 0.5% solution, or gel to wart bid for 3 days followed by 4-day rest for ≤4 cycles *or* Imiquimod, 5% cream, at hs 3 times a week for ≤16 wk Provider-applied: Cryotherapy with liquid nitrogen or cryoprobe *or* Podophyllin resin, 10%-25% in tincture of benzoin compound weekly (wash off in 1-4 hr). Repeat weekly as necessary *or* TCA or BCA 80%-90% weekly	Recommended for external genital warts: Client-applied Podofilox, 0.5% solution, or gel to wart bid for 3 days followed by 4-day rest for ≤4 cycles *or* Imiquimod, 5% cream, at hs 3 times a week for ≤16 wk Provider-applied: Cryotherapy with liquid nitrogen or cryoprobe *or* Podophyllin resin, 10%-25% in tincture of benzoin compound weekly (wash off in 1-4 hr). Repeat weekly as necessary *or* TCA or BCA 80%-90% weekly	Recommended for external genital warts: Provider applied: Cryotherapy with liquid nitrogen or cryoprobe *or* TCA or BCA 80%-90% weekly Imiquimod, podophyllin, and podofilox should not be used in pregnancy	Recommended for external genital warts: Provider applied: Cryotherapy with liquid nitrogen or cryoprobe *or* TCA or BCA 80%-90% weekly Imiquimod, podophyllin, and podofilox should not be used during lactation

BCA, Bichloroacetic acid; *hs,* at bedtime; *TCA,* trichloroacetic acid.

Gonorrhea

Gonorrhea is probably the oldest communicable disease in the United States. An estimated 600,000 American men and women contract gonorrhea each year (CDC et al., 2006). The incidence of drug-resistant cases of gonorrhea, in particular, penicillinase-producing *Neisseria gonorrhoeae* (PPNG), is increasing dramatically in the United States.

Gonorrhea is caused by the aerobic, gram-negative diplococcus, *N. gonorrhoeae.* Gonorrhea is almost exclusively transmitted by sexual contact. The principal means of communication is genital-to-genital contact; however, it also is spread by oral-to-genital and anal-to-genital contact. There also is evidence that infection may spread in females from vagina to rectum. Gonorrhea also can be transmitted to the newborn in the form of ophthalmia neonatorum during birth by direct contact with gonococcal organisms in the cervix.

Age is probably the most important risk factor associated with gonorrhea. In the United States, the highest reported rates of infection are among sexually active

table 8-2 **Sexually Transmitted Infections and Drug Therapies for Women*—cont'd**

DISEASE	NONPREGNANT WOMEN (13-17 YR)	NONPREGNANT WOMEN (>18 YR)	PREGNANT WOMEN	LACTATING WOMEN‡
Genital herpes simplex virus (HSV type I or 2)	*Primary infection:* Acyclovir, 400 mg orally tid for 7-10 days or Acyclovir, 200 mg orally 5 times a day for 7-10 days or Famciclovir, 250 mg orally tid for 7-10 days or Valacyclovir, I g orally bid for 7-10 days *Recurrent infection:* Acyclovir, 400 mg orally tid for 5 days or Acyclovir, 800 mg orally bid for 5 days or Acyclovir, 800 mg orally tid for 2 days or Famciclovir, 125 mg orally bid for 5 days or Valacyclovir, 500 mg orally bid for 5 days *Suppression therapy:* Acyclovir, 400 mg orally bid or Famciclovir, 250 mg orally bid or Valacyclovir, 500 mg orally once a day or Valacyclovir, I g orally once a day	*Primary infection:* Acyclovir, 400 mg orally tid for 7-10 days or Acyclovir, 200 mg orally 5 times a day for 7-10 days or Famciclovir, 250 mg orally tid for 7-10 days or Valacyclovir, I g orally bid for 7-10 days *Recurrent infection:* Acyclovir, 400 mg orally tid for 5 days or Acyclovir, 800 mg orally bid for 5 days or Acyclovir, 800 mg orally tid for 2 days or Famciclovir, 125 mg orally bid for 5 days or 1000 mg orally bid for I day or Valacyclovir, 500 mg orally bid for 5 days or I g orally once a day for 5 days *Suppression therapy:* Acyclovir, 400 mg orally bid or Famciclovir, 250 mg orally bid or Valacyclovir, 500 mg orally once a day or Valacyclovir, I g orally once a day	No increase in birth defects beyond the general population has been found with acyclovir use in pregnancy Acyclovir, 400 mg orally tid for 7 days for first episode or severe recurrent infection. May be given IV if infection is severe.	Acyclovir usually is considered compatible with breastfeeding Acyclovir, 400 mg tid for 7 days

tid, three times daily; *bid,* twice a day; *IV,* intravenous.
*These medications are usually compatible with breastfeeding.

teenagers, young adults, and African-Americans. The majority of those contracting gonorrhea are younger than age 20 years and engage in sexual activities with multiple partners (CDC, 2005b).

Women are often asymptomatic, with one third of infections in adolescent women going unnoticed; when symptoms are present, they are often less specific than are the symptoms in men. Women may have a purulent endocervical discharge, but discharge is usually minimal or absent. Menstrual irregularities may be the presenting symptom, or women may complain of pain—chronic or acute severe pelvic or lower abdominal pain or longer, more painful menses. Infrequently, dysuria, vague abdominal pain, or low backache prompts a woman to seek care. Gonococcal rectal infection may occur in women after anal intercourse, with 10% to 30% of urogenital infections accompanied by rectal infection. Individuals with rectal gonorrhea may be completely asymptomatic or, conversely, have severe symptoms with profuse purulent anal discharge, rectal pain, and blood in the stool. Rectal itching, fullness, pressure, and pain also are common symptoms, as is diarrhea. A diffuse vaginitis with vulvitis is the most common form of gonococcal infection in prepubertal girls. There may be few signs of infection, or vaginal discharge, dysuria, and swollen, reddened labia may be present.

Gonococcal infections in pregnancy potentially affect both mother and infant. In women with cervical gonorrhea, salpingitis may develop in the first trimester. Perinatal complications of gonococcal infection include premature rupture of membranes, preterm birth, chorioamnionitis, neonatal sepsis, intrauterine growth restriction, and maternal postpartum sepsis. Amniotic infection syndrome manifested by placental, fetal, and umbilical cord inflammation after premature rupture of the membranes may result from gonorrheal infections during pregnancy. Ophthalmia neonatorum, the most common manifestation of neonatal gonococcal infections, is highly contagious and, if untreated, may lead to blindness of the newborn (see Chapter 38).

Screening and Diagnosis

Because gonococcal infections in women often are asymptomatic, the CDC recommends screening all women at risk for gonorrhea (CDC et al., 2006). All pregnant women should be screened at the first prenatal visit, and infected women and those identified with risky behaviors rescreened at 36 weeks of gestation. Gonococcal infection cannot be diagnosed reliably by clinical signs and symptoms alone. Individuals may have "classic" symptoms, vague symptoms that may be attributed to a number of conditions, or no symptoms at all. Cultures with selective media are considered the gold standard for diagnosis of gonorrhea. Cultures should be obtained from the endocervix, the rectum, and when indicated, the pharynx. Thayer-Martin cultures are recommended to diagnose gonorrhea in women. Any woman suspected of having gonorrhea should have a chlamydial culture and serologic test for syphilis if one has not been done in the past 2 months, because coinfection is common.

Management

Management of gonorrhea is straightforward, and the cure is usually rapid with appropriate antibiotic therapy (see Table 8-2). Single-dose efficacy is a major consideration in selecting an antibiotic regimen for women with gonorrhea. Another important consideration is the high percentage (45%) of women with coexisting chlamydial infections. The treatment of choice for uncomplicated urethral, endocervical, and rectal infections in pregnant and nonpregnant women is cefixime (one oral dose of 400 mg) or ceftriaxone (125 mg intramuscularly [IM] once). The CDC recommends concomitant treatment for chlamydia because coinfection is common (CDC et al., 2006). All women with both gonorrhea and syphilis should be treated for syphilis according to CDC guidelines (see discussion of syphilis in this chapter).

Gonorrhea is a highly communicable disease. Recent (past 30 days) sexual partners should be examined, cultured, and treated with appropriate regimens. Most treatment failures result from reinfection. The client must be informed of this, as well as of the consequences of reinfection in terms of chronicity, complications, and potential infertility. Women are counseled to use condoms. All clients with gonorrhea should be offered confidential counseling and testing for HIV infection.

■ **LEGAL TIP** Reporting Communicable Diseases

Gonorrhea is a reportable communicable disease. Health care providers are legally responsible for reporting all cases to the health authorities, usually the local health department in the client's county of residence. Women should be informed that the case will be reported, told why, and informed of the possibility of being contacted by a health department epidemiologist.

Syphilis

Syphilis, one of the earliest described STIs, is caused by *Treponema pallidum,* a motile spirochete. Transmission is thought to be by entry in the subcutaneous tissue through microscopic abrasions that can occur during sexual intercourse. The disease also can be transmitted through kissing, biting, or oral-genital sex. Transplacental transmission may occur at any time during pregnancy; the degree of risk is related to the quantity of spirochetes in the maternal bloodstream.

Rates of syphilis in the United States declined among women and African-Americans since 1995 but in 2004 did not decrease. Rates of syphilis continue to be high in southern states (CDC, 2005b).

Syphilis is a complex disease that can lead to serious systemic disease and even death when untreated. Infection manifests itself in distinct stages with different symptoms and clinical manifestations. *Primary* syphilis is characterized by a primary lesion, the chancre, that appears 5 to 90 days after infection; this lesion often begins as a painless papule at the site of inoculation and then erodes to form a nontender, shallow, indurated, clean ulcer several millimeters to centimeters in size (Fig. 8-1). *Secondary* syphilis occurs 6 weeks to 6 months after the appearance of the chancre and is characterized by a widespread, symmetric maculopapular rash on the palms and soles and generalized lymphadenopathy. The infected individual also may experience fever, headache, and malaise.

Condylomata lata (broad, painless, pink-gray, wartlike infectious lesions) may develop on the vulva, the perineum, or the anus. If the woman is untreated, she enters a latent phase that is asymptomatic for the majority of individuals. If it is left untreated, tertiary syphilis will develop in about one third of these women. Neurologic, cardiovascular, musculoskeletal, or multiorgan system complications can develop in the third stage.

Screening and Diagnosis

All women who are diagnosed with another STI or with HIV should be screened for syphilis. All pregnant women should be screened for syphilis at the first prenatal visit and again in early third trimester and at the time of giving birth if high risk (CDC et al., 2006). Diagnosis is dependent on microscopic examination of primary and secondary lesion tissue and serology during latency and late infection. A test for antibodies may not be reactive in the presence of active

FIG. 8-1 Syphilis. **A,** Primary stage: chancre with inguinal adenopathy. **B,** Secondary stage: condylomata lata.

infection because it takes time for the body's immune system to develop antibodies to any antigens. Up to one third of people in early primary syphilis may have nonreactive serologic tests. Two types of serologic tests are used: nontreponemal and treponemal. Nontreponemal antibody tests such as the VDRL (Venereal Disease Research Laboratories) or RPR (rapid plasma reagin) are used as screening tests. False-positive results are not unusual, particularly when conditions such as acute infection, autoimmune disorders, malignancy, pregnancy, and drug addiction exist and after immunization or vaccination. The treponemal tests, fluorescent treponemal antibody absorbed (FTA-ABS) and microhemagglutination assays for antibody to *T. pallidum* (MHA-TP), are used to confirm positive results. Test results in clients with early primary or incubating syphilis may be negative. Seroconversion usually takes place 6 to 8 weeks after exposure, so testing should be repeated in 1 to 2 months when a suggestive genital lesion exists.

Tests for concomitant STIs (e.g., chlamydia and gonorrhea) should be done (e.g., wet preps and cultures) and HIV testing offered if indicated.

Management

Penicillin is the preferred drug for treating clients with syphilis (see Table 8-2). It is the only proven therapy that has been widely used for clients with neurosyphilis, congenital syphilis, or syphilis during pregnancy.

Intramuscular benzathine penicillin G (2.4 million units IM once) is used to treat primary, secondary, and early latent syphilis. Women with syphilis of longer than 1 year's duration (late latent or tertiary stages) require weekly treatment of 2.4 million units of benzathine penicillin G for 3 weeks. Although doxycycline, tetracycline, and erythromycin are alternative treatments for penicillin-allergic clients, both tetracycline and doxycycline are contraindicated in pregnancy, and erythromycin is unlikely to cure a fetal infection. Therefore pregnant women should, if necessary, receive skin testing and be treated with penicillin or be desensitized (CDC et al., 2006). Specific protocols are recommended by the CDC.

■ NURSE ALERT

Clients treated for syphilis may experience a Jarisch-Herxheimer reaction. This acute febrile reaction is often accompanied by headache, myalgias, and arthralgias that develop within the first 24 hours of treatment. The reaction may be treated symptomatically with analgesics and antipyretics. If the treatment precipitates this reaction in the second half of pregnancy women are at risk for preterm labor and birth. They should be advised to contact their health care provider if they notice any change in fetal movement or have any contractions.

Monthly follow-up is mandatory so that repeated treatment may be given if needed. The nurse should emphasize the necessity of long-term serologic testing even in the absence of symptoms. The woman should be advised to practice sexual abstinence until treatment is completed, all evidence of primary and secondary syphilis is gone, and serologic evidence of a cure is demonstrated. Women should be told to notify all partners who may have been exposed. They should be informed that the disease is reportable. Preventive measures should be discussed.

Pelvic Inflammatory Disease

Pelvic inflammatory disease (PID) is an infectious process that most commonly involves the uterine (fallopian) tubes (salpingitis), uterus (endometritis), and more rarely, the ovaries and peritoneal surfaces. Multiple organisms have been found to cause PID, and most cases are associated with more than one organism. In the past, the most common causative agent was thought to be *N. gonorrhoeae*; however, *C. trachomatis* is now estimated to cause half of all cases of PID. In addition to gonorrhea and chlamydia, a wide variety of anaerobic and aerobic bacteria are recognized to cause PID. PID encompasses a wide variety of pathologic processes; the infection can either be acute, subacute, or chronic and can have a wide range of symptoms.

Most PID results from ascending spread of microorganisms from the vagina and endocervix to the upper genital tract. This spread most frequently happens at the end of or just after menses following reception of an infectious agent. During the menstrual period, several factors facilitate the development of an infection: the cervical os is slightly open, the cervical mucus barrier is absent, and menstrual blood is an excellent medium for growth. PID also may develop after a miscarriage or an induced abortion, pelvic surgery, or childbirth.

CD: Animation: PID

Risk factors for acquiring PID are those associated with the risk of contracting an STI, including young age, nulliparity, multiple partners, high rate of new partners, and a history of STIs. Women who use intrauterine devices (IUDs) may be at increased risk for PID if they have more than one sexual partner or if the partner has other sexual partners, because they are at higher risk for acquiring an STI (World Health Organization [WHO], 2000). Most of this risk occurs in the first months after IUD insertion. PID tends to recur.

Women who have had PID are at increased risk for ectopic pregnancy, infertility, and chronic pelvic pain. After a single episode of PID, a woman's risk for ectopic pregnancy increases sevenfold compared with the risk for women who have never had PID. Other problems associated with PID include dyspareunia (painful intercourse), pyosalpinx (pus in the uterine tubes), tuboovarian abscess, and pelvic adhesions.

The symptoms of PID vary depending on whether the infection is acute, subacute, or chronic; however, pain is common to all clinical presentations. It may be dull, cramping, and intermittent (subacute) or severe, persistent, and incapacitating (acute). The woman with acute PID also may complain of intermenstrual bleeding. Physical examination reveals adnexal tenderness, with or without rebound, and exquisite tenderness with cervical movement (Chandelier sign). Pelvic tenderness is usually bilateral. There may or may not be a palpable adnexal swelling or thickening. A urethral or cervical discharge, often purulent, may be present. A fever of 39° C or above is characteristic. Significant laboratory data include an elevated white blood cell count and markedly elevated erythrocyte sedimentation rate. Fever and peritonitis are more characteristic of gonococcal PID; PID caused by other organisms is more likely to be "silent." Because PID caused by chlamydia is more commonly asymptomatic, it more often results in tubal obstruction from delayed diagnosis or inadequate treatment.

Subacute PID is far less dramatic, with great variety in the severity and extent of symptoms. At times these are so mild and vague that the woman ignores them. Symptoms that suggest subacute PID are chronic lower abdominal pain, dyspareunia, menstrual irregularities, urinary discomfort, low-grade fever, low backache, and constipation. Abdominal examination usually reveals no rebound tenderness; there is slight adnexal tenderness with cervical movement, and cervical or urethral discharge may be present.

Screening and Diagnosis

A careful history is necessary to distinguish between PID and other conditions that cause abdominal pain, such as an ectopic pregnancy or appendicitis. A menstrual history is useful in establishing the relation of onset of pain to menses and in identifying any variations from normal in the cycle. Other relevant history includes recent pelvic surgery, birth, induced abortion, or dilation of the cervix; purulent

vaginal discharge; irregular bleeding; and a longer, heavier menstrual period. A sexual history will assist in identifying possible increased risk for STI exposure. Symptoms of an STI in a woman's partner(s) also should be noted.

Vital signs are obtained, and a complete physical examination performed. Criteria for diagnosing PID include oral temperature greater than 38.3° C, abnormal cervical or vaginal discharge, elevated erythrocyte sedimentation rate, and laboratory documentation of cervical infection with *N. gonorrhoeae* or *C. trachomatis* (CDC et al., 2006). Physical findings of lower abdominal tenderness, bilateral adnexal tenderness, and cervical motion tenderness are important in making a clinical diagnosis of PID. Essential laboratory data are a complete blood count with differential and cervical cultures for gonorrhea and chlamydia.

Management

Perhaps the most important nursing intervention is prevention counseling. Primary prevention includes education in avoiding acquisition of STIs, whereas secondary prevention involves preventing a lower genital tract infection from ascending to the upper genital tract. Instructing women in self-protective behaviors such as practicing safer sex and using barrier methods is critical. Women using hormonal contraception or the IUD and those who have chosen tubal ligation must be reminded to use a condom with intercourse when indicated. Also important is the detection of asymptomatic gonorrheal and chlamydial infections through routine screening of women who practice risky behaviors or have specific risk factors such as young age. Partner notification when an STI is diagnosed is essential to prevent reinfection.

When and if women with PID are hospitalized varies. The CDC recommends hospitalization in the following situations (CDC et al., 2006):

- Surgical emergencies such as appendicitis cannot be excluded.
- The woman has a tuboovarian abscess.
- The woman is pregnant.
- Severe illness precludes outpatient management.
- The woman is unable to tolerate or follow an outpatient oral regimen.
- The woman has failed to respond to oral outpatient therapy.

Although many experts recommend that all women with PID be hospitalized so parenteral antibiotic treatment can be done, the CDC does not.

Although treatment regimens vary with the infecting organism, a broad-spectrum antibiotic generally is used. Several antimicrobial regimens have proved to be effective, and no single therapeutic regimen of choice exists (Table 8-3). The woman with acute PID should be on bed rest in a semi-Fowler's position. Comfort measures include analgesics for pain and all other nursing measures applicable to a client confined to bed. Few pelvic examinations should be done during the acute phase of the disease. During the recovery phase, the woman should restrict her

table 8-3	Treatment of Pelvic Inflammatory Disease

	TREATMENT OF CHOICE	ALTERNATIVES
Parenteral regimen	Cefotetan, 2 g IV every 12 hr or Cefoxitin, 2 g IV every 6 hr PLUS Doxycycline, 100 mg IV or orally every 12 hr	Clindamycin, 900 mg IV every 8 hr PLUS Gentamycin, loading dose IV or IM (2 mg/kg of body weight), followed by maintenance dose (1.5 mg/kg) every 8 hr. Single daily dosing may be substituted
Oral regimen	Ofloxacin, 400 mg orally bid for 14 days or Levofloxacin, 500 mg orally once a day for 14 days WITH OR WITHOUT Metronidazole, 500 mg orally twice a day for 14 days	Ceftriaxone, 250 mg IM in a single dose or Cefoxitin, 2 g IM AND Probenecid, 1 g orally in a single dose, concurrently or Other parenteral third-generation cephalosporin PLUS Doxycycline, 100 mg orally twice a day for 14 days WITH OR WITHOUT Metronidazole, 500 mg orally twice a day for 14 days

Source: Centers for Disease Control and Prevention et al., 2006. Sexually transmitted diseases treatment guidelines 2006. *MMWR Morbidity and Mortality Weekly Report, 55*(RR11), 1-94.
bid, Twice daily; *IM*, intramuscularly; *IV*, intravenously.

activity and make every effort to get adequate rest and a nutritionally sound diet. Follow-up laboratory work after treatment should include endocervical cultures for a test of cure.

Health education is central to effective management of PID. Nurses should explain the nature of the disease to women and should encourage them to comply with all therapy and prevention recommendations, emphasizing the necessity of taking all medication, even if symptoms disappear. Any potential problems (such as lack of money for prescriptions or lack of transportation to return to the clinic for follow-up appointments) that would prevent a woman from completing a course of treatment should be identified, referrals made for assistance as needed, and the importance of follow-up visits stressed. Women should be counseled to refrain from sexual intercourse until their treatment is completed. Contraceptive counseling should be provided, including barrier methods such as condoms, contraceptive sponge, or diaphragm. A woman with a history of PID should not choose an IUD as her contraceptive method.

The woman with PID may be acutely ill or have long-term discomfort. Either or both take an emotional toll. Pain in itself is debilitating and is compounded by the infectious process. The potential or actual loss of reproductive capabilities can be devastating and can adversely affect the woman's self-concept. Part of the nurse's role is to help the woman adjust her self-concept to fit reality and to accept alterations in a way that promotes health. Because PID is so closely tied to sexuality, body image, and self-concept, the woman diagnosed with it will need supportive care. Her feelings should be discussed and her partner(s) included when appropriate.

■ VIRAL SEXUALLY TRANSMITTED ■ INFECTIONS

Human Papillomavirus

Human papillomavirus (HPV) infections, also known as *condylomata acuminata*, or *genital warts*, is the most common viral STI seen in ambulatory health care settings. An estimated 20 million Americans are infected with HPV, and about 6.2 million new infections occur every year (CDC, 2005a). HPV, a double-stranded DNA virus, has more than 30 serotypes that can be sexually transmitted, five of which are known to cause genital wart formation, and eight of which are currently thought to have oncogenic potential (CDC et al., 2006). HPV is the primary cause of cervical neoplasia (American Cancer Society, 2006).

In women, HPV lesions (also called condylomata acuminata) are most frequently seen in the posterior part of the introitus; however, lesions also are found on the buttocks, the vulva, the vagina, the anus, and the cervix (Fig. 8-2). Typically the lesions are small—2 to 3 mm in diameter and 10 to 15 mm in height—soft, papillary swellings occurring singly or in clusters on the genital and anal-rectal region. Infections of long duration may appear as a cauliflower-like mass. In moist areas such as the vaginal introitus, the lesions may appear to have multiple, fine, fingerlike projections. Vaginal lesions are often multiple. Flat-topped papules, 1 to 4 mm in diameter, are seen most often on the cervix. Often these lesions are visualized only under magnification. Warts are usually flesh colored or slightly darker on Caucasian women, black on African-American women, and brownish on Asian women. Usually painless, the lesions also may be uncomfortable, particularly when very

FIG. 8-2 Human papillomavirus infection. Genital warts or condylomata acuminata.

large, inflamed, or ulcerated. Chronic vaginal discharge, pruritus, or dyspareunia can occur.

HPV infections are thought to be more frequent in pregnant than in nonpregnant women, with an increase in incidence from the first trimester to the third. Furthermore, a significant proportion of preexisting HPV lesions enlarge greatly during pregnancy, a proliferation presumably resulting from the relative state of immunosuppression present during pregnancy. Lesions may become so large during pregnancy that they affect urination, defecation, mobility, and fetal descent, although birth by cesarean is rarely necessary (Thomas, 2001). Cesarean birth may be performed when extensive growths are present. Initial observation of large growths can be misleading, suggesting that the entire vagina is involved; however, all of the growth may derive from one stalk, and in such cases, it may be possible to push the large mass to the side, allowing the baby to pass through. HPV infection may be acquired by the neonate during birth; the frequency of such transmission is unknown. The preventive value of cesarean birth is unknown, and it is not recommended solely to prevent transmission of HPV infection to newborns (American College of Obstetricians and Gynecologists [ACOG], 2005).

Screening and Diagnosis

A woman with HPV lesions may complain of symptoms such as a profuse, irritating vaginal discharge, itching, dyspareunia, or postcoital bleeding. She also may report "bumps" on her vulva or labia. History of a known exposure is important; however, because of the potentially long latency period and the possibility of subclinical infections in men, the lack of a history of known exposure cannot be used to exclude a diagnosis of HPV infection.

Physical inspection of the vulva, the perineum, the anus, the vagina, and the cervix is essential whenever HPV lesions are suspected or seen in one area. Because speculum examination of the vagina may block some lesions, it is important to rotate the speculum blades until all areas are visualized. When lesions are visible, the characteristic appearance previously described is considered diagnostic.

However, in many instances, cervical lesions are not visible, and some vaginal or vulvar lesions also may be unobservable to the naked eye. Because of the potential spread of vulvar or vaginal lesions to the anus, gloves should be changed between vaginal and rectal examinations.

Viral screening and typing for HPV is available but not standard practice. History, evaluation of signs and symptoms, Papanicolaou (Pap) test, and physical examination are used in making a diagnosis. The HPV-DNA test can be used in women over the age of 30 in combination with the Pap test to screen for types of HPV that are likely to cause cancer or in women with abnormal Pap test results (ACOG, 2005; ACS, 2006). The only definitive diagnostic test for presence of HPV is histologic evaluation of a biopsy specimen.

HPV lesions must be differentiated from molluscum contagiosum and condylomata lata. Molluscum contagiosum lesions are half-domed, smooth, flesh-colored to pearly white papules with depressed centers. Condylomata lata are a form of secondary syphilis and generally are flatter and wider than genital warts. A serologic test for syphilis would confirm the diagnosis of secondary syphilis.

Management

Untreated warts may resolve on their own in young women since their immune systems may be strong enough to fight the HPV infection. Treatment of genital warts, if needed, is often difficult. No therapy has been shown to eradicate HPV. The goal of treatment therefore is removal of warts and relief of signs and symptoms, not the eradication of HPV (CDC et al., 2006). The client often must make multiple office visits; frequently, many different treatment modalities will be used. Eradication of the virus is not considered conclusive even after there is no visible evidence of wart tissue because of the high incidence of recurrence.

Treatment of genital warts should be guided by preference of the woman, available resources, and experience of the health care provider. None of the treatments is superior to all other treatments, and no one treatment is ideal for all warts (CDC et al., 2006). Available treatments are outlined in Table 8-2. Imiquimod, podophyllin, and podofilox should not be used during pregnancy. Because the lesions can proliferate and become friable during pregnancy, many experts recommend their removal by using cryotherapy or various surgical techniques during pregnancy (CDC et al., 2006).

Women with discomfort associated with genital warts may find that bathing with an oatmeal solution and drying the area with a cool hair dryer will provide some relief. Keeping the area clean and dry will also decrease growth of the warts. Cotton underwear and loose-fitting clothes that decrease friction and irritation also may decrease discomfort. Women should be advised to maintain a healthy lifestyle to aid the immune system; women can be counseled regarding diet, rest, stress reduction, and exercise.

Client counseling is essential. Women must understand how the virus is transmitted, that no immunity is conferred with infection, and that reacquisition of the infection is likely with repeated contact. Women should know that their partners should be checked even if they are asymptomatic. Because HPV is highly contagious, the majority of women's partners will be infected and should be treated. All sexually active women with multiple partners or a history of HPV should be encouraged to use latex condoms for intercourse to decrease acquisition or transmission of condylomata.

Instructions for all medications and treatments must be detailed. Women should be informed before treatment of the possibility of posttreatment pain associated with specific therapies. The importance of thorough treatment of concurrent vaginitis or STI should be emphasized. The link between cervical cancer and HPV infections and the need for close follow-up should be discussed. Annual health examinations are recommended to assess disease recurrence and screening for cervical cancer. Women should be counseled to have regular Pap screening, as recommended for women without genital warts. The presence of genital warts is not an indication for a change in Pap test frequency or for cervical colposcopy (CDC et al., 2006).

Women with HPV infection may radically alter their sexual practices both from fear of transmission to and from a partner and from genital discomfort associated with treatment, which may have a negative impact on their sexual relationships. Unless the partner accepts and understands the necessary precautions, it may be difficult for the woman to follow the treatment regimen. The nurse can offer to discuss feelings that the woman may have. When indicated, joint counseling can be suggested.

Prevention

Preventive strategies that have been suggested include abstinence from all sexual activity, staying in a long-term monogamous relationship, and prophylactic vaccination (ACOG, 2005). A vaccine against HPV (types 6, 11, 16, 18) become available in 2006 and is recommended for females ages 9 to 26 years. Vaccines for other HPV types continue to be investigated (CDC et al., 2006). Practitioners should stay current with results of these clinical trials and make recommendations about vaccination based on the outcomes of the research.

Herpes Simplex Virus

Unknown until the middle of the twentieth century, herpes simplex virus (HSV) infection is now widespread in the United States, especially in women. HSV infection results in painful recurrent genital ulcers and is caused by two different antigen subtypes of herpes simplex virus: herpes simplex virus 1 (HSV-1) and herpes simplex virus 2 (HSV-2). HSV-2 is usually transmitted sexually, and HSV-1, nonsexually. Although HSV-1 is more commonly associated with gingivostomatitis and oral labial ulcers (fever blisters) and HSV-2 with genital lesions, neither type is exclusively associated with the respective sites.

Although HSV infection is not a reportable disease, it is estimated that about 50 million people in the United States are infected with genital herpes (CDC et al., 2006). Recurrent HSV infections are much more common. Most persons infected with HSV-2 have not been diagnosed, and most infections are transmitted by persons unaware that they are infected.

An initial HSV genital infection is characterized by multiple painful lesions, fever, chills, malaise, and severe dysuria and may last 2 to 3 weeks. Women generally have a more severe clinical course than men. Women with primary genital herpes have many lesions that progress from macules to papules, then forming vesicles, pustules, and ulcers that crust and heal without scarring (Fig. 8-3). These ulcers are extremely tender, and primary infections may be bilateral. Women also may have itching, inguinal tenderness, and lymphadenopathy. Severe vulvar edema may develop, and women may have difficulty sitting. HSV cervicitis also is common with initial HSV-2 infections. The cervix may appear normal or be friable, reddened, ulcerated, or necrotic. A heavy, watery-to-purulent vaginal discharge is common. Extragenital lesions may be present because of autoinoculation. Urinary retention and dysuria may occur secondary to autonomic involvement of the sacral nerve root.

Women with recurrent episodes of HSV infections commonly have only local symptoms that are usually less severe than those associated with the initial infection. Systemic symptoms are usually absent, although the characteristic prodromal genital tingling is common. Recurrent lesions are unilateral, are less severe, and usually last 5 to 7 days. Lesions begin as vesicles and progress rapidly to ulcers. Few women with recurrent disease have cervicitis.

During pregnancy, maternal infection with HSV-2 can have adverse effects on both the mother and fetus. Viremia occurs during the primary infection, and congenital infection is possible, though rare. Primary infections during the first trimester have been associated with increased miscarriage rates. The most severe complication of HSV infection is neonatal herpes, a potentially fatal or severely disabling disease occurring in 1 in 2000 to 1 in 10,000 live births.

FIG. 8-3 Herpes genitalis.

Most mothers of infants who contract neonatal herpes lack histories of clinically evident genital herpes. Risk of neonatal infection is highest among women with primary herpes infection who are near term and is low among women with recurrent herpes (CDC et al., 2006).

An association between cervical cancer and HSV-2 has been observed. It is theorized that genital herpes is a marker for high risk sexual behaviors that could transmit other STIs, including HPV (DiSaia & Creasman, 2002).

Screening and Diagnosis

A careful history provides much information when making a diagnosis of herpes. A history of exposure to an infected person is important, although infection from an asymptomatic individual is possible. A history of having viral symptoms such as malaise, headache, fever, or myalgia is suggestive. Local symptoms such as vulvar pain, dysuria, itching or burning at the site of infection, and painful genital lesions that heal spontaneously also are highly suggestive of HSV infections. The nurse should ask about a history of a primary infection, prodromal symptoms, vaginal discharge, and dyspareunia. Pregnant women should be asked whether they or their partner(s) have had genital lesions.

During the physical examination, the nurse should assess for inguinal and generalized lymphadenopathy and elevated temperature. The entire vulvar, perineal, vaginal, and cervical areas should be carefully inspected for vesicles or ulcerated or crusted areas. A speculum examination may be very difficult for the woman because of the extreme tenderness often associated with herpes infections. Any suggestive or recurrent lesions found during pregnancy should be cultured to verify HSV. Although a diagnosis of herpes infection may be suspected from the history and physical, it is confirmed by laboratory studies. A viral culture is obtained by swabbing exudate during the vesicular stage of the disease. In primary HSV infection, viral shedding is prolonged, and HSV is more easily isolated.

Management

Genital herpes is a chronic and recurring disease for which there is no known cure. Management is directed toward specific treatment during primary and recurrent infections, prevention, self-help measures, and psychologic support.

Systemic antiviral medications partially control the symptoms and signs of HSV infections when used for the primary or recurrent episodes or when used as daily suppressive therapy. However, these medications do not eradicate the infection, nor do they alter subsequent risk, frequency, or recurrences after the medication is stopped. Three antiviral medications provide clinical benefit: acyclovir, valacyclovir, and famciclovir. Treatment recommendations are given in Table 8-2. The safety of acyclovir, valacyclovir, and famciclovir therapy during pregnancy has not been established; however, acyclovir may be used to reduce the symptoms of HSV if the benefits to the woman

outweigh the potential harm to the fetus (CDC et al., 2006). Continued investigation of HSV therapy with these medications in pregnancy is needed.

Cleaning lesions twice a day with saline will help prevent secondary infection. Bacterial infection must be treated with appropriate antibiotics. Measures that may increase comfort for women when lesions are active include warm sitz baths with baking soda; keeping lesions dry by blowing the area dry with a hair dryer set on cool or patting dry with a soft towel; wearing cotton underwear and loose clothing; using drying aids such as hydrogen peroxide, Burow's solution, or oatmeal baths; applying cool, wet, black tea bags to lesions; and applying compresses with an infusion of cloves or peppermint oil and clove oil to lesions.

Oral analgesics such as aspirin or ibuprofen may be used to relieve pain and systemic symptoms associated with initial infections. Because the mucous membranes affected by herpes are extremely sensitive, any topical agents should be used with caution. Nonantiviral ointments, especially those containing cortisone, should be avoided. A thin layer of lidocaine ointment or an antiseptic spray may be applied to decrease discomfort, especially if walking is difficult.

A diet rich in vitamin C, B-complex vitamins, zinc, and calcium is thought to help prevent recurrences. The amino acid l-lysine has been used in doses of 750 to 1000 mg daily while lesions are active and 500 mg during asymptomatic periods. It is thought that l-lysine has an inhibitory effect on the multiplication of the HSV.

Counseling and education are critical components of the nursing care of women with herpes infections. Information regarding the etiology, signs and symptoms, transmission, and treatment should be provided. The nurse should explain that each woman is unique in her response to herpes and emphasize the variability of symptoms. Women should be helped to understand when viral shedding and thus transmission to a partner is most likely, and that they should refrain from sexual contact from the onset of prodrome until complete healing of lesions. Some authorities recommend consistent use of condoms for all persons with genital herpes. Condoms may not prevent transmission, particularly male-to-female transmission; however, this does not mean that the partners should avoid all intimacy. Women can be encouraged to maintain close contact with their partners while avoiding contact with lesions. Women should be taught how to look for herpetic lesions with a mirror and good light source and a wet cloth or finger covered with a finger cot to rub lightly over the labia. The nurse should ensure that women understand that when lesions are active, sharing intimate articles (e.g., washcloths, wet towel) that come into contact with the lesions should be avoided. Plain soap and water is all that is needed to clean hands that have come in contact with herpetic lesions; isolation is not necessary or appropriate.

The nurse should explain the role of precipitating factors in the reactivation of the latent virus and recurrent episodes. Stress, menstruation, trauma, febrile illnesses, chronic illness, and ultraviolet light have all been found to trigger genital herpes. Women may wish to keep a diary to identify stressors that seem to be associated with recurrent herpes attacks so that they can then avoid these stressors when possible. The role of exercise in reducing stress can be discussed. Referral for stress-reduction therapy, yoga, or meditation classes may be indicated. Avoiding excessive heat and sun and hot baths and using a lubricant during sexual intercourse to reduce friction also may be helpful. Women in their childbearing years should be counseled regarding the risk of herpes infection during pregnancy. They should be instructed to use condoms if there is any risk of contracting any STI from a sexual partner. If they become pregnant while taking acyclovir, the risk of birth defects does not appear to be higher than for the general population; however continued use should be based on whether the benefits for the woman outweigh the possible risks to the fetus. Acyclovir does enter breast milk but the amount of medication ingested during breastfeeding is very low and is usually not a health concern (Organization of Teratology Information Services, 2003.)

Because neonatal HSV infection is such a devastating disease, prevention is critical. Current recommendations include carefully examining and questioning all women about symptoms at onset of labor (CDC et al., 2006). If visible lesions are not present at onset of labor, vaginal birth is acceptable. Cesarean birth within 4 hours after labor begins or membranes rupture is recommended if visible lesions are present. Infants who are delivered through an infected vagina should be carefully observed and cultured (see Chapter 38). Because HSV infection may be associated with cervical dysplasia, women must be encouraged to have yearly Pap tests and gynecologic examinations.

The emotional impact of contracting herpes is considerable. Media publicity regarding this disease has made receiving a diagnosis of genital herpes a devastating experience. No cure is available, and most women will experience recurrences. At diagnosis, many emotions may surface–helplessness, anger, denial, guilt, anxiety, shame, or inadequacy. Women need the opportunity to discuss their feelings and help in learning to live with the disease. A woman can be encouraged to think of herself as a person who is not diseased but rather healthy and inconvenienced from time to time. Herpes can affect a woman's sexuality, her sexual practices, and her current and future relationships. She may need help in raising the issue with her partner or with future partners.

Viral Hepatitis

Five different viruses (hepatitis viruses A, B, C, D, and E) account for almost all cases of viral hepatitis in humans. Hepatitis viruses A, B, and C are discussed. Hepatitis D and E viruses, common among users of intravenous drugs and recipients of multiple blood transfusions, are not included in this discussion.

Hepatitis A

Hepatitis A virus (HAV) infection is acquired primarily through a fecal-oral route by ingestion of contaminated food, particularly milk, shellfish, or polluted water, or person-to-person contact. Women living in the western United States, Native-Americans, Alaska Natives, and children and employees in day care centers are at high risk. Hepatitis A, like other enteric infections, also can be transmitted during sexual activity.

HAV infection is characterized by flulike symptoms with malaise, fatigue, anorexia, nausea, pruritus, fever, and right upper quadrant pain. Serologic testing to detect the immunoglobulin M (IgM) antibody is done to confirm acute infections. The IgM antibody is detectable 5 to 10 days after exposure and can remain positive for up to 6 months. Because HAV infection is self-limited and does not result in chronic infection or chronic liver disease, treatment is usually supportive. Women who become dehydrated from nausea and vomiting or who have fulminating hepatitis A may need to be hospitalized. Medications that might cause liver damage or that are metabolized in the liver (e.g., acetaminophen, ethyl alcohol) should be avoided. A well-balanced diet is recommended. Hepatitis A vaccine is recommended for women at high risk for being exposed to HAV infection. The safety of the vaccine has not been established in pregnancy; therefore, immune globulin (gamma-globulin) or immune-specific globulin is indicated for a pregnant woman exposed to HAV. All household contacts of the woman also should receive gamma-globulin (CDC et al., 2006).

Hepatitis B

Hepatitis B virus (HBV) is the virus most threatening to the fetus and neonate. It is caused by a large DNA virus and is associated with three antigens and their antibodies: hepatitis B surface antigen (HBsAg), HBV antigen (HBeAg), and HBV core antigen (HBcAg), and antibody to HBsAg (anti-HBs), antibody to HBeAg (anti-HBe), and antibody to HBcAg (anti-HBc). Screening for active or chronic disease or disease immunity is based on testing for these antigens and their antibodies.

Populations at risk include women of Asian, Pacific Island (Polynesian, Micronesian, Melanesian), or Alaskan-Eskimo descent and women born in Haiti or sub-Saharan Africa. Women who have a history of acute or chronic liver disease, who work or receive treatment in a dialysis unit, or who have household or sexual contact with a hemodialysis client are at greater risk. Women who work or live in institutions for the mentally challenged are considered to be at risk, as are women with a history of multiple blood transfusions. Health care workers and public safety workers exposed to blood in the workplace are at risk. Behaviors such as multiple sexual partners and a history of intravenous drug use increase the risk of contracting HBV infections.

HBsAg has been found in blood, saliva, sweat, tears, vaginal secretions, and semen. Drug abusers who share needles are at risk, as are health care workers who are exposed to blood and needlesticks. Perinatal transmission most often occurs in infants of mothers who have acute hepatitis infection late in the third trimester or during the intrapartum or postpartum periods from exposure to HBsAg-positive vaginal secretions, blood, amniotic fluid, saliva, and breast milk. HBV has also been transmitted by artificial insemination. Although HBV can be transmitted via blood transfusion, the incidence of such infections has decreased significantly since testing of blood for HBsAg became routine.

HBV infection is a disease of the liver and is often a silent infection. In the adult, the course of the infection can be fulminating, and the outcome, fatal. Symptoms of HBV infection are similar to those of hepatitis A: arthralgias, arthritis, lassitude, anorexia, nausea, vomiting, headache, fever, and mild abdominal pain. Later the woman may have clay-colored stools, dark urine, increased abdominal pain, and jaundice. Between 5% and 10% of individuals with HBV have persistence of HBsAg and become chronic hepatitis B carriers.

Screening and Diagnosis. All women at high risk for contracting HBV should be screened on a regular basis. Screening only individuals at high risk may not identify up to 50% of HBsAg-positive women; therefore screening for the presence of HBsAg is recommended on all women at the first prenatal visit, regardless of whether they have been tested previously, and should be repeated later in pregnancy or on admission for labor and birth for women with high risk behaviors (USPSTF, 2005c).

Testing for HBV is complex. Clients with acute hepatitis B generally have detectable serum HBsAg levels in the late incubation phase of the disease, 2 to 5 weeks before symptoms appear. Anti-HBs with a negative HBsAg test signals immunity. Anti-HBs with a positive antigen denotes a chronic carrier state; during this time, the disease can be transmitted. During the recovery phase, the client may continue to be infectious even though HBsAg cannot be detected. This is called the "window phase" and is identified by anti-HBc in the absence of anti-Hbs. Women should be prepared for repeated testing because HBV screening tests also may be used to monitor the progression of the disease.

Components of the history to be obtained when hepatitis B is suspected include the inquiry about the symptoms of the disease and risk factors outlined earlier. Physical examination includes inspection of the skin for rashes, inspection of the skin and conjunctiva for jaundice, and palpation of the liver for enlargement and tenderness. Weight loss, fever, and general debilitation should be noted. If the HBsAg is positive, further laboratory studies may be ordered (anti-HBe, anti-HBc, serum glutamic-oxaloacetic transaminase [SGOT], alkaline phosphatase, and liver panel). If the HBsAg is negative in early pregnancy and the woman could be in the window phase or if high risk behaviors continue during pregnancy, a repeated HBsAg should be ordered in the third trimester.

Management. There is no specific treatment for hepatitis B. Recovery is usually spontaneous in 3 to 16 weeks. Pregnancies complicated by acute viral hepatitis are managed on an outpatient basis. Women should be advised to increase bed rest; eat a high-protein, low-fat diet; and increase their fluid intake. They should avoid medications metabolized in the liver, and alcohol. Pregnant women with a definite exposure to HBV should be given hepatitis B immune globulin and should begin the hepatitis B vaccine series within 14 days of the most recent contact to prevent infection (CDC et al., 2006). Vaccination during pregnancy is not thought to pose risks to the fetus.

All nonimmune women at high or moderate risk of hepatitis should be informed of the availability of hepatitis B vaccine. Vaccination is recommended for all individuals who have had multiple sex partners within the past 6 months (CDC et al., 2006). In addition, intravenous drug users, residents of correctional or long-term care facilities, persons seeking care for an STI, prostitutes, women whose partners are intravenous drug users or bisexual, and women whose occupation exposes them to high risk should be vaccinated. The vaccine is given in a series of three (four if rapid protection is needed) doses over a 6-month period, with the first two doses given at least 1 month apart. The vaccine is given in the deltoid muscle (CDC).

Client education includes explaining the meaning of hepatitis B infection, including transmission, state of infectivity, and sequelae. The nurse also should explain the need for immunoprophylaxis for household members and sexual contacts. To decrease transmission of the virus, women with hepatitis B or who test positive for HBV should be advised to maintain a high level of personal hygiene (e.g., wash hands after using the toilet; carefully dispose of tampons, pads, bandages in plastic bags; do not share razor blades, toothbrushes, needles, manicure implements; have male partner use a condom if unvaccinated and without hepatitis; avoid sharing saliva through kissing, or sharing of silverware or dishes; wipe up blood spills immediately with soap and water). They should inform all health care providers of their carrier state. Postpartum women should be reassured that breastfeeding is not contraindicated if their infants received prophylaxis at birth and are currently on the immunization schedule.

Hepatitis C

Hepatitis C virus (HCV) infection, the most common bloodborne infection in the United States, has become an important health problem as increasing numbers of persons acquire the disease with an estimated 3 million persons chronically infected (National Institutes of Health [NIH] Consensus Statement on Management of Hepatitis C, 2002). The most common risk factor for pregnant women is a history of injecting intravenous drugs. Other risk factors include STIs such as hepatitis B and HIV, multiple sexual partners, and a history of blood transfusions. Although the role of sexual activity in transmission of HCV is controversial, several studies have demonstrated that sexual activity is associated with HCV transmission, particularly with increasing numbers of sexual partners, failure to use a condom, history of STI such as hepatitis B and HIV, heterosexual sex with a male intravenous drug user , and sexual activities involving trauma (NIH; Terrault, 2002). No association has been documented between HCV and exposure resulting from medical, dental, or surgical procedures; tattooing; acupuncture; ear piercing; foreign travel; or military service (CDC, 2001).

Most clients with hepatitis C are asymptomatic or have general flulike symptoms similar to hepatitis A. About 10% have fatigue, nausea, and anorexia. HCV infection is confirmed by the presence of anti-C antibody during laboratory testing. Routine HCV testing is recommended for women who have ever injected drugs; women who received a blood transfusion prior to July 1992; children of HCV-positive women; health care, emergency, medical, and public safety workers; and women with chronic liver disease (CDC et al., 2006).

Interferon alfa-2b alone or with ribaviran for 6 to 12 months is the main therapy for HCV infection, although effectiveness of this treatment varies. In addition, drug-abuse treatment is an important adjunct for many persons with HCV (CDC et al., 2006).

Currently there is no vaccine to prevent hepatitis C. Transmission of HCV through breastfeeding has not been reported.

Human Immunodeficiency Virus

Although HIV has traditionally been thought to be a homosexual or gay disease, heterosexual transmission is now the most common means of transmission in women. Furthermore, women are now the fastest-growing population of individuals with HIV infection and acquired immunodeficiency syndrome (AIDS). An estimated 27% of new infections occur in women (CDC, 2006a). African-American women are estimated to have 50% of these infections, Hispanic women are estimated to have 15%, and Caucasian women have an estimated 32% (CDC, 2005a).

Transmission of HIV, a retrovirus, occurs primarily through exchange of body fluids (semen, blood or, less commonly, vaginal secretions). Severe depression of the cellular immune system associated with HIV infection characterizes AIDS. For both men and women, the most frequently reported opportunistic diseases are *Pneumocystis carinii* pneumonia (PCP), candida esophagitis, and wasting syndrome. Other viral infections such as HSV and cytomegalovirus infections seem to be more prevalent in women than men (Williams, 2003). PID may be more severe in HIV-infected women, and rates of HPV and cervical dysplasia may be higher. The clinical course of HPV infection in women with HIV infection is accelerated, and recurrence is more frequent.

Once HIV enters the body, seroconversion to HIV positivity usually occurs within 6 to 12 weeks. Although HIV seroconversion may be totally asymptomatic, it usually is accompanied by a viremic, influenza-like response.

CRITICAL THINKING EXERCISE

HIV Counseling

Estella is a 23-year-old Hispanic who has come for her first prenatal visit. She is about 11 weeks pregnant. As you interview her, you collect data that indicate she may be at risk for having a sexually transmitted infection (STI). You provide information and counseling about laboratory tests that are available to determine if she has HIV or another STI. She asks why she should have the test for HIV since there is nothing she can do about it if she tests positive. How would you respond?

1. Evidence: Is there sufficient evidence to draw conclusions about what advice the nurse should give to Estella?
2. Assumptions: Describe underlying assumptions about the following issues:
   a. Perinatal transmission of HIV
   b. Universal prenatal counseling and voluntary testing for HIV
   c. Antiviral therapy and elective cesarean birth to reduce perinatal transmission
3. What implications and priorities for nursing care can be made at this time?
4. Does the evidence objectively support your conclusion?
5. Are there alternative perspectives to your conclusion?

Symptoms include fever, headache, night sweats, malaise, generalized lymphadenopathy, myalgias, nausea, diarrhea, weight loss, sore throat, and rash.

Laboratory studies may reveal leukopenia, thrombocytopenia, anemia, and an elevated erythrocyte sedimentation rate. HIV has a strong affinity for surface-marker proteins on T lymphocytes. This affinity leads to significant T-cell destruction. Both clinical and epidemiologic studies have shown that declining CD_4 levels are strongly associated with increased incidence of AIDS-related diseases and death in many different groups of HIV-infected persons.

Transmission of the virus from mother to child can occur throughout the perinatal period. Exposure may occur to the fetus through the maternal circulation as early as the first trimester of pregnancy, to the infant during labor and birth by inoculation or ingestion of maternal blood and other infected fluids, or to the infant through breast milk (Lawrence & Lawrence, 2005; Riordan, 2005).

Screening and Diagnosis

Screening, teaching, and counseling regarding HIV risk factors, indications for being tested, and testing are major roles for nurses caring for women today. A number of behaviors place women at risk for HIV infection, including intravenous drug use, high risk sexual partners, multiple sex partners, and a previous history of multiple STIs. HIV infection is usually diagnosed by using HIV-1 and HIV-2 antibody tests. Antibody testing is first done with a sensitive screening test such as the enzyme immunoassay (EIA). Reactive screening tests must be confirmed by an additional test, such as the Western blot or an immunofluorescence assay. If a positive antibody test is confirmed by a supplemental test, it means that a woman is infected with HIV and is capable of infecting others. HIV antibodies are detectable in at least 95% of clients within 3 months after infection. Although a negative antibody test usually indicates that a person is not infected, antibody tests cannot exclude recent infection. Because HIV antibody crosses the placenta, definite diagnosis of HIV in children younger than 18 months is based on laboratory evidence of HIV in blood or tissues by culture, nucleic acid, or antigen detection (CDC et al., 2006).

The FDA has approved two methods of rapid testing for HIV. OraQuick Rapid HIV Antibody tests can use a blood sample obtained by fingerstick or venipuncture or an oral fluid sample to provide test results within 20 minutes, with an accuracy rate over 99%. If the results are reactive, further testing is done (Centers for Disease Control and Prevention, Divisions of HIV/AIDS Prevention, 2004; U.S. Food and Drug Administration [FDA], 2004). Quicker results mean that clients don't have to make extra visits for follow-up standard tests, and the oral test provides an option for clients who do not want to have a blood test.

The CDC and others (2006) and the USPSTF (2005a) recommend offering HIV testing to all women whose behavior places them at risk for HIV infection. It may be useful to allow women to self-select for HIV testing. On entry to the health care system, a woman can be handed written information about the risk factors for the AIDS virus and asked to inform the nurse if she believes she is at risk. She should be told that she does not have to say why she may be at risk, only that she thinks she might be.

All pregnant women should be offered counseling and HIV testing as early in pregnancy as possible (ACOG, 2004; CDC et al., 2006; USPSTF, 2005d). This recommendation is essential because of the available treatments that can reduce the likelihood of perinatal transmission and maintain the health of the woman. The ACOG and the CDC also recommend that HIV testing become a part of standard prenatal blood tests unless the woman declines or "opts out"; however, there are legal and ethical concerns related to not obtaining specific informed consent for HIV testing (USPSTF, 2005d). The ACOG and the CDC also recommend retesting in the third trimester for women known to be at high risk for HIV and rapid HIV testing in labor for women with unknown HIV status.

Counseling for HIV Testing

Counseling before and after HIV testing is standard nursing practice today. It is a nursing responsibility to assess a woman's understanding of the information such a test would provide and to be sure the client thoroughly understands the emotional, legal, and medical implications of a positive or negative test before she is ready to take an HIV test. One's life is profoundly altered by knowledge of HIV seropositivity. A unique stigma associated with HIV infection can have a profound impact on the quality of life of those infected. This stigma extends to those who are asymptomatic but seropositive (Black & Miles, 2002).

Given the strong social stigma attached to HIV infection, nurses must consider the issue of confidentiality and documentation before providing counseling and offering HIV testing to clients.

■ **LEGAL TIP** HIV Testing

If test results are placed in the woman's chart—the appropriate place for all health information—they are available to all who have access to the chart. The woman must be informed of this before testing. Informed consent must be obtained before an HIV test is performed. In some states, written consent is mandated.

■ **NURSE ALERT** Counseling for HIV Testing

Counseling associated with HIV testing has two components: pretest and posttest counseling. During pretest counseling, nurses conduct a personalized risk assessment, explain the meaning of positive and negative test results, obtain informed consent for HIV testing, and help women develop a realistic plan for reducing risk and preventing infection. Posttest counseling includes informing the woman of the test results, reviewing the meaning of the results, and reinforcing infection prevention messages. All pretest and posttest counseling should be documented.

Unless rapid testing is done, there is generally a 1-week to 3-week waiting period after testing for HIV, which can be a very anxious time for the woman. It is helpful if the nurse informs her that this time period between blood drawing and test results is routine. Test results, whatever they are, always must be communicated in person, and women need to be informed in advance that such is the procedure. Whenever possible, the person who provided the pretest counseling also should tell the woman her test results. Some women, when informed of negative results, may escalate their risk behaviors because of an equating of negativity with immunity. Others may believe that negative means "bad" and positive means "good." Women's reactions to a negative test should be explored, such as by asking, "How do you feel?" HIV-negative result counseling sessions are another opportunity to provide education. Emphasis can be placed on ways in which a woman can remain HIV free. She should be reminded that if she has been exposed to HIV in the past 6 months, she should be retested, and that if she continues high risk behaviors, she should have ongoing testing.

In posttest counseling to an HIV-positive woman, privacy with no interruptions is essential. Adequate time for the counseling sessions also should be provided. The nurse should make sure that the woman understands what a positive test means and review the reliability of the test results. Safer sex guidelines should be reemphasized. Referral for appropriate medical evaluation and follow-up should be made, and the need or desire for psychosocial or psychiatric referrals should be assessed.

The importance of early medical evaluation so that a baseline assessment can be made and prophylactic medication begun should be stressed. If possible, the nurse should make a referral or appointment for the woman at the posttest counseling session.

EVIDENCE-BASED PRACTICE

Prenatal HIV Screening: U.S. Preventive Services Task Force Review

BACKGROUND

- It is estimated that the mother-to-child transmission rate of human immunodeficiency virus (HIV) from an untreated HIV-positive mother giving birth vaginally is from 18% to 26%. Breastfeeding further increases transmission. In the United States, screening for HIV during pregnancy remains voluntary. Women who decline testing do not receive optimal prophylactic treatment to prevent mother-to-child (vertical) transmission. Prophylactic interventions include: prenatal treatment with antiviral medications; cesarean birth; avoidance of breastfeeding; and avoidance of risky behaviors such as smoking, unprotected intercourse, and drug abuse.

OBJECTIVES

- The U.S. Preventive Services Task Force commissioned a new review of available evidence of the risks and benefits of prenatal HIV screening. The major clinical outcome was mother-to-child transmission of HIV. Research questions regarded the effect of prenatal screening on perinatal outcomes, the accuracy of the tests, risks and benefits of screening and treatments, the utilization of the screening, the efficacy of drug regimens, and the effectiveness of promoting cesarean birth, formula feeding, and safer behavior.

METHODS

Search Strategy

- The reviewers searched available databases and sources. Randomized, controlled trials, cohort studies, diagnostic accuracy studies, and case-controlled studies were included if they met quality criteria. Each questions had its own relevant studies. Studies ranged from 1983 to 2004, and came predominantly from United States, Australia, Canada, and Western Europe, where HIV management is similar. The authors included research from Africa, Thailand, and the Bahamas on antiviral prophylaxis.

Statistical Analyses

- The data for each research question was meta-analyzed separately. A table was developed to analyze outcome predictions for low, medium, and high risk populations. These included estimates of the number needed to screen and needed to treat to prevent one case of vertical transmission. The confidence interval was set at 95% for each set of data.

FINDINGS

- Risk factors: High risk sexual behavior, intravenous drug use, and transfusion history between 1978 and 1985 increased risk for HIV.
- Antiviral medications: Serious side effects were rare. Multidrug regimens were more effective at preventing mother-to-child transmission. Lower maternal viral loads were less likely to result in vertical transmission than high viral loads. Longer duration of regimens was more effective than shorter duration. Long-term side effects for mother and baby were unknown, although one study showed no ill effects six years after ziduvodine.

- Avoidance of breastfeeding: Two meta-analyses showed a 14-16% increase in transmission with breastfeeding.
- Elective Cesarean birth (prior to rupture of membranes): Vertical transmission was reduced by 50% or more. This effect was dramatically enhanced when combined with antiviral therapy. Cesarean birth patients are subject to post-operative complications.
- Harm from screening: Positive results can cause anxiety, relationship strain, and discrimination. Initial false-positives caused unnecessary intervention. False-negatives could theoretically lead to risky behavior. One study showed no increase in intimate partner violence with a positive HIV diagnosis. Women were not more likely to seek abortion after a positive HIV result.
- Uptake of screening: Women were much more likely to accept screening if it was part of an "opt-out" policy (where HIV screening was the default).
- Accuracy of screening: The enzyme immunoassay, followed by the Western blot, is the gold standard, but the rapid tests were very accurate and well-accepted by women, and convenient for initiating prophylaxis immediately.
- Harm from treatment: Serious side effects were rare. No fetal abnormalities or low birth weights were noted after treatment. The evidence was equivocal on incidence of preterm births after therapy.

LIMITATIONS

- The heterogeneity of the studies and the breadth of the research questions made this a huge undertaking. The ethical problem remains: How to investigate with randomized, controlled trials when treatment might save lives. No trial linked prenatal HIV screening directly to health outcomes. Although cost was not addressed directly, the authors have calculated the number needed to screen and treat in order to stop one case of vertical transmission.

IMPLICATIONS FOR PRACTICE

- Prenatal HIV screening benefits infants. Prophylactic measures of early antiviral use, cesarean birth, and avoidance of breastfeeding reduces perinatal transmission of HIV from a high of 26% to a low of 1%-2%. "Opt-out" testing policies encourage prenatal screening for HIV. Rapid tests are convenient and well-accepted by women, and can facilitate timely prophylactic intervention, even during labor and birth.

IMPLICATIONS FOR FURTHER RESEARCH

- Well-designed trials are needed to directly establish prenatal HIV testing and outcomes. Counseling and risky behavior have not been adequately addressed. Investigators are still perfecting guidelines for ideal antiviral dosing, combinations, and timing. Cost is still the driving force behind treatment availability in developing countries. This review did not address the lingering controversy over whether breastfeeding's benefits outweigh its risks in developing countries with high infant and child mortality rates.

Reference: Chou, R., Smits, A., Huffman, L., Fu, R., & Korthius, P. (2005). Prenatal screening for HIV: A review of the evidence for the U. S. Preventive Services Task Force. *Annals of Internal Medicine, 143*(1), 38-54.

Management. During the initial contact with an HIV-infected woman, the nurse should establish what the woman knows about HIV infection and that she is being cared for by a medical practitioner or facility with expertise in caring for persons with HIV infections, including AIDS. Psychologic referral also may be indicated. Resources such as counseling for death and dying, suicide prevention, financial assistance, and legal advocacy may be appropriate. All women who are drug users should be referred to a substance-abuse program. A major focus of counseling is prevention of transmission of HIV to partners.

Nurses counseling seropositive women wishing contraceptive information may recommend oral contraceptives and latex condoms, or tubal sterilization or vasectomy and latex condoms. The IUD is not an ideal choice for the HIV-infected woman because of increased risk of infection. Insertion in a woman who is immunocompromised should be avoided (World Health Organization, 2000). Female condoms or abstinence can be offered to women whose partners refuse to use condoms.

Routine gynecologic care for HIV-positive women should include a pelvic examination every 6 months. Careful Pap screening is essential because of the greatly increased incidence of abnormal findings (Williams, 2003). In addition, HIV-positive women should be screened for syphilis, gonorrhea, chlamydia, and other vaginal infections.

No cure is available for HIV infection. Rare and unusual diseases are characteristic of HIV infection. Opportunistic infections and concurrent diseases should be managed vigorously with treatment specific to the infection or disease. Discussion of the medical care of HIV-positive women and women with AIDS is beyond the scope of this chapter. The reader is referred to the Centers for Disease Control and Prevention (www.cdc.gov), AIDS hotlines (800-342-2437), and Internet websites such as HIV/AIDS Treatment Information Service (www.hivatis.org) for the current information and recommendations.

HIV and Pregnancy

Perinatal transmission of HIV has decreased significantly in the past decade because of the administration of antiretroviral prophylaxis (e.g., zidovudine [ZDV, AZT, Retrovir]) to pregnant women in the prenatal and the perinatal periods. Treatment of HIV-infected women with the triple-drug antiviral therapy or highly active antiretroviral therapy (HAART) during pregnancy has been reported to decrease the mother-to-child transmission to 2% (Stephenson, 2005).

All HIV-infected women should be treated with zidovudine or HAART during pregnancy, regardless of their CD_4 counts (Perinatal HIV Guidelines Working Group, 2005). Antiviral therapy is administered orally, and usually is started after the first trimester and continued throughout pregnancy. The major side effect of this drug is bone marrow suppression; periodic hematocrit, white blood cell count, and platelet count assessments should be performed (Duff, 2002). Women who are HIV positive should also be vaccinated against hepatitis B, pneumococcal infection, *Haemophilus influenzae* type B, and viral influenza. To support any pregnant woman's immune system, appropriate counseling is provided about optimal nutrition, sleep, rest, exercise, and stress reduction. Use of condoms is encouraged to minimize further exposure to HIV if her partner is the source.

Key to preventing vertical transmission to the fetus is antiretroviral therapy and cesarean birth (ACOG, 2001; Perinatal HIV Guidelines Working Group, 2005). Women should be given the option of having a scheduled cesarean birth at 38 weeks of gestation to decrease this risk. Intravenous (IV) zidovudine is administered before the cesarean or during labor if the woman declines a cesarean birth. Avoidance of breastfeeding is recommended in the United States and most developed countries (Lawrence & Lawrence, 2005).

▬ VAGINAL INFECTIONS

Vaginal discharge and itching of the vulva and vagina are among the most frequent reasons a woman seeks help from a health care provider; more women complain of vaginal discharge than of any other gynecologic symptom. Vaginal discharge resulting from infection must be distinguished from normal secretions. Women who have adequate endogenous or exogenous estrogen will have vaginal secretions. Normal vaginal secretions, or leukorrhea, are clear to cloudy in appearance and may turn yellow after drying; the discharge is slightly slimy, is nonirritating, and has a mild, inoffensive odor. Normal vaginal secretions are acidic, with a pH range of 4 to 5. The amount of leukorrhea differs with phases of the menstrual cycle, with greater amounts occurring at ovulation and just before menses. Leukorrhea also is increased during pregnancy. Normal vaginal secretions contain lactobacilli and epithelial cells.

Vaginitis, or abnormal vaginal discharge, is an infection caused by a microorganism. The most common vaginal infections are bacterial vaginosis, candidiasis, and trichomoniasis. Vulvovaginitis, or inflammation of the vulva and vagina, may be caused by vaginal infection; copious leukorrhea, which can cause maceration of tissues; and chemical irritants, allergens, and foreign bodies, which may produce inflammatory reactions.

Bacterial Vaginosis

Bacterial vaginosis (BV), formerly called nonspecific vaginitis, *Haemophilus vaginitis,* or *Gardnerella,* is the most common type of vaginitis. BV is associated with preterm labor and birth. The exact etiology of BV is unknown. It is a syndrome in which normal H_2O_2-producing lactobacilli are replaced with high concentrations of anaerobic bacteria (*Gardnerella* and *Mobiluncus*). With the proliferation of anaerobes, the level of vaginal amines is increased, and the normal acidic pH of the vagina is altered. Epithelial cells slough, and numerous bacteria attach to their surfaces (clue cells). When the amines are volatilized, the characteristic odor of BV occurs.

CD: Resources

Screening and Diagnosis

A careful history may help distinguish BV from other vaginal infections if the woman is symptomatic. Women with previous occurrence of similar symptoms, diagnosis, and treatment should be queried, because women with BV often have been treated incorrectly because of misdiagnosis.

Most women with BV complain of a characteristic "fishy odor" in the vaginal area; however, not all note it. The odor may be noticed by the woman or her partner after heterosexual intercourse because semen releases the vaginal amines. When present, the BV discharge is usually profuse; thin; and white, gray, or milky in appearance. Some women also may have mild irritation or pruritus.

Microscopic examination of vaginal secretions is always done (Table 8-4). Both normal saline and 10% potassium hydroxide smears should be made. The presence of clue cells by wet smear is highly diagnostic because the phenomenon is specific to BV, but other criteria should be present as well (USPSTF, 2005a). Vaginal secretions should be tested for pH and amine odor. Nitrazine paper is sensitive enough to detect a pH of 4.5 or greater. The fishy odor of BV will be released when KOH is added to vaginal secretions on the lip of the withdrawn speculum.

Management

Treatment of bacterial vaginosis with oral metronidazole (Flagyl) is most effective (CDC et al., 2006). Table 8-5 outlines treatment guidelines. Side effects of metronidazole are numerous, including sharp, unpleasant metallic taste in the mouth, furry tongue, central nervous system reactions, and urinary tract disturbances. When oral metronidazole is taken, the woman is advised not to drink alcoholic beverages, or she will experience the severe side effects of abdominal distress, nausea, vomiting, and headache. Gastrointestinal symptoms are common whether alcohol is consumed or not. Treatment of sexual partners is not routinely recommended (CDC).

The medication is contraindicated if the woman is breastfeeding because high concentrations have been found in infants. If it is necessary to prescribe metronidazole for the lactating woman, she can suspend breastfeeding temporarily (pump and discard milk to maintain supply), and resume it 48 to 72 hours after taking the last dose.

Candidiasis

Vulvovaginal candidiasis (VVC), or yeast infection, is the second most common type of vaginal infection in the United States. Although vaginal candidiasis infections are common in healthy women, those seen in women with HIV infection are often more severe and persistent. Genital candidiasis lesions may be painful, coalescing ulcerations necessitating continuous prophylactic therapy.

The most common organism is *Candida albicans;* it is estimated that 80% to 95% of the yeast infections in women are caused by this organism. However, in the past 10 years, the incidence of non–*C. albicans* infections has increased steadily. Women with chronic or recurrent infections often are infected with a higher percentage of non–*C. albicans* species than are women with their first infection or are those who have few recurrences.

Numerous factors have been identified as predisposing a woman to yeast infections, including antibiotic therapy, particularly broad-spectrum antibiotics such as ampicillin, tetracycline, cephalosporins, and metronidazole; diabetes, especially when uncontrolled; pregnancy; obesity; diets high in refined sugars or artificial sweeteners; use of corticosteroids and exogenous hormones; and immunosuppressed states. Clinical observations and research have suggested that tight-fitting clothing and underwear or pantyhose made of nonabsorbent materials create an environment in which a vaginal fungus can grow.

The most common symptom of yeast infections is vulvar and possibly vaginal pruritus. The itching may be mild or intense, interfere with rest and activities, and occur during or after intercourse. Some women report a feeling of dryness. Others may have painful urination as the urine flows over the vulva; this usually occurs in women who have excoriations resulting from scratching. Most often the discharge is thick, white, lumpy, and cottage cheese–like. The discharge may be found in patches on the vaginal walls, cervix, and labia. Commonly the vulva is red and swollen, as are the labial folds, the vagina, and the cervix. Although there is no characteristic odor with yeast infections, sometimes a yeasty or musty smell occurs.

Screening and Diagnosis

In addition to a careful history of the woman's symptoms, their onset, and course, the history is a valuable screening tool for identifying predisposing risk factors. Physical

---

table 8-4 **Wet Smear Tests for Vaginal Infections**

INFECTION	TEST	POSITIVE FINDINGS
Trichomoniasis	Saline wet smear (vaginal secretions mixed with normal saline on a glass slide)	Presence of many white blood cell protozoa
Candidiasis	Potassium hydroxide (KOH) prep (vaginal secretions mixed with KOH on a glass slide)	Presence of hyphae and pseudohyphae (buds and branches of yeast cells)
Bacterial vaginosis	Normal saline smear	Presence of clue cells (vaginal epithelial cells coated with bacteria)
	Whiff test (vaginal secretions mixed with KOH)	Release of fishy odor

table 8-5 **Vaginal Infections and Drug Therapies for Women**

DISEASE	NONPREGNANT WOMEN 13-17 YEARS OF AGE	NONPREGNANT WOMEN >18 18 YEARS OF AGE	PREGNANT WOMEN	LACTATING WOMEN
Bacterial vaginosis	*Recommended:* Metronidazole, 500 mg bid for 7 days (no alcohol) *or* Metronidazole gel 0.75%, 5 g intravaginally bid for 7 days *or* Clindamycin cream 2%, 5 g intravaginally at bedtime for 7 days (less effective) *or* *Alternatives:* Clindamycin, 300 mg orally bid for 7 days (less effective) *or* Clindamycin ovules, 100 g intravaginally once at bedtime for 3 days	*Recommended:* Metronidazole, 500 mg bid for 7 days (no alcohol) *or* Metronidazole gel 0.75%, 5 g intravaginally bid for 7 days *or* Clindamycin cream 2%, 5 g intravaginally at bedtime for 7 days (less effective) *or* *Alternatives:* Clindamycin, 300 mg orally bid for 7 days (less effective) *or* Clindamycin ovules, 100 g intravaginally once at bedtime for 3 days	High risk asymptomatic or symptomatic women *Recommended:* Metronidazole, 500 mg orally bid for 7 days or Metronidazole, 250 mg orally tid for 7 days or Clindamycin, 300 mg orally bid for 7 days	*Recommended:* Clindamycin cream or ovules
Trichomoniasis	*Recommended:* Metronidazole, 2 g orally once Tinidazole, 2 g orally once *Alternative:* Metronidazole, 500 mg bid for 7 days	*Recommended:* Metronidazole, 2 g orally once *Alternative:* Metronidazole, 500 mg bid for 7 days	*Recommended:* Metronidazole, 2 g orally once	Metronidazole not recommended during lactation; stop lactation, treat, resume breastfeeding in 48 hr after drug completed Tinidazole stop and resume 3 days after treatment
Candidiasis	Numerous OTC topical intravaginal agents: butaconazole, clotrimazole, miconazole, tioconazole, terconazole; treatment with "azole" drugs more effective than nystatin Dose varies by agent from a single dose to 3 days to 7 to 14 days *Oral agent:* Fluconazole 150 mg oral tablet once	Numerous OTC topical intravaginal agents: butaconazole, clotrimazole, miconazole, tioconazole, terconazole; treatment with "azole" drugs more effective than nystatin Dose varies by agent from a single dose to 3 days to 7 to 14 days *Oral agent:* Fluconazole 150 mg oral tablet once	OTC topical "azole" intravaginal agents: butaconazole, clotrimazole, miconazole, terconazole Use for 7 days Oral agents not recommended	OTC topical "azole" intravaginal agents: butaconazole, clotrimazole, miconazole, terconazole Use for 7 days

Source: Centers for Disease Control and Prevention, et al. (2006). Sexually transmitted diseases treatment guidelines 2006. *MMWR Morbidity and Mortality Weekly Report, 55*(RR11), 1-94.
bid, Twice daily; *OTC,* over-the-counter; *tid,* three times daily.

examination should include a thorough inspection of the vulva and the vagina. A speculum examination is always done. Commonly saline and KOH wet smear and vaginal pH are obtained (see Table 8-4). Vaginal pH is normal with a yeast infection; if the pH is greater than 4.5, trichomoniasis or BV should be suspected. The characteristic pseudohyphae (bud or branching of a fungus) may be seen on a wet smear done with normal saline; however, they may be confused with other cells and artifacts.

Management

Exogenous *Lactobacillus* (in the form of dairy products or powder, tablet, capsule, or suppository supplements) has been suggested for prevention and treatment of vulvovaginal candidiasis, but research is inconclusive and no recommendation for use in practice has been made (Jeavons, 2003).

A number of antifungal preparations are available for the treatment of *C. albicans* (see Table 8-5). Many of these medications (e.g., miconazole [Monistat] and clotrimazole [Gyne-Lotrimin]) are available as over-the-counter (OTC) agents. The first time a woman suspects that she may have a yeast infection, she should see a health care provider for confirmation of the diagnosis and treatment recommendation. If she has another infection, she may wish to purchase an OTC preparation and self-treat. If she elects to do this, she should always be counseled regarding seeking care for numerous recurrent or chronic yeast infections. If vaginal discharge is extremely thick and copious, vaginal debridement with a cotton swab followed by application of vaginal medication may be useful.

Women who have extensive irritation, swelling, and discomfort of the labia and vulva may find sitz baths helpful in decreasing inflammation and increasing comfort. Adding Aveeno powder to the bath also may increase the woman's comfort. Not wearing underpants to bed may help decrease symptoms and prevent recurrences. Completing the full course of treatment prescribed is essential to removing the pathogen, and women are instructed to continue medication even during menstruation. They should be counseled not to use tampons during menses because the medication will be absorbed by the tampon. If possible, intercourse is avoided during treatment; if this is not feasible, the woman's partner should use a condom to prevent introduction of more organisms. Suggested measures to prevent genital tract infections are outlined in the Teaching for Self-Care box.

Trichomoniasis

Trichomoniasis is almost always a sexually transmitted infection. It also is a common cause of vaginal infection (up to 25% of all vaginitis) and discharge and thus is discussed in this section.

TEACHING FOR SELF-CARE

Prevention of Genital Tract Infections

- Practice genital hygiene.
- Choose underwear or hosiery with a cotton crotch.
- Avoid tight-fitting clothing (especially tight jeans).
- Select cloth car seat covers instead of vinyl.
- Limit time spent in damp exercise clothes (especially swimsuits, leotards, and tights).
- Limit exposure to bath salts or bubble bath.
- Avoid colored or scented toilet tissue.
- If sensitive, discontinue use of feminine hygiene deodorant sprays.
- Use condoms.
- Void before and after intercourse.
- Decrease dietary sugar.
- Drink yeast-active milk and eat yogurt (with lactobacilli).
- Do not douche.

Trichomoniasis is caused by *Trichomonas vaginalis*, an anaerobic one-celled protozoan with characteristic flagellae. Although trichomoniasis may be asymptomatic, commonly women have characteristically yellowish to greenish, frothy, mucopurulent, copious, malodorous discharge. Inflammation of the vulva, the vagina, or both may be present, and the woman may complain of irritation and pruritus. Dysuria and dyspareunia are often present. Typically, the discharge worsens during and after menstruation. Often the cervix and the vaginal walls will demonstrate the characteristic "strawberry spots" or tiny petechiae, and the cervix may bleed on contact. In severe infections, the vaginal walls, the cervix, and occasionally the vulva may be acutely inflamed.

Screening and Diagnosis

In addition to obtaining a history of current symptoms, a careful sexual history should be obtained. Any history of similar symptoms in the past and treatment used should be noted. The nurse should determine whether the client's partner(s) was treated and if she has had subsequent relations with new partners.

A speculum examination is always done, even though it may be very uncomfortable for the woman; relaxation techniques and breathing exercises may help the woman with the procedure. Any of the classic signs may be present on physical examination. The typical one-celled flagellate trichomonads are easily distinguished on a normal saline wet prep. Trichomoniasis also may be identified on Pap smears. Because trichomoniasis is an STI, once diagnosis is confirmed, appropriate laboratory studies for other STIs should be carried out.

Management

The recommended treatment is metronidazole, 2 g orally in a single dose (CDC et al., 2006) (see Table 8-5). Although the male partner is usually asymptomatic, it is recommended that he receive treatment also, because he often harbors the trichomonads in the urethra or prostate. It is important that nurses discuss the importance of partner treatment with their clients because if they are not treated, it is likely that the infection will recur.

Women with trichomoniasis need to understand the sexual transmission of this disease. The client must know that the organism may be present without symptoms being present, perhaps for several months, and that it is not possible to determine when she became infected. Women should be informed of the necessity for treating all sexual partners and helped with ways to raise the issue with their partner(s).

Group B Streptococcus

Group B streptococcus (GBS) may be considered a part of the normal vaginal flora in a woman who is not pregnant, and it is present in 9% to 23% of healthy pregnant women. GBS infection has been associated with poor pregnancy outcomes (Guise, Mahan, Aickin, Helfand, Peipert, & Westhoff, 2001). Furthermore, GBS infections are an important factor in neonatal morbidity and mortality, usually resulting from vertical transmission from the birth canal of the infected mother to the infant during birth.

Risk factors for neonatal GBS infection include positive prenatal culture for GBS in the current pregnancy; preterm birth of less than 37 weeks of gestation; premature rupture of membranes for a duration of 18 hours or more; intrapartum maternal fever higher than 38° C; and a positive history for early-onset neonatal GBS.

To decrease the risk of neonatal GBS infection, it is recommended that all women be screened at 36 to 37 weeks of gestation for GBS using a rectovaginal culture, and that intravenous antibiotic prophylaxis (IAP) be offered during labor to all who test positive. If a culture is not available at onset of labor or if a risk factor is present, IAP is also offered. IAP is not recommended before a cesarean birth if labor or rupture of membranes has not occurred. The recommended treatment is penicillin G, 5 million units IV loading dose, and then 2.5 million units IV every 4 hours during labor. Ampicillin, 2 g IV loading dose, followed by 1 g IV every 4 hours, is an alternative therapy (CDC, 2002).

EFFECTS OF SEXUALLY TRANSMITTED INFECTIONS ON PREGNANCY AND THE FETUS

Sexually transmitted infections in pregnancy are responsible for significant morbidity and mortality. Some consequences of maternal infection, such as infertility and sterility, last a lifetime. Congenitally acquired infection may affect a child's length and quality of life. Table 8-6 describes the effects of several common STIs on pregnancy

and the fetus. It is difficult to predict these effects with certainty. Factors such as coinfection with other STIs and when in pregnancy the infection was treated can affect outcomes.

TORCH Infections

TORCH infections can affect a pregnant woman and her fetus. *T*oxoplasmosis, *o*ther infections (e.g., hepatitis), *r*ubella virus, *c*ytomegalovirus (CMV), and *h*erpes simplex virus, known collectively as TORCH infections, form a group of organisms capable of crossing the placenta and adversely affecting the development of the fetus. Generally, all TORCH infections produce influenza-like symptoms in the mother, but fetal and neonatal effects are more serious. TORCH infections and their maternal and fetal effects are shown in Table 8-7. Neonatal effects are discussed in Chapter 38.

Toxoplasmosis

Toxoplasmosis is a protozoan infection associated with the consumption of infested raw or undercooked meat and with poor handwashing after handling infected cat litter. Pregnant women with HIV antibodies are at higher risk because toxoplasmosis is a common accompanying opportunistic infection. The presence of toxoplasmosis can be determined through blood studies, although laboratory diagnosis is difficult. Women at risk for infection should have toxoplasmosis titers evaluated. Acute infection in pregnancy produces influenza-like symptoms and lymphadenopathy in some women but no symptoms in others. Miscarriage may occur.

The treatment of choice for toxoplasmosis is spiramycin, sulfadine, or a combination of pyrimethamine and

table 8-6 Pregnancy and Fetal Effects of Common Sexually Transmitted Infections

INFECTION	PREGNANCY EFFECTS	FETAL EFFECTS
Chlamydia	Premature rupture of membranes Preterm labor	Preterm birth Conjunctivitis Pneumonia
Gonorrhea	Intraamniotic infection Preterm labor Premature rupture of membranes Postpartum endometritis Miscarriage	Preterm birth Sepsis Conjunctivitis
Group B streptococcus	Preterm labor Premature rupture of membranes Chorioamnionitis Postpartum sepsis Urinary tract infections	Preterm birth Early-onset sepsis
Herpes simplex	Rare: infection	Systemic infection
Human papillomavirus (HPV)	Dystocia from large lesions Excessive bleeding from lesions after birth trauma	Respiratory papillomatosis (rare) Preterm birth
Syphilis	Preterm labor Miscarriage	Stillbirth Congenital infection

Data from Cunningham, F., et al. (2005). *Williams obstetrics* (22nd ed.). New York: McGraw-Hill; Gilbert, E., & Harmon, J. (2003). *Manual of high risk pregnancy and delivery* (3rd ed.). St. Louis: Mosby; Yudkin, M., & Gonik, B. (2006). Perinatal infections. In R. Martin, A. Fanaroff, & M. Walsh (Eds.). *Fanaroff & Martin's neonatal-perinatal medicine: Diseases of the fetus and infant* (8th ed.). Philadelphia: Mosby.

sulfadiazine. Although pyrimethamine may be potentially harmful to the fetus, treatment of the parasitemia is essential (Lopez, Dietz, Wilson, Navin, & Jones, 2000).

Other Infections

The primary infection included in the category of other infections is hepatitis, which was discussed previously. Infections other than hepatitis also may be identified as "other" TORCH infections. These include GBS, varicella, and HIV.

Rubella

Rubella, also called German measles or 3-day measles, is a viral infection transmitted by droplets (such as from an infected person's sneeze). Rash, muscle aches, joint pain, and mild lymphedema are usually seen in the infected mother. Consequences for the fetus are much more serious and include miscarriage, congenital anomalies (referred to as congenital rubella syndrome), and death. Vaccination of pregnant women is contraindicated because a rubella infection may develop after the live vaccine is administered. Rubella vaccine is given to women who are not immune as part of preconception counseling or in the postpartum period prior to discharge, with instructions to use contraception for at least 1 month after vaccination (ACOG, 2002).

Cytomegalovirus

Maternal infection with CMV may begin as a mononucleosis-like syndrome. In most adults the onset of CMV infection is uncertain and asymptomatic; however, the disease may become a chronic persistent infection. Approximately 60% of the adult population has antibodies to CMV. This virus is primarily transmitted by close contacts but also has been isolated from semen, cervical and vaginal secretions, breast milk, placental tissue, urine, feces, and banked blood. Maternal CMV infection may be diagnosed by presence of CMV in urine or in serum, because many women have evidence of CMV infection. Women who show CMV infection in pregnancy (by positive viral titers) usually have chronic or recurrent infections (Yudkin & Gonik, 2006).

Women at risk for infection include those who work in or have children in day care centers, institutions for the mentally retarded, or certain health care settings (such as nursery, dialysis, laboratory, and oncology).

In the United States, 1% to 2% of infants have congenital CMV infection. Fetal infection can cause microcephaly; eye, ear, and dental defects; and mental retardation. No treatment is available during pregnancy.

Herpes Simplex Virus

The potential pregnancy effects of primary genital herpes infection include miscarriage, preterm labor, and intrauterine growth restriction. The main route of HSV transmission from mother to neonate is through an infected birth canal. The risk of maternal-infant transmission is greater during a primary HSV-2 infection than during a recurrent episode.

Cesarean birth is not recommended for all mothers with HSV; only mothers with clinical evidence of active lesions during labor should have cesarean birth. Prenatal HSV cultures do not predict the presence of a live virus at time of birth. Cultures in women with HSV lesions at or near term may be done to determine the absence of the virus at time of birth and increase the likelihood of a vaginal birth (see Table 8-2 for treatment guidelines).

■ CARE MANAGEMENT

Women may delay seeking care for STIs and other infections because they fear social stigma, have little accessibility to health care services, are asymptomatic, or are unaware that they have an infection.

■ Assessment and Nursing Diagnoses

A comprehensive assessment focuses on lifestyle issues that are often personal or sensitive. A culturally sensitive, nonjudgmental approach is essential to facilitate accurate data collection. Specific areas to address are listed in Box 8-3. A history that is accurate, comprehensive, and specific is crucial to diagnosis.

---

box 8-3 **Essential Areas of Assessment for a Woman at Risk for or Who Has a Sexually Transmitted Infection**

CURRENT PROBLEM
What symptoms are present?
- Vaginal discharge
- Lesions
- Rash
- Dysuria
- Fever
- Itching, burning
- Dyspareunia
- Malaise

MEDICAL HISTORY
- History of STIs
- Allergies, especially to medications

MENSTRUAL HISTORY
- Last menstrual period (possibility of pregnancy)

PERSONAL AND SOCIAL HISTORY
- Sexual history
  - Sexual preference
  - Number of partners (past, present)
  - Types of sexual activity
  - Frequency of sexual activity

LIFESTYLE BEHAVIORS
- Intravenous drug use (or use by partner)
- Smoking
- Alcohol use
- Inadequate/poor nutrition
- High levels of stress, fatigue

table 8-7 **Maternal Infection: TORCH**

INFECTION	MATERNAL EFFECTS	FETAL EFFECTS	COUNSELING: PREVENTION, IDENTIFICATION, AND MANAGEMENT
Toxoplasmosis (protozoa)	Acute infection similar to influenza, lymphadenopathy Woman immune after first episode (except in immunocompromised clients)	With maternal acute infection, parasitemia Less likely to occur with maternal chronic infection Miscarriage likely with acute infection early in pregnancy	Use good handwashing technique Avoid eating raw meat and exposure to litter used by infected cats; if cats in house, have toxoplasma titer checked If titer is rising during early pregnancy, abortion may be considered an option
Other Hepatitis A (infectious hepatitis) (virus)	Miscarriage, cause of liver failure during pregnancy Fever, malaise, nausea, and abdominal discomfort	Exposure during first trimester, fetal anomalies, fetal or neonatal hepatitis, preterm birth, intrauterine fetal death	Usually spread by droplet or hand contact, especially by culinary workers; gamma-globulin can be given as prophylaxis for hepatitis A; vaccine is available for populations at risk
Hepatitis B (serum hepatitis) (virus)	Symptoms variable: fever, rash, arthralgia, depressed appetite, dyspepsia, abdominal pain, generalized aching, malaise, weakness, jaundice, tender and enlarged liver	Infection occurs during birth Maternal vaccination during pregnancy presents no risk for fetus	Generally passed by contaminated needles, syringes, or blood transfusions, or sexually; also can be transmitted orally (but incubation period is longer); hepatitis B immune globulin can be given prophylactically after exposure Hepatitis B vaccinations recommendations: universal infant immunizations, universal immunizations of previously unvaccinated adolescents ages 11-12 yr, adolescents and adults at increased risk Populations at risk are women from Asia, Pacific Islands, Indochina, Haiti, South Africa, Alaska (women of Eskimo descent); other women at risk include health care providers, users of intravenous drugs, those sexually active with multiple partners or single partners with multiple risks

Source: Centers for Disease Control and Prevention (CDC) et al. (2006). Sexually transmitted diseases treatment guidelines 2006. *MMWR Morbidity and Mortality Weekly Report 55*(RR11), 1-94; Yudkin, M., & Gonik, B. (2006). Perinatal infections. In R. Martin, A. Fanaroff, & M. Walsh (Eds.). *Fanaroff & Martin's neonatal-perinatal medicine: Diseases of the fetus and infant* (8th ed.). Philadelphia: Mosby.
IUGR, Intrauterine growth restriction.

▬ History

Because many women are embarrassed or anxious, the history should be taken first, with the woman dressed. Information should be collected in a nonjudgmental manner, by using open-ended questions and avoiding assumptions of sexual preference. All partners should be referred to as partners and not by gender. A complete history is essential in identifying possible STIs. Factors that may influence the development and management of STIs in women include history of STI or PID, number of past or current sexual

table 8-7 **Maternal Infection: TORCH—cont'd**

INFECTION	MATERNAL EFFECTS	FETAL EFFECTS	COUNSELING: PREVENTION, IDENTIFICATION, AND MANAGEMENT
Rubella (3-day German measles) (virus)	Joint pain, muscle aches, rash, fever, mild symptoms; suboccipital lymph nodes may be swollen; some photophobia Occasionally arthritis or encephalitis Miscarriage	Incidence of congenital anomalies; first trimester 50%-90% Exposure during first 2 mo: malformations of heart, eyes, ears, or brain; abnormal dermatoglyphics Exposure after fourth mo: hearing loss, psychomotor retardation, systemic infection, hepatosplenomegaly, IUGR, rash, heart disease, cataracts	Vaccination of pregnant women contraindicated; pregnancy should be prevented for at least 1 mo after vaccination; pregnant women nonreactive to hemagglutinin-inhibition antigen can be safely vaccinated after giving birth
Cytomegalovirus (CMV) (a herpes virus)	Respiratory or sexually transmitted asymptomatic illness or mononucleosis-like syndrome, may have cervical discharge No immunity develops	Fetal death or severe, generalized disease: hemolytic anemia and jaundice, hydrocephaly or microcephaly, pneumonitis, hepatosplenomegaly, deafness, mental retardation	Virus may be reactivated and cause disease in utero or during birth in subsequent pregnancies; fetal infection may occur during passage through infected birth canal; disease is commonly progressive through infancy and childhood
Herpes genitalis (herpes simplex virus, type 2 [HSV-2])	Primary blisters, rash, fever, malaise, nausea, headache; pregnancy risks include miscarriage, preterm labor, stillbirths	Transmission occurs after rupture of membranes; congenital effects include skin lesions and scarring, IUGR, mental retardation, microcephaly Active HSV in first trimester: 20% to 50% miscarriage/stillbirth rate	Risk of transmission is greatest during vaginal birth if woman has active lesions Acyclovir may be given orally during pregnancy with first episode of HSV-2 or when benefit to woman is greater than risk to fetus. May also be treated symptomatically (see Table 8-2)

partners, and types of sexual activity. Women should be queried for specific lifestyle behaviors that place them at risk for STIs. Among these are intravenous drug use or partner intravenous drug use, smoking, alcohol use, inadequate or poor nutrition, and high levels of stress or fatigue.

■ **Physical Examination**

Before the actual physical examination is performed, the nurse should discuss the examination with the woman so she is prepared for it. A thorough assessment of symptoms including a comprehensive physical examination is essential to diagnosing STIs. Because the speculum usually is not lubricated before insertion into the vagina (cultures of vaginal secretions may have to be obtained), insertion may be more uncomfortable than usual. Women should be informed of this and reassured that every effort will be made to make the speculum examination as comfortable as possible.

▪ Laboratory Tests

Appropriate laboratory studies will be suggested, in part, by the history and physical examination results. Bacterial STIs are easily determined from genital tract, urine, and blood studies. Viral agents also can be cultured, but less successfully. Because women often are infected with more than one STI simultaneously, and many are asymptomatic, additional laboratory studies may be done, including Pap smear, wet mounts, gonococcal culture, and VDRL or RPR test for syphilis. Cultures for HSV are obtained when indicated by history or physical examination. The woman should be offered the HIV-antibody test. When indicated, a complete blood count, sedimentation rate, urinalysis, or urine culture and sensitivity should be obtained.

Nursing diagnoses are derived after carefully analyzing assessment findings, medical management, and health care provider directives. The following nursing diagnoses are representative of those used in a plan of care for women with STIs and other vaginal infections:

- *Anxiety/situational low self-esteem/disturbed body image related to*
  - perceived effects on sexual relationships and family processes
  - possible effects on pregnancy or fetus
  - long-term sequelae of infection
- *Deficient knowledge related to*
  - transmission/prevention of infection/reinfection
  - safer sex behaviors
  - management of infection
- *Acute pain/impaired tissue integrity related to*
  - effects of infection process
  - scratching (excoriation) of pruritic areas
  - hygiene practices
- *Sexual dysfunction related to*
  - effects of infection process
- *Social isolation and impaired social interaction related to*
  - perceived effects on relationships with others if STI status is unknown

▪ Expected Outcomes of Care

Care of the woman with an STI focuses on physical and psychologic needs. Avoidance of reinfection and harmful sequelae is critical. Measurable expected outcomes are mutually derived with the woman's input. Outcomes for the woman include that she will do the following:
- Be free of infection or, in the case of viral infection, have remission or stabilization of the infection.

- Identify and be able to discuss the etiology, management, and expected course of the infection and its prevention.
- Be able to identify her risky behaviors and discuss plans for decreasing her risk for infection.

▪ Plan of Care and Interventions

The woman with an STI will need encouragement to seek care at the earliest stage of symptoms. Counseling women about STIs is essential for (1) preventing new infections or reinfection; (2) increasing compliance with treatment and follow-up; (3) providing support during treatment; and (4) assisting women in discussions with their partner(s). Women must be made aware of the serious potential consequences of STIs and the behaviors that increase the likelihood of infection.

The nurse must make sure that the woman understands what infection she has, how it is transmitted, and why it must be treated (see Teaching for Self-Care box). Women should be given a brief description of the infection in language that they can understand. This description should include modes of transmission, incubation period, symptoms, infectious period, and potential complications. Effective treatment of STIs necessitates careful, thorough explanation of the treatment regimen and follow-up procedures. Thorough, careful instructions about medications must be provided, both verbally and in writing. Side effects, benefits, and risks of the medication should be discussed. Unpleasant side effects or early relief of symptoms may discourage women from completing their medication course. Clients should be strongly urged to take all the medication and not stop even if their symptoms diminish or disappear in a few days. Comfort measures to decrease symptoms such as pain, itching, or nausea should be suggested. Providing written information is a useful strategy because this is a time of high anxiety for many women, and they may not be able to hear or remember what they

---

TEACHING FOR SELF-CARE

Sexually Transmitted Infections

- Take your medication as directed.
- Use comfort measures for symptom relief as suggested by your health care provider.
- Keep your appointment for repeat cultures or checkups after your treatment to make sure your infection is cured.
- Inform your sexual partner(s) of the need to be tested and treated, if necessary.
- Abstain from sexual intercourse until your treatment is completed or for as long as you are advised by your health care provider.
- Use safer sex practices when sexual intercourse is resumed.
- Call your health care provider immediately if you notice bumps, sores, rashes, or discharges.
- Keep all future appointments with your health care provider, even if things appear normal.

were told. A number of booklets on STIs are available, or the nurse may wish to develop literature that is specific to the practice setting and clients.

In general, women will be advised to refrain from intercourse until all treatment is finished and a repeat culture, if appropriate, is done. After the infection is cured, women should be urged to continue using condoms to prevent repeat infections, especially if they have had one episode of PID or continue to have intercourse with new partners. Women may wish to avoid having sex with partners who have many other sexual partners. All women who have contracted an STI should be taught safer sex practices, if this has not been done already. Follow-up appointments should be made as needed.

Addressing the psychosocial component of STIs is essential. A woman may be afraid or embarrassed to tell her partner or to ask her partner to seek treatment. She may be embarrassed to admit her sexual practices, or she may be concerned about confidentiality. The nurse may need to help the woman deal with the impact of a diagnosis of an STI on a committed relationship, for the woman is now faced with the necessity of dealing with "uncertain monogamy."

In many instances, sexual partners should be treated; thus the infected woman is asked to identify and notify all partners who might have been exposed. Often she will find this difficult to do. Empathizing with the client's feelings and suggesting specific ways of talking with partners will help decrease anxiety and assist in efforts to control infection. For example, the nurse might suggest that the woman say, "I care about you and I'm concerned about you. That's why I'm calling to tell you that I have a sexually transmitted infection. My clinician is _____ and she will be happy to talk with you if you would like." Offering literature and role playing situations with the client also may be of assistance. It is often helpful to remind the woman that although this is an embarrassing situation, most persons would rather know than not know that they have been exposed. Health professionals who take time to counsel their clients on how to talk with their partner(s) can improve compliance and case finding.

Interrupting the transmission of infection is crucial to STI control. For treatable and vaccine-preventable STIs, further transmission and reinfection can be prevented with referral of sex partners. Many STIs are reportable;

---

plan of care ▸ **Sexually Transmitted Infections**

NURSING DIAGNOSIS Ineffective health maintenance related to practicing prevention of sexually transmitted infections as evidenced by client positive diagnosis of sexually transmitted infection

Expected Outcome *Woman will verbalize which health practices directly led to positive diagnosis of a sexually transmitted infection.*

Nursing Interventions/Rationales

- Inquire about woman's sexual history and sexual health practices *to provide database for current problem.*
- Use therapeutic communication for private, nonjudgmental discussion *to facilitate learning and promote self-esteem.*
- Provide emotional support *to indicate awareness of woman's feelings about this sensitive topic.*
- Provide information about transmission of disease, including cause, symptoms, and treatment for both partners *to enhance woman's knowledge base and correct any misinformation.*
- Discuss the use and importance of safe sexual practices *to raise woman's awareness and motivation to avoid future risk-taking behaviors.*
- Instruct woman and sexual partner to complete medication regimen *to completely eradicate transmitted organism.*

NURSING DIAGNOSIS Impaired social interaction related to diagnosis of sexually transmitted infection as evidenced by client verbal report

Expected Outcome *Woman will report increased incidences of social interaction.*

Nursing Interventions/Rationales

- Provide nonjudgmental, confidential therapeutic communication *to increase woman's feelings of self-worth.*
- Refer to support groups *to provide group interaction, discussion, and information.*

NURSING DIAGNOSIS Impaired tissue integrity related to effects of disease process as evidenced by client report of itching and vaginal discharge

Expected Outcome *Woman's tissue integrity will be restored.*

Nursing Interventions/Rationales

- Assess, monitor, and document characteristics of the damaged skin area, including color, lesions, drainage, and edema *to provide database.*
- Instruct woman in correct genital hygiene practices *to prevent further infection of damaged tissues with other organisms.*
- Provide warm soaks or sitz baths *to promote comfort, circulation, and healing.*
- Administer prescribed medications *to promote comfort and eradication of organism.*
- Provide written self-help materials and pamphlets *to prevent further skin integrity loss.*
- Teach woman to perform self-vulvar examination *to encourage participation in self-care.*

NURSING DIAGNOSIS Anxiety related to diagnosis of STI

Expected Outcome *Woman will report decreased level of anxiety.*

Nursing Interventions/Rationales

- Provide opportunity for therapeutic communication *to promote trust and expression of feelings.*
- Assist woman to identify effective coping mechanisms *to decrease anxiety.*
- Refer to support groups *to share feelings and common effective strategies.*

CD: Plan of Care: STIs

all states require that the five traditional STIs—gonorrhea, syphilis, chancroid, lymphogranuloma venereum, and granuloma inguinale—be reported to public health officials. Many other states require that other STIs such as chlamydial infections, genital herpes, and genital warts be reported. In addition, all states require that AIDS cases be reported; 35 states require that HIV infection be reported. The nurse is legally responsible for reporting all cases of those diseases identified as reportable and should know what the requirements are in the state in which she or he practices. The woman must be informed when a case will be reported and be told why. Failure to inform the woman that the case will be reported is a serious breach of professional ethics. Confidentiality is a crucial issue for many clients. When an STI is reportable, women must be told that they may be contacted by a health department epidemiologist. They should be assured that the information reported to and collected by health authorities is not available to anyone without their permission. Every effort, within the limits of one's public health responsibilities, should be made to reassure clients (see Plan of Care).

---

box 8-4 | Standard Precautions

Medical history and examination cannot reliably identify all persons infected with HIV or other blood-borne pathogens. Standard Precautions should therefore be used consistently in the care of all persons. These precautions apply to blood, body fluids, and all secretions and excretions, except sweat, nonintact skin, and mucous membranes. Standard Precautions are recommended to reduce the risk of transmission of microorganisms from known and unknown sources of infection (Bolyard, E. et al.,1998; CDC, 2001a).

1. Prompt and thorough handwashing is recommended between client contacts. Hands and other skin surfaces should be washed immediately and thoroughly if contaminated with blood or other body fluids. Hands should be washed immediately after gloves are removed.

2. In addition to handwashing, all health care workers should routinely use appropriate barrier precautions to prevent skin and mucous membrane exposure when contact with blood or other body fluids of any person is anticipated. *Latex gloves* should be worn for touching blood and body fluids, mucous membranes, or nonintact skin of all persons; for handling items or surfaces soiled with blood or body fluids; and for performing venipuncture and other vascular access procedures. Gloves should be changed after contact with each client. *Masks and protective eyewear* or face shields should be worn during procedures that are likely to generate droplets of blood or other body fluids to prevent exposure of mucous membranes of the mouth, nose, and eyes. *Gowns or aprons* should be worn during procedures that are likely to generate splashes of blood or other body fluids.

    Leg coverings, boots, or shoe covers also can be worn to provide protection against splashes and may be recommended for certain procedures such as surgery.

3. All health care workers should take precautions to prevent injuries caused by needles, scalpels, and other sharp instruments or devices during procedures; when cleaning used instruments; during disposal of used needles; and when handling sharp instruments after procedures. *To prevent needle-stick injuries,* needles should not be recapped, purposely bent or broken by hand, removed from disposable syringes, or otherwise manipulated by hand. After they are used, disposable syringes and needles, scalpel blades, and other sharp items should be immediately placed in a puncture-resistant container for disposal; puncture-resistant containers should be located as close as is practical to the use area.

4. Although saliva has not been implicated in HIV transmission, to minimize the need for emergency mouth-to-mouth resuscitation, mouthpieces, resuscitation bags, or other ventilation devices should be available for use in areas in which the need for resuscitation is predictable.

5. Health care workers who have exudative lesions or weeping dermatitis should refrain from all direct client care and from handling client care equipment until the condition resolves.

PRECAUTIONS FOR INVASIVE PROCEDURES

An invasive procedure is surgical entry into tissues, cavities, or organs; or repair of major traumatic injuries (1) in an operating or birthing room, emergency department, or out-of-hospital setting, including both physicians' and dentists' offices; and (2) a vaginal or cesarean birth or other invasive obstetric procedure during which bleeding may occur. Standard Precautions, combined with the following precautions, should serve as minimum precautions for all such invasive procedures:

1. All health care workers who participate in invasive procedures must routinely use appropriate barrier precautions to prevent skin and mucous membrane contact with blood and other body fluids of all clients. Gloves and surgical masks must be worn for all invasive procedures. Protective eyewear or face shields should be worn for procedures that commonly result in the generation of droplets, splashing of blood or other body fluids, or the generation of bone chips. Gowns or aprons made of materials that provide an effective barrier should be worn during invasive procedures that are likely to result in the splashing of blood or other body fluids. All health care workers who perform or assist in vaginal or cesarean births should wear gloves and gowns when handling the placenta or the infant until blood and amniotic fluid have been removed from the infant's skin. Gloves should be worn during infant eye prophylaxis, care of the umbilical cord, circumcision site, parenteral procedures, diaper changes, contact with colostrum, and postpartum assessments.

2. If a glove is torn or a needle stick or other injury occurs, the glove should be removed and a new glove used as promptly as client safety permits; the needle or instrument involved in the incident also should be removed from the sterile field.

3. Any needlestick or other injury should be reported and appropriate treatment obtained as specified by the health care facility.

Source: Bolyard, E., Tablan, O., Williams, W., Pearson, M., Shapiro, C., & Deitchmann, S. (1998). Guideline for infection control in healthcare personnel, 1998. Hospital Infection Control Practices Advisory Committee. *Infection Control and Hospital Epidemiology, 19*(6), 407-463; Centers for Disease Control and Prevention. (2001a). Updated U.S. Public Health Service guidelines for the management of occupational exposures to HBV, HCV, and HIV and recommendations for postexposure prophylaxis. *MMWR Morbidity and Mortality Weekly Report, 50*(RR-11), 1-52.

■ Infection Control

Infection-control measures are essential to protect care providers and to prevent nosocomial infection of clients, regardless of the infectious agent. The risk for occupational transmission varies with the disease. Even when the risk is low, as with HIV, the existence of any risk warrants reasonable precautions. Precautions against airborne disease transmission are available in all health care agencies. Standard Precautions (precautions to use in care of all persons for infection control) and additional precautions for labor and birth settings are listed in Box 8-4.

■ Evaluation

Evaluation is a continuous process. To be effective, evaluation is based on client-centered outcomes identified during the planning stage of nursing care. The nurse can be reasonably assured that care was effective to the extent that expected outcomes have been met.

community activity

Locate resources in your community for educating teens about STI prevention and safer sex practices (e.g., schools, churches, family planning/birth control clinics, health departments). Identify the interventions used by these resources. Determine if there is a need for more resources or for different types of programs.

key points

- Reproductive tract infections include STIs and common genital tract infections.
- Safer sex practices are key STI-prevention strategies.
- HIV is transmitted through body fluids, primarily blood, semen, and vaginal secretions.
- HPV is the most common viral STI.
- Syphilis has reemerged as a common STI.
- Chlamydia is the most common STI in women in the United States and the most common cause of PID.
- Viral hepatitis has several forms of transmission; HBV infections carry the greatest risk.
- Young, sexually active women who do not practice safer sex behaviors and have multiple partners are at greatest risk for STIs and HIV.
- STIs are responsible for substantial mortality and morbidity, great personal suffering, and heavy economic burden in the United States.
- STIs and vaginitis are biologic events for which all individuals have a right to expect objective, compassionate, and effective health care.
- Substance abuse can alter the body's immune system and possibly increase the risk for acquiring AIDS and associated conditions.
- Pregnancy confers no immunity against infection, and both mother and fetus must be considered when the pregnant woman contracts an infection.
- Because history and examination cannot reliably identify all persons with HIV or other blood-borne pathogens, blood and body-fluid precautions should be used consistently for everyone all the time.

REFERENCES

American Cancer Society (ACS). (2006). *Cancer facts and figures 2006.* New York: Author.

American College of Obstetricians and Gynecologists (ACOG). (2005). Human papillomavirus. ACOG Practice Bulletin No. 61. *Obstetrics and Gynecology, 105*(4), 905-912.

American College of Obstetricians and Gynecologists (ACOG). (2004). Prenatal and perinatal human immunodeficiency virus testing: Expanded recommendations. *Obstetrics and Gynecology, 104*(5 Pt 1), 1119-1124.

American College of Obstetricians and Gynecologists (ACOG). (2002). ACOG Committee Opinion. No. 281, December, 2002. Rubella vaccination. *Obstetrics and Gynecology, 100*(6), 1417.

American College of Obstetricians and Gynecologists (ACOG). (2001). ACOG Committee Opinion: Scheduled cesarean delivery and the prevention of vertical transmission of HIV infection. No. 234, May 2000. *International Journal of Gynaecology and Obstetrics, 73*(3), 279-281.

Black, B., & Miles, M. (2002). Calculating the risks and benefits of disclosure in African American women who have HIV. *Journal of Obstetric, Gynecologic, and Neonatal Nursing, 31*(6), 688-697.

Cates, W. (2004). Reproductive tract infections. In R. Hatcher, J. Trussell, F. Stewart, A. Nelson, W. Cates, F. Guest, et al. (2004). *Contraceptive technology* (18th revised ed.). New York: Ardent Media.

Centers for Disease Control and Prevention. (2001). *Viral hepatitis C prevention and control.* Accessed www.cdc.gov/ncidod/diseases/hepatitis/c/plan/HCV_infection.htm, February 20, 2006.

Centers for Disease Control and Prevention. (2002). Prevention of perinatal group B streptococcal disease: Revised guidelines from CDC. *MMWR Morbidity and Mortality Weekly Report, 51*(RR-11), 1-23.

Centers for Disease Control and Prevention, Workowski, K., & Berman, S. (2006). Sexually transmitted diseases treatment guidelines 2006. *MMWR Morbidity and Mortality Weekly Report, 55*(RR11), 1-94.

Centers for Disease Control and Prevention, Divisions of HIV/AIDS Prevention. (2004). *Frequently asked questions about the OraQuick Rapid HIV-1 Antibody Test.* Accessed www.cdc.gov/hiv/PUBS/faq/oraqckfaq.htm, February 22, 2006.

Centers for Disease Control and Prevention. (2005a). *HIV/AIDS Surveillance Report 2004,* Vol. 16. Atlanta, GA: U.S. Department of Health and Human Services.

Centers for Disease Control and Prevention. (2005b). *Sexually Transmitted Disease Surveillance Report, 2004.* Atlanta, GA: U.S. Department of Health and Human Services.

Centers for Disease Control and Prevention. (2006a). *HIV/AIDS Update: A glance at the epidemic.* Accessed www.cdc.gov/hiv/pubs/facts/at-a-glance.htm, February 22, 2006.

Centers for Disease Control and Prevention. (2006b). Trends in reportable sexually transmitted diseases in the United States, 2004. *STD Surveillance Report, 2004.* Accessed www.cdc.gov/std/stats/trends2004.htm.

DiSaia, P., & Creasman, W. (2002). *Clinical gynecologic oncology* (6th ed.). St. Louis: Mosby.

Duff, P. (2002). Maternal and perinatal infection. In S. Gabbe, J. Niebyl, & J. Simpson (Eds.), *Obstetrics: Normal and problem pregnancies* (4th ed.). New York: Churchill Livingstone.

Guest, F. (2004). HIV/AIDS and reproductive health. In R. Hatcher, J. Trussell, F. Stewart, A. Nelson, W. Cates, F. Guest, et al., (2004). *Contraceptive technology* (18th revised ed.). New York: Ardent Media.

Guise, J., Mahan, S., Aickin, M., Helfand, M., Peipert, J., & Westhoff, C. (2001). Screening for bacterial vaginosis in pregnancy. *American Journal of Preventive Medicine, 20*(3S), 62-72.

Hoffman, S., Mantell, J., Exner, T. & Stein, Z. (2004). The future of the female condom. *Perspectives on Sexual and Reproductive Health, 36*(3), 120-126.

Jeavons, H. (2003). Prevention and treatment of vulvovaginal candidiasis using exogenous lactobacillus. *Journal of Obstetric, Gynecologic, and Neonatal Nursing, 32*(3), 287-296.

Lawrence, R., & Lawrence, R. (2005). *Breastfeeding: A guide for the medical profession* (6th ed.). Philadelphia: Mosby.

Lopez, A., Dietz, V., Wilson, M., Navin, T., & Jones, J. (2000). Preventing congenital toxoplasmosis. *MMWR Morbidity and Mortality Weekly Report Recommendations and Reports, 49*(RR2), 59-68.

Murphy, P., Morgan, K., & Likis, F. (2006). Contraception. In K. Schuiling & F. Likis (Eds.). *Women's gynecological health.* Sudbury, MA: Jones & Bartlett.

NIH consensus statement on management of hepatitis C: 2002. (2002). *NIH Consensus and State of the Science Statements, 19*(3), 1-46.

Organization of Teratology Information Services. (2003). Acyclovir (Zovirax)/valacyclovir (Valtrex) in pregnancy. Accessed www.OTISpregnancy.org, June 12, 2006.

Perinatal HIV Guidelines Working Group. (2005). *Public Health Service Task Force recommendations for use of antiretroviral drugs in pregnant HIV-1-infected women for maternal health and interventions to reduce perinatal HIV-1 transmission in the United States.* [Online]. Accessed www.hivatis.org, February 22, 2006.

Rawlins, S. (2001). Nonviral sexually transmitted infections. *Journal of Obstetric, Gynecologic, and Neonatal Nursing, 30*(3), 324-331.

Riordan, J. (2005). *Breastfeeding and human lactation* (3rd ed.). Boston: Jones & Bartlett.

Stephenson, J. (2005). Reducing HIV vertical transmission scrutinized. *Journal of the American Medical Association, 293*(17), 2079-2081.

Terrault, A. (2002). Sexual activity as a risk factor for hepatitis C. *Hepatology, 36*(5 Suppl), S99-S105.

Thomas, D. (2001). Sexually transmitted viral infections: Epidemiology and treatment. *Journal of Obstetric, Gynecologic, and Neonatal Nursing, 30*(3), 316-323.

U.S. Food and Drug Administration (FDA). (2004). *FDA approves first oral fluid based rapid HIV test kit.* News release, March 26, 2004.

U.S. Preventive Services Task Force (USPSTF). (2005a). Screening for bacterial vaginosis in pregnancy. *The guide to clinical preventive services, 2005. Recommendations of the US Preventive Services Task Force.* Rockville, MD: Agency for Healthcare Research and Quality.

U.S. Preventive Services Task Force (USPSTF). (2005b). Screening for chlamydial infection. *The guide to clinical preventive services, 2005. Recommendations of the US Preventive Services Task Force.* Rockville, MD: Agency for Healthcare Research and Quality.

U.S. Preventive Services Task Force (USPSTF). (2005c). Screening for hepatitis B virus infection. *The guide to clinical preventive services, 2005. Recommendations of the US Preventive Services Task Force.* Rockville, MD: Agency for Healthcare Research and Quality.

U.S. Preventive Services Task Force (USPSTF). (2005d). Screening for HIV: Recommendations and rationale. *Annals of Internal Medicine, 143*(1), 32-37.

U.S. Preventive Services Task Force (USPSTF). (2005e). Screening for syphilis infection. *The guide to clinical preventive services, 2005. Recommendations of the US Preventive Services Task Force.* Rockville, MD: Agency for Healthcare Research and Quality.

Wilkinson, D., Ramjee, G., Tholandi, M., & Rutherford, G. (2002). Nonoxynol-9 spermicide for prevention of vaginally acquisition of HIV infection by women from men. In the *Cochrane Database of Systematic Reviews,* 2006, Issue 3. Chichester, UK: John Wiley & Sons.

Williams, A. (2003). Gynecologic care for women with HIV infection. *Journal of Obstetric, Gynecologic, and Neonatal Nursing, 32*(1), 87-93.

Workowski, K., Levine, W., & Wasserheit, J. (2002). U.S. Centers for Disease Control and Prevention guidelines for the treatment of sexually transmitted diseases: An opportunity to unify clinical and public health practice. *Annals of Internal Medicine, 137*(4), 255-262.

World Health Organization (WHO), Department of Reproductive Health and Research. (2000). *Improving access to quality care in family planning: Medical eligibility criteria for contraceptive use* (2nd ed.). Geneva: Author.

Yudkin, M., & Gonik, B. (2006). Perinatal infections. In R. Martin, A. Fanaroff, & M. Walsh (Eds.). *Fanaroff & Martin's neonatal-perinatal medicine: Diseases of the fetus and infant* (8th ed.). Philadelphia: Mosby.

Contraception and Abortion

learning objectives

- Compare the different methods of contraception.
- Identify the advantages and disadvantages of commonly used methods of contraception.
- Explain the common nursing interventions that facilitate contraceptive use.
- Examine the various ethical, legal, cultural, and religious considerations of contraception.
- Describe the techniques used for medical and surgical interruption of pregnancy.
- Discuss the various ethical and legal considerations of elective abortion.

electronic resources

Additional information related to the content in Chapter 9 can be found on

the companion website at *evolve*
http://evolve.elsevier.com/Lowdermilk/MWHC/
- NCLEX Review Questions
- WebLinks

or on the interactive companion CD
- NCLEX Review Questions
- Critical Thinking Exercise: Client Teaching – Contraception
- Plan of Care: Sexual Activity and Contraception

■ CONTRACEPTION

Contraception is the intentional prevention of pregnancy during sexual intercourse. *Birth control* is the device and/or practice to decrease the risk of conceiving, or bearing, off-spring. *Family planning* is the conscious decision on when to conceive, or to avoid pregnancy, throughout the reproductive years. With the wide assortment of birth control options available, it is possible for a woman to use several different contraceptive methods at various stages throughout her fertile years. Nurses interact with the woman to compare and contrast available options, reliability, relative cost, protection from sexually transmitted infections (STIs), the individual's comfort level, and partner's willingness to use a particular birth control method. Those who use contraception may still be at risk for pregnancy simply because their choice of contraceptive method is not perfect or is used inconsistently and/or incorrectly. Providing adequate instruction about how to use a contraceptive method, when to use a backup method, and when to use emergency contraception can decrease the chance of unintended pregnancy occurring (Stewart, Trussell, & Van Look, 2004b).

■ CARE MANAGEMENT

A multidisciplinary approach may assist a woman in choosing and correctly using an appropriate contraceptive method. Nurses, nurse-midwives, nurse practitioners, and other advanced practice nurses as well as physicians have the knowledge and expertise to assist a woman in making decisions about contraception that will satisfy the woman's personal, social, cultural, and interpersonal needs.

■ Assessment and Nursing Diagnoses

The woman's knowledge about contraception and commitment to any particular method are determined. Data are required about the frequency of coitus, number of sexual partners, level of contraceptive involvement, and her or her partner's objections to any methods. The woman's level of comfort and willingness to touch her genitals and cervical mucus are assessed. Myths are identified, and religious and cultural factors are determined. The woman's verbal and nonverbal responses to hearing about the various available methods are carefully noted. An individual's reproductive life plan must be considered. A history (including menstrual, contraceptive, and obstetric), physical examination (including pelvic examination), and laboratory tests are usually completed.

Informed consent is a vital component in the education of the client concerning contraception or sterilization. The nurse often has the responsibility of documenting information provided and the understanding of that information by the client. Use of the acronym *BRAIDED* may be useful (see Legal Tip).

▬ LEGAL TIP Informed Consent

B—Benefits: information about advantages and success rates
R—Risks: information about disadvantages and failure rates
A—Alternatives: information about other available methods
I— Inquiries: opportunity to ask questions
D—Decisions: opportunity to decide or to change mind
E—Explanations: information about method and how it is used
D—Documentation: information given and client's understanding

Nursing diagnoses reflect analysis of the assessment findings. Examples of nursing diagnoses that may emerge regarding contraception include those listed.

- *Decisional conflict related to*
  –contraceptive alternatives
  –partner's willingness to agree on contraceptive method
- *Fear related to*
  –contraceptive method side effects
- *Risk for infection related to*
  –unprotected sexual intercourse
  –type of contraceptive method used
  –broken skin or mucous membrane after surgery or intrauterine device (IUD) insertion
- *Ineffective sexuality patterns related to*
  –fear of pregnancy
- *Acute pain related to*
  –postoperative recovery after sterilization
- *Risk for spiritual distress related to*
  –discrepancy between religious or cultural beliefs and choice of contraception

▬ Expected Outcomes of Care

Planning is a collaborative effort among the woman, her sexual partner (when appropriate), the primary health care provider, and the nurse. The expected outcomes are determined and stated in client-centered terms and may include that the woman or couple will do the following:
- Verbalize understanding about contraceptive methods
- Verbalize understanding of all information necessary to give informed consent
- State comfort and satisfaction with the chosen method
- Use the contraceptive method correctly and consistently
- Experience no adverse sequelae as a result of the chosen method of contraception
- Prevent unplanned pregnancy or plan a pregnancy

▬ Plan of Care and Interventions

Unbiased client teaching is fundamental to initiating and maintaining any form of contraception. A care provider relationship based on trust is important for adherence by the client. To foster a safe environment for consultation, a private setting should be provided in which the client can feel free to be open. Distractions should be minimized, and samples of birth control devices for interactive teaching should be available. The nurse counters myths with facts, clarifies misinformation, and fills in gaps of knowledge. The ideal contraceptive should be safe, easily available, economical, acceptable, simple to use, and promptly reversible. Although no method may ever achieve all these objectives, significant advances in the development of new contraceptive technologies have occurred over the past 30 years (World Health Organization [WHO], 2004).

Contraceptive failure rate refers to the percentage of contraceptive users expected to have an unplanned pregnancy during the first year, even when they use a method consistently and correctly. Contraceptive effectiveness varies from couple to couple (Box 9-1) and depends on both the properties of the method and the characteristics of the user (Trussell, 2004). Failure rates decrease over time, either because a user gains experience and uses a method more appropriately or because the less effective users stop using the method.

CRITICAL THINKING EXERCISE

Choosing a Contraceptive

Joyce is a 45-year-old woman who has an appointment in the local health department family planning clinic. She is seeking information about which type of contraception would be best for her at this time in her life. She smokes a pack of cigarettes a day and has been having irregular periods.
1. Evidence—Is there sufficient evidence to draw conclusions about what response the nurse should give?
2. Assumptions—Describe underlying assumptions about the following issues:
   a. Personal considerations for choosing a birth control method
   b. Appropriate methods for perimenopausal women
3. What implications and priorities for nursing care can be made at this time?
4. Does the evidence objectively support your conclusion?
5. Are there alternative perspectives to your conclusion?

box 9-1 Factors Affecting Method Contraceptive Effectiveness

- Frequency of intercourse
- Motivation to prevent pregnancy
- Understanding of how to use the method
- Adherence to method
- Provision of short-term or long-term protection
- Likelihood of pregnancy for the individual woman
- Consistent use of method

Safety of a method depends on the woman's medical history. Barrier methods offer some protection from STIs, and oral contraceptives may reduce the incidence of ovarian and endometrial cancers but increase the risk of thromboembolic problems.

■ Methods of Contraception

The following discussion of contraceptive methods provides the nurse with information needed for client teaching. After implementing the appropriate teaching for contraceptive use, the nurse supervises return demonstrations and practice to assess client understanding (Fig. 9-1). The woman is given written instructions and telephone numbers for questions. If the woman has difficulty understanding written instructions, she (and her partner, if available) is offered graphic material and a telephone number to call as necessary, or is offered an opportunity to return for further instruction.

Coitus Interruptus

Coitus interruptus (withdrawal) involves the male partner withdrawing the penis from the woman's vagina before he ejaculates. Although coitus interruptus has been criticized as being an ineffective method of contraception, it is a good choice for couples who do not have another contraceptive available (Kowal, 2004). Effectiveness is similar to barrier methods and depends on the man's ability to withdraw his penis before ejaculation. The percentage of women who will experience an unintended pregnancy within the first year of typical use (failure rate) of withdrawal is about 19% (Trussell, 2004). Coitus interruptus does not protect against STIs or human immunodeficiency virus (HIV) infection.

Fertility Awareness Methods

Fertility awareness methods (FAMs) of contraception depend on identifying the beginning and end of the fertile period of the menstrual cycle. When women who want to use FAMs are educated about the menstrual cycle, three phases are identified:

1. Infertile phase: before ovulation
2. Fertile phase: about 5 to 7 days around the middle of the cycle, including several days before and during ovulation and the day afterward
3. Infertile phase: after ovulation

Although ovulation can be unpredictable in many women, teaching the woman about how she can directly observe her fertility patterns is an empowering tool. There are nearly a dozen categories of FAMs. To prevent pregnancy, each one uses a combination of charts, records, calculations, tools, observations, and either abstinence (natural family planning) or barrier methods of birth control during the fertile period in the menstrual cycle (Jennings, Arevalo, & Kowal, 2004). The charts and calculations associated with these methods can also be used to increase the likelihood of detecting the optimal timing of intercourse to achieve conception.

Advantages of these methods include low to no cost, absence of chemicals and hormones, and lack of alteration in the menstrual flow pattern. Disadvantages of FAMs include adherence to strict record-keeping, unintentional interference from external influences that may alter the woman's core body temperature and vaginal secretions, decreased effectiveness in women with irregular cycles (particularly adolescents who have not established regular ovulatory patterns), decreased spontaneity of coitus, and attending possibly time-consuming training sessions by qualified instructors (Jennings et al., 2004) (Box 9-2). The typical failure rate for most FAMs is 25% during the first year of use (Trussell, 2004). FAMs do not protect against STIs or HIV infection. A systematic review of randomized controlled trials of FAMs concluded that the efficacy of these methods is unknown (Grimes, Gallo, Grigorieva, Nanda, & Schulz, 2005).

FAMs involve several techniques to identify high risk, fertile days. The following discussion includes the most common techniques as well as some promising techniques for the future.

Periodic Abstinence. Periodic abstinence, or natural family planning (NFP), provides contraception by using methods that rely on avoidance of intercourse during

FIG. 9-1 Nurse counseling woman about contraceptive methods. (Courtesy Dee Lowdermilk, Chapel Hill, NC.)

---

box 9-2	**Potential Pitfalls of Using Fertility Awareness Methods of Contraception**

Potential pitfalls of using fertility awareness methods include the five *Rs*:
- **R**estriction on sexual spontaneity
- **R**igorous daily monitoring
- **R**equired training
- **R**isk of pregnancy during prolonged training period
- **R**isk of pregnancy high on unsafe days

Source: Hatcher, R., Zieman, M., Cwiak, C., Darney, P., Creinin, M., & Stosur, H. (2004). *A pocket guide to managing contraception.* Tiger, GA: Bridging the Gap Foundation.

fertile periods. NFP methods are the only contraceptive practices acceptable to the Roman Catholic Church. Signs and symptoms of fertility awareness most commonly used with abstinence are menstrual bleeding, cervical mucus, and basal body temperature (see later discussions) (Jennings et al., 2004).

The human ovum can be fertilized no later than 16 to 24 hours after ovulation. Motile sperm have been recovered from the uterus and the oviducts as long as 60 hours after coitus. However, their ability to fertilize the ovum probably lasts no longer than 24 to 48 hours. Pregnancy is unlikely to occur if a couple abstains from intercourse for 4 days before and for 3 or 4 days after ovulation (fertile period). Unprotected intercourse on the other days of the cycle (safe period) should not result in pregnancy. However, there are two principal problems with this method: the exact time of ovulation cannot be predicted accurately, and couples may find it difficult to exercise restraint for several days before and after ovulation. Women with irregular menstrual periods have the greatest risk of failure with this form of contraception.

Calendar Rhythm Method. Practice of the calendar rhythm method is based on the number of days in each cycle, counting from the first day of menses. With this method the fertile period is determined after accurately recording the lengths of menstrual cycles for 6 months. The beginning of the fertile period is estimated by subtracting 18 days from the length of the shortest cycle. The end of the fertile period is determined by subtracting 11 days from the length of the longest cycle (Jennings et al., 2004). If the shortest cycle is 24 days and the longest is 30 days, application of the formula to calculate the fertile period is as follows:

Shortest cycle: 24 − 18 = sixth day

Longest cycle: 30 − 11 = nineteenth day

To avoid conception the couple would abstain during the fertile period–days 6 through 19. If the woman has very regular cycles of 28 days each, the formula indicates the fertile days to be as follows:

Shortest cycle: 28 − 18 = tenth day

Longest cycle: 28 − 11 = seventeenth day

To avoid pregnancy, the couple abstains from day 10 through 17 because ovulation occurs on day 14 plus or minus 2 days. A major drawback of the calendar method is that one is trying to predict future events with past data. The unpredictability of the menstrual cycle also is not taken into consideration. The calendar rhythm method is most useful as an adjunct to the basal body temperature or the cervical mucus method.

Standard Days Method. The Standard Days Method (SDM) is essentially a modified form of the calendar rhythm method that has a "fixed" number of days of fertility for each cycle–that is, days 8 to 19 (Institute of Reproductive Health, 2003). A CycleBeads necklace–a color-coded string of beads–can be purchased as a concrete tool to track fertility (Fig. 9-2). Day 1 of the menstrual flow is counted as the first day to begin the counting. Women who use this device are taught to avoid unprotected intercourse on days 8 to 19 (white beads on CycleBeads™ necklace). Although this method is useful to women whose cycles are 26 to 32 days long, it is unreliable for those who have longer or shorter cycles (CycleBeads, 2003). The typical failure rate for the SDM is 12% during the first year of use (Sinai, Jennings, & Arevalo, 2004).

Ovulation Method. The cervical mucus ovulation-detection method (also called the Billings method and the Creighton model ovulation method) requires that the woman recognize and interpret the cyclic changes in the amount and consistency of cervical mucus that characterize her own unique pattern of changes (see Teaching for Self-Care box). The cervical mucus that accompanies ovulation is necessary for viability and motility of sperm. It alters the pH environment, neutralizing the acidity, to be more compatible for sperm survival. Without adequate cervical mucus, coitus does not result in conception. Women check quantity and character of mucus on the vulva or introitus with fingers or tissue paper each day for several months to learn the cycle. To ensure an accurate assessment of changes, the cervical mucus should be free from semen, contraceptive gels or foams, and blood or discharge from vaginal infections for at least one full cycle. Other factors that create difficulty in identifying mucus changes include douches and vaginal deodorants, being in the sexually aroused state (which thins the mucus), and taking medications such as antihistamines (which dry up the mucus). Intercourse is considered safe without restriction beginning the fourth day after the last day of wet, clear, slippery mucus (postovulation) (Hatcher, Zieman, Cwiak, Darney, Creinin, & Stosur, 2004).

Some women may find this method unacceptable if they are uncomfortable touching their genitals. Whether

FIG. 9-2 Cyclebeads™. Red bead marks the first day of the menstrual cycle. White beads mark days that are likely to be fertile days; therefore unprotected intercourse should be avoided. Brown beads are days when pregnancy is unlikely and unprotected intercourse is permitted. (Courtesy Dee Lowdermilk, Chapel Hill, NC.)

TEACHING FOR SELF-CARE

Cervical Mucus Characteristics

SETTING THE STAGE

- Show charts of menstrual cycle along with changes in the cervical mucus.
- Have woman practice with raw egg white.
- Supply her with a basal body temperature (BBT) log and graph if she does not already have one.
- Explain that assessment of cervical mucus characteristics is best when mucus is not mixed with semen, contraceptive jellies or foams, or discharge from infections. Douching should not be done before assessment.

CONTENT RELATED TO CERVICAL MUCUS

- Explain to woman (couple) how cervical mucus changes throughout the menstrual cycle.
  a. Postmenstrual mucus: scant.
  b. Preovulation mucus: cloudy, yellow or white, sticky
  c. Ovulation mucus: clear, wet, sticky, slippery
  d. Postovulation fertile mucus: thick, cloudy, sticky
  e. Postovulation, postfertile mucus: scant

- Right before ovulation, the watery, thin, clear mucus becomes more abundant and thick (Fig. A). It feels like a lubricant and can be stretched 5+ cm between the thumb and forefinger; this is called spinnbarkeit (Fig. B). This indicates the period of maximal fertility. Sperm deposited in this type of mucus can survive until ovulation occurs.

ASSESSMENT TECHNIQUE

- Stress that good handwashing is imperative to begin and end all self-assessment.
- Start observation from last day of menstrual flow.
- Assess cervical mucus several times a day for several cycles. Mucus can be obtained from vaginal introitus; no need to reach into vagina to cervix.
- Record findings on the same record on which BBT is entered.

Fig. A
Estrogens — Early follicular phase
Estrogens progesterone — Ovulation
Progesterone estrogens — Luteal phase

Fig. B
Day 10 — Spinnbarkeit 6 cm
Day 13 — Spinnbarkeit 12 cm
Day 16 — Spinnbarkeit 3 cm

or not the individual wants to use this method for contraception, it is to the woman's advantage to learn to recognize mucus characteristics at ovulation. Self-evaluation of cervical mucus can be highly accurate and can be useful diagnostically for any of the following purposes:

- To alert the couple to the reestablishment of ovulation while breastfeeding and after discontinuation of oral contraception
- To note anovulatory cycles at any time and at the commencement of menopause
- To assist couples in planning a pregnancy

Basal Body Temperature Method. The basal body temperature (BBT) is the lowest body temperature of a healthy person, taken immediately after waking and before getting out of bed. The BBT usually varies from 36.2° C to 36.3° C during menses and for about 5 to 7 days afterward (Fig. 9-3). At about the time of ovulation, a slight decrease in temperature (approximately 0.5° C) may occur in some women, but others may have no decrease at all. After ovulation, in concert with the increasing progesterone levels of the early luteal phase of the cycle, the BBT increases slightly (approximately 0.4° C to 0.8° C). The temperature remains on an elevated plateau until 2 to 4 days before menstruation, and then it decreases to the low levels recorded during the previous cycle, unless pregnancy has occurred and the temperature remains elevated. If ovulation fails to occur, the pattern of lower body temperature continues throughout the cycle.

FIG. 9-3 A, Special thermometer for recording basal body temperature, marked in tenths to enable person to read more easily. **B,** Basal temperature record shows drop and sharp rise at time of ovulation. Biphasic curve indicates ovulatory cycle.

To use this method, the fertile period is defined as the day of first temperature drop, or first elevation through 3 consecutive days of elevated temperature. Abstinence begins the first day of menstrual bleeding and lasts through 3 consecutive days of sustained temperature rise (at least 0.2° C). (Jennings et al., 2004). The decrease and subsequent increase in temperature are referred to as the *thermal shift.* When the entire month's temperatures are recorded on a graph, the pattern described is more apparent. It is more difficult to perceive day-to-day variations without the entire picture. Infection, fatigue, less than 3 hours sleep per night, awakening late, and anxiety may cause temperature fluctuations, altering the expected pattern. If a new BBT thermometer is purchased, this fact is noted on the chart, because the readings may vary slightly. Jet lag, alcohol and antipyretic medications taken the evening before, or sleeping in a heated waterbed also must be noted on the chart, because each affects the BBT. Therefore the BBT alone is not a reliable method of predicting ovulation (Jennings et al.).

Symptothermal Method. The symptothermal method is a tool for the woman to gain fertility awareness as she tracks the physiologic and psychologic symptoms that mark the phases of her cycle. This method combines at least two methods, usually cervical mucus changes with BBT, in addition to heightened awareness of secondary, cycle phase–related symptoms. Secondary symptoms may include increased libido, midcycle spotting, mittelschmerz, pelvic fullness or tenderness, and vulvar fullness. The woman is taught to palpate her cervix to assess for changes in texture, position, and dilation that indicate ovulation. During the preovulatory and ovulatory periods, the cervix softens, opens, rises in the vagina, and is more moist. During the postovulatory period the cervix drops, becomes

firm, and closes. The woman notes days on which coitus, changes in routine, illness, and so on have occurred (Fig. 9-4). Calendar calculations and cervical mucus changes are used to estimate the onset of the fertile period; changes in cervical mucus or the BBT are used to estimate its end.

Home Predictor Test Kits for Ovulation. All of the preceding methods discussed are indicative of but do not prove the occurrence and exact timing of ovulation. The urine predictor test for ovulation is a major addition to the NFP and fertility-awareness methods to help women who want to plan the time of their pregnancies and those who are trying to conceive (Fig. 9-5). The urine predictor test for ovulation detects the sudden surge of luteinizing hormone (LH) that occurs approximately 12 to 24 hours before ovulation. Unlike BBT, the test is not affected by illness, emotional upset, or physical activity. For home use, a test kit contains sufficient material for several days of testing during each cycle. A positive response indicative of an LH surge is noted by an easy-to-read color change. Directions for use of urine predictor test kits vary with the manufacturer. Saliva predictor tests for ovulation use dried, nonfoamy saliva as a tool to show fertility patterns. More research is needed to determine the efficacy of use of these tests for pregnancy prevention.

The Marquette Model (MM) is a natural family planning method that was developed through the Marquette University College of Nursing Institute for Natural Family Planning. The MM uses cervical monitoring along with the ClearPlan Easy Fertility Monitor. The ClearPlan Monitor is a handheld device that uses test strips to measure urinary metabolites of estrogen and LH. The monitor provides the user with "low," "high," and "peak" fertility readings. The MM incorporates the use of the monitor as an aid to learning NFP and fertility awareness. The MM is currently being tested at different sites in the United States for its effectiveness in helping couples avoid pregnancy (Institute for Natural Family Planning Services, 2005).

TwoDay Method of Family Planning. Based on monitoring and the recording of cervical secretions, a new algorithm for identifying the fertile window has been developed by the Institute for Reproductive Health at Georgetown University (Arevalo, Jennings, Nikula, & Sinai, 2004). The TwoDay Algorithm appears to be simpler to teach, learn, and use than current natural methods. Results suggest that the algorithm can be an effective alternative for low literacy populations or for programs that find current Natural Family Planning methods too time consuming or otherwise not feasible to incorporate into their services. Two questions are posed. Each day, the woman is to ask herself, (1) "Did I note secretions today?" and (2) "Did I note secretions yesterday?" If the answer to either is yes, she should avoid coitus or use a backup method of birth control. If the answer to both questions is no, her probability of getting pregnant is very low. Further studies are needed to determine the efficacy of the TwoDay Algorithm in avoiding pregnancy and to assess its acceptability to users and providers.

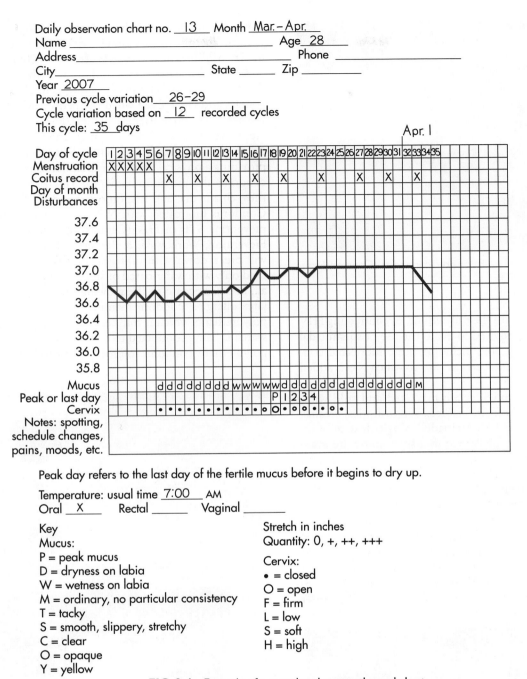

Daily observation chart no. __13__ Month __Mar.–Apr.__
Name _____ Age __28__
Address_____ Phone _____
City_____ State _____ Zip _____
Year _2007__
Previous cycle variation __26–29_____
Cycle variation based on __12__ recorded cycles
This cycle: _35_ days

FIG. 9-4 Example of a completed symptothermal chart.

Peak day refers to the last day of the fertile mucus before it begins to dry up.

Temperature: usual time _7:00__ AM
Oral __X__   Rectal _____   Vaginal _____

Key
Mucus:
P = peak mucus
D = dryness on labia
W = wetness on labia
M = ordinary, no particular consistency
T = tacky
S = smooth, slippery, stretchy
C = clear
O = opaque
Y = yellow

Stretch in inches
Quantity: 0, +, ++, +++

Cervix:
• = closed
O = open
F = firm
L = low
S = soft
H = high

Barrier Methods

Barrier contraceptives have gained in popularity not only as a contraceptive method but also as a protective measure against the spread of STIs, such as human papilloma virus (HPV) and herpes simplex virus (HSV). Some male condoms and female vaginal methods provide a physical barrier to several STIs, and some male condoms provide protection against HIV (Cates & Stewart, 2004; Warner, Hatcher, & Steiner, 2004). Spermicides serve as chemical barriers against the sperm.

Spermicides. Spermicides, such as nonoxynol-9 (N-9), work by reducing the sperm's mobility; the chemicals attack the sperm flagella and body, thereby preventing the sperm from reaching the cervical os. N-9, the most commonly used spermicidal chemical in the United States, is a surfactant that destroys the sperm cell membrane; however, data now suggest that frequent use (more than 2 times a day) of N-9, or use as a lubricant during anal intercourse, may increase the transmission of HIV and can cause lesions (Cates & Raymond, 2004). Women with high risk

FIG. 9-5 Examples of ovulation prediction tests. (Courtesy Shannon Perry, Phoenix, AZ.)

behaviors that increase their likelihood of contracting HIV and other STIs are advised to avoid the use of spermicidal products containing N-9, including those lubricated condoms, diaphragms, and cervical caps to which N-9 is added (WHO, 2004).

Intravaginal spermicides are marketed and sold without a prescription as foams, tablets, suppositories, creams, films, and gels (Fig. 9-6). Preloaded, single-dose applicators small enough to be carried in a small purse are available. Effectiveness of spermicides depends on consistent and accurate use. Caution clients against misunderstanding terms: contraceptive gel differs from fruit jelly, and cosmetics or hair products containing the nonspermicidal forms of nonoxynol are not adequate substitutes. The spermicide should be inserted high into the vagina so that it makes contact with the cervix. Some spermicide should be inserted at least 15 minutes before, and no longer than 1 hour before, sexual intercourse. Spermicide must be reapplied for each additional act of intercourse, even if a barrier

method is used. Studies have shown varying effectiveness rates for spermicidal use alone. Typical failure rate for spermicide use alone is about 29% (Trussell, 2004).

Condoms. The male condom is a thin, stretchable sheath that covers the penis before genital, oral, or anal contact and is removed when the penis is withdrawn from the partner's orifice after ejaculation (Fig. 9-7, *A*). Condoms are made of latex rubber, polyurethane (strong, thin plastic), or natural membranes (animal tissue). In addition to providing a physical barrier for sperm, nonspermicidal latex condoms also provide a barrier for STIs (particularly gonorrhea, chlamydia, and trichomonas) and HIV transmission. Condoms lubricated with N-9 are not recommended for preventing STIs or HIV (Centers for Disease Control and Prevention, Workowski, & Berman, 2006). Latex condoms will break down with oil-based lubricants and should be used only with water-based or silicone lubricants (Warner et al., 2004). Because of the growing number of people with latex allergies, condom manufacturers have begun using polyurethane, which is thinner and stronger than latex. Research is being conducted to determine the effectiveness of polyurethane condoms to protect against STIs and HIV.

FIG. 9-7 **A,** Mechanical barriers. From the top left corner, clockwise: female condom, male condom, cervical cap, diaphragm. **B,** Contraceptive sponge. (**A,** Courtesy Dee Lowdermilk, Chapel Hill, NC; **B,** Courtesy Allendale Pharmaceuticals, Inc., Allendale, NJ.)

FIG. 9-6 Spermicides. (Courtesy Marjorie Pyle, RNC, Lifecircle, Costa Mesa, CA.)

■ **NURSE ALERT**

All persons should be questioned about the potential for latex allergy. Latex condom use is contraindicated for people with latex sensitivity.

A small percentage of condoms are made from lamb cecum (natural skin). Natural skin condoms do not provide the same protection against STIs and HIV infection as latex condoms. Natural skin condoms contain small pores that could allow passage of viruses such as hepatitis B, HSV, and HIV. Condoms must be discarded after each single use. They are available without a prescription.

A functional difference in condom shape is the presence or absence of a sperm-reservoir tip. To enhance vaginal stimulation, some condoms are contoured and rippled or have ribbed or roughened surfaces (see Fig. 9-7, *A*). Thinner construction increases heat transmission and sensitivity; a variety of colors and flavors increase condoms' acceptability and attractiveness (Hatcher et al., 2004). A wet jelly or dry powder lubricates some condoms. Typical failure rate in the first year of male condom use is 15%

(Trussell, 2004). To prevent unintended pregnancy and the spread of STIs, it is essential that condoms be used consistently and correctly. Instructions, such as those listed in Box 9-3, can be used for client teaching.

The female condom is a lubricated vaginal sheath made of polyurethane and has flexible rings at both ends (see Fig. 9-7, *A*). The closed end of the pouch is inserted into the vagina and is anchored around the cervix, and the open ring covers the labia. Women whose partner will not wear a male condom can use this as a protective mechanical barrier. Rewetting drops or oil- or water-based lubricants can be used to help decrease the distracting noise that is produced while penile thrusting occurs. The female condom is available in one size, is intended for single use only, and is sold over the counter. Male condoms should not be used concurrently, because the friction from both sheaths can increase the likelihood of either or both tearing (Female Condom, 2004). Typical failure rate in the first year of female condom use is 21% (Trussell, 2004).

box 9-3　Male Condoms

MECHANISM OF ACTION
- Sheath is applied over the erect penis before insertion or loss of preejaculatory drops of semen. Used correctly, condoms prevent sperm from entering the cervix. Spermicide-coated condoms cause ejaculated sperm to be immobilized rapidly, thus increasing contraceptive effectiveness.

FAILURE RATE
- Typical users, 15%
- Correct and consistent users, 2%

ADVANTAGES
- Safe.
- No side effects.
- Readily available.
- Premalignant changes in cervix can be prevented or ameliorated in women whose partners use condoms.
- Method of male nonsurgical contraception.

DISADVANTAGES
- Must interrupt lovemaking to apply sheath.
- Sensation may be altered.
- If used improperly, spillage of sperm can result in pregnancy.
- Condoms occasionally may tear during intercourse.

STI PROTECTION
- If a condom is used throughout the act of intercourse and there is no unprotected contact with female genitals, a latex rubber condom, which is impermeable to viruses, can act as a protective measure against sexually transmitted infections.

NURSING CONSIDERATIONS
Teach man to do the following:
- Use a new condom (check expiration date) for each act of sexual intercourse or other acts between partners that involve contact with the penis.

Fig. A 　　　　 **Fig. B**

- Place condom after penis is erect and before intimate contact.
- Place condom on head of penis (Fig. A) and unroll it all the way to the base (Fig. B).
- Leave an empty space at the tip (Fig. A); remove any air remaining in the tip by gently pressing air out toward the base of the penis.
- If a lubricant is desired, use water-based products such as K-Y lubricating jelly. —Do not use petroleum-based products because they can cause the condom to break.
- After ejaculation, carefully withdraw the still-erect penis from the vagina, holding onto condom rim; remove and discard the condom.
- Store unused condoms in cool, dry place.
- Do not use condoms that are sticky, brittle, or obviously damaged.

STI, Sexually transmitted infection.

TEACHING FOR SELF-CARE

Use and Care of the Diaphragm

POSITIONS FOR INSERTION OF DIAPHRAGM

Squatting

- Squatting is the most commonly used position, and most women find it satisfactory.

Leg-up Method

- Another position is to raise the left foot (if right hand is used for insertion) on a low stool and, while in a bending position, insert the diaphragm.

Chair Method

- Another practical method for diaphragm insertion is to sit far forward on the edge of a chair.

Reclining

- You may prefer to insert the diaphragm while in a semi-reclining position in bed.

INSPECTION OF DIAPHRAGM

Your diaphragm must be inspected carefully before each use.

- The best way to do this is as follows:
  - Hold the diaphragm up to a light source. Carefully stretch the diaphragm at the area of the rim, on all sides, to make sure there are no holes. Remember, it is possible to puncture the diaphragm with sharp fingernails.
  - Another way to check for pinholes is carefully to fill the diaphragm with water. If there is any problem, it will be seen immediately.
  - If your diaphragm is puckered, especially near the rim, this could mean thin spots.
- The diaphragm should not be used if you see any of the above, consult your health care provider.

PREPARATION OF DIAPHRAGM

- Rinse off cornstarch. Your diaphragm must always be used with a spermicidal lubricant to be effective. Pregnancy cannot be prevented effectively by the diaphragm alone.
- Always empty your bladder before inserting the diaphragm. Place about 2 teaspoonfuls of contraceptive jelly or contraceptive cream on the side of the diaphragm that will rest against the cervix (or whichever way you have been instructed). Spread it around to coat the surface and the rim. This aids in insertion and offers a more complete seal. Many women also spread some jelly or cream on the other side of the diaphragm (Fig. A).

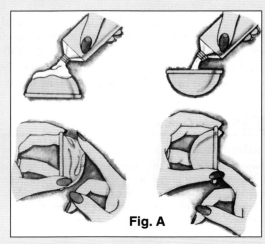

Fig. A

INSERTION OF DIAPHRAGM

- The diaphragm can be inserted as long as 6 hours before intercourse. Hold the diaphragm between your thumb and fingers. The dome can either be up or down, as directed by your health care provider. Place your index finger on the outer rim of the compressed diaphragm (Fig. B).

Fig. B

- Use the fingers of the other hand to spread the labia (lips of the vagina). This will assist in guiding the diaphragm into place.

Use and Care of the Diaphragm—cont'd

INSERTION OF DIAPHRAGM—cont'd

- Insert the diaphragm into the vagina. Direct it inward and downward as far as it will go to the space behind and below the cervix (Fig. C).

Fig. C

- Tuck the front of the rim of the diaphragm behind the pubic bone so that the rubber hugs the front wall of the vagina (Fig. D).

Fig. D

- Feel for your cervix through the diaphragm to be certain it is properly placed and securely covered by the rubber dome (Fig. E).

Fig. E

GENERAL INFORMATION

- Regardless of the time of the month, you must use your diaphragm every time intercourse takes place. Your diaphragm must be left in place for at least 6 hours after the last intercourse. If you remove your diaphragm before the 6-hour period, your chance of becoming pregnant could be greatly increased. If you have repeated acts of intercourse, you must add more spermicide for each act of intercourse.

REMOVAL OF DIAPHRAGM

- The only proper way to remove the diaphragm is to insert your forefinger up and over the top side of the diaphragm and slightly to the side.
- Next, turn the palm of your hand downward and backward, hooking the forefinger firmly on top of the inside of the upper rim of the diaphragm, breaking the suction (Fig. F).

Fig. F

- Pull the diaphragm down and out. This avoids the possibility of tearing the diaphragm with the fingernails. You should not remove the diaphragm by trying to catch the rim from below the dome.

CARE OF DIAPHRAGM

- When using a vaginal diaphragm, avoid using oil-based products, such as certain body lubricants, mineral oil, baby oil, vaginal lubricants, or vaginitis preparations during intercourse. These products can weaken the rubber.
- A little care means longer wear for your diaphragm. After each use, wash the diaphragm in warm water and mild soap. Do not use detergent soaps, cold-cream soaps, deodorant soaps, and soaps containing oil products, because they can weaken the rubber.
- After washing, dry the diaphragm thoroughly. All water and moisture should be removed with a towel. Then dust the diaphragm with cornstarch. Scented talc, body powder, baby powder, and the like should not be used because they can weaken the rubber.
- To clean the introducer (if one is used), wash with mild soap and warm water, rinse, and dry thoroughly.
- Place the diaphragm back in the plastic case for storage. Do not store it near a radiator or heat source or exposed to light for an extended period.

Diaphragms. The contraceptive diaphragm is a shallow, dome-shaped latex or silicone device with a flexible rim that covers the cervix (see Fig. 9-7, *A*). There are three types of diaphragms available: coil spring, arcing spring, and wide seal rim. Available in many sizes, the diaphragm should be the largest size the woman can wear without her being aware of its presence. Typical failure rate of the diaphragm combined with spermicide is 16% in the first year of use (Trussell, 2004). Effectiveness of the diaphragm is less when used without spermicide (Trussell). Women at high risk for HIV should avoid use of N-9 spermicides with the diaphragm (Cates & Raymond, 2004).

The woman is informed that she needs an annual gynecologic examination to assess the fit of the diaphragm. The device should be inspected before every use, replaced every 2 years, and may have to be refitted for a 20% weight fluctuation, after any abdominal or pelvic surgery, and after every pregnancy (Planned Parenthood, 2004). Because various types of diaphragms are on the market, the nurse uses the package insert for teaching the woman how to use and care for the diaphragm (see Teaching for Self-Care box).

Disadvantages of diaphragm use include the reluctance of some women to insert and remove the diaphragm. Although it can be inserted up to 6 hours before intercourse, a cold diaphragm and a cold gel temporarily reduce vaginal response to sexual stimulation if insertion of the diaphragm occurs immediately before intercourse. Some women or couples object to the messiness of the spermicide. These annoyances of diaphragm use, along with failure to insert the device once foreplay has begun, are the most common reasons for failures of this method. Side effects may include irritation of tissues related to contact with spermicides. The diaphragm is not a good option for women with poor vaginal muscle tone or recurrent urinary tract infections. For proper placement, the diaphragm must rest behind the pubic symphysis and completely cover the cervix. To decrease the chance of exerting urethral pressure, the woman should be reminded to empty her bladder before diaphragm insertion and immediately after intercourse. Diaphragms are contraindicated for women with pelvic relaxation (uterine prolapse) or a large cystocele. Women with a latex allergy should not use latex diaphragms.

Toxic shock syndrome (TSS), although reported in very small numbers, can occur in association with the use of the contraceptive diaphragm and cervical caps (Cates & Stewart, 2004). The nurse should instruct the woman about ways to reduce her risk for TSS. These measures include prompt removal 6 to 8 hours after intercourse, not using the diaphragm or cervical caps during menses, and learning and watching for danger signs of TSS.

■ **NURSE ALERT**

The nurse should alert the woman about signs of TSS in women who use a diaphragm or cervical cap as a contraceptive method. The most common signs include a sunburn type of rash, diarrhea, dizziness, faintness, weakness, sore throat, aching muscles and joints, sudden high fever, and vomiting (Planned Parenthood, 2004).

Cervical Caps. Three types of cervical caps are available; two come in varying sizes and one is one-size-fits-all. They are made of rubber or latex-free silicone and have soft domes and firm brims (see Fig. 9-7, *A*). The cap fits snugly around the base of the cervix close to the junction of the cervix and vaginal fornices. It is recommended that the cap remain in place no less than 6 hours and not more than 48 hours at a time. It is left in place at least 6 hours after the last act of intercourse. The seal provides a physical barrier to sperm: spermicide inside the cap adds a chemical barrier. The extended period of wear may be an added convenience for women.

TEACHING FOR SELF-CARE

Use of the Cervical Cap

• Push cap up into vagina until it covers cervix.

• Press rim against cervix to create a seal.

• To remove, push rim toward right or left hip to loosen from cervix, and then withdraw.

• The woman can assume several positions to insert the cervical cap. See the four positions shown for inserting the diaphragm.

Instructions for the actual insertion and use of the cervical cap closely resemble the instructions for the use of the contraceptive diaphragm. Some of the differences are that the cervical cap can be inserted hours before sexual intercourse without a need for additional spermicide later, no additional spermicide is required for repeated acts of intercourse when the cap is used, and the cervical cap requires less spermicide than the diaphragm when initially inserted. The angle of the uterus, the vaginal muscle tone, and the shape of the cervix may interfere with the cervical cap's ease of fitting and use. Correct fitting requires time, effort, and skill from both the woman and the clinician. The woman must check the cap's position before and after each act of intercourse (see Teaching for Self-Care box).

Because of the potential risk of TSS associated with the use of the cervical cap, another form of birth control is recommended for use during menstrual bleeding and up to at least 6 weeks postpartum. The cap should be refitted after any gynecologic surgery or birth and after major weight losses or gains. Otherwise, the size should be checked at least once a year.

Women who are not good candidates for wearing the cervical cap include those with abnormal Papanicolaou (Pap) test results, those who cannot be fitted properly with the existing cap sizes, those who find the insertion and removal of the device too difficult, those with a history of TSS, those with vaginal or cervical infections, and those who experience allergic responses to the latex cap or spermicide. Failure rates the first year of use are 16% in nulliparous and 32% in multiparous women (Trussell, 2004).

Contraceptive Sponge. The vaginal sponge is a small, round, polyurethane sponge that contains N-9 spermicide (see Fig. 9-7, *B*). It is designed to fit over the cervix (one size fits all). The side that is placed next to the cervix is concave for better fit. The opposite side has a woven polyester loop to be used for removal of the sponge.

The sponge must be moistened with water before it is inserted. It provides protection for up to 24 hours and for repeated instances of sexual intercourse. The sponge should be left in place for at least 6 hours after the last act of intercourse. Wearing it longer than 24 to 30 hours may put the woman at risk for TSS (Cates & Stewart, 2004).

Typical failure rate in the first year of use is 40% for parous women and 20% for nulliparous women (Trussell, 2004).

Hormonal Methods

More than 30 different contraceptive formulations are available in the United States today. General classes are described in Table 9-1. Because of the wide variety of preparations available, the woman and the nurse must read the package insert for information about specific products prescribed. Formulations include combined estrogen-progestin medications and progestational agents. The formulations are administered orally, transdermally, vaginally, by implantation, or by injection.

Combined Estrogen-Progestin Contraceptives

Oral Contraceptives. The normal menstrual cycle is maintained by a feedback mechanism. Follicle-stimulating hormone (FSH) and LH are secreted in response to fluctuating levels of ovarian estrogen and progesterone. Regular ingestion of combined oral contraceptive pills (COCs) suppresses the action of the hypothalamus and anterior pituitary, leading to insufficient secretion of FSH and LH; therefore follicles do not mature, and ovulation is inhibited.

Other contraceptive effects are induced by the combined steroids. Maturation of the endometrium is altered, making it a less favorable site for implantation. COCs also have a direct effect on the endometrium, so that from 1 to 4 days after the last COC is taken, the endometrium sloughs and bleeds as a result of hormone withdrawal. The withdrawal bleeding is usually less profuse than that of normal menstruation and may last only 2 to 3 days. Some women have no bleeding at all. The cervical mucus remains thick from the effect of the progestin (Hatcher & Nelson, 2004).

Cervical mucus under the effect of progesterone does not provide as suitable an environment for sperm penetration as does the thin, watery mucus at ovulation. The possible effect, if any, of altered tubal and uterine motility induced by COCs is not clear.

Monophasic pills provide fixed dosages of estrogen and progestin. Multiphasic pills (e.g., biphasic and triphasic oral contraceptives) alter the amount of progestin

table 9-1 Hormonal Contraception		
COMPOSITION	**ROUTE OF ADMINISTRATION**	**DURATION OF EFFECT**
Combination estrogen and progestin (synthetic estrogens and progestins in varying doses and formulations)	Oral Transdermal Vaginal ring insertion Intramuscular injection	24 hours; extended cycle—12 weeks 7 days 3 weeks 1 month*

Progestin only
  Norethindrone, norgestrel
  Medroxyprogesterone acetate
  Levonorgestrel
  Progestin etonogestrel
	Oral
	Intramuscular injection
	Intrauterine device
	Subdermal implant
		24 hours
		3 months
		Up to 5 years
		3 to 5 years*

* Not currently available in the United States.

and sometimes the amount of estrogen within each cycle. These preparations reduce the total dosage of hormones in a single cycle without sacrificing contraceptive efficacy (Hatcher & Nelson, 2004). To maintain adequate hormonal levels for contraception and enhance compliance, COCs should be taken at the same time each day.

Advantages. Because taking the pill does not relate directly to the sexual act, its acceptability may be increased. Improvement in sexual response may occur once the possibility of pregnancy is not an issue. For some women, it is convenient to know when to expect the next menstrual flow.

Evidence of noncontraceptive benefits of oral contraceptives is based on studies of high-dose pills (50 mg estrogen). Few data exist on noncontraceptive benefits of low-dose oral contraceptives (less than 35 mg estrogen) (Hatcher & Nelson, 2004). The noncontraceptive health benefits of COCs include decreased menstrual blood loss and decreased iron-deficiency anemia, regulation of menorrhagia and irregular cycles, and reduced incidence of dysmenorrhea and premenstrual syndrome (PMS). Oral contraceptives also offer protection against endometrial cancer and ovarian cancer, reduce the incidence of benign breast disease, improve acne, protect against the development of functional ovarian cysts and salpingitis, and decrease the risk of ectopic pregnancy. Oral contraceptives are considered a safe option for nonsmoking women until menopause. Perimenopausal women can benefit from regular bleeding cycles, a regular hormonal pattern, and the noncontraceptive health benefits of oral contraceptives (Hatcher & Nelson).

Women taking combined oral contraceptives are examined before the medication is prescribed and yearly thereafter. The examination includes medical and family history, weight, blood pressure, general physical and pelvic examinations, and screening cervical cytologic analysis (Pap test). Consistent monitoring by the health care provider is valuable in the detection of disorders that are not contraception related as well, so that timely treatment can be initiated. Most health care providers assess the woman 3 months after beginning COCs to detect any complications.

Use of oral hormonal contraceptives is initiated on one of the first days of the menstrual cycle (day 1 of the cycle is the first day of menses) or after childbirth or abortion. With a "Sunday start," women begin taking pills on the first Sunday after the start of their menstrual period. If contraceptives are to be started at any time other than during normal menses, or within 3 weeks after birth, miscarriage, or induced abortion, another method of contraception should be used throughout the first week to avoid the risk of pregnancy (Hatcher & Nelson, 2004). Taken exactly as directed, oral contraceptives prevent ovulation, and pregnancy cannot occur; the overall effectiveness rate is almost 100%. Almost all failures (i.e., pregnancy occurs) are caused by omission of one or more pills during the regimen. The typical failure rate of COCs due to omission is 8% (Trussell, 2004).

Disadvantages and Side Effects. Since hormonal contraceptives have come into use, the amount of estrogen and progestational agent contained in each tablet has been reduced considerably. This is important because adverse effects are, to a degree, dose related.

Women must be screened for conditions that present absolute or relative contraindications to oral contraceptive use. Contraindications for COC use include a history of thromboembolic disorders, cerebrovascular or coronary artery disease, breast cancer, estrogen-dependent tumors, pregnancy, impaired liver function, liver tumor, lactation less than 6 weeks postpartum, smoking if older than 35 years, headaches with focal neurologic symptoms, surgery with prolonged immobilization or any surgery on the legs, hypertension (160/100 mm Hg), and diabetes mellitus (of more than 20 years' duration) with vascular disease (Hatcher & Nelson, 2004).

Certain side effects of COCs are attributable to estrogen, progestin, or both. Serious adverse effects documented with high doses of estrogen and progesterone include stroke, myocardial infarction, thromboembolism, hypertension, gallbladder disease, and liver tumors (Hatcher & Nelson, 2004). Common side effects of estrogen excess include nausea, breast tenderness, fluid retention, and chloasma. Side effects of estrogen deficiency include early spotting (days 1 to 14), hypomenorrhea, nervousness, and atrophic vaginitis leading to painful intercourse (dyspareunia). Side effects of progestin excess include increased appetite, tiredness, depression, breast tenderness, vaginal yeast infection, oily skin and scalp, hirsutism, and postpill amenorrhea. Side effects of progestin deficiency include late spotting and breakthrough bleeding (days 15 to 21), heavy flow with clots, and decreased breast size. One of the most common side effects of combined COCs is bleeding irregularities (Hatcher & Nelson).

In the presence of side effects, especially those that are bothersome to the woman, a different product, a different drug content, or another method of contraception may be required. The "right" product for a woman contains the lowest dose of hormones that prevents ovulation and that has the fewest and least harmful side effects. There is no way to predict the right dosage for any particular woman. Issues to consider in prescribing oral contraceptives include history of oral contraceptive use, side effects during past use, menstrual history, and drug interactions (Hatcher & Nelson, 2004).

Large prospective studies have not shown a relation between oral contraceptive use and diabetes or glucose intolerance (Hatcher & Nelson, 2004). The risks and benefits should be assessed before prescribing oral contraceptives for diabetic women.

The effectiveness of oral contraceptives can be negatively influenced when the following medications are taken simultaneously (Hatcher & Nelson, 2004):

- *Anticonvulsants:* barbiturates, oxcarbazepine, phenytoin, phenobarbital, felbamate, carbamazepine, primidone, and topiramate

- *Systemic antifungals:* griseofulvin
- *Antituberculosis drugs:* rifampicin and rifabutin
- *Anti-HIV protease inhibitors:* e.g., nelfinavir, amprenavir

■ **NURSE ALERT**

Over-the-counter medications, as well as some herbal supplements (such as St John's wort) can alter the effectiveness of COCs. Women should be asked about their use when COCs are being considered for contraception.

No strong pharmacokinetic evidence exists that shows a relation between broad-spectrum antibiotic use and altered hormonal levels among oral contraceptive users, although potential antibiotic interaction can occur (Hatcher & Nelson, 2004). Metaanalysis of studies on the incidence of breast cancer in COC users has not found a significant increase of breast cancer in women who use COCs (Marchbanks et al., 2002).

After discontinuing oral contraception, return to fertility usually happens quickly, but fertility rates are slightly lower the first 3 to 12 months after discontinuation (Hatcher & Nelson, 2004). Many women ovulate the next month after stopping oral contraceptives. Women who discontinue oral contraception for a planned pregnancy commonly ask whether they should wait before attempting to conceive. Studies indicate that these infants have no greater chance of being born with any type of birth defect than do infants born to women in the general population, even if conception occurred in the first month after the medication was discontinued. Little evidence suggests that oral contraceptives cause postpill amenorrhea. Amenorrhea after oral contraceptive use is probably related to the woman's menstrual cycle before taking the pill (Hatcher & Nelson).

Nursing Considerations. Many different preparations of oral hormonal contraceptives are available. The nurse reviews the prescribing information in the package insert with the woman. Because of the wide variations, each woman must be clear about the unique dosage regimen for the preparation prescribed for her. Directions for care after missing one or two tablets also vary (Fig. 9-8).

Withdrawal bleeding tends to be short and scanty when some combination pills are taken. A woman may see no fresh blood at all. A drop of blood or a brown smudge on a tampon or the underwear counts as a menstrual period.

Only about 68% of women who start taking oral contraceptives are still taking them after 1 year (Trussell, 2004). It therefore is important that nurses recommend that all women choosing to use oral contraceptives be provided with a second method of birth control and that women be instructed and comfortable with this backup method. Most women stop taking oral contraceptives for nonmedical reasons.

The nurse also reviews the signs of potential complications associated with the use of oral contraceptives (see Signs of Potential Complications box). Oral contraceptives

---

signs of potential complications

Oral Contraceptives

Before oral contraceptives (OCs) are prescribed and periodically throughout hormone therapy, alert the woman to stop taking the pill and to report any of the following symptoms to the health care provider immediately. The word *ACHES* helps in retention of this list:

A—Abdominal pain may indicate a problem with the liver or gallbladder.

C—Chest pain or shortness of breath may indicate possible clot problem within lungs or heart.

H—Headaches (sudden or persistent) may be caused by cardiovascular accident or hypertension.

E—Eye problems may indicate vascular accident or hypertension.

S—Severe leg pain may indicate a thromboembolic process.

---

do not protect a woman against STIs or HIV. A barrier method such as condoms and spermicide should be used for protection.

Oral Contraceptives 91-Day Regimen. An extended-cycle oral contraceptive was approved by the U.S. Food and Drug Administration (FDA) in 2003. Levonorgestrel/ethinyl estradiol (Seasonale) contains both estrogen and progestin and is taken in 3-month cycles of 12 weeks of active pills followed by 1 week of inactive pills. Menstrual periods occur during the thirteenth week of the cycle. There is no protection from sexually transmitted infections, and risks are similar to COCs. Available only by prescription, Seasonale must be taken on a daily schedule, regardless of the frequency of intercourse. Since users will have fewer menstrual flows, they should consider the possibility of pregnancy if they do not experience their thirteenth-week flows. Typical failure rate in the first year of Seasonale use is less than 2% (FDA, 2003).

Transdermal Contraceptive System. Available by prescription only, the contraceptive transdermal patch delivers continuous levels of norelgestromin (progesterone) and ethinyl estradiol. The patch can be applied to intact skin of the upper outer arm, the upper torso (front and back, excluding the breasts), the lower abdomen, or the buttocks (Fig. 9-9). Application is on the same day once a week for 3 weeks, followed by a week without the patch. Withdrawal bleeding occurs during the "no-patch" week. Mechanism of action, efficacy, contraindications, skin reactions, and side effects are similar to those of COCs. The typical failure rate during the first year of use is under 2% in women weighing less than 198 pounds (FDA, 2003).

Vaginal Contraceptive Ring. Available only with a prescription, the vaginal contraceptive ring is a flexible ring (made of ethylene vinyl acetate copolymer) worn in the vagina to deliver continuous levels of etonorgestrel (progesterone) and ethinyl estradiol (see Fig. 9-9). One vaginal ring is worn for 3 weeks, followed by a week without the ring. The ring is inserted by the woman and does not have

Flowchart for Missed *Active* Oral Contraceptive Pills

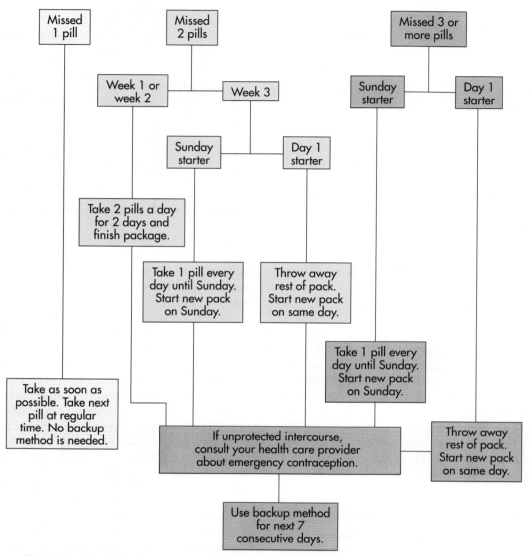

FIG. 9-8 Flowchart for missed contraceptive pills. (Courtesy Patsy Huff, PharmD, Chapel Hill, NC.)

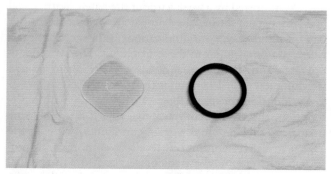

FIG. 9-9 Hormonal contraceptive transdermal patch and vaginal ring. (Courtesy Dee Lowdermilk, Chapel Hill, NC.)

to be fitted. Some wearers may experience vaginitis, leukorrhea, and vaginal discomfort (Hatcher & Nelson, 2004). Withdrawal bleeding occurs during the "no-ring" week. If the woman or partner notices discomfort during coitus, the ring can be removed from the vagina for no longer than 3 hours to still be effective. Mechanism of action, efficacy, contraindications, and side effects are similar to those of COCs. The typical failure rate of the vaginal contraceptive ring is reportedly under 2% during the first year of use (FDA, 2003).

Progestin-Only Contraceptives. Progestin-only methods impair fertility by inhibiting ovulation, thickening and decreasing the amount of cervical mucus, thinning the endometrium, and altering cilia in the uterine tubes (Hatcher, 2004).

Oral Progestins (Minipill). Failure rate of progestin-only pills for typical users is about 8% in the first year of use (Trussell, 2004). Effectiveness is increased if minipills are taken correctly. Because minipills contain such a low dose of progestin, the minipill must be taken at the same time every day (Hatcher, 2004). Users often complain of irregular vaginal bleeding.

Injectable Progestins. Depot medroxyprogesterone acetate (DMPA or Depo-Provera), 150 mg, is given intramuscularly in the deltoid or the gluteus maximus muscle. A 21- to 23-gauge needle, 2.5 to 4 cm long, should be used. DMPA should be initiated during the first 5 days of the menstrual cycle and administered every 11 to 13 weeks.

■ NURSE ALERT

When administering an intramuscular injection of progestin (e.g., Depo-Provera), do NOT massage the site after the injection, because this action can hasten the absorption and shorten the period of effectiveness.

Advantages of DMPA include a contraceptive effectiveness comparable to that of combined oral contraceptives, long-lasting effects, requirement of injections only 4 times a year, and the unlikeliness of lactation being impaired (Hatcher, 2004). Side effects at the end of a year include decreased bone mineral density, weight gain, lipid changes, increased risk of venous thrombosis and thromboembolism, irregular vaginal spotting, decreased libido, and breast changes (Contraception Online, 2003). Other disadvantages include no protection against STIs (including HIV). Return to fertility may be delayed as long as up to 18 months after discontinuing DMPA. Typical failure rate is 3% in the first year of use (Trussell, 2004).

■ NURSE ALERT

Women who use DMPA may lose significant bone mineral density with increasing duration of use. It is unknown if this effect is reversible. It is unknown if use of DMPA during adolescence or early adulthood, a critical period of bone accretion, will reduce peak bone mass and increase the risk of osteoporotic fracture in later life. Women who receive DMPA should be counseled about calcium intake and exercise (Hatcher, 2004; Robinson, 2005).

Implantable Progestins. The Norplant system consisted of six flexible, nonbiodegradable polymeric silicone (Silastic) capsules implanted subdermally in the inner aspect of the nondominant upper arm. These capsules contained levonorgestrel that provided up to 5 years of contraception, dependent upon the client's weight and age. The system is no longer available in the United States (it was discontinued in 2002 in part, due to limited supplies of component materials and some concerns about efficacy), and women who have the system will need to have them removed when the 5 years is up or if they develop problems before that time.

A single-rod implant (Implanon) that is effective for up to 3 years is available in Europe and Australia, and was approved for use in the United States in July, 2006. A two-rod implant may also be available. Like Norplant, these implants will prevent some, but not all, ovulatory cycles and will thicken cervical mucus. Other advantages include reversibility and long-term continuous contraception that is not related to frequency of coitus. Irregular menstrual bleeding is the most common side effect. Less common side effects include headaches, nervousness, nausea, skin changes, and vertigo. No STI protection is provided with the implant method, so condoms should be used for protection.

Emergency Contraception

Emergency contraception (EC) is available in over 100 countries, and in about one third of these countries it is available without a prescription. In the United States, Plan B has been the only EC method available without a prescription and only in limited pharmacies and clinics in pharmacy access states (states where legislation has been passed to allow this practice)—Alaska, California, Hawaii, Maine, Massachusetts, New Hampshire, New Mexico, Vermont, and Washington. However on August 24, 2006, the FDA approved Plan B for over-the-counter sale to women ages 18 and older (FDA, 2006).

Plan B contains 2 doses of levonorgestrel. Other options that the FDA has determined to be safe for emergency contraception include high doses of oral estrogen or COCs (termed emergency contractive pills [ECPs] and insertion of the copper IUD (Stewart, Trussell, & Van Hook, 2004b). These options will continue to be available by prescription only. Plan B will be prescription only for women under the age of 18 except in those designated pharmacy access states (FDA, 2006).

Emergency contraception should be taken by a woman as soon as possible but within 120 hours of unprotected intercourse, or birth control mishap (broken condom, dislodged ring or cervical cap, missed OCPs, late for injection, and so on) to prevent unintended pregnancy (American College of Obstetricians and Gynecologists [ACOG], 2005). If taken before ovulation, emergency contraception prevents ovulation by inhibiting follicular development. If taken after ovulation occurs, there is little effect on ovarian hormone production or the endometrium. Recommended oral medication regimens with ECPs are presented in Table 9-2. To minimize the side effect of nausea that occurs with high doses of estrogen and progestin, the woman can be advised to take an over-the-counter antiemetic 1 hour before each dose. Women with contraindications for estrogen use should use progestin-only emergency contraception. No medical contraindications for emergency contraception exist, except pregnancy and undiagnosed abnormal vaginal bleeding (Stewart et al. 2004b). If the woman does not begin menstruation within 21 days after taking the pills, she should be evaluated for pregnancy (Stewart et al., 2004b). Emergency contraception is ineffective if the woman is pregnant, since the pills do not disturb an implanted pregnancy. Risk of pregnancy is reduced by as much as 75% and 89% if the woman takes ECPs (Stewart et al., 2004b).

table 9-2 Emergency Contraceptive Pills Dosages		
BRAND NAMES	**FIRST DOSE (WITHIN 120 HR)**	**SECOND DOSE (12 HR LATER)**
COMBINED ORAL CONTRACEPTIVES*		
Ovral	2 white pills	2 white pills
Ogestrel	2 white pills	2 white pills
Cryselee	2 white pills	2 white pills
Portia	2 pink pills	2 pink pills
Seasonale	4 pink pills	4 pink pills
Lo/Ovral	4 white pills	4 white pills
Low-Ogestrel	4 white pills	4 white pills
Enpresse	4 orange pills	4 orange pills
Nordette	4 light orange pills	4 light orange pills
Levlen	4 light orange pills	4 light orange pills
Levora	4 white pills	4 white pills
Trivora	4 yellow pills	4 yellow pills
Triphasil	4 yellow pills	4 yellow pills
Tri-Levlen	4 yellow pills	4 yellow pills
Alesse	5 pink pills	5 pink pills
Levlite	5 pink tablets	5 pink tablets
Aviane	5 orange pills	5 orange pills
Lutera	5 white pills	5 white pills
PROGESTIN ONLY		
Ovrette	20 yellow tablets	20 yellow tablets
Plan B†	1 white tablet	1 white tablet

* Antinausea medications needed for any of the combined oral contraceptives.
† May take both pills at same time.
Sources: American College of Obstetricians and Gynecologists. (2005). Emergency contraception: ACOG Practice Bulletin No. 69. *Obstetrics and Gynecology 106*, (6), 1443-1452; Stewart, F., Trussell, J., and Van Look, P. (2004b). Emergency contraception. In R. Hatcher, et al. (Eds.). *Contraceptive technology* (18th rev. ed.). New York: Ardent Media.

■ **NURSE ALERT**

Emergency contraception will not protect the woman against pregnancy if she engages in unprotected intercourse in the days or weeks that follow treatment. Because ingestion of emergency contraceptive pills may delay ovulation, caution the woman that she needs to establish a reliable form of birth control in order to prevent unintended pregnancy (Stewart et al. 2004b). Information about emergency contraception method options and access to providers are available on the web at **www.NOT-2-LATE.com** or by calling 1-888-NOT-2-LATE.

IUDs containing copper (see later discussion) provide another emergency contraception option. The IUD should be inserted within 8 days of unprotected intercourse (Stewart, Trussell, & Van Look, 2004). This method is suggested only for women who wish to have the benefit of long-term contraception. The risk of pregnancy is reduced by as much as 99% with emergency insertion of the copper-releasing IUD.

Contraceptive counseling should be provided to all women requesting emergency contraception, including a discussion of modification of risky sexual behaviors to prevent STIs and unwanted pregnancy.

Intrauterine Devices

An IUD is a small, T-shaped device with bendable arms for insertion through the cervix (Fig. 9-10). Once the trained

FIG. 9-10 Intrauterine devices (IUDs). **A,** Copper T 380A. **B,** Levonorgestrel-releasing IUD.

health care provider inserts the IUD against the uterine fundus, the arms open near the fallopian tubes to maintain position of the device and to adversely affect the sperm motility and irritate the lining of the uterus. Two strings hang from the base of the stem through the cervix and protrude into the vagina for the woman to feel for assurance that the device has not been dislodged (Grimes, 2004). The client should have had a negative pregnancy test, treatment for dysplasia if present, cervical cultures to rule out STIs, and a consent form signed before IUD insertion. Advantages to choosing this method of contraception include long-term protection from pregnancy and immediate return to fertility when removed. Disadvantages include increased risk of pelvic inflammatory disease (PID) shortly after placement, unintentional expulsion of the device, infection, and possible uterine perforation. IUDs offer no protection against HIV or other STIs. Therefore, women who are in mutually monogamous relationships are the best candidates for this device.

There are two FDA-approved IUDs. The ParaGard T380A (copper IUD) is made of radiopaque polyethylene and fine solid copper and is approved for 10 years of use. The copper primarily serves as a spermicide and inflames the endometrium, preventing fertilization (Grimes, 2004). Sometimes women experience more bleeding and cramping within the first year after insertion, but nonsteroidal antiinflammatory drugs (NSAIDs) may be taken for pain relief. The typical failure rate in the first year of use of the copper IUD is less than 1% (Trussell, 2004).

The hormonal intrauterine system releases levonorgestrel from its vertical reservoir. Effective for up to 5 years, it impairs sperm motility, irritates the lining of the uterus, and has some anovulatory effects (Grimes, 2004). Uterine cramping and uterine bleeding is usually decreased with this device, although irregular spotting is common in the first few months following insertion. The typical failure rate in the first year of use is less than 1% (Trussell, 2004).

Nursing Considerations. The woman should be taught to check for the presence of the IUD strings after menstruation to rule out expulsion of the device. If pregnancy occurs with the IUD in place, an ultrasound should confirm that it is not ectopic. Early removal of the IUD helps decrease the risk of spontaneous miscarriage or preterm labor. The woman should report any signs of flulike

signs of potential complications

Intrauterine Devices (IUDs)

Signs of potential complications related to IUDs can be remembered in the following manner (Hatcher et al., 2004):

P— Period late, abnormal spotting or bleeding
A—Abdominal pain, pain with intercourse
I—Infection exposure, abnormal vaginal discharge
N—Not feeling well, fever, or chills
S— String missing; shorter or longer

illness, since this may indicate a septic miscarriage (Grimes, 2004). In some women who are allergic to copper, a rash develops, necessitating the removal of the copper-bearing IUD. Signs of potential complications to be taught to the woman are listed in the accompanying box (Signs of Potential Complications box).

Sterilization

Sterilization refers to surgical procedures intended to render the person infertile. Most procedures involve the occlusion of the passageways for the ova and sperm (Fig. 9-11).

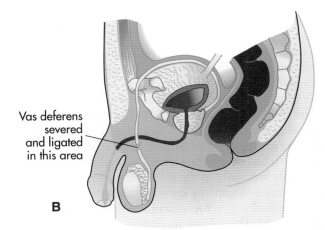

FIG. 9-11 Sterilization. **A,** Uterine tubes severed and ligated (tubal ligation). **B,** Sperm duct severed and ligated (vasectomy).

For the woman, the oviducts (uterine tubes) are occluded; for the man, the sperm ducts (vas deferens) are occluded. Only surgical removal of the ovaries (oophorectomy) or uterus (hysterectomy) or both will result in absolute sterility for the woman. All other sterilization procedures have a small but definite failure rate; that is, pregnancy may result.

Female Sterilization. Female sterilization (bilateral tubal ligation [BTL]) may be done immediately after childbirth (within 24 to 48 hours), concomitant with abortion, or as an interval procedure (during any phase of the menstrual cycle). If sterilization is performed as an interval procedure, the health care provider must be certain that the woman is not pregnant. Half of all female sterilization procedures are performed immediately after a pregnancy (Pollack, Carignan, & Jacobstein, 2004). Sterilization procedures can be safely done on an outpatient basis.

Tubal Occlusion. A laparoscopic approach or a minilaparotomy may be used for tubal ligation (Fig. 9-12), tubal electrocoagulation, or the application of bands or clips. Electrocoagulation and ligation are considered to be permanent methods. Use of the bands or clips has the theoretic advantage of possible removal and return of tubal patency.

For the minilaparotomy, the woman is admitted the morning of surgery, having received nothing by mouth since midnight. Preoperative sedation is given. The procedure may be carried out with a local anesthetic, but a regional or general anesthetic also may be used. A small incision is made in the abdominal wall below the umbilicus. The woman may experience sensations of tugging, but no pain, and the operation is completed within 20 minutes. She may be discharged several hours later if she has recovered from anesthesia. Any abdominal discomfort usually can be controlled with a mild analgesic (e.g., acetaminophen). Within days the scar is almost invisible

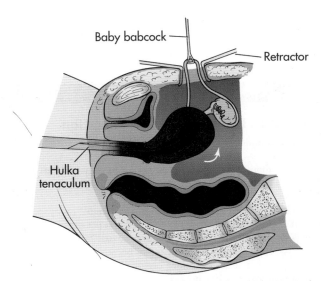

FIG 9-12 Use of minilaparotomy to gain access to uterine tubes for occlusion procedures. Tenaculum is used to lift uterus (arrow) toward incision.

(see Teaching for Self-Care box). As with any surgery, there is always a possibility of complications of anesthesia, infection, hemorrhage, and trauma to other organs.

Transcervical Sterilization. Still considered experimental, hysteroscopic techniques can be used to inject occlusion agents into the uterine tubes. One FDA-approved device is the Essure System, an interval sterilization method (not intended for the postpartum period). A trained health care professional inserts a small catheter holding the polyester fibers through the vagina and cervix and places the small metallic implants into each uterine tube. The device works by stimulating the woman's own scar tissue formation to occlude the uterine tubes and prevent conception (FDA, 2003). An advantage is the nonhormonal form of contraception can be inserted during an office procedure without anesthesia. Analgesia is recommended to decrease mild to moderate discomfort associated with tubal spasm. Particularly convenient for obese women, or those with abdominal adhesions, the transcervical approach eliminates the need for abdominal surgery. Since the procedure is not immediately effective, it is essential that the woman and her partner use another form of contraception until tubal blockage is proven. It may take up to 3 months for tubal occlusion to fully occur, and success must be confirmed by hysterosalpingogram. Other disadvantages include expulsion and perforation. Typical failure rate during the first year of use of the Essure System is less than 1% (Essure, 2004). Long-term efficacy and safety rates are unknown (Pollack et al., 2004).

Tubal Reconstruction. Restoration of tubal continuity (reanastomosis) and function is technically feasible except after laparoscopic tubal electrocoagulation. Sterilization reversal, however, is costly, difficult (requiring microsurgery), and uncertain. The success rate varies with the extent of tubal destruction and removal. The risk of ectopic pregnancy after tubal reanastomosis is increased by 2% to 12.5% (Pollack et al., 2004).

Male Sterilization. *Vasectomy* is the sealing, tying, or cutting of a man's vas deferens so that the sperm cannot travel from the testes to the penis (FDA, 2003). It is considered the easiest and most commonly used operation for male sterilization. Vasectomy can be carried out with local anesthesia on an outpatient basis. Pain, bleeding, infection, and other postsurgical complications are considered the disadvantages to the surgical procedure (FDA). It is considered a permanent method of sterilization because reversal is generally unsuccessful.

Two methods are used for scrotal entry: conventional and no-scalpel vasectomy. The surgeon identifies and immobilizes the vas deferens through the scrotum. Then the vas is ligated or cauterized (see Fig. 9-11, *B*). Surgeons vary in their techniques to occlude the vas deferens: ligation with sutures, division, cautery, application of clips, excision of a segment of the vas, fascial interposition, or some combination of these methods (Pollack et al., 2004).

The man is instructed in self-care to promote a safe return to routine activities. To reduce swelling and relieve discomfort, ice packs are applied to the scrotum intermittently for a few hours after surgery. A scrotal support may be applied to decrease discomfort. Moderate inactivity for about 2 days is advisable because of local scrotal tenderness. The skin suture can be removed 5 to 7 days after surgery. Sexual intercourse may be resumed as desired; however, sterility is not immediate. Some sperm will remain in the proximal portions of the sperm ducts after vasectomy. One week to several months are required to clear the ducts of sperm; therefore some form of contraception is needed until the sperm count in the ejaculate on two consecutive tests is down to zero (Pollack et al., 2004).

Vasectomy has no effect on potency (ability to achieve and maintain erection) or volume of ejaculate. Endocrine production of testosterone continues, so secondary sex characteristics are not affected. Sperm production continues, but sperm are unable to leave the epididymis and are lysed by the immune system. Men occasionally may develop a hematoma, infection, or epididymitis (Pollack et al., 2004). Less common are painful granulomas from accumulation of sperm.

Complications after bilateral vasectomy are uncommon and usually not serious. They include bleeding (usually external), suture reaction, and reaction to anesthetic agent. Failure rate for male sterilization is 0.15% (Trussell, 2004).

Tubal Reconstruction. Microsurgery to reanastomose (restoration of tubal continuity) the sperm ducts can be accomplished successfully in more than 90% of cases (i.e., sperm in the ejaculate); however, the fertility rate is only about 50% (Pollack et al., 2004). The rate of success decreases as the time since the procedure increases. The vasectomy may result in permanent changes in the testes that leave men unable to father children. The changes are those ordinarily seen only in the elderly (e.g., interstitial fibrosis [scar tissue between the seminiferous tubules]). In some men, antibodies develop against their own sperm (autoimmunization). The role of antisperm antibodies in fertility after vasectomy reversal has not been completely determined. Additional research is needed to explore a possible link between vasectomy and prostate cancer.

TEACHING FOR SELF-CARE

What to Expect After Tubal Ligation

- You should expect no change in hormones and their influence.
- Your menstrual period will be about the same as before the sterilization.
- You may feel pain at ovulation.
- The ovum disintegrates within the abdominal cavity.
- It is highly unlikely that you will become pregnant.
- You should not have a change in sexual functioning; you may enjoy sexual relations more because you will not be concerned about becoming pregnant.
- Sterilization offers no protection against sexually transmitted infections (STIs); therefore, you may need to use condoms.

Laws and Regulations. All states have strict regulations for informed consent. Many states permit voluntary sterilization of any mature, rational woman without reference to her marital or pregnancy status. Although the partner's consent is not required by law, the woman is encouraged to discuss the situation with the partner, and health care providers may request the partner's consent. Sterilization of minors or mentally incompetent individuals is restricted by most states and often requires the approval of a board of eugenicists or other court-appointed individuals (see Legal Tip).

▬ LEGAL TIP Sterilization

- If federal funds are used for sterilization, the person must be aged 21 years or older.
- Informed consent must include an explanation of the risks, benefits, and alternatives; a statement that describes sterilization as a permanent, irreversible method of birth control; and a statement that mandates a 30-day waiting period between giving consent and the sterilization.
- Informed consent must be in the person's native language, or an interpreter must be provided to read the consent form to the person.

Nursing Considerations. The nurse plays an important role in assisting people with decision making so all requirements for informed consent are met. The nurse also provides information about alternatives to sterilization, such as contraception. The nurse acts as a "sounding board" for people who are exploring the possibility of choosing sterilization and their feelings about and motivation for this choice. The nurse records this information, which may be the basis for referral to a family-planning clinic, a psychiatric social worker, or another professional health care provider.

Information must be given about what is entailed in various procedures, how much discomfort or pain can be expected, and what type of care is needed. Many individuals fear sterilization procedures because of the imagined effect on their sex life. They need reassurance concerning the hormonal and psychologic basis for sexual function and that uterine tube occlusion or vasectomy has no biologic sequelae in terms of sexual adequacy (Pollack et al., 2004).

Preoperative care includes health assessment, which includes a psychologic assessment, physical examination, and laboratory tests. The nurse assists with the health assessment, answers questions, and confirms the client's understanding of printed instructions (e.g., nothing by mouth after midnight). Ambivalence and extreme fear of the procedure are reported to the physician.

Postoperative care depends on the procedure performed (e.g., laparoscopy, laparotomy for tubal occlusion, or vasectomy). General care includes recovery after anesthesia, monitoring of vital signs and fluid and electrolyte balance (intake and output, laboratory values), prevention of or early identification and treatment for infection or hemorrhage, control of discomfort, and assessment of emotional response to the procedure and recovery.

Discharge planning depends on the type of procedure performed. In general, the client is given written instructions about observing for and reporting symptoms and signs of complications, the type of recovery to be expected, and the date and time for a follow-up appointment.

Breastfeeding: Lactational Amenorrhea Method

Lactational Amenorrhea Method (LAM) can be a highly effective, *temporary* method of birth control. It is more popular in underdeveloped countries and traditional societies, where breastfeeding is used to prolong birth intervals. The method has seen limited use in the United States since only about half of new mothers initiate breastfeeding, and most American women do not establish breastfeeding patterns that provide maximum protection against pregnancy (Kennedy & Trussell, 2004).

When the infant suckles at the mother's breast, a surge of prolactin hormone is released, which inhibits estrogen production and suppresses ovulation and the return of menses. LAM works best if the mother is exclusively or almost exclusively breastfeeding, if the woman has not had a menstrual flow since giving birth, and if the infant is under 6 months of age. Effectiveness is enhanced by frequent feedings at intervals of less than 4 hours during the day and no more than 6 hours during the night, long duration of each feeding, and no bottle supplementation or limited supplementation by spoon or cup. The woman should be counseled that disruption of the breastfeeding pattern or supplementation can increase the risk of pregnancy. The typical failure rate is 2% (Kennedy & Trussell, 2004).

Future Trends

Contraceptive options are more limited in the United States and Canada than in some other industrialized countries. Lack of funding for research, governmental regulations, conflicting values about contraception, and high costs of liability coverage for contraception have been cited as blocks to new and improved methods. Existing methods of contraception are being improved, however, and a variety of new methods are being developed.

Lower-dose COCs (15 micrograms of ethinyl estradiol) are available in Europe. Female barrier methods (new female condoms, client-fitted diaphragms, and new vaginal sponges) are being tested. Vaginal delivery systems including progestin-only vaginal rings and progesterone daily suppositories are under investigation. Two new IUDs and spermicidal microbicides are being evaluated. Male hormonal methods are also being investigated, including hormonal injections (testosterone), gonadotropin-releasing hormone antagonists, antisperm compounds, immunologic methods, and contraceptive vaccines (Hatcher et al., 2004).

▬ Evaluation

The nurse can be reasonably assured that care was effective when the client-centered expected outcomes have been achieved: the woman and her partner learn about

CD: Plan of Care: Sexual Activity and Contraception

| plan of care | Sexual Activity and Contraception |

NURSING DIAGNOSIS Decisional conflict related to contraceptive alternatives

Expected Outcomes *Woman and partner will verbalize understanding of different methods of contraception and will choose the method best suited for their needs.*

Nursing Interventions/Rationales
- Provide information regarding reliability, use, indications, contraindications, and side effects of different methods of contraception *to facilitate the decision-making process.*
- Utilize privacy and therapeutic communication during discussion of sexual activity and methods of contraception *to provide clarification of information and client trust of caregiver.*

NURSING DIAGNOSIS Risk for infection related to ongoing sexual activity as evidenced by client history

Expected Outcome *Woman and her partner will remain free of sexually transmitted infections.*

Nursing Interventions/Rationales
- Provide information regarding safer sex practices, use of spermicides and barrier methods *to raise client awareness of methods to prevent infection.*

NURSING DIAGNOSIS Ineffective health maintenance related to unfamiliarity with contraceptive method

Expected Outcome *Woman and partner will verbalize intent to utilize chosen contraception correctly.*

Nursing Interventions/Rationales
- Review information given regarding use, reliability, and side effects of chosen contraceptive method *to ensure woman's and partner's understanding.*
- Provide list of informational resources *to promote consistency of use of chosen method.*
- Encourage ongoing effective communication with health care provider *to promote trust.*

the various methods of contraception; the couple achieves pregnancy only when planned; and they have no adverse sequelae as a result of the chosen method of contraception (see Plan of Care).

▬ INDUCED ABORTION

Induced abortion is the purposeful interruption of a pregnancy before 20 weeks of gestation. (Spontaneous abortion [miscarriage] is discussed in Chapter 31.) If the abortion is performed at the woman's request, the term *elective abortion* is used; if performed for reasons of maternal or fetal health or disease, the term *therapeutic abortion* applies. Many factors contribute to a woman's decision to have an abortion. Indications include (1) preservation of the life or health of the mother, (2) genetic disorders of the fetus, (3) rape or incest, and (4) the pregnant woman's request. The control of birth, dealing as it does with human sexuality and the question of life and death, is one of the most emotional components of health care and has been the most controversial social issue in the last half of the twentieth century and continues to be so today. Regulations exist to protect the mother from the complications of abortion.

Abortion is regulated in most countries, including the United States. Before 1970, legal abortion was not widely available in the United States. However, in January 1973, the U.S. Supreme Court set aside previous antiabortion laws and legalized abortion. This decision established a trimester approach to abortion. In the first trimester, abortion is permissible, the decision is between the woman and her health care provider, and a state has little right to interfere (Stewart, Ellertson, & Cates, 2004a). In the second trimester, abortion was left to the discretion of the individual states to regulate procedures as long as they are reasonably related to the woman's health. In the third trimester, abortions may be limited or even prohibited by state regulation unless the restriction interferes with the life or health of the pregnant woman (Stewart et al., 2004a).

In 1992, the U.S. Supreme Court made another landmark ruling, this time allowing states to restrict early abortion services as long as the restrictions did not place an "undue burden" on the woman's ability to choose abortion. Since then many bills have been introduced to limit access and funds for women seeking abortion. In 2006, several states introduced bills to ban most abortions; the U.S. Supreme Court will again play a major role in deciding the future of abortions.

The laws for abortion in Canada have also changed over the last 35 years, from being very restricted before 1969 to unrestricted in 1988. Today Canada is one of the only countries in the world without abortion regulation. Abortion is available throughout pregnancy, although more than 90% are performed in the first trimester and only 2% to 3% are performed after 16 weeks (Wikipedeia, 2006).

▬ LEGAL TIP   Induced Abortion

It is important for nurses to know the laws regarding abortion in their country or state of practice before they offer abortion counseling or nursing care to a woman choosing an abortion. Many states enforce a mandatory delay or state-directed counseling before a woman may legally obtain an abortion.

Incidence

The number of abortions performed in the United States in 2002 was 854,122 (Strauss, Herndon, Chang, Parker, Bowens, & Berg, 2005). About 88% of all abortions are performed in the first trimester, with about 60% in the first 8 weeks after the last menstrual period. Most women who are having an elective abortion are Caucasian, younger than 24 years of age, and unmarried (Strauss et al., 2005). In 2002, 105,154 abortions reportedly were performed in Canada (National Campus Life Network, 2005).

Decision to Have an Abortion

A woman who is deciding whether or not to have an abortion is often ambivalent. She needs information and an opportunity to discuss her feelings about pregnancy, abortion, and the impact of either choice on her future. She needs to make her decision without feeling coerced (Robinson, Dollins, & McConlogue-O'Shaughnessy, 2000).

Nurses and other health care providers often struggle with the same values and moral convictions as those of the pregnant woman. The conflicts and doubts of the nurse can be readily communicated to women who are already anxious and overly sensitive. Regardless of personal views on abortion, nurses who provide care to women seeking abortion have an ethical responsibility to counsel women about their options and to make appropriate referrals (Goss, 2002).

The Association of Women's Health, Obstetric and Neonatal Nurses (AWHONN, 1999) continues to support a nurse's right to choose to participate or not in abortion procedures in keeping with his or her "personal, moral, ethical, or religious beliefs." AWHONN also advocates that "nurses have an obligation to inform their employers, at the time of employment, of any attitudes and beliefs that may interfere with essential job functions."

> ### LEGAL TIP Institutional Policies for Nurses' Rights and Responsibilities Related to Abortion
>
> Nurses' rights and responsibilities related to caring for abortion clients should be protected through policies that describe how the institution will accommodate the nurse's ethical or moral beliefs and what the nurse should do to avoid client abandonment in such situations. Nurses should know what policies are in place in their institutions and encourage such policies to be written if there are none (AWHONN, 1999; Joint Commission on Accreditation for Healthcare Organizations [JCAHO], 2000).

CARE MANAGEMENT

Assessment and Nursing Diagnoses

A thorough assessment is conducted through history, physical examination, and laboratory tests. The length of pregnancy and the condition of the woman must be determined to select the appropriate type of abortion procedure. An ultrasound examination should be performed before a second trimester abortion is done. If the woman is Rh negative, she is a candidate for prophylaxis against Rh isoimmunization. She should receive $Rh_o(D)$ immune globulin within 72 hours after the abortion if she is D negative and if Coombs' test results are negative (if the woman is unsensitized or isoimmunization has not developed).

The woman's understanding of alternatives, the types of abortions, and expected recovery is assessed. Misinformation and gaps in knowledge are identified and corrected. The record is reviewed for the signed informed consent, and the client's understanding is verified. General preoperative, operative, and postoperative assessments are performed.

Analysis of data leads to identification of the appropriate nursing diagnoses for the woman undergoing elective abortion. Potential nursing diagnoses are listed.

- *Decisional conflict related to*
  - value system
- *Fear related to*
  - abortion procedure
  - potential complications
  - implications for future pregnancies
  - what others might think
- *Anticipatory grieving related to*
  - distress at loss or feelings of guilt
- *Risk for infection related to*
  - effects of the procedure
  - lack of understanding of preoperative and postoperative self-care
- *Acute pain related to*
  - effects of the procedure or postoperative events

Expected Outcomes of Care

Planning is a collaborative effort among the woman, her sexual partner (as appropriate), the physician, and the nurse. Expected outcomes are established collaboratively, should be stated in client-centered terms, and may include that the woman will do the following:

- Verbalize understanding of the information necessary to give informed consent
- Undergo a successful procedure and uneventful recovery
- Continue to be satisfied with the decision for induced abortion, the procedure, and her experience with the health care team

Plan of Care and Interventions

Counseling about abortion includes help for the woman in identifying how she perceives the pregnancy, information about the choices available (i.e., having an abortion or carrying the pregnancy to term and then either keeping the infant or placing the baby for adoption), and information about the types of abortion procedures.

First-Trimester Abortion

Methods for performing early abortion (less than 9 weeks of gestation) include surgical (aspiration) and medical methods (mifepristone with misoprostol, and methotrexate with misoprostol).

Aspiration. Aspiration (vacuum or suction curettage) is the most common procedure in the first trimester, with almost 95% of all procedures being performed by this method (Strauss et al., 2005). Aspiration abortion is usually performed under local anesthesia in the physician's office, the clinic, or the hospital. The suction procedure for performing an early elective abortion (ideal time is 8 to 12 weeks since the last menstrual period) usually requires less than 5 minutes.

EVIDENCE-BASED PRACTICE

Comparing Medical and Surgical Abortions

BACKGROUND

- Abortion has been practiced for millennia. Approximately 53 million abortions are performed each year. An estimated one third of these are performed in unsafe circumstances, mostly in developing countries, and account for one out of eight maternal deaths worldwide. Surgical abortion in safe settings has the lowest complication rates. Complications are 2.3 times higher for dilation and curettage (D&C) as compared with vacuum aspiration. Complications of surgical abortion include infection, incomplete evacuation, cervical trauma, uterine perforation, hemorrhage, complications with anesthesia, and possible associations with infertility, miscarriages, and low birth weight in subsequent pregnancies. Medical abortions use pharmaceuticals to terminate pregnancy growth or stimulate expulsion of uterine contents. Four protocols are commonly used: misoprostol (prostaglandin E_1), mifepristone, mifepristone with misoprostol, and methotrexate with misoprostol. Methotrexate stops rapid cell replication. Misoprostol causes uterine contractions. Both methotrexate and misoprostol are teratogenic. Side effects of medical abortion are moderate to heavy bleeding, pain, nausea, vomiting, diarrhea, and more observed blood loss and passage of tissue.

OBJECTIVES

- The reviewers compared medical versus surgical methods of first-trimester abortion.
- Outcomes were efficacy, side effects, and acceptability of the procedure. Primary outcomes included incomplete abortion, pelvic infection, blood transfusion, blood loss or hemoglobin drop, uterine perforation, cervical injury, and readmission. Secondary outcomes included hospital stay exceeding 24 hours, duration of bleeding, use of uterotonic or antibiotic drugs not routinely given, pain or analgesia use, vomiting, diarrhea, and dissatisfaction.

METHODS

Search Strategy

- The authors searched Cochrane, MEDLINE, and POPLINE, and contacted experts at the World Health Organization (WHO). Search keywords included abortion, pregnancy termination, first trimester, vacuum aspiration, suction, dilation and curettage, D&C, mifepristone, misoprostol, prostaglandin, methotrexate, and RU 486.
- Five randomized trials comparing medical versus surgical abortion were chosen. The trials represented 989 women from Sweden, Denmark, the United Kingdom, the United States, and a WHO multicenter trial from India, Vietnam, Slovenia, Zambia, China, Sweden, and Hungary. The trials were published from 1984 to 2000.

Statistical Analyses

- Outcomes of each medical abortion protocol were compared with outcomes of vacuum aspiration, the surgical treatment of choice for first-trimester abortion.

FINDINGS

- *Misoprostol alone, versus vacuum aspiration:* The misoprostol group resulted in significantly more incomplete abortions and increased bleeding and pain, compared with vacuum aspiration. No significant differences were found between groups in infection rates.
- *Mifepristone alone, versus vacuum aspiration:* No significant differences were found between groups in infection rates, incomplete abortions, or perforations.
- *Mifepristone plus misoprostol, versus vacuum aspiration:* No difference in blood loss occurred, but the medical group had significantly longer duration of bleeding.
- *Methotrexate plus misoprostol, versus vacuum aspiration:* Duration of bleeding and use of analgesia for pain were both significantly greater in the medical abortion group. No differences between groups were found in incomplete abortion rates.
- Overall efficacy rate for medical abortions was 76% to 97%, and for surgical abortions it was 94% to 100%. Mifepristone alone had the lowest efficacy, at 76%. One perforation occurred in the surgical groups. Medical intervention groups experienced more days of bleeding than surgical clients. The medical group also experienced more pain, which may reflect the use of analgesia during the surgical procedure. The longer the gestation, the less acceptable the medical procedure was to the women. In one study, 63% of the medical group would choose that method again, whereas 92% of the surgical group would opt to repeat the surgical procedure, should the need arise. Overall, vacuum aspiration may be more effective than misoprostol alone and seems to be associated with less pain and bleeding.

LIMITATIONS

- The small number of trials and small sample sizes limit the generalizability of the results to the larger population. Many women were lost to follow-up.

IMPLICATIONS FOR PRACTICE

- The decision between a medical or a surgical abortion carries trade-offs. Careful counseling is necessary to prepare the woman for realistic expectations of each protocol, with careful attention to the attitude toward pregnancy and abortion. The setting may dictate one procedure over another, depending on whether a safe surgical procedure is available, or the proximity of a woman to a health facility for the duration of the medical abortion.

IMPLICATIONS FOR FURTHER RESEARCH

- Larger studies about women's preferences for methods of abortion, and the efficacy of the methods, are needed. More information about the pain experienced in abortion, preparation techniques, precounseling, alternative therapies, and presence of a support person would be useful.

Reference: Say, L., Kulier, R., Culmezoglo, M., & Campana, A. (2002). Medical versus surgical methods for first trimester termination of pregnancy. In *The Cochrane Database of Systematic Reviews,* 2006, Issue 3. Chichester, UK: John Wiley & Sons.

A bimanual examination is done before the procedure to assess uterine size and position. A speculum is inserted and the cervix is anesthetized with a local anesthetic agent. The cervix is dilated if necessary and a cannula connected to suction is inserted into the uterine cavity. The products of conception are evacuated from the uterus.

During the procedure the nurse or physician keeps the woman informed about what to expect next (e.g., menstrual-like cramping, sounds of the suction machine). The nurse assesses the woman's vital signs. The aspirated uterine contents must be carefully inspected to ascertain whether all fetal parts and adequate placental tissue have been evacuated. After the abortion the woman rests on the table until she is ready to stand. Then she remains in the recovery area or waiting room for 1 to 3 hours for detection of excessive cramping or bleeding; then she is discharged.

Bleeding after the operation is normally about the equivalent of a heavy menstrual period, and cramps are rarely severe. Excessive vaginal bleeding and infection, such as endometritis or salpingitis, are the most common complications of elective abortion. Retained products of conception are the primary cause of vaginal bleeding. Evacuation of the uterus, uterine massage, and administration of oxytocin or methylergonovine (Methergine) or both may be necessary. Prophylactic antibiotics to decrease the risk of infection are commonly prescribed (Stewart et al., 2004a). Postabortion pain may be relieved with NSAIDs such as ibuprofen.

Postabortion instructions differ among health care providers (e.g., tampons should not be used for at least 3 days or should be avoided for up to 3 weeks, and resumption of sexual intercourse may be permitted within 1 week or discouraged for 2 weeks). The woman may shower daily. Instruction is given to watch for excessive bleeding and other signs of complications (see Signs of Potential Complications box) and to avoid douches of any type. The woman may expect her menstrual period to resume 4 to 6 weeks from the day of the procedure. Information about the birth control method the woman prefers is offered, if this has not been done previously during the counseling interview that usually precedes the decision to have an abortion. Some methods can be initiated immediately such as an IUD insertion. Hormonal methods may be started immediately or within a week (Stewart et al., 2004a). The woman must be strongly encouraged to return for her follow-up visit so complications can be detected. A pregnancy test may also be performed at that time to determine whether the pregnancy was successfully terminated (Stenchever, Droegemueller, Herbst, & Mishell, 2001).

Medical Abortion. Early medical abortion has been popular in Canada and Europe for more than 15 years, but it is a relatively new procedure in the United States. Medical abortions are available for use in the United States for up to 9 weeks after the last menstrual period. Methotrexate, misoprostol, and mifepristone are the drugs used in the current regimens to induce early abortion. About 5% of all reported abortion procedures in 2002 were medical procedures (Strauss et al., 2005).

Methotrexate is a cytotoxic drug that causes early abortion by blocking folic acid in fetal cells so that they cannot divide. Misoprostol (Cytotec) is a prostaglandin analog that acts directly on the cervix to soften and dilate and on the uterine muscle to stimulate contractions. Mifepristone, formerly known as RU 486, was approved by the FDA in 2000. It works by binding to progesterone receptors and blocking the action of progesterone, which is necessary for maintaining pregnancy (Kahn et al., 2000; Taylor & Hwang, 2004).

Methotrexate and Misoprostol. There is no standard protocol, but methotrexate is given intramuscularly or orally (usually mixed with orange juice). Vaginal placement of misoprostol follows in 3 to 7 days. The woman returns for a follow-up visit to confirm the abortion is complete. If not, the woman is offered an additional dose of misoprostol, or vacuum aspiration is performed (Kahn et al., 2000).

Mifepristone and Misoprostol. Mifepristone can be taken up to 7 weeks after the last menstrual period. The FDA-approved regimen is that the woman takes 600 mg of mifepristone orally; 48 hours later she returns to the office and takes 400 mcg of misoprostol orally (unless abortion has already occurred and been confirmed). Two weeks after the administration of mifepristone, the woman must return to the office for a clinical examination or ultrasound to confirm that the pregnancy has been terminated. In 1% to 5% of cases, the drugs do not work, and surgical abortion (aspiration) is needed (Kahn et al., 2000).

Research has demonstrated a more effective regimen that has fewer side effects. This regimen can be given up to 9 weeks after the last menstrual period and includes administration of 200 mg mifepristone orally followed by misoprostol 800 mcg vaginally in 24 to 48 hours. This vaginal insertion can be done at home by the woman. A

---

signs of potential complications

Induced Abortion

Call your health care provider if you have any of the following signs:
- Fever greater than 38° C (100.4° F)
- Chills
- Bleeding greater than two saturated pads in 2 hours or heavy bleeding lasting a few days
- Foul-smelling vaginal discharge
- Severe abdominal pain, cramping, or backache
- Abdominal tenderness (when pressure applied)
- No return of menstrual period within 6 weeks

Reference: Stewart, F., Ellertson, C., & Cates, W. (2004a). Abortion. In R. Hatcher, J. Trussell, F. Stewart, S. Nelson, W. Cates, F. Guest, et al. (Eds.), *Contraceptive technology* (18th rev. ed.). New York: Ardent Media.

follow-up visit is in 4 to 8 days (National Abortion Federation, 2003).

With any medical abortion regimen, the woman usually will experience bleeding and cramping. Side effects of the medications include nausea, vomiting, diarrhea, headache, dizziness, fever, and chills. These are attributed to misoprostol and usually subside in a few hours after administration (Taylor & Hwang, 2004).

▬ Second-Trimester Abortion

Second-trimester abortion is associated with more complications and costs than first-trimester abortions. Dilation and evacuation accounts for almost all procedures performed in the United States. Induction of uterine contractions with hypertonic solutions (e.g., saline, urea) injected directly into the uterus and uterotonic agents (e.g., misoprostol, dinoprostone) account for only about 0.8% of all abortions (Strauss et al., 2005).

Dilation and Evacuation. Dilation and evacuation (D&E) can be performed at any point up to 20 weeks of gestation although it is most commonly performed between 13 and 16 weeks of gestation (Stewart et al., 2004a). The cervix requires more dilation because the products of conception are larger. Often, osmotic dilators (e.g., laminaria) are inserted several hours or several days before the procedure, or misoprostol can be applied to the cervix. The procedure is similar to vaginal aspiration except a larger cannula is used and other instruments may be needed to remove the fetus and placenta. Nursing care includes monitoring vital signs, providing emotional support, administering analgesics, and postoperative monitoring. Disadvantages of D&E may include possible long-term harmful effects on the cervix.

▬ Nursing Considerations

The woman will need help exploring the meaning of the various alternatives and consequences to herself and her significant others. It is often difficult for a woman to express her true feelings (e.g., what abortion means to her now and in the future and what support or regret her friends and peers may demonstrate). A calm, matter-of-fact approach on the part of the nurse can be helpful (e.g., "Yes, I know you are pregnant. I am here to help. Let's talk about alternatives."). Listening to what the woman has to say and encouraging her to speak are essential. Neutral responses such as "Oh," "Uh-huh," and "Umm," and nonverbal encouragement such as nodding, maintaining eye contact, and use of touch are helpful in setting an open, accepting environment. Clarifying, restating, and reflecting statements, open-ended questions, and feedback are communication techniques that can be used to maintain a realistic focus on the situation and bring the woman's problems into the open.

Information about alternatives to abortion such as referral to adoption agencies or to support services if the woman chooses to keep her baby is provided. If a decision is made to have an abortion, the woman must be assured of continued support. Information about what is entailed in various procedures, how much discomfort or pain can be expected, and what type of care is needed must be given. A discussion of the various feelings including depression, guilt, regret, and relief that the woman might experience after the abortion is needed. Information about community resources for postabortion counseling may be needed (Goss, 2002). If family or friends cannot be involved, scheduling time for nursing personnel to give the necessary support is an essential component of the care plan.

After the abortion, studies have indicated that most women report relief, but some have temporary distress or mixed emotions. Evidence of long-term depression after elective abortion has been inconclusive (Schmiege & Russo, 2005; Stewart et al., 2004a). Guilt and anxiety may occur more with young women, women with poor social support, multiparous women, and women with a history of psychiatric illness. Women having second-trimester abortions may have more emotional distress than women having abortions in the first trimester (Williams, 2000). Also, women feeling pressure to have an abortion had symptoms of short-term grief in the study reported by Williams. Because symptoms can vary among women who have had abortions, nurses must assess women for grief reactions and facilitate the grieving process through active listening and nonjudgmental support and care.

▬ Evaluation

The nurse can be reasonably sure that care was effective when the expected outcomes have been met: the woman understands all information necessary to give informed consent; the procedure is successful; recovery is uneventful; and the woman continues to be satisfied with the decision for elective abortion, the procedure, and the experience with the health care team.

---

community activity

- Visit a pharmacy (freestanding or service within a grocery or discount store). Where are the OTC contraceptives located? Are they easy to access, and is it easy to compare among brands? Are there generic brands as well as name brands? If so, how do the costs compare? Is there counseling available? If so, is there privacy for the counseling? Does the pharmacy provide emergency contraception? If not, is information made available on where it can be obtained? Is information/counseling available in languages other than English?
- Locate the facilities (freestanding and hospital-based) that offer abortion counseling and procedures in your community. What types of counseling are offered, for example, alternatives to abortion? What types of procedures are performed? Is there any follow-up to determine if the woman had any psychologic effects?

key points

- A variety of contraceptive methods are available with various effectiveness rates, advantages, and disadvantages.
- Women and their partners should choose the contraceptive method or methods best suited to them.
- Effective contraceptives are available through both prescription and nonprescription sources.
- A variety of techniques are available to enhance the effectiveness of periodic abstinence in motivated couples who prefer this natural method.
- Hormonal contraception includes both precoital and postcoital prevention through various modalities and requires thorough client education.
- The barrier methods of diaphragm and cervical cap provide safe and effective contraception for women or couples motivated to use them consistently and correctly.

- Proper, concurrent use of spermicides and latex condoms provides protection against STIs.
- Tubal ligations and vasectomies are permanent sterilization methods used by increasing numbers of women and men.
- Induced abortion performed in the first trimester is safer than an abortion performed in the second trimester.
- The most common complications of induced abortion include infection, retained products of conception, and excessive vaginal bleeding.
- Major psychologic sequelae of induced abortion are rare.

REFERENCES

American College of Obstetricians and Gynecologists (ACOG). (2005). Emergency contraception: ACOG Practice Bulletin No. 69. *Obstetrics and Gynecology, 106*(6), 143-149.

Arevalo, M., Jennings, V., Nikula, M., & Sinai, I. (2004). Efficacy of the new TwoDay method of family planning. *Fertility and Sterility, 82*(4), 885-892.

Association of Women's Health, Obstetric, and Neonatal Nurses (AWHONN). (1999). *Nurses' rights and responsibilities related to abortion and sterilization.* Policy Position Statement. Accessed www.awhonn.org, February 25, 2006.

Cates, W., & Raymond, E. (2004). Vaginal spermicide. In R. Hatcher, J. Trussell, F. Stewart, S. Nelson, W. Cates, F. Guest, et al. (Eds.), *Contraceptive technology* (18th rev. ed.). New York: Ardent Media.

Cates, W., & Stewart, F. (2004). Vaginal barriers. In R. Hatcher, J. Trussell, F. Stewart, S. Nelson, W. Cates, F. Guest, et al. (Eds.), *Contraceptive technology* (18th rev. ed.). New York: Ardent Media.

Centers for Disease Control and Prevention, Workowski, K., & Berman, S. (2006) Guideline, 2006. MMWR 55(RR11), 1-94. Sexually transmitted disease treatment guidelines. *MMWR Morbidity and Mortality Weekly Report.*

Contraception Online. (2003). Facts about injectable contraception. *The Contraception Report, 14*(3). Accessed www.contraceptiononline.org/contrareport/article01.cfm?art=256, February 25, 2006.

CycleBeads (2003). *Frequently asked questions.* Accessed http://cyclebeads.com/February 23, 2006.

Essure. (2004). *Patient information booklet.* Accessed www.essure.com/Patient_Information_Booklet.pdf, February 25, 2006.

Female Condom: The Product. Accessed www.femalehealth.com/theproduct.html, November 28, 2004.

Goss, G. (2002). Pregnancy termination: Understanding and supporting women who undergo medical abortion. *AWHONN Lifelines, 6*(1), 46-50.

Grimes, D. (2004). Intrauterine devices (IUDs). In R. Hatcher, J. Trussell, F. Stewart, S. Nelson, W. Cates, F. Guest, et al. (Eds.), *Contraceptive technology* (18th rev. ed.). New York: Ardent Media.

Grimes, D., Gallo, M., Grigorieva, V., Nanda, K., & Schulz, K. (2005a). Fertility awareness-based methods for contraception: Systematic review of randomized controlled trials. *Contraception, 72*(2), 85-90.

Grimes, D., Lopez, L., Raymond, E., Halpern, V., Nanda, K., & Schulz, K. (2005). Spermicide used alone for contraception. *The Cochrane Database of Systematic Reviews, 2006,* Issue 3, Chichester, UK: John Wiley & Sons.

Hatcher, R. (2004). Depo provera injections, implants and progestin only pills. In R. Hatcher, J. Trussell, F. Stewart, S. Nelson, W. Cates, F. Guest, et al. (Eds.), *Contraceptive technology* (18th rev. ed.). New York: Ardent Media.

Hatcher, R., & Nelson, A. (2004). Combined hormonal contraceptive methods. In R. Hatcher, J. Trussell, F. Stewart, S. Nelson, W. Cates, F. Guest, et al. (Eds.), *Contraceptive technology* (18th rev. ed.). New York: Ardent Media.

Hatcher, R., Zieman, M., Cwiak, C., Darney, P., Creinin, M., & Stosur, H. (2004). *A pocket guide to managing contraception.* Tiger, GA: Bridging the Gap Foundation.

Institute for Natural Family Planning Services. (2005). *Definition of natural family planning. Marquette method.* Accessed www.marquette.edu/nursing/nfp, February 23, 2006.

Institute of Reproductive Health. (March 2003). *Standard days method.* Accessed www.irh.org, February 23, 2006.

Jennings, V., Arevalo, M., & Kowal, D. (2004). Fertility awareness-based methods. In R. Hatcher, J. Trussell, F. Stewart, S. Nelson, W. Cates, F. Guest, et al. (Eds.), *Contraceptive technology* (18th rev. ed.). New York: Ardent Media.

Joint Commission on Accreditation for Healthcare Organizations (JCAHO). (2006). Standards, intents, and examples for managing staff requests. In *Comprehensive accreditation manual for hospitals. The official handbook.* Oakbrook Terrace, IL: JCAHO.

Kahn, J. Becker, B., McIsaa, L., Amor, J., Neuhous, L., Olkin, L., et al. (2000). The efficacy of medical abortion: A meta-analysis. *Contraception, 61*(1), 29-40.

Kennedy, K., & Trussell, J. (2004). Postpartum contraception and lactation. In: R. Hatcher, J. Trussell, F. Stewart, S. Nelson, W. Cates, F. Guest, et al. (Eds.), *Contraceptive technology,* (18th rev. ed.). New York: Ardent Media.

Kowal, D. (2004). Coitus interruptus. In R. Hatcher, J. Trussell, F. Stewart, S. Nelson, W. Cates, F. Guest, et al. (Eds.), *Contraceptive technology* (18th rev. ed.). New York: Ardent Media.

Marchbanks, P., McDonald, J., Wilson, H., Folger, S., Mandel, M., Daling, J., et al. (2002). Oral contraceptives and the risk of breast cancer. *New England Journal of Medicine, 346*(26), 2025-2032.

National Abortion Federation. (2003). *Clinical policy guidelines.* Washington, DC: Author.

National Campus Life Network. (2005). *Frequently asked questions. How many abortions are performed in Canada?* Accessed www.ncln.ca/resources, February 25, 2006.

Planned Parenthood. (2004). *Diaphragms, caps and shields* (Updated December, 2005). Accessed www.plannedparenthood.org, February 25, 2006.

Pollack, A., Carignan, C., & Jacobstein, R. (2004). Female and male sterilization. In R. Hatcher, J. Trussell, F. Stewart, S. Nelson, W. Cates, F. Guest, et al. (Eds.), *Contraceptive technology* (18th rev. ed.). New York: Ardent Media.

Robinson, D., Dollins, A., & McConlogue-O'Shaughnessy, L. (2000). Care of the woman before and after an elective abortion. *American Journal of Nurse Practitioners, 4*(3), 17-29.

Robinson, K. (2005). Depo-provera: New concerns—same issues? *AWHONN Lifelines, 9*(3), 214-217.

Schmiege, S., & Russo, N. (2005). Depression and unwanted first pregnancy: Longitudinal cohort study. *BMJ, 331*(7528), 1303-1307.

Sinai, I., Jennings, V., & Arevalo, M. (2004). The importance of screening and monitoring the standard day method and cycle regularity. *Contraception, 69*(3), 201-206.

Stenchever, M., Droegemueller, W., Herbst, A., & Mishell, D. (2001). *Comprehensive gynecology* (4th ed.). St. Louis: Mosby.

Stewart, F., Ellertson, C., & Cates, W. (2004a). Abortion. In R. Hatcher, J. Trussell, F. Stewart, S. Nelson, W. Cates, F. Guest, et al. (Eds.), *Contraceptive technology* (18th rev. ed.). New York: Ardent Media.

Stewart, F., Trussell, J., & Van Look, P. (2004b). Emergency contraception. In R. Hatcher, J. Trussell, F. Stewart, S. Nelson, W. Cates, F. Guest, et al. (Eds.), *Contraceptive technology* (18th rev. ed.). New York: Ardent Media.

Strauss, L., Herndon, J., Chang, J., Parker, W., Bowens, S., & Berg, C. (2005). Abortion surveillance—United States, 2002. *MMWR Morbidity and Mortality Weekly Report—Surveillance Summaries, 54*(7), 1-31.

Taylor, D., & Hwang, A. (2004). Mifepristone for medical abortion: Exploring new options for nurse practitioners. *AWHONN Lifelines, 7*(6), 524-529.

Trussell, J. (2004). Contraceptive efficacy. In R. Hatcher, J. Trussell, F. Stewart, S. Nelson, W. Cates, F. Guest, et al. (Eds.), *Contraceptive technology* (18th rev. ed.). New York: Ardent Media.

U.S. Food and Drug Administration. (2003). *Birth control guide.* Accessed www.fda.gov/fdac/features/1997/babytable.html, February 25, 2006.

U.S. Food and Drug Administration. (2006). FDA approves over-the-counter access for Plan B for women 18 and older. Prescription remains required for those 17 and under. *FDA News.* Accessed www.fda.gov/bbs/topics/NEWS/2006/NEW01436.html.

Warner, L., Hatcher, R., & Steiner, M. (2004). Male condoms. In R. Hatcher, J. Trussell, F. Stewart, S. Nelson, W. Cates, F. Guest, et al. (Eds.), *Contraceptive technology* (18th rev. ed.). New York: Ardent Media.

Wikipedeia. (2006). *Abortion in Canada.* Accessed http://en.wikipedia.org/wiki/Abortion_in_Canada , June 14, 2006.

Williams, G. (2000). Grief after elective abortion: Exploring nursing interventions for another kind of perinatal loss. *AWHONN Lifelines, 4*(2), 37-40.

World Health Organization (WHO), Department of Reproductive Health and Research. (2004). *Medical criteria for contraceptive use* (3rd ed.). Geneva: Author.

Deitra Leonard Lowdermilk

Infertility

learning objectives

- List common causes of infertility.
- Investigate the psychologic impact of infertility.
- Describe common diagnoses and treatments for infertility.
- Identify reproductive alternatives for infertile couples.
- Examine the various ethical and legal considerations of infertility.

electronic resources

Additional information related to the content in Chapter 10 can be found on

the companion website at **evolve**
http://evolve.elsevier.com/Lowdermilk/MWHC/
- NCLEX Review Questions
- WebLinks

or on the interactive companion CD
- NCLEX Review Questions
- Plan of Care: Infertility

THIS chapter addresses infertility, associated tests, and common therapies. The available alternatives and the psychosocial implications of infertility are discussed.

■ INCIDENCE

Infertility is a serious medical concern that affects quality of life and is a problem for 10% to 15% of reproductive-age couples (American Society for Reproductive Medicine [ASRM], 2006a; Nelson & Marshall, 2004). The term *infertility* implies subfertility, a prolonged time to conceive, as opposed to *sterility,* which means inability to conceive. Normally, a fertile couple has approximately a 20% chance of conception in each ovulatory cycle. Primary infertility applies to a woman who has never been pregnant; secondary infertility applies to a woman who has been pregnant in the past.

The prevalence of infertility is relatively stable among the overall population but increases with the age of the woman, particularly in those older than 40 years (Stenchever, Droegemueller, Herbst, & Mishell, 2001). Probable causes include the trend toward delaying pregnancy until later in life, when fertility decreases naturally and the prevalence of diseases such as endometriosis and ovulatory dysfunction increases. There is some controversy regarding whether there has been an increase in male infertility,

or whether male infertility is being more readily identified because of improvements in diagnosis.

Diagnosis and treatment of infertility require considerable physical, emotional, and financial investment over an extended period. Men and women often perceive infertility differently, with women having more stress from tests and treatments, placing greater importance on having children, being more accepting of indicated treatments, and wanting children more than men (Sherrod, 2004).

In the United States, feelings connected with infertility are many and complex. The origins of some of these feelings are myths, superstitions, misinformation, or magical thinking about the causes of infertility. Other feelings arise from the need to undergo many tests and examinations and from a perception of being "different" from others (RESOLVE, 2006). The attitude, the sensitivity, and the caring nature of those who are involved in the assessment of infertility lay the foundation for the clients' ability to cope with the subsequent therapy and management. Team members also must respect affected individuals' and couples' desires in choosing to stop treatment and to select other alternatives, such as adoption. RESOLVE (www.resolve.org) is an organization that provides support, advocacy, and education about infertility for the infertility community as well as health care providers (Isaacs, 2005) (Critical Thinking Exercise).

CRITICAL THINKING EXERCISE

Infertility Counseling

Jenny, age 38 years, is a lawyer and has a history of endometriosis. Brad is a 39-year-old emergency department physician. Jenny has been trying to get pregnant for 2 years and seems very concerned about her lack of success. She has come to the Women's Clinic seeking help. She states that she has read about the success of assisted reproductive therapies and wants to know if she can have in vitro fertilization (IVF). What response by the nurse would be appropriate?

1. Evidence—Is there sufficient evidence to draw conclusions about what response the nurse should give?
2. Assumptions—Describe underlying assumptions about the following issues:
   a. Causes of male and female infertility
   b. Age and fertility
   c. Infertility as a major life stressor
3. What implications and priorities for nursing care can be made at this time?
4. Does the evidence objectively support your conclusion?
5. Are there alternative perspectives to your conclusion?

▬ FACTORS ASSOCIATED
▬ WITH INFERTILITY

Many factors, both male and female, contribute to normal fertility. A normally developed reproductive tract in both the male and female partner is essential. Normal functioning of an intact hypothalamic-pituitary-gonadal axis supports gametogenesis—the formation of sperm and ova. The life spans of the sperm and the ovum are short. Although sperm remain viable in the female's reproductive tract for 48 hours or more, probably only a few retain fertilization potential for more than 24 hours. Ova remain viable for about 24 hours, but the optimal time for fertilization may be no more than 1 to 2 hours (Cunningham, Leveno, Hauth, Gilstrap, & Wenstrom, 2005); thus timing of intercourse becomes critical.

An alteration in one or more of these structures, functions, or processes results in some degree of impaired fertility. Causes of impaired fertility are sometimes difficult to assign to either the male or female. In general, about 20% of couples will have unexplained or idiopathic causes of infertility. Among the 80% of couples who have an identifiable cause of infertility, about 40% are related to factors in the female partner, 40% are related to factors in the male partner, and 20% are related to factors in both partners (Nelson & Marshall, 2004; Stenchever et al., 2001). Boxes 10-1 and 10-2 list factors affecting female and male infertility.

Infertility also may be caused by something as simple as poor timing or inadequate frequency of intercourse. The couple should be taught about the menstrual cycle and the way to detect ovulation (see Chapters 5 and 9).

Female Infertility
Congenital or Developmental Factors

Congenital factors rarely cause impaired fertility. If the woman has abnormal external genitals, surgical

---

box 10-1 Factors Affecting Female Fertility

OVARIAN FACTORS
- Developmental anomalies
- Anovulation, primary
  - Pituitary or hypothalamic hormone disorder
  - Adrenal gland disorder
  - Congenital adrenal hyperplasia
- Anovulation, secondary
  - Disruption of hypothalamic-pituitary-ovarian axis
  - Amenorrhea after discontinuing oral contraceptive pills
  - Premature ovarian failure
- Increased prolactin levels

UTERINE, TUBAL, AND PERITONEAL FACTORS
- Developmental anomalies
- Tubal motility reduced
- Inflammation within the tube
- Tubal adhesions
- Endometrial and myometrial tumors
- Asherman syndrome (uterine adhesions or scar tissue)
- Endometriosis
- Chronic cervicitis
- Hostile or inadequate cervical mucus

OTHER FACTORS
- Nutritional deficiencies (e.g., anemia)
- Thyroid dysfunction
- Idiopathic condition

---

box 10-2 Factors Affecting Male Fertility

STRUCTURAL OR HORMONAL DISORDERS
- Undescended testes
- Hypospadias
- Varicocele
- Obstructive lesions of the vas deferens or epididymis
- Low testosterone levels
- Hypopituitarism
- Endocrine disorders
- Testicular damage caused by mumps
- Retrograde ejaculation

OTHER FACTORS
- Sexually transmitted infections
- Exposure to workplace hazards such as radiation or toxic substances
- Exposure of scrotum to high temperatures
- Nutritional deficiencies
- Antisperm antibodies
- Substance abuse
  - Changes in sperm—cigarette smoking, heroin, marijuana, amyl nitrate, butyl nitrate, ethyl chloride, methaqualone
  - Decrease in libido—heroin, methadone, selective serotonin reuptake inhibitors (SSRIs), and barbiturates
  - Impotence—alcohol, antihypertensive medications
- Idiopathic condition

reconstruction of abnormal tissue and construction of a functional vagina may permit normal intercourse. However, if internal reproductive tract structures are absent, there is no hope of fertility. Vaginal and uterine anomalies and their surgical repair vary from individual to individual. If a functional uterus can be reconstructed, pregnancy may be possible.

Hormonal and Ovulatory Factors

Anovulation may be primary or secondary. Primary anovulation may be caused by a pituitary or hypothalamic hormone disorder or an adrenal gland disorder such as congenital adrenal hyperplasia. It is usually seen in adolescents. Secondary anovulation, usually seen in young to midlife women, is relatively common and is caused by the disruption of the hypothalamic-pituitary-ovarian axis. In amenorrheic states and instances of anovulatory cycles, hormone studies usually reveal the problem.

Although it is a relatively rare occurrence, amenorrhea after the discontinuation of oral contraceptives is seen more frequently in women with histories of menstrual dysfunction before initiation of contraceptive use. Because most clients resume menstruating within 6 months, the workup should be delayed until that time in the absence of other symptoms.

Occasionally, women experience menopause before they are 40 years old. In a vast majority of cases of early menopause, the ovaries do not respond to ovulation-inducing drugs.

Increased prolactin levels may cause anovulation and amenorrhea. Many drugs affect the secretion of prolactin, including phenothiazine, opiates, diazepam, reserpine, methyldopa, and tricyclic antidepressants. In general, these agents are thought to inhibit the release of prolactin-inhibiting factor from the hypothalamus. Stress also can inhibit the release of prolactin-inhibiting factor, thereby causing the release of excess prolactin. Physical stressors such as surgery, cranial lesions, or injury also may initiate this response. Another common cause of hyperprolactinemia is benign pituitary adenoma, which is diagnosed through sophisticated radiographic techniques or computed tomographic (CT) scan.

Age-Related Infertility. The rate of fertility declines dramatically after the age of 35, and by 40 the total number of ovarian follicles is diminishing and the quality of remaining eggs is poor. Abnormalities of oocytes are thought to be the primary reason for age-associated infertility. By age 42, it is estimated that 90% of a woman's eggs have chromosomal abnormalities (Forbus, 2005).

Tubal/Peritoneal Factors

The motility of the tube and its fimbriated end may be reduced or absent as a result of infections, adhesions, scarring, or tumors. Chlamydial infection negatively influences tubal function and impedes fertility (Thomas, Coughlin, Mannion, & Haddad, 2000). In rare instances, one tube may be congenitally absent. One tube may be relatively

shorter than the other, which is often associated with an abnormally developed uterus.

Inflammation within the tube or involving the exterior of the tube or the fimbriated ends represents a major cause of impaired fertility. Tubal adhesions resulting from pelvic infections (e.g., ruptured appendix, sexually transmitted infections [STIs]) may impair fertility. When infection with purulent discharge heals, scar tissue adhesions form. In the process, the tube may be blocked anywhere along its length. It can be closed off at the fimbriated end, or it can be distorted and kinked by adhesions. Adhesions may permit the tiny sperm to pass through the tube but may prevent a fertilized egg from completing the journey into the intrauterine cavity. This results in an ectopic pregnancy that may completely destroy the tube. In other cases, adhesions of the tubes to the ovary or the bowel may follow endometriosis (see Chapter 7). Endometriosis is more commonly seen in women who delay childbearing until they are older than 30 years. Women who have a first-degree relative with a history of endometriosis also have a slightly higher risk.

Uterine Factors

Abnormalities of the uterus are more common than might be expected. Minor developmental anomalies of the uterus are fairly common; major anomalies occur rarely. Hysterosalpingography may reveal double uteri or other anomalous congenital variations (Fig. 10-1). Endometrial and myometrial tumors (e.g., polyps or myomas) may also be revealed by x-ray studies of infertile women. These anomalies can affect implantation and the maintenance of a pregnancy.

Asherman syndrome (uterine adhesions or scar tissue) is characterized by hypomenorrhea. The adhesions, which may partially or totally obliterate the uterine cavity, are sequelae to surgical interventions such as too vigorous curettage (scraping) after an elective abortion or miscarriage. The hysteroscope is useful in the verification of intrauterine anomalies.

Endometritis (inflammation of the endometrium) may result from any of the causes of infection of the cervix or uterine tubes (e.g., *Chlamydia*). Women who have numerous sexual partners are more susceptible to endometrial infection than are women in monogamous relationships.

FIG. 10-1 Abnormal uterus. **A,** Complete bicornuate uterus with vagina divided by a septum. **B,** Complete bicornuate uterus with normal vagina. **C,** Partial bicornuate uterus with normal vagina. **D,** Unicornuate uterus.

monthly menstruation is inadequate to conclude that ovulation is occurring and is optimal for conception.

procedure is used to visualize pelvic tissues for a variety of reasons (e.g., to identify abnormalities such as fibroid

transducer. *H,* Horizontal; *V,* vertical.

tumors and ovarian cysts, to verify follicular development and maturity, and to assess thickness of the endometrium around the time of ovulation).

Timed Endometrial Biopsy. Endometrial biopsy is scheduled after ovulation, during the luteal phase of the menstrual cycle. Late in the menstrual cycle, 2 to 3 days before expected menses, a small cannula is introduced into

immobilize the uterus and tubes, kink the tubes, and surround the ovaries.

Hysterosalpingography is scheduled 2 to 5 days after menstruation to avoid flushing a potential fertilized ovum out through a uterine tube into the peritoneal cavity. No open vessels exist at this time, and all menstrual debris has been discharged. This decreases the risk of embolism or of forcing menstrual debris out through the tubes into the peritoneal cavity.

box 10-5 **Assessment of the Woman**

HISTORY	PHYSICAL EXAMINATION

1. Age
2. Duration of infertility: length of contraceptive and non-contraceptive exposure
3. Obstetric
   a. Number of pregnancies, miscarriages, and abortions
   b. Length of time required to initiate each pregnancy
	1. General: complete physical examination
	2. Genital tract: state of hymen (full penetration); clitoris; vaginal infection, including trichomoniasis and candidiasis; cervical tears, polyps, infection, patency of os, accessibility to insemination; uterus, including size and position, mobility; adnexae, tumors, evidence of endometriosis

FIG. 10-3   Hysterosalpingography. Note that contrast medium flows through intrauterine cannula and out through the uterine tubes.

Referred shoulder pain may occur during this procedure. The referred pain is indicative of subphrenic irritation from the contrast media if it is spilled out of the patent uterine tubes. The discomfort can be managed with position change and mild analgesics. Pain usually subsides within 12 to 14 hours. Women with blocked tubes may have cramping for up to 48 hours.

This procedure may be both therapeutic and diagnostic. The passage of contrast medium may clear tubes of mucous plugs, straighten kinked tubes, or break up adhesions within the tubes (caused by salpingitis). The procedure may stimulate cilia in the lining of the tubes to facilitate transport of the ovum. It also may aid healing as a result of the bacteriostatic effect of the iodine within the contrast medium.

Laparoscopy. Laparoscopy is usually scheduled early in the menstrual cycle. During the procedure, a small endoscope is inserted through a small incision in the anterior abdominal wall. Cold fiberoptic light sources allow superior visualization of the internal pelvic structures (Fig. 10-4). The woman is usually admitted shortly before surgery,

having taken nothing by mouth (NPO) for 8 hours. She voids before surgery. A general anesthetic is usually given, and the woman is placed in the lithotomy position. A needle is inserted, and carbon dioxide gas is pumped into the peritoneum to elevate the abdominal wall from the organs, thereby creating an empty space that permits visualization and exploration with the laparoscope. If tubal patency is being assessed, a cannula is used to instill a dye contrast medium through the cervix.

Visualization of the peritoneal cavity in infertile women may reveal endometriosis, pelvic adhesions, tubal occlusion, leiomyomas (fibroids), or polycystic ovaries. Fulguration (destruction of tissue by means of electricity) of small endometrial implants, lysis of adhesions, and taking ovarian biopsies are some of the procedures possible with a laparoscope.

After surgery, deflation of most gas is done by direct expression. Trocar and needle sites are closed with a single subcuticular absorbable suture or skin clip, and an adhesive bandage is applied. Postoperative recovery requires taking vital signs, assessing level of consciousness, preventing aspiration, monitoring intravenous fluids, and reassuring the client regarding referred shoulder discomfort. Discharge from the hospital usually occurs in 4 to 6 hours. Referred shoulder pain or subcostal discomfort usually lasts only 24 hours and is relieved with a mild analgesic. Severe pain may be relieved when the woman assumes a knee-chest position. The woman must be cautioned against heavy lifting or strenuous activity for 4 to 7 days, at which time she is usually asymptomatic.

▬ Assessment of Male Infertility

The systematic investigation of infertility in the male client begins with a thorough history and physical examination (Box 10-7). Assessment of the male client proceeds in a manner similar to that of the female client, starting with noninvasive tests.

Semen Analysis. The basic test for male infertility is the semen analysis. A complete semen analysis, study of the effects of cervical mucus on sperm forward motility and survival, and evaluation of the sperm's ability to penetrate an ovum provide basic information. Semen is collected by ejaculation into a clean container or a plastic sheath that does not contain a spermicidal agent. The specimen is usually collected by masturbation after 2 to 5 days of abstinence from ejaculation. The semen is taken to the laboratory in a sealed container within 2 hours of ejaculation. Exposure to excessive heat or cold is avoided. Commonly accepted values based on the World Health Organization (WHO) criteria for semen characteristics are given in Box 10-8. If results are in the fertile range, no further sperm evaluation is necessary. If results are not within this range, the test is repeated. If subsequent results are still in the subfertile range, further evaluation is needed to identify the problem (Nelson & Marshall, 2004).

Seminal deficiency may be attributable to one or more of a variety of factors. The male is assessed for these

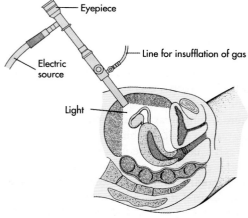

FIG. 10-4   Laparoscopy.

box 10-7 **Assessment of the Man**

HISTORY

1. Age
2. Fertility in this and other sexual relationships
3. Medical: General medical history, including infections (such as STIs, mononucleosis), mumps, orchitis after adolescence, chronic diseases, recent fever, medications, weight changes, undescended testes after age 3 mo, normal sexual development at puberty
4. Surgical: Herniorrhaphy, injuries to genitals, or other surgery in genital area
5. Occupational and environmental exposure to chemicals or radiation, physical nature of occupation and hobbies, vacations, and work habits
6. Previous tests and therapy done for study of infertility, duration of infertility in this and previous relationships
7. Sex history in detail: libido, coital history (such as frequency and ability to ejaculate), adequacy of erection, number of lifetime sex partners, attitudes toward masturbation
8. Personal: Motivation for childbearing; attitude toward partner; support system available, reason for seeking advice regarding infertility at this time; amount of exercise and stress level; use of alcohol, recreational drugs, caffeine, tobacco, anabolic steroids

PHYSICAL EXAMINATION

1. General: Complete physical examination, with special attention given to physical condition and fat and hair distribution
2. Genital tract: Penis and urethra; scrotal size; position, size, and consistency of testes; epididymides and vasa deferentia; prostate size and consistency
3. Careful search for varicocele, with man in both supine and upright positions

LABORATORY DATA

1. Routine urine test, gonorrhea and *Chlamydia* tests; serologic test for syphilis
2. Complete semen analysis (see Box 10-8)
3. Additional laboratory studies as indicated
   a. Basic endocrine studies indicated in men with oligospermia or aspermia:
      (1) Serum FSH, LH, and testosterone levels
      (2) T_3, T_4, TSH
      (3) Test for sperm antibodies, autoimmunization: autoimmune antibodies (produced by the man against his own sperm) agglutinate or immobilize sperm in <5% of men who have infertility problems
      (4) 17-Hydroxycorticoids and 17-ketosteroids
      (5) Buccal smear and chromosome studies (e.g., Klinefelter syndrome, XXY sex chromosomes)
   b. Testicular biopsy where correct interpretation is available (may give a more accurate diagnosis and prognosis in cases of azoospermia and severe oligospermia), vasography if indicated and available

FSH, Follicle-stimulating hormone; *LH,* luteinizing hormone; *STIs,* sexually transmitted infections; T_3, triiodothyronine; T_4, thyroxine; *TSH,* thyroid-stimulating hormone.

factors: hypopituitarism; nutritional deficiency; debilitating or chronic disease; trauma; exposure to environmental hazards such as radiation and toxic substances; use of tobacco, alcohol, and marijuana; gonadotropic inadequacy; and obstructive lesions of the epididymis and vas deferens. Congenital absence of the vas deferens can occur more frequently in men with the gene for cystic fibrosis. Genetic

testing for this and other anomalies is a common clinical practice (ASRM, 2001; Weber, Dohle, and Romijn, 2005). Hormone analyses are done for testosterone, gonadotropin, FSH, and LH. The sperm penetration assay and other alternative tests may be used to evaluate the ability of sperm to penetrate an egg (ASRM, 2001; Weber et al.). In addition, testicular biopsy may be warranted.

Ultrasonography. Scrotal ultrasound is used to examine the testes for presence of varicoceles and to identify abnormalities in the scrotum and spermatic cord. Transrectal ultrasound is used to evaluate the ejaculatory ducts, seminal vesicles, and the vas deferens (Zahalsky & Nagler, 2001).

■ *Assessment of the Couple*

Postcoital Test. The postcoital test (PCT) is one method used to test for adequacy of coital technique, cervical mucus, sperm, and degree of sperm penetration through cervical mucus. The test is performed within several hours after ejaculation of semen into the vagina. A specimen of cervical mucus is obtained from the cervical os and examined under a microscope. The quality of mucus and the number of forward-moving sperm are noted. A PCT with good mucus and motile sperm is associated with fertility.

Intercourse is synchronized with the expected time of ovulation (as determined from evaluation of BBT, cervical

box 10-8 **Semen Analysis**

- Liquefaction usually complete within 10 to 20 min
- Semen volume 2 to 6 ml
- Semen pH 7.2 to 8.0
- Sperm density 20 to 200 million/ml
- Total sperm count 40 million/ml
- Normal morphology 30% (normal oval)
- Motility (important consideration in sperm evaluation); percentage of forward-moving sperm estimated with respect to abnormally motile and nonmotile sperm 50%
- White cell count 1 million/ml
- Ovum penetration test (may be done if further evaluation necessary)

NOTE: These values are not absolute but are only relative to final evaluation of the couple as a single reproductive unit. Values also differ according to source used as a reference.
Values are based on the following: World Health Organization (WHO). (1992). *Laboratory manual for the examination of semen and sperm-cervical mucus interaction.* Geneva: Author.

mucus changes, and usual length of menstrual cycle or use of LH detection kit to determine LH surge) (see Fig. 9-5). It is performed only in the absence of vaginal infection. Couples may experience some difficulty abstaining from intercourse for 2 to 4 days before expected ovulation and then having intercourse with ejaculation on schedule. Sex on demand may strain the couple's interpersonal relationship. A problem may arise if the expected day of ovulation occurs when facilities or the physician is unavailable (such as over a weekend or holiday).

Nursing diagnoses are derived from the database. Examples of nursing diagnoses related to impaired fertility include the following:

- *Anxiety related to*
  -unknown outcome of diagnostic workup
- *Disturbed body image or situational low self-esteem related to*
  -impaired fertility
- *Ineffective coping related to*
  -methods used in the investigation of impaired fertility
  -alternatives to therapy: childfree living or adoption
- *Interrupted family processes related to*
  -unmet expectations for pregnancy
- *Acute pain related to*
  -effects of diagnostic tests (or surgery)
- *Ineffective sexuality patterns related to*
  -loss of libido secondary to medically imposed restrictions
- *Deficient knowledge related to*
  -preconception risk factors
  -factors surrounding ovulation
  -factors surrounding fertility

▬ Expected Outcomes of Care

Planning requires sensitivity to the couple's needs. Equipped with a knowledge of impaired fertility, the nurse can help develop a plan of care for the couple. The expected outcomes are phrased in client-centered terms and may include that the couple will do the following:

- Verbalize understanding of the anatomy and physiology of the reproductive system.
- Verbalize understanding of treatment for any abnormalities identified through various tests and examinations (e.g., infections, blocked uterine tubes, sperm allergy, and varicocele) and be able to make an informed decision about treatment.
- Verbalize understanding of their potential to conceive.
- Resolve guilt feelings and not need to focus blame.
- Conceive or, failing to conceive, decide on an alternative acceptable to both of them (e.g., childfree living or adoption).
- Demonstrate acceptable methods for handling pressure they may feel from peers and relatives regarding their childless state.

▬ Plan of Care and Interventions
▬ *Psychosocial*

Infertility is recognized as a major life stressor that can affect self-esteem, relations with the spouse, family, and friends, and careers. Couples often need assistance in separating their concepts of success and failure related to treatment for infertility from personal success and failure. Recognizing the significance of infertility as a loss and resolving these feelings are crucial to putting infertility into perspective, even if treatment is successful (ASRM, 2006b; Forbus, 2005; Nelson & Marshall, 2004).

Nurses can help couples express and discuss their feelings as honestly as possible. Ventilation may help couples to unburden themselves of negative feelings. Referral for mental health counseling may be beneficial.

Psychologic responses to a diagnosis of infertility may tax a couple's giving and receiving of physical and sexual closeness. The prescriptions and proscriptions for achieving conception may add tension to a couple's sexual functioning. Couples may report decreased desire for intercourse, orgasmic dysfunction, or midcycle erectile disorders.

To be able to deal comfortably with a couple's sexuality, nurses must be comfortable with their own sexuality so that they can better help couples understand why the private act of lovemaking must be shared with health care professionals. Nurses need up-to-date factual knowledge about human sexual practices and must be accepting of the preferences and activities of others without being judgmental, skilled in interviewing and in therapeutic use of self, sensitive to the nonverbal cues of others, and knowledgeable regarding each couple's sociocultural and religious beliefs.

The woman or couple facing infertility exhibits behaviors of the grieving process that are associated with other types of loss (Table 10-2). The loss of one's genetic continuity with the generations to come leads to a loss of self-esteem, to a sense of inadequacy as a woman or a man, to a loss of control over one's destiny, and to a reduced sense of self (Applegarth, 2000). Infertile individuals have impaired self-concept and greater dissatisfaction with their marriages (Newton, 2000). The investigative process leads to a loss of spontaneity and control over the couple's marital relationship and sometimes to a loss of control over progress toward career and life goals. All people do not have all the reactions described, nor can it be predicted how long any reaction will last for an individual.

The support systems of the couple with impaired fertility must be explored. This exploration should include persons available to assist, their relationship to the couple, their ages, their availability, and the available cultural or religious support.

If the couple conceives, nurses must be aware that the concerns and problems of the previously infertile couple may not be over. Many couples are overjoyed with the pregnancy; however, some are not. Some couples rearrange their lives, sense of self, and personal goals within their

table 10-2 Nursing Actions in Response to Behavior Associated with Impaired Fertility

BEHAVIORAL CHARACTERISTIC	NURSING ACTIONS
Surprise: Each person assumes she or he is fertile and that pregnancy is an option	Point out resemblance to grieving process—a normal, expected reaction to loss. Refer to support group.*
	Prepare clients for length of time it may take to grieve and for types of feelings (psychologic, somatic) to expect.
	Encourage and allow time to talk of past and present feelings of sexuality, self-image, and self-esteem.
Denial: "It can't happen to me!"	Allow time for denial, because it gives the body and mind time to adjust a little at a time.
	Do not feed into the client's denial; instead say, "It must be hard to believe such a devastating report."
Anger: Toward others (perhaps even the nurse) or themselves	Explain that the reaction to loss of control and to a feeling of helplessness is often anger, which can easily be projected onto another person. Anger is a natural feeling.
	Allow time to express anger at losing sense of control over bodies and destinies.
	A helpful approach may be, "It's OK to be angry . . . at those who are pregnant, at people who want abortions, at self, at mate, at caregivers" and so forth.
Bargaining: "If I get pregnant, I'll dedicate the child to God."	Accept bargaining statements without comment
Depression: Isolation: Personal	Allow time for both woman and man to talk about how it feels whenever a sight, event, or word serves as a reminder of his or her own state of impaired fertility.
	Develop role-playing situations to practice interactions with others under various circumstances to increase the couple's ability to cope and to solve problems (increases their self-confidence).
	The nurse may say, "You must feel so terribly alone sometimes."
Guilt or unworthiness	Allow time to identify feelings that may be related to earlier behaviors (such as abortion, premarital sex, contact with sexually transmitted infections [STIs]).
Acceptance (resolution)	Couple or person comes to the realization that "unworthiness" and impaired fertility are unrelated.
	Clients need to know that grief feelings are never laid away forever; they may be activated by special reminders (such as anniversaries).

*RESOLVE, Inc., 1310 Broadway, Somerville, MA 02144. www.resolve.org.

acceptance of their infertile state. The couple may feel that those who worked with them to identify and treat impaired fertility expect them to be happy with the pregnancy. The couple may be shocked to find that they feel resentment because the pregnancy, once a cherished dream, now necessitates another change in goals, aspirations, and identities. The normal ambivalence toward pregnancy may be perceived as reneging on the original choice to become parents. The couple might choose to abort the pregnancy at this time. Other couples worry about miscarriage. If the couple wishes to continue with the pregnancy, they will need the care other expectant couples need. The couple may need extra preparation for the realities of pregnancy, labor, and parenthood because they developed fantasies about childbearing when they thought it was beyond their reach. A history of impaired fertility is considered to be a risk factor for pregnancy.

If the couple does not conceive, they are assessed regarding their desire to be referred for help with adoption, therapeutic intrauterine insemination, other reproductive alternatives, or choosing a childfree state. The couple may find a list of agencies, support groups, and other resources in their community helpful such as ASRM (www.asrm.org) and RESOLVE (www.resolve.org).

■ Nonmedical

Simple changes in lifestyle may be effective in the treatment of subfertile men. Only water-soluble lubricants should be used during intercourse, because many commonly used lubricants contain spermicides or have spermicidal properties. High scrotal temperatures may be caused by daily hot-tub bathing or saunas in which the testes are kept at temperatures too high for efficient spermatogenesis. It must be remembered that these conditions lead to only lessened fertility and should not be used as a means of contraception.

Treatment is available for women who have immunologic reactions to sperm. The use of condoms during genital intercourse for 6 to 12 months will reduce female antibody production in most women who have elevated antisperm antibody titers. After the serum reaction subsides, condoms are used at all times except at the expected time of ovulation. Approximately one third of couples with this problem conceive by following this course of action.

Changes in nutrition and habits may increase fertility for both men and women. For example, a well-balanced diet, exercise, decreased alcohol intake, not smoking or abusing drugs, and stress management may be effective.

■ Herbal Alternative Measures

Most herbal remedies have not been proven clinically to promote fertility or to be safe in early pregnancy and should be taken by the woman only as prescribed by a physician or nurse-midwife who has expertise in herbology. Relaxation, osteopathy, stress management (e.g., aromatherapy, yoga), and nutritional and exercise counseling have been reported to increase pregnancy rates in some women (Tiran & Mack, 2000). Herbal remedies that reportedly promote fertility in general include red clover flowers, nettle leaves, dong quai, St John's wort, chasteberry, and false unicorn root (Weed, 1986). Vitamin C, calcium, and magnesium may promote fertility and conception (Tiran & Mack). Vitamins E and C, glutathione, and coenzyme Q10 are antioxidants that have proven beneficial effects for male infertility (Sheweita et al, 2005). Herbs to avoid while trying to conceive include licorice root, yarrow, wormwood, ephedra, fennel, goldenseal, lavender, juniper, flaxseed, pennyroyal, passionflower, wild cherry, cascara, sage, thyme, and periwinkle (Sampey, Bourque, & Wren, 2004).

■ Medical

Pharmacologic therapy for female infertility is often directed at treating ovulatory dysfunction either by stimulating ovulation or by enhancing ovulation so that more oocytes mature. These medications include clomiphene citrate, human menopausal gonadotropin (HMG), FSH, recombinant FSH (rFSH), and human chorionic gonadotropin (hCG). Gonadotropin-releasing hormone (GnRH) agonists, progesterone, and bromocriptine (Parlodel) also are used (Leibowitz & Hoffman, 2000; Nelson & Marshall, 2004). Table 10-3 describes common medications used for treating female infertility. These medications are extremely potent and require daily monitoring with ovarian ultrasonography and monitoring of estradiol levels to prevent hyperstimulation. The prevalence of multiple pregnancy with the use of these medications is greater than 25%. When ovulation is caused either by hypothalamic-pituitary dysfunction or failure, or failure to respond to clomiphene, GnRH may be used. Thyroid-stimulating hormone (Synthroid) is indicated if the woman has hypothyroidism.

The woman who has low estrogen levels may be a candidate for conjugated estrogens and medroxyprogesterone. A hypoestrogenic condition may result from a high stress level or decreased percentage of body fat as a result of an eating disorder (e.g., anorexia nervosa) or excessive exercise. Hydroxyprogesterone supplementation with vaginal suppositories or intramuscular injection is used to treat luteal phase defects. The nurse may encounter other medications as well. In the presence of adrenal hyperplasia, prednisone, a glucocorticoid, is taken orally. Treatment of endometriosis may include danazol, progesterones, combined oral contraceptives, or GnRH agonists (Leibowitz & Hoffman, 2000; Stenchever et al., 2001) (see Table 10-3). Infections are treated with appropriate antimicrobial formulations.

Drug therapy may be indicated for male infertility. Problems with the thyroid or adrenal glands are corrected with appropriate medications. Infections are identified and treated promptly with antimicrobials. FSH, HMG, and clomiphene may be used to stimulate spermatogenesis in men with hypogonadism (Leibowitz & Hoffman, 2000).

The primary care provider is responsible for informing clients fully about the prescribed medications. However, the nurse must be ready to answer clients' questions and to confirm their understanding of the drug, its administration, potential side effects, and expected outcomes. Because information varies with each drug, the nurse must consult the medication package inserts, pharmacology references, the physician, and the pharmacist as necessary.

■ Surgical

A number of surgical procedures can be used for problems causing female infertility. Ovarian tumors must be excised. Whenever possible, functional ovarian tissue is left intact. Scar tissue adhesions caused by chronic infections may cover much or all of the ovary. These adhesions usually necessitate surgery to free and expose the ovary so that ovulation can occur.

Hysterosalpingography is useful for identification of tubal obstruction and also for the release of blockage. During laparoscopy, delicate adhesions may be divided and removed, and endometrial implants may be destroyed by electrocoagulation or laser. Laparotomy and even microsurgery may be required to do extensive repair of the damaged tube. Prognosis is dependent on the degree to which tubal patency and function can be restored (Stenchever et al., 2001).

Reconstructive surgery (e.g., the unification operation for bicornuate uterus) often improves a woman's ability to conceive and carry the fetus to term. Surgical removal of tumors or fibroids involving the endometrium or uterus often improves the woman's chance of conceiving and maintaining the pregnancy to viability. Surgical treatment of uterine tumors or maldevelopment that results in successful pregnancy usually requires birth by cesarean surgery near term gestation because the uterus may rupture as a result of weakness of the area of reconstructive surgery.

Chemocautery (destruction of tissue with chemicals) or thermocautery (destruction of tissue with heat, usually electrical) of the cervix, cryosurgery (destruction of tissue by application of extreme cold, usually liquid nitrogen), or conization (excision of a cone-shaped piece of tissue from the endocervix) is effective in eliminating chronic inflammation and infection. However, when the cervix has been deeply cauterized or frozen, or when extensive conization has been performed, extreme limitation of mucus production by the cervix may result. Sperm migration may be difficult or impossible because of the absence of a mucus bridge from the vagina to the uterus. Therapeutic intrauterine insemination may be necessary to carry the sperm directly through the internal os of the cervix.

table 10-3 Medications Used in the Treatment of Infertility

DRUG	INDICATION	MECHANISM OF ACTION	DOSAGE	COMMON SIDE EFFECTS
Clomiphene citrate	Ovulation induction, treatment of luteal-phase inadequacy	Thought to bind to estrogen receptors in the pituitary, blocking them from detecting estrogen	Tablets, starting with 50 mg/day by mouth for 5 days beginning on fifth day of menses; if ovulation does not occur, may increase dose next cycle-variable dosage	Vasomotor flushes, abdominal discomfort, nausea and vomiting, breast tenderness, ovarian enlargement
Menotropins (human menopausal gonadotropins)	Ovarian follicular growth and maturation	LH and FSH in 1:1 ratio, direct stimulation of ovarian follicle; given sequentially with hCG to induce ovulation	IM injections, dosage regimen variable based on ovarian response. Initial dose is 75 international units of FSH and 75 international units of LH (1 ampoule) daily for 7-12 days followed by 10,000 international units hCG	Ovarian enlargement, ovarian hyperstimulation, local irritation at injection site, multifetal gestations
Follitropins (purified FSH)	Treatment of polycystic ovarian disease; follicle stimulation for assisted reproductive techniques	Direct action on ovarian follicle	Subcutaneous or IM injections, dosage regimen variable	Ovarian enlargement, ovarian hyperstimulation, local irritation at injection site, multifetal gestations
Human chorionic gonadotropin (hCG)	Ovulation induction	Direct action on ovarian follicle to stimulate meiosis and rupture of the follicle	5000-10,000 international units IM 1 day after last dose of menotropins; dosage regimen variable	Local irritation at injection site; headaches, irritability, edema, depression, fatigue
Androgens (danazol)	Treatment of endometriosis	Combination of estrogen and androgen suppresses ovarian activity, eliminating stimulation to endometrial glands and stroma, with resultant shrinkage and disappearance	200-800 mg/day by mouth for 3 to 6 mo	Mild hirsutism, acne, edema and weight gain, increase of liver enzyme levels
GnRH agonists (nafarelin acetate, leuprolide acetate)	Treatment of endometriosis, uterine fibroids	Desensitization and downward regulation of GnRH receptors of pituitary, resulting in suppression of LH, FSH, and ovarian function	Nafarelin, 200 mcg (1 spray) intranasally twice daily for 6 mo; leuprolide acetate 3.75 mg IM every 28 days for 6 mo	Nafarelin irritation, nosebleeds; both nafarelin and leuprolide—hot flashes, vaginal dryness, myalgia and arthralgia, headaches, mild bone loss (usually reversible within 12-18 mo after treatment)
Progesterone (natural progesterone in oil, gel, or micronized powder)	Treatment of luteal-phase inadequacy	Direct stimulation of endometrium	Vaginal or rectal suppositories, 50 to 100 mg daily; progesterone capsules, 100 mg by mouth 3 times daily, IM—25 to 100 mg a day; vaginal gel 8%—1 to 2 prefilled applicators per day	Breast tenderness, local irritation, headaches
GnRH antagonists (ganirelix acetate, cetrorelix acetate)	Controlled ovarian stimulation for infertility treatment	Suppresses gonadotropin secretion; inhibits premature LH surges in women undergoing ovarian hyperstimulation	250 mcg daily subcutaneously usually in the early to midfollicular phase of the menstrual cycle; usually followed by hCG administration	Abdominal pain, headache, vaginal bleeding, irritation at the injection site

References: Clinical Pharmacology. (2005). *Nafarelin and Leuprolide*. Gold Standard Multimedia. Accessed http://cp.gsm.com, June 24, 2005; Leibowitz, D., & Hoffman, J. (2000). Fertility drug therapies: Past, present, and future. *Journal of Obstetric, Gynecologic, and Neonatal Nursing, 29*(2), 201-210; Weiner, C., & Buhimschi, C. (2004). *Drugs for pregnant and lactating women*. Philadelphia: Churchill Livingstone.
hCG, Human chorionic gonadotropin; *FSH*, follicle-stimulating hormone; *GnRH*, gonadotropin-releasing hormone; *IM*, intramuscularly; *LH*, luteinizing hormone.

EVIDENCE-BASED PRACTICE

Tubal Flushing: Diagnosis Plus Treatment for Infertility

BACKGROUND

- Fertility requires patent fallopian tubes. A blockage in the fallopian tube can prevent transport of sperm to egg, or prevent the fertilized ovum from traveling to implant in the uterus. For more than half a century, tubal patency has been evaluated using dye or liquid medium injected into the uterus and forced out into the fallopian tubes. The resulting flow was visible directly using laparoscopy, or radiographic imaging (hysterosalpingogram). Physicians and researchers noticed that the diagnostic procedure of tubal flushing increased the odds of pregnancy and live birth. Oil-soluble contrast media (OSCM) was eventually replaced with water-soluble contrast media (WSCM), which permitted better tube imaging, faster filling, less cost, and less risk of inflammation and anaphylaxis than OSCM. However, OSCM offered other benefits: the slower filling time allowed visualization of slow peritoneal spillage, sharper image of the uterus, less pain, and an increased pregnancy rate.

OBJECTIVES

- The authors decided to systematically evaluate the fertility outcomes of infertile women undergoing tubal flushing.

METHODS

Search Strategy

- The reviewers thoroughly searched the scientific literature for fertility-enhancing effects of tubal flushing. Eleven randomized trials, dated 1986 to 2004, met the criteria. The trials represented 2163 women from Canada, China, Denmark, Holland, Japan, New Zealand, the United Kingdom, and the United States.

Statistical Analyses

- Similar data were pooled. Reviewers calculated risk ratios for dichotomous (categoric) data, such as pregnancies and live births. Differences between groups outside the 95% confidence interval were accepted as significant.

FINDINGS

- OSCM improved the odds of pregnancy and live birth significantly over no treatment (no trials compared WSCM to no treatment). OSCM caused less bleeding and pain than WSCM. Infection rates were similar. There was a greater risk for extravasation (media escaping into surrounding tissues) with OSCM, but no serious harm resulted.
- The pregnancy rate was slightly higher for OSCM than WSCM, an effect that has held across three such metaanalyses. This could be because OSCM is more effective at removing debris from fallopian tubes. It could decrease peritoneal inflammation and phagocytosis of sperm, or improve uterine or cervical conditions. Mechanically, the pressure of the media may straighten tortuous tubes or disrupt adhesions.

LIMITATIONS

- Some studies had notable losses to follow-up. Randomization too far in advance led to some losses to follow-up, changed minds, and withdrawals due to conception. It was not possible to analyze by intention to treat (analyzing the subject's data in the group originally assigned, for statistical purposes, which strengthens the generalizability of the study). Two of the trials were funded by a manufacturer of contrast media. None of the trials mentioned blinding, which would have been possible at least for the subjects.

IMPLICATIONS FOR PRACTICE

- Nurses who work with infertile couples should know the various tests and treatments that are available, and be sensitive to increasing invasiveness. Tubal flushing is a very invasive diagnostic test, but has a long track record of increasing pregnancy outcomes. In an era where in vitro fertilization is seen as standard treatment, tubal flushing retains its place as a simpler and economical way of improving outcomes. For safety, the authors recommend confirming tubal patency before flushing.

IMPLICATIONS FOR FURTHER RESEARCH

- Explanations for why OSCM enhances fertility are still speculative. The therapeutic effect may enhance fertility in some nontubal occlusion cases. Blinding may decrease bias and placebo effect. Live births should be the standard outcome in future studies.

Reference: Johnson, N., Vanderkerkhove, P., Watson, A., Lilford, R., Harada, T., & Hughes, E. (2005). Tubal flushing for subfertility. In *The Cochrane Database of Systematic Reviews*, 2006, Issue 3. Chichester, UK: John Wiley & Sons.

Surgical procedures also may be used for problems causing male infertility. Surgical repair of varicocele has been relatively successful in increasing sperm count but not fertility rates.

Microsurgery to reanastomose (restore tubal continuity) the sperm ducts after vasectomy can restore fertility (Nagler & Rotman, 2002).

■ Assisted Reproductive Therapies

Although remarkable developments have occurred in reproductive medicine, assisted reproductive therapies (ARTs) account for less than 1% of all U.S. births (Van Voorhis, 2006) and less than 3% of infertility treatment (ASRM, 2006a) (www.asrm.org). They are associated with many ethical and legal issues (Box 10-9). The lack of information or misleading information about success rates and the risks and benefits of treatment alternatives prevents couples from making informed decisions. Nurses can provide information so that couples have an accurate understanding of their chances for a successful pregnancy and live birth. Nurses also can provide anticipatory guidance about the moral and ethical dilemmas regarding the use of ARTs. Some of the ARTs for treatment of infertility include in vitro fertilization-embryo transfer (IVF-ET), gamete intrafallopian transfer (GIFT), zygote intrafallopian transfer (ZIFT), ovum transfer (oocyte donation), embryo adoption, embryo hosting and surrogate parenting, and therapeutic donor insemination (TDI). Table 10-4

box 10-9 Issues to Be Addressed by Infertile Couples Before Treatment

- Risks of multiple gestation
- Possible need for multifetal reduction
- Possible need for donor oocytes, sperm, or embryos, or for gestational carrier (surrogate mother)
- Whether to or how to disclose facts of conception to offspring
- Freezing embryos for later use
- Possible risks of long-term effects of medications and treatment on women, children, and families

FIG. 10-5   Gamete intrafallopian transfer. **A,** Through laparoscopy, a ripe follicle is located and fluid containing the egg is removed. **B,** The sperm and egg are placed separately in the uterine tube, where fertilization occurs.

describes these procedures and the possible indications for the ARTs. Other options using micromanipulation include intracytoplasmic sperm injection and assisted hatching. Adoption is an option for couples who choose not to have infertility treatments or who decide to adopt after infertility treatments have failed.

In Vitro Fertilization-Embryo Transfer. In vitro fertilization-embryo transfer (IVF-ET) is a common approach for women with blocked or absent uterine tubes or with unexplained infertility and for men with very low sperm counts. About 99% of all ARTs use this procedure (Van Voorhis, 2006). Generally only three or fewer embryos are transferred, to minimize the risk of multiple pregnancy. When more than three embryos develop in the culture media, the extra embryos can be cryopreserved. If necessary, they can be thawed in a subsequent cycle for later uterine transfer.

■ LEGAL TIP   Cryopreservation of Human Embryos

Couples who have excess embryos frozen for later transfer must be fully informed before consenting to the procedure, to make decisions regarding the disposal of embryos in the event of (1) death, (2) divorce, or (3) the decision that the couple no longer wants the embryos at a later time.

Success rates for pregnancy and for live births vary widely from center to center. Each couple's physical status and age factor into their individual chances for pregnancy as well as whether the embryos are fresh or frozen and from donor or nondonor eggs (Van Voorhis, 2006) (Table 10-5). Costs vary by treatment and by region of the country: one cycle of IVF-ET averages $12,400 (ASRM, 2006a).

Gamete Intrafallopian Transfer. Gamete intrafallopian transfer (GIFT) is similar to IVF-ET. GIFT requires women to have at least one normal uterine tube. Ovulation is induced as in IVF-ET, and the oocytes are aspirated from follicles via laparoscopy (Fig. 10-5, *A*). Semen is collected before laparoscopy, and sperm are capacitated by the same technique used for IVF-ET. The ova and sperm are then transferred to one uterine tube (Fig. 10-5, *B*), permitting natural fertilization and cleavage. Less than 1% of all ARTs use this technique (Van Voorhis, 2006).

Zygote Intrafallopian Transfer. Zygote intrafallopian transfer (ZIFT) is similar to GIFT except that in ZIFT,

after in vitro fertilization the ova are placed in the uterine tube during the zygote stage. ZIFT accounts for less than 1% of all ART procedures (Van Voorhis, 2006).

Complications. Other than the established risks associated with laparoscopy and general anesthesia, few risks are associated with IVF-ET, GIFT, and ZIFT. The more common transvaginal needle aspiration requires only local or intravenous analgesia. Congenital anomalies occur no more frequently than among naturally conceived embryos. Multiple gestations are more likely and are associated with increased risks for both the mother and fetuses (Wright, Schieve, Reynolds, Jeng, & Kissin, 2004). However, ectopic pregnancies do occur more often, and these carry a significant maternal risk. No increase in maternal or perinatal complications occurs with TDI; the same frequencies of anomalies (about 5%) and obstetric complications (between 5% and 10%) that accompany natural insemination (through sexual intercourse) apply also to TDI.

Oocyte Donation. Women who have ovarian failure or oophorectomy, who have a genetic defect, or who fail to achieve pregnancy with their own oocytes may be eligible for the use of donor oocytes. Oocyte donation is usually done by women who are younger than 35 years and healthy, and who are recruited and paid to undergo ovarian stimulation and oocyte retrieval. The donor eggs are then fertilized in the laboratory with the male partner's sperm. The recipient woman undergoes hormonal stimulation to allow development of the uterine lining. Embryos are then transferred. The psychosocial issues are similar to those in therapeutic donor insemination. Historically the courts have upheld the gestational mother as the legal mother. It is expected that the egg donor will have no rights or responsibilities in relation to the offspring (Hahn & Craft-Rosenberg, 2002).

Embryo Donation. On occasion, a couple decide that they do not want their frozen embryos, and they release these for "adoption" by other infertile couples. Infertility centers are struggling to develop guidelines and protocols to address the various legal and ethical issues associated with these procedures. Extensive medical testing of both

table 10-4 **Assisted Reproductive Therapies**

PROCEDURE	DEFINITION	INDICATIONS
In vitro fertilization-embryo transfer (IVF-ET)	A woman's eggs are collected from her ovaries, fertilized in the laboratory with sperm, and transferred to her uterus after normal embryo development has occurred.	Tubal disease or blockage; severe male infertility; endometriosis; unexplained infertility; cervical factor; immunologic infertility
Gamete intrafallopian transfer (GIFT)	Oocytes are retrieved from the ovary, placed in a catheter with washed motile sperm, and immediately transferred into the fimbriated end of the uterine tube. Fertilization occurs in the uterine tube.	Same as for IVF-ET, except there must be normal tubal anatomy, patency, and absence of previous tubal disease in at least one uterine tube
IVF-ET and GIFT with donor sperm	This process is the same as described above except in cases where the male partner's fertility is severely compromised and donor sperm can be used; if donor sperm are used, the woman must have indications for IVF-ET or GIFT.	Severe male infertility; azoospermia; indications for IVF-ET or GIFT
Zygote intrafallopian transfer (ZIFT)	This process is similar to IVF-ET; after in vitro fertilization the ova are placed in one uterine tube during the zygote stage.	Same as for GIFT
Donor oocyte	Eggs are donated by an IVF procedure, and the donated eggs are inseminated. The embryos are transferred into the recipient's uterus, which is hormonally prepared with estrogen/progesterone therapy.	Early menopause; surgical removal of ovaries; congenitally absent ovaries; autosomal or sex-linked disorders; lack of fertilization in repeated IVF attempts because of subtle oocyte abnormalities or defects in oocyte-spermatozoa interaction
Donor embryo (embryo adoption)	A donated embryo is transferred to the uterus of an infertile woman at the appropriate time (normal or induced) of the menstrual cycle.	Infertility not resolved by less aggressive forms of therapy; absence of ovaries; male partner is azoospermic or is severely compromised
Gestational carrier (embryo host); surrogate mother	A couple undertakes an IVF cycle, and the embryo(s) is transferred to the uterus of another woman (the carrier) who has contracted with the couple to carry the baby to term. The carrier has no genetic investment in the child. Surrogate motherhood is a process by which a woman is inseminated with semen from the infertile woman's partner and then carries the fetus until birth.	Congenital absence or surgical removal of uterus; a reproductively impaired uterus, myomas, uterine adhesions, or other congenital abnormalities; a medical condition that might be life threatening during pregnancy, such as diabetes, immunologic problems, or severe heart, kidney, or liver disease
Therapeutic donor insemination (TDI)	Donor sperm are used to inseminate the female partner.	Male partner is azoospermic or has a very low sperm count; couple has a genetic defect; male partner has antisperm antibodies
Intracytoplasmic sperm injection	Selection of one sperm cell that is injected directly into the egg to achieve fertilization. Used with IVF.	Same as TDI
Assisted hatching	The zona pellucida is penetrated chemically or manually to create an opening for the dividing embryo to hatch and implant into uterine wall.	Recurrent miscarriages; to improve implantation rate in women with previously unsuccessful IVF attempts; advanced age

Data from American Society for Reproductive Medicine (ASRM). (2006a). *Frequently asked questions about infertility.* Accessed www.asrm.org, March 31, 2006; Stenchever, M., Droegemueller, W., Herbst, A., & Mishell, D. (2001). *Comprehensive gynecology* (4th ed.). St. Louis: Mosby; Van Voorhis, B. (2006). Outcomes from assisted reproductive technology. *Obstetrics and Gynecology, 107*(1), 183-200.

table 10-5 2003 Assisted Reproductive Technology Success Rates

TYPE OF CYCLE	AGE OF WOMAN (YR)			
	35	35-37	38-40	41-42
FRESH EMBRYOS FROM NONDONOR EGGS				
Number of cycles	39,852	20,056	18,660	8,185
Percentage of cycles resulting in pregnancies	43.1	36.2	27.0	18.5
Percentage of cycles resulting in live births	37.3	30.2	20.2	11.0
Percentage of transfers resulting in live births	43.2	36.6	26.1	15.1
Average number of embryos transferred	2.6	2.9	3.1	3.5
Percentage of pregnancies with twins	33.3	27.6	22.6	14.5
Percentage of pregnancies with triplets or more	6.4	6.2	5.4	2.8
Percentage of live births having multiple infants	38.4	32.1	26.1	17.4
FROZEN EMBRYOS FROM NONDONOR EGGS				
Number of transfers	8,353	3,678	2,455	728
Percentage of transfers resulting in live births	29.4	28.2	22.6	16.5
Average number of embryos transferred	2.7	2.7	2.8	3.0

DONOR EGGS	ALL AGES COMBINED	
	FRESH EMBRYOS	FROZEN EMBRYOS
Number of transfers	8,970	4,026
Percentage of transfers resulting in live births	50.8	30.1
Average number of embryos transferred	2.6	2.8

Source: Centers for Disease Control and Prevention. (2005). 2003 *Assisted reproductive technology (ART) report: National summary.* Accessed http://apps.nccd.cdc.gov/ART2003/nation03.asp, June 19, 2006.

partners is required as well (ASRM Ethics Committee, 2004; Hershberger, 2004).

Surrogate Mothers/Embryo Hosts. Surrogate motherhood can be achieved by two methods. The first is for the surrogate mother to be inseminated with semen from the infertile woman's partner and to carry the baby until the birth. The baby is then formally adopted by the infertile couple. A less common method is to retrieve an ovum from the infertile woman, fertilize it with her partner's sperm, and place it into the uterus of a surrogate, who becomes an embryo host or gestational carrier. These interventions raise considerable legal and ethical issues that require extensive counseling of couples and the women to choose to become pregnant.

Therapeutic Donor Insemination. Therapeutic donor insemination (TDI), previously referred to as artificial insemination by donor, is used when the male partner has no sperm or a very low sperm count (less than 20 million motile sperm per milliliter), the couple has a genetic defect, or the male partner has antisperm antibodies. Couples need to be counseled extensively regarding the mutuality of their decision, their ability (particularly of the male partner) to grieve the loss of a biologic child, and long-term issues relating to parenting the child conceived through TDI (Boivin et al., 2001; Van Voorhis, 2006). Couples also must be aware of the legal status of TDI in their state.

In TDI, donor semen is subjected to laboratory testing to reduce the possibility of life-threatening illnesses for the recipient and her fetus, as well as for factors that could

jeopardize the woman's future fertility or compromise the chance of the success of the procedure. Donor semen is tested for syphilis (serology testing), serum hepatitis B antigen, *Neisseria gonorrhoeae, Chlamydia trachomatis,* cytomegalovirus antibodies, and human immunodeficiency virus (HIV) antibodies (U.S. Food and Drug Administration, 2004).

The procedure is done in the physician's office or clinic, usually the day after the woman has an LH surge. The sperm are loaded into a catheter that is then inserted in the vagina, through the cervix, and placed high in the uterine cavity. The sperm are injected slowly, and the catheter is removed. The woman lies flat for a few minutes and then can get up and resume her usual activities (Stenchever et al., 2001).

Assuming normal female fertility, intrauterine TDI at or about the time of ovulation has resulted in pregnancy in as many as 70% of cases. If pregnancy has not occurred within six cycles of well-timed insemination, further investigation of the female partner is warranted. The couple must know that there is no guarantee of pregnancy and that the miscarriage rate is approximately the same as in a control population.

Micromanipulation. Techniques to improve fertilization, embryo growth, and genetic testing are improving at a rapid pace. *Micromanipulation* allows the handling of individual eggs and sperm through the use of specific instruments and controls. Intracytoplasmic sperm injection (ICSI) is a technique that makes it possible to achieve fertilization or to correct abnormal fertilization by introducing sperm beneath the zona pellucida directly into the egg. ICSI offers the opportunity to enhance the chances of fertilization in cases of a severe male factor (i.e., poor sperm quality) (Van Voorhis, 2006). It is commonly used as the insemination technique in IVF therapy (Georgia Reproductive Specialists, 2005).

Preimplantation genetic diagnosis (PGD) is a form of early genetic testing designed to eliminate embryos with serious genetic defects before implantation through one of the ARTs and to avoid future termination of pregnancy for genetic reasons. Micromanipulation allows removal of a single cell from a multicellular embryo for genetic study (i.e., embryo biopsy) (Georgia Reproductive Specialists, 2005; Kearnes et al., 2005). Various techniques are used to test the cell for numerical and structural chromosomal abnormalities as well as for disease-specific DNA mutations. In more than 20 worldwide centers, PGD is being used clinically. Couples must be counseled about their options and choices, as well as the implications of their choices, when genetic analysis is considered. For example, the transfer of only embryos that are free from abnormalities can increase the implantation rate and decrease the miscarriage rate and may increase the likelihood of the birth of a healthy infant (Kearnes et al.).

Another micromanipulation option is assisted hatching. In some instances, the zona pellucida is thick or tough and the embryo cannot break through or "hatch" through this coating in the blastocystic phase of development. An infared laser is used to create a hole in the zona pellucida so that the embryo can break through and implant. This procedure is considered experimental and research continues (Georgia Reproductive Specialists, 2005) (www.ivf. com).

Adoption. Couples may choose to build their family through adoption of children who are not their own biologically. With increased availability of birth control and abortion and increasing numbers of single mothers keeping their babies, however, the adoption of Caucasian infants is extremely limited. Minority infants and infants with special needs, older children, and foreign adoptions are other options (ASRM, 2003).

Most adults assume that they will be able to have children of their own. The discovery that they are unable to do so is often accompanied by feelings of inferiority, doubts about masculinity or femininity, and feelings of guilt or blame in relation to the partner. These feelings and frustrations, combined with the anxiety of waiting for pregnancies, feelings of loss, and the multiple medical procedures to investigate infertility create a unique situation for the adoptive couple preparing for parenthood (Salzer, 2000).

Couples who decide to adopt a child have decided that being a parent and having a child is more important than the actual process of birthing the child. The birth process is a very small aspect of having a baby and becoming a parent.

---

plan of care ▶ Infertility

CD Plan of Care: Infertility

NURSING DIAGNOSIS Deficient knowledge related to lack of understanding of the reproductive process with regard to conception as evidenced by client questions

Expected Outcome *Client and partner will verbalize understanding of the components of the reproductive process, common problems leading to infertility, usual infertility testing, and the importance of completing testing in a timely manner.*

Nursing Interventions/*Rationales*
- Assess client's current level of understanding of the factors promoting conception *to identify gaps or misconceptions in knowledge base.*
- Provide information in a supportive manner regarding factors promoting conception, including common factors leading to infertility of either partner *to raise client's awareness and promote trust in caregiver.*
- Identify and describe the basic infertility tests and the rationale for precise scheduling *to enhance completion of the diagnostic phase of the infertility workup.*

NURSING DIAGNOSIS Ineffective coping related to inability to conceive as evidenced by client and partner statements

Expected Outcome *Client and partner will identify situational stressors and positive coping methods to deal with testing and unknown outcomes.*

Nursing Interventions/*Rationales*
- Provide opportunities through therapeutic communication to discuss feelings and concerns *to identify common feelings and perceived stressors.*
- Evaluate couple's support system, including support of each other during this process, *to identify any barriers to effective coping.*
- Identify support groups and refer as needed *to enhance coping by sharing experiences with other couples experiencing similar problems.*

NURSING DIAGNOSIS Hopelessness related to inability to conceive as evidenced by woman's and partner's statements

Expected Outcome *Woman and partner will verbalize a realistic plan to decrease feelings of hopelessness.*

Nursing Interventions/*Rationales*
- Provide support for couple while grieving for loss of fertility *to allow couple to work through feelings.*
- Assess for behaviors indicating possible depression, anger, and frustration *to prevent impending crisis.*
- Refer to support groups *to promote a common bond with other couples during expression of feelings and concerns.*

So much emphasis is placed on being pregnant and having a child composed of one's own genetic makeup that the focus of the reason to have a child becomes cloudy. The question to be answered by couples who want to adopt is, "Do you want to have a baby, or do you want to become parents?"

Salzer (2000) describes five emotional stages that adoptive parents travel through as they make the decision to adopt. These include (1) initial consideration of adoption as an option, (2) forming a decision as a couple, (3) soul searching (questioning personal beliefs, needs, and fears), (4) grieving over the unborn biologic child, and (5) gathering information. These stages do not always happen in a straightforward manner and are not mutually exclusive but are pieces of the path toward parenthood. Nurses should have information on options for adoption available for couples or refer to community resources for further assistance.

Evaluation

Evaluation of the effectiveness of care of the couple with impaired fertility is based on the previously stated outcomes (see Plan of Care).

community activity

What resources are available in your community for couples experiencing infertility for the following:
  a. Assessment and diagnosis
  b. Treatment including ARTS
  How well are these resources publicized in the community? What costs are associated with these resources? What is covered by insurance? Is there a support network and, if so, how do couples gain access?

key points

- Infertility is the inability to conceive and carry a child to term gestation when the couple has chosen to do so.
- Infertility affects between 10% and 15% of otherwise healthy adults. Infertility increases as the woman ages, especially after age 40 years.
- In the United States, about 20% of infertility causes are unexplained; of the 80% that causative factors are known, about 40% is related to female causes, 40% is related to male causes, and 20% is attributable to both male and female causes.
- Common etiologic factors of infertility include decreased sperm production, ovulation disorders, tubal occlusion, and endometriosis.

- The investigation of infertility is conducted systematically and simultaneously for both male and female partners.
- The couple's relationship dynamics, sexuality, and ability to cope with the psychologic and emotional effects caused by diagnostic procedures and treatment of infertility must be considered in the plan of care.
- Most infertility cases are treated with conventional medical and surgical therapies; less than 3% are treated with in vitro fertilization.
- Reproductive alternatives for family building include IVF-ET, GIFT, ZIFT, oocyte donation, embryo donation, TDI, surrogate motherhood, and adoption.

REFERENCES

American Society for Reproductive Medicine (ASRM). (2001). *Patient's fact sheet: Diagnostic testing for male factor infertility.* Accessed www.asrm.org, June 20, 2006.

American Society for Reproductive Medicine (ASRM). (2003). *Patient's fact sheet: Adoption.* Accessed www.asrm.org, June 20, 2006.

American Society for Reproductive Medicine (ASRM). (2006a). *Frequently asked questions about infertility.* Accessed http://www.asrm. org, June 20, 2006.

American Society for Reproductive Medicine (ASRM). (2006b). *Frequently asked questions. The psychological component of infertility.* Accessed http://www.asrm.org, June 20, 2006.

American Society for Reproductive Medicine (ASRM) Ethics Committee. (2004). Informing offspring of their conception by gamete donation. *Fertility and Sterility, 81*(3), 527-531.

Applegarth, L. (2000). Individual counseling and psychotherapy. In L. Burns & S. Covington (Eds.), *Infertility counseling: A comprehensive handbook for clinicians.* New York: Parthenon Publishing Group.

Boivin, J., Appleton, T., Baetens, P., Baron, J., Bitzer, J., Corrigan, E., et al. (2001). Guidelines for counseling in infertility: Outline version. *Human Reproduction, 16*(6), 1301-1304.

Cunningham, F., Leveno, K., Hauth, J., Gilstrap, L., & Wenstrom, K. (2005). *Williams obstetrics* (22nd ed.). New York: McGraw-Hill.

Forbus, S. (2005). Age-related infertility. Tuning in to the ticking clock. *AWHONN Lifelines, 9*(2), 126-132.

Georgia Reproductive Specialists. (2005). *Micromanipulation. Accessed* www.ivf.com, June 20, 2006.

Hahn, S., & Craft-Rosenberg, M. (2002). The disclosure decisions of parents who conceive children using donor eggs. *Journal of Obstetric, Gynecologic, and Neonatal Nursing, 31*(3), 283-293.

Hershberger, P. (2004). Recipients of oocyte donation: An integrative review. *Journal of Obstetric, Gynecologic, and Neonatal Nursing, 33*(5), 610-621.

Hruska, K., Furth, P., Seifer, D., Sharara, F., & Flaws, J. (2000). Environmental factors in infertility. *Clinics in Obstetrics and Gynecology, 43*(4), 821-829.

Isaacs, J. (2005). The patient voice in infertility. *AWHONN Lifelines, 9*(5), 363-364.

Kearnes, W., Pen, R., Graham, J., Han, T., Carter, J., Moyer, M., et al. (2005). Preimplantation genetic diagnosis and screening. *Seminars in Reproductive Medicine, 23*(4), 336-347.

Kunzle, R., Mueller, M., Hanggi, W., Birkhauser, M., Drescher, H., & Bersinger, N. (2003). Semen quality of male smokers and nonsmokers in infertile couples. *Fertility and Sterility, 79*(2 Pt 1), 675-676.

Leibowitz, D., & Hoffman, J. (2000). Fertility drug therapies: Past, present, and future. *Journal of Obstetric, Gynecologic, and Neonatal Nursing, 29*(2), 201-210.

Muthusami, K., & Chinnaswamy, P. (2005). Effect of chronic alcoholism on male fertility hormones and semen quality. *Fertility and Sterility, 84*(4), 919-924.

Nagler, H., & Rotman, M. (2002). Predictive parameters for microsurgical reconstruction. *The Urology Clinics of North America, 29*(4), 913-919, ix.

Nelson, A., Marshall, J., Trussell, J., Stewart, F., Nelson, S., Cates, W., Guest, F., et al. (2004). Impaired fertility. In R. Hatcher et al. (Eds.), *Contraceptive technology* (18th ed.). New York: Ardent Media.

Newton, C. (2000). Counseling the infertile couple. In H. Burns & S. Covington (Eds.), *Infertility counseling: A comprehensive handbook for clinicians.* New York: Parthenon Publishing Group.

RESOLVE. (2006). *Demystifying infertility.* Accessed www.resolve.org, June 20, 2006.

Salzer, L. (2000). Adoption after infertility. In H. Burns & S. Covington (Eds.), *Infertility counseling: A comprehensive handbook for clinicians.* New York: Parthenon Publishing Group.

Sampey, A., Bourque, J., & Wren, K. (2004). Learning scope: Herbal medicines. *Advance for Nurses, 6*(25), 13-19.

Sherrod, R. (2004). Understanding the emotional aspects of infertility: Implications for nursing practice. *Journal of Psychosocial Nursing and Mental Health Services, 42*(3), 40-49.

Sheweita, S., Tilmisany, A., & Al-Sawaf, H. (2005). Mechanisms of male infertility: Role of antioxidants. *Current Drug Metabolism, 6*(5), 495-501.

Stenchever, M., Droegemueller, W., Herbst, A., & Mishell, D. (2001). *Comprehensive gynecology* (4th ed.). St. Louis: Mosby.

Thomas, K., Coughlin, L., Mannion, P., & Haddad, N. (2000). The value of *Chlamydia trachomatis* antibody testing as part of routine infertility investigations. *Human Reproduction, 15*(5), 1079-1082.

Tiran, D., & Mack, S. (2000). *Complementary therapies for pregnancy and childbirth.* Edinburgh: Baillière Tindall.

U.S. Food and Drug Administration. (2004). *Eligibility determination for donors of human cells, tissues, and other cellular and tissue-based products.* Accessed www.fda.gov/cber/rules/suitdonor.pdf, March 31, 2006.

Van Voorhis, B. (2006). Outcomes from assisted reproductive technology. *Obstetrics and Gynecology, 107*(1), 183-200.

Weber, R., Dohle, G., & Romijn, J. (2005). Clinical laboratory evaluation of male subfertility. *Advances in Clinical Chemistry, 40*, 317-364.

Weed, S. (1986). *Wise woman herbal for the childbearing year.* Woodstock, NY: Ash Tree.

Wright, V., Schieve, L., Reynolds, M., Jeng, G., & Kissin, D. (2004). Assisted reproductive technology surveillance–United States, 2000. *MMWR Morbidity and Mortality Weekly Report Surveillance Summary, 53*(1), 1-20.

Zahalsky, M., & Nagler, H. (2001). Ultrasound and infertility: Diagnostic and therapeutic uses. *Current Urology Report, 2*(6), 437-442.

Angela Sammarco

Problems of the Breast

learning objectives

- Discuss the pathophysiology of selected benign and malignant breast disorders found in women.
- Explain the emotional effect of benign and malignant neoplasms.
- Design a nursing plan of care for the woman with a breast disorder.

- Evaluate treatment alternatives for women with breast cancer.
- Integrate critical elements for teaching clients who have undergone medical-surgical management of benign or malignant neoplasms of the breast.

electronic resources

Additional information related to the content in Chapter 11 can be found on

the companion website at **evolve**
http://evolve.elsevier.com/Lowdermilk/MWHC/
- NCLEX Review Questions
- Case Study: Breast Cancer
- WebLinks

or on the interactive companion CD
- NCLEX Review Questions
- Case Study: Breast Cancer
- Plan of Care: The Woman After Breast Conserving Surgery and Axillary Node Dissection

APPROXIMATELY 50% of women have a breast problem at some point in their adult lives. The most common sign of a breast problem is a palpable mass. Most of these lumps are benign, although finding them may produce anxiety for the woman, who may fear she has cancer. Cancer of the breast is the most frequently diagnosed cancer in women in the United States (American Cancer Society [ACS], 2006). The development of breast cancer can have a far-reaching impact on the woman and her family. Beyond the obvious physiologic alterations, the woman also may experience threats to her self-concept and her ability to cope. The condition and its treatments can affect a woman's concept of herself as a sexual being. A woman's family is also challenged in the way it responds to her diagnosis. When breast cancer occurs during or after pregnancy, it adds to the complexity of both physical and emotional responses to childbearing.

Nurses have important roles in teaching women about early detection and treatment and in providing supportive care to clients and their families. This chapter presents information that will assist the nurse in providing care for women with benign breast conditions or breast cancer. Nursing care concepts related to early detection, treatment methods, and education are included. The ongoing investigations of new drug therapies to prevent breast cancer are also introduced.

■ BENIGN CONDITIONS OF THE BREAST

Fibrocystic Changes

The most common benign breast problem is fibrocystic change, found in varying degrees in healthy women's breasts. Fibrocystic changes are palpable thickenings in the breast usually associated with pain and tenderness. The pain and tenderness fluctuate with the menstrual cycle and can become progressively worse until menopause (Miers, 2001).

Except for proliferative change or atypia, which confers an increased risk of breast cancer, the histologic findings associated with fibrocystic changes are considered part of the spectrum of normal involutional patterns of the breast and, thus, a "nondisease" (Smith, Pruthi, & Fitzpatrick, 2004).

Etiology

Fibrocystic changes tend to appear most commonly in women in their second and third decades of life. No known etiologic agent is responsible for benign breast disease, although an imbalance of estrogen and progesterone may be responsible. One theory is that estrogen excess and progesterone deficiency in the luteal phase of the menstrual cycle may cause changes in breast tissue. Risk factors associated with benign breast disease include nulliparity, low parity, late menopause, and estrogen therapy (Smith et al., 2004).

Clinical Manifestations and Diagnosis

The usual clinical presentation of fibrocystic change is lumpiness in both breasts; however, single simple cysts also may occur. Symptoms usually develop about a week before menstruation begins and subside about a week after menstruation ends. They include dull, heavy pain and a sense of fullness and tenderness that increases in the premenstrual period. The woman with fibrocystic change may form cysts that manifest as painful enlarging lumps in her breasts. Cysts are common in premenopausal women who are not receiving estrogen therapy. The cysts are soft on palpation, well differentiated, and movable. Deeper cysts, especially aggregations of cysts, are indistinguishable by palpation from carcinomas, which are malignant growths that infiltrate surrounding tissue.

A first step in the workup of a breast lump is ultrasonography to determine if it is fluid-filled or solid. Fluid-filled cysts are aspirated, and the woman is monitored on a routine basis for development of other cysts. If the lump is solid and the woman is older than 35 years, mammography is obtained. A fine-needle aspiration (FNA) is performed, regardless of the woman's age, to determine the nature of the lump. In some cases, a core biopsy may be needed after FNA to harvest adequate amounts of tissue for pathologic examination (Lucas & Cone, 2003).

Therapeutic Management

Treatment for fibrocystic changes is usually conservative, traditionally including diuretic administration and restriction of salt and fluid. Vitamin E supplements also have been recommended, although megadose therapy should be avoided. Even though no research support has been found, some advocate eliminating dimethylxanthines, such as caffeine. Some symptom relief may be achieved by avoiding smoking and the consumption of alcohol. Recommended pain-relief measures include taking analgesics or nonsteroidal antiinflammatory drugs (NSAIDs) such as ibuprofen, wearing a supportive bra, and applying heat to the breasts. Danazol may be prescribed to relieve breast pain and tenderness. Some women report relief while taking oral contraceptives, but others report worsening of symptoms (Smith et al., 2004). It is important to stress that women may need to try several approaches for a number of months before improvement is noted.

Surgical removal of nodules is attempted only in selected cases. In the presence of multiple nodules, the surgical approach involves multiple incisions and tissue manipulation and may not prevent the development of more nodules.

Fibroadenomas

The next most common benign condition of the breast is a fibroadenoma. Fibroadenomas occur in women from puberty through menopause. Masses are solid, encapsulated, nontender, and most often found in the upper, outer quadrant of the breast (Pruthi, 2001).

The cause of fibroadenomas is unknown. Fibroadenomas are characterized by discrete, usually solitary lumps less than 3 cm in diameter. Occasionally the woman with a fibroadenoma will have tenderness in the tumor during the menstrual cycle. Fibroadenomas increase in size during pregnancy and shrink as the woman ages. Fibroadenomas do not increase in size in response to the menstrual cycle (in contrast to fibrocystic cysts). The mass tends to remain the same size or increase in size slowly over time (Pruthi, 2001).

Diagnosis is made by a review of the client history and physical examination. Mammography, ultrasonography, or magnetic resonance imaging (MRI) may be used to determine the type of lesion, and FNA may be used to determine the underlying disorder. Surgical excision may be necessary if the lump is suspicious or if the symptoms are severe. Fibroadenomas do not respond to either dietary changes or hormonal therapy. Periodic observation of masses by professional physical examination or mammography may be all that is necessary for those masses not requiring surgical intervention (Osuch, 2002).

Lipomas

A lipoma is a soft tumor composed of fat and has discrete borders. The cause of lipomas is unknown. Lipomas are often found in women older than 45 years. They are usually located on the chest wall and breast. The physical characteristics of lipomas are noted as being palpable soft masses that are mobile and nontender. Diagnosis of lipomas is achieved via mammography. Biopsy usually is not required; however, lipomas can be surgically excised if removal is desired.

Nipple Discharge

Nipple discharge is a common occurrence that concerns many women. While most nipple discharge is physiologic, each woman who presents with this problem must be evaluated carefully, because in a small percentage of women, nipple discharge may be related to a serious endocrine disorder or malignancy. Bilateral serous discharge expressed during nipple stimulation can be considered a normal finding (Osuch, 2002). Client education and reassurance are indicated.

Galactorrhea is another form of nipple discharge that is unrelated to malignancy. Galactorrhea manifests as a bilaterally spontaneous, milky, sticky discharge. It is a normal finding in pregnancy. Galactorrhea also may occur as the result of elevated prolactin levels. Increased prolactin levels may be a result of a thyroid disorder, pituitary tumor, coitus, eating, stress, trauma, or chest wall surgery. Certain medications may precipitate galactorrhea, and thus it is essential to have a complete medication history on each woman (Osuch, 2002). Oral contraceptives and neuroleptic drugs are known to cause galactorrhea in some instances (Leung & Pacund, 2004). See Box 11-1 for other classes of drugs that may be associated with galactorrhea.

The optimal time to draw blood to assess a prolactin level is between 8 and 10 AM. Ideally, prolactin levels should not be drawn directly after a breast examination, sexual activity, or exercise session. Other diagnostic tests that may be indicated include a microscopic analysis of the discharge from each breast, a thyroid profile, a pregnancy test, and a mammogram.

Mammary Duct Ectasia

Mammary duct ectasia is an inflammation of the ducts behind the nipple. The cause of mammary duct ectasia is unknown, although chronic inflammation and dilation of the lactiferous ducts has been suggested. This condition occurs most often in perimenopausal women and is characterized by a thick, sticky nipple discharge that is white, brown, green, or purple in color. Frequently the woman will experience a burning pain, itching, or a palpable mass behind the nipple.

box 11-1 Drugs Associated with Galactorrhea

- Estrogens, including oral contraceptives
- Phenothiazines
- Cimetidine
- Methyldopa
- Opiates
- Antiemetics
- Long-term use of alcohol
- Marijuana

The diagnostic workup consists of a mammogram, aspiration of fluid, and culture of fluid. Duct ectasia is usually self-limiting, requiring only reassurance of the woman. An infection in the inflamed area can occur and requires antibiotic therapy. If an abscess develops, an incision and drainage may be necessary. Treatment may also include a local excision of the affected duct or ducts if the woman has no future plans to breastfeed.

Intraductal Papilloma

Intraductal papilloma is a rare, benign condition that develops in the terminal nipple ducts. The cause is unknown. It usually occurs in women between ages 30 and 50 years. Papillomas are usually too small to be palpated (less than 0.5 cm), and present with the characteristic sign of serous, serosanguineous, or bloody nipple discharge. The discharge is unilateral and spontaneous (Osuch, 2002). After the possibility of malignancy is eliminated, treatment for papillomas includes excision of the affected segments of the ducts and breasts. Table 11-1 compares common manifestations of benign breast masses.

Macromastia and Micromastia

Macromastia, or breast hyperplasia, is a condition in which the woman has very large breasts. The size and weight of the breasts can cause chronic pain in the breast, back, neck, and shoulders, as well as significant disruption in psychosocial functioning and body image. Macromastia also can cause thoracic kyphosis, headache, paresthesia of the upper extremities, and shoulder grooving from brassiere straps. Macromastia is treated by reduction mammoplasty, in which the plastic surgeon removes breast tissue to reduce the size and weight of the breasts. Women who have had breast reduction surgery have significant improvement of preoperative signs and symptoms and their quality of life (Smith & Kent, 2002). However, risks associated with the surgery include the potential to affect the woman's ability to breastfeed an infant in the future, infection, decreased nipple sensation, and scarring (Grassley, 2002). Breast reduction surgery is considered reconstructive surgery when done to relieve symptoms of macromastia and may be

table 11-1 Comparison of Common Manifestations of Benign Breast Masses

FIBROCYSTIC CHANGES	FIBROADENOMA	LIPOMA	INTRADUCTAL PAPILLOMA	MAMMARY DUCT ECTASIA
Multiple lumps	Single lump	Single lump	Single or multiple	Mass behind nipple
Nodular	Well delineated	Well delineated	Not well delineated	Not well delineated
Palpable	Palpable	Palpable	Nonpalpable	Palpable
Movable	Movable	Movable	Nonmobile	Nonmobile
Round, smooth	Round, lobular	Round, lobular	Small, ball-like	Irregular
Firm or soft	Firm	Soft	Firm or soft	Firm
Tenderness influenced by menstrual cycle	Usually asymptomatic	Nontender	Usually nontender	Painful, burning, itching
Bilateral	Unilateral	Unilateral	Unilateral	Unilateral
May or may not have nipple discharge	No nipple discharge	No nipple discharge	Serous or bloody nipple discharge	Thick, sticky nipple discharge

covered by health insurance policies. Women considering reduction mammoplasty should review their health insurance policies to determine exact coverage (Grassley).

Although it is not a breast disorder, micromastia, or having very small breasts, may negatively influence a woman's body image. Augmentation mammoplasty may be done to increase the size of the breasts. The plastic surgeon inserts implants filled with normal saline between the breast tissue and the chest wall. Silicone gel–filled implants are not available for breast augmentation done for cosmetic reasons (Smith & Kent, 2002) (see later discussion on breast reconstruction). Breast augmentation surgery is considered cosmetic surgery and is usually not covered by health insurance policies. Breast implants do not last; most must be replaced in 10 to 15 years or sooner. About 25% of women who have breast implants will have them removed within 3 years of insertion because of complications (Zuckerman, 2002).

Collaborative Care

Assessment should include a careful client history and physical examination. The history should focus on risk factors for breast diseases, events related to the breast mass, and health maintenance practices. Risk factors for breast cancer are discussed later in this chapter. Information related to the breast mass should include how, when, and by whom the mass was discovered. The interval between discovery and seeking care is crucial. Answers to these questions can give clues about breast self-examination (BSE) practice and access to care. The nurse should document the following client information: presence of pain, whether symptoms increase with menses, dietary habits, smoking habits, use of oral contraceptives, regularity of BSE, and the examination technique used. The woman's emotional status, including her stress level, fears, and concerns, and her ability to cope also should be assessed.

Physical examination may include assessment of the breasts for symmetry, masses (size, number, consistency, mobility), and nipple discharge.

Nursing actions might include the following:
- Demonstrate correct BSE technique (see Chapter 5, p. 94).
- Discuss the intervals for and facets of breast screening, including professional examination and mammography (see Table 11-3). Women with breast implants may need special views of the breast, and precautions might have to be taken not to rupture the implant during mammography.
- Provide written educational materials.
- Encourage the verbalization of fears and concerns about treatment and prognosis.
- Provide specific information regarding the woman's condition and treatment, including dietary changes, drug therapy, comfort measures, stress management, and surgery.
- Describe pain-relieving strategies in detail, and collaborate with the primary health care provider to ensure effective pain control.

- Encourage discussion of feelings about body image.
- Refer to a support group or stress management resource if needed to cope with long-term consequences of benign breast conditions.

■ MALIGNANT CONDITIONS OF THE BREAST

The United States has one of the highest rates of breast carcinoma in the world. In one in eight American women, breast cancer will develop in her lifetime. Statistics released from the American Cancer Society (ACS, 2005) indicate that breast cancer incidence increased about 4% per year between 1980 and 1997 and about 0.3% from 1987 to 2002. The continued incidence may be related to better detection of early-stage breast cancer, obesity, and postmenopausal hormonal therapy (ACS). The incidence of breast cancer is higher in Caucasian women than in African-American women, but the mortality rate for African-American women with breast cancer is higher. More African-American women are initially diagnosed with a later stage of breast cancer (Figs. 11-1 and 11-2) (ACS).

Incidence and Etiologies

Although the exact cause of breast cancer continues to elude investigators, certain factors that increase a woman's risk for developing a malignancy have been identified. These factors are listed in Box 11-2.

Evolve/CD Case Study: Breast Cancer

box 11-2 Risk Factors for Breast Cancer*

- Age (risk increases with age)
- Family history of breast cancer, especially a mother or sister (particularly significant if premenopausal)
- Personal history of breast cancer
- Inherited genetic mutations for BRCA1 and BRCA2
- Previous history of benign breast disease with epithelial hyperplasia
- High breast tissue density
- High-dose radiation to the chest
- Previous history of ovarian, endometrial, colon, or thyroid cancer
- Early menarche (before age 12)
- Late menopause (after age 55)
- Nulliparity or first pregnancy after age 30
- Race (Caucasian women have highest incidence)
- High socioeconomic status
- Sedentary lifestyle
- Use of hormone replacement therapy
- Obesity after menopause
- Drinking more than one alcoholic beverage a day
- Never breastfed a child
- Recent use of oral contraceptives

Sources: American Cancer Society (ACS). (2005). *Breast cancer facts and figures 2005-2006.* Atlanta: Author; American Cancer Society (ACS). (2006). *Cancer facts and figures 2006.* Atlanta: Author.
*Risk factors are cumulative—the more risk factors present, the greater the likelihood of breast cancer occurring.

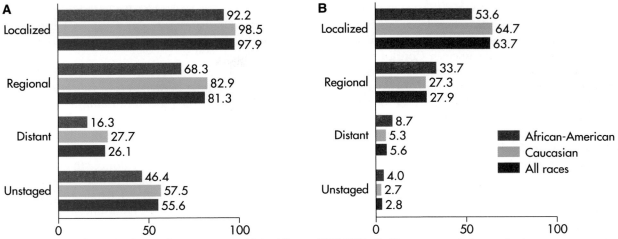

FIG. 11-1 Female breast cancer—United States, 1995-2001. **A,** Five-year survival rates by stage at diagnosis and race (%). **B,** Percentage diagnosed by stage and race. (Courtesy American Cancer Society, Surveillance Research, 2005.)

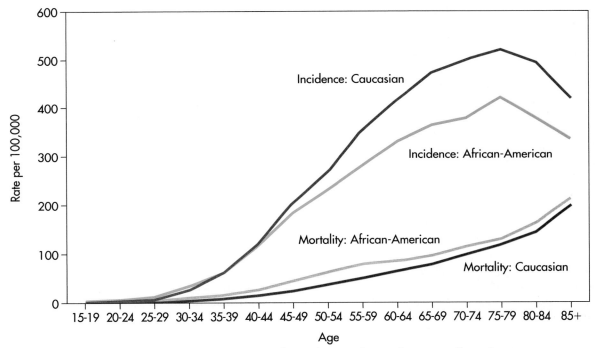

FIG. 11-2 Female breast cancer age-specific incidence and mortality rates—Caucasian versus African-American women, United States, 1998-2002. (Courtesy American Cancer Society, Surveillance Research, 2005.)

The most important predictor of risk for breast cancer is age. Each woman's risk of breast cancer increases as her age increases. Most of the other risk factors involve the effects of the menstrual-reproductive cycle (probably the effect of estrogen or progesterone) on the development of breast cancer. Fewer menstrual cycles and early childbearing appear to have produced a lower risk (Sakorafas, 2003).

Although most breast cancers are not related to genetic factors, the identification of the BRCA1 and BRCA2 genes demonstrated the role of heredity and genetic mutations in this disease. Only about 5% to 10% of breast cancers are

due to a specific, inherited mutation that confers a high risk of developing breast cancer. The American Society of Clinical Oncology has identified the following as factors that place a woman at high risk for genetically transmitted breast cancer: a family with more than two breast cancer cases and one or more ovarian cancer cases diagnosed at any age; a family with more than three breast cancer cases diagnosed before 50 years of age; and sister pairs that have been diagnosed before age 50 with two breast cancers, or two ovarian cancers, or a breast and ovarian cancer (Sakorafas, 2003).

Ethical Considerations of Genetic Testing

Although knowing whether one is hereditarily predisposed to breast cancer may have benefits, the extent to which an individual can benefit remains unclear. Confirming one's mutation status may provide a sense of control in life plans, yet may alternatively create high levels of anxiety and distress. Genetic testing can alter decisions regarding family and intimate relationships, childbearing, body image, and quality of life. Regardless of whether results are positive or negative in testing for BRCA1 and BRCA2 mutations, they can have a highly negative impact on women's lives. Genetic counseling may not be an adequate measure for relieving the ensuing psychologic distress. Women at increased risk for breast cancer need comprehensive information about the benefits and limitations of genetic testing, in addition to alternatives, to ensure that informed decisions can be made about genetic testing. Nurses and other health care professionals should tailor care to women who have undergone genetic testing for hereditary breast cancer or those who plan to undergo testing, and they should impart current information related to these women's specific emotional and medical needs. Since decisions regarding genetic testing, genetic counseling, and breast cancer risk assessment are highly individualized, health care professionals should be careful regarding any generalizations about women at risk for breast cancer (Hutson, 2003).

Research has been ongoing to identify possible environmental factors that may represent significant risk for developing breast cancer. Some known and suspected environmental risk factors include exposure to organochlorine pesticides and other synthetic chemicals, hormonal factors (both exogenous and endogenous), diet, tobacco and alcohol use, and magnetic fields; however, definitive links between these factors and development of breast cancer have not been established (Calle, Frumkin, Henley, Savitz, & Thun, 2002; Hindle, 2002a). Prolonged exposure to radiation has been associated with increased breast cancer risk (McReady, 2003).

A comprehensive review of the research discussion about possible links between breast cancer and hormonal therapy revealed such a confounding range of variables that it has been impossible to draw definitive conclusions about hormonal replacement therapy and the risk of breast cancer. Observational data suggest that long-term use of estrogen replacement therapy (longer than 10 years) may slightly increase the risk, but the risk decreases after discontinuing use (Marsden, 2002). Clinical outcomes of the Women's Health Initiative randomized controlled trial to assess the risks and benefits of estrogen and progestin in healthy postmenopausal women were released in May 2002. The safety monitoring board recommended the trial be stopped because the overall health risks exceeded the benefits. These risks included 290 cases of breast cancer in the study group of about 8500 women (Writing Group for the Women's Health Initiative Investigators, 2002). Further evidence supports that combined estrogen and progestin increased the risk of breast cancer more than estrogen alone among healthy users (Peterson, Thacker, Corso, Marchbanks, & Koplan, 2004). Women considering hormonal replacement therapy should be cautious and consult with their health care providers to determine their suitability for hormonal therapy.

Information about breast cancer risks can be confusing, and women can overestimate or underestimate their risks. The Breast Cancer Risk Assessment Tool can be used by women and health professionals to calculate risk. This tool was developed and verified by the National Cancer Institute (NCI) to predict the risk of breast cancer in 5 years and over the lifetime (to age 90 years) of a woman. The risk factors used are listed in Box 11-3. The tool is available at the website **www.nci.nih.gov**.

An accurate estimation of risk for breast cancer is needed in order that women may be given rational management recommendations. During breast cancer risk counseling, facts should be presented to women by their physicians in a supportive, nondirective way, without personal opinions or preferences. Discussion should also include treatment options and prognosis of breast cancer, as well as risks and benefits of alternative methods of prevention and early diagnosis. A woman's recognition of having increased

---

CRITICAL THINKING EXERCISE

Breast Cancer Treatment Options

Carolyn is a 39-year-old woman with stage I breast cancer. She is divorced, has three school-age children, and is employed full-time as an administrative office assistant. She states that she does not want to have a mastectomy but thinks she should because she has heard that is the best treatment for long-term survival. How would you respond to this statement?

1. Evidence: Is there sufficient evidence to draw conclusions about what the nurse should say?
2. Assumptions: What assumptions can be made about the following issues?
   a. Differences between breast-conserving surgery and mastectomy for stage I cancer
   b. Adjuvant therapy with tamoxifen
   c. Psychosocial and socioeconomic needs of single parent facing breast cancer treatment
3. What implications and priorities for nursing care can be made at this time?
4. Does the evidence objectively support your conclusion?
5. Are there alternative perspectives to your conclusion?

---

box 11-3 **Risk Factors Included in the Breast Cancer Risk Assessment Tool**

- Woman's age
- Number of first-degree relatives affected
- Age of woman at menarche
- Age of woman at first live birth
- Number of breast biopsies
- History of abnormal hyperplasia in biopsy specimens

breast cancer risk can carry psychologic consequences such as anxiety, guilt, depression, and reduced self-esteem. Enormous guilt may be experienced by high risk women who pass specific genetic mutations on to their children. Psychologic intervention should be considered to assist these individuals in coping with these significant adverse sequelae (Sakorafas, 2003).

Chemoprevention

Ongoing studies by the NCI and other groups are investigating the role of tamoxifen, raloxifene, and anastrazole in the prevention of breast cancer (NCI, 2006; Vogel, Costantino, Wickerham, Cronin, & Wolmark, 2002). Raloxifene, in postmenopausal women, prevents osteoporosis without the possible increased cancer risks of estrogen therapy. This medication may be an ideal choice for the woman at high risk for both osteoporosis and breast cancer. Tamoxifen has already been shown to reduce the recurrence of breast cancer in women with prior breast malignancies. The current prevention studies are attempting to identify which women would most benefit from administration of these chemopreventive drugs. Although many women may want to start chemopreventive drugs for breast cancer prevention, the risk of occasional serious side effects demands careful consideration before prescribing these drugs (Kissinger, Harris, Woolf, Sox, & Lohr, 2002; Sakorafas, 2003) (see later discussion).

Pathophysiology

Breast cancer occurs when there are genetic alterations in the deoxyribonucleic acid (DNA) of breast epithelial cells. Many types of breast cancer exist. Genetic alterations, either inherited or spontaneous, are found in the epithelial cells, compromising ductal or lobular tissue. Researchers are investigating which oncogenes (potentially cancer-inducing genes) may cause breast cancer or change its growth pattern and how the process can be stopped.

Breast cancer begins in the epithelial cells lining the mammary ducts of the breast. The rate of breast cancer growth depends on the effect of estrogen and progesterone. These cancers can be either invasive (infiltrating) or noninvasive (in situ). Invasive or infiltrating breast cancers can grow into the wall of the mammary duct and into the surrounding tissues. By far the most frequently occurring cancer of the breast is invasive ductal carcinoma. Ductal carcinoma originates in the lactiferous ducts and invades surrounding breast structures. The tumor is usually unilateral, not well delineated, solid, nonmobile, and nontender. Lobular carcinoma originates in the lobules of the breasts. It is usually bilateral and nonpalpable. Nipple carcinoma *(Paget's disease)* originates in the nipple. It usually occurs with invasive ductal carcinoma and can cause bleeding, oozing, and crusting of the nipple.

Breast cancer can invade surrounding tissues in such a way that the primary tumor can have tentacle-like projections. This invasive growth pattern can result in the irregular tumor border felt on palpation. As the tumor grows, fibrosis develops around it and can shorten Cooper's ligaments. When Cooper's ligaments are shortened, the result is the characteristic peau d'orange (orange peel-like skin) changes and edema associated with some breast cancers. If the breast cancer invades the lymphatic channels, tumors can develop in the regional lymph nodes, often occupying the axillary lymph nodes. The tumor may invade the outer layers of skin, creating ulcerations.

Metastasis results from seeding of the breast cancer cells into the blood and lymph systems, leading to tumor development in the bones, the lungs, the brain, and the liver (Table 11-2).

Clinical Manifestations and Diagnosis

Breast cancer in its earliest form can be detected on a mammogram before it can be felt by the woman or her health care provider. It is estimated, however, that 90% of all breast lumps are detected by the woman. Of this 90%, only 20% to 25% are malignant. More than half of all lumps are discovered in the upper, outer quadrant of the breast (Fig. 11-3). The most common initial symptom is a

table 11-2 Staging for Breast Cancer*

STAGE	DEFINITION
Stage 0	Carcinoma in situ (Tis-N0-M0)
Stage I	Tumor <2 cm with negative nodes (T1-N0-M0) (includes microinvasive T1, <0.1 cm)
Stage IIA	Tumor 0 to 2 cm with positive nodes (including micrometastasis N1, or <0.2 cm), or 2 to 5 cm with negative nodes (T0-N1, T1-N1, T2-N0, all M0)
Stage IIB	Tumor 2 to 5 cm with positive nodes or >5 cm with negative nodes (T2-N1, T3-N0, all M0)
Stage IIIA	No evidence of primary tumor or tumor <2 cm with involved fixed lymph nodes, or tumor >5 cm with involved movable or nonmovable nodes (T0-N2, T1-N2, T2-N2, T3-N1, T3-N2, all M0)
Stage IIIB	Tumor of any size with direct extension to chest wall or skin, with or without involved lymph nodes, or any size tumor with involved internal mammary lymph nodes (T4-any N, any T-N3, all M0)
Stage IV	Any distant metastasis (includes ipsilateral supraclavicular nodes) (all M1)

From National Comprehensive Cancer Network (NCCN). (2005). *Breast cancer treatment guidelines for patients* [on-line]. Accessed www.nccn.org, March 4, 2006.
*Breast cancer is most frequently staged according to the *TNM classification system*, which evaluates the tumor size (*T*), involvement of regional lymph nodes (*N*), and distant spread of the disease or metastases (*M*).

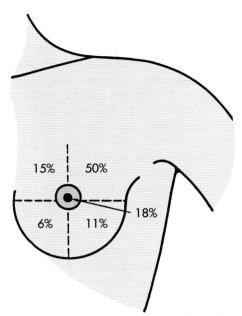

FIG. 11-3 Relative location of malignant lesions of the breast. (Modified from DiSaia, P., & Creasman, W. [2002]. *Clinical gynecologic oncology* [6th ed.]. St. Louis: Mosby.)

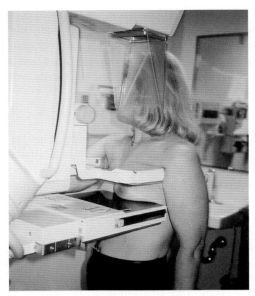

FIG. 11-4 Mammography. (Courtesy Shannon Perry, Phoenix, AZ.)

lump or thickening of the breast. The lump may feel hard and fixed or soft and spongy. It may have well-defined or irregular borders. It may be fixed to the skin, causing dimpling to occur. A bloody or clear nipple discharge also may be present.

Unilateral and spontaneous discharge (without nipple manipulation) is associated with mastitis, intraductal papilloma, and cancer. The discharge is usually intermittent and persistent and may be clear, serous, green-gray, purulent, serosanguineous, or sanguineous. Women with these findings need a complete diagnostic workup to determine the actual cause of their symptoms.

As a general principle, any unilateral breast symptom (i.e., mass, discharge, pain, or itching) is a more ominous finding than a bilateral symptom. However, all findings must be carefully followed up to avoid missing a serious diagnosis such as cancer. Any delay in treatment may adversely affect the woman's subsequent prognosis and treatment options.

Early detection and diagnosis reduce the mortality rate because cancer is found when it is smaller, lesions are more localized, and there tends to be a lower percentage of positive nodes. Therefore it is imperative that protocols for assessment and diagnosis be established. In addition to regular BSE from midadolescence on, the use of clinical examination by a qualified health care provider and screening mammography (x-ray filming of the breast) (Fig. 11-4) may aid in the early detection of breast cancers. Table 11-3 lists the 2006 recommendations of the American Cancer Society (ACS) for breast cancer screening.

Research has suggested that the major obstacles to breast cancer screening include older age; fiscal barriers (e.g., expense, lack of health insurance); knowledge, attitudinal,

table 11-3 Screening Guidelines for Breast Cancer Detection in Asymptomatic Women Recommended by the American Cancer Society

AGE (YR)	EXAMINATION	FREQUENCY
20-39	Breast self-examination (BSE)	Monthly
	Clinical breast examination	Every 3 yr
40 and older	BSE	Monthly
	Clinical breast examination	Yearly
	Mammography	Yearly

Source: American Cancer Society. (2006). *Cancer facts and figures, 2006.* Atlanta: Author.

and behavioral barriers (e.g., fear, ignorance, lack of motivation); and organizational barriers (e.g., scheduling problems, lack of availability of mammography services, lack of physician referral) (Coleman et al., 2003; Partin & Slater, 2003; Yarbrough, 2004). Strategies that may be helpful to health care providers in improving screening for breast cancer include education and encouragement of older women, continuing education of providers, provision of information about new, affordable screening options, use of reminder systems in office practice, use of client-directed literature, and interventions that will reward, support, and prompt desired screening behaviors (Coleman et al.; Partin & Slater; Yarbrough). In addition, it is important for a practitioner to assess a woman's BSE technique and frequency at the annual visit.

Cultural factors may influence a woman's decision to participate in breast cancer screening. Knowledge of these factors and use of culturally sensitive, tailored messages and materials that appeal to the unique concerns, beliefs, and reading abilities of target groups of underutilizers may assist the nurse in helping women overcome barriers to seeking care (see Cultural Considerations box).

cultural considerations

Breast Screening Practices

Certain minority women tend to have low compliance rates in the use of early screening methods for breast cancer. Many factors play a role in influencing the screening practices of these women. African-American women reported not participating in early breast cancer screening because of discomfort with impersonal care from providers, lack of health care insurance, lack of funds to pay for mammograms, lack of awareness of community assistance within the health care system, lack of access to transportation, and feelings of fatalism, fear, helplessness, and powerlessness. Hispanic women cited lack of a regular physician, lack of health insurance coverage, inaccessibility of screening facilities, lack of access to transportation, and being unable to obtain time off from work. Asian women cited unawareness of mammography tests, gender and modesty concerns unique to their cultural beliefs, and fear resulting from a sense of vulnerability to breast cancer.

Interventions that will encourage minority women to participate in early breast cancer screening practices begin with the development of culturally sensitive community education programs designed to help women overcome barriers to reaching optimal levels of health. Programs should be designed to educate small groups of woman about risk factors of breast cancer, prevention strategies, and early detection methods. Recruitment of women may be communicated through fliers in neighborhoods, women's groups, churches, clubs, and organizations. Use of incentives to reward participation may be helpful. Nurses and guest speakers of similar ethnicity as the attending group who are breast cancer survivors would be valuable in providing meaningful information and support, and providing past, present, and future perspective to the educational content.

Source: Kelley, M., & Comley, A. (2001). Breast cancer among minority women: Current knowledge and efforts in early detection programs. *American Journal of Nursing, 101*(Suppl), 13-15.

Screen-film mammography is thought of as the gold standard for breast cancer screening. New technologies that are considered for breast cancer screening must equal or exceed the performance of screen-film mammography to be accepted as screening tools for breast cancer. In other words, new technologies must demonstrate identification of more breast cancers that are missed by screen-film mammography, such as a higher fraction of early-stage cancers (stages 0 and 1), and be cost-effective, noninvasive, and available and acceptable to clients. One recently improved technology for breast cancer screening is full-field digital mammography. In addition, computer-aided detection and diagnosis (CAD) has been developed to aid radiologists in detecting suspicious breast lesions. This method digitizes screen-film mammograms and analyzes them for abnormalities. The overall detection rate using CAD has increased from 3.2 to 3.8 cancers per 1000 women screened (Smith, Cokkinides, Eyre, & ACS, 2003).

Ultrasound has become a valuable screening adjunct to mammography, especially for women with significant breast density. It is cost-effective, noninvasive, and widely available. Ultrasound has been helpful in distinguishing between fluid-filled masses and solid masses, and also between benign and malignant masses. It has also been useful in performing image-guided biopsies (Smith et al., 2003).

MRI of the breast has also become a valuable screening adjunct to mammography and ultrasound. MRI of the breast has shown an overall sensitivity to breast cancer of 96%. However, factors such as cost, lack of standardized exam technique and interpretation criteria, insensitivity to microcalcifications, and higher rate of false-positive results than mammography have caused concern regarding the potential of breast MRI as a screening method (Smith et al., 2003).

When a suspicious finding on a mammogram is noted or a lump is detected, diagnosis is confirmed by FNA, core needle biopsy, or needle localization biopsy (Fig. 11-5). The latter procedure requires the collaborative efforts of both the radiologist and the surgeon. This often requires that the procedure take place in two different environments (radiology and surgery), so clients need specific information regarding procedures, duration, and outcomes.

Cytologic analysis of cells from aspirated breast tissue is extremely useful as an adjunct to the clinical evaluation of a palpable mass. If the mass resolves after aspiration, malignancy is unlikely. However, if the mass remains after aspiration, it should be biopsied, because there is a greater chance of cancer being present (Lucas & Cone, 2003).

Laboratory diagnosis of breast cancer and possible cancer metastasis includes complete blood count, liver enzyme levels, serum calcium level, and alkaline phosphatase level. Elevated liver enzyme levels indicate possible liver metastasis, and increased serum calcium and alkaline phosphatase levels may indicate bone metastasis.

Prognosis

Major advances have been made in the understanding of the biology of cancer. Breast cancer is thought to be a systemic disease, which means that micrometastasis could be present at the initial presentation with or without nodal involvement. The area in which affected lymph nodes are located also is prognostic. The involvement of axillary lymph nodes worsens the prognosis of breast cancer. Nodal involvement and tumor size, however, remain the most significant prognostic criteria for long-term survival (Fig. 11-6).

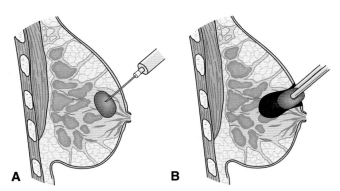

FIG. 11-5 Diagnosis. **A,** Needle aspiration. **B,** Open biopsy.

FIG. 11-6 Lymphatic spread of breast cancer.

Other biologic factors have been shown to be helpful in predicting response to therapy or survival. These biologic factors include estrogen receptor assay, progesterone receptor assay, tumor *ploidy* (the amount of DNA in a tumor cell compared with that in a normal cell), S-phase index or growth rate (the percentage of cells in the S phase of cellular division done by flow cytometric determinations of the S-phase fraction), and histologic or nuclear grade (Crane-Okada, 2001). Estrogen and progesterone receptors are proteins in the cell cytoplasm and surface of some breast cancer cells. When these receptors are present, they bind to estrogen or progesterone, and binding promotes growth of the cancer cell. A breast cancer can have estrogen or progesterone receptors (ERs, PRs) or both types. It is valuable to know the estrogen receptor status of the cancer to predict which clients will respond to hormone therapy (McReady, 2003).

Molecular and biologic factors are valuable indicators for prognosis and treatment of breast cancer. Human epidermal growth factor receptor 2 (HER2), which is associated with cell growth, is overexpressed in 30% of all breast cancers and is associated with loss of cell regulation and uncontrolled cell proliferation. Thus, a positive HER2 status is associated with aggressive tumors, poor prognosis, and resistance to certain chemotherapeutic drugs (McReady, 2003).

Therapeutic Management

Medical management of breast cancer includes surgery, breast reconstruction, radiation therapy, adjuvant hormone therapy, and chemotherapy.

Surgery

After a diagnosis of breast cancer is made, surgical treatment options are offered to the woman. The most frequently recommended surgical approaches for the treatment of breast cancer are lumpectomy and modified radical mastectomy. A lumpectomy (Fig. 11-7) involves the removal of the breast tumor and a small amount of surrounding tissue, leaving the pectoralis major muscle intact. Partial mastectomy (see Fig 11-7, *B*) includes *tylectomy, wide excision,* and *quadrantectomy* or *segmental mastectomy* and involves removal of differing amounts of tissue along with the tumor. Sampling of axillary lymph nodes is usually done through a separate incision at the time of these procedures, and surgery is usually followed by radiation therapy to the remaining breast tissue (Crane-Okada, 2001; DiSaia & Creasman, 2002). These procedures are used for the primary treatment of women with early-stage (I or II) breast cancer. Lumpectomy offers survival equivalent to that with modified radical mastectomy (DiSaia & Creasman).

Axillary dissection is performed as a standard part of breast cancer treatment in order to obtain prognostic information and maintain local control in the axilla, and it is helpful in determining the need for adjunctive systemic treatment by indicating whether nodes are positive for metastatic cells. Lymphatic mapping and sentinel node biopsy is a minimally invasive technique that identifies women with axillary node involvement. The sentinel node is the first node that receives lymphatic drainage from the tumor, and is identified by injecting vital blue dye or radioactive dye in the area surrounding the tumor. A small incision in the axilla allows for identification of the blue-stained lymphatic channel leading to the blue sentinel node, either visually or by gamma probe. This node then can be removed and examined for the presence of tumor cells, as opposed to an entire axillary dissection. Clinical trials have reported identification of the sentinel node in more than 95% of cases, with false-negative rates for predicting axillary nodal metastases of less than 5% (Morrow & Gradishar, 2002).

Total mastectomy (see Fig 11-7, *C*) (also called *simple mastectomy*) is the removal of all breast tissue, the nipple and areola; the axillary nodes and pectoral muscles are not removed. Modified radical mastectomy is the removal of the entire breast and a sample of axillary lymph nodes, sparing the pectoral muscles. A radical mastectomy (see Fig 11-7, *D*), although rarely performed, removes the entire breast, axillary nodes, and the pectoral muscles. Mastectomy is used for the treatment of early-stage breast cancer when the woman fits the criteria listed in Box 11-4. Women

---

box 11-4 **Contraindications for Breast Conserving Treatment**

- Presence of multiple tumors, especially in different parts of the breast
- Tumor removal alone would produce a cosmetically unacceptable result
- Previous breast radiation
- Pregnancy in the first or second trimester
- Persistent positive margins after reasonable surgery
- Possible history of collagen-vascular disease

Sources: DiSaia, P., & Creasman, W. (2002). *Clinical gynecologic oncology* (6th ed.). St. Louis: Mosby; Shuster, T., et al. (2000). Multidisciplinary care for patients with breast cancer. *Surgical Clinics of North America, 80*(2), 505-533.

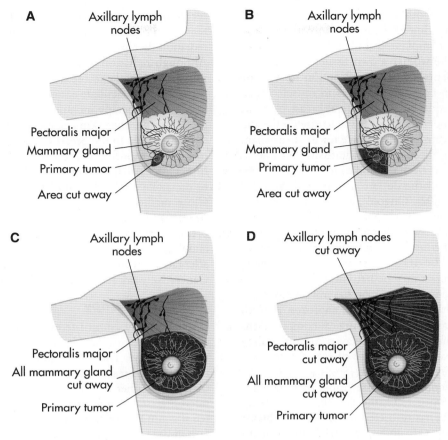

FIG. 11-7 Surgical alternatives for breast cancer. **A,** Lumpectomy. **B,** Partial mastectomy. **C,** Total (simple) mastectomy. **D,** Radical mastectomy.

who are found to have metastatic breast cancer at the time of diagnosis usually do not have a mastectomy because it does not offer increased chances of survival. Women who have these surgeries experience cosmetic changes. Change in shape (because of lumpectomy) or loss of a breast results in a change in body image, which can cause significant alterations in perceptions of femininity and sexual image and interest (Morrow et al., 2002).

Breast Reconstruction. The goals of surgical breast reconstruction are achievement of symmetry and preservation of body image. Surgical reconstruction can be done immediately or at a later date. Immediate reconstruction at the time of mastectomy does not change survival rates or interfere with therapy or the treatment of recurrent disease (Osuch, 2002). It is important that women be aware of this information. Women choosing surgical reconstruction offer the following rationale for reconstructive surgery: the need to feel complete again, to avoid using an external prosthesis, to achieve symmetry, to decrease self-consciousness about appearance, and to enhance femininity (Resnick & Belcher, 2002).

Autologous flap reconstruction involves the use of the woman's own tissue to create a breast. Using the woman's own tissue results in a more natural shape. There are three types of autologous flaps: the latissimus dorsi flap, the transverse rectus abdominis myocutaneous (TRAM) flap,

and the inferior gluteus free flap. The latissimus dorsi and TRAM flaps are the most common. The latissimus flap consists of skin, fat, and muscle separated from the upper back, tunneled subcutaneously to an incision in the chest area, and attached to this area (Sandau, 2002). The TRAM flap consists of a portion of skin and fat harvested from the abdominal wall and used to reconstruct the chest area (Resnick & Belcher, 2002). When these flaps are used for reconstruction, they can be pedicled (attached to its blood supply) or free flaps (cut completely from the donor site); adequate blood supply to the reconstructed tissue is a major concern (Sandau). For this reason, plastic surgeons are careful not to offer this option to women who may be at high risk for complications. Women at high risk for complications include those with extensive, locally invasive breast cancers, extensive chest wall disease, metastatic breast cancer, diabetes mellitus, poorly controlled pulmonary disease, or hypertension. Women who smoke tobacco, are obese, or have had preoperative chemotherapy or radiation therapy also are at high risk for complications (Resnick & Belcher; Sandau). After the reconstruction is done, postoperative care specific to the procedure focuses on monitoring the skin flap for signs of decreased capillary refill, hematoma, infection, and necrosis. Standard mastectomy activity restrictions and client education points also are followed.

Breast Implants. Another method of surgical reconstruction involves creating a breast mound with a saline-filled tissue expander implanted under the muscle or an autologous flap of the woman's own tissue. Breast reconstruction using implants is not a good option for women with inadequate skin coverage, changes in muscle innervation, or a large, pendulous contralateral breast. A tissue expander is placed under the chest tissue to stretch the surrounding tissue to create adequate space for the permanent implant. Through an injection port, the tissue expander is slowly filled with saline, over a period of months, to stretch the skin gradually until the desired symmetry is attained (Resnick & Belcher, 2002). Ongoing emotional support is needed for women who choose this option because they often become impatient waiting for the implant to be totally filled or are self-conscious about the uneven appearance of their breasts. Use of cotton padding to equalize the appearance of the breasts may be helpful during this time. After each saline injection, the woman has mild discomfort, which is easily relieved with ibuprofen or naproxen. As with all implantation procedures, risks of surgical complications such as hematoma, infection, and delayed wound healing are possible, as well as the possibility of capsular contractions from, or leakage of, the implant (Resnick & Belcher).

The safety of silicone gel breast implants continues to be controversial. Since 1992, the U.S. Food and Drug Administration (FDA) has restricted use of silicone breast implants to women who are undergoing reconstruction after mastectomy, who have had severe breast injuries, who have birth defects that affect the breasts, who have a medical condition causing a severe breast abnormality, or who need to replace an existing implant (FDA, 2004). Women interested in these implants should be informed of all the risks before making a decision (Resnick & Belcher, 2002).

After the woman has recovered from initial reconstructive surgery, she may choose to have nipple and areolar reconstruction. Nipple reconstruction is achieved by using an autologous skin graft to construct a nipple, either from tissue from the remaining nipple or from a donor site. Tiny flaps from the new breast itself also may be used. This outpatient procedure requires local anesthesia, intravenous sedation, or a combination of both, depending on how much sensation has returned to the breast. The procedure lasts about an hour and, 4 weeks later, tattooing may be used to create an areola and match the color of the natural nipple (Sandau, 2002).

Radiation

As mentioned, the conservative approach to treatment involves lumpectomy followed by radiation therapy as standard therapy for early-stage breast cancer. Radiation to the breast destroys tumor cells remaining after manipulation and handling of the tumor during surgery. The total recommended radiation dose is 4500 to 5000 cGy over a 6- to 8-week period. A booster dose of up to 1000 cGy may be prescribed with the use of either implants or external beam irradiation (Morrow et al., 2002). The risk of local

recurrence depends on several treatment factors such as extent of breast resection, tumor margins, technical details of radiation therapy, and the use of adjuvant systemic therapy. Although radiation after lumpectomy surgery is standard protocol, some large breast tumors may be irradiated before surgery to facilitate easier surgical removal. Side effects of radiation therapy include swelling and heaviness in the breast, sunburnlike skin changes in the treated area, and fatigue. Changes to the breast tissue and skin usually resolve in 6 to 12 months. The breast may become smaller and firmer after radiation therapy. Radiation therapy in the area of the axilla can cause lymphedema of the ipsilateral arm. Close medical follow-up is important after conservative surgery and radiation. Recommended guidelines include a breast physical examination every 4 to 6 months for 5 years, and then yearly. A mammogram is recommended 6 months after radiation and then annually (National Comprehensive Cancer Network [NCCN], 2005).

Adjuvant Therapy

Chemotherapy administered soon after initial diagnosis and surgical removal of the tumor is referred to as adjuvant chemotherapy. The role of adjuvant chemotherapy in the treatment of breast cancer (chemotherapy and endocrine therapy) is either to eradicate or to impede the growth of micrometastatic (microscopic cell metastasis) disease. Often it is not possible to detect the presence of micrometastasis at the time of initial treatment, and when it is present, mutations can occur in the tumor cells. These mutations make tumor cells resistant to the effects of chemotherapeutic agents despite tumor sensitivity to drug therapy being greatest when the tumor burden is small. Consequently, the prediction cannot be made with confidence that all tumors of 1 cm or less can be cured with initial local and regional treatment. The early introduction of systemic adjuvant therapy, as determined by the estimated risk of tumor recurrence in certain subsets of women with node-negative disease, is a prudent course of treatment. Research findings suggest that adjuvant chemotherapy significantly reduces the risks for recurrence and mortality in women with node-positive disease (Osuch, 2002).

Hormonal Therapy. To determine whether a woman is a candidate for hormonal therapy, a receptor assay is done. After the entire tumor or a portion is removed by biopsy or excision, cancer cells are examined by a pathologist for ERs and PRs.

The presence of a receptor on the cell wall indicates that the woman is positive for that type of hormone receptor. If these receptors are present, the growth of the woman's breast cancer may be influenced by estrogen, progesterone, or both. It is unknown exactly how these hormones affect breast cancer growth. Bilateral oophorectomy has been noted to benefit women diagnosed with their first breast cancer before age 50 years by reducing exposure to endogenous estrogen. Oophorectomy reduces the risk of breast cancer by approximately 50% in BRCA1 carriers (Morrow & Gradishar, 2002). Thus, oophorectomy is an option that helps decrease the odds of recurrence and improve length of survival. In addition to or instead of oophorectomy, medications may be given to stop tumor growth that is influenced by hormones.

Tamoxifen is an oral antiestrogen medication that mimics progesterone and estrogen. Tamoxifen attaches to the hormone receptors on cancer cells and prevents natural hormones from attaching to the receptors. When tamoxifen fits into the receptors, the cell is unable to grow. Research has demonstrated a clear benefit for use of tamoxifen in all age groups (Riggs & Hartmann, 2003). Adjuvant hormonal therapy with tamoxifen is recommended for all postmenopausal women with breast cancer. In this age group, adjuvant tamoxifen therapy improves disease-free survival and, in some cases, length of survival. Use of hormonal therapy for 5 years in premenopausal women with breast cancer significantly reduces recurrence and mortality rates. The NCCN Guidelines recommend adjuvant hormonal therapy be given to women with hormone receptor–positive breast cancer regardless of menopause status, age, or HER2/neu status, with the exception of women with lymph node–negative cancers less than or equal to 0.5 cm, or 0.6 to 1.0 cm in diameter with favorable prognostic features. Women treated with hormonal therapy should receive therapy for at least 5 years (NCCN, 2005). Use beyond 5 years in node-positive women results in a reduction in beneficial effects with an increase in toxicity, although the optimal duration of tamoxifen administration is under investigation (Riggs & Hartmann, 2003). The side effects of hormonal therapy include hot flashes, nausea, vomiting, fluid retention, weight gain, and thrombocytopenia. Tamoxifen therapy also increases the risk of endometrial cancer and deep vein thrombosis (Simpson & Rosenzweig, 2002) (see Medication Guide box).

---

medication guide

Tamoxifen (Nolvadex)

ACTION ▬ Antiestrogenic effects; attaches to hormone receptors on cancer cells and prevents natural hormones from attaching to the receptors.

INDICATION ▬ For treatment of metastatic breast cancer; treatment of breast cancer in postmenopausal women after breast cancer surgery and radiation therapy; to reduce the incidence of breast cancer in women at high risk.

DOSAGE AND ROUTE ▬ 20 to 40 mg orally, daily. Dosages greater than 20 mg should be given in divided doses (AM and PM).

ADVERSE REACTIONS ▬ Common side effects include hot flashes, nausea, vomiting, vaginal bleeding or discharge, menstrual irregularities, and rash. Hair loss is an uncommon effect. Serious side effects include deep vein thrombosis, increased risk of endometrial cancer, and stroke.

NURSING CONSIDERATIONS ▬ The medication may be taken on an empty stomach or with food. Missed doses should be taken as soon as possible, but taking two doses at once is not recommended. A barrier or nonhormonal form of contraception is recommended in premenopausal women because tamoxifen may be harmful to the fetus.

Aromatase inhibitors markedly suppress plasma estrogen levels in postmenopausal women by inhibiting or inactivating aromatase, the enzyme responsible for synthesizing estrogens from androgenic substrates (Smith & Dowsett, 2003). Aromatase inhibitors such as anastrozole, letrozole, and exemestane have shown to be effective agents in hormonal therapy for breast cancer. Clinical trials indicate that letrozole is convincingly better than tamoxifen in treating advanced disease in postmenopausal women, and anastrozole is at least as good. In early-stage breast cancer, adjuvant therapy with anastrozole appears to be superior to adjuvant therapy with tamoxifen in reducing recurrence in postmenopausal women. In preoperative therapy, letrozole appears to be more effective than tamoxifen. The aromatase inhibitors appear to be well tolerated with lower incidence of adverse effects as compared to tamoxifen. The adverse effects of aromatase inhibitors include hot flashes, vaginal dryness, musculoskeletal pain, and headache (Smith & Dowsett).

Chemotherapy. Chemotherapy drugs are most often given in combination regimens, which have been shown to improve or increase the disease-free survival time after therapy. The most common chemotherapy regimens used for adjuvant treatment of node-positive and node-negative tumors are the following:

- CMF (cyclophosphamide, methotrexate, fluorouracil)
- CAF (cyclophosphamide, doxorubicin, fluorouracil)
- AC (doxorubicin, cyclophosphamide)
- A → CMF (doxorubicin followed by CMF)
- AC → T (doxorubicin, cyclophosphamide, followed by a taxane)
- AT (doxorubicin and a taxene) (DiSaia & Creasman, 2002; Osuch, 2002)

Adjuvant chemotherapy has been found to be most useful in premenopausal women who have breast cancer with positive nodes, regardless of hormone receptor status (Osuch, 2002). It is postulated that younger women often have tumors with a higher S-phase fraction and proliferative rate, which makes the tumors more sensitive to chemotherapy. While adjuvant chemotherapy effectively decreases the risks for recurrence and mortality in premenopausal women with node-positive disease, postmenopausal women can also be offered chemotherapy, depending on the cancer size, nodal involvement, and morphologic and biologic factors/markers of the particular cancer (Hindle, 2002b).

Chemotherapy with multiple drug combinations is used in the treatment of recurrent and advanced breast cancer with positive results. First-line single agents for women with locally advanced or metastatic breast cancer include paclitaxel, docetaxel, epirubicin, doxorubicin, pegylated liposomal doxorubicin, capecitabine, vinorelbine, and gemcitabine. Combination regimens and sequential single agents may be used (NCCN, 2005). Capecitabine is an oral chemical precursor of 5-fluorouracil and is given as a treatment for metastatic breast cancer unresponsive to paclitaxel and an anthracycline-containing regimen. It also is given if breast cancers are resistant to paclitaxel and further anthracycline therapy is contraindicated (Wagstaff, Ibbotson, & Goa, 2003). Trastuzumab, another drug used in advanced breast cancer, is a recombinant, humanized monoclonal antibody. Trastuzumab is used for advanced tumors that demonstrate overexpression of HER2/neu (NCCN). These chemotherapeutic agents provide additional treatment options for women with metastatic breast cancer.

Because chemotherapy drugs are designed to kill rapidly reproducing cells, normal body cells that rapidly reproduce (red and white blood cells, gastric mucosa, and hair) also can be affected during treatment. Thus chemotherapy can cause leukopenia, neutropenia, thrombocytopenia, anemia, gastrointestinal side effects (nausea, vomiting, anorexia, mucositis), and partial or full hair loss.

Chemotherapy treatments are usually administered in ambulatory care settings once or twice per month. During the informed consent process, before the treatment is selected, the woman and her family members should be educated about the names of the medications, routes of administration, treatment schedule, timing and ordering of medications, length of time of administration, reimbursed and unreimbursed costs of therapy, potential side effects, management of side effects, possible changes in body image (e.g., full or partial hair loss), recovery time after treatment (necessitating lost work time), and need for a caregiver to transport the woman to treatment and care for her afterward. Depending on the medications used, the treatments may include intravenous, subcutaneous, and oral medications. Often a long-term central venous catheter is inserted when the women will be receiving chemotherapy for an extended period or when she will receive medications that may damage the vein. Presence of a central venous catheter, hair loss, loss of part or all of her breast, menopause, and possible infertility all have the potential to cause a change in body image and increase emotional distress for the woman with breast cancer.

Breast cancer treatment with chemotherapy, hormonal therapy, or a combination of the two often causes changes in reproductive function. The premenopausal woman may experience these changes along with symptoms of menopause and possible infertility. It is not known whether hormonal therapy to ease the effects of menopause is safe for women with breast cancer; therefore it is not recommended. For this reason, the nurse must use other measures to help the client cope with menopause (see Chapter 7). The young woman with breast cancer may become devastated by early and abrupt menopausal symptoms and the possibility of jeopardized reproductive function. The postmenopausal woman must cope with unpleasant side effects from chemotherapy and loss of part or all of her breast, and frequently, with treatment side effects superimposed upon the presence of comorbidities that develop with aging.

Women receiving chemotherapy and their partners must understand that chemotherapy is a *mutagen* and a *teratogen*. Any woman who is of childbearing age and receiving chemotherapy, even though no longer menstruating, must use birth control. Birth control pills are not recommended because they contain hormones that may assist in the growth of cancer. A birth control method must be chosen with the assistance of the gynecologist and the medical oncologist, and it must be used before chemotherapy begins and continue to be used until the medical oncologist and gynecologist believe it is safe to discontinue.

With the advance in monoclonal antibody technology, it is now possible to test for residual disease with a serum tumor marker, *CA 15-3,* if it is secreted by the client's tumor. From 75% to 80% of women with breast cancer secrete this tumor marker. If the level of *CA 15-3* is elevated at the time of diagnosis, circulating levels of *CA 15-3* can be checked periodically through the treatment course to measure response. This technology is used to determine effectiveness of therapy for cancer without the need for second-look diagnostic surgery.

High-Dose Chemotherapy and Transplant. High-dose chemotherapy followed by *autologous bone marrow transplant (ABMT)* or *peripheral blood stem cell transplant (PSCT)* may be offered to women with breast cancer who have a high risk of relapse or metastatic disease (Crane-Okada, 2001). Although initial studies showed a favorable impact on disease-free survival in women who had metastatic disease, definitive analysis of the benefits or limitations of these treatments is not available (Hinterberger-Fischer & Hinterberger, 2001). PSCT may be preferred to ABMT because it seems to have lower morbidity and mortality and may cost less. Clinical trials continue to evaluate the effectiveness of these procedures.

■ CARE MANAGEMENT

■ Assessment and Nursing Diagnoses

The nurse takes a client history of symptoms, including timing of detection of lump, size, changes, location, nipple discharge, and breast symmetry.

In addition to taking a history and palpating the breast lump, a clinician should compare past and present mammographic findings with physical assessment findings. The mass should be described in terms of location (by using the clock-dial method), shape, size, consistency, and fixation to the surrounding tissues. Skin changes, such as dimpling, peau d'orange, increased vascularity, nipple retraction, or ulceration, may indicate advanced disease, so their presence should be recorded. Physical examination includes palpation of the infraclavicular, supraclavicular, and axillary lymph nodes. Pain and soreness in the affected breast and arm should be evaluated. Often a diagram of the breast is drawn, and findings are recorded in the client record. Psychosocial assessment should include not only the client's present emotional state but also the reaction of her family and significant others and history of handling crises. The nurse should determine what the diagnosis of cancer means to the woman and her family.

Nursing diagnoses for women with a diagnosis of breast cancer might include the following:

- *Fear/anxiety related to*
  - diagnosis of breast cancer
  - treatment choices
  - choice of reconstructive procedure
- *Decisional conflict related to*
  - choices of and controversies about treatment options
- *Sexual dysfunction related to*
  - altered body image
  - side effects of therapy
- *Compromised/disabled family coping related to*
  - diagnosis and prognosis
- *Anticipatory grieving related to*
  - loss of breast or diagnosis of advanced cancer
- *Fatigue related to*
  - cancer treatments
- *Acute pain related to*
  - incision or metastatic cancer
- *Impaired skin integrity related to*
  - surgery or radiation
- *Disturbed body image related to*
  - loss of breast
  - hair loss (chemotherapy)

▬ Expected Outcomes of Care

Planning realistic outcomes in collaboration with the woman might include that the woman will do the following:

- Experience a reasonable level of anxiety related to diagnosis that does not interfere with use of healthy coping mechanisms.
- Elicit appropriate support from significant others.
- Choose among alternative treatment options and verbalize satisfaction with the decision-making process.
- Report satisfactory sexual functioning after surgery.
- Demonstrate necessary self-care techniques correctly.
- Accept a change in body image and demonstrate a positive self-concept.

Other expected outcomes include the following:

- The family will adapt to the diagnosis and provide appropriate support through all stages of treatment.
- The woman's skin will remain intact and will heal without complications.
- The woman will continue usual activities as tolerated during treatment.

▬ Plan of Care and Interventions

Nursing actions that will best assist the woman in achieving her expected outcomes are selected, such as the following:

- Provide time to discuss the diagnosis, answer questions, and listen to concerns.

- Encourage ventilation of feelings by the woman and family in a nonjudgmental atmosphere.
- Offer information about support groups or individual therapy for the woman and the family members, including children.

▬ Emotional Support After Diagnosis

When a woman is confronted with a diagnosis of cancer, she faces not only possible major changes in appearance but also the possibility of death. The emotional reaction to the diagnosis of cancer is always intense, and the many disruptions caused by the disease challenge the woman's and family's ability to cope. Disruptions may be caused by costs of treatment, loss of role function, lack of stress-relieving activities, spouse's or child's reaction to the diagnosis, change in body image and sexual function, disability, and pain. The woman may feel despair, fear, and shame. Sexuality issues related to breast cancer include a change in body image, changes in sexual function (such as decreased vaginal lubrication caused by hormonal therapy), and relational distress. Health care providers are responsible for discussing the influence of breast cancer on the woman's life and in assisting the woman and her family in coping effectively with these changes. Nurses need to be especially aware of the individual quality of life needs of their clients and deliver interventions that improve quality of life outcomes within the context of the breast cancer survivor's personal history, life cycle concerns, and psychosocial life stage (National Women's Health Resource Center, 2005; Sammarco, 2003).

Women and their families often undergo a period of distress after the diagnosis of cancer. It is difficult to accept the diagnosis of cancer when the woman may feel and look well. This period is characterized by anguish and shock followed by disbelief and denial. During this time, absorbing information and education can be difficult, and the nurse should be sensitive as to how this may affect decision-making abilities. Flexibility is the key to sensitive nursing care. As the woman and family begin to accept the diagnosis of breast cancer, more and more information can be shared, and care planning with full client participation can take place, including the following:

- Validate and reinforce accurate information processing by the woman and her family.
- Assist in client decision making and arrange for the woman to speak with breast cancer survivors who have chosen a variety of treatment options (Box 11-5).
- Suggest approaches the woman might take to deal with the sexual concerns of her significant other.
- Discuss the application of alternative therapies to alleviate stress and promote healing, such as exercise, guided imagery, meditation, and progressive muscle relaxation.
- Refer the woman to the ACS's Reach to Recovery program.
- Refer the woman to a cancer rehabilitation program, such as ENCORE, a program run by the YWCA.

box 11-5 **Decision-Making Questions to Ask**

1. What kind of breast cancer is it (invasive or noninvasive)?
2. What is the stage of the cancer (i.e., how extensive is the spread)?
3. Did the cancer test positive for hormone (estrogen)? (May be slower growing).
4. What further tests are recommended?
5. What are the treatment options? (Pros and cons of each, including side effects)?
6. If surgery is recommended, what will the scar look like?
7. If a mastectomy is done, can breast reconstruction be done (at the time of surgery or later)?
8. How long will the client be in the hospital? What kind of postoperative care will the client need?
9. How long will treatment last if radiation or chemotherapy is recommended? What effects can the client expect from these treatments?
10. What community resources are available for support?

Source: National Women's Health Resource Center. (1999). Breast health. *National Women's Health Report, 17*(5), 1-11.

The National Comprehensive Cancer Network (NCCN) (www.nccn.org) and the ACS (www.cancer.org) now provide specific, up-to-date recommendations on breast cancer treatments on the Internet. This is an invaluable resource for women to learn about scientifically tested treatment protocols for each stage of breast cancer (ACS, 2006).

After assisting the woman with accepting the diagnosis and obtaining support, consider nursing care in the preoperative, postoperative, and convalescent periods. The discussion that follows is pertinent to the care required by a woman who is having a modified radical mastectomy.

■ *Preoperative Care*

General preoperative teaching and care are given, including expectations regarding physical appearance, pain management, equipment to be used (e.g., intravenous therapy, drains), and emotional support. Some emotional support may be obtained by arranging for a visit from a member of an organization such as Reach for Recovery. The woman is reminded that when she awakens after surgery, her arm on the affected side will feel tight.

■ *Immediate Postoperative Care*

After recovery from anesthesia, the woman is returned to her room. Special precautions must be observed to prevent or to minimize lymphedema of the affected arm.

■ NURSE ALERT

When vital signs are taken, never apply the blood pressure cuff to the affected arm.

The affected arm is elevated with pillows above the level of the right atrium. Blood is not drawn from this arm, and this arm is not used for intravenous therapy. Early arm movement is encouraged. Any increase in the circumference of that arm is reported immediately.

Nursing care of the wound involves observation for signs of hemorrhage (dressing, drainage tubes, and Hemovac or Jackson-Pratt drainage reservoirs are emptied at least every 8 hours and more frequently as needed), shock, and infection. Dressings are reinforced as necessary. The woman is asked to turn (alternating between unaffected side and back), cough (while the nurse or the woman applies support to the chest), and deep breathe every 2 hours. Breath sounds are auscultated every 4 hours. Active range of motion (ROM) exercise of legs is encouraged. Parenteral fluids are given until adequate oral intake is possible. Emotional support is continued.

Care given during the immediate postoperative period is continued as necessary. Most women who undergo lumpectomy have surgery as ambulatory clients and return home a few hours after surgery. Women are discharged 24 to 48 hours after modified radical mastectomy. Because of the short time spent in the hospital, thorough teaching is important. It is best to do as much teaching as possible before surgery if the outcome is known. If this is not possible, discharge teaching should be done with the woman's caregiver present. This is to acknowledge the possibility that emotional stress or recovery from anesthesia may cause the woman to forget some of the discharge instructions. Printed information also should be provided for the woman and family to refer to at home.

Women who have had breast surgery are usually seen by their surgeon within 5 days of surgery. This follow-up visit is important because it allows the physician to assess the outcome of surgical treatment as well as to provide reinforcement of education and emotional support.

Mobility is a key subject to be addressed with women having breast surgery. Early ambulation is encouraged to improve circulation and ventilation and to prevent loss of calcium from bone. The psychologic benefits of early mobility include resumption of self-care and activities of daily living that serve to reinforce the woman's control over her life and help her move from a sick role to the role of breast cancer survivor.

Arm exercises are encouraged at least 4 times daily (Box 11-6). Exercise is increased as tolerated and is stopped at the point of pain. Initially the woman alternately clenches and extends her fingers and then progresses to wrist and elbow exercises, gradually abducting her arm and raising it to and over her head. She is encouraged to exercise by assisting with her care—washing her face, brushing her teeth, and eating with her hand and arm on the affected side. Physical therapy may be prescribed to improve strength and mobility of the affected arm.

BSE of the unaffected breast, bilateral axillae, and remaining breast in women who have had a lumpectomy is another key teaching subject. Written client education materials are available from the American Cancer Society

EVIDENCE-BASED PRACTICE

Complementary and Alternative Medicine with Early-Stage Breast Cancer Therapy

BACKGROUND

- By many accounts, most women with early-stage breast cancer are very likely to supplement their conventional therapy with some form of complementary and alternative medicine (CAM), but less than half discuss this with their oncologist. CAM is defined as therapies not used in mainstream, conventional medicine. Women using CAM therapies tend to be younger, educated, affluent, and better equipped to self-advocate for holistic care. The prevailing beliefs among clients about CAM is that it will work by stimulating the immune system, detoxify, potentiate the anticancer therapy, and alleviate unpleasant cancer symptoms and drug side effects.

OBJECTIVES

- The reviewers envisioned a systematic evaluation of the risks and benefits of the most popular CAM therapies used by women with early-stage breast cancer. Outcomes included cancer prevention, recurrence of cancer, quality of life, and survival rates.

METHODS

Search Strategy

- After a comprehensive review of the literature for each therapy chosen, the authors identified clinical trials, and human and animal cell culture studies, dated 1995 to 2005. The number of subjects and their countries was not reported.

Statistical Analyses

- Similar data were pooled. Reviewers calculated relative risks for dichotomous (categoric) data, and weighted mean differences for continuous data. Differences between groups that fell outside the 95% confidence interval were considered to be significant differences.

FINDINGS

- *Mistletoe:* Mice data showed anticancer, antimetastatic, and proapoptic (timed natural death of tumor cells) properties of mistletoe, but possible damage of healthy tissue. There was evidence of increased quality of life and increased immune status, but no increased survival rates were found.
- *Phytoestrogens:* Found in soy, wheat, flax seed, fruits and vegetables, phytoestrogens can have either an estrogenic or an antiestrogenic effect. In vitro breast cancer cells proliferated at low doses, but paradoxically were inhibited at high doses. Phytoestrogens, especially soy, were frequently used for perimenopausal symptoms, but soy may have increased tumor growth in estrogen-sensitive organs (such as breast and endometrium).
- *Vitamins A, B, and E:* Although data showed antioxidant and anti–free radical, and anticancer effects in vitro, there was still no evidence that vitamins prevented cancer. However, there

was a decrease in recurrence of breast cancer in premenopausal breast cancer survivors. There were no recommendations for vitamins and mineral supplements for clients with healthy diets, except in conditions related to malabsorption.
- *Trace elements:* Known to enhance killer cells and interferon, selenium prevents some prostate and gastric cancers, but not breast cancer. It may have reduced sensitivity to chemotherapy. Copper and zinc protected against free radicals, but zinc may have increased tumor growth. No increase in prevention, quality of life, or survival were noted with trace elements.
- *Coenzyme Q10:* Claims of remission using Q10, an antioxidant, have not been supported by trials, but it increased quality of life by decreasing cancer symptoms and drug side effects. Q10 may have decreased the efficacy of radiation therapy.
- *Herbal therapy:* Some biologic effects of herbs included antioxidant, endocrine, immune stimulation, and antitumor activities. However, herbs may have had anticoagulant, hepatotoxic, nephrotoxic, tumorigenic and carcinogenic effects, and unknown interactions with cancer drugs. Green tea use may have benefited cancer remission and survival rates. Chinese herbal mixtures have shown anticancer activity in vitro, but no trials have been performed.
- *Acupuncture:* Acupuncture was beneficial for symptoms of nausea, menopause, or pain.
- *Hypnosis/psychologic therapies:* Decreasing stress may increase immune system functioning.

LIMITATIONS

- Randomization was lacking; one study reported that only 6% of its breast cancer clients were willing to be randomized, reflecting the strong opinions clients may hold about CAM. Interactions between combinations of CAMs, and between CAMs and cancer drugs, are still unknown.

IMPLICATIONS FOR PRACTICE

- The authors of this review do not see enough evidence to warrant recommending CAM as adjuvant therapy for early-stage breast cancer. However, health care providers should examine the objective evidence for specific client concerns. Women are more likely to discuss their use of CAM with a nurse or general practitioner than a specialist, such as an oncologist, but all healthcare providers should ask about CAM use.

IMPLICATIONS FOR FURTHER RESEARCH

- More research is especially needed to resolve the doubts about the safety of herbs, and the interaction of CAM and medical cancer treatments. Randomized controlled trials of sufficient power will help to establish safe, useful dosages and combinations of CAM. Resolving the gaps in medical care that make CAM seem necessary is the biggest challenge.

Reference; Gerber, B., Scholz, C., Reimer, T., Briese, V., & Janni, W. (2006). Complementary and alternative therapeutic approaches in patients with early breast cancer: A systematic review. *Breast Cancer Research and Treatment, 95*(3), 199-209.

box 11-6 Arm Exercises After Lymph Node Dissection

Check with your health care provider before performing these range of motion exercises. Perform exercises slowly to stretch the muscle gently. Repeat exercises several times a day, with time to rest in between.

EXERCISE: CLIMBING THE WALL
1. Stand facing wall with toes close to wall.
2. Bend elbows and place palms of hands against wall at shoulder level.
3. Move both hands parallel to each other up the wall as far as possible until incisional pull or pain occurs.
4. Move both hands down to starting position either by sliding them back down or walking them back down.
5. Goal is to reach all the way up with arm in complete extension with elbow straight. Repeat several times.
6. Perform activities that use the same action: reaching top shelves, washing windows, blow-drying hair.

EXERCISE: ROPE PULL
1. Attach a 6-foot rope over a shower rod or a hook at the top of a door.

2. Grasp one end of the rope in each hand, and extend your arms to your sides. Pull down on one end while raising the other arm, raising arm as high as you can (on affected side to a point of incisional pull or pain). Reverse the exercise, with the raised arm being lowered and raising the lower arm.
3. Shorten rope over time until arm on affected side is raised almost directly overhead.

EXERCISE: ELBOW SPREAD
1. Clasp hands behind neck.
2. Raise elbows to chin level, holding head erect; move slowly and rest when incisional pull or pain occurs.
3. Gradually spread elbows apart; rest when pull or pain occurs. Repeat several times.

EXERCISE: ARM OVER HEAD
1. Lie down with your arms by your side.
2. Raise the arm on the surgery side straight up and reach over your head. Repeat several times.

and National Cancer Institute and should be shared with the woman and her family.

It is important to discuss the appearance of the woman's breast if dressings have not been removed before discharge. Some women may not want to view their surgical site, but it is important to give them the opportunity to do so and

to provide emotional support at that time. The woman should be encouraged to express her emotions and verbalize her feelings. The woman needs to know that it will take time to become accustomed to her change of appearance.

An option for restoration of body image is choosing an external prosthesis to replace the lost breast or portion of

TEACHING FOR SELF-CARE

After a Mastectomy

- Wash hands well before and after touching incision area or drains.
- Empty surgical drains twice a day and as needed, recording the date, time, drain site (if more than one drain is present), and amount of drainage in milliliters in the diary you will take to each surgical checkup until your drains are removed. (Before discharge, you may receive a graduated container for emptying drains and measuring drainage.)
- Avoid driving, lifting more than 10 pounds, or reaching above your head until given permission by surgeon.
- Take medications for pain as soon as pain begins.
- Perform arm exercises as directed.
- Call physician if inflammation of incision or swelling of the incision or the arm occurs.
- Avoid tight clothing, tight jewelry, and other causes of decreased circulation in the affected arm.
- Until drains are removed, wear loose-fitting underwear (camisole or half-slip) and clothes, pinning surgical drains inside of clothing. (You will be taught how to do this safely.)
- After drains are removed and surgical sites are healing and still tender, wear a mastectomy bra or camisole with a cotton-filled, muslin temporary prosthesis. Temporary prostheses of this type are often available from Reach to Recovery.
- Avoid depilatory creams, strong deodorants, and shaving of affected chest area, axilla, and arm.

- Sponge bathe until drains are removed.
- Return to the surgeon's office for incision check, drain inspection, and possible drain removal as directed.
- Contact Reach to Recovery for assistance in obtaining external prosthesis and lingerie when dressings, drains, and staples are removed and wound is healing and nontender.
- Contact insurance company for information about coverage of prosthesis and wig if needed. Obtain prescriptions for prosthesis and wig to submit with receipts of purchase for these items to the insurance company. If insurance does not pay for these items, contact hospital or agency social worker or local American Cancer Society for assistance.
- Continue with monthly BSE of unaffected side and affected surgical site and axilla.
- Keep follow-up visits for professional examination, mammography, and testing to detect recurrent breast cancer.
- Expect decreased sensation and tingling at incision sites and in the affected arm for weeks to months after surgery.
- Resume sexual activities as desired.
- Participate in breast cancer survivor support group if desired.
- Encourage mother, sisters, and daughters (if applicable) to learn and practice monthly BSE and to have annual professional breast examinations and mammography (if appropriate).

breast tissue. The external prosthesis is inserted into the bra. Women who choose to use a partial external prosthesis after lumpectomy or full external prosthesis after mastectomy need information about where to obtain prostheses and appropriate bra. Women need to be advised on how to submit the cost of the prosthesis to their insurance company. Volunteers of the American Cancer Society's Reach to Recovery program are able to provide this information, as well as a list of sources for prostheses and lingerie. They can offer helpful hints and suggestions for coping with prostheses and wearing apparel. Some women find that an external prosthesis does not restore body image and seek surgical reconstruction of the missing or disfigured breast (see previous discussion).

■ *Discharge Planning and Follow-up Care*

Before discharge, considerable time should be spent counseling the woman and her family about the aspects of self-care. These instructions are summarized in the Teaching for Self-Care box. Printed instructions should be given to the woman and her family. A referral for home nursing care may be made if the woman needs assistance caring for her incision.

■ *Teaching Needs for the Client and Family Undergoing Adjuvant Therapies*

It is important that the woman and her family be given thorough instructions regarding side effects and avoidance of possible complications of adjuvant treatment. A common

---

plan of care ▶ **Woman After Breast Conserving Surgery and Axillary Node Dissection**

NURSING DIAGNOSIS Acute pain related to surgical incision and surgical drains, as evidenced by client verbalizations

Expected Outcome *Woman will report minimal intensity and decreased number of painful episodes.*

Nursing Interventions/Rationales
- Use pain scale to assess type and intensity of pain *to provide accurate database.*
- Administer analgesics as ordered *to decrease perception of pain.*
- Teach and reinforce use of relaxation techniques *to reduce anxiety and provide distraction that may decrease the perception of pain.*
- Reposition woman with affected arm elevated *to promote comfort and lymphatic channel return.*

NURSING DIAGNOSIS Risk for infection related to disruption of skin integrity and removal of lymph nodes

Expected Outcome *Woman will experience no clinical manifestations of infection.*

Nursing Interventions/Rationales
- Assess clinical manifestations of infection at the incision and drain sites that may include redness, swelling, localized heat, fever, increasing pain, and foul-smelling drainage *to facilitate prompt treatment.*
- Demonstrate the procedure for emptying and recording the amount of drainage from the Jackson-Pratt drain(s) *to provide information to the surgeon as to the appropriate removal time of drains. Drains are usually removed when drainage in 24 hours is less than 30 ml of fluid.*
- Explain the need to avoid trauma or irritation to the affected arm *to reinforce to the woman that alterations in sensation and removal of some lymph nodes may affect ability to sense irritation or prevent infection.*
- Reinforce to the woman the need to protect arm from injury and to avoid blood drawing or blood pressures to be taken on the affected arm *to avoid trauma and infection, because decreased sensation may be present as well as decreased lymphatic return.*

- Explain the importance of reporting any clinical manifestations of infection to the caregiver as soon as possible *to provide identification and treatment of problem.*

NURSING DIAGNOSIS Disturbed body image related to loss of all or part of a breast as evidenced by client statements

Expected Outcomes *Woman will report acceptance of herself as she is and regain a positive body image.*

Nursing Interventions/Rationales
- Provide opportunity through therapeutic communication to express feelings about body image changes *to clarify and validate feelings.*
- Provide information about breast prostheses and other cosmetic devices *to assist in maintaining an intact body image.*
- Encourage woman to speak to physician about the possibility of breast reconstructive surgery *to provide additional resources for body image enhancement.*
- Refer to support groups *to facilitate verbalization of feelings with women who have similar concerns.*

NURSING DIAGNOSIS Impaired physical mobility related to pain and tissue trauma

Expected Outcome *The woman will return to her preoperative level of mobility.*

Nursing Interventions/Rationales
- Encourage woman to do hand, arm, and wrist exercises that can be performed in the immediate postoperative period *to enhance fluid return and prevent muscle atrophy.*
- Encourage woman to perform activities of daily living as much as possible *to encourage woman to focus on her strengths rather than her limitations.*
- Teach woman exercises to be performed after the drains are removed *to promote range of motion in the arm that had the axillary nodes dissected.*
- Teach woman to do exercises slowly and gently *to prevent injury and pain.*
- Caution woman not to lift anything heavier than 10 pounds for 4 to 6 weeks *to avoid exerting strain on affected arm.*

CD: Plan of Care: Breast Conserving Surgery

side effect of radiation therapy is skin irritation and breakdown. The woman should avoid using lotions, powders, or ointments on the skin at the radiation site unless instructed by the radiologist. The skin should be cleansed gently with mild soap and water, rinsed thoroughly, and patted dry. Skin markings that direct the placement of the radiation beam should not be removed. Soft, nonirritating clothing should be worn over the site, and the skin should be protected from exposure to sun and heat.

Common side effects of chemotherapy include alopecia, fatigue, nausea, vomiting, mouth sores, and immunosuppression. The woman planning to receive chemotherapy that produces hair loss should be encouraged to obtain a wig matching her own hair color and style before beginning treatments so that she is prepared when hair loss begins. The American Cancer Society can assist the woman in obtaining a wig and head coverings designed for women experiencing hair loss from chemotherapy. The woman should be taught the importance of rest periods when fatigue occurs. The woman and her family will need to know that work and family schedules may need adjustment to accommodate needed rest. Nausea and vomiting should be reported to the physician and are treated with antiemetics. Mouth sores may be very painful, and the woman should be instructed to maintain good oral hygiene and avoid trauma to the oral mucosa. The mouth should be rinsed frequently with water or saline,

and mouthwashes containing alcohol or glycerine should be avoided. Spicy or irritating foods should be avoided. Topical anesthetic medications may be prescribed by the physician. The woman with immunosuppression should be instructed to use frequent handwashing and avoid crowds and other large gatherings of people, especially during cold and flu season. She should be taught to avoid eating raw fruits and vegetables (low-bacteria diet) and maintain strict personal hygiene. The woman should be taught the signs and symptoms of infection and to report them to the physician immediately.

■ Evaluation

Evaluation is based on the client-centered expected outcomes. The nurse can be assured that care was effective to the extent that the goals for care have been achieved (see Plan of Care).

---

community activity

Contact the nearest American Cancer Society office to assess the resources available for women with breast cancer (e.g., pamphlets, support groups for breast cancer survivors), and what breast cancer screening is recommended for early detection. How can women get access to American Cancer Society information? What resources and information are available in your community?

---

key points

- The most common benign breast problems are fibrocystic changes and fibroadenomas.
- The development of breast neoplasms, whether benign or malignant, can have a significant physical and emotional effect on the woman and her family.
- The risk of American women developing cancer of the breast is one in eight.
- An estimated 90% of all breast lumps are detected by the woman during BSE.
- Monthly BSE, routine screening mammography, and yearly breast examinations by practitioners are recommended for early detection of breast cancer.

- The primary therapy for most women with stage I or stage II breast cancer is breast conserving surgery followed by radiation therapy.
- Adjuvant chemotherapy is most helpful to premenopausal women with breast cancer that has spread to the lymph nodes.
- Tamoxifen, along with raloxifene and anastrazole, provides the first real hope for the prevention of breast cancer.
- The emotional diagnosis of breast cancer is always intense, and the many disruptions caused by the disease challenge the woman's and her family's ability to cope.

REFERENCES

American Cancer Society (ACS). (2005). *Breast cancer facts and figures 2005-2006.* Atlanta: Author.

American Cancer Society (ACS). (2006). *Cancer facts and figures 2006.* Atlanta: Author.

Calle, E., Frumkin, H., Henley, S., Savitz, D., & Thun, M. (2002). Organochlorines and breast cancer risk. *CA: A Cancer Journal for Clinicians, 52*(5), 301-309.

Coleman, E., Lord, J., Heard, J., Coon, S., Cartrell, M., Mohrmann, C., et al. (2003). The delta project: Increasing breast cancer screening among rural minority and older women by targeting rural healthcare providers. *Oncology Nursing Forum, 30*(4), 669-677.

Crane-Okada, R. (2001). Breast cancers. In S. Otto (Ed.), *Oncology nursing* (4th ed.). St. Louis: Mosby.

DiSaia, P., & Creasman, W. (2002). *Clinical gynecologic oncology* (6th ed.). St. Louis: Mosby.

Grassley, B. (2002). Breast reduction surgery: What every woman needs to know. *AWHONN Lifelines, 6*(3), 244-249.

Hindle, W. (2002a). Breast cancer prevention and surveillance. *Clinical Obstetrics and Gynecology, 45*(3), 778-783.

Hindle, W. (2002b). Treatment of invasive breast cancer. *Clinical Obstetrics and Gynecology, 45*(3), 767-769.

Hinterberger-Fischer, M., & Hinterberger, T. (2001). Blood stem cell transplantation for breast cancer: New approaches using pre-peripost-transplant immunotherapy. *Expert Opinion in Biologic Therapy, 1*(6), 1029-1048.

Hutson, S. (2003). Attitudes and psychological impact of genetic testing, genetic counseling, and breast cancer risk assessment among women at increased risk. *Oncology Nursing Forum, 30*(2), 241-246.

Kissinger, L., Harris, R., Woolf, S., Sox, H., & Lohr, K. (2002). Chemoprevention of breast cancer: A summary of the evidence for the U.S. Preventive Services Task Force. *Annals of Internal Medicine, 137*(1), 59-69.

Leung, A., & Pacund, D. (2004). Diagnosis and management of galactorrhea. *American Family Physician, 70*(3), 543-550.

Lucas, J., & Cone, L. (2003). Breast cyst aspiration. *American Family Physician, 68*(10), 1983-1986.

Marsden, J. (2002). Hormone-replacement therapy and breast cancer. *Lancet Oncology, 3*(5), 303-311.

McReady, T. (2003). Management of patients with breast cancer. *Nursing Standard, 17*(41), 45-55.

Miers, M. (2001). Understanding benign breast disorders and disease. *Nursing Standard, 15*(50), 45-55.

Morrow, M., & Gradishar, W. (2002). Breast cancer. *BMJ, 324*(7334), 410-414.

Morrow, M., Strom, E., Bassett, L., Dershaw, S., Fowble, B., Guiliano, A., et al. (2002). Standard for breast conservation therapy in the management of invasive breast carcinoma. *CA: A Cancer Journal for Clinicians, 52*(5), 277-300.

National Cancer Institute (NCI). (2006). *Cancer trials information* [online]. Accessed www.nci.nih.gov/clinicaltrials/, March 4, 2006.

National Comprehensive Cancer Network (NCCN). (2005). *Breast cancer treatment guidelines for patients* [on-line]. Accessed www.nccn.org, March 4, 2006.

National Women's Health Resource Center. (2005). Women and living with breast cancer today. *National Women's Health Report, 25*(5), 1-8.

Osuch, J. (2002). Breast health and disease over a lifetime. *Clinical Obstetrics and Gynecology, 45*(4), 1140-1161.

Partin, M., & Slater, J. (2003). Promoting repeat mammography use: Insights from a systematic needs assessment. *Health Education & Behavior, 30*(1), 97-112.

Peterson, H., Thacker, S., Corso, P., Marchbanks, P., & Koplan, J. (2004). Hormone therapy: Making decisions in the face of uncertainty. *Archives of Internal Medicine, 164*(21), 2308-2312.

Pruthi, S. (2001). Detection and evaluation of a palpable breast mass. *Mayo Clinic Proceedings, 76*(6), 641-648.

Resnick, B., & Belcher, A. (2002). Breast reconstruction. *American Journal of Nursing, 102*(4), 26-33.

Riggs, B., & Hartmann, L. (2003). Drug therapy: Selective estrogen-receptor modulators—mechanisms of action and application to clinical practice. *The New England Journal of Medicine, 348*(7), 618-629.

Sakorafas, G. (2003). The management of women at high risk for breast cancer: Risk estimation and prevention strategies. *Cancer Treatment Reviews, 29*(2), 79-89.

Sammarco, A. (2003). Quality of life of older survivors of breast cancer. *Cancer Nursing, 26*(6), 431-438.

Sandau, K. (2002). Free TRAM flap breast reconstruction. *American Journal of Nursing, 102*(4), 36-43.

Simpson, J., & Rosenzweig, M. (2002). Treatment considerations for the elderly person with cancer. *AACN Clinical Issues, 13*(1), 43-60.

Smith, I., & Dowsett, M. (2003). Drug therapy: Aromatase inhibitors in breast cancer. *The New England Journal of Medicine, 348*(24), 2431-2442.

Smith, M., & Kent, K. (2002). Breast concerns and lifestyles of women. *Clinical Obstetrics and Gynecology, 45*(4), 1129-1139.

Smith, R., Cokkinides, V., Eyre, H., & ACS. (2003). American Cancer Society guidelines for breast cancer screening: Update 2003. *CA: A Cancer Journal for Clinicians, 53*(3), 141-169.

Smith, R., Pruthi, S., & Fitzpatrick, L. (2004). Evaluation and management of breast pain. *Mayo Clinic Proceedings, 79*(3), 353-372.

U.S. Food and Drug Administration (FDA). (2004). *FDA breast implant consumer handbook-2004.* Accessed www.fda.gov/cdrh/breast-implants/, March 4, 2006.

Vogel, V., Costantino, J., Wickerham, D., Cronin, W., & Wolmark, N. (2002). The study of tamoxifen and raloxifene: Preliminary enrollment data from a randomized breast cancer risk reduction trial. *Clinical Breast Cancer, 3*(2), 153-159.

Wagstaff, A., Ibbotson, T., & Goa, K. (2003). Capecitabine: A review of its pharmacology and therapeutic efficacy in the management of advanced breast cancer. *Drugs, 63*(2), 217-236.

Writing Group for the Women's Health Initiative Investigators. (2002). Risks and benefits of estrogen plus progestin in healthy postmenopausal women: Principal results from the Women's Health Initiative randomized controlled trial. *Journal of the American Medical Association, 288*(3), 366-368.

Yarbrough, S. (2004). Older women and breast cancer screening: Research synthesis. *Oncology Nursing Forum, 31*(1), E9-E15.

Zuckerman, D. (2002). The breast cancer information gap. *RN, 65*(2), 39-41.

CHAPTER 12

Deitra Leonard Lowdermilk

Structural Disorders and Neoplasms of the Reproductive System

learning objectives

- Describe the various structural disorders of the uterus and vagina.
- Discuss the pathophysiology of selected benign and malignant neoplasms of the female reproductive tract.
- Compare the common medical and surgical therapies for selected benign gynecologic conditions.
- Examine the emotional impact of benign and malignant neoplasms.
- Develop a nursing plan of care for a woman with endometrial cancer who has had a hysterectomy.
- Explain diagnostic procedures in client-centered terms.

- Differentiate treatments for preinvasive and invasive conditions.
- Investigate health-promoting behaviors that reduce cancer risk.
- Assess the impact of benign and malignant neoplasms on pregnancy.
- Discuss the development and sequelae of gestational trophoblastic neoplasia.
- Identify critical elements for teaching clients with selected benign or malignant neoplasms.

electronic resources

Additional information related to the content in Chapter 12 can be found on

the companion website at *evolve*
http://evolve.elsevier.com/Lowdermilk/MWHC/
- NCLEX Review Questions
- WebLinks

or on the interactive companion CD
- NCLEX Review Questions
- Plan of Care: Hysterectomy for Endometrial Cancer

WOMEN are at risk for structural disorders and neoplastic diseases of the reproductive system from the age of menarche through menopause and the older years. Problems may include structural disorders of the uterus and vagina related to pelvic relaxation and urinary incontinence. Benign neoplasms of the reproductive organs, such as fibroids and cysts, and malignant neoplasms of the reproductive system also may occur. Benign tumors usually do not endanger life, tend to grow slowly, and are not invasive. Malignant tumors (cancers) grow rapidly in a disorganized manner and invade surrounding tissues. The development of structural disorders and benign or malignant neoplasms can have far-reaching effects for the woman and her family. Beyond the obvious physiologic alterations, the woman also experiences threats to her self-concept and her ability to cope. A woman's concept of herself as a sexual being can be affected by the condition and its treatments. A woman's family also is challenged in the way it responds to her diagnosis. When cancer occurs with pregnancy, it adds to the complexity of both physical and emotional responses to childbearing.

Nurses have important roles in teaching women about early detection and treatment and in providing supportive care to women and their families. This chapter presents information that will assist the nurse in assessing and identifying problems associated with structural problems or benign or malignant reproductive neoplasms. Nursing care concepts related to early detection, treatment methods, and education are included.

▌ STRUCTURAL DISORDERS OF THE UTERUS AND VAGINA

Alterations in Pelvic Support

Uterine Displacement and Prolapse

The round ligaments normally hold the uterus in anteversion, and the uterosacral ligaments pull the cervix backward and upward (see Fig. 5-3). Uterine displacement is a variation of this normal placement. The most common type of displacement is posterior displacement, or retroversion, in which the uterus is tilted posteriorly, and the

FIG. 12-1 Types of uterine displacement. **A,** Anterior displacement. **B,** Retroversion (backward displacement of the uterus).

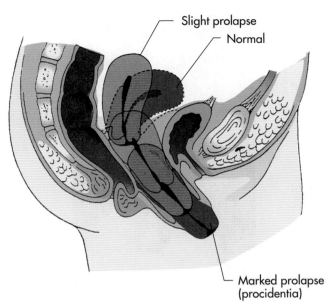

FIG. 12-2 Prolapse of uterus.

cervix rotates anteriorly. Other variations include retroflexion and anteflexion (Fig. 12-1).

By 2 months postpartum, the ligaments should return to normal length, but in about one third of women, the uterus remains retroverted. This condition is rarely symptomatic, but conception may be difficult because the cervix points toward the anterior vaginal wall and away from the posterior fornix, where seminal fluid pools after coitus. If symptoms occur, they may include pelvic and low back pain, dyspareunia, and exaggeration of premenstrual symptoms.

Uterine prolapse is a more serious type of displacement. The degree of prolapse can vary from mild to complete. In complete prolapse, the cervix and body of the uterus protrude through the vagina, and the vagina is inverted (Fig. 12-2).

Uterine displacement and prolapse can be caused by congenital or acquired weakness of the pelvic support structures (often referred to as pelvic relaxation). In many cases, problems can be a delayed but direct result of childbearing. Although extensive damage may be noted and

repaired shortly after birth, symptoms related to pelvic relaxation most often appear during the perimenopausal period, when the effects of ovarian hormones on pelvic tissues are lost, and atrophic changes begin. Pelvic trauma, stress and strain, and the aging process also are contributing factors. Other causes of pelvic relaxation include reproductive surgery and pelvic radiation.

Clinical Manifestations. Symptoms of pelvic relaxation generally relate to the structure involved: urethra, bladder, uterus, vagina, cul-de-sac, or rectum. The most common complaints are pulling and dragging sensations, pressure, protrusions, fatigue, and low backache. Symptoms may be worse after prolonged standing or deep penile penetration during intercourse. Urinary incontinence may be present.

Cystocele and Rectocele

Cystocele and rectocele almost always accompany uterine prolapse, causing the uterus to sag even farther backward and downward into the vagina. Cystocele (Fig. 12-3, *A*) is the protrusion of the bladder downward into the vagina that develops when supporting structures in the vesicovaginal septum are injured. Anterior wall relaxation gradually develops over time as a result of congenital defects of support structures, childbearing, obesity, or advanced age. When the woman stands, the weakened anterior vaginal wall cannot support the weight of the urine in the bladder; the vesicovaginal septum is forced downward, the bladder is stretched, and its capacity is increased. With time the cystocele enlarges until it protrudes into the vagina. Complete emptying of the bladder is difficult because the cystocele sags below the bladder neck. Rectocele is the herniation of the anterior rectal wall through the relaxed or ruptured vaginal fascia and rectovaginal septum; it appears as a large bulge that may be seen through the relaxed introitus (Fig. 12-3, *B*).

FIG. 12-3 **A,** Cystocele. **B,** Rectocele. (From Seidel, H., Ball, J., Dains, J., & Benedict, G. [2006]. *Mosby's guide to physical examination* [6th ed.]. St. Louis: Mosby.)

Clinical Manifestations. Cystoceles and rectoceles often are asymptomatic. If symptoms of cystocele are present, they may include complaints of a bearing-down sensation or that "something is in my vagina." Other symptoms include urinary frequency, retention, and/or incontinence, and possible recurrent cystitis and urinary tract infections (UTIs). Pelvic examination will reveal a bulging of the anterior wall of the vagina when the woman is asked to bear down. Unless the bladder neck and urethra are damaged, urinary continence is unaffected. Women with large cystoceles complain of having to push upward on the sagging anterior vaginal wall to be able to void.

Rectoceles may be small and produce few symptoms, but some are so large that they protrude outside of the vagina when the woman stands. Symptoms are absent when the woman is lying down. A rectocele causes a disturbance in bowel function, the sensation of "bearing down," or the sensation that the pelvic organs are falling out. With a very large rectocele, it may be difficult to have a bowel movement. Each time the woman strains during bowel evacuation, the feces are forced against the thinned rectovaginal wall, stretching it more. Some women facilitate evacuation by applying digital pressure vaginally to hold up the rectal pouch.

Urinary Incontinence

Urinary incontinence (UI) affects young and middle-aged women, with the prevalence increasing as the woman ages (Sampselle, 2003). More than one third of women over the age of 60 in the United States have some form of urinary incontinence (Mallett, 2005). Although nulliparous women can have UI, the incidence is higher in women who have given birth and also increases with parity (Sampselle). Conditions that disturb urinary control include stress incontinence due to sudden increases in intraabdominal pressure (such as that due to sneezing or coughing); urge incontinence, caused by disorders of the bladder and urethra, such as urethritis and urethral stricture, trigonitis, and cystitis; neuropathies, such as multiple sclerosis, diabetic neuritis, and pathologic conditions of the spinal cord; and congenital and acquired urinary tract abnormalities.

Stress incontinence may follow injury to bladder neck structures. A sphincter mechanism at the bladder neck compresses the upper urethra, pulls it upward behind the

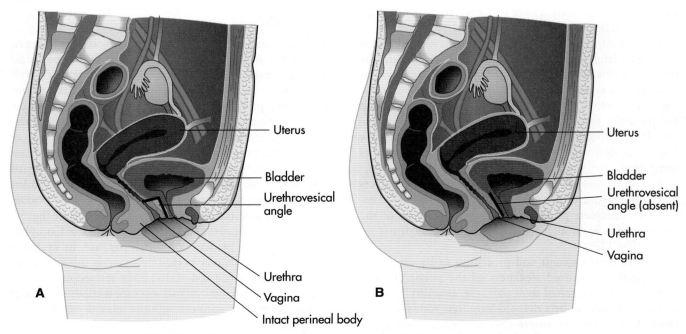

FIG. 12-4 Urethrovesical angle. **A,** Normal angle. **B,** Widening (absence) of angle.

symphysis, and forms an acute angle at the junction of the posterior urethral wall and the base of the bladder (Fig. 12-4). To empty the bladder, the sphincter complex relaxes, and the trigone contracts to open the internal urethral orifice and pull the contracting bladder wall upward, forcing urine out. The angle between the urethra and the base of the bladder is lost or increased if the supporting pubococcygeus muscle is injured; this change, coupled with urethrocele, causes incontinence. Urine spurts out when the woman is asked to bear down or cough in the lithotomy position.

Clinical Manifestations. Involuntary leaking of urine is the main sign. Episodes of leaking are common during coughing, laughing, and exercise.

Genital Fistulas

Genital fistulas are perforations between genital tract organs. Most occur between the bladder and the genital tract (e.g., vesicovaginal); between the urethra and the vagina (urethrovaginal); and between the rectum or sigmoid colon and the vagina (rectovaginal) (Fig. 12-5). Genital fistulas also may be a result of a congenital anomaly, gynecologic surgery, obstetric trauma, cancer, radiation therapy, gynecologic trauma, or infection (e.g., in the episiotomy).

Clinical Manifestations. Signs and symptoms of vaginal fistulas depend on the site but may include presence of urine, flatus, or feces in the vagina; odors of urine or feces in the vagina; and irritation of vaginal tissues.

Collaborative Care

Assessment for problems related to structural disorders of the uterus and vagina focuses primarily on the genitourinary tract, the reproductive organs, bowel elimination, and psychosocial and sexual factors. A complete health history,

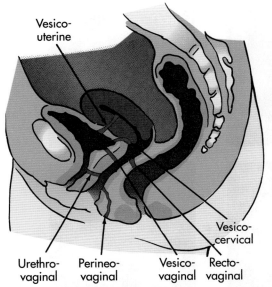

FIG. 12-5 Types of fistulas that may develop in the vagina, uterus, or rectum. (From Phipps, W., Monohan, F., Sands, J., Marek, J., & Neighbors, M. [2003]. *Medical-surgical nursing: Health and illness perspectives* [7th ed.]. St. Louis: Mosby.)

a physical examination, and laboratory tests are done to support the appropriate medical diagnosis. The nurse must assess the woman's knowledge of the disorder, its management, and possible prognosis. Possible nursing diagnoses for structural problems of the uterus and vagina include the following:

- *Deficient knowledge related to*
  –causes of structural disorders and treatment options
- *Constipation or diarrhea related to*
  –anatomic changes
- *Acute pain related to*
  –relaxation of pelvic support or elimination difficulties
- *Ineffective coping related to*
  –changes in body image
- *Interrupted family processes related to*
  –the woman's anatomic and functional changes
- *Risk for injury related to*
  –lack of skill in self-care procedures
  –lack of understanding of the reasons for the need to comply with therapy
- *Social isolation, spiritual distress, disturbed body image, or chronic low self-esteem related to*
  –changes in anatomy and function
- *Anxiety related to*
  –surgical procedure
  –prognosis

The health care team works together to treat the disorders related to alterations in pelvic support and to assist the woman in management of her symptoms. In general, nurses working with these women can provide information and self-care education to prevent problems before they occur, to manage or reduce symptoms and promote comfort and hygiene if symptoms are already present, and to recognize when further intervention is needed. This information can be part of all postpartum discharge teaching or can be provided at postpartum follow-up visits in clinics or physician/nurse-midwife offices, during postpartum home visits, or during gynecologic health examinations. In addition, information on how to prevent or recognize problems can be a topic for workshops for women or health fairs in community settings.

Besides providing information about prevention, nurses participate in a team effort to prepare the woman for surgery and self-care after discharge. Preoperative teaching involves the primary nurse, operating room nurse, surgeon, and anesthesiologist. Postoperatively, a nurse in the health promotion setting may be most aware of the woman's living circumstances, physical limitations, and social problems and therefore may be best suited to coordinate continuity of care after discharge.

Interventions for specific problems depend on the problem and the severity of the symptoms. If discomfort related to uterine displacement is a problem, several interventions can be implemented to treat uterine displacement. Kegel exercises (see p. 120) can be performed several times daily to increase muscle strength. A knee-chest position performed for a few minutes several times a day can correct a mildly retroverted uterus. A fitted pessary to support the uterus and hold it in the correct position (Fig. 12-6) may be inserted in the vagina. Usually a pessary is used only for a short time because it can lead to pressure necrosis and vaginitis. Good hygiene is important; some women can be taught to remove the pessary at night, cleanse it, and replace it in the morning. If the pessary is always left in place, regular douching with commercially prepared solutions or weak white vinegar solutions (1 tablespoon to 1 quart of water) to remove increased secretions and keep the vaginal pH at 4 to 4.5 are suggested. After a period of treatment, most women are free of symptoms and do not require the pessary. Surgical correction is rarely indicated.

Treatment for uterine prolapse depends on the degree of prolapse. Pessaries may be useful in mild prolapse. Estrogen therapy also may be used in the older woman to improve tissue tone. If these conservative treatments do not correct the problem, or if there is a significant degree of prolapse, abdominal or vaginal hysterectomy (see p. 286) is usually recommended.

Mild to moderate UI can be significantly decreased or relieved in many women by bladder training and pelvic muscle (Kegel) exercises (Klausner 2005; Sampselle, 2003). Other management strategies include pelvic flow support devices (i.e., pessaries), vaginal estrogen therapy, serotonin-norepinephrine reuptake inhibitors, electrical stimulation, insertion of an artificial urethral sphincter, and surgery (e.g., anterior repair) (Dwyer & Kreder, 2005; Kielb, 2005; Miller, 2005).

Nursing care for women with urinary incontinence includes assessment for depression that can result from decreased quality of life and functional status (Melville, Delaney, Newton, & Katon, 2005). Women also may need guidance about changes in lifestyle (e.g., losing weight) and education about pelvic muscle exercises.

Treatment for a cystocele includes use of a vaginal pessary or surgical repair. Pessaries may not be effective. *Anterior repair (colporrhaphy)* is the usual surgical procedure and is usually done for large, symptomatic cystoceles. This involves a surgical shortening of pelvic muscles to provide better support for the bladder. An anterior repair is often combined with a vaginal hysterectomy.

Small rectoceles may not require treatment. The woman with mild symptoms may derive relief from a high-fiber diet and adequate fluid intake, stool softeners, or mild laxatives. Vaginal pessaries usually are not effective. Large rectoceles that are causing significant symptoms are usually repaired surgically. A *posterior repair (colporrhaphy)* is the usual procedure. This surgery is performed vaginally and involves shortening the pelvic muscles to provide better support for the rectum. Anterior and posterior repairs may be performed at the same time and with a vaginal hysterectomy.

Management of genital fistulas depends on the location. Surgical repair is the usual treatment; however, it may not be successful.

Nursing care of the woman with a cystocele, rectocele, or fistula requires great sensitivity, because the woman's reactions are often intense. She may become withdrawn or hostile because of embarrassment caused by odors and soiling of her clothing that are beyond her control. She may have concerns about engaging in sexual activities because her partner is repelled by these problems. The nurse may tactfully suggest hygiene practices that reduce odor. Commercial deodorizing douches are available, or noncommercial solutions, such as chlorine solution

FIG. 12-6 Examples of pessaries. **A,** Smith. **B,** Hodge without support. **C,** Incontinence dish without support. **D,** Ring without support. **E,** Cube. **F,** Gellhorn. (Courtesy Milex Products, Inc., a division of CooperSurgical, Trumbull, CT.)

(1 teaspoon of household chlorine bleach to 1 quart of water) may be used. The chlorine solution also is useful for external perineal irrigation. Sitz baths and thorough washing of the genitals with unscented, mild soap and warm water help. Sparse dusting with deodorizing powders can be useful. If a rectovaginal fistula is present, enemas given before leaving the house may provide temporary relief from oozing of fecal material until corrective surgery is performed. Irritated skin and tissues may benefit from use of the heat lamp or application of an emollient ointment. Hygienic care is time consuming and may need to be repeated frequently throughout the day; protective pads or pants may have to be worn. All of these activities can be demoralizing to the woman and frustrating to her and her family. If surgical repair is performed, nursing care focuses on preventing infection and helping the woman avoid putting stress on the surgical site.

▬ BENIGN NEOPLASMS

Benign neoplasms include a variety of nonmalignant cysts and tumors of the ovaries, the uterus, the vulva, and other organs of the reproductive system.

Ovarian Cysts

Functional ovarian cysts (Fig. 12-7) are dependent on hormonal influences associated with the menstrual cycle. These cysts may be classified as follicular cysts, corpus luteum cysts, theca-lutein cysts, endometrial cysts, and polycystic ovarian syndrome. Other benign ovarian neoplasms include dermoid cysts and ovarian fibromas.

Follicular Cysts

Follicular cysts develop most commonly in normal ovaries of young women as a result of the mature graafian follicle failing to rupture, or when an immature follicle does not reabsorb fluid after ovulation. A cyst is usually asymptomatic unless it ruptures, in which case, it causes severe pelvic pain. If the cyst does not rupture, it usually shrinks after two or three menstrual cycles.

FIG. 12-7 Ovarian cyst. (From Seidel, H., Ball, J., Dains, J., & Benedict, G. [2006]. *Mosby's guide to physical examination* [6th ed.]. St. Louis: Mosby.)

Corpus Luteum Cysts

Corpus luteum cysts occur after ovulation and are possibly caused by an increased secretion of progesterone that results in an increase of fluid in the corpus luteum. Clinical manifestations associated with a corpus luteum cyst include pain, tenderness over the ovary, delayed menses, and irregular or prolonged menstrual flow. A rupture can cause intraperitoneal hemorrhage. Corpus luteum cysts usually disappear without treatment within one or two menstrual cycles.

Theca-lutein Cysts

Theca-lutein cysts are uncommon and in up to 50% of cases are associated with hydatidiform mole (see Chapter 31). Theca-lutein cysts develop as a result of prolonged stimulation of the ovaries by human chorionic gonadotropin (hCG). They also may occur if the woman has taken ovulation induction drugs; if she is pregnant and a large placenta is present, such as in the presence of a multiple gestation; or if the woman has diabetes (Stenchever, Droegemueller, Herbst, & Mishell, 2001). The cysts are almost always bilateral. A feeling of pelvic fullness may be noted by the woman if the ovary is enlarged, but most women are asymptomatic.

Polycystic Ovarian Syndrome

Polycystic ovarian syndrome (PCOS) occurs when an endocrine imbalance results in high levels of estrogen, testosterone, and luteinizing hormone (LH) and decreased secretion of follicle-stimulating hormone. This syndrome is associated with a variety of problems in the hypothalamic-pituitary-ovarian axis and with androgen-producing tumors. The condition can be transmitted as an X-linked dominant or autosomal dominant trait (Stein-Leventhal syndrome). Multiple follicular cysts develop on one or both ovaries and produce excess estrogen. The ovaries often double in size. Clinical manifestations include obesity, hirsutism (excessive hair growth), irregular menses or amenorrhea, and infertility. Impaired glucose tolerance and hyperinsulinemia occur in about 45% of women with PCOS (Stenchever et al., 2001). Affected women are at high risk for developing type 2 diabetes mellitus and possibly cardiovascular diseases (Buggs & Rosenfield, 2005; Sheehan, 2004). The prevalence in Mexican-American women is twice that of other ethnic groups (Goodarzi, Quinones, Azziz, Rotter, Hsueh, & Yang, 2005). It is often diagnosed in adolescence when menstrual irregularities and other symptoms appear (Buggs & Rosenfield).

Collaborative Care

A variety of interventions may be implemented for the woman with a functional cyst. If expectant management is the treatment, the woman is advised to keep appointments for pelvic examinations to monitor the changes in size of the cyst (enlarging or shrinking). Pharmacologic interventions such as analgesics may be prescribed for pain management. Oral contraceptives may be ordered for several months to suppress ovulation for functional cysts. Large cysts (greater than 8 cm) or cysts that do not shrink may be removed surgically (cystectomy). Corpus luteum cysts are treated similarly. Theca-lutein cysts are usually managed conservatively (they usually regress) or by removal of the hydatidiform mole (Stenchever et al., 2001).

Nursing care focuses on educating the woman regarding treatment options as well as pain management with analgesics or comfort measures such as heat to the abdomen or relaxation techniques. If surgery is performed, the nurse provides preoperative and postoperative care. Discharge teaching includes signs of infection, postoperative incision care, the possibility of recurrence, and advice regarding follow-up appointments.

The treatment for PCOS depends on what symptoms are of greatest concern to the woman. Lifestyle modifications (e.g., losing weight) and management of presenting symptoms such as infertility, irregular menses, and hirsutism are the focus. Oral contraceptives (OCs) are the usual treatment for irregular menses, if pregnancy is not desired, because they inhibit LH and decrease testosterone levels. OCs can also lessen acne to some degree. Gonadotropin-releasing hormone (GnRH) analogues may be used to treat hirsutism if oral contraceptives do not improve this condition. If pregnancy is desired, ovulation-inducing medications are given (Jackson, 2004-2005; Sheehan, 2004). Metformin and other insulin medications for type 2 diabetes also are used to lower insulin, testosterone, and glucose levels which, in turn, can reduce acne, hirsutism, abdominal obesity, amenorrhea, and other symptoms in women with PCOS (American College of Obstetricians and Gynecologists [ACOG], 2002); Lord & Wilkin, 2004; Teede, Meyer, & Norman, 2005).

Nurses can provide information and counseling for women with PCOS. Information may be needed about the syndrome or about its long-term effects on the woman's health. Women may need to discuss their feelings about the physical manifestations of PCOS and may need emotional support if they have self-image problems related to the symptoms. Teaching about lifestyle modifications such as exercise and diet may be needed as well as education about the medications that are prescribed. Information about finding a support group or information on the Internet may be useful.

Other Benign Ovarian Cysts and Neoplasms

Two other ovarian neoplasms that must be discussed include dermoid cysts and ovarian fibromas. Dermoid cysts are germ cell tumors, usually occurring in childhood. These cysts contain substances such as hair, teeth, sebaceous secretions, and bones. Unless the cyst is large enough to put pressure on other organs, it is usually asymptomatic. Dermoid cysts may develop bilaterally and are often attached to the ovary. Treatment is usually surgical removal.

Ovarian fibromas are solid ovarian neoplasms developing from connective tissue and most often occurring after menopause. Fibromas range in size from small nodules to large masses weighing more than 23 kg. Most fibromas are unilateral. They are usually asymptomatic, but if large enough, they may cause ascites, feelings of pelvic pressure, or abdominal enlargement. Treatment is usually surgical removal.

Nursing care of women treated for dermoid cysts and ovarian fibromas is similar to that described for functional ovarian cysts.

Uterine Polyps

Uterine polyps may be endometrial or cervical in origin. They are tumors that are on pedicles (stalks) arising from the mucosa (Fig. 12-8). The etiology is unknown, although they may develop in response to hormonal stimulus or be the result of inflammation. Polyps are the most common benign lesions of the cervix and endometrium that occur during the reproductive years. These polyps may be single or multiple. Endocervical polyps are most common in multiparous women older than 40 years. The woman may be asymptomatic or she may have premenstrual or postmenstrual bleeding or postcoital bleeding (Stenchever et al., 2001).

Collaborative Care

Clinical management of endometrial polyps is by surgical removal. Cervical polyps are usually removed in an office or clinic procedure without anesthesia. The polyp is grasped with a clamp and twisted or cut off. All polyps should be sent for pathologic examination. Endometrial sampling (may require local anesthesia) should be done to determine if other pathologic conditions are present (Stenchever et al., 2001).

Nursing care includes preparing the woman for what to expect during the removal procedure and encouraging relaxation and breathing exercises and providing support during the procedure. After the procedure, the woman is

FIG. 12-8 Endometrial polyps.

advised to avoid use of tampons, sexual intercourse, and douching for up to 1 week or until the site is healed. She is taught how to identify signs of infection and to notify her health care provider if she experiences heavy bleeding (more than one pad in 1 hour). Polyps rarely recur after removal (Stenchever et al., 2001).

Leiomyomas

Leiomyomas, also known as fibroid tumors, fibromas, myomas, or fibromyomas, are slow-growing benign tumors arising from the muscle tissue of the uterus (Stenchever et al., 2001). They are the most common benign tumors of the reproductive system, occurring most often after age 50 years. They tend to occur more often in African-American women and women who have never been pregnant (Stenchever et al., 2001). They rarely become malignant. Because their growth is influenced by ovarian hormones, these benign tumors can become quite large when the woman is taking birth control pills, is pregnant, or is receiving hormone therapy. They spontaneously shrink after menopause when circulating ovarian hormones are diminished (Cook & Walker, 2004).

Clinical Manifestations and Diagnosis

The cause of leiomyomas remains unknown, although genetic factors may be involved in their development. Most of the tumors are found in the body of the uterus. Leiomyomas are classified according to the location in the uterine wall. *Subserous* leiomyomas develop beneath the peritoneal surface of the uterus and appear as small or large masses that protrude from the outer uterine surface (Fig. 12-9, *A*). *Intramural* leiomyomas are tumors that develop within the wall of the uterus (Fig. 12-9, *B*). *Submucosal* leiomyomas are the least common tumors, but often they cause the most symptoms. These tumors develop in the endometrium and protrude into the uterine cavity (Fig. 12-9, *C*). Leiomyomas also can develop in the cervix and on the broad ligaments (Fig. 12-9, *D*). They also can grow on pedicles or stalks (Fig. 12-9, *E*). Occasionally these break off the pedicle and attach to other tissues (become parasitic).

Most women are asymptomatic; abnormal uterine bleeding is the most common symptom of fibroids. If the tumor is very large, pelvic circulation may be compromised, and surrounding viscera may be displaced. A woman may complain of backache, low abdominal pressure, constipation, urinary incontinence, or dysmenorrhea (painful menstruation). Nausea and vomiting may occur if the tumor is obstructing the intestines. The woman also may notice an abdominal mass if the tumor is large. Anemia may be present if the woman has excessive bleeding. Pedunculated tumors can twist and become necrotic, causing pain.

The tumors appear to be influenced by the presence of estrogen; during pregnancy, the tumors may produce complications such as preterm labor, miscarriage, or dystocia (difficult labor). The severity of the symptoms seems to be directly related to the size and location of the tumors.

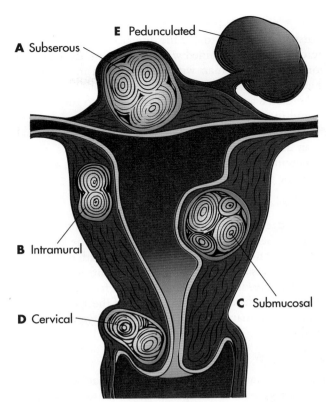

FIG. 12-9 Types of leiomyomas. **A,** Subserous. **B,** Intramural. **C,** Submucosal. **D,** Cervical. **E,** Pedunculated.

■ CARE MANAGEMENT

■ Assessment and Nursing Diagnoses

Assessment should include a history of symptoms (which might include abnormal bleeding, abdominal pain, dysmenorrhea, pelvic fullness or heaviness, or problems with elimination) and a pelvic examination. Diagnosis is usually accomplished by a process of elimination. A pelvic examination usually identifies the presence of uterine enlargement. Negative pregnancy tests will rule out pregnancy as the cause of the symptoms. Laparoscopy may be used to differentiate ovarian masses from uterine masses. Ultrasound examination can differentiate between inflammatory masses or endometriosis and subserous fibroids.

Possible nursing diagnoses for a woman with a leiomyoma include the following:

- *Anxiety related to*
  - –uncertain diagnosis
  - –fear of malignancy
  - –potential surgical treatment
- *Acute or chronic pain related to*
  - –leiomyomas
- *Sexual dysfunction related to*
  - –dyspareunia

▬ Expected Outcomes of Care

Nursing diagnoses provide the direction for care. Expected outcomes are determined with the woman. Expected outcomes for the woman with a leiomyoma might include that the woman will do the following:

* Verbalize a decrease in anxiety related to the diagnosis and therapeutic regimen.
* Verbalize understanding of treatment options to make an informed decision.
* Report no compromise in sexual functioning as a result of the therapeutic intervention.

▬ Plan of Care and Interventions

Knowledge of the medical-surgical management of leiomyomas is essential in planning nursing care. The knowledge enables the nurse to work collaboratively with other health care providers and to meet the woman's informational and emotional needs. Clinical management for benign tumors of the uterus depends on the severity of the symptoms, the age of the woman, and her desire to preserve childbearing potential.

▬ *Medical Management*

If symptoms are mild, regular checkups may suffice to observe for growth or changes in size. Nonsteroidal antiinflammatory drugs (NSAIDs) may be prescribed for pain; oral contraceptives inhibit ovulation and may relieve symptoms; and GnRH agonists such as leuprolide acetate (Lupron, Synarel) may be prescribed to reduce the size of the leiomyoma. Other medications used include medroxyprogesterone acetate (Depo-Provera), danazol (Danocrine) and mifepristone (RU-486; Mifeprex) (DeLeo et al., 2002; Sharts-Hopko, 2001). Selective estrogen receptor modulators (SERMs) (e.g., raloxifene) also may be beneficial for treating uterine fibroids, but more clinical trials are needed (Ohara, 2005).

The woman who prefers medical treatment will need information about the various medications, their actions and side effects, and routes of administration. A woman who is receiving GnRH agonists to decrease the size of the fibroid must understand that regrowth will occur after the treatment is stopped. She also must know that a small loss in bone mass and changes in lipid levels can occur; therefore long-term use is not recommended. Adding raloxifene to GnRH administration has been effective in preventing these effects in premenopausal women (Palomba et al., 2004). Amenorrhea may occur; however, women who wish to avoid pregnancy should use a nonhormonal or barrier method of contraception. A discussion of administration methods for GnRH agonists, including subcutaneous and intramuscular injections, intranasal administration, and subcutaneous implantation, will assist the woman in making a decision about her preferred method of administration (see Table 10-3).

Uterine Artery Embolization. Uterine artery embolization (UAE) is a treatment during which polyvinyl alcohol (PVA) pellets are injected into selected blood vessels to block the blood supply to the fibroid and cause shrinkage and resolution of symptoms (Society of Obstetricians and Gynaecologists of Canada [SOGC], 2005). The procedure is done under local anesthesia and conscious sedation. An incision is made into the groin, and a catheter is threaded into the femoral artery to the uterine artery. An arteriogram identifies the vessels supplying the fibroid. Most fibroids are reduced in size by 50% within 3 months. Temporary amenorrhea or early menopause can occur in some women. Although symptom improvement occurs for most women, data are lacking about the effects on future fertility and pregnancy outcomes. Long-term effects of the procedure are unknown (SOGC, 2005; Spies, Myers, Worthington-Kirsch, Mulgund, Goodwin, & Mauro, 2005).

Preoperative teaching includes advising the woman not to drink alcohol or smoke and not to take aspirin or anticoagulant medications 24 hours before the procedure. The woman is told to expect cramping during injection of the PVA pellets. Explanations about what to expect postoperatively include that pelvic pain, fever, malaise, and nausea and vomiting may be caused by acute fibroid degeneration. Pain may be controlled with a patient-controlled analgesia pump. Postoperative nursing assessments include checking for bleeding in the groin, taking vital signs, assessing pain level, and checking the pedal pulse and neurovascular condition of the affected leg (Hiller, Miller, & Stavas, 2005; Todd, 2002). Discharge teaching includes signs of possible complications and when to notify the physician, self-care instructions, and follow-up advice (see Teaching for Self-Care box). An ultrasound or magnetic resonance imaging (MRI) examination may be done after the UAE to determine the effectiveness of the procedure (Nicholson, 2004).

▬ *Surgical Management*

Laser Surgery. Laser surgery or electrocauterization can be used to destroy small fibroids through a laparoscopic (abdominal) or hysteroscopic (vaginal) approach.

TEACHING FOR SELF-CARE

Home Care After Uterine Artery Embolization

* Take prescribed medications as ordered.
* Call your physician if you have any of the following symptoms:
  - Bleeding
  - Pain
  - Swelling or hematoma at the puncture site
  - Fever of 39° C
  - Urinary retention
  - Abnormal vaginal drainage (foul odor, brown color, tissue)
* Eat a normal diet including fluids and fiber.
* Do not use tampons, douche, or have vaginal intercourse for at least 4 weeks.
* Avoid straining during bowel movements.
* Keep your follow-up appointment.

EVIDENCE-BASED PRACTICE

Uterine-Conserving Treatments Versus Hysterectomy for Uterine Fibroids

BACKGROUND

- Benign tumors of the uterine smooth muscle, or leiomyomata, are thought to occur in nearly one third of women aged 25 to 45 years. The risk of uterine fibroids is almost three times higher for African-American women than the general population. Although frequently present without symptoms, fibroids can cause abnormal bleeding and pain, as well as urinary frequency and constipation due to pelvic mass. Fibroids are also associated with pregnancy complications and infertility.
- Treatments vary considerably. Medical therapies include nonsteroidal antiinflammatory drugs and hormonal therapies. Uterine-sparing surgical procedures include uterine artery embolization, coagulation using cautery or laser, and myomectomy. Uterine fibroids are the most common reason for hysterectomy.

OBJECTIVES

- The reviewers set out to compare the efficacy, the risks for complications, and the benefits of treatments for uterine fibroids. Outcomes were to include physiologic, symptomatic, pregnancy rates and complications, quality of life, adverse outcomes, and need for additional treatment.

METHODS

Search Strategy

- After a comprehensive search of health databases and reference lists, the authors identified few randomized controlled trials or prospective cohort studies, the two highest quality studies. Therefore, they also accepted large cohort studies, retrospective reviews, and large case studies, which had to meet certain internal and external validity criteria. The dates, countries, and numbers of studies or subjects were not noted.

Statistical Analyses

- Data also came from a survey of 1,000 hospitals (or 20% of all U.S. hospitals), and from the hospital administration of Duke University Medical Center, for statistics on client trends and costs. Similar data were pooled. Differences between groups that exceeded the 95% confidence interval were accepted as significant.

FINDINGS

- African-American women were more likely than Caucasian women to receive hysterectomy or myomectomy. Hyster-

ectomies led to favorable outcomes and symptomatic relief, even two years out. Complications of myomectomy increased with additional fibroids, while a single fibroid lowered the risk of recurrence. Use of GnRH agonists, (e.g., Lupron) before surgery led to decreased blood loss. In pregnancy, fibroids were associated with increased preterm labor, placental abruption, cesarean birth, and breech presentation. Ovarian hormone levels may have been altered by removal of the uterus, even when the ovaries were spared. Hysterectomy did not adversely affect sexual functioning, and may have improved it, in severely symptomatic women.

- The lowest cost treatment for symptomatic fibroids was nonsteroidal antiinflammatory drugs, at around $60 a month, followed by oral contraceptives at $90 a month, and GnRH inhibitors at $500 for a standard 3-month course. Myomectomies cost less than hysterectomies.

LIMITATIONS

- There were insufficient data to compare the risks and benefits of myomectomy versus hysterectomy, or to recommend the most appropriate treatment for asymptomatic clients. Randomized controlled data were sparse.

IMPLICATIONS FOR PRACTICE

- Although hysterectomy is the second most common major surgical procedure performed in the United States, there is little evidence upon which to base recommendations for interventions and alternatives for management of leiomyomata. Hysterectomy had the best record of long-term symptom relief. Nurses can question clients about their history of fibroids, and alert them to the increased concerns for pregnancy. Uterus-preserving interventions may be cost effective and preserve fertility.

IMPLICATIONS FOR FURTHER RESEARCH

- There is a need for research on the genetics and long-term natural history of fibroids. Randomized controlled trials with standardized measures comparing medical versus surgical interventions would facilitate metaanalysis and therefore the power of research to allow comparison of outcomes and recommendations for management. Researchers need to address costs, quality of life, and racial disparities of health care access of fibroid management.

Reference: Management of uterine fibroids: Summary, evidence report/technology assessment: Number 34. (2001). *AHRQ Publication No. 01-E051*. Rockville, MD: Agency for Healthcare Research and Quality.

Hysteroscopic uterine *ablation* (vaporization of tissues) can be performed under local or general anesthesia, usually as an outpatient procedure. Medical therapy using GnRH agonists to control bleeding temporarily and to suppress endometrial tissue may be given for 8 to 12 weeks before surgery. Although the uterus remains in place, the vaporization process can cause scarring and adhesions in the uterine cavity, affecting future fertility. Thus this procedure is for women who wish to retain their uterus but no longer desire childbearing potential (Lefebvre et al., 2003). Risks

of the procedure include uterine perforation, cervical injury, and fluid overload (caused by the leaking into blood vessels of fluid used to expand the uterus during surgery). The woman may experience postoperative cramping and a slight vaginal discharge for a few days. Before discharge, the following information is given:

- Analgesics or NSAIDs may be used for pain relief as needed.
- Normal activities may be resumed within several days.
- Vaginal discharge is to be expected for 4 to 6 weeks.

- Use of tampons or vaginal intercourse should be avoided for 2 weeks.
- The next menstrual period may be irregular.
- The woman should be reminded about the effects of ablation on her fertility, if appropriate.
- The physician should be called if the woman has heavy bleeding or signs of infection.

Myomectomy. If the tumor is near the outer wall of the uterus, the uterine size is no larger than that at 12 to 14 weeks of gestation, and symptoms are significant, myomectomy (removal of the tumor) may be performed. Myomectomy can be performed through a laparoscopic or abdominal incision approach or a vaginal (hysteroscopic) approach (ACOG, 2005a; Stenchever et al., 2001). Myomectomy leaves the uterine muscle walls relatively intact, thereby preserving the uterus and allowing the possibility of future pregnancies (Lefebvre et al., 2003). It is usually performed in the proliferative phase of the menstrual cycle to avoid interrupting a possible pregnancy. GnRH therapy may be given before surgery to reduce the size of the fibroid. Fibroids may recur after myomectomy; further treatment may be needed (Lethaby, Vollenhoven, & Sowter, 2001).

Hysterectomy. Hysterectomy (removal of the entire uterus) is the treatment of choice if bleeding is severe or if the fibroid is obstructing normal function of other organs. An abdominal or vaginal surgical approach depends on the size and location of the tumors. For example, abdominal hysterectomy is usually performed for leiomyomas larger than a uterus would be at 12 to 14 weeks of gestation or for multiple leiomyomas. The uterus is removed through either a vertical or transverse incision. In some circumstances, the cervix may not be removed. Vaginal approaches can be used for smaller tumors. In both abdominal and vaginal approaches, the uterus is removed from the supporting ligaments (broad, round, and uterosacral). These ligaments are then attached to the vaginal cuff, allowing maintenance of normal depth of the vagina (Fig. 12-10). Alternatives to these procedures are the *laparoscopic assisted vaginal hysterectomy (LAVH)* and the laparoscopic supracervical hysterectomy (LSH). LAVH converts an abdominal procedure to a vaginal one by using a laparoscope in the abdomen to assist with removal of the uterus. LSH allows the cervix to remain. Both are associated with a quicker recovery and fewer postoperative complications (ACOG, 2005a; Johnson, Barlow, Lethaby, Tavender, Curr, & Garry, 2005).

Preoperative Care. Assessments needed before surgery include the woman's knowledge of treatment options, her desire for future fertility if she is premenopausal, the benefits and risks of each procedure, preoperative and postoperative procedures (Boxes 12-1 and 12-2), and the recovery process (Wade, Pletsch, Morgan, & Menting, 2000). If the woman can demonstrate understanding of this information, she can make an informed decision about treatment and feel a sense of control over the surgical experience (Lindberg & Nolan, 2001). Resources on helping women to make decisions about treatment may be found at the

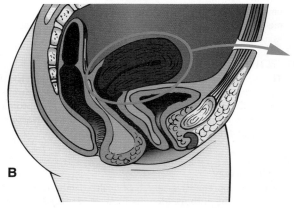

FIG. 12-10   Hysterectomy. **A,** Vaginal. **B,** Abdominal.

website for the Fibroid Treatment Collective, www.fibroid.org.

Psychologic assessment is essential, particularly for a woman who is scheduled for a hysterectomy. Areas to be explored include the significance of the loss of the uterus for the woman, misconceptions about effects of surgery, and adequacy of her support system. Women who have not completed their childbearing, who believe that their

---

box 12-1 | **Questions for the Woman to Ask to Ensure Informed Consent**

- Why is this procedure proposed for my condition/problem?
- What are the risks/benefits of the proposed surgery?
- Are there alternatives to this surgery? If so, what are the risks and benefits of these alternatives?
- How many times have you performed this surgery?
- How long will I be hospitalized? (or, Can the procedure be done in an outpatient setting?) How long will it take to recover?
- What types of anesthesia can be used?
- What hospital and surgical procedures can I expect?
- How will the surgery affect me (e.g., any changes in physical function, sexual function, or childbearing ability)?

Source: Wade, J., Pletsch, P., Morgan, S., & Menting, S. (2000). Hysterectomy: What do women need and want to know? *Journal of Obstetric, Gynecologic, and Neonatal Nursing, 29*(1), 33-42.

---

box 12-2 **Preoperative Procedures for Hysterectomy**

- Vaginal examination or physical examination
- Laboratory tests
  - Complete blood count, type, and crossmatch
  - Urinalysis
- Chest radiograph
- Electrocardiogram
- Teaching for postoperative routines
  - Turning, coughing, deep breathing
  - Passive and active leg exercises
  - Need for early ambulation
  - Pain relief options
- Nothing by mouth after midnight
- Enema if ordered
- Douche if ordered
- Abdominal: mons or perineal shave if ordered
- Removal of makeup, nail polish
- Removal of glasses, contact lenses, dentures, etc.
- Identification band in place
- Signed consent form in chart
- Have woman empty bladder immediately before surgery

---

self-concept is related to having a uterus (to be a complete woman), who feel that sexual functioning is related to having a uterus, or who have too little or too much anxiety about the surgery may be at risk for postoperative emotional reactions (Kim & Lee, 2001). However, Roussis, Waltrous, Kerr, Robertazzi, and Cabbad (2004) found that postoperatively, most women had positive feelings about femininity, their body image, and sexual responses.

Postoperative Care. Postoperative assessments and care after myomectomy and abdominal hysterectomy are similar to those for other abdominal surgery (Box 12-3). Assessments specific to abdominal and vaginal hysterec-

tomy include assessment for vaginal bleeding (one perineal pad saturated in less than 1 hour is excessive), urinary retention (especially after vaginal hysterectomy), perineal pain after vaginal hysterectomy, and psychologic assessments (depression is the most common emotional reaction) (Kjerulff, Langenberg, Rhodes, Harvey, Guzinski, & Stolley, 2000).

Discharge Planning and Teaching. Discharge planning and teaching are similar for myomectomy and hysterectomy (see Teaching for Self-Care box). Myomectomy and vaginal hysterectomy may be performed in an ambulatory setting, and women may be discharged the evening of the surgery. Women who have an abdominal hysterectomy

---

TEACHING FOR SELF-CARE

Care After Myomectomy or Hysterectomy

- Eat foods high in protein, iron, and vitamin C to aid in tissue healing; include foods with high fiber content; and drink six to eight 8-oz glasses of water daily.
- Rest when tired; resume activities as comfort level permits. Avoid vigorous exercise and heavy lifting for 6 weeks. Avoid sitting for long periods. Resume driving when comfort allows or on advice from health care provider.
- Avoid tub baths, intercourse (vaginal rest), and douching until after the follow-up examination.
- When vaginal intercourse is resumed, use of water-soluble lubricants may decrease discomfort.
- Report the following symptoms to your health care provider: vaginal bleeding, gastrointestinal changes, persistent postoperative symptoms (cramping, distention, change in bowel habits), and signs of wound infection (redness, swelling, heat, or pain at incision site).
- Keep your follow-up appointment with your health care provider.

---

box 12-3 **Postoperative Care After Hysterectomy**

- Monitor vital signs every 15 min until stable; then every 4 hr for 48 hr
- Maintain unobstructed airway
- Turn, cough, deep breathe every 2 hr for 24 hr
  - Assist woman to splint incision with hands or pillow
- Incentive spirometry if ordered
- Leg exercises every 2-4 hr until ambulatory Assess Homans sign
- Assess bleeding
  - Abdominal: assess dressing or incision
  - Vaginal: perineal pad count (one saturated pad in less than 1 hour is excessive; vaginal bleeding is usually minimal)
- Check laboratory values, especially hematocrit
- Assess lungs
- Assess bowel sounds and monitor bowel function
- Monitor intake and output
  - Foley catheter may be in place for 24 hr after abdominal surgery
  - After vaginal hysterectomy, urinary retention may be a problem because of manipulation of the urethra during surgery

- Assess abdominal incision or vagina for signs of infection
- Observe for signs of complications
  - Abdominal hysterectomy: assess for signs of wound evisceration, pulmonary embolism, thrombophlebitis, pneumonia, bowel obstruction, bleeding (incisional or vaginal)
  - Vaginal hysterectomy: assess for signs of urinary tract infection, urinary retention, wound infection, vaginal bleeding
- Pain relief
  - Pharmacologic measures: Patient-controlled analgesia (PCA) or epidural narcotics may be ordered for the first 24 hr, followed by oral analgesics and nonsteroidal antiinflammatory drugs
  - Nonpharmacologic measures: breathing and relaxation exercises, position changes, guided imagery, application of heat to the abdomen, and sitz baths or ice packs for the perineum; ambulation may relieve gas pains
- Psychologic assessments
  - Assess for depression or other emotional reactions
  - Assess support systems
  - Assess sexual concerns

may have a 1- to 2-day stay in the hospital before being discharged.

If a hysterectomy was performed, the woman is reminded that she will experience cessation of menses. If the woman is premenopausal, she will not experience menopause at this time unless her ovaries also were removed. In this case, there will be no reason for her to consider hormone replacement therapy. If the ovaries are removed, the woman will need the most current information on the risks and benefits of hormone replacement therapy (see Chapter 7). Other symptoms she may experience include pain, sleep disturbance, fatigue, anxiety, and depression. The level of severity of symptoms is influenced by physiologic, psychologic, and social factors (Kim & Lee, 2001).

Vaginal intercourse may be uncomfortable at first, especially after vaginal procedures. Use of water-soluble lubricants, relaxation exercises, and positions that control penile penetration may be beneficial (Katz, 2002). Women can be assured that this discomfort will decrease over time (Hartmann, Ma, Lamvu, Langenberg, Steege, & Kjerulff, 2004).

The schedule for follow-up care depends on the procedure performed, but usually a postoperative visit is scheduled within a week. Vaginal screening with cytology/ Papanicolaou (Pap) test after total hysterectomy for a nonmalignant reason is not recommended (American Cancer Society [ACS], 2006a; National Comprehensive Cancer Network [NCCN], 2004); however, general practice varies from testing yearly to testing every 2 to 3 years to assess for vaginal cancer (DiSaia & Creasman, 2002).

▬ Evaluation

The nurse evaluates the care of the woman who has had treatment of uterine leiomyomas by using the outcome criteria.

Vulvar Neoplasms
Bartholin Cysts

Bartholin cysts are the most common benign lesions of the vulva. They arise from obstruction of the Bartholin duct, which causes it to enlarge. Small cysts often are asymptomatic; however, large cysts or infected cysts cause symptoms such as vulvar pain, dyspareunia (painful intercourse), and a feeling of a mass in the vulvar area.

Collaborative Care. If the woman is asymptomatic, no treatment is necessary. If the cyst is symptomatic or infected, surgical incision and drainage may provide temporary relief. Cysts tend to recur; therefore a permanent opening for drainage may be recommended. This procedure is called *marsupialization* and is the formation of a new duct opening for drainage.

Nursing care after surgery includes teaching the woman about pain-relief measures such as sitz baths, heat lamps to the perineum, and use of analgesics. The woman is taught to assess the incision site for signs of healing and infection and to take antibiotics, if prescribed, for prevention of infection.

▬ MALIGNANT NEOPLASMS

Malignant neoplasms of the reproductive system include cancers of the endometrium, the cervix, the ovary, the vulva, the vagina, and the uterine tubes. Every year, over 80,000 women in the United States are diagnosed with a gynecologic cancer (National Women's Health Resource Center [NWHRC], 2004).

Cancer of the Endometrium
Incidence and Etiology

Endometrial cancer is the most common malignancy of the reproductive system (ACS, 2006a). It is most commonly seen in perimenopausal and postmenopausal women between ages 50 and 65 years. Certain risk factors have been associated with the development of endometrial cancer, including obesity, nulliparity, infertility, late onset of menopause, diabetes mellitus, hypertension, polycystic ovarian syndrome, and family history of ovarian or breast disease. There appears to be an increase in risk for endometrial cancer in families with hereditary nonpolyposis colorectal cancer (HNPCC). Hormone imbalance, however, seems to be the most significant risk factor (ACOG, 2005c; NWHRC, 2004). Numerous studies have correlated the use of exogenous estrogens (unopposed stimulation, i.e., absence of progesterone) in postmenopausal women with an increased incidence of uterine cancer. Tamoxifen taken by women for breast cancer also has been related to an increase in endometrial cancer (DiSaia & Creasman, 2002). Pregnancy and use of low-dose oral contraceptive pills appear to offer some protection (ACS). The incidence of endometrial cancer among Caucasian women is higher than that among African-American women; however, the mortality rates are more than one and a half times higher in African-American women (Reis et al., 2004).

Endometrial cancer is slow-growing and for that reason has a good prognosis if diagnosed at a localized stage. Most endometrial cancers are adenocarcinomas that develop from endometrial hyperplasia. The tumor usually develops in the fundus of the uterus and can spread directly to the myometrium and cervix, as well as to the reproductive organs. Metastasis (spread of cancer from its original site) is through the lymphatic system in the pelvis and through the blood to the liver, the lungs, and the brain.

▬ CARE MANAGEMENT

▬ Assessment and Nursing Diagnoses

Assessment includes a history of physical symptoms. The cardinal sign of endometrial cancer is abnormal uterine bleeding (e.g., postmenopausal bleeding and premenopausal recurrent metrorrhagia). Thirty percent of postmenopausal bleeding is caused by carcinoma. Late signs include a mucosanguineous vaginal discharge, low back pain, or low pelvic pain. A pelvic examination may reveal the presence of a uterine enlargement or mass.

■ NURSE ALERT

Women can be informed that they can identify their own risk for developing endometrial as well as ovarian, cervical, and breast cancers by filling out a confidential cancer risk assessment survey that is available on-line at the American Cancer Society website—www.cancer.org.

Histologic examination is used for diagnosis. A Pap smear of cellular material obtained by aspiration of the endocervix will identify only one third to one half of cases. Fractional curettage or endometrial biopsy yields the most accurate results. Fractional curettage involves scraping the endocervix and endometrium for histologic evaluation to determine the grade of neoplasm and its stage (extent). Perforation of the uterus is a possible complication of this procedure. Endometrial biopsy will identify about 90% of cases (DiSaia & Creasman, 2002). It is usually done on an outpatient basis under local anesthesia. A suction-type curette is used to remove tissue for sampling. It is recommended that women at risk for HNPCC have an annual biopsy beginning at age 35 years (ACOG, 2005c; NWHRC, 2004). Other diagnostic tests that may be useful include hysteroscopy (examination of the uterus through an endoscope) and vaginal ultrasonography. Other tests may be done to determine the spread of cancer. These include liver function tests, renal function tests, chest x-ray, intravenous pyelography (IVP), barium enema, computed tomography (CT), MRI, bone scans, and biopsy of suggestive tissues. Testing for the CA-125 antigen (tumor marker) may suggest metastasis for some endometrial cancers if high levels are found (NCCN, 2005b). The International Federation of Gynecology and Obstetrics (FIGO) classification system is used to describe the stages of endometrial carcinoma (Table 12-1).

Possible nursing diagnoses that would apply to a woman with endometrial cancer include the following:

- *Deficient knowledge related to*
  –diagnosis, treatment, and prognosis
- *Decisional conflict related to*
  –treatment options
- *Fear/anxiety related to*
  –diagnosis of cancer, loss of uterus
- *Impaired skin integrity related to*
  –surgery or radiation therapy
- *Acute or chronic pain related to*
  –cancer
  –surgical procedure
- *Disturbed body image related to*
  –loss of uterus
- *Sexual dysfunction related to*
  –anatomic and functional changes caused by cancer or its treatment

■ Expected Outcomes of Care

Planning for care of the woman with endometrial cancer depends on the stage of cancer and the treatment selected.

table 12-1 FIGO Classification of Endometrial Carcinoma*

STAGE	DESCRIPTION
Ia G123	Tumor limited to endometrium
Ib G123	Invasion of less than half of the myometrium
Ic G123	Invasion of more than half of the myometrium
IIa G123	Endocervical glandular involvement only
IIb G123	Cervical stromal invasion
IIIa G123	Tumor invades serosa and/or adnexae and/or positive peritoneal cytology
IIIb G123	Vaginal metastases
IIIc G123	Metastases to pelvic and/or paraaortic lymph nodes
IVa G123	Tumor invasion of bladder and/or bowel mucosa
IVb	Distant metastases, including intraabdominal and/or inguinal lymph node

Histopathology: Degree of differentiation

Cases of carcinoma of the corpus should be grouped according to the degree of differentiation of the adenocarcinoma as follows:

G1 = ≤5% of a nonsquamous or nonmorular solid growth pattern

G2 = 6% to 50% of a nonsquamous or nonmorular solid growth pattern

G3 = >50% of a nonsquamous or nonmorular solid growth pattern

*Approved by FIGO, October 1988, Rio de Janeiro. From DiSaia, P., & Creasman, W. (2002). *Clinical gynecologic oncology* (6th ed.). St. Louis: Mosby.

Examples of expected outcomes are that the woman will do the following:

- Demonstrate understanding of her diagnosis of endometrial cancer, the treatments available, and her prognosis.
- Make informed decisions about treatment options.
- Describe a decrease in anxiety and fear.
- Report that pain is reduced or manageable.
- Experience no skin breakdown or infection related to treatment.
- State that she understands the effects of cancer and treatment on her body image and that her concerns are reduced.
- Report that she and her partner expect to be able to resume mutually satisfying sexual relations after treatment.

■ Plan of Care and Interventions
■ *Therapeutic Management*

Collaborative efforts from various health disciplines are needed to work with the woman with endometrial cancer. All must have an understanding of the treatments that may be used.

For stage I adenocarcinoma of the endometrium, total abdominal hysterectomy (TAH) and bilateral salpingo-oophorectomy (BSO) are the usual treatments of choice. A radical hysterectomy (abdominal hysterectomy plus pelvic node dissection) usually is performed for stage II endometrial cancer. Removal of the upper third of the vagina and parametrium also may be done. Radiation use in stage I is controversial: it can reduce the risk of recurrence, but evidence does not demonstrate improved survival rates or reduce metastasis to distant sites. External radiation therapy to the whole pelvis (see p. 299) usually is given when there is extensive uterine disease or metastasis outside the uterus (DiSaia & Creasman, 2002). Treatment is usually 4 to 5 days a week for 6 weeks as an outpatient. Internal radiation therapy or brachytherapy (placement of an applicator loaded with a radiation source into the uterine cavity) also may be used (see p. 299). Treatment is usually 1 to 3 days for an inpatient but also may be given in a special outpatient unit in a shorter time by using higher doses of radiation (DiSaia & Creasman, 2002). Radiation therapy may cause skin ulcerations, cystitis, enteritis, and delayed complications such as genital fistulas.

Chemotherapy is used to treat advanced and recurrent disease, although no effective treatment regimen has been established (Stenchever et al., 2001). Agents that have been somewhat effective include cisplatin, doxorubicin (Adriamycin), carboplatin (Paraplatin), cyclophosphamide (Cytoxan), 5-fluorouracil (5-FU), vincristine (Oncovin), and paclitaxel (Taxol) (NCCN, 2005b). Chemotherapy may cause hair loss, anemia, and bone marrow depression, as well as other side effects (see Table 12-2).

Progestational therapy—use of medroxyprogesterone (Depo-Provera) and megestrol (Megace)—may be effective for estrogen-dependent cancers. These drugs usually do not cause acute side effects. Tamoxifen (Tamofen) (see Medication Guide p. 267). is an antiestrogen that is being investigated for its effectiveness against recurrent endometrial cancer. It may cause hot flashes and nausea and vomiting (DiSaia & Creasman, 2002; Stenchever et al., 2001).

■ Nursing Management

Nursing care is individualized to the woman and her specific situation and diagnosis. Interventions for the woman having surgery are directed by assessment of her perception of the anticipated surgery, her knowledge of what to expect after surgery, and any preoperative special procedures, such as cleansing enemas or douches. In today's practice of short hospital stays even for radical surgery, many of these preoperative procedures are performed at home before admission, so assessment of understanding becomes a critical nursing action (see Cultural Considerations box).

Preoperative Care. The nurse working with the woman preparing for a radical hysterectomy should explain any preoperative procedures to be done, (see Box 12-2, p. 287). Additional teaching is needed regarding possible postsurgical events (e.g., drainage tubes). The woman should be prepared to have a suprapubic drain that will remain in place for several days to a week.

Postoperative Care. Assessment of vital signs usually follows a postanesthesia protocol, gradually decreasing in frequency to 4 times a day. Intravenous fluids are

---

cultural considerations

Meaning of Cancer

A woman's culture influences the meaning she attaches to cancer. Her response to the diagnosis must be appropriate to her cultural context for it to be acceptable to her. For example, body image issues (e.g., loss of uterus), the meaning of death, and pain responses (e.g., stoic or expressive) are influenced by cultural beliefs and values. In making assessments about these issues, the nurse takes into account the influence of culture before developing a plan of care.

---

table 12-2 **Common Side Effects of Chemotherapy Agents Used for Gynecologic Cancers**

		SIDE EFFECTS*				
AGENT	ALOPECIA	MYELOSUPPRESSION, LEUKOPENIA, THROMBOCYTOPENIA	NAUSEA AND VOMITING	STOMATITIS	NEUROTOXICITY	STERILITY
Cisplatin	−	+	+	−	+	−
Doxorubicin	+	+	+	+	−	−
Paclitaxel	+	+	+	−	+	−
Bleomycin	+	−	+	+	−	−
5-fluorouracil (5-FU)	+	−	+	+	−	−
Carboplatin	−	+	+	−	+	−
Mitomycin	+	+	+	+	−	−
Ifosfamide	+	+	+	−	+	−
Cyclophosphamide	+	+	+	+	−	+ (temp)
Methotrexate	+	+	+	+	+	−
Vincristine	+	+	+	+	+	−

Sources: Facts and Comparisons. (2006). *Drug facts and comparisons.* St Louis: Wolters Kluwer; National Comprehensive Cancer Network Inc. (2005b). *NCCN practice guidelines in oncology. Uterine cancers. Version 1.2005.* Accessed www.nccn.org, January 12, 2006; Otto, S. (2001). Gynecologic cancers. In S. Otto, *Oncology nursing.* St. Louis: Mosby.
*Incidence and seriousness of side effects may be dose related.

maintained at a rate rapid enough to maintain hydration and electrolyte balance. Diet is gradually resumed as bowel sounds are heard and flatus is passed. A nasogastric tube may be in place to prevent distention. Intake and output are monitored.

The woman should turn and take deep breaths with assistance as needed. Breath sounds are assessed, and any deviations from normal are reported immediately. The most significant single cause of morbidity and prolonged hospitalization after major procedures is respiratory complications. Anesthesia and surgery alter breathing patterns and ability to cough. Atelectasis, pneumonia, and pulmonary embolus may occur.

Hemorrhage is always a possible complication after surgery. The wound drainage tube is emptied as needed or every 4 hours, and the amount and character of drainage is recorded. Drainage from any tube is assessed for bleeding. Vaginal drainage, if any, should be serosanguineous. Hematuria is noted and recorded. The primary health care provider is kept apprised of any deviations from normal expectations.

Paralytic ileus may occur after surgery in which the intestinal tract has been manipulated. Use of a nasogastric tube, limiting oral fluids, and early ambulation all support the return of gastrointestinal function. An enema or suppository may bring relief of flatus and stimulate the return of bowel function. Oral laxatives should not be given until lower bowel function has returned.

Sitting may result in pelvic congestion, so the high Fowler's position is avoided. Pelvic congestion is discouraged by avoiding use of the knee gatch (or pillow). Nursing measures such as massages, repositioning, fresh linen, regular perineal care, and emotional support are all helpful adjuncts to pharmacologic control of discomfort.

Discharge Planning and Teaching. Because the inhospital convalescent period is generally short, close observation by the nurse and attention to detail are critical. Nursing actions appropriate to this period include monitoring for urinary retention after the catheter is removed, monitoring the woman's appetite and diet, monitoring bowel function, and encouraging progressive ambulation and self-care.

Estrogen therapy after hysterectomy for endometrial cancer is controversial, but may be an option for women with low risk of recurrence (NCCN, 2005b). If prescribed, estrogen is usually started as soon as the woman can take oral fluids. The nurse can take this opportunity to remind the woman that she will no longer have menstrual periods (if she was premenopausal) and to encourage her to verbalize questions or concerns she may have about the risks and benefits (Stenchever et al., 2001). If estrogen therapy is not given, the woman will need information on how to decrease her risk for osteoporosis (e.g., exercise and calcium), and how to combat menopausal symptoms (e.g., diet, herbal therapy, and water-based lubricants for vaginal dryness) (Otto, 2001).

Discharge planning and teaching is done throughout the preoperative and postoperative phases and culminates during the convalescent phase. Discharge teaching topics for the woman with a radical hysterectomy are similar to those for the woman who has had a hysterectomy for leiomyomas and can be found in the Teaching for Self-Care box on p. 287 (also see Plan of Care box).

Care for the woman who has had external or internal radiation therapy is the same as that described for the woman with cervical cancer (p. 299).

Nursing care for the woman undergoing chemotherapy will depend on the type of drug given. If alopecia is likely, the nurse can suggest wigs, scarves, or other kinds of head coverings. If the therapy affects the appetite or causes gastrointestinal side effects, suggestions such as those in Box 12-4 may be useful.

After discharge, the woman may require continued nursing care or monitoring of her physical status or advice for management of effects of treatment or the cancer. The family is likely to have to provide much of the woman's care. Nurses must identify what families see as their greatest need so that interventions are planned that best use the family's resources (Lowdermilk & Germino, 2000).

Psychologic care for the woman with endometrial cancer is essential. A women needs to be able to discuss her concerns about having cancer and the potential for recurrence. She may have fears of death; permanent disfigurement and change in functioning; altered feelings of self as a woman; concerns regarding her femininity, sexuality, and loss of reproductive capacity. She may have questions arising from things she has heard about posthysterectomy changes, radiation therapy, or chemotherapy. Significant others should be encouraged to express their questions and concerns as well. The woman may benefit from a referral to a community cancer support group (see American Cancer Society [ACS] website, www.cancer.org).

■ Evaluation

The nursing care of a woman with endometrial cancer is evaluated by using the expected outcomes and measurable criteria to ascertain the degree to which the outcomes were met.

Cancer of the Ovary
Incidence and Etiology

Cancer of the ovary is the second most frequently occurring reproductive cancer and causes more deaths than any other female genital tract cancer (ACS, 2006a). Because the symptoms of this type of cancer are vague and definitive screening tests do not exist, ovarian cancer is often diagnosed in an advanced stage. The 5-year survival rate for cancer diagnosed at a localized stage is about 94%; however, only about 19% of all ovarian cancers are found at this stage. For advanced stages, the rate is about 25% (ACS). Malignant neoplasia of the ovaries occurs at all ages, including in infants and children. However, the greatest number of cases is found in women between ages 50 and 59 years.

Major histologic cell types occur in different age groups, with malignant germ cell tumors most common in women

CD: Plan of Care: Hysterectomy for Endometrial Cancer

---

plan of care ▶ **Hysterectomy for Endometrial Cancer**

NURSING DIAGNOSIS Anxiety related to lack of understanding of diagnosis, treatment, and prognosis of endometrial cancer as evidenced by woman's questions and concerns

Expected Outcomes *Woman will identify source of anxiety and verbalize understanding of diagnosis, effects of hysterectomy, and prognosis.*

Nursing Interventions/Rationales
- Assess woman's level of understanding of procedure and its effects *to correct any misunderstanding, provide clarification, and identify starting point for further information.*
- Provide information about cancer of the endometrium, individualizing information to woman's situation *to provide clarification concerning treatment regimen.*
- Provide preoperative and postoperative teaching *to give anticipatory guidance and rationales for upcoming events.*

NURSING DIAGNOSIS Fear related to diagnosis of endometrial cancer as evidenced by woman's questions and concerns

Expected Outcome *Woman will be able to verbalize that fears have diminished after the procedure.*

Nursing Interventions/Rationales
- Through therapeutic communication, encourage verbalization of fears *to provide clarification and validation of feelings.*
- Encourage woman to identify support system *to have resources readily available as needed.*

NURSING DIAGNOSIS Acute pain related to surgical procedure as evidenced by woman's verbal and nonverbal behaviors

Expected Outcome *Woman will verbalize decrease in intensity and number of painful episodes after interventions.*

Nursing Interventions/Rationales
- Assess the location and intensity of pain by using a pain scale *to use appropriate treatment.*
- Administer prescribed analgesics *to decrease perception of pain.*
- Use nonpharmacologic techniques such as distraction, relaxation, position changes, and heat *to decrease perception of pain.*
- Monitor effectiveness of interventions *to modify interventions if needed.*

NURSING DIAGNOSIS Risk for infection related to surgical incision and impaired skin integrity

Expected Outcome *Woman will experience no infection after the procedure.*

Nursing Interventions/Rationales
- Assess for clinical manifestations of infection: fever, drainage, redness, swelling at the incision site *to provide prompt treatment.*
- Encourage a diet high in protein, vitamin C, and calories *to promote wound healing.*
- Teach woman to maintain aseptic technique when performing dressing changes, such as good handwashing *to decrease chance of introducing microorganisms at the incision site.*

NURSING DIAGNOSIS Disturbed body image related to loss of uterus as evidenced by woman's statements of fears or concerns

Expected Outcome *Woman will maintain a positive body image.*

Nursing Interventions/Rationales
- Encourage expression of feelings through therapeutic communication *to provide clarification of and validity to feelings.*
- Encourage woman to share feelings with significant other *to obtain emotional support.*
- Assist woman to identify support systems *to be available in case of client need to ventilate feelings.*

NURSING DIAGNOSIS Sexual dysfunction related to perceived loss of femininity

Expected Outcome *Woman will resume usual sexual relationship with partner.*

Nursing Interventions/Rationales
- Encourage verbalization of feelings related to sexuality *to provide clarification.*
- Provide opportunity for role-playing *to alleviate fears about interactions with partner.*
- Encourage communication with partner *to address concerns about resumption of sexual relations.*
- Refer to sexual counselor *to provide in-depth intervention as needed.*

---

between 20 and 40 years of age and epithelial cancers occurring in the perimenopausal age groups. The spread of ovarian cancer is by direct extension to adjacent organs, but distal spread can occur through lymphatic spread to the liver and the lungs.

The cause of ovarian cancer is unknown; however, a number of risk factors have been identified. These factors include nulliparity, infertility, previous breast cancer, family history of ovarian or breast cancer, and history of HNPCC. Although BRCA1 and BRCA2 mutations have been found in some families with a history of ovarian cancer, the disease is not inherited for most women (DiSaia & Creasman, 2002). Women of North American or northern European descent have the highest incidence of ovarian cancers. Genital exposure to talc, a diet high in fat, lactose intolerance, and use of fertility drugs have been suggested as risk factors, but research findings are inconclusive (DiSaia & Creasman, 2002; Furniss, 2000). Pregnancy and use of oral contraceptives seem to have some protective benefits against ovarian cancer, whereas use of postmenopausal estrogen may increase the risk (ACS, 2006a).

Clinical Manifestations and Diagnosis

Ovarian cancer has been called a silent disease because early warning symptoms that would send a woman to her health care provider are absent (e.g., no bleeding or other discharge and no pain). Vague lower abdominal discomfort and mild digestive complaints are the early symptoms for

---

box 12-4 **Nutritional Management for Common Problems Related to Gynecologic Cancer or Treatment**

ALTERED TASTE
- Perform mouth care after meals
- Use extra seasoning
- Use sauces and marinades for meats
- Eat fish or chicken instead of red meat
- Eat tart foods to stimulate taste buds

ANOREXIA
- Eat with family, friends
- Try new foods, recipes
- Use smaller servings
- Eat high-calorie snacks
- Serve protein shakes
- Exercise before meals to stimulate appetite
- Eat when hungry

NAUSEA AND VOMITING
- Drink clear liquids
- Avoid carbonated fluids
- Avoid sweet, rich, fatty foods
- Eat cool foods rather than hot or warm foods
- Eat small meals
- Consume a high-calorie, high-protein diet
- Eat toast, bland foods
- Take antiemetics before meals

STOMATITIS: MILD TO MODERATE
- Eat small meals
- Eat soft, bland foods
- Drink 3 L of fluids a day

- Avoid citrus fruits, spicy foods
- Avoid alcohol
- Avoid very hot or very cold foods
- Add nutritional supplements, as needed

SEVERE STOMATITIS
- Eat liquid or pureed foods
- Enteral or total parenteral nutrition may be needed

CONSTIPATION
- Increase fiber (bran, fresh fruits and vegetables)
- Increase fluid intake (3 L/day)
- Eat natural laxative foods (prunes, apples)
- Avoid cheese products

DIARRHEA
- Avoid milk products
- Avoid high-fiber, spicy foods
- Eat foods high in potassium
- Increase fluid intake (3 L/day); avoid caffeine and carbonated fluids
- Add nutmeg to food to decrease gastric motility
- Eat a high-protein, high-carbohydrate diet

POSTOPERATIVE RECOVERY
- Eat food high in iron
- Eat high-protein foods
- Eat foods high in vitamins C, B complex, and K
- Drink 6 to 8 glasses of fluids a day (1.5 to 2L a day)

Sources: American Cancer Society. (2006a.). *Cancer facts and figures* 2006. New York: Author; Lowdermilk, D. (1995). Home care of the patient with gynecologic cancer. *Journal of Obstetric, Gynecologic, and Neonatal Nursing, 24*(2), 159.

---

some. An ovary enlarged 5 cm or more than normal that is found during routine examination requires careful diagnostic workup. The accompanying increase in abdominal girth (caused by ovarian enlargement or ascites) is usually attributed to an increase in weight or a shift in weight that is seen commonly in women entering their middle years. Pelvic pain, anemia, and general weakness and malnutrition are signs of late-stage disease.

Early diagnosis of ovarian cancer is uncommon. Attempts at early detection have not proven to be reliable. Taking a family history is important because it may reveal cancer of the uterus or breast. Transvaginal ultrasound, CA-125 antigen (a tumor-associated antigen) testing, and frequent pelvic examinations have all been used without a great deal of success because these tumors grow quickly and painlessly. Research is in progress on the use of proteomics (study of proteins in blood) to identify ovarian cancer in its earlier stages (ACS, 2006a; NWHRC, 2004).

Transvaginal ultrasound and CA-125 screening currently are not recommended for routine screening in the general population but are recommended for women who are BRCA1 mutation carriers (ACS, 2006a). Routine pelvic examination continues to be the only practical screening method for detecting early disease, even though few cancers are detected in women without symptoms. Any ovarian enlargement should be considered highly suggestive and needs further evaluation by laparoscopy or laparotomy. Responsibility for diagnosis rests with the pathologist. The size of the tumor is not indicative of the severity of disease. Clinical staging is done surgically and gives direction to treatment and prognosis (DiSaia & Creasman, 2002).

Therapeutic Management

Treatment is dictated by the stage of the disease at the time of initial diagnosis. Surgical removal of as much of the tumor as possible is the first step in therapy. This may involve just the removal of one ovary and tube or the radical excision of uterus, ovaries, tubes, and omentum. Cytoreductive surgery (the debulking of the poorly vascularized larger tumors) also is done. The smaller the volume of tumor remaining, the better the response to adjuvant therapy. Because about three fourths of women are in stage II, III, or IV disease at the time of diagnosis, surgical cure is not possible; therefore after tumor reduction surgery is performed, women with epithelial cell carcinoma will receive chemotherapy. Many institutions use a multiagent approach. Combinations of antineoplastic drugs such as cyclophosphamide (Cytoxan) and cisplatin or cisplatin and doxorubicin (Adriamycin) are common. Intravenous paclitaxel (Taxol) with cisplatin and other platinum drugs is the standard therapy in the United States. A combination of intravenous paclitaxel and peritoneal cisplatin and paclitaxel has improved survival rates in women with stage III ovarian cancer who have undergone surgical removal (debulking) of most of the tumor (Armstrong et al., 2006).

Combining immunotherapy with chemotherapy is being investigated (DiSaia & Creasman, 2002). Women being treated with chemotherapy are followed up closely with laboratory and radiologic tests and CA-125 levels to monitor their response to the therapy.

Second-look surgery is a technique used to determine the response of the disease to chemotherapy and to determine whether treatment should be continued; however, this is no longer a widely used practice.

Radiation has been used as a palliative measure, and some women have had long-term survival after debulking surgery followed by radiation therapy (NCCN, 2005a). More research is needed regarding the role of radiation therapy in treatment of ovarian cancer.

Nursing Implications

The woman diagnosed with ovarian cancer has concerns similar to those described for the woman with endometrial and cervical cancer. Nursing interventions for the woman having surgery, chemotherapy, or external radiation therapy are described in other sections of this chapter.

Women with advanced ovarian cancer have a significant rate of recurrence. Follow-up for 5 years must be intensive. When a cure or remission cannot be achieved, palliative measures are initiated that alleviate symptoms of the progressing disease and provide comfort and maximal function. As the disease progresses, nutritional support, including enteral feedings and parenteral hyperalimentation, may be needed because of the effects of both the disease and the treatments on the gastrointestinal tract. The goal of nursing care is assisting the woman to maintain quality of life.

Because the period between a focus on cure and a focus on palliation is often prolonged, the woman with ovarian cancer is apt to experience most of the grief stages described by Kübler-Ross and to need support through each. After diagnosis, the woman often experiences denial and then anger. As treatment begins, she may "bargain" for a cure. If treatment is successful and death is forestalled by remission or cure, the process of adjustment to dying ceases, and the woman again focuses on life and its challenges. When treatment fails to secure a cure or remission ends, the woman must turn again to the task of adjustment (see Legal Tip).

■ **LEGAL TIP** Advance Directives
Nurses who work with clients in hospitals with federal funding must know that because of the Patient Self-Determination Act, all clients must be asked if they have knowledge of Advance Directives and be provided with the information if desired. This is important to nurses working in gynecology-oncology settings, where decisions about living wills and "no codes" may be issues.

Family and friends also have diverse feelings. When grieving is prolonged, as it often is when the woman has cancer, the stress can be enormous and can interfere with other interpersonal relationships. If the woman is hospitalized, the environment may further intrude on relationships, limiting privacy and access to the woman and hindering opportunities for caring gestures. The nurse can assist the woman and her family to share their feelings with each other and help them to develop a support network. Referral to a cancer support group may be useful (see National Ovarian Cancer Coalition, www.ovarian.org).

Cancer of the Cervix
Incidence and Etiology

Cancer of the cervix is the third most common reproductive cancer. The accessible location of the cervix to both cell and tissue study and direct examination have led to a refinement of diagnostic techniques, contributing to improved management of these disorders. The incidence of invasive cancer has decreased by 50% over the last 30 years, reducing mortality rates. However, the incidence of preinvasive cancer has increased, and more women in their twenties and thirties are being diagnosed with preinvasive cervical lesions (ACS, 2006a).

Cancer of the cervix begins as neoplastic changes in the cervical epithelium. Terms that have been used to describe these epithelial changes or preinvasive lesions include dysplasia and cervical intraepithelial neoplasia (CIN). Mild cervical dysplasia and CIN 1 refer to abnormal cellular proliferation in the lower one third of the epithelium; this dysplasia tends to be self-limiting and generally regresses to normal. Moderate dysplasia and CIN 2 involve the lower two thirds of the epithelium and may progress to carcinoma in situ. Severe dysplasia and CIN 3 involve the full thickness of the epithelium and often progress to carcinoma in situ. Carcinoma in situ (CIS) is diagnosed when the full thickness of epithelium is replaced with abnormal cells (Fig. 12-11). Newer terms to describe neoplastic changes

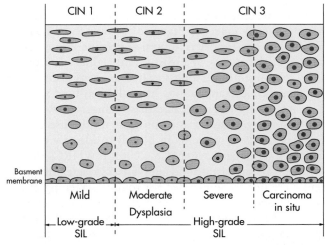

FIG. 12-11 Diagram of cervical epithelium showing progressive changes and various terminology.

are low-grade and high-grade squamous intraepithelial lesions (SILs); however, CIN continues to be a common term used in clinical practice.

Preinvasive lesions are limited to the cervix and usually originate in the squamocolumnar junction or transformation zone (Fig. 12-12). Intensive study of the cervix and the cellular changes that take place has shown that most cervical tumors have a gradual onset rather than an explosive one. Preinvasive conditions may exist for years before the development of invasive disease. These preinvasive conditions are highly treatable in many cases.

Invasive carcinoma is the diagnosis when abnormal cells penetrate the basement membrane and invade the stroma. There are two types of invasive carcinoma of the cervix: microinvasive and invasive. Microinvasive carcinoma is defined as one or more lesions that penetrate no more than 3 mm into the stroma below the basement membrane with no areas of lymphatic or vascular invasion (DiSaia & Creasman, 2002). Invasive carcinoma describes invasion that goes beyond these parameters. The staging of invasive carcinoma extends from stage 0 (CIS) to stage IVb (distant metastasis or disease outside the true pelvis). A number of substages within each stage also exist. Clinical stages for cancer of the cervix are shown in Table 12-3.

Approximately 90% of cervical malignancies are squamous cell carcinomas; 10% are adenocarcinoma. Squamous cell carcinomas can spread by direct extension to the vaginal mucosa, the pelvic wall, the bowels, and the bladder. Metastasis usually occurs in the pelvis, but it can occur to the lungs and the brain through the lymphatic system.

The average age range for the occurrence of cervical cancer is 40 to 50 years; however, preinvasive conditions may exist for 10 to 15 years before the development of an invasive carcinoma. About 90% of cervical cancers are caused by human papillomavirus (HPV) (Kahn, 2005). A strong link has been established between HPV types 16 and 18 and cervical neoplasia. Eighteen other types have been associated with genital tract infections and also may be associated with CIN (ACOG, 2005b; DiSaia & Creasman, 2002). Other sexually transmitted infections that are identified as risk factors are herpes simplex virus II and possibly cytomegalovirus (DiSaia & Creasman, 2002). Other risk factors include early age at first coitus (younger than

table 12-3 FIGO Classification of Cervical Carcinoma

STAGE	DESCRIPTION
0	Carcinoma in situ, intraepithelial carcinoma
I	The carcinoma is strictly confined to the cervix (extension to the corpus should be disregarded)
Ia	Invasive cancer identified only microscopically; all gross lesions, even with superficial invasion, are stage Ib cancers. Invasion is limited to measured stromal invasion with maximum depth of 5.0 mm and no wider than 7.0 mm
Ia1	Measured invasion of stroma 3.0 mm in depth and no wider than 7.0 mm
Ia2	Measured invasion of stroma >3.0 mm and 5.0 mm and no wider than 7.0 mm. The depth of invasion should not be >5.0 mm taken from the base of the epithelium, surface or glandular, from which it originates. Vascular space involvement, venous or lymphatic, should not alter the staging
Ib	Clinical lesions confined to the cervix or preclinical lesions greater than stage Ia
Ib1	Clinical lesions 4.0 cm
Ib2	Clinical lesions >4.0 cm
II	Involvement of the vagina but not the lower third, or infiltration of the parametria but not out to the side wall
IIa	Involvement of the vagina, but no evidence of parametrial involvement
IIb	Infiltration of the parametria, but not out to the side wall
III	Involvement of the lower third of the vagina or extension to the pelvic side wall. All cases with a hydronephrosis or nonfunctioning kidney should be included, unless they are known to be attributable to other cause
IIIa	Involvement of the lower third of the vagina but not out to the pelvic side wall if the parametria are involved
IIIb	Extension onto the pelvic side wall and/or hydronephrosis or nonfunctional kidney
IV	Extension outside the reproductive tract
IVa	Involvement of the mucosa of the bladder or the rectum
IVb	Distant metastasis or disease outside the true pelvis

From DiSaia, P., & Creasman, W. (2002). *Clinical gynecologic oncology* (6th ed.). St. Louis: Mosby.

20 years); multiple sexual partners (more than two); a sexual partner with a history of multiple sexual partners; and belonging to a lower socioeconomic group (ACS, 2006a; DiSaia & Creasman). Other potential factors include use of oral contraceptives, cigarette smoking, and intrauterine exposure to diethylstilbestrol (DES). Vitamins A, C, E, and folate may be protective (Furniss, 2000).

The incidence of cervical cancer in the United States is highest in Hispanic women and lowest in Native-American women, whereas the highest mortality occurs in African-American women (ACS, 2006a). Factors that may influence cervical screening behaviors for these groups include lack of a health promotion or disease prevention perspective,

FIG. 12-12 Location of squamocolumnar junction according to age. The location where the endocervical glands meet the squamous epithelium becomes progressively higher with age. **A,** Puberty. **B,** Reproductive years. **C,** Postmenopausal.

lack of knowledge about Pap smears and availability of services, financial barriers, and failure of health care providers to recommend screening (Giarratano, Bustamante-Forest, & Carter, 2005). There also is a high rate of CIN in human immunodeficiency virus–positive women, suggesting that altered immune status is a risk factor.

Clinical Manifestations and Diagnosis

Preinvasive cancer of the cervix is often asymptomatic. Abnormal bleeding, especially postcoital bleeding, is the classic symptom of invasive cancer. Other late symptoms include rectal bleeding, hematuria, back pain, leg pain, and anemia. Diagnosis includes taking a history that includes menstrual and sexual activity information, particularly a history of sexually transmitted infections and abnormal bleeding episodes (Adams, 2002). A pelvic examination usually will be normal except in late-stage cancer.

The single most reliable method to detect preinvasive cancer is the Pap test. The Pap test will detect 90% of early cervical changes. The U.S. Preventive Services Task Force (USPSTF) and the ACS recommend Pap tests to begin about 3 years after a woman becomes sexually active but not later than age 21. Annual screening is recommended to age 30 (with conventional Pap test; every 2 years if liquid-based Pap tests). After age 30 and three negative Pap tests, screening may be done every 2 to 3 years in consultation with the health care provider. Women ages 65 to 70 with no abnormal tests in the previous 10 years may choose to stop screenings (ACS, 2006a; USPSTF, 2005). Women in high risk categories should have more frequent Pap tests.

Pap test results in the past have been recorded by using several different classification systems. The reporting system most often used today is the Bethesda system, one that reports on gynecologic cytology as well as histology of cervical lesions (Box 12-5). Changes secondary to inflammation, treatment (e.g., radiation), and contraceptive devices can be reported, as well as changes caused by infections. Epithelial cell abnormalities are described in three categories: atypias, or atypical squamous cells (ASC); low-grade squamous intraepithelial lesions (LSILs); and high-grade squamous intraepithelial lesions (HSILs). Several options for follow-up of a finding of ASC of undetermined significance (ASC-US) are suggested. These include repeating cytology at 6 months and 12 months, colposcopy, or HPV testing and referral for colposcopy if test is positive (ACOG, 2005b; NCCN, 2004; Wright et al., 2003). A finding of LSIL may include HPV, mild dysplasia, and CIN 1. Colposcopy is recommended for evaluation of LSIL except in adolescents. These teens can be followed with cytology tests at 6 and 12 months or a single HPV test at 12 months, followed by colposopy if there is an abnormal cytology result or positive HPV test. HSILs include lesions described as moderate dysplasia (CIN 2), severe dysplasia (CIN 3), and carcinoma in situ (CIS). Follow-up for a report of HSIL includes colposcopy and directed biopsy of any visual lesions (ACOG, 20005b; DiSaia & Creasman, 2002; NCCN, 2004).

---

box 12-5 **2001 Bethesda System for Reporting Cervical Cytology Results**

RESULTS/INTERPRETATIONS

Negative for Intraepithelial Malignancy
- Organisms (e.g., *trichomoniasis*, bacterial vaginosis)
- Other nonneoplastic findings (e.g., inflammation, atrophy)
- Other (e.g., endometrial cells)

EPITHELIAL CELL ABNORMALITIES

Squamous Cell
- Atypical squamous cells of undetermined significance (ASC-US)
- Atypical cells and cannot exclude HSIL (ASC-H)
- Low-grade squamous intraepithelial lesion (LSIL); includes human papillomavirus (HPV), mild dysplasia, and cervical intraepithelial neoplasia (CIN) 1
- High-grade squamous intraepithelial lesion (HSIL); includes moderate and severe dysplasia, carcinoma in situ (CIS), CIN 2, and CIN 3
- Squamous cell carcinoma

Glandular Cell
- Atypical cells including endocervical, endometrial, and glandular or not otherwise specified
- Atypical cells including endocervical or glandular, suggestive of neoplasia (endocervical or not otherwise specified)
- Endocervical adenocarcinoma in situ
- Adenocarcinoma (endocervical, endometrial, extrauterine, or not otherwise specified)

Other Malignant Neoplasms

Modified from: National Comprehensive Cancer Network Inc. (2004). *NCCN practice guidelines in oncology. Cervical screening. Version 1.2005.* Accessed www.nccn.org, January 12, 2006; Soloman, D., Davey, D., Kurman, R., Moriarty, A., O'Connor, D., Prey, M. et al., (2002). The 2001 Bethesda System: Terminology for reporting results of cervical cytology. *Journal of the American Medical Association, 287*(16), 2114-2119.

HPV testing has been suggested as an alternative to these methods of follow-up for abnormal Pap results. A consensus conference sponsored by the American Society for Colposcopy and Cervical Pathology published guidelines for management of women with cervical cytology abnormalities. Repeated Pap testing, colposcopy, and DNA HPV tests are all safe and effective. However, if a Pap result shows ASC-US, DNA testing for high risk types of HPV is preferred, particularly if the Pap test was done by using liquid-based screening (Wright et al., 2003).

Colposcopy is the examination of the cervix with a stereoscopic binocular microscope that magnifies the view of the cervix. Usually a solution of 3% acetic acid is applied to the cervix for better visualization of the epithelium and to identify areas for biopsy. Colposcopy is not an invasive procedure and is usually well tolerated by the woman. However, the woman who is scheduled for colposcopy because of an abnormal Pap test may be anxious about the procedure and may need explanations or written information about what to expect during the procedure.

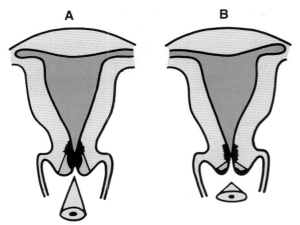

A   **B**

FIG. 12-13   A, Cone biopsy for endocervical disease. Limits of lesion were not seen colposcopically. **B,** Cone biopsy for cervical intraepithelial neoplasia of the exocervix. Limits of lesion were identified colposcopically. (From DiSaia, P., & Creasman, W. [2002]. *Clinical gynecologic oncology* [6th ed.]. St. Louis: Mosby.)

Biopsy is the removal of cervical tissue for study, and several techniques can be used. An endocervical curettage is an effective diagnostic tool in about 90% of cases. It can be performed as an outpatient procedure with little or no anesthesia. It may be uncomfortable, and interventions to help the woman relax and cope with the pain may be needed.

Conization and loop electrosurgical excision procedure (LEEP) (p. 298) can be done as outpatient procedures, although neither is usually done unless the biopsy is positive or the results of the colposcopy are unsatisfactory. Conization involves removal of a cone of tissue from the exocervix and endocervix (Fig. 12-13). It can be done as a cold knife procedure, a laser excision, or an electrosurgical excision (see discussion on p. 298). There are two advantages to a cone biopsy. It can be used (1) to establish the diagnosis and (2) to effect a cure. If CIS is diagnosed, and if the woman wishes to retain her childbearing capacity, conization removes the abnormal tissue; further treatment (e.g., hysterectomy) is unnecessary. The woman is monitored with Pap tests and colposcopy when indicated.

If invasive cancer is diagnosed, other diagnostic tests are done to assess the extent of spread (see earlier discussion under endometrial cancer). Once the extent of the cancer is known, treatment begins.

▬ CARE MANAGEMENT

▬ Assessment and Nursing Diagnoses

For the woman diagnosed with invasive carcinoma of the cervix, pretherapy assessment includes physical, psychologic, and educational components, regardless of whether surgery or radiation is the method of treatment. Physical assessment includes a review of current medications, because medications for other medical problems may have to be continued. Skin is assessed to identify potential pressure points; respiratory and gastrointestinal status and state

of nutrition are important factors to assess. Urinalysis and complete blood count also are commonly performed. An electrocardiogram and a chest x-ray examination may be done if use of a general anesthetic is anticipated for surgery or placement of internal applicators.

Psychologic assessment is important because frequently these women are emotionally distressed about the diagnosis and anticipated treatment (i.e., fear of being radioactive and fear of pain) and fear that family or significant others will become distant.

Educational assessment involves identifying the woman's current knowledge base regarding the diagnosis and proposed therapeutic regimen. Nursing diagnoses for the woman having surgery for cervical cancer are similar to those identified for the woman having a hysterectomy for endometrial cancer (see p. 292). Nursing diagnoses that might arise from an assessment for the woman who is to have external or internal radiation therapy for treatment of cervical cancer include the following:

- *Deficient knowledge related to*
  –treatment procedures
- *Fear/anxiety related to*
  –diagnosis
  –anticipated pain
  –concerns about radioactivity
  –the response of the significant other or family
- *Disturbed sensory perception related to*
  –internal radiation therapy
  –restricted contact with visitors and nursing staff
- *Risk for impaired skin integrity related to*
  –external radiation exposure
  –immobility and bed rest (internal radiation therapy)
- *Risk for injury related to*
  –dislodgment of radiation source
- *Acute pain related to*
  –internal applicators
- *Sexual dysfunction related to*
  –treatment or concerns of significant other

▬ Expected Outcomes of Care

Mutually determined outcomes for the woman undergoing radiation therapy for cervical cancer related to the identified nursing diagnoses might include that the woman will do the following:

- Verbalize an understanding of the proposed treatment and accompanying procedures.
- Verbalize her fears regarding diagnosis, treatment, and response of significant others and family.
- Maintain contact with family and friends through short visits or by telephone if internal radiation therapy is done.
- Remain free from skin breakdown.
- Identify methods to maintain skin hygiene.
- Remain on strict bed rest on her back to prevent dislodgment of the internal applicators if internal radiation therapy is done.

- Verbalize control of pain.
- Resume a satisfactory sexual relationship with her partner.

▬ Plan of Care and Interventions
▬ *Preinvasive Lesions*

Once a diagnosis has been identified, a course of treatment is planned. For preinvasive lesions, several techniques are used. As stated earlier, because many preinvasive conditions are detected in younger women who may wish to continue childbearing, treatment is geared toward eradicating abnormal cells while attempting to preserve the structure of the cervix. The techniques currently available for preinvasive lesions are cryotherapy, laser therapy, and LEEP. These three techniques have comparable success rates in treating CIN successfully (ACOG, 2005b). Treatment for invasive cancer includes surgery, radiation therapy, and chemotherapy.

Cryosurgery. Cryosurgery uses a freezing technique that freezes abnormal cells, and when sloughing occurs, normal tissue is regenerated. Side effects occurring after treatment are usually few and not of a serious nature. A profuse watery discharge can persist for 2 to 4 weeks. Follow-up examination and a Pap test are scheduled in 4 to 6 months. Endocervical cells are thought to regenerate, leaving a normal cervical canal in most instances. Spotting or cervical stenosis are rare complications. Surveillance with frequent Pap tests and colposcopic examination must continue indefinitely after this type of conservative therapy. Persistent abnormal cells require reevaluation, and plans are made for repeated cryosurgery or other therapy.

Laser Ablation. Laser ablation uses a laser mounted on a colposcope that allows precise direction of a beam of light (heat) to remove diseased tissue. An endometrial sampling is recommended before ablation to avoid removal of unrecognized invasive cancer. For treatment of the cervix (relatively insensitive tissue), the woman may need no anesthesia. Some women complain of a burning or cramping sensation that is tolerable for most women. The cervix treated with CO_2 laser will show epithelial regrowth beginning by 2 days afterward. The site is usually healed in 4 to 6 weeks. The original architecture of the cervix is preserved, and the squamocolumnar junction remains visible; however, there may be more damage to normal tissues than with other treatments. Women usually have less vaginal discharge than with cryosurgery, but there may be more discomfort after the procedure (Stenchever et al., 2001).

Electrosurgical Excision. The LEEP is a standard treatment for cervical dysplasia in the United States. This procedure uses a wire loop electrode that can excise and cauterize with minimal tissue damage (Fig. 12-14). Healing is rapid, and there is only a mild discharge afterward. Possible complications include bleeding, cervical stenosis, infertility, and loss of cervical mucus (ACOG, 2005b).

▬ *Invasive Cancer of the Cervix*

Once the cancer is staged, treatment is begun. Microinvasive cancer is usually treated with conization, but a hysterectomy is often done if childbearing is not desired. The choice of treatment for early-stage invasive cancer is by either surgery or radiation therapy, because survival rates are comparable (DiSaia & Creasman, 2002). Locally advanced

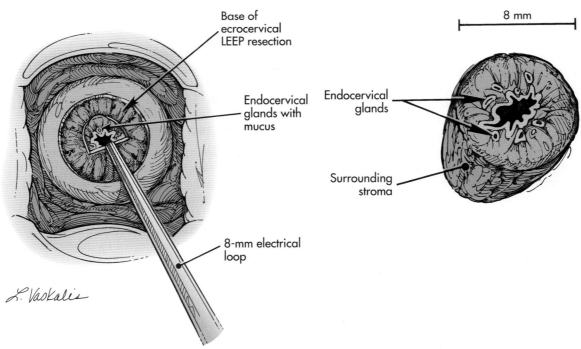

FIG. 12-14 Electrosurgical excision. The electric loop vaporizes quickly and removes cone of tissue. (From Nichols, D., & Clark-Pearson, D. [2000]. *Gynecologic, obstetric, and related surgery* [2nd ed.]. St. Louis: Mosby.)

CRITICAL THINKING EXERCISE

Informed Decision-Making for Cervical Cancer Treatment

Betsy, a 34-year-old married Caucasian, has just been diagnosed with moderate dysplasia (cervical intraepithelial neoplasia [CIN 2]). She has expressed concern about the treatment since she does not want to have a hysterectomy and her friends have told her that she will probably have to have one. What response by the nurse would be appropriate?

1. Evidence: Is there sufficient evidence to draw conclusions about what the nurse should say?
2. Assumptions: What assumptions can be made about the following issues?
   a. Differences between dysplasia and invasive cervical cancer
   b. Differences between conization and hysterectomy as cervical cancer treatments
3. What implications and priorities for nursing care can be made at this time?
4. Does the evidence objectively support your conclusion?
5. Are there alternative perspectives to your conclusion?

stages of cervical cancer usually are treated with radiation therapy, both external and internal. A radical hysterectomy is performed if the cancer has extended beyond the cervix but not to the pelvic wall. Late stages may be treated with radiation and chemotherapy (ACS, 2006a).

Radical Hysterectomy. *Radical hysterectomy* involves removal of the uterus, the tubes, the ovaries, the upper third of the vagina, the entire uterosacral and uterovesical ligaments, and all of the parametrium on each side, along with pelvic node dissection encompassing the four major pelvic lymph node chains: ureteral, obturator, hypogastric, and iliac. Dissection serves to preserve the bladder, the rectum, and the ureters while removing as much of the remaining tissue of the pelvis as is feasible. Women with positive pelvic nodes usually receive postoperative whole pelvis irradiation, although there is little evidence that it alters the incidence of recurrence in the pelvic area (DiSaia & Creasman, 2002).

Nursing Management. Nursing care for the woman having a radical hysterectomy was discussed in the previous section on endometrial cancer (p. 290).

Radiation Therapy. Radiation may be delivered by internal radium applications to the cervix or external radiation therapy that includes lymphatics of the pelvic side wall. In preparation for radiation therapy, the woman must maintain good nutritional status and a high-protein, high-vitamin, and high-calorie diet. Anemia, if present, should be corrected before the initiation of radiotherapy.

External radiation therapy and internal radiation therapy are given in various combinations for the best results and are tailored to each woman and her particular lesion. For example, external radiation may be given first to treat regional pelvic nodes and to shrink the tumor. External irradiation is usually an outpatient procedure given 5 days

a week for 4 to 6 weeks. Internal radiation therapy consists of one or two intracavitary treatments at least 2 weeks apart (DiSaia & Creasman, 2002).

External irradiation is provided by megavoltage machines such as cobalt, and supervoltage machines such as linear accelerators and betatron, all which have the distinct advantage of providing a more homogeneous dose to the pelvis. Before treatment begins, a localization procedure is done to determine the best way to deliver the treatments. Markings or small tattoos are placed on the body to make sure the woman is positioned correctly to get the treatment (Iwamoto, 2001).

For internal radiation therapy, the woman may be treated in the hospital or in a special outpatient unit. If treatment is done in the hospital, the woman is taken to the operating room, and while she is under general or spinal anesthesia, a specially designed applicator is placed into her vagina and cervix. X-rays are taken to make sure the applicator is correctly placed. The woman is returned to her room, where the radioactive source is placed into the applicator (Fig. 12-15). The source remains in place from 12 hours to 3 days. If treatment is in the outpatient setting, the applicator is inserted into the uterus in a treatment room; use of high-dose implants shortens the treatment time (DiSaia & Creasman, 2002).

In advanced carcinoma of the cervix, conventional intracavitary applicators are not applicable. Interstitial therapy uses a template to guide the transperineal insertion of a group of 18-gauge hollow steel needles into the lesion (Fig. 12-16). After the needles are placed, the iridium wires are inserted when the woman is returned to her room.

Nursing Management. Nursing actions for external and internal radiation differ, so they are discussed separately.

External Therapy. Before external radiation therapy, the woman's anxiety may be so high that information given by the radiologist may not be processed. The nurse should reinforce or fill in gaps, especially related to the following: the equipment, which is similar to that used for x-ray examination except larger; the hyperbaric oxygen chamber,

FIG. 12-15 Intracavitary implant. Applicator in place in uterus is loaded with radium source.

FIG. 12-16 Interstitial-intracavitary implant.

which may be used to increase cellular oxygen and thus make tumor cells more radiosensitive; the radiotherapist, who will be behind a shield, but still close by and in communication with her; the position she will be put in and asked to maintain for some minutes; and the therapy, which is painless.

During the course of the therapy, the woman is counseled regarding maintaining general good health. To maintain good skin care, the woman is taught to assess her skin often; avoid soaps, ointments, cosmetics, and deodorants if the axilla is being irradiated, and so on, because these may contain metals that would alter the dose she receives and could lead to skin breakdown; wear loose clothing over the area and cotton underwear (or no underwear); use an air mattress or cover the mattress with foam pads or sheepskin; avoid exposing the irradiated areas to temperature extremes (e.g., hot tubs); and especially avoid removing the markings made by the radiologist. If her skin becomes red or itchy, treat it with remedies recommended by the radiologist (e.g., aloe vera lotion, Aquaphor, or warm sitz baths). To treat skin that is broken or desquamating, the woman is shown how to use remedies prescribed by the radiologist (e.g., irrigation with equal parts peroxide and saline, application of antibiotic or lanolin ointment, exposure to air, and application of a loose dressing). The use of adhesive (or any) tape directly on the target area of skin should be avoided (Iwamoto, 2001; Stenchever et al., 2001).

■ **NURSE ALERT**

If a woman is receiving chemotherapy during radiation therapy, she is at a higher risk for developing a skin infection (Iwamoto, 2001).

To maintain good nutrition, the woman is reminded to maintain a daily record of weight; use high-protein supplements; eat small, attractive, appetizing meals that are more bland than spicy; and keep the environment light, airy, clean, and quiet (especially before and after meals). A dietitian consult may be needed to help the woman and her family plan to meet the woman's nutritional needs. If the woman is ill enough to be hospitalized, she may need total parenteral nutrition or tube feedings. Nausea interferes with adequate intake; therefore the woman may take antiemetics, as necessary. High daily fluid intake (2 to 3 L) should be suggested if not contraindicated. To increase her comfort, minimize infection, and promote adequate food intake, the woman is encouraged to perform frequent oral hygiene. Box 12-4 (p. 293) provides other suggestions for nutritional problems associated with radiation treatment.

The nurse explains, as necessary, the need for routine blood studies to monitor white blood cell count (to determine degree of immunosuppression). The woman and her family will need information about neutropenia, thrombocytopenia, and anemia and precautions to be taken. Because the woman is more vulnerable to infection, she is reminded of general measures to avoid infection (e.g., practice good hygiene, avoid people with infection, avoid large crowds, keep environment clean).

After the radiation treatment is completed, the woman needs information for self-care (see Teaching for Self Care box). She should also be informed that side effects of the treatment can continue for weeks after the therapy is completed.

Internal Therapy. Internal radiation therapy may require hospitalization or be done in a special outpatient unit. Radiation safety officers determine the precautions to be observed in each situation. This discussion focuses on treatment in the hospital setting, but similar precautions would be used in the outpatient setting. Printed instruction sheets are usually available stating precautions to be followed for each type of radiation substance used. A precaution sign is placed on the door of the woman's room.

TEACHING FOR SELF-CARE

Care After External Radiation Therapy

- Avoid infection and report symptoms of infection to health care provider immediately.
- Maintain good nutrition and fluid intake.
- Anticipate possible effects of radiation for 10 to 14 days after last treatment.
- Expect signs of healing to occur in about 3 weeks.
- Maintain good skin and mouth care to support a sense of well-being and prevent infection.
- Report the following symptoms to your health care provider:
  Continued gastrointestinal symptoms (nausea, vomiting, anorexia, diarrhea)
  Increasing skin irritation at the site of therapy (redness, swelling, pain, pruritus)
- Take medications as prescribed, and avoid any medications not prescribed or approved by health care provider.

■ NURSE ALERT

Personnel who come in direct contact with anyone receiving radiation therapy should wear a film badge or other device to monitor the amount of exposure received.

Nurses must protect themselves from overexposure to radiation. Precautions include the following behaviors (Iwamato, 2001):

- Careful isolation techniques: wearing gloves while handling bodily fluids and observing good handwashing technique. These behaviors reflect knowledge that alpha and beta rays cannot pass through skin but may be in body fluids and excrement.
- Careful planning of nursing activity to limit time (to 30 minutes or less per 8 hours) spent in close proximity to the woman to avoid exposure to gamma rays, which can penetrate several inches of lead.

Exposure to radiation is controlled in three ways: distance, time, and shielding (with lead). For the woman with sealed radiotherapy, a movable lead screen can be placed between the area in which the therapeutic applicator is located and the personnel. The lead screen also is used to protect visitors from radiation. Increasing the distance from the source also decreases exposure (Iwamoto, 2001).

Familiarity with applicators is a must for all nurses working with people receiving radiotherapy so that if a "strange object" is found in the linen or on the floor, it is not touched. Today most hospital protocols include having a lead container and forceps in the room for use if a radioactive implant is dislodged.

The woman is prepared for insertion with the following care, which is accompanied by an explanation for each activity. To reduce the need for an enema or attention to bowel elimination for a few days, the gastrointestinal tract is usually prepared by using low-residue diet, enemas, and sometimes bowel sedation. The vaginal vault is usually prepared with an antiseptic douche, such as povidone-iodine.

An indwelling urinary bladder catheter is inserted, as ordered, to prevent urinary distention that could dislodge the applicator. Nothing is taken by mouth the night before the procedure in anticipation of general anesthesia. Preoperative medications may be ordered for the morning of the procedure. Deep-breathing exercises, range of motion exercises, and positioning are all demonstrated before the procedure to minimize the effects of immobilization afterward. An intravenous (IV) solution will probably be started before the procedure, and IV therapy may be continued if nausea prevents good intake of oral fluids. The woman is assured that pain will be managed.

Explanations about restricted visitation of personnel and visitors also are given in the preinsertion phase. Women are often encouraged to bring reading materials to the hospital to combat the boredom that isolation imposes on them (Iwamoto, 2001). In addition many units are equipped with television, CD, and video/DVD players.

The applicator is inserted into the woman's vaginal vault during surgery and after the usual postanesthesia recovery care, the woman is returned to her room, where the applicators are loaded with the radioactive substance.

A lead shield is placed next to the bed in line with the woman's pelvic area to protect the care givers and visitors. Vital signs are monitored every 4 hours. Active range of motion and deep-breathing exercises are encouraged every 2 hours; the woman is positioned on her back and may not be permitted to turn from side to side, although logrolling may be done occasionally to relieve back pressure. The head of the bed may or may not be elevated slightly (Iwamoto, 2001).

The woman's diet is changed from clear liquid to low residue, as ordered. Many women have difficulty eating while lying flat or even if the bed is elevated slightly. The nurse arranges the food so that it is easy to reach. Finger foods or liquids are generally more manageable. Parenteral or oral fluids are given, up to 3 L daily.

The urinary catheter remains in the bladder while the implant is in place. However, no perineal or catheter care is given. Intake and output are measured. The woman is given a partial bath, washing only above her waist. Massage is restricted to her shoulders and neck. Linen is changed only as absolutely necessary. Any linen or equipment used is retained in the room until therapy is complete to prevent loss of an applicator or seed. If vaginal or rectal bleeding or hematuria occurs, the physician is notified immediately.

Emotional support is provided by planning to be with the woman for short periods; encouraging her to verbalize concerns and needs; and encouraging family members, clergy, or others to visit for short periods daily or to communicate by telephone. Pregnant women and children are not permitted to visit.

Many women undergoing internal radiation treatment are given medication to prevent complications and to promote comfort during the procedure. Such medications might include antibiotics to prevent bladder infections, heparin injections to prevent thrombophlebitis, sedatives for relaxation, antiemetics for nausea, and narcotics for pain. The woman is considered radioactive during the time the internal sources are in place (Iwamoto, 2001).

After the radium is removed, the Foley catheter is removed, and the woman is assisted in getting out of bed the first time. She is usually discharged the same day. Discharge teaching can be found in the Teaching for Self-Care box. The woman and her family are reassured that she is not radioactive after the treatment.

Posttreatment complications range from those arising from immobilization, such as thrombophlebitis, pulmonary embolism, and pneumonia, to those arising from the treatment itself, such as hemorrhage, skin reactions (rashes or inflammation), diarrhea, cramping, dysuria, and vaginal stenosis. The woman is assessed for any of these complications before discharge.

The woman may experience altered patterns of sexuality related to treatment side effects. A decrease in vaginal secretions and sensation may occur, as well as vaginal stenosis. These can contribute to decreased sexual desire,

TEACHING FOR SELF-CARE

Care After Internal Radiation Therapy

- Eat three balanced meals a day, and increase fluid to 3 L daily.
- Rest when tired, and resume normal activities as comfort permits.
- Maintain good hygiene (e.g., daily showers and daily douches until discharge stops).
- Use vaginal dilator if needed for vaginal stenosis. Sexual intercourse may be resumed in 7 to 10 days or as recommended by physician.
- Understand that sterility and cessation of menstruation usually occur with this procedure if you are premenopausal.
- Report any of the following to your health care provider: bleeding (vaginal, rectal, or in the urine), foul-smelling vaginal discharge, fever, abdominal distention, or pain.
- Take any prescribed medications as directed.
- Call your health care provider or clinic if there are concerns or problems.
- Plan follow-up visits to determine emotional as well as physical recovery.

because pain and discomfort during intercourse can affect the desire to resume sexual activities. The nurse can initiate a discussion with the woman and her partner, offer information about the effects of radiation on the ability to have sexual intercourse, and offer suggestions for specific problems, such as using a water-based lubricant for vaginal dryness and using a vaginal dilator 3 times a week for a year or more. If necessary, the couple can be referred to other resources (Iwamoto, 2001; Wilmoth & Spinelli, 2000).

Complications of Radiation Therapy. Morbidity as a direct result from properly conducted therapy is usually minimal. Some of the morbidity seen may be caused by the uncontrolled tumor and not by the therapy. Acute treatment complications occurring during or shortly after therapy include irritation of the rectum, the small bowel, and the bladder; reactions in the skin folds; and mild bone marrow suppression. Dysuria and frequency may occur. Late complications, although not common, include genital fistulas and necrosis (Stenchever et al., 2001).

▬ *Recurrent and Advanced Cancer of the Cervix*

Approximately one third of women with invasive cervical cancer will have recurrent or persistent disease after therapy (Stenchever et al., 2001). Prognosis is discouraging, with a 1-year survival rate between 10% and 15% (DiSaia & Creasman, 2002). Irradiation of metastatic areas is commonly successful in providing local control and symptomatic relief. Irradiation for recurrent disease may be considered for women who were initially treated with surgery. Further radiation may not be effective for those women who were initially treated with radiation.

Pelvic Exenteration. The woman who has recurrence only within the pelvis may be considered for pelvic

exenteration if a cure is thought to be possible. A total exenteration involves removal of the perineum, the pelvic floor, the levator muscles, and all reproductive organs. Additionally, pelvic lymph nodes, rectum, sigmoid colon, urinary bladder, and distal ureters are removed, and a colostomy and ileal conduit are constructed (Fig. 12-17, *A*). In very select cases, the procedure can be modified to either an anterior or a posterior exenteration. In anterior pelvic exenteration, all of the previously mentioned pelvic viscera are removed except the rectosigmoid, which is preserved. Urine is rerouted through an ileal conduit (Fig. 12-17, *B*). In the posterior pelvic exenteration procedure, all pelvic viscera with the exception of the bladder are removed. The

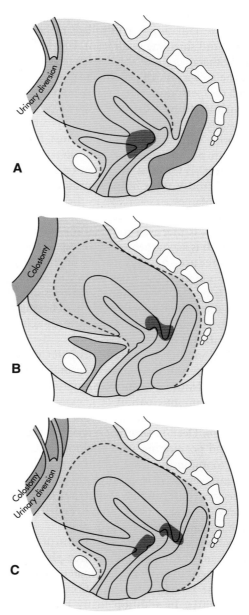

FIG. 12-17 Pelvic exenteration procedures. **A,** Anterior exenteration. **B,** Posterior exenteration. **C,** Total exenteration. (From DiSaia, P., & Morrow, C. [1973]. *California Medicine, 118,* p. 13, Feb.)

feces are rerouted through a colostomy (Fig. 12-17, *C*). A neovagina (new vagina) may be constructed.

Women are carefully selected for this procedure; 5-year survival rates range from 20% to 62% (DiSaia & Creasman, 2002). Many of the complications that follow this surgery are those that follow any form of major surgery, for example, pulmonary embolism, pulmonary edema, myocardial infarction, and cerebrovascular accident. These complications are seen immediately after surgery. Infection originating in the pelvic cavity usually occurs later, if it occurs.

Nursing Management. Nursing care of the woman having a pelvic exenteration depends on what is removed. General preoperative considerations include assessments similar to those for a woman having a radical hysterectomy. Additionally, a thorough sexual assessment is needed because of the drastic changes involved. The woman needs information about the construction of a neovagina if that is an option. She will need to be assessed for stoma site selection and information about management of colostomy or ileal conduit if appropriate. Extensive preoperative bowel preparation is needed before surgery. Pain management is discussed, as is what to expect postoperatively (e.g., nasogastric tubes, arterial catheters). Significant others should be included in preoperative discussions when possible, because their postoperative support is essential.

Postoperative care usually begins in an intensive care unit until the woman's condition is stable. She is monitored for signs of complications, including shock, hemorrhage, pulmonary embolus and other pulmonary complications, fluid and electrolyte imbalance, and urinary complications (Otto, 2001). Nursing care continues after the woman is stabilized and moved back to her room. Wound care consists of irrigation with half-strength normal saline, followed by drying of the area with either a hair dryer on cool setting or a heat lamp placed at least 12 inches from the perineal area. The woman is taught how to care for her colostomy or ileal conduit when she is able to begin self-care. Assessment for psychologic reactions is important. The woman will probably experience a grief reaction over her mutilated body. She may become depressed during the long convalescence.

The woman may be discharged to a long-term care facility or to her home. She will need assistance in her physical care for at least 6 months. Teaching needed for home care includes colostomy or ureterostomy care; dietary needs for healing; perineal care, including use of perineal pads to protect clothing from discharge; range of motion exercises and physical activities permitted by her health care provider; and signs of complication, especially infection and bowel obstruction (Otto, 2001).

Because the woman will have sexual disruption and the possibility of not being able to have vaginal intercourse (if the vagina is not reconstructed), counseling about sexual activity is needed. Usually even with a vaginal reconstruction, vaginal intercourse is not advised until healing has taken place, usually 12 to 18 months. Women with neovaginas may complain of decreased vaginal sensations or chronic discharge, or that the vagina is too short or too long. Women with colostomies or ureterostomies may worry about leakage or odors during sexual activities. Women may be concerned about their change in appearance. They may need counseling about alternative activities for sexual expression for themselves and their partners. The woman and her partner may need referral for further sexual counseling (Wilmoth & Spinelli, 2000).

Chemotherapy. Chemotherapy may be used in advanced cancer of the cervix to reduce tumor size before surgery or as adjuvant therapy for poor-prognosis tumors. In general, no long-term benefits are derived with chemotherapy, although giving chemotherapy concurrent with radiation therapy may improve survival (ACS, 2006a). Cisplatin and 5-FU are the most effective; other chemotherapeutic agents used singly or in combination include ifosfamide, carboplatin, doxorubicin, methotrexate, vinblastine, bleomycin, and paclitaxel (Iwamoto, 2001). Chemotherapy is beneficial as a pain-relief method (DiSaia & Creasman, 2002).

■ Evaluation

The nurse can be reasonably assured that care was effective to the extent that the expected outcomes of care for the woman who has had radiation therapy or other treatment have been achieved.

Cancer of the Vulva
Incidence and Etiology

Vulvar carcinoma accounts for about 5% of all female genital malignancies and is the fourth most commonly occurring gynecologic cancer. It appears most frequently in older women in their middle sixties to seventies; DNA testing of these women often shows mutation of the p53 tumor suppressor gene (ACS, 2006b). Fifteen percent of vulvar cancers occur in women under 40 years of age: HPV infection is thought to be responsible for most of these cancers (ACS). Women who have a history of genital warts (condylomata acuminata) and who smoke have an increased risk of developing vulvar cancer (ACS).

By far the majority (90%) of vulvar carcinoma is squamous cell; other vulvar neoplasms are attributed to Paget's disease, adenocarcinoma of Bartholin glands, fibrosarcoma and melanoma, and basal cell carcinoma. Vulvar intraepithelial neoplasia (VIN) is the first neoplastic change. VIN progresses over time to CIS, and then to invasive cancer. Metastatic spread is by direct extension and lymphatic spread.

Prognosis depends on the size of the lesion and the tumor grade at the time of diagnosis. Fifty percent of women have symptoms for 2 to 16 months before seeking treatment. Fortunately, vulvar cancer grows slowly, extends slowly, and metastasizes fairly late. Even with a pattern of delayed diagnosis, survival rates are greater than 90% for all stages if nodes are negative. Survival rates plummet to less than 50%, however, if lymph node metastasis has occurred (DiSaia & Creasman, 2002).

Clinical Manifestations and Diagnosis

The most common site for vulvar lesions is on the labia majora. The vulvar lesion is usually asymptomatic until it is 1 to 2 cm in diameter. When it is symptomatic, women may complain of vulvar pruritus or burning or pain. Necrosis and infection of the lesion result in ulceration with bleeding or watery discharge.

VINs are usually multifocal in young women. Unifocal lesions are associated with invasive cancer and are more common in older women. Initially, growth is superficial but later extends into the urethra, the vagina, and the anus. In approximately 50% of late cases, superficial inguinal and femoral lymph nodes become involved.

Simple biopsy with histologic evaluation reveals the diagnosis. The areas of pathologic involvement are identified by staining the vulva with toluidine blue (1%), allowing an absorption time of 3 to 5 minutes, and then washing with acetic acid (2% to 3%); abnormal tissue retains the dye. Biopsy is necessary to rule out such conditions as sexually transmitted infections (e.g., chancroid, granuloma inguinale, syphilis), basal cell carcinoma, and CIS. In situ malignancies are initially small, red, white, or pigmented friable papules. In Paget's disease, the lesions are red, moist, and elevated. Melanomas appear as bluish-black, pigmented, or papillary lesions. Melanomas metastasize through the bloodstream and lymphatics.

Collaborative Care

Therapeutic Management. Treatment varies, depending on the extent of the disease. Laser surgery, cryosurgery, or electrosurgical excision may be used to treat VIN. A disadvantage to these treatments is that healing is slow, and the treated area is painful. A local wide excision may be performed for localized lesions.

There are several types of vulvectomy procedures used for CIS and invasive cancer. A *skinning vulvectomy* involves removal of the superficial vulvar skin; however, this procedure is rarely done (ACS, 2006b).

A *simple vulvectomy* involves removal of part or all of the vulva (external genital organs including the mons pubis, labia majora and minora, and possibly the clitoris). The clitoris usually can be saved if there is not cancer present.

For invasive disease, a *partial* or *complete radical vulvectomy* is performed. A partial vulvectomy is the removal of part of the vulva and deep tissues; a complete vulvectomy includes the removal of the whole vulva, deep tissues, and the clitoris (Fig. 12-18).

Skin grafts may be done if a large area of skin is removed during the vulvectomy; however, most surgeries can be closed without grafts. If grafts are needed, a surgeon who performs reconstruction surgery may be consulted (ACS, 2006b).

The inguinal nodes may be removed through an inguinal (groin) node dissection. Usually only lymph nodes on the same side as the cancer are removed; however nodes on both sides may be removed if the cancer is in the mid-

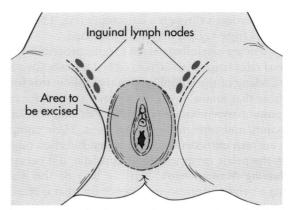

FIG. 12-18 Radical vulvectomy. Note dotted lines denoting vulvectomy incision and inguinal groin incisions.

dle (see Fig. 12-18). Swelling of the leg often is a problem after this surgery.

A *sentinel node biopsy* may be done instead of the inguinal node dissection. This procedure involves injecting blue dye or radioactive material into the tumor site. A scan is performed to identify the sentinel (first) node to pick up the dye or radioactive material. The node is removed for microscopic study. If cancer cells are found, the rest of the lymph nodes will be removed, but if cancer is not found, further lymph node removal is not done. This procedure continues to be studied (ACS, 2006b).

External radiation therapy can be used to shrink tumors before surgery, but it is not used as the primary treatment. Postoperative external radiation therapy may be used for women who are at risk for recurrence. Radiation treatment causes dermatitis and ulceration that are uncomfortable for the woman.

Chemotherapy has not been very effective as a treatment except for the topical application of 5-FU for VIN or CIS. This treatment is painful and not used often. Chemotherapy continues to be investigated in combination with radiation as an adjunct to surgery in advanced cancer of the vulva (ACS, 2006b; Gynecologic Cancer Foundation, 2005).

Nursing Management. Nursing care for the woman with vulvar cancer is similar to that for the woman with other gynecologic malignancies. A history of symptoms and a physical examination should be done. An assessment of the woman's understanding of the surgical procedure and her emotional state also should be done. Nursing diagnoses for women with vulvar cancer are similar to those for other gynecologic cancers; possible nursing diagnoses specific to problems with vulvar cancer treatment include the following:

- *Risk for infection related to*
  –surgical incision
- *Sexual dysfunction related to*
  –vulvectomy

• Disturbed body image related to
  −loss of sexual organ
  −perceived or actual disfigurement
  −altered patterns of elimination as a result of surgery

Interventions for the woman treated with laser therapy include applying topical steroids to the area, administering sitz baths and drying the area with a hair dryer, applying local anesthetics, or giving oral pain medication as needed. Women need to be informed that pain may get worse 3 to 4 days after the treatment.

A woman undergoing radical vulvectomy requires some special nursing actions in addition to the routine postoperative care given (see Teaching for Self-Care box). Additional nursing actions focused on the prevention of infection include the following:

- Irrigate the surgical site with half-strength normal saline or other recommended solution after each elimination.
- Dry the area thoroughly by using a hair dryer on cool setting or a heat lamp.
- Use a bed cradle or other means to lift the bed covers and allow air to circulate around the wound.
- Give stool softeners to decrease straining and disruption of the suture line.
- Note any change in color of the surgical site.
- Note any drainage or foul odor and, if present, notify primary health care provider.
- Perform catheter care as needed.
- Provide and instruct woman in the use of sitz baths.

The woman is at high risk for sexual dysfunction related to the effects of the surgery. For example, the woman may have concerns that her partner will be repulsed by the scarring and loss of the vulva. She also may have concerns about reaching orgasm and vaginal numbness or painful

---

TEACHING FOR SELF-CARE

Care After Radical Vulvectomy

- Avoid sexual activity for 4 to 6 weeks or as health care provider directs.
- Rest frequently.
- Avoid crossing legs, sitting, or standing for long periods.
- Avoid tight, constricting clothing, and wear cotton underwear.
- Keep perineal area clean and dry. Wash perineum with a solution of peroxide and water after each elimination, and pat dry.
- Report to your health care provider any swelling, redness, unusual tenderness, drainage, or foul odor of incision site.
- Report any temperature over 38.4° C.
- Eat a well-balanced diet to promote healing.
- Take all medications as prescribed.
- Elevate legs periodically to prevent pelvic congestion.
- Call your health care provider or clinic if there are concerns or problems.

---

vaginal penetration. Nursing actions that focus on minimizing these risks include the following:

- Encouraging verbalization of feelings
- Providing privacy for discussion
- Encouraging open communication between woman and partner
- Discussing when sexual activity can be safely resumed
- Discussing alternative methods to achieve sexual satisfaction
- Providing information about use of vaginal dilators and water-soluble lubricants for painful vaginal intercourse
- Providing resources for counseling if necessary

Cancer of the Vagina

Vaginal carcinomas account for only 1% to 2% of gynecologic malignancy, with a peak incidence between 50 and 70 years of age. Most lesions are squamous cell carcinomas, and most are secondary carcinomas of the vagina rather than primary tumors. Vaginal intraepithelial neoplasia (VAIN) is uncommon, and clear-cell adenocarcinoma is even rarer. It is found primarily in young women (aged 15 to 30 years) and is related to intrauterine exposure to DES. Sarcoma botryoides (embryonal rhabdomyosarcoma) occurs in infants and children.

The etiology is unknown, but vaginal cancer may be caused by chronic vaginal irritation, vaginal trauma, and genital viruses. Women with VAIN often have had cancer or currently have cancer of another part of the genital tract (DiSaia & Creasman, 2002). Vaginal lesions, usually seen in the upper one third of the vagina, often extend into the bladder and the rectum in late stages. Metastasis can occur early because of the rich lymphatic drainage in the vaginal area.

Some women with vaginal cancer are asymptomatic. Diagnosis often comes after an abnormal Pap test. Symptoms that have been associated with vaginal cancer include bleeding after coitus or examination, dyspareunia, and watery discharge. Bladder involvement results in urinary frequency or urgency; rectal extension causes painful defecation. A pelvic examination may reveal a single lesion, although multiple lesions are common.

Colposcopy examination and biopsy of Schiller-stained areas disclose the diagnosis. Therapy for vaginal cancer is directed by the extent of the lesion and the age and condition of the woman. Local excision is the preferred therapy for localized lesions. Topical application of 5-FU cream has been used with varying results. Laser surgery may be used to treat VAIN. Radical hysterectomy and removal of the upper vagina with dissection of the pelvic nodes or internal and external radiation are options for invasive cancer. Radiation therapy is the usual treatment of choice. If a vaginectomy is performed, sexual function will be lost without reconstructive surgery. Chemotherapy has not been effective in treatment of vaginal cancer, although studies are being conducted on the effectiveness of chemotherapy in combination with radiation. In early-stage cancer, 5-year survival rates approach 70% to 80%, with stage II survival rates in the 50% range (DiSaia & Creasman, 2002).

Nursing care for the woman with vaginal cancer is similar to that for other gynecologic cancers. Sexual counseling or referral may be needed.

Cancer of the Uterine Tubes

Primary carcinoma of the uterine (fallopian) tube (usually the distal one third) is rare (less than 1%), with a peak incidence between ages 50 and 60 years. The cause is unknown. Most women are asymptomatic in the early stages of tubal cancer. Vaginal bleeding is the most common symptom of tubal cancer, but clear vaginal discharge and lower abdominal pain also occur frequently. An enlarging unilateral pelvic mass or ascites may occur and is often misdiagnosed as ovarian carcinoma or endometrial carcinoma. Differential diagnosis of tubal cancer is usually made postoperatively. It is currently recommended that therapy guidelines parallel those established for ovarian carcinoma; therefore tumor-reducing surgery such as a total abdominal hysterectomy with bilateral salpingo-oophorectomy and omentectomy (removal of connective tissue covering the organs) is performed. Postoperative therapy consists of chemotherapy with cisplatin or other platinum-based drugs, sometimes followed by second-look surgery to determine whether further treatment is needed. Radiation therapy also may be used if the disease is limited to the tube, ovary, and uterus, although reports of its effectiveness vary (DiSaia & Creasman, 2002). Nursing care for the woman with uterine tube cancer is similar to that of the woman with ovarian cancer.

▬ CANCER AND PREGNANCY

Cancer occurs with relative infrequency during the reproductive years. Approximately one of every 1000 pregnant women also will have cancer (Berman, DiSaia, & Tewari, 2004). These malignancies may be responsible for up to one third of maternal deaths. Although all forms of neoplasms have been documented in conjunction with pregnancy, the most frequently occurring types are breast cancer, cervical cancer, melanomas, ovarian cancer, leukemia and lymphomas, tubal cancers, and thyroid cancers. Bone, colorectal, vulvar, uterine, and vaginal cancers are rarely diagnosed during pregnancy. When pregnancy and cancer coincide, therapeutic issues are complex, and intense reactions occur in the woman, her family, and the health care team. Women are confronted with issues such as continuing or terminating the pregnancy. The selection and timing of therapies such as chemotherapy, radiation, and surgery are all affected by the pregnancy. Add to this the conflicting feelings the woman has (i.e., the joy of pregnancy versus the fear and anxiety associated with cancer), and the task of providing comprehensive care for the woman and her family presents a formidable challenge to the health care team. A brief discussion of the most frequent types of cancers that occur during pregnancy and the current therapies associated with them follows.

Cancer of the Breast

Approximately 2% to 3% of women are pregnant or lactating at the time of diagnosis of cancer of the breast (Copeland & Landon, 2002). Breast cancer complicates about one in 3000 pregnancies. The survival rate for women who are diagnosed with breast cancer while pregnant may be as low as 15% to 20% because the disease is generally in the advanced stages when first diagnosed (DiSaia & Creasman, 2002). Diagnosis is often delayed because breast engorgement may obscure the mass from palpation, and increased density of the tissue makes mammographic visualization more difficult. In addition, increased vascularity and lymphatic drainage in the breast of a pregnant woman may increase the speed of metastasis. Treatment is the same as for the nonpregnant woman, although surgery is usually the treatment of choice for breast cancer in pregnancy (Leslie & Lange, 2005). If an invasive tumor is found, it must be determined whether the tissue is positive or negative for estrogen receptors (ERs). ER-negative tumors spread more rapidly than ER-positive tumors and are more common in pregnancy.

Maternal-fetal management involves consideration of the gestational age of the fetus, the extent of disease, the tumor growth potential, and the proposed treatment. Termination of the pregnancy in early stages of the disease appears to have no impact on survival. There is little evidence to suggest that pregnancy affects the malignant process. Therapeutic abortion may become an issue in the presence of advanced disease and may be deemed necessary to achieve effective palliation. Lumpectomy or partial mastectomy is the most commonly used surgical procedure, but radical mastectomy is tolerated well in these women. For advanced disease in the second or third trimester, alkylating agents, 5-FU, and vincristine are relatively safe for the fetus (DiSaia & Creasman, 2002). Radiation therapy is avoided if at all possible until after the birth, because even with careful shielding, the fetus may still receive sufficient radiation to produce detrimental effects (Psyrri & Burtness, 2005).

There is no agreement about whether a postpartum woman with breast cancer should breastfeed, although many surgeons recommend formula feeding (Berman et al., 2004). There are theoretic concerns that if one of the oncogenes for breast cancer is a virus, as many have postulated, the remaining breast may be contaminated, and the virus may be passed to the newborn, possibly acting as a latent inducer of breast carcinoma. Another reason is that lactation increases vascularity in the remaining breast, which may contain a neoplasm as well.

Breastfeeding after lumpectomy is possible, but the site of the incision may interrupt the milk ducts or prevent the nipple from extending during feeding (DiSaia & Creasman, 2002). Breastfeeding is contraindicated if the woman is receiving chemotherapy.

Pregnancy incidence after mastectomy is influenced by many factors, including prior treatment and duration of survival. About 7% of women will have one or more pregnancies within the first 5 years after mastectomy. In general, women with good prognoses (e.g., no positive nodes) are likely to be counseled to wait at least 3 years before attempting pregnancy (DiSaia & Creasman, 2002).

Cancer of the Cervix

The incidence of cervical cancer concurrent with pregnancy is reported to be 3% to 7%, or about one in 2000 pregnancies, making it the most common reproductive tract cancer associated with pregnancy (Copeland & Landon, 2002). Birth can be accomplished by either the vaginal or the cesarean route; however, there is some concern regarding vaginal birth in the presence of invasive disease, because the risk of hemorrhage and metastatic seeding from local trauma may be increased (DiSaia & Creasman, 2002). The outcome for the woman with cervical cancer is roughly the same as that for the nonpregnant woman (DiSaia & Creasman, 2002).

Cervical abnormalities are diagnosed during pregnancy with an abnormal Pap test. If the report suggests that the pregnant woman has a squamous intraepithelial lesion, a colposcopy, possibly with directed biopsy, is done. If invasive disease is not found, treatment is delayed until after the woman gives birth. Colposcopy is repeated in the third trimester and again postpartum. Cryosurgery has been performed with little effect on the pregnancy; however, conization is not advised during pregnancy unless necessary to rule out invasive cancer because it is associated with bleeding, miscarriage, and preterm birth.

The therapy of invasive carcinoma of the cervix during pregnancy is affected by many factors. The stage of the disease and the trimester in which the cancer is diagnosed are important. Equally important are the beliefs and desires of the woman and her family in terms of initiating therapy that can interrupt the pregnancy, as opposed to postponing the therapy until fetal viability is achieved. If the woman chooses not to continue the pregnancy, external radiation to the pelvis is done. Miscarriage usually occurs, and then internal radiation is done. If miscarriage does not occur, a modified radical hysterectomy may be performed. If the woman desires to continue the pregnancy, treatment of early-stage invasive cervical cancer can be delayed until fetal viability is reached, without harmful effects on the woman. Cesarean birth is usually performed, followed by radiation therapy (Copeland & Landon, 2002).

Leukemia

The average age for pregnant women with acute leukemia is 28 years; incidence during pregnancy is not specified, but the incidence in the general population in the United States is 10 in 100,000. Pregnancy seems to have no specific effect on the course of the disease, except that vigorous therapy is detrimental to early gestation. Preterm labor and postpartum hemorrhage are associated with acute leukemia (DiSaia & Creasman, 2002). Acute

myelocytic leukemia (90% of cases) has a more fulminant course and requires immediate therapy; in the presence of chronic myelocytic leukemia, therapy can be delayed somewhat. Some pregnant women with the chronic form of the disease who had chemotherapy and radiation therapy directed at the spleen have given birth to apparently healthy infants. The decision to terminate the pregnancy rests with the woman and her family; however, prompt, aggressive therapy is always advisable if remission is to be achieved. Decisions may be influenced by the aggressiveness of the disease.

Hodgkin's Disease

Hodgkin's disease is a malignant lymphoma that affects many younger people and complicates about one in 6000 pregnancies. Younger women (younger than 40 years) have a better prognosis.

Pregnancy appears to have no effect on the disease and vice versa, other than those effects resulting from therapy. Radiation therapy of the nodes and multiagent chemotherapy result in about a 75% cure rate. Unless gestation is well into the third trimester, delay in initiating therapy should be minimal, which brings up the dilemma of therapeutic abortion. Radiation therapy to diseased areas above the diaphragm can be initiated during the third trimester with proper shielding of the fetus. Chemotherapy is strongly contraindicated during the first trimester and is relatively contraindicated in the second and third trimesters. Termination of the pregnancy during the course of the disease is not definitely indicated, although treatment is easier (DiSaia & Creasman, 2002).

Melanoma

Malignant melanoma may be one of the rare cancers that can be affected by pregnancy. This is suggested by reports in which pregnancy has been shown to induce or exacerbate a melanoma. These suggestions are based on changes that occur naturally during pregnancy and include hyperpigmentation, an increase in melanocyte-stimulating hormone (MSH), and increased production of estrogen. ERs have been identified in about half of all melanomas (DiSaia & Creasman, 2002).

Although pregnancy has been implicated in the more rapid metastases to regional lymph nodes, stage for stage there does not seem to be a significant difference in the survival of pregnant and nonpregnant women. As a result, most authorities recommend that women who have histories of malignant melanoma delay pregnancy for about 3 years after surgical excision, because this is the period of highest risk for recurrence (DiSaia & Creasman, 2002).

Diagnosis is established by biopsy. Therapy consists of radical local excision. For most other malignancies, the placenta is unexplainably resistant to invasion by maternal cancer. Although melanoma accounts for few cases of malignant disease during pregnancy, almost 50% of the placental metastases and almost 90% of fetal metastases occur from maternal melanoma (DiSaia & Creasman, 2002).

Thyroid Cancer

The incidence of thyroid cancer in pregnancy is not established. Normally the thyroid gland enlarges during pregnancy, and an asymptomatic nodular mass is a common finding. Diagnosis is usually by cytologic testing of fine-needle aspirate. Treatment is usually nonsurgical until after the birth. Thyroid suppression is the preferred treatment during pregnancy (DiSaia & Creasman, 2002).

Bone Tumors

Bone tumors are rare in pregnancy. Ewing sarcoma and osteogenic sarcoma and osteocystoma are the most common primary malignant bone tumors seen in pregnancy. Usually the areas involved are the clavicle, the sternum, the spine, the humerus, and the femur. A lump or mass, local pain, and disability are characteristic manifestations.

Osteogenic sarcoma affects areas of high bone turnover (especially during growth spurts); Ewing sarcoma is a rare condition that develops within bone marrow. Pregnancy does not affect and is not affected by the disease.

Surgical excision is usually well tolerated during pregnancy; adjuvant chemotherapy is delayed until after birth if the cancer is diagnosed near term. If the disease recurs, it usually does so within 3 years; therefore women are counseled to defer pregnancy during this time (DiSaia & Creasman, 2002).

Other Gynecologic Cancers
Cancer of the Vulva

The diagnosis of preinvasive (VIN) disease during pregnancy is rare. Therapy is postponed until the postpartum period. If invasive disease (a rare occurrence) is diagnosed during the first trimester, vulvectomy with bilateral groin dissection may be done after the fourteenth week. When it is diagnosed in the third trimester, local wide excision is done, deferring definitive surgery until after birth. Pregnancy does not alter the course of the disease.

After radical vulvectomy and bilateral inguinal node dissection, a woman who becomes pregnant again can carry the pregnancy to term and give birth vaginally. If vaginal stenosis is present and could impede birth, cesarean birth may be more appropriate.

Cancer of the Vagina

Except for clear-cell adenocarcinoma of DES-exposed women, cancer of the vagina is rare. If clear-cell adenocarcinoma of the cervix and vagina or sarcoma is found in the upper vagina, the preferred surgery is radical hysterectomy, upper vaginectomy, and bilateral pelvic lymphadenectomy, followed by chemotherapy. Radiation is usually not advocated during pregnancy. Pregnancy does not seem to affect the course of the disease or the prognosis.

Cancer of the Uterus

Endometrial carcinoma during pregnancy is very rare; only a few cases have been documented since 1900. Diagnosis was usually an incidental finding after therapeutic abortion or surgery, and the lesions were minimally or not invasive. Recommended therapy is total abdominal hysterectomy and bilateral salpingo-oophorectomy (TAH-BSO) and adjuvant radiotherapy (DiSaia & Creasman, 2002).

Cancer of the Uterine Tube

With a peak incidence between 50 and 55 years of age, concurrent pregnancy is only a remote possibility. Should it occur, the recommended therapy (TAH-BSO with postoperative radiotherapy or chemotherapy) is the same as that for the nonpregnant woman. Removal of the uterine tube is an alternative treatment (DiSaia & Creasman, 2002).

Cancer of the Ovary

Cancer of the ovary is the second most frequent reproductive cancer that occurs with pregnancy. Still, ovarian malignancy is relatively rare, being reported to occur in one per 10,000 to 25,000 births (DiSaia & Creasman, 2002).

Ovarian masses occur frequently during pregnancy. Because corpus luteum cysts account for a high percentage of these masses and because 99% of these resolve by the fourteenth week, any mass smaller than 5 cm may simply be observed until the end of the first trimester. Any mass larger than 5 cm, one that is growing, or one that does not resolve after the fourteenth week warrants further investigation. Abdominal palpation and ultrasound are the diagnostic tools of choice during pregnancy. However, in many cases, laparotomy is necessary to confirm the diagnosis. Laparotomy after 16 weeks of gestation has negligible fetal wastage associated with the procedure and is therefore considered safe.

An ovarian tumor may be first diagnosed at birth or after birth because the enlarged uterus obscured its presence. Definitive diagnosis is needed before treatment is selected. For stage I tumors, treatment includes conservative surgery (unilateral oophorectomy and salpingectomy) and use of chemotherapy. If diagnosis occurs in the second or third trimester, treatment choices are difficult to make. They include interrupting the pregnancy and starting chemotherapy immediately, preserving pregnancy and starting chemotherapy with the fetus in utero (controversial), or delaying chemotherapy until the fetus is more mature and early scheduled birth is a low risk to the fetus (DiSaia & Creasman, 2002).

Cancer Therapy and Pregnancy

Decisions about the type and timing of therapy for cancer in the pregnant woman evoke moral and philosophic dilemmas, as well as complex medical judgments and intense emotional responses.

Ethical Considerations

When a pregnant woman has cancer and her survival is contingent on treatment that will harm the fetus, the health care team must work with the woman and her significant others to make decisions about how to proceed with her care. If a one-client model of ethical decision making is used, the risk-benefit analysis is applied to the maternal-fetal unit. The pregnant woman decides what is best for her and the fetus. The woman may accept or refuse treatment. If a two-client model is used for decision making, more weight is given to fetal well-being, but the pregnant woman cannot be forced to accept harm to herself for the sake of the fetus. Thus she could elect to accept treatment.

The fetus is at risk with either chemotherapy or radiation therapy. The impact of cancer therapy on the fetus can include death, miscarriage, teratogenesis, alteration in growth and development, alterations in function, and genetic mutation. The long-term effects on the fetus are unknown. However, the long-term experiences of young women exposed to DES in utero make very real the possibility of long-term effects associated with cancer therapy. These theoretic dangers must be weighed against the potential detrimental effects to the mother if treatment is withheld (Blackwell, Elam, & Blackwell, 2000).

Timing of Therapy

Timing of therapy also is an important issue to discuss. Because most cancer therapy (except surgery) is geared toward having a differential and noxious effect on rapidly growing tissue, the fetus is most at risk during the first trimester, when organogenesis and rapid tissue growth occur. Surgery offers the least potential risk to the fetus; however, the risk of miscarriage and preterm labor may be increased.

Chemotherapy is avoided in the first trimester if at all possible. Although use of most chemotherapeutic agents has had isolated reports of fetal abnormalities, data on the agents used after the first trimester have recorded surprisingly few fetal abnormalities. The placenta may act as a barrier against the chemotherapeutic agents; therefore although risk still exists, the judicious use of chemotherapy after the first trimester can result in live births with few congenital abnormalities. Acute drug toxicities may occur if treatment has occurred just before birth. Breastfeeding by women who are taking cytotoxic drugs is not recommended because these drugs may be excreted in breast milk (Copeland & Landon, 2002).

Radiation therapy presents its own set of issues. During embryonic development, tissues are extremely radiosensitive. If cells are genetically altered or killed during this time, the child either will fail to survive or will be deformed. From a radiologic stance, there are three significant periods in embryonic development (DiSaia & Creasman, 2002):

1. Preimplantation: If irradiation does not destroy the fertilized egg, it probably does not affect it significantly.
2. Critical period of organogenesis: During this period, especially between days 18 and 38, the organism is most vulnerable; microcephaly, anencephaly, eye damage, growth restriction, spina bifida, and foot damage may occur.
3. After day 40: Large doses may still cause observable malformation and damage to the central nervous system.

Pregnancy After Cancer Treatment

If cancer therapy has not included the removal of the uterus, ovaries, or uterine (fallopian) tubes, there is a possibility that the woman may still be able to become pregnant. Although a woman's menstrual cycle may have resumed, pregnancy may be difficult to achieve. Therapy that has affected the pituitary or thyroid gland may make conception difficult. Radiation appears to have the most deleterious effects on the endocrine system. The use of chemotherapy may result in temporary or permanent sterility, depending on the drug, the dose, and the length of time since the therapy was completed. Alkylating agents are most commonly associated with infertility (DiSaia & Creasman, 2002).

Of growing concern is the increase in the number of childhood and adolescent cancer survivors. Long-term effects of therapy on fertility, including incidence of congenital anomalies, are not well known. The newly diagnosed client must be counseled on the potential effects of treatment on later reproductive function (Blackwell et al., 2000).

For recovery from the disease and treatment to be complete, a delay of at least 2 years from the end of therapy to conception often is advised (Berman et al., 2004). Before conception, a woman who has had cancer should have a complete physical examination to rule out complications that may place her or a fetus in jeopardy. Cardiac, pulmonary, hematologic, neurologic, renal, or gonadal function may be impaired. The woman and the potential father (if partnered) may be referred for reproductive and genetic counseling as well.

■ GESTATIONAL TROPHOBLASTIC ■ DISEASE

Gestational trophoblastic disease (GTD) is a term that encompasses a spectrum of disorders arising from the placental trophoblast. It includes hydatidiform mole (see Chapter 31), invasive mole, and choriocarcinoma. Gestational trophoblastic neoplasia (GTN) refers to persistent trophoblastic tissue that is presumed to be malignant (DiSaia & Creasman, 2002).

Box 12-6 describes the clinical classifications of GTN. For several reasons, GTN is recognized as the most curable gynecologic malignancy. There is a sensitive marker produced by the tumor (hCG); the tumor is extremely sensitive to various chemotherapeutic agents; high risk factors in the disease process can be identified, allowing individualized therapy; and the aggressive use of multiple treatment methods is possible.

Malignant disease follows normal pregnancy in about 50% of cases and hydatidiform mole in about 25% of cases. Miscarriage or ectopic pregnancy or another gestational event precedes about 25% of cases (DiSaia & Creasman, 2002). Metastasis occurs most often in the lungs, the vagina, the liver, and the brain.

Continued bleeding after evacuation of a hydatidiform mole is usually the most suggestive symptom of GTN.

box 12-6 **Classification of Gestational Trophoblastic Neoplasia**

I. Nonmetastatic disease: No evidence of disease outside uterus
II. Metastatic disease: Any disease outside uterus
  A. Good-prognosis metastatic disease
    1. Short duration (last pregnancy <4 months)
    2. Low pretreatment hCG titer (<100,000 international units/24 hr or 40,000 milliinternational units/ml)
    3. No metastasis to brain or liver
    4. No significant prior chemotherapy
  B. Poor-prognosis metastatic disease
    1. Long duration (last pregnancy >4 mo)
    2. High pretreatment hCG titer (>100,000 international units/24 hr or >40,000 milliinternational units/ml)
    3. Brain or liver metastasis
    4. Significant prior chemotherapy
    5. Term pregnancy

From DiSaia, P., & Creasman, W. (2002). *Clinical gynecologic oncology* (6th ed.). St. Louis: Mosby.

Other clinical signs include abdominal pain and uterine and ovarian enlargement. Signs of metastasis include pulmonary symptoms (e.g., dyspnea, cough). The diagnosis is usually confirmed by increasing or plateauing hCG levels after evacuation of a molar pregnancy. Once diagnosis is confirmed, other clinical studies (e.g., CT scan of lungs and brain, chest x-ray, pelvic ultrasound, and liver scan) are done to determine the extent of the disease (Soper, Mutch, Schink, & ACOG, 2004).

For women who wish to preserve their fertility, single-agent chemotherapy is chosen. Methotrexate has been the treatment of choice for years (Soper et al., 2004). High-dose methotrexate followed by folinic acid "rescue" within 24 hours also has shown excellent results and causes fewer toxic effects (DiSaia & Creasman, 2002). Dactinomycin also has been used with equally good results and is used for women with liver or renal disease, both of which are contraindications for methotrexate. Hysterectomy with adjuvant chemotherapy is often the choice of treatment for nonmetastatic tumors in women who have completed their childbearing (Soper et al.).

Women who have metastasis are classified as having either a good or poor prognosis, depending on the absence or presence of brain or liver metastasis, unsuccessful prior chemotherapy, symptoms lasting longer than 4 months, and serum β-hCG levels greater than 40,000 milliinternational units/ml. Treatment progresses from single-agent chemotherapy in the good-prognosis metastatic GTN to multiple-agent chemotherapy and multiple methods of treatment for the poor-prognosis group. Cure rates for the good-prognosis group are almost as positive as for those with nonmetastatic disease, both approaching 100% (DiSaia & Creasman, 2002; Soper et al., 2004).

Therapy is continued until negative hCG levels are obtained. After successful chemotherapy, follow-up by serum hCG levels varies. One schedule is to obtain levels every 2 weeks for 3 months, every month for 3 months, every other month for 6 months, and then every 6 months indefinitely (DiSaia & Creasman, 2002). ACOG recommends obtaining levels at 2-week intervals for the first 3 months of remission followed by screening at 1-month intervals until 1 year of normal hCG levels have been demonstrated (Soper et al., 2004). Physical examinations are done at least yearly, and chest radiographs are done if indicated. Contraception is needed until the woman has been in remission for 6 months (DiSaia & Creasman, 2002) to 1 year (Soper et al.). Oral contraceptives are preferred, but barrier methods are acceptable if oral contraceptives are contraindicated. During a subsequent pregnancy, pelvic ultrasonography is recommended, because the woman is at higher risk (1% to 2%) to develop another molar pregnancy. Serum hCG levels should be obtained 6 weeks after the birth (DiSaia & Creasman).

community activity

Check in your community for resources that provide information for public awareness about cervical cancer prevention and diagnostic services for low income and minority women. Assess how differences for age, culture, and education level are addressed.

key points

- Gynecologic disorders diminish the quality of life for affected women and their families.
- Structural disorders of the uterus and vagina related to pelvic relaxation and urinary incontinence may be a delayed result of childbearing, but they may be seen in young or childless women.
- Bladder training and pelvic muscle exercises can significantly decrease or relieve mild to moderate urinary incontinence.

- The development of neoplasms, whether benign or malignant, can have a significant physical and emotional impact on the woman and her family.
- Abnormal uterine bleeding is the most common symptom of leiomyomas or fibroid tumors.
- Various alternatives to hysterectomy exist for structural and benign disorders of the uterus; women need to be informed

key points—cont'd

about the risks and benefits to make an informed decision about treatment.

- Endometrial cancer is the most common reproductive system malignancy.
- Hysterectomy is the usual treatment for early-stage endometrial cancer.
- Human papillomavirus infection is the primary cause of cervical cancer and is linked to vulvar cancer in women under 40 years of age.
- The squamocolumnar junction is an important landmark identified with neoplastic changes of the cervix.
- Preinvasive cancer of the cervix may be treated with techniques such as electrosurgical excision, cryotherapy, and laser therapy to save the structure of the cervix, particularly in women who desire to retain childbearing ability.
- External and internal radiation therapy in combination are as successful as surgery in treating early stages of cancer of the cervix.

- The Pap test will detect approximately 90% of early cervical dysplasias.
- Cancer of the ovary causes more deaths than any other female genital tract cancer.
- Nurses can control their exposure to radiation in three ways: by increasing the distance from the radiation source, by limiting the time of exposure, and by using lead shielding.
- Cancer is relatively infrequent during pregnancy, occurring about once in every 1000 pregnancies.
- Radiation or chemotherapy treatment of the pregnant woman who has cancer places the fetus at risk for death, miscarriage, teratogenesis, and alterations in growth and development.
- Gestational trophoblastic neoplasms are highly curable but require close monitoring of hCG levels after treatment.

REFERENCES

Adams, K. (2002). Confronting cervical cancer: Screening is the key to stopping this killer. *AWHONN Lifelines, 6*(3), 216-222.

American Cancer Society (ACS). (2006a). *Cancer facts and figures 2006.* New York: Author.

American Cancer Society (ACS). (2006b). Vulvar cancer. *Cancer reference information.* Accessed www.cancer.org, January 16, 2006.

American College of Obstetricians and Gynecologists (ACOG). (2002). Polycystic ovary syndrome. ACOG Practice Bulletin: Clinical management guidelines for obstetrician-gynecologists. No. 41. *Obstetrics and Gynecology, 100*(6), 1389-1401.

American College of Obstetricians and Gynecologists (ACOG). (2005a). Appropriate use of laparoscopically assisted vaginal hysterectomy. ACOG Committee Opinion No. 311. *Obstetrics and Gynecology, 105*(4), 929-930.

American College of Obstetricians and Gynecologists (ACOG). (2005b). Management of abnormal cervical cytology and histology. ACOG Practice Bulletin: Clinical management guidelines for obstetrician-gynecologists. No. 66. *Obstetrics and Gynecology, 106*(3), 645-664.

American College of Obstetricians and Gynecologists (ACOG). (2005c). Management of endometrial cancer. ACOG Practice Bulletin: Clinical management guidelines for obstetrician-gynecologists. No. 65. *Obstetrics and Gynecology, 106*(2), 413-425.

Armstrong, D., Bundy, B., Wenzel, L., Huang, H., Baergen, R., Lele, S., et al. (2006). Intraperitoneal cisplatin and paclitaxel in ovarian cancer. *New England Journal of Medicine, 354*(1), 34-43.

Berman, M., DiSaia, P., & Tewari, K. (2004). Pelvic malignancies, gestational trophoblastic neoplasia, and non-pelvic malignancies. In R. Creasy, R. Resnick, & J. Iams (Eds.), *Maternal-fetal medicine: Principles and practice* (5th ed.). Philadelphia: Saunders.

Blackwell, D., Elam, S., & Blackwell, J. (2000). Cancer and pregnancy: A health care dilemma. *Journal of Obstetric, Gynecologic, and Neonatal Nursing, 29*(4), 405-412.

Buggs, C., & Rosenfield, R. (2005). Polycystic ovary syndrome in adolescence. *Endocrinology and Metabolism Clinics of North America, 34*(3), 677-705.

Cook, J., & Walker, C. (2004). Treatment strategies for uterine leiomyoma: The role of hormonal modulation. *Seminars in Reproductive Medicine, 22*(2), 105-111.

Copeland, L., & Landon, M. (2002). Malignant disease and pregnancy. In S. Gabbe, J. Niebyl, & J. Simpson (Eds.), *Obstetrics: Normal and problem pregnancies* (4th ed.). New York: Churchill Livingstone.

De Leo, V., Morgante, G., La Marca, A., Musacchhio, M., Sorace, M., Cavicchioli, C., et al. (2002). A benefit-risk assessment of medical treatment for uterine leiomyomas. *Drug Safety, 25*(11), 759-779.

DiSaia, P., & Creasman, W. (2002). *Clinical gynecologic oncology* (6th ed.). St. Louis: Mosby.

Dwyer, N., & Kreder, K. (2005). Conservative strategies for the treatment of stress urinary incontinence. *Current Urology Report, 6*(5), 371-375.

Furniss, K. (2000). Tomatoes, Pap smears, and tea? Adopting behaviors that may prevent reproductive cancers and improve health. *Journal of Obstetric, Gynecologic, and Neonatal Nursing, 29*(6), 641-652.

Giarratano, G., Bustamante-Forest, R., & Carter, C. (2005). A multicultural and multilingual outreach program for cervical and breast cancer screening. *Journal of Obstetric, Gynecologic, and Neonatal Nursing, 34*(3), 395-402.

Goodarzi, M., Quinones, M., Azziz, R., Rotter, J., Hsueh, W., & Yang, H. (2005). Polycystic ovary syndrome in Mexican-Americans: Prevalence and association with the severity of insulin resistance. *Fertility and Sterility, 84*(3), 766-769.

Gynecologic Cancer Foundation. (2005). *State of the state of gynecologic cancers. Third annual report to the women of America.* Accessed www.wcn.org, February 1, 2006.

Hartmann, K., Ma, C., Lamvu, G., Langenberg, P., Steege, J., & Kjerulff, K. (2004). Quality of life and sexual function after hysterectomy in women with preoperative pain and depression. *Obstetrics and Gynecology, 104*(4), 701-709.

Hiller, J., Miller, M., & Stavas, J. (2005). Uterine artery embolization: A minimally invasive option to end fibroid symptoms. *Advance for Nurse Practitioners, 13*(10), 20-26.

Iwamoto, R. (2001). Radiation therapy. In S. Otto, *Oncology nursing* (4th ed.). St. Louis: Mosby.

Jackson, M. (2005). Polycystic ovarian syndrome. What nurses need to know about this misunderstood disorder. *AWHONN Lifelines 8*(6), 511-518.

Johnson, N., Barlow, D., Lethaby, A., Tavender, E., Curr, E., & Garry, R. (2005). Surgical approach to hysterectomy for benign gynaecological disease. *Cochrane Database of Systematic Reviews,* 2006, Issue 2. Chichester, UK: John Wiley & Sons.

Kahn, J. (2005). Vaccination as a prevention strategy for human papillomavirus-related diseases. *Journal of Adolescent Health, 27*(6 Suppl), S10-S16.

Katz, A. (2002). Sexuality after hysterectomy. *Journal of Obstetric, Gynecologic, and Neonatal Nursing, 31*(3), 256-262.

Kielb, S. (2005). Stress incontinence: Alternatives to surgery. *International Journal of Fertility and Women's Medicine, 50*(1), 24-29.

Kim, K., & Lee, K. (2001). Symptom experience in women after hysterectomy. *Journal of Obstetric, Gynecologic, and Neonatal Nursing, 30*(5), 472-480.

Kjerulff, K., Langenberg, P., Rhodes, J., Harvey, L., Guzinski, G., & Stolley, P. (2000). Effectiveness of hysterectomy. *Obstetrics and Gynecology, 95*(3), 319-326.

Klausner, T. (2005). The best kept secret. Pelvic floor muscle therapy for urinary incontinence. *Advance for Nurse Practitioners, 13*(7), 43-46, 48.

Lefebvre, G., Vilos, G., Allaire, C., Jeffry, J., Arneja, J., Birch, C. et al. (2003). The management of uterine leiomyomas. *Journal of Obstetrics and Gynecology, 25*(5), 396-418.

Leslie, K., & Lange, C. (2005). Breast cancer and pregnancy. *Obstetric and Gynecologic Clinics of North America, 32*(4), 547-558.

Lethaby, A., Vollenhoven, B., & Sowter, M. (2001). Pre-operative GnRH analogue therapy before hysterectomy or myomectomy for uterine fibroids. *Cochrane Database of Systematic Reviews,* 2006, Issue 2. Chichester, UK: John Wiley & Sons.

Lindberg, C., & Nolan, L. (2001). Women's decision making regarding hysterectomy. *Journal of Obstetric, Gynecologic, and Neonatal Nursing, 30*(6), 607-616.

Lord, J., & Wilkin, T. (2004). Metformin in polycystic ovary syndrome. *Current Opinions in Obstetrics and Gynecology, 16*(6), 481-486.

Lowdermilk, D., & Germino, B. (2000). Helping women and their families cope with the impact of gynecologic cancer. *Journal of Obstetric, Gynecologic, and Neonatal Nursing, 29*(6), 653-660.

Mallett, V. (2005). Female urinary incontinence: What the epidemiologic data tell us. *International Journal of Fertility and Women's Medicine, 50*(10), 12-17.

Melville, J., Delaney, K., Newton, K., & Katon, W. (2005). Incontinence severity and major depression in incontinent women. *Obstetrics and Gynecology, 106*(3), 585-592.

Miller, K. (2005). Stress urinary incontinence in women: Review and update on neurological control. *Journal of Women's Health, 14*(7), 595-608.

National Comprehensive Cancer Network (NCCN). (2004). *NCCN practice guidelines in oncology. Cervical screening. Version 1.2005.* Accessed www.nccn.org, January 12, 2006.

National Comprehensive Cancer Network (NCCN). (2005a). *NCCN practice guidelines in oncology. Ovarian cancer. Version 1.2005.* Accessed www.nccn.org, January 12, 2006.

National Comprehensive Cancer Network (NCCN). (2005b). *NCCN practice guidelines in oncology. Uterine cancers. Version 1.2005.* Accessed www.nccn.org, January 12, 2006.

National Women's Health Resource Center (NWHRC). (2004). Gynecologic cancers and women's health. *National Women's Health Report, 26*(4), 1-7.

Nicholson, T. (2004). Outcome in patients undergoing unilateral artery embolization for symptomatic fibroids. *Clinical Radiology, 59*(2), 186-191.

Ohara, N. (2005). Selective estrogen receptor modulator and selective progesterone receptor modulator: Therapeutic efficacy in the treatment of uterine leiomyoma. *Clinical and Experimental Obstetrics and Gynecology, 32*(1), 9-11.

Otto, S. (2001). Gynecologic cancers. In S. Otto, *Oncology nursing.* St. Louis: Mosby.

Palomba, S., Orio, F., Fusso, T., Falbo, A., Cascella, T., Doldo, P., et al. (2004). Long-term effectiveness and safety of GnRH agonist plus raloxifene administration in women with uterine leiomyomas. *Human Reproduction, 19*(6), 1308-1314.

Psyrri, A., & Burtness, B. (2005). Pregnancy-associated breast cancer. *Cancer Journal, 11*(2), 83-95.

Reis, L., Eisner, M., Kosary, C., Hankey, B., Miller, B., Clegg, L., et al. (2004). *SEER cancer statistics review, 1975-2001.* Bethesda MD: National Cancer Institute. Accessed http:seer.cancer.gov/csr/1975_2001/, January 25, 2006.

Roussis, N., Waltrous, L., Kerr, A., Robertazzi, R., & Cabbad, M. (2004). Sexual response in the patient after hysterectomy: Total abdominal versus supracervical versus vaginal procedure. *American Journal of Obstetrics and Gynecology, 190*(5), 1427-1428.

Sampselle, C. (2003). Behavioral interventions in young and middle-aged women: Simple interventions to combat a complex problem. *American Journal of Nursing, 103*(Suppl), March, 9-19.

Sharts-Hopko, N. (2001). Hysterectomy for nonmalignant conditions. *American Journal of Nursing, 101*(9), 32-40.

Sheehan, M. (2004). Polycystic ovarian syndrome: Diagnosis and management. *Clinics in Medical Research, 2*(1), 13-27.

Society of Obstetricians and Gynaecologists of Canada (SOGC). (2005). SOGC clinical guidelines: Uterine fibroid embolization (UFE). *International Journal of Gynaecologists and Obstetricians, 89*(3), 305-318.

Soper, J., Mutch, D., Schink, J., & the American College of Obstetricians and Gynecologists (ACOG). (2004). ACOG Practice Bulletin Diagnosis and treatment of gestational trophoblastic disease; No. 53. *Gynecologic Oncology, 93*(3), 575-585.

Spies, J., Myers, E., Worthington-Kirsch, R., Mulgund, J., Goodwin, S., & Mauro, M. (2005). The FIBROID registry: Symptom and quality-of-life status 1 year after therapy. *Obstetrics and Gynecology, 106*(6), 1309-1318.

Stenchever, M., Droegemueller, W., Herbst, A., & Mishell, D. (2001). *Comprehensive gynecology* (4th ed.). St. Louis: Mosby.

Teede, H., Meyer, C., & Norman, R. (2005). Insulin–sensitisers in the treatment of polycystic ovary syndrome. *Expert Opinion on Pharmacotherapy, 6*(14), 2419-2427.

Todd, A. (2002). An alternative to hysterectomy. *RN, 65*(3), 30-35.

U.S. Preventive Services Task Force (USPTF). (2005). *The guide to clinical preventive services 2005. Screening for cervical cancer.* AHRQ Publication No. 05-0570, June 2005. Rockville, MD: Agency for Healthcare Research and Quality.

Wade, J., Pletsch, P., Morgan, S., & Menting, S. (2000). Hysterectomy: What do women need and want to know? *Journal of Obstetric, Gynecologic, and Neonatal Nursing, 29*(1), 33-42.

Wilmoth, M., & Spinelli, A. (2000). Sexual implications of gynecologic cancer treatments. *Journal of Obstetric, Gynecologic, and Neonatal Nursing, 29*(4), 413-421.

Wright, T., Cox, J., Massad, L., Carlson, J., Twiggs, L., & Wilkinson, E., et al. (2003). 2001 consensus guidelines for the management of women with cervical cytology abnormalities. *American Journal of Obstetrics and Gynecology, 189*(1), 295-304.

Conception and Fetal Development

learning objectives

- Summarize the process of fertilization.
- Describe the development, structure, and functions of the placenta.
- Describe the composition and functions of the amniotic fluid.
- Identify three organs or tissues arising from each of the three primary germ layers.

- Summarize the significant changes in growth and development of the embryo and fetus.
- Identify the potential effects of teratogens during vulnerable periods of embryonic and fetal development.

electronic resources

Additional information related to the content in Chapter 13 can be found on

the companion website at **evolve**
http://evolve.elsevier.com/Lowdermilk/MWHC/
- NCLEX Review Questions
- WebLinks

or on the interactive companion CD
- NCLEX Review Questions
- Anatomy Review: Fetal Circulation
- Animations: Maternal and Fetal Circulation, Trimesters

*T*HIS chapter presents an overview of the process of fertilization and the development of the normal embryo and fetus.

■ CONCEPTION

Conception, defined as the union of a single egg and sperm, marks the beginning of a pregnancy. Conception occurs not as an isolated event but as part of a sequential process. This sequential process includes gamete (egg and sperm) formation, ovulation (release of the egg), fertilization (union of the gametes), and implantation in the uterus.

Cell Division

Cells are reproduced by two different methods: mitosis and meiosis. In mitosis, body cells replicate to yield two cells with the same genetic makeup as the parent cell. First the cell makes a copy of its deoxyribonucleic acid (DNA), and then it divides; each daughter cell receives one copy of the genetic material. Mitotic division facilitates growth and development or cell replacement.

Meiosis, the process by which germ cells divide and decrease their chromosomal number by half, produces gametes (eggs and sperm). Each homologous pair of chromosomes contains one chromosome received from the mother and one from the father; thus meiosis results in cells that contain one of each of the 23 pairs of chromosomes. Because these germ cells contain 23 single chromosomes, half of the genetic material of a normal somatic cell, they are called *haploid*. This halving of the genetic material is accomplished by replicating the DNA once and then dividing twice. When the female gamete (egg or ovum) and the male gamete (spermatozoon) unite to form the zygote, the diploid number of human chromosomes (46, or 23 pairs) is restored.

The process of DNA replication and cell division in meiosis allows different alleles (genes on corresponding loci that code for variations of the same trait) for genes to be distributed at random by each parent and then rearranged on the paired chromosomes. The chromosomes then separate and proceed to different gametes. Many combinations of genes are possible on each chromosome because parents have genotypes derived from four different grandparents. This random mixing of alleles accounts for the variation of traits seen in the offspring of the same two parents.

Gametogenesis

When a male reaches puberty, his testes begin the process of spermatogenesis. The cells that undergo meiosis in the male are called *spermatocytes*. The primary spermatocyte, which undergoes the first meiotic division, contains the diploid number of chromosomes. The cell has already copied its DNA before division, so four alleles for each gene are present. The cell is still considered diploid because the copies are bound together (i.e., one allele plus its copy on each chromosome).

During the first meiotic division, two haploid secondary spermatocytes are formed. Each secondary spermatocyte contains 22 autosomes and one sex chromosome; one contains the X chromosome (plus its copy), and the other, the Y chromosome (plus its copy). During the second meiotic division, the male produces two gametes with an X chromosome and two gametes with a Y chromosome, all of which will develop into viable sperm (Fig. 13-1, *A*).

Oogenesis, the process of egg (ovum) formation, begins during fetal life in the female. All the cells that may undergo meiosis in a woman's lifetime are contained in her ovaries at birth. The majority of the estimated 2 million primary oocytes (the cells that undergo the first meiotic division) degenerate spontaneously. Only 400 to 500 ova will mature during the approximately 35 years of a woman's reproductive life. The primary oocytes begin the first meiotic division (i.e., they replicate their DNA) during fetal life but remain suspended at this stage until puberty (Fig. 13-1, *B*). Then usually monthly, one primary oocyte matures and completes the first meiotic division, yielding two unequal cells: the secondary oocyte and a small polar body. Both contain 22 autosomes and one X sex chromosome.

At ovulation the second meiotic division begins; however, the ovum does not complete the second meiotic division unless fertilization occurs. At fertilization, when the sperm is united with the mature ovum, a second polar body and the zygote (the united egg and sperm) are produced (Fig. 13-1, *C*). The three polar bodies degenerate. If fertilization does not occur, the ovum also degenerates.

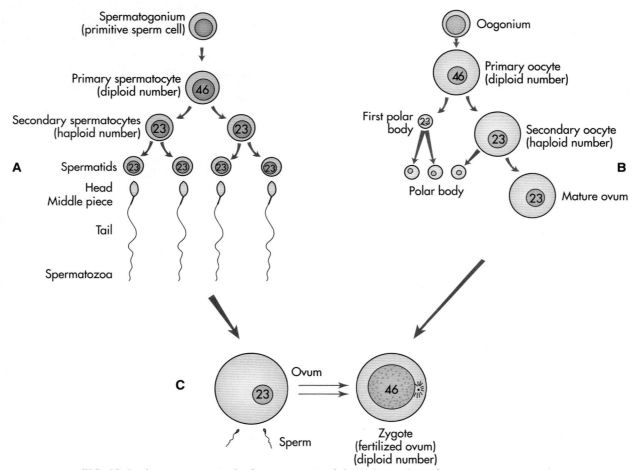

FIG. 13-1 Spermatogenesis. **A,** Gametogenesis of the male produces four mature gametes, the sperm. **B,** Oogenesis. Gametogenesis in the female produces one mature ovum and three polar bodies. Note the relative difference in overall size between the ovum and sperm. **C,** Fertilization results in the single-cell zygote and the restoration of the diploid number of chromosomes.

Ovum

Meiosis occurs in the female in the ovarian follicles and produces an egg, or ovum. Each month, one ovum matures with a host of surrounding supportive cells. At ovulation the ovum is released from the ruptured ovarian follicle. High estrogen levels increase the motility of the uterine tubes so their cilia are able to capture the ovum and propel it through the tube toward the uterine cavity. An ovum cannot move by itself.

Two protective layers surround the ovum (Fig. 13-2). The inner layer is a thick, acellular layer, the *zona pellucida*. The outer layer, the *corona radiata*, is composed of elongated cells.

Ova are considered fertile for about 24 hours after ovulation. If unfertilized by a sperm, the ovum degenerates and is reabsorbed.

Sperm

Ejaculation during sexual intercourse normally propels about a teaspoon of semen, containing as many as 200 to 500 million sperm, into the vagina. The sperm swim propelled by the flagellar movement of their tails. Some sperm can reach the site of fertilization within 5 minutes, but average transit time is 4 to 6 hours. Sperm remain viable within the woman's reproductive system for an average of 2 to 3 days. Most sperm are lost in the vagina, within the cervical mucus, or in the endometrium, or they enter the uterine tube that contains no ovum.

As the sperm travel through the female reproductive tract, enzymes are produced to aid in their capacitation. *Capacitation* is a physiologic change that removes the protective coating from the heads of the sperm. Small perforations then form in the *acrosome* (a cap on the sperm) and allow enzymes (e.g., hyaluronidase) to escape (see Fig. 13-2). These enzymes are necessary for the sperm to penetrate the protective layers of the ovum before fertilization.

Fertilization

Fertilization takes place in the ampulla (outer third) of the uterine tube. When a sperm successfully penetrates the membrane surrounding the ovum, both sperm and ovum are enclosed within the membrane, and the membrane becomes impenetrable to other sperm; this process is termed the *zona reaction*. The second meiotic division of the secondary oocyte is then completed, and the ovum nucleus becomes the female pronucleus. The head of the sperm enlarges to become the male pronucleus, and the tail degenerates. The nuclei fuse, and the chromosomes combine, restoring the diploid number (46) (Fig. 13-3). Conception, the formation of the zygote (the first cell of the new individual), has been achieved.

Mitotic cellular replication, called *cleavage*, begins as the zygote travels the length of the uterine tube into the uterus. This transit takes 3 to 4 days. Because the fertilized egg divides rapidly with no increase in size, successively smaller cells, *blastomeres*, are formed with each division. A 16-cell morula, a solid ball of cells, is produced within 3 days and is still surrounded by the protective zona pellucida (Fig. 13-4, *A*). Further development occurs as the morula floats freely within the uterus. Fluid passes through the zona pellucida into the intercellular spaces between the blastomeres, separating them into two parts, the trophoblast (which gives rise to the placenta) and the embryoblast (which gives rise to the embryo). A cavity forms within the cell mass as the spaces come together, forming a structure called the *blastocyst cavity*. When the cavity becomes recognizable, the whole structure of the developing embryo is known as the blastocyst. Stem cells are derived from the inner cell mass of the blastocyst. The outer layer of cells surrounding the blastocyst cavity is the *trophoblast*.

Implantation

The zona pellucida degenerates, the trophoblast cells displace endometrial cells at the implantation site, and the blastocyst embeds in the endometrium, usually in the anterior or posterior fundal region. Between 6 and 10 days after conception, the trophoblast secretes enzymes that

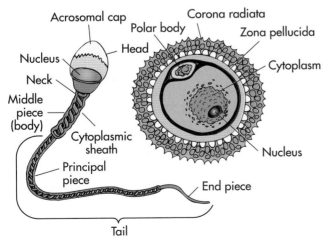

FIG. 13-2 Sperm and ovum.

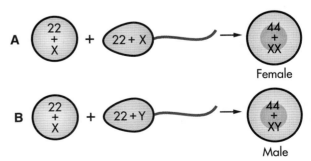

FIG. 13-3 Fertilization. **A,** Ovum fertilized by X-bearing sperm to form female zygote. **B,** Ovum fertilized by Y-bearing sperm to form male zygote.

FIG. 13-4 First weeks of human development. **A,** Follicular development in the ovary, ovulation, fertilization, and transport of the early embryo down the uterine tube and into the uterus, where implantation occurs. **B,** Blastocyst embedded in endometrium. Germ layers forming. (*A* from Carlson, B. [2004]. *Human embryology and developmental biology* (ed 3). Philadelphia: Mosby; *B* adapted from Langley, L., et al. [1980]. *Dynamic human anatomy and physiology* [5th ed.]. New York: McGraw-Hill.)

nutrients from the maternal bloodstream and dispose of carbon dioxide and waste products into the maternal blood.

After implantation, the endometrium is termed the *decidua.* The portion directly under the blastocyst, where the chorionic villi tap into the maternal blood vessels, is the decidua basalis. The portion covering the blastocyst is the *decidua capsularis,* and the portion lining the rest of the uterus is the *decidua vera* (Fig. 13-5).

■ EMBRYO AND FETUS

Pregnancy lasts approximately 10 lunar months, 9 calendar months, 40 weeks, or 280 days. Length of pregnancy is computed from the first day of the last menstrual period (LMP) until the day of birth. However, conception occurs approximately 2 weeks after the first day of the LMP; thus the postconception age of the fetus is 2 weeks less, for a total of 266 days or 38 weeks. Postconception age is used in the discussion of fetal development.

Intrauterine development is divided into three stages: ovum or preembryonic, embryo, and fetus (Fig. 13-6). The stage of the ovum lasts from conception until day 14. This period covers cellular replication, blastocyst formation, initial development of the embryonic membranes, and establishment of the primary germ layers.

Primary Germ Layers

During the third week after conception, the embryonic disk differentiates into three primary germ layers: the ectoderm, the mesoderm, and the endoderm (or entoderm) (see Fig. 13-4, *B*). All tissues and organs of the embryo develop from these three layers.

The upper layer of the embryonic disk, the *ectoderm,* gives rise to the epidermis, the glands (anterior pituitary, cutaneous, and mammary), the nails and hair, the central and peripheral nervous systems, the lens of the eye, the tooth enamel, and the floor of the amniotic cavity.

The middle layer, the *mesoderm,* develops into the bones and teeth, the muscles (skeletal, smooth, and cardiac), the dermis and connective tissue, the cardiovascular system and spleen, and the urogenital system.

The lower layer, the *endoderm,* gives rise to the epithelium lining the respiratory and digestive tracts, and the glandular cells of associated organs, including the oropharynx, the liver and pancreas, the urethra, the bladder, and the vagina. The endoderm forms the roof of the yolk sac.

Development of the Embryo

The stage of the embryo lasts from day 15 until approximately 8 weeks after conception, when the embryo measures 3 cm from crown to rump. This embryonic stage is the most critical time in the development of the organ systems and the main external features. Developing areas with rapid cell division are the most vulnerable to malformation caused by environmental teratogens (substances or exposure that causes abnormal development). At the end of

enable it to burrow into the endometrium until the entire blastocyst is covered. This is termed implantation. Endometrial blood vessels erode, and some women have slight implantation bleeding (slight spotting or bleeding at the time of the first missed menstrual period). Chorionic villi, fingerlike projections, develop out of the trophoblast and extend into the blood-filled spaces of the endometrium. These villi are vascular processes that obtain oxygen and

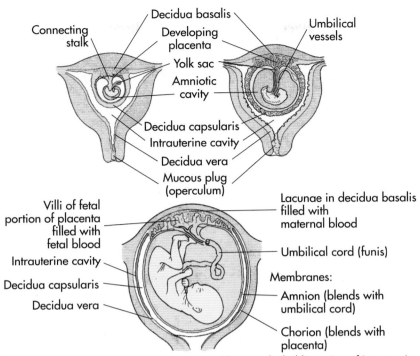

FIG. 13-5 Development of the fetal membranes. Note gradual obliteration of intrauterine cavity as decidua capsularis and decidua vera meet. Also note thinning of uterine wall. Chorionic and amniotic membranes are in apposition to each other but may be peeled apart.

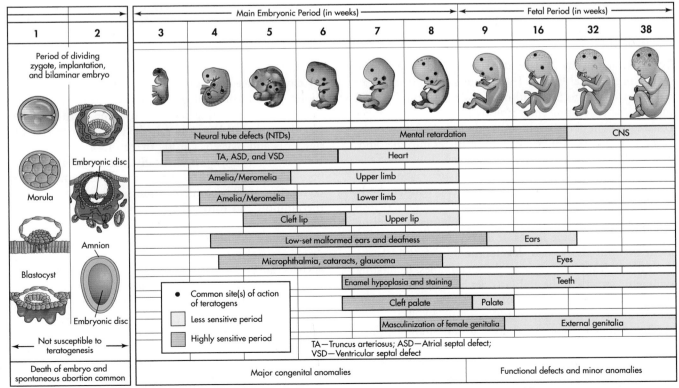

FIG. 13-6 Sensitive or critical periods in human development. Dark color denotes highly sensitive periods; light color indicates stages that are less sensitive to teratogens. (From Moore, K., & Persaud, T. [2003]. *Before we are born: Essentials of embryology and birth defects* (6th ed.). Philadelphia: Saunders.

the eighth week, all organ systems and external structures are present, and the embryo is unmistakably human (see Fig. 13-6 and Visible Embryo, www.visembryo.com, for a pictorial view of normal and abnormal development).

Membranes

At the time of implantation, two fetal membranes that will surround the developing embryo begin to form. The *chorion* develops from the trophoblast and contains the chorionic villi on its surface. The villi burrow into the decidua basalis and increase in size and complexity as the vascular processes develop into the placenta. The chorion becomes the covering of the fetal side of the placenta. It contains the major umbilical blood vessels as they branch out over the surface of the placenta. As the embryo grows, the decidua capsularis stretches. The chorionic villi on this side atrophy and degenerate, leaving a smooth chorionic membrane.

The inner cell membrane, the *amnion,* develops from the interior cells of the blastocyst. The cavity that develops between this inner cell mass and the outer layer of cells (trophoblast) is the *amniotic cavity* (see Fig. 13-4, *B*). As it grows larger, the amnion forms on the side opposite the developing blastocyst (see Figs. 13-4 and 13-5). The developing embryo draws the amnion around itself, forming a fluid-filled sac. The amnion becomes the covering of the umbilical cord and covers the chorion on the fetal surface of the placenta. As the embryo grows larger, the amnion enlarges to accommodate the embryo/fetus and the surrounding amniotic fluid. The amnion eventually comes in contact with the chorion surrounding the fetus.

Amniotic Fluid

The amniotic cavity initially derives its fluid by diffusion from the maternal blood. The amount of fluid increases weekly, and 800 to 1200 ml of transparent liquid is normally present at term. The amniotic fluid volume changes constantly. The fetus swallows fluid, and fluid flows into and out of the fetal lungs. The fetus urinates into the fluid, greatly increasing its volume.

Many functions for the embryo/fetus are served by amniotic fluid. Amniotic fluid helps maintain a constant body temperature. It serves as a source of oral fluid and a repository for waste. It cushions the fetus from trauma by blunting and dispersing outside forces. It allows freedom of movement for musculoskeletal development. The fluid keeps the embryo from tangling with the membranes, facilitating symmetric growth. If the embryo does become tangled with the membranes, amputations of extremities or other deformities can occur from constricting amniotic bands.

The volume of amniotic fluid is an important factor in assessing fetal well-being. Having less than 300 ml of amniotic fluid (*oligohydramnios*) is associated with fetal renal abnormalities. Having more than 2 L of amniotic fluid (*hydramnios*) is associated with gastrointestinal and other malformations.

Amniotic fluid contains albumin, urea, uric acid, creatinine, lecithin, sphingomyelin, bilirubin, fructose, fat, leukocytes, proteins, epithelial cells, enzymes, and lanugo hair. Study of fetal cells in amniotic fluid through amniocentesis yields much information about the fetus. Genetic studies (karyotyping) provide knowledge about the sex and the number and structure of chromosomes (see Chapter 3). Other studies, such as lecithin/sphingomyelin ratio, determine the health or maturity of the fetus (see Chapter 29).

Yolk Sac

When the amniotic cavity and amnion are forming, another blastocyst cavity forms on the other side of the developing embryonic disk (see Fig. 13-4, *B*). This cavity becomes surrounded by a membrane, forming the yolk sac. The yolk sac aids in transferring maternal nutrients and oxygen, which have diffused through the chorion, to the embryo. Blood vessels form to aid transport. Blood cells and plasma are manufactured in the yolk sac during the second and third weeks, while uteroplacental circulation is being established and is forming primitive blood cells until hematopoietic activity begins. At the end of the third week, the primitive heart begins to beat and circulate the blood through the embryo, the connecting stalk, the chorion, and the yolk sac.

The folding in of the embryo during the fourth week results in incorporation of part of the yolk sac into the embryo's body as the primitive digestive system. Primordial germ cells arise in the yolk sac and move into the embryo. The shrinking remains of the yolk sac degenerate (see Fig. 13-5). By the fifth or sixth week, the remnant has separated from the embryo.

Umbilical Cord

By day 14 after conception, the embryonic disk, the amniotic sac, and the yolk sac are attached to the chorionic villi by the connecting stalk. During the third week, the blood vessels develop to supply the embryo with maternal nutrients and oxygen. During the fifth week, the embryo has curved inward on itself from both ends, bringing the connecting stalk to the ventral side of the embryo. The connecting stalk becomes compressed from both sides by the amnion and forms the narrower umbilical cord (see Fig. 13-5). Two arteries carry blood from the embryo to the chorionic villi, and one vein returns blood to the embryo. Approximately 1% of umbilical cords contain only two vessels: one artery and one vein. This occurrence is sometimes associated with congenital malformations.

The cord rapidly increases in length. At term, the cord is 2 cm in diameter and ranges from 30 to 90 cm long (with an average of 55 cm). It twists spirally on itself and loops around the embryo/fetus. A true knot is rare, but false knots occur as folds or kinks in the cord and may jeopardize circulation to the fetus. Connective tissue called *Wharton's jelly* prevents compression of the blood vessels and ensures continued nourishment of the embryo/fetus.

Compression can occur if the cord lies between the fetal head and the maternal pelvis or is twisted around the fetal body. When the cord is wrapped around the fetal neck, it is called a nuchal cord.

Because the placenta develops from the chorionic villi, the umbilical cord is usually located centrally. A peripheral location is less common and is termed *battledore placenta.* The blood vessels are arrayed out from the center to all parts of the placenta.

Placenta

Structure. The placenta begins to form at implantation. During the third week after conception, the trophoblast cells of the chorionic villi continue to invade the decidua basalis. As the uterine capillaries are tapped, the endometrial spiral arteries fill with maternal blood. The chorionic villi grow into the spaces with two layers of cells: the outer syncytium and the inner cytotrophoblast. A third layer develops into anchoring septa, dividing the projecting decidua into separate areas called *cotyledons.* In each of the 15 to 20 cotyledons, the chorionic villi branch out, and a complex system of fetal blood vessels forms. Each cotyledon is a functional unit. The whole structure is the placenta (Fig. 13-7).

The maternal-placental-embryonic circulation is in place by day 17, when the embryonic heart starts beating. By the end of the third week, embryonic blood is circulating between the embryo and the chorionic villi. In the intervillous spaces, maternal blood supplies oxygen and nutrients to the embryonic capillaries in the villi (Fig. 13-8). Waste products and carbon dioxide diffuse into the maternal blood.

The placenta functions as a means of metabolic exchange. Exchange is minimal at this time because the two cell layers of the villous membrane are too thick. Permeability increases as the cytotrophoblast thins and disappears; by the fifth month, only the single layer of syncytium is left between the maternal blood and the fetal capillaries. The syncytium is the functional layer of the placenta. By the eighth week, genetic testing may be done on a sample of chorionic villi by aspiration biopsy; however, limb defects have been associated with chorionic villus sampling done before 10 weeks. The structure of the placenta is complete by the twelfth week. The placenta continues to grow wider until 20 weeks, when it covers approximately half of the uterine surface. It then continues to grow thicker. The branching villi continue to develop within the body of the placenta, increasing the functional surface area.

Functions. One of the early functions of the placenta is as an endocrine gland that produces four hormones necessary to maintain the pregnancy and support the embryo and fetus. The hormones are produced in the syncytium.

The protein hormone human chorionic gonadotropin (hCG) can be detected in the maternal serum by 8 to 10 days after conception, shortly after implantation. This hormone is the basis for pregnancy tests. The hCG preserves the function of the ovarian corpus luteum, ensuring the

FIG. 13-7 Term placenta. **A,** Maternal (or uterine) surface, showing cotyledons and grooves. **B,** Fetal (or amniotic) surface, showing blood vessels running under amnion and converging to form umbilical vessels at attachment of umbilical cord. **C,** Amnion and smooth chorion are arranged to show that they are (1) fused and (2) continuous with margins of placenta. (Courtesy Marjorie Pyle, RNC, Lifecircle, Costa Mesa, CA.)

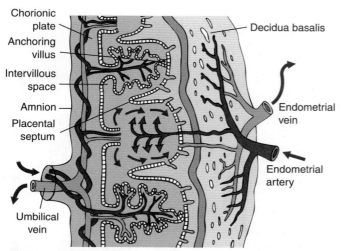

Chorionic plate
Anchoring villus
Intervillous space
Amnion
Placental septum
Umbilical vein
Decidua basalis
Endometrial vein
Endometrial artery

FIG. 13-8 Schematic drawing of placenta illustrating how it supplies oxygen and nutrition to embryo and removes its waste products. Deoxygenated blood leaves fetus through the umbilical arteries and enters the placenta, where it is oxygenated. Oxygenated blood leaves the placenta through the umbilical vein, which enters the fetus via the umbilical cord.

continued supply of estrogen and progesterone needed to maintain the pregnancy. Miscarriage occurs if the corpus luteum stops functioning before the placenta is producing sufficient estrogen and progesterone. The amount of hCG reaches its maximal level at 50 to 70 days and then begins to decrease.

The other protein hormone produced by the placenta is human chorionic somatomammotropin (hCS), or human placental lactogen (hPL). This substance is similar to a growth hormone and stimulates the maternal metabolism to supply nutrients needed for fetal growth. This hormone increases the resistance to insulin, facilitates glucose transport across the placental membrane, and stimulates breast development to prepare for lactation.

The placenta eventually produces more of the steroid hormone progesterone than the corpus luteum does during the first few months of pregnancy. Progesterone maintains the endometrium, decreases the contractility of the uterus, and stimulates maternal metabolism and development of breast alveoli.

By 7 weeks after fertilization, the placenta is producing most of the maternal estrogens, which are steroid hormones. The major estrogen secreted by the placenta is estriol, whereas the ovaries produce mostly estradiol. Estriol levels may be measured to determine placental functioning. Estrogen stimulates uterine growth and uteroplacental blood flow. It causes a proliferation of the breast glandular tissue and stimulates myometrial contractility. Placental estrogen production increases greatly toward the end of pregnancy. One theory for the cause of the onset of labor is the decrease in circulating levels of progesterone and the increased levels of estrogen.

The metabolic functions of the placenta are respiration, nutrition, excretion, and storage. Oxygen diffuses from the

maternal blood across the placental membrane into the fetal blood, and carbon dioxide diffuses in the opposite direction. In this way, the placenta functions as lungs for the fetus.

Carbohydrates, proteins, calcium, and iron are stored in the placenta for ready access to meet fetal needs. Water, inorganic salts, carbohydrates, proteins, fats, and vitamins pass from the maternal blood supply across the placental membrane into the fetal blood, supplying nutrition. Water and most electrolytes with a molecular weight less than 500 readily diffuse through the membrane. Hydrostatic and osmotic pressures aid the flow of water and some solutions. Facilitated and active transport assist in the transfer of glucose, amino acids, calcium, iron, and substances with higher molecular weights. Amino acids and calcium are transported against the concentration gradient between the maternal blood and fetal blood.

The fetal concentration of glucose is lower than the glucose level in the maternal blood because of its rapid metabolism by the fetus. This fetal requirement demands larger concentrations of glucose than simple diffusion can provide. Therefore maternal glucose moves into the fetal circulation by active transport.

Pinocytosis is a mechanism used for transferring large molecules, such as albumin and gamma globulins, across the placental membrane. This mechanism conveys the maternal immunoglobulins that provide early passive immunity to the fetus.

Metabolic waste products of the fetus cross the placental membrane from the fetal blood into the maternal blood. The maternal kidneys then excrete them. Many viruses can cross the placental membrane and infect the fetus. Some bacteria and protozoa first infect the placenta and then infect the fetus. Drugs also can cross the placental membrane and may harm the fetus. Caffeine, alcohol, nicotine, carbon monoxide, and other toxic substances in cigarette smoke, as well as prescription and recreational drugs (such as cocaine and marijuana) readily cross the placenta (Box 13-1).

Although no direct link exists between the fetal blood in the vessels of the chorionic villi and the maternal blood in the intervillous spaces, only one cell layer separates them. Breaks occasionally occur in the placental membrane. Fetal erythrocytes then leak into the maternal circulation, and the mother may develop antibodies to the fetal red blood cells. This is often the way an Rh-negative mother becomes sensitized to the erythrocytes of her Rh-positive fetus. (See discussions of isoimmunization in Chapters 23 and 39.)

Although the placenta and the fetus are analogous to living tissue transplants, they are not destroyed by the host mother (Silver, Peltier, & Branch, 2004). Either the placental hormones suppress the immunologic response, or the tissue evokes no response.

Placental function depends on the maternal blood pressure supplying circulation. Maternal arterial blood, under pressure in the small uterine spiral arteries, spurts into the intervillous spaces (see Fig. 13-8). As long as rich arterial blood continues to be supplied, pressure is exerted on the blood

box 13-1 **Developmentally Toxic Exposures in Humans**

- Aminopterin
- Androgens
- Angiotensin-converting enzyme inhibitors
- Carbamazepine
- Cigarette smoking
- Cocaine
- Coumarin anticoagulants
- Cytomegalovirus
- Diethylstilbestrol
- Ethanol (>1 drink/day)
- Etretinate
- Hyperthermia
- Iodides
- Ionizing radiation (>10 rads)
- Isotretinoin
- Lead
- Lithium
- Methimazole
- Methyl mercury
- Parvovirus B19
- Penicillamine
- Phenytoin
- Radioiodine
- Rubella
- Syphilis
- Tetracycline
- Thalidomide
- Toxoplasmosis
- Trimethadione
- Valproic acid
- Varicella

already in the intervillous spaces, pushing it toward drainage by the low-pressure uterine veins. At term gestation, 10% of the maternal cardiac output goes to the uterus.

If there is interference with the circulation to the placenta, the placenta cannot supply the embryo or fetus. Vasoconstriction, such as that caused by hypertension and cocaine use, diminishes uterine blood flow. Decreased maternal blood pressure or cardiac output also diminishes uterine blood flow.

When a woman lies on her back with the pressure of the uterus compressing the vena cava, blood return to the right atrium is diminished (see discussion of supine hypotension in Chapters 16 and 21; see Fig. 21-5). Excessive maternal exercise that diverts blood to the muscles away from the uterus compromises placental circulation. Optimal circulation is achieved when the woman is lying at rest on her side. Decreased uterine circulation may lead to intrauterine growth restriction of the fetus and to infants who are small for gestational age.

Braxton Hicks contractions appear to enhance the movement of blood through the intervillous spaces, aiding placental circulation. Prolonged contractions or too-short intervals between contractions during labor, however, reduce blood flow to the placenta.

Fetal Maturation

The stage of the fetus lasts from 9 weeks (when the fetus becomes recognizable as a human being) until the pregnancy ends. Changes during the fetal period are not so dramatic, because refinement of structure and function are taking place. The fetus is less vulnerable to teratogens, except for those affecting central nervous system functioning.

Viability refers to the capability of the fetus to survive outside the uterus. In the past, the earliest age at which fetal survival could be expected was 28 weeks after conception. With modern technology and advancements in maternal and neonatal care, viability is now possible at 20 weeks after conception (22 weeks after LMP, fetal weight of 500 g or more). The limitations on survival outside the uterus are based on central nervous system function and the oxygenation capability of the lungs.

Fetal Circulatory System

The cardiovascular system is the first organ system to function in the developing human. Blood vessel and blood cell formation begins in the third week and supplies the embryo with oxygen and nutrients from the mother. By the end of the third week, the tubular heart begins to beat, and the primitive cardiovascular system links the embryo, connecting stalk, chorion, and yolk sac. During the fourth and fifth weeks, the heart develops into a four-chambered organ. By the end of the embryonic stage, the heart is developmentally complete.

The fetal lungs do not function for respiratory gas exchange, so a special circulatory pathway, the ductus arteriosus, bypasses the lungs. Oxygen-rich blood from the placenta flows rapidly through the umbilical vein into the fetal abdomen (Fig. 13-9). When the umbilical vein reaches the liver, it divides into two branches; one branch circulates some oxygenated blood through the liver. Most of the blood passes through the ductus venosus into the inferior vena cava. There it mixes with the deoxygenated blood from the fetal legs and abdomen on its way to the right atrium. Most of this blood passes straight through the right atrium and through the foramen ovale, an opening into the left atrium. There it mixes with the small amount of deoxygenated blood returning from the fetal lungs through the pulmonary veins.

The blood flows into the left ventricle and is squeezed out into the aorta, where the arteries supplying the heart, head, neck, and arms receive most of the oxygen-rich blood. This pattern of supplying the highest levels of oxygen and nutrients to the head, neck, and arms enhances the cephalocaudal (head-to-rump) development of the embryo/fetus.

Deoxygenated blood returning from the head and arms enters the right atrium through the superior vena cava. This blood is directed downward into the right ventricle, where it is squeezed into the pulmonary artery. A small amount of blood circulates through the resistant lung tissue, but the majority follows the path with less resistance through the ductus arteriosus into the aorta,

CD: Anatomy Review: Fetal Circulation

CD: Animations

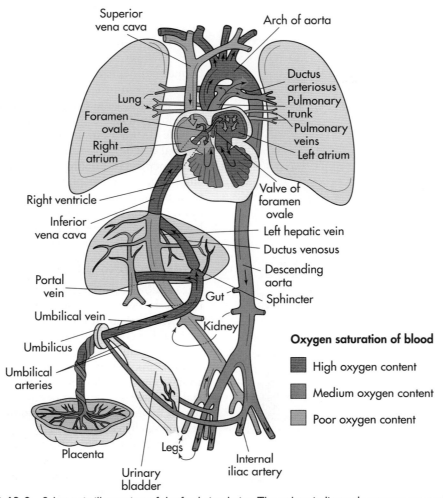

FIG. 13-9 Schematic illustration of the fetal circulation. The colors indicate the oxygen saturation of the blood, and the arrows show the course of the blood from the placenta to the heart. The organs are not drawn to scale. Observe that three shunts permit most of the blood to bypass the liver and lungs: (1) ductus venosus, (2) foramen ovale, and (3) ductus arteriosus. The poorly oxygenated blood returns to the placenta for oxygen and nutrients through the umbilical arteries. (From Moore, K., & Persaud, T. [2003]. *Before we are born: Essentials of embryology and birth defects* [6th ed]. Philadelphia: Saunders)

distal to the point of exit of the arteries supplying the head and arms with oxygenated blood. The oxygen-poor blood flows through the abdominal aorta into the internal iliac arteries, where the umbilical arteries direct most of it back through the umbilical cord to the placenta. There the blood gives up its wastes and carbon dioxide in exchange for nutrients and oxygen. The blood remaining in the iliac arteries flows through the fetal abdomen and legs, ultimately returning through the inferior vena cava to the heart.

The following three special characteristics enable the fetus to obtain sufficient oxygen from the maternal blood:

- Fetal hemoglobin carries 20% to 30% more oxygen than maternal hemoglobin.
- The hemoglobin concentration of the fetus is about 50% greater than that of the mother.
- The fetal heart rate is 110 to 160 beats/min, making the cardiac output per unit of body weight higher than that of an adult.

Hematopoietic System

Hematopoiesis, the formation of blood, occurs in the yolk sac (see Fig. 13-4, *B*) beginning in the third week. Hematopoietic stem cells seed the fetal liver during the fifth week, and hematopoiesis begins there during the sixth week. This accounts for the relatively large size of the liver between the seventh and ninth weeks. Stem cells seed the fetal bone marrow, spleen, thymus, and lymph nodes between weeks 8 and 11 (for more information about stem cells see http:// stemcells.nih.gov/index.asp).

The antigenic factors that determine blood type are present in the erythrocytes soon after the sixth week. For this reason, the Rh-negative woman is at risk for isoimmunization in any pregnancy that lasts longer than 6 weeks after fertilization.

Gastrointestinal System

During the fourth week, the shape of the embryo changes from being almost straight to a C shape, as both ends fold in toward the ventral surface. A portion of the yolk sac is incorporated into the body from head to tail as the primitive gut (digestive system).

The foregut produces the pharynx, part of the lower respiratory tract, the esophagus, the stomach, the first half of the duodenum, the liver, the pancreas, and the gallbladder. These structures evolve during the fifth and sixth weeks. The malformations that can occur in these areas are esophageal atresia, hypertrophic pyloric stenosis, duodenal stenosis or atresia, and biliary atresia.

The midgut becomes the distal half of the duodenum, the jejunum and the ileum, the cecum and the appendix, and the proximal half of the colon. The midgut loop projects into the umbilical cord between weeks 5 and 10. A malformation (omphalocele) results if the midgut fails to return to the abdominal cavity, causing the intestines to protrude from the umbilicus. Meckel diverticulum, the most common malformation of the midgut, occurs when a remnant of the yolk stalk that has failed to degenerate attaches to the ileum, leaving a blind sac.

The hindgut develops into the distal half of the colon, the rectum and parts of the anal canal, the urinary bladder, and the urethra. Anorectal malformations are the most common abnormalities of the digestive system.

The fetus swallows amniotic fluid beginning in the fifth month. Gastric emptying and intestinal peristalsis occur. Fetal nutrition and elimination needs are taken care of by the placenta. As the fetus nears term, fetal waste products accumulate in the intestines as dark green to black, tarry meconium. Normally, this substance is passed through the rectum within 24 hours of birth. Sometimes with a breech presentation or fetal hypoxia, meconium is passed in utero into the amniotic fluid. The failure to pass meconium after birth may indicate atresia somewhere in the digestive tract, an imperforate anus, or meconium ileus, in which a firm meconium plug blocks passage (seen in infants with cystic fibrosis).

The metabolic rate of the fetus is relatively low, but the infant has great growth and development needs. Beginning in week 9, the fetus synthesizes glycogen for storage in the liver. Between 26 and 30 weeks, the fetus begins to lay down stores of brown fat in preparation for extrauterine cold stress. Thermoregulation in the neonate requires increased metabolism and adequate oxygenation.

The gastrointestinal system is mature by 36 weeks. Digestive enzymes (except pancreatic amylase and lipase) are present in sufficient quantity to facilitate digestion. The neonate cannot digest starches or fats efficiently. Little saliva is produced.

Hepatic System

The liver and biliary tract develop from the foregut during the fourth week of gestation. Hematopoiesis begins during the sixth week and requires that the liver be large. The embryonic liver is prominent, occupying most of the abdominal cavity. Bile, a constituent of meconium, begins to form in the twelfth week.

Glycogen is stored in the fetal liver beginning at week 9 or 10. At term, glycogen stores are twice those of the adult. Glycogen is the major source of energy for the fetus and neonate stressed by in utero hypoxia, extrauterine loss of the maternal glucose supply, the work of breathing, or cold.

Iron also is stored in the fetal liver. If the maternal intake is sufficient, the fetus can store enough iron to last for 5 months after birth.

During fetal life, the liver does not have to conjugate bilirubin for excretion because the unconjugated bilirubin is cleared by the placenta. Therefore the glucuronyl transferase enzyme needed for conjugation is present in the fetal liver in amounts less than those required after birth. This predisposes the neonate, especially the preterm infant, to hyperbilirubinemia.

Coagulation factors II, VII, IX, and X cannot be synthesized in the fetal liver because of the lack of vitamin K synthesis in the sterile fetal gut. This coagulation deficiency persists after birth for several days and is the rationale for the prophylactic administration of vitamin K to the newborn.

Respiratory System

The respiratory system begins development during embryonic life and continues through fetal life and into childhood. The development of the respiratory tract begins in week 4 and continues through week 17 with formation of the larynx, the trachea, the bronchi, and the lung buds. Between 16 and 24 weeks, the bronchi and terminal bronchioles enlarge, and vascular structures and primitive alveoli are formed. Between 24 weeks and term birth, more alveoli form. Specialized alveolar cells, type I and type II cells, secrete pulmonary surfactants to line the interior of the alveoli. After 32 weeks, sufficient surfactant is present in developed alveoli to provide infants with a good chance of survival.

Pulmonary Surfactants. The detection of the presence of pulmonary surfactants, surface-active phospholipids, in amniotic fluid has been used to determine the degree of fetal lung maturity, or the ability of the lungs to function after birth. Lecithin (L) is the most critical alveolar surfactant required for postnatal lung expansion. It is detectable at approximately 21 weeks and increases in amount after week 24. Another pulmonary phospholipid, sphingomyelin (S), remains constant in amount. Thus the measure of lecithin in relation to sphingomyelin, or the L/S ratio, is used to determine fetal lung maturity. When the L/S ratio reaches 2:1, the infant's lungs are considered to be mature. This occurs at approximately 35 weeks of gestation (Mercer, 2004).

Certain maternal conditions that cause decreased maternal blood flow, such as maternal hypertension, placental dysfunction, infection, or corticosteroid use, accelerate fetal lung maturity. This apparently is caused by the resulting fetal hypoxia, which stresses the fetus and increases the blood levels of corticosteroids that accelerate alveolar and surfactant development.

EVIDENCE-BASED PRACTICE

Pregnancy Outcomes with Folic Acid Supplementation Throughout Pregnancy

BACKGROUND

- It is well-accepted that folic acid supplements, taken before and after conception, can prevent neural tube defects, which occur around week 5 post-conception, when failure of the neural tube to fold in on itself can lead to spina bifida and anencephaly. Folic acid is essential to cell division. Folate deficiency in pregnancy is associated with preterm birth, low birth weight, and antepartal hemorrhage, so supplementation is conventionally continued throughout pregnancy. More recently, elevated maternal homocysteine levels have been associated with neural tube defects, pregnancy loss, and placental abnormalities. Homocysteine may damage the endothelial lining and cause the inflammation and vasoconstriction of gestational hypertension. Folate supplementation lowers the homocysteine levels, but there are no studies of whether this improves pregnancy outcomes.

OBJECTIVES

- The authors sought information regarding the effects of folic acid supplementation on pregnancy outcomes. The defined outcomes were the following: preterm birth as occurring before 37 weeks of gestation; low birth weight as being less than 2500 gm; and antepartal hemorrhage as occurring after 28 weeks of gestation (excluding placenta previa). Other outcomes included preeclampsia, placental weight, gestational age, fetal abnormalities, and perinatal death.

METHODS

Search Strategy

- The reviewers combined data of the 1960s' Aberdeen Folate Supplementation Trial, representing 2797 U.S. women, with a 2003 Cochrane Review on prenatal folic acid supplementation, representing 6425 women from Australia, Canada, France, Hungary, Ireland, Israel, the United Kingdom, and the former USSR, 1981 to 1994. The goal of the review was to compare outcomes for women randomized to daily doses of 200 mcg, 5 mg, or none throughout their pregnancy.

Statistical Analyses

- Standardization of doses facilitated metaanalysis. Compliance in the three groups was confirmed using serum folate levels. The reviewers used weighted mean differences for continuous data, such as birth weight, and calculated relative risks for dichotomous data, such as treatment group. They combined the 200 mcg and the 5 mg group into a "treated" group, to compare outcomes with "untreated." They also used the 5 mg group to compare with other studies that used 5 mg doses.

FINDINGS

- There were no significant differences between groups for gestational age at birth or placental weight, but there was a nonsignificant increase in preterm birth in the treated groups when compared to the controls. Mean birth weight was not significantly different between groups, but starting folic acid early in pregnancy (before 17 weeks) helped prevent low birth weights. There was a trend of increased risk of antenatal hemorrhage with the 200 mcg dose, but decreased risk in the 5 mg dose group. Preeclampsia was decreased in the treated group, compared to the control group, but not significantly. There was a modest risk of increased fetal abnormalities in the 200 mcg group, but not the 5 mg group, and there were more perinatal deaths in the treated groups than the controls.

LIMITATIONS

- None of the differences was significant, and therefore they could have been due to chance alone. The confidence interval for categoric statistics was wide. There was no conclusion in this review as to whether placental weights were related to birth outcomes.

IMPLICATIONS FOR PRACTICE

- There appear to be no adverse effects of folic acid use in pregnancy. The authors were not able to establish benefits of late folic acid supplementation. However, early folate supplementation, which is already recommended, may also be beneficial for the early rapid growth of the placenta, preventing low birth weight, and decreasing the risk of preeclampsia, especially at higher doses.

IMPLICATIONS FOR FURTHER RESEARCH

- Folate use to prevent gestational hypertension looks promising. Placental development measurements have to be standardized and studied, comparing early versus late folate supplementation.

Reference: Charles, D., Ness, A., Campbell, D., Smith, G., Whitley, E., & Hall, M. (2005). Folic acid supplements in pregnancy and birth outcome: Reanalysis of a large randomized controlled trial and update of Cochrane review. *Paediatric and Perinatal Epidemiology, 19*(2), 112-124.

Conditions such as gestational diabetes and chronic glomerulonephritis can retard fetal lung maturity. The use of intrabronchial synthetic surfactant in the treatment of respiratory distress syndrome in the newborn has greatly improved the chances of survival for preterm infants.

Fetal respiratory movements have been seen on ultrasound examination as early as week 11. These fetal respiratory movements may aid in development of the chest wall muscles and regulate lung fluid volume. The fetal lungs produce fluid that expands the air spaces in the lungs. The fluid drains into the amniotic fluid or is swallowed by the fetus.

Before birth, secretion of lung fluid decreases. The normal birth process squeezes out approximately one third of the fluid. Infants of cesarean births do not benefit from this squeezing process; thus they may have more respiratory difficulty at birth. The fluid remaining in the lungs at birth is usually reabsorbed into the infant's bloodstream within 2 hours of birth.

Renal System

The kidneys form during the fifth week and begin to function approximately 4 weeks later. Urine is excreted into the amniotic fluid and forms a major part of the amniotic fluid volume. Oligohydramnios is indicative of renal dysfunction. Because the placenta acts as the organ of excretion and maintains fetal water and electrolyte balance, the fetus does not need functioning kidneys while in utero. At birth, however, the kidneys are required immediately for excretory and acid-base regulatory functions.

A fetal renal malformation can be diagnosed in utero. Corrective or palliative fetal surgery may treat the malformation successfully, or plans can be made for treatment immediately after birth.

At term, the fetus has fully developed kidneys. However, the glomerular filtration rate (GFR) is low, and the kidneys lack the ability to concentrate urine. This makes the newborn more susceptible to both overhydration and dehydration.

Most newborns void within 24 hours of birth. With the loss of the swallowed amniotic fluid and the metabolism of nutrients provided by the placenta, voidings for the first days of life are scanty until fluid intake increases.

Neurologic System

The nervous system originates from the ectoderm during the third week after fertilization. The open neural tube forms during the fourth week. It initially closes at what will be the junction of the brain and spinal cord, leaving both ends open. The embryo folds in on itself lengthwise at this time, forming a head fold in the neural tube at this junction. The cranial end of the neural tube closes, and then the caudal end closes. During week 5, different growth rates cause more flexures in the neural tube, delineating three brain areas: the forebrain, the midbrain, and the hindbrain.

The forebrain develops into the eyes (cranial nerve II) and the cerebral hemispheres. The development of all areas of the cerebral cortex continues throughout fetal life and into childhood. The olfactory system (cranial nerve I) and the thalamus also develop from the forebrain. Cranial nerves III and IV (oculomotor and trochlear) form from the midbrain. The hindbrain forms the medulla, the pons, the cerebellum, and the remainder of the cranial nerves. Brain waves can be recorded on an electroencephalogram by week 8.

The spinal cord develops from the long end of the neural tube. Another ectodermal structure, the neural crest, develops into the peripheral nervous system. By the eighth week, nerve fibers traverse throughout the body. By week 11 or 12, the fetus makes respiratory movements, moves all extremities, and changes position in utero. The fetus can suck his or her thumb and swim in the amniotic fluid pool, turn somersaults, and sometimes ties a knot in the umbilical cord. Box 13-2 describes the major types of fetal movements. Sometime between 16 and 20 weeks, when the movements are strong enough to be perceived by the mother as "the baby moving," quickening has occurred. The perception of movement occurs earlier in the multipara than in the primipara. The mother also becomes aware of the sleep and wake cycles of the fetus.

---

box 13-2 Major Types of Fetal Movements

General movements. These slow gross movements involve the whole body. Their duration is from several seconds to a minute.

Startle movements. These quick (less than 1 second), generalized movements always start in the limbs and may spread to the trunk and neck.

Hiccups. These are repetitive phasic contractions of the diaphragm. A bout may last several minutes.

Fetal breathing movements. These are paradoxic movements in which the thorax moves inward and the abdomen outward with each contraction of the diaphragm.

Isolated arm or leg movements. These movements of extremities occur without movement of the trunk.

Hand-face contact. This occurs any time the moving hand makes contact with the face or mouth.

Retroflexion of the head. This is a slow-to-jerky backward bending of the head.

Lateral rotation of the head. This involves isolated turning of the head from side to side.

Anteflexion of the head. This is a normally slow forward bending of the head.

Opening of the mouth. This isolated movement may be accompanied by protrusion of the tongue.

Yawn. The mouth is slowly opened and rapidly closed after a few seconds.

Sucking. This burst of rhythmic jaw movements is sometimes followed by swallowing. With this movement the fetus may be drinking amniotic fluid.

Stretch. This complex movement involves overextension of the spine, retroflexion of the head, and elevation of the arms.

From Carlson, B. (2004). *Human embryology and developmental biology* (3rd ed.). Philadelphia: Mosby.

Sensory Awareness. Purposeful movements of the fetus have been demonstrated in response to a firm touch transmitted through the mother's abdomen. Because it can feel, the fetus requires anesthesia when invasive procedures are done.

Fetuses respond to sound by 24 weeks. Different types of music evoke different movements. The fetus can be soothed by the sound of the mother's voice. Acoustic stimulation can be used to evoke a fetal heart rate response. The fetus becomes accustomed (i.e., habituates) to noises heard repeatedly. Hearing is fully developed at birth.

The fetus is able to distinguish taste. By the fifth month, when the fetus is swallowing amniotic fluid, a sweetener added to the fluid causes the fetus to swallow faster. The fetus also reacts to temperature changes. A cold solution placed into the amniotic fluid can cause fetal hiccups.

The fetus can see. Eyes have both rods and cones in the retina by the seventh month. A bright light shone on the mother's abdomen in late pregnancy causes abrupt fetal movements. During sleep time, rapid eye movements have been observed similar to those occurring in children and adults while dreaming.

At term, the fetal brain is approximately one fourth the size of an adult brain. Neurologic development continues.

Stressors on the fetus and neonate (e.g., chronic poor nutrition or hypoxia, drugs, environmental toxins, trauma, disease) cause damage to the central nervous system long after the vulnerable embryonic time for malformations in other organ systems. Neurologic insult can result in cerebral palsy, neuromuscular impairment, mental retardation, and learning disabilities.

Endocrine System

The thyroid gland develops along with structures in the head and neck during the third and fourth weeks. The secretion of thyroxine begins during the eighth week. Maternal thyroxine does not readily cross the placenta; therefore the fetus that does not produce thyroid hormones will be born with congenital hypothyroidism. If untreated, hypothyroidism can result in severe mental retardation. Screening for hypothyroidism is typically included in the testing when screening for phenylketonuria (PKU) after birth.

The adrenal cortex is formed during the sixth week and produces hormones by the eighth or ninth week. As term approaches, the fetus produces more cortisol. This is believed to aid in initiation of labor by decreasing the maternal progesterone and stimulating production of prostaglandins.

The pancreas forms from the foregut during the fifth through eighth weeks. The islets of Langerhans develop during the twelfth week. Insulin is produced by week 20. In infants of mothers with uncontrolled diabetes, maternal hyperglycemia produces fetal hyperglycemia, stimulating hyperinsulinemia and islet cell hyperplasia. This results in a macrosomic (large) fetus. The hyperinsulinemia also blocks lung maturation, placing the neonate at risk for respiratory distress and hypoglycemia when the maternal glucose source is lost at birth. Control of the maternal glucose level before and during pregnancy minimizes problems for the fetus and infant.

Reproductive System

Sex differentiation begins in the embryo during the seventh week. Female and male external genitalia are indistinguishable until after the ninth week. Distinguishing characteristics appear around the ninth week and are fully differentiated by the twelfth week. When a Y chromosome is present, testes are formed. By the end of the embryonic period, testosterone is being secreted and causes formation of the male genitalia. By week 28, the testes begin descending into the scrotum. After birth, low levels of testosterone continue to be secreted until the pubertal surge.

The female, with two X chromosomes, forms ovaries and female external genitalia. By the sixteenth week, oogenesis has been established. At birth, the ovaries contain the female's lifetime supply of ova. Most female hormone production is delayed until puberty. However, the fetal endometrium responds to maternal hormones, and withdrawal bleeding or vaginal discharge (pseudomenstruation) may occur at birth when these hormones are lost. The high level of maternal estrogen also stimulates mammary engorgement and secretion of fluid ("witch's milk") in newborn infants of both sexes.

Musculoskeletal System

Bones and muscles develop from the mesoderm by the fourth week of embryonic development. At that time, the cardiac muscle is already beating. The mesoderm next to the neural tube forms the vertebral column and ribs. The parts of the vertebral column grow toward each other to enclose the developing spinal cord. Ossification, or bone formation, begins. If there is a defect in the bony fusion, various forms of spina bifida may occur. A large defect affecting several vertebrae may allow the membranes and spinal cord to pouch out from the back, producing neurologic deficits and skeletal deformity.

The flat bones of the skull develop during the embryonic period, and ossification continues throughout childhood. At birth, connective tissue sutures exist where the bones of the skull meet. The areas where more than two bones meet (called *fontanels*) are especially prominent. The sutures and fontanels allow the bones of the skull to mold, or move during birth, enabling the head to pass through the birth canal.

The bones of the shoulders, arms, hips, and legs appear in the sixth week as a continuous skeleton with no joints. Differentiation occurs, producing separate bones and joints. Ossification will continue through childhood to allow growth. Beginning during the seventh week, muscles contract spontaneously. Arm and leg movements are visible on ultrasound examination, although the mother does not perceive them until sometime between 16 and 20 weeks.

CRITICAL THINKING EXERCISE

Ultrasound Examination During Pregnancy

Melanie is 12 weeks pregnant. Because of her family history of neural tube defects, she has taken a folic acid supplement since before she was pregnant. She has requested that no ultrasound examination be done to try to detect anomalies since, with her religious beliefs, she would not consider having an abortion. However, she has many questions for the nurse: What would the fetus look like now? What fetal structures would be apparent on ultrasound if she had one? Would any structural anomalies be apparent at 12 weeks? Are there reasons other than for detecting anomalies that an ultrasound examination would be done? What are the risks and benefits of having such an examination? Of not having the examination?

What information should the nurse provide Melanie?

1. Evidence: Is there sufficient evidence to draw conclusions about what information the nurse should provide Melanie?
2. Assumptions: What assumptions can be made about the following factors:
   a. Melanie's motivation to learn about fetal development
   b. Melanie's concern for her fetus
   c. Melanie's knowledge about ultrasound examinations
   d. Melanie's right to refuse an examination
3. What implications and priorities for nursing care can be made at this time?
4. Does the evidence objectively support your conclusion?
5. Are there alternative perspectives to your conclusion?

Integumentary System

The epidermis begins as a single layer of cells derived from the ectoderm at 4 weeks. By the seventh week, there are two layers of cells. The cells of the superficial layer are sloughed and become mixed with the sebaceous gland secretions to form the white, cheesy *vernix caseosa*, the material that protects the skin of the fetus. The vernix is thick at 24 weeks but becomes scant by term.

The basal layer of the epidermis is the germinal layer, which replaces lost cells. Until 17 weeks, the skin is thin and wrinkled, with blood vessels visible underneath. The skin thickens, and all layers are present at term. After 32 weeks, as subcutaneous fat is deposited under the dermis, the skin becomes less wrinkled and red in appearance.

By 16 weeks, the epidermal ridges are present on the palms of the hands, the fingers, the bottom of the feet, and the toes. These handprints and footprints are unique to that infant.

Hairs form from hair bulbs in the epidermis that project into the dermis. Cells in the hair bulb keratinize to form the hair shaft. As the cells at the base of the hair shaft proliferate, the hair grows to the surface of the epithelium. Very fine hairs, called *lanugo*, appear first at 12 weeks on the eyebrows and upper lip. By 20 weeks, they cover the entire body. At this time, the eyelashes, eyebrows, and scalp hair are beginning to grow. By 28 weeks, the scalp hair is longer than the lanugo, which thins and may disappear by term gestation.

Fingernails and toenails develop from thickened epidermis at the tips of the digits beginning during the tenth week. They grow slowly. Fingernails usually reach the fingertips by 32 weeks, and toenails reach toetips by 36 weeks.

Immunologic System

During the third trimester, albumin and globulin are present in the fetus. The only immunoglobulin that crosses the placenta, immunoglobulin G (IgG), provides passive acquired immunity to specific bacterial toxins. The fetus produces IgM by the end of the first trimester. These are produced in response to blood group antigens, gram-negative enteric organisms, and some viruses. IgA is not produced by the fetus; however, colostrum, the precursor to breast milk, contains large amounts of IgA and can provide passive immunity to the neonate who is breastfed.

The normal term neonate can fight infection but not so effectively as an older child. The preterm infant is at much greater risk for infection.

Table 13-1 summarizes embryonic and fetal development.

Multifetal Pregnancy
Twins

The incidence of twinning is 1 in 43 pregnancies (Benirschke, 2004). There has been a steady rise in multiple births since 1973. This is partly attributed to delayed childbearing. The use of ovulation-enhancing drugs is also a factor.

Dizygotic Twins. When two mature ova are produced in one ovarian cycle, both have the potential to be fertilized by separate sperm. This results in two zygotes, or dizygotic twins (Fig. 13-10). There are always two amnions, two chorions, and two placentas, which may be fused. These dizygotic, or fraternal, twins may be the same sex or different sexes and are genetically no more alike than siblings born at different times. Dizygotic twinning occurs in families, more often among African-American women than among Caucasian women, and least often among Asian women. Dizygotic twinning increases in frequency with maternal age up to 35 years, with parity, and with the use of fertility drugs.

Monozygotic Twins. Identical twins, or monozygotic twins, develop from one fertilized ovum, which then divides (Fig. 13-11). They are the same sex and have the same genotype. If division occurs soon after fertilization, two embryos, two amnions, two chorions, and two placentas that may be fused will develop. Most often, division occurs between 4 and 8 days after fertilization, and there are two embryos, two amnions, one chorion, and one placenta. Rarely, division occurs after the eighth day after fertilization. In this case, there are two embryos within a common amnion and a common chorion with one placenta. This often causes circulatory problems because the umbilical cords may tangle together, and one or both fetuses may die. If division occurs very late, cleavage may not be complete, and conjoined twins could result. Monozygotic twinning occurs in approximately 1 of 250 births (Benirschke, 2004). There is no association with race, heredity, maternal age, or parity. Fertility drugs increase the incidence of monozygotic twinning.

Two chorions   Two amnions

FIG. 13-10 Formation of dizygotic twins, with fertilization of two ova, two implantations, two placentas, two chorions, and two amnions.

table 13-1 Milestones in Human Development Before Birth Since Last Menstrual Period

	4 WEEKS	8 WEEKS	12 WEEKS
EXTERNAL APPEARANCE	Body flexed, C-shaped; arm and leg buds present; head at right angles to body	Body fairly well formed; nose flat, eyes far apart; digits well formed; head elevating; tail almost disappeared; eyes, ears, nose, and mouth recognizable	Nails appearing; resembles a human; head erect but disproportionately large; skin pink, delicate
CROWN-TO-RUMP MEASUREMENT; WEIGHT	0.4-0.5 cm; 0.4 g	2.5-3 cm; 2 g	6-9 cm; 19 g
GASTROINTESTINAL SYSTEM	Stomach at midline and fusiform; conspicuous liver; esophagus short; intestine a short tube	Intestinal villi developing; small intestines coil within umbilical cord; palatal folds present; liver very large	Bile secreted; palatal fusion complete; intestines have withdrawn from cord and assume characteristic positions
MUSCULOSKELETAL SYSTEM	All somites present	First indication of ossification—occiput, mandible, and humerus; fetus capable of some movement; definitive muscles of trunk, limbs, and head well represented	Some bones well outlined, ossification spreading; upper cervical to lower sacral arches and bodies ossify; smooth muscle layers indicated in hollow viscera
CIRCULATORY SYSTEM	Heart develops, double chambers visible, begins to beat; aortic arch and major veins completed	Main blood vessels assume final plan; enucleated red cells predominate in blood	Blood forming in marrow
RESPIRATORY SYSTEM	Primary lung buds appear	Pleural and pericardial cavities forming; branching bronchioles; nostrils closed by epithelial plugs	Lungs acquire definite shape; vocal cords appear
RENAL SYSTEM	Rudimentary ureteral buds appear	Earliest secretory tubules differentiating; bladder-urethra separates from rectum	Kidney able to secrete urine; bladder expands as a sac
NERVOUS SYSTEM	Well-marked midbrain flexure; no hindbrain or cervical flexures; neural groove closed	Cerebral cortex begins to acquire typical cells; differentiation of cerebral cortex, meninges, ventricular foramina, cerebrospinal fluid circulation; spinal cord extends entire length of spine	Brain structural configuration almost complete; cord shows cervical and lumbar enlargements; fourth ventricle foramina are developed; sucking present
SENSORY ORGANS	Eye and ear appearing as optic vessel and otocyst	Primordial choroid plexuses develop; ventricles large relative to cortex; development progressing; eyes converging rapidly; internal ear developing; eyelids fuse	Earliest taste buds indicated; characteristic organization of eye attained
GENITAL SYSTEM	Genital ridge appears (fifth week)	Testes and ovaries distinguishable; external genitalia sexless but begin to differentiate	Sex recognizable; internal and external sex organs specific

table 13-1 Milestones in Human Development Before Birth Since Last Menstrual Period—cont'd

16 WEEKS	20 WEEKS	24 WEEKS
EXTERNAL APPEARANCE		
Head still dominant; face looks human; eyes, ears, and nose approach typical appearance on gross examination; arm/leg ratio proportionate; scalp hair appears	Vernix caseosa appears; lanugo appears; legs lengthen considerably; sebaceous glands appear	Body lean but fairly well proportioned; skin red and wrinkled; vernix caseosa present; sweat glands forming
CROWN-TO-RUMP MEASUREMENT; WEIGHT		
11.5-13.5 cm; 100 g	16-18.5 cm; 300 g	23 cm; 600 g
GASTROINTESTINAL SYSTEM		
Meconium in bowel; some enzyme secretion; anus open	Enamel and dentine depositing; ascending colon recognizable	
MUSCULOSKELETAL SYSTEM		
Most bones distinctly indicated throughout body; joint cavities appear; muscular movements can be detected	Sternum ossifies; fetal movements strong enough for mother to feel	
CIRCULATORY SYSTEM		
Heart muscle well developed; blood formation active in spleen		Blood formation increases in bone marrow and decreases in liver
RESPIRATORY SYSTEM		
Elastic fibers appear in lungs; terminal and respiratory bronchioles appear	Nostrils reopen; primitive respiratory-like movements begin	Alveolar ducts and sacs present; lecithin begins to appear in amniotic fluid (weeks 26 to 27)
RENAL SYSTEM		
Kidney in position; attains typical shape and plan		
NERVOUS SYSTEM		
Cerebral lobes delineated; cerebellum assumes some prominence	Brain grossly formed; cord myelination begins; spinal cord ends at level of first sacral vertebra (S1)	Cerebral cortex layered typically; neuronal proliferation in cerebral cortex ends
SENSORY ORGANS		
General sense organs differentiated	Nose and ears ossify	Can hear
GENITAL SYSTEM		
Testes in position for descent into scrotum: vagina open		Testes at inguinal ring in descent to scrotum

Continued

table 13-1 **Milestones in Human Development Before Birth Since Last Menstrual Period—cont'd**

28 WEEKS	30-31 WEEKS	36 AND 40 WEEKS
EXTERNAL APPEARANCE		
Lean body, less wrinkled and red; nails appear	Subcutaneous fat beginning to collect; more rounded appearance; skin pink and smooth; has assumed birth position	**36 Weeks** Skin pink, body rounded; general lanugo disappearing; body usually plump **40 Weeks** Skin smooth and pink; scant vernix caseosa; moderate to profuse hair; lanugo on shoulders and upper body only; nasal and alar cartilage apparent
CROWN-TO-RUMP MEASUREMENT; WEIGHT		
27 cm; 1100 g	31 cm; 1800-2100 g	**36 Weeks** 35 cm; 2200-2900 g **40 Weeks** 40 cm; 3200+ g
MUSCULOSKELETAL SYSTEM		
Astragalus (talus, ankle bone) ossifies; weak, fleeting movements, minimum tone	Middle fourth phalanxes ossify; permanent teeth primordia seen; can turn head to side	**36 Weeks** Distal femoral ossification centers present; sustained, definite movements; fair tone; can turn and elevate head **40 Weeks** Active, sustained movement; good tone; may lift head
RESPIRATORY SYSTEM		
Lecithin forming on alveolar surfaces	L/S ratio = 1.2:1	**36 Weeks** L/S ratio >2:1 **40 Weeks** Pulmonary branching only two thirds complete
RENAL SYSTEM		
		36 Weeks Formation of new nephrons ceases
NERVOUS SYSTEM		
Appearance of cerebral fissures, convolutions rapidly appearing; indefinite sleep-wake cycle; cry weak or absent; weak suck reflex		**36 Weeks** End of spinal cord at level of third lumbar vertebra (L3); definite sleep-wake cycle **40 Weeks** Myelination of brain begins; patterned sleep-wake cycle with alert periods; cries when hungry or uncomfortable; strong suck reflex
SENSORY ORGANS		
Eyelids reopen; retinal layers completed, light-receptive; pupils capable of reacting to light	Sense of taste present; aware of sounds outside mother's body	
GENITAL SYSTEM		
	Testes descending to scrotum	**40 Weeks** Testes in scrotum; labia majora well developed

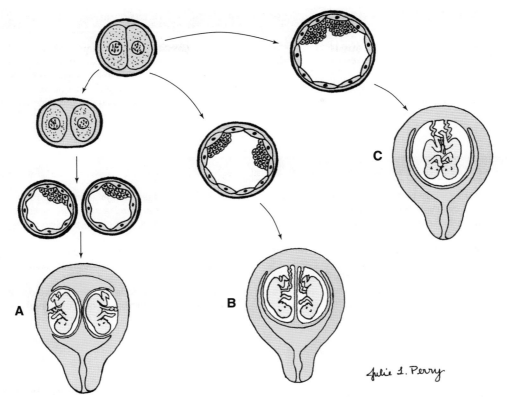

FIG. 13-11 Formation of monozygotic twins. **A,** One fertilization: blastomeres separate, resulting in two implantations, two placentas, and two sets of membranes. **B,** One blastomere with two inner cell masses, one fused placenta, one chorion, and separate amnions. **C,** One blastomere with incomplete separation of cell mass, resulting in conjoined twins.

Other Multifetal Pregnancies

The occurrence of multifetal pregnancies with three or more fetuses has increased with the use of fertility drugs and in vitro fertilization. Triplets occur in approximately 1 of 1341 pregnancies (Benirschke, 2004). They can occur from the division of one zygote into two, with one of the two dividing again, producing identical triplets. Triplets also can be produced from two zygotes, one dividing into a set of identical twins, and the second zygote developing as a single fraternal sibling, or from three zygotes. Quadruplets, quintuplets, sextuplets, and so on, likewise have similar possible derivations.

■ NONGENETIC FACTORS
■ INFLUENCING DEVELOPMENT

Congenital disorders may be inherited, may be caused by environmental factors, or by inadequate maternal nutrition. *Congenital* means that the condition was present at birth. Some congenital malformations may be the result of teratogens, that is, environmental substances or exposures that result in functional or structural disability. In contrast to other forms of developmental disabilities, disabilities

caused by teratogens are theoretically totally preventable. Known human teratogens are drugs and chemicals, infections, exposure to radiation, and certain maternal conditions such as diabetes and PKU (see Box 13-1). A teratogen has the greatest effect on the organs and parts of an embryo during its periods of rapid growth and differentiation. This occurs during the embryonic period, specifically from days 15 to 60. During the first 2 weeks of development, teratogens either have no effect or have effects so severe that they cause miscarriage. Brain growth and development continue during the fetal period, and teratogens can severely affect mental development throughout gestation (see Fig. 13-6).

In addition to the genetic makeup and the influence of teratogens, the adequacy of maternal nutrition influences development. The embryo and fetus must obtain the nutrients they need from the mother's diet; they cannot tap the maternal reserves. Malnutrition during pregnancy produces low-birth-weight newborns who are susceptible to infection. Malnutrition also affects brain development during the latter half of gestation and may result in learning disabilities in the child. Inadequate folic acid is associated with neural tube defects.

Using your preferred search engine, find resources on fetal development. Select two of the Web addresses and access the sites.

Compare and contrast the appearance, the readability, and the information contained in the sites.

- To whom would you recommend these sites?
- Is the information contained culturally relevant?
- Is information available in languages other than English?
- What information would parents need?
- As a nurse, how could you use this information?

key points

- Mitosis is the process by which body cells replicate for growth and development and cell replacement of the organism.
- Meiosis is the process by which gametes are formed for reproduction of the organism.
- Human gestation lasts approximately 280 days after the last menstrual period or 266 days after conception.
- Fertilization occurs in the uterine tube within 24 hours of ovulation. The zygote undergoes mitotic divisions, creating a 16-cell morula.

- Implantation begins 6 days after fertilization.
- The organ systems and external features develop during the embryonic period, that is, the third to the eighth week after fertilization.
- Refinement of structure and function occurs during the fetal period, and the fetus becomes capable of extrauterine survival.
- During critical periods in human development, the embryo and fetus are vulnerable to environmental teratogens.

REFERENCES

Benirschke, K. (2004). Multiple gestation. The biology of twinning. In R. Creasy, R. Resnik, & J. Iams (Eds.). *Maternal-fetal medicine: Principles and practice* (5th ed.). Philadelphia: Saunders.

Mercer, B. (2004). Assessment and induction of fetal pulmonary maturity. In R. Creasy, R. Resnik, & J. Iams (Eds.). *Maternal-fetal medicine: Principles and practice* (5th ed.). Philadelphia: Saunders.

Silver, R., Peltier, M., & Branch, E. (2004). The immunology of pregnancy. In R. Creasy, R. Resnik, J. Iams (Eds.). *Maternal-fetal medicine: Principles and practice* (5th ed.). Philadelphia: Saunders.

Anatomy and Physiology of Pregnancy

learning objectives

- Determine gravidity and parity by using the five- and four-digit systems.
- Describe the various types of pregnancy tests including the timing of tests and interpretation of results.
- Explain the expected maternal anatomic and physiologic adaptations to pregnancy for each body system.
- Differentiate among presumptive, probable, and positive signs of pregnancy.

- Compare normal adult laboratory values with values for pregnant women.
- Identify the maternal hormones produced during pregnancy, their target organs, and their major effects on pregnancy.
- Compare the characteristics of the abdomen, the vulva, and the cervix of the nullipara and the multipara.

electronic resources

Additional information related to the content in Chapter 14 can be found on

the companion website at *evolve*
http://evolve.elsevier.com/Lowdermilk/MWHC/
- NCLEX Review Questions
- WebLinks

or on the interactive companion CD
- NCLEX Review Questions

THE goal of maternity care is a healthy pregnancy with a physically safe and emotionally satisfying outcome for mother, infant, and family. Consistent health supervision and surveillance are of utmost importance in achieving this outcome. However, many maternal adaptations are unfamiliar to pregnant women and their families. Helping the pregnant woman recognize the relation between her physical status and the plan for her care assists her in making decisions and encourages her to participate in her own care.

■ GRAVIDITY AND PARITY

An understanding of the following terms used to describe pregnancy and the pregnant woman is essential to the study of maternity care:
- **gravida:** a woman who is pregnant
- **gravidity:** pregnancy
- **multigravida:** a woman who has had two or more pregnancies
- **multipara:** a woman who has completed two or more pregnancies to 20 or more weeks of gestation

- **nulligravida:** a woman who has never been pregnant
- **nullipara:** a woman who has not completed a pregnancy with a fetus or fetuses who have reached 20 weeks of gestation
- **parity:** the number of pregnancies in which the fetus or fetuses have reached 20 weeks of gestation when they are born, not the number of fetuses (e.g., twins) born. Whether the fetus is born alive or is stillborn (fetus who shows no signs of life at birth) does not affect parity
- **postdate** or **postterm:** a pregnancy that goes beyond 42 weeks of gestation
- **preterm:** a pregnancy that has reached 20 weeks of gestation but ends before completion of 37 weeks of gestation
- **primigravida:** a woman who is pregnant for the first time
- **primipara:** a woman who has completed one pregnancy with a fetus or fetuses who have reached 20 weeks of gestation
- **term:** a pregnancy from the beginning of week 38 of gestation to the end of week 42 of gestation
- **viability:** capacity to live outside the uterus; about 22 to 25 weeks of gestation

Gravidity and parity information is obtained during history-taking interviews. Obtaining and documenting this information accurately is important in making a plan of care for the pregnant woman. Information may be recorded in client records in a variety of ways because there is no one standardized system. It is important that the nurse understands the documentation system used by the health care facility. Gravidity and parity may be described with only 2 digits: the first digit represents the number of pregnancies the woman has had, including the present one; and parity is the number of pregnancies that have reached viability. For example, if the woman had twins at 36 weeks with her first pregnancy, parity would still be counted as one birth (gravida 1, para 1) (Cunningham, Leveno, Bloom, Hauth, Gilstrap, & Wenstrom, 2005). Another system, which consists of five digits separated with hyphens, is commonly used in maternity centers. This system provides more specific information about the woman's obstetric history although it may not provide accurate information about parity since it provides information about births and not pregnancies reaching viability (Beebe, 2005). The first digit represents gravidity; the second digit represents the total number of term births; the third indicates the number of preterm births; the fourth identifies the number of abortions (miscarriage or elective termination of pregnancy); and the fifth is the number of children currently living. The acronym *GTPAL* (gravidity, term, preterm, abortions, living children) may be helpful in remembering this system of notation. For example, if a woman pregnant only once gives birth at week 34 and the infant survives, the abbreviation that represents this information is "1-0-1-0-1." During her next pregnancy, the abbreviation is "2-0-1-0-1." Additional examples are given in Table 14-1.

▬ PREGNANCY TESTS

Early detection of pregnancy allows early initiation of care. Human chorionic gonadotropin (hCG) is the earliest biochemical marker for pregnancy, and pregnancy tests are based on the recognition of hCG or a beta (β) subunit of hCG. Production of β-hCG begins as early as the day of implantation and can be detected as early as 7 to

10 days after conception (Stewart, 2004). The level of hCG increases until it peaks at about 60 to 70 days of gestation and then declines until about 80 days of pregnancy. It remains stable until about 30 weeks and then gradually increases until term. Higher than normal levels of hCG may indicate abnormal gestation (e.g., fetus with Down syndrome) or multiple gestation; an abnormally slow increase or a decrease in hCG levels may indicate ectopic pregnancy or impending miscarriage (Buster & Carson, 2002; Cunningham et al., 2005).

Serum and urine pregnancy tests are performed in clinics, offices, women's health centers, and laboratory settings, and urine pregnancy tests may be performed at home. Both serum and urine tests can provide accurate results. A 7- to 10-ml sample of venous blood is collected for serum testing. Most urine tests require a first-voided morning urine specimen because it contains levels of hCG approximately the same as those in serum. Random urine samples usually have lower levels. Urine tests are less expensive and provide more immediate results than do serum tests (Stewart, 2004).

Many different pregnancy tests are available (Fig. 14-1). The wide variety of tests precludes discussion of each; however, several categories of tests are described here. The

FIG. 14-1 Many pregnancy test products are available over the counter. (Courtesy Dee Lowdermilk, Chapel Hill, NC.)

table 14-1 Gravidity and Parity Using Five-Digit (GTPAL) System and Two-Digit System (G/P)

CONDITION	G GRAVIDITY	T TERM BIRTHS	P PRETERM BIRTHS	A ABORTIONS AND MISCARRIAGES	L LIVING CHILDREN	TWO DIGIT G/P
Shauna is pregnant for the first time.	1	0	0	0	0	1/0
She carries the pregnancy to 34 weeks, and the neonate survives.	1	0	1	0	1	1/1
She becomes pregnant again.	2	0	1	0	1	2/1
Her second pregnancy ends in miscarriage at 10 weeks.	2	0	1	1	1	2/1
During her third pregnancy, she gives birth at 38 weeks.	3	1	1	1	2	3/2

nurse should read the manufacturer's directions for the test to be used.

Radioimmunoassay (RIA) pregnancy tests for the beta subunit of hCG in serum or urine samples use radioactively labeled markers and are usually performed in a laboratory. These tests are accurate with low hCG levels (5 milliinternational units/ml) and can confirm pregnancy as soon as 1 week after conception. Results are available within a few hours (Stewart, 2004).

Radioreceptor assay (RRA) is a serum test that measures the ability of a blood sample to inhibit the binding of radiolabeled hCG to receptors. The test is 90% to 95% accurate from 6 to 8 days after conception (Pagana & Pagana, 2003).

Enzyme-linked immunosorbent assay (ELISA) testing is the most popular method of testing for pregnancy. It uses a specific monoclonal antibody (anti-hCG) with enzymes to bond with hCG in urine. As an office or home procedure, it requires minimal time and offers results in less than 5 minutes. A positive test result is indicated by a simple color-change reaction. Depending on the specific test, levels of hCG as low as 25 milliinternational units/ml can be detected as early as 7 days after conception (Stewart, 2004).

ELISA technology is the basis for most over-the-counter home pregnancy tests. With these one-step tests, the woman usually applies urine to a strip and reads the results. The test kits come with directions for collection of the specimen, the testing procedure, and reading of the results. Most manufacturers of the kits provide a toll-free telephone number to call if users have concerns and questions about test procedures or results (see Teaching for Self-Care box). The most common error in performing home pregnancy tests is performing the test too early in pregnancy (Stewart, 2004). Cole, Khanlian, Sutton, Davies, and Rayburn (2004) found that a sensitivity of 12.5 milliinternational units/ml hCG was needed to detect 95% of pregnancies at the time of the missed period. Only one home pregnancy test out of 18 studied had this sensitivity. Less than half (44%) of the tests studied gave clear positive

CRITICAL THINKING EXERCISE

Pregnancy Testing

Blanca is a 16-year-old high school junior who thought her menstrual period was 5 days late. She used a home pregnancy test and the results were negative. At school the next day, she tells the school nurse that she is relieved that the test was negative because she did not want to be pregnant. How should the nurse respond to Blanca's statement?

1. Evidence—Is there sufficient evidence to draw conclusions about how the nurse should respond?
2. Assumptions—What assumptions can be made about the following issues?
   a. hCG levels during pregnancy
   b. Accuracy of home pregnancy tests
   c. Adolescent development, specifically menstrual cycles
3. What implications and priorities for nursing care can be made at this time?
4. Does the evidence objectively support your conclusion?
5. Are there alternative perspectives to your conclusion?

results at 100 milliinternational units/ml hCG. At this level of specificity, about 16% of pregnancies would be detected at the time of missed menses.

Interpreting the results of pregnancy tests requires some judgment. The type of pregnancy test and its degree of sensitivity (ability to detect low levels of a substance) and specificity (ability to discern the absence of a substance) must be considered in conjunction with the woman's history (Sadler, Dynes, Daley, Ickovics, Leventhal, & Reynolds, 2004). This includes the date of her last menstrual period (LMP), her usual cycle length, and results of previous pregnancy tests. It is important to know if the woman is a substance abuser and what medications she is taking, because medications such as anticonvulsants and tranquilizers can cause false-positive results, whereas diuretics and promethazine can cause false-negative results (Pagana & Pagana, 2003). Improper collection of the specimen, hormone-producing tumors, and laboratory errors also may cause false results. Whenever there is any question, further evaluation or retesting may be appropriate.

■ ADAPTATIONS TO PREGNANCY

Maternal physiologic adaptations are attributed to the hormones of pregnancy and to mechanical pressures arising from the enlarging uterus and other tissues. These adaptations protect the woman's normal physiologic functioning, meet the metabolic demands pregnancy imposes on her body, and provide a nurturing environment for fetal development and growth. Although pregnancy is a normal phenomenon, problems can occur.

Signs of Pregnancy

Some of the physiologic adaptations are recognized as signs and symptoms of pregnancy. Three commonly used categories of signs and symptoms of pregnancy are

TEACHING FOR SELF-CARE

Home Pregnancy Testing

- Follow the manufacturer's instructions carefully. Do not omit steps.
- Review the manufacturer's list of foods, medications, and other substances that can affect the test results.
- Use a first-voided morning urine specimen.
- If the test done at the time of your missed period is negative, repeat the test in 1 week if you still have not had a period.
- If you have questions about the test, contact the manufacturer.
- Contact your health care provider for follow-up if the test result is positive, or if the test result is negative and you still have not had a period.

presumptive (those changes felt by the woman—e.g., amenorrhea, fatigue, nausea and vomiting, breast changes); probable (those changes observed by an examiner—e.g., Hegar sign, ballottement, pregnancy tests); and positive (those signs that are attributable only to the presence of the fetus—e.g., hearing fetal heart tones, visualization of the fetus, and palpating fetal movements). Table 14-2 summarizes these signs of pregnancy in relation to when they might occur and other causes for their occurrence.

Reproductive System and Breasts
Uterus

Changes in Size, Shape, and Position. The phenomenal uterine growth in the first trimester is stimulated by high levels of estrogen and progesterone. Early uterine enlargement results from increased vascularity and dilation of blood vessels, hyperplasia (production of new muscle fibers and fibroelastic tissue) and hypertrophy (enlargement of preexisting muscle fibers and fibroelastic tissue), and development of the decidua. By 7 weeks of gestation, the uterus is the size of a large hen's egg; by 10 weeks of gestation, it is the size of an orange (twice its nonpregnant size);

and by 12 weeks of gestation, it is the size of a grapefruit. After the third month, uterine enlargement is primarily the result of mechanical pressure of the growing fetus.

As the uterus enlarges, it also changes in shape and position. At conception the uterus is shaped like an upside-down pear. During the second trimester, as the muscular walls strengthen and become more elastic, the uterus becomes spherical or globular. Later, as the fetus lengthens, the uterus becomes larger and more ovoid and rises out of the pelvis into the abdominal cavity.

The pregnancy may "show" after the fourteenth week, although this depends to some degree on the woman's height and weight. Abdominal enlargement may be less apparent in the nullipara with good abdominal muscle tone (Fig. 14-2). Posture also influences the type and degree of abdominal enlargement that occurs. In normal pregnancies, the uterus enlarges at a predictable rate. As the uterus grows, it may be palpated above the symphysis pubis some time between the twelfth and fourteenth weeks of pregnancy (Fig. 14-3). The uterus rises gradually to the level of the umbilicus at 22 to 24 weeks of gestation and nearly reaches the xiphoid process at term. Between weeks 38 and

table 14-2 Signs of Pregnancy

TIME OF OCCURRENCE (GESTATIONAL AGE)	SIGN	OTHER POSSIBLE CAUSE
PRESUMPTIVE SIGNS		
3-4 wk	Breast changes	Premenstrual changes, oral contraceptives
4 wk	Amenorrhea	Stress, vigorous exercise, early menopause, endocrine problems, malnutrition
4-14 wk	Nausea, vomiting	Gastrointestinal virus, food poisoning
6-12 wk	Urinary frequency	Infection, pelvic tumors
12 wk	Fatigue	Stress, illness
16-20 wk	Quickening	Gas, peristalsis
PROBABLE SIGNS		
5 wk	Goodell sign	Pelvic congestion
6-8 wk	Chadwick sign	Pelvic congestion
6-12 wk	Hegar sign	Pelvic congestion
4-12 wk	Positive result of pregnancy test (serum)	Hydatidiform mole, choriocarcinoma
6-12 wk	Positive result of pregnancy test (urine)	False-positive results may be caused by pelvic infection, tumors
16 wk	Braxton Hicks contractions	Myomas, other tumors
16-28 wk	Ballottement	Tumors, cervical polyps
POSITIVE SIGNS		
5-6 wk	Visualization of fetus by real-time ultrasound examination	No other causes
6 wk	Fetal heart tones detected by ultrasound examination	No other causes
16 wk	Visualization of fetus by radiographic study	No other causes
8-17 wk	Fetal heart tones detected by Doppler ultrasound stethoscope	No other causes
17-19 wk	Fetal heart tones detected by fetal stethoscope	No other causes
19-22 wk	Fetal movements palpated	No other causes
Late pregnancy	Fetal movements visible	No other causes

FIG. 14-2 Comparison of abdomen, vulva, and cervix in nullipara **(A)** and multipara **(B)** at the same stage of pregnancy.

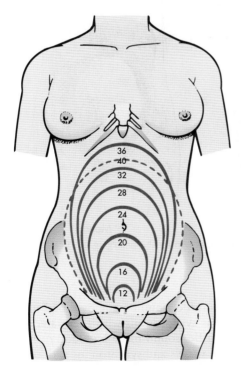

FIG. 14-3 Height of fundus by weeks of normal gestation with a single fetus. Dashed line, height after lightening. (From Seidel, H., Ball, J., Dains, J., & Benedict, G. [2006]. *Mosby's guide to physical examination* [6th ed.]. St. Louis: Mosby.)

40, fundal height drops as the fetus begins to descend and engage in the pelvis (lightening) (see Fig. 14-3, *dashed line*). Generally, lightening occurs in the nullipara about 2 weeks before the onset of labor and at the start of labor in the multipara.

Uterine enlargement is determined by measuring fundal height, a measurement commonly used to estimate the duration of pregnancy. However, variation in the position of the fundus or the fetus, variations in the amount of amniotic fluid present, the presence of more than one fetus, maternal obesity, and variation in examiner techniques can reduce the accuracy of this estimation of the duration of pregnancy.

The uterus normally rotates to the right as it elevates, probably because of the presence of the rectosigmoid colon on the left side, but the extensive hypertrophy (enlargement) of the round ligaments keeps the uterus in the midline. Eventually the growing uterus touches the anterior abdominal wall and displaces the intestines to either side of the abdomen (Fig. 14-4). Whenever a pregnant woman is standing, most of her uterus rests against the anterior abdominal wall, and this contributes to altering her center of gravity.

At approximately 6 weeks of gestation, softening and compressibility of the lower uterine segment (the uterine isthmus) occur (Hegar sign) (Fig. 14-5). This results in exaggerated uterine anteflexion during the first 3 months of pregnancy. In this position, the uterine fundus presses on the urinary bladder, causing the woman to have urinary frequency.

Changes in Contractility. Soon after the fourth month of pregnancy, uterine contractions can be felt through the abdominal wall. These contractions are referred to as the Braxton Hicks sign. Braxton Hicks contractions are irregular and painless and occur intermittently throughout pregnancy. These contractions facilitate uterine blood flow through the intervillous spaces of the placenta and thereby promote oxygen delivery to the fetus. Although Braxton Hicks contractions are not painful, some women complain that they are annoying. After the twenty-eighth week, these contractions become much more definite, but they usually cease with walking or exercise. Braxton Hicks contractions can be mistaken for true labor; however, they do not increase in intensity or frequency or cause cervical dilation.

Uteroplacental Blood Flow. Placental perfusion depends on the maternal blood flow to the uterus. Blood flow increases rapidly as the uterus increases in size. Although uterine blood flow increases twentyfold, the fetoplacental unit grows more rapidly. Consequently, more oxygen is extracted from the uterine blood during the latter part of pregnancy (Cunningham et al., 2005). In a normal term pregnancy, one sixth of the total maternal blood volume is within the uterine vascular system. The rate of blood flow through the uterus averages 500 ml/min, and oxygen consumption of the gravid uterus increases to meet fetal needs. A low maternal arterial pressure, contractions of the uterus,

4 Months 6 Months 9 Months

4 Months 6 Months 9 Months

FIG. 14-4 Displacement of internal abdominal structures and diaphragm by the enlarging uterus at 4, 6, and 9 months of gestation.

and maternal supine position are three factors known to decrease blood flow. Estrogen stimulation may increase uterine blood flow. Doppler ultrasound examination can be used to measure uterine blood flow velocity, especially in pregnancies at risk because of conditions associated with decreased placental perfusion such as hypertension, intrauterine growth restriction, diabetes mellitus, and multiple gestation (Harman, 2004). By using an ultrasound device or a fetal stethoscope, the health care provider may hear the uterine souffle (sound made by blood in the uterine arteries that is synchronous with the maternal pulse) or the funic souffle (sound made by blood rushing through the umbilical vessels and synchronous with the fetal heart rate).

Cervical Changes. A softening of the cervical tip called Goodell sign may be observed about the beginning of the sixth week in a normal, unscarred cervix. This sign is brought about by increased vascularity, slight hypertrophy,

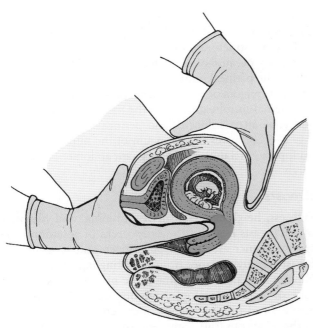

FIG. 14-5 Hegar sign. Bimanual examination for assessing compressibility and softening of the isthmus (lower uterine segment) while the cervix is still firm.

FIG. 14-6 Internal ballottement (18 weeks).

and hyperplasia (increase in number of cells) of the muscle and its collagen-rich connective tissue, which becomes loose, edematous, highly elastic, and increased in volume. The glands near the external os proliferate beneath the stratified squamous epithelium, giving the cervix the velvety appearance characteristic of pregnancy. *Friability* (tissue is easily damaged) is increased and may cause slight bleeding after coitus with deep penetration or after vaginal examination. Pregnancy also can cause the squamocolumnar junction, the site for obtaining cells for cervical cancer screening, to be located away from the cervix. Because of all these changes, evaluation of abnormal Papanicolaou (Pap) tests during pregnancy can be complicated. However, careful assessment of all pregnant women is important, because about 3% of all cervical cancers are diagnosed during pregnancy (Berman, DiSaia, & Tewari, 2004).

The cervix of the nullipara is rounded. Lacerations of the cervix almost always occur during the birth process. With or without lacerations, however, after childbirth, the cervix becomes more oval in the horizontal plane, and the external os appears as a transverse slit (see Fig. 14-2).

Changes Related to the Presence of the Fetus. Passive movement of the unengaged fetus is called ballottement and can be identified generally between the sixteenth and eighteenth week. Ballottement is a technique of palpating a floating structure by bouncing it gently and feeling it rebound. In the technique used to palpate the fetus, the examiner places a finger in the vagina and taps gently upward, causing the fetus to rise. The fetus then sinks, and a gentle tap is felt on the finger (Fig. 14-6).

The first recognition of fetal movements, or "feeling life," by the multiparous woman may occur as early as the fourteenth to sixteenth week. The nulliparous woman may not notice these sensations until the eighteenth week or later. Quickening is commonly described as a flutter and is difficult to distinguish from peristalsis. Fetal movements gradually increase in intensity and frequency. The week when quickening occurs provides a tentative clue in dating the duration of gestation.

Vagina and Vulva

Pregnancy hormones prepare the vagina for stretching during labor and birth by causing the vaginal mucosa to thicken, the connective tissue to loosen, the smooth muscle to hypertrophy, and the vaginal vault to lengthen. Increased vascularity results in a violet-bluish color of the vaginal mucosa and cervix. The deepened color, termed the Chadwick sign, may be evident as early as the sixth week but is easily noted at the eighth week of pregnancy (Monga & Sanborn, 2004).

Leukorrhea is a white or slightly gray mucoid discharge with a faint musty odor. This copious mucoid fluid occurs in response to cervical stimulation by estrogen and progesterone. The fluid is whitish because of the presence of many exfoliated vaginal epithelial cells caused by the hyperplasia of normal pregnancy. This vaginal discharge is never pruritic or blood stained. Because of the progesterone effect, ferning usually does not occur in the dried cervical mucus smear, as it would in a smear of amniotic fluid. Instead, a beaded or cellular crystallizing pattern is seen in the dried mucus (Gibbs, Sweet, & Duff, 2004). The mucus fills the endocervical canal, resulting in the formation of the mucous plug (operculum) (Fig. 14-7). The operculum acts as a barrier against bacterial invasion during pregnancy.

During pregnancy, the pH of vaginal secretions is more acidic (ranging from about 3.5 to 6 [normal 4 to 7]). This change is due to increased production of lactic acid caused by *Lactobacillus acidophilus* action on glycogen in the vaginal epithelium, probably resulting from increased estrogen levels (Cunningham et al., 2005). While this acidic environment provides more protection from some organisms, the pregnant woman is more vulnerable to other infections, especially yeast infections because the glycogen-rich environment is more susceptible to *Candida albicans* (Gibbs et al., 2004).

FIG. 14-7   A, Cervix in nonpregnant woman. **B,** Cervix during pregnancy.

The increased vascularity of the vagina and other pelvic viscera results in a marked increase in sensitivity. The increased sensitivity may lead to a high degree of sexual interest and arousal, especially during the second trimester of pregnancy. The increased congestion plus the relaxed walls of the blood vessels and the heavy uterus may result

in edema and varicosities of the vulva. The edema and varicosities usually resolve during the postpartum period.

External structures of the perineum are enlarged during pregnancy because of an increase in vasculature, hypertrophy of the perineal body, and deposition of fat (Fig. 14-8). The labia majora of the nullipara approximate and obscure the vaginal introitus; those of the parous woman separate and gape after childbirth and perineal or vaginal injury. Fig. 14-2 compares the perineum of the nullipara and the multipara in relation to the pregnant abdomen, vulva, and cervix.

Breasts

Fullness, heightened sensitivity, tingling, and heaviness of the breasts begin in the early weeks of gestation in response to increased levels of estrogen and progesterone. Breast sensitivity varies from mild tingling to sharp pain. Nipples and areolae become more pigmented, secondary pinkish areolae develop, extending beyond the primary areolae, and nipples become more erectile. Hypertrophy of the sebaceous (oil) glands embedded in the primary areolae, called Montgomery tubercles (see Fig. 5-6), may be seen around the nipples. These sebaceous glands may have a protective role in that they keep the nipples lubricated for breastfeeding.

The richer blood supply causes the vessels beneath the skin to dilate. Once barely noticeable, the blood vessels become visible, often appearing in an intertwining blue network beneath the surface of the skin. Venous congestion in the breasts is more obvious in primigravidas. Striae gravidarum may appear at the outer aspects of the breasts.

During the second and third trimesters, growth of the mammary glands accounts for the progressive breast enlargement. The high levels of luteal and placental hormones in pregnancy promote proliferation of the lactiferous ducts and lobule-alveolar tissue, so that palpation of the breasts reveals a generalized, coarse nodularity. Glandular tissue

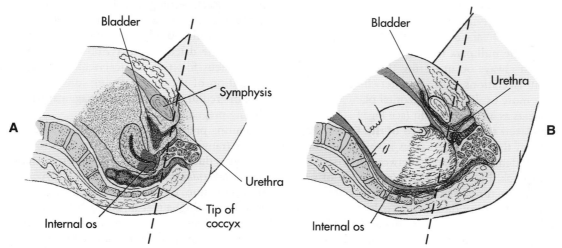

FIG. 14-8   A, Pelvic floor in nonpregnant woman. **B,** Pelvic floor at end of pregnancy. Note marked hypertrophy and hyperplasia below dotted line joining tip of coccyx and inferior margin of symphysis. Note elongation of bladder and urethra as a result of compression. Fat deposits are increased.

displaces connective tissue, and as a result, the tissue becomes softer and looser.

Although development of the mammary glands is functionally complete by midpregnancy, lactation is inhibited until a decrease in estrogen level occurs after the birth. A thin, clear, viscous secretory material (precolostrum) can be found in the acini cells by the third month of gestation. Colostrum, the creamy, white-to-yellowish-to-orange premilk fluid, may be expressed from the nipples as early as 16 weeks of gestation (Lawrence & Lawrence, 2004). See Chapter 27 for discussion of lactation.

General Body Systems
Cardiovascular System

Maternal adjustments to pregnancy involve extensive changes in the cardiovascular system, both anatomic and physiologic. Cardiovascular adaptations protect the woman's normal physiologic functioning, meet the metabolic demands pregnancy imposes on her body, and provide for fetal developmental and growth needs.

Slight cardiac hypertrophy (enlargement) is probably secondary to the increased blood volume and cardiac output that occurs. The heart returns to its normal size after childbirth. As the diaphragm is displaced upward by the enlarging uterus, the heart is elevated upward and rotated forward to the left (Fig. 14-9). The apical impulse, a point of maximal intensity (PMI), is shifted upward and laterally about 1 to 1.5 cm. The degree of shift depends on the duration of pregnancy and the size and position of the uterus.

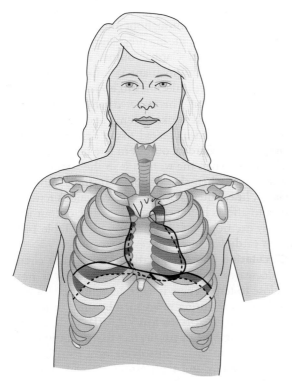

FIG. 14-9 Changes in position of heart, lungs, and thoracic cage in pregnancy. *Broken line,* nonpregnant; *solid line,* change that occurs in pregnancy.

The changes in heart size and position and increases in blood volume and cardiac output contribute to auscultatory changes common in pregnancy. There is more audible splitting of S_1 and S_2, and S_3 may be readily heard after 20 weeks of gestation. In addition, systolic and diastolic murmurs may be heard over the pulmonic area in some women. These are transient and disappear shortly after the woman gives birth (Cunningham et al., 2005).

Between 14 and 20 weeks of gestation, the pulse increases about 10 to 15 beats/min, which then persists to term. Palpitations may occur. In twin gestations the maternal heart rate increases significantly in the third trimester (Malone & D'Alton, 2004).

The cardiac rhythm may be disturbed. The pregnant woman may experience sinus arrhythmia, premature atrial contractions, and premature ventricular systole. In the healthy woman with no underlying heart disease, no therapy is needed; however, women with preexisting heart disease will need close medical and obstetric supervision during pregnancy (see Chapter 33).

Blood Pressure. Arterial blood pressure (brachial artery) is affected by age, activity level, presence of health problems, and circadian rhythm (Hermida, Ayala, Mojon, & Fernandez, 2001). Additional factors must be considered during pregnancy. These factors include maternal anxiety, maternal position, and size and type of blood pressure apparatus.

Maternal anxiety can elevate readings. If an elevated reading is found, the woman is given time to rest, and the reading is repeated.

Maternal position affects readings. Brachial blood pressure is highest when the woman is sitting, lowest when she is lying in the lateral recumbent position, and intermediate when she is supine, except for some women who experience supine hypotensive syndrome (see later discussion). Therefore at each prenatal visit, the reading should be obtained in the same arm and with the woman in the same position. The position and arm used should be recorded along with the reading (Gonik & Foley, 2004).

The proper-size cuff is absolutely necessary for accurate readings. The cuff should be 20% wider than the diameter of the arm around which it is wrapped, or about 12 to 14 cm for average-sized individuals and 18 to 20 cm for obese persons. Too small a cuff yields a false high reading; too large a cuff yields a false low reading. Caution also should be used when comparing auscultatory and oscilatory blood pressure readings, because discrepancies can occur (Pickering, 2002).

Systolic blood pressure usually remains the same as the prepregnancy level but may decrease slightly as pregnancy advances. Diastolic blood pressure begins to decrease in the first trimester, continues to drop until 24 to 32 weeks, then gradually increases and returns to prepregnancy levels by term (Blackburn, 2003; Monga, 2004).

Calculating the *mean arterial pressure (MAP)* (mean of the blood pressure in the arterial circulation) can increase the diagnostic value of the findings. Normal MAP readings in the nonpregnant woman are 86.4 mm Hg ± 7.5 mm Hg. MAP readings for a pregnant woman are slightly higher (Gonik & Foley, 2004). One way to calculate a MAP is illustrated in Box 14-1. Some degree of compression of the vena cava occurs in all women who lie flat on their backs during the second half of pregnancy (see Fig. 21-5). Some women experience a decrease in their systolic blood pressure of more than 30 mm Hg. After 4 to 5 minutes a reflex bradycardia is noted, cardiac output is reduced by half, and the woman feels faint. This condition is referred to as *supine hypotensive syndrome* (Cunningham et al., 2005).

Compression of the iliac veins and inferior vena cava by the uterus causes increased venous pressure and reduced blood flow in the legs (except when the woman is in the lateral position). These alterations contribute to the dependent edema, varicose veins in the legs and vulva, and hemorrhoids that develop in the latter part of term pregnancy (Fig. 14-10).

Blood Volume and Composition. The degree of blood volume expansion varies considerably. Blood volume increases by approximately 1500 ml, or 40% to 45% above nonpregnancy levels (Cunningham et al., 2005). This increase consists of 1000 ml plasma plus 450 ml red

box 14-1 Calculation of Mean Arterial Pressure

Blood pressure: 106/70 mm Hg

Formula: $\dfrac{\text{(systolic)} + 2\text{(diastolic)}}{3}$

$$\dfrac{(106) + 2(70)}{3}$$

$$\dfrac{106 + 140}{3}$$

$$246/3 = 82 \text{ mm Hg}$$

FIG. 14-10 Hemorrhoids. (Courtesy Marjorie Pyle, RNC, Lifecircle, Costa Mesa, CA.)

blood cells (RBCs). The blood volume starts to increase at about the tenth to twelfth week, peaks at about the thirty-second to thirty-fourth week, and then decreases slightly at the fortieth week. The increase in volume of a multiple gestation is greater than that for a pregnancy with a single fetus (Malone & D'Alton, 2004). Increased volume is a protective mechanism. It is essential for meeting the blood volume needs of the hypertrophied vascular system of the enlarged uterus, for adequately hydrating fetal and maternal tissues when the woman assumes an erect or supine position, and for providing a fluid reserve to compensate for blood loss during birth and the puerperium. Peripheral vasodilation maintains a normal blood pressure despite the increased blood volume in pregnancy.

During pregnancy there is an accelerated production of RBCs (normal, 4.2 to 5.4 million/mm³). The percentage of increase depends on the amount of iron available. The RBC mass increases by about 20% to 30% (Monga, 2004).

Because the plasma increase exceeds the increase in RBC production, there is a decrease in normal hemoglobin values (12 to 16 g/dl blood) and hematocrit values (37% to 47%). This state of hemodilution is referred to as *physiologic anemia*. The decrease is more noticeable during the second trimester, when rapid expansion of blood volume takes place faster than RBC production. If the hemoglobin value decreases to 10 g/dl or less or if the hematocrit decreases to 35% or less, the woman is considered anemic.

The total white cell count increases during the second trimester and peaks during the third trimester. This increase is primarily in the granulocytes; the lymphocyte count stays about the same throughout pregnancy. See Table 14-3 for laboratory values during pregnancy.

Cardiac Output. Cardiac output increases from 30% to 50% over the nonpregnant rate by the thirty-second week of pregnancy; it declines to about a 20% increase at 40 weeks of gestation. This elevated cardiac output is largely a result of increased stroke volume and heart rate and occurs in response to increased tissue demands for oxygen (Monga, 2004). Cardiac output in late pregnancy is appreciably higher when the woman is in the lateral recumbent position than when she is supine. In the supine position the large, heavy uterus often impedes venous return to the heart and affects blood pressure. Cardiac output increases with any exertion, such as labor and birth. Table 14-4 summarizes cardiovascular changes in pregnancy.

Circulation and Coagulation Times. The circulation time decreases slightly by week 32. It returns to near normal close to term. There is a greater tendency for blood to coagulate (clot) during pregnancy because of increases in various clotting factors (factors VII, VIII, IX, X, and fibrinogen). This, combined with the fact that fibrinolytic activity (the splitting up or the dissolving of a clot) is depressed during pregnancy and the postpartum period, provides a protective function to decrease the chance of bleeding but also makes the woman more vulnerable to thrombosis, especially after cesarean birth.

table 14-3 Laboratory Values for Pregnant and Nonpregnant Women

VALUES	NONPREGNANT	PREGNANT
HEMATOLOGIC		
Complete Blood Count (CBC)		
Hemoglobin, g/dl	12-16*	>11*
Hematocrit, packed cell volume (PCV), %	37-47*	>33*
Red blood cell (RBC) volume, per ml	1600	1500-1900
Plasma volume, per ml	2400	3700
RBC count, million per mm^3	4.2-5.4	5-6.25
White blood cells, total per mm^3	5000-10,000	5000-15,000
Neutrophils, %	55-70	60-85
Lymphocytes, %	20-40	15-40
Erythrocyte sedimentation rate, mm/hr	20	Elevated in second and third trimesters
Mean corpuscular hemoglobin concentration (MCHC), g/dl packed RBCs	32-36	No change in hemoglobin concentration
Mean corpuscular hemoglobin (MCH), pg	27-31	No change per pg (less than 1 ng)
Mean corpuscular volume (MCV), cubic micrometer	80-95	No change per cubic micrometer
Blood Coagulation and Fibrinolytic Activity†		
Factor VII	65-140	Increase in pregnancy, return to normal in early puerperium
Factor VIII	55-145	Increases during pregnancy and immediately after birth
Factor IX	60-140	See Factor VII
Factor X	45-155	See Factor VII
Factor XI	65-135	Decrease in pregnancy
Factor XII	50-150	See Factor VII
Prothrombin time (PT), sec	11-12.5	Slight decrease in pregnancy
Partial thromboplastin time (PTT), sec	60-70	Slight decrease in pregnancy and decrease during second and third stage of labor (indicates clotting at placental site)
Bleeding time, min	1-9 (Ivy test)	No appreciable change
Coagulation time, min	6-10 (Lee/White test)	No appreciable change
Platelets, per mm^3	150,000-400,000	No significant change until 3-5 days after birth and then a rapid increase (may predispose woman to thrombosis) and gradual return to normal
Fibrinolytic activity	Normal	Decreases in pregnancy and then abruptly returns to normal (protection against thromboembolism)
Fibrinogen, mg/dl	200-400	Increased levels late in pregnancy
Mineral and Vitamin Concentrations		
Vitamin B$_{12}$, folic acid, ascorbic acid	Normal	Moderate decrease
Serum Proteins		
Total, g/dl	6.4-8.3	5.5-7.5
Albumin, g/dl	3.5-5	Slight increase
Globulin, total, g/dl	2.3-3.4	3-4
Blood Glucose		
Fasting, mg/dl	70-105	Decreases
2-hr postprandial, mg/dl	<140	<140 after a 100-g carbohydrate meal is considered normal
Acid-Base Values in Arterial Blood		
Po$_2$, mm Hg	80-100	104-108 (increased)
Pco$_2$, mm Hg	35-45	27-32 (decreased)
Sodium bicarbonate (HCO$_3$), mEq/L	21-28	18-31 (decreased)
Blood pH	7.35-7.45	7.40-7.45 (slightly increased, more alkaline)

From Gordon, M. (2002). Maternal physiology in pregnancy. In S. Gabbe, J. Niebyl, & J. Simpson (Eds.), *Obstetrics: Normal and problem pregnancies* (4th ed.). New York: Churchill Livingstone; Pagana, K., & Pagana, T. (2003). *Mosby's diagnostic and laboratory test reference* (6th ed.). St. Louis: Mosby.
*At sea level. Permanent residents of higher altitudes (e.g., Denver, CO) require higher levels of hemoglobin.
†Pregnancy represents a hypercoagulable state.

Continued

table 14-3	Laboratory Values for Pregnant and Nonpregnant Women—cont'd	
VALUES	**NONPREGNANT**	**PREGNANT**
HEPATIC		
Bilirubin, total, mg/dl	<1	Unchanged
Serum cholesterol, mg/dl	120-200	Increases from 16 to 32 weeks of pregnancy; remains at this level until after birth
Serum alkaline phosphatase, units/L	30-120	Increases from week 12 of pregnancy to 6 weeks after birth
Serum albumin, g/dl	3.5-5	Slight increase
RENAL		
Bladder capacity, ml	1300	1500
Renal plasma flow (RPF), ml/min	490-700	Increase by 25%-30%
Glomerular filtration rate (GFR), ml/min	88-128	Increase by 30%-50%
Nonprotein nitrogen (NPN), mg/dl	25-40	Decreases
Blood urea nitrogen (BUN), mg/dl	10-20	Decreases
Serum creatinine, mg/dl	0.5-1.1	Decreases
Serum uric acid, mg/dl	2.7-7.3	Decreases
Urine glucose	Negative	Present in 20% of pregnant women
Intravenous pyelogram (IVP)	Normal	Slight to moderate hydroureter and hydronephrosis; right kidney larger than left kidney

table 14-4	Cardiovascular Changes in Pregnancy
Heart rate	Increases 10-15 beats/min
Blood pressure	Remains at prepregnancy levels in first trimester (systolic)
	Slight decrease in second trimester (systolic and diastolic)
	Returns to prepregnancy levels in late third trimester (diastolic)
Blood volume	Increases by 1500 ml or 40%-50% above prepregnancy level
Red blood cell mass	Increases 17%
Hemoglobin	Decreases
Hematocrit	Decreases
White blood cell count	Increases in second and third trimesters
Cardiac output	Increases 30%-50%

Respiratory System

Structural and ventilatory adaptations occur during pregnancy to provide for maternal and fetal needs. Maternal oxygen requirements increase in response to the acceleration in the metabolic rate and the need to add to the tissue mass in the uterus and breasts. In addition, the fetus requires oxygen and a way to eliminate carbon dioxide.

Elevated levels of estrogen cause the ligaments of the rib cage to relax, permitting increased chest expansion (see Fig. 14-9). The transverse diameter of the thoracic cage increases by about 2 cm, and the circumference increases by 6 cm (Cunningham et al., 2005). The costal angle increases, and the lower rib cage appears to flare out. The chest may not return to its prepregnant state after birth (Seidel, Ball, Dains, & Benedict, 2006).

The diaphragm is displaced by as much as 4 cm during pregnancy. As pregnancy advances, thoracic (costal) breathing replaces abdominal breathing, and it becomes less possible for the diaphragm to descend with inspiration. Thoracic breathing is accomplished primarily by the diaphragm rather than by the costal muscles (Whitty & Dombrowski, 2004).

The upper respiratory tract becomes more vascular in response to elevated levels of estrogen. As the capillaries become engorged, edema and hyperemia develop within the nose, pharynx, larynx, trachea, and bronchi. This congestion within the tissues of the respiratory tract gives rise to several conditions commonly seen during pregnancy, including nasal and sinus stuffiness, epistaxis (nosebleed), changes in the voice, and a marked inflammatory response that can develop into a mild upper respiratory infection.

Increased vascularity of the upper respiratory tract also can cause the tympanic membranes and eustachian tubes to swell, giving rise to symptoms of impaired hearing, earaches, or a sense of fullness in the ears.

Pulmonary Function. Respiratory changes in pregnancy are related to the elevation of the diaphragm and to chest wall changes. Changes in the respiratory center result in a lowered threshold for carbon dioxide. The actions of progesterone and estrogen are presumed responsible for the increased sensitivity of the respiratory center to carbon dioxide. In addition, pregnant women become more aware of the need to breathe; some may even complain of dyspnea at rest, especially in the third trimester (Blackburn, 2003) (see Table 14-5 for respiratory changes in pregnancy). Although pulmonary function is not impaired by pregnancy, diseases of the respiratory tract may be more serious during this time (Cunningham et al., 2005). One important factor responsible for this may be the increased oxygen requirement.

Basal Metabolic Rate. The basal metabolic rate (BMR) increases during pregnancy. This increase varies considerably depending on the prepregnancy nutritional status of

table 14-5	Respiratory Changes in Pregnancy
Respiratory rate	Unchanged or slightly increased
Tidal volume	Increased 30%-40%
Vital capacity	Unchanged
Inspiratory capacity	Increased
Expiratory volume	Decreased
Total lung capacity	Unchanged to slightly decreased
Oxygen consumption	Increased 15%-20%

the woman and fetal growth (Blackburn, 2003). The BMR returns to nonpregnant levels by 5 to 6 days after birth. The elevation in BMR during pregnancy reflects increased oxygen demands of the uterine-placental-fetal unit and greater oxygen consumption because of increased maternal cardiac work. Peripheral vasodilation and acceleration of sweat gland activity help dissipate the excess heat resulting from the increased BMR during pregnancy. Pregnant women may experience heat intolerance, which is annoying to some women. Lassitude and fatigability after only slight exertion are experienced by many women in early pregnancy. These feelings, along with a greater need for sleep, may persist and may be caused in part by the increased metabolic activity.

Acid-Base Balance. By about the tenth week of pregnancy, there is a decrease of about 5 mm Hg in the partial pressure of carbon dioxide (PCO_2). Progesterone may be responsible for increasing the sensitivity of the respiratory center receptors, so that tidal volume is increased, PCO_2 decreases, the base excess (HCO_3 or bicarbonate) decreases, and pH increases slightly. These alterations in acid-base balance indicate that pregnancy is a state of compensatory respiratory alkalosis (Blackburn, 2003). These changes also facilitate the transport of CO_2 from the fetus and O_2 release from the mother to the fetus (see Table 14-3).

Renal System

The kidneys are responsible for maintaining electrolyte and acid-base balance, regulating extracellular fluid volume, excreting waste products, and conserving essential nutrients.

Anatomic Changes. Changes in renal structure during pregnancy result from hormonal activity (estrogen and progesterone), pressure from an enlarging uterus, and an increase in blood volume. As early as the tenth week of pregnancy, the renal pelves and the ureters dilate. Dilation of the ureters is more pronounced above the pelvic brim, in part because they are compressed between the uterus and the pelvic brim. In most women, the ureters below the pelvic brim are of normal size. The smooth-muscle walls of the ureters undergo hyperplasia, hypertrophy, and muscle tone relaxation. The ureters elongate, become tortuous, and form single or double curves. In the latter part of pregnancy, the renal pelvis and ureter are dilated more on the right side than on the left because the heavy uterus is displaced to the right by the sigmoid colon.

Because of these changes, a larger volume of urine is held in the pelves and ureters, and urine flow rate is slowed.

The resulting urinary stasis or stagnation has the following consequences:
- A lag occurs between the time urine is formed and when it reaches the bladder. Therefore clearance test results may reflect substances contained in glomerular filtrate several hours before.
- Stagnated urine is an excellent medium for the growth of microorganisms. In addition, the urine of pregnant women contains more nutrients, including glucose, thereby increasing the pH (making the urine more alkaline). This makes pregnant women more susceptible to urinary tract infection.

Bladder irritability, nocturia, and urinary frequency and urgency (without dysuria) are commonly reported in early pregnancy. Near term, bladder symptoms may return, especially after lightening occurs.

Urinary frequency results initially from increased bladder sensitivity and later from compression of the bladder (see Fig. 14-8). In the second trimester, the bladder is pulled up out of the true pelvis into the abdomen. The urethra lengthens to 7.5 cm as the bladder is displaced upward. The pelvic congestion that occurs in pregnancy is reflected in hyperemia of the bladder and urethra. This increased vascularity causes the bladder mucosa to be traumatized and bleed easily. Bladder tone may decrease, which increases the bladder capacity to 1500 ml. At the same time, the bladder is compressed by the enlarging uterus, resulting in the urge to void even if the bladder contains only a small amount of urine.

Functional Changes. In normal pregnancy, renal function is altered considerably. Glomerular filtration rate (GFR) and renal plasma flow (RPF) increase early in pregnancy (Cunningham et al., 2005). These changes are caused by pregnancy hormones, an increase in blood volume, the woman's posture, physical activity, and nutritional intake. The woman's kidneys must manage the increased metabolic and circulatory demands of the maternal body and the excretion of fetal waste products. Renal function is most efficient when the woman lies in the lateral recumbent position and least efficient when the woman assumes a supine position. A side-lying position increases renal perfusion, which increases urinary output and decreases edema. When the pregnant woman is lying supine, the heavy uterus compresses the vena cava and the aorta, and cardiac output decreases. As a result, blood flow to the brain and heart is continued at the expense of other organs, including the kidneys and uterus.

Fluid and Electrolyte Balance. Selective renal tubular reabsorption maintains sodium and water balance regardless of changes in dietary intake and losses through sweat, vomitus, or diarrhea. From 500 to 900 mEq of sodium is normally retained during pregnancy to meet fetal needs. To prevent excessive sodium depletion, the maternal kidneys undergo a significant adaptation by increasing tubular reabsorption. Because of the need for increased maternal intravascular and extracellular fluid volume, additional sodium is needed to expand fluid volume and to maintain an isotonic state. As efficient as the renal system is, it can be overstressed by excessive dietary sodium intake or restriction or by use of diuretics. Severe hypovolemia and reduced placental perfusion are two consequences of using diuretics during pregnancy.

The capacity of the kidneys to excrete water during the early weeks of pregnancy is more efficient than it is later in pregnancy. As a result, some women feel thirsty in early pregnancy because of the greater amount of water loss. The pooling of fluid in the legs in the latter part of pregnancy decreases renal blood flow and GFR. This pooling of blood in the lower legs is sometimes referred to as *physiologic edema* or dependent edema and requires no treatment. The normal diuretic response to the water load is triggered when the woman lies down, preferably on her side, and the pooled fluid reenters general circulation.

Normally the kidney reabsorbs almost all of the glucose and other nutrients from the plasma filtrate. In pregnant women, however, tubular reabsorption of glucose is impaired, so that glucosuria occurs at varying times and to varying degrees. Normal values range from 0 to 20 mg/dl, meaning that during any day, the urine is sometimes positive and sometimes negative for glucose. In nonpregnant women, blood glucose levels must be at 160 to 180 mg/dl before glucose is "spilled" into the urine (not reabsorbed). During pregnancy, glucosuria (glycosuria) occurs when maternal glucose levels are lower than 160 mg/dl. Why glucose, as well as other nutrients such as amino acids, is wasted during pregnancy is not understood, nor has the exact mechanism been discovered. Although glucosuria may be found in normal pregnancies (2+ levels may be seen with increased anxiety states), the possibility of diabetes mellitus and gestational diabetes must be kept in mind.

Proteinuria usually does not occur in normal pregnancy except during labor or after birth (Cunningham et al., 2005). However, the increased amount of amino acids that must be filtered may exceed the capacity of the renal tubules to absorb it, so that small amounts of protein are then lost in the urine. Values of trace to 1+ protein (dipstick assessment) or less than 300 mg per 24 hours are acceptable during pregnancy (Gordon, 2002). The amount of protein excreted is not an indication of the severity of renal disease, nor does an increase in protein excretion in a pregnant woman with known renal disease necessarily indicate a progression in her disease. However, a pregnant woman with hypertension and proteinuria must be carefully evaluated because she may be at greater risk for an adverse pregnancy outcome (see Table 14-3).

Integumentary System

Alterations in hormonal balance and mechanical stretching are responsible for several changes in the integumentary system during pregnancy. Hyperpigmentation is stimulated by the anterior pituitary hormone melanotropin, which is increased during pregnancy. Darkening of

the nipples, the areolae, the axillae, and the vulva occurs about the sixteenth week of gestation. Facial melasma, also called chloasma or mask of pregnancy, is a blotchy, brownish hyperpigmentation of the skin over the cheeks, nose, and forehead, especially in dark-complexioned pregnant women. Chloasma appears in 50% to 70% of pregnant women, beginning after the sixteenth week and increasing gradually until term. The sun intensifies this pigmentation in susceptible women. Chloasma caused by normal pregnancy usually fades after birth.

The linea nigra (Fig. 14-11) is a pigmented line extending from the symphysis pubis to the top of the fundus in the midline; this line is known as the *linea alba* before hormone-induced pigmentation. In primigravidas the extension of the linea nigra, beginning in the third month, keeps pace with the rising height of the fundus; in multigravidas, the entire line often appears earlier than the third month. Not all pregnant women develop linea nigra, and some women notice hair growth along the line with or without the change in pigmentation.

Striae gravidarum, or stretch marks (seen over lower abdomen in Fig. 14-11), which appear in 50% to 90% of pregnant women during the second half of pregnancy, may be caused by action of adrenocorticosteroids. Striae reflect separation within the underlying connective (collagen) tissue of the skin. These slightly depressed streaks tend to occur over areas of maximal stretch (i.e., abdomen, thighs, and breasts). The stretching sometimes causes a sensation that resembles itching. The tendency to develop striae may be familial. After birth they usually fade, although they never disappear completely. Color of striae varies depending on the pregnant woman's skin color. The striae appear pinkish on a woman with light skin and are lighter than surrounding skin in dark-skinned women. In the multipara, in addition to the striae of the present pregnancy, glistening silvery lines (in light-skinned women) or purplish lines (in dark-skinned women) are commonly seen. These represent the scars of striae from previous pregnancies.

FIG. 14-11 Striae gravidarum and linea nigra in a dark-skinned woman. (Courtesy Shannon Perry, Phoenix, AZ.)

Angiomas are commonly referred to as *vascular spiders*. They are tiny, star-shaped or branched, slightly raised and pulsating end-arterioles usually found on the neck, thorax, face, and arms. They occur as a result of elevated levels of circulating estrogen. The spiders are bluish in color and do not blanch with pressure. Vascular spiders appear during the second to the fifth month of pregnancy in almost 65% of Caucasian women and 10% of African-American women. The spiders usually disappear after birth (Blackburn, 2003).

Pinkish-red, diffuse mottling or well-defined blotches are seen over the palmar surfaces of the hands in about 60% of Caucasian women and 35% of African-American women during pregnancy (Blackburn, 2003). These color changes, called palmar erythema, are related primarily to increased estrogen levels.

■ **NURSE ALERT**

Because integumentary system changes vary greatly among women of different racial backgrounds, the color of a woman's skin should be noted along with any changes that may be attributed to pregnancy when performing physical assessments.

Some dermatologic conditions have been identified as unique to pregnancy or as having an increased incidence during pregnancy. Pruritus is a relatively common dermatologic symptom in pregnancy, with *cholestasis of pregnancy* being the most common cause of pruritic rash. Other forms are uncommon or rare (Rapini, 2004) (Box 14-2). The goal of management is to relieve the itching. Topical steroids are the usual treatment, although systemic steroids may be needed. The problem usually resolves in the postpartum period (Cunningham et al., 2005). Preexisting skin diseases may complicate pregnancy or be improved (see Chapter 33 for further discussion of skin disorders in pregnancy).

■ **NURSE ALERT**

Women with severe acne taking isotretinoin (Accutane) should avoid pregnancy while receiving the treatment because it is teratogenic and is associated with major malformations.

Gum hypertrophy may occur. An epulis (gingival granuloma gravidarum) is a red, raised nodule on the gums that bleeds easily. This lesion may develop around the third month and usually continues to enlarge as pregnancy

---

box 14-2 **Frequency of Dermatologic Disorders of Pregnancy**

- Cholestasis of pregnancy: Common—1.5%-2%
- Pruritic urticarial papules and plaques of pregnancy (PUPPP): Common—0.25% to 1%
- Prurigo of pregnancy: Uncommon—0.3%
- Herpes gestationis: Rare—0.002%
- Impetigo herpetiformis: Very rare

Sources: Cunningham, F., Leveno, K., Bloom, S., Hauth, J., Gilstrap, L., & Wenstrom, K. (2005). *Williams obstetrics* (22nd ed.). New York: McGraw-Hill; Rapini, R. (2004). The skin and pregnancy. In R. Creasy, R. Resnik, & J. Iams (Eds.), *Maternal-fetal medicine: Principles and practice* (5th ed.). Philadelphia: Saunders.

---

progresses. It is usually managed by avoiding trauma to the gums (e.g., using a soft toothbrush). An epulis usually regresses spontaneously after birth.

Nail growth may be accelerated. Some women may notice thinning and softening of the nails. Oily skin and acne vulgaris may occur during pregnancy. For some women, the skin clears and looks radiant. Hirsutism, the excessive growth of hair or growth of hair in unusual places, is commonly reported. An increase in fine hair growth may occur but tends to disappear after pregnancy; however, growth of coarse or bristly hair does not usually disappear. The rate of scalp hair loss slows during pregnancy, and increased hair loss may be noted in the postpartum period.

Increased blood supply to the skin leads to increased perspiration. Women feel hotter during pregnancy, a condition possibly related to a progesterone-induced increase in body temperature and the increased BMR.

Musculoskeletal System

The gradually changing body and increasing weight of the pregnant woman cause noticeable alterations in her posture (Fig. 14-12) and the way she walks. The great abdominal distention that gives the pelvis a forward tilt, decreased abdominal muscle tone, and increased weight bearing require a realignment of the spinal curvature late in pregnancy. The woman's center of gravity shifts forward. An increase in the normal lumbosacral curve (lordosis) develops, and a compensatory curvature in the cervicodorsal region (exaggerated anterior flexion of the head) develops to help her maintain her balance. Aching, numbness, and weakness of the upper extremities may result. Large breasts and a stoop-shouldered stance will further accentuate the lumbar and dorsal curves. Walking is more difficult, and the waddling gait of the pregnant woman, called "the proud walk of pregnancy" by Shakespeare, is commonly seen. The ligamentous and muscular structures of the middle and lower spine may be severely stressed. These and related changes often cause musculoskeletal discomfort, especially in older women or those with a back disorder or a faulty sense of balance.

Slight relaxation and increased mobility of the pelvic joints are normal during pregnancy. These adaptations permit enlargement of pelvic dimensions to facilitate labor and birth. The degree of relaxation varies, but considerable separation of the symphysis pubis and the instability of the sacroiliac joints may cause pain and difficulty in walking. Obesity and multifetal pregnancy tend to increase the pelvic instability. Peripheral joint laxity also increases as pregnancy progresses, but the cause is not known (Cunningham et al., 2005).

The muscles of the abdominal wall stretch and ultimately lose some tone. During the third trimester, the rectus abdominis muscles may separate (Fig. 14-13), allowing abdominal contents to protrude at the midline. The umbilicus flattens or protrudes. After birth, the muscles gradually regain tone; however, separation of the muscles (diastasis recti abdominis) may persist.

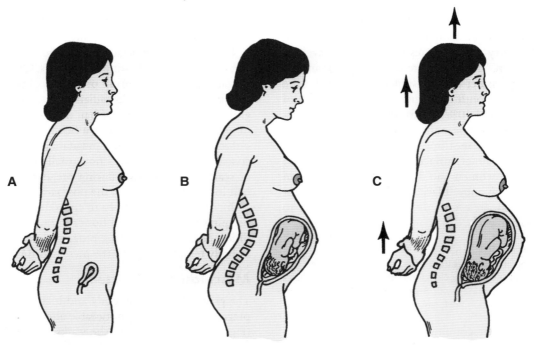

FIG. 14-12 Postural changes during pregnancy. **A,** Nonpregnant. **B,** Incorrect posture during pregnancy. **C,** Correct posture during pregnancy.

FIG. 14-13 Possible change in rectus abdominis muscles during pregnancy. **A,** Normal position in nonpregnant woman. **B,** Diastasis recti abdominis in pregnant woman.

Neurologic System

Little is known regarding specific alterations in function of the neurologic system during pregnancy, aside from hypothalamic-pituitary neurohormonal changes. Specific physiologic alterations resulting from pregnancy may cause the following neurologic or neuromuscular symptoms:

- Compression of pelvic nerves or vascular stasis caused by enlargement of the uterus may result in sensory changes in the legs.
- Dorsolumbar lordosis may cause pain because of traction on nerves or compression of nerve roots.

- Edema involving the peripheral nerves may result in carpal tunnel syndrome during the last trimester (Padua et al., 2001). The syndrome is characterized by paresthesia (abnormal sensation such as burning or tingling) and pain in the hand, radiating to the elbow. The sensations are caused by edema that compresses the median nerve beneath the carpal ligament of the wrist. Smoking and alcohol consumption can impair the microcirculation and may worsen the symptoms (Padua et al., 2001). The dominant hand is usually affected most, although as many as 80% of women experience symptoms in both hands. Symptoms usually regress after pregnancy. In some cases, surgical treatment may be necessary (Aminoff, 2004).
- Acroesthesia (numbness and tingling of the hands) is caused by the stoop-shouldered stance (see Fig. 14-12, *B*) assumed by some women during pregnancy. The condition is associated with traction on segments of the brachial plexus.
- Tension headache is common when anxiety or uncertainty complicates pregnancy. However, vision problems, sinusitis, or migraine also may be responsible for headaches.
- "Light-headedness," faintness, and even syncope (fainting) are common during early pregnancy. Vasomotor instability, postural hypotension, or hypoglycemia may be responsible.
- Hypocalcemia may cause neuromuscular problems such as muscle cramps or tetany.

Gastrointestinal System

Appetite. During pregnancy, the woman's appetite and food intake fluctuate. Early in pregnancy, some women have nausea with or without vomiting (morning sickness), possibly in response to increasing levels of hCG and altered carbohydrate metabolism (Gordon, 2002). Morning sickness or nausea and vomiting of pregnancy (NVP) appears at about 4 to 6 weeks of gestation and usually subsides by the end of the third month (first trimester) of pregnancy. Severity varies from mild distaste for certain foods to more severe vomiting. The condition may be triggered by the sight or odor of various foods. By the end of the second trimester, the appetite increases in response to increasing metabolic needs. Rarely does NVP have harmful effects on the embryo, fetus, or the woman; some beneficial effects may be that these pregnancies may be less likely to result in miscarriage, preterm labor, or intrauterine growth restriction (Furneaux, Langley-Evans, & Langley-Evans, 2001). Whenever the vomiting is severe or persists beyond the first trimester, or when it is accompanied by fever, pain, or weight loss, further evaluation is necessary, and medical intervention is likely.

Women also may have changes in their sense of taste, leading to cravings and changes in dietary intake. Some women have nonfood cravings (called *pica*), such as for ice, clay, and laundry starch. Usually the subjects of these cravings, if consumed in moderation, are not harmful to the pregnancy if the woman has adequate nutrition with appropriate weight gain (Gordon, 2002). See Chapter 15 for a discussion of nutrition in pregnancy.

Mouth. The gums become hyperemic, spongy, and swollen during pregnancy. They tend to bleed easily because the increasing levels of estrogen cause selective increased vascularity and connective tissue proliferation (a nonspecific gingivitis). Epulis (discussed in the section on the integumentary system) may develop at the gumline. Some pregnant women complain of ptyalism (excessive salivation), which may be caused by the decrease in unconscious swallowing by the woman when nauseated or from stimulation of salivary glands by eating starch (Cunningham et al., 2005).

Esophagus, Stomach, and Intestines. Herniation of the upper portion of the stomach (hiatal hernia) occurs after the seventh or eighth month of pregnancy in about 15% to 20% of pregnant women. This condition results from upward displacement of the stomach, which causes the hiatus of the diaphragm to widen. It occurs more often in multiparas and older or obese women.

Increased estrogen production causes decreased secretion of hydrochloric acid; therefore peptic ulcer formation or flare-up of existing peptic ulcers is uncommon during pregnancy and symptoms may improve (Winbery & Blaho, 2001).

Increased progesterone production causes decreased tone and motility of smooth muscles, resulting in esophageal regurgitation, slower emptying time of the stomach, and reverse peristalsis. As a result, the woman may experience "acid indigestion" or heartburn (pyrosis) beginning as early as the first trimester and intensifying through the third trimester.

Iron is absorbed more readily in the small intestine in response to increased needs during pregnancy. Even when the woman is deficient in iron, it will continue to be absorbed in sufficient amounts for the fetus to have a normal hemoglobin level.

Increased progesterone (causing loss of muscle tone and decreased peristalsis) results in an increase in water absorption from the colon and may cause constipation. Constipation also may result from hypoperistalsis (sluggishness of the bowel), food choices, lack of fluids, iron supplementation, decreased activity level, abdominal distention by the pregnant uterus, and displacement and compression of the intestines. If the pregnant woman has hemorrhoids (see Fig. 14-10) and is constipated, the hemorrhoids may become everted or may bleed during straining at stool.

Gallbladder and Liver. The gallbladder is quite often distended because of its decreased muscle tone during pregnancy. Increased emptying time and thickening of bile caused by prolonged retention are typical changes. These features, together with slight hypercholesterolemia from increased progesterone levels, may account for the development of gallstones during pregnancy.

Hepatic function is difficult to appraise during pregnancy; however, only minor changes in liver function develop. Occasionally, intrahepatic cholestasis (retention and accumulation of bile in the liver, caused by factors within the liver) occurs late in pregnancy in response to placental steroids and may result in pruritus gravidarum (severe itching) with or without jaundice. These distressing symptoms subside soon after birth.

Abdominal Discomfort. Intraabdominal alterations that can cause discomfort include pelvic heaviness or pressure, round ligament tension, flatulence, distention and bowel cramping, and uterine contractions. In addition to displacement of intestines, pressure from the expanding uterus causes an increase in venous pressure in the pelvic organs. Although most abdominal discomfort is a consequence of normal maternal alterations, the health care provider must be constantly alert to the possibility of disorders such as bowel obstruction or an inflammatory process.

Appendicitis may be difficult to diagnose in pregnancy because the appendix is displaced upward and laterally, high and to the right, away from McBurney's point (Fig. 14-14).

Endocrine System

Profound endocrine changes are essential for pregnancy maintenance, normal fetal growth, and postpartum recovery.

Pituitary and Placental Hormones. During pregnancy, the elevated levels of estrogen and progesterone

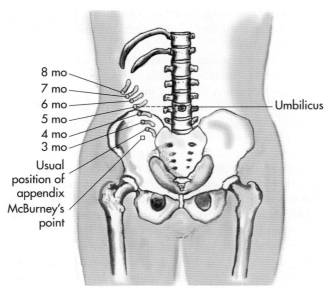

8 mo
7 mo
6 mo
5 mo
4 mo
3 mo

Umbilicus

Usual
position of
appendix
McBurney's
point

FIG. 14-14 Change in position of appendix in pregnancy. Note McBurney's point.

(produced first by the corpus luteum in the ovary until about 14 weeks of gestation and then by the placenta) suppress secretion of follicle-stimulating hormone (FSH) and luteinizing hormone (LH) by the anterior pituitary. The maturation of a follicle and ovulation do not occur. Although the majority of women have amenorrhea (absence of menses), at least 20% have some slight, painless spotting during early gestation. Implantation bleeding and bleeding after intercourse related to cervical friability can occur. Most of the women experiencing slight gestational bleeding continue to term and have normal infants; however, all instances of bleeding should be reported and evaluated.

After implantation, the fertilized ovum and the chorionic villi produce hCG, which maintains the production by the corpus luteum of estrogen and progesterone until the placenta takes over production (Buster & Carson, 2002).

Progesterone is essential for maintaining pregnancy by relaxing smooth muscles, resulting in decreased uterine contractility and prevention of miscarriage. Progesterone and estrogen cause fat to deposit in subcutaneous tissues over the maternal abdomen, back, and upper thighs. This fat serves as an energy reserve for both pregnancy and lactation. Estrogen also promotes the enlargement of the genitals, the uterus, and the breasts and increases vascularity, causing vasodilation. Estrogen causes relaxation of pelvic ligaments and joints. It also alters metabolism of nutrients by interfering with folic acid metabolism, increasing the level of total body proteins, and promoting retention of sodium and water by kidney tubules. Estrogen may decrease secretion of hydrochloric acid and pepsin, which may be responsible for digestive upsets such as nausea.

Serum prolactin produced by the anterior pituitary begins to increase early in the first trimester and increases progressively to term. It is responsible for initial lactation; however, the high levels of estrogen and progesterone inhibit lactation by blocking the binding of prolactin to breast tissue until after birth (Liu, 2004).

Oxytocin is produced by the posterior pituitary in increasing amounts as the fetus matures. This hormone can stimulate uterine contractions during pregnancy, but high levels of progesterone prevent contractions until near term. Oxytocin also stimulates the let-down or milk-ejection reflex after birth in response to the infant's sucking at the mother's breast.

Human chorionic somatomammotropin (hCS), previously called human placental lactogen, is produced by the placenta and has been suggested to act as a growth hormone and contribute to breast development. It also may decrease the maternal metabolism of glucose and increase the amount of fatty acids for metabolic needs; however, its function is poorly understood (Liu, 2004).

Thyroid Gland. During pregnancy, gland activity and hormone production increase. The increased activity is reflected in a moderate enlargement of the thyroid gland caused by hyperplasia of the glandular tissue and increased vascularity (Cunningham et al., 2005). Thyroxine-binding globulin (TBG) increases as a result of increased estrogen levels. This increase begins at about 20 weeks of gestation. The level of total (free and bound) thyroxine (T_4) increases between 6 and 9 weeks of gestation and plateaus at 18 weeks of gestation. Free thyroxine (T_4) and free triiodothyronine (T_3) return to nonpregnant levels after the first trimester. Despite these changes in hormone production, hyperthyroidism usually does not develop in the pregnant woman (Cunningham et al., 2005).

Parathyroid Gland. Parathyroid hormone controls calcium and magnesium metabolism. Pregnancy induces a slight hyperparathyroidism, a reflection of increased fetal requirements for calcium and vitamin D. The peak level of parathyroid hormone occurs between 15 and 35 weeks of gestation, when the needs for growth of the fetal skeleton are greatest. Levels return to normal after birth.

Pancreas. The fetus requires significant amounts of glucose for its growth and development. To meet its need for fuel, the fetus not only depletes the store of maternal glucose but also decreases the mother's ability to synthesize glucose by siphoning off her amino acids. Maternal blood glucose levels decrease. Maternal insulin does not cross the placenta to the fetus. As a result, in early pregnancy the pancreas decreases its production of insulin.

As pregnancy continues, the placenta grows and produces progressively greater amounts of hormones (i.e., hCS, estrogen, and progesterone). Cortisol production by the adrenals also increases. Estrogen, progesterone, hCS, and cortisol collectively decrease the mother's ability to use insulin. Cortisol stimulates increased production of insulin but also increases the mother's peripheral resistance to insulin (i.e., the tissues cannot use the insulin). Decreasing the mother's ability to use her own insulin is a protective mechanism that ensures an ample supply of glucose for the needs of the fetoplacental unit. The result is an added demand for insulin by the mother that continues to increase at a steady rate until term. The normal beta cells of the islets of Langerhans in the pancreas can meet this demand for insulin.

Adrenal Glands. The adrenal glands change little during pregnancy. Secretion of aldosterone is increased, resulting in reabsorption of excess sodium from the renal tubules. Cortisol levels also are increased (Blackburn, 2003).

community activity

Visit a chain drug store (e.g., Walgreen's), an independently (locally) owned pharmacy (e.g., Edwards Pharmacy), and a super discount store with a pharmacy (e.g., Walmart) in your community. Select two home pregnancy tests that are sold in all three stores; if possible one should be a generic or store brand and one a trade name brand. Compare how convenient it is to find the tests in the stores, the costs of the tests, and the availability of someone to discuss use of the test with consumers. What languages other than English do the directions come in for the tests?

Since many teenagers use home pregnancy tests when they suspect they are pregnant, discuss strategies for improving/changing access for these consumers to tests and information in these stores. Explore the feasibility of posting information where pregnant teens can seek assistance.

key points

- The biochemical, physiologic, and anatomic adaptations that occur during pregnancy are profound and revert to the nonpregnant state after birth and lactation.
- Maternal adaptations are attributed to the hormones of pregnancy and to mechanical pressures exerted by the enlarging uterus and other tissues.
- ELISA testing, with monoclonal antibody technology, is the most popular method of pregnancy testing and is the basis for most over-the-counter home pregnancy tests.
- Presumptive, probable, and positive signs of pregnancy aid in the diagnosis of pregnancy; only positive signs (identification of a fetal heartbeat, verification of fetal movements, and visualization of the fetus) can establish the diagnosis of pregnancy.

- Adaptations to pregnancy protect the woman's normal physiologic functioning, meet the metabolic demands pregnancy imposes, and provide for fetal development and growth needs.
- Although the pH of the pregnant woman's vaginal secretions is more acidic, she is more vulnerable to some vaginal infections, especially yeast infections.
- Increased vascularity and sensitivity of the vagina and other pelvic viscera may lead to a high degree of sexual interest and arousal.
- Some adaptations to pregnancy result in discomforts such as fatigue, urinary frequency, nausea, and breast sensitivity.
- As pregnancy progresses, balance and coordination are affected by changes in the woman's joints and her center of gravity.

REFERENCES

Aminoff, M. (2004). Neurologic disorders. In R. Creasy, R. Resnik, & J. Iams (Eds.), *Maternal-fetal medicine: Principles and practice* (5th ed.). Philadelphia: Saunders.

Beebe, K. (2005). The perplexing parity puzzle. *AWHONN Lifelines, 9*(5), 394-399.

Berman, M., DiSaia, P., & Tewari, K. (2004). Pelvic malignancies, gestational trophoblastic neoplasia, and nonpelvic malignancies. In R. Creasy, R. Resnik, & J. Iams (Eds.), *Maternal-fetal medicine: Principles and practice* (5th ed.). Philadelphia: Saunders.

Blackburn, S. (2003). *Maternal, fetal, & neonatal physiology: A clinical perspective* (2nd ed.). St. Louis: Saunders.

Buster, J., & Carson, S. (2002). Endocrinology and diagnosis of pregnancy. In S. Gabbe, J. Niebyl, & J. Simpson (Eds.), *Obstetrics: Normal and problem pregnancies* (4th ed.). New York: Churchill Livingstone.

Cole, L., Khanlian, S., Sutton, J., Davies, S., & Rayburn, W. (2004). Accuracy of home pregnancy tests at the time of missed menses. *American Journal of Obstetrics and Gynecology, 190*(1), 100-105.

Cunningham, F., Leveno, K., Bloom, S., Hauth, J., Gilstrap, L., & Wenstrom, K. (2005). *Williams obstetrics* (22nd ed.). New York: McGraw-Hill.

Furneaux, E., Langley-Evans, A., & Langley-Evans, S. (2001). Nausea and vomiting of pregnancy: Endocrine basis and contribution to

pregnancy outcome. *Obstetrical and Gynecological Survey, 56*(12), 775-782.

Gibbs, R., Sweet, R., & Duff, W. (2004). Maternal and fetal infectious disorders. In R. Creasy, R. Resnik, & J. Iams (Eds.), *Maternal-fetal medicine: Principles and practice* (5th ed.). Philadelphia: Saunders.

Gonik, B., & Foley, M. (2004). Intensive care monitoring of the critically ill pregnant patient. In R. Creasy, R. Resnik, & J. Iams (Eds.), *Maternal-fetal medicine: Principles and practice* (5th ed.). Philadelphia: Saunders.

Gordon, M. (2002). Maternal physiology in pregnancy. In S. Gabbe, J. Niebyl, & J. Simpson (Eds.), *Obstetrics: Normal and problem pregnancies* (4th ed.). New York: Churchill Livingstone.

Harman, C. (2004). Assessment of fetal health. In R. Creasy, R. Resnik, & J. Iams (Eds.), *Maternal-fetal medicine: Principles and practice* (5th ed.). Philadelphia: Saunders.

Hermida, R., Ayala, D., Mojon, A., & Fernandez, J. (2001). Time-qualified reference values for ambulatory blood pressure monitoring in pregnancy. *Hypertension, 38*(3 Pt 2), 746-752.

Lawrence, R., & Lawrence, R. (2004). The breast and the physiology of lactation. In R. Creasy, R. Resnik, & J. Iams (Eds.), *Maternal-fetal medicine: Principles and practice* (5th ed.). Philadelphia: Saunders.

Liu, J. (2004). Endocrinology of pregnancy. In R. Creasy, R. Resnik, & J. Iams (Eds.), *Maternal-fetal medicine: Principles and practice* (5th ed.). Philadelphia: Saunders.

Malone, F., & D'Alton, M. (2004). Multiple gestation: Clinical characteristics and management. In R. Creasy, R. Resnik, & J. Iams (Eds.), *Maternal-fetal medicine: Principles and practice* (5th ed.). Philadelphia: Saunders.

Monga, M. (2004). Maternal cardiovascular and renal adaptation to pregnancy. In R. Creasy, R. Resnik, & J. Iams (Eds.), *Maternal-fetal medicine: Principles and practice* (5th ed.). Philadelphia: Saunders.

Monga, M., & Sanborn, M. (2004). Biology and physiology of the reproductive tract and control of myometrial contraction. In R. Creasy, R. Resnik, & J. Iams (Eds.), *Maternal-fetal medicine: Principles and practice* (5th ed.). Philadelphia: Saunders.

Padua, L., Aprile, I., Caliandro, P., Carboni, T., Meloni, A., Massi, S., et al. (2001). Symptoms and neurophysical picture of carpal tunnel syndrome in pregnancy. *Clinical Neurophysiology, 112*(10), 1946-1951.

Pagana, K., & Pagana, T. (2003). *Mosby's diagnostic and laboratory test reference* (6th ed.). St. Louis: Mosby.

Pickering, T. (2002). Principles and techniques of blood pressure measurement. *Cardiology Clinics, 20*(2), 207-223.

Rapini, R. (2004). The skin and pregnancy. In R. Creasy, R. Resnik, & J. Iams (Eds.), *Maternal-fetal medicine: Principles and practice* (5th ed.). Philadelphia: Saunders.

Sadler, L., Dynes, M., Daley, A., Ickovics, J., Leventhal, J., & Reynolds, H. (2004). Use of home pregnancy tests among adolescent women. *MCN American Journal of Maternal/Child Nursing, 29*(1), 50-55.

Seidel, H., Ball, J., Dains, J., & Benedict, G. (2006). *Mosby's guide to physical examination* (6th ed.). St. Louis: Mosby.

Stewart, F. (2004). Pregnancy testing and management of early pregnancy. In R. Hatcher, J. Trussell, F. Stewart, A. Nelson, W. Cates, F. Guest, et al. (Eds.), *Contraceptive technology* (18th ed.). New York: Ardent Media.

Whitty, J., & Dombrowski, M. (2004). Respiratory diseases in pregnancy. In R. Creasy, R. Resnik, & J. Iams (Eds.), *Maternal-fetal medicine: Principles and practice* (5th ed.). Philadelphia: Saunders.

Winbery, S., & Blaho, K. (2001). Dyspepsia in pregnancy. *Obstetrics and Gynecology Clinics of North America, 28*(2), 333-350.

Maternal and Fetal Nutrition

learning objectives

- Explain recommended maternal weight gain during pregnancy.
- State the recommended level of intake of energy sources, protein, and key vitamins and minerals during pregnancy and lactation.
- Give examples of the food sources that provide the nutrients required for optimal maternal nutrition during pregnancy and lactation.
- Examine the role of nutritional supplements during pregnancy.

- List five nutritional risk factors during pregnancy.
- Compare the dietary needs of adolescent and mature pregnant women.
- Analyze examples of eating patterns of two women from different ethnic or cultural backgrounds, and identify potential dietary problems.
- Assess nutritional status during pregnancy.

electronic resources

Additional information related to the content in Chapter 15 can be found on

the companion website at ***evolve***
http://evolve.elsevier.com/Lowdermilk/MWHC/
- NCLEX Review Questions
- WebLinks

or on the interactive companion CD

- NCLEX Review Questions
- Critical Thinking Exercise: Nutrition Education
- Plan of Care: Nutrition During Pregnancy

NUTRITION is one of many factors that influence the outcome of pregnancy (Fig. 15-1). However, maternal nutritional status is an especially significant factor, both because it is potentially alterable and because good nutrition before and during pregnancy is an important preventive measure for a variety of problems. These problems include birth of low-birth-weight (LBW; birth weight of 2500 g or less) and preterm infants. Neonatal and infant death rates for moderately LBW infants (1500 to 2499 g) are five times higher than that of infants born weighing >2500 g; the risk for very LBW (VLBW) infants (<1500 g) is more than 100 times that of infants born weighing 2500 g or more (Hoyert, Mathews, Menacker, Strobino, & Guyer, 2006). VLBW infants surviving the first year of life are much more likely to have serious health impairments than infants weighing more than 2500 g at birth. Thus it is essential that the importance of good nutrition be emphasized to all women of childbearing potential. Therefore the nurse must have a thorough understanding of nutrient needs before and during pregnancy, and nutrition assessment, intervention, and evaluation must be an integral part of the nursing care given to all pregnant women.

■ NUTRIENT NEEDS BEFORE CONCEPTION

The first trimester of pregnancy is a crucial one in terms of embryonic and fetal organ development. A healthful diet before conception is the best way to ensure that adequate nutrients are available for the developing fetus. Folate or folic acid intake is of particular concern in the periconceptual period. "Folate" is the form in which this vitamin is found naturally in foods, and "folic acid" is the form used in fortification of grain products and other foods and in vitamin supplements. Neural tube defects, or failures in closure of the neural tube, are more common in infants of women with poor folic acid intake. Proper closure of the neural tube is required for normal formation of the spinal cord, and the neural tube begins to close within the

FIG. 15-1   Factors that affect the outcome of pregnancy.

first month of gestation, often before the woman realizes that she is pregnant. It is estimated that the incidence of neural tube defects could be decreased as much as 70% if all women had an adequate folate intake during the periconceptual period (Cornel, Smit, & de Jong-van den Berg, 2005). All women capable of becoming pregnant are advised to consume 0.4 mg (400 micrograms) of fo-

lic acid daily in fortified foods (ready-to-eat cereals and enriched grain products) or supplements, in addition to a diet rich in folate-containing foods: green leafy vegetables, whole grains, and fruits (Box 15-1) (Institute of Medicine, 2003).

Both maternal and fetal risks in pregnancy are increased when the mother is significantly underweight or

---

box 15-1   **Food Sources of Folate**

FOODS PROVIDING 500 MICROGRAMS OR MORE PER SERVING
Liver: chicken, turkey, goose (3.5 oz [100 g])

FOODS PROVIDING 200 MICROGRAMS OR MORE PER SERVING
Liver: lamb, beef, veal (3.5 oz [100 g])

FOODS PROVIDING 100 MICROGRAMS OR MORE PER SERVING
Legumes, cooked (½ cup)
  Peas: black-eyed, chickpea (garbanzo)
  Beans: black, kidney, pinto, red, navy
  Lentils
Vegetables (½ cup)
  Asparagus
  Spinach, cooked
Papaya (1 medium)
Breakfast cereal, ready-to-eat (½-1 cup)
Wheat germ (¼ cup)

FOODS PROVIDING 50 MICROGRAMS OR MORE PER SERVING
Vegetables (½ cup)
  Broccoli
  Beans: lima, baked, or pork and beans
  Greens: collard or mustard, cooked
  Spinach, raw
Fruits (½ cup)
  Avocado
  Orange or orange juice
Pasta, cooked (1 cup)
Rice, cooked (1 cup)

FOODS PROVIDING 20 MICROGRAMS OR MORE PER SERVING
Bread (1 slice)
Egg (1 large)
Corn (½ cup)

overweight when pregnancy begins. Ideally all women would achieve their desirable body weights before conception.

NUTRIENT NEEDS DURING PREGNANCY

Nutrient needs are determined, at least in part, by the stage of gestation, in that the amount of fetal growth varies during the different stages of pregnancy. During the first trimester, the synthesis of fetal tissues places relatively few demands on maternal nutrition; therefore during the first trimester, when the embryo or fetus is very small, the needs are only slightly greater than those before pregnancy. In contrast, the last trimester is a period of noticeable fetal growth, when most of the fetal stores of energy and minerals are deposited. Therefore as fetal growth progresses during the second and third trimesters, the pregnant woman's need for some nutrients increases greatly. Factors that contribute to the increase in nutrient needs include the following:

- The uterine-placental-fetal unit
- Maternal blood volume and constituents: During pregnancy the total blood volume increases by about 40%–50% over normal. The plasma volume increases by 50% in women in their first pregnancies and more than this in multifetal pregnancies. Although red blood cell (RBC) production also is stimulated, the expansion of RBC mass is not as great as that of plasma volume.
- Maternal mammary development
- Metabolic needs: Basal metabolic rates, when expressed as kilocalories (kcal) per minute, are approximately 20% higher in pregnant women than in nonpregnant women. This increase includes the energy cost for tissue synthesis.

The Food and Nutrition Board of the National Academies of Sciences publishes recommendations for the people of the United States, the Dietary Reference Intakes or DRIs (www.iom.edu). The DRIs consist of Recommended Dietary Allowances (RDAs) and Adequate Intakes (AIs), as well as Upper Limits (ULs), guidelines for avoiding excessive intakes of nutrients that may be toxic if consumed in excess. RDAs for some nutrients have been available for many years, and they have been revised periodically. RDAs are recommendations for daily nutritional intakes that meet the needs of almost all (97% to 98%) of the healthy members of the population. AIs are similar to the RDAs and are believed to cover the needs for virtually all healthy individuals in a group, except that they deal with nutrients for which there are not enough data to be certain of their requirements. The RDAs and AIs include a wide variety of nutrients and food components, and they are divided into age, sex, and life-stage categories (e.g., infancy, pregnancy, and lactation). They can be used as goals in planning the diets of individuals (Table 15-1).

Energy Needs

Energy (kilocalories or kcal) needs are met by carbohydrate, fat, and protein in the diet. No specific recommendations exist for the amount of carbohydrate and fat in the diet of the pregnant woman, but the intake of these nutrients should be adequate to support the recommended weight gain. Although protein can be used to supply energy, its primary role is to provide amino acids for the synthesis of new tissues (see discussion later in chapter). The estimated energy expenditure for the first trimester is the same as in the prepregnant state; during the second trimester of pregnancy, the RDA is 340 kcal greater than the prepregnancy needs, and during the third trimester it is 462 kcal more than the prepregnant need (Institute of Medicine, 2003). Longitudinal assessment of weight gain during pregnancy is the best way to determine whether the kilocalorie intake is adequate; very underweight or active women may require more than the recommended increase in kcal to sustain the desired rate of weight gain.

Weight Gain

The optimal weight gain during pregnancy is not known precisely. It is known, however, that the amount of weight gained by the mother during pregnancy has an important bearing on the course and outcome of the pregnancy. Although an adequate weight gain does not necessarily indicate that the diet is nutritionally adequate, it is associated with a reduced risk of giving birth to a small-for-gestational age (SGA) or preterm infant (Centers for Disease Control and Prevention, 2005).

The desirable weight gain during pregnancy varies among women. The primary factor to consider in making a weight gain recommendation is the appropriateness of the prepregnancy weight for the woman's height, that is, whether the woman's weight was normal before pregnancy, or whether she was underweight or overweight. Maternal and fetal risks in pregnancy are increased when the mother is significantly underweight or overweight before pregnancy and when weight gain during pregnancy is either too low or too high. Severely underweight women are more likely to have preterm labor and to give birth to LBW infants. Both normal-weight and underweight women with inadequate weight gain have an increased risk of giving birth to an infant with intrauterine growth restriction (IUGR). Greater-than-expected weight gain during pregnancy may occur for many reasons, including multiple gestation, edema, gestational hypertension, and overeating. When obesity is present (either preexisting obesity or obesity that develops during pregnancy), there is an increased likelihood of macrosomia and fetopelvic disproportion; operative birth; emergency cesarean birth; postpartum hemorrhage; wound, genital tract, or urinary tract infection; birth trauma; and late fetal death (Kabiru & Raynor, 2004; Linne, 2004; Vahratian, Siega-Riz, Savitz, & Zhang, 2005). Obese women are more likely than normal-

CD: Critical Thinking Exercise: Nutrition Education

table 15-1 Recommendations for Daily Intakes of Selected Nutrients During Pregnancy and Lactation

NUTRIENT (UNITS)	RECOMMENDATION FOR NONPREGNANT WOMAN	RECOMMENDATION FOR PREGNANCY*	RECOMMENDATION FOR LACTATION*	ROLE IN RELATION TO PREGNANCY AND LACTATION	FOOD SOURCES
Energy (kilocalories [kcal] or kilojoules [kJ])†	Variable	1st trimester, same as nonpregnant; second trimester, nonpregnant needs + 81 kcal (340 kJ); 3rd trimester, nonpregnant needs + 108 kcal (452 kJ)	1st 6 months, nonpregnant needs + 79 kcal (330 kJ); 2nd 6 months, nonpregnant needs + 55 kcal (230 kJ)	Growth of fetal and maternal tissues; milk production	Carbohydrate, fat, and protein
Protein (g)	46	1st trimester, same as nonpregnant; 2nd and 3rd trimesters, nonpregnant needs + 25 g‡	Nonpregnant needs + 25 g	Synthesis of the products of conception; growth of maternal tissue and expansion of blood volume; secretion of milk protein during lactation	Meats, eggs, cheese, yogurt, legumes (dry beans and peas, peanuts), nuts, grains
Water (L)	2.7 total (2.2 in beverages)	3 total (2.3 in beverages)	3.8 total (3.1 in beverages)	Expansion of blood volume, excretion of wastes; milk secretion	Water and beverages made with water, milk, juices; all foods, especially frozen desserts, fruits, lettuce and other fresh vegetables
Fiber (g)	25	28	29	Promote regular bowel elimination; reduce long-term risk of heart disease, diverticulosis, and diabetes	Whole grains, bran, vegetables, fruits, nuts and seeds
MINERALS					
Calcium (mg)	1300/1000	1300/1000	1300/1000	Fetal and infant skeleton and tooth formation; maintenance of maternal bone and tooth mineralization	Milk, cheese, yogurt, sardines or other fish eaten with bones left in, deep green leafy vegetables except spinach or Swiss chard, calcium-set tofu, baked beans, tortillas
Iron (mg)	15/18	30	10/9	Maternal hemoglobin formation, fetal liver iron storage	Liver, meats, whole grain or enriched breads and cereals, deep green leafy vegetables, legumes, dried fruits
Zinc (mg)	9/8	12/11	13/12	Component of numerous enzyme systems, possibly important in preventing congenital malformations	Liver, shellfish, meats, whole grains, milk
Iodine (mcg)	150	220	290	Increased maternal metabolic rate	Iodized salt, seafood, milk and milk products, commercial yeast breads, rolls, and donuts

Nutrient				Function	Food Sources
Magnesium (mg)	360/310-320	400/350-360	360/310-320	Involved in energy and protein metabolism, tissue growth, muscle action	Nuts, legumes, cocoa, meats, whole grains
FAT-SOLUBLE VITAMINS					
A (mcg)	700	750/770	1200/1300	Essential for cell development, tooth bud formation, bone growth	Deep green leafy vegetables; dark yellow vegetables; and fruits, chili peppers; liver, fortified margarine and butter
D (mcg)	5	5	5	Involved in absorption of calcium and phosphorus, improves mineralization	Fortified milk and margarine, egg yolk, butter, liver, seafood
E (mg)	15	15	19	Antioxidant (protects cell membranes from damage), especially important for preventing breakdown of RBCs	Vegetable oils, green leafy vegetables, whole grains, liver, nuts and seeds, cheese, fish
WATER SOLUBLE VITAMINS					
C (mg)	65/75	80/85	115/120	Tissue formation and integrity, formation of connective tissue, enhancement of iron absorption	Citrus fruits, strawberries, melons, broccoli, tomatoes, peppers, raw deep green leafy vegetables
Folate (mcg)	400	600	500	Prevention of neural tube defects, support for increased maternal RBC formation	Fortified ready-to-eat cereals and other grain products, green leafy vegetables, oranges, broccoli, asparagus, artichokes, liver
B₆ or pyridoxine (mg)	1.2/1.3	1.9	2	Involved in protein metabolism	Meats, liver, deep green vegetables, whole grains
B₁₂ (mcg)	2.4	2.6	2.8	Production of nucleic acids and proteins, especially important in formation of RBC and neural functioning	Milk and milk products, eggs, meats, liver, fortified soy milk

Sources: Institute of Medicine. (2002). Dietary reference intakes for energy, carbohydrate, fiber, fat, fatty acids, cholesterol, protein, and amino acids. Washington, DC: National Academies Press; Institute of Medicine. (2003). Dietary reference intakes: Applications in dietary planning. Washington, DC: National Academies Press; Institute of Medicine. (2004). Dietary reference intakes for water, potassium, sodium, chloride, and sulfate. Washington, DC: National Academies Press.
RBCs, Red blood cells.
* When two values appear, separated by a diagonal slash, the first is for females younger than 19 years, and the second is for those 19 to 50 years of age.
† The international metric unit of energy measurement is the joule (J). 1 kcal = 4.184 kJ.
‡ Add an additional 25 g in twin pregnancies.

weight women to have preeclampsia and gestational diabetes (Kabiru & Raynor).

A commonly used method of evaluating the appropriateness of weight for height is the body mass index (BMI), which is calculated by the following formula:

$$BMI = Weight \div Height^2$$

where the weight is in kilograms and height is in meters. Thus for a woman who weighed 81 kg before pregnancy and is 1.68 m tall:

$$BMI = 81 \text{ kg} \div (1.68 \text{ m})^2 = 28.7$$

Prepregnant BMI can be classified into the following categories: less than 19.8, underweight or low; 19.8 to 26, nor-

table 15-2 **Body Mass Index (BMI)**

	HEIGHT IN INCHES																		
	58	59	60	61	62	63	64	65	66	67	68	69	70	71	72	73	74	75	76
	BODY WEIGHT (POUNDS)																		
BMI																			
Normal																			
19	91	94	97	100	104	107	110	114	118	121	125	128	132	136	140	144	148	152	156
20	96	99	102	106	109	113	116	120	124	127	131	135	139	143	147	151	155	160	164
21	100	104	107	111	115	118	122	126	130	134	138	142	146	150	154	159	163	168	172
22	105	109	112	116	120	124	128	132	136	140	144	149	153	157	162	166	171	176	180
23	110	114	118	122	126	130	134	138	142	146	151	155	160	165	169	174	179	184	189
24	115	119	123	127	131	135	140	144	148	153	158	162	167	172	177	182	186	192	197
Overweight																			
25	119	124	128	132	136	141	145	150	155	159	164	169	174	179	184	189	194	200	205
26	124	128	133	137	142	146	151	156	161	166	171	176	181	186	191	197	200	208	213
27	129	133	138	143	147	152	157	162	167	172	177	182	188	196	199	204	210	216	221
28	134	138	143	148	153	158	163	168	173	178	184	189	195	200	206	212	218	224	230
29	138	143	148	153	158	163	169	174	179	185	190	196	202	208	213	219	225	232	238
Obese																			
30	143	148	153	158	164	169	174	180	186	191	197	203	209	215	221	227	233	240	246
31	148	153	158	164	169	175	180	186	192	198	203	209	216	222	228	235	241	248	254
32	153	158	163	169	175	180	186	192	198	204	210	216	222	229	235	242	249	256	263
33	158	163	168	174	180	186	192	198	204	211	216	223	229	236	242	250	256	264	271
34	162	168	174	180	186	191	197	204	210	217	223	230	236	243	250	257	264	272	279
35	167	173	179	185	191	197	204	210	216	223	230	236	243	250	258	265	272	279	287
36	172	178	184	190	196	203	209	216	223	230	236	243	250	257	265	272	280	287	295
37	177	183	189	195	202	208	215	222	229	236	243	250	257	265	272	280	287	295	304
38	181	188	194	201	207	214	221	228	235	242	249	257	264	272	279	288	295	303	312
39	186	193	199	206	213	220	227	234	241	249	256	263	271	279	287	295	303	311	320
Extreme Obesity																			
40	191	198	204	211	218	225	232	240	247	255	262	270	278	286	294	302	311	319	328
41	196	203	209	217	224	231	238	246	253	261	269	277	285	293	302	310	319	327	336
42	201	208	215	222	229	237	244	252	260	268	276	284	292	301	309	318	326	335	344
43	205	212	220	227	235	242	250	258	266	274	282	291	299	308	316	325	334	343	353
44	210	217	225	232	240	248	256	264	272	280	289	297	306	315	324	333	342	351	361
45	215	222	230	238	246	254	262	270	278	287	295	304	313	322	331	340	350	359	369
46	220	227	235	243	251	259	267	276	284	293	302	311	320	329	338	348	358	367	377
47	224	232	240	248	256	265	273	282	291	299	308	318	327	338	346	355	365	375	385
48	229	237	245	254	262	270	279	288	297	306	315	324	334	343	353	363	373	383	394
49	234	242	250	259	267	278	285	294	303	312	322	331	341	351	361	371	381	391	402
50	239	247	255	264	273	282	291	300	309	319	328	338	348	358	368	378	389	399	410
51	244	252	261	269	278	287	296	306	315	325	335	345	355	365	375	386	396	407	418
52	248	257	266	275	284	293	302	312	322	331	341	351	362	372	383	393	404	415	426
53	253	262	271	280	289	299	308	318	328	338	348	358	369	379	390	401	412	423	435
54	258	267	276	285	295	304	314	324	334	344	354	365	376	386	397	408	420	431	443

From the National Heart, Lung, and Blood Institute (2006). Body mass index table. Accessed Sept. 12, 2006, www.nhlbi.nih.gov/guidelines/obesity/bmi_tbl.htm.
To use this table, find the appropriate height under the first row labeled 'Height" and then find the weight closest to the person's weight on the rows below. The number in the first column is the BMI for that height and weight.

Age (at conception) _____
Prepregnant weight _____
Height (w/o shoes) _____
Desirable weight _____
% Desirable weight _____
Body mass index _____
Term weight goal _____

WEIGHT GAIN (KILOGRAMS)

WEEKS GESTATION

FIG. 15-2 Prenatal weight-gain chart for plotting weight gain of normal-weight women. NOTE: Young adolescents, African-American women, and smokers should aim for the upper end of the recommended range; short women (<157 cm or 5 feet 2 inches) should strive for gains at the lower end of the range.

mal; 26 to 29, overweight or high; and greater than 29, obese (Institute of Medicine, 1992). Table 15-2 provides a tool for estimating the BMI without the need for calculation.

For women with single fetuses, current recommendations are that women with normal BMI should gain 11.5 to 16 kg during pregnancy (Fig. 15-2); underweight women should gain 12.5 to 18 kg; overweight women should gain 7 to 11.5 kg; and obese women should gain at least 7 kg (Institute of Medicine, 1992). Adolescents are encouraged to strive for weight gains at the upper end of the recommended range for their BMI, because it appears that the fetus and the still-growing mother compete for nutrients. The risk of mechanical complications at birth is reduced if the weight gain of short adult women (shorter than 157 cm) is near the lower end of their recommended range.

For twin gestations, it has been suggested that the total weight gain at term should be 21 to 28 kg for women who are underweight before conception, 17 to 24.5 kg for normal-weight women, 16.4 to 20.4 kg for overweight women, and 12 to 17.7 kg for obese women (Luke, 2005).

Pattern of Weight Gain

Weight gain should take place throughout pregnancy. The risk of giving birth to an SGA infant is greater when the weight gain early in pregnancy has been poor. The likelihood of preterm birth is greater when the gains during the

last half of pregnancy have been inadequate. These risks exist even when the total gain for the pregnancy is in the recommended range.

The optimal rate of weight gain depends on the stage of pregnancy. During the first and second trimesters, growth takes place primarily in maternal tissues; during the third trimester, growth occurs primarily in fetal tissues. During the first trimester of singleton pregnancy, the average total weight gain is only 1 to 2.5 kg; thereafter the recommended weight gain increases to approximately 0.4 kg per week for a woman of normal weight (see Fig. 15-2). The recommended weekly weight gain for overweight women during the second and third trimesters is 0.3 kg, and it is 0.5 kg for underweight women.

In multiple gestation, weight gain during the first half of pregnancy appears to be especially important (Luke, 2005). For the first trimester of twin gestation, a gain of 0.3 to 0.8 kg a week has been associated with good outcomes. This general goal should be adjusted for prepregnancy weight, i.e., 0.6 to 0.8 kg weekly for underweight women and 0.3 to 0.6 kg weekly for obese women. Similarly, during midpregnancy in twin gestation, recommended weekly weight gains are 0.45 to 0.9 kg, with the lower value for obese women and the higher for underweight women. During late pregnancy, weekly gains of 0.3 to 0.6 kg are recommended for the woman pregnant with twins (Luke).

The recommended energy (kcal) intake corresponds to the recommended pattern of gain (see Table 15-1). There is no increment for the first trimester; an additional 340 and 462 kcal per day over the prepregnant intake is recommended during the second and third trimesters, respectively. These recommendations are most appropriate for singleton pregnancy and may need to be adjusted in multiple gestation. The amount of food providing the needed increase in energy intake is not great. The 340 additional kcal needed during the second trimester can be provided by one additional serving from each of the following groups: milk, yogurt, or cheese (all skim milk products); fruits; vegetables; and bread, cereal, rice, or pasta.

The reasons for an inadequate weight gain (less than 1 kg per month for normal-weight women or less than 0.5 kg per month for obese women during the last two trimesters) or excessive weight gain (more than 3 kg per month) should be thoroughly evaluated. Possible reasons for deviations from the expected rate of weight gain, besides inadequate or excessive dietary intake, include measurement or recording errors, differences in the weight of clothing, the time of day, and the accumulation of fluids. An exceptionally high gain is likely to result from the accumulation of fluids, and a gain of more than 3 kg in a month, especially after the twentieth week of gestation, often indicates the development of preeclampsia.

Hazards of Restricting Adequate Weight Gain

An obsession with thinness and dieting pervades the North American culture. Figure-conscious women may find it difficult to make the transition from guarding against weight

table 15-3 Tissues Contributing to Maternal Weight Gain at 40 Weeks of Gestation

TISSUE	KILOGRAMS	POUNDS
Fetus	3-3.9	7-8.5
Placenta	0.9-1.1	2-2.5
Amniotic fluid	0.9	2
Increase in uterine tissue	0.9	2
Breast tissue	0.5-1.8	1-4
Increased blood volume	1.8-2.3	4-5
Increased tissue fluid	1.4-2.3	3-5
Increased stores (fat)	1.8-2.7	4-6

gain before pregnancy to valuing weight gain during pregnancy. In counseling these women, the nurse can emphasize the positive effects of good nutrition, as well as the adverse effects of maternal malnutrition (manifested by poor weight gain) on infant growth and development. This counseling includes information on the components of weight gain during pregnancy (Table 15-3) and the amount of this weight that will be lost after the birth. Because lactation can help to reduce maternal energy stores gradually, this also provides an opportunity to promote breastfeeding.

Pregnancy is not a time for a weight reduction diet. Even overweight or obese pregnant women need to gain at least enough weight to equal the weight of the products of conception (fetus, placenta, and amniotic fluid). If they limit their energy intake to prevent weight gain, they also may excessively limit their intake of important nutrients. Moreover, dietary restriction results in the catabolism of fat stores, which in turn augments the production of ketones. The long-term effects of mild ketonemia during pregnancy are not known, but ketonuria has been found to be correlated with the occurrence of preterm labor. It should be stressed to obese women, and all pregnant women for that matter, that the quality of the weight gain is important, with emphasis placed on the consumption of nutrient-dense foods and the avoidance of empty-calorie foods.

Weight gain is important, but pregnancy is not an excuse for uncontrolled dietary indulgence. The old saying that the pregnant woman is "eating for two" should not be interpreted to mean that the food intake should be doubled. Instead the woman should place an emphasis on the quality of her food intake as she considers her needs and those of her fetus. Excessive weight gained during pregnancy may be difficult to lose after pregnancy, thus contributing to chronic overweight or obesity, an etiologic factor in a host of chronic diseases, including hypertension, diabetes mellitus, and arteriosclerotic heart disease. The woman who gains 18 kg or more is especially at risk. Food energy intake and particularly intake of fat is likely to be high among pregnant women, especially low-income women.

Protein

Protein, with its essential constituent nitrogen, is the nutritional element basic to growth. An adequate protein intake is essential to meet increasing demands in pregnancy.

These demands arise from the rapid growth of the fetus; enlargement of the uterus and its supporting structures, the mammary glands, and the placenta; increase in the maternal circulating blood volume and the subsequent demand for increased amounts of plasma protein to maintain colloidal osmotic pressure; and formation of amniotic fluid.

Milk, meat, eggs, and cheese are complete protein foods with a high biologic value. Legumes (dried beans and peas), whole grains, and nuts also are valuable sources of protein. In addition, these protein-rich foods are a source of other nutrients such as calcium, iron, and B vitamins; plant sources of protein often provide needed dietary fiber. The recommended daily food plan (Table 15-4) is a guide to the amounts of these foods that would supply the quantities of protein needed. The recommendations provide for only a modest increase in protein intake over the prepregnant levels in adult women. Protein intake in many people in the United States is relatively high, and thus many women may not need to increase their protein intake at all during pregnancy. Three servings of milk, yogurt, or cheese (four for adolescents) and two servings (5 to 6 oz [140 to 168 g]) of meat, poultry, or fish would supply the recommended protein for the pregnant woman. Additional protein would be provided by vegetables and breads, cereals, rice, or pasta. Pregnant adolescents, women from impoverished backgrounds, and women adhering to unusual diets, such as a macrobiotic (highly restricted vegetarian) diet, are those whose protein intake is most likely to be inadequate. The use of high-protein supplements is not recommended, because they have been associated with an increased incidence of preterm births.

Pregnant and nursing women should be especially careful when choosing fish to select those that are low in mercury.

■ NURSE ALERT

High levels of mercury can harm the developing nervous system of the fetus or young child, and certain fish are especially high in mercury. Women who may become pregnant, women who are pregnant or nursing, and young children need to follow some precautions: (1) avoid eating shark, swordfish, king mackerel, and tilefish; (2) check local advisories about the safety of fish caught by family and friends in local bodies of water, but if no advisory is available, limit intake of these fish to 6 ounces and eat no other fish that week; and (3) eat as much as 12 ounces a week of a variety of commercially-caught fish and shellfish low in mercury, such as shrimp, salmon, pollock, catfish, and canned light tuna (but limit intake of albacore or "white" tuna and tuna steaks, which contain more mercury, to 6 ounces per week). Additional information about mercury levels in a variety of commercial fish is available at **www.cfsan.fda.gov/~frf/sea-mehg.html**.

Fluid

Essential during the exchange of nutrients and waste products across cell membranes, water is the main substance of cells, blood, lymph, amniotic fluid, and other vital body fluids. It also aids in maintaining body temperature. A

table 15-4 Daily Food Guide for Pregnancy and Lactation

FOOD GROUP	DAILY AMOUNT OF FOOD RECOMMENDED FOR WOMEN*	SERVING SIZE
GRAINS	6 ounce-equivalents At least half of grain servings should be whole grains. *Whole grains* are those that contain the entire grain kernel (bran, germ, endosperm), e.g., whole wheat or cornmeal, oatmeal, and brown rice. *Refined grains* have been milled to remove the bran and germ, e.g., white flour, white bread, degermed cornmeal, white rice, and corn or flour tortillas.	1 ounce-equivalent = 1 slice bread, 1 cup ready-to-eat cereal, or ½ cup cooked rice or pasta or cooked cereal
VEGETABLES Vary the vegetables consumed to take advantage of the different nutrients they offer.	2.5 cups Weekly intake should include at least the following: 3 cups dark green vegetables (e.g., spinach or greens, broccoli, bok choy, romaine lettuce); 2 cups orange vegetables (e.g., carrots; acorn, butternut, or hubbard squash; sweet potatoes); 3 cups dry beans or peas (e.g., black, navy, or kidney beans; chickpeas; black-eyed peas; split peas; lentils; soy beans; tofu); 3 cup starchy vegetables (corn, green peas, potatoes); and 6.5 cups of other vegetables (e.g., artichokes, asparagus, bean sprouts, Brussels sprouts, green beans, cauliflower, cucumber, tomatoes, iceberg or head lettuce, vegetable juice).	1 cup = 2 cups raw leafy greens; 1 cup of other vegetables, raw or cooked; or 1 cup of vegetable juice
FRUITS	1.5 cups	1 cup = 1 cup raw, frozen or canned fruit; 1 cup 100% juice; or ½ cup dried fruit
MILK, YOGURT, AND CHEESE (MILK GROUP)	3 cups for nonpregnant and pregnant; 4 for lactation Most milk group choices should be fat-free or low-fat.	1 cup = 1 cup milk or yogurt; 1.5 ounces natural cheese; 2 ounces processed cheese (such as American); 2 cups cottage cheese; 1.5 cups ice cream (choose fat-free or low-fat most often)
MEAT, POULTRY, FISH, DRY BEANS, EGGS, AND NUTS (MEAT AND BEANS† GROUPS)	5 ounce-equivalents Most meat and poultry choices should be lean or low-fat. Fish, nuts, and seeds contain healthy oils, so choose these foods frequently instead of meat or poultry.	1 ounce-equivalent = 1 ounce (30 g) meat, poultry, or fish; ¼ cup cooked dry beans;† 1 egg; 1 tablespoon (15 ml) peanut butter; ½ ounce nuts or seeds
OILS	6 teaspoons (30 ml) Choose oils rather than solid fats. Solid fats are fats that are solid at room temperature, such as butter, shortening, stick margarine, and pork, chicken, or beef fat. Read the label: choose products with no *trans* fats, limit intake of saturated fats, and choose oils high in monounsaturated and polyunsaturated fats.	1 teaspoon = 1 teaspoon liquid oil (olive, canola, sunflower, safflower, peanut, soybean, cottonseed, etc.) or soft margarine (tub or squeeze bottle); 1 tablespoon mayonnaise or Italian salad dressing; ¾ tablespoon Thousand Island salad dressing; 8 large olives; ⅙ medium avocado; ⅓ ounce dry roasted peanuts, mixed nuts, cashews, sunflower seeds†

*These are approximate amounts, based on a relatively sedentary lifestyle, and should be individualized. For example, intake may have to be increased for women with a more active lifestyle or multiple gestation, those who are underweight before pregnancy, or those exhibiting poor gestational weight gain. Needs during lactation may also be greater than these recommendations.
†Beans are also part of the vegetable group; avocados are also part of the fruit group, and nuts and seeds are part of the meat and beans group.

CRITICAL THINKING EXERCISE

Imbalanced Nutrition

Lisa is a 25-year-old woman who is G1, P0 at 20 weeks of gestation. She is seen for her regular appointment and is noted to have gained 18 lb (8.2 kg) since the beginning of her pregnancy.

1. Evidence—Is there sufficient evidence to draw conclusions about her diagnosis and preferred treatment?
2. Assumptions—What assumptions can be made about the following items?
   a. Possible diagnoses for Lisa
   b. Client history, physical assessment, laboratory tests, and diagnostic procedures that will be needed to make a diagnosis
   c. Lisa's concern for her fetus
   d. Therapy for her problem
3. What implications and priorities for nursing care can be made at this time?
4. Does the evidence objectively support your conclusion?
5. Are there alternative perspectives to your conclusion?

good fluid intake promotes regular bowel function, which is sometimes a problem during pregnancy. The recommended daily intake is about 8 to 10 glasses (2.3 L) of fluid. Water, milk, and fruit juices are good sources. Foods in the diet should supply an additional 700 ml or more of fluid. Dehydration may increase the risk of cramping, contractions, and preterm labor.

Caffeine in moderate amounts has not been proved to cause adverse effects during pregnancy. However, women who consume more than 300 mg of caffeine daily (equivalent to about 3 cups of coffee) may be at increased risk of miscarriage and of giving birth to infants with IUGR. The ill effects of caffeine have been proposed to result from vasoconstriction of the blood vessels supplying the uterus or from interference with cell division in the developing fetus. Consequently, caffeine-containing products, including caffeinated coffee, tea, soft drinks, and cocoa beverages, should be avoided or consumed only in limited quantities. Some authorities recommend consumption of no more than 150 mg caffeine daily, and others recommend no more than 300 mg caffeine per day (California Diabetes & Pregnancy Program, rev 2004; National Toxicology Program Center for the Evaluation of Risks to Human Reproduction, 2005). Regardless of the exact amount, caffeine intake should be limited to no more than moderate use until further information is available. There does not seem to be any evidence that moderate amounts of caffeine interfere with conception (National Toxicology Program Center for the Evaluation of Risks to Human Reproduction).

Aspartame (Nutrasweet, Equal), acesulfame potassium (Sunett), and sucralose (Splenda), artificial sweeteners commonly used in low- or no-calorie beverages and low-calorie food products, have not been found to have adverse effects on the normal mother and fetus and are therefore approved by the U.S. Food and Drug Administration (FDA) for use during pregnancy. Aspartame, which contains phenylalanine, should be avoided by the pregnant woman with phenylketonuria (PKU), however. Stevia (stevioside) is a sweetener that has not been approved by the FDA.

Minerals and Vitamins

In general, the nutrient needs of pregnant women, with perhaps the exception of folate and iron, can be met through dietary sources. Counseling about the need for a varied diet rich in vitamins and minerals should be a part of the early prenatal care of every pregnant woman and should be reinforced throughout pregnancy. However, supplements of certain nutrients (listed in the following discussion) are recommended whenever the woman's diet is very poor or whenever significant nutritional risk factors are present. Nutritional risk factors in pregnancy are listed in Box 15-2.

Iron

Iron is needed both to allow transfer of adequate iron to the fetus and to permit expansion of the maternal RBC mass. Beginning in the latter part of the first trimester, the blood volume of the mother increases steadily, peaking at about 1500 ml more than that in the nonpregnant state. In twin gestations, the increase is at least 500 ml greater than that in pregnancies with single fetuses. Plasma volume increases more than RBC mass, with the difference between plasma and RBCs being greatest during the second trimester. The relative excess of plasma causes a modest decrease in the hemoglobin concentration and hematocrit, known as physiologic anemia of pregnancy. This is a normal adaptation during pregnancy.

However, poor iron nutriture, which can result in iron deficiency anemia, is relatively common among women in the childbearing years. Iron deficiency (not necessarily anemia) is estimated to affect approximately 10% of nonpregnant women in the childbearing years in the United States. Anemic women are poorly prepared to tolerate hemorrhage at the time of birth. In addition, women who have iron deficiency anemia during early pregnancy are at increased risk of preterm birth (Scholl, 2005). Iron deficiency during the third trimester apparently does not carry the same risk. In the United States, anemia is most com-

box 15-2 Indicators of Nutritional Risk in Pregnancy

- Adolescence
- Frequent pregnancies: three within 2 years
- Poor fetal outcome in a previous pregnancy
- Poverty
- Poor diet habits with resistance to change
- Use of tobacco, alcohol, or drugs
- Weight at conception under or over normal weight
- Problems with weight gain
  Any weight loss
  Weight gain of less than 1 kg/mo after the first trimester
  Weight gain of more than 3 kg/month after the first trimester
- Multifetal pregnancy
- Low hemoglobin and/or hematocrit values

mon among adolescents, African-American women, and women of lower socioeconomic status.

The Institute of Medicine (1992) recommended that all pregnant women receive a supplement of 30 mg of ferrous iron daily, starting by 12 weeks of gestation. (Iron supplements may be poorly tolerated during the nausea prevalent in the first trimester.) Iron supplementation of women with iron deficiency can improve maternal hematologic indices and appears to reduce LBW births (Scholl, 2005). If maternal iron-deficiency anemia is present (preferably diagnosed by measurement of serum ferritin, a storage form of iron), increased iron dosages (60 to 120 mg daily) are recommended. Certain foods taken with an iron supplement can promote or inhibit the absorption of iron from the supplement. See the Teaching for Self-Care box regarding iron supplementation. Even when a woman is taking an iron supplement, however, she also should include good food sources of iron in her daily diet (see Table 15-1).

Iron supplementation during pregnancy enhances maternal iron status, producing increases in hemoglobin, serum iron, mean red cell volume, saturation of the iron transport protein transferrin, and serum ferritin. However, there is concern that routine supplementation of all women, regardless of iron status, results in a median iron intake above the tolerable upper limit for a substantial number of women. Women with the highest levels of ferritin have been found to be at increased risk of gestational diabetes mellitus in some investigations (Scholl, 2005).

Calcium

There is no increase in the DRI of calcium during pregnancy and lactation, in comparison to the recommendation for the nonpregnant woman (see Table 15-1). The DRI (1000 mg daily for women 19 years and older and 1300 mg for those younger than 19 years) appears to provide sufficient calcium for fetal bone and tooth development to proceed while maintaining maternal bone mass. Milk and yogurt are especially rich sources of calcium, providing approximately 300 mg per cup (240 ml). Nevertheless, many women do not consume these foods or do not consume adequate amounts to provide the recommended intakes of calcium. One problem that can interfere with milk consumption is lactose intolerance, the inability to digest milk sugar (lactose) because of the lack of the enzyme lactase in the small intestine. It is relatively common in adults, particularly African-Americans, Asians, Native Americans, and Inuits (Alaska Natives). Milk consumption may cause abdominal cramping, bloating, and diarrhea in such people, although many lactose-intolerant individuals can tolerate small amounts of milk without symptoms. Yogurt, sweet acidophilus milk, buttermilk, cheese, chocolate milk, and cocoa may be tolerated even when fresh fluid milk is not. Commercial lactase supplements (e.g., Lactaid) are widely available to consume with milk, and many supermarkets stock lactase-treated milk. The lactase in these products hydrolyzes, or digests, the lactose in the milk, making it possible for lactose-intolerant people to drink milk.

In some cultures, it is uncommon for adults to drink milk. For example, Puerto Ricans and other Hispanic people may use it only as an additive in coffee. Pregnant women from these cultures may need to consume nondairy sources of calcium. Vegetarian diets also may be lacking in calcium (Box 15-3). If calcium intake appears low

---

TEACHING FOR SELF-CARE

Iron Supplementation

- Vitamin C (in citrus fruits, tomatoes, melons, and strawberries) and heme iron (in meats) increase the absorption of iron supplement; therefore include these in the diet often.
- Bran, tea, coffee, milk, oxalates (in spinach and Swiss chard), and egg yolk decrease iron absorption. Avoid consuming them at the same time as the supplement.
- Iron is absorbed best if it is taken when the stomach is empty; that is, take it between meals with a beverage other than tea, coffee, or milk.
- Iron can be taken at bedtime if abdominal discomfort occurs when it is taken between meals.
- If an iron dose is missed, take it as soon as it is remembered if that is within 13 hours of the scheduled dose. Do not double up on the dose.
- Keep the supplement in a childproof container and out of the reach of any children in the household.
- The iron may cause stools to be black or dark green.
- Constipation is common with iron supplementation. A diet high in fiber with adequate fluid intake is recommended.

---

box 15-3 Calcium Sources for Women Who Do Not Drink Milk

Each of the following provides approximately the same amount of calcium as 1 cup of milk:

FISH
3-oz can of sardines
4½-oz can of salmon (if bones are eaten)

BEANS AND LEGUMES
3 c of cooked dried beans
2½ c of refried beans
2 c of baked beans with molasses
1 c of tofu (calcium added in processing)

GREENS
1 c of collards
1½ c of kale or turnip greens

BAKED PRODUCTS
3 pieces of cornbread
3 English muffins
4 slices of French toast
2 (7-inch diameter) waffles

FRUITS
11 dried figs
1⅛ c of orange juice with calcium added

SAUCES
3 oz of pesto sauce
5 oz of cheese sauce

| box 15-4 | **Complementary and Alternative Therapies** |

Bone meal, which is sometimes used as a calcium source by pregnant women, is frequently found to be contaminated with lead. Lead freely crosses the placenta and thus regular maternal intake of bone meal may result in high levels of lead in the fetus.

Reference: Shannon, M. (2003). Severe lead poisoning in pregnancy. *Ambulatory Pediatrics, 3*(1), 37-39.

and the woman does not change her diet habits despite counseling, a supplement containing 600 mg of elemental calcium may be needed daily. Calcium supplements also may be recommended when a pregnant woman has leg cramps that are caused by an imbalance in the calcium-phosphorus ratio. Bone meal supplements are not recommended in pregnancy (Box 15-4).

Other Minerals and Electrolytes

Magnesium. Diets of women in the childbearing years are likely to be low in magnesium, and as many as half of pregnant and lactating women may have inadequate intakes (Institute of Medicine, 2004). Adolescents and low income women are especially at risk. Dairy products, nuts, whole grains, and green leafy vegetables are good sources of magnesium.

Sodium. During pregnancy, the need for sodium increases slightly, primarily because the body water is expanding (e.g., the expanding blood volume). Sodium is essential for maintaining body water balance. In the past, dietary sodium was routinely restricted in an effort to control the peripheral edema that commonly occurs during pregnancy. It is now recognized, however, that moderate peripheral edema is normal in pregnancy, occurring as a response to the fluid-retaining effects of elevated levels of estrogen. Sodium is not routinely restricted in pregnancy, and restriction has not proved effective in reducing the rates of preeclampsia. Severe sodium restriction also may make it difficult for pregnant women to achieve an adequate diet. Grain, milk, and meat products, which are good sources of the nutrients needed during pregnancy, are significant sources of sodium. Additionally, sodium restriction may stress the adrenal glands and kidneys as they attempt to retain adequate sodium. In general, sodium restriction is necessary only if the woman has a medical condition such as renal or liver failure or hypertension that warrants such a restriction.

On the other hand, excessive sodium intake is unwarranted because it may contribute to development of hypertension in salt-sensitive individuals. An adequate sodium intake for pregnant and lactating women, as well as nonpregnant women in the childbearing years, is estimated to be 1.5 g/day, with a recommended upper limit of intake of 2.3 g/day (Institute of Medicine, 2003). Table salt (sodium chloride) is the richest source of sodium,

with approximately 2.3 g sodium contained in 1 teaspoon (6 g) of salt. Most canned foods contain added salt, unless the label states otherwise. Large amounts of sodium also are found in many processed foods, including meats (e.g., smoked or cured meats, cold cuts, and corned beef), frozen entrees and meals, baked goods, mixes for casseroles or grain products, soups, and condiments. Products low in nutritive value and excessively high in sodium include pretzels, potato and other chips (except salt-free), pickles, catsup, prepared mustard, steak and Worcestershire sauces, some soft drinks, and bouillon. A moderate sodium intake can usually be achieved by salting food lightly during cooking, adding no additional salt at the table, and avoiding low nutrient–high sodium foods.

Potassium. Diets including adequate intakes of potassium are associated with reduced risk of hypertension. Potassium has been identified as one of the nutrients most likely to be lacking in the diets of women of childbearing years (Institute of Medicine, 2004). A diet including 8 to 10 servings of unprocessed fruits and vegetables daily, along with moderate amounts of low-fat meats and dairy products, has been effective in reducing sodium intake while providing adequate amounts of potassium.

Zinc. Zinc is a constituent of numerous enzymes involved in major metabolic pathways. Zinc deficiency is associated with malformations of the central nervous system in infants. When large amounts of iron and folic acid are consumed, the absorption of zinc is inhibited, and the serum zinc levels are reduced as a result. Because iron and folic acid supplements are commonly prescribed during pregnancy, pregnant women should be encouraged to consume good sources of zinc daily (see Table 15-1). Women with anemia who receive high-dose iron supplements also need supplements of zinc and copper.

Fluoride. There is no evidence that prenatal fluoride supplementation reduces the child's likelihood of tooth decay during the preschool years. No increase in fluoride intake over the nonpregnant DRI is currently recommended during pregnancy (Institute of Medicine, 2003).

Fat-Soluble Vitamins

The fat-soluble vitamins include vitamins A, D, E, and K. These are of special concern during pregnancy because vitamin E intake is among the nutrients most likely to be lacking in the diets of women of childbearing age, and intake of vitamins A and D is also low in the diets of some women (Institute of Medicine, 2004). Fat-soluble vitamins are stored in the body tissues; in the event of prolonged overdoses, these vitamins can reach toxic levels. Because of the high potential for toxicity, pregnant women are advised to take fat-soluble vitamin supplements only as prescribed. Toxicity from dietary sources is very unlikely, however.

Vitamin E is needed for protection against oxidative stress, and pregnancy is associated with increased oxidative stress. Indeed, oxidative stress has been proposed as an explanation for the etiology of preeclampsia (Allen, 2005). Vegetable oils and nuts are especially good sources of

EVIDENCE-BASED PRACTICE

Prevention of Preeclampsia with Antioxidants

BACKGROUND

- Preeclampsia is gestational hypertension with proteinuria, and is caused by oxidative damage and inflammation (see Chapter 30). In its extreme form, it can cause seizures, hemolysis-elevated liver enzymes-low platelets syndrome (HELLP), and maternal death. For the fetus, the poor uteroplacental perfusion of preeclampsia is associated with intrauterine growth restriction, small-for-gestational-age (SGA), preterm births, perinatal death, and long-term poor growth and risk for diabetes and hypertension.
- Antioxidant therapy protects healthy cells from damage by inhibiting the oxidative process and scavenging the free radicals that are released by oxidation. Vitamins C, E, and A are free radical scavengers, and may be a cost-effective, low-technology intervention for the prevention of preeclampsia.

OBJECTIVES

- The authors' task was to determine the efficacy and safety of antioxidant supplementation on preeclampsia, SGA, maternal and perinatal morbidity and mortality, and long-term outcomes.

METHODS

Search Strategy

- The reviewers investigated databases, expert recommendations, and reference lists for studies, and found six randomized, or quasi-randomized, controlled trials that met their criteria. Two of the trials were double-blinded, so neither subject nor evaluator knew their treatment allocations. Five of the studies were dated 1999 to 2003, representing 1069 women from China, India, South Africa, Venezuela, and the United States. The People's League Study was an extraordinary example of dedication to research: it was a quasi-randomized study, representing 5515 pregnant women, seen 1938 to 1939, of whom 494 were lost to follow-up when they were evacuated from London during World War II. The study was completed and published in 1942.

Statistical Analyses

- Reviewers calculated relative risks for categoric data. Subgroup analyses were made of the varying ranges of vitamin C, with the understanding that the circulating concentration of vitamin C is maximized at doses above 400 mg. Most of the women were of moderate to low (6%) risk for developing preeclampsia, although four studies recruited women with risk factors who were classified as being at high (19%) risk. Differences between groups outside the 95% confidence interval were accepted as significant.

FINDINGS

- Antioxidant therapy of any kind was associated with a 39% reduction in relative risk for preeclampsia, or an absolute risk reduction of 3%. Antioxidant use was associated with greater risk for preterm birth, but no adverse neonatal outcomes resulted from those births. There was a lower risk for SGA with antioxidant use, as well as greater birth weight. There were no differences between groups in maternal bleeding, nor stillbirths. No side effects nor adverse outcomes were reported in any of the trials.

LIMITATIONS

- The studies varied on doses, combinations, gestational age at onset of treatment, and even the definition of preeclampsia. There was not enough evidence to determine the additive effects of the antioxidants, or of other nutritional supplements. Only the People's League study assessed the nutritional status of their subjects (half were deficient in vitamin C) at intake. It was the largest study, but was quasi-randomized, involved other nutritional interventions, and was conducted in a time of stress and scarcity.

IMPLICATIONS FOR PRACTICE

- Antioxidants are inexpensive and readily available, making them a low-technology way to prevent preeclampsia in low-resource, high risk populations, especially in developing countries. However, the reviewers stopped short of recommending their routine use until their benefits (for preeclampsia and SGA) and risks (for preterm birth) are better established. In the meantime, nurses can confirm the benefits of dietary advice for fresh vegetables and fruit as sources of antioxidants.

IMPLICATIONS FOR FURTHER RESEARCH

- Information is needed to clarify the prematurity noted with antioxidant use. Further research is needed to determine if other nutritional supplements, such as calcium or fish oil, help or hinder the beneficial effects of antioxidants. Aspirin is frequently studied as a promising adjunct therapy to prevent preeclampsia (see Evidence-Based Practice box for Chapter 34, "Can Aspirin Prevent Preeclampsia?"). Further information is needed about identifying women who could benefit, dosing and timing of antioxidants, and dietary advice. Much more information is needed to measure the onset and severity of hypertension, and short- and long-term outcomes for mother and baby.

Reference: Rumbold, A., Duley, L., Crowther, C., & Haslam, R. (2005). Antioxidants for preventing pre-eclampsia. *The Cochrane Database of Systematic Reviews,* 2006, Issue 3. Chichester, UK: John Wiley & Sons.

vitamin E, and whole grains and leafy green vegetables are moderate sources.

Adequate intake of vitamin A is needed so that sufficient amounts of the vitamin can be stored in the fetus; however, a well-chosen diet including adequate amounts of deep yellow and deep green vegetables and fruits such as leafy greens, broccoli, carrots, cantaloupe, and apricots provides sufficient amounts of carotenes that can be converted in the body to vitamin A. Congenital malformations have occurred in infants of mothers who took excessive amounts of preformed vitamin A (from supplements) during pregnancy, and thus supplements are not recommended routinely for pregnant women. Vitamin A analogs (e.g., isotretinoin [Accutane]), which are prescribed for the treatment of cystic acne, are a special concern. Isotretinoin use during early pregnancy has been associated with an increased incidence of heart malformations, facial abnormalities, cleft palate, hydrocephalus, and deafness and blindness in the infant, as well as an increased risk of miscarriage. Topical agents such as tretinoin (Retin-A) do not appear to enter the circulation in substantial amounts, but their safety in pregnancy has not been confirmed.

Vitamin D plays an important role in the absorption and metabolism of calcium. The main food sources of this vitamin are enriched or fortified foods such as milk and ready-to-eat cereals. Vitamin D also is produced in the skin by the action of ultraviolet light (in sunlight). A severe deficiency may lead to neonatal hypocalcemia and tetany, as well as to hypoplasia of the tooth enamel. Women with lactose intolerance and those who do not include milk in their diet for any reason are at risk for vitamin D deficiency. Other risk factors for deficiency are dark skin, with African-American women being at high risk of deficiency; habitual use of clothing that covers most of the skin (e.g., Moslem women with extensive body covering); and living in northern latitudes where sunlight exposure is limited, especially during the winter. Use of recommended amounts of sunscreen with an SPF rating of 15 or greater reduces skin vitamin D production by as much as 99%, thus bringing about a need for regular intake of fortified foods or a supplement.

Water-Soluble Vitamins

Body stores of water-soluble vitamins are much smaller than those of fat-soluble vitamins, and the water-soluble vitamins, in contrast to the fat-soluble ones, are readily excreted in the urine. Therefore good sources of these vitamins must be consumed frequently, and toxicity with overdose is less likely than it is in people taking fat-soluble vitamins.

Folate/Folic Acid. Because of the increase in RBC production during pregnancy, as well as the nutritional requirements of the rapidly growing cells in the fetus and placenta, pregnant women should consume about 50% more folic acid than nonpregnant women, or about 0.6 mg (600 micrograms) daily. In the United States, all enriched grain products (which include most white breads, flour, and pasta) must contain folic acid at a level of 1.4 mg/kg flour. This level of fortification is designed to supply approximately 0.1 mg folic acid daily in the average American diet and has significantly increased folic acid consumption in the population as a whole. All women of childbearing potential need careful counseling about including good sources of folate in their diets (see Box 15-1). Supplemental folic acid is usually prescribed to ensure that intake is adequate. Women who have borne a child with a neural tube defect are advised to consume 4 mg of folic acid daily, and a supplement is required for them to achieve this level of intake.

Pyridoxine. Pyridoxine, or vitamin B_6, is involved in protein metabolism. Although levels of a pyridoxine-

containing enzyme have been reported to be low in women with preeclampsia, there is no evidence that supplementation prevents or eradicates the condition. No supplement is recommended routinely, but women with poor diets and those at nutritional risk (see Box 15-2) may need a supplement providing 2 mg/day (Institute of Medicine, 1992). Pyridoxine has been effective in reducing the nausea and vomiting of early pregnancy in some trials (Jewell & Young, 2003).

Vitamin C. Vitamin C, or ascorbic acid, plays an important role in tissue formation and enhances the absorption of iron. The vitamin C needs of most women are readily met by a diet that includes at least one or two daily servings of citrus fruit or juice or another good source of the vitamin (see Table 15-1), but women who smoke need more. A supplement of 50 mg/day is recommended for women determined to be at nutritional risk (Institute of Medicine, 1992); however, if the mother should take excessive doses of this vitamin during pregnancy, vitamin C deficiency may develop in the infant after birth.

Multivitamin-Multimineral Supplements During Pregnancy

Food can and should be the normal vehicle to meet the additional nutrient needs imposed by pregnancy, except for iron (Institute of Medicine, 1992). In addition, the recommended folate/folic acid intake may be difficult for some women to achieve. Some women habitually consume diets that are deficient in necessary nutrients and, for whatever reason, may be unable to change this intake. For these women, a multivitamin-multimineral supplement should be considered to ensure that they consume the RDA for most known vitamins and minerals. It is important that the pregnant woman understand that the use of a vitamin-mineral supplement does not lessen the need to consume a nutritious, well-balanced diet.

Pica and Food Cravings

Pica, which is the practice of consuming nonfood substances (e.g., clay, soil, and laundry starch) or excessive amounts of foodstuffs low in nutritional value (e.g., ice or freezer frost, baking powder or soda, and cornstarch), often is influenced by the woman's cultural background (Fig. 15-3). In the United States, it appears to be most common among African-American and Hispanic women, women from rural areas, and women with a family history of pica. In some studies, pica has been reported in almost 40% of pregnant women (Corbett, Ryan, & Weinrich, 2003). One problem with pica is that regular and heavy consumption of low-nutrient products may cause more nutritious foods to be displaced from the diet. As an example, cornstarch ingestion is popular among African-American women. It is a source of "empty" calories; half a cup (64 g) provides 240 kcal (57 kJ) but almost no vitamins, minerals, or protein. In addition, the pica items consumed may interfere with the absorption of nutrients, especially minerals (Ukaonu, Hill, & Christensen, 2003). Women with pica

FIG. 15-3 Nonfood substances consumed in pica: red clay from Georgia, Nzu from East Nigeria, baking powder, corn starch, baking soda, laundry starch, and ice. Some individuals practice *poly-pica*, consuming more than one of these or other nonfood substances. (Courtesy Shannon Perry, Phoenix, AZ.)

have been found to have lower hemoglobin levels than do those without pica.

Moreover, there is a risk that nonfood items will be contaminated with heavy metals or other toxic substances. Among Mexican-American women, consumption of "tierra" includes both soil and pulverized Mexican pottery (Klitzman, Sharma, Nicaj, Vitkevich, & Leighton, 2002; Shannon, 2003). Lead contamination of soils and soil-based products has caused high levels of lead in both pregnant women and their newborns (Klitzman, Sharma, Nicaj, Vitkevich, & Leighton; Shannon; Ukaonu, Hill, & Christensen). Regular household use of Mexican pottery in cooking or serving food or ingestion of ground pottery must be included in interviews or questionnaires regarding nutritional intake of pregnant women. The possibility of pica must be considered when pregnant women are found to be anemic, and the nurse should provide counseling about the health risks associated with pica.

The existence of pica, as well as details of the types and amounts of products ingested, is likely to be discovered only by the sensitive interviewer who has developed a relationship of trust with the woman. It has been proposed that pica and food cravings (i.e., the urge to have ice cream, pickles, or pizza, for example) during pregnancy are caused by an innate drive to consume nutrients missing from the diet. However, research has not supported this hypothesis.

Adolescent Pregnancy Needs

Many adolescent females have diets that provide less than the recommended intakes of key nutrients, including energy, calcium, and iron. Pregnant adolescents and their infants are at increased risk of complications during pregnancy and parturition. Growth of the pelvis is delayed in comparison to growth in stature, and this helps to explain why cephalopelvic disproportion and other mechanical problems associated with labor are common among young adolescents. Com-

petition between the growing adolescent and the fetus for nutrients also may contribute to some of the poor outcomes apparent in teen pregnancies. Pregnant adolescents are encouraged to choose a weight-gain goal at the upper end of the range for their BMI (Institute of Medicine, 1992). The goal is to reduce the prevalence of LBW among infants of teen mothers. Adolescent pregnancy increases the woman's risk of obesity later in life; thus the adolescent mother needs careful teaching regarding nutritional intake and physical activity to control body weight in the postpartum period.

Efforts to improve the nutritional health of pregnant adolescents focus on improving the nutrition knowledge, meal planning, and food preparation and selection skills of young women; promoting access to prenatal care; developing nutrition interventions and educational programs that are effective with adolescents; and striving to understand the factors that create barriers to change in the adolescent population.

Preeclampsia

The cause of preeclampsia is not known. There has been speculation that the poor intake of several nutrients, including calcium, magnesium, vitamin B_6, and protein, might foster its development, but there is no definite evidence that nutritional deficiencies are causes or that nutritional supplements can help prevent it. At present, a diet adequate in the recommended nutrients (see Table 15-1) appears to be the best means of reducing the risk of preeclampsia.

Physical Activity During Pregnancy

Moderate exercise during pregnancy yields numerous benefits, including improving muscle tone, potentially shortening the course of labor, and promoting a sense of well-being. If no medical or obstetric problems contraindicate physical activity, pregnant women should obtain a minimum of 30 minutes of moderate physical exercise on most, if not all, days of the week (American College of Obstetricians and Gynecologists, 2002). Two nutritional concepts are especially important for women who choose to exercise during pregnancy. First, a liberal amount of fluid should be consumed before, during, and after exercise, because dehydration can trigger premature labor. Second, the calorie intake should be sufficient to meet the increased needs of pregnancy and the demands of exercise.

▬ NUTRIENT NEEDS DURING LACTATION

Nutritional needs during lactation are similar in many ways to those during pregnancy (see Table 15-1). Needs for energy (calories), protein, calcium, iodine, zinc, the B vitamins (thiamin, riboflavin, niacin, pyridoxine, and vitamin B_{12}), and vitamin C remain greater than nonpregnant needs. The recommendations for some of these (e.g., vitamin C, zinc, and protein) are slightly to moderately higher than those during pregnancy (see Table 15-1). This allowance covers the amount of the nutrient released in the milk, as well as needs of the mother for tissue maintenance. In the case of iron and folic acid, the recommendation during lactation is lower than that during pregnancy. Both of these nutrients are essential for RBC formation and thus for maintaining the increase in the blood volume that occurs during pregnancy. With the decrease in maternal blood volume to nonpregnant levels after birth, maternal iron and folic acid needs also decrease. Many lactating women have a delay in the return of menses, and this also conserves blood cells and reduces iron and folic acid needs. It is especially important that the calcium intake be adequate; if it is not and the woman does not respond to diet counseling, a supplement of 600 mg of calcium per day may be needed.

The recommended energy intake is an increase of 330 kcal for first 6 months more than the woman's nonpregnant intake. It becomes difficult to obtain adequate nutrients for the maintenance of lactation if total caloric intake is less than 1800 kcal. Because of the deposition of energy stores, the woman who has gained the optimal amount of weight during pregnancy is heavier after birth than at the beginning of pregnancy. As a result of the caloric demands of lactation, however, the lactating mother usually has a gradual but steady weight loss. Most women rapidly lose several kilograms during the first month after birth, whether they breastfeed or not. After the first month, the average loss during lactation is 0.5 to 1 kg per month, and a woman who is overweight may be able to lose up to 2 kg without decreasing her milk supply.

Fluid intake also must be adequate to maintain milk production, but the mother's level of thirst is the best guide to the right amount. There is no need to consume more fluids than those needed to satisfy thirst.

Smoking and alcohol and excessive caffeine intake should be avoided during lactation. Smoking not only may impair milk production, but it also exposes the infant to the risk of passive smoking. It is speculated that the infant's psychomotor development may be affected by maternal alcohol use, and alcoholic beverages (two drinks per day) may impair the milk-ejection reflex. Caffeine intake can lead to a reduced iron concentration in milk and consequently contribute to the development of anemia in the infant. The caffeine concentration in milk is only approximately 1% of the mother's plasma level, but caffeine seems to accumulate in the infant. Breastfed infants of mothers who drink large amounts of coffee or caffeine-containing soft drinks may be unusually active and wakeful.

▬ CARE MANAGEMENT

During pregnancy, nutrition plays a key role in achieving an optimal outcome for the mother and her unborn baby. The motivation to learn about nutrition is usually greater during pregnancy because parents strive to "do what's right for the baby." Optimal nutrition cannot eliminate all the problems that may arise during pregnancy, but it does establish a good foundation for supporting the needs of the mother and her unborn baby.

▬ Assessment and Nursing Diagnoses

Assessment is based on a diet history (a description of the woman's usual food and beverage intake and factors affecting her nutritional status, such as medications being taken and the adequacy of income to allow her to purchase the necessary foods) obtained from an interview and review of the woman's health records, physical examination, and laboratory results. Ideally a nutritional assessment is performed before conception so that any recommended changes in diet, lifestyle, and weight can be undertaken before the woman becomes pregnant.

▬ Diet History

Obstetric and Gynecologic Effects on Nutrition. Nutritional reserves may be depleted in the multiparous woman or in the one who has had frequent pregnancies (especially three pregnancies within 2 years). A history of preterm birth or birth of an LBW or SGA infant may indicate inadequate dietary intake. Preeclampsia also may be a factor in poor maternal nutrition. Birth of a large-for-gestational age (LGA) infant often indicates the existence of maternal diabetes mellitus. Previous contraceptive methods also may affect reproductive health. Increased menstrual blood loss often occurs during the first 3 to 6 months after placement of an intrauterine contraceptive device; consequently the user may have low iron stores or even iron deficiency anemia. Oral contraceptive agents conversely are associated with decreased menstrual losses and increased iron stores; however, oral contraceptives may interfere with folic acid metabolism.

Medical History. Chronic maternal illnesses such as diabetes mellitus, renal disease, liver disease, cystic fibrosis or other malabsorptive disorders, seizure disorders and the use of anticonvulsant agents, hypertension, and PKU may affect a woman's nutritional status and dietary needs. In women with illnesses that have resulted in nutritional deficits or that require dietary treatment (e.g., diabetes mellitus or PKU), it is extremely important for nutritional care to be started and for the condition to be optimally controlled before conception. The registered dietitian can provide in-depth counseling for the woman who requires medical nutrition therapy during pregnancy and lactation.

Usual Maternal Diet. The woman's usual food and beverage intake, the adequacy of her income and other resources to meet her nutritional needs, any dietary modifications, food allergies and intolerances, and all medications and nutrition supplements being taken, as well as pica and cultural dietary requirements, should be ascertained. In addition, the presence and severity of nutrition-related discomforts of pregnancy such as morning sickness, constipation, and pyrosis (heartburn) should be determined. The nurse should be alert to any evidence of eating disorders such as anorexia nervosa, bulimia, and frequent and rigorous dieting before or during pregnancy.

The impact of food allergies and intolerances on nutritional status ranges from very important to almost nil. Lactose intolerance is of special concern in pregnant and lactating women because no other food group equals milk and milk products in terms of calcium content. If a woman has lactose intolerance, the interviewer should explore her intake of other calcium sources (see Box 15-3).

The assessment must include an evaluation of the woman's financial resources and her knowledge of sound dietary practices. The quality of the diet improves with increasing socioeconomic status and educational level. Poor women may not have access to adequate refrigeration and cooking facilities and may find it difficult to obtain adequate nutritious food. Pregnancy rates are high among homeless women, and many such women cannot or do not take advantage of services such as food stamps.

Box 15-5 provides a simple tool for obtaining diet history information. When potential problems are identified, they should be followed up with a careful interview.

---

box 15-5 **Food Intake Questionnaire**

Which of the following did you eat or drink yesterday? If the way you ate yesterday wasn't the way you usually eat, choose a recent day that was typical for you.

FOOD OR DRINK	NUMBER OF SERVINGS	FOOD OR DRINK	NUMBER OF SERVINGS
Beer, wine, other alcoholic drinks	_____	Orange or grapefruit juice	_____
Tea	_____	Fruit juice other than orange or grapefruit	_____
Coffee		Soft drinks	_____
Caffeinated	_____	Milk	_____
Decaffeinated	_____	Cereal with milk	_____
Fruit drink	_____	Yogurt	_____
Water	_____	Pizza	_____
Cheese	_____	Melon (such as watermelon, cantaloupe, honeydew)	_____
Macaroni and cheese	_____	Berries (kind _____)	_____
Other foods with cheese (such as lasagna, enchiladas, cheeseburgers)	_____	Apples	_____
Orange or grapefruit	_____	Other fruit	_____
Bananas	_____	Broccoli	_____
Peaches or apricots	_____	Green beans	_____
Green salad	_____	Potatoes (other than fried)	_____
Spinach or greens	_____	Corn	_____
Green peas	_____	Other vegetables	_____
Sweet potatoes	_____	Chicken or turkey	_____
Carrots	_____	Egg	_____
Meat	_____	Nuts	_____
Fish	_____	Hot dog	_____
Peanut butter	_____	Cold cuts (e.g., bologna)	_____
Dried beans or peas	_____	Roll/bagel	_____
Bacon or sausage	_____	Noodles	_____
Bread	_____	Chips	_____
Rice	_____	Cake	_____
Spaghetti or other pasta	_____	Donut or pastry	_____
Tortillas	_____		
French fries	_____		
Cookie	_____		
Pie	_____		

Are you often bothered by any of the following? (Circle all that apply)
    Nausea   Vomiting   Heartburn   Constipation

Are you on a special diet? No _____ Yes _____ If yes, what kind? _____

Do you try to limit the amount or kind of food you eat to control your weight? No _____ Yes _____

Do you avoid any foods for health or religious reasons? No _____ Yes _____ If yes, what foods? _____

Do you take any prescribed drugs or medications? No_____ Yes _____

If yes, what are they? _____

Do you take any over-the-counter medications (such as aspirin, cold medicines, Tylenol)?

    No _____ Yes _____ If yes, what are they? _____

Do you take any herbal supplements?

    No _____ Yes _____ If yes, what are they? _____

Do you ever have trouble affording the food you need? No _____ Yes _____

Do you have any help getting the food you need? No _____ Yes _____

    Food stamps   WIC   School lunch or breakfast

    Food from a food pantry, soup kitchen, or food bank

■ *Physical Examination*

Anthropometric (body) measurements provide short- and long-term information on a woman's nutritional status and are thus essential to the assessment. At a minimum, the woman's height and weight must be determined at the time of her first prenatal visit, and her weight should be measured at every subsequent visit (see earlier discussion of BMI).

A careful physical examination can reveal objective signs of malnutrition (Table 15-5). It is important to note, however, that some of these signs are nonspecific, and the physiologic changes of pregnancy may complicate the interpretation of physical findings. For example, lower-extremity edema often occurs when caloric and protein deficiencies are present, but it also may be a normal finding in the third trimester. The interpretation of physical findings is made easier by a thorough health history and by laboratory testing, if indicated.

■ *Laboratory Testing*

The only nutrition-related laboratory test necessary for most pregnant women is a hematocrit or hemoglobin measurement to screen for the presence of anemia. Because of the physiologic anemia of pregnancy, the reference values

table 15-5 Physical Assessment of Nutritional Status

SIGNS OF GOOD NUTRITION	SIGNS OF POOR NUTRITION
GENERAL APPEARANCE	
Alert, responsive, energetic, good endurance	Listless, apathetic, cachectic, easily fatigued, looks tired
MUSCLES	
Well developed, firm, good tone, some fat under skin	Flaccid, poor tone, tender, "wasted" appearance
GASTROINTESTINAL FUNCTION	
Good appetite and digestion, normal regular elimination, no palpable organs or masses	Anorexia, indigestion, constipation or diarrhea, liver or spleen enlargement
CARDIOVASCULAR FUNCTION	
Normal heart rate and rhythm, no murmurs, normal blood pressure for age	Rapid heart rate, enlarged heart, abnormal rhythm, elevated blood pressure
HAIR	
Shiny, lustrous, firm, not easily plucked, healthy scalp	Stringy, dull, brittle, dry, thin and sparse, depigmented, can be easily plucked
SKIN (GENERAL)	
Smooth, slightly moist, good color	Rough, dry, scaly, pale, pigmented, irritated, easily bruised, petechiae
FACE AND NECK	
Skin color uniform, smooth, pink, healthy appearance; no enlargement of thyroid gland; lips not chapped or swollen	Scaly, swollen, skin dark over cheeks and under eyes, lumpiness or flakiness of skin around nose and mouth; thyroid enlarged; lips swollen, angular lesions or fissures at corners of mouth
ORAL CAVITY	
Reddish-pink mucous membranes and gums; no swelling or bleeding of gums; tongue healthy pink or deep reddish in appearance, not swollen or smooth, surface papillae present; teeth bright and clean, no cavities, no pain, no discoloration	Gums spongy, bleed easily, inflamed or receding; tongue swollen, scarlet and raw, magenta color, beefy, hyperemic and hypertrophic papillae, atrophic papillae; teeth with unfilled caries, absent teeth, worn surfaces, mottled
EYES	
Bright, clear, shiny, no sores at corners of eyelids, membranes moist and healthy pink color, no prominent blood vessels or mound of tissue (Bitot's spots) on sclera, no fatigue circles beneath	Eye membranes pale, redness of membrane, dryness, signs of infection, redness and fissuring of eyelid corners, dryness of eye membrane, dull appearance of cornea, blue sclerae
EXTREMITIES	
No tenderness, weakness, or swelling; nails firm and pink	Edema, tender calves, tingling, weakness; nails spoon-shaped, brittle
SKELETON	
No malformations	Bowlegs, knock-knees, chest deformity at diaphragm, beaded ribs, prominent scapulas

for hemoglobin and hematocrit must be adjusted during pregnancy. The lower limit of the normal range for hemoglobin during pregnancy is 11 g/dl in the first and third trimesters and 10.5 g/dl in the second trimester (compared with 12 g/dl in the nonpregnant state). The lower limit of the normal range for hematocrit is 33% during the first and third trimesters and 32% in the second trimester (compared with 36% in the nonpregnant state). Cutoff values for anemia are higher in women who smoke or live at high altitudes, because the decreased oxygen-carrying capacity of their RBCs causes them to produce more RBCs than other women (Institute of Medicine, 1992).

A woman's history or physical findings may indicate the need for additional testing, such as a complete blood cell count with a differential to identify megaloblastic or macrocytic anemia and the measurement of levels of specific vitamins or minerals believed to be lacking in the diet. The assessment gives a basis for making appropriate nursing diagnoses, such as the following:

- *Imbalanced nutrition: less than body requirements related to*
  - –inadequate information about nutritional needs and weight gain during pregnancy
  - –misperceptions regarding normal body changes during pregnancy and inappropriate fear of becoming fat
  - –inadequate income or skills in meal planning and preparation
- *Imbalanced nutrition: more than body requirements related to*
  - –excessive intake of energy (kcal) or decrease in activity during pregnancy
  - –use of unnecessary dietary supplements, especially supplements of fat-soluble vitamins, protein (if diet is adequate in protein), and therapeutic amounts of iron (in the absence of iron deficiency anemia)
- *Constipation related to*
  - –decrease in gastrointestinal (GI) motility because of elevated progesterone levels
  - –compression of intestines by enlarging uterus
  - –oral iron supplementation
- *Deficient knowledge related to*
  - –inadequate information regarding nutritional needs during pregnancy

■ Expected Outcomes of Care

An individualized nursing plan of care based on the nursing diagnoses should be developed in collaboration with the woman. For many women with uncomplicated pregnancies, the nurse can serve as the primary source of nutrition education during pregnancy. The registered dietitian, who has specialized training in diet evaluation and planning, nutritional needs during illness, and ethnic and cultural food patterns, as well as in translating nutrient needs into food patterns, frequently serves as a consultant. Pregnant women with serious nutritional problems, those

with intervening illnesses such as diabetes (either preexisting or gestational), and any others requiring in-depth nutrition counseling should be referred to the dietitian. The nurse, dietitian, physician, and nurse-midwife collaborate in helping the woman achieve nutrition-related expected outcomes. Some common nutrition-related outcomes require the woman to take the following actions:

- Achieve an appropriate weight gain during pregnancy—an appropriate goal for weight gain takes into account such factors as the woman's prepregnancy weight, whether she is overweight/obese or underweight, and whether the pregnancy is single or multifetal.
- Consume adequate nutrients from the diet and supplements to meet estimated needs.
- Cope successfully with the nutrition-related discomforts associated with pregnancy, such as pyrosis (heartburn), morning sickness, and constipation.
- Avoid or reduce potentially harmful practices such as smoking, alcohol consumption, and caffeine intake.
- Return to prepregnancy weight (or an appropriate weight for height) within 6 months of giving birth.

■ Plan of Care and Interventions

Nutritional care and teaching generally involve (1) acquainting the woman with the nutritional needs during pregnancy and the characteristics of an adequate diet, if necessary; (2) helping her to individualize her diet so that she achieves an adequate intake while conforming to her personal, cultural, financial, and health circumstances; (3) acquainting her with strategies for coping with the nutrition-related discomforts of pregnancy; (4) helping her use nutrition supplements appropriately; and (5) consulting with and making referrals to other professionals or services as indicated. Two programs that provide nutrition services are the food stamp program and the Special Supplemental Program for Women, Infants, and Children (WIC), which provides vouchers for selected foods to pregnant and lactating women, as well as infants and children at nutritional risk.

■ *Adequate Dietary Intake*

Nutrition teaching can take place in a one-on-one interview or in a group setting. In either case, teaching should emphasize the importance of choosing a varied diet composed of readily available foods (rather than specialized diet supplements). Good nutrition practices (and the avoidance of poor practices such as smoking and alcohol or drug use) are essential content for prenatal classes designed for women in early pregnancy.

MyPyramid (Fig. 15-4) can be used as a guide to making daily food choices during pregnancy and lactation, just as it is during other stages of the life cycle. Additional individualized information and resources for professionals are available from the website www.mypyramid.gov. The importance of consuming adequate amounts from the milk, yogurt, and cheese group must be emphasized, especially for adolescents and women younger than 25 years who are

CD: Resources

MyPyramid
STEPS TO A HEALTHIER YOU
MyPyramid.gov

GRAINS	VEGETABLES	FRUITS	OILS	MILK	MEAT & BEANS
Make half your grains whole	Vary your veggies	Focus on fruits		Get your calcium-rich foods	Go lean with protein

GRAINS	VEGETABLES	FRUITS	MILK	MEAT & BEANS
Eat at least 3 oz. of whole-grain cereals, breads, crackers, rice, or pasta every day 1 oz. is about 1 slice of bread, about 1 cup of breakfast cereal, or ½ cup of cooked rice, cereal, or pasta	Eat more dark-green veggies like broccoli, spinach, and other dark leafy greens Eat more orange vegetables like carrots and sweet potatoes Eat more dry beans and peas like pinto beans, kidney beans, and lentils	Eat a variety of fruit Choose fresh, frozen, canned, or dried fruit Go easy on fruit juices	Go low-fat or fat-free when you choose milk, yogurt, and other milk products If you don't or can't consume milk, choose lactose-free products or other calcium sources such as fortified foods and beverages	Choose low-fat or lean meats and poultry Bake it, broil it, or grill it Vary your protein routine — choose more fish, beans, peas, nuts, and seeds

For a 2,000-calorie diet, you need the amounts below from each food group. To find the amounts that are right for you, go to MyPyramid.gov.

Eat 6 oz. every day	Eat 2½ cups every day	Eat 2 cups every day	Get 3 cups every day; for kids aged 2 to 8, it's 2	Eat 5½ oz. every day

Find your balance between food and physical activity
- Be sure to stay within your daily calorie needs.
- Be physically active for at least 30 minutes most days of the week.
- About 60 minutes a day of physical activity may be needed to prevent weight gain.
- For sustaining weight loss, at least 60 to 90 minutes a day of physical activity may be required.
- Children and teenagers should be physically active for 60 minutes every day, or most days.

Know the limits on fats, sugars, and salt (sodium)
- Make most of your fat sources from fish, nuts, and vegetable oils.
- Limit solid fats like butter, margarine, shortening, and lard, as well as foods that contain these.
- Check the Nutrition Facts label to keep saturated fats, *trans* fats, and sodium low.
- Choose food and beverages low in added sugars. Added sugars contribute calories with few, if any, nutrients.

MyPyramid.gov
STEPS TO A HEALTHIER YOU

U.S. Department of Agriculture
Center for Nutrition Policy and Promotion
April 2005
CNPP-15

USDA

USDA is an equal opportunity provider and employer.

FIG. 15-4   MyPyramid plan for guiding nutrition choices. Each part of the figure is designed to remind consumers to make wise choices. Additional information, along with interactive nutrition and activity analysis, is available at **www.mypyramid.gov**. (Courtesy U.S. Department of Agriculture, Washington, DC.)

still actively adding calcium to their skeletons; adolescents need at least 3 to 4 cups from the milk group daily.

Pregnancy. The pregnant woman must understand what an adequate weight gain during pregnancy means, recognize the reasons for its importance, and be able to evaluate her own gain in terms of the desirable pattern. Many women, particularly those who have worked hard to control their weight before pregnancy, may find it difficult to understand the reason the weight gain goal is so high when a newborn is so small. The nurse can explain that the maternal weight gain consists of increments in the weight of many tissues, not just the growing fetus (see Table 15-3).

Dietary overindulgence, conversely, which may result in excessive fat stores that persist after giving birth, should be discouraged. Nevertheless, it is best not to focus unduly on weight gain, which can result in feelings of stress and guilt in the woman who does not observe the preferred pattern of gain. Teaching regarding weight gain during pregnancy is summarized in the Box 15-6.

Postpartum. The need for a varied diet consisting of a representation of foods from all the food groups continues throughout lactation. As mentioned previously, the lactating woman should be advised to consume at least 1800 kcal daily, and she should receive counseling if her diet appears to be inadequate in any nutrients. Special attention should be given to her zinc, vitamin B_6, and folic acid intake, because the recommendations for these remain higher than those for nonpregnant women (see Table 15-1). Sufficient calcium is needed to allow for both milk formation and maintenance of maternal bone mass. It may be difficult for lactating women to consume enough of these nutrients without careful diet planning.

The woman who does not breastfeed will lose weight gradually if she consumes a balanced diet that provides slightly less than her daily energy expenditure. A reasonable weight loss goal for nonlactating women is 0.5 to 0.9 kg per week; a loss of 1 kg per month is recommended for most lactating women. On average, at 6 weeks postpartum,

women retain 3 to 7 kg of the weight gained during pregnancy, and two thirds of them weigh more than they did before pregnancy (Walker, Sterling, & Timmerman, 2005). Those at risk for obesity and overweight need follow-up to ensure that they know how to make wise food choices, primarily from fruits, vegetables, whole grains, lean meats, and low-fat dairy products. An hour of moderately vigorous physical activity (walking, jogging, swimming, cycling, aerobic dance, etc.) most days of the week will improve the ability of the woman to lose weight gradually and maintain the weight loss.

Daily Food Guide and Menu Planning. The daily food plan (see Table 15-4 and Fig. 15-4) can be used as a guide for educating the woman about nutritional needs during pregnancy and lactation. This food plan is general enough to be used by women from a wide variety of cultures, including women following a vegetarian diet. One of the more helpful teaching strategies is to help the woman plan daily menus that follow the food plan and are affordable, are realistic in terms of preparation time, and are compatible with personal preferences and cultural practices. Information regarding cultural food patterns is provided later in this chapter.

Medical Nutrition Therapy. During pregnancy and lactation, the food plan for women receiving special medical nutrition therapy may have to be modified. The registered dietitian can instruct these women about their diets and assist them in meal planning. However, the nurse should understand the basic principles of the diet and be able to reinforce the teaching.

The nurse should be especially aware of the dietary modifications necessary for women with diabetes mellitus (gestational or preexisting) because this disease is relatively common and because fetal morbidity and mortality occur more often in pregnancies complicated by hyperglycemia or hypoglycemia. Every effort should be made to maintain blood glucose levels in the normal range throughout pregnancy. The food plan of the woman with diabetes usually includes four to six meals and snacks daily, with the daily carbohydrate intake distributed fairly evenly among the meals and snacks. The complex carbohydrates—fibers and starches—should be well represented in the diet. To maintain strict control of the blood glucose level, the pregnant woman with diabetes usually must monitor her own blood glucose daily (American Diabetes Association, 2004). The nurse must therefore teach the woman how to monitor her own blood glucose level, unless she has already been doing this before pregnancy (see Chapter 32).

Counseling About Iron Supplementation. As mentioned earlier, the nutritional supplement most commonly needed during pregnancy is iron; however, a variety of dietary factors can affect the completeness of absorption of an iron supplement. Bran, milk, egg yolks, coffee, tea, or oxalate-containing vegetables such as spinach and Swiss chard consumed at the same time as iron will inhibit iron absorption. Conversely, iron absorption is promoted by a diet rich in vitamin C (e.g., citrus fruits or melons) or

---

box 15-6 Weight Gain During Pregnancy

- Progressive weight gain during pregnancy is essential to ensure normal fetal growth and development and the deposition of maternal stores that promote successful lactation.
- Recommended weight gain during pregnancy is determined largely by prepregnancy weight for height: Normal-weight women, 11.5-16 kg; underweight women, 12.5-18 kg; overweight women, 7-11.5 kg.
- Weight gain should be achieved through a balanced diet of regular foods chosen from all the different food groups (see Table 15-4).
- The pattern of weight gain is important: approximately 0.4 kg per week during the second and third trimesters for normal-weight women; 0.5 kg per week for underweight women; and 0.3 kg per week for overweight women.

"heme iron" (found in meats, fish, and poultry). Iron supplements are best absorbed on an empty stomach, and thus they can be taken between meals with beverages other than milk, tea, or coffee. Some women have gastrointestinal discomfort when they take the supplement on an empty stomach; therefore a good time for them to take the supplement is just before bedtime. Constipation is common with iron supplementation (see below). Iron supplements should be kept away from any children in the household because their ingestion could result in acute iron poisoning and even death. The Teaching for Self-Care box on p. 363 summarizes important points regarding iron supplementation.

▬ Coping with Nutrition-Related Discomforts of Pregnancy

The most common nutrition-related discomforts of pregnancy are nausea and vomiting or "morning sickness," constipation, and pyrosis.

Nausea and Vomiting. Nausea and vomiting are most common during the first trimester. Most of the time the nausea and vomiting cause only mild to moderate problems nutritionally, although they may be a source of substantial discomfort. Antiemetic medications, vitamin B_6, or ginger may be effective in reducing the severity of nausea (Borrelli, Capasso, Aviello, Pittler, & Izzo, 2005; Jewell & Young, 2003; Smith, Crowther, Willson, Hotham, & McMillian, 2004). Whether or not P6 acupressure is effective is not clear (Jewell & Young). In addition, the pregnant woman may find the following suggestions helpful in alleviating the problems:

- Eat dry, starchy foods such as dry toast, melba toast, or crackers on awakening in the morning and at other times when nausea occurs.
- Avoid consuming excessive amounts of fluids early in the day or when nauseated (but compensate by drinking fluids at other times).
- Eat small amounts frequently (every 2 to 3 hours) and avoid large meals that distend the stomach.
- Avoid skipping meals and thus becoming extremely hungry, which may worsen nausea. Have a snack such as cereal with milk, a small sandwich, or yogurt before bedtime.
- Avoid sudden movements. Get out of bed slowly.
- Decrease intake of fried and other fatty foods. Good choices are starches, such as pastas, rice, and breads, and low-fat protein foods (skinless broiled or baked poultry, cooked dried beans or peas, lean meats, and broiled or canned fish).
- Breathe fresh air to help relieve nausea. Keep the environment well ventilated (e.g., open a window), go for a walk outside, or decrease cooking odors by using an exhaust fan.
- Eat foods served at cool temperatures and foods that give off little aroma.
- Avoid brushing teeth immediately after eating.

- Try salty and tart foods (e.g., potato chips and lemonade) during periods of nausea.
- Try herbal teas such as those made with raspberry leaf or peppermint to decrease nausea.

Hyperemesis gravidarum, or severe and persistent vomiting causing weight loss, dehydration, and electrolyte abnormalities, occurs in up to approximately 1% of pregnant women. Intravenous fluid and electrolyte replacement is usually necessary for those women who lose 5% of their body weight. Often this is followed by improved tolerance to the oral intake of food; therapy then consists of the frequent consumption of small amounts of low-fat foods. Enteral tube feeding by means of small-bore nasogastric tubes has been successful in some women. Because the pulmonary aspiration of the feeding is a potential complication if vomiting occurs, antiemetic medications are sometimes administered in conjunction with the tube feedings. Tube feedings may be used to supplement oral intake, with the volume of the tube feeding gradually being decreased as oral intake improves. In some instances, total parenteral nutrition (balanced intravenous feedings of amino acids, carbohydrates, lipids, vitamins, and minerals) has been used to nourish women with hyperemesis gravidarum when their nutritional status has been severely impaired. None of the interventions already mentioned for morning sickness (i.e., antihistamines, vitamin B_6, ginger) have shown any benefit in hyperemesis gravidarum (Jewell & Young, 2003).

Constipation. Improved bowel function generally results from increasing the intake of fiber (e.g., bran and whole grain products, popcorn, and raw or lightly steamed vegetables) in the diet, because fiber helps to retain water within the stool, creating a bulky stool that stimulates intestinal peristalsis. The recommendation for pregnant woman for fiber is 28 g. An adequate fluid intake (at least 50 ml/kg/day) helps to hydrate the fiber and increase the bulk of the stool. Making a habit of participating in physical activity that uses large muscle groups (walking, swimming, cycling) also helps to stimulate bowel motility.

Pyrosis. Pyrosis, or heartburn, is usually caused by the reflux of gastric contents into the esophagus. This condition can be minimized by the consumption of small, frequent meals, rather than two or three larger meals daily. Because fluids further distend the stomach, they should not be consumed with foods. The woman needs to be sure to drink adequate amounts between meals, however. Avoiding spicy foods may help alleviate the problem. Lying down immediately after eating and wearing clothing that is tight across the abdomen can contribute to the problem of reflux.

▬ Cultural Influences and Vegetarian Diets

Consideration of a woman's cultural food preferences enhances communication, providing a greater opportunity for compliance with the agreed-on pattern of intake. Women in most cultures are encouraged to eat a diet typical for them. The nurse needs to be aware of what constitutes a typical diet for different cultural or ethnic groups; however, within one cultural group, several variations may occur. Thus careful exploration of individual preferences is needed. Although ethnic and cultural food beliefs may seem, at first glance, to conflict with the dietary instruction provided by physicians, nurses, and dietitians, it is often possible for the empathic health care provider to identify cultural beliefs that are congruent with the modern understanding of pregnancy and fetal development. Many cultural food practices have some merit, or the culture would not have survived. Food cravings during pregnancy are considered normal by many cultures, but the kinds of cravings often are culturally specific. In most cultures, women crave acceptable foods, such as chicken, fish, and greens among African-Americans. Cultural influences on food intake usually lessen if the woman and her family become more integrated into the dominant culture. Nutritional beliefs and the practices of selected cultural groups are summarized in Table 15-6.

Vegetarian diets represent another cultural effect on nutritional status. Foods basic to almost all vegetarian diets are vegetables, fruits, legumes, nuts, seeds, and grains, but with many variations. Semivegetarians, as opposed to true vegetarians, include fish, poultry, eggs, and dairy products in their diets but do not eat beef or pork. Such a diet can be completely adequate for pregnant women. Another type of vegetarians, ovolactovegetarians, consume eggs and dairy products in addition to plant products. Iron and zinc intake may not be adequate in these women, but such diets can be otherwise nutritionally sound. Strict vegetarians, or vegans, consume only plant products. Because vitamin B_{12} is found only in foods of animal origin, this diet is therefore deficient in vitamin B_{12}. As a result, strict vegetarians should take a supplement or consume vitamin B_{12}-fortified foods (e.g., soy milk) regularly. Vitamin B_{12} deficiency can result in megaloblastic anemia, glossitis (inflamed red tongue), and neurologic deficits in the mother. Infants born to affected mothers are likely to have megaloblastic anemia and to exhibit neurodevelopmental delays. Iron, calcium, zinc, and vitamin B_6 intake also may be low in women on this diet, and some strict vegetarians have excessively low caloric intakes. The protein intake should be assessed especially carefully, because plant proteins tend to be "incomplete," in that they lack one or more amino acids required for growth and the maintenance of body tissues. However, the daily consumption of a variety of different plant proteins—grains, dried beans and peas, nuts, and seeds—helps to provide all of the essential amino acids.

▬ Evaluation

It is essential to set concrete, measurable outcomes; evaluate the woman's progress toward these outcomes regularly; and revise the plan of care if the outcomes are not achieved. In evaluating the adequacy of nutritional intake during pregnancy, the woman's weight gain can be compared with standardized grids showing recommended patterns (see Fig. 15-2). These grids are based on mean data and do not always take into account factors such as ethnic or racial variations. To evaluate the adequacy of the woman's diet, compare her diet with the plan in Table 15-4. Again, it is essential that individual factors affecting nutritional needs and dietary intake be considered. Physical examination and laboratory testing (see section on assessment) can be used as a means of confirming that a woman's nutritional status is adequate. If an inadequate weight gain is found or nutritional deficits appear, it is essential that the nurse reassess the woman and her understanding of her nutritional needs, reinforce teaching as needed, make referrals as indicated, and continue to reevaluate her nutritional status regularly (Plan of Care).

---

community activity

Visit a public health clinic and a private obstetric practice. Assess educational materials and teaching regarding the need for folic acid supplementation prior to and during pregnancy. Are there discrepancies in availability of materials and education efforts in the two settings? What resources in the community can be used to alert teens and other women in the childbearing years to the benefits of folic acid supplementation?

---

key points

- A woman's nutritional status before, during, and after pregnancy contributes, to a significant degree, to her well-being and that of her developing fetus and newborn.
- Many physiologic changes occurring during pregnancy influence the need for additional nutrients and the efficiency with which the body uses them.
- Both the total maternal weight gain and the pattern of weight gain are important determinants of the outcome of pregnancy.
- The appropriateness of the mother's prepregnancy weight for height (BMI) is a major determinant of her recommended weight gain during pregnancy.
- Nutritional risk factors include adolescent pregnancy; bizarre or faddish food habits; abuse of nicotine, alcohol, or drugs; a low or high weight for height; and frequent pregnancies.
- Iron supplementation is usually recommended routinely during pregnancy, even though there is some controversy regarding its beneficial effects on successful outcome of pregnancy. Other supplements may be recommended when nutritional risk factors are present.
- The nurse and client are influenced by cultural and personal values and beliefs during nutrition counseling.
- Pregnancy complications that may be nutrition related include anemia, gestational hypertension, gestational diabetes, and intrauterine growth restriction (IUGR).
- Dietary adaptation can be effective for some of the common discomforts of pregnancy, including nausea and vomiting, constipation, and heartburn.

table 15-6 Popular Foods of Various Cultural and Ethnic Groups and Their Place in MyPyramid

CULTURAL OR ETHNIC GROUP OR EATING PATTERN	FOOD GROUPS				
	GRAINS	VEGETABLE	FRUIT	MILK	MEAT AND BEANS
Mexican	Tortilla Taco shell Posole (corn soup) Rice Postres (pastries)*	*Other vegetables:* Chayote (Mexican squash) Jicama (root vegetable) Nopales (cactus leaves) Tomato Corn	Avocado Mango Papaya Plantano (cooking banana) Zapote (sweet, yellowish fruit)	Queso blanco (white Mexican cheese) Custard (1 cup = 1 cup milk serving) Leche (milk)	Chorizo (sausage)* Chicken, beef, goat, or pork Beans, dry, cooked
African-American soul food (Southern-style cooking)	Biscuit Cornbread Grits, rice, macaroni, or noodles Hominy Crackers Hush puppies	*Dark green:* Collard, kale, mustard, or turnip greens *Orange:* Sweet potatoes *Other:* Okra Snap, pole, lima, and butter beans Turnips Summer squash (yellow or zucchini) Coleslaw	Blackberries Melons Muscadines (grapes) Peaches	Buttermilk	Pork (cured ham and uncured cuts), chicken, beef, fish Peas or beans (black-eyed, crowder, purple-hull, or cream)
Vegetarian	Whole-grain bread Cereal, cooked or ready-to-eat Brown rice Whole-grain pasta Bagel	All	All	Milk and cheese (lactovegetarians) Soy milk, calcium-fortified Soy cheese	Cooked dry beans or peas Tofu (soybean curd) or tempeh (fermented soy) Nuts or seeds Peanut butter Egg (ovovegetarians)
Italian	Bread sticks, breads Gnocchi (dumplings) Polenta (corn meal mush) Risotto (creamy rice dish) Pastas	*Dark green:* Spinach *Other:* Artichoke Eggplant Mushrooms Marinara sauce	Berries Figs Pomegranate	Cheeses (mozzarella, Parmesan, Romano, ricotta, etc.) Gelato (Italian ice cream)	Veal or beef Fish Sausage* Luncheon meats* Lentils Squid Almonds, pistachios
Chinese	Rice or millet Rice vermicelli (thin rice pasta) Cellophane noodles (bean thread) Steamed rolls Rice congee (soup) Rice sticks	*Other:* Pea pods Yard-long beans Baby corn Bamboo shoots Straw mushrooms Eggplant Bitter melon	Guava Lychee Persimmon Pummelo Kumquat Star fruit	Soy milk	Pork, fish, chicken Shrimp, crab, lobster Tofu or tempeh

Cultural group	Breads/Grains	Vegetables	Fruits	Milk products	Protein/Meat
Indian (south Asia)	Breads: roti (chapati), naan, paratha, batura, puris, dosa, idli Rice or rice pilau Pooha, upma, sabudana	*Dark green:* Saag (mixed greens and potatoes) Spinach *Other:* Green peppers Cabbage Eggplant Green beans Methi (fenugreek leaves) Cucumbers Chutney or vegetable pickles	Mango Dates Raisins Melons Figs Fruit juices and nectars	Yogurt	Dal (lentils, mung beans, other dried beans) Beef, chicken (some are vegetarian)
Native American†	Bread Fry bread Wild rice or oats Popcorn Tortilla Mush (cooked cereal)	*Orange:* Winter squash (hard outer shell) *Starchy:* Potato Corn *Other:* Rhubarb	Berries Cherries Plums Apples Peaches		Wild game (deer, rabbit, elk, beaver) Lamb Salmon and other fish Clams, mussels Crab Duck or quail
Middle Eastern	Rice or bulgur (cracked wheat) Couscous Bread Pita	*Yellow:* Pumpkin or winter squash (butternut) *Other:* Peppers Tomatoes Grape leaves Cucumbers Fava beans Eggplant	Apricots Grapes Melons Dried fruits: dates, raisins, apricots	Yogurt	Lamb, goat, fish Almonds Pistachio nuts Dried beans and peas, lentils Eggs

*High-fat; use sparingly.
†Varies widely depending on tribal grouping and locale.

CD: Plan of Care: Nutrition During Pregnancy

NURSING DIAGNOSIS Deficient knowledge related to nutritional requirements during pregnancy

Expected Outcomes *The woman will describe nutritional requirements and exhibit evidence of incorporating requirements into diet.*

Nursing Interventions/*Rationales*

- Review basic nutritional requirements for a healthy diet by using recommended dietary guidelines and the food guide pyramid *to provide knowledge baseline for discussion.*
- Discuss increased nutrient needs (calories, protein, minerals, vitamins) that occur as a result of being pregnant *to increase knowledge needed for altered dietary requirements.*
- Discuss the relation between weight gain and fetal growth *to reinforce interdependence of fetus and mother.*
- Calculate the appropriate total weight gain range during pregnancy using the woman's body mass index as a guide, and discuss recommended rates of weight gain during the various trimesters of pregnancy *to provide concrete measures of dietary success.*
- Review food preferences, cultural eating patterns or beliefs, and prepregnancy eating patterns *to enhance integration of new dietary needs.*
- Discuss how to fit nutritional needs into usual dietary patterns and how to alter any identified nutritional deficits or excesses *to increase chances of success with dietary alterations.*
- Discuss food aversions or cravings that may occur during pregnancy and strategies to deal with these if they are detrimental to fetus (e.g., pica) *to ensure well-being of fetus.*
- Have woman keep a food diary delineating eating habits, dietary alterations, aversions, and cravings *to track eating habits and potential problem areas.*

NURSING DIAGNOSIS Imbalanced nutrition: more than body requirements related to excessive intake and/or inadequate activity levels

Expected Outcome *The woman's weekly weight gain will be reduced to the appropriate rate using her body mass index (BMI) and recommended weight gain ranges as guidelines.*

Nursing Interventions/*Rationales*

- Review recent diet history (including food cravings) using a food diary, 24-hour recall, or food frequency approach *to ascertain food excesses contributing to excess weight gain.*
- Review normal activity and exercise routines *to determine level of energy expenditure;* discuss eating patterns and reasons that lead to increased food intake (e.g., cultural beliefs or myths, increased stress, boredom) *to identify habits that contribute to excess weight gain.*
- Review optimal weight gain guidelines and their rationale *to ensure that woman is knowledgeable about healthful weight gain rates.*
- Set target weight gains for the remaining weeks of the pregnancy *to establish set goals.*
- Discuss with the woman what changes can be made in diet, activity, and lifestyle *to enhance chances of meeting weight gain goals and dietary needs.* (Weight-reduction diets should be avoided, because they may deprive mother and fetus of needed nutrients and lead to ketonemia.)

NURSING DIAGNOSIS Imbalanced nutrition: less than body requirements related to inadequate intake of needed nutrients

Expected Outcome *The woman's weekly weight gain will be increased to the appropriate rate using her BMI and recommended weight gain ranges as guidelines.*

Nursing Interventions/*Rationales*

- Review recent diet history (including food aversions) using a food diary, 24-hour recall, or food frequency approach *to ascertain dietary inadequacies contributing to lack of sufficient weight gain.*
- Review normal activity and exercise routines *to determine level of energy expenditure;* discuss eating patterns and reasons that lead to decreased food intake (e.g., morning sickness, pica, fear of becoming fat, stress, boredom) *to identify habits that contribute to inadequate weight gain.*
- Review optimal weight gain guidelines and their rationale *to ensure that woman is knowledgeable about healthful weight gain rates.*
- Set target weight gains for the remaining weeks of the pregnancy *to establish set goals.*
- Review increased nutrient needs (calories, protein, minerals, vitamins) that occur as a result of being pregnant *to ensure woman is knowledgeable about altered dietary requirements.*
- Review relation between weight gain and fetal growth *to reinforce that adequate weight gain is needed to promote fetal well-being.*
- Discuss with woman what changes can be made in diet, activity, and lifestyle *to enhance chances of meeting set weight gain goals and nutrient needs of mother and fetus.*
- If woman has fear of being fat, if symptoms of an eating disorder are evident, or if problems in adjusting to a changing body image surface, refer woman to the appropriate mental health professional for evaluation, *because intensive treatment and follow-up may be required to ensure fetal health.*

NURSING DIAGNOSIS Nausea related to physiologic alterations of the first trimester of pregnancy

Expected Outcome *Nausea will not be so severe that it interferes with adequate nutrient intake or substantially reduces quality of life.*

Nursing Interventions/*Rationales*

- Assess state of hydration to ensure that the woman does not have deficient fluid volume and assess pattern of weight gain during pregnancy *to ensure that nausea is not causing inadequate energy intake.*
- Review the nausea history (i.e., frequency of episodes of nausea, the likelihood of nausea progressing to vomiting, factors precipitating or associated with nausea, and any relief measures that the woman has tried) *to determine the severity of the problem and to begin to identify effective and ineffective measures for coping with nausea.*
- Review measures for prevention or relief of morning sickness *to ensure that the woman is knowledgeable about measures that are often effective in alleviating morning sickness.*
- Discuss with the woman what relief measures she will try *to determine whether she understands how to implement the measures.*

REFERENCES

Allen, L. (2005). Multiple micronutrients in pregnancy and lactation: An overview. *American Journal of Clinical Nutrition, 81*(5), 1206S-1212S.

American College of Obstetricians and Gynecologists (ACOG). (2002). Exercise during pregnancy and the postpartum period. ACOG committee opinion No. 267. *Obstetrics and Gynecology, 99*(1), 171-173.

American Diabetes Association. (2004). Gestational diabetes mellitus. *Diabetes Care, 27*(Suppl 1), S88-S91.

Borrelli, F., Capasso, R., Aviello, G., Pittler, M., & Izzo, A. (2005). Effectiveness and safety of ginger in the treatment of pregnancy-induced nausea and vomiting. *Obstetrics and Gynecology, 105*(4), 849-856.

California Diabetes & Pregnancy Program. (rev 2004). Sweet success guidelines for care—2002. Accessed www.regionalperinatalprogram. org, July 20, 2005.

Centers for Disease Control and Prevention. (2005, April 11). Pediatric and pregnancy nutrition surveillance tables. Accessed http://www. cdc.gov/pednss/pnss_tables/tables_health_indicators.htm, July 18, 2005.

Corbett, R., Ryan, C., & Weinrich, S. (2003). Pica in pregnancy: Does it affect pregnancy outcomes? *MCN American Journal of Maternal/ Child Nursing, 28*(3), 183-189.

Cornel, M., Smit, D., & de Jong-van den Berg, L. (2005). Folic acid— the scientific debate as a base for public health policy. *Reproductive Toxicology, 20*(3), 411-415.

Hoyert, D., Mathews, T., Menacker, F., Strobino, D., & Guyer, B. (2006). Annual summary of vital statistics: 2004. *Pediatrics, 117*(1), 168-183.

Institute of Medicine. (1992). *Nutrition during pregnancy and lactation: An implementation guide.* Washington, DC: National Academies Press.

Institute of Medicine. (2003). *Dietary reference intakes: Applications in dietary planning.* Washington, DC: National Academies Press.

Institute of Medicine. (2004). *Proposed criteria for selecting the WIC food packages: A preliminary report of the committee to review the WIC food packages.* Washington, DC: National Academies Press.

Jewell, D., & Young, G. (2003). Interventions for nausea and vomiting in early pregnancy. *The Cochrane Database of Systematic Reviews,* 2006, Issue 3, Chichester, UK: John Wiley & Sons.

Kabiru, W., & Raynor, B. (2004). Obstetric outcomes associated with increase in BMI category during pregnancy. *American Journal of Obstetrics and Gynecology, 191*(3), 928-932.

Klitzman, S., Sharma, A., Nicaj, L., Vitkevich, R., & Leighton, J. (2002). Lead poisoning among pregnant women in New York City: Risk factors and screening practices. *Journal of Urban Health, 79*(2), 225-237.

Linne, Y. (2004). Effects of obesity on women's reproduction and complications during pregnancy. *Obesity Review, 5*(3), 137-143.

Luke, B. (2005). Nutrition in multiple gestations. *Clinics in Perinatology, 32*(2), 403-429, vii.

National Toxicology Program Center for the Evaluation of Risks to Human Reproduction. (2005). *Caffeine.* Accessed http://cerhr. niehs.nih.gov/common/caffeine.html, September 12, 2006.

Scholl, T. (2005). Iron status during pregnancy: Setting the stage for mother and infant. *American Journal of Clinical Nutrition, 81*(5), 1218S-1222S.

Shannon, M. (2003). Severe lead poisoning in pregnancy. *Ambulatory Pediatrics, 3*(1), 37-39.

Smith, C., Crowther, C., Willson, K., Hotham, N., & McMillian, V. (2004). A randomized controlled trial of ginger to treat nausea and vomiting in pregnancy. *Obstetrics and Gynecology, 103*(4), 639-645.

Ukaonu, C., Hill, D., & Christensen, F. (2003). Hypokalemic myopathy in pregnancy caused by clay ingestion. *Obstetrics and Gynecology, 102*(5 Pt 2), 1169-1171.

Vahratian, A., Siega-Riz, A., Savitz, D., & Zhang, J. (2005). Maternal pre-pregnancy overweight and obesity and the risk of cesarean delivery in nulliparous women. *Annals of Epidemiology, 15*(7), 467-474.

Walker, L., Sterling, B., & Timmerman, G. (2005). Retention of pregnancy-related weight in the early postpartum period: Implications for women's health services. *Journal of Obstetric, Gynecologic, and Neonatal Nursing, 34*(4), 418-427.

Nursing Care During Pregnancy

learning objectives

- Describe the process of confirming pregnancy and estimating the date of birth.
- Summarize the physical, psychosocial, and behavioral changes that usually occur as the mother and other family members adapt to pregnancy.
- Discuss the benefits of prenatal care and problems of accessibility for some women.
- Outline the patterns of health care used to assess maternal and fetal health status at the initial and follow-up visits during pregnancy.

- Identify the typical nursing assessments, diagnoses, interventions, and methods of evaluation in providing care for the pregnant woman.
- Discuss education needed by pregnant women to understand physical discomforts related to pregnancy and to recognize signs and symptoms of potential complications.
- Examine the impact of culture, age, parity, and number of fetuses on the response of the family to the pregnancy and on the prenatal care provided.

electronic resources

Additional information related to the content in Chapter 16 can be found on

the companion website at 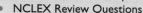 *evolve*
http://evolve.elsevier.com/Lowdermilk/MWHC/
- NCLEX Review Questions
- Case Study: First Trimester
- Case Study: Second Trimester
- Case Study: Third Trimester
- WebLinks

or on the interactive companion CD
- NCLEX Review Questions
- Assessment Video: Chest wall, breast, abdomen/fundal height, fetal lie, presentation, position, fetal heart rate
- Case Study: First Trimester
- Case Study: Second Trimester
- Case Study: Third Trimester
- Critical Thinking Exercise: Teenage Pregnancy
- Critical Thinking Exercise: Discomforts of Pregnancy
- Plan of Care: Adolescent Pregnancy
- Plan of Care: Discomforts of Pregnancy and Warning Signs

THE prenatal period is a time of physical and psychologic preparation for birth and parenthood. Becoming a parent is considered one of the maturational milestones of adult life. It is a time of intense learning for both parents and those close to them. The prenatal period provides a unique opportunity for nurses and other members of the health care team to influence family health. During this period, essentially healthy women seek regular care and guidance. The nurse's health promotion interventions can affect the well-being of the woman, her unborn child, and the rest of her family for many years.

Regular prenatal visits, ideally beginning soon after the first missed menstrual period, offer opportunities to ensure the health of the expectant mother and her infant. Prenatal health care permits diagnosis and treatment of maternal disorders that may have preexisted or may develop during the pregnancy. Care is designed to monitor the growth and development of the fetus and to identify abnormalities that may interfere with the course of normal labor. Education and support for self-care and parenting can be provided.

Pregnancy spans 9 months, but health care providers, in contrast to using the familiar monthly calendar to ascertain fetal age or discuss the pregnancy, use the concept of lunar months, which last 28 days, or 4 weeks. Normal pregnancy, then, lasts about 10 lunar months, which is the same as 40 weeks or 280 days. Health care providers also refer to early, middle, and late pregnancy as trimesters. The first trimester lasts from weeks 1 through 13; the second, from weeks 14 through 26; and the third, from weeks 27 through 40. A pregnancy is considered to be at term if it advances to 38 to 40 weeks. The focus of this chapter is on meeting the health needs of the expectant family over the course of pregnancy, which is known as the prenatal period.

▬ DIAGNOSIS OF PREGNANCY

Women may suspect pregnancy when they miss a menstrual period. Many women come to the first prenatal visit after a positive home pregnancy test; however, the clinical diagnosis of pregnancy before the second missed period may be difficult in some women. Physical variations, obesity, or tumors, for example, may confound even the experienced examiner. Accuracy is important, however, because emotional, social, medical, or legal consequences of an inaccurate diagnosis, either positive or negative, can be extremely serious. A correct date for the *last (normal) menstrual period (LMP or LNMP)* and for the date of intercourse and a basal body temperature (BBT) record may be of great value in the accurate diagnosis of pregnancy (see Chapter 9).

Signs and Symptoms

Great variability is possible in the subjective and objective symptoms of pregnancy; therefore the diagnosis of pregnancy may be uncertain for a time. Many of the indicators of pregnancy are clinically useful in the diagnosis of pregnancy, and they are classified as presumptive, probable, or positive.

Presumptive indicators of pregnancy include subjective symptoms and objective signs. Subjective symptoms are reported by the woman and may include amenorrhea, nausea and vomiting (morning sickness), breast tenderness, urinary frequency, and fatigue. Quickening, the mother's first perception of fetal movement, may be noted between weeks 16 and 20. Objective signs that may be validated by the examiner include elevation of BBT, breast and abdominal enlargement, and changes in the uterus and vagina. Other visible changes occur in the skin, such as striae gravidarum, deeper pigmentation of the areola, chloasma (mask of pregnancy), and linea nigra (pigmented line on the abdomen) (see Table 14-2).

The presumptive indicators of pregnancy can be caused by conditions other than gestation. For example, amenorrhea may be caused by illness or excessive exercise; fatigue may signify anemia or infection; a tumor may cause enlargement of the abdomen; and nausea or vomiting may be caused by a gastrointestinal (GI) upset or food allergy. Therefore these signs alone are not reliable for diagnosis. Probable indicators of pregnancy are detected by an examiner and are related mainly to physical changes in the uterus. Objective signs include uterine enlargement, Braxton Hicks contractions, uterine souffle, ballottement, and a positive pregnancy test. When combined with presumptive signs and symptoms, they strongly suggest pregnancy, but they are not conclusive. For example, uterine enlargement may be due to the presence of tumors; unusual bowel sounds may be misinterpreted; or positive results on a pregnancy test may be due to a malignant tumor that secretes the hormone human chorionic gonadotropin (hCG).

---

box 16-1	**Use of Nägele's Rule**

July 10, 2006, is the first day of the last menstrual period.

	7	10	2006
	−3	+7	
EDB =	4	17	2007

The estimated date of birth (EDB) is April 17, 2007.

The positive indicators of pregnancy are directly attributed to the fetus and include the presence of a fetal heartbeat distinct from that of the mother, fetal movement felt by someone other than the mother, and visualization of the fetus with a technique such as ultrasound examination. The fetal heartbeat can be detected as early as 6 weeks of gestation with Doppler techniques, but ultrasound examination becomes 100% reliable only at 8 to 9 weeks of gestation. However, the fetal heartbeat usually cannot be detected with a fetoscope until weeks 16 to 20. An examiner may palpate fetal movements with increasing reliability after 20 to 24 weeks.

Estimating Date of Birth

After the diagnosis of pregnancy, the woman's first question usually concerns when she will give birth. This date has traditionally been termed the *estimated date of confinement (EDC)*, although *estimated date of delivery (EDD)* also has been used (Katz, Farmer, Tufariello, & Carpenter, 2001). To promote a more positive perception of both pregnancy and birth, however, the term *estimated date of birth (EDB)* is suggested. Because the precise date of conception generally is unknown, several formulas have been suggested for calculating the EDB. None of these guides is infallible, but Nägele's rule is reasonably accurate and is usually used.

Nägele's rule is as follows: After determining the first day of the LMP, subtract 3 calendar months, add 7 days and 1 year; or alternatively, add 7 days to the LMP and count forward 9 calendar months. Box 16-1 demonstrates use of Nägele's rule.

Nägele's rule assumes that the woman has a 28-day menstrual cycle and that pregnancy commenced on the fourteenth day. An adjustment is in order if the woman's cycle is longer or shorter than 28 days. With the use of Nägele's rule, only about 5% of pregnant women give birth spontaneously on the EDB (Katz et al., 2001). Most women give birth during the period extending from 7 days before to 7 days after the EDB.

▬ ADAPTATION TO PREGNANCY

Pregnancy affects all family members, and each family member must adapt to the pregnancy and interpret its meaning in light of his or her own needs. This process of family adaptation to pregnancy takes place within a cultural environment influenced by societal trends. Dramatic changes have occurred in Western society in recent years, and the nurse must be prepared to support not only traditional families in the childbirth experience but also single-parent families, reconstituted families, dual-career families, and alternative families.

Much of the investigation of family dynamics in pregnancy by scholars in the United States and Canada has been done with Caucasian, middle-class nuclear families, and findings may not apply to families who do not fit the traditional North American model. Adaptation of terms is appropriate to avoid embarrassment to the nurse and offense to the family. Additional research is needed on a variety of families to determine if study findings generated in traditional families are applicable to others.

Maternal Adaptation

Women of all ages use the months of pregnancy to adapt to the maternal role, a complex process of social and cognitive learning. Early in pregnancy, nothing seems to be happening, and a woman may spend much time sleeping secondary to the increased fatigue of this stage. With the perception of fetal movement in the second trimester, the woman turns her attention inward to her pregnancy and to relationships with her mother and other women who have been or who are pregnant.

Pregnancy is a maturational milestone that can be stressful but also rewarding as the woman prepares for a new level of caring and responsibility. Her self-concept changes in readiness for parenthood as she prepares for her new role. She moves gradually from being self-contained and independent to being committed to a lifelong concern for another human being. This growth requires mastery of certain developmental tasks: accepting the pregnancy, identifying with the role of mother, reordering the relationships between herself and her mother and between herself and her partner, establishing a relationship with the unborn child, and preparing for the birth experience. The partner's emotional support is an important factor in the successful accomplishment of these developmental tasks. Single women with limited support may have difficulty making this adaptation.

Accepting the Pregnancy

The first step in adapting to the maternal role is accepting the idea of pregnancy and assimilating the pregnant state into the woman's way of life. Mercer (1995) described this process as *cognitive restructuring* and credited Reva Rubin (1984) as the nurse theorist who pioneered our understanding of maternal role attainment. The degree of acceptance is reflected in the woman's emotional responses. Many women are dismayed initially at finding themselves pregnant, especially if the pregnancy is unintended. Eventual acceptance of pregnancy parallels the growing acceptance of the reality of a child. Nonacceptance of the pregnancy, however, should not be equated with rejection of the child, for a woman may dislike being pregnant but feel love for the child to be born.

Women who are happy and pleased about their pregnancy often view it as biologic fulfillment and part of their life plan. They have high self-esteem and tend to be confident about outcomes for themselves, their babies, and other family members. Despite a general feeling of well-being, many women are surprised to experience emotional lability, that is, rapid and unpredictable changes in mood. These swings in emotions and increased sensitivity to others are disconcerting to the expectant mother and those around her. Increased irritability, explosions of tears and anger, and feelings of great joy and cheerfulness alternate, apparently with little or no provocation.

Profound hormonal changes that are part of the maternal response to pregnancy may be responsible for mood changes. Other reasons such as concerns about finances and changed lifestyle contribute to this seemingly erratic behavior.

Pregnant women are affected emotionally by changes that occur in the physical contours and functions of their bodies. During the first trimester, body shape changes little, but by the second trimester, obvious bulging of the abdomen, thickening of the waist, and enlargement of the breasts proclaim the state of pregnancy. A feeling develops of an overall increase in the size of her body and occupying more space.

The woman's attitude about her body is influenced by her values, weight before pregnancy and ethnicity. This attitude often changes as pregnancy progresses and may fluctuate throughout pregnancy (Johnson, Burrows, & Williamson, 2004; Schmied & Lupton, 2001). A positive body image usually is expressed during the first trimester. As the pregnancy advances, however, the feelings may become more negative. For most women, the feeling of liking or not liking their bodies in the pregnant state is temporary and does not cause permanent changes in their self-perceptions (Schmied & Lupton).

Most women have ambivalent feelings during pregnancy whether the pregnancy was intended or not. Ambivalence—having conflicting feelings simultaneously—is considered a normal response for people preparing for a new role. During pregnancy, women may, for example, feel great pleasure that they are fulfilling a lifelong dream, but they also may feel great regret that life as they now know it is ending.

Even women who are pleased to be pregnant may experience feelings of hostility toward the pregnancy or unborn child from time to time. Such incidents as a partner's chance remark about the attractiveness of a slim, nonpregnant woman or news of a colleague's promotion can give rise to ambivalent feelings. Body sensations, feelings of dependence, or the realization of the responsibilities of child care also can generate such feelings.

Intense feelings of ambivalence that persist through the third trimester may indicate an unresolved conflict with the motherhood role (Mercer, 1995). After the birth of a healthy child, memories of these ambivalent feelings usually are dismissed. If the child is born with a defect, however, a woman may look back at the times when she did not want the pregnancy and feel intensely guilty. She may believe that her ambivalence caused the birth defect. She then will need assurance that her feelings were not responsible for the problem.

Identifying with the Mother Role

The process of identifying with the mother role begins early in each woman's life when she is being mothered as a child. Her social group's perception of what constitutes the feminine role can subsequently influence her toward choosing between motherhood or a career, being married or single, being independent rather than interdependent, or being able to manage multiple roles. Practice roles, such as playing with dolls, babysitting, and taking care of siblings, may increase her understanding of what being a mother entails.

Many women have always wanted a baby, liked children, and looked forward to motherhood. Their high motivation to become a parent promotes acceptance of pregnancy and eventual prenatal and parental adaptation. Other women apparently have not considered in any detail what motherhood means to them. During pregnancy, conflicts such as not wanting the pregnancy and child-related or career-related decisions must be resolved.

Reordering Personal Relationships

Close relationships of the pregnant woman undergo change during pregnancy as she prepares emotionally for the new role of mother. As family members learn their new roles, periods of tension and conflict may occur. An understanding of the typical patterns of adjustment can help the nurse to reassure the pregnant woman and explore issues related to social support. Promoting effective communication patterns between the expectant mother and her own mother and between the expectant mother and her partner are common nursing interventions provided during the prenatal visits.

The woman's own relationship with her mother is significant in adaptation to pregnancy and motherhood. Important components in the pregnant woman's relationship with her mother are the mother's availability (past and present), her reactions to the daughter's pregnancy, respect for her daughter's autonomy, and the willingness to reminisce (Mercer, 1995).

The mother's reaction to the daughter's pregnancy signifies her acceptance of the grandchild and of her daughter. If the mother is supportive, the daughter has an opportunity to discuss pregnancy and labor and her feelings of joy or ambivalence with a knowledgeable and accepting woman (Fig. 16-1). Reminiscing about the pregnant woman's early childhood and sharing the prospective grandmother's account of her childbirth experience help the daughter to anticipate and prepare for labor and birth.

Although the woman's relationship with her mother is significant in considering her adaptation in pregnancy, the most important person to the pregnant woman is usually the father of her child. The support and concern of a partner during pregnancy have positive consequences for a woman's desire to carry out the pregnancy (Kroelinger & Oths, 2000), and she has fewer emotional and physical symptoms, fewer labor and childbirth complications, and an easier postpartum adjustment. Women express two major needs within this relationship during pregnancy: feeling loved and valued and having the child accepted by the partner.

FIG. 16-1 A pregnant woman and her mother enjoying their walk together. (Courtesy Michael S. Clement, MD, Mesa, AZ.)

The marital or committed relationship is not static but evolves over time. The addition of a child changes forever the nature of the bond between partners. This may be a time when couples grow closer, and the pregnancy has a maturing effect on the partners' relationship as they assume new roles and discover new aspects of one another. Partners who trust and support each other are able to share mutual-dependency needs (Mercer, 1995).

Sexual expression during pregnancy is highly individual. The sexual relationship is affected by physical, emotional, and interactional factors, including myths about sex during pregnancy, sexual dysfunction, and physical changes in the woman. Myths about body functions and fantasies about the influence of the fetus as a third party in lovemaking are commonly expressed. An individual may also inaccurately attribute anomalies, mental retardation, and other injuries to the fetus and mother to sexual relations during pregnancy. Some couples fear that the woman's genitals will be drastically changed by the birth process. Couples may not express their concerns to the health care provider because of embarrassment or because they do not want to appear foolish.

As pregnancy progresses, changes in body shape, body image, and levels of discomfort influence both partners' desire for sexual expression. During the first trimester, the woman's sexual desire may decrease, especially if she has breast tenderness, nausea, fatigue, or sleepiness. As she progresses into the second trimester, however, her sense of well-being combined with the increased pelvic congestion that occurs at this time may increase her desire for sexual release. In the third trimester, somatic complaints and physical bulkiness may increase her physical discomfort and again diminish her interest in sex. As a woman's pregnancy progresses, her enlarging gravid abdomen may limit the use of the man-on-top position for intercourse. Therefore other positions (e.g., side to side or the woman on top) may allow intercourse and minimize pressure on the woman's abdomen (Westheimer & Lopater, 2005).

Partners need to feel free to discuss their sexual responses during pregnancy with each other and with their health care provider. Their sensitivity to each other and willingness to share concerns can strengthen their sexual relationship. Partners who do not understand the rapid physiologic and emotional changes of pregnancy can become confused by the other's behavior. By talking to each other about the changes they are experiencing, couples can define problems and then offer the needed support. Nurses can facilitate communication between partners by talking to expectant couples about possible changes in feelings and behaviors they may experience as pregnancy progresses.

Establishing a Relationship with the Fetus

Emotional attachment—feelings of being tied by affection or love—begins during the prenatal period as women use fantasizing and daydreaming to prepare themselves for motherhood (Rubin, 1975). They think of themselves as mothers and imagine maternal qualities they would like to possess. Expectant parents desire to be warm, loving, and close to their child. They try to anticipate changes that the child will bring in their lives and wonder how they will react to noise, disorder, reduced freedom, and caregiving activities. The mother-child relationship progresses through pregnancy as a developmental process that unfolds in three phases.

In phase 1 the woman accepts the biologic fact of pregnancy. She needs to be able to state, "I am pregnant" and incorporate the idea of a child into her body and self-image. The woman's thoughts center around herself and the reality of her pregnancy. The child is viewed as part of herself, not a separate and unique person.

In phase 2 the woman accepts the growing fetus as distinct from herself, usually accomplished by the fifth month. She can now say, "I am going to have a baby." This differentiation of the child from the woman's self permits the beginning of the mother-child relationship that involves not only caring but also responsibility. Attachment of a mother to her child is enhanced by experiencing a planned pregnancy, and it increases when ultrasound examination and quickening confirm the reality of the fetus.

With acceptance of the reality of the child (hearing the heart beat and feeling the child move) and an overall feeling of well-being, the woman enters a quiet period and becomes more introspective. A fantasy child becomes precious to the woman. As the woman seems to withdraw and to concentrate her interest on the unborn child, her partner sometimes feels left out. If there are children in the family, they may become more demanding in their efforts to redirect the mother's attention to themselves.

During phase 3 of the attachment process, the woman prepares realistically for the birth and parenting of the child. She expresses the thought, "I am going to be a mother"

and defines the nature and characteristics of the child. She may, for example, speculate about the child's sex (if she has not had an ultrasound that confirms the sex) and personality traits based on patterns of fetal activity.

Although the mother alone experiences the child within, both parents and siblings believe the unborn child responds in a very individualized, personal manner. Family members may interact a great deal with the unborn child by talking to the fetus and stroking the mother's abdomen, especially when the fetus shifts position. The fetus may have a nickname used by family members.

Preparing for Childbirth

Many women actively prepare for birth by reading books, viewing films, attending parenting classes, and talking to other women. They seek the best caregiver possible for advice, monitoring, and caring. The multipara has her own history of labor and birth, which influences her approach to preparation for this childbirth experience.

Anxiety can arise from concern about a safe passage for herself and her child during the birth process (Mercer, 1995; Rubin, 1975). This concern may not be expressed overtly, but cues are given as the nurse listens to plans women make for care of the new baby and other children in case "anything should happen." These feelings persist despite statistical evidence about the safe outcome of pregnancy for mothers and their infants. Many women fear the pain of childbirth or mutilation because they do not understand anatomy and the birth process. Education by the nurse can alleviate many of these fears. Women also express concern over what behaviors are appropriate during the birth process and whether caregivers will accept them

---

CRITICAL THINKING EXERCISE

Deciding About a Home Birth

Millie, 28 years old and gravida 1, para 0, is interested in having a home birth. She is currently 14 weeks pregnant, and her pregnancy is progressing normally. According to an ultrasound examination she has one fetus, which is of appropriate size for gestational age with no detectable anomalies. She asks a nurse in the obstetric clinic how to find a midwife who will attend a home birth.

1. Evidence—Is there sufficient evidence to draw conclusions about the safety of a home birth for Millie?
2. Assumptions—Describe the underlying assumptions for each of the following issues:
   a. Assessments that are necessary to identify whether it is feasible and safe for Millie to have a home birth
   b. Supports necessary for a home birth
   c. How to identify providers who are willing to attend a home birth
   d. Ethics of the nurse assisting Millie to find a midwife who will attend a home birth
3. What implications and priorities for nursing care can be made at this time?
4. Does the evidence objectively support your conclusion?
5. Are there alternative perspectives to your conclusion?

and their actions. The best preparation for childbirth is "a healthy sense of the realistic—an awareness of work, pain, and risk balanced by a sense of excitement and expectation of the final reward" (Lederman, 1996). Childbirth education is further discussed in Chapter 17.

Toward the end of the third trimester, breathing is difficult, and fetal movements become vigorous enough to disturb the woman's sleep. Backaches, frequency and urgency of urination, constipation, and varicose veins can become troublesome. The bulkiness and awkwardness of her body interfere with the woman's ability to care for other children, perform routine work-related duties, and assume a comfortable position for sleep and rest. By this time, most women become impatient for labor to begin, whether the birth is anticipated with joy, dread, or a mixture of both. A strong desire to see the end of pregnancy, to be over and done with it, makes women at this stage ready to move on to childbirth.

Paternal Adaptation

The father's beliefs and feelings about the ideal mother and father and his cultural expectation of appropriate behavior during pregnancy affect his response to his partner's need for him. One man may engage in nurturing behavior. Another may feel lonely and alienated as the woman becomes physically and emotionally engrossed in the unborn child. He may seek friends and relationships outside the home or become interested in a new hobby or involved with his work. Some men view pregnancy as proof of their masculinity and their dominant role. To others, pregnancy has no meaning in terms of responsibility to either mother or child. However, for most men, pregnancy can be a time of preparation for the parental role with intense learning.

Accepting the Pregnancy

The ways fathers adjust to the parental role has been the subject of considerable research. In older societies the man enacted the ritual couvade; that is, he behaved in specific ways and respected taboos associated with pregnancy and giving birth so the man's new status was recognized and endorsed. Today, some men experience pregnancy-like symptoms, such as nausea, weight gain, and other physical symptoms. This phenomenon is known as the couvade syndrome. Changing cultural and professional attitudes in the past 30 years in North America have encouraged fathers' participation in the birth experience.

A man's readiness for fatherhood may be reflected in the way he views the couple's relative financial security and the stability of the couple relationship and in the way he deals with the realization that the upcoming birth marks the end of the childless period. Many men express concern for the family's economic security. Today, most women are employed outside the home but have a period of unemployment for childbearing and child care. The length of unemployment is determined by the couple's economic status, the policies of the woman's employer, and the couple's value system. Some men compensate for anticipated needs by keeping their current jobs even though they had planned a change, by working overtime, or by taking on extra work. Some men acquire new or additional insurance at this time.

The man's emotional responses to becoming a father, his concerns, and his informational needs change during the course of pregnancy. Phases of the developmental pattern become apparent. May (1982) described three phases characterizing the developmental tasks experienced by the expectant father:

- The *announcement phase* may last from a few hours to a few weeks. The developmental task is to accept the biologic fact of pregnancy. Men react to the confirmation of pregnancy with joy or dismay, depending on whether the pregnancy is desired or unplanned or unwanted. Ambivalence in the early stages of pregnancy is common.

  If pregnancy is unplanned or unwanted, some men find the alterations in life plans and lifestyles difficult to accept. Some men engage in extramarital affairs for the first time during their partner's pregnancy. Others batter their wives for the first time or escalate the frequency of battering episodes (Martin, Mackie, Kupper, Buescher, & Moracco, 2001). Chapter 6 provides information about violence against women and offers guidance on assessment and intervention.

- The second phase, the *moratorium phase*, is the period when he adjusts to the reality of pregnancy. The developmental task is to accept the pregnancy. Men appear to put conscious thought of the pregnancy aside for a time. They become more introspective and engage in many discussions about their philosophy of life, religion, childbearing, and childrearing practices and their relationships with family members, particularly with their father. Depending on the man's readiness for the pregnancy, this phase may be relatively short or persist until the last trimester.

- The third phase, the *focusing phase*, begins in the last trimester and is characterized by the father's active involvement in both the pregnancy and his relationship with his child. The developmental task is to negotiate with his partner the role he is to play in labor and to prepare for parenthood. In this phase the man concentrates on his experience of the pregnancy and begins to think of himself as a father.

Identifying with the Father Role

Each man brings to pregnancy attitudes that affect the way in which he adjusts to the pregnancy and parental role. His memories of the fathering he received from his own father, the experiences he has had with child care, and the perceptions of the male and father roles within his social group will guide his selection of the tasks and responsibilities he will assume. Some men are highly motivated to nurture and love a child. They may be excited and pleased about the anticipated role of father (Fig. 16-2). Others may be more detached or even hostile to the idea of fatherhood.

FIG. 16-2 Prospective mother and father walk together. Women respond positively to their partner's interest and concern. (Courtesy Marjorie Pyle, RNC, Lifecircle, Costa Mesa, CA.)

Reordering Personal Relationships

The partner's main role in pregnancy is to nurture and respond to the pregnant woman's feelings of vulnerability. The partner also must deal with the reality of the pregnancy. The partner's support indicates involvement in the pregnancy and preparation for attachment to the child.

Some aspects of a partner's behavior may indicate rivalry, and it may be especially evident during sexual activity. For example, men may protest that fetal movements prevent sexual gratification or that they are being watched by the fetus during sexual activity. However, feelings of rivalry may be unconscious and not verbalized, but expressed in subtle behaviors.

The woman's increased introspection may cause her partner to feel uneasy as she becomes preoccupied with thoughts of the child and of her motherhood, with her growing dependence on her physician or midwife, and with her reevaluation of the couple's relationship. Couples who are told early in the pregnancy that ambivalence, anxiety, and increased tensions are common experiences for expectant couples then can devote energy to managing the changes. Perinatal educators are in an especially favorable position to incorporate needs of prospective fathers as well as mothers in their class presentations and discussions.

Establishing a Relationship with the Fetus

The father-child attachment can be as strong as the mother-child relationship, and fathers can be as competent as mothers in nurturing their infants. The father-child attachment also begins during pregnancy. A father may rub or kiss the maternal abdomen, try to listen, talk, or sing to the fetus, or play with the fetus as he notes movement. Calling the unborn child by name or nickname helps to confirm the reality of pregnancy and promote attachment.

Men prepare for fatherhood in many of the same ways as women do for motherhood—by reading and by fantasizing about the baby. Daydreaming about their role as father is common in the last weeks before the birth; however, men rarely describe their thoughts unless they are reassured that such daydreams are normal.

Nurses can help fathers identify concerns and prepare for the reality of a baby by asking questions such as the following:

- What do you expect the baby to look and act like?
- What do you think being a father will be like?
- Have you thought about the baby's crying? Changing diapers? Burping the baby? Being awakened at night? Sharing your partner with the baby?

The father may not wish to answer such questions when he is asked but may need time to think them through or discuss them with his partner.

As the birth date approaches, men have more questions about fetal and newborn behaviors. Some men are shocked or amazed at the smallness of clothes and furniture for the baby. If an expectant father can imagine only an older child and has difficulty visualizing or talking about an infant, this situation must be explored. The nurse can tell the father about the unborn child's ability to respond to light, sound, and touch and encourage him to feel and talk to the fetus. A tour of a newborn nursery or discussions with new fathers, as in childbirth classes, may be welcomed.

Some men become involved by picking the child's name and anticipating the child's sex, if it is not already known. Some couples select the name of the child as early as the first month of pregnancy. Family tradition, religious customs and the continuation of the parent's name or names of relatives or friends are important in the selection process.

Parents may occasionally show or voice disappointment over the sex of the child. The parents may experience grief and a sense of loss at birth as they release their fantasized image of the child and begin to accept the real child. However, these negative responses are usually temporary. Providing an accepting environment for parental reactions facilitates the parent's ability to move beyond disappointment to acceptance.

Preparing for Childbirth

The days and weeks immediately before the expected day of birth are characterized by anticipation and anxiety. Boredom and restlessness are common as the couple focuses on the birth process; however, during the last 2 months of pregnancy, many expectant fathers experience a surge of creative energy at home and on the job. They may become dissatisfied with their present living space. If possible, they tend to act on the need to alter the environment (remodeling, painting, etc.). This activity may be overt evidence of their sharing in the childbearing experience. They are able to channel the anxiety and other feelings experienced during the final weeks before birth into productive activities. This behavior earns recognition and compliments from friends, relatives, and their partners.

Major concerns for the man are getting the woman to a medical facility in time for the birth and not appearing ignorant. Many men want to be able to recognize labor and determine when it is appropriate to leave for the hospital or call the physician or midwife. They may fantasize different situations and plan what they will do in response to them, or they may rehearse taking various routes to the hospital, timing each route at different times of the day.

Some prospective fathers have questions about the labor suite's furniture and equipment, nursing staff, and location, as well as the availability of the physician and anesthesiologist. Others want to know what is expected of them when their partners are in labor. The man also may have fears concerning safe passage of his child and partner and the possible death or complications of his partner and child. It is important he verbalize these fears, otherwise he cannot help his mate deal with her own unspoken or overt apprehension.

With the exception of childbirth preparation classes, a man has few opportunities to learn ways to be an involved and active partner in this rite of passage into parenthood. The tensions and apprehensions of the unprepared, unsupportive father are readily transmitted to the mother and may increase her fears.

The same fears, questions, and concerns may affect birth partners who are not the biologic fathers. Birth partners need to be kept informed, supported, and included in all activities in which the mother desires their participation. The nurse can do much to promote pregnancy and birth as a family experience.

Sibling Adaptation

Sharing the spotlight with a new brother or sister may be the first major crisis for a child. The older child often experiences a sense of loss or feels jealous at being "replaced" by the new sibling. Some of the factors that influence the child's response are age, the parents' attitudes, the role of the father, the length of separation from the mother, the hospital's visitation policy, and the way the child has been prepared for the change.

A mother with other children must devote time and effort to reorganizing her relationships with them. She needs to prepare siblings for the birth of the baby (see Fig. 17-4 and Box 17-4) and begin the process of role transition in the family by including the children in the pregnancy and being sympathetic to older children's concerns about losing their places in the family hierarchy. No child willingly gives up a familiar position.

Siblings' responses to pregnancy vary with their age and dependency needs. The 1-year-old infant seems largely unaware of the process, but the 2-year-old child notices the change in his or her mother's appearance and may comment that "Mommy's fat." Toddlers' need for sameness in the environment makes children aware of any change. They may exhibit more clinging behavior and revert to dependent behaviors in toilet training or eating.

FIG. 16-3 Four-year-old likes to examine the pregnant abdomen of his mother. (Courtesy Kara George, Phoenix, AZ.)

By age 3 or 4 years, children like to be told the story of their own beginning and accept its being compared with the present pregnancy. They like to listen to the fetal heart beat and feel the baby moving in utero (Fig. 16-3). Sometimes they worry about how the baby is being fed and what it wears.

School-age children take a more clinical interest in their mother's pregnancy. They may want to know in more detail, "How did the baby get in there?" and "How will it get out?" Children in this age-group notice pregnant women in stores, churches, and schools and sometimes seem shy if they need to approach a pregnant woman directly. On the whole, they look forward to the new baby, see themselves as "mothers" or "fathers," and enjoy buying baby supplies and readying a place for the baby. Because they still think in concrete terms and base judgments on the here and now, they respond positively to their mother's current good health.

Early and middle adolescents preoccupied with the establishment of their own sexual identity may have difficulty accepting the overwhelming evidence of the sexual activity of their parents. They reason that if they are too young for such activity, certainly their parents are too old. They seem to take on a critical parental role and may ask, "What will people think?" or "How can you let yourself get so fat?" or "How can you let yourself get pregnant?" Many pregnant women with teenage children will confess that the attitudes of their teenagers are the most difficult aspect of their current pregnancy.

Late adolescents do not appear to be unduly disturbed. They are busy making plans for their own lives and realize that they soon will be gone from home. Parents usually report they are comforting and act more as other adults than as children.

Grandparent Adaptation

Every pregnancy affects all family relationships. For expectant grandparents, a first pregnancy in a child is undeniable evidence that they are growing older. Many think of a grandparent as old, white-haired, and becoming feeble of mind and body; however, some people face grandparenthood while still in their 30s or 40s. Parents-to-be announcing their pregnancy to their parents may be greeted by a negative response, indicating that they are not ready to be grandparents. The parents-to-be may be hurt by this initial response.

In some family units, expectant grandparents are nonsupportive and may also inadvertently decrease the self-esteem of the parents-to-be. Mothers may talk about their terrible pregnancies; fathers may discuss the endless cost of rearing children; and mothers-in-law may complain that their sons are neglecting them because their concern is now directed toward the pregnant daughters-in-law.

However, most grandparents are delighted at the prospect of a new baby in the family. It reawakens the feelings of their own youth, the excitement of giving birth, and their delight in the behavior of the parents-to-be when they were infants. They set up a memory store of the child's first smiles, first words, and first steps, which they can use later for "claiming" the newborn as a member of the family. These behaviors provide a link between the past and present for the parents- and grandparents-to-be.

In addition, the grandparent is the historian who transmits the family history, a resource person who shares knowledge based on experience; a role model; and a support person. The grandparent's presence and support can strengthen family systems by widening the circle of support and nurturance (Fig. 16-4).

Many women report that their pregnancies bridged the final gap between them and their own mothers. The estrangement that began in adolescence disappears as the now-pregnant daughter experiences joys, concerns, and anxieties similar to those felt by her mother before her.

Expectant grandparenthood also can represent a maturational milestone for the parent of an expectant parent. To be truly family oriented, maternity care must include the grandparent in the implementation of the nursing process

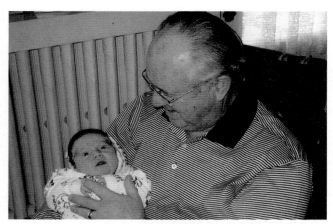

FIG. 16-4 Grandfather getting to know his grandson. (Courtesy Nicole Larson, Eden Prairie, MN.)

with the whole childbearing family. A class for grandparents is one method of incorporating the grandparents into the family system and encouraging communication between the generations.

Grandparents' anxieties and concerns and their relationships with expectant parents and grandchildren should be discussed during courses for expectant parents. The expectant parents may use this opportunity to begin to resolve conflicts and perceived differences with their parents, a task that can also enhance their ability to relate to their own children.

CARE MANAGEMENT

The purpose of prenatal care is to identify existing risk factors and other deviations from normal so that pregnancy outcomes may be enhanced (Johnson & Niebyl, 2002). Major emphasis is placed on preventive aspects of care, primarily to motivate the pregnant woman to practice optimal self-care and to report unusual changes early so that problems can be prevented or minimized. If health behaviors must be modified in early pregnancy, nurses need to understand psychosocial factors that may influence the woman. In holistic care, nurses provide information and guidance about not only the physical changes but also the psychosocial impact of pregnancy on the woman and members of her family. The goals of prenatal nursing care, therefore, are to foster a safe birth for the infant and to promote satisfaction of the mother and family with the pregnancy and birth experience.

Advances have been made in the number of women in the United States who receive adequate prenatal care. In 2003, 84% of all women received care in the first trimester and 3.5% had late or no prenatal care. There is disparity in use of prenatal care in the first trimester by race and ethnicity: 89% of non-Hispanic whites, 76% of non-Hispanic blacks, and 78% of Hispanic women receive care in the first trimester (Hoyert, Mathews, Menacker, Strobino, & Guyer, 2006). Although prenatal care is sought routinely by women of middle or high socioeconomic status, women living in poverty or who lack health insurance may have difficulty using public medical services or gaining access to private care. Lack of culturally sensitive care providers and barriers in communication resulting from differences in language also interfere with access to care (Shaffer, 2002). Likewise, immigrant women who come from cultures in which prenatal care is not emphasized may not know to seek routine prenatal care. Birth outcomes in these populations are therefore less positive, with higher rates of maternal and fetal or newborn complications. Problems with low birth weight (LBW; less than 2500 g) and infant mortality have in particular been associated with lack of adequate prenatal care.

Barriers to obtaining health care during pregnancy include lack of transportation, unpleasant clinic facilities or procedures, inconvenient clinic hours, and personal attitudes (Boyle, Banks, Petrizzi, & Larimore, 2003; Chandler, 2002; Handler, Rosenberg, Raube, & Lyons, 2003; Sword, 2003). The availability and accessibility of prenatal care may be improved by the increasing use of advanced practice nurses in collaborative practice with physicians (Boyle et al.). The effectiveness of a regular schedule of home visiting by nurses during pregnancy also has been validated (Fetrick, Christensen, & Mitchell, 2003).

The current model for provision of prenatal care has been used for more than a century. The initial visit usually occurs in the first trimester, with monthly visits through week 28 of pregnancy. Thereafter, visits are scheduled every 2 weeks until week 36, and then every week until birth (see Box 16-3). This model is currently being questioned, and in some practices there is a growing tendency to have fewer visits with women who are at low risk for complications (Villar, Carroli, Khan-Neelofur, Piaggio, & Gulmezoglu, 2001). Health care providers are challenged to create a system of prenatal care that has minimal barriers and a focus on individualized care.

In response to the call of the United States Public Health Service (1989) to develop new models of prenatal care, Rising (1998), a certified nurse-midwife, developed an innovative approach that emphasizes the assessment of risk, education, and support in a group setting using a holistic and comprehensive focus. In this centering pregnancy (CP) approach, women have over 20 contact hours with a health care provider during pregnancy and postpartum. Eight to 12 women are placed in gestational age cohort groups; group sessions begin at 12 to 16 weeks of gestation and end with an early postpartum meeting (Carlson & Lowe, 2006).

Before groups begin, each woman has an individual assessment, physical examination, and history. At the beginning of the group meeting, women measure their own blood pressure, weigh themselves, and test their own urine using dipsticks, and record the results. Fundal height and the fetal heart rate are assessed individually and privately. Individual follow-up is scheduled as needed (Carlson & Lowe, 2006).

Results assessing the effectiveness of this approach have been promising; in a study of adolescents, the incidence of low birth weight was reduced and rates of breastfeeding were increased (Grady & Bloom, 2004). Other studies of CP are ongoing.

In recent years the concept of preconception care has been recognized as an important contributor to good pregnancy outcomes (see Chapter 17). If women can be taught and demonstrate healthy lifestyle behaviors preconceptually—specifically good nutrition, adequate intake of folic acid, avoidance of alcohol and tobacco use, prevention of sexually transmitted infections (STIs) and other health hazards—a healthier pregnancy may result. Likewise, women who have health problems related to chronic diseases such as diabetes mellitus can be counseled regarding their special needs, with the intent to minimize maternal and fetal complications.

Prenatal care is ideally a multidisciplinary activity in which nurses work with physicians or midwives, nutritionists, social workers, and others. Collaboration among these individuals is necessary to provide holistic care. The case management model, which makes use of care maps and critical pathways, is one system that promotes comprehensive care with limited overlap in services. To emphasize the nursing role, care management here is organized around the central elements of the nursing process: assessment, nursing diagnoses, expected outcomes, plan of care and interventions, and evaluation.

▆ Assessment and Nursing Diagnoses

Once the presence of pregnancy has been confirmed and the woman's desire to continue the pregnancy has been validated, prenatal care is begun. The assessment process begins at the initial prenatal visit and is continued throughout the pregnancy. Assessment techniques include the interview, physical examination, and laboratory tests. Because the initial visit and follow-up visits are distinctly different in content and process, they are described separately.

▆ *Initial Visit*

The pregnant woman and family members who may be present should be told that the first prenatal visit is more lengthy and detailed than future visits. The initial evaluation includes a comprehensive health history emphasizing the current pregnancy, previous pregnancies, the family, a psychosocial profile, a physical assessment, diagnostic testing, and an overall risk assessment. A prenatal history form (Fig. 16-5) is the best way to document information obtained.

Interview. The therapeutic relationship between the nurse and the woman is established during the initial assessment interview. It is a time for planned, purposeful communication that focuses on specific content. The data collected are of two types: the woman's subjective appraisal of her health status and the nurse's objective observations. During the interview the nurse observes the woman's affect, posture, body language, skin color, and other physical and emotional signs.

Often the pregnant woman is accompanied by one or more family members. The nurse needs to build a relationship with these people as part of the social context of the client. With her permission, those accompanying the woman can be included in the initial prenatal interview, and the observations and information about the woman's family form part of the database (Fig. 16-6, p. 394.). For example, if the woman is accompanied by small children, the nurse can ask about her plans for child care during the time of labor and birth. Special needs are noted at this time (e.g., wheelchair access, assistance in getting on and off the examining table, and cognitive deficits).

Reason for Seeking Care. Although pregnant women are scheduled for "routine" prenatal visits, they often come to the health care provider seeking information or

Text continued on p. 394.

Patient Addressograph

DATE _____

NAME _____
        LAST   FIRST   MIDDLE

ID # _____ HOSPITAL OF DELIVERY _____

NEWBORN'S PHYSICIAN _____ REFERRED BY _____

| FINAL EDD _____ | PRIMARY PROVIDER/GROUP _____ |

BIRTH DATE AGE RACE MARITAL STATUS MONTH DAY YEAR S M W D SEP	ADDRESS
OCCUPATION EDUCATION (LAST GRADE COMPLETED)	ZIP PHONE (H) (O)
LANGUAGE	INSURANCE CARRIER/MEDICAID #
HUSBAND/DOMESTIC PARTNER PHONE	POLICY #
FATHER OF BABY PHONE	EMERGENCY CONTACT PHONE

TOTAL PREG	FULL TERM	PREMATURE	AB. INDUCED	AB. SPONTANEOUS	ECTOPICS	MULTIPLE BIRTHS	LIVING

MENSTRUAL HISTORY

LMP ☐ DEFINITE ☐ APPROXIMATE (MONTH KNOWN) MENSES MONTHLY ☐ YES ☐ NO FREQUENCY: Q _____ DAYS MENARCHE _____ (AGE ONSET)

☐ UNKNOWN ☐ NORMAL AMOUNT/DURATION PRIOR MENSES _____ DATE ON BCP AT CONCEPT ☐ YES ☐ NO hCG + ___/___/___

☐ FINAL _____

PAST PREGNANCIES (LAST SIX)

DATE MONTH/ YEAR	GA WEEKS	LENGTH OF LABOR	BIRTH WEIGHT	SEX M/F	TYPE DELIVERY	ANES.	PLACE OF DELIVERY	PRETERM LABOR YES/NO	COMMENTS/ COMPLICATIONS

MEDICAL HISTORY

	O Neg. + Pos.	DETAIL POSITIVE REMARKS INCLUDE DATE & TREATMENT		O Neg. + Pos.	DETAIL POSITIVE REMARKS INCLUDE DATE & TREATMENT
1. DIABETES			17. D (Rh) SENSITIZED		
2. HYPERTENSION			18. PULMONARY (TB, ASTHMA)		
3. HEART DISEASE			19. SEASONAL ALLERGIES		
4. AUTOIMMUNE DISORDER			20. DRUG/LATEX ALLERGIES/ REACTIONS		
5. KIDNEY DISEASE/UTI					
6. NEUROLOGIC/EPILEPSY			21. BREAST		
7. PSYCHIATRIC			22. GYN SURGERY		
8. DEPRESSION/POSTPARTUM DEPRESSION					
9. HEPATITIS/LIVER DISEASE			23. OPERATIONS/ HOSPITALIZATIONS (YEAR & REASON)		
10. VARICOSITIES/PHLEBITIS					
11. THYROID DYSFUNCTION			24. ANESTHETIC COMPLICATIONS		
12. TRAUMA/VIOLENCE			25. HISTORY OF ABNORMAL PAP		
13. HISTORY OF BLOOD TRANSFUS.			26. UTERINE ANOMALY/DES		

	AMT/DAY PREPREG	AMT/DAY PREG	# YEARS USE	27. INFERTILITY		
14. TOBACCO				28. RELEVANT FAMILY HISTORY		
15. ALCOHOL						
16. ILLICIT/RECREATIONAL DRUGS				29. OTHER		

COMMENTS _____

Vertical text right margin: ACOG ANTEPARTUM RECORD (FORM A)

Version 5. Copyright © 2003 The American College of Obstetricians and Gynecologists, 409 12th Street, SW, PO Box 96920, Washington, DC 20090-6920   AA129   12345/76543

FIG. 16-5 A sample prenatal history form. (Copyright © 2003 The American College of Obstetricians and Gynecologists, 409 12th Street, SW, P.O. Box 96920, Washington, DC, 20090-6920.)

Patient Addressograph

SYMPTOMS SINCE LMP

GENETIC SCREENING/TERATOLOGY COUNSELING
INCLUDES PATIENT, BABY'S FATHER, OR ANYONE IN EITHER FAMILY WITH:

	YES	NO		YES	NO
1. PATIENT'S AGE ≥35 YEARS AS OF ESTIMATED DATE OF DELIVERY			12. HUNTINGTON'S CHOREA		
2. THALASSEMIA (ITALIAN, GREEK, MEDITERRANEAN, OR ASIAN BACKGROUND): MCV <80			13. MENTAL RETARDATION/AUTISM		
			IF YES, WAS PERSON TESTED FOR FRAGILE X?		
3. NEURAL TUBE DEFECT (MENINGOMYELOCELE, SPINA BIFIDA, OR ANENCEPHALY)			14. OTHER INHERITED GENETIC OR CHROMOSOMAL DISORDER		
4. CONGENITAL HEART DEFECT			15. MATERNAL METABOLIC DISORDER (EG, TYPE 1 DIABETES, PKU)		
5. DOWN SYNDROME			16. PATIENT OR BABY'S FATHER HAD A CHILD WITH BIRTH DEFECTS NOT LISTED ABOVE		
6. TAY-SACHS (EG, JEWISH, CAJUN, FRENCH CANADIAN)			17. RECURRENT PREGNANCY LOSS, OR A STILLBIRTH		
7. CANAVAN DISEASE			18. MEDICATIONS (INCLUDING SUPPLEMENTS, VITAMINS, HERBS OR OTC DRUGS)/ILLICIT/RECREATIONAL DRUGS/ALCOHOL SINCE LAST MENSTRUAL PERIOD		
8. SICKLE CELL DISEASE OR TRAIT (AFRICAN)					
9. HEMOPHILIA OR OTHER BLOOD DISORDERS			IF YES, AGENT(S) AND STRENGTH/DOSAGE		
10. MUSCULAR DYSTROPHY					
11. CYSTIC FIBROSIS			19. ANY OTHER		

COMMENTS/COUNSELING _____

_____

INFECTION HISTORY	YES	NO		YES	NO
1. LIVE WITH SOMEONE WITH TB OR EXPOSED TO TB			4. HISTORY OF STD, GONORRHEA, CHLAMYDIA, HPV, SYPHILIS		
2. PATIENT OR PARTNER HAS HISTORY OF GENITAL HERPES			5. OTHER (See Comments)		
3. RASH OR VIRAL ILLNESS SINCE LAST MENSTRUAL PERIOD					

COMMENTS _____

INTERVIEWER'S SIGNATURE _____

INITIAL PHYSICAL EXAMINATION

DATE _____/_____/_____   HEIGHT _____   BP _____

1. HEENT	□ NORMAL	□ ABNORMAL	12. VULVA	□ NORMAL	□ CONDYLOMA	□ LESIONS
2. FUNDI	□ NORMAL	□ ABNORMAL	13. VAGINA	□ NORMAL	□ INFLAMMATION	□ DISCHARGE
3. TEETH	□ NORMAL	□ ABNORMAL	14. CERVIX	□ NORMAL	□ INFLAMMATION	□ LESIONS
4. THYROID	□ NORMAL	□ ABNORMAL	15. UTERUS SIZE	_____ WEEKS		□ FIBROIDS
5. BREASTS	□ NORMAL	□ ABNORMAL	16. ADNEXA	□ NORMAL	□ MASS	
6. LUNGS	□ NORMAL	□ ABNORMAL	17. RECTUM	□ NORMAL	□ ABNORMAL	
7. HEART	□ NORMAL	□ ABNORMAL	18. DIAGONAL CONJUGATE	□ REACHED	□ NO	_____ CM
8. ABDOMEN	□ NORMAL	□ ABNORMAL	19. SPINES	□ AVERAGE	□ PROMINENT	□ BLUNT
9. EXTREMITIES	□ NORMAL	□ ABNORMAL	20. SACRUM	□ CONCAVE	□ STRAIGHT	□ ANTERIOR
10. SKIN	□ NORMAL	□ ABNORMAL	21. SUBPUBIC ARCH	□ NORMAL	□ WIDE	□ NARROW
11. LYMPH NODES	□ NORMAL	□ ABNORMAL	22. GYNECOID PELVIC TYPE	□ YES	□ NO	

COMMENTS (Number and explain abnormals) _____

_____

EXAM BY _____

ACOG ANTEPARTUM RECORD (FORM B)

FIG. 16-5, cont'd   A sample prenatal history form. (Copyright © 2003 The American College of Obstetricians and Gynecologists, 409 12th Street, SW, P.O. Box 96920, Washington, DC, 20090-6920.)

Continued

Patient Addressograph

NAME _____
        LAST   FIRST   MIDDLE

DRUG ALLERGY	LATEX ALLERGY		

IS BLOOD TRANSFUSION ACCEPTABLE IN AN EMERGENCY?   ☐ YES   ☐ NO   ANESTHESIA CONSULT PLANNED   ☐ YES   ☐ NO

PROBLEMS/PLANS

1. _____
2. _____
3. _____
4. _____
5. _____
6. _____

MEDICATION LIST   Start date   Stop date

1. _____ ___/___/___ ___/___/___
2. _____ ___/___/___ ___/___/___
3. _____ ___/___/___ ___/___/___
4. _____ ___/___/___ ___/___/___
5. _____ ___/___/___ ___/___/___
6. _____ ___/___/___ ___/___/___

EDD CONFIRMATION

INITIAL EDD
LMP ___/___/___ = EDD ___/___/___
INITIAL EXAM ___/___/___ = ___ WKS = EDD ___/___/___
ULTRASOUND ___/___/___ = ___ WKS = EDD ___/___/___
INITIAL EDD ___/___/___ INITIALED BY _____

18–20-WEEK EDD UPDATE

QUICKENING ___/___/___ +22 WKS = ___/___/___
FUNDAL HT. AT UMBIL. ___/___/___ +20 WKS = ___/___/___
ULTRASOUND ___/___/___ = ___ WKS = ___/___/___
FINAL EDD ___/___/___ INITIALED BY _____

PREPREGNANCY WEIGHT _____

WEEKS GEST. (BEST EST.)	FUNDAL HEIGHT (CM)	PRESENTATION	FHR	FETAL MOVEMENT	PRETERM LABOR SIGNS/SYMPTOMS + = PRESENT o = ABSENT	CERVIX EXAM (DIL/EFF/STA.) ULTRASOUND LENGTH	BLOOD PRESSURE	WEIGHT	URINE (ALBUMIN/GLUCOSE)	NEXT APPOINTMENT	PROVIDER (INITIALS)	COMMENTS

PROBLEMS _____

COMMENTS _____

FIG. 16-5, cont'd   A sample prenatal history form. (Copyright © 2003 The American College of Obstetricians and Gynecologists, 409 12th Street, SW, P.O. Box 96920, Washington, DC, 20090-6920.)

ACOG ANTEPARTUM RECORD (FORM C)

Patient Addressograph

LABORATORY AND EDUCATION

INITIAL LABS	DATE	RESULT	REVIEWED
BLOOD TYPE	/ /	A B AB O	
D (Rh) TYPE	/ /		
ANTIBODY SCREEN	/ /		
HCT/HGB	/ /	_____ % _____ g/dL	
PAP TEST	/ /	NORMAL/ABNORMAL _____	
RUBELLA	/ /		
VDRL	/ /		
URINE CULTURE/SCREEN	/ /		
HBsAg	/ /		
HIV COUNSELING/TESTING*	/ /	POS. NEG. DECLINED	

OPTIONAL LABS	DATE	RESULT	REVIEWED
HGB ELECTROPHORESIS	/ /	AA AS SS AC SC AF $\uparrow A_2$	
PPD	/ /		
CHLAMYDIA	/ /		
GONORRHEA	/ /		
GENETIC SCREENING TESTS (SEE FORM B)	/ /		
OTHER			

8–18-WEEK LABS (WHEN INDICATED/ELECTED)	DATE	RESULT	
ULTRASOUND	/ /		
MSAFP/MULTIPLE MARKERS	/ /		
AMNIO/CVS	/ /		
KARYOTYPE	/ /	46,XX OR 46,XY/OTHER _____	
AMNIOTIC FLUID (AFP)	/ /	NORMAL _____ ABNORMAL _____	

24–28-WEEK LABS (WHEN INDICATED)	DATE	RESULT	
HCT/HGB	/ /	_____ % _____ g/dL	
DIABETES SCREEN	/ /	1 HOUR _____	
GTT (IF SCREEN ABNORMAL)	/ /	_____ FBS _____ 1 HOUR _____ 2 HOUR _____ 3 HOUR	
D (Rh) ANTIBODY SCREEN	/ /		
ANTI-D IMMUNE GLOBULIN (RhIG) GIVEN (28 WKS)	/ /	SIGNATURE _____	

32–36-WEEK LABS	DATE	RESULT	
HCT/HGB	/ /	_____ % _____ g/dL	
ULTRASOUND (WHEN INDICATED)	/ /		
VDRL (WHEN INDICATED)	/ /		
GONORRHEA (WHEN INDICATED)	/ /		
CHLAMYDIA (WHEN INDICATED)	/ /		
GROUP B STREP	/ /		

COMMENTS/ADDITIONAL LABS

*Check state requirements before recording results.

PROVIDER SIGNATURE (AS REQUIRED) _____

ACOG ANTEPARTUM RECORD (FORM D)

FIG. 16-5, cont'd A sample prenatal history form. (Copyright © 2003 The American College of Obstetricians and Gynecologists, 409 12th Street, SW, P.O. Box 96920, Washington, DC, 20090-6920.)

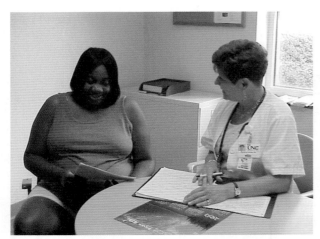

FIG. 16-6 Prenatal interview. (Courtesy Dee Lowdermilk, Chapel Hill, NC.)

reassurance about a particular concern. When the client is asked a broad, open-ended question such as, "How have you been feeling?" she may reveal problems that could otherwise be overlooked. The woman's chief concerns should be recorded in her own words to alert other personnel to the priority of needs as identified by her. At the initial visit the desire for information about what is normal in the course of pregnancy is typical.

Current Pregnancy. The presumptive signs of pregnancy may be of great concern to the woman. A review of symptoms she is experiencing and how she is coping with them helps to establish a database to develop a plan of care. Some early teaching may be provided at this time.

Obstetric and Gynecologic History. Data are gathered on the woman's age at menarche, menstrual history, and contraceptive history; the nature of any infertility or gynecologic conditions; her history of any STIs; her sexual history; and a detailed history of all her pregnancies, including the present pregnancy, and their outcomes. The date of the last Papanicolaou (Pap) test and the result are noted. The date of her LMP is obtained to establish the EDB.

▬ Prenatal Interview

Medical History. The medical history includes those medical or surgical conditions that may affect the pregnancy or that may be affected by the pregnancy. For example, a pregnant woman who has diabetes, hypertension, or epilepsy requires special care. Because most women are anxious during the initial interview, the nurse's reference to cues, such as a MedicAlert bracelet, prompts the woman to explain allergies, chronic diseases, or medications being taken (e.g., cortisone, insulin, or anticonvulsants).

The nature of previous surgical procedures also should be described. If a woman has undergone uterine surgery or extensive repair of the pelvic floor, a cesarean birth may be necessary; appendectomy rules out appendicitis as a cause of right lower quadrant pain in pregnancy; and spinal surgery may contraindicate the use of spinal or epidural anesthesia. Any injury involving the pelvis is noted.

Often women who have chronic or handicapping conditions forget to mention them during the initial assessment because they have become so adapted to them. Special shoes or a limp may indicate the existence of a pelvic structural defect, which is an important consideration in pregnant women. The nurse who observes these special characteristics and inquires about them sensitively can obtain individualized data that will provide the basis for a comprehensive nursing care plan. Observations are vital components of the interview process because they prompt the nurse and woman to focus on the specific needs of the woman and her family.

Nutritional History. The woman's nutritional history is an important component of the prenatal history because her nutritional status has a direct effect on the growth and development of the fetus. A dietary assessment can reveal special dietary practices, food allergies, eating behaviors, the practice of pica (Corbett, Ryan, & Weinrich, 2003), and other factors related to her nutritional status (see Box 15-5). Pregnant women are usually motivated to learn about good nutrition and respond well to nutritional advice generated by this assessment.

History of Drug and Herbal Preparations Use. A woman's past and present use of drugs, both legal (over-the-counter [OTC] and prescription medications; herbal preparations; caffeine; alcohol; nicotine) and illegal (e.g., marijuana, cocaine, heroin), must be assessed because many substances cross the placenta and may therefore harm the developing fetus. Periodic urine toxicology screening tests are often recommended during the pregnancies of women who have a history of illegal drug use. Results of such tests have been used for criminal prosecution, which results in a breach in client-provider relationship and in ethical responsibilities to the client (Foley, 2002; Harris & Paltrow, 2003). Nurses may have ethical concerns if pregnant women are not informed of the possibility of random urine testing for presence of drugs. The other side of this concern is the unborn child and whether the mother has a duty not to harm him or her. Today, increased numbers of individuals are using herbal preparations, and this usage includes pregnant women. Therefore, it is important for health care providers to question prenatal women regarding the use of herbal preparations and document the woman's responses. Further investigation in this area is needed.

▬ LEGAL TIP Screening for Drug Use
Hospitals must obtain informed consent from a pregnant woman before she can be tested for drug use (Kehringer, 2003).

Family History. The family history provides information about the woman's immediate family, including parents, siblings, and children. These data help identify familial or genetic disorders or conditions that could affect the present health status of the woman or her fetus.

Social, Experiential, and Occupational History. Situational factors such as the family's ethnic and cultural background and socioeconomic status are assessed while the history is obtained. The following information may be obtained in several encounters. The woman's perception of this pregnancy is explored by asking questions such as the following: Is this pregnancy planned or not, wanted or not? Is the woman pleased, displeased, accepting, or non-accepting? What problems related to finances, career, or living accommodations may arise as a result of the pregnancy? The family support system is determined by asking the following questions: What primary support is available to her? Are changes needed to promote adequate support? What are the existing relationships among the mother, father or partner, siblings, and in-laws? What preparations are being made for her care and that of dependent family members during labor and for the care of the infant after birth? Is financial, educational, or other support needed from the community? What are the woman's ideas about childbearing, her expectations of the infant's behavior, and her outlook on life and the female role?

Other questions that should be asked include the following: What does the woman think it will be like to have a baby in the home? How is her life going to change by having a baby? What plans are interrupted by having a baby? During interviews throughout the pregnancy the nurse should remain alert to the appearance of potential parenting problems, such as depression, lack of family support, and inadequate living conditions. The nurse must assess the woman's attitude toward health care, particularly during childbearing, her expectations of health care providers, and her view of the relationship between herself and the nurse.

Coping mechanisms and patterns of interacting also are identified. Early in the pregnancy the nurse should determine the woman's knowledge in various areas: of pregnancy, maternal changes, fetal growth, self-care, and care of the newborn, including feeding. Asking about attitudes toward unmedicated or medicated childbirth and about her knowledge of the availability of parenting skills classes is important. Before planning for nursing care, the nurse needs information about the woman's decision-making abilities and living habits (e.g., exercise, sleep, diet, diversional interests, personal hygiene, clothing). Common stressors during childbearing include the baby's welfare, labor and birth process, behaviors of the newborn, the woman's relationship with the baby's father and her family, changes in body image, and physical symptoms.

Attitudes concerning the range of acceptable sexual behavior during pregnancy also should be explored by asking questions such as the following: What has your family (partner, friends) told you about sex during pregnancy? The woman's sexual self-concept is given more emphasis by asking questions such as the following: How do you feel about the changes in your appearance? How does your partner feel about your body now? How do you feel about wearing maternity clothes?

Women should be questioned regarding their occupation—past and present, since this may adversely affect maternal and fetal health. For some women, heavy lifting and exposure to chemicals and radiation may be part of their daily work, and these activities may negatively affect the pregnancy.

History of Physical Abuse. All women should be assessed for a history or risk of physical abuse, particularly because the likelihood of abuse increases during pregnancy. Although visual cues from the woman's appearance or behavior may suggest the possibility, if questioning is limited to those women who fit the supposed profile of the battered woman, many women will be missed. Identification of abuse and immediate clinical intervention that includes information about safety can result in behaviors that may prevent future abuse and increase the safety and well-being of the woman and her infant (McFarlane, Parker, & Cross, 2001). During pregnancy, the target body parts change during abusive episodes. Women report physical blows directed to the head, breasts, abdomen, and genitalia. Sexual assault is common.

Battering and pregnancy in teenagers constitutes a particularly difficult situation. Adolescents may be trapped in the abusive relationship because of their inexperience. Many professionals and the adolescents themselves ignore the violence because it may not be believable, because relationships are transient, and because the jealous and controlling behavior is interpreted as love and devotion. Routine screening for abuse and sexual assault is recommended for pregnant adolescents. Because pregnancy in young adolescent girls is commonly the result of sexual abuse, the nurse should assess the desire to maintain the pregnancy (see Chapter 6 for further discussion).

Review of Systems. During this portion of the interview, the woman is asked to identify and describe preexisting or concurrent problems in any of the body systems, and her mental status is assessed. The woman is questioned about physical symptoms she has experienced, such as shortness of breath or pain. Pregnancy affects and is affected by all body systems; therefore information on the present status of the body systems is important in planning care. For each sign or symptom described, the following additional data should be obtained: body location, quality, quantity, chronology, aggravating or alleviating factors, and associated manifestations (onset, character, course) (Seidel, Ball, Dains, & Benedict, 2006).

Physical Examination. The initial physical examination provides the baseline for assessing subsequent changes. The examiner should determine the woman's needs for basic information regarding reproductive anatomy and provide this information, along with a demonstration of the equipment that may be used and an explanation of the procedure itself. The interaction requires an unhurried, sensitive, and gentle approach with a matter-of-fact attitude.

The physical examination begins with assessment of vital signs and height and weight (for calculation of body mass index [BMI]). The bladder should be empty before pelvic examination. A urine specimen may be obtained to test for protein, glucose, or leukocytes or other urine tests.

Each examiner develops a routine for proceeding with the physical examination; most choose the head-to-toe progression. Heart and lung sounds are evaluated, and

Evolve/CD: Case Study: First Trimester

extremities are examined. Distribution, amount, and quality of body hair are of particular importance because the findings reflect nutritional status, endocrine function, and attention to hygiene. The thyroid gland is assessed carefully. The height of the fundus is noted if the first examination is done after the first trimester of pregnancy. During the examination the examiner must remain alert to the woman's cues that give direction to the remainder of the assessment and that indicate imminent untoward response such as supine hypotension—low blood pressure (BP) that occurs while the woman is lying on her back, causing feelings of faintness. See Chapter 5 for a detailed description of the physical examination.

Whenever a pelvic examination is performed, the tone of the pelvic musculature and the woman's knowledge of Kegel exercises are assessed. Particular attention is paid to the size of the uterus because this is an indication of the duration of gestation. The nurse present during the examination can coach the woman in breathing and relaxation techniques at this time, as needed. One vaginal examination during pregnancy is recommended, but another is usually not done unless medically indicated.

Laboratory Tests. The laboratory data yielded by the analysis of the specimens obtained during the examination provide important information concerning the symptoms of pregnancy and the woman's health status.

Specimens are collected at the initial visit so that the cause of any abnormal findings can be treated (Table 16-1). Blood is drawn for a variety of tests; RPR (rapid plasma reagent)/VDRL (Venereal Disease Research Laboratory) test for syphilis; complete blood cell count (CBC) with hematocrit, hemoglobin, and differential values; tests for blood type and Rh factor; antibody screen, rubella, toxoplasmosis, and anti-Rh; and measurement of folate level, when indicated. The woman is tested for hepatitis B surface antigen (HBsAg) and hepatitis B surface antibody (HBsAb), if she has not received hepatitis B vaccine. A varicella (chickenpox) titer may be drawn for women who are unsure of their chickenpox immune status. A sickle cell screen is recommended for women of African, Asian, or Middle Eastern descent, and testing for antibody to the human immunodeficiency virus (HIV) is strongly recommended for all pregnant women (Centers for Disease Control and Prevention, Workowski, & Berman, 2006) (Box 16-2). In addition, pregnant women and fathers with a family history of cystic fibrosis and of Caucasian ethnicity may elect to have blood drawn for testing to ascertain if they are a cystic fibrosis carrier (Fries, Bashford, Workowsky, & Berman, 2006 & Numes, 2005). Urine is tested for glucose (diabetes), protein (preeclampsia), and nitrites and leukocytes (urinary tract infection). Urine specimens are usually tested by dipstick; culture and sensitivity tests are ordered as necessary. A purified protein derivative

table 16-1 Laboratory Tests in Prenatal Period

LABORATORY TEST	PURPOSE
Hemoglobin, hematocrit, WBC, differential	Detects anemia; detects infection
Hemoglobin electrophoresis	Identifies women with hemoglobinopathies (e.g., sickle cell anemia, thalassemia)
Blood type, Rh, and irregular antibody	Identifies those fetuses at risk for developing erythroblastosis fetalis or hyperbilirubinemia in neonatal period
Rubella titer	Determines immunity to rubella
Tuberculin skin testing; chest film after 20 weeks of gestation in women with reactive tuberculin tests	Screens for exposure to tuberculosis
Urinalysis, including microscopic examination of urinary sediment; pH, specific gravity, color, glucose, albumin, protein, RBCs, WBCs, casts, acetone; hCG	Identifies women with unsuspected diabetes mellitus, renal disease, hypertensive disease of pregnancy; infection; occult hematuria
Urine culture	Identifies women with asymptomatic bacteriuria
Renal function tests: BUN, creatinine, electrolytes, creatinine clearance, total protein excretion	Evaluates level of possible renal compromise in women with a history of diabetes, hypertension, or renal disease
Pap test	Screens for cervical intraepithelial neoplasia, herpes simplex type 2, and HPV
Vaginal or rectal smear for Neisseria gonorrhoeae, Chlamydia, HPV, GBS	Screens high risk population for asymptomatic infection; GBS done at 35-37 weeks
RPR, VDRL, or FTA-ABS	Identifies women with untreated syphilis
HIV* antibody, hepatitis B surface antigen, toxoplasmosis	Screens for specific infections
1-hr glucose tolerance	Screens for gestational diabetes; done at initial visit for women with risk factors; done at 24-28 weeks for all pregnant women
3-hr glucose tolerance	Screens for diabetes in women with elevated glucose level after 1-hr test; must have two elevated readings for diagnosis
Cardiac evaluation: ECG, chest x-ray film, and echocardiogram	Evaluates cardiac function in women with a history of hypertension or cardiac disease

BUN, Blood urea nitrogen; *ECG*, electrocardiogram; *FTA-ABS*, fluorescent treponemal antibody absorption test; *GBS*, group B streptococcus; *hCG*, human chorionic gonadotropin; *HIV*, human immunodeficiency virus; *HPV*, human papillomavirus; *RBC*, red blood cell; *RPR*, rapid plasma reagin; *VDRL*, Venereal Disease Research Laboratory; *WBC*, white blood cell.
*With client permission.

box 16-2 **HIV Screening**

- Pregnant women are ethically obligated to seek reasonable care during pregnancy and to avoid causing harm to the fetus. Maternity nurses should be advocates for the fetus while accepting of the pregnant woman's decision regarding testing and/or treatment for HIV.
- The incidence of perinatal transmission from an HIV-positive mother to her fetus ranges from 25% to 35%. Zidovudine decreases perinatal transmission and the risk of infant death.* Elective cesarean birth significantly reduces the risk of transmission from the mother to child. Thus testing has the potential to identify HIV positive women who can then be treated. Health care providers have an obligation to ensure that pregnant women are well informed about HIV symptoms, testing, and methods of decreasing maternal-fetal transmission. However, mandatory HIV screening involves ethical issues related to privacy invasion, discrimination, social stigma, and reproductive risks to the pregnant woman.

*Source: Brocklehurst, P., & Volmink, J. (2002). Antiretrovirals for reducing the risk of mother-to-child transmission of HIV infection. *The Cochrane Database for Systematic Reviews,* 2006, Issue 3. Chichester, UK: John Wiley & Sons,

(PPD) tuberculin test may be administered to assess exposure to tuberculosis. During the pelvic examination, cervical and vaginal smears may be obtained for cytologic studies and for diagnosis of infection (e.g., *Chlamydia,* gonorrhea, group B streptococcus [GBS]).

The finding of risk factors during pregnancy may indicate the need to repeat some tests at other times. For example, exposure to tuberculosis or an STI would necessitate repeat testing. STIs are common in pregnancy and may have negative effects on mother and fetus. Careful assessment and screening are essential.

■ *Follow-Up Visits*

Monthly visits are scheduled routinely during the first and second trimesters, although additional appointments may be made as the need arises. During the third trimester, however, the possibility for complications increases, and closer monitoring is warranted. Starting with week 28, maternity visits are scheduled every 2 weeks until week 36, and then every week until birth, unless the health care provider individualizes the schedule. Individual needs, complications, and risks of the pregnant woman may warrant visits more or less often. The pattern of interviewing the woman first and then assessing physical changes and performing laboratory tests is maintained.

Interview. Follow-up visits are less intensive than the initial prenatal visit. At each of these follow-up visits, the woman is asked to summarize relevant events that have occurred since the previous visit. She is asked about her general emotional and physiologic well-being, complaints, problems, and questions she may have. Personal and family needs also are identified and explored.

Because the woman's emotional state affects her and her family's general well-being, the emotional adjust-ment for all is assessed at each visit. Because emotional changes are expected during pregnancy, the nurse logically asks whether the woman has had any mood swings; reactions to changes in her body image, bad dreams, or worries. Positive feelings (her own and those of her family) are also noted. The reactions of family members to the pregnancy and the woman's progression through the developmental tasks of pregnancy also are assessed and recorded.

During the third trimester, current family situations and their effect on the woman are assessed (e.g., partners', siblings', and grandparents' responses to the pregnancy and the coming child). In addition, the following questions are addressed:

- What anticipatory planning is in progress concerning new parenting responsibilities, sibling rivalry, recuperation from pregnancy and birth, and fertility management?
- What successes or frustrations with diet, rest and relaxation, sexuality, and emotional support is the woman experiencing?
- What is the woman's understanding of her family's needs in relation to the pregnancy and the unborn child?
- How well prepared are the parents for coping with an emergency? That is, does the woman know the warning signs (e.g., bleeding, abdominal pain, signs of preeclampsia), understand what they represent, and know how and to whom to report them?
- Does the woman know the signs of preterm and term labor?
- What is the woman's understanding of the labor process and expectations of herself and others during labor?
- Does she know when to come and what to bring to the hospital or birthing center?
- What plans have the woman and her family made for labor?
- What anxieties are the woman or her family experiencing regarding labor or the unborn child?
- What does the woman wish to know about the control of discomfort during labor?
- Is the woman (and her partner or support person) planning to attend any parent education classes?
- Does the woman have questions about fetal development and methods to assess fetal well-being?

A review of the woman's physical systems is appropriate at each prenatal visit, and any suspicious signs or symptoms are assessed in depth. Discomforts reflecting adaptations to pregnancy are identified. Special inquiries are made about possible infections (e.g., genitourinary tract, respiratory tract). The woman's knowledge of and success with self-care measures are assessed, as well as outcomes of prescribed therapy.

Physical Examination. Reevaluation is a constant aspect of a pregnant woman's care. Each woman reacts differently to pregnancy. As a result, careful monitoring of the pregnancy and her reactions to care is vital. The database is updated at each time of contact with the pregnant woman. Physiologic changes are documented as the pregnancy progresses and reviewed for possible deviations from normal progress.

At each visit, physical parameters are measured. Ideally, BP is taken by using the same arm at every visit, with the woman sitting, using a cuff of appropriate size (which is noted on her chart). Her weight is assessed, and the appropriateness of the gestational weight gain is evaluated in relationship to her BMI. Urine may be checked by dipstick, and the presence and degree of edema are noted. For examination of the abdomen, the woman lies on her back with her arms by her side and head supported by a pillow. The bladder should be empty. Abdominal inspection is followed by measurement of the height of the fundus. While the woman lies on her back, the nurse should be alert for the occurrence of supine hypotension (see Emergency box).

The findings revealed during the interview and physical examination reflect the status of maternal adaptations. When any of the findings is suspicious, an in-depth examination is performed. For example, careful interpretation of BP is important in the risk factor analysis of all pregnant women. BP is evaluated on the basis of absolute values and the length of gestation and is interpreted in light of modifying factors.

Individuals whose systolic BP (SBP) is 120 to 139 mm Hg or whose diastolic BP (DBP) is 80 to 89 mm Hg are viewed as prehypertensive (National High Blood Pressure Education Program [NHBPEP], 2003). Hypertension is defined by the NHBPEP Working Groups as a systolic BP of 140 mm Hg or more and a diastolic BP of 90 mm Hg or more after 20 weeks of gestation in women with previously normal blood pressure (American College of Obstetricians and Gynecologists [ACOG], 2002a).

An absolute SBP of 140 mm Hg or more and a DBP of 90 mm Hg or more suggests the presence of hypertension. An SBP ≥125 mm Hg or a DBP ≥75 mm Hg in midpregnancy or an SBP ≥130 mm Hg or DBP ≥85 in later pregnancy are indicative of problems and should be reported to the primary health care provider immediately (Peters & Flack, 2004).

A rise in SBP of 30 mm Hg or more over the baseline pressure, or rise in the DBP of 15 mm Hg more than the baseline pressure, is also a significant finding regardless of the absolute values and should be closely monitored (ACOG, 2002a). To prevent chronic health problems such as cardiovascular disease, elevated BP readings require health-promoting lifestyle modifications (NHBPEP, 2003). See Chapter 30 for an in-depth discussion of problems associated with hypertension.

The pregnant woman is monitored continuously for a range of signs and symptoms that indicate potential complications in addition to hypertension. For example, persistent and excessive vomiting and ketonuria may indicate the development of hyperemesis gravidarum. Uterine cramping and vaginal bleeding are signs of threatened miscarriage. Chills and fever are symptoms of infection. Discharge from the vagina may be amniotic fluid or may be associated with infection (see Signs of Potential Complications box).

Fetal Assessment. Toward the end of the first trimester, before the uterus is an abdominal organ, the fetal heart tones (FHTs) can be heard with an ultrasound fetoscope or an ultrasound stethoscope. To hear the FHTs, place the instrument in the midline, just above the symphysis pubis, and apply firm pressure. The woman and her family should be offered the opportunity to listen to the FHTs. The health status of the fetus is assessed at each visit for the remainder of the pregnancy by assessing FHT and fetal movement. One method for assessment of fetal movement is to count kicks for one hour following a meal, with a minimum number of 4 fetal movements being indicative of fetal well-being.

Fundal Height. During the second trimester, the uterus becomes an abdominal organ. The fundal height, measurement of the height of the uterus above the symphysis pubis, is used as one indicator of fetal growth. The measurement also provides a gross estimate of the duration of pregnancy. From gestational weeks (GW) 18 to 32, the height of the fundus in centimeters is approximately the same as the number of weeks of gestation (±2 GW), with an empty bladder at the time of measurement (Cunningham, Leveno, Bloom, Hauth, Gilstrap, & Wenstrom, 2005). For example, a woman of 28 weeks of gestation, with an empty bladder, would measure from 26 to 30 cm. In addition, the fundal height measurement may aid in the identification of high risk factors. A stable or decreased fundal height may indicate the presence of intrauterine growth restriction (IUGR); an excessive increase could indicate the presence of multifetal gestation (more than one fetus) or hydramnios.

A paper tape typically is used to measure fundal height. To increase the reliability of the measurement, the same person examines the pregnant woman at each of her prenatal visits, but often this is not possible. All clinicians who examine a particular pregnant woman should be consistent in their measurement technique. Ideally, a protocol should be established for the health care setting in which the measurement technique is explicitly set forth, and the woman's position on the examining table, the measuring device, and method of measurement used are specified. Conditions under which the measurements are taken also can be

CD: Assessment Video

EMERGENCY

Supine Hypotension

SIGNS AND SYMPTOMS
- Pallor
- Dizziness, faintness, breathlessness
- Tachycardia
- Nausea
- Clammy (damp, cool) skin; sweating

INTERVENTIONS
- Position woman on her side until her signs and symptoms subside and vital signs stabilize within normal limits (WNL).

First, Second, and Third Trimesters

FIRST TRIMESTER

SIGNS AND SYMPTOMS	POSSIBLE CAUSES
Severe vomiting	Hyperemesis gravidarum
Chills, fever	Infection
Burning on urination	Infection
Diarrhea	Infection
Abdominal cramping; vaginal bleeding	Miscarriage, ectopic pregnancy

SECOND AND THIRD TRIMESTERS

SIGNS AND SYMPTOMS	POSSIBLE CAUSES
Persistent, severe vomiting	Hyperemesis gravidarum, hypertension, preeclampsia
Sudden discharge of fluid from vagina before 37 wk	Premature rupture of membranes (PROM)
Vaginal bleeding, severe abdominal pain	Miscarriage, placenta previa, abruptio placentae
Chills, fever, burning on urination, diarrhea	Infection
Severe backache or flank pain	Kidney infection or stones; preterm labor
Change in fetal movements: absence of fetal movements after quickening, any unusual change in pattern or amount	Fetal jeopardy or intrauterine fetal death
Uterine contractions; pressure; cramping before 37 wk	Preterm labor
Visual disturbances: blurring, double vision, or spots	Hypertensive conditions, preeclampsia
Swelling of face or fingers and over sacrum	Hypertensive conditions, preeclampsia
Headaches: severe, frequent, or continuous	Hypertensive conditions, preeclampsia
Muscular irritability or convulsions	Hypertensive conditions, preeclampsia
Epigastric or abdominal pain (perceived as severe stomachache)	Hypertensive conditions, preeclampsia, abruptio placentae
Glycosuria, positive glucose tolerance test reaction	Gestational diabetes mellitus

A   B

FIG. 16-7 Measurement of fundal height from symphysis that **(A)**, includes the upper curve of the fundus and **(B)**, does not include the upper curve of the fundus. Note position of hands and measuring tape. (Courtesy Chris Rozales, San Francisco, CA.)

described in the woman's records, including whether the bladder was empty and whether the uterus was relaxed or contracted at the time of measurement.

Various positions for measuring fundal height have been described. The woman can be supine, have her head elevated, have her knees flexed, or have both her head elevated and knees flexed. Measurements obtained with the woman in the various positions differ, making it even more important to standardize the fundal height measurement technique. The bladder must be empty before the measurement is taken. As much as a 3-cm variation is possible if the bladder is full (Cunningham et al., 2005).

Placement of the tape measure also can vary. The tape can be placed in the middle of the woman's abdomen and the measurement made from the upper border of the symphysis pubis to the upper border of the fundus, with the tape measure held in contact with the skin for the entire length of the uterus (Fig. 16-7, *A*). In another measurement technique, the upper curve of the fundus is not included in the measurement. Instead, one end of the tape measure is held at the upper border of the symphysis pubis with one hand, and the other hand is placed at the upper border of the fundus. The tape is placed between the middle and index fingers of the other hand, and the point where these fingers intercept the tape measure is taken as the measurement (Fig. 16-7, *B*).

Gestational Age. In an uncomplicated pregnancy, fetal gestational age is estimated after the duration of pregnancy and the EDB are determined. Fetal gestational age is determined from the menstrual history, contraceptive history, pregnancy test result, and the following findings obtained during the clinical evaluation:

- First uterine evaluation: date, size
- Fetal heart (FH) first heard: date, method (Doppler stethoscope, fetoscope)
- Date of quickening
- Current fundal height, estimated fetal weight (EFW)
- Current week of gestation by history of LMP and/or ultrasound examination
- Ultrasound examination: date, week of gestation, biparietal diameter (BPD)
- Reliability of dates

Quickening ("feeling of life") refers to the mother's first perception of fetal movement. It usually occurs between 16 and 20 weeks of gestation and is initially experienced as a fluttering sensation. The mother's report should be recorded. Multiparas often perceive fetal movement earlier than primigravidas.

Routine use of ultrasound examination (also called a *sonogram*) in early pregnancy has been recommended, and many health care providers have this equipment available in the office. This procedure may be used to establish the duration of pregnancy if the woman cannot give a precise date for her LMP or if the size of the uterus does not conform to the EDB as calculated by Nägele's rule. Ultrasound also provides information about the well-being of the fetus. However, the routine use of ultrasound has not been found to substantively improve fetal outcome (Neilson, 2002). Nurses performing ultrasound have a valuable opportunity to provide both education and support to the pregnant woman and her family.

Health Status. The assessment of fetal health status includes consideration of fetal movement. The mother is instructed to note the extent and timing of fetal movements and to report immediately if the pattern changes or if movement ceases. Regular movement has been found to be a reliable indicator of fetal health (Cunningham et al., 2005).

The fetal heart rate (FHR) is checked on routine visits once it has been heard (Fig. 16-8, *A*). Early in the second trimester, the heartbeat may be heard with a Doppler stethoscope (Fig. 16-8, *B*). To detect the heartbeat before the fetal position can be palpated by Leopold maneuvers (see Fig. 27-5), the scope is moved around the abdomen until the heartbeat is heard. Each nurse develops a set pattern for searching the abdomen for the heartbeat—for example, starting first in the midline about 2 to 3 cm above the symphysis, then moving to the left lower quadrant, and so on. The heartbeat is counted for 1 minute, and the quality and rhythm noted. Later in the second trimester, the

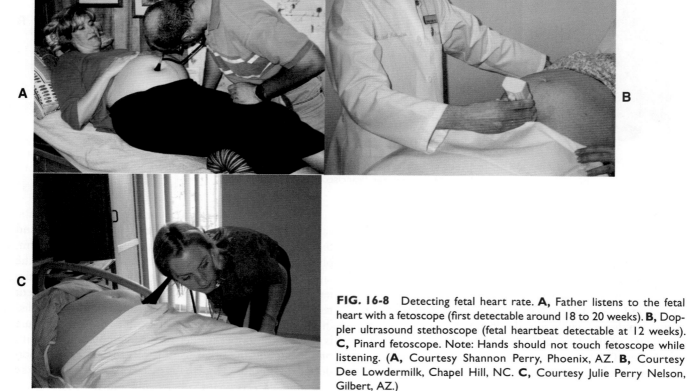

FIG. 16-8 Detecting fetal heart rate. **A,** Father listens to the fetal heart with a fetoscope (first detectable around 18 to 20 weeks). **B,** Doppler ultrasound stethoscope (fetal heartbeat detectable at 12 weeks). **C,** Pinard fetoscope. Note: Hands should not touch fetoscope while listening. (**A,** Courtesy Shannon Perry, Phoenix, AZ. **B,** Courtesy Dee Lowdermilk, Chapel Hill, NC. **C,** Courtesy Julie Perry Nelson, Gilbert, AZ.)

FHR can be determined with a fetoscope or a Pinard fetoscope (Fig. 16-8, *A* and *C*). A normal rate and rhythm are other good indicators of fetal health. Once the heart beat is noted, its absence is cause for immediate investigation.

Fetal health status is investigated intensively if any maternal or fetal complications arise (e.g., gestational hypertension, IUGR, premature rupture of membranes [PROM], irregular or absent FHR, or absence of fetal movements after quickening). Careful, precise, and concise recording of client responses and laboratory results contributes to the continuous supervision vital to ensuring the well-being of the mother and fetus.

Laboratory Tests. The number of routine laboratory tests done during follow-up visits in pregnancy is limited. A clean-catch urine specimen is obtained to test for glucose, protein, nitrites, and leukocytes at each visit. Urine specimens for culture and sensitivity, as well as blood samples, are obtained only if signs and symptoms warrant.

It is recommended that the maternal serum alphafetoprotein (MSAFP) screening be done between 15 and 22 GW, ideally between 16 and 18 weeks of gestation (Jenkins & Wapner, 2004). Elevated levels are associated with open neural tube defects and multiple gestations, whereas low levels are associated with Down syndrome. Abnormal levels are followed by second trimester ultrasonography for a more indepth investigation (Benn, Egan, Fang, & Smith-Bindman, 2004). The multiple-marker, or triple-screen, blood test is also recommended (Graves, Miller, & Sellers, 2002). Done between 16 and 18 weeks of gestation, it measures the MSAFP, hCG, and unconjugated estriol, the levels of which are combined to yield one value. Low levels may be associated with Down syndrome and other chromosomal abnormalities (Cunningham et al., 2005). Other blood tests are repeated as necessary: RPR/VDRL test for syphilis; CBC with hematocrit, hemoglobin, and differential values; antibody screen, rubella, toxoplasmosis, anti-Rh, HIV; sickle cell; and level of folate when indicated. Cervical and vaginal smears are repeated as necessary.

If not done earlier in pregnancy, a glucose screen is obtained. A glucose challenge is usually done between 24 and 28 weeks of gestation. GBS testing is done between 35 and 37 weeks of gestation; cultures collected earlier will not accurately predict GBS status at time of birth (Box 16-3) (Himmelberger, 2002). GBS testing may be done also at the initial physical to identify and treat women who are GBS positive who may give birth before 35 weeks of gestation.

---

box 16-3 Risk Factors Indicating Need for GBS Prophylaxis

- Previous infant with a group B streptococcus infection
- GBS bacteriuria during this pregnancy
- Membranes ruptured or onset of labor before 37 wk of gestation

Data from Himmelberger, S. (2002). Preventing group B strep in newborns. *AWHONN Lifelines, 6*(4), 339-342.

Other Tests. Other diagnostic tests are available to assess the health status of both the pregnant woman and the fetus. Ultrasonography, for example, may be performed to determine the status of the pregnancy and to confirm gestational age of the fetus. Amniocentesis, a procedure used to obtain amniotic fluid for analysis, may be needed to evaluate the fetus for genetic disorders or gestational maturity. These and other tests that are used to determine health risks for the mother and infant are described in Chapter 29.

After obtaining information through the assessment process, the data are analyzed to identify deviations from the norm and unique needs of the pregnant woman and her family. Although comprehensive health care requires collaboration among professionals from several disciplines, nurses are in an excellent position to formulate diagnoses that can be used to guide independent interventions. The following are examples of the nursing diagnoses that may be appropriate in the prenatal period.

- *Anxiety related to*
  - –physical discomforts of pregnancy
  - –ambivalent and labile emotions
  - –changes in family dynamics
  - –fetal well-being
  - –ability to manage anticipated labor
- *Constipation related to*
  - –progesterone relaxation of GI smooth muscle
  - –dietary behaviors
- *Imbalanced nutrition: less than body requirements related to*
  - –morning sickness (nausea and vomiting)
  - –fatigue
- *Disturbed body image related to*
  - –anatomic and physiologic changes of pregnancy
  - –changes in the couple relationship
- *Disturbed sleep patterns related to*
  - –discomforts of late pregnancy
  - –anxiety about approaching labor

▄ Expected Outcomes of Care

The plan of nursing care for women and their families during pregnancy is guided by the diagnoses that have been formulated during prenatal visits. Individualized plans that are developed mutually with the pregnant woman or couple are more likely to result in desirable outcomes than are those developed by the nurse for the woman. Measured outcomes of prenatal care include not only physical outcomes but also developmental and psychosocial outcomes.

The following are examples of outcomes that the pregnant woman may be expected to achieve:

- Verbalize decreased anxiety about the health of her fetus and herself.
- Verbalize improved family dynamics.
- Show appropriate weight gain patterns per trimester.
- Report increasing acceptance of changes in body image.

- Demonstrate knowledge for self-care.
- Seek clarification of information about pregnancy and birth.
- Report signs and symptoms of complications.
- Describe appropriate measures taken to relieve physical discomforts.
- Develop a realistic birth plan.

Plan of Care and Interventions

The nurse-client relationship is critical in setting the tone for further interaction. The techniques of listening with an attentive expression, touching, and using eye contact have their place, as does recognizing the woman's feelings and her right to express these feelings. The interaction may occur in various formal or informal settings. The clinic, home visits, or telephone conversations all provide opportunities for contact and can be used effectively.

In supporting a woman, the nurse must remember that both the nurse and the woman are contributing to the relationship. The nurse has to accept the woman's responses as a factor in trying to be of help. An example of one nurse-client relationship is as follows:

> Keisha has been very forthright in saying that this pregnancy was unplanned but had countered this observation with comments such as, "All things happen for the best," and "Children bring their own love." Over time, as our relationship developed to one of mutual trust, she complained increasingly of her fear of pain, of hating to wear maternity clothes, and of having to give up helping the family. Finally I ventured to say, "Sometimes when a pregnancy is unplanned, women resent it and are angry about it." Her relief was evident. She said, "You don't know how angry I've been." As a result, the whole tenor of support being offered changed, and the plan was adjusted to meet her real needs.

The nurse also must accept that the woman must be a willing partner in a purely voluntary relationship. As such, the relationship can be refused or terminated at any time by the pregnant woman or her family.

Supportive care involves developing, augmenting, or changing the mechanisms used by women and their families in coping with stress. The nurse tries to promote active participation by the people in the solution of their own problems. The nurse can help a woman gather pertinent information, explore options, decide on a course of action, and assume responsibility for the outcomes. These outcomes may include living with a problem as it is, easing the effects of a problem so that it can be accepted more readily, or eliminating the problem by effecting change.

At other times a successful outcome can be documented readily. For example, a woman who early in her pregnancy had predicted a severe depressive state in the postbirth period was elated when such a state did not materialize. She remarked to the nurse who had provided support during the pregnancy and birth, "You're the best nerve medicine I've ever had!"

Care Paths

Better coordination of prenatal care services for childbearing families is emphasized in current health care systems. Because a large number of health care professionals can be involved in care of the expectant mother, unintentional gaps or overlaps in care may occur. Care paths can be used to improve the consistency of care and to reduce costs. Although the Care Path on p. 403 focuses only on prenatal education, it is one example of the type of form that might be developed to guide health care providers in carrying out the appropriate assessments and interventions in a timely way. Use of care paths also may contribute to improved satisfaction of families with the prenatal care provided, and members of the health care team may function more efficiently and effectively.

Education About Maternal and Fetal Changes

Expectant parents are typically curious about the growth and development of the fetus and the subsequent changes that occur in the mother's body. Mothers in particular are sometimes more tolerant of the discomforts related to the continuing pregnancy if they understand the underlying causes. Educational literature that describes fetal and maternal changes is available and can be used in explaining changes as they occur. The nurse's familiarity with any material shared with pregnant families is essential to effective client education. Educational material may include electronic and written materials appropriate to the pregnant woman's or couple's literacy level and experience and the agency's resources. It is important that available educational materials reflect the pregnant woman's or couple's ethnicity, culture, and literacy level to be most effective.

Education for Self-Care

The expectant mother needs information about many subjects. The nurse who is observant, listens, and knows typical concerns of expectant parents can anticipate questions that will be asked and prompt mothers and partners to discuss what is on their minds. Many times, printed literature can be given to supplement the individualized teaching the nurse provides, and women often avidly read books and pamphlets related to their own experience. When nurses read the literature before they distribute it, they have an opportunity to point out areas that may not correspond with local health care practices. Since family members are common sources for health information, it is also important to include them in the health education endeavors (Lewallen, 2004). In addition, as more individuals use the computer for information, the pregnant woman or couple may have questions from their Internet reviews. Nurses may also share recommended electronic sites from reliable sources.

Pregnant women who receive conflicting advice or instruction are likely to grow increasingly frustrated with members of the health care team and the care provided. Several topics that may cause concerns in pregnant women are discussed in the following sections.

care path ▶   **Prenatal Care Pathway**

PRENATAL EDUCATION CLINICAL PATHWAY

INITIAL VISIT AND ORIENTATION: _____   SOCIAL SERVICE: _____   DIETITIAN: _____

I. EARLY PREGNANCY (WEEKS 1-20) (Initial and date after education given)

Fetal growth and development _____	Testing: Labs _____	Ultrasound _____
Maternal changes _____	Possible Complications:	
Lifestyle: Exercise/stress/nutrition _____	a. Threatened miscarriage _____	
Drugs, OTC, tobacco, alcohol	b. Diabetes _____	
STIs _____	c. _____ _____	
Psychologic/social adjustments:	Introduction to breastfeeding _____	
FOB involved/accepts _____	Acceptance of pregnancy and childbirth	
Baby for adoption _____	preparation _____	
	Dietary follow-up _____	

II. MIDPREGNANCY (WEEKS 21-27) (Initial and date after education given)

Fetal growth and development _____	Breastfeeding or bottle feeding _____
Maternal changes _____	Birth plan initiated _____
Daily fetal movement _____	Childbirth preparation _____
Possible complications:	_____
a. Preterm labor prevention _____	Dietary follow-up _____
b. Preeclampsia symptoms _____	
c. _____	

III. LATE PREGNANCY (WEEKS 28-40) (Initial and date after education given)

Fetal growth and development _____	Childbirth preparation:
Fetal evaluation:	S/S of labor; labor process _____
Daily movement _____ NSTs _____	Pain management: natural childbirth,
Kick counts _____ BPPs _____	medications, epidural _____
Maternal changes _____	Cesarean; VBAC _____
Possible complications:	Birth plan complete _____
a. Preterm labor prevention _____	Review hospital policies _____
b. Preeclampsia symptoms _____	Parenting preparation:
c. _____ _____	Pediatrician _____ Child care _____
Breastfeeding preparation:	Siblings _____ Immunizations _____
Nipple assessment _____	Car seat/safety _____
Dietary follow-up _____	Postpartum
	PP care and checkup _____
	Emotional changes _____
	BC options _____
	Safer sex and STIs _____

Signature: _____

BC, Birth control; *BPP,* biophysical profile; *FOB,* father of baby; *NST,* nonstress test; *OTC,* over-the-counter preparations; *PP,* postpartum; *S/S,* signs and symptoms; *STI,* sexually transmitted infection; *VBAC,* vaginal birth after cesarean.

Nutrition. Good nutrition is important for the maintenance of maternal health during pregnancy and the provision of adequate nutrients for embryonic and fetal development (American Dietetic Association [ADA], 2002). Assessing a woman's nutritional status and providing information on nutrition are part of the nurse's responsibilities in providing prenatal care. This includes assessment of weight gain during pregnancy as well as prenatal nutrition. Teaching may include discussion about foods high in iron, encouragement to take prenatal vitamins, and recommendations to moderate or limit caffeine intake. In some settings a registered dietitian conducts classes for pregnant women on the topics of nutritional status and nutrition during pregnancy, or interviews them to assess their knowledge of these topics. Nurses can refer women to a registered dietitian if a need is revealed during the nursing assessment. (For detailed information concerning maternal and fetal nutritional needs and related nursing care, see Chapter 15.)

Personal Hygiene. During pregnancy, the sebaceous (sweat) glands are highly active because of hormonal influences, and women often perspire freely. They may be reassured that the increase is normal and that their previous patterns of perspiration will return after the postpartum period. Baths and warm showers can be therapeutic because they relax tense, tired muscles, help counter insomnia, and make the pregnant woman feel fresh. Tub bathing is permitted even in late pregnancy because little water enters the vagina unless under pressure. However, late in pregnancy, when the woman's center of gravity lowers, she is at risk for falling. Tub bathing is contraindicated after rupture of the membranes.

Prevention of Urinary Tract Infections. Because of physiologic changes that occur in the renal system during pregnancy (see Chapter 14), urinary tract infections are common but they may be asymptomatic. Women should be instructed to inform their health care provider if blood or pain occurs with urination. These infections pose a risk to the mother and fetus; therefore the prevention or early treatment of these infections is essential.

The nurse can assess the woman's understanding and use of good handwashing techniques before and after urinating and the importance of wiping the perineum from front to back. Soft, absorbent toilet tissue, preferably white and unscented, should be used; harsh, scented, or printed toilet paper may cause irritation. Bubble bath or other bath oils should be avoided because these may irritate the urethra. Women should wear cotton-crotch underpants and panty hose and avoid wearing tight-fitting slacks or jeans for long periods; anything that allows a buildup of heat and moisture in the genital area may foster the growth of bacteria.

Some women do not consume enough fluid and food. After discovering the woman's food preferences, the nurse should advise her to drink at least 2 L (eight glasses) of liquid a day, preferably water, to maintain an adequate fluid intake that ensures frequent urination. Pregnant women should not limit fluids in an effort to reduce the frequency of urination. Women need to know that if urine looks dark (concentrated), they must increase their fluid intake. The consumption of yogurt and acidophilus milk also may help prevent urinary tract and vaginal infections. The nurse should review healthy urination practices with the woman. Women are told not to ignore the urge to urinate because holding urine lengthens the time bacteria are in the bladder and allows them to multiply. Women should plan ahead when they are faced with situations that may normally require them to delay urination (e.g., a long car ride). They always should urinate before going to bed at night. Bacteria can be introduced during intercourse;

therefore, women are advised to urinate before and after intercourse, and then drink a large glass of water to promote additional urination. Although frequently recommended, there is conflicting evidence regarding the effectiveness of cranberry juice and, in particular, the effective dosage in the prevention of urinary tract infections (Jepson, Mihaljevic, & Craig, 2004; Kiel, Nashelsky, Robbins, & Bondi, 2003; Raz, Chazan, & Dan, 2004).

Kegel Exercises. Kegel exercises, deliberate contraction and relaxation of the pubococcygeus muscle, strengthen the muscles around the reproductive organs and improve muscle tone. Many women are not aware of the muscles of the pelvic floor until it is pointed out that these are the muscles used during urination and sexual intercourse that can be consciously controlled. The muscles of the pelvic floor encircle the vaginal outlet, and they need to be exercised, because an exercised muscle can then stretch and contract readily at the time of birth. Practice of pelvic muscle exercises during pregnancy also results in fewer complaints of urinary incontinence in late pregnancy and postpartum (Sampselle, 2003).

Several ways of performing Kegel exercises have been described. The method described in the Teaching for Self-Care box in Chapter 5 demonstrates evidence-based nursing care. This method was developed by nurses involved in a research utilization project for continence in women. Teaching has been effective if the woman reports an increased ability to control urine flow and greater muscular control during sexual intercourse.

Preparation for Breastfeeding. Pregnant women are usually eager to discuss their plans for feeding the newborn. Breast milk is the food of choice, in part because breastfeeding is associated with a decreased incidence of perinatal morbidity and mortality. The American Academy of Pediatrics recommends breastfeeding for at least a year. However, a deep-seated aversion to breastfeeding on the part of the woman or partner, the woman's need for certain medications or use of street drugs, and certain life-threatening illnesses and medical complications, such as HIV infection, are contraindications to breastfeeding (Lawrence & Lawrence, 2005). Although hepatitis B antigen has not been shown to be transmitted through breast milk, as an added precaution, it is recommended that infants born to HBsAg–positive women receive the hepatitis B vaccine and hepatitis B immune globulin (HBIg) immediately after birth. Women who are HIV positive are discouraged from nursing because the risk of HIV transmission outweighs the risk of the infant dying from another cause (Lawrence & Lawrence).

A woman's decision about the method of infant feeding often is made before pregnancy; therefore the education of women of childbearing age about the benefits of breastfeeding is essential. If undecided, the pregnant woman and her partner are encouraged to choose which method of feeding is suitable for them (Pavill, 2002). Once the couple has been given information about the advantages and

Evolve/CD: Case Study: Third Trimester

disadvantages of bottle feeding and breastfeeding, they can make an informed choice. Health care providers support their decisions and provide any needed assistance.

Women with inverted nipples need special consideration if they are planning to breastfeed. The pinch test is done to determine whether the nipple is everted or inverted (Fig. 16-9). The nurse shows the woman the way to perform the pinch test. It involves having the woman place her thumb and forefinger on her areola and gently press inward. This action will cause her nipple either to stand erect or to invert. Most nipples will stand erect.

Exercises to break the adhesions that cause the nipple to invert do not work and may precipitate uterine contractions (Lawrence & Lawrence, 2005). The use of breast shells, small plastic devices that fit over the nipples, may be recommended for women who have flat or inverted nipples (Fig. 16-10). Breast shells work by exerting a continuous, gentle pressure around the areola that pushes the nipple through a central opening in the inner shield. Breast shells should be worn for 1 to 2 hours daily during the last trimester of pregnancy. They should be worn for gradually increasing lengths of time (Lawrence & Lawrence). Breast

FIG. 16-10 Breast shell in place inside bra to evert nipple. (Courtesy Michael S. Clement, MD, Mesa, AZ.)

stimulation is contraindicated in women at risk for preterm labor; therefore the decision to suggest the use of breast shells to women with flat or inverted nipples must be made judiciously. Continuous support and guidance must be given to the woman as part of the nursing plan of care.

The woman is taught to cleanse the nipples with warm water to keep the ducts from being blocked with dried colostrum. Soap, ointments, alcohol, and tinctures should not be applied because they remove protective oils that keep the nipples supple. The use of these substances may cause the nipples to crack during early lactation (Lawrence & Lawrence, 2005).

The woman who plans to breastfeed should purchase a nursing bra that will accommodate her increased breast size during the last few months of pregnancy and during lactation. If her breasts are very heavy, or if the woman feels uncomfortable with the weight unsupported, the bra can be worn day and night.

Dental Care. Dental care during pregnancy is especially important because nausea during pregnancy may lead to poor oral hygiene, allowing dental caries to develop. A fluoride toothpaste should be used daily. Inflammation and infection of the gingival and periodontal tissues may occur (Carl, Roux, & Matacale, 2000). Research links periodontal disease with preterm births and LBW (Lopez, 2005) and an increased risk for preeclampsia (Boggess, Lieff, Murtha, Moss, Beck, & Offenbacher, 2003).

Because calcium and phosphorus in the teeth are fixed in enamel, the old adage "for every child a tooth" is not true. There is no scientific evidence to support the belief that filling teeth or even dental extraction involving the administration of local or nitrous oxide–oxygen anesthesia precipitates miscarriage or premature labor. However, antibacterial therapy should be considered for sepsis, especially in pregnant women who have had rheumatic heart disease or nephritis. Emergency dental surgery is not contraindicated during pregnancy. However, the risks

A

B

FIG. 16-9 **A,** Normal nipple everts with gentle pressure. **B,** Inverted nipple inverts with gentle pressure. (Modified from Lawrence, R., and Lawrence, R. [2005]. *Breastfeeding: A guide for the medical profession* [6th ed.]. Philadelphia: Mosby.)

and benefits of dental surgery must be explained. If dental treatment is necessary, the woman will be most comfortable during the second trimester because the uterus is now outside the pelvis but not so large as to cause discomfort while she sits in a dental chair (Carl et al., 2000).

Physical Activity. Physical activity promotes a feeling of well-being in the pregnant woman. It improves circulation, promotes relaxation and rest, and counteracts boredom, as it does in the nonpregnant woman (ACOG, 2002b). Detailed exercise tips for pregnancy are presented in the Teaching for Self-Care box. Exercises that help relieve the low back pain that often arises during the second trimester because of the increased weight of the fetus are demonstrated in Fig. 16-11.

Posture and Body Mechanics. Skeletal and musculature changes and hormonal changes (relaxin) in pregnancy

may predispose the woman to backache and possible injury. As pregnancy progresses, the pregnant woman's center of gravity changes, pelvic joints soften and relax, and stress is placed on abdominal musculature. Poor posture and body mechanics contribute to the discomfort and potential for injury. To minimize these problems, women can learn good body posture and body mechanics (Fig. 16-12). Strategies to prevent or relieve backache are presented in the Teaching for Self-Care box.

Rest and Relaxation. The pregnant woman is encouraged to plan regular rest periods, particularly as pregnancy advances. The side-lying position is recommended because it promotes uterine perfusion and fetoplacental oxygenation by eliminating pressure on the ascending vena cava and descending aorta, which can lead to supine hypotension (Fig. 16-13). The mother also should be shown the

FIG. 16-11 Exercises. **A-C,** Pelvic rocking relieves low backache (excellent for relief of menstrual cramps as well). **D,** Abdominal breathing aids relaxation and lifts abdominal wall off uterus.

FIG. 16-12 Correct body mechanics. **A,** Squatting. **B,** Lifting. (Courtesy Michael S. Clement, MD, Mesa, AZ.)

TEACHING FOR SELF-CARE

Exercise Tips for Pregnant Women

- *Consult your health care provider* when you know or suspect you are pregnant. Discuss your medical and obstetric history, your current exercise regimen, and the exercises you would like to continue throughout pregnancy.
- *Seek help* in determining an exercise routine that is well within your limit of tolerance, especially if you have not been exercising regularly.
- *Consider decreasing weight-bearing exercises* (jogging, running) and concentrating on non–weight bearing activities such as swimming, cycling, or stretching. If you are a runner, starting in your seventh month, you may wish to walk instead.
- *Avoid risky activities* such as surfing, mountain climbing, sky-diving, and racquetball because such activities, which require precise balance and coordination, may be dangerous. Avoid activities that require holding your breath and bearing down (Valsalva maneuver). Jerky, bouncy motions also should be avoided.
- *Exercise regularly* every day if possible, as long as you are healthy, to improve muscle tone and increase or maintain your stamina. Exercising sporadically may put undue strain on your muscles. Thirty minutes of moderate physical exercise is recommended. This activity can be broken up into shorter segments with rest in between. For example, exercise for 10 to 15 minutes, rest for 2 to 3 minutes, then exercise for another 10 to 15 minutes.
- *Decrease your exercise level* as your pregnancy progresses. The normal alterations of advancing pregnancy, such as decreased cardiac reserve and increased respiratory effort, may produce physiologic stress if you exercise strenuously for a long time.
- *Take your pulse* every 10 to 15 minutes while you are exercising. If it is more than 140 beats/min, slow down until it returns to a maximum of 90 beats/min. You should be able to converse easily while exercising. If you cannot, you need to slow down.
- *Avoid becoming overheated* for extended periods. It is best not to exercise for more than 35 minutes, especially in hot, humid weather. As your body temperature rises, the heat is transmitted to your fetus. Prolonged or repeated elevation of fetal temperature may result in birth defects, especially during the first 3 months. Your temperature should not exceed 38° C.
- *Avoid the use of hot tubs and saunas.*
- *Warm-up and stretching exercises* prepare your joints for more strenuous exercise and lessen the likelihood of strain or injury to your joints. After the fourth month of gestation, you should not perform exercises flat on your back.
- *A cool-down period* of mild activity involving your legs after an exercise period will help bring your respiration, heart, and metabolic rates back to normal and prevent the pooling of blood in the exercised muscles.
- *Rest for 10 minutes after exercising*, lying on your side. As the uterus grows, it puts pressure on a major vein in your abdomen, which carries blood to your heart. Lying on your side removes the pressure and promotes return circulation from your extremities and muscles to your heart, thereby increasing blood flow to your placenta and fetus. You should rise gradually from the floor to prevent dizziness or fainting (orthostatic hypotension).
- *Drink two or three 8-oz glasses of water* after you exercise to replace the body fluids lost through perspiration. While exercising, drink water whenever you feel the need.
- *Increase your caloric intake* to replace the calories burned during exercise and provide the extra energy needs of pregnancy. (Pregnancy alone requires an additional 340-452 kcal/day.) Choose such high-protein foods as fish, milk, cheese, eggs, and meat.
- *Take your time.* This is not the time to be competitive or train for activities requiring speed or long endurance.
- *Wear a supportive bra.* Your increased breast weight may cause changes in posture and put pressure on the ulnar nerve.
- *Wear supportive shoes.* As your uterus grows, your center of gravity shifts and you compensate for this by arching your back. These natural changes may make you feel off balance and more likely to fall.
- *Stop exercising immediately* if you experience shortness of breath, dizziness, numbness, tingling, pain of any kind, more than four uterine contractions per hour, decreased fetal activity, or vaginal bleeding, and consult your health care provider.

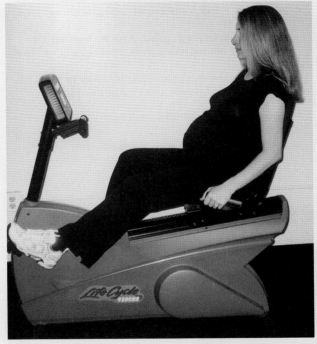

Riding a recumbent bicycle provides exercise while supplying back support. (Courtesy Shannon Perry, Phoenix, AZ.)

Sources: American College of Obstetricians and Gynecologists (ACOG). (2002). Exercise during pregnancy and the postpartum period. ACOG Committee Opinion No. 267. *Obstetrics & Gynecology, 99*(1), 171-173; Kramer, M. (2002). Aerobic exercise for women during pregnancy. *The Cochrane Database for Systematic Reviews, 2006*, Issue 3. Chichester, UK: John Wiley & Sons; Morris, S., & Johnson, N. (2005). Exercise in pregnancy: A critical appraisal of the literature. *Journal of Reproductive Medicine, 50*(3), 181-188.

TEACHING FOR SELF-CARE

Posture and Body Mechanics

TO PREVENT OR RELIEVE BACKACHE

Do pelvic tilt:
- Pelvic tilt (rock) on hands and knees (see Fig. 16-11, A) and while sitting in straight-back chair.
- Pelvic tilt (rock) in standing position against a wall, or lying on floor (see Fig. 16-11, B and C).
- Perform abdominal muscle contractions during pelvic tilt while standing, lying, or sitting to help strengthen rectus abdominis muscle (see Fig. 16-11, D).
- Use good body mechanics.
- Use leg muscles to reach objects on or near floor. Bend at the knees, not from the back. Knees are bent to lower body to squatting position. Feet are kept 12 to 18 inches apart to provide a solid base to maintain balance (see Fig. 16-12, A).
- Lift with the legs. To lift heavy object (e.g., young child), one foot is placed slightly in front of the other and kept flat as woman lowers herself onto one knee. She lifts the weight holding it close to her body and never higher than the chest. To stand up or sit down, she places one leg slightly behind the other as she raises or lowers herself (see Fig. 16-12, B).

TO RESTRICT THE LUMBAR CURVE
- For prolonged standing (e.g., ironing, employment), place one foot on low footstool or box; change positions often.
- Move car seat forward so that knees are bent and higher than hips. If needed, use a small pillow to support low back area.
- Sit in chairs low enough to allow both feet to be placed on floor, preferably with knees higher than hips.

TO PREVENT ROUND LIGAMENT PAIN AND STRAIN ON ABDOMINAL MUSCLES
- Implement suggestions given in Table 16-2.

way to rise slowly from a side-lying position to prevent placing strain on the back and to minimize the orthostatic hypotension caused by changes in position common in the latter part of pregnancy. To stretch and rest back muscles at home or work, the nurse can show the woman the way to do the following exercises:

Stand behind a chair. Support and balance self by using the back of the chair (Fig. 16-14). Squat for 30 seconds; stand for 15 seconds. Repeat 6 times, several times per day, as needed. Then, while sitting in a chair, lower head to knees for 30 seconds. Raise head. Repeat 6 times, several times per day, as needed.

Conscious relaxation is the process of releasing tension from the mind and body through deliberate effort and practice. The ability to relax consciously and intentionally can be beneficial for the following reasons:
- To relieve the normal discomforts related to pregnancy
- To reduce stress and therefore diminish pain perception during the childbearing cycle
- To heighten self-awareness and trust in one's own ability to control responses and functions
- To help cope with stress in everyday life situations, whether the woman is pregnant or not

The techniques for conscious relaxation are numerous and varied. Guidelines are given in Box 16-4.

Employment. Employment of pregnant women usually has no adverse effects on pregnancy outcomes. Job discrimination that is based strictly on pregnancy is illegal. However, some job environments pose potential risk to the fetus (e.g., dry-cleaning plants, chemistry laboratories, parking garages). Excessive fatigue is usually the deciding

FIG. 16-13 Side-lying position for rest and relaxation. Some women prefer to support upper part of leg with pillows. (Courtesy Julie Perry Nelson, Gilbert, AZ.)

FIG. 16-14 Squatting for muscle relaxation and strengthening and for keeping leg and hip joints flexible. (Courtesy Michael S. Clement, MD, Mesa, AZ.)

box 16-4 | Conscious Relaxation Tips

- *Preparation:* Loosen clothing, assume a comfortable sitting or side-lying position with all parts of body well supported with pillows.
- *Beginning:* Allow yourself to feel warm and comfortable. Inhale and exhale slowly, and imagine peaceful relaxation coming over each part of the body, starting with the neck and working down to the toes. Often people who learn conscious relaxation speak of feeling relaxed even if some discomfort is present.
- *Maintenance:* Use imagery (fantasy or daydream) to maintain the state of relaxation. Using active imagery, imagine yourself moving or doing some activity and experiencing its sensations. Using passive imagery, imagine yourself watching a scene, such as a lovely sunset.
- *Awakening:* Return to the wakeful state gradually. Slowly begin to take in stimuli from the surrounding environment.
- *Further retention and development of the skill:* Practice regularly for some periods each day, for example, at the same hour for 10 to 15 minutes each day, to feel refreshed, revitalized, and invigorated.

TEACHING FOR SELF-CARE

Safety During Pregnancy

Changes in the body resulting from pregnancy include relaxation of joints, alteration to center of gravity, faintness, and discomforts. Problems with coordination and balance are common. Therefore, the woman should follow these guidelines:

- Use good body mechanics.
- Use safety features on tools and vehicles (safety seat belts, shoulder harnesses, headrests, goggles, helmets) as specified.
- Avoid activities requiring coordination, balance, and concentration.
- Take rest periods; reschedule daily activities to meet rest and relaxation needs.

Embryonic and fetal development is vulnerable to environmental teratogens. Many potentially dangerous chemicals are present in the home, yard, and workplace: cleaning agents, paints, sprays, herbicides, and pesticides. The soil and water supply may be unsafe. Therefore the woman should follow these guidelines:

- Read all labels for ingredients and proper use of product.
- Ensure adequate ventilation with clean air.
- Dispose of wastes appropriately.
- Wear gloves when handling chemicals.
- Change job assignments or workplace as necessary.
- Avoid travel to high-altitude regions, which could jeopardize oxygen intake.

factor in the termination of employment. Strategies to improve safety during pregnancy are described in the Teaching for Self-Care box.

Women with sedentary jobs need to walk around at intervals to counter the usual sluggish circulation in the legs. They also should neither sit nor stand in one position for long periods, and they should avoid crossing their legs at the knees, because all of these activities can foster the development of varices and thrombophlebitis. Standing for long periods also increases the risk of preterm labor. The pregnant woman's chair should provide adequate back support. Use of a footstool can prevent pressure on veins, relieve strain on varicosities, minimize edema of feet, and prevent backache.

Clothing. Some women continue to wear their usual clothes during pregnancy as long as they fit and feel comfortable. If maternity clothing is needed, outfits may be purchased new or found at thrift shops or garage sales in good condition. Comfortable, loose clothing is recommended. Tight bras and belts, stretch pants, garters, tight-top knee socks, panty girdles, and other constrictive clothing should be avoided because tight clothing over the perineum encourages vaginitis and miliaria (heat rash), and impaired circulation in the legs can cause varicosities.

Maternity bras are constructed to accommodate the increased breast weight, chest circumference, and the size of breast tail tissue (under the arm). These bras also have drop-flaps over the nipples to facilitate breastfeeding. A good bra can help prevent neckache and backache.

Maternal support hose give considerable comfort and promote greater venous emptying in women with large varicose veins. Ideally, support stockings should be put on before the woman gets out of bed in the morning. Figure 16-15 demonstrates a position for resting the legs and reducing swelling and varicosities.

Comfortable shoes that provide firm support and promote good posture and balance also are advisable. Very high heels and platform shoes are not recommended because of the changes in the pregnant woman's center of gravity, and the hormone relaxin, which softens pelvic joints in later pregnancy, all of which can cause her to lose her balance. In addition, in the third trimester, the woman's pelvis tilts

FIG. 16-15 Position for resting legs and for reducing edema and varicosities. Encourage woman with vulvar varicosities to include pillow under her hips. (Courtesy Julie Perry Nelson, Gilbert, AZ.)

forward, and her lumbar curve increases. The resulting leg aches and cramps are aggravated by nonsupportive shoes. Exercises to relieve legs cramps are depicted in Fig. 16-16.

Travel. Travel is not contraindicated in low risk pregnant women. However, women with high risk pregnancies are advised to avoid long-distance travel after fetal viability has been reached to avert possible economic and psychologic consequences of giving birth to a preterm infant far from home. Travel to areas in which medical care is poor, water is untreated, or malaria is prevalent should be avoided if possible. Women who contemplate foreign travel should be aware that many health insurance carriers do not cover a birth in a foreign setting or even hospitalization for preterm labor. In addition, vaccinations for foreign travel may be contraindicated during pregnancy.

Pregnant women who travel for long distances should schedule periods of activity and rest. While sitting, the woman can practice deep breathing, foot circling, and alternately contracting and relaxing different muscle groups. She should avoid becoming fatigued. Although travel in itself is not a cause of adverse outcomes such as miscarriage or preterm labor, certain precautions are recommended while traveling in a car. For example, women riding in a car should wear automobile restraints and stop and walk every hour.

Maternal death as a result of injury is the most common cause of fetal death. The next most common cause is placental separation (abruptio placentae) that occurs because body contours change in reaction to the force of a collision. The uterus as a muscular organ can adapt its shape to that of the body, but the placenta is not resilient. At the impact of collision, placental separation can occur. A combination lap belt and shoulder harness is the most effective automobile restraint, and both should be used (Fig. 16-17). The lap belt should be worn low across the pelvic bones and as snug as is comfortable. The shoulder harness should be worn above the gravid uterus and below the neck to prevent chafing. The pregnant woman should sit upright. The headrest should be used to prevent whiplash injury.

Pregnant women traveling in high-altitude regions have lowered oxygen levels that may cause fetal hypoxia, especially if the pregnant woman is anemic. However, the current information on this condition is limited, and recommendations are not standardized.

Airline travel in large commercial jets usually poses little risk to the pregnant woman, but policies vary from airline to airline. The pregnant woman is advised to inquire about restrictions or recommendations from her carrier. Most health care providers allow air travel up to 36 weeks of gestation in women without medical or pregnancy complications. Metal detectors used at airport security checkpoints are not harmful to the fetus. The 8% humidity at which the cabins of commercial airlines are maintained may result in

A

B

FIG. 16-16 Relief of muscle spasm (leg cramps). **A,** Another person dorsiflexes foot with knee extended. **B,** Woman stands and leans forward, thereby dorsiflexing foot of affected leg. (Courtesy Shannon Perry, Phoenix, AZ.)

FIG. 16-17 Proper use of seat belt and headrest. (Courtesy Brian and Mayannyn Sallee, Las Vegas, NV.)

some water loss; hydration (with water) should therefore be maintained under these conditions. Sitting in the cramped seat of an airliner for prolonged periods may increase the risk of superficial and deep thrombophlebitis; therefore a pregnant woman is encouraged to take a 15-minute walk around the aircraft during each hour of travel to minimize this risk. However, women who are pilots, flight attendants, or frequent flyers expose themselves to in-flight radiation that exceeds recommended levels (Barish, 2004). Resources from the U.S. Federal Aviation Administration (www.faa.gov) will assist the health care provider in determining safe levels for those women at high risk for radiation exposure.

Medications and Herbal Preparations. Although much has been learned in recent years about fetal drug toxicity, the possible teratogenicity of many medications, both prescription and OTC, is still unknown. This is especially true for new medications and combinations of drugs. Moreover, certain subclinical errors or deficiencies in intermediate metabolism in the fetus may cause an otherwise harmless drug to be converted into a hazardous one. The greatest danger of drug-caused developmental defects in the fetus extends from the time of fertilization through the first trimester, a time when the woman may not realize she is pregnant. Self-treatment must be discouraged. The use of all drugs, including OTC medications, herbs, and vitamins, should be limited and a careful record kept of all therapeutic and nontherapeutic agents used.

Immunizations. Some concern has been raised over the safety of various immunization practices during pregnancy. Immunization with live or attenuated live viruses is contraindicated during pregnancy because of its potential teratogenicity but should be part of postpartum care (ACOG, 2003). Live-virus vaccines include those for measles (rubeola and rubella), chickenpox, and mumps, as well as the Sabin (oral) poliomyelitis vaccine (no longer used in the United States) (ACOG). Vaccines consisting of killed viruses may be used. Those that may be administered during pregnancy include tetanus, diphtheria, recombinant hepatitis B, and rabies vaccines.

Alcohol, Cigarette Smoke, Caffeine, and Drugs. A safe level of alcohol consumption during pregnancy has not yet been established. Although the consumption of occasional alcoholic beverages may not be harmful to the mother or her developing embryo or fetus, complete abstinence is strongly advised. Maternal alcoholism is associated with high rates of miscarriage and fetal alcohol syndrome; the risk for miscarriage in the first trimester is dose related (three or more drinks per day). Growing evidence indicates that the pattern of drinking (frequency, timing, and duration), especially in the first trimester, is more predictive of fetal damage than is the amount. Considerably less alcohol use is reported among pregnant women than in nonpregnant women, but a high prevalence of some alcohol use among pregnant women still exists. Such a finding underscores the need for more systematic public health efforts to educate women about the hazards of alcohol consumption during pregnancy.

Cigarette smoking or continued exposure to second-hand smoke (even if the mother does not smoke) is associated with IUGR and an increase in perinatal and infant morbidity and mortality. Smoking is associated with an increased frequency of preterm labor, PROM, abruptio placentae, placenta previa, and fetal death, possibly resulting from decreased placental perfusion. Smoking cessation activities should be incorporated into routine prenatal care (Todd, LaSala, & Neil-Urban, 2001; Yu, Park, & Schwalberg, 2002).

All women who smoke should be strongly encouraged to quit or at least reduce the number of cigarettes they smoke. Pregnant women need to be told about the negative effects of even second-hand smoke on the fetus and encouraged to avoid such environments (Andres, 2004). Efforts focused on preventing girls and women from beginning to smoke should be intensified.

Most studies of human pregnancy have revealed no association between caffeine consumption and birth defects or LBW (Andres, 2004). In contrast, some studies have documented an increased risk for miscarriage with caffeine intake greater than 300 mg/day (Giannelli, Doyle, Roman, Pelerin, & Hermon, 2003) or fetal growth restriction with caffeine intake greater than 223 mg/day (Vit, Bakketeig, Trygg, Lund-Larsen, & Jacobsen, 2003). Because other effects are unknown, however, pregnant women are advised to limit their caffeine intake, particularly coffee intake, as it has a high caffeine content per unit of measure. Therefore health care providers often encourage pregnant women to limit caffeine intake to no more than 3 cups of coffee or cola per day (ADA, 2002).

Any drug or environmental agent that enters the pregnant woman's bloodstream has the potential to cross the placenta and harm the fetus. Marijuana, heroin, and cocaine are common examples of such substances. Although the problem of substance abuse in pregnancy is considered a major public health concern and comprehensive care of drug-addicted women improves maternal and neonatal outcomes, few facilities are available for treatment of these women (see Chapters 35 and 38).

Normal Discomforts. Pregnant women have physical symptoms that would be considered abnormal in the nonpregnant state. Women pregnant for the first time have an increased need for explanations of the causes of the discomforts and for advice on ways to relieve them. The discomforts of the first trimester are fairly specific. Information about the physiology and prevention of and self-care for discomforts experienced during the three trimesters is given in Table 16-2. Box 16-5 on p. 416 lists alternative and complementary therapies and why they might be used in pregnancy (see also Figs. 4-4 and 4-5). Nurses can do much to allay a first-time mother's anxiety about such symptoms by telling her about them in advance and using terminology that the woman (or couple) can understand. Understanding the rationale for treatment promotes their participation in their care. Interventions should be individualized, with attention given to the woman's lifestyle and culture.

Text continued on p. 414.

CD: Critical Thinking Exercise: Discomforts of Pregnancy

table 16-2 Discomforts Related to Pregnancy

DISCOMFORT	PHYSIOLOGY	EDUCATION FOR SELF-CARE
FIRST TRIMESTER		
Breast changes, new sensation: pain, tingling, tenderness	Hypertrophy of mammary glandular tissue and increased vascularization, pigmentation, and size and prominence of nipples and areolae caused by hormonal stimulation	Wear supportive maternity bras with pads to absorb discharge, may be worn at night; wash with warm water and keep dry; breast tenderness may interfere with sexual expression or foreplay but is temporary
Urgency and frequency of urination	Vascular engorgement and altered bladder function caused by hormones; bladder capacity reduced by enlarging uterus and fetal presenting part	Empty bladder regularly; perform Kegel exercises; limit fluid intake before bedtime; wear perineal pad; report pain or burning sensation to primary health care provider
Languor and malaise; fatigue (early pregnancy, most commonly)	Unexplained; may be caused by increasing levels of estrogen, progesterone, and hCG or by elevated BBT; psychologic response to pregnancy and its required physical and psychologic adaptations	Rest as needed; eat well-balanced diet to prevent anemia
Nausea and vomiting, morning sickness—occurs in 50%-75% of pregnant women; starts between first and second missed periods and lasts until about fourth missed period; may occur any time during day; fathers also may have symptoms	Cause unknown; may result from hormonal changes, possibly hCG; may be partly emotional, reflecting pride in, ambivalence about, or rejection of pregnant state	Avoid empty or overloaded stomach; maintain good posture—give stomach ample room; stop smoking; eat dry carbohydrate on awakening; remain in bed until feeling subsides, or alternate dry carbohydrate every other hour with fluids such as hot herbal decaffeinated tea, milk, or clear coffee until feeling subsides; eat five to six small meals per day; avoid fried, odorous, spicy, greasy, or gas-forming foods; consult primary health care provider if intractable vomiting occurs
Ptyalism (excessive salivation) may occur starting 2 to 3 weeks after first missed period	Possibly caused by elevated estrogen levels; may be related to reluctance to swallow because of nausea	Use astringent mouthwash, chew gum, eat hard candy as comfort measures
Gingivitis and epulis (hyperemia, hypertrophy, bleeding, tenderness of the gums); condition will disappear spontaneously 1 to 2 months after birth	Increased vascularity and proliferation of connective tissue from estrogen stimulation	Eat well-balanced diet with adequate protein and fresh fruits and vegetables; brush teeth gently and observe good dental hygiene; avoid infection; see dentist
Nasal stuffiness; epistaxis (nosebleed)	Hyperemia of mucous membranes related to high estrogen levels	Use humidifier; avoid trauma; normal saline nose drops or spray may be used
Leukorrhea: often noted throughout pregnancy	Hormonally stimulated cervix becomes hypertrophic and hyperactive, producing abundant amount of mucus	Not preventable; do not douche; wear perineal pads; perform hygienic practices such as wiping front to back; report to primary health care provider if accompanied by pruritus, foul odor, or change in character or color
Psychosocial dynamics, mood swings, mixed feelings	Hormonal and metabolic adaptations; feelings about female role, sexuality, timing of pregnancy, and resultant changes in life and lifestyle	Participate in pregnancy support group; communicate concerns to partner, family, and health care provider; request referral for supportive services if needed (financial assistance)

BBT, Basal body temperature; *hCG,* human chorionic gonadotropin.

table 16-2 Discomforts Related to Pregnancy—cont'd

DISCOMFORT	PHYSIOLOGY	EDUCATION FOR SELF-CARE
SECOND TRIMESTER		
Pigmentation deepens; acne, oily skin	Melanocyte-stimulating hormone (from anterior pituitary)	Not preventable; usually resolves during puerperium
Spider nevi (angiomas) appear over neck, thorax, face, and arms during second or third trimester	Focal networks of dilated arterioles (end arteries) from increased concentration of estrogens	Not preventable; they fade slowly during late puerperium; rarely disappear completely
Pruritus (noninflammatory)	Unknown cause; various types as follows: nonpapular; closely aggregated pruritic papules	Keep fingernails short and clean; contact primary health care provider for diagnosis of cause
	Increased excretory function of skin and stretching of skin possible factors	Not preventable; use comfort measures for symptoms such as Keri baths; distraction; tepid baths with sodium bicarbonate or oatmeal added to water; lotions and oils; change of soaps or reduction in use of soap; loose clothing; see health care provider if mild sedation is needed
Palpitations	Unknown; should not be accompanied by persistent cardiac irregularity	Not preventable; contact primary health care provider if accompanied by symptoms of cardiac decompensation
Supine hypotension (vena cava syndrome) and bradycardia	Induced by pressure of gravid uterus on ascending vena cava when woman is supine; reduces uteroplacental and renal perfusion	Side-lying position or semisitting posture, with knees slightly flexed (see supine hypotension, p. 398)
Faintness and, rarely, syncope (orthostatic hypotension) may persist throughout pregnancy	Vasomotor lability or postural hypotension from hormones; in late pregnancy may be caused by venous stasis in lower extremities	Moderate exercise, deep breathing, vigorous leg movement; avoid sudden changes in position and warm crowded areas; move slowly and deliberately; keep environment cool; avoid hypoglycemia by eating five or six small meals per day; wear elastic hose; sit as necessary; if symptoms are serious, contact primary health care provider
Food cravings	Cause unknown; craving influenced by culture or geographic area	Not preventable; satisfy craving unless it interferes with well-balanced diet; report unusual cravings to primary health care provider
Heartburn (pyrosis or acid indigestion): burning sensation, occasionally with burping and regurgitation of a little sour-tasting fluid	Progesterone slows GI tract motility and digestion, reverses peristalsis, relaxes cardiac sphincter, and delays emptying time of stomach; stomach displaced upward and compressed by enlarging uterus	Limit or avoid gas-producing or fatty foods and large meals; maintain good posture; sip milk for temporary relief; drink hot herbal tea; primary health care provider may prescribe antacid between meals; contact primary health care provider for persistent symptoms
Constipation	GI tract motility slowed because of progesterone, resulting in increased resorption of water and drying of stool; intestines compressed by enlarging uterus; predisposition to constipation because of oral iron supplementation	Drink 8 to 10 glasses of water per day; include roughage in diet; engage in moderate exercise; maintain regular schedule for bowel movements; use relaxation techniques and deep breathing; do not take stool softener, laxatives, mineral oil, other drugs, or enemas without first consulting primary health care provider

GI, Gastrointestinal.

Continued

table 16-2 Discomforts Related to Pregnancy—cont'd

DISCOMFORT	PHYSIOLOGY	EDUCATION FOR SELF-CARE
SECOND TRIMESTER—cont'd		
Flatulence with bloating and belching	Reduced GI motility because of hormones, allowing time for bacterial action that produces gas; swallowing air	Chew foods slowly and thoroughly; avoid gas-producing foods, fatty foods, large meals; exercise; maintain regular bowel habits
Varicose veins (varicosities): may be associated with aching legs and tenderness; may be present in legs and vulva; hemorrhoids are varicosities in perianal area	Hereditary predisposition; relaxation of smooth muscle walls of veins because of hormones causing tortuous dilated veins in legs and pelvic vasocongestion; condition aggravated by enlarging uterus, gravity, and bearing down for bowel movements; thrombi from leg varices rare but may occur in hemorrhoids	Avoid obesity, lengthy standing or sitting, constrictive clothing, and constipation and bearing down with bowel movements; moderate exercise; rest with legs and hips elevated (see Fig. 16-15); wear support stockings; thrombosed hemorrhoid may be evacuated; relieve swelling and pain with warm sitz baths, local application of astringent compresses
Leukorrhea: often noted throughout pregnancy	Hormonally stimulated cervix becomes hypertrophic and hyperactive, producing abundant amount of mucus	Not preventable; do not douche; maintain good hygiene; wear perineal pads; report to primary health care provider if accompanied by pruritus, foul odor, or change in character or color
Headaches (through week 26)	Emotional tension (more common than vascular migraine headache); eye strain (refractory errors); vascular engorgement and congestion of sinuses resulting from hormone stimulation	Conscious relaxation; contact primary health care provider for constant "splitting" headache, to assess for preeclampsia
Carpal tunnel syndrome (involves thumb, second, and third fingers, lateral side of little finger)	Compression of median nerve resulting from changes in surrounding tissues; pain, numbness, tingling, burning; loss of skilled movements (typing); dropping of objects	Not preventable; elevate affected arms; splinting of affected hand may help; regressive after pregnancy; surgery is curative
Periodic numbness, tingling of fingers (acrodysesthesia) occurs in 5% of pregnant women	Brachial plexus traction syndrome resulting from drooping of shoulders during pregnancy (occurs especially at night and early morning)	Maintain good posture; wear supportive maternity bra; condition will disappear if lifting and carrying baby does not aggravate it
Round ligament pain (tenderness)	Stretching of ligament caused by enlarging uterus	Not preventable; rest, maintain good body mechanics to avoid overstretching ligament; relieve cramping by squatting or bringing knees to chest; sometimes heat helps
Joint pain, backache, and pelvic pressure; hypermobility of joints	Relaxation of symphyseal and sacroiliac joints because of hormones, resulting in unstable pelvis; exaggerated lumbar and cervicothoracic curves caused by change in center of gravity resulting from enlarging abdomen	Maintain good posture and body mechanics; avoid fatigue; wear low-heeled shoes; abdominal supports may be useful; conscious relaxation; sleep on firm mattress; apply local heat or ice; get back rubs; do pelvic tilt exercises; rest; condition will disappear 6 to 8 weeks after birth

■ **NURSE ALERT**

Although complementary and alternative medications (CAM) may benefit the woman during pregnancy, some practices should be avoided because they may cause miscarriage or preterm labor. It is important to ask the woman what therapies she may be using.

Recognizing Potential Complications. One of the most important responsibilities of care providers is to alert the pregnant woman to signs and symptoms that indicate a potential complication of pregnancy. The woman needs to know how and to whom to report such warning signs. Therefore the pregnant woman and her family can be reassured if they receive and use a printed form written at the appropriate literacy level, in their language and reflective of their culture, listing the signs and symptoms that warrant an investigation and the telephone numbers to call with questions or in an emergency.

The nurse must answer questions honestly as they arise during pregnancy. Pregnant women often have difficulty

table 16-2 Discomforts Related to Pregnancy—cont'd

DISCOMFORT	PHYSIOLOGY	EDUCATION FOR SELF-CARE
THIRD TRIMESTER		
Shortness of breath and dyspnea occur in 60% of pregnant women	Expansion of diaphragm limited by enlarging uterus; diaphragm is elevated about 4 cm; some relief after lightening	Good posture; sleep with extra pillows; avoid overloading stomach; stop smoking; contact health care provider if symptoms worsen to rule out anemia, emphysema, and asthma
Insomnia (later weeks of pregnancy)	Fetal movements, muscle cramping, urinary frequency, shortness of breath, or other discomforts	Reassurance; conscious relaxation; back massage or effleurage; support of body parts with pillows; warm milk or warm shower before retiring
Psychosocial responses: mood swings, mixed feelings, increased anxiety	Hormonal and metabolic adaptations; feelings about impending labor, birth, and parenthood	Reassurance and support from significant other and health care providers; improved communication with partner, family, and others
Urinary frequency and urgency return	Vascular engorgement and altered bladder function caused by hormones; bladder capacity reduced by enlarging uterus and fetal presenting part	Empty bladder regularly, Kegel exercises; limit fluid intake before bedtime; reassurance; wear perineal pad; contact health care provider for pain or burning sensation
Perineal discomfort and pressure	Pressure from enlarging uterus, especially when standing or walking; multifetal gestation	Rest, conscious relaxation, and good posture; contact health care provider for assessment and treatment if pain is present
Braxton Hicks contractions	Intensification of uterine contractions in preparation for work of labor	Reassurance; rest; change of position; practice breathing techniques when contractions are bothersome; effleurage; differentiate from preterm labor
Leg cramps (gastrocnemius spasm), especially when reclining	Compression of nerves supplying lower extremities because of enlarging uterus; reduced level of diffusible serum calcium or elevation of serum phosphorus; aggravating factors: fatigue, poor peripheral circulation, pointing toes when stretching legs or when walking, drinking more than 1 L (1 qt) of milk per day	Check for Homans sign; if negative, use massage and heat over affected muscle; dorsiflex foot until spasm relaxes (see Fig. 16-16); stand on cold surface; oral supplementation with calcium carbonate or calcium lactate tablets; aluminum hydroxide gel, 30 ml, with each meal removes phosphorus by absorbing it (consult primary health care provider before taking these remedies)
Ankle edema (nonpitting) to lower extremities	Edema aggravated by prolonged standing, sitting, poor posture, lack of exercise, constrictive clothing, or hot weather	Ample fluid intake for natural diuretic effect; put on support stockings before arising; rest periodically with legs and hips elevated (see Fig. 16-15); exercise moderately; contact health care provider if generalized edema develops; diuretics are contraindicated

deciding when to report signs and symptoms. The mother is encouraged to refer to the printed list of potential complications and to listen to her body. If she senses that something is wrong, she should call her care provider. Several signs and symptoms must be discussed more extensively. These include vaginal bleeding, alteration in fetal movements, symptoms of gestational hypertension, rupture of membranes, and preterm labor (see Signs of Potential Complications box on p. 399).

Recognizing Preterm Labor. Teaching each expectant mother to recognize preterm labor is necessary for early diagnosis and treatment. Preterm labor occurs after the twentieth week but before the thirty-seventh week of pregnancy and consists of uterine contractions that, if untreated, cause the cervix to open earlier than normal and result in preterm birth.

Although the exact etiology of preterm labor is unknown, it is assumed to have multiple causes. An increased

box 16-5 **Complementary and Alternative Therapies Used in Pregnancy**

MORNING SICKNESS AND HYPEREMESIS
- Acupuncture
- Acupressure (see Figs. 4-4 and 4-5)
- Shiatzu
- Herbal remedies*
  - Lemon balm
  - Peppermint
  - Spearmint
  - Ginger root
  - Raspberry leaf
  - Fennel
  - Chamomile
  - Hops
  - Meadowsweet
  - Wild yam root

RELAXATION AND MUSCLE-ACHE RELIEF
- Yoga
- Biofeedback
- Reflexology
- Therapeutic touch
- Massage

From Beal, M. (1998). Women's use of complementary and alternative therapies in reproductive health. *Journal of Nurse-Midwifery, 43*(3), 224-233; Schirmer, G. (1998). *Herbal medicine*. Bedford, TX: MED2000; Tiran, D., & Mack, S. (2000). *Complementary therapies for pregnancy and childbirth* (2nd ed.). Edinburgh: Baillière Tindall; Smith, C., Crowther, C., Willson, K., Hotham, N., & McMillian, V. (2004). A randomized controlled trial of ginger to treat nausea and vomiting in pregnancy. *Obstetrics & Gynecology, 103*(4), 639-645.
*Some herbs can cause miscarriage, preterm labor, or fetal or maternal injury. Pregnant women should discuss use with pregnancy health care provider, as well as an expert qualified in the use of the herb.

incidence of preterm birth is associated with sociodemographic factors such as poverty, low educational level, lack of social support, smoking, domestic violence, and stress (Freda, 2003; Freda & Patterson, 2003; Moos, 2004). Other risk factors include a previous preterm labor (McPheeters et al., 2005), current multifetal gestation, and some uterine and cervical variations (March of Dimes Birth Defects Foundation, 2005). The rate is almost twice as high in the

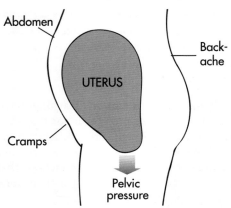

FIG. 16-18 Symptoms of preterm labor.

TEACHING FOR SELF-CARE

How to Recognize Preterm Labor

- Because the onset of preterm labor is subtle and often hard to recognize, it is important to know how to feel your abdomen for uterine contractions. You can feel for contractions in the following way:
  - While lying down, place your fingertips on the top of your uterus. A contraction is the periodic tightening or hardening of your uterus.
  - If your uterus is contracting, you will actually feel your abdomen get tight or hard and then feel it relax or soften when the contraction is over.
- If you think you are having any of the other signs and symptoms of preterm labor, empty your bladder, drink three to four glasses of water for hydration, lie down tilted toward your side, and place a pillow at your back for support.
- Check for contractions for 1 hour. To tell how often contractions are occurring, check the minutes that elapse from the beginning of one contraction to the beginning of the next.
- It is *not normal* to have frequent uterine contractions (every 10 minutes or more often for 1 hour).
- Contractions of labor are regular, frequent, and hard. They also may be felt as a tightening of the abdomen or a backache. This type of contraction causes the cervix to efface and dilate.
- Call your doctor, nurse-midwife, clinic, or labor and birth unit, or go to the hospital if any of the following signs occur:
  - You have uterine contractions every 10 minutes or more often for 1 hour, or
  - You have any of the other signs and symptoms for 1 hour, or
  - You have any bloody spotting or leaking of fluid from your vagina
- It is often difficult to identify preterm labor. Accurate diagnosis requires assessment by the health care provider, usually in the hospital or clinic.
- Post these instructions where they can be seen by everyone in the family.

African-American population as in Caucasians. The pathology associated with preterm labor also is unclear, and more research is necessary to identify the pathophysiology of preterm labor and effective treatment strategies.

If a woman knows the warning signs and symptoms of preterm labor and seeks care early enough, prevention of preterm birth may be possible. Warning signs and symptoms of preterm labor are given in the Teaching for Self-Care box. Figure 16-18 shows the possible locations of symptoms in the body. See discussion in Chapter 36.

Sexual Counseling

Sexual counseling of expectant couples includes countering misinformation, providing reassurance of normality, and suggesting alternative behaviors. The uniqueness of each couple is considered within a biopsychosocial framework (see the Teaching for Self-Care box on p. 418.). Nurses can initiate discussion about sexual adaptations

EVIDENCE-BASED PRACTICE

Tocolytics to Delay Preterm Labor

BACKGROUND

- Preterm birth is the second leading cause of perinatal mortality, frequently resulting in respiratory distress syndrome (RDS) and bronchopulmonary dysplasia, brain hemorrhage, sepsis, necrotizing enterocolitis (NEC), cerebral palsy, blindness, and deafness. It often afflicts vulnerable populations who are least able to cope with its costs and complicated care. Preterm birth may arise from genetic factors, stress, inflammatory responses, hemorrhage, and mechanical factors. Tocolytic drugs inhibit labor, allowing additional time to administer a course of corticosteroids to mature the fetal lungs and to transfer the woman to a tertiary care facility that can care for the high risk preterm infant. Calcium channel blockers, antiprostaglandins, magnesium sulfate, nitric oxide, and oxytocin receptor antagonists have been used. Betamimetics (such as terbutaline and ritodrine) have been used for two decades, especially in low-resource areas, and are effective at inhibiting labor. Maternal beta-adrenergic side effects include palpitations, tremor, nausea and vomiting, headaches, anxiety, hyperglycemia, hypokalemia, and pulmonary edema. Adverse fetal effects include tachycardia and hypoglycemia. Recent improvements in perinatal mortality may be due to tocolytic therapy, corticosteroid use, or neonatal intensive care units.

OBJECTIVES

- The reviewers' task was to assess the risks and benefits of tocolytic use of betamimetics on fetal and maternal outcomes.

METHODS

Search Strategy

- The authors searched the Cochrane Pregnancy and Childbirth Group trials register and reference lists. They identified 11 randomized, controlled trials, dated 1966 to 1992, comparing betamimetics with placebo, representing 1332 women from Australia, Canada, Denmark, the Netherlands, and the United States. Publication dates ranged from 1966 to 1992. Five additional trials, dated 1978 to 1996, compared ritodrine to other betamimetics in 948 women.

Statistical Analyses

- Similar data were pooled. Reviewers calculated relative risk for dichotomous (categoric) data, such as type of birth, and weighted mean difference for continuous data, such as time until birth. Differences between groups outside the

95% confidence interval were accepted as significant. All were analyzed in their original randomly assigned "intention to treat" categories.

FINDINGS

- Birth was significantly delayed at least 48 hours in the betamimetic group, when compared with placebo/no treatment. However, betamimetics did not reduce perinatal mortality, RDS, cerebral palsy, or NEC. Women experienced significant side effects from betamimetics; incidence of fetal tachycardia was also significant. One case of maternal pulmonary edema was noted.
- Calcium channel blockers were superior to betamimetics for prolonging gestation and reducing RDS, NEC, jaundice, and maternal side effects. Magnesium sulfate was ineffective at delaying birth, and difficult to titrate to avoid respiratory depression and hyporeflexia.

LIMITATIONS

- All the trials were conducted before 1990, before corticosteroids were widely used to speed fetal lung maturity. Although 48 hours provides sufficient time to transfer to a high risk center, the trials were conducted on women already being treated in a tertiary care center. Actually transferring the women may have resulted in different outcomes. Most of the participants were past 32 weeks of gestation. It is possible that increasing gestational age in later pregnancy has no advantage for certain outcomes. Some pregnancy conditions may be dangerous if prolonged. Although the studies used reasonably similar definitions of preterm labor, there was some disparity about the definition of RDS.

IMPLICATIONS FOR PRACTICE

- Although betamimetics delay labor, many maternal and fetal side effects, some life threatening, are cause for alert nursing assessment. Calcium channel blockers are associated with better fetal outcomes and fewer side effects. Magnesium sulfate is widely used, but is not evidence-based practice.

IMPLICATIONS FOR FURTHER RESEARCH

- Future research should include clinically meaningful outcomes from low-resource areas. The outcomes of the use of tocolytics when transferring women to high risk centers need further study. Calcium channel blockers look promising.

Reference: Anotayanonth, S., Subhedar, N., Garner, P., Neilson, J., & Harigopal, S. (2004). Betamimetics for inhibiting preterm labour. *The Cochrane Database of Systematic Reviews*, 2006, Issue 3. Chichester, UK: John Wiley & Sons.

that must be made during pregnancy, but they themselves need a sound knowledge base about the physical, social, and emotional responses to sex during pregnancy. Not all maternity nurses are comfortable dealing with the sexual concerns of their clients; therefore those nurses who are aware of their personal strengths and limitations in dealing with sexual content are better prepared to make referrals if necessary (Westheimer & Lopater, 2005).

Many women merely need permission to be sexually active during pregnancy. Many other women, however, need to be given information about the physiologic changes

that occur during pregnancy, have the myths that are associated with sex during pregnancy dispelled, and participate in open discussions of positions for intercourse that decrease pressure on the gravid abdomen (Westheimer & Lopater, 2005). Such tasks are within the purview of the nurse and should be an integral component of the health care rendered.

Some couples need to be referred for sex therapy or family therapy. Couples with long-standing problems with sexual dysfunction that are intensified by pregnancy are candidates for sex therapy. Whenever a sexual problem is

TEACHING FOR SELF-CARE

Sexuality in Pregnancy

- Be aware that maternal physiologic changes, such as breast enlargement, nausea, fatigue, abdominal changes, perineal enlargement, leukorrhea, pelvic vasocongestion, and orgasmic responses, may affect sexuality and sexual expression.
- Discuss responses to pregnancy with your partner.
- Keep in mind that cultural prescriptions ("dos") and proscriptions ("don'ts") may affect your responses.
- Although your libido may be depressed during the first trimester, it often increases during the second and third trimesters.
- Discuss and explore with your partner:
  - Alternative behaviors (e.g., mutual masturbation, foot massage, cuddling)
  - Alternative positions (e.g., female superior, side-lying) for sexual intercourse
- Intercourse is safe as long as it is not uncomfortable. There is no correlation between intercourse and miscarriage, but observe the following precautions:
  - Abstain from intercourse if you experience uterine cramping or vaginal bleeding; report event to your caregiver as soon as possible.
  - Abstain from intercourse (or any activity that results in orgasm) if you have a history of cervical incompetence, until the problem is corrected.
- Continue to use "safer sex" behaviors. Women at risk for acquiring or conveying STIs are encouraged to use condoms during sexual intercourse throughout pregnancy.

STI, Sexually transmitted infection.

a symptom of a more serious relationship problem, the couple would benefit from family therapy.

Using the History. The couple's sexual history provides a basis for counseling, but history taking also is an ongoing process. The couple's receptivity to changes in attitudes, body image, partner relationships, and physical status are relevant topics throughout pregnancy. The history reveals the woman's knowledge of female anatomy and physiology and her attitudes about sex during pregnancy, as well as her perceptions of the pregnancy, the health status of the couple, and the quality of their relationship.

Countering Misinformation. Many myths and much of the misinformation related to sex and pregnancy are masked by seemingly unrelated issues. For example, a discussion about the baby's ability to hear and see in utero may be prompted by questions about the baby being an "unseen observer" of the couple's lovemaking. The counselor must be extremely sensitive to the questions behind such questions when counseling in this highly charged emotional area.

Suggesting Alternative Behaviors. Research has not demonstrated conclusively that coitus and orgasm are contraindicated at any time during pregnancy for the obstetrically and medically healthy woman (Cunningham et al., 2005). However, a history of more than one miscarriage; a threatened miscarriage in the first trimester; impending miscarriage in the second trimester; and PROM, bleeding,

or abdominal pain during the third trimester warrant caution when it comes to coitus and orgasm.

Solitary and mutual masturbation and oral-genital intercourse may be used by couples as alternatives to penile-vaginal intercourse. Partners who enjoy cunnilingus (oral stimulation of the clitoris or vagina) may feel "turned off" by the normal increase in the amount and odor of vaginal discharge during pregnancy. Couples who practice cunnilingus should be cautioned against the blowing of air into the vagina, particularly during the last few weeks of pregnancy when the cervix may be slightly open. An air embolism can occur if air is forced between the uterine wall and the fetal membranes and enters the maternal vascular system through the placenta.

Showing the woman or couple pictures of possible variations of coital position often is helpful (Fig. 16-19). The female-superior, side-by-side, rear-entry, and side-lying positions are possible alternative positions to the traditional male-superior position. The woman astride (superior position) allows her to control the angle and depth of penile penetration, as well as to protect her breasts and abdomen. The side-by-side position or any position that places less pressure on the pregnant abdomen and requires less energy

FIG. 16-19 Positions for sexual intercourse during pregnancy. **A,** Female superior. **B,** Side by side. **C,** Rear entry. **D,** Side-lying, facing each other.

may be preferred during the third trimester (Westheimer & Lopater, 2005).

Multiparous women sometimes have significant breast tenderness in the first trimester. A coital position that avoids direct pressure on the woman's breasts and decreased breast fondling during love play can be recommended to such couples. The woman also should be reassured that this condition is normal and temporary.

Some women complain of lower abdominal cramping and backache after orgasm during the first and third trimesters. A back rub can often relieve some of the discomfort and provide a pleasant experience. A tonic uterine contraction, often lasting up to a minute, replaces the rhythmic contractions of orgasm during the third trimester. Changes in the FHR without fetal distress also have been reported.

The objective of "safer sex" is to provide prophylaxis against the acquisition and transmission of STIs (e.g., herpes simplex virus [HSV], HIV). Because these diseases may be transmitted to the woman and her fetus, the use of condoms is recommended throughout pregnancy if the woman is at risk for acquiring an STI.

Well-informed nurses who are comfortable with their own sexuality and the sexual counseling needs of expectant couples can offer information and advice in this valuable but often neglected area. They can establish an open environment in which couples can feel free to introduce their concerns about sexual adjustment and seek support and guidance.

Psychosocial Support

Esteem, affection, trust, concern, consideration of cultural and religious responses, and listening are all components of the emotional support given to the pregnant woman and her family. The woman's satisfaction with her relationships—partner and familial—and their support, her feeling of competence, and her sense of being in control are important issues to be addressed in the third trimester. A discussion of fetal responses to stimuli, such as sound and light, as well as patterns of sleeping and waking, can be helpful. Other issues of concern that may arise for the pregnant woman and couple include fear of pain, loss of control, and possible birth of the infant before reaching the hospital; anxieties about parenthood; parental concerns about the safety of the mother and unborn child; siblings and their acceptance of the new baby; social and economic responsibilities; and parental concerns arising from conflicts in cultural, religious, or personal value systems. In addition, the father's or partner's commitment to the pregnancy and to the couple's relationship and concerns about sexuality and its expression are topics for discussion for many couples. Providing the prospective mother and father with an opportunity to discuss their concerns and validating the normality of their responses can meet their needs to varying degrees. Nurses also must recognize that men feel more vulnerable during their partner's pregnancy. Anticipatory guidance and health promotion strategies can help partners cope with their concerns. Health care providers can stimulate and encourage open dialogue between the expectant father and mother.

Evaluation

Evaluation of the effectiveness of the care of the woman during pregnancy is based on the previously stated outcomes. More effort is needed in evaluating outcomes of nursing care during the prenatal period. A formal systematic follow-up on quality of care is not common but should be developed and incorporated in all settings (see Plan of Care).

CD: Plan of Care: Discomforts of Pregnancy

---

plan of care ▶ **Discomforts of Pregnancy and Warning Signs**

FIRST TRIMESTER
NURSING DIAGNOSIS Anxiety related to deficient knowledge about schedule of prenatal visits throughout pregnancy as evidenced by woman's questions and concerns

Expected Outcome *Woman will verbalize correct appointment schedule for the duration of the pregnancy and feelings of being "in control."*

Nursing Interventions/Rationales
- Provide information regarding schedule of visits, tests, and other assessments and interventions that will be provided throughout the pregnancy *to empower woman to function in collaboration with the caregiver and diminish anxiety.*
- Allow woman time to describe level of anxiety *to establish basis for care.*
- Provide information to woman regarding prenatal classes and labor area tours *to decrease feelings of anxiety about the unknown.*

NURSING DIAGNOSIS Imbalanced nutrition: less than body requirements, related to nausea and vomiting as evidenced by woman's report and weight loss

Expected Outcome *Woman will gain 1 to 2.5 kg during the first trimester.*

Nursing Interventions/Rationales
- Verify prepregnant weight *to plan a realistic diet according to individual woman's nutritional needs.*
- Obtain diet history *to identify current meal patterns and foods that may be implicated in nausea.*
- Advise woman to consume small frequent meals and avoid having empty stomach *to avoid further nausea episodes.*
- Suggest that woman eat a simple carbohydrate such as dry crackers before arising in the morning *to avoid empty stomach and decrease incidence of nausea and vomiting.*
- Advise woman to call health care provider if vomiting is persistent and severe *to identify possible incidence of hyperemesis gravidarum.*

Continued

NURSING DIAGNOSIS Fatigue related to hormonal changes in the first trimester as evidenced by woman's complaints

Expected Outcome *Woman will report a decreased number of episodes of fatigue.*

Nursing Interventions/*Rationales*
- Rest as needed *to avoid increasing feeling of fatigue.*
- Eat a well-balanced diet *to meet increased metabolic demands and avoid anemia.*
- Discuss the use of support systems to help with household responsibilities *to decrease workload at home and decrease fatigue.*
- Reinforce to woman the transitory nature of first trimester fatigue *to provide emotional support.*
- Explore with the woman a variety of techniques *to prioritize roles to decrease family expectations.*

SECOND TRIMESTER
NURSING DIAGNOSIS Constipation related to progesterone influence on GI tract as evidenced by woman's report of altered patterns of elimination

Expected Outcome *Woman will report a return to normal bowel elimination pattern after implementation of interventions.*

Nursing Interventions/*Rationales*
- Provide information to woman regarding pregnancy-related causes: progesterone slowing gastrointestinal motility, growing uterus compressing intestines, and influence of iron supplementation *to provide basic information for self-care during pregnancy.*
- Assist woman to plan a diet that will promote regular bowel movements, such as increasing amount of oral fluid intake to at least 8 glasses of water a day, increasing the amount of fiber in daily diet, and maintaining moderate exercise program *to promote self-care.*
- Reinforce for woman that she should not take any laxatives, stool softeners, or enemas without first consulting the health care provider *to prevent any injuries to woman or fetus.*

NURSING DIAGNOSIS Anxiety related to deficient knowledge about course of first pregnancy as evidenced by woman's questions regarding possible complications of second and third trimesters

Expected Outcomes *Woman will correctly list signs of potential complications that can occur during the second and third trimesters and exhibit no overt signs of stress.*

Nursing Interventions/*Rationales*
- Provide information concerning the potential complications or warning signs that can occur during the second and third trimesters, including possible causes of signs and the importance of calling the health care provider immediately, *to ensure identification and treatment of problems in a timely manner.*
- Provide a written list of complications *to have a reference list for emergencies.*

THIRD TRIMESTER
NURSING DIAGNOSIS Fear related to deficient knowledge regarding onset of labor and the processes of labor related to inexperience as evidenced by woman's questions and statement of concerns

Expected Outcomes *Woman will verbalize basic understanding of signs of labor onset and when to call the health care provider, identify resources for childbirth education, and express increasing confidence in readiness to cope with labor.*

Nursing Interventions/*Rationales*
- Provide information regarding signs of labor onset, when to call the health care provider, and give written information regarding local childbirth education classes *to empower and promote self-care.*
- Promote ongoing effective communication with health care provider *to promote trust and decrease fear of unknown.*
- Provide the woman with decision-making opportunities *to promote effective coping.*
- Provide opportunity for woman to verbalize fears regarding childbirth *to assist in decreasing fear through discussion.*

NURSING DIAGNOSIS Disturbed sleep patterns related to discomforts or insomnia of third trimester as evidenced by woman's report of inadequate rest

Expected Outcome *Woman will report an improvement of quality and quantity of rest and sleep.*

Nursing Interventions/*Rationales*
- Assess current sleep pattern and review need for increased requirement during pregnancy *to identify need for change in sleep patterns.*
- Suggest change of position to side-lying with pillows between legs or to semi-Fowler's position *to increase support and decrease any problems with dyspnea or heartburn.*
- Reinforce the possibility of the use of various sleep aides such as relaxation techniques, reading, and decreased activity before bedtime *to decrease the possibility of anxiety or physical discomforts before bedtime.*

NURSING DIAGNOSIS Ineffective sexuality patterns related to changes in comfort level and fatigue

Expected Outcomes *Woman will verbalize feelings regarding changes in sexual desire, and woman and her partner will express satisfaction with sexual activities.*

Nursing Interventions/*Rationales*
- Assess couple's usual sexuality patterns *to determine how patterns have been altered by pregnancy.*
- Provide information regarding expected changes in sexuality patterns during pregnancy *to correct any misconceptions.*
- Allow the couple to express feelings in a nonjudgmental atmosphere *to promote trust.*
- Refer couple for counseling as appropriate *to assist the couple to cope with sexuality pattern changes.*
- Suggest alternative sexual positions *to decrease pressure on enlarging abdomen of woman and increase sexual comfort and satisfaction of couple.*

GI, Gastrointestinal.

▬ VARIATIONS IN PRENATAL CARE

The course of prenatal care described thus far may seem to suggest that the experiences of childbearing women are similar and that nursing interventions are uniformly consistent across all populations. Although typical patterns of response to pregnancy are easily recognized and many aspects of prenatal care indeed are consistent, pregnant women enter the health care system with individual concerns and needs. The nurse's ability to assess unique needs and to tailor interventions to the individual is the hallmark of expertise in providing care. Variations that influence prenatal care include culture, age, and number of fetuses.

Cultural Influences

Prenatal care as we know it is a phenomenon of Western medicine. In the U.S. biomedical model of care, women are encouraged to seek prenatal care as early as possible in their pregnancy by visiting a physician, and/or a nurse-midwife. Such visits are usually routine and follow a systematic sequence, with the initial visit followed by monthly, then semimonthly, and then weekly visits. Monitoring weight and BP; testing blood and urine; teaching specific information about diet, rest, and activity; and preparing for childbirth are common components of prenatal care. This model not only is unfamiliar but also seems strange to women of other cultures. Different models for providing prenatal care for women throughout the world are being explored (Chalmers, Mangiaterra, & Porter, 2001).

Many cultural variations are found in prenatal care. Even if the prenatal care described is familiar to a woman, some practices may conflict with the beliefs and practices of a subculture group to which she belongs. Because of these and other factors, such as lack of money, lack of transportation, and language barriers, women from diverse cultures may not participate in the prenatal care system, for instance by keeping prenatal appointments (Shaffer, 2002). Such behavior may be misinterpreted by nurses as uncaring, lazy, or ignorant.

A concern for modesty also is a deterrent to many women seeking prenatal care. For some women, exposing body parts, especially to a man, is considered a major violation of their modesty. For many women, invasive procedures, such as a vaginal examination, may be so threatening that they cannot be discussed even with their own husbands; therefore many women prefer a female health care provider. Too often, health care providers assume women lose this modesty during pregnancy and labor, but actually most women value and appreciate efforts to maintain their modesty.

For many cultural groups, a physician is deemed appropriate only in times of illness, and because pregnancy is considered a normal process and the woman is in a state of health, the services of a physician are considered inappropriate. Even if what are considered problems with pregnancy by standards of Western medicine do develop, they may not be perceived as problems by members of other cultural groups.

Although pregnancy is considered normal by many, certain practices are expected of women of all cultures to ensure a good outcome. Cultural prescriptions tell women what to do, and cultural proscriptions establish taboos. The purposes of these practices are to prevent maternal illness resulting from a pregnancy-induced imbalanced state and to protect the vulnerable fetus. Prescriptions and proscriptions regulate the woman's emotional response, clothing, activity and rest, sexual activity, and dietary practices. Exploration of the woman's beliefs, perceptions of the meaning of childbearing, and health care practices may help health care providers foster her self-actualization, promote attainment of the maternal role, and positively influence her relationship with her spouse.

To provide culturally sensitive care, the nurse must be knowledgeable about practices and customs, although it is not possible to know all there is to know about every culture and subculture or the many lifestyles that exist. It is important to learn about the varied cultures in which specific nurses practice. When exploring cultural beliefs and practices related to childbearing, the nurse can support and nurture those beliefs that promote physical or emotional adaptation. However, if potentially harmful beliefs or activities are identified, the nurse should carefully provide education and propose modifications.

Emotional Response

Virtually all cultures emphasize the importance of maintaining a socially harmonious and agreeable environment for a pregnant woman. A lifestyle with minimal stress is important in ensuring a successful outcome for the mother and baby. Harmony with other people must be fostered, and visits from extended family members may be required to demonstrate pleasant and noncontroversial relationships. If discord exists in a relationship, it is usually dealt with in culturally prescribed ways.

Besides proscriptions regarding food, other proscriptions involve forms of magic. For example, some Mexicans believe that pregnant women should not witness an eclipse of the moon because it may cause a cleft palate in the infant. They also believe that exposure to an earthquake may precipitate preterm birth, miscarriage, or even a breech presentation. In some cultures a pregnant woman must not ridicule someone with an affliction for fear her child might be born with the same handicap. A mother should not hate a person lest her child resemble that person, and dental work should not be done because it may cause a baby to have a "harelip." A widely held folk belief in some cultures is that the pregnant woman should refrain from raising her arms above her head, because such movement ties knots in the umbilical cord and may cause it to wrap around the baby's neck. Another belief is that placing a knife under the bed of a laboring woman will "cut" her pain.

Clothing

Although most cultural groups do not prescribe specific clothing to be worn during pregnancy, modesty is an expectation of many. Some Mexican women of the Southwest and women of Central America wear a cord beneath the breasts and knotted over the umbilicus. This cord, called a muñeco, is thought to prevent morning sickness and ensure a safe birth. Amulets, medals, and beads also may be worn to ward off evil spirits.

Physical Activity and Rest

Norms that regulate the physical activity of mothers during pregnancy vary tremendously. Many groups, including Native Americans and some Asian groups, encourage women to be active, to walk, and to engage in normal, although not strenuous, activities to ensure that the baby is healthy and not too large. Conversely, other groups such as Filipinos believe that any activity is dangerous, and others willingly take over the work of the pregnant woman. Some Filipinos believe that this inactivity protects the mother and child. The mother is encouraged simply to produce the succeeding generation. If health care providers do not know of this belief, they could misinterpret this behavior as laziness or noncompliance with the desired prenatal health care regimen. It is important for the nurse to find out the way each pregnant woman views activity and rest.

Sexual Activity

In most cultures, sexual activity is not prohibited until the end of pregnancy. Some Latinos view sexual activity as necessary to keep the birth canal lubricated. Conversely, some Vietnamese may have definite proscriptions against sexual intercourse, requiring abstinence throughout the pregnancy because it is thought that sexual intercourse may harm the mother and fetus.

Diet

Nutritional information given by Western health care providers also may be a source of conflict for many cultural groups. Such a conflict commonly is not known by health care providers unless they understand the dietary beliefs and practices of the people for whom they are caring. For example, Muslims have strict regulations regarding preparation of food, and if meat cannot be prepared as prescribed, they may omit meats from their diets. Many cultures permit pregnant women to eat only warm foods.

Age Differences

The age of the childbearing couple may have a significant influence on their physical and psychosocial adaptation to pregnancy. Normal developmental processes that occur in both very young and older mothers are interrupted by pregnancy and require a different type of adaptation to pregnancy than that of the woman of typical childbearing age. Although the individuality of each pregnant woman is recognized, special needs of expectant mothers 15 years of age or younger or those 35 years of age or older are summarized.

Adolescents

Teenage pregnancy is a worldwide problem (Cherry, Dillon, & Rugh, 2001). About 1 million adolescent females in the United States, or 4 out of every 10 girls, become pregnant each year. Most of the pregnancies are unintended; 56% end in live birth; 29% end in induced abortion; and 15% in miscarriage (Arias, MacDorman, Strobino, & Guyer, 2003). Adolescents are responsible for almost 500,000 births in the United States annually. Hispanic adolescents currently have the highest birth rate, although the rate for African-American adolescents also is high. Of girls who become pregnant, 21% are repeat pregnancies (Hoyert et al., 2006). Most of these young women are unmarried, and many are not ready for the emotional, psychosocial, and financial responsibilities of parenthood.

Despite these alarming statistics and the fact that the United States has the highest adolescent birth rate in the industrialized world, the birth rate for adolescents has steadily declined since 1991 (Hoyert et al., 2006). Concentrated national efforts have generated a host of adolescent pregnancy-prevention programs that have had varying degrees of success (Ford, Weglicki, Kershaw, Schram, Hoyer, & Jacobson, 2002). Characteristics of programs that make a difference are those that have sustained commitment to adolescents over a long time, involve the parents and other adults in the community, promote abstinence and personal responsibility, and assist adolescents to develop a clear strategy for reaching future goals such as a college education or a career.

When adolescents do become pregnant and decide to give birth, they are much less likely than older women to receive adequate prenatal care, with many receiving no care at all (Ford et al., 2002). These young women also are more likely to smoke and less likely to gain adequate weight during pregnancy. As a result of these and other factors, babies born to adolescents are at greatly increased risk of LBW, of serious and long-term disability, and of dying during the first year of life.

Delayed entry into prenatal care may be the result of late recognition of pregnancy, denial of pregnancy, or confusion about the available services. Such a delay in care may leave an inadequate time before birth to attend to correctable problems. The very young pregnant adolescent is at higher risk for each of the confounding variables associated with poor pregnancy outcomes (e.g., socioeconomic factors) and for those conditions associated with a first pregnancy regardless of age (e.g., gestational hypertension). However, when prenatal care is initiated early and consistently, and confounding variables are controlled, very young pregnant adolescents are at no greater risk (nor are their infants) for an adverse outcome than are older pregnant women. The role of the nurse in reducing the risks and consequences of adolescent pregnancy is therefore twofold: first, to encourage early and continued prenatal care, and second, to refer the adolescent, if necessary, for appropriate social support services, which can help reverse the effects of a negative socioeconomic environment (Fig. 16-20) (see Plan of Care).

CD: Critical Thinking Exercise: Teenage Pregnancy

plan of care > Adolescent Pregnancy

NURSING DIAGNOSIS Imbalanced nutrition: less than body requirements related to intake insufficient to meet metabolic needs of fetus and adolescent client

Expected Outcomes *Adolescent will gain weight as prescribed by age, take prenatal vitamins and iron as prescribed, and maintain normal hematocrit and hemoglobin.*

Nursing Interventions/*Rationales*

- Assess current diet history and intake *to determine prescriptions for additions or changes in present dietary pattern.*
- Compare prepregnancy weight with current weight *to determine if pattern is consistent with appropriate fetal growth and development.*
- Provide information concerning food prescriptions for appropriate weight gain, considering preferences for "fast food" and peer influences *to correct any misconceptions and increase chances for compliance with diet.*
- Include adolescent's immediate family or support system during instruction *to ensure that person preparing family meals receives information.*

NURSING DIAGNOSIS Risk for injury, maternal or fetal, related to inadequate prenatal care and screening

Expected Outcomes *Adolescent will experience uncomplicated pregnancy and give birth to a healthy fetus at term.*

Nursing Interventions/*Rationales*

- Provide information using therapeutic communication and confidentiality *to establish relationship and build trust.*
- Discuss importance of ongoing prenatal care and possible risks to adolescent client and fetus *to reinforce that ongoing assessment is crucial to health and well-being of client and fetus, even if client feels well. The adolescent client is at greater risk for certain complications that may be avoided or managed early if prenatal visits are maintained.*
- Discuss risks of alcohol, tobacco, and recreational drug use during pregnancy *to minimize risks to client and fetus, because adolescent client has a higher abuse rate than the rest of the pregnant population.*
- Assess for evidence of sexually transmitted infection (STI) and provide information regarding safer sexual practice *to minimize risk to client and fetus, because adolescent is at greater risk for STIs.*
- Screen for preeclampsia on an ongoing basis *to minimize risk, because adolescent population is at greater risk for preeclampsia.*

NURSING DIAGNOSIS Social isolation related to body image changes of pregnant adolescent as evidenced by client statements and concerns

Expected Outcomes *Adolescent will identify support systems and report decreased feelings of social isolation.*

Nursing Interventions/*Rationales*

- Establish a therapeutic relationship *to listen objectively and establish trust.*
- Discuss with adolescent changes in relationships that have occurred as a result of the pregnancy *to determine extent of isolation from family, peers, and father of the baby.*

- Provide referrals and resources appropriate for developmental stage of adolescent *to give information and support.*
- Provide information regarding parenting classes, breastfeeding classes, and childbirth-preparation classes *to give further information and group support, which lessens social isolation.*

NURSING DIAGNOSIS Interrupted family processes related to adolescent pregnancy

Expected Outcome *Adolescent will reestablish relationship with her mother and father of baby.*

Nursing Interventions/*Rationales*

- Encourage communication with mother *to clarify roles and relationships related to birth of infant.*
- Encourage communication with father of baby (if she desires continued contact) *to ascertain level of support to be expected of father of baby.*
- Refer to support group *to learn more effective ways of problem solving and reduce conflict within the family.*

NURSING DIAGNOSIS Disturbed body image related to situational crisis of pregnancy

Expected Outcome *Pregnant adolescent will verbalize positive comments regarding her body image during the pregnancy.*

Nursing Interventions/*Rationales*

- Assess pregnant adolescent's perception of self related to pregnancy *to provide basis for further interventions.*
- Give information regarding expected body changes occurring during pregnancy *to provide a realistic view of these temporary changes.*
- Provide opportunity to discuss personal feelings and concerns *to promote trust and support.*

NURSING DIAGNOSIS Risk for impaired parenting related to immaturity and lack of experience in new role of adolescent mother

Expected Outcome *Parents will demonstrate parenting roles with confidence.*

Nursing Interventions/*Rationales*

- Provide information on growth and development *to enhance knowledge so that adolescent mother can have basis for caring for her infant.*
- Refer to parenting classes *to enhance knowledge and obtain support for providing appropriate care to newborn and infant.*
- Initiate discussion of child care *to assist adolescent in problem solving for future needs.*
- Assess parenting abilities of adolescent mother and father *to provide baseline for education.*
- Provide information on parenting classes that are appropriate for parents' developmental stage *to give opportunity to share common feelings and concerns.*
- Assist parents to identify pertinent support systems *to give assistance with parenting as needed.*

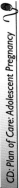

CD: Plan of Care: Adolescent Pregnancy

FIG. 16-20 Pregnant adolescents reviewing fetal development. (Courtesy Marjorie Pyle, RNC, Lifecircle, Costa Mesa, CA.)

Women Older Than 35 Years

Two groups of older parents have emerged in the population of women having a child late in their childbearing years. One group consists of women who have many children or who have an additional child during the menopausal period. The other group consists of women who have deliberately delayed childbearing until their late 30s or early 40s.

Multiparous Women. Multiparous women may have never used contraceptives because of personal choice or lack of knowledge concerning contraceptives. They also may be women who have used contraceptives successfully during the childbearing years, but as menopause approaches, they may cease menstruating regularly or stop using contraceptives and consequently become pregnant. The older multiparous woman may feel that pregnancy separates her from her peer group and that her age is a hindrance to close associations with young mothers. Other parents welcome the unexpected infant as evidence of continuing maternal and paternal roles.

Primiparous Women. The number of first-time pregnancies in women between the ages of 35 and 40 years has increased significantly over the past three decades (Tough, Newburn-Cook, Johnston, Svenson, Rose, & Belik, 2002). Seeing women in their late 30s or 40s during their first pregnancy is no longer unusual for health care providers. Reasons for delaying pregnancy include a desire to obtain advanced education, career priorities, and use of better contraceptive measures. Women who are infertile do not delay pregnancy deliberately but may become pregnant at a later age as a result of fertility studies and therapies.

These women choose parenthood. They often are successfully established in a career and a lifestyle with a partner that includes time for self-attention, the establishment of a home with accumulated possessions, and freedom to travel. When asked the reason they chose pregnancy later in life, many reply, "Because time is running out."

The dilemma of choice includes the recognition that being a parent will have positive and negative consequences. Couples should discuss the consequences of childbearing and childrearing before committing themselves to this lifelong venture. Partners in this group seem to share the preparation for parenthood, planning for a family-centered birth, and desire to be loving and competent parents; however, the reality of child care may prove difficult for such parents.

First-time mothers older than 35 years select the "right time" for pregnancy; this time is influenced by their awareness of the increasing possibility of infertility or of genetic defects in the infants of older women. Such women seek information about pregnancy from books, friends, and electronic resources. They actively try to prevent fetal disorders and are careful in searching for the best possible maternity care. They identify sources of stress in their lives. They have concerns about having enough energy and stamina to meet the demands of parenting and their new roles and relationships.

If older women become pregnant after treatment for infertility, they may suddenly have negative or ambivalent feelings about the pregnancy. They may experience a multifetal pregnancy that may create emotional and physical problems. Adjusting to parenting two or more infants requires adaptability and additional resources.

During pregnancy, parents explore the possibilities and responsibilities of changing identities and new roles. They must prepare a safe and nurturing environment during pregnancy and after birth. They must integrate the child into an established family system and negotiate new roles (parent roles, sibling roles, grandparent roles) for family members.

Adverse perinatal outcomes are more common in older primiparas than in younger women, even when they receive good prenatal care. Tough and colleagues (2002) reported that women aged 35 years and older are more likely than are younger primiparas to have LBW infants, premature birth, and multiple births. The occurrence of these complications is quite stressful for the new parents, and nursing interventions that provide information and psychosocial support are needed, as well as care for physical needs. In addition, in women aged 35 years or older there is an increased risk of maternal mortality. Pregnancy-related deaths are from hemorrhage, infection, embolisms, hypertensive disorders of pregnancy, cardiomyopathy, and strokes (Callaghan & Berg, 2003).

Multifetal Pregnancy

When the pregnancy involves more than one fetus, both the mother and fetuses are at increased risk for adverse outcomes. The maternal blood volume is increased, resulting in an increased strain on the maternal cardiovascular system. Anemia often develops because of a greater demand for iron by the fetuses. Marked uterine distention and increased pressure on the adjacent viscera and pelvic vasculature and diastasis of the two rectus abdominis muscles (see Fig. 14-13) may occur. Placenta previa develops more commonly in multifetal pregnancies because of the large size or placement of the placentas (Clark, 2004). Premature separation of the placenta may occur before the second and any subsequent fetuses are born.

Twin pregnancies often end in prematurity. Spontaneous rupture of membranes before term is common. Congenital malformations are twice as common in monozygotic twins as in singletons, although there is no increase in the incidence of congenital anomalies in dizygotic twins. In addition, two-vessel cords—that is, cords with a vein and a single umbilical artery instead of two—occur more often in twins than in singletons, but this abnormality is most common in monozygotic twins. The clinical diagnosis of multifetal pregnancy is accurate in about 90% of cases. The likelihood of a multifetal pregnancy is increased if any one or a combination of the following factors is noted during a careful assessment:

- History of dizygous twins in the female lineage
- Use of fertility drugs
- More rapid uterine growth for the number of weeks of gestation
- Hydramnios
- Palpation of more than the expected number of small or large parts
- Asynchronous fetal heart beats or more than one fetal electrocardiographic tracing
- Ultrasonographic evidence of more than one fetus

The diagnosis of multifetal pregnancy can come as a shock to many expectant parents, and they may need additional support and education to help them cope with the changes they face. The mother needs nutrition counseling so that she gains more weight than that needed for a singleton birth, counseling that maternal adaptations will probably be more uncomfortable, and information about the possibility of a preterm birth.

If the presence of more than three fetuses is diagnosed, the parents may receive counseling regarding selective reduction of the pregnancies to reduce the incidence of premature birth and improve the opportunities for the remaining fetuses to grow to term gestation (Malone & D'Alton, 2004). This situation poses an ethical dilemma for many couples, especially those who have worked hard to overcome problems with infertility and those who harbor strong values regarding the right to life (Strong, 2003). Nurse-initiated discussions to identify what resources could help the couple (e.g., a minister, priest, or mental health counselor) can make the decision-making process somewhat less traumatic.

The prenatal care given women with multifetal pregnancies includes changes in the pattern of care and modifications in other aspects such as the amount of weight gained and the nutritional intake necessary. The prenatal visits of these women are scheduled at least every 2 weeks in the second trimester and weekly thereafter. In twin gestations the recommended weight gain is 16 to 20 kg. Iron and vitamin supplementation is desirable. Since preeclampsia and eclampsia are increased in multifetal pregnancies, nurses aggressively work to prevent, identify, and treat these complications of pregnancy.

The considerable uterine distention involved can cause the backache commonly experienced by pregnant women to be even worse. Maternal support hose may be worn to control leg varicosities. If risk factors such as premature dilation of the cervix or bleeding are present, abstinence from orgasm and nipple stimulation during the last trimester is recommended to help avert preterm labor. Frequent ultrasound examinations, nonstress tests, and FHR monitoring will be performed. Some practitioners recommend bed rest beginning at 20 weeks in women carrying multiple fetuses to prevent preterm labor. Other practitioners question the value of prolonged bed rest. If bed rest is recommended, the mother assumes a lateral position to promote increased placental perfusion. If birth is delayed until after the thirty-sixth week, the risk of morbidity and mortality decreases for the neonates.

Multiple newborns will likely place a strain on finances, space, workload, and the woman's and family's coping capability. Lifestyle changes may be necessary. Parents will need assistance in making realistic plans for the care of the babies (e.g., whether to breastfeed and whether to raise them as "alike" or as separate persons). Parents should be referred to national organizations such as Parents of Twins and Triplets (www.potatonet.org). Mothers of Twins (www.nomotc.org), and the La Leche League (www.lalecheleague.org) for further support.

CD: Resources

community activity

Select an immigrant or other minority group in your community and identify childbirth-related beliefs and practices that are unique to that group. Are there stores in the area that sell items that meet the needs of that group? Does the community center have activities or classes that are directed toward that group? Are there childbirth education programs available that provide essential information while incorporating cultural patterns? As a nurse, what could you contribute to the community that would help meet the needs of that group?

key points

- The prenatal period is a period of significant psychosocial adaptation for all members of the expectant family as they anticipate changes in roles and responsibilities.
- Prenatal care is common among women of middle and high socioeconomic status, but women living in poverty or those who lack health insurance may have difficulty using public medical services or gaining access to private care.
- Prenatal care is ideally a multidisciplinary activity that fosters a safe birth and promotes satisfaction of the woman and family with the pregnancy and birth experience.
- Important components of the initial prenatal visit include an in-depth interview to determine the presence of potential complications, a comprehensive physical examination, and selected laboratory tests.

Continued

key points—cont'd

- Follow-up visits are shorter than the initial visit but are important for monitoring the health of the mother and fetus and providing anticipatory guidance as needed.
- Individualized care may be implemented through the assessment process, the formulation of nursing diagnoses, and planning mutually derived outcomes with the woman and her family when appropriate; evaluation of care is an ongoing process.
- The nurse has an important role in teaching the pregnant woman and her family about the physical changes and discomforts of pregnancy and self-care measures that can be implemented.
- Each woman needs to know how to recognize and report preterm labor and other warning signs and symptoms.
- Culture, age, parity, and multiple pregnancy may have a significant impact on the course and outcome of the pregnancy.

REFERENCES

American College of Obstetricians and Gynecologists (ACOG). (2002a). Diagnosis and management of preclampsia and eclampsia. Practice Bulletin No. 53. *Obstetrics and Gynecology* (99)1, 159-167.

American College of Obstetricians and Gynecologists (ACOG). (2002b). Exercise during pregnancy and the postpartum period, ACOG Committee Opinion No. 267. *Obstetrics and Gynecology, 99*(1), 171-173.

American College of Obstetricians and Gynecologists (ACOG). (2003). Immunization during pregnancy *ACOG Committee Opinion No. 282, Obstetrics and Gynecology* 101(1), 207-212.

American Dietetic Association (ADA). (2002). Position of the American Dietetic Association: Nutrition and lifestyle for a healthy pregnancy. *Journal of the American Dietetic Association, 102*(10), 1479-1490.

Andres, R. (2004). Effects of therapeutic, diagnostic, and environmental agents and exposure to social and illicit drugs. In R. Creasy, R. Resnik, & J. Iams (Eds.), *Maternal-fetal medicine: Principles and practice* (5th ed.). Philadelphia: Saunders.

Arias, E., MacDorman, M., Strobino, D., & Guyer, B. (2003). Annual summary of vital statistics–2002. *Pediatrics, 112*(6), 1215-1230.

Barish, R. (2004). In-flight radiation exposure during pregnancy. *Obstetrics and Gynecology, 103*(6), 1326-1330.

Barron, M. (2001). Antenatal care. In K. Simpson & P. Creehan (Eds.), *Perinatal nursing* (2nd ed.). Philadelphia: Lippincott.

Benn, P., Egan, J., Fang, M., & Smith-Bindman, R. (2004) Changes in the utilization of prenatal diagnosis. *Obstetrics and Gynecology, 103*(6), 1255-1260.

Boggess, K., Lieff, S., Murtha, A., Moss, K., Beck, J., & Offenbacher, S. (2003). Maternal periodontal disease is associated with an increased risk for preeclampsia. *Obstetrics and Gynecology, 101*(2), 227-231.

Boyle, G., Banks, J., Petrizzi, M., & Larimore, W. (2003). Sharing maternity care. *Family Practice Management, 10*(3), 37-40.

Callaghan, W., & Berg, C. (2003). Pregnancy related mortality among women aged 35 years and older, United States, 1991-1997. *Obstetrics and Gynecology, 102*(5 Part 1), 1015-1021.

Carl, D., Roux, G., & Matacale, R. (2000). Exploring dental hygiene and perinatal outcomes: Oral health implications for pregnancy and early childhood. *AWHONN Lifelines, 4*(1), 22-27.

Carlson, N., & Lowe, N. (2006). Centering pregnancy: A new approach to prenatal care. *MCN American Journal of Maternal/Child Nursing, 31*(4), 218-223.

Chalmers, B., Mangiaterra, V., & Porter, R. (2001). WHO principles of prenatal care: The essential antenatal, perinatal, and postpartum care course. *Birth, 28*(3), 202-207.

Centers for Disease Control and Prevention, Worhowsky, K., & Berman, S. (2006). Sexually transmitted diseases treatment guidelines, 2006. *MMWR Morbidity and Mortality Weekly Report, 55* (RR-11), 1-94.

Cherry, A., Dillon, M., & Rugh, D. (2001). *Teenage pregnancy: A global view.* Westport: Greenwood Press.

Clark, S. (2004). Placenta previa and abruption placentae. In R. Creasy, R. Resnik, & J. Iams (Eds.), *Maternal-Fetal medicine: Principles and practice* (5th ed.). Philadelphia: Saunders.

Corbett, R., Ryan, C., & Weinrich, S. (2003). Pica in pregnancy: Does it affect pregnancy outcomes? *MCN American Journal of Maternal/Child Nursing, 28*(3), 183-191.

Cunningham, F., Leveno, K., Bloom, S., Hauth, J., Gilstrap, L., & Wenstrom, K. (2005). *Williams obstetrics* (22nd ed.). New York: McGraw Hill.

Fetrick, A., Christensen, M., & Mitchell, C. (2003). Does public health nurse home visitation make a difference in the health outcomes of pregnant clients and their offspring? *Public Health Nursing, 20*(3), 184-189.

Foley, E. (2002). Drug screening and criminal prosecution of pregnant women. *Journal of Obstetric, Gynecologic, and Neonatal Nursing, 33*(2), 133-137.

Ford, K., Weglicki, L., Kershaw, T., Schram, C., Hoyer, P., & Jacobson, M. (2002). Effects of a prenatal care intervention for adolescent mothers on birth weight, repeat pregnancy, and educational outcomes at one year postpartum. *Journal of Perinatal Education, 11*(1), 35-38.

Freda, M. (2003). Nursing's contribution to the literature on preterm labor and birth. *Journal of Obstetric, Gynecologic, and Neonatal Nursing, 32*(5), 659-667.

Freda, M., & Patterson, E. (2003). *Preterm labor and birth: Prevention and nursing management* (3rd ed.) (Nursing Module). New York: March of Dimes Birth Defects Foundation.

Fries, M., Bashford, M., & Nunes, M. (2005). Implementing prenatal screening for cystic fibrosis in routine obstetric practice. *American Journal of Obstetrics and Gynecology, 192*(2), 527-534.

Giannelli, M., Doyle, P., Roman, E., Pelerin, M., & Hermon, C. (2003). The effect of caffeine consumption and nausea on the risk of miscarriage. *Paediatric and Perinatal Epidemiology, 17*(4), 316-323.

Grady, M., & Bloom, K. (2004). Pregnancy outcomes of adolescents enrolled in a Centering Pregnancy program. *Journal of Midwifery & Womens Health, 49*(5), 412-420.

Graves, J., Miller, K., & Sellers, A. (2002). Maternal serum triple analyte screening in pregnancy. *American Family Physician, 65*(5), 915-920.

Handler, A., Rosenberg, D., Raube, K., & Lyons, S. (2003). Prenatal care characteristics and African-American women's satisfaction with care in a managed care organization. *Women's Health Issues, 13*(3), 93-103.

Harris, L., & Paltrow, L. (2003). The status of pregnant women and fetuses in U.S. criminal law, *Journal of the American Medical Association, 289*(13), 1697-1699.

Himmelberger, S. (2002). Preventing group B strep in newborns. *AWHONN Lifelines, 6*(4), 339-342.

Hoyert, D., Mathews, T., Menacker, F., Strobino, D., & Guyer, B. (2006). Annual summary of vital statistics: 2004. *Pediatrics, 117*(1), 168-183.

Jenkins, T. & Wapner, R., (2004). Prenatal diagnosis of congenital disorders. In R. Creasy, R. Resnik, & J. Iams (Eds.), *Maternal-fetal medicine: Principles and practice* (5th ed.). Philadelphia: Saunders

Jepson, R., Mihaljevic, L., & Craig, J. (2004). Cranberries for preventing urinary tract infections. *The Cochrane Database for Systematic Reviews*, 2006, Issue 3. Chichester, UK: John Wiley & Sons.

Johnson, S., Burrows, A., & Williamson, I. (2004). 'Does my bump look big in this?' The meaning of bodily changes for first-time mothers-to-be. *Journal of Health Psycholology, 9*(3), 361-74.

Johnson, T., & Niebyl, J. (2002). Preconception and prenatal care: Part of the continuum. In S. Gabbe, J. Niebyl, & J. Simpson (Eds.), *Obstetrics: Normal and problem pregnancies* (4th ed.). New York: Churchill Livingstone.

Katz, V., Farmer, R., Tufariello, J., & Carpenter, M. (2001). Why we should eliminate the due date: A truth in jest. *Obstetrics and Gynecology, 98*(6), 1127-1129.

Kehringer, K. (2003). Informed consent: Hospitals must obtain informed consent prior to drug testing pregnant patients. *The Journal of Law, Medicine, & Ethics, 32*(3), 455-457.

Kiel, R., Nashelsky, J., Robbins, B., & Bondi, S. (2003). Does cranberry juice prevent or treat urinary tract infection? *The Journal of Family Practice, 52*(2), 154-155.

Kroelinger, C., & Oths, K. (2000). Partner support and pregnancy wantedness. *Birth, 27*(2), 112-119.

Lawrence, R., & Lawrence, R. (2005). *Breastfeeding: A guide for the medical profession* (6th ed.). Philadelphia: Mosby.

Lederman, R. (1996). *Psychosocial adaptation in pregnancy* (2nd ed.). New York: Springer.

Lewallen, L. (2004). Healthy behaviors and sources of health information among low-income pregnant women. *Public Health Nursing, 21*(3), 200-206.

Lopez, R. (2005). Peridontal disease, preterm birth, and low birth weight. *Evidence-based dentistry, 6*(4), 90-91.

Malone, F., & D'Alton, M. (2004). Multiple gestation. Clinical characteristics and management. In R. Creasy, R. Resnik, & J. Iams (Eds.), *Maternal-fetal medicine: Principles and practice* (5th ed.). Philadelphia: Saunders.

March of Dimes Birth Defects Foundation. (2005). *PeriStats (2005): Born too soon and too small in the United States.* Accessed www.marchofdimes.com/peristats, May 15, 2005.

Martin, S., Mackie, L., Kupper, L., Buescher, P., & Moracco, K. (2001). Physical abuse of women before, during, and after pregnancy. *Journal of the American Medical Association, 285*(12), 1581-1584.

May, K. (1982). Three phases of father involvement in pregnancy. *Nursing Research, 31*(6), 337-342.

McFarlane, J., Parker, B., & Cross, B. (2001). *Abuse during pregnancy: A protocol for prevention and intervention* (2nd ed.) (Nursing Module). New York: March of Dimes Birth Defects Foundation.

McPheeters, M., Miller, W., Hartman, K., Savitz, D., Kaufman, J., Garrett, J., et al. (2005). The epidemiology of threatened preterm labor: A prospective cohort study. *American Journal of Obstetrics and Gynecology, 192*(4), 1325-1330.

Mercer, R. (1995). *Becoming a mother.* New York: Springer.

Moos, M. (2004). Understanding prematurity: Sorting fact from fiction. *AWHONN Lifelines, 8*(1), 32-37.

National High Blood Pressure Education Program (NHBPEP). (2003). *Seventh report of the Joint National Committee on Prevention, Detection,* *Evaluation, and Treatment of High Blood Pressure,* Bethesda, MD: U.S. Department of Health and Human Services, National Institutes of Health, National Heart, Lung, and Blood Institute.

Neilson, J. (2000). Ultrasound for fetal assessment in early pregnancy. *The Cochrane Database for Systematic Reviews*, 2006, Issue 3. Chichester, UK: John Wiley & Sons.

Pavill, B. (2002). Fathers and breastfeeding: Consider these ways to get dad involved. *AWHONN Lifelines, 6*(4), 324-331.

Peters, R., & Flack, J. (2004). Hypertensive disorders of pregnancy. *Journal of Obstetric, Gynecologic, and Neonatal Nursing, 33*(2), 209-220.

Raz, R., Chazan, B., & Dan, M. (2004). Cranberry juice and urinary tract infection. *Clinical Infectious Diseases, 38*(10), 1413-1419.

Rising, S. (1998). Centering pregnancy. An interdisciplinary model of empowerment. *Journal of Nurse-Midwifing, 43*(1), 46-54.

Rubin, R. (1975). Maternal tasks in pregnancy. *Maternal-Child Nursing Journal, 4*(3), 143-153.

Rubin, R. (1984). *Maternal identity and the maternal experience.* New York: Springer.

Sampselle, C. (2003). Behavior interventions in young and middle-aged women: Simple interventions to combat a complex problem. *American Journal of Nursing, 103*(Suppl), 9-19.

Schmied, V., & Lupton, D. (2001). The externality of the inside: Body images of pregnancy. *Nursing Inquiry, 8*(1), 32-40.

Seidel, H., Ball, J., Dains, J., & Benedict, G. (2006). *Mosby's guide to physical examination* (6th ed.). St. Louis: Mosby.

Shaffer, C. (2002). Factors influencing the access to prenatal care by Hispanic pregnant women. *Journal of the American Academy of Nurse Practitioners, 14*(2), 93-98.

Strong, C. (2003). Too many twins, triplets, quadruplets, and so on: A call for new priorities. *Journal of Law, Medicine & Ethics, 31*(2), 272-282.

Sword, W. (2003). Prenatal care use among women of low income: A matter of "taking care of self." *Qualitative Health Research, 13*(3), 319-332.

Todd, S-J., LaSala, K., & Neil-Urban, S. (2001). An integrated approach to prenatal smoking cessation interventions. *MCN American Journal of Maternal/Child Nursing, 26*(4), 185-191.

Tough, S., Newburn-Cook, C., Johnston, D., Svenson, L., Rose, S., & Belik, J. (2002). Delayed childbearing and its impact on population rate changes in lower birth weight, multiple birth, and preterm delivery. *Pediatrics, 109*(3), 399-403.

Villar, J., Carroli, G., Khan-Neelofur, D., Piaggio, G., & Gulmezoglu, M. (2001). Patterns of routine antenatal care for low-risk pregnancy. *The Cochrane Database for Systematic Reviews*, 2006, Issue 3. Chichester, UK: John Wiley & Sons.

Vit, T., Bakketeig, L., Trygg, K., Lund-Larsen, K., & Jacobsen, G. (2003). High caffeine consumption in the third trimester of pregnancy: Gender-specific effects on fetal growth. *Paediatric and Perinatal Epidemiology, 17*(4), 324-331.

Westheimer, R., & Lopater, S. (2005). *Human sexuality: A psychosocial perspective* (2nd ed.). Philadelphia: Lippincott Williams & Wilkins.

Yu, S., Park, C., & Schwalberg, R. (2002). Factors associated with smoking cessation among U.S. pregnant women. *Maternal and Child Health Journal, 6*(2), 89-97.

Childbirth and Perinatal Education

learning objectives

- Determine the scope of childbirth and perinatal education in the community.
- Compare philosophies underlying maternal choices for childbirth.
- Contrast the different choices of care providers.

- Differentiate among four settings in which birth may be given.
- Interpret the role and benefits of a doula.
- List the community-based provider organizations for childbirth and perinatal educators.

electronic resources

Additional information related to the content in Chapter 17 can be found on

the companion website at **evolve**
http://evolve.elsevier.com/Lowdermilk/MWHC/
- NCLEX Review Questions
- WebLinks

or on the interactive companion CD
- NCLEX Review Questions

A goal of childbirth and perinatal education is to assist individuals and their family members to make informed, safe decisions about pregnancy, birth, and early parenthood. A specific focus is to assist them to comprehend the long-lasting potential that birth experiences, which achieve an empowering nature, can have in the lives of women. Additionally it is to convey the impact that early parenting experiences have on the development of children and the family. Overall, it is to facilitate wise choices. Perinatal education programs are an expansion of the earlier childbirth education movement that originally only offered a set of classes in the third trimester of pregnancy to prepare parents for birth. Today childbirth education programs may also be called perinatal education programs and may consist of a menu of class series and activities from preconception through pregnancy, childbirth, and the early months of parenting.

■ THE IMPORTANCE OF CHILDBIRTH EXPERIENCES IN THE LIVES OF WOMEN
The Need for Childbirth Education

For women who conceive, childbirth experiences have been described as some of the most important experiences in their lives. Historically, in psychoanalytic theory,

pregnancies and childbirth have long been proposed as developmental milestones for females in that they constitute a developmental crisis in the life cycle out of which, in favorable circumstances, new psychic structures are created and mental functioning is integrated (Deutch, 1945; Holmes, 2000). Newman (2004) refers to childbirth as a developmental transition. This perspective is consistent with the more general theory of flow experiences. Flow experiences are defined as achievable events which require enough internal focus to mentally remove one from outside events and which can lead to a reintegration of one's internal self (Csikszentmihalyi, 1990). Thus when a woman is prepared and well supported to give birth actively, as opposed to being delivered passively, the event can present a unique and powerful opportunity to find her core strength in a manner that forever changes her self-perception. In addition, childbirth can offer a woman an experience in trusting her body wisdom in a way that may alter how she responds throughout life to other health challenges to herself and her family. However, the full benefits of a positive childbirth experience are not optimally documented nor well understood either among the general public or among health professionals. It takes a well-informed, articulate childbirth educator to teach consumer-oriented childbirth classes today. Optimally these classes help women trust their bodies and offer women a way to take full advantage of the opportunities presented by a prepared-for and well supported childbirth experience.

For the new family, prior experience related to the pregnancy and birth of others or in the care of younger siblings or relatives is increasingly uncommon, given the small size of many American families. As a result, many individuals facing parenthood may have little information about what to expect and thus do not have the important skills necessary to deal effectively with pregnancy, childbirth, or parenthood. Perinatal education classes can partially fill this void.

Empowering Pregnant Women and Their Partners

For many decades, research has consistently shown that perceived control in childbirth is an important aspect of birth satisfaction for women. Control in labor has been shown to consist of (1) control of what the staff does to you, (2) feeling in control of your own behavior, and (3) feeling in control during contractions. All three types of control in childbirth have been shown to contribute to a satisfying experience as well as to positive psychologic outcomes for women (Green & Baston, 2004). Among women who experienced low control in labor, resultant distress was frequent. This was regardless of whether the women initially reported either a high or a low desire for situation control (Baron, Cusumano, & Evans, 2004). In summary, low control equaled low birth satisfaction across both groups. Similarly, for Swedish women, a more negative birth experience included lack of control, lack of support during labor as well as administration of obstetric analgesia (Waldenstrom, Hildingsson, Rubertsson, & Radestad, 2004). Mozingo, Davis, and Thomas (2002) interviewed women with full-term vaginal births who had anger related to their birth experiences. Anger resulted when their expectations for trust, power, control, and being kept informed were not met.

Researchers consistently state that women need to be treated as full participants in the decision-making process to facilitate their having a good birth experience. Preparing expectant parents to play their part well as knowledgeable and skilled participants takes skill on the part of the educator, especially if the parents are interacting with health care providers who do not highly value consumer input into decisions made.

Prenatal Support and Partner Relationships

Prenatal stress and depression are linked to negative birth outcomes such as low-birth-weight or preterm infants. However, a Cochrane review of 16 trials did not find that social support during pregnancy was a strong enough intervention to overcome premature birth rates for those with a lifetime of disadvantage or long-standing pregnancy complications (Hodnett & Fredericks, 2000). Thus perinatal education alone is not likely to resolve long-standing issues of lack of support or partner problems.

For families with support issues of a less serious nature, perinatal education early in the pregnancy may make a difference. Hill (2002) reported a study that supported the long-held belief that having a supportive intimate partner present throughout the labor experience reduced maternal anxiety, although reduced anxiety did not influence many aspects of physiologic labor outcomes. However mothers targeted for extra support as part of their care were less likely to have a cesarean birth, less likely to report being worried about their babies, less likely to be dissatisfied with their antenatal care, and less likely to complain of lack of help at home (Hodnett, Gates, Hofmeyr, & Sakala, 2003). Thus, early perinatal or preconception education can include helping the woman and her partner to build a strong social support network to carry them through the perinatal year and beyond.

Pregnancy is a time when the partner relationship can be strengthened or stressed. Pregnancy, birth, and parenthood are major developmental tasks that slowly move new partners to becoming a family of three or more. In addition to the physical changes during pregnancy, the pregnant woman and her partner face significant emotional, social, and cognitive changes. Expectant fathers may be concerned about finances, their role as a father, sexuality, and the child's effect on the couple's relationship. Fathers or partners often worry about their role during childbirth classes and labor and birth, as well as the safety of their partner and baby during the birth (Pollack, Amankwaa, & Amankwaa, 2005). Both the pregnant woman and her partner benefit from an assessment of the symptoms and changes they are experiencing and their individual coping styles. Discussions with couples in educational programs acknowledge the many changes they are experiencing. Teaching exercises and skills to keep the lines of communication open may be used.

Theoretical Framework

Theoretical frameworks that have been used for childbirth education include Adaptation Theory, Crisis Theory Competence Model, the Health Education Model and Orem's Self-Care Theory. No one model has been shown to be best. However, using a theoretic framework assists the childbirth educator to organize facts into sets of meaningful and related concepts and thus furthers the effort to increase expectant parents' understanding, problem solving, and decision making related to these facts.

■ CHILDBIRTH EDUCATION: HISTORY ■ AND RECENT ADVANCES

Historically, women have always shared information about and assisted each other in childbirth. Until the late nineteenth century, childbirth was a family and social event in which women gave birth at home, often with the help of a midwife and a group of friends. The Industrial Revolution, with its urban crowding and associated health problems, led to higher rates of maternal and infant mortality from puerperal fever, sepsis, and infant diarrhea (Wertz & Wertz, 1979). The weakened family bonds consequent to industrialization and the emergence of obstetrics, drugs, and medication for pain and infection control in birth moved childbirth from being "women's work" and controlled by nature into the hospital (Lindell, 1988).

During these changes, women sought to have some choice in the management of birth. During the late nineteenth century, women organized the National Twilight Sleep Association to promote the use of the new technique of giving morphine and scopolamine to control labor pain. By the early twentieth century, most women had accepted centralized and routine birth practices over which they had little or no control in the unsubstantiated belief that childbirth would be safer for themselves and their babies. Not until the midtwentieth century did women (energized by the consumer rights movement, women's movement, and increased availability of certified nurse-midwives) begin to question the rigid policies, the preemption of the process by the medical profession, and the regimentation of birth. The childbirth education movement began in the 1950s and grew. Prepared childbirth classes are now recommended for all expectant parents by most caregivers and by the nation's health goals in *Healthy People 2010* (U.S. Department of Health and Human Services [USDHHS], 2000).

Early Methods of Childbirth Education

An English physician, Grantly Dick-Read, published two books in which he theorized that pain in childbirth is socially conditioned and caused by a fear-tension-pain syndrome. His first book, *Natural Childbirth,* was published in 1933. Dick-Read's second book, *Childbirth without Fear,* was published in the United States in 1944. The work of Dick-Read became the foundation for organized programs of preparation for childbirth and teacher training throughout the United States, Canada, Great Britain, and South Africa. In 1960 those prepared through such programs established the International Childbirth Education Association (ICEA). The Grantly Dick-Read method, referred to as *Childbirth without Fear,* initially recommended deep abdominal breathing during early first-stage contractions, shallow breathing for later first stage, and sustained pushing with breath holding (Dick-Read, 1987). Women were taught to relax different muscle groups through the entire body, consciously and progressively, until a high degree of skill at relaxation was achieved. Consequently a woman was taught to relax completely between contractions and keep all muscles except the uterus relaxed during contractions.

During the 1960s the Lamaze method, originally known as the psychoprophylactic method (PPM), gained popularity in the United States. PPM offered new perspectives on preparation for childbirth by emphasizing control by using the mind. Marjorie Karmel introduced PPM to the United States in her book *Thank You, Dr. Lamaze,* which was published in the United States in 1959. PPM combined controlled muscular relaxation and breathing techniques. Active relaxation was an integral part of the Lamaze method. The woman was taught to contract specific muscle groups (neuromuscular control) while relaxing the remainder of her body. The goal was to be able to relax the uninvolved muscles in her body while her uterine muscle contracted. Rather than tensing during uterine contractions, women were conditioned to respond with relaxation and breathing patterns.

In 1960 the American Society for Psychoprophylaxis in Obstetrics (ASPO) was formed in New York and became a national organization to promote use of the Lamaze method and prepare teachers of the method. It continues to be an active organization, known since 1998 as Lamaze International and dedicated to advancing normal birth. Lamaze's Institute of Normal Birth publishes reviews of research related to normal birth. In the official Lamaze *Guide to Giving Birth with Confidence,* the authors state that "Mothers do know how to give birth, simply. And doctors, hospitals and technology have not made normal birth safer" (Lothian & Devries, 2005). They further state that women need to rediscover birth as a natural part of life based on research that confirms that interfering in the normal birth process is harmful unless there is clear evidence that interference provides benefits.

A third, early advocate of prepared childbirth was the Denver obstetrician, Robert Bradley, who published *Husband-Coached Childbirth* in 1965. He advocated what he called true "natural" childbirth, without any form of anesthesia or analgesia and with a husband-coach and breathing techniques for labor. The American Academy of Husband-Coached Childbirth (AAHCC) was founded to make the Bradley method available and to prepare teachers (www.bradleybirth.com). This method of partner-coached childbirth used breath control, abdominal breathing, and general body relaxation. Working in harmony with the body was emphasized (Bradley, 1965). Bradley's technique emphasized environmental variables such as darkness, solitude, and quiet to make childbirth a more natural experience. Women using the Bradley method may appear to be sleeping during labor because they are in such a deep state of mental relaxation.

These three organizations continue to exist, but are now less focused on a "method" approach. Rather, women are assisted to develop their birth philosophy and inner knowledge and then offered many skills from which to choose. Many childbirth educators teach a plethora of techniques that originated in several different organizations or publications. Women are encouraged to choose the techniques that work for them. Other childbirth educator organizations that have come onto the scene include: *Birthworks, Association of Childbirth Educators and Labor Assistants (ALACE), Birthing from Within, Childbirth and Postpartum Association (CAPPA),* and *Hypnobirth* to name a few.

Selecting a Certified Childbirth Educator

When couples choose a childbirth educator, they should look for one who is certified though a national organization. This insures that the educator has met some criteria for knowledge and skills. Classes for parents should be small enough to be interactive and sufficiently long to cover the content. For the content on childbirth itself, 12 to 15 hours are commonly recommended. There are no common standards set for the length of other classes such as breastfeeding education, preconception classes, or early pregnancy classes. Furthermore, there are currently no commonly recognized standards for what content is covered in each of the many classes that may be offered throughout the perinatal year.

Certified childbirth educators are an interdisciplinary, postprofessional specialty group made up largely of nurses joined by physical therapists, social workers, teachers, psychologists, and others who have taken course work to prepare specifically for this role. The field of childbirth education has benefited from the rich tapestry of interaction from its interdisciplinary membership with their many perspectives. Regardless of the original professional background, the competencies of a childbirth educator include skills that enable them to do the following:

- Promote the childbearing experience as a normal, natural, healthy process that profoundly affects women and their families
- Assist women and families to discover and use strategies that facilitate normal, natural, healthy pregnancy, birth, breastfeeding, and early parenting
- Help women and their families to understand how interventions and complications influence the normal course of pregnancy, birth, breastfeeding, and early parenting
- Provide information and support that encourage attachment between babies and their families
- Assist women and their families to make informed decisions for childbearing
- Act as an advocate to promote normal, natural, healthy, fulfilling childbirth experiences for women and their families
- Design, teach, and evaluate a course that increases a woman's confidence and ability to give birth (Lamaze International, 2005)

For many educators, this education takes place in a classroom and is conducted for couples in evening or weekend classes. However, some low-income, high risk women are taught in the waiting room of a clinic where the primary focus may be pregnancy health behavior and the prevention of preterm infants (Tiedje, 2004).

The Coalition to Improve Maternity Services

In 1994, under the leadership of Lamaze International, a summit meeting of maternity organizations was held, which in 1996 became a new independent organization: *The Coalition to Improve Maternity Services (CIMS)*

(www.motherfriendly.org). The group drafted standards for normal birth, entitled the *Mother Friendly Childbirth Initiative (MFCI)*. This document was ratified by Lamaze International (www.lamaze-childbirth.com), La Leche League (www.lalecheleague.org), Birth Works (www.birthworks.org), the AAHCC, the American College of Nurse-Midwives (ACNM) (www.midwife.org), The Association of Women's Health, Obstetric and Neonatal Nurses (AWHONN) (www.awhonn.org), International Childbirth Education Association (ICEA) (www.icea.org), Midwife Alliance of North America (MANA) (www.mana.org), and Physicians for Midwifery Care, to name a few of the more than 50 early endorsers.

CIMS adopted the Lamaze International philosophy of birth as follows:
- Birth is normal, natural, and healthy.
- The experience of birth profoundly affects women and their families.
- Women's inner wisdom guides them through birth.
- Women's confidence and ability to give birth is either enhanced or diminished by the care provider and place of birth.
- Women have a right to give birth free from routine medical interventions.
- Birth can safely take place in birth centers and homes and hospitals.
- Childbirth education empowers women to make informed choices in health care, to assume responsibility for their health, and to trust their inner wisdom (Lothian & Devries, 2005).

This philosophy has become an ideal for many childbirth education organizations in the United States. It fits closely with the principles of perinatal care put forth by the World Health Organization (WHO, 1998), which states that care for normal pregnancy and birth should be removed from total control of doctors, based on the use of appropriate technology (as opposed to overuse), evidence based, regionalized, multidisciplinary, holistic, family centered, culturally appropriate, should involve women in decision making, and should respect the privacy, dignity, and confidentiality of women (Cultural Considerations box).

A Guide to Effective Care in Pregnancy and Childbirth (Enkin et al., 2000) presents the evidence basis for effective care in pregnancy and childbirth based on systematic reviews from the Cochrane Pregnancy and Childbirth Group. The authors describe effects of maternity interventions. Free web access is available (www.maternitywise.org) to this book. How the childbirth educator uses this evidence in education programs depends on the population who attend classes as well as the care provider practices in the community. Expectant parents cannot and should not be taught to manage all details of medical interventions that are listed. Expectant parents can, however, ask their care providers if they are familiar with this database and if they use it to discontinue routines that have been found to be useless or harmful. In the role as advocate, the

cultural considerations

Culturally Competent Perinatal Education

Cultural competency is particularly significant in perinatal education because childbirth, as one of life's most significant events, is culturally shaped and socially constructed. Because of the multicultural composition of the North American population, great diversity exists in attitudes, expectations, and behaviors judged appropriate during pregnancy and early parenthood. No one approach can meet all needs. For example, classes for new immigrants are particularly effective when taught in class members' primary language. For classes to be meaningful, childbirth educators must understand the value systems in other cultures and their influences on issues such as nutrition, early prenatal care, maternal weight gain, and infant feeding practices. Educators must establish rapport, be understood, and build on cultural practices, reinforcing the positive and promoting change only if a practice is directly harmful.

Most childbirth education classes in the United States are attended by the pregnant woman and her partner, although a friend, teenage daughter, or parent may be the selected support person, or more than one support person may attend classes. Where family-centered care is practiced, other family members may be present for the birth. These decisions are often cultural in nature and should be addressed with sensitivity.

Reference: Ottani, P. (2002). Embracing global similarities: A framework for cross-cultural obstetric care. *Journal of Obstetric, Gynecologic, and Neonatal Nursing, 31*(1), 33-38.

childbirth educator can let families know that items on the list of ineffective or harmful care routines might affect their choice of care provision.

The Maternity Center Association released a survey report in 2002 conducted by Harris Interactive from the Harris Poll group entitled *Listening to Mothers* which is available at www.maternitywise.org/listeningtomothers/. This is the first national U.S. survey of women's childbearing experiences. A total of 136 mothers were interviewed by telephone and 1,447 completed a written survey. In Table 17-1, the recommendations from the Cochrane collaboration are compared to the frequency of use of interventions according to the *Listening to Mothers Survey* (Declercq, Sakala, Corry, Applebaum, & Risher, 2002). The results suggest that a large percentage of mothers giving birth receive interventions that are not evidence based. It takes skill, judgment, and tact for the childbirth educator to assist consumers to make choices about their desired care without undermining medical colleagues, when local routine care frequently lacks an evidence base.

The Lamaze Institute for Normal Birth

Lamaze International recently established the Lamaze Institute for Normal Birth (LINB). It is an evidence-based resource for new and expectant parents and childbirth professionals, whether they practice from a medical, nursing, or midwifery model of care. Its foundation

table 17-1 A Comparison of Rates of Recommended Interventions with Actual Experiences of Mothers in Childbirth

INTERVENTIONS IN CHILDBIRTH	EVIDENCE-BASED RATING: A GUIDE TO EFFECTIVE CARE IN PREGNANCY AND CHILDBIRTH (ENKIN ET AL., 2000)	EXPERIENCED RECENTLY DURING CHILDBIRTH BY MOTHERS: LISTENING TO MOTHERS SURVEY RESULTS (DECLERCQ ET AL., 2002)
Shaving	Ineffectiveness or harm demonstrated by clear evidence	Nearly 20% of women
Enemas	Ineffectiveness or harm demonstrated by clear evidence	Less than 5% of women
Intravenous (IV) lines	Forms of care unlikely to be beneficial	Nearly half of women
Withholding nourishment and water	Forms of care unlikely to be beneficial	Not allowed to drink: 66% Almost 90% not allowed to eat
Early rupture of bag of waters (RBOW)	Forms of care of unknown effectiveness	Over half of the mothers had RBOW after labor began; nearly 60% of mothers for induction
Electronic fetal monitoring	Ineffectiveness or harm demonstrated by clear evidence	Over 90% of mothers
Induction	Forms of care with a trade-off between beneficial and adverse effects	Almost 60% for medical reasons Nearly 20% of mothers for nonmedical reasons
Episiotomy	Forms of care that are likely to be ineffective or harmful	Over 33% reported episiotomies
Cesarean rate	The optimal rate is not known, but from national data available, little improvement in outcome appears to occur when rates rise above about 7%	Reported by 25% which is consistent with national statistics (in 2002)
Vaginal birth after cesarean (VBAC) rate	Forms of care that are likely to be beneficial	Only 25% had VBAC Nearly 50% requested and were denied the opportunity to try VBAC

Adapted from Hotelling, B., & Humenick, S. (2005). Tools for teaching: Advancing normal birth: organizations, goals and research. *Journal of Perinatal Education, 14*(2), 40-48.

comprises six care principles modified from the WHO recommendations:

1. Labor to begin on its own
2. Freedom of movement throughout labor
3. Continuous labor support
4. No routine interventions
5. Nonsupine (e.g., upright or side-lying) positions for birth
6. No separation of mother and baby after birth, with unlimited opportunity for breastfeeding

Brief papers documenting the research supporting each of these care principles is available at www.lamaze.org. Additionally LINB produces a free web-based newsletter that reviews recent studies that address some aspect of normal birth. Thus all perinatal educators, perinatal care providers, and consumers can have ready access to current research on the subject of normal birth.

■ THE SCOPE OF PERINATAL
■ EDUCATION IN THE COMMUNITY
Preconceptual and Early Pregnancy Classes

Prenatal care ideally begins preconceptually because early decisions lay a foundation for the entire perinatal year. If at all possible, education continues in each trimester of pregnancy, and extends through the early postpartum weeks. Traditionally, women who intended to become pregnant did so without specific preconception planning with a health care provider. Some health care providers today promote preconception care as an important component of perinatal services. This care ideally begins by fostering conscious conception and healthy behaviors for the woman and her potential fetus and fosters risk management, as needed. Preconception education is preferable because parents welcome children best when they consciously prepare their own bodies, minds, and spirits for pregnancy and birth and think of conception as a deep commitment between themselves and the baby (The Alliance for Transforming the Lives of Children [aTLC], 2001).

Even when pregnancy is unplanned, as many are, parents can create a healthy, nurturing environment for their unborn child. Thus many perinatal education programs offer preconception and early pregnancy classes as part of their comprehensive program series. Once a family has decided to have a baby, or has achieved pregnancy, the next decisions involve choosing a health care provider based on competence, care philosophy, and associated birth-site choices, with consideration to limits on choice available to many women. Additional choices include desired birth experiences and plans for infant feeding and infant care.

Maternity care providers are typically split into two ideologic groups, with the medical model more oriented toward intervention and the midwifery model inclined to be more holistic and natural. There are many gradations between the two models of care; however, the emphasis on the former is on the use of technology versus an emphasis on health promotion and problem prevention by the latter (Moore, 2005). Early education is an important component of contemporary maternity services that enable parents to sort through how they feel about these approaches to care. Perinatal educators can assist aspiring or newly expectant parents to choose knowledgeably between preferred models of prenatal care. Development and understanding of their own philosophy and desires will enable expectant parents to choose compatible care providers and the place of giving birth. These early decisions will strongly influence the remaining choices in their perinatal experiences.

All women of reproductive age should be considered as having a potential for pregnancy and be advised about anticipatory activities that are important in preconception care (Riskin-Mashiah, 2004). In order to reach women most in need of preconception education, nurses in roles offering interaction with young women can reach out creatively beyond the offices of traditional care providers. School nurses and college health service nurses can arrange to be guest lecturers in appropriate high school and college classes. Community health nurses can develop displays for community health fairs or offer programs through day care centers where they would encounter young women who may conceive again. Nurses in family planning agencies can be alert to the benefits of reaching out with preconception education to women who may become pregnant, intentionally or unintentionally.

If a couple is planning a pregnancy, the perinatal educator or the primary health care provider may assist them in the timing of conception after implementing lifestyle recommendations for their health. These recommendations could include diet and weight management, physical conditioning, immunizations, and genetic counseling. Fostering normal adaptations to an ever-changing physiology should be a focus of a preconception curriculum or plan of care. Teaching stress reduction through relaxation, guided imagery, moderate exercise, and rest also is useful in promoting behaviors appropriate for early pregnancy (Tiran & Chummun, 2004). Expectant fathers may not yet have established a source of health care as adults. Thus, they too can be encouraged to have a physical examination and to care for their own health. Polomeno (1998) describes how selected aspects of health education and health screening for expectant fathers can be woven into perinatal education classes.

By the end of the eighth week after conception, and certainly by the end of the first trimester, any major structural anomalies in the fetus are already present. Thus the period of greatest danger from intrauterine environmental hazards for the developing fetus is between 17 and 56 days after fertilization. Because many women do not realize that they are pregnant, do not have their pregnancy confirmed, or do not seek prenatal care until well into the first trimester, the rapidly growing fetus may be exposed to many intrauterine environmental hazards during this vulnerable developmental phase. Preconception and early pregnancy education, therefore, fosters behaviors in women planning pregnancies to do the following:

- Establish lifestyle behaviors to maintain optimal health (e.g., eating a healthy diet including sources of folic acid; getting enough rest and exercise; and avoiding alcohol use, smoking, and other drugs)
- Prepare psychologically for pregnancy and the responsibilities that come with parenthood, and build a support system to sustain the new family throughout the perinatal year

- Identify, minimize, or treat risk factors before conception (e.g., medical conditions such as diabetes mellitus, substance abuse, use of medications for chronic illness, or infections, including those sexually transmitted)
- Screen for health hazards in the workplace or home
- Obtain, when warranted, genetic counseling to identify carriers of inherited diseases (e.g., Tay-Sachs disease, sickle-cell disease, or thalassemia)
- Compare the quality and philosophic bases of the perinatal care options available

EVIDENCE-BASED PRACTICE

Smoking Reduction During Pregnancy

BACKGROUND

- Smoking causes harm in pregnancy and is associated with low birth weight (less than 2500 grams), prematurity, perinatal death, and sudden infant death syndrome. In addition, smoking is associated with low breastfeeding initiation and duration, as well as higher rates of childhood lung disease and ear infections. Approximately one out of eight pregnant women smoke. Smoking is more prevalent for women of lower income and education, white race, young age, single status, increased parity, and Medicaid assistance. Psychosocial markers for smoking include depression, stress, intimate partner violence, and lack of community practical support. Pregnancy is often a "golden moment" for quitting, since the woman may feel protective of her future child and herself as its mother. This may still not be motivation enough for heavily addicted smokers, who may erroneously believe that a small baby will make for an easy delivery. Smokers live with guilt, anxiety, and stress because of the continuation of smoking during pregnancy. Self-report of smoking is notoriously unreliable.

OBJECTIVES

- The authors sought to update a previous review of smoking cessation to determine what kinds of information and support given to pregnant women can facilitate reduction of smoking. They wished to investigate pregnancy outcomes and smoking recidivism.

METHODS

Search Strategy

- A thorough search of medical and psychologic databases and relevant reference lists identified 51 randomized controlled trials and six cluster-randomized trials, representing over 28,000 women, published 1976 to 2003. The countries of origin were Argentina, Australia, Brazil, Canada, Cuba, Denmark, Holland, Ireland, Mexico, the Netherlands, New Zealand, Norway, Scotland, Sweden, the United Kingdom, and the United States.

Statistical Analyses

- Although interventions varied greatly and have intensified over the last 3 decades, the reviewers were able to metaanalyze 48 trials by pooling all interventional data and comparing to all "usual care," or control, data. Categoric data, such as pregnancy outcomes, were calculated using risk ratio; and continuous data, such as number of cigarettes or birth weight,

were calculated using weighted means. Differences between groups that fell outside the 95% confidence interval were accepted as significant.

FINDINGS

- Various interventions included information about the risks of smoking for fetus and mother, timetables for quitting, recommendations about benefits and strategies of quitting, rewards, social and peer support, and nicotine replacement therapy. The interventions were significantly effective at reducing smoking in late pregnancy, and resulted in an absolute reduction of 6% of women who continued to smoke. Perinatal outcomes that improved included close to 20% fewer low-birth-weight infants and fewer preterm births.

LIMITATIONS

- Randomization and the elimination of cointerventions are difficult in the "real world" settings, where caregivers are striving for optimum outcome on each subject, but this is not a new problem in research. The control groups were exposed to background smoking messages that increased over time. Some trials excluded women with perinatal deaths, thus limiting important outcome data.

IMPLICATIONS FOR PRACTICE

- A comprehensive program of information on the risks of smoking to mother and fetus and effects of passive smoke on growing children, combined with long-term rewards, smoking cessation for partners and other caretakers, and practical support, is recommended in all maternity settings. Nicotine replacement therapy is still not recommended until questions about safety in pregnancy are resolved.

IMPLICATIONS FOR FURTHER RESEARCH

- Standardizing measures, such as salivary or urinary cotinine, are available now to confirm nonsmoking status. Long-term studies can provide information about growth, learning, and cognition in childhood and even adulthood. Telephone quitlines and on-line smoking cessation interventions have shown promise. Information is needed on the safety in pregnancy of nicotine replacement and antidepressant therapies. Outcomes may vary by gestational age at which smoking ceased. Accounting for all pregnancy outcomes, including early pregnancy loss, will give a better picture of the true risks of smoking.

Reference: Lumley, J., Oliver, S., Chamberlain, C., & Oakley, L. (2004). Interventions for promoting smoking cessation during pregnancy (review). *The Cochrane Database of Systematic Reviews*, 2006, Issue 3. Chichester, UK: John Wiley & Sons.

The components of general preconception education such as health promotion, risk assessment, and interventions, are outlined in Box 17-1.

In many communities, preconception or early pregnancy classes also emphasize health-promoting behavior as well as choices of care. For example, an adequate maternal intake of folic acid (400 mcg/day preconceptually; 600 mcg/day during pregnancy) decreases the risk of having a child with a neural tube defect (NTD). For those women who have had a previous pregnancy affected by NTD, an intake of 4 mg/day of folic acid from 1 month before conception through the first trimester has been recommended since 1999 (American Academy of Pediatrics [AAP], 1999). All health-promoting education should be provided in a context that emphasizes how well designed

box 17-1 Components of Preconception Care

HEALTH PROMOTION: GENERAL TEACHING
- Nutrition
  - Healthy diet, including folic acid
  - Optimal weight
- Exercise and rest
- Avoidance of substance abuse (tobacco, alcohol, "recreational" drugs)
- Use of safer sex practices
- Attending to family and social needs

RISK FACTOR ASSESSMENT
- Medical history
  - Immune status (e.g., rubella)
  - Family history (e.g., genetic disorders)
  - Illnesses (e.g., infections)
  - Current use of medication (prescription, nonprescription, herbal)
- Reproductive history
  - Contraceptive
  - Obstetric
- Psychosocial history
  - Spouse/partner and family situation, including domestic violence
  - Availability of family or other support systems
  - Readiness for pregnancy (e.g., age, life goals, stress)
- Financial resources
- Environmental (home, workplace) conditions
  - Safety hazards
  - Toxic chemicals
  - Radiation

INTERVENTIONS AS INDICATED
- Anticipatory guidance/teaching
- Treatment of medical conditions and results
  - Medications
  - Cessation/reduction in substance use/abuse
  - Immunizations (e.g., rubella, hepatitis)
- Nutrition, diet, and weight management
- Exercise
- Referral for genetic counseling
- Referral to and use of other services
  - Family planning services
  - Family and social needs management

a healthy body is to adapt to the changes that accompany pregnancy. Without this context of health, routine care and testing for risks may contribute to a mindset of families that pregnancy is a pathologic as opposed to a healthy mind-body-spirit event (Strong, 2002).

Individualized education, as an aspect of early perinatal education, is especially important for women who have had a problem with a previous pregnancy (e.g., miscarriage or preterm birth) (Lamb, 2002). Supporting preconception health care may minimize fetal malformations through identification and treatment of problems. For example, women with insulin-dependent diabetes mellitus who maintain excellent control of blood sugar at the time of conception could reduce the risk for congenital anomalies (malformations) in the fetus. However, these mothers may need assistance in maintaining a balanced perspective that includes the positive aspects of pregnancy rather than a focus only on the difficulties of maintaining a blood sugar safe for both mother and baby (Berg, 2005). In an example related to preconception care, women who have systemic lupus erythematosus are at high risk for miscarriage or preterm labor; planning a pregnancy during a remission period can increase the chances of a healthy pregnancy. (A preconception assessment that identifies areas to be explored is provided in Box 17-2.)

Demographic information such as age and race also suggest areas where early education and care is important. Women younger than 15 or older than 35 years are at a higher risk for negative pregnancy outcomes than are women aged 16 to 34 years. Some ethnic groups have special risks; for example, African-Americans and Southeast Asians are at risk for sickle cell disease, and people of Jewish descent are at risk for Tay-Sachs disease. Once care is established, parents have additional decisions to make including the use and frequency of ultrasound examination and amniocentesis, if recommended. A Cochrane review of fetal assessment in early pregnancy concludes that ultrasound in early pregnancy appears to enable better gestational age assessment, thus reducing rates of induction of labor for postterm pregnancy, increasing diagnosis of multiple pregnancy, and diagnosing fetal anomaly at a time when termination of pregnancy is an option (Neilson, 2000).

There are a multitude of environmental drugs and chemical and physical agents that have been documented to produce congenital malformations (Brent, 2004). Fortunately only a small percentage of birth defects are known to occur as a result of environmental factors, and these may be amenable to educational awareness. Families can be taught that cleanliness, ventilation, adherence to manufacturer's directions for use and disposal of materials, use of protective gear to shield against known and unknown hazards, and avoidance of exposure to radiation are examples of strategies to reduce risk. In some instances, safer materials can be substituted for potentially hazardous ones. For example, most household cleaning needs can be met with baking soda, table salt, distilled white vinegar, lemon juice, trisodium phosphate (TSP, which does not emit fumes), a plunger, and

---

box 17-2 **Preconception Assessment**

INTERVIEW
- Lifestyle
  Nutrition
  Exercise, rest
  Substance use: alcohol, tobacco, cocaine, other
  Occupation
  Psychosocial: stress, anxiety, depression; support from partner, family, friends; domestic violence
  Financial resources
- Immunization status
  Rubella
  Hepatitis B
  Toxoplasmosis (not universal)
- Medications
  Over-the-counter, nonprescription (e.g., aspirin)
  Herbal remedies
  Prescription
  Medical conditions: review of systems
  Hypertension, cardiovascular disease
  Seizure disorders
  Diabetes mellitus
  Renal disease
  Autoimmune disorders (e.g., lupus, rheumatoid arthritis)
  Tuberculosis, asthma, allergies
- Reproductive system
  Fertility problems, endometriosis
  Contraceptive history
  Obstetric history (e.g., prior pregnancies, miscarriages, child with a disorder)
  Abnormal Papanicolaou (Pap) smear results
  Sexually transmitted infections (STIs)
  Sexual practices

- Family history, including father of baby
  Medical conditions
  Genetic conditions (e.g., sickle cell disease, Tay-Sachs disease, cystic fibrosis, bleeding disorders, phenylketonuria [PKU])
  Birth defects
- Treatment history
  Previous abdominal reproductive surgery
  Trauma
  Previous blood transfusion(s)
- Environmental history—exposure to teratogens such as organic solvents, pesticides, and ionizing radiation
  Work exposures
  Home exposures

PHYSICAL EXAMINATION
- General medical with following emphasis:
  Thyroid gland
  Breasts
  Pelvic structures

LABORATORY STUDIES
- General: CBC, urinalysis, blood type and Rh, rubella titer, STIs (e.g., syphilis, gonorrhea, *Chlamydia*), hepatitis B surface antigen, Pap smear, and cervical culture
- Depending on risk:
  PPD
  HIV
  Toxicology screen
  Thalassemia

CBC, Complete blood count; *HIV,* human immunodeficiency virus; *PPD,* purified protein derivative test (for tuberculosis).

---

some common sense. These substances can be used to clean drains, wash windows, degrease, prevent mold and mildew, disinfect, and scour. Nurses must be alert to conditions in the workplace that may affect the reproductive health of workers and their partners. As private citizens, nurses should become involved in professional and political organizations to promote and support legislation to control pollution of the environment. Nurses can teach about alternative ways to clean the home and care for yards and gardens to reduce exposure to potentially harmful substances.

Evaluation of short-term results of environmental consciousness is possible only when observing outcomes in large populations over the years. The birth of a healthy baby with no apparent disorder or disease, the uncomplicated recovery of the new mother, continued fertility, and demonstration of a lifestyle that supports good reproductive health are some expected outcomes when preconception and pregnancy care are effective. However, long-term effects may not be known for many years or generations.

Perinatal Provider and Care Choices

The environment in which a woman gives birth is equally as influential as educating her how to listen to and work with her body during childbirth. Thus perinatal education

ideally includes informing women about that choice. CIMS produced a document to assist women in selecting their perinatal care. In the document, after some explanation of choices, women are encouraged to ask potential perinatal care providers the following questions:
- Who can be with me during labor and birth?
- What happens during a normal labor and birth in your setting?
- How do you allow for differences in culture and beliefs?
- Can I walk and move around during labor? What position do you suggest for birth?
- How do you make sure everything goes smoothly when my nurse, doctor, midwife, or agency work with each other?
- What things do you normally do to a woman in labor?
- How do you help mothers stay as comfortable as they can be? Besides drugs, how do you help mothers relieve the pain of labor?
- What if my baby is born early or has special problems?
- Do you circumcise babies?
- How do you help mothers who want to breastfeed?

The entire document can be obtained at www. motherfriendly.org. CIMS has also produced a Mother

Friendly Childbirth Initiative with guidelines for identifying and designating "mother-friendly" birth sites including hospitals, birth centers, and home-birth services. This information is available at the same website. CIMS identified several principles for mother-friendly services. They should do the following:

- Promote birth as a normal, natural, and healthy process
- Empower a woman to develop confidence in her ability to give birth and care for her baby
- Give the woman autonomy to make informed choices about the care she and her baby receive
- Do no harm by applying only medically necessary interventions
- Take responsibility for the quality of care provided, based on the needs of the mother and child

These principles give expectant parents an idea of what they have a right to expect in their perinatal care and may influence how they make choices when interacting with the health care system throughout their lives. The educator can provide information about the different types of health care providers described below and in general the kind of care to anticipate from each type.

Physicians

Physicians (obstetricians and family practice physicians) attended about 91.4% of births in hospitals in the United States in 2003, although this number has decreased slightly over the last decade as births attended by midwives increased to 8% in 2003 (Martin, Hamilton, Sutton, Ventura, Menacker, & Munson, 2005). Physicians see low and high risk clients. Care often includes pharmacologic and medical management of problems and the early use of technologic procedures such as ultrasound examination and amniocentesis. Family practice physicians may need backup by obstetricians if a specialist is needed for a problem such as a cesarean birth. Almost all physicians manage births in a hospital setting.

Nurse-Midwives

Nurse-midwives are registered nurses with additional education and training in the care of obstetric clients. Throughout history, midwives have held a holistic view of childbirth. Midwives provide care for about 8% of the births in the United States (Martin et al., 2005) and 95% of these are nurse-midwives who attended births primarily in hospitals. A few nurse-midwives manage births in home settings. Certified nurse-midwives may practice with physicians or independently with an arrangement for physician backup. They usually see low risk obstetric clients. Care in a midwifery model is noninterventional in orientation, and the woman and family are usually encouraged to be active participants in their care. However, not all nurse-midwives practice using a strictly midwifery model, just as not all physicians practice using an intervention focus for maternity care. Nurse-midwives refer clients with complications to physicians.

Direct-Entry Midwives

Direct-entry midwives (also called certified professional midwives) are trained through self-study, apprenticeship, midwifery schools, or universities as a profession distinct from nursing. However, their certification process is administered by the American College of Nurse-Midwives. They manage slightly less than 1% of births in the United States. They also refer the clients in whom problems develop to physicians. A majority (61%) of births attended by these midwives take place in the home setting. Because of underreporting of direct-entry midwife-attended births, these data should be considered lower estimates of actual numbers of midwife-attended births. Jungblom (2003) contrasted the care of 52 women between these midwives and obstetricians. She found no difference in postpartum depression rates, but those women in the midwifery group reported receiving more education, more social support, and having better relationships with their health care providers. Similar results were found by Smook (2001).

Doulas

Whereas the caregivers discussed previously provide medical and health supervision and manage the birth, doulas provide a support service. A certified doula is professionally trained to provide labor support, including physical, emotional, and informational support, to women and their partners during labor and birth. The doula role does not include becoming involved with clinical tasks. Some childbirth educators serve in the doula role for those who attend their classes. Today, many couples, no matter which type of childbirth classes they take, also employ a doula for labor support. A Cochrane synopsis of 15 trials involving 12,791 women found that "continuous labor support like that provided by doulas reduces a woman's likelihood of having pain medication, increases her satisfaction and chances for spontaneous birth, and has no known risks" (Hodnett et al., 2003).

A doula typically meets with the woman and her husband or partner before labor. At this meeting, she ascertains the woman's expectations and desires for the birth experience. With this information as her guide during labor and birth, the doula focuses her efforts on assisting the woman to achieve her goals. Doulas work collaboratively with other health care providers and the husband or other supportive individuals, but their primary goal is assisting the woman.

Doulas may be found through community contacts, other health care providers, or childbirth educators; a number of organizations offer information or referral services. It is important that the expectant mother be comfortable with the doula who will be attending her. See Box 17-3 for a list of questions to ask when arranging for a doula. Doulas of North America (DONA) is an organization that certifies doulas (www.dona.com). Although the doula role originally developed as an assistant during labor, some women benefit from assistance during the postpartum box 17-3 **Questions to Ask When Choosing a Doula**

To discover the specific training, experience, and services offered by anyone who provides labor support, potential clients, nursing supervisors, physicians, midwives, and others should ask the following questions of that person:
- What training have you had?
- Tell me about your experience with birth, personally and as a doula.
- What is your philosophy about childbirth and supporting women and their partners through labor?
- May we meet to discuss our birth plans and the role you will play in supporting me through childbirth?
- May we call you with questions or concerns before and after the birth?
- When do you try to join women in labor? Do you come to our home or meet us at the hospital?
- Do you meet with us after the birth to review the labor and answer questions?
- Do you work with one or more backup doulas for times when you are not available? May we meet them?
- What are your fees and your refund policy?

From Simkin, P., Young, D., The Director of Publications and the 2005 International Board of Directors (2005). DONA Position Paper: *The doula's contributions to modern maternity care,* ed 2, Seattle: Doulas of North America.

period. There are small but growing numbers of postnatal doulas, who provide assistance to the new mother as she develops competence with infant care, feeding, and other maternal tasks.

Birth Plans

Once the maternity care provider is chosen, there are numerous other decisions to be made over the course of the perinatal year. Many prenatal care providers and childbirth educators encourage expectant parents to develop a birth plan to identify their options and set priorities. The birth plan is a natural evolution of a contemporary wellness-oriented lifestyle in which clients assume a level of responsibility for their own health. For some, beginning this approach to perinatal care will influence their approach to health care throughout their lives. The birth plan is a tool with which parents can explore their childbirth options and choose those that are most important to them. The plan must be viewed as tentative since the realities of what is feasible may change as the actual labor and birth unfold. It is understood to be a preference list based on a best case scenario.

The birth plan can be conceptualized as an advance directive similar in purpose to end-of-life directives (Philipsen & Haynes, 2005). (Some care providers may be more accepting of birth plans if they view them in the same context as advance directives, a term that is more widely accepted although still a flexible one.) Many parents already indicate some of their birthing preferences by the type of health care provider and birth setting (hospital, free-standing birth center, or home) they have chosen. Some pregnant women enlist the services of a health care provider only after an interview and a tour of the birth facility. Others do not give

conscious thought to the conduct of their pregnancies, the labor and birth process, recovery, and early parenthood. These women may benefit from further help with making decisions according to their preferences.

After the confirmation of pregnancy, couples tend to be focused on the reality of their situation and their emotional responses. However, it is useful for the nurse in a prenatal clinic setting to initiate a discussion of choices and birth planning during the first and second prenatal visits. Some maternity clinics provide printed material describing available options and giving answers to commonly asked questions, and tours of the birth setting are offered by almost all birthing facilities. The nurse can provide couples with pertinent information so they can begin making informed decisions, alerting them to various options for care and the advantages and consequences of each. Early plans can be modified as the couple learns more details in their childbirth class.

The birth plan can serve as a means of open communication between the pregnant woman and her partner and also between the couple and health care providers. An early introduction to the idea of a birth plan allows the couple time to think about events or situations that could make their childbearing experience more meaningful and those they would prefer to avoid. For most, a discussion of the birth plan should take place in an accepting atmosphere in which women can see themselves as unique and yet normal. The educator should assess clients' readiness to learn and avoid overloading them too rapidly with information. Some health care providers provide birth plan templates. A discussion of the printed template can assist the couples to start thinking about, discussing, and identifying what is important to them. The options of women with a high risk pregnancy or those in whom complications develop during labor may be more limited. Berg, Lundgren, and Lindmark (2003) found that for women with complications during pregnancy, the use of a birth plan appeared to intensify their negative feelings related to being more vulnerable, and thus birth plans should be used with caution for such women.

There are numerous interactive programs on the Internet which will assist couples to create their birth plans. However, childbirth educators should screen any such programs before referring couples to them since some contain advertising that is contrary to promoting good health.

Topics for birth plan discussion and decision making may include any or all of the following:
- Partner's participation: Attend prenatal visits? Childbirth and parent education classes? Present during labor? During birth? During cesarean birth?
- Birth setting: Hospital delivery room or birthing room (if available)? A birthing center? Home?
- Labor management: Walk around during labor? Use a rocking chair? Use a shower? Use a Jacuzzi, if available? Intermittent versus continuous use of an electronic fetal monitor? Have music or dimmed lighting? Have older children or other people present? Is telemetry

monitoring available? Consider stimulation of labor? Consider medication—what kind?

- Birth: Positions—Side-lying? On hands and knees, kneeling, or squatting? Use a birthing bed? Or delivery table? Will you be photographing, videotaping, or recording any of the labor or birth? Who would you like to be present—partner, older siblings, other family members, or friends? What do you know about the use of forceps? Episiotomies? Will your partner want to cut the umbilical cord?
- Immediately after birth: Do you want to hold the baby right away? Breastfeed immediately?
- Postpartum care: What kind of care do you anticipate—labor, delivery, recovery, postpartum room; mother-baby coupling? How long does your insurance company provide coverage for you to stay? Would you like to attend self-care classes, or do you prefer to get such information from videotapes? On which subjects?

Birth Setting Choices

An important choice of the expectant couple is the birth setting. With careful thought, the concept of natural, family, or woman-centered maternity care can be implemented in any setting. The three primary options for birth settings today are the hospital, the birth center, and home. Women consider several factors in choosing a setting for childbirth, including the preference of their health care provider, characteristics of the birthing unit, and preference of their third-party payer. Approximately 99% of all births in the United States took place in a hospital setting in 2003 (Martin et al., 2005). However, the types of labor and birth services available in hospitals vary greatly, from the traditional labor and delivery rooms with separate postpartum and newborn units to in-hospital birthing centers where all or almost all care takes place in a single unit.

Hospital Labor, Delivery, Recovery, and Postpartum (Birthing) Rooms

Labor, delivery, recovery (LDR) and labor, delivery, recovery, postpartum (LDRP) rooms offer families a single, comfortable, private space for all facets of childbirth. In contrast, women who are admitted to LDR units, labor and give birth and only spend the first 1 to 2 hours there for immediate postpartum recovery and for having time with their families to bond with their newborns (Fig. 17-1). After this period of recovery, the mothers and newborns are transferred to a postpartum unit and nursery or mother-baby unit for the duration of their stay. Care is provided by different nursing staff (e.g., labor and delivery nurses, postpartum nurses, nursery nurses). In some hospitals, the same nurse provides care for both mothers and newborns.

In LDRP units, total care is provided from admission for labor through postpartum discharge in the same room, usually by the same nursing staff. The woman and her family may stay in this unit for 6 to 48 hours after giving birth. The units are furnished similar to LDR units but have accommodations for family members to stay overnight.

FIG. 17-1 **A,** LDR unit. **B,** LDRP unit. (**A,** Courtesy Marjorie Pyle, RNC, Lifecircle, Costa Mesa, CA. **B,** Courtesy Dee Lowdermilk, Chapel Hill, NC.)

Both units are equipped with fetal monitors, emergency resuscitation equipment for both mother and newborn, and heated cribs or warming units for the newborn. Often this equipment is out of sight in cabinets or closets when it is not being used.

Birth Centers

In 2003, of the 1% of births that occurred outside of hospitals, 27% were in a free-standing birth center (Martin et al., 2005). Freestanding birth centers are usually built in locations separate from the hospital but may be located in close proximity in case the transfer of the woman or newborn is needed. These birth centers are intended to offer families an alternative to home or hospital birth, providing a third choice that is a safe and cost-effective compromise. Nurse-midwives or physicians who also have privileges at the local hospital usually staff the centers. Clients are evaluated carefully as a measure to ensure that only women who are at low risk for complications are included for care. This is a requirement of the standards of the Commission on Accreditation of Free-Standing Birth Centers.

Birth centers typically have homelike accommodations; including perhaps a double bed for the couple and a crib for the newborn (Fig. 17-2). Emergency equipment is available but ideally stored out of view. Many centers have an

FIG. 17-2 Birth center. **A,** Note double bed, baby crib, and birthing stool. **B,** Lounge and kitchen. (**A,** Courtesy Dee Lowdermilk, Chapel Hill, NC. **B,** Courtesy Michael S. Clement, MD, Mesa, AZ. Photo location: Bethany Birth Center, Phoenix, AZ.)

early-labor lounge or a living room, and a small kitchen may be available. The family is admitted to the birth center for labor and birth and will remain there until discharge, often within 6 hours of the birth.

Other services provided by free-standing birth centers include those necessary for safe management during the childbearing cycle. In addition, attendance at childbirth and parenting classes is often required of all clients. Prenatal discussions with the woman, whose nutritional and health status must be good and who must be experiencing a low risk pregnancy, begins in the first trimester. Women are ideally presented with situations that may require transfer to a hospital and must agree to abide by those guidelines. These expectant families do develop birth plans.

Birth centers as well as a hospital with a comprehensive birthing program may more likely have resources such as a lending library for parents, reference files on related topics, recycled maternity clothes and baby clothes and equipment, and supplies and reference materials for childbirth educators. The centers also may have referral files for community resources that offer services related to childbirth and early parenting, including support groups (such as for single parents, postbirth support group, and parents of twins), genetic counseling, women's issues, and consumer action.

When births occur in a birth center or a home setting, they should be located close to a major hospital so that quick transfer to that institution is possible when necessary. Ambulance service and emergency procedures must be readily available. Fees vary with the services provided but typically are less than or equal to those charged by local hospitals. Some centers base fees on the ability of the family to pay (reduced-fee sliding scale). Several third-party payers, Medicaid, and TRICARE/CHAMPUS (the armed services insurance) recognize and reimburse these centers; however, clients should check with their health care payers regarding reimbursement for prenatal care and birth in a birth center.

Home Birth

Home birth has always been popular in certain countries such as Sweden and the Netherlands. In developing countries, hospitals or adequate lying-in facilities are often unavailable to most pregnant women, and home birth is a necessity. In North America, home births account for less than 1% of births (Martin et al., 2005) but account for about 65% of out-of-hospital births. National groups supporting home birth are the Home Oriented Maternity Experience (HOME) and the National Association of Parents for Safe Alternatives in Childbirth (NAPSAC) (www.napsac.org). These groups work to foster more humane childbearing practices at all levels, integrating the alternatives for childbirth to meet the needs of the total population.

Over time, many studies have documented the safety of home births. For example, Schlenzka (1999) examined 816,000 California births in 1989 through 1990. After comparing both low risk and high risk births outside and inside the hospital, he found that each approach produced the same perinatal mortality outcomes for both high and low risk births. He additionally noted that the out-of-the-hospital approach shows significant advantage with respect to lower maternity care costs as well as reduced morbidity from unnecessary cesareans and other obstetric interventions, and significant benefits from avoiding negative long-term consequences from unnecessary obstetric interventions and procedures. Similarly, Olsen and Jewell (2000) reported a metaanalysis of observational studies that found that planned home birth is safe, with fewer interventions than planned hospital births. Most recently, the surveillance and risk assessment division in the Public Health Agency of Canada conducted a prospective cohort study involving certified professional midwives of 5418 births across the United Sates and Canada. Substantially lower rates of epidurals, episiotomies, forceps, vacuum extractions, and cesarean births occurred among them, including the 12% who were transferred to the hospital. No mothers died and infant mortality was similar to rates of other low risk home and hospital births. Thus although home births are considered countercultural by many in the United States, there is no evidence base to discourage low risk couples who desire a carefully planned out-of-the-hospital birth (Johnson & Daviss, 2005).

One advantage of home birth is that the family is in control of the experience. Another is that the birth may be more physiologically normal in familiar surroundings. The mother may be more relaxed than she would be in the hospital environment. Care providers who participate in home births tend to be more support oriented and less intervention oriented. The family can assist in and be a part of the happy event, and contact with the newborn is immediate and sustained. In addition, home birth may be less expensive than a hospital confinement. Serious infection may be less likely, assuming strict aseptic principles are followed, because people generally are relatively immune to their own home bacteria.

Components of Perinatal Education Programs

In addition to preparing families for childbirth, perinatal educators promote many aspects of perinatal wellness. Pregnancy is a time of personal growth, during which most couples are open to making changes in lifestyle and habits. Information on infant care, feeding, and stimulation and couple and family adjustments also is incorporated into many prenatal programs. A variety of approaches to perinatal education beyond preparation for birth have evolved as educators attempt to meet learning and support needs of expectant parents and to capitalize on the openness to learning they exhibit. For example, prenatal and new-mother weekly exercise classes can offer both physiologic and social support for a mixture of expectant and new mothers who may even elect to stay connected with e-mail for support between weekly classes. However, *it is important that a focus on preparation for birth not become lost* in all the topics that could be offered to expectant parents. Some of the additional topics mentioned below might fit well into a second trimester class as part of an organized series for the perinatal year.

Refresher classes are frequently available for parents with previous birth experience who just want to review coping techniques for labor and birth. In areas with sufficient population, there may be classes designed specifically for pregnant adolescents and their partners or parents or classes designed for groups with special learning needs, such as first-time mothers over 35 years of age, single women, adoptive parents, parents of multiples or women with handicaps such as those who are visually impaired or deaf.

Pain Management as an Aspect of Childbirth Education

Before birth, fear of pain in labor is a key issue and a reason many women give for attending childbirth education classes. Numerous studies show that women who have received childbirth preparation later report no less pain but consistently do report greater ability to cope with the pain during labor and birth and increased birth satisfaction compared to unprepared women. Thus although pain management strategies are an essential component of childbirth education, total pain eradication is not the primary source of birth satisfaction nor a goal, any more than it is in training for an intense athletic event. Eliminating suffering, however, is a realistic goal. As described above, control in childbirth, meaning participation in decision making, has been repeatedly found to be the primary source of birth satisfaction. The advantages and disadvantages of pain medication for coping with labor are covered in detail in Chapter 19.

In a study of prenatal women, the prenatal childbirth-related fears of 8000 women who gave birth in a hospital setting that offers modern obstetrics and alternative birth methods were as follows: fear for the child's health (50%), fear of pain (40%), and fear of dealing with medical intervention such as operative birth, anesthesia, and nerve blockage and of being at the mercy of obstetric practices (12%) (Geissbuehler & Eberhard, 2002). Birth preparation classes are limited in their ability to reduce all these childbirth fears, some of which are reality based. Classes can, however, work to bring any fears out into the open, dispel those that are myths, discuss coping strategies, and create confidence related to those that are real.

There are many differences in beliefs related to pain control choices in childbirth. Whether they take birth preparation classes or not, the majority of women today plan to have epidural medication. Heinze and Sleigh (2003) studied this decision and found that women who chose to give birth with an epidural had higher fear of childbirth, a more external locus of control for childbirth, and more of a desire for passive compliance in the childbirth process. They lacked the confidence in their own ability that childbirth education classes attempt to instill. Results also showed that women who labored without an epidural had lower fear of childbirth, a more internal locus of control for childbirth, and a stronger desire to actively participate in the childbirth process, as well as higher knowledge of risks associated with epidural use. Based on the most recent Cochrane review, in 11 studies of 3157 women, epidural analgesia is very effective in reducing pain but is also associated with longer labors, greater incidence of fetal malposition, greater use of oxytocin, and greater use of forceps or vacuum extractions (Anim-Somuah, Smyth, & Howell, 2005). Epidurals have not been shown to be associated with greater satisfaction with birth experiences.

Anesthesia and analgesics used in childbirth affect the levels of oxytocin released during and right after birth for several days (Uvnäs-Moberg, 2005). The hormone oxytocin has noticeable effects in making a mother calm and relaxed while breastfeeding. In addition to leading to greater birth satisfaction, a well-supported, nonmedicated birth has potential for a positive impact on initiating breastfeeding. In summary there are numerous advantages for having a birth with low or no medication. However, women can be assured that within the bounds of safety, the choice rightfully belongs to the birthing mother. Birthing with low or no medication takes planning for skills, resources, and a support team. Even among strong normal birth advocates, there is no thought that mothers should be made to suffer. Beck (2004) concludes that among mothers who perceived that their births were traumatic, their clinicians often viewed them as routine. Some of the themes she found that are underlying birth trauma were related to care, communication, and safety and included feelings of betrayal and powerlessness. Thus as emphasized earlier, every effort should be made to help an expectant mother create a support system that will provide her with the most choices feasible within the bounds of safety.

Education for Labor and Childbirth

Childbearing couples are taught to recognize labor's start, what to expect, and when to start using coping skills such as relaxation, conscious breathing, and other nonpharmacologic strategies. The concept of coaching a woman in labor by "calling the plays" has been replaced by the concept of supporting a woman who knows how to give birth and benefits from support and encouragement. Supportive techniques may include reassurance, massage, pressure on the palms or soles of the feet, applications of heat or cold, hydrotherapy, conscious breathing, and focusing of attention. Additional techniques to increase coping and decrease the distress from labor pain include vocalization or "sounding" to relieve tension, subdued lighting, warm water for showers or bathing during labor, and aromatherapy.

Relaxation

Relaxation or reduction of body tension is a technique suggested by virtually all childbirth education organizations. Learning relaxation in childbirth education classes can help couples with the stresses of pregnancy, childbirth, and adjustment to parenting and can be a form of stress management throughout life (Fig. 17-3). A review of research across many studies found that relaxation skill is reported to be the most effective nonpharmacologic strategy for coping with the stress of labor. Relaxation is ideally combined with activity such as walking, slow dancing, rocking, and position changes that help the baby rotate through the pelvis. Rhythmic motion stimulates mechanoreceptors in the brain, which decreases pain perception.

Imagery and Visualization

Imagery and visualization also are taught in classes during preparation for birth. Although research on their use in childbirth is scant, clinical reports suggest that imagery and visualization can be used to produce a sense of well-being during pregnancy as well as assist with cervical dilation and decrease the experience of pain and tension during labor. A variety of skills taught in childbirth classes augment relaxation during pregnancy as well as in labor. All can be taught as lifetime skills useful to the couple and can be used to teach their children to cope with the stresses of life.

Conscious Breathing

Using conscious breathing patterns is a visible technique and thus is frequently used in the media to characterize childbirth preparation. Relaxed individuals automatically slow their breathing, and conversely, slowing one's breathing serves to increase one's relaxation. During labor, nursing support includes guiding couples in the application of breathing and relaxation methods and adapting methods to their particular needs.

Biofeedback

The use of observation in class (informal biofeedback) helps couples develop awareness of their bodies and learn strategies to change their responses to stress. During preparation for birth, formal biofeedback (which uses machines prenatally to detect skin temperature, blood flow, or muscle tension) can prepare women to perfect their relaxation response. Biofeedback *machines* per se are not routinely needed for childbirth classes, but weekly feedback to the expectant mother on relaxation progress is beneficial.

Energy Work, Massage, Music and Acupressure

Energy work such as therapeutic touch or healing touch involves energy fields around the body and can be taught in class for use during labor to decrease anxiety and pain and to increase relaxation. Certified practitioners in energy work are consulted throughout pregnancy and during childbirth by some women who have access to such care.

Music promotes relaxation (Browning, 2001) and has been known for centuries to be generally therapeutic. Acupressure, which consists of applying pressure to various pressure points, has been correlated with relief of dizziness, headaches, back pain, nausea, and leg cramps, as well as labor pain. Massage has been shown in a randomized trial to decrease pain and anxiety during labor, and the husbands' participation in massage positively increases the experience for the woman (Chang, Wang, & Chen, 2002).

FIG. 17-3 Childbirth class: Learning relaxation with the whole family. (Courtesy Marjorie Pyle, RNC, Lifecircle, Costa Mesa, CA.)

Preparation for Cesarean Birth

Given that almost 30% of births in the United States is cesarean surgery, this is an important topic for birth preparation education (www.childbirth.org/section/ICAN). Education regarding cesarean birth is threefold in nature. The first component is helping expectant parents know what they can do to avoid the necessity of a cesarean birth. Cesarean birth rates vary widely by care provider and care setting. Cesarean births are more common in women who choose epidurals, in part because the powers of the mother's muscles do not effectively assist the infant in rotation through the pelvis; in part because if given early, epidurals prolong labor; and in part because the mother has less urge to push. In a setting where nursing support during labor is low and care provider rate of cesarean birth is high, women should be aware that their chances of a cesarean birth are increased.

Expectant parents can be encouraged to inquire about the cesarean rates of both their care provider and their planned birth site. Healthy mothers also can be encouraged to refrain from being admitted to the hospital before they are in active labor (can still independently walk and talk through contractions), because the longer their hospitalization, the greater the tendency for them and their care providers to become impatient with their progress and resort to cesareans. Recently there has been a move by some care providers to offer, and for expectant parents to request, elective cesarean births. For those considering an elective cesarean, the risks involved for both mothers and fetus should be well described. Childbirth educators should explore the reason a woman might elect nonnecessary surgery and determine if the basis is rooted in fear, misinformation, or perceived convenience. Currently there is not enough evidence to evaluate fully the risks and benefits of cesarean birth on mother's request (Mennick, 2006).

In the second approach, the effort can be to prevent the need for a subsequent cesarean or preparing for it when it is inevitable or highly likely. Women with a prior cesarean birth can be encouraged to explore the availability of a vaginal birth, with the exception of those who have a history of classic vertical or unknown uterine incisions or those with medical contraindication. Women with a prior cesarean birth can be informed on how to obtain access to their medical records to understand the reason it occurred and the implications for a subsequent birth. In many communities, there are vaginal birth after cesarean (VBAC) support groups, physicians who are known to be supportive, and special childbirth classes for those attempting a VBAC. In contrast, in larger communities, there are likely to be special classes for women who know they will have medical need of a cesarean birth.

The third educational aspect is to prepare all mothers for the differences in postpartum recovery for women after a cesarean birth. Their hospital stay will be longer, their need for assistance at home will be greater, and they may need extra support to establish breastfeeding comfortably.

CRITICAL THINKING EXERCISE

Elective Cesarean Birth

Tracy is a teacher and has planned her pregnancy so that she will give birth soon after the semester ends. She plans to request a cesarean birth so that the infant will be born at the beginning of the summer and she will have 3 months of time with the baby before returning to teaching in the fall. Her mother expresses serious misgivings about this plan, stating that when a baby is ready to be born, it will be born. This difference of opinion has resulted in a serious disagreement between Tracy and her mother. Tracy has asked you to convince her mother that her plan is best for her and her baby.

1. Evidence—Is there sufficient evidence to draw conclusions about the wisdom and safety of a cesarean birth as an elective procedure?
2. Assumptions—Describe the underlying assumptions for each of the following issues:
   a. Assessments that are necessary to identify whether it is feasible and safe for Tracy to have an elective cesarean birth
   b. Risks of a cesarean birth
   c. How to deal with Tracy's request that you convince her mother that her plan is best for her and her baby
   d. Education of Tracy to prepare her for a cesarean birth
3. What implications and priorities for nursing care can be made at this time?
4. Does the evidence objectively support your conclusion?
5. Are there alternative perspectives to your conclusion?

Sibling Classes

Many perinatal education programs include classes that can be attended by siblings whether or not their parents intend for siblings to attend the birth. Siblings experience transitions when a new baby enters the family. Parents need to know about sibling regression and ways to help older children adapt to a new brother or sister. Sibling classes that offer a tour of the birthing unit, show a birth film, and help the children talk about the changes that are apt to occur, such as Mommy being busy with the baby, offer valuable interventions (Fig. 17-4; Box 17-4). When siblings are being prepared to attend the birth, it is important that plans be made to have an adult present whose sole focus is on meeting the needs of the sibling.

FIG. 17-4 Sibling class of preschoolers learning infant care by using dolls. (Courtesy Michael S. Clement, MD, Mesa, AZ.)

box 17-4 Tips for Sibling Preparation

PRENATAL

1. Adjust the timing and content of information about an anticipated infant to the age and understanding of the older child.
2. Take your child on a prenatal visit. Let the child listen to the fetal heartbeat and feel the baby move.
3. Involve the child in preparations for the baby, such as helping decorate the baby's room.
4. Move the child to a bed (if still sleeping in a crib) at least 2 months before the baby is due.
5. Read books, show videos, or take child to sibling preparation classes, including a hospital tour.
6. Answer your child's questions about the coming birth, what babies are like, and any other questions.
7. Take your child to the homes of friends who have babies so that the child has realistic expectations of what babies are like.

DURING THE HOSPITAL STAY

1. Have someone bring the child to the hospital to visit you and the baby (unless you plan to have the child attend the birth or have a home birth).
2. Do not force interactions between the child and the baby. Often the child will be more interested in seeing you and being reassured of your love.

3. Help the child explore the infant by showing how and where to touch the baby.
4. Give the child a gift (from you or from you, the father, and the baby).

GOING HOME

1. Leave the child at home with a relative or babysitter.
2. Have someone else carry the baby from the car so that you can hug the child right away.

ADJUSTMENT AFTER THE BABY IS HOME

1. Arrange for a special time with the child alone with each parent.
2. Do not exclude the child during infant feeding times. The child can sit with you and the baby and feed a doll or drink juice or milk with you or sit quietly with a game.
3. Prepare small gifts for the child so that when the baby gets gifts, the sibling will not feel left out. The child also can help open the baby gifts.
4. Praise the child for acting age appropriately (so that being a baby does not seem better than being older).

Grandparent Classes

Grandparents benefit from classes that help them learn strategies for assisting the couple's transition to parenthood. Grandparents can be a valuable asset, especially if they help with household chores and the care of any older siblings and provide social support. Grandparents may need to be cautioned about taking over caring for the baby themselves instead of allowing the new parents time to develop parenting skills, criticizing the parents' care taking, questioning whether the baby is being adequately breastfed, or other activities that would undermine new parents' adjustment. Grandparents also can benefit by learning about childrearing practices that have changed since they had infants, including infant sleep positions and breastfeeding support.

Parenting

During the perinatal period, parents can be assisted to develop a general connection approach to parenting that will foster resilience in their child throughout childhood. Corwin (1999) describes an integration of childbirth preparation with parenting. Effective parenting is an art that can be learned, so making parents aware of resources about children's developmental stages, temperament, and individuality will help parents make informed decisions and serve as advocates of the child's well-being. Parents also can be taught to carry the baby in the arms or in a sling through the day to provide the near-constant movement that optimizes brain development as well as the touch, safety, and comfort essential to secure bonding (aTLC, 2001).

Childbearing couples who have grown up in large families or have had exposure to infants from babysitting may already be aware of the "24-7" care and feeding needs of a newborn. However, many couples, are surprised by the needs of an infant in the first 2 months, no matter how much others have told them. They also may be surprised at their own response to fatigue after several weeks of lacking uninterrupted sleep. Bringing in parents of a recent newborn to a childbirth class to describe their early parenting experiences is an effective way to help expectant parents envision the task ahead. Informing parents that the newborn's stomach is roughly the size of a walnut can help them understand why the typical infant initially needs to breastfeed 8 to 10 times a day.

Many communities have support or new parents' groups that are helpful to couples making the transition to parenthood. Besides the routine mother-baby classes after birth, some organizations have begun to offer father-baby classes in which new fathers spend time with their babies learning about babies' unique characteristics and the basics of infant care. Childbirth educators also have an opportunity with new families to introduce issues such as the effects on the environment of disposable diapers vs. cloth diapers.

Breastfeeding

The American Academy of Pediatrics has joined the call by many nursing and breastfeeding organizations for infants to be exclusively breastfed for 6 months and breastfed for a year or longer, based on the long list of benefits to mother and child (Gartner, Morton, Lawrence, Naylor,

O'Hare, & Schanler, 2005). Childbirth educators present breastfeeding as a choice with important consequences. The prenatal breastfeeding presentation to expectant couples should refrain from being overly detailed with problem-solving techniques lest the parents be overwhelmed and left with the impression that breastfeeding is too complex and fraught with problems. The focus is to present basic information so that breastfeeding is portrayed as both desirable and readily achievable. The information presented prenatally in classes should be designed to do the following:

- *Motivate:* ensure that pregnant mothers and their immediate supporters know why breastfeeding is a desirable, worthwhile effort, and minimize their barriers to breastfeeding.
- *Explicate*: provide a basic overview of breastfeeding to expectant parents.
- *Initiate:* educate parents on basic techniques and the optimal characteristics of postpartum care for the launching of breastfeeding.
- *Maintain*: educate parents on the techniques to promote lactation and the available resources to assist them in making the adjustments commonly needed in early weeks of breastfeeding.
- *Sustain*: introduce families to strategies to develop the environment and support system that will encourage mothers to sustain breastfeeding through the first year and beyond.

It may be discouraging before birth to review a long list of potential breastfeeding problems and solutions. Rather it is important to make certain that a good source of 24-hours-a-day support is available, including hotlines, friends, family, literature, and professionals. For example, in some communities, the postpartum staff will take calls in the night from mothers who recently gave birth at their hospital.

Infant Massage

Many parents do not know about their infant's capabilities to see and hear in the early weeks of life. It is helpful for parents to realize that the senses are the primary source of information for babies during the first 6 months of life. *Infant massage* is one technique that expectant parents can learn to soothe and comfort the infant, promote relaxation and lessen irritability and crying, and provide a mechanism for positive interaction between parents and infants. Giving the father this role in relating to the infant may prevent some fathers from inadvertently and unintentionally sabotaging breastfeeding by pressuring the mother to let him feed the baby.

Couple Sexuality

The role of the childbirth educator in sexuality is to promote the couple's understanding of the sexual changes of pregnancy and the postpartum period and to facilitate their choices for meeting sexual needs during this time.

The following is a summary of what couples need to learn from class discussions:

- Information and basic understanding about the process of human sexual response and the effect of pregnancy on this response
- Reassurance regarding the safety of sexual activities
- Awareness of their own needs, likes, and dislikes as well as those of their partner
- Strategies to maintain an intimate relationship
- Ways to enhance their sexual relationship
- Effective communication skills to make their needs known to each other
- Comfortable ways to provide feedback to each other

To hold class discussions on this subject, the childbirth educator must be aware of his or her own values and attitudes regarding human sexuality. He or she also must develop an adequate knowledge base about sexuality in general and the changes during the perinatal year. The pregnancy, postpartum resumption, and challenges related to breastfeeding bring an ever-changing set of sexual adjustments during the perinatal year. Finally, he or she must develop skills and methods for integrating this content into childbirth classes.

Family Adjustments to Parenthood

Couples making the transition to parenthood experience challenges that can threaten the quality and stability of their relationships and the health of family members. The movement in health care systems to be involved in strengthening marriage and family life is already under way, and the focus of perinatal education can be expanded to include helping parents create stronger, more stable relationships that will improve the physical and psychologic health of children and adults throughout their lives (Hawkins, Gilliland, Christiaens, & Carroll, 2002). The addition of a baby brings change to all members of the family. The workload increases significantly as parents add the demands of the new infant to their other responsibilities. Childbirth educators help expectant parents anticipate these changes. An example of one technique involves an exercise in working through the family workload, in which parents project the way they will divide their responsibilities after birth. Both new fathers and mothers may be highly focused on their own needs and not understand the needs of the other. Family-centered support providers could miss these needs if not alert to that potential.

If both partners work outside the home, a discussion about negotiating maternity and paternity leaves and plans for returning to work is important. Couples who do not have family or friends available for child care must find competent child care providers. Discussions on the way to select licensed child care providers and federal and state guidelines regarding rights to maternity and paternity leaves are important. Couples also need information about the intensity and length of emotional and physiologic recovery from childbirth and the demands of adapting to parenthood. This knowledge should lead to more realistic planning for household help during the early days or weeks and more appropriate expectations of when women are typically ready to return to work. An understanding of the impact of returning to work on infant well-being and breastfeeding may result in some couples arranging to prolong the mother's time at home.

▬ CHILDBIRTH EDUCATION OUTCOMES

Researchers studying childbirth education outcomes have not adopted a standard set of operational definitions of childbirth education or a theoretical frame work that acknowledges that multiple factors, as opposed to childbirth education alone, impact the outcomes (Koehn, 2002). Research on the influence of childbirth education on biologic birth outcomes has not accounted for the management mindset of those providing care during labor.

However, the research findings on positive childbirth education outcomes have been consistent over many decades. In a review of studies between 1995 and 2001, Koehn (2002) found that the three studies that investigated health promotion all found positive changes in selected health behaviors among class attendees. Examples were communication with partner, relaxation, interpersonal support, and health responsibility. A frequent finding across 12 studies was more prenatal confidence in ability to cope with birth by the end of the class. These findings are similar to those of a decade ago that found that childbirth education "promotes positive attitudes towards labor and delivery and fosters early maternal-infant attachment" (Lindell, 1988). Jones (1983), in a metaanalysis of 58 studies published between 1960 and 1981, examined the effects of childbirth education. Significant effect sizes were found for less maternal fear and anxiety, increases in women's self-esteem, positive mother's relationship with her infant, and on marital relationships, plus a reduced number of medical interventions.

The effects of childbirth education have consistently been shown to be in birth satisfaction, building confidence, and building relationships. Physiologic outcomes are not demonstrated to be strongly influenced by educating expectant parents. Many researchers have treated childbirth education as a direct influence on the birth without considering the mediating influence of care providers' philosophy and their usual type of care. If considered, a more accurate evaluation of childbirth education influence on birth outcomes might be obtained.

Pregnancy is a time when expectant parents expect change in their lives and are open to many types of education. This education can enhance their health and coping in pregnancy, childbirth, and early parenting. It also can influence how they relate to health professionals over a lifetime, how they problem solve with each other, and how they launch their new family. It is an opportunity for nurses to engage in meaningful health promotion and the building of resilience and connection in families.

community activity

Pretend you are a woman contemplating conception who wants to choose her maternity care providers, childbirth educator, and place of birth knowledgeably. Search for information on relevant resources in your community. For example, you might search through the Internet, the phone directory, and the newspaper and call local hospitals. How readily available is the information? How informative is the information that you found? Does this community need a more systematic organization of resources to enable women to make informed decisions? Are there resources for women who do not speak English?

key points

- The experience of birth profoundly affects women and their families, and positive outcomes of childbirth education have consistently been found to be improved confidence, birth satisfaction, and better family relationships.
- Childbirth education teaches tuning into the body's inner wisdom and coping strategies that enhance women's ability to know how to give birth.
- Preconception care stresses healthy behavior that promotes the health of the woman and her fetus, as well as decisions to be made that will influence her entire perinatal year.
- Childbirth education should be available to all pregnant women and their families in a culturally sensitive format.
- Stress and pain management strategies are valuable family tools throughout life.
- Childbirth education strives to promote healthier pregnancies and family lifestyles.
- Active support and choice during labor and birth, directed toward achieving the woman's goals, promotes personal satisfaction and adaptation to the maternal role.

REFERENCES

American Academy of Pediatrics (AAP). (1999). Folic acid for the prevention of neural tube defects. *Pediatrics, 104*(2), 325-327.

Anim-Somuah, M., Smyth, R., & Howell, C. (2005). Epidural versus no-epidural or no analgesia in labor. *The Cochrane Database of Systematic Reviews*, 2006, Issue 3. Chichester, UK: John Wiley & Sons.

aTLC (The Alliance for Transforming the Lives of Children). (2001). A blueprint for transforming the lives of children. *Journal of Perinatal Education, 10*(4), iv-50. [On-line]. Accessed www.atlc.org, April 21, 2006.

Baron, R., Cusumano, M., & Evans, D. (2004). The effect of desired control and anticipated control of the stress of childbirth. *Basic & Applied Social Psychology, 26*(4), 249-261.

Beck, C. (2004). Birth trauma: In the eye of the beholder. *Nursing Research, 53*(1), 28-35.

Berg, M. (2005). Pregnancy and diabetes: How women handle the challenge. *Journal of Perinatal Education, 14*(3), 23-32.

Berg, M., Lundgren, I., & Lindmark, G. (2003). Childbirth experience in women at high risk: Is it improved by use of a birth plan? *Journal of Perinatal Education, 12*(2), 1-15.

Bradley, R. (1965). *Husband-coached childbirth*. New York: HarperCollins.

Brent, R. (2004). Environmental causes of human congenital malformations: The pediatrician's role in dealing with these complex clinical problems caused by a multiplicity of environmental and genetic factors. *Pediatrics, 113*(4 Suppl), 957-968.

Browning, C. (2001). Music therapy in childbirth: Research in practice. *Music Therapy Perspectives, 19*(2), 74-81.

Chang, M., Wang, S., & Chen, C. (2002). Effects of massage on pain and anxiety during labour; A randomized controlled trial in Taiwan. *Journal of Advanced Nursing, 38*(1), 68-73.

Corwin, A. (1999). Integrating preparation for parenting into childbirth education: Part II, a study. *Journal of Perinatal Education, 8*(1), 22-28.

Csikszentmihalyi, M. (1990) *Flow: The psychology of optimal experience.* New York, Harper Perennial.

Declercq, E., Sakala, C., Corry, M., Applebaum, S., & Risher, P. (2002). *Listening to mothers: Report of the first national U.S. survey of women's childbearing experiences.* New York Maternity Center Association. Accessed http://maternitywise.org/pdfs/LtMreport.pdf, April 21, 2006.

Deutch, H. (1945). *The psychology of women: A psychoanalytic interpretation* (2 vols). New York: Grune & Stratton.

Dick-Read, G. (1987). *Childbirth without fear* (5th ed.). New York: Harper & Collins.

Enkin, M., Keirse, J., Neilson, J., Crowther, C., Duley, L., Hodnett, E., et al. (2000). *A guide to effective care in pregnancy and childbirth* (3rd ed.). Oxford: Oxford University Press.

Gardner, P. (2003). Previous traumatic birth: An impetus for requested cesarean birth. *Journal of Perinatal Education, 12*(1), 1-50.

Gartner, L., Morton, J., Lawrence, R., Naylor, A., O'Hare, D., Schanler, R., et al. (2005). Breastfeeding and the use of human milk. *Pediatrics, 115*(2), 496-506.

Geissbuehler, V., & Eberhard, J. (2002). Fear of childbirth during pregnancy: A study of more than 8000 pregnant women. *Journal of Psychosomatic Obstetrics & Gynecology, 23*(4), 229-335.

Green, J., & Baston, H. (2004). Feeling in control during labor: Concepts, correlates and consequences. *Birth: Issues in Perinatal Care, 30*(4), 235-247.

Hawkins, A., Gilliland, T., Christiaens, G., & Carroll, J. (2002) Integrating marriage education into perinatal education. *Journal of Perinatal Education, 11*(4), 1-10.

Heinze, S., & Sleigh, M. (2003). Epidural or no epidural anaesthesia: Relationships between beliefs about childbirth and pain control choices. *Journal of Reproductive & Infant Psychology, 21*(4), 323-333.

Hill, T. (2002). The impact of relationship factors and anxiety on the maternal childbirth experience. *Dissertation Abstracts International: Section B: The Sciences & Engineering, 62*(12-B), 5965.

Hodnett, E., & Fredericks, S. (2000). Support during pregnancy for women at increased risk of low birthweight babies. *The Cochrane Database of Systematic Reviews,* 2006, Issue 3. Chichester, UK: John Wiley & Sons.

Hodnett, E., Gates, S., Hofmeyr, G., & Sakala, C. (2003). Continuous support for women during childbirth. *The Cochrane Database of Systematic Reviews,* 2006, Issue 3. Chichester, UK: John Wiley & Sons.

Holmes, L. (2000). Childbirth as a developmental milestone. *Modern Psychoanalysis, 25*(1), 109-133.

Johnson, K., & Daviss, B. (2005). Outcomes of planned home births and certified professional midwives: Large prospective study in North America. *BMJ, 330*(7505), 1416.

Jones, L. (1983). *A meta-analytic study of the effects of childbirth education research from 1960 to 1981.* Unpublished doctoral dissertation, Texas A & M University.

Jungblom, R. (2003). Lay midwives and obstetricians: Alternative models of care and postpartum psychological adjustment. *Dissertation Abstracts International: Section B: The Sciences & Engineering, 64*(1-B), 43.

Karmel, M. (1959). *Thank you, Dr. Lamaze.* New York: Harper & Row.

Koehn, M. (2002). Childbirth education outcomes: An integrated review of literature. *Journal of Perinatal Education, 11*(3), 10-19.

Lamaze International. (2005). *About Lamaze International, Inc.* [Online]. Accessed www.lamazechildbirth.com/fact_sheet.html, April 21, 2006.

Lamb, E. (2002). The impact of previous perinatal loss on subsequent pregnancy and parenting. *Journal of Perinatal Education, 11*(2), 33-40.

Lindell, S. (1988). Education for childbirth: A time for change. *Journal of Obstetric, Gynecologic, and Neonatal Nursing, 17*(2), 108-112.

Lothian, J., & Devries, C. (2005). *The official Lamaze guide: Giving birth with confidence.* New York: Meadowbrook Press.

Martin, J., Hamilton, B., Sutton, P., Ventura, S., Menacker, F., & Munson, L. (2005). Births: Final data for 2003. *National Vital Statistics Report, 54*(2), 1-116.

Mennick, F. (2006). Cesarean section on demand. *American Journal of Nursing, 106*(6), 19-20.

Moore, M. (2005). Guest editorial—Increasing cesarean birth rates: A clash of cultures? *Journal of Perinatal Education, 14*(1), 5-8.

Mozingo, J., Davis, M., & Thomas, S. (2002). "I felt violated": Women's experience of childbirth-associated anger. *MCN American Journal of Maternal/Child Nursing, 27*(6), 342-348.

Neilson, J. (2000). Ultrasound for fetal assessment in early pregnancy. *The Cochrane Database of Systematic Reviews,* 2006, Issue 3. Chichester, UK: John Wiley & Sons.

Newman, R. (2004). Toward a new era of childbirth education. *Journal of Prenatal & Perinatal Psychology & Health, 18*(4), 327-337.

Olsen, O., & Jewell, M. (2000). Home versus hospital birth. *The Cochrane Database of Systematic Reviews,* 2006, Issue 3. Chichester, UK: John Wiley & Sons.

Philipsen, N., & Haynes, D. (2005). Ask an expert—The similarities between birth plans and living wills. *Journal of Perinatal Education, 14*(4), 46-48.

Pollack, M., Amankwaa, L., & Amankwaa, A. (2005). First-time fathers and stressors in the postpartum period. *Journal of Perinatal Education, 14*(2), 19-25.

Polomeno, V. (1998). An exemplary service: Health promotion for expectant fathers: Part II. Practical considerations. *Journal of Perinatal Education, 7*(2), 27-36.

Riskin-Mashiah, S. (2004). Preconception counseling—for all. *Harefuah, 143*(7), 530-536.

Schlenzka, P. (1999). Safety of alternative approaches to childbirth. *Dissertation Abstracts International* (Accession number AAG 9924602). Palo Alto, CA: Stanford University.

Smook, R. (2001). Birthing options: Women's experiences with obstetrical and midwifery models of care. *Dissertation Abstracts International: Section B: The Sciences & Engineering, 62*(4-B), 2079.

Strong, T. (2002). *Expecting trouble: The myth of prenatal care in America.* New York: New York University Press.

Tiedje, L. (2004). Teaching is more than telling: Education about prematurity in a prenatal clinic waiting room. *MCN American Journal of Maternal/Child Nursing, 29*(6), 373-379.

Tiran, D., & Chummun, H. (2004). Complementary therapies to reduce physiological stress in pregnancy. *Complementary Therapies in Nursing & Midwifery, 10*(3), 162-167.

United States Department of Health and Human Services. (2000). *Healthy People 2010: Conference edition.* Volume II. Washington, DC: U.S. Government Printing Office.

Uvnäs-Moberg, K. (2005). The psychobiology of emotion: The role of the oxytocinergic system. *International Journal of Behavioral Medicine, 12*(2), 59-65.

Waldenstrom, U., Hildingsson, I., Rubertsson, C., & Radestad, I. (2004). A negative birth experience: Prevalence and risk factors in a national sample. *Birth: Issues in Perinatal Care, 31*(1), 17-27.

Wertz, R., & Wertz, D. (1979). *Lying-in: A history of childbirth in America.* New York: Shocken Books.

World Health Organization (WHO). (1998). *Workshop on perinatal care proceedings.* Venice, April 16-18. Geneva: Author.

Labor and Birth Processes

learning objectives

- Explain the five major factors that affect the labor process.
- Describe the anatomic structure of the bony pelvis.
- Recognize the normal measurements of the diameters of the pelvic inlet, cavity, and outlet.
- Explain the significance of the size and position of the fetal head during labor and birth.

- Summarize the cardinal movements of the mechanism of labor for a vertex presentation.
- Examine the maternal anatomic and physiologic adaptations to labor.
- Describe fetal adaptations to labor.

electronic resources

Additional information related to the content in Chapter 18 can be found on

the companion website at **evolve**
http://evolve.elsevier.com/Lowdermilk/MWHC/
- NCLEX Review Questions
- WebLinks

or on the interactive companion CD
- NCLEX Review Questions
- Critical Thinking Exercise: Fetal Presentation

*D*URING late pregnancy the woman and fetus prepare for the labor process. The fetus has grown and developed in preparation for extra-uterine life. The woman has undergone various physiologic adaptations during pregnancy that prepare her for birth and motherhood. Labor and birth represent the end of pregnancy, the beginning of extrauterine life for the newborn, and a change in the lives of the family. This chapter discusses the factors affecting labor, the process involved, the normal progression of events, and the adaptations made by both the woman and fetus.

■ FACTORS AFFECTING LABOR

At least five factors affect the process of labor and birth. These are easily remembered as the five *P*s: *p*assenger (fetus and placenta), *p*assageway (birth canal), *p*owers (contractions), *p*osition of the mother, and *p*sychologic response. The first four factors are presented here as the basis of understanding the physiologic process of labor. The fifth factor is discussed in Chapter 19. Other factors that may be a part of the woman's labor experience may be important as well. VandeVusse (1999) identified external forces including place of birth, preparation, type of provider (especially

nurses), and procedures. Physiology (sensations) was identified as an internal force. These factors are discussed generally in Chapter 21 as they relate to nursing care during labor. Further research investigating essential forces of labor is recommended.

~ Passenger

The way the passenger, or fetus, moves through the birth canal is determined by several interacting factors: the size of the fetal head, fetal presentation, fetal lie, fetal attitude, and fetal position. Because the placenta also must pass through the birth canal, it can be considered a passenger along with the fetus; however, the placenta rarely impedes the process of labor in normal vaginal birth, except in cases of placenta previa.

Size of the Fetal Head

Because of its size and relative rigidity, the fetal head has a major effect on the birth process. The fetal skull is composed of two parietal bones, two temporal bones, the frontal bone, and the occipital bone (Fig. 18-1, *A*). These bones are united by membranous sutures: sagittal, lambdoidal, coronal, and frontal (Fig. 18-1, *B*). Membrane-filled spaces called fontanels are located where the sutures intersect.

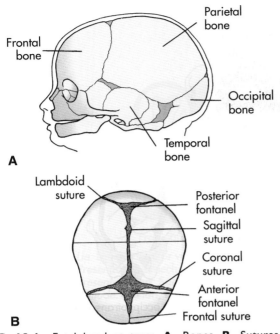

FIG. 18-1   Fetal head at term. **A,** Bones. **B,** Sutures and fontanels.

During labor, after rupture of membranes, palpation of fontanels and sutures during vaginal examination reveals fetal presentation, position, and attitude.

The two most important fontanels are the anterior and posterior ones (see Fig. 18-1, *B*). The larger of these, the anterior fontanel, is diamond shaped, is about 3 cm by 2 cm, and lies at the junction of the sagittal, coronal, and frontal sutures. It closes by 18 months after birth. The posterior fontanel lies at the junction of the sutures of the two parietal bones and the occipital bone, is triangular, and is about 1 cm by 2 cm. It closes 6 to 8 weeks after birth.

Sutures and fontanels make the skull flexible to accommodate the infant brain, which continues to grow for some time after birth. However, because the bones are not firmly united, slight overlapping of the bones, or molding of the shape of the head, occurs during labor. This capacity of the bones to slide over one another also permits adaptation to the various diameters of the maternal pelvis. Molding can be extensive, but the heads of most newborns assume their normal shape within 3 days after birth.

Although the size of the fetal shoulders may affect passage, their position can be altered relatively easily during labor, so one shoulder may occupy a lower level than the other. This creates a shoulder diameter that is smaller than the skull, facilitating passage through the birth canal. The circumference of the fetal hips is usually small enough not to create problems.

Fetal Presentation

Presentation refers to the part of the fetus that enters the pelvic inlet first and leads through the birth canal during labor. The three main presentations are cephalic presentation (head first), occurring in 96% of births (Fig. 18-2); breech presentation (buttocks or feet first), occurring in 3% of births (Fig. 18-3, *A-C*); and shoulder presentation, seen in 1% of births (Fig. 18-3, *D*). The presenting part is that part of the fetal body first felt by the examining finger during a vaginal examination. In a cephalic presentation the presenting part is usually the occiput; in a breech presentation it is the sacrum; in the shoulder presentation it is the scapula. When the presenting part is the occiput, the presentation is noted as vertex (see Fig. 18-2). Factors that determine the presenting part include fetal lie, fetal attitude, and extension or flexion of the fetal head.

Fetal Lie

Lie is the relation of the long axis (spine) of the fetus to the long axis (spine) of the mother. The two primary lies are longitudinal, or vertical, in which the long axis of the fetus is parallel with the long axis of the mother (see Fig. 18-2); and transverse, horizontal, or oblique, in which the long axis of the fetus is at a right angle diagonal to the long axis of the mother (see Fig. 18-3, *D*). Longitudinal lies are either cephalic or breech presentations, depending on the fetal structure that first enters the mother's pelvis. Vaginal birth cannot occur when the fetus stays in a transverse lie. An oblique lie, one in which the long axis of the fetus is lying at an angle to the long axis of the mother, is less common and usually converts to a longitudinal or transverse lie during labor (Cunningham, Leveno, Bloom, Hauth, Gilstrap, & Wenstrom, 2005).

Fetal Attitude

Attitude is the relation of the fetal body parts to each other. The fetus assumes a characteristic posture (attitude) in utero partly because of the mode of fetal growth and partly because of the way the fetus conforms to the shape of the uterine cavity. Normally the back of the fetus is rounded so that the chin is flexed on the chest, the thighs are flexed on the abdomen, and the legs are flexed at the knees. The arms are crossed over the thorax, and the umbilical cord lies between the arms and the legs. This attitude is termed general flexion (see Fig. 18-2).

Deviations from the normal attitude may cause difficulties in childbirth. For example, in a cephalic presentation, the fetal head may be extended or flexed in a manner that presents a head diameter that exceeds the limits of the maternal pelvis, leading to prolonged labor, forceps- or vacuum-assisted birth, or cesarean birth.

Certain critical diameters of the fetal head are usually measured. The biparietal diameter, which is about 9.25 cm at term, is the largest transverse diameter and an important indicator of fetal head size (Fig. 18-4, *B*). In a well-flexed cephalic presentation, the biparietal diameter will be the widest part of the head entering the pelvic inlet. Of the several anteroposterior diameters, the smallest and the most critical one is the suboccipitobregmatic diameter (about 9.5 cm at term). When the head is in complete flexion, this diameter allows the fetal head to pass through

CD: Critical Thinking Exercise: Fetal Presentation

FIG. 18-8   Pelvic cavity. **A,** Inlet and midplane. Outlet now shown. **B,** Cavity of true pelvis. **C,** Note curve of sacrum and axis of birth canal.

FIG. 18-9   Estimation of angle of subpubic arch. With both thumbs, examiner externally traces descending rami down to tuberosities. (From Barkauskas, V., Baumann, L., & Darling-Fisher, C. [2002]. *Health and physical assessment* [3rd ed.]. St. Louis: Mosby.)

Engagement is the term used to indicate that the largest transverse diameter of the presenting part (usually the biparietal diameter) has passed through the maternal pelvic brim or inlet into the true pelvis and usually corresponds to station 0. Engagement often occurs in the weeks just before labor begins in nulliparas and may occur before labor or during labor in multiparas. Engagement can be deter-

table 18-1 Obstetric Measurements

PLANE	DIAMETER	MEASUREMENTS

Inlet (superior strait)
Conjugates
  Diagonal
  Obstetric: measurement that determines whether presenting part can engage or enter superior strait
  True (vera) (anteroposterior)
	12.5-13 cm
	1.5-2 cm less than diagonal (radiographic)
	
	≥11 cm (12.5) (radiographic)
		
		Length of diagonal conjugate (solid colored line), obstetric conjugate (broken colored line), and true conjugate (blue line)*

Midplane
  Transverse diameter (interspinous diameter)
  The midplane of the pelvis normally is its largest plane and the one of greatest diameter
	10.5 cm	Measurement of interspinous diameter*

Outlet
  Transverse diameter (intertuberous diameter) (biischial)
  The outlet presents the smallest plane of the pelvic canal
	≥8 cm	
		Use of Thom's pelvimeter to measure intertuberous diameter*

* From Seidel, H., Ball, J., Dains, J., & Benedict, G. (2006). Mosby's guide to physical examination (6th ed.). St. Louis: Mosby.

table 18-2 Comparison of Pelvic Types

	GYNECOID (50% OF WOMEN)	ANDROID (23% OF WOMEN)	ANTHROPOID (24% OF WOMEN)	PLATYPELLOID (3% OF WOMEN)
Brim	Slightly ovoid or transversely rounded	Heart-shaped, angulated	Oval, wider anteroposteriorly	Flattened anteroposteriorly, wide transversely
	◯ Round	♡ Heart	◯ Oval	⬭ Flat
Depth	Moderate	Deep	Deep	Shallow
Side walls	Straight	Convergent	Straight	Straight
Ischial spines	Blunt, somewhat widely separated	Prominent, narrow interspinous diameter	Prominent, often with narrow interspinous diameter	Blunted, widely separated
Sacrum	Deep, curved	Slightly curved, terminal portion often beaked	Slightly curved	Slightly curved
Subpubic arch	Wide	Narrow	Narrow	Wide
Usual mode of birth	Vaginal Spontaneous Occipitoanterior position	Cesarean Vaginal Difficult, with forceps	Vaginal Forceps Spontaneous Occipitoposterior or occipitoanterior position	Vaginal Spontaneous

are approximate. Precise bony pelvis measurements can be determined by use of computed tomography, ultrasound, or x-ray films. However, radiographic examination is rarely done during pregnancy because the x-rays may damage the developing fetus.

Soft Tissues

The soft tissues of the passageway include the distensible lower uterine segment, the cervix, the pelvic floor muscles, the vagina, and the introitus. Before labor begins, the uterus is composed of the uterine body (corpus) and the cervix (neck). After labor has begun, uterine contractions cause the uterine body to have a thick and muscular upper segment and a thin-walled, passive, muscular lower segment. A physiologic *retraction ring* separates the two segments (Fig. 18-10). The lower uterine segment gradually distends to accommodate the intrauterine contents as the wall of the upper segment thickens and its accommodating capacity is reduced. The contractions of the uterine body thus exert downward pressure on the fetus, pushing it against the cervix.

The cervix effaces (thins) and dilates (opens) sufficiently to allow the first fetal portion to descend into the vagina. As the fetus descends, the cervix is actually drawn upward and over this first portion.

The pelvic floor is a muscular layer that separates the pelvic cavity above from the perineal space below. This structure helps the fetus rotate anteriorly as it passes through the birth canal. As noted earlier, the soft tissues of the vagina develop throughout pregnancy until at term the vagina can dilate to accommodate the fetus and permit passage of the fetus to the external world.

Powers

Involuntary and voluntary powers combine to expel the fetus and the placenta from the uterus. Involuntary uterine contractions, called the *primary powers*, signal the beginning of labor. Once the cervix has dilated, voluntary bearing-down efforts by the woman, called the *secondary powers*, augment the force of the involuntary contractions.

Primary Powers

The involuntary contractions originate at certain pacemaker points in the thickened muscle layers of the upper uterine segment. From the pacemaker points, contractions move downward over the uterus in waves, separated by short rest periods. Terms used to describe these involuntary contractions include *frequency* (the time from the beginning of one contraction to the beginning of the next), *duration* (length of contraction), and *intensity* (strength of contraction).

The primary powers are responsible for the effacement and dilation of the cervix and descent of the fetus. Effacement of the cervix means the shortening and thinning of the cervix during the first stage of labor. The cervix, normally 2 to 3 cm long and about 1 cm thick, is obliterated or "taken up" by a shortening of the uterine muscle bundles during the thinning of the lower uterine segment that occurs in advancing labor. Only a thin edge of the cervix can be palpated when effacement is complete. Effacement generally is advanced in first-time term pregnancy before more than slight dilation occurs. In subsequent pregnancies, effacement and dilation of the cervix tend to progress together. Degree of effacement is expressed in percentages from 0% to 100% (e.g., a cervix is 50% effaced) (Fig. 18-11, *A-C*).

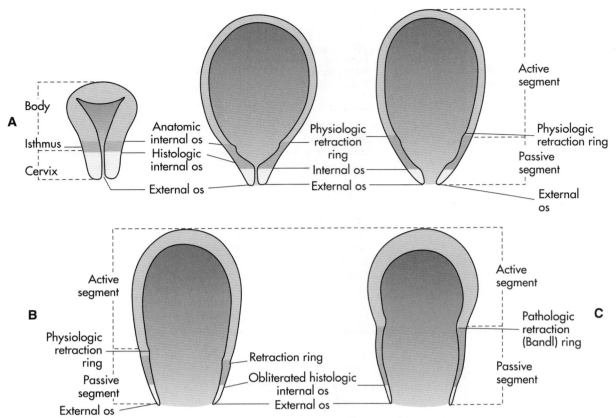

FIG. 18-10 **A,** Uterus in normal labor in early first stage, and **B,** in second stage. Passive segment is derived from lower uterine segment (isthmus) and cervix, and physiologic retraction ring is derived from anatomic internal os. **C,** Uterus in abnormal labor in second-stage dystocia. Pathologic retraction (Bandl) ring that forms under abnormal conditions develops from the physiologic ring.

Dilation of the cervix is the enlargement or widening of the cervical opening and the cervical canal that occurs once labor has begun. The diameter of the cervix increases from less than 1 cm to full dilation (approximately 10 cm) to allow birth of a term fetus. When the cervix is fully dilated (and completely retracted), it can no longer be palpated (Fig. 18-11, *D*). Full cervical dilation marks the end of the first stage of labor.

Dilation of the cervix occurs by the drawing upward of the musculofibrous components of the cervix, caused by strong uterine contractions. Pressure exerted by the amniotic fluid while the membranes are intact or by the force applied by the presenting part also can promote cervical dilation. Scarring of the cervix as a result of prior infection or surgery may slow cervical dilation.

In the first and second stages of labor, increased intrauterine pressure caused by contractions exerts pressure on the descending fetus and the cervix. When the presenting part of the fetus reaches the perineal floor, mechanical stretching of the cervix occurs. Stretch receptors in the posterior vagina cause release of endogenous oxytocin that triggers the maternal urge to bear down, or the Ferguson reflex.

Uterine contractions are usually independent of external forces. For example, laboring women who are paralyzed because of spinal cord lesions above T-12 will have normal but painless uterine contractions (Cunningham et al., 2005). However, uterine contractions may decrease temporarily in frequency and intensity if narcotic analgesic medication is given early in labor. Studies of effects of epidural analgesia have demonstrated prolonged length of labor for nulliparas both in the active phase of first-stage labor and in the second stage (Salim, Nachum, Moscovici, Lavee, & Shalev, 2005; Schiessl, Janni, Jundt, Rammel, Peschers, & Kainer, 2005; Sharma & Leveno, 2003).

Secondary Powers

As soon as the presenting part reaches the pelvic floor, the contractions change in character and become expulsive. The laboring woman experiences an involuntary urge to push. She uses secondary powers (bearing-down efforts) to aid in expulsion of the fetus as she contracts her diaphragm and abdominal muscles and pushes. These bearing-down efforts result in increased intraabdominal pressure that compresses the uterus on all sides and adds to the power of the expulsive forces.

The secondary powers have no effect on cervical dilation, but they are of considerable importance in the expulsion of the infant from the uterus and vagina after the cervix is fully dilated. Studies have shown that pushing in the second stage is more effective and the woman is less fatigued

A
Internal os
Cavity of cervix
External os

B
Internal os
External os

C
Internal os
External os

D
Internal os
External os

FIG. 18-11   Cervical effacement and dilation. Note how cervix is drawn up around presenting part (internal os). Membranes are intact, and head is not well applied to cervix. **A,** Before labor. **B,** Early effacement. **C,** Complete effacement (100%). Head is well applied to cervix. **D,** Complete dilation (10 cm). Cranial bones overlap somewhat, and membranes are still intact.

when she begins to push only after she has the urge to do so rather than beginning to push when she is fully dilated without an urge to do so (Roberts, 2002; Roberts, 2003).

When and how a woman pushes in the second stage is a much-debated topic. Studies have investigated the effects of spontaneous bearing-down efforts, directed pushing, delayed pushing, Valsalva maneuver (closed glottis and prolonged bearing down), and open-glottis pushing (Hansen, Clark, & Foster, 2002; Mayberry, Wood, Strange, Lee, Heisler, & Neilsen-Smith, 2000; Simpson & James, 2005). Although no significant differences have been found in the duration of second-stage labor, adverse effects of certain types of pushing techniques have been reported. For example, fetal hypoxia and subsequent acidosis have been associated with prolonged breath holding and forceful pushing efforts, whereas delayed pushing results in less fetal oxygen desaturation (Roberts, 2002; Simpson & James). Perineal trauma has been associated with prolonged second-stage labor (Myles & Santolaya, 2003). Continued study is needed to determine the effectiveness and appropriateness of strategies used by nurses to teach pushing techniques, the suitability and effectiveness of various pushing techniques related to nonreassuring fetal heart patterns, and the standards for duration of pushing in terms of maternal and fetal outcomes (Roberts, 2003).

⌐ Position of the Laboring Woman

Position affects the woman's anatomic and physiologic adaptations to labor. Frequent changes in position relieve fatigue, increase comfort, and improve circulation. Therefore a laboring woman should be encouraged to find positions that are most comfortable for her (Fig. 18-12, *A*).

An upright position (walking, sitting, kneeling, or squatting) offers a number of advantages. Gravity can promote the descent of the fetus. Uterine contractions are generally stronger and more efficient in effacing and dilating the cervix, resulting in shorter labor (Gupta, Hofmeyr, & Smyth, 2006; Simkin & Ancheta, 2000).

An upright position also is beneficial to the mother's cardiac output, which normally increases during labor as uterine contractions return blood to the vascular bed. The increased cardiac output improves blood flow to the uteroplacental unit and the maternal kidneys. Cardiac output is compromised if the descending aorta and ascending vena cava are compressed during labor. Compression of these major vessels may result in supine hypotension that decreases placental perfusion. With the woman in an upright position, pressure on the maternal vessels is reduced, and compression is prevented. If the woman wishes to lie down, a lateral position is suggested (Blackburn, 2003).

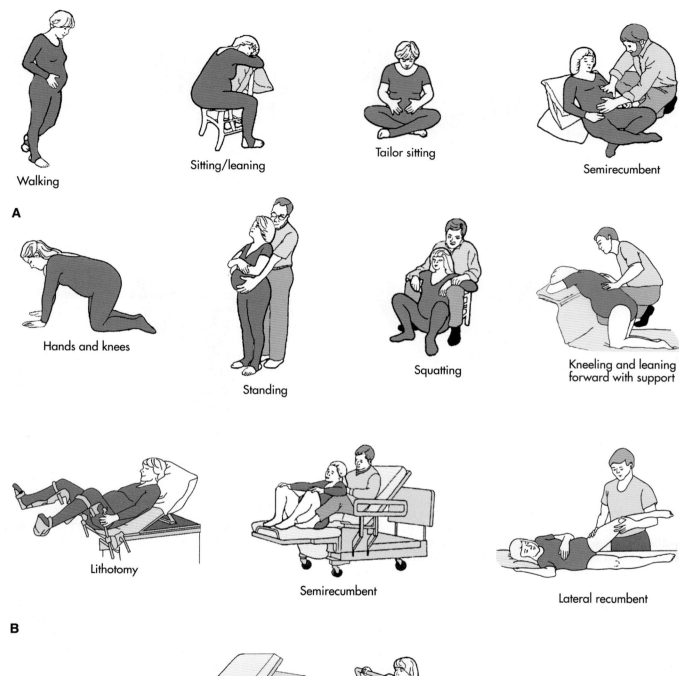

A

Walking

Sitting/leaning

Tailor sitting

Semirecumbent

Hands and knees

Standing

Squatting

Kneeling and leaning forward with support

B

Lithotomy

Semirecumbent

Lateral recumbent

Squatting

FIG. 18-12 Positions for labor and birth. **A,** Positions for labor. **B,** Positions for birth.

The "all fours" position (hands and knees) may be used to relieve backache if the fetus is in an occipitoposterior position and may assist in anterior rotation of the fetus and in cases of shoulder dystocia (Hofmeyr & Kulier, 2005; Simkin & Ancheta, 2000).

Positioning for second-stage labor (Fig. 18-12, *B*) may be determined by the woman's preference, but it is constrained by the condition of the woman and fetus, the environment, and the health care provider's confidence in assisting with a birth in a specific position (Simkin & Ancheta, 2000). The predominant position in the United States in physician-attended births is the lithotomy position. Alternative positions and position changes that result in more births over an intact perineum are more commonly practiced by nurse-midwives (Shorten, Donsante, & Shorten, 2002).

A woman who pushes in a semirecumbent position needs adequate body support to push effectively because her weight will be on her sacrum, moving the coccyx forward and causing a reduction in the pelvic outlet. In a sitting or squatting position, abdominal muscles work in greater synchrony with uterine contractions during bearing-down efforts. Kneeling or squatting moves the uterus forward and aligns the fetus with the pelvic inlet and can facilitate the second stage of labor by increasing the pelvic outlet (Simkin & Ancheta, 2000).

The lateral position can be used by the woman to help rotate a fetus that is in a posterior position. It also can be used when there is a need for less force to be used during bearing down, such as when there is a need to control the speed of a precipitate birth (Simkin & Ancheta, 2000).

Upright positions for women who have epidural analgesia are associated with a reduced labor duration (Roberts, Algert, Cameron, & Torvaldsen, 2005).

CRITICAL THINKING EXERCISE

Positions for Second Stage Labor

During your clinical experience in the labor and birth unit, you are assigned to an 18-year-old having her first baby. She does not have an epidural. Her cervix is 10 cm dilated and 100% effaced, the fetus is in a vertex presentation, and the presenting part is at station 0. The woman has been pushing in a lithotomy position for 1 hour with no noticeable fetal descent. You suggest that she change her position but she responds that she doesn't want to change positions because it must be the best position for pushing since that is the way it's done in all the TV programs when women are having babies. How would you respond?

1. Evidence—Is there sufficient evidence to draw conclusions about what response should be made?
2. Assumptions—Describe underlying assumptions about the following issues:
   a. Positions for second-stage labor
   b. Prolonged second-stage labor
3. What implications and priorities for nursing care can be made at this time?
4. Does the evidence objectively support your conclusion?
5. Are there alternative perspectives to your conclusion?

No evidence exists that any of these positions suggested for second-stage labor increases the need for use of operative techniques (e.g., forceps- or vacuum-assisted birth, cesarean birth, episiotomy) or causes perineal trauma. No evidence has been found that use of any of these positions adversely affects the newborn (Mayberry et al., 2000; Roberts et al., 2005).

■ PROCESS OF LABOR

The term *labor* refers to the process of moving the fetus, placenta, and membranes out of the uterus and through the birth canal. Various changes take place in the woman's reproductive system in the days and weeks before labor begins. Labor itself can be discussed in terms of the mechanisms involved in the process and the stages the woman moves through.

Signs Preceding Labor

In first-time pregnancies, the uterus sinks downward and forward about 2 weeks before term, when the fetus's presenting part (usually the fetal head) descends into the true pelvis. This settling is called lightening, or "dropping," and usually happens gradually. After lightening, women feel less congested and breathe more easily, but usually more bladder pressure results from this shift, and consequently a return of urinary frequency occurs. In a pregnancy in a multiparous woman, lightening may not take place until after uterine contractions are established and true labor is in progress.

The woman may complain of persistent low backache and sacroiliac distress as a result of relaxation of the pelvic joints. She may identify strong and frequent but irregular uterine (Braxton Hicks) contractions.

The vaginal mucus becomes more profuse in response to the extreme congestion of the vaginal mucous membranes. Brownish or blood-tinged cervical mucus may be passed (bloody show). The cervix becomes soft (ripens) and partially effaced and may begin to dilate. The membranes may rupture spontaneously.

Other phenomena are common in the days preceding labor: (1) loss of 0.5 to 1.5 kg in weight, caused by water loss resulting from electrolyte shifts that in turn are produced by changes in estrogen and progesterone levels; and (2) a surge of energy. Women speak of having a burst of energy that they often use to clean the house and put everything in order. Less commonly, some women have diarrhea, nausea, vomiting, and indigestion. Box 18-1 lists signs that may precede labor.

Onset of Labor

The onset of true labor cannot be ascribed to a single cause. Many factors, including changes in the maternal uterus, cervix, and pituitary gland, are involved. Hormones produced by the normal fetal hypothalamus, pituitary, and adrenal cortex probably contribute to the onset of labor. Progressive uterine distention, increasing intrauterine pressure, and aging of the placenta seem to be associated with increasing myometrial irritability. This is a result of

box 18-1 Signs Preceding Labor

- Lightening
- Return of urinary frequency
- Backache
- Stronger Braxton Hicks contractions
- Weight loss 0.5-1.5 kg
- Surge of energy
- Increased vaginal discharge; bloody show
- Cervical ripening
- Possible rupture of membranes

increased concentrations of estrogen and prostaglandins, as well as decreasing progesterone levels. The mutually coordinated effects of these factors result in the occurrence of strong, regular, rhythmic uterine contractions. The outcome of these factors working together is normally the birth of the fetus and the expulsion of the placenta; however, how certain alterations trigger others and how proper checks and balances are maintained is not known.

Fetal fibronectin (fFN) is a protein found in plasma and cervicovaginal secretions of pregnant women before the onset of labor. Assessment for the presence of fetal fibronectin is being used to predict the likelihood of preterm labor in women who are at increased risk for this complication, including those women with twin gestations (Goldenberg et al., 2003; Ruiz, Fullerton, & Brown, 2004). The value of detection of fetal fibronectin in management of women with preterm labor has yet to be determined, and therefore the test is not indicated for screening for preterm labor in low risk pregnant women (Bernhardt & Dorman, 2004).

Stages of Labor

The course of labor at or near term gestation in a woman without complications and a fetus in vertex presentation consists of (1) regular progression of uterine contractions, (2) effacement and progressive dilation of the cervix, and (3) progress in descent of the presenting part. Four stages of labor are recognized. These stages are discussed in greater detail, along with nursing care for the laboring woman and family, in Chapter 21.

The first stage of labor is considered to last from the onset of regular uterine contractions to full dilation of the cervix. Commonly the onset of labor is difficult to establish because the woman may be admitted to the labor unit just before birth, and the beginning of labor may be only an estimate. The first stage is much longer than the second and third combined. Great variability is the rule, however, depending on the factors discussed previously in this chapter. Parity has a strong effect on the duration of first-stage labor (Gross, Drobnic, & Keirse, 2005). Full dilation may occur in less than 1 hour in some multiparous pregnancies. In first-time pregnancy, complete dilation of the cervix can take up to 20 hours. Variations may reflect differences in the client population (e.g., risk status, age) or in clinical management of the labor and birth.

The first stage of labor has been divided into three phases: a latent phase, an active phase, and a transition phase. During the latent phase, there is more progress in effacement of the cervix and little increase in descent. During the active phase and the transition phase, there is more rapid dilation of the cervix and increased rate of descent of the presenting part. Maternal prepregnancy overweight and obesity can cause the active phase of labor to be longer than for women of normal weight (Liao, Buhimschi, & Norwitz, 2005; Vahratian, Zhang, Troendle, Savitz, & Siega-Riz, 2004).

The second stage of labor lasts from the time the cervix is fully dilated to the birth of the fetus. The second stage takes an average of 20 minutes for a multiparous woman and 50 minutes for a nulliparous woman. Labor of up to 2 hours has been considered within the normal range for the second stage, but Cesario (2004) found a wider range of normal was still associated with no adverse effects on the mother or infant. Cheng, Hopkins, & Caughey (2004) found that a prolonged second stage was associated with increased rates of operative births and maternal morbidity. Epidural analgesia will likely prolong the second stage (Decca et al., 2004; Salim et al., 2005; Schiessl et al., 2005). Ethnicity may shorten the length of the second-stage labor for African-American and Puerto Rican women (Diegmann, Andrews, & Niemczura, 2000).

Simkin and Ancheta (2000) describe the latent and active phases of second-stage labor. The latent phase is a period that begins about the time of complete dilation of the cervix, when the contractions are weak or not noticeable and the woman is not feeling the urge to push, is resting, or is exerting only small bearing-down efforts with contractions. The active phase is a period when contractions resume, the woman is making strong bearing-down efforts, and the fetal station is advancing.

The third stage of labor lasts from the birth of the fetus until the placenta is delivered. The placenta normally separates with the third or fourth strong uterine contraction after the infant has been born. After it has separated, the placenta can be delivered with the next uterine contraction. The duration of the third stage may be as short as 3 to 5 minutes, although up to 1 hour is considered within normal limits. The risk of hemorrhage increases as the length of the third stage increases (Cunningham et al., 2005).

The fourth stage of labor arbitrarily lasts about 2 hours after delivery of the placenta. It is the period of immediate recovery, when homeostasis is reestablished. It is an important period of observation for complications, such as abnormal bleeding (see Chapter 37).

Mechanism of Labor

As already discussed, the female pelvis has varied contours and diameters at different levels, and the presenting part of the passenger is large in proportion to the passage. Therefore for vaginal birth to occur, the fetus must adapt to the birth canal during the descent. The turns and other adjustments necessary in the human birth process are termed the mechanism of labor (Fig. 18-13). The seven cardinal

EVIDENCE-BASED PRACTICE

Reversing Breech Presentation by Facilitating External Cephalic Version

BACKGROUND

- Breech presentation may delay the birth of the head, complicating delivery. Breech presentation is associated with an increased risk for childhood handicap. Clear benefit is seen when birth is via cesarean section. External cephalic version (ECV) is the procedure whereby the breech fetus is manually repositioned for vaginal birth. At term, ECV has been supported by various interventions to improve its success, which is at about 60%. Tocolytic drugs relax the uterus, but may cause maternal and fetal tachycardia. Vibroacoustic stimulation to the maternal abdomen may cause the fetus to change positions due to startle or avoidance. Epidural or spinal analgesia greatly improves the success of ECV, but may cause maternal hypotension or headache, and may lead to fetal trauma if the mother cannot feel any pain from the force applied externally by the clinician. Finally, increasing amniotic fluid volume, either directly transabdominally or indirectly via maternal intravenous fluid bolus, may enable fetal position change, but increases the risk of infection and ruptured membranes.

OBJECTIVES

- The reviewers' task was to compare the outcomes of perinatal and maternal morbidity and mortality for these four interventions facilitating ECV: tocolysis, vibroacoustic stimulation, analgesia, and amnioinfusion. Potential outcomes included failed ECV, maternal and fetal adverse effects, presentation at birth, and type of birth.

METHODS

Search Strategy

- After an extensive search of research literature, the reviewers identified six randomized controlled trials of tocolysis, dated 1989 to 2003, representing 617 women. The authors added two trials from 2000 and 2003, totaling 109 women, in which sublingual nitric oxide was administered as a tocolytic drug. One small (26 women) randomized controlled trial with a crossover design, dated 1995, explored the effects of vibroacoustic stimulation. In five randomized controlled trials, dated 1997 to 2003, researchers compared success of ECV with and without epidural/spinal analgesia for 456 women. No trials for amnioinfusion were identified. No countries of origin were noted for the studies selected.

Statistical Analyses

- Similar data were pooled. Reviewers calculated risk ratios for dichotomous data, such as successful ECV. Differences between groups outside the 95% confidence interval were considered significant.

FINDINGS

- Tocolysis improved the risk of ECV success. Fetal bradycardia was less frequent in the tocolysis than placebo, and there were fewer cesarean births after ECV with tocolysis.
- Nitric oxide, on the other hand, decreased the success of ECV, and was associated with headaches and hypotension.
- Vibroacoustic stimulation was very effective at facilitating ECV in the one small trial.
- The results of using epidural or spinal analgesia before ECV were equivocal. Two trials of epidural analgesia showed benefit for ECV success, while three trials found no improvement using spinal analgesia. There were no adverse affects for the fetus.
- No trials for amnioinfusion were identified that met the pre-established criteria for the review.

LIMITATIONS

- Few high-quality, randomized controlled trials have addressed these procedures, even though they are in widespread use. All the trials were small, leading to small power to predict, even in metaanalysis. Although there were no studies of amnioinfusion that met criteria for inclusion, the routine preloading with intravenous fluid bolus before epidural/spinal administration, plus the extra time needed for the epidural to take effect, may have increased amniotic fluid volume, which may have contributed to ECV success.

IMPLICATIONS FOR PRACTICE

- The authors support the use of tocolysis to augment the success of ECV. Nitric oxide was not recommended. There is not yet enough evidence to recommend vibroacoustic stimulation, which is new and possibly controversial. Epidural/spinal analgesia shows promise, but equivocal results prevent any recommendations for its use.

IMPLICATIONS FOR FURTHER RESEARCH

- More research is needed to determine if the success of tocolysis and vibroacoustic stimulation may be due to less force being necessary for ECV, and therefore less trauma resulting. Research may also determine if amnioinfusion is the beneficial factor in epidural analgesia protocols, which routinely call for fluid bolus. Trials should be designed to investigate short- and long-term maternal and fetal outcomes when tocolysis and vibroacoustic stimulation are used.

Reference: Hofmeyr, G., & Gyte, G. (2004). Interventions to help external cephalic version for breech presentation at term. In *The Cochrane Database of Systematic Reviews*, 2006, Issue 3. Chichester, UK: John Wiley & Sons.

movements of the mechanism of labor that occur in a vertex presentation are engagement, descent, flexion, internal rotation, extension, external rotation (restitution), and finally birth by expulsion. Although these movements are discussed separately, in actuality a combination of movements occurs simultaneously. For example, engagement involves both descent and flexion.

Engagement

When the biparietal diameter of the head passes the pelvic inlet, the head is said to be engaged in the pelvic inlet (Fig. 18-13, *A*). In most nulliparous pregnancies, this occurs before the onset of active labor because the firmer abdominal muscles direct the presenting part into the pelvis. In multiparous pregnancies, in which the

FIG. 18-13 Cardinal movements of the mechanism of labor. Left occipitoanterior (LOA) position. **A,** Engagement and descent. **B,** Flexion. **C,** Internal rotation to occipitoanterior position (OA). **D,** Extension. **E,** External rotation beginning (restitution). **F,** External rotation.

abdominal musculature is more relaxed, the head often remains freely movable above the pelvic brim until labor is established.

Asynclitism. The head usually engages in the pelvis in a synclitic position—one that is parallel to the anteroposterior plane of the pelvis. Frequently asynclitism occurs (the head is deflected anteriorly or posteriorly in the pelvis), which can facilitate descent because the head is being positioned to accommodate to the pelvic cavity (Fig. 18-14). Extreme asynclitism can cause cephalopelvic disproportion, even in a normal-size pelvis, because the head is positioned so that it cannot descend.

Descent

Descent refers to the progress of the presenting part through the pelvis. Descent depends on at least four forces: (1) pressure exerted by the amniotic fluid, (2) direct pressure exerted by the contracting fundus on the fetus, (3) force of the contraction of the maternal diaphragm and abdominal muscles in the second stage of labor, and (4) extension and straightening of the fetal body. The effects of these forces are modified by the size and shape of the maternal pelvic

planes and the size of the fetal head and its capacity to mold.

The degree of descent is measured by the station of the presenting part (see Fig. 18-6). As mentioned, little descent occurs during the latent phase of the first stage of labor. Descent accelerates in the active phase when the cervix has dilated to 5 to 7 cm. It is especially apparent when the membranes have ruptured.

In a first-time pregnancy, descent is usually slow but steady; in subsequent pregnancies descent may be rapid. Progress in descent of the presenting part is determined by abdominal palpation (Leopold maneuvers) and vaginal examination until the presenting part can be seen at the introitus.

Flexion

As soon as the descending head meets resistance from the cervix, pelvic wall, or pelvic floor, it normally flexes, so that the chin is brought into closer contact with the fetal chest (see Fig. 18-13, *B*). Flexion permits the smaller suboccipitobregmatic diameter (9.5 cm) rather than the larger diameters to present to the outlet.

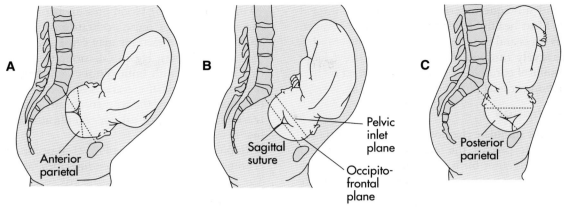

FIG. 18-14   Synclitism and asynclitism. **A,** Anterior asynclitism. **B,** Normal synclitism. **C,** Posterior asynclitism.

Internal Rotation

The maternal pelvic inlet is widest in the transverse diameter; therefore the fetal head passes the inlet into the true pelvis in the occipitotransverse position. The outlet is widest in the anteroposterior diameter; for the fetus to exit, the head must rotate. Internal rotation begins at the level of the ischial spines but is not completed until the presenting part reaches the lower pelvis. As the occiput rotates anteriorly, the face rotates posteriorly. With each contraction, the fetal head is guided by the bony pelvis and the muscles of the pelvic floor. Eventually the occiput will be in the midline beneath the pubic arch. The head is almost always rotated by the time it reaches the pelvic floor (see Fig. 18-13, *C*). Both the levator ani muscles and the bony pelvis are important for achieving anterior rotation. A previous childbirth injury or regional anesthesia may compromise the function of the levator sling.

Extension

When the fetal head reaches the perineum for birth, it is deflected anteriorly by the perineum. The occiput passes under the lower border of the symphysis pubis first, and then the head emerges by extension: first the occiput, then the face, and finally the chin (see Fig. 18-13, *D*).

Restitution and External Rotation

After the head is born, it rotates briefly to the position it occupied when it was engaged in the inlet. This movement is referred to as *restitution* (see Fig. 18-13, *E*). The 45-degree turn realigns the infant's head with her or his back and shoulders. The head can then be seen to rotate further. This external rotation occurs as the shoulders engage and descend in maneuvers similar to those of the head (see Fig. 18-13, *F*). As noted earlier, the anterior shoulder descends first. When it reaches the outlet, it rotates to the midline and is delivered from under the pubic arch. The posterior shoulder is guided over the perineum until it is free of the vaginal introitus.

Expulsion

After birth of the shoulders, the head and shoulders are lifted up toward the mother's pubic bone and the trunk of the baby is born by flexing it laterally in the direction of the symphysis pubis. When the baby has completely emerged, birth is complete, and the second stage of labor ends.

■ PHYSIOLOGIC ADAPTATION TO LABOR

In addition to the maternal and fetal anatomic adaptations that occur during birth, physiologic adaptations must occur. Accurate assessment of the laboring woman and fetus requires knowledge of these expected adaptations.

Fetal Adaptation

Several important physiologic adaptations occur in the fetus. These changes occur in fetal heart rate (FHR), fetal circulation, respiratory movements, and other behaviors.

Fetal Heart Rate

FHR monitoring provides reliable and predictive information about the condition of the fetus related to oxygenation. The average FHR at term is 140 beats/min. The normal range is 110 to 160 beats/min. Earlier in gestation the FHR is higher, with an average of approximately 160 beats/min at 20 weeks of gestation. The rate decreases progressively as the maturing fetus reaches term. However, temporary accelerations and slight early decelerations of the FHR can be expected in response to spontaneous fetal movement, vaginal examination, fundal pressure, uterine contractions, abdominal palpation, and fetal head compression. Stresses to the uterofetoplacental unit result in characteristic FHR patterns (see Chapter 20 for further discussion).

Fetal Circulation

Fetal circulation can be affected by many factors, including maternal position, uterine contractions, blood pressure, and umbilical cord blood flow. Uterine contractions during labor tend to decrease circulation through the spiral arterioles and subsequent perfusion through the intervillous space. Most healthy fetuses are well able to compensate for this stress and exposure to increased pressure while moving passively through the birth canal during labor. Usually umbilical cord blood flow is undisturbed by uterine contractions or fetal position (Tucker, 2004).

Fetal Respiration

Certain changes stimulate chemoreceptors in the aorta and carotid bodies to prepare the fetus for initiating respirations immediately after birth (Blackburn, 2003; Gilstrap, 2004). These changes occur during labor and include the following:

- Fetal lung fluid is cleared from the air passages during labor and (vaginal) birth.
- Fetal oxygen pressure (PO_2) decreases.
- Fetal arterial carbon dioxide pressure (PCO_2) increases.
- Fetal arterial pH decreases.
- Fetal bicarbonate level decreases.
- Fetal respiratory movements decrease during labor.

Maternal Adaptation

As the woman progresses through the stages of labor, various body system adaptations cause the woman to exhibit both objective signs and subjective symptoms (Box 18-2).

Cardiovascular Changes

During each contraction, an average of 400 ml of blood is emptied from the uterus into the maternal vascular system. This increases cardiac output by about 12% to 31% in the first stage and by about 50% in the second stage. The heart rate increases slightly (Monga, 2004).

Changes in the woman's blood pressure also occur. Blood flow, which is reduced in the uterine artery by contractions, is redirected to peripheral vessels. As a result, peripheral resistance increases, and blood pressure increases (Monga, 2004). During the first stage of labor, uterine contractions cause systolic readings to increase by about

---

| box 18-2 | **Maternal Physiologic Changes During Labor** |

- Cardiac output increases 10%-15% in first stage; 30%-50% in second stage.
- Heart rate increases slightly in first and second stages.
- Systolic blood pressure increases during uterine contractions in first stage; systolic and diastolic pressures increase during uterine contractions in second stage.
- White blood cell (WBC) count increases.
- Respiratory rate increases.
- Temperature may be slightly elevated.
- Proteinuria may occur.
- Gastric motility and absorption of solid food is decreased; nausea and vomiting may occur during transition to second-stage labor.
- Blood glucose level decreases.

---

10 mm Hg; assessing blood pressure between contractions therefore provides more accurate readings. During the second stage, contractions may cause systolic pressures to increase by 30 mm Hg and diastolic readings to increase by 25 mm Hg, with both systolic and diastolic pressures remaining somewhat elevated even between contractions (Monga). Therefore the woman already at risk for hypertension is at increased risk for complications such as cerebral hemorrhage.

Supine hypotension (see Fig. 21-5) occurs when the ascending vena cava and descending aorta are compressed. The laboring woman is at greater risk for supine hypotension if the uterus is particularly large because of multifetal pregnancy, hydramnios, or obesity or if the woman is dehydrated or hypovolemic. In addition, anxiety and pain, as well as some medications, can cause hypotension.

The woman should be discouraged from using the Valsalva maneuver (holding one's breath and tightening abdominal muscles) for pushing during the second stage. This activity increases intrathoracic pressure, reduces venous return, and increases venous pressure. The cardiac output and blood pressure increase and the pulse slows temporarily. During the Valsalva maneuver, fetal hypoxia may occur. The process is reversed when the woman takes a breath.

The white blood cell (WBC) count can increase (Pagana & Pagana, 2006). Although the mechanism leading to this increase in WBCs is unknown, it may be secondary to physical or emotional stress or to tissue trauma. Labor is strenuous, and physical exercise alone can increase the WBC count.

Some peripheral vascular changes occur, perhaps in response to cervical dilation or to compression of maternal vessels by the fetus passing through the birth canal. Flushed cheeks, hot or cold feet, and eversion of hemorrhoids may result.

Respiratory Changes

Increased physical activity with greater oxygen consumption is reflected in an increase in the respiratory rate. Hyperventilation may cause respiratory alkalosis (an increase in pH), hypoxia, and hypocapnia (decrease in carbon dioxide). In the unmedicated woman in the second stage, oxygen consumption almost doubles. Anxiety also increases oxygen consumption.

Renal Changes

During labor, spontaneous voiding may be difficult for various reasons: tissue edema caused by pressure from the presenting part, discomfort, analgesia, and embarrassment. Proteinuria of 1+ is a normal finding because it can occur in response to the breakdown of muscle tissue from the physical work of labor.

Integumentary Changes

The integumentary system changes are evident, especially in the great distensibility (stretching) in the area of the vaginal introitus. The degree of distensibility varies with the individual. Despite this ability to stretch, even in the absence of episiotomy or lacerations, minute tears in the skin around the vaginal introitus do occur.

Musculoskeletal Changes

The musculoskeletal system is stressed during labor. Diaphoresis, fatigue, proteinuria (1+), and possibly an increased temperature accompany the marked increase in muscle activity. Backache and joint ache (unrelated to fetal position) occur as a result of increased joint laxity at term. The labor process itself and the woman's pointing her toes can cause leg cramps.

Neurologic Changes

Sensorial changes occur as the woman moves through phases of the first stage of labor and as she moves from one stage to the next. Initially she may be euphoric. Euphoria gives way to increased seriousness, then to amnesia between contractions during the second stage, and finally to elation or fatigue after giving birth. Endogenous endorphins (morphinelike chemicals produced naturally by the body) raise the pain threshold and produce sedation. In addition, physiologic anesthesia of perineal tissues, caused by pressure of the presenting part, decreases perception of pain.

Gastrointestinal Changes

During labor, gastrointestinal motility and absorption of solid foods are decreased, and stomach-emptying time is slowed. Nausea and vomiting of undigested food eaten after onset of labor are common. Nausea and belching also occur as a reflex response to full cervical dilation. The woman may state that diarrhea accompanied the onset of labor, or the nurse may palpate the presence of hard or impacted stool in the rectum.

Endocrine Changes

The onset of labor may be triggered by decreasing levels of progesterone and increasing levels of estrogen, prostaglandins, and oxytocin. Metabolism increases, and blood glucose levels may decrease with the work of labor.

Accurate assessment of the mother and fetus during labor and birth depends on knowledge of these expected adaptations so that appropriate interventions can be implemented.

---

community activity

Attend a local childbirth class specifically on the process of labor. Evaluate the presentation, especially the audiovisuals used to depict the birth process. Assess the level of the presentation in terms of the education level of the audience. How does the presentation address the range of ages in the class? Identify the positive aspects of the class as well as those that need improvement. Suggest how the class could be improved.

---

key points

- Labor and birth are affected by the five Ps: *passenger, passageway, powers, position* of the woman, and *psychologic* responses.
- Because of its size and relative rigidity, the fetal head is a major factor in determining the course of birth.
- The diameters at the plane of the pelvic inlet, the midpelvis, and the outlet, plus the axis of the birth canal, determine whether vaginal birth is possible and the manner in which the fetus passes down the birth canal.
- Involuntary uterine contractions act to expel the fetus and placenta during the first stage of labor; these are augmented by voluntary bearing-down efforts of the woman during the second stage.
- The first stage of labor lasts from the time dilation begins to the time when the cervix is fully dilated. The second stage of labor lasts from the time of full dilation to the birth of the infant. The third stage of labor lasts from the infant's birth to the expulsion of the placenta. The fourth stage is the first 2 hours after birth.
- The cardinal movements of the mechanism of labor are engagement, descent, flexion, internal rotation, extension, restitution and external rotation, and expulsion of the infant.
- Although the events precipitating the onset of labor are unknown, many factors, including changes in the maternal uterus, cervix, and pituitary gland, are thought to be involved.
- A healthy fetus with an adequate uterofetoplacental circulation will be able to compensate for the stress of uterine contractions.
- As the woman progresses through labor, various body systems adapt to the birth process.

REFERENCES

Bernhardt, J., & Dorman, K. (2004). Pre-term birth risk assessment tools: Exploring fetal fibronectin and cervical length for validating risk. *AWHONN Lifelines, 8*(1), 38-44.

Blackburn, S. (2003). *Maternal, fetal, and neonatal physiology: A clinical perspective* (2nd ed.). St. Louis: Saunders.

Cesario, S. (2004). Reevaluation of Friedman's labor curve: A pilot study. *Journal of Obstetric, Gynecologic, and Neonatal Nursing, 33*(6), 713-722.

Cheng, Y., Hopkins, L., & Caughey, A. (2004). How long is too long: Does a prolonged second stage of labor in nulliparous women affect maternal and neonatal outcomes? *American Journal of Obstetrics and Gynecology, 191*(3), 933-938.

Cunningham, F., Leveno, K., Bloom, S., Hauth, J., Gilstrap, L., & Wenstrom, K. (2005). *Williams obstetrics* (22nd ed.). New York: McGraw-Hill.

Decca, L., Daldoss, C., Fratelli, N., Lojacono, A., Slompo, M., Stegher, C., et al. (2004). Labor course and delivery in epidural analgesia: A case-control study. *Journal of Maternal, Fetal, and Neonatal Medicine, 16*(2), 115-118.

Diegmann, E., Andrews, C., & Niemczura, C. (2000). The length of the second stage of labor in uncomplicated, nulliparous African American and Puerto Rican women. *Journal of Midwifery & Women's Health, 45*(1), 67-71.

Gilstrap, L. (2004). Fetal acid-base balance. In R. Creasy, R. Resnik, & J. Iams (Eds.), *Maternal-fetal medicine: Principles and practice* (5th ed.). Philadelphia: Saunders.

Goldenberg, R., Iams, J., Mercer, B., Meis, P., Moawad, A., Das, A., et al. (2003). What have we learned about the predictors of preterm birth? *Seminars in Perinatology, 27*(3), 185-193.

Gross, M., Drobnic, S., & Keirse, M. (2005). Influence of fixed and time-dependent factors on duration of normal first stage labor. *Birth, 32*(1), 27-33.

Gupta, J., Hofmeyr, G., & Smyth, R. (2006). Position in the second stage of labour for women without epidural anaesthesia (Cochrane Review). In *The Cochrane Database of Systematic Reviews*, 2006, Issue 3. Chichester, UK: John Wiley & Sons.

Hansen, S., Clark, S., & Foster, J. (2002). Active pushing versus passive fetal descent in the second stage of labor: A randomized controlled trial. *Obstetrics and Gynecology, 99*(1), 29-34.

Hofmeyr, G., & Kulier, R. (2005). Hands and knees posture in late pregnancy or labour for fetal malposition (lateral or posterior) (Cochrane Review). In *The Cochrane Database of Systematic Reviews*, 2006, Issue 3. Chichester, UK: John Wiley & Sons.

Liao, J., Buhimschi, D., & Norwitz, E. (2005). Normal labor: Mechanism and duration. *Obstetric and Gynecologic Clinics of North America, 32*(2), 145-164.

Mayberry, L., Wood, S., Strange, L., Lee, L., Heisler, D., & Neilsen-Smith, K. (2000). *Second-stage labor management: Promotion of evidence-based practice and a collaborative approach to patient care.* Washington, DC: Association of Women's Health, Obstetric and Neonatal Nurses.

Monga, M. (2004). Maternal cardiovascular and renal adaptations to pregnancy. In R. Creasy, R. Resnik, & J. Iams (Eds.), *Maternal-fetal medicine: Principles and practice* (5th ed.). Philadelphia: Saunders.

Myles, T., & Santolaya, K. (2003). Maternal and neonatal outcomes in patients with a prolonged second stage of labor. *Obstetrics and Gynecology 102*(1), 52-58.

Pagana, K., & Pagana, T. (2006). *Mosby's manual of diagnostic and laboratory tests* (3rd ed.). St. Louis: Mosby.

Roberts, J. (2002). The "push" for evidence: Management of the second stage. *Journal of Midwifery & Women's Health, 47*(1), 2-15.

Roberts, J. (2003). A new understanding of the second stage of labor: Implications for nursing care. *Journal of Obstetric, Gynecologic, and Neonatal Nursing, 32*(6), 794-801.

Roberts, C., Algert, C., Cameron, C., & Torvaldsen, S. (2005). A meta-analysis of upright positions in the second stage to reduce instrumental deliveries in women with epidural analgesia. *Acta Obstetricia et Gynecologogica Scandinavica, 84*(8), 794-798.

Ruiz, R., Fullerton, J., & Brown, C. (2004). The utility of fFN for the prediction of preterm birth in twin gestations. *Journal of Obstetric, Gynecologic, and Neonatal Nursing, 33*(4), 446-454.

Salim, R., Nachum, Z., Moscovici R., Lavee, M., & Shalev, E. (2005). Continuous compared with intermittent epidural infusion on progress of labor and patient satisfaction. *Obstetrics and Gynecology, 106*(2), 301-306.

Schiessl, B., Janni, W., Jundt, K., Rammel, G., Peschers, U., & Kainer, F. (2005). Obstetrical parameters influencing the duration of second stage labor. *European Journal of Obstetric and Gynecologic Reproductive Biology, 118*(1), 17-20.

Sharma, S., & Leveno, K. (2003). Regional analgesia and progress of labor. *Clinical Obstetrics and Gynecology, 46*(3), 633-645.

Shorten, A., Donsante, J., & Shorten, B. (2002). Birth position, accoucheur, and perineal outcomes: Informing women about choices for vaginal birth. *Birth, 29*(1), 18-27.

Simkin, P., & Ancheta, R. (2000). *The labor progress handbook: Early interventions to prevent and treat dystocia.* Oxford: Blackwell Science.

Simpson, K., & James, D. (2005). Effects of immediate versus delayed pushing during second-stage labor on fetal well-being: A randomized clinical trial. *Nursing Research, 54*(3), 149-157.

Tucker, S. (2004). *Pocket guide to fetal monitoring and assessment* (5th ed.). St. Louis: Mosby.

Vahratian, A., Zhang, J., Troendle, J., Savitz, D., & Siega-Riz, A. (2004). Maternal prepregnancy overweight and obesity and the pattern of labor progression in term nulliparous women. *Obstetrics and Gynecology, 104*(5 Part 1), 943-951.

VandeVusse, L. (1999). The essential forces of labor revisited: 13 *P*s reported in women's birth stories. *MCN American Journal of Maternal/Child Nursing, 24*(4), 176-184.

Management of Discomfort

learning objectives

- Analyze the various childbirth preparation methods.
- Describe breathing and relaxation techniques used for each stage of labor.
- Identify nonpharmacologic strategies to enhance relaxation and decrease discomfort during labor.
- Compare pharmacologic methods used to relieve discomfort in different stages of labor and for vaginal or cesarean birth.

- Discuss the use of naloxone (Narcan).
- Apply the nursing process to the management of the discomfort of a woman in labor.
- Summarize the nursing responsibilities appropriate for a woman receiving analgesia or anesthesia during labor.

electronic resources

Additional information related to the content in Chapter 19 can be found on

the companion website at **evolve**
http://evolve.elsevier.com/Lowdermilk/MWHC/
- NCLEX Review Questions
- WebLinks

or on the interactive companion CD
- NCLEX Review Questions
- Critical Thinking Exercise: Patient Receiving Epidural Block
- Plan of Care: Nonpharmacologic Management of Discomfort

*P*AIN is an unpleasant, complex, highly individualized phenomenon with both sensory and emotional components. Pregnant women commonly worry about the pain they will experience during labor and birth and about how they will react to and deal with that pain. Many physiologic, psychosocial, and environmental factors influence the nature and degree of pain experienced by the laboring woman and how she will respond to and cope with the pain (Lowe, 2002). A variety of nonpharmacologic and pharmacologic methods can help the woman or the couple cope with the discomforts of labor. The methods selected depend on the situation, availability, and the preferences of the woman and her health care provider.

■ DISCOMFORT DURING
■ LABOR AND BIRTH

Neurologic Origins

The pain and discomfort of labor have two origins, visceral and somatic (Lowe, 2002). During the first stage of labor, uterine contractions cause cervical dilation and effacement.

Uterine ischemia (decreased blood flow and therefore local oxygen deficit) results from compression of the arteries supplying the myometrium during uterine contractions. Pain impulses during the first stage of labor are transmitted via the T-1 to T-12 spinal nerve segment and accessory lower thoracic and upper lumbar sympathetic nerves. These nerves originate in the uterine body and cervix.

The pain from cervical changes, distention of the lower uterine segment, and uterine ischemia that predominates during the first stage of labor is visceral pain. It is located over the lower portion of the abdomen. Referred pain occurs when the pain that originates in the uterus radiates to the abdominal wall, lumbosacral area of the back, iliac crests, gluteal area, and down the thighs. The woman usually has discomfort only during contractions and is free of pain between contractions, although some women have continuous contraction-related low back pain, even in the interval between contractions (Lowe, 2002; Trout, 2004).

During the second stage of labor, the woman has somatic pain, which is often described as intense, sharp, burning, and well localized. Pain results from stretching and distention of perineal tissues and the pelvic floor to allow passage of the fetus, from distention and traction on the peritoneum and uterocervical supports during contractions, and from lacerations of soft tissue (e.g., cervix, vagina, perineum). Discomfort also can be produced by expulsive forces or by pressure exerted by the presenting part on the bladder, the bowel, or other sensitive pelvic structures. Pain impulses during the second stage of labor are transmitted via the pudendal nerve through S2 to S4 spinal nerve segments and the parasympathetic system (Lowe, 2002).

Pain experienced during the third stage of labor and the afterpains of the early postpartum period are uterine, similar to the pain experienced early in the first stage of labor. Areas of discomfort during labor are shown in Fig. 19-1.

Perception of Pain

Although the pain threshold is remarkably similar in all persons regardless of gender, social, ethnic, or cultural differences, these differences play a definite role in the person's perception of and behavioral responses to pain. The effects of factors such as culture, counterstimuli, and distraction in coping with pain are not fully understood. The meaning of pain and the verbal and nonverbal expressions given to pain are apparently learned from interactions within the primary social group. Cultural influences may impose certain behavioral expectations regarding acceptable and unacceptable behavior when experiencing pain. For instance, women from some cultures or groups (e.g., Asian, Amish) believe it shameful and counterproductive to scream or show pain, and therefore avoid outward expressions when they are in pain (Trout, 2004).

Expression of Pain

Pain results in physiologic effects and sensory and emotional (affective) responses. During childbirth, pain gives rise to identifiable physiologic effects. Sympathetic nervous system activity is stimulated in response to intensifying pain, resulting in increased catecholamine levels. Blood pressure and heart rate increase. Maternal respiratory patterns change in response to an increase in oxygen consumption. Hyperventilation, sometimes accompanied by respiratory alkalosis, can occur as pain intensifies. Pallor and diaphoresis may be seen. Gastric acidity increases, and nausea and vomiting are common in the active phase of labor. Placental perfusion may decrease, and uterine activity may diminish, potentially prolonging labor and affecting fetal well-being.

The sensory quality of visceral and somatic pain has been described as prickling, stabbing, burning, bursting, aching, heavy, pulling, throbbing, sharp, shooting, stinging, or cramping. The emotional (affective) quality of pain has been described as tiring, exhausting, annoying, sickening, and nauseating (Lowe, 2002).

Certain emotional (affective) expressions of pain often are seen. Such changes include increasing anxiety with

FIG. 19-1 Discomfort during labor. **A,** Distribution of labor pain during first stage. **B,** Distribution of labor pain during transition and early phase of second stage. **C,** Distribution of pain during late second stage and actual birth. (*Gray areas* indicate mild discomfort; *light pink areas* indicate moderate discomfort; *dark red areas* indicate intense discomfort).

lessened perceptual field, writhing, crying, groaning, gesturing (hand clenching and wringing), and excessive muscular excitability throughout the body. Cultural expression of pain may vary. For example, Chinese women often use soft voices and calm demeanors to cope with pain as a means of conserving energy during labor whereas Mayan women may repeat a mantra and call out to the Lord to cope with pain and enhance the labor process (Callister, Khalaf, Semenic, Kartchner, & Vehvilainen-Julkunen, 2003).

Factors Influencing Pain Response

Pain during childbirth is unique to each woman. How she perceives or interprets that pain is influenced by a variety of physiologic, psychologic, emotional, social, cultural, and environmental factors (Trout, 2004). Women who approach pain as a challenge for which they have sufficient resources to cope effectively are unlikely to equate pain with suffering. In contrast, women without sufficient self-confidence and coping strategies may feel threatened and view their pain experience as suffering (Lowe, 2004; Simkin & Bolding, 2004).

Physiologic Factors

A variety of physiologic factors can affect the intensity of pain experienced by women during childbirth. Women with a history of dysmenorrhea may experience increased pain during childbirth as a result of higher prostaglandin levels. Back pain associated with menstruation also may increase the likelihood of contraction-related low back pain. Upright positions, when assumed during labor, seem to result in decreased pain and an overall increase in comfort when compared with the supine position. Women also report that being able to move freely to find a position of comfort is an important factor in reducing pain and muscle tension and maintaining control during labor. Finally, the relation of fetal size to the dimensions of the maternal pelvis may influence pain intensity (Lowe, 2002; Simkin & O'Hara, 2002).

Endorphins are endogenous opioids secreted by the pituitary gland that act on the central and peripheral nervous systems to reduce pain. Beta-endorphin is the most potent of the endorphins. The physiologic role of endorphins is not completely understood. It is thought that endorphin levels increase during pregnancy and birth in humans. Higher endorphin levels may increase the ability of women in labor to tolerate acute pain and may reduce their irritability and anxiety. Levels of beta-endorphins are higher when a woman experiences a spontaneous, natural childbirth (Righard, 2001).

Culture

The obstetric population reflects the increasingly multicultural nature of U.S. society. As nurses care for women and families from a variety of cultural backgrounds, they must have knowledge and understanding of how culture mediates pain. Although all women expect to experience at least some pain and discomfort during childbirth, it is their culture and religious belief system that determines how they will perceive, interpret, and respond to and manage the pain. For example, women with strong religious beliefs often accept pain as a necessary and inevitable part of bringing a new life into the world (Callister et al., 2003; Mattson, 2000). An understanding of the beliefs, values, expectations, and practices of various cultures will narrow the cultural gap and help the nurse to assess the laboring woman's pain experience more accurately. This will enable the nurse to provide culturally sensitive care

---

cultural considerations

Some Cultural Beliefs About Pain

The following are examples of how women of different cultural backgrounds may react to pain. Because they are generalizations, the nurse must assess each woman experiencing pain related to childbirth.

- Chinese women may not exhibit reactions to pain, although it is acceptable to exhibit pain during childbirth. They consider it impolite to accept something when it is first offered; therefore pain interventions must be offered more than once. Acupuncture may be used for pain relief.
- Arab or Middle Eastern women may be vocal in response to labor pain. They may prefer medication for pain relief.
- Japanese women may be stoic in response to labor pain, but they may request medication when pain becomes severe.
- Southeast Asian women may endure severe pain before requesting relief.
- Hispanic women may be stoic until late in labor, when they may become vocal and request pain relief.
- Native-American women may use medications or remedies made from indigenous plants. They are often stoic in response to labor pain.
- African-American women may express pain openly. Use of medication for pain relief varies.

---

by using appropriate pain relief measures that preserve the woman's sense of control and self-confidence (see Cultural Considerations box; see Table 21-2). It is important for the nurse to recognize that although a woman's behavior in response to pain may vary according to her cultural background, it may not accurately reflect the intensity of the pain she is experiencing. The nurse must assess the woman for the physiologic effects of pain and must listen to the words the woman uses to describe the sensory and affective qualities of her pain (Lowe, 2002).

Anxiety

Anxiety is commonly associated with increased pain during labor. Mild anxiety is considered normal for a woman during labor and birth. However, excessive anxiety and fear cause more catecholamine secretion, which increase the stimuli to the brain from the pelvis because of decreased blood flow and increased muscle tension; this in turn magnifies pain perception (Lowe, 2002). Thus as anxiety and fear heighten, muscle tension increases, the effectiveness of uterine contractions decreases, the experience of discomfort increases, and a cycle of increased fear and anxiety begins. Ultimately this cycle will slow the progress of labor. The woman's "self-efficacy" or confidence in her ability to cope with pain will be diminished, potentially resulting in reduced effectiveness of pain relief measures being used.

Previous Experience

Previous experience with pain and childbirth may affect a woman's description of her pain and her ability to cope with the pain. Childbirth, for a healthy young adult woman, may be her first experience with significant pain, and as a result, she may not have developed effective pain coping strategies. She may describe the intensity of even early labor pain as pain "as bad as it can be." The nature of previous childbirth experiences also may affect a woman's responses to pain. For women who have had a difficult and painful previous birth experience, anxiety and fear from this past experience may lead to an increased perception of pain. Conversel__ _____ has experienced a labor and birth __ ____ _____ __ ____ __ matched her expectatio__ ___ __ _____ ____ __ ___ successful may exp_____ _ _____ ____ __ pride in her ac_____ __ _____ __ _____iety will incre___ ___ _____ __ _____ ___ _____ ffective duri__ _____

S____ ____ ___ ____ _____ _____ reater than ___ _____ __ ___ _____ ___ ____ (dilation ___ _____ ___ ____ ____ _____ struc-tures ___ _____ ___ _____ _____ of the first s__ __ _____ _____ __ ___ __ labor, multipa__ ____ _____ ____ ___ _____sory pain than null__ _____ _____ _____ ___ upple tissue increases th__ ____ __ _____ __ ___ __ereby intensi-fies pain. The h__ __ _____ __ous women results in a slower, more gradual descent. Affective pain is usually greater for nulliparous women throughout the first stage of labor but decreases for both nulliparous and multiparous women during the second stage of labor (Lowe, 2002).

Fatigue and sleep deprivation magnify pain. Parity may affect perception of labor pain because nulliparous women often have longer labors and therefore greater fatigue, causing a vicious cycle of increased pain, fatigue, reduced ability to cope, and a more likely use of pharmacologic support.

Gate-Control Theory of Pain

Even particularly intense pain stimuli can, at times, be ignored. This is possible because certain nerve cell groupings within the spinal cord, brainstem, and cerebral cortex have the ability to modulate the pain impulse through a blocking mechanism. This gate-control theory of pain helps explain the way hypnosis and the pain relief techniques taught in childbirth preparation classes work to relieve the pain of labor. According to this theory, pain sensations travel along sensory nerve pathways to the brain, but only a limited number of sensations, or messages, can travel through these nerve pathways at one time. Using distraction techniques such as massage or stroking, music, focal points, and imagery reduce or completely block the capacity of nerve pathways to transmit pain. These distractions are thought to work by closing down a hypothetic gate in the spinal cord, thus preventing pain signals from reaching the brain. The perception of pain is thereby diminished.

In addition, when the laboring woman engages in neuromuscular and motor activity, activity within the spinal cord itself further modifies the transmission of pain. Cognitive work involving concentration on breathing and relaxation requires selective and directed cortical activity that activates and closes the gating mechanism as well. As labor intensifies, more complex cognitive techniques are required to maintain effectiveness. The gate-control theory underscores the need for a supportive birth setting that allows the laboring woman to relax and use various higher mental activities.

Comfort

Although the predominant medical approach to labor is that it is painful, and the pain must be removed, an alternative view is that labor is a natural process, and women can experience comfort and transcend the discomfort or pain to reach the joyful outcome of birth. Having needs and desires met engenders a feeling of comfort. Comfort may be viewed as strengthening (Koehn, 2000). The most helpful interventions in enhancing comfort are a caring nursing approach and supportive presence.

Support

A woman's satisfaction with her childbirth experience is primarily influenced by the attitudes and behaviors of her caregivers, including the caregivers' ability to communicate and to be helpful, supportive, accepting, and kind. In addition, satisfaction is influenced by the degree to which she was able to stay in control of her labor and to participate in decision making regarding her labor, including the pain relief measures to be used (Hodnett, 2002).

The continuous supportive presence of a person (e.g., women with or without special training including doulas, childbirth educators, family members, friends, nurses) who provides physical comforting, emotional support, facilitation of communication, and information and guidance to the woman in labor is a beneficial form of care. Continuous support begun early in labor significantly relieves pain, improves outcomes, decreases interventions (e.g., use of pharmacologic pain relief measures) and complication rates (e.g., cesarean births) associated with labor, and enhances overall maternal satisfaction. Interestingly, a more positive effect was achieved when the continuous support was provided by a woman who was not part of the staff of the hospital (Enkin et al., 2000; Hodnett, Gates, Hofmeyr, & Sakala, 2003; Righard, 2001; Simkin & Bolding, 2004; Simkin & O'Hara, 2002).

Environment

According to Lowe (2002), environment should be viewed in terms of the persons present (e.g., how they communicate, their philosophy of care, practice policies, and quality of support) and the physical space in which the labor occurs. The quality of the environment can influence a woman's ability to cope with the pain of labor. Women prefer to be cared for by familiar caregivers in a comfortable, homelike setting (Hodnett, 2002). An environment should be safe and private, allowing a woman to feel free to be herself as she tries out different comfort measures. Stimuli including light, noise, and temperature should be adjusted according to the woman's preferences. There should be space for movement, and equipment should be readily available for a variety of nonpharmacologic pain relief measures such as birth balls, comfortable chairs, tubs, and showers. The familiarity of the environment can be enhanced by bringing items from home such as pillows, objects for a focal point, music, and videos or DVDs.

NONPHARMACOLOGIC MANAGEMENT OF DISCOMFORT

The alleviation of pain is important. Commonly it is not the amount of pain the woman experiences, but whether she meets her goals for herself in coping with the pain, that influences her perception of the birth experience as "good" or "bad." The observant nurse looks for clues to the woman's desired level of control in the management of pain and its relief. Nonpharmacologic measures are often simple, safe, and relatively inexpensive and provide the woman with a sense of control over her childbirth as she makes choices about the measures that are best for her. During the prenatal period, the woman should explore a variety of nonpharmacologic measures. Techniques she finds helpful in relieving stress and enhancing relaxation (e.g., music, meditation, massage, warm baths) also may be very effective as components of a plan for managing labor pain. The woman should be encouraged to communicate to her health care providers her preferences for relaxation and pain relief measures and to actively participate in their implementation.

Many of the nonpharmacologic methods for relief of discomfort are taught in different types of prenatal preparation classes, or the woman or couple may have read various books and magazine articles on the subject in advance. Many of these methods require practice for best results (e.g., hypnosis, patterned breathing and controlled relaxation techniques, biofeedback), although the nurse may use some of them successfully without the woman or couple having prior knowledge (e.g., slow-paced breathing, massage and touch, effleurage, counterpressure). Women should be encouraged to try a variety of methods and to seek alternatives, including pharmacologic methods, if the measure being used is no longer effective (Box 19-1). The analgesic effect of many nonpharmacologic measures is comparable to or even superior to opioids that are administered parenterally. None of these measures, however, are more effective than methods of epidural analgesia. Nonpharmacologic measures are relatively inexpensive and safe with few, if any, major adverse reactions, and they can be used throughout labor. A major drawback regarding nonpharmacologic measures is the lack of evidence to support their effectiveness in relieving the pain of childbirth (Simkin & Bolding, 2004).

Childbirth Preparation Methods

Most health care providers recommend or offer childbirth preparation classes to expectant parents. The major methods taught in the United States are the Dick-Read method,

---

box 19-1 Nonpharmacologic Strategies to Encourage Relaxation and Relieve Pain

CUTANEOUS STIMULATION STRATEGIES
- Counterpressure*
- Effleurage (light massage)*
- Therapeutic touch and massage*
- Walking*
- Rocking*
- Changing positions*
- Application of heat or cold*
- Transcutaneous electrical nerve stimulation
- Acupressure
- Water therapy (showers, whirlpool baths)
- Intradermal water block

SENSORY STIMULATION STRATEGIES
- Aromatherapy
- Breathing techniques*
- Music (see p. 474)
- Imagery*
- Use of focal points*

COGNITIVE STRATEGIES
- Childbirth education*
- Hypnosis
- Biofeedback

From Enkin, M., Keirse, M., Neilson, J., Crowther, C., Duley, L., Hodnett, E., et al. (2001). Effective care in pregnancy and childbirth: A synopsis. *Birth 28*(1), 41-51.
*Forms of care likely to be beneficial.

---

the Lamaze (psychoprophylaxis) method; and the Bradley (husband-coached childbirth) method (Koehn, 2002).

Gaining popularity are methods developed and promoted by Birthing From Within and Birthworks. These methods offer classes and other services which focus on fostering a woman's confidence in her innate ability to give birth. The woman or couple is helped to recognize the uniqueness of their pregnancy and childbirth experience (see Resources on student CD for contact information). Childbirth preparation methods are discussed in more detail in Chapter 17.

CD: Resources

Relaxing and Breathing Techniques
Focusing and Relaxation

By reducing tension and stress, focusing and relaxation techniques allow a woman in labor to rest and to conserve energy for the task of giving birth. *Attention-focusing* and *distraction* techniques are forms of care likely to be beneficial in relieving labor pain (Enkin et al., 2000). Some women bring a favorite object such as a photograph or stuffed animal to the labor room and focus their attention on this object during contractions. Others choose to fix their attention on some object in the labor room. As the contraction begins, they focus on their chosen object and perform a breathing technique to reduce their perception of pain.

With *imagery,* the woman focuses her attention on a pleasant scene, a place where she feels relaxed, or an activity she enjoys. She can imagine walking through a restful garden or breathing in light, energy, and healing color and breathing out worries and tension. Choosing the subject for the imagery and practicing the technique during pregnancy will enhance effectiveness during labor (Koehn, 2002).

These techniques, coupled with feedback relaxation, help the woman work with her contractions rather than against them. The support person monitors this process, telling the woman when to begin the breathing techniques (Fig. 19-2).

During childbirth preparation classes, the coach can learn how to palpate a woman's body to detect tense and contracted muscles. The woman then learns how to relax the tense muscle in response to the gentle stroking of the muscle by the coach (Fig. 19-3). In a common feedback

FIG. 19-2 Expectant parents learning relaxation techniques. (Courtesy Marjorie Pyle, RNC, Lifecircle, Costa Mesa, CA.)

FIG. 19-3 Laboring woman using focusing and breathing techniques during a uterine contraction with coaching from her partner. (Courtesy Marjorie Pyle, RNC, Lifecircle, Costa Mesa, CA.)

mechanism, the woman and her coach say the word "relax" at the onset of each contraction and throughout it as needed. With practice, the coach can effectively use support, feedback, and touch to facilitate the woman's relaxation and thereby reduce tension and stress and enhance the progress of labor (Humenick, Schrock, & Libresco, 2000). The nurse can assist the woman by providing a quiet environment and offering cues as needed.

Breathing Techniques

Different approaches to childbirth preparation stress varying breathing techniques to provide distraction, thereby reducing the perception of pain and helping the woman maintain control throughout contractions. In the first stage of labor, such breathing techniques can promote relaxation of the abdominal muscles and thereby increase the size of the abdominal cavity. This lessens discomfort generated by friction between the uterus and abdominal wall during contractions. Because the muscles of the genital area also become more relaxed, they do not interfere with fetal descent. In the second stage, breathing is used to increase abdominal pressure and thereby assist in expelling the fetus. Breathing also can be used to relax the pudendal muscles to prevent precipitate expulsion of the fetal head.

For couples who have prepared for labor by practicing relaxing and breathing techniques, occasional reminders may be all that are necessary to help them along. For those who have had no preparation, instruction in simple breathing and relaxation can be given early in labor and often is surprisingly successful. Motivation is high, and readiness to learn is enhanced by the reality of labor.

There are various breathing techniques for controlling pain during contractions (Box 19-2). The nurse needs to ascertain what, if any, techniques the laboring couple knows before giving them instruction. Simple patterns are more easily learned. Paced breathing is the technique most associated with prepared childbirth and includes slow-paced, modified-paced, and patterned-paced breathing techniques. Each labor is different, and nursing support includes assisting couples to adapt breathing techniques to their individual labor experience.

All patterns begin with a deep relaxing cleansing breath to "greet the contraction" and end with another deep breath exhaled to "gently blow the contraction away." In general, *slow-paced breathing,* at approximately half the woman's normal breathing rate, is initiated when the woman can no longer walk or talk through contractions. She should continue to use this technique for as long as it is effective in reducing the perception of pain and maintaining control. As contractions increase in frequency and intensity, the woman often needs to change to a more complex breathing technique, which is shallower and approximately twice her normal rate of breathing. This *modified-paced breathing* pattern requires more concentration and therefore blocks more painful stimuli than the simpler slow-paced breathing pattern (Nichols, 2000; Perinatal Education Associates, 2006 [www.birthsource.com]).

box 19-2 Paced Breathing Techniques

CLEANSING BREATH
- Relaxed breath in through nose and out mouth. Used at the beginning and end of each contraction.

SLOW-PACED BREATHING (APPROXIMATELY 6 TO 8 BREATHS PER MINUTE)
- Not less than half the normal breathing rate (number of breaths per minute divided by 2)
- IN-2-3-4/OUT-2-3-4/IN-2-3-4/OUT-2-3-4 . . .

MODIFIED-PACED BREATHING (APPROXIMATELY 32 TO 40 BREATHS PER MINUTE)
- Not more than twice the normal breathing rate (number of breaths per minute multiplied by 2)
- IN-OUT/IN-OUT/IN-OUT/IN-OUT . . .
- For more flexibility and variety, the woman may combine the slow and modified breathing by using the slow breathing for beginnings and ends of contractions and modified breathing for more intense peaks. This technique conserves energy, lessens fatigue, and decreases the chance of hyperventilation.

PATTERNED-PACED BREATHING (SAME RATE AS MODIFIED)
- Enhances concentration
  3:1 Patterned breathing IN-OUT/IN-OUT/IN-OUT/IN-BLOW (repeat through contraction)
  4:1 Patterned breathing IN-OUT/IN-OUT/IN-OUT/IN-OUT/IN-BLOW (repeat through contraction)

Source: Nichols, F. (2000). Paced breathing techniques. In F. Nichols & S. Humenick (Eds.), *Childbirth education: Practice, research, and theory* (2nd ed.). Philadelphia: Saunders; Perinatal Education Associates. (2006). *Breathing.* Accessed www.birthsource.com, July 18, 2006.

CRITICAL THINKING EXERCISE

Childbirth Classes and Epidural Analgesia

Sandra, a primigravida at 20 weeks of gestation, tells the nurse that she is not going to participate in the recommended childbirth classes offered at the hospital where she will be giving birth. She explains that she has heard that most women get epidurals during labor and are pain free, so "Why should I spend the time and money learning how to breathe?" How should the nurse respond to Sandra's plan for her labor?

1. Evidence—Is there sufficient evidence to draw conclusions about what advice the nurse should give to Sandra about her plan to use an epidural during labor and not attend childbirth classes?
2. Assumptions—What assumptions can be made about the following issues related to childbirth classes and epidural analgesia?
   a. Benefits of attending childbirth classes
   b. Effect of prepared childbirth techniques on promotion of comfort and relaxation
   c. Advantage of combining both childbirth classes and epidural analgesia
3. How should the nurse address Sandra's belief that her labor will be pain free if she uses epidural analgesia?
4. Does the evidence objectively support your response to Sandra's belief?
5. Are there alternative perspectives to your conclusion?

The most difficult time to maintain control during contractions comes when the cervix dilates from 8 cm to 10 cm. This phase is called the *transition phase* of the first stage of labor. Even for the woman who has prepared for labor, concentration on breathing techniques is difficult to maintain. The *patterned-paced breathing* technique is suggested for use during this phase. It may be the 4:1 pattern: breath, breath, breath, breath, blow (as though gently blowing out a candle). This ratio may be increased to 6:1 or 8:1. An undesirable side effect of this type of breathing is hyperventilation. The woman and her support person must be aware of and watch for symptoms of the resultant respiratory alkalosis: light-headedness, dizziness, tingling of the fingers, or circumoral numbness. Respiratory alkalosis may be eliminated by having the woman breathe into a paper bag held tightly around the mouth and nose. This enables her to rebreathe carbon dioxide and replace the bicarbonate ion. The woman also can breathe into her cupped hands if no bag is available. Maintaining a breathing rate that is no more than twice the normal rate will lessen chances of hyperventilation. The partner can help the woman maintain her breathing rate with visual, tactile, or auditory cues (Nichols, 2000).

As the fetal head reaches the pelvic floor, the woman may feel the urge to push and may automatically begin to exert downward pressure by contracting her abdominal muscles. During second-stage pushing, the woman should find a breathing pattern that is relaxing and feels good to her and her baby. Any regular or rhythmic breathing that avoids prolonged breath holding during pushing should maintain a good oxygen flow to the fetus (Perinatal Education Associates, 2006).

The woman can control the urge to push by taking panting breaths or by slowly exhaling through pursed lips. This type of breathing can be used to overcome the urge to push when the cervix is not fully prepared (e.g., less than 8 cm dilated, not retracting) and to facilitate a slow birth of the fetal head.

Effleurage and Counterpressure

Effleurage (light massage) and counterpressure have brought relief to many women during the first stage of labor. The gate-control theory may supply the explanation for the effectiveness of these measures. Effleurage is light stroking, usually of the abdomen, in rhythm with breathing during contractions. It is used to distract the woman from contraction pain. Often the presence of monitor belts makes it difficult to perform effleurage on the abdomen; thus a thigh or the chest may be used. As labor progresses, hyperesthesia may make effleurage uncomfortable and thus less effective.

Counterpressure is steady pressure applied by a support person to the sacral area with the fist or heel of the hand. This technique helps the woman cope with the sensations of internal pressure and pain in the lower back. It is especially helpful when back pain is caused by pressure of the occiput against spinal nerves when the fetal head is in a posterior position. Counterpressure lifts the occiput off these nerves, thereby providing pain relief. Although not an evidenced-based practice, pressure also may be applied bilaterally to the hips or knees to reduce low back pain (Simkin & Ancheta, 2000). The support person will need to be relieved occasionally because application of counterpressure is hard work.

Music

Music, recorded or live, can enhance relaxation and lift spirits during labor, thereby reducing the woman's level of stress, anxiety, and perception of pain. It can be used to promote relaxation in early labor and to stimulate movement as labor progresses (Browning, 2000; Simkin & Bolding, 2004). Women should be encouraged to prepare their musical preferences in advance and to bring a compact disc player or iPod to the hospital or birthing center. Use of a headset or earphones may increase the effectiveness of the music because other sounds will be shut out. Live music provided at the bedside by a support person may also be very helpful in transmitting energy that decreases tension

and elevates mood. Changing the tempo of the music to coincide with the rate and rhythm of each breathing technique may facilitate proper pacing (Gentz, 2001). While promising, there is insufficient evidence at the present time to support the effectiveness of music as a method of pain relief during labor. Further research is recommended (Smith, Collins, Cyna, & Crowther, 2005).

Water Therapy (Hydrotherapy)

Bathing, showering, and jet hydrotherapy (whirlpool baths) with warm water (e.g., at or below body temperature) are nonpharmacologic measures that can be used to promote comfort and relaxation during labor (Fig. 19-4). Sitting in a tub of water up to the shoulders or lower has several immediate benefits. Buoyancy in the water results in general body relaxation and temporary relief from discomfort and pain (Cluett, Nikodem, McCandlish, & Burns, 2004). This reduces the woman's anxiety and enhances a feeling of well-being. Catecholamine production decreases. This triggers an increase in the levels of oxytocin (to stimulate uterine contractions) and endorphins (to reduce pain perception). In addition, the bubbles and gentle lapping of the water stimulate the nipples, also triggering an increase

A

B

C

FIG. 19-4 Water therapy during labor. **A,** Use of shower during labor. **B,** Woman experiencing back labor relaxes as partner sprays warm water on her back. **C,** Laboring woman relaxes in Jacuzzi. Note that fetal monitoring can continue during time in the Jacuzzi. (**A** and **B,** Courtesy Marjorie Pyle, RNC, Lifecircle, Costa Mesa, CA; **C,** Courtesy Spacelabs Medical, Redmond, WA.)

in oxytocin production; this has not been observed to cause uterine hyperstimulation. The cervix has often been observed to dilate 2 to 3 cm in 30 minutes of whirlpool therapy. Whirlpool baths in labor also have been found to have positive effects on analgesia requirements, instrumentation rates, condition of the perineum, and personal satisfaction with labor (Simkin & Bolding, 2004; Simkin & O'Hara, 2002). However, there is no clear evidence that these effects can be attributed solely to hydrotherapy (Benfield, 2002).

If the woman is having "back labor" as the result of an occiput posterior or transverse position, she is encouraged to assume the hands-and-knees or the side-lying position in the tub. Because these positions decrease pain and increase relaxation and production of oxytocin, the fetus can then rotate spontaneously to the occiput anterior position. Less effort is needed when the woman changes positions in the water.

In some settings, jet hydrotherapy must be approved by the woman's primary health care provider. The woman's vital signs must be within normal limits, and she should be in the active phase of the first stage of labor (e.g., cervix at least 5 cm dilated). If she is in the latent phase, her contractions could slow (Mackey, 2001).

Fetal heart rate (FHR) monitoring is done by Doppler device, fetoscope, or wireless external monitor device (see Fig. 19-4, *C*). Placement of internal electrodes is contraindicated for jet hydrotherapy. The woman's membranes may be intact or ruptured. If they are ruptured, the fluid must be clear or only lightly stained with meconium (Mackey, 2001).

There is no limit to the time women can stay in the bath, and often women are encouraged to stay in it as long as desired. However, most women use jet hydrotherapy for 30 to 60 minutes at a time. During the bath, if the woman's temperature and the FHR increase, if the labor process becomes less effective (e.g., slows or becomes too intense), or if relief of pain is reduced, the woman can come out of the bath and return at a later time. Repeated baths with occasional breaks may be more effective in relieving pain in long labors than extended amounts of time in the water. Fluids to maintain hydration and a cool face cloth for comfort are offered during the bath (Mackey, 2001; Simkin & O'Hara, 2002). The recommended temperature for the bath is between 36° and 38° C to avoid harmful effects (Florence & Palmer, 2003).

Transcutaneous Electrical Nerve Stimulation

Transcutaneous electrical nerve stimulation (TENS) involves the placing of two pairs of flat electrodes on either side of the woman's thoracic and sacral spine (Fig. 19-5). These electrodes provide continuous low-intensity electrical impulses or stimuli from a battery-operated device. During a contraction, the woman increases the stimulation from low to high intensity by turning control knobs on the device. High intensity should be maintained for at least 1 minute to facilitate release of endorphins. Women

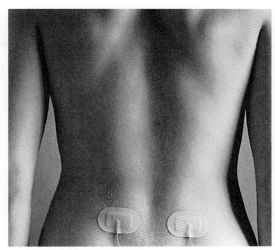

FIG. 19-5   Placement of transcutaneous electrical nerve stimulation (TENS) electrodes on back for relief of labor pain.

describe the resulting sensation as a tingling or buzzing and the pain relief as good or very good. TENS is most useful for lower back pain during the early first stage of labor. Using TENS poses no risk to the mother or fetus, and it is credited with a modest reduction in pain and the use of analgesics and with increasing the woman's perception of control over the experience (Simkin & Bolding, 2004). It may be effective because of the placebo effect; that is, confidence in the effectiveness of TENS may stimulate the release of endogenous opiates (endorphins) in the woman's body, especially if begun early in labor, and thus alleviate the discomfort (Gentz, 2001). TENS is now considered a form of care with insufficient quality data to recommend its use (Enkin et al., 2000). The nurse assists the woman in using TENS by explaining the device and its use, by carefully placing and securing the electrodes, and by closely evaluating its effectiveness.

Acupressure and Acupuncture

Acupressure and acupuncture techniques can be used in pregnancy and labor and postpartum to relieve pain and other discomforts. Pressure, heat, or cold is applied to acupuncture points called *tsubos*. These points have an increased density of neuroreceptors and increased electrical conductivity. The effectiveness of acupressure has been attributed to the gate-control theory of pain and an increase in endorphin levels (Tiran & Mack, 2000). Acupressure is best applied over the skin without using lubricants. Pressure is usually applied with the heel of the hand, fist, or pads of the thumbs and fingers (Fig. 19-6). Tennis balls or other devices also may be used to apply pressure. Pressure is applied with contractions initially and then continuously as labor progresses to the transition phase at the end of the first stage of labor (Koehn, 2000). Synchronized breathing by the caregiver and the woman is suggested for greater effectiveness. Acupressure points are found on the neck, the shoulders, the wrists, the lower back including sacral

FIG. 19-6 Ho-Ku acupressure point (back of hand where thumb and index finger come together) used to enhance uterine contractions without increasing pain. (Courtesy Julie Perry Nelson, Gilbert, AZ.)

points, the hips, the area below the kneecaps, the ankles, the nails on the small toes, and the soles of the feet.

Acupuncture is the insertion of fine needles into specific areas of the body to restore the flow of *qi* (energy) and to decrease pain, which is thought to be obstructing the flow of energy. It should be done by a trained certified therapist. Current evidence indicates that acupuncture may be beneficial for relief of labor pain; however, further study is indicated (Florence & Palmer, 2003; Smith et al., 2005).

Application of Heat and Cold

Warmed blankets, warm compresses, heated rice bags, a warm bath or shower, or a moist heating pad can enhance relaxation and reduce pain during labor. Heat relieves muscle ischemia and increases blood flow to the area of discomfort. Heat application is effective for back pain caused by a posterior presentation or general backache from fatigue (Simkin & O'Hara, 2002).

Cold application such as cool cloths or ice packs applied to the back, the chest, and/or the face during labor may be effective in increasing comfort when the woman feels warm. They also may be applied to areas of pain. Cooling relieves pain by reducing the muscle temperature and relieving muscle spasms. A woman's culture may make the use of cold during labor unacceptable (Simkin & Bolding, 2004).

Heat and cold may be used alternately for a greater effect. Neither heat nor cold should be applied over ischemic or anesthetized areas because tissues can be damaged. One or two layers of cloth should be placed between the skin and a hot or cold pack to prevent damage to the underlying integument (Simkin & Bolding, 2004).

Touch and Massage

Touch and massage have been an integral part of the traditional care process for women in labor. They are likely to be beneficial in relieving labor pain (Enkin et al., 2000).

Touch can be as simple as holding the woman's hand, stroking her body, and embracing her. When using touch to communicate caring, reassurance, and concern, it is important that the woman's preferences for touch (e.g., who can touch her, where they can touch her, and how they can touch her) and responses to touch be determined. A woman with a history of sexual abuse or certain cultural beliefs may be uncomfortable with touch (Simkin & O'Hara, 2002; Trout, 2004). Touch also can involve very specialized techniques that require manipulation of the human energy field. Therapeutic touch (TT) uses the concept of energy fields within the body called *prana*. Prana are thought to be deficient in some people who are in pain. TT uses laying-on of hands by a specially trained person to redirect energy fields associated with pain (Schieber & Selby, 2000). Research has demonstrated effectiveness of TT to enhance relaxation, reduce anxiety, and relieve pain (Marks, 2000); however, little is known about the use or effectiveness of TT for relieving labor pain.

Healing touch (HT) is another energy-based healing modality. Whereas TT emphasizes a single sequence of energy modulation, HT combines a variety of techniques from a series of disciplines. This gives the practitioner an array of "tools" to use with clients. Practitioners are taught energetic diagnosis and treatment forms and the means of documenting the client's response and progress. These techniques are said to align and balance the human energy field, thereby enhancing the body's ability to heal itself. HT has been used in labor management, but no studies have been published about its effectiveness (Hover-Kramer, Mentgen, & Scandrett-Hibdon, 2001) (see Fig. 4-6).

Head, hand, back, and foot massage may be very effective in reducing tension and enhancing comfort. Hand and foot massage may be especially relaxing in advanced labor when hyperesthesia limits a woman's tolerance for touch on other parts of her body. The woman and her partner should be encouraged to experiment with different types of massage during pregnancy to determine what might feel best and be most relaxing during labor.

Hypnosis

Hypnosis, although not commonly used for pain management in the United States, is associated with shorter labors and less analgesia (Tiran & Mack, 2000). Current evidence suggests that hypnosis may relieve pain, increase the likelihood of vaginal birth, reduce the use of oxytocin, and enhance maternal satisfaction. Further research is required to confirm these potentially promising outcomes (Simkin & Bolding, 2004; Smith et al., 2005). Hypnosis techniques used for labor and birth place an emphasis on enhancing relaxation and diminishing fear, anxiety, and perception of pain. The woman may be given direct suggestions about pain relief or indirect suggestions that she is experiencing diminished sensations (Ketterhagen, VandeVusse, & Berner, 2002). The woman receives posthypnotic suggestions, such as, "You will be able to push the baby out easily," to increase her confidence. To be successful, the woman must be educated regarding hypnosis and practice the techniques during the prenatal period (Gentz, 2001).

Biofeedback

Biofeedback may provide another relaxation technique that can be used for labor. Biofeedback is based on the theory that if a person can recognize physical signals, certain internal physiologic events can be changed (i.e., whatever signs the woman has that are associated with her pain). For biofeedback to be effective, the woman must be educated during the prenatal period to become aware of her body and its responses and how to relax. The woman must learn how to use thinking and mental processes (e.g., focusing) to control body responses and functions. Informational biofeedback helps couples develop awareness of their bodies and use strategies to change their responses to stress. If the woman responds to pain during a contraction with tightening of muscles, frowning, moaning, and breath holding, her partner uses verbal and touch feedback to help her relax. Formal biofeedback, which uses machines to detect skin temperature, blood flow, or muscle tension, also can prepare women to intensify their relaxation responses (DiFranco, 2000; Gentz, 2001; Snyder & Lindquist, 2000).

Aromatherapy

Aromatherapy uses oils distilled from plants, flowers, herbs, and trees to promote health and well-being and treat illnesses. The use of herbal teas and vapors is reported to have good effects in pregnancy and labor for some women (Tiran & Mack, 2000). Rose, lavender, frankincense, and bergamot oils can promote relaxation and reduce pain. Oils are used by adding a few drops to a warm bath, to warm water used for soaking compresses that can be applied to the body, to an aromatherapy lamp to vaporize a room, or to oil for a back massage. Drops of essential oils can also be put on a pillow or on a woman's brow or palms (Simkin & Bolding, 2004; Tiran & Mack). Certain odors or scents can evoke pleasant memories and feelings of love and security. As a result, it would be helpful for a woman to choose the scents that she will use (Trout, 2004). Currently, there is insufficient evidence to support the effectiveness of aromatherapy for pain relief in labor although its use has elicited promising results (Smith et al., 2005).

▬ NURSE ALERT

Caution: Never apply the essential oils used for aromatherapy in full strength directly to the skin. Most oils should be diluted in a vegetable oil base before use. In addition, essential oils vary in terms of safe use during pregnancy. Inhaling vapors from the oils can lead to unpleasant side effects including nausea or headaches (Gentz, 2001).

Intradermal Water Block

An intradermal water block involves the injection of small amounts of sterile water (e.g., 0.05 to 0.1 ml) by using a fine needle (e.g., 25 gauge) into four locations on the lower back to relieve low back pain (Fig. 19-7). It may be effective in early labor and in an effort to delay the initiation of pharmacologic pain relief measures. Stinging will occur for about 20 to 30 seconds after injection, but back pain will be relieved for approximately 45 minutes to 2 hours.

FIG. 19-7 Intradermal injections of 0.1 ml of sterile water in the treatment of women with back pain during labor. Sterile water is injected into four locations on the lower back, two over each posterior superior iliac spine (PSIS) and two 3 cm below and 1 cm medial to the PSIS. The injections should raise a bleb on the skin. Simultaneous injections administered by two clinicians will decrease the pain of the injections. (Source: Leeman, L., Fontaine, P., King, V., Klein, M., & Ratcliffe, S. (2003). The nature and management of labor pain: part I. Nonpharmacologic pain relief. *American Family Physician* 68(6), 1109-1112.

Effectiveness of this method may be related to the mechanisms of counterirritation (i.e., reducing localized pain in one area by irritating the skin in an area nearby), gate control, or an increase in the level of endogenous opioids (endorphins). When the effect wears off, the treatment can be repeated, or another method of pain relief can be used (Gentz, 2001; Simkin & O'Hara, 2002).

▬ PHARMACOLOGIC MANAGEMENT OF DISCOMFORT

Pharmacologic measures for pain management should be implemented before pain becomes so severe that catecholamines increase and labor is prolonged. Pharmacologic and nonpharmacologic measures, when used together, increase the level of pain relief and create a more positive labor experience for the woman and her family. Nonpharmacologic measures can be used for relaxation and pain relief, especially in early labor. Pharmacologic measures can be implemented as labor becomes more active and discomfort and pain intensify. Less pharmacologic intervention often is required because nonpharmacologic measures enhance relaxation and potentiate the analgesic's effect (Faucher & Brucker, 2000). However, from 1981 to 2001, more women took advantage of pharmacologic measures to relieve their pain during labor and birth and fewer opted for no pharmacologic support. The largest increase was noted in the use of epidural forms of analgesia (Bucklin, Hawkins, Anderson, & Ullrich, 2005).

Sedatives

Sedatives relieve anxiety and induce sleep. They may be given to a woman experiencing a prolonged latent phase of labor and if there is a need to decrease anxiety or promote sleep. They may also be given to augment analgesics and reduce nausea when an opioid is used. Barbiturates such as secobarbital sodium (Seconal) can cause undesirable side effects including respiratory and vasomotor depression affecting the woman and newborn. These effects are increased if a barbiturate is administered with another central nervous system (CNS) depressant such as an opioid analgesic. However, pain will be magnified if a barbiturate is given without an analgesic to women experiencing pain. Because of these disadvantages, barbiturates are seldom used (Faucher & Brucker, 2000; Hawkins, Chestnut, & Gibbs, 2002).

Phenothiazines (e.g., promethazine [Phenergan], hydroxyzine [Vistaril]) do not relieve pain but decrease anxiety and apprehension, increase sedation, and potentiate opioid analgesic effects. This potentiation effect causes the two drugs to work together more effectively, so the opioid dose can be reduced. In addition, they can be used to reduce the nausea and vomiting that often accompany opioid use (Florence & Palmer, 2003; McCool, Packman, & Zwerling, 2004). Metoclopramide (Reglan) is an antiemetic that also can be used for this purpose.

Benzodiazepines (e.g., diazepam [Valium], lorazepam [Ativan]), when given with an opioid analgesic, seem to enhance pain relief and reduce nausea and vomiting, although the increased sedation experienced may be unacceptable to women in labor (Bricker & Lavender, 2002; Lehne, 2004).

Analgesia and Anesthesia

The use of analgesia and anesthesia was not generally accepted as part of obstetric management until Queen Victoria used chloroform during the birth of her son in 1853. Since then, much study has gone into the development of pharmacologic measures for controlling discomfort during the birth period. The goal of researchers is to develop methods that will provide adequate pain relief to women without increasing maternal or fetal risk or affecting the progress of labor.

Nursing management of obstetric analgesia and anesthesia combines the nurse's expertise in maternity care with a knowledge and understanding of anatomy and physiology and of medications and their therapeutic effects, adverse reactions, and methods of administration.

Anesthesia encompasses analgesia, amnesia, relaxation, and reflex activity. Anesthesia abolishes pain perception by interrupting the nerve impulses to the brain. The loss of sensation may be partial or complete, sometimes with the loss of consciousness.

The term analgesia refers to the alleviation of the sensation of pain or the raising of the threshold for pain perception without loss of consciousness.

The type of analgesic or anesthetic chosen is determined in part by the stage of labor of the woman and by the method of birth planned (Box 19-3).

Systemic Analgesia

Systemic analgesia as a pharmacologic method for relieving pain has been declining, although it still remains the major pharmacologic method for relieving the pain of labor when personnel trained in regional analgesia (e.g., epidural analgesia) are not available (Bricker & Lavender, 2002; Bucklin et al., 2005; Caton et al., 2002). It is a form of care with a trade-off between beneficial and adverse

---

box 19-3 **Pharmacologic Control of Discomfort by Stage of Labor and Method of Birth**

FIRST STAGE
- Systemic analgesia
  Opioid agonist analgesics
  Opioid agonist-antagonist analgesics
- Epidural (block) analgesia
- Combined spinal-epidural (CSE) analgesia
- Paracervical block (rarely used)
- Nitrous oxide

SECOND STAGE
- Nerve block analgesia and anesthesia
  Local infiltration anesthesia
  Pudendal block
  Spinal (block) anesthesia
  Epidural (block) analgesia
  Combined spinal-epidural (CSE) analgesia
- Nitrous oxide

VAGINAL BIRTH
- Local infiltration anesthesia
- Pudendal block
- Epidural (block) analgesia and anesthesia
- Spinal (block) anesthesia
- CSE analgesia and anesthesia
- Nitrous oxide

CESAREAN BIRTH
- Spinal (block) anesthesia
- Epidural (block) anesthesia
- General anesthesia

---

effects (Enkin et al., 2000). Systemic analgesics cross the maternal blood-brain barrier to provide central analgesic effects. They also cross through the placenta. Once transferred to the fetus, analgesics cross the fetal blood-brain barrier more readily than the maternal blood-brain barrier. The duration of action also will be longer because the systemic analgesics used during labor have a significantly longer half-life in the fetus and newborn. Effects on the fetus and newborn can be profound (e.g., respiratory depression, decreased alertness, delayed sucking), depending on the characteristics of the specific systemic analgesic used, the dosage given, and the route and timing of administration. Intravenous (IV) administration is preferred to intramuscular (IM) administration because the medication's onset of action is faster and more predictable; as a result, a higher level of pain relief usually occurs. IV patient-controlled analgesia (PCA) is now available for use during labor. With this method, the woman self-administers small doses of an opioid analgesic by using a pump programmed for dose and frequency. Overall, a lower total amount of analgesic is used, and maternal satisfaction is high (Bricker & Lavender, 2002). Classifications of analgesic drugs used to relieve the pain of childbirth include opioid (narcotic) agonists and opioid (narcotic) agonist-antagonists. Choice of which medication to use is often dependent upon preferences of the primary health care provider and characteristics of the laboring woman. Types of systemic analgesics used may also vary from one obstetric unit to another.

Opioid Agonist Analgesics. Opioid agonist analgesics such as hydromorphone hydrochloride (Dilaudid), meperidine (Demerol), fentanyl (Sublimaze), and sufentanil citrate (Sufenta) are effective for relieving severe, persistent, or recurrent pain. As pure opioid agonists, they stimulate both major opioid receptors, mu and kappa. They have no amnesic effect but create a feeling of well-being or euphoria. These analgesics decrease gastric emptying and increase nausea and vomiting. Bladder and bowel elimination can be inhibited. Because heart rate (e.g., bradycardia, tachycardia), blood pressure (e.g., hypotension), and respiratory effort (e.g., depression) can be adversely affected, opioid analgesics should be used cautiously in women with respiratory and cardiovascular disorders (Lehne, 2004). Safety precautions should be taken because sedation and dizziness can occur after administration, increasing the risk for injury (Lehne). Research findings suggest that women who receive opioids for their labor pain have less effective pain relief and are less satisfied with their pain management method than women whose pain is managed by using epidural analgesia. In a 2002 national survey of women's childbearing experiences, nearly 40% of women who received opioids parenterally during labor rated them as not being very helpful or not helpful at all. Conversely, opioid use is associated with shorter labors, less oxytocin augmentation, and fewer instrumental vaginal births (e.g., forceps-assisted, or vacuum-assisted birth) when compared with epidural analgesia (Bricker & Lavender, 2002; Caton et al., 2002; Leighton & Halpern, 2002; Maternity Center Association, 2002).

Hydromorphone hydrochloride (Dilaudid) is a potent opioid agonist analgesic that can be administered by IV or IM route during labor. After IV administration the onset of action occurs within 10 to 15 minutes, the peak effect is reached in 15 to 30 minutes, and the duration of action is approximately 2 to 3 hours. IM administration has an onset of action in 15 minutes, with a peak in 30 to 60 minutes and a duration of action approximately 4 to 5 hours (see Medication Guide).

Meperidine hydrochloride (Demerol) used to be the most commonly used opioid agonist analgesic for women in labor, but it is no longer the preferred choice because other medications have fewer side effects. Also, its short half-life requires more frequent administration, increasing the risk for adverse reactions (e.g., dysphoria, irritability, seizures, tremors) related to the accumulation of a toxic metabolite (Florence & Palmer, 2003; Lehne, 2004). After IV administration, the onset of action is rapid (30 to 60 seconds), the peak effect is reached in 5 to 7 minutes, and the duration of action is approximately 2 to 4 hours. The onset of action begins in 10 to 15 minutes after an IM injection of meperidine; the peak is reached in 30 to 50 minutes; and the duration of action is 2 to 4 hours (Lehne, 2004) (see Medication Guide).

Ideally, birth should occur less than 1 hour or more than 4 hours after administration of an opioid agonist an-

---

medication guide

Opioid-Agonist Analgesics
Meperidine hydrochloride (Demerol)
Hydromorphone hydrochloride (Dilaudid)

ACTION ■ Opioid agonist analgesics; stimulate mu and kappa opioid receptors to decrease transmission of pain impulses

INDICATION ■ Moderate to severe labor pain and postoperative pain after cesarean birth

DOSAGE AND ROUTE ■ *Meperidine hydrochloride:* 25 mg IV; 50 to 100 mg IM; may repeat in 1-3 hr
■ *Hydromorphone hydrochloride:* 1 mg IV every 3 hours as needed; 1 to 2 mg IM, may repeat in 3-6 hr if needed; or 3 to 4 mg, may repeat in 4-6 hours if needed

ADVERSE EFFECTS ■ Nausea and vomiting, sedation, confusion, drowsiness, tachycardia or bradycardia, hypotension, dry mouth, pruritus, urinary retention, respiratory depression (woman and newborn), decreased fetal heart rate (FHR) variability, decreased uterine activity if given in early labor

NURSING CONSIDERATIONS ■ Assess maternal vital signs, degree of pain, fetal heart rate and pattern, and uterine activity before and after administration; observe for maternal respiratory depression, notifying primary health care provider if maternal respirations are ≤12 breaths/minute; encourage voiding every 2 hours and palpate for bladder distention; administer with a phenothiazine or benzodiazepine, if ordered, to potentiate the analgesic effect, enhance sedation, and decrease nausea and vomiting; if birth occurs within 1-4 hr of dose, observe newborn for respiratory depression; have naloxone available as antidote; implement safety measures as appropriate, including use of side rails and assistance with ambulation; continue use of nonpharmacologic pain relief measures

IM, Intramuscular; *IV,* intravenous.

---

algesic so that neonatal CNS depression resulting from the opioid is minimized.

Fentanyl citrate (Sublimaze) and sufentanil citrate (Sufenta) are potent, short-acting opioid agonist analgesics. Sufentanil use is increasing since it is has a more potent analgesic action than fentanyl when given epidurally. Also, less sufentanil will cross the placenta resulting in reduced fetal exposure. Onset of action after IV injection of either fentanyl or sufentanil occurs within 2 to 5 minutes; the action peaks in 3 to 5 minutes; and the duration of action is about 30 to 60 minutes. More frequent dosing is required with fentanyl and sufentanil because of their relatively short duration of action. As a result, these opioids are most commonly administered intrathecally or epidurally, alone or in combination with a local anesthetic agent (e.g., bupivacaine) (Faucher & Brucker, 2000; Florence & Palmer, 2003; Lehne, 2004) (see Medication Guide).

Opioid Agonist-Antagonist Analgesics. An agonist is an agent that activates or stimulates a receptor to act; an antagonist is an agent that blocks a receptor or a medication designed to activate a receptor. Opioid agonist-antagonist analgesics such as butorphanol (Stadol) and nalbuphine (Nubain) are agonists at kappa opioid receptors and are either antagonists or weak agonists at mu opioid receptors. In the doses used during labor, these mixed opioids provide adequate analgesia without causing significant m e d i c a t i o n   g u i d e

Opioid Agonist Analgesics for Intrathecal and Epidural Use

Fentanyl citrate (Sublimaze)
Sufentanil citrate (Sufenta)

ACTION ▬ Opioid agonist analgesics that stimulate both mu and kappa opioid receptors to decrease the transmission of pain impulses, rapid action with short duration (0.5-1 hr IV; 1-2 hr epidural); sufentanil citrate has a more potent analgesic action than fentanyl citrate with less passage across the placenta to the fetus

INDICATION
▬ Because of their short duration of action when given intravenously, they are most commonly administered epidurally or intrathecally, alone or in combination with a local anesthetic agent, to relieve moderate to severe labor pain and postoperative pain after cesarean birth

DOSAGE AND ROUTE
▬ *Fentanyl citrate:* 25 to 50 mg IV; 1 to 2 mg with 0.125% bupivacaine at rate of 8 to 10 ml/hr epidurally
▬ *Sufentanil citrate:* 1 mg with 0.125% bupivacaine at rate of 10 ml/hr

ADVERSE EFFECTS
▬ Dizziness, drowsiness, allergic reactions, rash, pruritus, maternal and fetal/neonatal respiratory depression, nausea and vomiting, urinary retention

NURSING CONSIDERATIONS
▬ Assess for respiratory depression; naloxone should be available as antidote

IV, Intravenous.

m e d i c a t i o n   g u i d e

Opioid Agonist-Antagonist Analgesics

Butorphanol tartrate (Stadol)
Nalbuphine hydrochloride (Nubain)

ACTION
▬ Mixed agonist-antagonist analgesics; stimulate kappa opioid receptors and blocks or weakly stimulates mu opioid receptors, resulting in good analgesia but with less respiratory depression and nausea and vomiting when compared with opioid agonist analgesics

INDICATION
▬ Moderate to severe labor pain and postoperative pain after cesarean birth

DOSAGE AND ROUTE
▬ *Butorphanol tartrate:* 1 mg (range 0.5 to 2 mg) IV every 3-4 hr as needed; 2 mg (range 1 to 4 mg) IM every 3-4 hr as needed
▬ *Nalbuphine hydrochloride:* 10 mg IV; 10 to 20 mg IM every 3-4 hours as needed

ADVERSE EFFECTS
▬ Confusion, sedation, drowsiness, headache, dizziness, nervousness, sweating; maternal palpitations/tachycardia or bradycardia; transient nonpathologic sinusoidal-like FHR rhythm; respiratory depression; nausea and vomiting; difficulty with urination (retention, urgency)

NURSING CONSIDERATIONS
▬ See opioid agonist analgesics; may precipitate withdrawal symptoms in opioid-dependent women and their newborns

IM, Intramuscular; *IV,* intravenous.

s i g n s   o f   p o t e n t i a l   c o m p l i c a t i o n s

Maternal Opioid Abstinence Syndrome (Opioid Withdrawal)

- Yawning, rhinorrhea (runny nose), sweating, lacrimation (tearing), mydriasis (dilation of pupils)
- Anorexia
- Irritability, restlessness, generalized anxiety
- Tremor
- Chills and hot flashes
- Piloerection ("gooseflesh")
- Violent sneezing
- Weakness, fatigue, and drowsiness
- Nausea and vomiting
- Diarrhea, abdominal cramps
- Bone and muscle pain, muscle spasm, kicking movements

respiratory depression in the mother or neonate. They are less likely to cause nausea and vomiting, but sedation may be as great or greater when compared with pure opioid agonists. As a result of these effects, parenteral opioid agonist-antagonist analgesics are used more commonly during labor than the opioid agonist analgesics. Both IM and IV routes of administration can be used, but the IV route is preferred. This classification of opioid analgesics, especially nalbuphine, is not suitable for women with an opioid dependence because the antagonist activity could precipitate withdrawal symptoms (abstinence syndrome) in both the mother and her newborn (Florence & Palmer, 2003; Hawkins et al., 2002; Lehne, 2004) (see Medication Guide and Signs of Potential Complications box).

Opioid Antagonists. Opioids such as hydromorphone, meperidine, and fentanyl can cause excessive CNS depression in the mother, the newborn, or both, though today's practice of giving lower doses of opioids intravenously has reduced the incidence and severity of opioid-induced CNS depression. Opioid antagonists such as naloxone (Narcan) can promptly reverse the CNS depressant effects, especially respiratory depression. In addition, the antagonist counters the effect of the stress-induced levels of endorphins. An opioid antagonist is especially valuable if labor is more rapid than expected and birth is anticipated when the opioid is at its peak effect. The antagonist may be given through the woman's IV line, or it can be administered intramuscularly (see Medication Guide). The woman should be told that the pain that was relieved with the use of the opioid analgesic will return with the administration of the opioid antagonist. Some authorities believe that unless maternal CNS depression is severe enough to affect her well-being and that of her fetus, the woman should not receive naloxone just before birth in an attempt to prevent neonatal CNS depression. Placental transfer of naloxone is unpredictable; the newborn may not require treatment with an opioid antagonist; and the sudden return of severe pain could have adverse physiologic and psychologic effects on the mother (Hawkins et al., 2002; Lehne, 2004).

medication guide

Opioid Antagonist

Naloxone hydrochloride (Narcan)

ACTION ■ Opioid antagonist which blocks both mu and kappa opioid receptors from the effects of opioid agonists

INDICATION ■ Reverses opioid-induced respiratory depression in woman or newborn; may be used to reverse pruritus from epidural opioids

DOSAGE AND ROUTE

ADULT ■ Opioid overdose: 0.4 to 2 mg IV, may repeat IV at 2- to 3-min intervals up to 10 mg; if IV route unavailable, IM or SC administration may be used

■ Postoperative opioid depression: Initial dose 0.1 to 0.2 mg IV at 2- to 3-min intervals up to 3 doses to desired degree of reversal obtained; may repeat dose in 1 to 2 hours if needed

NEWBORN ■ Opioid-induced depression: Initial dose is 0.1 mg/kg IV, IM, or SC; may be repeated at 2- to 3-min intervals up to 3 doses until desired degree of reversal obtained

ADVERSE EFFECTS ■ Maternal hypotension and hypertension, tachycardia, hyperventilation, nausea and vomiting, sweating, and tremulousness

NURSING CONSIDERATOINS ■ Woman should delay breastfeeding until medication is out of system; do not give to mother or newborn if woman is opioid dependent—may cause abrupt withdrawal in woman and newborn if given to woman for reversal of respiratory depression caused by opioid analgesic, pain will return suddenly

IM, Intramuscular; *IV,* intravenous; *SC,* subcutaneous.

■ NURSE ALERT

An opioid antagonist is containdicated for an infant of an opioid-dependent woman because it may precipitate abstinence syndrome (withdrawal symptoms) (see Signs of Potential Complications box).

An opioid antagonist can be given to the newborn as one part of the treatment for neonatal narcosis, which is a state of CNS depression in the newborn produced by an opioid. Prophylactic administration of naloxone is controversial. Affected infants may exhibit respiratory depression, hypotonia, lethargy, and a delay in temperature regulation. Risk for hypoxia, hypercarbia, and acidosis increases if neonatal narcosis is not treated promptly. Treatment involves ventilation, administration of oxygen, and gentle stimulation. Naloxone is administered, if still required, to reverse CNS depression. More than one dose of naloxone may be required because its half-life is shorter than the half-life of opioids. Alterations in neurologic and behavioral responses may be evident in the newborn for as long as 2 to 4 days after birth. Some depression of attention and social responsiveness can be evident for up to 6 weeks after birth. The significance of these neurobehavioral changes is unknown (Hawkins et al., 2002; Lehne, 2004).

Nerve Block Analgesia and Anesthesia

A variety of local anesthetic agents are used in obstetrics to produce regional analgesia (some pain relief and motor block) and anesthesia (complete pain relief and motor block). Most of these agents are related chemically to cocaine and end with the suffix *-caine.* This helps to identify a local anesthetic.

The principal pharmacologic effect of local anesthetics is the temporary interruption of the conduction of nerve impulses, notably pain. Examples of common agents given are bupivacaine, chloroprocaine, lidocaine, ropivacaine, and mepivacaine. The solution strength of the local anesthetic agent and the amount used will depend on the type of nerve block being performed (Florence & Palmer, 2003).

Rarely, people are sensitive (allergic) to one or more local anesthetics. Such a reaction may include respiratory depression, hypotension, and other serious adverse effects. Epinephrine, antihistamines, oxygen, and supportive measures should reverse these effects. Sensitivity may be identified by administering minute amounts of the drug to be used to test for an allergic reaction.

Local Perineal Infiltration Anesthesia. Local perineal infiltration anesthesia may be used when an episiotomy is to be performed or when lacerations must be sutured after birth in a woman who does not have regional anesthesia. Rapid anesthesia is produced by injecting approximately 10 to 20 ml of 1% lidocaine or 2% chloroprocaine into the skin and then subcutaneously into the region to be anesthetized. Epinephrine often is added to the solution to localize and intensify the effect of the anesthesia in a region and to prevent excessive bleeding and systemic absorption by constricting local blood vessels (Lehne, 2004). Repeated injection will prolong the anesthesia as long as needed.

Pudendal Nerve Block. Pudendal nerve block, administered late in the second stage of labor, is useful if an episiotomy is to be performed or if forceps or a vacuum extractor is to be used to facilitate birth. It can also be administered during the third stage of labor if an episiotomy or lacerations have to be repaired. Its use has declined as a result of the increased use of epidural anesthesia (McCool et al., 2004). Although it does not relieve the pain from uterine contractions, it does relieve pain in the lower vagina, the vulva, and the perineum (Fig. 19-8, *A*). A pudendal nerve block must be administered 10 to 20 minutes before perineal anesthesia is needed.

The pudendal nerve traverses the sacrosciatic notch just medial to the tip of the ischial spine on each side. Injection of an anesthetic solution at or near these points anesthetizes the pudendal nerves peripherally (Fig. 19-9). The transvaginal approach is generally used because it is less painful for the woman, has a higher rate of success in blocking pain, and tends to cause fewer fetal complications (Hawkins et al., 2002). Pudendal block does not change maternal hemodynamic or respiratory functions, vital signs, or the FHR. However, the bearing-down reflex is lessened or lost completely.

Spinal Anesthesia (Block). In spinal anesthesia (block), an anesthetic solution containing a local anesthetic alone or in combination with fentanyl is injected

A   **B**

FIG. 19-8 Pain pathways and sites of pharmacologic nerve blocks. **A,** Pudendal nerve block: suitable during second and third stages of labor and for repair of episiotomy or lacerations. **B,** Epidural block: suitable for all stages of labor and types of birth, and for repair of episiotomy and lacerations.

FIG. 19-9 Pudendal nerve block. Use of needle guide (Iowa trumpet) and Luer-Lok syringe to inject medication.

through the third, fourth, or fifth lumbar interspace into the subarachnoid space (Fig. 19-10, *A* and *B*), where the anesthetic solution mixes with cerebrospinal fluid (CSF). The use of this technique has increased for both elective and emergent cesarean births and is more common than epidural anesthesia for these types of births (Bucklin et al., 2005). Low spinal anesthesia (block) may be used for vaginal birth, but it is not suitable for labor. Spinal anesthesia (block) used for cesarean birth provides anesthesia from the nipple (T6) to the feet. If it is used for vaginal birth, the anesthesia level is from the hips (T10) to the feet (Fig. 19-10, *C*).

For spinal anesthesia (block), the woman is sitting or lying on her side (e.g., modified Sims position) with back curved to widen the intervertebral space to facilitate

insertion of a small-gauge spinal needle and injection of the anesthetic solution. The nurse supports the woman because she must remain still during the placement of the spinal needle. The insertion is made between contractions. After the anesthetic solution has been injected, the woman may be positioned upright to allow the heavier (hyperbaric) anesthetic solution to flow downward to obtain the lower level of anesthesia suitable for a vaginal birth. She may be positioned supine with head and shoulders slightly elevated and the uterus displaced with a wedge under one of her hips to obtain the higher level of anesthesia desired for cesarean birth. The anesthetic effect usually begins 1 to 2 minutes after the anesthetic solution is injected and lasts 1 to 3 hours, depending on the type of agent used (Hawkins et al., 2002) (Fig. 19-11).

Marked hypotension, impaired placental perfusion, and an ineffective breathing pattern may occur during spinal anesthesia. Before induction of the spinal anesthetic (block), the woman's fluid balance is assessed, and IV fluid usually is administered to decrease the potential for hypotension caused by sympathetic blockade (vasodilation with pooling of blood in the lower extremities decreases cardiac output). After induction of the anesthetic, maternal blood pressure, pulse, and respirations and fetal heart rate and pattern must be checked and documented every 5 to 10 minutes. If signs of serious maternal hypotension (e.g., a drop in the baseline blood pressure of more than 20%) or fetal distress (e.g., bradycardia, diminished variability, late decelerations) develop, emergency care must be given (see Emergency box).

EMERGENCY

Maternal Hypotension with Decreased Placental Perfusion

SIGNS AND SYMPTOMS
- Maternal hypotension (20% decrease from preblock baseline level or 100 mm Hg systolic)
- Fetal bradycardia
- Decreased beat-to-beat fetal heart rate variability

INTERVENTIONS
- Turn woman to lateral position or place pillow or wedge under hip (see Fig. 21-5) to displace uterus.
- Maintain IV infusion at rate specified, or increase "as-needed" administration per hospital protocol.
- Administer oxygen by face mask at 10 to 12 L/min or per protocol.
- Elevate the woman's legs.
- Notify the primary health care provider, anesthesiologist, and/or nurse anesthetist.
- Administer IV vasopressor (e.g., ephedrine 5 to 10 mg) per protocol if above measures are ineffective.
- Remain with woman; continue to monitor maternal blood pressure and fetal heart rate every 5 minutes until her condition is stable or per primary health care provider's order.

IV, Intravenous.

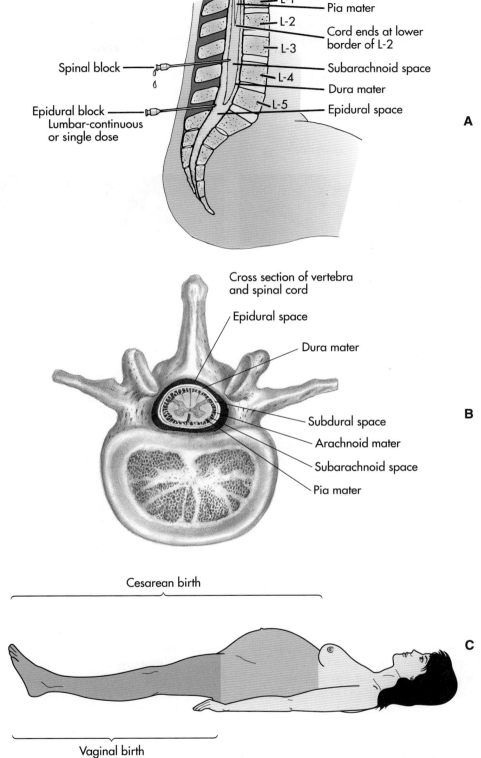

FIG. 19-10   **A,** Membranes and spaces of spinal cord and levels of sacral, lumbar, and thoracic nerves. **B,** Cross section of vertebra and spinal cord. **C,** Level of anesthesia necessary for cesarean birth and for vaginal births.

FIG. 19-11 Positioning for spinal and epidural blocks. **A,** Lateral position. **B,** Upright position. **C,** Catheter for epidural is taped to woman's back with port segment located near her shoulder. (**B** and **C,** Courtesy Michael S. Clement, MD, Mesa, AZ.)

Because the woman is unable to sense her contractions, she must be instructed when to bear down during a vaginal birth. Use of a combination of local anesthetic agent and an opioid reduces the degree of motor function loss, thereby enhancing a woman's ability to push effectively. If the birth occurs in a delivery room (rather than a labor, delivery, recovery room), the woman will need assistance in the transfer to a recovery bed after expulsion of the placenta.

Advantages of spinal anesthesia include ease of administration and absence of fetal hypoxia with maintenance of normotension. Maternal consciousness is maintained, excellent muscular relaxation is achieved, and blood loss is not excessive.

Disadvantages of spinal anesthesia include medication reactions (e.g., allergy), hypotension, and an ineffective breathing pattern; cardiopulmonary resuscitation may be needed. When a spinal anesthetic is given, the need for operative birth (e.g., episiotomy, forceps-assisted birth, vacuum-assisted birth) tends to increase because voluntary expulsive efforts are reduced or eliminated. After birth, the incidence of bladder and uterine atony, as well as postspinal headache, is higher.

Leakage of cerebrospinal fluid (CSF) from the site of puncture of the dura mater (membranous covering of the spinal cord) is thought to be the major causative factor in postdural puncture headache (PDPH). Presumably postural changes cause the diminished volume of CSF to exert traction on pain-sensitive CNS structures. Characteristically, assuming an upright position triggers or intensifies the headache, whereas assuming a supine position achieves relief in 30 minutes or less (Govenar, 2000). The resulting headache, auditory problems (e.g., tinnitus) and visual problems (e.g., blurred vision, photophobia) begin within 2 days of the puncture and may persist for days or weeks.

The likelihood of headache after dural puncture can be reduced, however, if the anesthesiologist uses a small-gauge spinal needle and avoids making multiple punctures of the meninges. Positioning the woman flat in bed (with only a small, flat pillow for her head) for at least 8 hours after spinal anesthesia also has been recommended to prevent headache, but no definitive evidence shows that this measure is effective. Positioning the woman on her abdomen, a difficult if not impossible position after a cesarean birth, is thought to decrease the loss of CSF through the puncture site. Hydration has been claimed to be of value in preventing and treating headache, but no compelling evidence supports its use (Cunningham, Leveno, Bloom, Hauth, Gilstrap, & Wenstrom, 2005). Initial treatment for a postdural puncture headache usually includes oral analgesics, bed rest in a quiet dimly lit or dark room, caffeine, and increased fluid intake (Govenar, 2000; Hawkins et al., 2002).

An autologous epidural blood patch is the most rapid, reliable, and beneficial relief measure for PDPH. The woman's blood (i.e., 10 to 20 ml) is injected slowly into the lumbar epidural space, creating a clot that patches the tear or hole in the dura mater around the spinal cord. It is considered if the headache does not resolve spontaneously or after use of more conservative, noninvasive techniques (Govenar, 2000) (Fig. 19-12).

FIG. 19-12 Blood-patch therapy for spinal headache.

After the blood-patch procedure, the woman should be observed for alteration of vital signs, pallor, clammy skin, and leakage of CSF. A bandage and cold pack are placed on the puncture site, and the woman rests in bed for approximately 1 hour. Discharge instructions include resting in bed for 24 to 48 hours, applying cold packs to the site as needed for comfort, avoiding analgesics that affect platelet aggregation (e.g., nonsteroidal antiinflammatory drugs [NSAIDs]) for 2 days, drinking plenty of fluids, and observing for signs of infection at the site and for neurologic symptoms such as pain, numbness and tingling in legs, and difficulty with walking or elimination. The woman should be cautioned to avoid lifting, straining at stool, coughing, tub bathing, or swimming for at least 2 days (Govenar, 2000; Hawkins et al., 2002).

Epidural Anesthesia or Analgesia (Block). Relief from the pain of uterine contractions and birth (vaginal and cesarean) can be relieved by injecting a suitable local anesthetic agent (e.g., bupivacaine, ropivacaine), an opioid analgesic (e.g., fentanyl, sufentanil), or both into the epidural (peridural) space, usually between the fourth and fifth lumbar vertebrae (see Figs. 19-8, *B*, and 19-10, *A*). Depending on the type and amount of medication(s) used, an anesthetic or analgesic effect will occur with varying degrees of motor impairment. The combination of an opioid with the local anesthetic agent reduces the dose of anesthetic required, thereby preserving a greater degree of motor function (McCool et al., 2004).

Lumbar Epidural Anesthesia and Analgesia. Lumbar epidural anesthesia and analgesia (block) is the most effective pharmacologic pain relief method for labor currently available. As a result, it is the most commonly used method for relieving pain during labor in the United States, and its use has been increasing. Nearly two thirds of American women choose epidural analgesia for their plan of pain care during labor (Bucklin et al., 2005; Lieberman & O'Donoghue, 2002). For relieving the discomfort of labor

and vaginal birth, a block from T-10 to S-5 is required. For cesarean birth, a block from at least T-8 to S-1 is essential. The diffusion of epidural anesthesia depends on the location of the catheter tip, the dose and volume of the anesthetic agent used, and the woman's position (e.g., horizontal or head-up position). It is essential that the woman cooperate and maintain her position without moving during the insertion of the epidural catheter in order to prevent misplacement, neurologic injury, or hematoma formation. Administration of an opioid analgesic may be necessary to decrease pain and enhance her ability to remain still during the procedure (Cunningham et al., 2005; Mahlmeister, 2003).

For the induction of a lumbar epidural block, the woman is positioned as for a spinal block. She may sit with her back curved or she may assume a modified Sims position with her shoulders parallel, legs slightly flexed, and back arched (see Fig. 19-11).

After the epidural has been started, the woman is positioned preferably on her side so that the uterus does not compress the ascending vena cava and descending aorta, which can impair venous return, reduce cardiac output and blood pressure, and decrease placental perfusion. Her position should be alternated from side to side every hour. Upright positions and ambulation may be encouraged, depending on the degree of motor impairment. Oxygen should be available if hypotension occurs despite maintenance of hydration with IV fluid and displacement of the uterus to the side. Ephedrine (a vasopressor used to increase maternal blood pressure) and increased IV fluid infusion may be needed (see Emergency box). The fetal heart rate and pattern, and progress in labor must be monitored carefully, because the woman in labor may not be aware of changes in the strength of the uterine contractions or the descent of the presenting part.

Several methods can be used for an epidural block. An intermittent block is achieved by using repeated injections of anesthetic solution; it is the least common method. The most commonly used method is the continuous block, achieved by using a pump to infuse the anesthetic solution through an indwelling plastic catheter. Patient-controlled epidural analgesia (PCEA) is the newest method; it uses an indwelling catheter and a programmed pump that allows the woman to control the dosing. This method enhances a woman's sense of control over her labor and has been found to decrease the total amount of medication used.

The advantages of an epidural block are numerous: the woman remains alert and is more comfortable and able to participate, good relaxation is achieved, airway reflexes remain intact, only partial motor paralysis develops, gastric emptying is not delayed, and blood loss is not excessive. Fetal complications are rare but may occur in the event of rapid absorption of the medication or marked maternal hypotension. The dose, volume, and type of medication(s) used can be modified to allow the woman to push, to assume upright positions and even to walk, to produce

CD: Critical Thinking Exercise: Patient Receiving Epidural Block

EVIDENCE-BASED PRACTICE

Outcomes of Epidural Analgesia

BACKGROUND

- The need for pain relief in labor depends on the physical, psychosocial, and emotional status of the woman, as well as labor onset and birth interventions. Pain experience during labor can affect bonding and breastfeeding. For about 60 years, health care providers have been injecting anesthetic into the epidural space in the lower spinal column, blocking pain from the uterus. The choice of drugs impacts the degree of motor function preserved. Recently, combined spinal-epidural (CSE) combines the rapid relief of a single injection into the spinal column with the ongoing pain relief of an epidural catheter. Usage of epidural analgesia varies greatly by region. Recently, nonpharmacologic pain relief methods, such as distraction, relaxation, acupressure and acupuncture, massage, water immersion, hypnosis, and aromatherapy and audiotherapy have shown promise.

- Problems with epidurals include vasodilation and hypotension, which occur when the sympathetic nerve is anesthetized. To avoid compromising uteroplacental perfusion, most institutions routinely administer a fluid bolus before epidural placement. Epidural catheters can become kinked and cause uneven pain relief. Urinary retention may necessitate a urinary catheter. Puncture of the dura can lead to headache and immobility. Epidurals may also prolong labor, compromise the maternal ability to push, and increase the use of oxytocin and instrumental births. Babies born to mothers with epidurals may have higher cord pH, need for resuscitation, and low blood sugar.

OBJECTIVES

- The task of the reviewers was to compare the efficacy and adverse effects of epidural analgesia with other pain relief interventions or no intervention. Their primary outcomes included women's perception of pain and satisfaction, instrumental or surgical birth, and fetal outcomes.

METHODS

Search Strategy

- The authors searched the Cochrane Pregnancy and Childbirth Group Trials Register. Twenty-one randomized controlled trials, reported in 48 publications dated 1974 to 2003, met the inclusion criteria. These trials represented 6,664 women from Australia, Canada, China, Denmark, Finland, France, India, Mexico, Sweden, the United Kingdom, and the United States. Most were low risk women laboring at term.

Statistical Analyses

- Similar data were pooled. Reviewers calculated relative risk for dichotomous (categoric) data, such as type of birth, and weighted mean difference for continuous data, such as pain scale. Differences between groups outside the 95% confidence interval were accepted as significant. All were analyzed in their original randomly assigned "intention to treat" categories, even if they changed their minds.

FINDINGS

- The epidural analgesia group experienced significantly greater pain relief than controls, as well as decreased need for additional pain relief, in first- and second-stage labor. There was a greater risk of instrumental birth in the epidural group when compared to the nonepidural group. Second-stage labor was prolonged and oxytocin more frequently used for the epidural group. There was more hypotension, motor blockage, urinary retention, and fever in the epidural group. The epidural group had fewer neonates with cord pH less than 7.2. No differences were found for cesarean birth rates, maternal satisfaction, backache, malposition, meconium staining, neonatal Apgar scores, or admission to the neonatal intensive care unit.

LIMITATIONS

- The trials span 3 decades. The interventions include different combinations of nerve blockers and dosing, and improvements in drug delivery, such as patient-controlled pumps. Nonepidural interventions covered opioids as well as nonpharmacologic techniques, which have only recently attained research status. Blinding was not possible. Women did not always stay with their assigned intervention, or labored too rapidly to receive it. The measures of women's satisfaction and pain were not standardized.

IMPLICATIONS FOR PRACTICE

- Epidural analgesia in labor offers better pain relief than nonepidural methods, but can lead to a cascade of interventions: instrumental birth, prolonged labor, and increased use of oxytocin. Epidurals can cause hypotension, which can be prevented with a fluid bolus. No adverse outcomes were found for the neonates.

IMPLICATIONS FOR FURTHER RESEARCH

- More information is needed on maternal and long-term fetal side effects of epidural analgesia. Standardization of dosing and agents would increase the power to generalize the results. Most of the studies were on term, low risk labor clients, which may not be generalizable to higher risk or preterm labor clients. Information on dosing and drug delivery would be helpful. Nonpharmacologic pain-relief therapies may complement epidural or other pain-relief methods, but information on combinations and specific protocols will be needed.

Reference: Anim-Soumah, M., Smyth, R., & Howell, C. (2005). Epidural versus non-epidural or no analgesia in labour. *The Cochrane Database of Systematic Reviews, 2006,* Issue 3. Chichester, UK: John Wiley & Sons.

perineal anesthesia, and to permit forceps-assisted, vacuum-assisted, or cesarean birth if required (Cunningham et al., 2005; McCool et al., 2004).

The disadvantages of epidural block also are numerous. The woman's ability to move freely and to maintain control of her labor is limited, related to the use of numerous medical interventions (e.g., an intravenous infusion and electronic monitoring) and the occurrence of orthostatic hypotension and dizziness, sedation, and weakness of the legs. CNS effects such as excitation, bizarre behavior, tinnitus, disorientation, paresthesia, and convulsions can occur if a solution containing a local anesthetic agent is accidentally injected into a blood vessel. Respiratory arrest can occur if the relatively high dosage used with an epidural block is accidentally injected into the subarachnoid space. Women who receive an epidural have a higher rate of fever (i.e., intrapartum temperature of 38° C or higher), especially when labor lasts longer than 12 hours; the temperature elevation most likely is related to thermoregulatory changes, although infection cannot be ruled out. The elevation in temperature can result in fetal tachycardia and neonatal workup for sepsis, whether or not signs of infection are present.

Severe hypotension (more than a 20% decrease in baseline blood pressure) as a result of sympathetic blockade can be an outcome of an epidural block (see Emergency Box). It can result in a significant decrease in uteroplacental perfusion and oxygen delivery to the fetus (Anim-Somuah, Smyth, & Howell, 2005). Urinary retention and stress incontinence can occur in the immediate postpartum period. This temporary difficulty in urinary elimination could be related not only to the effects of the epidural block but also to the increased duration of labor and need for instrumental birth associated with the block (Lieberman & O'Donoghue, 2002). Pruritus (itching) is a side effect associated with the use of an opioid, especially fentanyl. A relation between epidural analgesia and longer second-stage labor, increased incidence of fetal malposition, use of oxytocin, and forceps-assisted or vacuum-assisted birth has been documented. Research findings have been unable to demonstrate a significant increase in cesarean birth associated with epidural analgesia (Anim-Somuah et al., 2005; Lieberman & O'Donoghue, 2002; Sharma & Leveno, 2003). Occasionally a PDPH can occur after accidental perforation of the dura mater during the administration of the epidural block. Because a larger needle is used for an epidural block, the risk for greater CSF loss and resultant severe headache is high (Hawkins et al., 2002). For some women, the epidural block is not effective, and a second form of analgesia is required to establish effective pain relief. When women progress rapidly in labor, pain relief may not be obtained before birth occurs.

Combined Spinal-Epidural Analgesia.
Using opioids such as fentanyl and sufentanil to potentiate the effects of local anesthetic agents has resulted in the reduction of the amount of the local anesthetic used, thereby reducing motor blockade. A combined spinal-epidural (CSE) technique is an increasingly popular approach that can be used to block pain transmission without compromising motor ability. There is a high concentration of opioid receptors along the pain pathway in the spinal cord, in the brainstem, and in the thalamus. Because these receptors are highly sensitive to opioids, a small quantity of an opioid-agonist analgesic produces marked pain relief lasting for several hours. The opioid is injected into the subarachnoid space for rapid activation of the opioid receptors. A catheter is left in place in the epidural space to extend the duration of the analgesia by using a lower dose of a local anesthetic agent alone or in combination with an opioid agonist analgesic (Hawkins et al., 2002). Although women can walk (hence the term "walking epidural"), they often choose not to do so because of sedation and fatigue, abnormal sensations in and weakness of the legs, and a feeling of insecurity. Often health care providers are reluctant to encourage or assist women to ambulate for fear of injury (Mayberry, Clemmens, & De, 2002). However, women can be assisted to change positions and use upright positions during labor and birth. Enhanced motor function facilitates more effective bearing-down efforts, thereby reducing the risk for forceps- or vacuum-assisted birth (Mayberry, Strange, Suplee, & Gennaro, 2003; McCool et al., 2004).

CSE analgesia may be associated with fetal bradycardia, necessitating close assessment of fetal heart rate and pattern. Also, since it involves both the puncture of the dura and the placement of a catheter in the epidural space, there is a higher risk for infection and PDPH (Lieberman & O'Donoghue, 2002; McCool et al., 2004).

Epidural and Intrathecal Opioids.
Opioids also can be used alone, eliminating the effect of a local anesthetic altogether. The use of epidural or intrathecal (spinal) opioids without the addition of a local anesthetic agent during labor has several advantages. Opioids administered in this manner do not cause maternal hypotension or affect vital signs. The woman feels contractions but not pain. Her ability to bear down during the second stage of labor is preserved because the pushing reflex is not lost, and her motor power remains intact.

Fentanyl, sufentanil, or preservative-free morphine may be used. Fentanyl and sufentanil produce short-acting analgesia (i.e., 1.5 to 3.5 hours), and morphine may provide pain relief for 4 to 7 hours. Morphine may be combined with fentanyl or sufentanil. It would be appropriate to use short-acting opioids with multiparous women, and morphine with nulliparous women or women with a history of long labor. For most women, intrathecal opioids do not provide adequate analgesia for second-stage labor pain, episiotomy, or birth (Cunningham et al., 2005). Pudendal nerve blocks or local perineal infiltration anesthesia may be necessary.

A more common indication for the administration of epidural or intrathecal analgesics is the relief of postoperative pain. For example, women who give birth by cesarean can receive fentanyl or morphine through a catheter. The catheter may then be removed, and the women are usually free of pain for 24 hours. Occasionally the catheter is left in place in the epidural space in case another dose is needed.

Women receiving epidurally administered morphine after the cesarean birth are up soon after surgery with surprising ease and are able to care for their newborns. The early ambulation and freedom from pain also facilitate bladder emptying, enhance peristalsis, and prevent clot formation in the lower extremities (e.g., thrombophlebitis). To those women who have had a previous cesarean birth and have had the usual postoperative pain, the effects of this approach seem miraculous. However, the mother may not understand why she may have pain after the opioid effect wears off.

Side effects of opioids administered by the epidural and intrathecal routes include nausea, vomiting, pruritus, urinary retention, and delayed respiratory depression. These effects are more common when morphine is administered. Antiemetics, antipruritics, and opioid antagonists are used to relieve these symptoms. For example, naloxone (Narcan), promethazine (Phenergan), or metoclopramide (Reglan) may be administered. Hospital protocols should provide specific instructions for the treatment of these side effects. Use of epidural opioids is not without risks. Respiratory depression is a serious concern; for this reason, the woman's respiratory rate should be assessed and documented every hour for 24 hours, or as designated by hospital protocol. Naloxone should be readily available for use if the respiratory rate decreases to less than 10 breaths per minute or if the oxygen saturation rate decreases to less than 89%. Administration of oxygen by face mask also may be initiated, and the anesthesiologist should be notified.

Contraindications to Subarachnoid and Epidural Blocks. Some contraindications to epidural analgesia include the following (Hawkins et al., 2002; McCool et al., 2004):

- Active antepartum hemorrhage. Acute hypovolemia leads to increased sympathetic tone to maintain the blood pressure. Any anesthetic technique that blocks the sympathetic fibers can produce significant hypotension that can endanger the mother and baby.
- Anticoagulant therapy or bleeding disorder. If a woman is receiving anticoagulant therapy or has a bleeding disorder, injury to a blood vessel may cause the formation of a hematoma that may compress the cauda equina or the spinal cord and lead to serious CNS complications.
- Infection at the injection site. Infection can be spread through the peridural or subarachnoid spaces if the needle traverses an infected area.
- Allergy to the anesthetic drug.
- Maternal refusal or inability to cooperate.
- Some types of maternal cardiac conditions.

Epidural Block Effects on Neonate. Debate persists concerning the effects of epidural anesthesia and analgesia on the newborn's neurobehavioral responses. Findings from studies that examine associations between neurobehavioral outcome and epidural block are far from consistent. For example, studies comparing the neonatal neurobehavioral scores for infants born to mothers who did and mothers who did not receive epidural analgesia either have shown little or no difference in the scores or have shown that the infants of mothers who received epidural anesthesia did not score as well on neurobehavioral tests. In one research study, infants exposed to an epidural block tended to have less muscle tone but were better able to orient and habituate to sound when compared with infants whose mother received opioids during labor (Lieberman & O'Donoghue, 2002).

Nitrous Oxide for Analgesia

Nitrous oxide mixed with oxygen can be inhaled in a low concentration (50% or less) to reduce but not eliminate pain during the first and second stages of labor. At the lower doses used for analgesia, the woman remains awake, and the danger of aspiration is avoided because the laryngeal reflexes are unaffected. It can be used in combination with other nonpharmacologic and pharmacologic measures for pain relief.

A face mask or mouthpiece is used to self-administer the gas. The woman should place the mask over her mouth and nose or insert the mouthpiece 30 seconds before the onset of a contraction (if regular) or as soon as a contraction begins (if irregular). When she inhales, a valve opens, and the gas is released. She should continue to inhale the gas slowly and deeply until the contraction starts to subside. When inhalation stops, the valve closes. Onset of action is 50 seconds; therefore beginning the inhalation process 30 seconds before the onset of a contraction provides the best pain relief. During the interval between contractions, the woman should remove the device and breathe normally (Rosen, 2002).

Approximately half of women who use nitrous oxide obtain adequate pain relief and are satisfied with the method, but it can be difficult to coordinate adequate inhalation and placement of the mask or mouthpiece (McCool et al., 2004). The nurse should observe the woman for nausea and vomiting, drowsiness, dizziness, hazy memory, and loss of consciousness. Loss of consciousness is more likely to occur if opioids are used with the nitrous oxide. The use of nitrous oxide does not appear to depress uterine contractions or cause adverse reactions in the fetus and newborn (Rosen, 2002).

Nitrous oxide for pain relief during labor is more readily available in Canada and European countries than in the United States (Caton et al., 2002).

General Anesthesia

General anesthesia rarely is used for uncomplicated vaginal birth and is infrequently used for elective cesarean birth. It may be necessary if there is a contraindication to a spinal or epidural block or if indications necessitate rapid birth (vaginal or emergent cesarean) without sufficient time or available personnel to perform a block (Bucklin et al., 2005). In addition, being awake and aware during major surgery may be unacceptable for some women having a cesarean birth.

If general anesthesia is being considered, the nurse gives the woman nothing by mouth and ensures that an IV infusion is in place. If time allows, the nurse premedicates the woman with a nonparticulate (clear) oral antacid (e.g., sodium citrate, Bicitra, Alka-Seltzer) to neutralize the acidic contents of the stomach. Aspiration of highly acidic gastric contents will damage lung tissue. Some anesthesiologists and physicians also order the administration of a histamine (H_2)-receptor blocker such as cimetidine (Tagamet) to decrease the production of gastric acid and metoclopramide (Reglan) to increase gastric emptying (Hawkins et al., 2002). Before the anesthesia is given, a wedge should be placed under one of the woman's hips to displace the uterus. Uterine displacement prevents aortocaval compression, which interferes with placental perfusion.

Trachea

Esophagus   Cricoid cartilage   Thyroid
            (cricoid ring)   cartilage

FIG. 19-13 Technique of applying pressure on cricoid cartilage to occlude esophagus to prevent pulmonary aspiration of gastric contents during induction of general anesthesia.

Thiopental, a short-acting barbiturate, or ketamine is administered intravenously to render the woman unconscious, and then succinylcholine, a muscle relaxer, is administered to facilitate passage of an endotracheal tube. Sometimes the nurse is asked to assist with applying cricoid pressure before intubation as the woman begins to lose consciousness. This maneuver blocks the esophagus and prevents aspiration should the woman vomit or regurgitate (Fig. 19-13). Pressure is released once the endotracheal tube is securely in place.

After the woman is intubated, nitrous oxide and oxygen in a 50:50 mixture are administered. A low concentration of a volatile halogenated agent (e.g., isoflurane) also may be administered to increase pain relief and to reduce maternal awareness and recall (Hawkins et al., 2002). In higher concentrations, isoflurane or methoxyflurane relaxes the uterus quickly and facilitates intrauterine manipulation, version, and extraction. However, at higher concentrations, these agents cross the placenta readily and can produce narcosis in the fetus and could reduce uterine tone after birth, increasing the risk for hemorrhage.

Priorities for recovery room care are to maintain an open airway and cardiopulmonary function and to prevent postpartum hemorrhage. Routine postpartum care is organized to facilitate parent-infant attachment as soon as possible and to answer the mother's questions. When appropriate, the nurse assesses the mother's readiness to see the baby, as well as her response to the anesthesia and to the event that necessitated general anesthesia (e.g., emergency cesarean birth when vaginal birth was anticipated).

▪ CARE MANAGEMENT

The choice of pain relief depends on a combination of factors, including the woman's special needs and wishes, the availability of the desired method(s), the knowledge and expertise in nonpharmacologic and pharmacologic methods of the health care providers involved in the woman's care, and the phase and stage of labor.

▪ Assessment and Nursing Diagnoses

The assessment of the woman, her fetus, and her labor is a joint effort of the nurse and the primary health care providers, who consult with the woman regarding their findings and recommendations. The needs of each woman are different, and many factors must be considered before deciding whether nonpharmacologic methods, pharmacologic methods, or a combination of both will be used to manage labor pain. It is critical that the nurse take note of all pain characteristics including location, intensity, quality, frequency, duration, and effectiveness of relief measures. The nurse should never assume that because a woman is in labor, her pain must be uterine in origin. Because pain is a subjective phenomenon, the nurse must listen to the woman's description of her pain. One self-assessment tool that can be used is a visual analog scale (VAS). The VAS allows the woman to indicate on a line how severe or intense she perceives her pain to be from "no pain" to "pain as bad as it could possibly be." The McGill Pain Questionnaire provides a more complete picture of the pain experience because the woman is able to describe the sensory and emotional or affective dimensions of her pain rather than just its intensity (Lowe, 2002). Self-assessment is recommended to ensure that pain management is based on the subjective nature of the woman's pain rather than just on the nurse's judgment. It is not unusual for a nurse to overestimate or underestimate the pain being experienced by the woman. When there are major cultural differences between the health care provider and the client, inaccurate interpretation of pain intensity often occurs (Lowe).

▪ History

The woman's prenatal record is read and relevant information identified. This includes the woman's parity, estimated date of birth, and complications and medications during pregnancy, and conditions that would contraindicate the use of specific pharmacologic methods. If the woman has a history of allergies, this is noted, and a warning is displayed in a prominent place on her chart and she is provided with an appropriate ID band that indicates her allergy (Mahlmeister, 2003). A history of smoking and neurologic and spinal disorders also is noted.

▪ Interview

Interview data consist of the time of the woman's last meal and the type of food and fluid consumed; the nature of any existing respiratory condition (e.g., cold, asthma); and unusual reactions (e.g., allergy) to medications, cleansing agents, or tape. The woman is asked whether she attended childbirth preparation classes. The extent of her preparation and her preferences for management of discomfort including a birth plan are reviewed. Her knowledge of the options for the management of discomfort also is assessed. Information on the woman's perception of discomfort and her expressed need for medication is added to the database. Relevant events that have occurred since the woman's last contact with her primary health care provider also are reviewed (e.g., infections, diarrhea, a change in fetal movement patterns). If verbal and physical signs indicate the existence of substance abuse (e.g., opioids, alcohol), the nurse should ask the woman to identify the type of substance used, the last time it was taken, and the method of administration.

▬ Physical Examination

The character and status of the labor and fetal response are assessed during a physical examination. The nurse evaluates the woman's hydration status by assessing intake and output measurements, the moistness of the mucous membranes, skin turgor, and concentration of urine. Bladder distention is noted. Any evidence of skin infection near sites of possible needle insertion is recorded and reported. Signs of apprehension such as fist clenching and restlessness also are noted.

If the woman is in labor, the status of maternal vital signs, fetal heart rate and pattern, uterine contractions, amniotic membranes and fluid, cervical effacement and dilation, and fetal descent is determined before any pharmacologic administration. Following administration, ongoing assessment of the maternal-fetal unit and the progress of labor should be performed according to agency protocol and professional standards (Association of Women's Health, Obstetric, and Neonatal Nurses [AWHONN], 2001; Mahlmeister, 2003). The anticipated time until birth is estimated if possible. The length of labor and degree of fatigue are other important considerations. If pharmacologic methods are to be used, the type of analgesia or anesthesia chosen will vary depending on the status of the maternal-fetal unit, the progress of labor, and the method of birth planned (see Box 19-3).

▬ Laboratory Tests

The results of laboratory tests are reviewed to determine whether the woman is experiencing anemia (hemoglobin and hematocrit), a coagulopathy or bleeding disorder (clotting studies and platelet count), or infection (white blood cell count and differential).

▬ Signs of Potential Problems

Any medication can cause a minor or severe allergic reaction. As part of the assessment for such allergic reactions, the nurse should monitor the woman's vital signs, respiratory status, cardiovascular status, integument, and platelet and white blood cell count. The woman is observed for side effects of drug therapy, especially drowsiness. Minor reactions can consist of a rash, rhinitis, fever, asthma, or pruritus. Management of the less acute allergic response is not an emergency (Lehne, 2004).

Severe reactions may occur suddenly and lead to shock. The most dramatic form of anaphylaxis is sudden severe bronchospasm, vasospasm, severe hypotension, and death. Signs of anaphylaxis are largely caused by contraction of smooth muscles and may begin with irritability, extreme weakness, nausea, and vomiting. This may lead to dyspnea, cyanosis, convulsions, and cardiac arrest. An acute allergic reaction (anaphylaxis) must be diagnosed and treated immediately. Treatment usually consists of 1:1000 epinephrine injected subcutaneously or intramuscularly, followed by parenteral administration of antihistamines. Supportive care is given to alleviate the symptoms; the type of care is determined by the rapidly assessed cardiovascular and respiratory response of the woman to the primary interventions (Lehne, 2004). Cardiopulmonary resuscitation may be necessary.

▬ NURSE ALERT

Complications may occur with epidural analgesia, including injection-related emergencies and compression problems. These complications can require immediate interventions. Nurses must be prepared to provide safe and effective care during the emergency situation. Clear procedures or protocols should be in place in labor and birth units delineating responsibilities and actions needed (Mahlmeister, 2003).

The nurse also must be alert for changes in fetal well-being; nonreassuring changes in fetal heart rate and pattern should be noted and reported to the primary health care provider.

The following nursing diagnoses are relevant in the management of discomfort during labor and birth:

- *Acute pain related to*
  - –processes of labor and birth
- *Ineffective tissue perfusion related to*
  - –effects of analgesia or anesthesia
  - –maternal position
- *Hypothermia related to*
  - –effects of analgesia or anesthesia
- *Situational low self-esteem related to*
  - –negative perception of the woman's (or her family's) behavior
- *Fear related to deficient knowledge of*
  - –procedure for epidural analgesia
  - –expected sensation during spinal anesthesia
- *Risk for maternal injury related to*
  - –effects of analgesia and anesthesia on sensation and motor control

▬ Expected Outcomes of Care

The expected outcomes of nursing care in the management of the discomfort of labor and birth include the following:
- The woman will promptly report the characteristics of her pain and discomfort.
- The woman will verbalize understanding of her needs and rights with regard to pain relief management that uses a variety of nonpharmacologic and pharmacologic methods reflecting her preferences.
- The woman will have adequate pain relief without adding maternal risk (e.g., through the use of appropriate nonpharmacologic methods and appropriate medication, including the appropriate dose, timing, and route of administration).

- The fetus will maintain well-being, and the newborn will adjust to extrauterine life.

■ Plan of Care and Interventions

A plan of care is developed for each woman to address her particular clinical and nursing problems. The nurse collaborates with the primary health care provider and laboring woman in selecting those aspects of care relevant to the woman and her family.

■ *Nonpharmacologic Interventions*

The nurse supports and assists the woman as she uses nonpharmacologic interventions for pain relief and relaxation. During labor, the nurse should ask the woman how she feels to evaluate the effectiveness of the specific pain management techniques used. Appropriate interventions can then be planned or continued for effective care, such as trying other nonpharmacologic methods or combining nonpharmacologic methods with medications (see Plan of Care).

The woman's perception of her behavior during labor is of utmost importance. If she planned an unmedicated birth but then needs and accepts medication, her self-esteem may falter. Verbal and nonverbal acceptance of her behavior is given as necessary by the nurse and reinforced by discussion and reassurance after birth. Providing explanations about the fetal response to maternal discomfort, the effects of maternal stress and fatigue on the progress of labor, and the medication itself is a supportive measure. The woman also may experience anxiety and stress related to anticipated or actual pain. Stress can cause increased maternal catecholamine production. Increased levels of catecholamines have been linked to dysfunctional labor and fetal and neonatal distress and illness. Nurses must be able to implement strategies aimed at reducing this stress (Hodnett, 2002; Lowe, 2002).

■ *Informed Consent*

Pregnant women have the right to be active participants in determining the best pain care approach to use during labor and birth (Lowe, 2004). The primary health care provider and anesthesia care provider are responsible for fully informing women of the alternative methods of pharmacologic pain relief available in the hospital. A description of the various anesthetic techniques and what they entail is essential to informed consent, even if the woman received

---

plan of care ▶   **Nonpharmacologic Management of Discomfort**

NURSING DIAGNOSIS Anxiety related to lack of confidence in ability to cope effectively with pain during labor

Expected Outcomes *Woman will express decrease in anxiety and experience satisfaction with her labor and birth performance.*

Nursing Interventions/Rationales
- Assess whether woman and significant other have attended childbirth classes, their knowledge of labor process, and their current level of anxiety *to plan supportive strategies that address this couple's specific needs.*
- Encourage support person to remain with woman in labor *to provide support and increase probability of response to comfort measures.*
- Teach or review nonpharmacologic techniques available to decrease anxiety and pain during labor (e.g., focusing, relaxation and breathing techniques, effleurage, and sacral pressure) *to enhance chances of success in using techniques.*
- Explore other techniques that the woman or significant other may have learned in childbirth classes (e.g., hypnosis, yoga, acupressure, biofeedback, therapeutic touch, aromatherapy, imaging, music) *to provide largest repertoire of coping strategies.*
- Explore use of hydrotherapy if ordered by the primary health care provider and if woman meets use criteria (i.e., vital signs within normal limits [WNL], cervix 4 to 5 cm dilated, active phase of first-stage labor) *to aid relaxation and stimulate production of natural oxytocin.*
- Explore use of transcutaneous nerve stimulation if ordered by the primary health care provider *to provide an increased perception of control over pain and an increase in release of endogenous opiates.*
- Assist woman to change positions and to use pillows *to reduce stiffness, aid circulation, and promote comfort.*

- Assess bladder for distention and encourage voiding often *to avoid bladder distention and subsequent discomfort.*
- Encourage rest between contractions *to minimize fatigue.*
- Keep woman and significant other informed about progress *to allay anxiety.*
- Guide couple through the labor stages and phases, helping them use and modify comfort techniques that are appropriate to each phase, *to ensure greatest effectiveness of techniques employed.*
- Support couple if pharmacologic measures are required to increase pain relief, explaining safety and effectiveness, *to reduce anxiety and maintain self-esteem and sense of control over labor process.*

NURSING DIAGNOSIS Health-seeking behavior (labor) related to desire for a healthy outcome of labor and birth

Expected Outcome *Woman will participate in care planning for labor.*

Nursing Interventions/Rationales
- Discuss woman's birth plan and knowledge about the birth process *to collect data for plan of care.*
- Provide information about the labor process *to correct any misconceptions.*
- Inform woman about her labor status and fetus's well-being *to promote comfort and confidence.*
- Discuss rationales for all interventions *to incorporate woman into plan of care.*
- Incorporate nonpharmacologic interventions into plan of care *to increase woman's sense of control during labor.*
- Provide emotional support and ongoing positive feedback *to enhance positive coping mechanisms.*

CD: Plan of Care: Nonpharmacologic Management of Discomfort

information about analgesia and anesthesia earlier in her pregnancy. The initial discussion of pain management options ideally should take place in the third trimester so the woman has time to consider alternatives. Nurses play a part in the informed consent by clarifying and describing procedures or by acting as the woman's advocate and asking the primary health care provider for further explanations. There are three essential components of an informed consent. First, the procedure and its advantages and disadvantages must be thoroughly explained. Second, the woman must agree with the plan of labor pain care as explained to her. Third, her consent must be given freely without coercion or manipulation from her health care provider (Lowe).

■ **LEGAL TIP** Informed Consent for Anesthesia

The woman receives (in an understandable manner) the following:
- Explanation of alternative methods of anesthesia and analgesia available
- Description of the anesthetic, including its effects and the procedure for its administration
- Description of the benefits, discomforts, risks, and consequences for the mother and the fetus
- Explanation of how complications can be treated
- Information that the anesthetic is not always effective
- Indication that the woman may withdraw consent at any time
- Opportunity to have any question answered
- Opportunity to have components of the consent explained in the woman's own words

Consent form will
- Be written or explained in the woman's primary language
- Have the woman's signature
- Have the date of consent
- Carry the signature of anesthesia care provider, certifying that the woman has received and appears to understand the explanation

■ Timing of Administration

It is often the nurse who notifies the primary health care provider that the woman is in need of pharmacologic measures to relieve her discomfort. Orders may be written for the administration of pain medication as needed by the woman and based on the nurse's clinical judgment. To avoid suppressing the progress of labor, pharmacologic measures for pain relief are generally not implemented until labor has advanced to the active phase of the first stage of labor and the cervix is dilated approximately 4 to 5 cm (see Box 19-3). Conversely, nonpharmacologic measures can be used to relieve pain in early labor while relieving stress and enhancing progress.

■ Preparation for Procedures

The methods of pain relief available to the woman are reviewed and information is clarified as necessary. The procedure and what will be asked of the woman (e.g., to maintain flexed position during insertion of epidural needle) must be explained. The woman also can benefit from knowing the way that the medication is to be given, the in-

terval before the medication takes effect, and the expected pain relief from the medication. Skin-preparation measures are described, and an explanation is given for the need to empty the bladder before the analgesic or anesthetic is administered and the reason for keeping the bladder empty. When an indwelling catheter is to be threaded into the epidural space, the woman should be told that she may have a momentary twinge down her leg, hip, or back, and that this feeling is not a sign of injury.

■ Administration of Medication

Accurate monitoring of the progress of labor forms the basis for the nurse's judgment that a woman needs pharmacologic control of discomfort. Knowledge of the medications used during childbirth is essential. The most effective route of administration is selected for each woman; then the medication is prepared and administered correctly.

Intravenous Route. The preferred route of administration of medications such as hydromorphone, butorphanol, fentanyl, or nalbuphine is through IV tubing, administered into the port nearest the woman while the infusion of the IV solution is stopped. The medication is given slowly, in small doses, during a contraction. It may be given over the period of three to five consecutive contractions to complete the dose, if necessary. It is given during contractions to decrease fetal exposure to the medication because uterine blood vessels are constricted during contractions and the medication stays within the maternal vascular system for several seconds before the uterine blood vessels reopen. When the medication is infused, the IV infusion is then restarted slowly to prevent a bolus of medication from being administered. With this method of injection, along with smaller but more frequent dosing, the amount of medication crossing the placenta to the fetus is reduced while the woman's degree of pain relief is maximized. The IV route is associated with the following advantages:
- The onset of pain relief is more predictable.
- Pain relief is obtained with small doses of the drug.
- The duration of effect is more predictable.

Intramuscular Route. IM injections of analgesics, although still used, are not the preferred route for administration for women in labor. Identified disadvantages of the IM route include the following:
- The onset of pain relief is delayed.
- Higher doses of medication are required.
- Medication from muscle tissue is released at an unpredictable rate and is available for transfer across the placenta to the fetus.

The maternal plasma level of the medication necessary to bring pain relief usually is reached 45 minutes after IM injection, followed by a decline in plasma levels. The maternal medications levels (after IM injections) also are unequal because of uneven distribution (maternal uptake) and metabolism. The advantage of using the IM route is quick administration by the health care provider. IM injections given in the upper arm (deltoid muscle) seem to result in more rapid absorption and higher blood levels of the medication (Bricker & Lavender, 2002). If regional anesthesia is planned later in labor, the autonomic blockade from the regional (e.g., epidural) anesthesia increases blood flow to the gluteal region and accelerates absorption of medication that may be sequestered there.

Spinal Nerve Blocks. An intravenous infusion is usually established before the induction of spinal nerve blocks (e.g., epidural, subarachnoid). Anesthesia protocols often include the prophylactic administration of IV fluid before epidural and spinal anesthesia for blood volume expansion to prevent maternal hypotension. However, routine preloading with IV fluids before epidural analgesia is a form of care with a trade-off between beneficial and adverse effects (Enkin et al., 2000).

Lactated Ringer's or normal saline solutions are commonly used infusion solutions. Infusion solutions without dextrose are preferred, especially when the solution must be infused rapidly (e.g., to treat dehydration or to maintain blood pressure) because solutions containing dextrose rapidly increase maternal blood glucose levels. The fetus responds to high blood glucose levels by increasing insulin production; neonatal hypoglycemia may result. In addition, dextrose changes the osmotic pressure so that fluid is excreted from the kidneys more rapidly.

According to professional standards (AWHONN, 2002), the nonanesthetist registered nurse is permitted to monitor the status of the woman, the fetus and the progress of labor, replace empty infusion syringes or bags with the same medication and concentration, stop the infusion and initiate emergency measures if the need arises, and remove the catheter if properly educated to do so. Only qualified, licensed anesthesia care providers are permitted to insert a catheter and initiate epidural anesthesia, verify catheter placement, inject medication through the catheter, or alter the medication(s) including the type, the amount, or the rate of infusion.

Because spinal nerve blocks can reduce bladder sensation, resulting in difficulty voiding, the woman should empty her bladder before the induction of the block and should be encouraged to void at least every 2 hours thereafter. The nurse should palpate for bladder distention and measure urinary output to ensure that the bladder is being completely emptied. A distended bladder can inhibit uterine contractions and fetal descent, resulting in a slowing of the progress of labor. The status of the maternal-fetal unit and the progress of labor must be established before the block is performed. The nurse or the woman's partner must assist the woman to assume and maintain the correct position for induction of epidural and spinal anesthesia (see Fig. 19-10, *A* and *B*).

After a spinal nerve block is administered, the woman is protected from injury by raising the side rails if required, and safety is ensured by placing a call bell within easy reach when the nurse is not in attendance. Oxygen and suction should be readily available at the bedside. Since catheter-related infections (e.g., meningitis, abscess formation) seem

to increase in frequency, if a catheter is in place for continuous or patient controlled epidural analgesia, the insertion site should be maintained using strict asepsis according to agency protocol (Birnbach, 2005; Mahlmeister, 2003). The woman should be assessed and the insertion site inspected for signs of infection (e.g., fever; pain, erythema, and swelling at the site) during the infusion and after it is discontinued. The nurse must make sure there is no prolonged pressure on an anesthetized part (e.g., lying on one side with weight on one leg, tight linen on feet). If stirrups are used for birth, the nurse should pad them, adjust both stirrups to the same level and angle, place both of the woman's legs into them simultaneously while avoiding putting pressure on the popliteal angle, and apply restraints (if used) without restricting circulation.

Depending on the level of motor blockade, the woman should be assisted to remain as mobile as possible. When in bed, her position should be alternated from side to side every hour to ensure adequate distribution of the anesthetic solution and to maintain circulation to the uterus and placenta. Assisting the woman to assume upright positions such as sitting (e.g., modified throne position in which the woman sits on the bed with the bottom part lowered to place her feet below her body) (Fig. 19-14), tug-of-war position (woman tugs on towel or sheet that is tied to the bar on the bed or held by the nurse), and squatting by using the head of the bed for support will facilitate fetal descent and enhance bearing-down efforts (Gilder, Mayberry, Gennaro, & Clemmons, 2002). Upright positions are very important in the prevention of operative births (e.g., forceps or vacuum-assisted birth) and should be encouraged when the woman has a low-dose epidural or CSE (Mayberry et al., 2003). To prevent injury, the nurse must assess the level of motor function (e.g., woman takes three unassisted steps with accompaniment; woman stands and closes eyes while the nurse notes ability to maintain

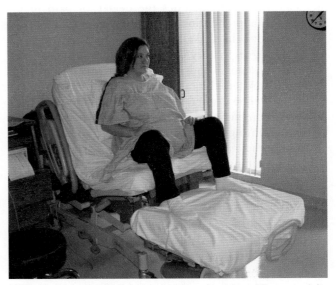

FIG. 19-14 Modified throne position for labor. (Courtesy Julie Perry Nelson, Gilbert, AZ.)

balance; woman is able to move feet and flex knees and ankles; woman is able to rise from a supine position), level of sensation in legs (e.g., degree of numbness), and level of sedation before the woman is assisted out of bed and periodically thereafter (Mahlmeister, 2003; Mayberry et al., 2002). The woman should sit on the side of the bed before standing to determine if orthostatic hypotension occurs. If she is not dizzy or lightheaded, then she can stand at the side of the bed and even walk.

Health care providers should recognize that the second stage of labor may be prolonged in women who use epidural analgesia for pain management. Research evidence indicates that as long as the well-being of the maternal-fetal unit is established, a period of "laboring down" can be implemented to allow the fetus to passively descend and rotate with uterine contractions until the woman perceives the urge to bear down and her fetus reaches a +1 station and is rotating to an anterior position. She is encouraged to use a self-directed, open-glottis pushing technique and is assisted to assume an upright position (e.g., squatting or sitting upright) (Mayberry et al., 2002; Mayberry et al., 2003; Simpson & James, 2005). Fetal well-being along with less maternal fatigue, fever, and perineal trauma and fewer operative vaginal births are beneficial outcomes of this approach for the management of the second stage of labor for women with epidural analgesia. There is insufficient evidence to support the practice of discontinuing epidural analgesia during the second stage in an effort to enhance the effectiveness of bearing-down efforts and decrease the risk for forceps- or vacuum-assisted birth. This practice does result in an increase in the woman's level of pain (Torvaldsen, Roberts, Bell, & Raynes-Greenow, 2005). (See Chapter 21 for a full discussion of second stage labor management.)

▬ *Safety and General Care*

The nurse monitors and records the woman's response to nonpharmacologic pain relief methods and to medication(s). This includes the degree of pain relief, the level of apprehension, the return of sensations and perception of pain, and allergic or adverse reactions (e.g., hypotension, respiratory depression, hypothermia, fever, pruritus, and nausea and vomiting). The nurse continues to monitor maternal vital signs and fetal heart rate and pattern at frequent intervals, the strength and frequency of uterine contractions, changes in the cervix and station of the presenting part, the presence and quality of the bearing-down reflex, bladder filling, and state of hydration. Determining the fetal response after administration of analgesia or anesthesia is vital (AWHONN, 2001). The woman is asked if she (or the family) has any questions. The nurse also assesses the woman's and her family's understanding of the need for ensuring her safety (e.g., keeping side rails up, calling for assistance as needed).

The time that elapses between the administration of an opioid and the baby's birth is documented. Medications given to the newborn to reverse opioid effects are recorded. After birth, the woman who has had spinal, epidural, or

general anesthesia is assessed for return of sensory and motor function in addition to the usual postpartum assessments. Both the nurse and the anesthesia provider are responsible for documenting assessments and care in relation to the epidural (Mahlmeister, 2003).

▬ Evaluation

Evaluation of the effectiveness of care of the woman needing management of discomfort during labor and birth is based on the previously stated outcomes (see Plan of Care).

---

community activity

1. Survey your community for services that provide pregnant women with instruction in complementary or alternative nonpharmacologic methods (e.g., hypnosis, TENS, biofeedback, touch and massage, aromatherapy, etc.) to relieve and cope with pain during labor. Use your survey to create a booklet that could be provided to women during a prenatal visit or class. Include the following information on each method you include in your booklet:
   a. Description of the method, including how it works and evidence available to validate its effectiveness. Quotes from women who used the method and found it helpful could also be included.
   b. Agencies providing instruction in this method, including contact information (e.g., contact person, address, phone number, email), cost of the classes or service, and credentials of persons providing instruction.
   c. When instruction should begin during pregnancy and level of preparation and practice that will be necessary to facilitate effectiveness during labor.

---

key points

- The expected outcome of preparation for childbirth and parenting is "education for choice."
- Nonpharmacologic pain and stress management strategies are valuable for managing labor discomfort alone or in combination with pharmacologic methods.
- The gate-control theory of pain and the stress response are the bases for many of the nonpharmacologic methods of pain relief.
- The type of analgesic or anesthetic to be used is determined in part by the stage of labor and the method of birth.
- Sedatives may be appropriate for women in prolonged early labor when there is a need to decrease anxiety or to promote sleep or therapeutic rest.
- Phenothiazines and benzodiazepines can be used during labor to decrease anxiety and apprehension, increase sedation, potentiate opioid analgesic effects, and reduce nausea and vomiting.
- Naloxone (Narcan) is an opioid antagonist that can reverse opioid effects, especially respiratory depression.
- Pharmacologic control of discomfort during labor requires collaboration among the health care providers and the laboring woman.

- The nurse must understand medications, their expected effects, their potential adverse reactions, and their methods of administration.
- Maintenance of maternal fluid balance is essential during spinal and epidural nerve blocks.
- Maternal analgesia or anesthesia potentially affects neonatal neurobehavioral response.
- The use of opioid agonist-antagonist analgesics in women with preexisting opioid dependence may cause symptoms of abstinence syndrome (opioid withdrawal).
- General anesthesia is rarely used for vaginal birth but may be used for cesarean birth or whenever rapid anesthesia is needed in an emergency.

REFERENCES

Anim-Somuah, M., Smyth, R., & Howell, C. (2005). Epidural versus non-epidural or no analgesia in labor. *The Cochrane Database of Systematic Reviews,* 2006, Issue 3. Chichester, UK: John Wiley & Sons.

Association of Women's Health, Obstetric, and Neonatal Nurses (AWHONN). (2001). *Evidence-based clinical practice guidelines: Nursing care of the woman receiving regional analgesia/anesthesia in labor.* Washington, DC: Author.

Association of Women's Health, Obstetric, and Neonatal Nurses (AWHONN). (2002). *The role of the registered nurse (RN) in the care of pregnant women receiving analgesia/anesthesia by catheter techniques (epidural, intrathecal, spinal, PCEA catheters).* Clinical Position Statement. Accessed http://www.awhonn.org, November 20, 2005.

Benfield, R. (2002). Hydrotherapy in labor. *Image: Journal of Nursing Scholarship, 34*(4), 347-352.

Birnbach, D. (2005). Committee on obstetrical anesthesia greets future with guarded optimism. *ASA Newsletter, 69*(4). Accessed http://www.asahq.org/Newsletters, November 15, 2005.

Bricker, L., & Lavender, T. (2002). Parenteral opioids for labor pain relief: A systematic review. *American Journal of Obstetrics and Gynecology, 186*(5), S94-S109.

Browning, C. (2000). Using music during childbirth. *Birth, 27*(4), 272-276.

Bucklin, B., Hawkins, J., Anderson, J., & Ullrich, F. (2005). Obstetric anesthesia workforce survey. *Anesthesiology, 103*(3), 645-653.

Callister, L., Khalaf, I., Semenic, S., Kartchner, R., & Vehvilainen-Julkunen, K. (2003). The pain of childbirth: Perceptions of culturally diverse women. *Pain Management Nursing, 4*(4), 145-154.

Caton D., Corry, M., Frigoletto, F., Hopkins, D., Lieberman, E., Mayberry, L., et al. (2002). The nature and management of labor pain: Executive summary. *American Journal of Obstetrics and Gynecology, 186*(5), S1-S15.

Cluett, E., Nikodem, V., McCandlish, R., & Burnes, E. (2004). Immersion in water in pregnancy, labour, and birth. *The Cochrane Database of Systematic Reviews,* 2006, Issue 3. Chichester, UK: John Wiley & Sons.

Cunningham, F., Leveno, K., Bloom, S., Hauth, J., Gilstrap, L., & Wenstrom, K. (2005). *Williams obstetrics* (22nd ed.). New York: McGraw-Hill.

DiFranco, J. (2000). Biofeedback. In F. Nichols & S. Humenick, *Childbirth education: Practice, research, and theory* (2nd ed.). Philadelphia: Saunders.

Enkin, M., Keirse, M., Neilson, J., Crowther, C., Duley, L., Hodnett, E., et al. (2000). *A guide to effective care in pregnancy and childbirth* (3rd ed.). Oxford, NY: Oxford University Press.

Faucher, M., & Brucker, M. (2000). Intrapartum pain: Pharmacologic management. *Journal of Obstetric, Gynecologic, and Neonatal Nursing, 29*(2), 169-180.

Florence, D., & Palmer, D. (2003). Therapeutic choices for the discomforts of labor. *Journal of Perinatal and Neonatal Nursing, 17*(4), 238-249.

Gentz, B. (2001). Alternative therapies for the management of pain in labor and delivery. *Clinical Obstetrics and Gynecology, 44*(4), 704-732.

Gilder, K., Mayberry, L., Gennaro, S., & Clemmons, D. (2002). Maternal positions in labor with epidural analgesia: Results from a multi-site survey. *AWHONN Lifelines, 6*(1), 40-45.

Govenar, J. (2000). Handling headache after dural puncture. *RN, 63*(12), 26-31.

Hawkins, J., Chestnut, D., & Gibbs, C. (2002). Obstetric anesthesia. In S. Gabbe, J. Niebyl, & J. Simpson (Eds.), *Obstetrics: Normal and problem pregnancies* (4th ed.). Philadelphia: Churchill Livingstone.

Hodnett, E. (2002). Pain and women's satisfaction with the experience of childbirth: A systematic review. *American Journal of Obstetrics and Gynecology, 186*(5), S160-S172.

Hodnett, E., Gates, S., Hofmeyr, G., & Sakala, C. (2003). Continuous support for women during childbirth. *The Cochrane Database of Systematic Reviews,* 2006, Issue 3. Chichester, UK: John Wiley & Sons.

Hover-Kramer, D., Mentgen, J., & Scandrett-Hibdon, S. (2001). *Healing touch: A resource for health care professionals.* Albany, NY: Delmar.

Humenick, S., Schrock, P., & Libresco, M. (2000). Relaxation. In F. Nichols & S. Humenick. (Eds.), *Childbirth education: Practice, research, and theory* (2nd ed.). Philadelphia: Saunders.

Ketterhagen, D., VandeVusse, L., & Berner, M. (2002). Self-hypnosis: Alternative anesthesia for childbirth. *MCN American Journal of Maternal/Child Nursing, 27*(6), 335-340.

Koehn, M. (2000). Alternative and complementary therapies for labor and birth: An application of Kolcaba's theory of holistic comfort. *Holistic Nursing Practice, 15*(1), 66-77.

Koehn, M. (2002). Childbirth education outcomes: An integrated review. *Journal of Perinatal Education, 11*(3), 10-19.

Lehne, R. (2004). *Pharmacology for nursing care* (5th ed.). Philadelphia: Saunders.

Leighton, B., & Halpern, S. (2002). The effects of epidural analgesia on labor, maternal, and neonatal outcomes: A systematic review. *American Journal of Obstetrics and Gynecology, 186*(5), S69-S77.

Lieberman, E., & O'Donoghue, C. (2002). Unintended effects of epidural anesthesia during labor: A systematic review. *American Journal of Obstetrics and Gynecology, 186*(5), S31-S68.

Lowe, N. (2002). The nature of labor pain. *American Journal of Obstetrics and Gynecology, 186*(5), S16-S24.

Lowe, N. (2004). Context and process of informed consent for pharmacologic strategies in labor pain care. *Journal of Midwifery & Women's Health, 49*(3), 250-259.

Mackey, M. (2001). Use of water in labor and birth. *Clinical Obstetrics and Gynecology, 44*(4), 733-749.

Mahlmeister, L. (2003). Nursing responsibilities in preventing, preparing for, and managing epidural emergencies. *Journal of Perinatal and Neonatal Nursing, 17*(1), 19-32.

Marks, G. (2000). Alternative therapies. In F. Nichols & S. Humenick. (Eds.), *Childbirth education: Practice, research, and theory* (2nd ed.). Philadelphia: Saunders.

Maternity Center Association. (2002). *Listening to mothers: Report of the first national U.S. survey of women's childbearing experiences executive summary and recommendations issued by the Maternity Center Association.* New York: Maternity Center Association. Accessed http://www.maternitywise.org, September 11, 2005.

Mattson, S. (2000). Striving for cultural competence: Providing care for the changing face of the U.S. *AWHONN Lifelines, 4*(3), 48-52.

Mayberry, L., Clemmens, D., & De, A. (2002). Epidural analgesia side effects, co-interventions, and care of women during childbirth: A systematic review. *American Journal of Obstetrics and Gynecology, 186*(5), S81-S93.

Mayberry, L., Strange, L., Suplee, P., & Gennaro, S. (2003). Use of upright positioning with epidural analgesia: Findings from an observational study. *MCN American Journal of Maternal/Child Nursing, 28*(3), 152-159.

McCool, W., Packman, J., & Zwerling, A. (2004). Obstetric anesthesia: Changes and choices. *Journal of Midwifery & Women's Health, 49*(6), 505-513.

Nichols, F. (2000). Paced breathing techniques. In F. Nichols & S. Humenick (Eds.), *Childbirth education: Practice, research, and theory* (2nd ed.). Philadelphia: Saunders.

Perinatal Education Associates. (2006). *Breathing.* Accessed http://www.birthsource.com, July 18, 2006.

Righard, L. (2001). Making childbirth a normal process. *Birth, 28*(1), 1-4.

Rosen, M. (2002). Nitrous oxide for relief of labor pain: A systematic review. *American Journal of Obstetrics and Gynecology, 186*(5), S110-S126.

Scheiber, B., & Selby, C. (Eds.). (2000). *Therapeutic touch.* New York: Prometheus Books.

Sharma, S., & Leveno, K. (2003). Regional anesthesia and progress in labor. *Clinical Obstetrics and Gynecology, 46*(3), 633-645.

Simkin, P., & Ancheta, R. (2000). *The labor progress handbook: Early interventions to prevent and treat dystocia.* Malden, MA: Blackwell Science.

Simkin, P., & Bolding, A. (2004). Update on nonpharmacologic approaches to relieve labor pain and prevent suffering. *Journal of Midwifery & Women's Health, 49*(6), 489-504.

Simkin, P., & O'Hara, M. (2002). Nonpharmacologic relief of pain during labor: Systematic reviews of five methods. *American Journal of Obstetrics & Gynecology, 186*(5), S131-S159.

Simpson, K., & James, D. (2005). Effects of immediate versus delayed pushing during second-stage labor on fetal well-being: A randomized clinical trial. *Nursing Research, 54*(3), 149-157.

Smith, C., Collins, C., Cyna, A., & Crowther, C. (2005). Complementary and alternative therapies for pain management in labour. *The Cochrane Database of Systematic Reviews,* 2006, Issue 3. Chichester, UK: John Wiley & Sons.

Snyder, M., & Lindquist, R. (Eds.). (2000). *Complementary/alternative therapies in nursing* (4th ed.). New York: Springer.

Tiran, D., & Mack, S. (2000). *Complementary therapies for pregnancy and childbirth* (2nd ed.). Edinburgh: Bailliere-Tindall.

Torvaldsen, S., Roberts, C., Bell, J., & Raynes-Greenow, C. (2005). Discontinuation of epidural analgesia late in labour for reducing the adverse delivery outcomes associated with epidural analgesia. *The Cochrane Database of Systematic Reviews,* 2006, Issue 3. Chichester, UK: John Wiley & Sons.

Trout, K. (2004). The neuromatrix theory of pain: Implications for selected nonpharmacologic methods of pain relief for labor. *Journal of Midwifery & Women's Health, 49*(6), 482-488.

CHAPTER 20

Margaret Wagoner Gilliam and Linda Fowler Shahzad

Fetal Assessment During Labor

learning objectives

- Identify typical signs of nonreassuring fetal heart rate (FHR) patterns.
- Compare FHR monitoring done by intermittent auscultation with external and internal electronic methods.
- Explain the baseline FHR and evaluate periodic changes.
- Describe nursing measures that can be used to maintain FHR patterns within normal limits.

- Differentiate among the nursing interventions used for managing specific FHR patterns, including tachycardia and bradycardia; increased and decreased variability; and late and variable decelerations.
- Review the application of the monitor.
- Review the documentation of the monitoring process necessary during labor.

electronic resources

Additional information related to the content in Chapter 20 can be found on

the companion website at *evolve*
http://evolve.elsevier.com/Lowdermilk/MWHC/
- NCLEX Review Questions
- WebLinks

or on the interactive companion CD
- NCLEX Review Questions
- Plan of Care: Electronic Fetal Monitoring During Labor

THE ability to assess the fetus by auscultation of fetal heart sounds was initially described more than 300 years ago. With the advent of the fetoscope and stethoscope after the turn of the twentieth century, the listener could hear clearly enough to count the fetal heart rate (FHR). When electronic FHR monitoring made its debut for clinical use in the early 1970s, it was anticipated that its use would effect a decrease in cerebral palsy and be more sensitive than stethoscopic auscultation in predicting and preventing fetal compromise (Simpson & Knox, 2000). Clinical implementation of electronic fetal monitoring (EFM) rapidly expanded, such that EFM supplanted intrauterine auscultation within 15 years of its introduction (Dildy, 2005). Despite the widespread use of electronic fetal heart rate monitoring and a fivefold increase in the cesarean birth rate over the same period of time, the rate of cerebral palsy has not decreased in developed countries over the past 30 years (Clark & Hankins, 2003), and many researchers and clinicians are of the opinion that EFM interpretation is subjective and difficult, often leading to erroneous assessment of the fetal physiologic condition (Dildy). Furthermore, although decreased variability and increased late decelerations are associated with decreasing umbilical arterial pH and base excess, EFM was unable to identify fetuses in whom cerebral white matter

injury was later diagnosed in preterm neonates (Althaus, Petersen, Fox, Holcroft, & Graham, 2005).

Still, electronic fetal monitoring is a useful tool for visualizing FHR patterns on a monitor screen or printed tracing and continues to be the primary mode of intrapartum fetal assessment. Pregnant women should be informed about the equipment and procedures used and the risks, benefits, and limitations of intermittent auscultation (IA) and EFM. This chapter discusses the basis for fetal monitoring, the types of monitoring, and nursing assessment and management of nonreassuring fetal status.

■ BASIS FOR MONITORING

Fetal Response

Because labor is a period of physiologic stress for the fetus, frequent monitoring of fetal status is part of the nursing care during labor. The fetal oxygen supply must be maintained during labor to prevent fetal compromise and to promote newborn health after birth. The fetal oxygen supply can decrease in a number of ways:

1. Reduction of blood flow through the maternal vessels as a result of maternal hypertension (chronic hypertension or gestational hypertension), hypotension (caused by supine maternal position, hemorrhage, or epidural

analgesia or anesthesia), or hypovolemia (caused by hemorrhage)

2. Reduction of the oxygen content in the maternal blood as a result of hemorrhage or severe anemia

3. Alterations in fetal circulation, occurring with compression of the umbilical cord (transient–during uterine contractions [UCs]; or prolonged–resulting from cord prolapse), placental separation or complete abruption, or head compression (head compression causes increased intracranial pressure and vagal nerve stimulation with an accompanying decrease in the FHR)

4. Reduction in blood flow to the intervillous space in the placenta secondary to uterine hypertonus (generally caused by excessive exogenous oxytocin) or secondary to deterioration of the placental vasculature associated with maternal disorders such as hypertension or diabetes mellitus

Fetal well-being during labor can be assessed by the response of the FHR to UCs. In general, reassuring FHR patterns are characterized by the following:

- A baseline FHR in the normal range of 110 to 160 beats/min with no periodic decelerations and a moderate baseline variability

- Accelerations with fetal movement

A normal uterine activity pattern in labor is characterized by contractions occurring every 2 to 5 minutes and lasting less than 90 seconds; such contractions are moderate to strong in intensity, as evidenced by palpation, or intensity is less than 100 mm Hg, as measured by an intrauterine pressure catheter (IUPC); 30 seconds or more should elapse between the end of one contraction and the beginning of the next contraction; between contractions, uterine relaxation should be detected by palpation or by an average intrauterine pressure of 15 mm Hg or less.

Fetal Compromise

The goals of intrapartum FHR monitoring are to identify and differentiate the reassuring patterns from the nonreassuring patterns, which can be indicative of fetal compromise.

Nonreassuring FHR patterns are those associated with fetal hypoxemia, which is a deficiency of oxygen in the arterial blood. If uncorrected, hypoxemia can deteriorate to severe fetal hypoxia, which is an inadequate supply of oxygen at the cellular level. Nonreassuring FHR patterns include the following:

- Progressive increase or decrease in baseline rate
- Tachycardia of 160 beats/min or more
- Progressive decrease in baseline variability
- Severe variable decelerations (FHR less than 60 beats/min lasting longer than 30 to 60 seconds, with rising baseline, decreasing variability, or slow return to baseline)
- Late decelerations of any magnitude, especially those that are repetitive and uncorrectable
- Absence of FHR variability
- Prolonged deceleration (greater than 60 to 90 seconds)
- Severe bradycardia (less than 70 beats/min)

The nurse's role is to assess whether the FHR pattern is reassuring, which reflects adequate fetal oxygenation, or nonreassuring. The nursing interventions to be taken when encountering nonreassuring patterns are described in detail in this chapter.

■ MONITORING TECHNIQUES

The ideal method of fetal assessment during labor continues to be debated. Results from multiple research studies indicate that both intermittent auscultation (IA) of the FHR and electronic FHR monitoring are associated with similar fetal outcomes (Wood, 2003). Although IA is a high-touch, low-technology method of assessing fetal status during labor that places fewer restrictions on maternal activity, more than 85% of laboring women in the United States are monitored electronically for at least part of their labor (Martin, Hamilton, Sutton, Ventura, Menacker, & Munson, 2005). The continued use of EFM in place of IA is thought to be due to concerns about liability and the increased nurse-to-client ratio required with IA (Wood). Since all surveillance methods, including EFM, have limitations, some feel the evidence supports a return to the use of IA for low risk laboring women (Dildy, 2005).

Intermittent Auscultation

Intermittent auscultation (IA) uses listening to fetal heart sounds at periodic intervals to assess the FHR. IA of the fetal heart can be performed with a Leff scope, a DeLee-Hillis fetoscope, or an ultrasound device. If a Leff scope is used, the domed side should be opened to the connective tubing to the earpieces. The domed side is then applied to the maternal abdomen. The fetoscope is applied over the listener's head because bone conduction amplifies the fetal heart sounds for counting. The ultrasound device transmits ultrahigh-frequency sound waves reflecting movement of the fetal heart and converts these sounds into an electronic signal that can be counted (Fig. 20-1).

FIG. 20-1 A, Ultrasound fetoscope. B, Ultrasound stethoscope. C, DeLee-Hillis fetoscope. (Courtesy Michael S. Clement, MD, Mesa, AZ.)

One procedure for performing auscultation is as follows:

1. Perform Leopold maneuvers (see p. 535 by palpating the maternal abdomen to identify fetal presentation and position.
2. Place the listening device over the area of maximal intensity and clarity of the fetal heart sounds to obtain the clearest and loudest sound, which is easiest to count.
3. Palpate the abdomen for the absence of uterine activity to be able to count the FHR between contractions.
4. Count the maternal radial pulse at the same time as listening to the FHR to differentiate it from the fetal rate. "The regular rhythm of the FHR must be distinguished from the somewhat similar sounds produced by the maternal vessels (uterine bruit or uterine souffle), sounds that are synchronous with the maternal pulse" (Association of Women's Health, Obstetric and Neonatal Nurses [AWHONN], 2003).
5. Count the FHR for 30 to 60 seconds between contractions to identify the baseline rate. This rate can be assessed only during the absence of uterine activity.
6. Auscultate the FHR during a contraction and for 30 seconds after the end of the contraction to identify any increases or decreases in FHR in response to the contraction.

By using IA, the nurse can assess the FHR baseline rate, rhythm, and increases and decreases from baseline. The method and frequency of fetal surveillance during labor will vary depending on maternal-fetal risk factors and the preference of the facility (Table 20-1). In addition, the FHR is assessed before and after ambulation, rupture of membranes, administration of medications and anesthesia, and more frequently when nonreassuring fetal heart rates or rhythms are heard (AWHONN, 2003; Tucker, 2004).

▬ NURSE ALERT

When the FHR is auscultated and documented, it is inappropriate to use the descriptive terms associated with EFM (e.g., moderate variablility, variable deceleration) because most of the terms are visual descriptions of the patterns produced on the monitor tracing. Terms that are numerically defined, however, such as bradycardia and tachycardia, can be used. Fetal heart rate when auscultated should be described as a baseline number or range and as having a regular or irregular rhythm, and the presence or absence of accelerations or decelerations both during and after contractions should be noted (AWHONN, 2003).

Every effort should be made to use the method of fetal assessment the woman desires, if possible. However, auscultation of the FHR in accordance with the frequency guidelines just given may be difficult in today's busy labor and birth units. When used as the primary method of fetal assessment, auscultation requires a 1:1 nurse-to-client staffing ratio. If acuity and census change so that auscultation standards are no longer met, the nurse must inform the physician or nurse-midwife that continuous EFM will be used until staffing can be arranged to meet the standards.

The woman can become anxious if the examiner cannot readily count the fetal heartbeats. It often takes time for the inexperienced listener to locate the heartbeat and find the area of maximal intensity. To allay the mother's concerns, she can be told that the nurse is "finding the spot where the sounds are loudest." If it takes considerable time

---

table 20-1 **Frequency of Auscultation: Recommended Assessment and Documentation**

	LATENT PHASE	ACTIVE PHASE	SECOND STAGE
ACOG[a]			
Low risk	—	q30 minutes	q15 minutes
High risk	—	q15 minutes	q5 minutes
AWHONN[b]			
Low risk	—	q30 minutes	q15 minutes
High risk	—	q15 minutes	q5 minutes
SOGC[c]	Regularly after rupture of membranes or other clinically significant change	q15 minutes	q5 minutes once pushing is initiated

Assess FHR before
- Initiation of labor-enhancing procedures (e.g., amniotomy)
- Ambulation
- Administration of medications
- Administration or initiation of analgesia or anesthesia
- Transfer or discharge of client

Assess FHR after
- Admission of client
- Artificial or spontaneous rupture of membranes
- Vaginal examination
- Ambulation
- Recognition of abnormal uterine activity patterns
- Administration of medication

From Association of Women's Health, Obstetric and Neonatal Nurses (AWHONN). (2003). *Fetal heart monitoring principles and practice* (3rd ed.). Dubuque, IA: Kendall/Hunt.
[a]American College of Obstetricians and Gynecologists. (1995). *Fetal heart rate patterns: Monitoring, interpretation, and management. Technical Bulletin No. 207.* Washington DC: Author.
[b]Association of Women's Health, Obstetric and Neonatal Nurses. (2000). *Fetal assessment* (Clinical Position Statement). Washington, DC: Author
[c]Society of Obstetricians and Gynecologists of Canada. (2002). Fetal health surveillance in labour. (SOGC Clinical Practice Guidelines No. 112. *Journal of Obstetrics and Gynaegology in Canada, 112* (March), 1-13.

to locate the fetal heartbeats, the examiner can reassure the mother by offering her an opportunity to listen to them, too. If the examiner cannot locate the fetal heartbeat, assistance should be requested. In some cases, ultrasound can be used to help locate the fetal heartbeat. Seeing the fetal heart beat on the ultrasound screen will be reassuring to the mother if there was initial difficulty in locating the best area for auscultation.

When using IA, uterine activity is assessed by palpation. The examiner should keep his or her fingertips placed over the fundus before, during, and after contractions. The contraction intensity is usually described as mild, moderate, or strong. The contraction duration is measured in seconds, from the beginning to the end of the contraction. The frequency of contractions is measured in minutes, from the beginning of one contraction to the beginning of the next contraction. The examiner should keep his or her hand on the fundus after the contraction is over to evaluate uterine resting tone or relaxation between contractions. Resting tone between contractions is usually described as soft or relaxed (AWHONN, 2003) (see Chapter 21 for further discussion).

Accurate and complete documentation of fetal status and uterine activity is especially important when IA and palpation are being used, because no paper tracing record of these assessments is provided as is by continuous EFM. Labor flow records or computer charting systems that prompt notations of all assessments are useful for ensuring such comprehensive documentation.

Electronic Fetal Monitoring

The purpose of electronic FHR monitoring is the ongoing assessment of fetal oxygenation. FHR tracings are analyzed for characteristic patterns that suggest specific hypoxic and nonhypoxic events (King & Parer, 2000). The two modes of electronic fetal monitoring include the external mode, which uses external transducers placed on the maternal abdomen to assess FHR and pattern and uterine activity, and the internal mode, which uses a spiral electrode applied to the fetal presenting part to assess the FHR and an intrauterine pressure catheter to assess uterine activity and pressure. The differences between the external and internal modes of EFM are summarized in Table 20-2.

External Monitoring

Separate transducers are used to monitor the FHR and UCs (Fig. 20-2). The ultrasound transducer works by reflecting high-frequency sound waves off a moving interface: in this case, the fetal heart and valves. It is sometimes difficult to reproduce a continuous and precise record of the FHR because of artifacts introduced by fetal and maternal movement. The FHR is printed on specially formatted monitor paper. The standard paper speed is 3 cm/min. After performing Leopold maneuvers to determine fetal position and locating the area of maximal intensity of the FHR, conductive gel is applied to the surface of the ultrasound transducer, and the transducer is then positioned over this area.

The tocotransducer (tocodynamometer) measures uterine activity transabdominally. The device is placed over the fundus above the umbilicus. UCs or fetal movements depress a pressure-sensitive surface on the side next to the abdomen. The tocotransducer can measure and record the frequency, regularity, and approximate duration of UCs but not their intensity. This method is especially valuable for measuring uterine activity during the first stage of labor in women with intact membranes or for antepartum testing. Because the tocotransducer of most electronic fetal monitors is designed for assessing uterine activity in the term pregnancy, it may not be sensitive enough to detect

table 20-2	External and Internal Modes of Monitoring

EXTERNAL MODE	INTERNAL MODE
FHR	
Ultrasound transducer: High-frequency sound waves reflect mechanical action of the fetal heart. Noninvasive. Does not require rupture of membranes or cervical dilation. Used during both the antepartum and intrapartum periods.	*Spiral electrode:* This electrode converts the fetal ECG as obtained from the presenting part to the FHR via a cardiotachometer. This method can be used only when membranes are ruptured and the cervix is sufficiently dilated during the intrapartum period. Electrode penetrates into fetal presenting part by 1.5 mm and must be attached securely to ensure a good signal.
UTERINE ACTIVITY	
Tocotransducer: This instrument monitors frequency and duration of contractions by means of pressure-sensing device applied to the maternal abdomen. Used during both the antepartum and intrapartum periods.	*Intrauterine pressure catheter (IUPC):* This instrument monitors the frequency, duration, and intensity of contractions. The two types of IUPCs are a fluid-filled system and a solid catheter. Both measure intrauterine pressure at the catheter tip and convert the pressure into millimeters of mercury on the uterine activity panel of the strip chart. Both can be used only when membranes are ruptured and the cervix is sufficiently dilated during the intrapartum period.

ECG, Electrocardiogram; *FHR,* fetal heart rate.

FIG. 20-2 **A,** External noninvasive fetal monitoring with to-cotransducer and ultrasound transducer. **B,** Ultrasound transducer is placed below umbilicus, over the area where fetal heart rate is best heard, and tocotransducer is placed on uterine fundus. (Courtesy Marjorie Pyle, RNC, Costa Mesa, CA.)

preterm uterine activity. When monitoring the woman in preterm labor, remember that the fundus may be located below the level of the umbilicus. The nurse may need to rely on the woman to indicate when uterine activity is occurring and should use palpation as an additional way of assessing contraction frequency and validating the monitor tracing.

The external transducer is easily applied by the nurse, but it must be repositioned as the woman or fetus changes position (see Fig. 20-2, *B*). The woman is asked to assume a semi-sitting position or lateral position. The equipment is removed periodically to wash the applicator sites and to give back rubs. Use of an external transducer confines the woman to bed or chair. Portable telemetry monitors allow observation of the FHR and uterine contraction patterns by means of centrally located electronic display stations. These portable units permit the woman to walk around

during electronic monitoring. Other monitoring equipment can be used when the woman is submerged in water (see Fig. 19-4).

Internal Monitoring

The technique of continuous internal monitoring provides a more accurate appraisal of fetal well-being during labor than external monitoring since it is not interrupted by fetal or maternal movement (Fig. 20-3). For this type of monitoring, the membranes must be ruptured, the cervix sufficiently dilated, and the presenting part low enough to allow placement of the electrode. A small spiral electrode attached to the presenting part shows a continuous FHR on the fetal monitor strip.

Internal monitoring of the FHR may be implemented without internal monitoring of uterine activity. To monitor uterine activity, a solid or fluid-filled intrauterine pressure catheter or IUPC is introduced into the uterine cavity. The solid catheter has a pressure-sensitive tip that measures changes in intrauterine pressure. A fluid-filled catheter detects pressure changes in the sterile water through a strain gauge. As the catheter is compressed during a contraction, pressure is placed on the pressure transducer or strain gauge; this pressure is then converted into a pressure reading in millimeters of mercury. The average pressure during a contraction ranges from 50 to 85 mm Hg. The IUPC can measure the frequency, the duration, and the intensity of UCs.

Display

The FHR and uterine activity (UA) are displayed on the monitor paper with the FHR in the upper section and UA in the lower section. Fig. 20-4 contrasts the internal and

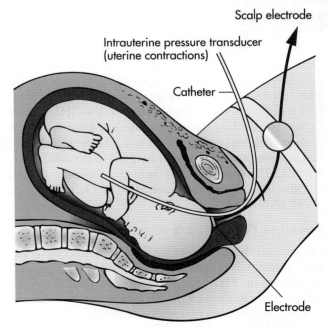

FIG. 20-3 Diagrammatic representation of internal invasive fetal monitoring with intrauterine pressure catheter and spiral electrode in place (membranes ruptured and cervix dilated).

FIG. 20-4 Display of fetal heart rate and uterine activity on monitor paper. **A,** External mode with ultrasound and tocotransducer as signal source. **B,** Internal mode with spiral electrode and intrauterine catheter as signal source. Frequency of contractions is measured from the beginning of one contraction to the beginning of the next. (From Tucker, S. [2004]. *Pocket guide to fetal monitoring and assessment* [5th ed.]. St. Louis: Mosby.)

external modes of electronic monitoring. Note that each small square represents 10 seconds; each larger box of six squares equals 1 minute (when paper is moving through the monitor at 3 cm/min).

▬ FETAL HEART RATE PATTERNS

Characteristic FHR patterns are associated with fetal and maternal physiologic processes and have been identified for many years, but some variations in descriptions, definitions, and interpretations have limited the study of the validity and effectiveness of electronic FHR monitoring. In 1997 the National Institute of Child Health and Human Development (NICHD) published a proposed nomenclature system for EFM interpretation with standardized definitions for FHR monitoring (NICHD, 1997). Concerns regarding the enhancement of communication among caregivers and client safety (Simpson, 2004), as well as about research validity, have led to the adoption of the NICHD terminology by both the American College of Obstetricians and Gynecologists (ACOG) (2005) and AWHONN (2003).

Baseline Fetal Heart Rate

The intrinsic rhythmicity of the fetal heart, the central nervous system (CNS), and the fetal autonomic nervous system control the FHR. An increase in sympathetic response results in acceleration of the FHR, whereas an augmentation in parasympathetic response produces a slowing of the FHR. Usually a balanced increase of sympathetic and parasympathetic response occurs during contractions, with no observable change in the baseline FHR.

Baseline fetal heart rate is the average rate during a 10-minute segment that excludes periodic or episodic changes, periods of marked variability, and segments of the baseline that differ by more than 25 beats/min (NICHD, 1997). The normal range at term is 110 to 160 beats/min.

Variability of the FHR can be described as irregular fluctuations in the baseline FHR of two cycles per minute or greater (NICHD, 1997). Variability has been described as short-term (beat to beat) (STV) or long-term (rhythmic waves or cycles from baseline) (LTV). The current definition for research does not distinguish between short-term and long-term variability because in actual practice, they are viewed together (NICHD); however, this definition does identify four ranges of variability as seen in Fig. 20-5. These are based on visualization of the amplitude of the FHR in the peak-to-trough segment in beats/min and include the following:

- Absent or undetected variability
- Minimal variability (greater than undetected but not more than 5 beats/min)
- Moderate variability (6 to 25 beats/min)
- Marked variability (greater than 25 beats/min)

Absence of or undetected variability is considered nonreassuring. Diminished variability can result from fetal hypoxemia and acidosis, as well as from certain drugs that depress the CNS, including analgesics, narcotics (meperidine [Demerol]), barbiturates (secobarbital [Seconal] and pentobarbital [Nembutal]), tranquilizers (diazepam [Valium]), ataractics (promethazine [Phenergan]), and general anesthetics. In addition, a temporary decrease in variability can occur when the fetus is in a sleep state. These sleep states do not usually last longer than 30 minutes.

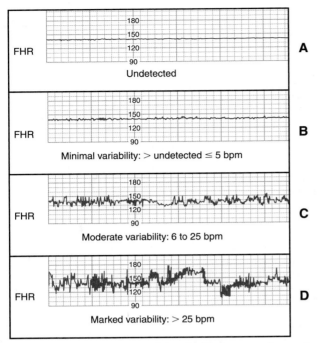

FIG. 20-5 Fetal heart rate variability. **A,** Absent or undetected. **B,** Minimal. **C,** Moderate. **D,** Marked. (Modified from Tucker, S. [2004]. *Pocket guide to fetal monitoring and assessment* [5th ed.]. St. Louis: Mosby.)

Table 20-3 contrasts key differences between increased and decreased variability.

A sinusoidal pattern, a regular smooth, undulating wavelike pattern, is not included in the current research definition of FHR variability. This uncommon pattern occurs when fetal hypoxia results from Rh isoimmunization or fetal anemia (Fig. 20-6).

Tachycardia is a baseline FHR greater than 160 beats/min for a duration of 10 minutes or longer. It can be considered an early sign of fetal hypoxemia, especially when associated with late decelerations and minimal or absent variability. Fetal tachycardia can result from maternal or fetal infection, such as prolonged rupture of membranes with amnionitis; from maternal hyperthyroidism or fetal anemia; or in response to drugs such as atropine, hydroxyzine

FIG. 20-6 Sinusoidal fetal heart rate. Note the rhythmic, undulating pattern. (From Tucker, S. [2004]. *Pocket guide to fetal monitoring and assessment* [5th ed.]. St. Louis: Mosby.)

(Vistaril), terbutaline, or illicit drugs such as cocaine or methamphetamines.

Bradycardia is a baseline FHR less than 110 beats/min for a duration of 10 minutes or longer. (Bradycardia should be distinguished from prolonged deceleration patterns, which are periodic changes described later in this chapter.) It can be considered a later sign of fetal hypoxia and is known to occur before fetal death. Bradycardia can result from placental transfer of drugs such as anesthetics, prolonged compression of the umbilical cord, maternal hypothermia, and maternal hypotension. Maternal supine hypotension syndrome, caused by the weight and pressure of the gravid uterus on the inferior vena cava, decreases the return of blood flow to the maternal heart, which then reduces maternal cardiac output and blood pressure. These responses in the mother subsequently result in a decrease in the FHR and fetal bradycardia. Table 20-4 contrasts tachycardia with bradycardia.

Changes in Fetal Heart Rate

Changes in FHR from the baseline are categorized as periodic or episodic. Periodic changes are those that occur with uterine contractions. Episodic changes (nonperiodic changes) are those that are not associated with uterine contractions. These patterns include accelerations and decelerations (NICHD, 1997).

Accelerations

Acceleration of the FHR is defined as a visually apparent abrupt increase in FHR above the baseline rate. The increase is 15 beats/min or greater and lasts 15 seconds or more, with the return to baseline less than 2 minutes from the beginning of the acceleration. In preterm gestations, the definition of an acceleration is a peak of 10 beats/min or more above baseline for at least 10 seconds. Acceleration of the FHR for more than 10 minutes is considered a change in baseline rate.

CRITICAL THINKING EXERCISE

Interpretation of FHR Patterns

While admitting a woman who is at 40 weeks of gestation in early labor, you identify fetal tachycardia and a pattern of recurrent FHR decelerations from the baseline FHR. How would you respond in this situation?

1. Evidence—Is there sufficient evidence to draw conclusions about how to respond in this situation?
2. Assumptions—Describe an underlying assumption about the following issues related to
   a. Causes of tachycardia
   b. Late versus variable decelerations of the FHR
   c. Intrauterine resuscitation for nonreassuring FHR patterns
3. What implications and priorities for responding to this woman can be made at this time?
4. Does the evidence objectively support your conclusion?
5. Are there alternative perspectives to your conclusion?

table 20-3 Increased and Decreased Variability

INCREASED VARIABILITY	DECREASED VARIABILITY
CAUSE	
Early mild hypoxemia Fetal stimulation by the following: 　–Uterine palpation 　–Uterine contractions 　–Fetal activity 　–Maternal activity Drugs 　Illicit drugs (e.g., cocaine and methamphetamines) 　Sympathomimetics (e.g., terbutaline and asthma 　　drugs)	Hypoxia or acidosis CNS depressants Analgesics or narcotics 　Meperidine (Demerol) 　Morphine 　Pentazocine (Talwin) Barbiturates 　Secobarbital (Seconal) 　Pentobarbital (Nembutal) 　Amobarbital (Amytal) Tranquilizers 　Diazepam (Valium) Ataractics 　Promethazine (Phenergan) 　Propiomazine (Largon) 　Hydroxyzine (Vistaril) 　Promazine (Sparine) Parasympatholytics 　Atropine General anesthetics Prematurity: <24 wk Fetal sleep cycles Congenital abnormalities Fetal cardiac dysrhythmias
CLINICAL SIGNIFICANCE	
Significance of marked variability not known; increased variability from a previous average variability is earliest FHR sign of mild hypoxemia.	Benign when associated with periodic fetal sleep states, which last 20 to 30 min; if caused by drugs, variability usually increases as drugs are excreted. Decreased variability is not reassuring and is considered a sign of fetal stress unless it has an identifiable temporary (e.g., fetal sleep) or correctable cause. Decreased variability associated with uncorrectable late decelerations indicates presence of fetal acidosis and can result in low Apgar scores.
NURSING INTERVENTION	
Priority depends on cause: Observe FHR tracing carefully for any nonreassuring patterns, including decreasing variability and late decelerations; if using external mode of monitoring, consider using internal mode (spiral electrode) for a more accurate tracing. Intervention usually not required unless nonreassuring FHR pattern develops.	Dependent on cause; intervention not warranted if associated with fetal sleep states or temporarily associated with CNS depressants; consider performing external stimulation or scalp stimulation during a vaginal examination to elicit an acceleration of FHR or return to moderate variability; consider application of spiral electrode; assist health care provider with fetal oxygen saturation monitoring if ordered; prepare for birth if so indicated by the primary health care provider.

From Tucker, S. (2004). *Pocket guide to fetal monitoring and assessment* (5th ed.). St. Louis: Mosby.
CNS, Central nervous system; *FHR*, fetal heart rate.

Accelerations can be periodic or episodic. Periodic accelerations are caused by dominance of the sympathetic nervous response and are usually encountered with breech presentations (Fig. 20-7, *A*). Pressure of the contraction applied to the fetal buttocks results in accelerations, whereas pressure applied to the head results in decelerations. However, accelerations may occur during the second stage of labor in cephalic presentations. Episodic accelerations of the FHR (Fig. 20-7, *B*) occur during fetal movement and are indications of fetal well-being.

Decelerations

A deceleration (caused by dominance of a parasympathetic response) may be benign or nonreassuring. Three types of decelerations are encountered during labor: *early, late,* and *variable.* FHR decelerations are described by their visual relation to the onset and end of a contraction and by their shape.

Early Decelerations. *Early deceleration* of the FHR is a visually apparent gradual (onset to lowest point 30 seconds or more) decrease in FHR and return to baseline in response

FIG. 20-7 A, Acceleration of fetal heart rate (FHR) with uterine contractions. **B,** Acceleration of FHR with fetal movement. (From Tucker, S. [2004]. *Pocket guide to fetal monitoring and assessment* [5th ed.]. St. Louis: Mosby.)

to fetal head compression. It is a normal and benign finding (Fig. 20-8, *A*) (NICHD, 1997). The deceleration generally starts before the peak of the uterine contraction, with the lowest point of deceleration occurring at the same time as the peak of the contraction, and the FHR returning to the baseline at the same time as the uterine contraction returns to its baseline. Early decelerations may occur during uterine contractions, during vaginal examinations, as a result of fundal pressure, and during placement of the internal mode of fetal monitoring. When present, they usually occur dur-

ing the first stage of labor when the cervix is dilated 4 to 7 cm. Early decelerations sometimes are seen during the second stage when the woman is pushing.

Because early decelerations are considered to be benign, interventions are not necessary. The value of identifying early decelerations is so that they can be distinguished from late or variable decelerations, which can be nonreassuring and for which interventions are appropriate. The different characteristics of accelerations of the FHR and early decelerations are contrasted in Table 20-5.

table 20-4 Tachycardia and Bradycardia

TACHYCARDIA	BRADYCARDIA
DEFINITION	
FHR >160 beats/min lasting >10 min	FHR <110 beats/min lasting >10 min
CAUSE	
Early fetal hypoxemia	Late fetal hypoxemia/hypoxia
Maternal fever	β-Adrenergic blocking drugs (propranolol; anesthetics for
Parasympatholytic drugs (atropine, hydroxyzine)	epidural, spinal, caudal, and pudendal blocks)
β-Sympathomimetic drugs (ritodrine, isoxsuprine)	Maternal hypotension
Maternal hyperthyroidism	Prolonged umbilical cord compression
Fetal anemia	Fetal congenital heart block
Fetal heart failure	Maternal hypothermia
Fetal cardiac arrhythmias	Prolonged maternal hypoglycemia
Illicit drugs (cocaine, methamphetamines)	
CLINICAL SIGNIFICANCE	
Persistent tachycardia in absence of periodic changes does not appear serious in terms of neonatal outcome (especially true if tachycardia is associated with maternal fever); tachycardia is a nonreassuring sign when associated with late decelerations, severe variable decelerations, or absence of variability.	Bradycardia with moderate variability and absence of periodic changes is not a sign of fetal compromise if FHR remains >80 beats/min; bradycardia caused by hypoxia is a nonreassuring sign when associated with loss of variability and late decelerations.
NURSING INTERVENTION	
Dependent on cause; reduce maternal fever with antipyretics as ordered and cooling measures; oxygen at 8 or 10 L/min by face mask may be of some value; carry out health care provider's orders based on alleviating cause.	Dependent on cause; intervention not warranted in fetus with heart block diagnosed by ECG; oxygen at 8 to 10 L/min by face mask may be of some value; carry out health care provider's orders based on alleviating cause. Scalp stimulation may be performed to determine whether the fetus has the ability to compensate physiologically for stress (FHR will accelerate).

ECG, Electrocardiogram; *FHR,* fetal heart rate.

FIG. 20-8 Decelerations patterns. **A,** Early decelerations caused by head compression. **B,** Late decelerations caused by uteroplacental insufficiency. **C,** Variable decelerations caused by cord compression. (From Tucker, S. [2004]. *Pocket guide to fetal monitoring and assessment* [5th ed.]. St. Louis: Mosby.)

Late Decelerations. Uteroplacental insufficiency causes late decelerations. *Late deceleration* of the FHR is a visually apparent gradual (onset to lowest point 30 sec or more) decrease in FHR and return to baseline (NICHD, 1997). The deceleration begins after the contraction has started, and the lowest point of the deceleration occurs after the peak of the contraction. The deceleration usually does not return to baseline until after the contraction is over (Fig. 20-8, *B*).

Persistent and repetitive late decelerations usually indicate the presence of fetal hypoxemia stemming from insufficient placental perfusion. They can be associated with fetal hypoxemia progressing to hypoxia, and acidemia progressing to acidosis. They should be considered an ominous sign when they are uncorrectable, especially if they are associated with decreased variability and tachycardia. Late decelerations caused by the maternal supine hypotension syndrome are usually correctable when the woman turns on her side to displace the weight of the gravid uterus off the inferior vena cava. Such lateral positioning allows better return of maternal blood flow to the heart, which in turn increases cardiac output and blood pressure.

Late decelerations caused by uteroplacental insufficiency can result from uterine hyperstimulation with oxytocin, preeclampsia, postdate or postterm pregnancy, amnionitis, small-for-gestational-age (SGA) fetus, maternal diabetes, placenta previa, abruptio placentae, conduction anesthetics (producing maternal hypotension), maternal cardiac disease, and maternal anemia. The clinical significance and nursing interventions are described in Table 20-6.

Variable Decelerations. *Variable deceleration* is defined as a visual abrupt (onset to lowest point in less than 30 sec) decrease in FHR below the baseline. The decrease is 15 beats/min or more, lasts at least 15 seconds, and returns to baseline in less than 2 minutes from the time of onset (NICHD, 1997). Variable decelerations occur any time during the uterine contracting phase and are caused by compression of the umbilical cord. Table 20-6 contrasts late deceleration with variable deceleration.

The pattern of variable decelerations differs from those of early and late decelerations, which closely approximate the shape of the corresponding uterine contraction. Instead, variable decelerations have a U, V, or W shape, characterized by a rapid descent and ascent to and from the nadir (or depth) of the deceleration (Fig. 20-8, *C*). Some variable decelerations are preceded and followed by brief accelerations of the FHR, known as "shoulders," which is an appropriate compensatory response to compression of the umbilical cord.

Variable decelerations may be related to partial, brief compression of the cord. If encountered in the first stage of labor, they usually can be resolved by changing the woman's position, for example from one side to the other. Oxygen administration by face mask to the woman is

table 20-5 Accelerations and Early Decelerations

	ACCELERATION	EARLY DECELERATIONS
Description	Transitory increase of fetal heart rate (FHR) above baseline (see Fig. 20-7)	Transitory decrease of FHR below baseline concurrent with uterine contractions (see Fig. 20-8, A)
Shape	May resemble shape of uterine contraction or be spikelike	Uniform shape; mirror image of uterine contraction
Onset	Onset to peak (30 sec; often precedes or occurs simultaneously with uterine contraction)	Early in contraction phase before peak of contraction
Recovery	Less than 2 min from onset	By end of contraction as uterine pressure returns to its resting tone
Amplitude	Usually 15 beats/min above baseline	Usually proportional to amplitude of contraction; rarely, decelerations to <100 beats/min
Baseline	Usually associated with average baseline variability	Usually associated with average baseline variability
Occurrence	Variable; may be repetitive with each contraction	Repetitious (occurs with each contraction); usually occurs between 4- and 7-cm dilation and in second stage of labor
Cause	Spontaneous fetal movement Vaginal examination Electrode application Scalp stimulation Reaction to external sounds Breech presentation Occiput posterior position Uterine contractions Fundal pressure Abdominal palpation	Head compression resulting from the following: • Uterine contractions • Vaginal examination • Fundal pressure • Placement of internal mode of monitoring
Clinical significance	Acceleration with fetal movement signifies fetal well-being representing fetal alertness or arousal states	Reassuring pattern not associated with fetal hypoxemia, acidemia, or low Apgar scores
Nursing intervention	None required	None required

table 20-6	**Late Decelerations and Variable Decelerations**	
	LATE DECELERATIONS	**VARIABLE DECELERATIONS**
Description	Transitory gradual decrease in fetal heart rate (FHR) below baseline rate in contracting phase (see Fig. 20-8, B)	Abrupt decrease in FHR that is variable in duration, intensity, and timing related to onset of contractions (see Fig. 20-8, C)
Shape	Uniform; mirror image of uterine contraction; may be deep or shallow	Variable; characterized by sudden decrease in FHR in V, U, or W shape
Onset	Late in contraction phase; after peak of contraction; nadir of deceleration occurs after peak of contraction	Onset of deceleration to the beginning of nadir, <30 sec; decrease in FHR baseline is ≥15 beats/min, lasting ≥15 sec; variable times in contracting phase; often preceded by transitory acceleration
Recovery	Well after end of contraction	Return to baseline is rapid and <2 min from onset, sometimes with transitory acceleration or acceleration immediately before and after deceleration (shouldering or "overshoot"); slow return to baseline with severe variable decelerations
Deceleration	Usually proportional to amplitude of contraction; rarely decelerates to <100 beats/min; however, shallow late decelerations have the same significance	*Mild:* decelerates to any level, <30 sec with abrupt return to baseline *Moderate:* decelerates to <70 beats/min for 30 to 60 sec or <70 to 80 beats/min for >60 sec *Severe:* decelerates to <70 beats/min for >60 sec, with slow return to baseline
Baseline	Often associated with loss of variability and increasing baseline rate	Mild variables usually associated with average baseline variability; moderate and severe variables often associated with decreasing variability and increasing baseline rate
Occurrence	Occurs with each contraction; may be observed at any time during labor	Variable; commonly observed late in labor with fetal descent and pushing
Cause	Uteroplacental insufficiency caused by the following: —Uterine hyperactivity or hypertonicity —Maternal supine hypotension —Epidural or spinal anesthesia —Placenta previa —Abruptio placentae —Hypertensive disorders —Postmaturity —Intrauterine growth restriction —Diabetes mellitus —Intraamniotic infection	Umbilical cord compression caused by the following: —Maternal position with cord between fetus and maternal pelvis —Cord around fetal neck, arm, leg, or other body part —Short cord —Knot in cord —Prolapsed cord
Clinical significance	Nonreassuring pattern associated with fetal hypoxemia, acidemia, and low Apgar scores; considered ominous if persistent and uncorrected, especially when associated with fetal tachycardia and loss of variability	Variable decelerations occur in ~50% of all labors and usually are transient and correctable *Reassuring* variable decelerations last <45 sec and abruptly return to the FHR baseline; normal baseline rate continues; variability does not decrease *Nonreassuring* variable decelerations decrease to ≤70 beats/min for ≥60 sec and have a prolonged return to baseline; baseline rate increases, variability is absent Nonreassuring variable decelerations are associated with fetal acidemia, hypoxemia, and low Apgar scores; severe variable decelerations with average baseline variability just before birth are usually well tolerated

From Tucker, S. (2004). *Pocket guide to fetal monitoring and assessment* (5th ed.). St. Louis: Mosby.   *Continued*

sometimes helpful. Variable decelerations can result from decreased amniotic fluid or oligohydramnios, more often seen in postterm pregnancies. Amnioinfusion of warmed saline through an intrauterine pressure catheter may be used to alleviate the compression of the cord (see later dis-

cussion). Variable decelerations are also more common in preterm labor (Simpson, 2004) and are often seen during the second stage of labor as a result of umbilical cord compression during fetal descent (Freeman, Garite, & Nageotte, 2003). If repetitive variable decelerations occur during the

table 20-6 Late Decelerations and Variable Decelerations—cont'd

	LATE DECELERATIONS	VARIABLE DECELERATIONS
Nursing interventions	The usual priority is —Change maternal position (lateral) —Correct maternal hypotension by elevating legs —Increase rate of maintenance IV solution —Palpate uterus to assess for hyperstimulation —Discontinue oxytocin if infusing —Administer oxygen at 8-10 L/min with tight face mask —Consider internal monitoring for a more accurate fetal and uterine assessment —Fetal scalp or acoustic stimulation —Assist with fetal oxygen saturation monitoring if ordered —Assist with birth (cesarean or vaginal assisted) if pattern cannot be corrected	The usual priority is —Change maternal position (side to side, knee chest); if decelerations are severe, proceed with following measures: a. Discontinue oxytocin if infusing b. Administer oxygen at 8-10 L/min with tight face mask c. Assist with vaginal or speculum examination to assess for cord prolapse d. Assist with amnioinfusion if ordered e. Assist with fetal oxygen saturation monitoring if ordered f. Assist with birth (vaginal assisted or cesarean) if pattern cannot be corrected

IV, intravenous.

second stage, it is important to discourage the woman from pushing with every contraction so that the fetus has time to recover. Variable decelerations are associated with neonatal depression only when cord compression is severe or prolonged (i.e., tight nuchal cord, short cord, knot in cord, prolapsed cord). Further descriptions of the types of variable decelerations, their clinical significance, and nursing interventions are given in Table 20-6.

Prolonged Decelerations. A prolonged deceleration is a visually apparent decrease in FHR below the baseline 15 beats/min or more and lasting more than 2 minutes but less than 10 minutes. A deceleration lasting more than 10 minutes is considered a baseline change (NICHD, 1997). Generally the benign causes are pelvic examination, application of a spiral electrode, rapid fetal descent, and sustained maternal Valsalva maneuver. Other, less benign causes are progressive severe variable decelerations, sudden umbilical cord prolapse, hypotension produced by spinal or epidural analgesia or anesthesia, paracervical anesthesia, tetanic contraction, placental hemorrhage, uterine rupture, and maternal hypoxia, which may occur during a seizure. When the deceleration lasts longer than 1 to 2 minutes, a loss of variability with rebound tachycardia usually occurs. Occasionally a period of late decelerations follows. Prolonged decelerations usually are isolated events that end spontaneously. However, when a prolonged deceleration is seen late in the course of severe variable decelerations or during a prolonged series of late decelerations, the prolonged deceleration may occur just before fetal death.

■ NURSE ALERT
Nurses should notify the physician or nurse-midwife immediately and initiate appropriate treatment of nonreassuring patterns when they see a prolonged deceleration.

■ CARE MANAGEMENT

The care given to women being monitored by auscultation or EFM is the same as that given to the woman having a low risk labor. Care of the woman being monitored by internal methods may vary. FHR and pattern recognition and intervention may require a nurse to have additional education and clinical experience.

■ Assessment and Nursing Diagnoses

The assessment of the woman includes the maternal temperature, pulse, respiratory rate, blood pressure, position, comfort, voiding pattern, status of membranes, uterine contraction pattern, cervical effacement and dilation, and emotional status. The fetal assessment includes the fetal presentation, fetal position, FHR, and identification of both reassuring and nonreassuring FHR patterns. A checklist may be used by the nurse to assess the FHR when EFM is being used (Box 20-1). All of the assessment information must be documented in the woman's medical record.

Evaluation of the EFM equipment also must be done to ensure that the equipment is working properly and to allow an accurate assessment of the woman and fetus. A checklist for fetal monitoring equipment can be used to evaluate the equipment functions (Box 20-2).

Nursing diagnoses for the woman who is being monitored electronically for fetal status are based on assessment findings. Possible diagnoses include the following:

- *Decreased maternal cardiac output related to*
  –supine hypotension secondary to maternal position
- *Anxiety related to*
  –lack of knowledge concerning fetal monitoring during labor
  –restriction of mobility or movement during EFM
- *Impaired fetal gas exchange related to*
  –umbilical cord compression
  –placental insufficiency
- *Acute pain related to*
  –use of belts to position transducers
  –maternal position
  –vaginal examinations associated with application of maternal or fetal internal monitoring equipment or fetal blood sampling

- *Risk for fetal injury related to*
  - unrecognized hypoxemia, hypoxia, or anoxia
  - infection secondary to internal monitoring or scalp blood sampling

▬ Expected Outcomes of Care

The primary goals of nursing care are to have a healthy fetal and maternal outcome. The interventions implemented to achieve these outcomes are determined by knowledge

---

box 20-1 **Checklist for Fetal Heart Rate and Uterine Activity Assessment with EFM**

Client's name _____
Date/time _____

1. What is the baseline fetal heart rate (FHR)?
   _____ Beats/min
   Check one of the following as observed on the monitor strip:
   _____ Average baseline FHR (110 to 160 beats/min)
   _____ Tachycardia (>160 beats/min)
   _____ Bradycardia (<110 beats/min)
2. What is the baseline variability?
   _____ Absence of variability
   _____ Minimal variability (barely detectable up to 5 beats/min)
   _____ Moderate variability (6 to 25 beats/min)
   _____ Marked variability (>25 beats/min)
3. Are there any periodic or episodic changes in FHR?
   _____ Accelerations with fetal movement
   _____ Repetitive accelerations with each contraction
   _____ Early decelerations (head compression)
   _____ Late decelerations (uteroplacental insufficiency)
   _____ Variable decelerations (cord compression)
       _____ Reassuring (<30 to 45 seconds, abrupt return to baseline, normal baseline, moderate variability)
       _____ Nonreassuring (>60 seconds, slow return to baseline, increasing baseline rate, absence of variability)
   _____ Prolonged deceleration (>2 minutes to 10 minutes)
4. What is the uterine activity (UA)/contraction (UC) pattern?
   _____ Frequency (beginning to beginning of UC)
   _____ Duration (beginning to end of UC)
   Abdominal palpation method
   _____ Strength (mild, moderate, strong)
   _____ Resting time (from end of one contraction to beginning of next one)
   Internal monitoring (IUPC)
   _____ Intensity (mm Hg pressure)
   _____ Resting tone (mm Hg pressure)
COMMENTS: _____
_____
PANEL NUMBER: _____
WHAT CAN BE OR SHOULD HAVE BEEN DONE?
_____
_____
_____
_____

Modified from Tucker, S. (2004). *Pocket guide to fetal monitoring and assessment* (5th ed.). St. Louis: Mosby.

---

box 20-2 **Checklist for Fetal Monitoring Equipment**

PREPARATION OF MONITOR
1. Is the paper inserted correctly?
2. Are transducer cables plugged into the appropriate outlet of the monitor?
3. Is paper speed set to 3 cm/min?

ULTRASOUND TRANSDUCER
1. Has ultrasound transmission gel been applied to the transducer?
2. Was the fetal heart rate (FHR) compared to maternal pulse and noted on the monitor paper?
3. Does a signal light flash or an audible beep occur with each heartbeat?
4. Is the belt secure and snug but comfortable for the laboring woman?

TOCOTRANSDUCER
1. Is the tocotransducer firmly positioned at the site of the least maternal tissue?
2. Has it been applied without gel or paste?
3. Was the uterine activity (UA) reference knob pressed between contractions to adjust the UA baseline to print at the 20 mm Hg line?
4. Is the belt secure and snug but comfortable for the laboring woman?

SPIRAL ELECTRODE
1. Is the connector attached firmly to the leg plate?
2. Is the spiral electrode attached to the presenting part of the fetus?
3. Is the inner surface of the leg plate covered with electrode gel (if necessary)?
4. Is the leg plate properly secured to the woman's thigh?

INTERNAL CATHETER/STRAIN GAUGE
1. Is the length line on the catheter visible at the introitus?
2. Is it noted on the monitor paper that a UA test or calibration was done?
3. Has the monitor been set to zero according to manufacturer's directions?
4. Is the IUPC properly secured to the woman's thigh?

Modified from Tucker, S. (2004). *Pocket guide to fetal monitoring and assessment* (5th ed.). St. Louis: Mosby.

---

of fetal status and by standards for care. The planning process includes accommodating the wishes of the woman and family, answering questions, and explaining nursing interventions.

Expected outcomes for the pregnant woman and family and the fetus include the following:

- The pregnant woman and family will verbalize their understanding of the need for monitoring.
- The pregnant woman and the family will recognize and avoid situations that compromise maternal and fetal circulation.
- The fetus will not have any hypoxemic, hypoxic, or anoxic episodes.
- Should fetal compromise occur, it will be identified promptly, and appropriate nursing interventions such as

intrauterine resuscitation will be initiated and the physician or nurse-midwife notified.

▬ Plan of Care and Interventions

It is the responsibility of the nurse providing care to women in labor to assess FHR and patterns, implement independent nursing interventions, document observations and actions according to the established standard of care, and report nonreassuring patterns to the primary care provider (e.g., physician, certified nurse-midwife). See Box 20-3 for a sample protocol for FHR monitoring, which contains guidelines for the care of the woman being monitored by IA or EFM for fetal status during labor.

Although the use of EFM can be reassuring to many parents, it can be a source of anxiety to some. Therefore the nurse must be particularly sensitive to and respond appropriately to the emotional, informational, and comfort needs of the woman in labor and those of her family (Fig. 20-9 and Box 20-4).

▬ *Electronic Fetal Monitoring Pattern Recognition*

Nurses must evaluate many factors to determine whether a FHR pattern is reassuring or nonreassuring. A complete description of FHR tracings includes both qualitative and quantitative descriptions of baseline rate and variability, presence of accelerations, periodic or episodic decelerations, and changes in the FHR and pattern over time (NICHD, 1997). Nurses evaluate these factors based on other obstetric complications, progress in labor, and analgesia or

---

box 20-3 **Protocol for Fetal Heart Rate Monitoring**

MATERNAL/FETAL ASSESSMENTS
- Obtain a 20-min strip of EFM for all clients admitted to labor unit.

Low Risk Client
- Auscultate or assess tracing every 30 min in active phase of first stage of labor.
- Auscultate or assess tracing every 15 min in second stage.

High Risk Client
- Auscultate or assess tracing every 15 min in active phase and every 5 min in second stage.

Auscultation: All Clients
- Count baseline FHR in between contractions.
- Assess FHR during the contraction and for 30 sec after the contraction.
- Note increases or decreases of FHR.
- Assess FHR before ambulation.
- Interpret FHR data, nursing interventions, and client responses.
- Notify primary health care provider of nonreassuring signs.

EFM: All Clients
- Assess and interpret baseline FHR, variability of FHR, and presence or absence of decelerations and accelerations.

Assessments for All Clients
- Assess uterine activity for frequency and duration, the intensity of contractions, and uterine resting tone.
- Assess FHR immediately after rupture of membranes, vaginal examinations, and any invasive procedure.

MATERNAL CARE
- Assist woman to a comfortable position other than supine.
- Change maternal position at least every 2 hr.

EXTERNAL MONITORING
Ultrasound Transducer
Function
- Monitors FHR with high-frequency sound waves.

Nursing Care
- Tap transducer before use to ensure sound transmission.
- Apply ultrasound transmission gel to transducer, clean abdomen and transducer, and reapply gel every 2 hr and as needed.
- Auscultate FHR with stethoscope or fetoscope if in doubt as to validity of tracing.
- Position and reposition transducer as needed to ensure receipt of clear, interpretable FHR data.

Tocotransducer
Function
- Monitors uterine activity via a pressure-sensing device placed on the maternal abdomen.

Nursing Care
- Position and reposition every 2 hr and as needed on the fundus, where there is the least maternal tissue.
- Keep abdominal strap snug but comfortable for the laboring woman.
- Adjust knob between contractions to print between 10 and 20 mm Hg on the monitor strip paper.
- Palpate fundus every 30 to 60 min to assess strength of contraction; only frequency and duration of contractions can be assessed with tocotransducer.
- Do not attempt to determine woman's need for analgesia based on uterine activity displayed on monitor strip.

INTERNAL MONITORING
Spiral Electrode
Function
- Obtains fetal ECG from presenting part and converts it into FHR.

Nursing Care
- Ensure that the connector to the scalp electrode is appropriately attached to leg plate.
- Reapply electrode paste to leg plate when needed.
- Observe FHR tracing on monitor strip for variability.
- Turn electrode counterclockwise to remove; never pull straight out from presenting part.
- Administer perineal care after the woman voids during labor and as needed.

ECG, Electrocardiogram; *EFM,* electronic fetal monitoring, *FHR,* fetal heart rate.

Continued

| box 20-3 | **Protocol for Fetal Heart Rate Monitoring—cont'd** |

Intrauterine Catheter

Function

- Catheter (solid or fluid filled) that monitors intraamniotic pressure internally.

Nursing Care

- Ensure that the length line on catheter is visible at introitus.
- For closed-system catheters, set baseline rate between uterine contractions when uterus is relaxed.
- Flush open-system catheter with sterile water before insertion and as needed.
- For open-system catheters, turn stopcock off to woman, then with pressure valve of strain gauge released, flush strain gauge, remove syringe, and set stylus to 0 line of chart paper; test further according to manufacturer's instructions every 3 hr and as needed.
- Check proper functioning by tapping catheter, asking woman to cough, or applying fundal pressure; observe appropriate inflection on strip chart.
- Keep catheter or cable secured to woman's leg to prevent dislodgment.

REPORTABLE CONDITIONS

- Presence of nonreassuring patterns:
  - Severe variable decelerations
  - Late decelerations
  - Absence of variability
  - Prolonged deceleration
  - Severe bradycardia
- Worsening of any pattern
- Presence of identifiable fetal arrhythmias
- Difficulty in obtaining adequate FHR tracing or inadequate audible FHR

EMERGENCY MEASURES

- Implement the following measures immediately in the event of the nonreassuring patterns:
  - Reposition client in lateral position to increase uteroplacental perfusion or relieve cord compression

- Administer oxygen at 8 to 10 L/min or per hospital protocol by face mask
- Discontinue oxytocin if infusing
- Correct maternal hypovolemia by increasing IV rate per protocol or as ordered
- Assess for bleeding or other cause of pattern change, such as maternal hypotension
- Notify primary health care provider
- Assist with other methods of assessment such as fetal oxygen saturation monitoring or interventions such as amnioinfusion
- Anticipate emergency preparation for surgical intervention if nonreassuring pattern continues despite interventions

DOCUMENTATION*

Client Record: Auscultation

- FHR baseline, rate and rhythm, increases or decreases

Client Record: EFM

- Method of monitoring, change in method, and adjustments to equipment
- FHR range, variability, presence of decelerations or accelerations
- Uterine activity as determined by palpation or by external or internal monitoring
- Interpretation of FHR data, nursing interventions, and client responses
- Notification of primary health care provider

Monitor Strip

- Client identification data
- Assessments, procedures, and interventions (medications, etc.)
- Notification of primary health care provider
- Significant occurrences (sterile vaginal examination, rupture of membranes, etc.)
- Adjustments of the monitor equipment

* If computer charting system is used, follow institutional policies and system guidelines/protocols.

FIG. 20-9 Nurse explains electronic fetal monitoring as ultrasound transducer monitors the fetal heart rate. (Courtesy Marjorie Pyle, RNC, Lifecircle, Costa Mesa, CA.)

anesthesia. They also must consider the estimated time interval until birth. Interventions are therefore based on clinical judgment of a complex, integrated process (Simpson & James, 2005).

▬ **LEGAL TIP** Fetal Monitoring Standards

Nurses who care for women during childbirth are legally responsible for correctly interpreting FHR patterns, initiating appropriate nursing interventions based on those patterns, and documenting the outcomes of those interventions. Perinatal nurses are responsible for the timely notification of the physician or nurse-midwife in the event of nonreassuring FHR patterns. Perinatal nurses also are responsible for initiating the institutional chain of command should differences in opinion arise among health care providers concerning the interpretation of the FHR pattern and the intervention required.

Nursing Management of Nonreassuring Patterns.
The term intrauterine resuscitation is sometimes used to

box 20-4 **Client/Family Teaching When Electronic Fetal Monitor Is Used**

The following guidelines relate to client teaching and the functioning of the monitor:

- Explain the purpose of monitoring.
- Explain each procedure.
- Provide rationale for maternal position other than supine.
- Explain that fetal status can be continuously assessed by electronic fetal monitoring (EFM), even during contractions.
- Explain that the lower tracing on the monitor strip paper shows uterine activity; the upper tracing shows the fetal heart rate (FHR).
- Reassure woman and partner that prepared childbirth techniques can be implemented without difficulty.
- Explain that, during external monitoring, effleurage can be performed on sides of abdomen or upper portion of thighs.
- Explain that breathing patterns based on the time and intensity of contractions can be enhanced by the observation of uterine activity on the monitor strip paper, which shows the onset of contractions.
- Note peak of contraction; knowing that contraction will not get stronger and is half over is usually helpful.
- Note diminishing intensity.
- Coordinate with appropriate breathing and relaxation techniques.
- Reassure woman and partner that the use of internal monitoring does not restrict movement, although she is confined to bed.*
- Explain that use of external monitoring usually requires the woman's cooperation during positioning and movement.
- Reassure woman and partner that use of monitoring does not imply fetal jeopardy.
- Reassure woman that the equipment is removed periodically to permit the applicator sites to be washed and other care to be given.

*Portable telemetry monitors allow the FHR and uterine contraction patterns to be observed on centrally located display stations. These portable units permit ambulation during electronic monitoring.

refer to those interventions initiated when a nonreassuring FHR pattern is noted; they are directed primarily toward improving uterine and intervillous space blood flow and secondarily toward increasing maternal oxygenation and cardiac output (Simpson & James, 2005). For example, oxytocin always should be infused as a piggyback connection near the indwelling needle. If FHR patterns change for any reason, oxytocin stimulation of the uterine muscle is usually discontinued. This consists of turning off the IV line from the piggyback (containing oxytocin) and opening the primary infusion line.

Nurses must assign priorities to interventions to maximize the efficacy of the intrauterine resuscitation. The *first priority* is to open the maternal and fetal vascular systems; the *second priority* is to increase blood volume; and the *third priority* is to optimize oxygenation of the circulating blood volume. For example, to relieve an acute FHR deceleration, the nurse can do the following:

- Assist the woman to the side-lying position if she is not already in a lateral position.

- Increase the maternal blood volume by increasing the rate of the primary IV infusion or by raising the woman's legs. Blood pooled in the legs, especially that occurring as the result of sympathetic blockade (e.g., epidural anesthesia), will then drain quickly into the central venous circulation, and this will augment the intravascular volume (Parilla, 2006).
- Provide oxygen by face mask at 8 to 10 L/min.

Some interventions are specific to the FHR pattern. Nursing interventions appropriate for the management of tachycardia and bradycardia are given in Table 20-4, and those appropriate for the management of increased or decreased variability are given in Table 20-3. No specific nursing interventions are required for the management of FHR acceleration or early deceleration (see Table 20-5). However, late and some variable FHR decelerations require aggressive intervention (see Table 20-6). The primary health care provider decides whether medical intervention should be instituted, what intervention is indicated, or whether immediate vaginal or cesarean birth should be performed.

■ Other Methods of Assessment and Intervention

Other methods of assessment and intervention are designed to be used in conjunction with EFM in an effort to identify and intervene in the presence of a nonreassuring FHR or pattern. These methods include FHR response to stimulation, fetal oxygen saturation monitoring, fetal blood sampling, amnioinfusion, and tocolysis. Umbilical cord acid-base determination is an assessment technique that is a useful adjunct to the Apgar score in assessing the immediate condition of the newborn.

Fetal Heart Rate Response to Stimulation. Stimulation of the fetus is done to elicit an acceleration of the FHR of 15 beats/min for at least 15 seconds (Tucker, 2004). The two methods of fetal stimulation currently in practice are scalp stimulation (using digital pressure during a vaginal examination) and vibroacoustic stimulation (using an artificial larynx or fetal acoustic stimulation device over the fetal head for 1 to 2 seconds). An FHR acceleration response to this stimulation usually indicates fetal well-being. If the fetus does not have an acceleration, it does not necessarily indicate fetal compromise; however, further evaluation of fetal well-being is needed.

Fetal Oxygen Saturation Monitoring. Continuous monitoring of fetal oxygen saturation ($FSpO_2$) or fetal pulse oximetry (FPO) is a method of fetal assessment that was approved for clinical use by the Food and Drug Administration in May 2000 (Dildy, 2004). FPO works in a way similar to the pulse oximetry used in children and adults. A specially designed sensor is inserted next to the fetal cheek or temple area to assess oxygen saturation. The sensor is then connected to a monitor, and the data are displayed on the uterine activity panel of the fetal monitor tracing. The normal range of oxygen saturation in the adult is 95% to 100%. The normal range for the healthy fetus is

30% to 70%, with the cutoff value for the critical threshold of $FSpO_2$ at 30% (Dildy).

FPO may be used if certain criteria are met, including a single fetus at least 36 weeks of gestation in a vertex presentation with a nonreassuring FHR pattern. The membranes should be ruptured, the cervix dilated at least 2 cm, and the fetal station at least a −2 or less (Garite et al., 2000). The value of $FSpO_2$ monitoring is that in the event of nonreassuring FHR patterns, it could support the decision about whether labor should continue or whether to intervene with an expeditious assisted vaginal or cesarean birth of the fetus. The American College of Obstetricians and Gynecologists has not endorsed the use of FPO in clinical practice and recommends further clinical research (ACOG, 2005).

If FPO becomes more widely used, the labor nurse's role will expand to include this type of monitoring in practice. Simpson and Porter (2001) suggested that nurses will be in-volved in identifying potential candidates for monitoring, inserting the sensor (according to state nurse practice acts and institutional policies), interpreting data, documenting findings, and communicating with the primary health care provider.

Fetal Scalp Blood Sampling. Sampling of the fetal scalp blood was designed to assess the fetal pH, PO_2, and PCO_2. The procedure is performed by obtaining a sample of fetal scalp blood through the dilated cervix after the membranes have ruptured. The scalp is swabbed with a disinfecting solution before making the puncture, and the sample is then collected. However, the blood gas values vary so rapidly with transient circulatory changes that fetal blood sampling is seldom performed. When used, it is usually in tertiary centers with the capability for repetitive sampling and rapid report of results. The circulatory changes that cause the variability and thus undermine the

---

EVIDENCE-BASED PRACTICE

Vibroacoustic Fetal Stimulation

BACKGROUND
- Tests of prenatal well-being rely on fetal movement and heart rate reactivity to assess adequate muscular and myocardial oxygenation and hence, uteroplacental perfusion. Popular tests correlating fetal movement to well-being include non-stress tests, kick counts, ultrasounds, and biophysical profiles. If the fetus is in a sleeping period, the tests may look falsely abnormal, which may trigger unnecessary or prolonged testing, parental anxiety, and expense. To awaken the fetus, health care providers may change maternal position or activity, manually manipulate the fetus, use light, or use a vibroacoustic stimulator to transmit a sharp sound through the maternal abdominal wall to the fetus. Possible adverse effects may include fetal compromise, vigorous fetal movement which could tighten a nuchal cord, bradycardia, and subsequent cesarean birth.

OBJECTIVES
- The reviewers sought to investigate the benefits and adverse effects of vibroacoustic stimulation to improve efficiency of prenatal tests of fetal well-being and decrease falsely abnormal results. Outcomes were to include perinatal outcomes, maternal satisfaction, cost savings, shorter testing time, and fetal hearing and neurologic tests.

METHODS
Search Strategy
- The authors searched the Cochrane Pregnancy and Child-birth Group trials register, as well as conference proceedings. They located nine randomized controlled trials dated 1986 to 2003, representing 4838 women from Australia, Greece, Turkey, Mexico, and the United States.

Statistical Analyses
- Similar data were pooled. Reviewers calculated relative risk for dichotomous (categoric) data, such as type of birth, and weighted mean difference for continuous data, such as heart rate. Differences between groups outside the 95% confidence interval were accepted as significant.

FINDINGS
- Vibroacoustic stimulation increased the accuracy of nonstress tests by decreasing the number of nonreactive (abnormal) tests, when compared to groups receiving mock stimulation or nothing. Test time was shorter with vibroacoustic stimulation. Fetal movement increased significantly in response to vibroacoustic stimulation. No difference was found between manual manipulation and vibroacoustic stimulation. There were too few numbers to draw conclusions about fetal compromise. No trial measured fetal hearing or neurologic damage.

LIMITATIONS
- Most trials could not double-blind participants or evaluators, leading to possible bias. The frequency, intensity, and duration of the stimulation varied, or were not noted.

IMPLICATIONS FOR PRACTICE
- Fetal reactivity is an important determinant of fetal well-being, and an active fetus will make testing more accurate and efficient. Research has not yet established the safety of vibro-acoustic stimulation, particularly for fetal distress, neurologic and hearing impairment, and perinatal mortality. The nurse can safely try gentle manual manipulation and maternal position and activity changes, as well as light and sound stimulation, to stimulate the fetus.

IMPLICATIONS FOR FURTHER RESEARCH
- Future research should first establish the safety of vibroacoustic stimulation for the outcomes of fetal distress, perinatal death, cesarean birth, and hearing and neurologic impairment. Double-blinding is possible, with mock stimulators and blinded evaluators. If safety is established, optimal frequency, intensity, duration, and location of the vibroacoustic stimulation can be investigated for various gestational ages. Researchers should include maternal satisfaction in their outcomes.

Reference: Tan, K., & Smyth, R. (2001). Fetal vibroacoustic stimulation for facilitation of tests of fetal wellbeing. *The Cochrane Database of Systematic Reviews* 2006, Issue 3. Chichester, UK: John Wiley & Sons.

utility of this procedure are maternal acidosis or alkalosis, caput succedaneum, the stage of labor, and the time relation of scalp sampling to UCs.

Amnioinfusion. Amnioinfusion is used during labor either to supplement the amount of amniotic fluid to reduce the severity of variable decelerations caused by cord compression or to dilute meconium-stained amniotic fluid with saline or lactated Ringer's solution (Hofmeyr, 2002). The procedure to supplement amniotic fluid is indicated for clients with oligohydramnios, secondary to uteroplacental insufficiency, premature rupture of membranes, or postmaturity, who are at risk for variable decelerations because of umbilical cord compression.

Oligohydramnios is an abnormally small amount of amniotic fluid or the absence of amniotic fluid. Without the buffer of amniotic fluid, the umbilical cord can easily become compressed during contractions or fetal movement, diminishing the flow of blood between the fetus and placenta, as evidenced by variable decelerations. Amnioinfusion replaces the "cushion" for the cord and relieves both the frequency and intensity of variable decelerations.

Amnioinfusion also is indicated in the presence of moderate to thick meconium to dilute and flush out the meconium with the intent of avoiding meconium-aspiration syndrome in the neonate (Hofmeyr, 2002; Parer & Nageotte, 2004).

Risks of amnioinfusion are overdistention of the uterine cavity and increased uterine tone. Techniques of amnioinfusion treatment vary, but usually fluid is administered through an IUPC. The woman's membranes must be ruptured for the IUPC placement. The fluid is administered by attaching plastic (IV) tubing to a liter of normal saline or lactated Ringer's solution through a port in the IUPC. Double-lumen IUPCs are preferred because the IUP can be monitored without stopping the procedure. The fluid can be warmed with a blood warmer before administration for the preterm or SGA fetus (refer to institutional policies/protocols). The fluid can be infused by bolus or continuous flow or by a combination of these two methods.

Intensity and frequency of UCs should be continually assessed during the procedure. The recorded uterine resting tone during amnioinfusion will appear higher than normal because of resistance to outflow and turbulence at the end of the catheter. The true resting tone can be checked by discontinuing the amnioinfusion when using a single-lumen IUPC (Tucker, 2004).

Tocolytic Therapy. Tocolysis (relaxation of the uterus) can be achieved through the administration of drugs that inhibit UCs. This therapy can be used as an adjunct to other interventions in the management of fetal stress when the fetus is exhibiting nonreassuring patterns associated with increased uterine activity. Tocolysis improves blood flow through the placenta by inhibiting UCs. Tocolysis may be considered by the primary health care provider and implemented when other interventions to reduce uterine activity, such as maternal position change, hydration, and discontinuance of an oxytocin infusion, have no effect on diminishing the UCs. A tocolytic drug such as magnesium sulfate or terbutaline can be administered by IV to decrease uterine activity. If the FHR pattern improves, the woman may be allowed to continue labor; if there is no improvement, immediate surgical intervention for birth may be needed.

Umbilical Cord Acid-Base Determination. In assessing the immediate condition of the newborn after birth, a sample of cord blood is a useful adjunct to the Apgar score. The procedure is generally done by withdrawing blood from the umbilical artery and having the blood tested for pH, P_{CO_2}, and P_{O_2}. Umbilical cord gas measurements reflect the acid-base status of the newborn at birth, a measurement not reflected in the Apgar score (Gilstrap, 2004). If acidosis is present, the type—respiratory, metabolic, or mixed—is determined by analyzing blood gas values (Table 20-7).

■ *Client and Family Teaching*

Part of the nurse's role includes acting as a partner with the woman to achieve a high-quality birthing experience. In addition to teaching and supporting the woman and her family with understanding of the laboring and birth process, breathing techniques, use of equipment, and pain management techniques, the nurse can assist with two factors that have an effect on fetal status: pushing and positioning. The nurse should provide information and support to the woman in regard to these two factors.

table 20-7 **Types of Acidosis**

BLOOD GASES*	RESPIRATORY	METABOLIC	MIXED
pH	↓ (<7.1)	↓ (<7.1)	↓ (<7.1)
P_{CO_2} (mm Hg)	↑ (>60)	Normal (<60)	↑ (>60)
H_{CO_3} (mEq/L)	Normal (16-24)	↓ (<16)	↓ (<16)
Base	Normal (<12)	↑ (>12)	↑ (>12)

Sources: Gilstrap, L. (2004). Fetal acid-base balance. In R. Creasy, R. Resnik, & J. Iams (Eds.). *Maternal-fetal medicine: Principles and practice* (5th ed.). Philadelphia: Saunders; Pagana, K., & Pagana, T. (2006). *Mosby's manual of diagnostic and laboratory tests* (3rd ed.). St. Louis: Mosby; Tucker, S. (2004). *Pocket guide to fetal monitoring and assessment* (5th ed.). St. Louis: Mosby.
*Arterial values.

Maternal Positioning. Maternal supine hypotensive syndrome is caused by the weight and pressure of the gravid uterus on the ascending vena cava when the woman is in a supine position (see Fig. 21-5). This decreases venous return to the woman's heart and cardiac output and subsequently reduces her blood pressure. The low maternal blood pressure decreases intervillous space blood flow during UCs and results in fetal hypoxemia. This is reflected on the fetal monitor as a nonreassuring FHR pattern, usually late decelerations. The nurse should solicit the woman's cooperation in avoiding the supine position. The woman should be encouraged to maintain a side-lying position or semi-Fowler's position with a lateral tilt to the uterus. Previously it was thought that the left lateral maternal position preferentially promoted maternal cardiac output, thereby enhancing blood flow to the fetus. However, it is now known that either the right or left lateral maternal position effectively enhances uteroplacental blood flow.

Discouraging the Valsalva Maneuver. The Valsalva maneuver can be described as the process of making a forceful bearing-down attempt while holding one's breath with a closed glottis and tightening the abdominal muscles. This process stimulates the parasympathetic division of the autonomic nervous system, producing a vagal response, and results in the decrease of the maternal heart rate and blood pressure. Prolonged pushing in this manner can decrease placental blood flow, alter maternal and fetal oxygenation, decrease the fetal pH and PO_2, increase the fetal PCO_2, and increase the likelihood of fetal hypoxemia, as reflected in FHR pattern changes.

During the second stage of labor, when the woman needs to push, an alternative to breath holding with a closed glottis is to perform the open-mouth and open-glottis breathing-pushing technique. The nurse should instruct the woman to keep her mouth and glottis open and to let air escape from the lungs during the pushing process. This may result in an audible grunting sound and will prevent the Valsalva maneuver (see Chapter 21).

Some providers of care prefer the laboring-down process or delayed pushing, which is to refrain from pushing in the early second stage of labor. The natural forces of labor contractions are used to move the fetus down the birth canal, and then focused pushing is used for a short period to expel the fetus from the birth canal.

▬ Documentation

Clear and complete documentation on the woman's monitor strip is started before the initiation of monitoring and consists of identifying information plus other relevant data. This documentation is continued and updated according to institutional protocol as monitoring progresses. In some institutions, observations noted and interventions implemented are recorded on the monitor strip to produce a comprehensive document that chronicles the course of labor and the care rendered. In other institutions, this documentation is confined to the labor flow record or computer chart. Advocates of documenting on both the medical record and the EFM strip cite advantages of this approach: the ease of writing directly on the strip while at the bedside or inputting the data on a computer-based documentation system, and the improved accuracy in documenting critical events and the interventions implemented. Others believe that charting on the EFM strip constitutes duplication—documentation of the same information noted in the medical record—and thus unnecessary additional paperwork for the nurse.

One way of documenting that frequent maternal-fetal assessments have been done at the bedside is either to initial the EFM strip or to depress the "mark" button during these assessments. Data-entry devices are now available

---

box 20-5 **Documentation**

OBSERVATIONS
Maternal
- Vital signs: BP, TPR
- Oxygen saturation if monitored
- Uterine activity: frequency, duration, intensity, resting tone
- Behavior: anxiety, irritability, fear of losing control
- Breathing pattern
- Position; activity (ambulating, BRP, use of birth ball, etc.)
- Rupture of membranes; time, color, amount, odor
- Voidings; nausea, vomiting
- Urge to push; bearing down; pushing

Fetal
- FHR, variability, periodic/episodic changes
- Fetal movement
- Oxygen saturation if monitored
- Presentation, position, station

ADJUSTMENTS
- Relocation of transducers
- Replacement of electrode
- Replacement of IUPC
- Adjustment or flushing of IUPC
- Testing of monitor
- Monitor paper changes; time lapse
- Interruption/removal of monitoring equipment

INTERVENTIONS
- Maternal position change
- Administration of oxygen
- Parenteral fluids; changes in flow rate
- Amnioinfusion
- Fetal scalp stimulation
- Medication administration
  Oxytocin
  Analgesics
  Anesthetics
  Tocolytics
- Primary health care provider notification, reason, and response
- Birth data

BP, Blood pressure; *BRP,* bathroom privileges; *FHR,* fetal heart rate; *IUPC,* intrauterine pressure catheter; *TPR,* temperature, pulse, respiration.

with some EFM systems; assessments are keyed in and subsequently printed on the strip. A disadvantage of documenting on both the EFM strip and the medical record is that frequently the times noted for events and interventions on the EFM strip do not correlate with what is later documented in the medical record. These discrepancies can lead those involved in the retrospective review process carried out during litigation to infer that documentation errors have occurred. Therefore if institutional policy mandates documentation on both the monitor strip and the medical record, it is critically important for the nurse to make sure the times and notations of events and inter-

ventions recorded in each place agree. No one method of documentation is right; rather the nurse must be aware of and follow individual institutional policies, as well as participate in formulating such policies (McCartney, 2002). Many of the aspects of care and events that can be documented on the client's medical record or the monitor strip are listed in Box 20-5.

■ Evaluation

Evaluation is a continuous process. The nurse can assume that care was effective when the outcomes for care have been achieved (see Plan of Care).

---

plan of care ▶   **Electronic Fetal Monitoring During Labor**

NURSING DIAGNOSIS Maternal anxiety related to lack of knowledge about use of electronic monitor

Expected Outcome *The woman will exhibit increased understanding about fetal monitoring and signs of reduced anxiety (i.e., absence of physical indicators, absence of perceived threat, and absence of feelings of dread).*

Nursing Interventions/Rationales
- Explain and demonstrate to woman and labor support partner how the electronic monitor (internal or external) works in assessing FHR and in detecting and assessing quality of uterine contractions *to remove fear of unknown and ensure that woman can move with the monitor.*
- When making adjustment to the monitor, explain to the couple what is being done and why, *because information increases understanding and allays anxiety.*
- Explain that although a side-lying position or Fowler's position provides for optimal monitoring, position changes decrease discomfort; therefore encourage frequent changes in position (other than supine) and explain any monitoring adjustments that are being made as a result *to reduce discomfort and allay anxiety.*

NURSING DIAGNOSIS Risk for fetal injury related to inaccurate placement of transducers/electrodes, misinterpretation of results, or failure to use other assessment techniques to monitor fetal well-being

Expected Outcomes *Fetal well-being is adequately assessed. Any fetal compromise is identified with appropriate interventions implemented.*

Nursing Interventions/Rationales
- Carefully follow guidelines and checklist for application and initiation of monitoring *to ensure proper placement of monitoring devices and production of accurate output from monitoring device.*
- Check placement throughout monitoring process *to ensure that devices remain correctly placed.*
- Regularly assess and record results of EFM (FHR and variability, decelerations, accelerations, uterine activity, contractions, uterine resting tone) *to provide consistent and timely evaluation of fetal well-being and progress of labor.*
- Auscultate FHR and palpate contractions on a regular basis *to provide a cross-check on the EFM output and ensure fetal well-being.*

NURSING DIAGNOSIS Risk for maternal injury related to incorrect placement of external or internal monitors or misinterpretation of contraction pattern

Expected Outcomes *Maternal well-being is assessed per standards of care/agency guidelines for women having EFM.*
Any alterations in maternal status are identified promptly and appropriate interventions implemented.

Nursing Interventions/Rationales
- Palpate uterine contractions *to correlate data with electronic monitoring results.*
- Periodically recheck placement *to verify that all monitoring devices are accurately placed.*
- Assess uterine activity, contraction pattern, and baseline *to provide ongoing evaluation and basis for further interventions.*
- Use correct aseptic technique for insertion of internal monitors *to prevent infection.*
- Monitor maternal temperature, as well as color, odor, and amount of amniotic fluid, *to determine indicators of infection.*

NURSING DIAGNOSIS Risk for impaired physical mobility related to restriction of movement with monitoring devices

Expected Outcomes *The woman will be able to change positions and ambulate at intervals.*
The woman will have no physical impairments related to use of EFM.

Nursing Interventions/Rationales
- Discontinue continuous external EFM at intervals *to encourage ambulation, (e.g. out of bed to the bathroom, up in chair, to shower or tub).*
- Use external monitor or handheld Doppler monitoring device intermittently *to collect data while woman is out of bed.*
- Encourage woman who is not able to get out of bed to change position at least every 2 hours and as needed *to decrease complications of immobility.*
- Assist and encourage range of motion exercises while the woman is in bed *to decrease complications of immobility.*

EFM, Electronic fetal monitoring; *FHR,* fetal heart rate.

CD: Plan of Care: EFM During Labor

community activity

Survey area providers of obstetric care including private obstetricians, nurse-midwives, prenatal clinics (both public and private), and area hospitals regarding client education provided on electronic fetal monitoring (EFM).

- What content is covered, and how is it delivered to the client and her partner? Are written materials given to the client? Is the option of intermittent auscultation discussed? Are intermittent auscultation and EFM discussed in prenatal classes?
- When admitting the laboring client, does the nurse document education provided regarding EFM? Is the education provided in different languages? Is a signed consent required before applying EFM?
- Do local providers think low risk obstetric clients have the right to refuse EFM? Is the client given a choice when in labor if no risk factors are present? What percentage of clients in area hospitals are monitored by intermittent auscultation?

key points

- Fetal well-being during labor is gauged by the response of the FHR to uterine contractions.
- FHR characteristics include the baseline FHR, and variability and periodic/episodic changes in the FHR.
- The monitoring of fetal well-being includes FHR assessment, watching for meconium-stained amniotic fluid, and assessment of maternal vital signs and uterine activity.
- It is the responsibility of the nurse to assess FHR and patterns, implement independent nursing interventions, and report nonreassuring patterns to the physician or nurse-midwife.
- The Association of Women's Health, Obstetric, and Neonatal Nurses (AWHONN) and the American College of Obstetricians and Gynecologists (ACOG) have established and published health care provider standards and guidelines for fetal heart monitoring.
- The emotional, informational, and comfort needs of the woman and her family must be addressed when the mother and her fetus are being monitored.
- Documentation of fetal assessment is initiated and updated according to institutional protocol.

REFERENCES

Althaus, J., Petersen, S., Fox, H., Holcroft, C., & Graham, E. (2005). Can electronic fetal monitoring identify preterm neonates with cerebral white matter injury? *Obstetrics and Gynecology, 105*(3), 458-465.

American College of Obstetricians and Gynecologists (ACOG). (2005). Intrapartum fetal heart rate monitoring. ACOG Practice Bulletin, No. 70. *Obstetrics and Gynecology, 106*(6), 1453-1461.

Association of Women's Health, Obstetric and Neonatal Nurses (AWHONN). (2003). *Fetal heart monitoring principles and practice* (3rd ed.). Dubuque, IA: Kendall/Hunt.

Clark, S., & Hankins, G. (2003). Temporal and demographic trends in cerebral palsy—fact and fiction. *American Journal of Obstetrics and Gynecology, 188*(3), 628-633.

Dildy, G. (2004). Fetal pulse oximetry: A critical appraisal. *Best Practice & Research Clinical Obstetrics and Gynecology, 18*(3), 477-484.

Dildy, G. (2005). Intrapartum assessment of the fetus: Historical and evidence-based practice. *Obstetrics and Gynecology Clinics of North America, 32*(2), 255-271.

Freeman, R., Garite, T., & Nageotte, M. (2003). *Fetal heart rate monitoring* (3rd ed.). Philadelphia: Lippincott Williams & Wilkins.

Garite, T., Dilday, G., McNamara, H., Nageotte, M., Boehm, F., Dellinger, et al. (2000). A multicenter controlled trial of fetal pulse oximetry in the intrapartum management of nonreassuring fetal heart rate patterns. *American Journal of Obstetrics and Gynecology, 183*(5), 1049-1058.

Gilstrap, L. (2004). Fetal acid-base balance. In R. Creasy, R. Resnik, & J. Iams (Eds.), *Maternal-fetal medicine: Principles and practice* (5th ed.). Philadelphia: Saunders.

Hofmeyr, G. (2002). Amnioinfusion for meconium-stained liquor in labour. (Cochrane Review). *The Cochrane Database of Systematic Reviews, 2006,* Issue 3. Chichester, UK: John Wiley & Sons.

King, T., & Parer, J. (2000). The physiology of fetal heart rate patterns and perinatal asphyxia. *Journal of Perinatal and Neonatal Nursing, 14*(3), 19-39.

Martin, J., Hamilton, B., Sutton, P., Ventura, S., Menacker, F., & Munson, M. (2005). Births: Final data for 2003. *National Vital Statistics Report, 54*(2), 1-116.

McCartney, P. (2002). Electronic fetal monitoring and the legal medical record. *MCN American Journal of Maternal/Child Nursing, 27*(4), 249.

National Institute of Child Health and Human Development (NICHD) Research Planning Workshop. (1997). Electronic fetal heart rate monitoring: Research guidelines for interpretation. *American Journal of Obstetrics and Gynecology, 177*(6), 1385-1390.

Parer, J., & Nageotte, M. (2004). Intrapartum fetal surveillance. In R. Creasy, R. Resnik, & J. Iams (Eds.), *Maternal-fetal medicine: Principles and practice* (5th ed.). Philadelphia: Saunders.

Parilla, B. (2006). Estimation of fetal well-being. Part 2. Evaluation of the intrapartum fetus. In R. Martin, A. Fanaroff, & M. Walsh (Eds.)., *Fanaroff and Martin's neonatal-perinatal medicine: Diseases of the fetus and infant* (8th ed.). St. Louis: Mosby.

Simpson, K. (2004). Standardized language for electronic fetal heart rate monitoring. *MCN American Journal of Maternal/Child Nursing, 29*(5), 336.

Simpson, K., & James, D. (2005). Efficacy of intrauterine resuscitation techniques in improving fetal oxygen status during labor. *Obstetrics and Gynecology, 105*(6), 1362-1368.

Simpson, K., & Knox, G. (2000). Risk management and electronic fetal monitoring: Decreasing risk of adverse outcomes and liability exposure. *Journal of Perinatal and Neonatal Nursing, 14*(3), 40-52.

Simpson, K., & Porter, M. (2001). Fetal oxygen saturation monitoring: Using this new technology for fetal assessment during labor. *AWHONN Lifelines, 5*(2), 26-33.

Tucker, S. (2004). *Pocket guide to fetal monitoring and assessment* (5th ed.). St. Louis: Mosby.

Wood, S. (2003). Should women be given a choice about fetal assessment in labor? *MCN American Journal of Maternal/Child Nursing, 28*(5), 292-298.

Karen A. Piotrowski

Nursing Care During Labor

learning objectives

- Review the factors included in the initial assessment of the woman in labor.
- Describe the ongoing assessment of maternal progress during the first, second, and third stages of labor.
- Recognize the physical and psychosocial findings indicative of maternal progress during labor.
- Describe fetal assessment during labor.
- Identify signs of developing complications during labor and birth.
- Develop a comprehensive plan of care relevant to each stage of labor.
- Analyze the influence of cultural and religious beliefs and practices on the process of labor and birth.

- Evaluate research findings on the importance of support (family, partner, doula, nurse) in facilitating maternal progress during labor and birth.
- Describe the role and responsibilities of the nurse during an emergency childbirth situation.
- Evaluate the impact of perineal trauma on the woman's reproductive and sexual health.
- Discuss ways the nurse can use evidence-based practices to enhance the quality of care a woman receives during labor and birth.

electronic resources

Additional information related to the content in Chapter 21 can be found on

the companion website at **evolve**
http://evolve.elsevier.com/Lowdermilk/MWHC/
- NCLEX Review Questions
- Case Study: First Stage of Labor
- Case Study: Second/Third Stages of Labor
- WebLinks

or on the interactive companion CD
- NCLEX Review Questions
- Animations: Vaginal birth, breech exam, breech birth, cord prolapse, shoulder dystocia
- Assessment Video: Leopold maneuvers
- Case Study: First Stage of Labor
- Case Study: Second/Third Stages of Labor
- Critical Thinking Exercise: Positioning During Labor
- Plan of Care: Labor and Birth
- Video: Childbirth (cesarean and vaginal)

THE labor process is an exciting and anxious time for the woman and her significant others (support persons, family). In a relatively short period, they experience one of the most profound changes in their lives.

For most women, labor begins with the first uterine contraction, continues with hours of hard work during cervical dilation and birth, and ends as the woman and her significant others begin the attachment process with the newborn. Nursing care management focuses on assessment and support of the woman and her significant others throughout labor and birth, with the goal of ensuring the best possible outcome for all involved.

■ FIRST STAGE OF LABOR

■ CARE MANAGEMENT

The first stage of labor begins with the onset of regular uterine contractions and ends with full cervical effacement and dilation. The first stage of labor consists of the following three phases: the latent phase (up to 3 cm of dilation), the active phase (4 to 7 cm of dilation), and the transition phase (8 to 10 cm of dilation). Most nulliparous women seek admission to the hospital in the latent phase because they have not experienced labor before and are unsure of the "right" time to come in. Multiparous women usually do not come to the hospital until they are in the active phase. Even though no two labors are identical, women who have given birth before appear less anxious about the process, unless their previous experience has been negative.

A woman often has lingering impressions of her childbirth experience. Satisfaction with childbirth hinges on the woman's ability to maintain a sense of control. Caregivers who encourage a woman to be actively involved in decision making and who are respectful, supportive, available, protective, encouraging, kind, patient, professional, calm, and comforting help the woman to remember her childbirth experience in positive terms. A satisfactory view of childbirth contributes to a woman's self-esteem and sense of accomplishment with her performance. Adaptation to her role as a mother may also be enhanced. Frustrations a woman feels regarding her childbirth experience stem from unmet expectations, poorly managed pain, loss of control, lack of knowledge, or the negative behaviors of some caregivers. A woman who perceives her childbirth to be unsatisfactory or traumatic could be at risk for postpartum depression and cesarean birth for a subsequent pregnancy (Goodman, Mackey, & Tavakoli, 2004; Hanson, VandeVusse, & Harrod, 2001; Tumblin & Simkin, 2001).

▬ Assessment and Nursing Diagnoses

Assessment begins at the first contact with the woman, whether by telephone or in person. Many women call the hospital or birthing center first to receive validation that it is all right for them to come in for evaluation or admission. The manner in which the nurse communicates with the woman during this first contact can set the tone for a positive birth experience. A caring attitude by the nurse encourages the woman to verbalize questions and concerns. If possible, the nurse should have the woman's prenatal record in hand when speaking to her or admitting her for evaluation of labor. Copies of records are often filed on the perinatal unit at some time during the woman's third trimester. The nurse should ask the woman for a description of what she is experiencing that signals to her that she is in labor. A study by Gross, Haunschild, Stoexen, Methner, and Guenter (2003) found that women may describe a variety of signs and symptoms which signal to them that labor has begun. These signs and symptoms can include recurrent or nonrecurrent pain, watery or blood-stained fluid from the vagina, gastrointestinal symptoms (e.g., vomiting, stomachache, diarrhea), emotional upheaval (e.g., anxiety), and sleep disturbances.

Certain factors are assessed initially to determine whether the woman is in true or false labor and whether she should come for further assessment or admission (see Teaching for Self-Care box).

The pregnant woman may call her primary health care provider or come to the hospital while in false labor or early in the latent phase of the first stage of labor. She may feel discouraged, angry, or confused on learning that the contractions that feel so strong and regular to her are

---

TEACHING FOR SELF-CARE

How to Distinguish True Labor from False Labor

TRUE LABOR
- Contractions
  - Occur regularly, becoming stronger, lasting longer, and occurring closer together
  - Become more intense with walking
  - Usually felt in lower back, radiating to lower portion of abdomen
  - Continue despite use of comfort measures
- Cervix (by vaginal examination)
  - Shows progressive change (softening, effacement, and dilation signaled by the appearance of bloody show)
  - Moves to an increasingly anterior position
- Fetus
  - Presenting part usually becomes engaged in the pelvis. This results in increased ease of breathing; at the same time, the presenting part presses downward and compresses the bladder, resulting in urinary frequency.

FALSE LABOR
- Contractions
  - Occur irregularly or become regular only temporarily
  - Often stop with walking or position change
  - Can be felt in the back or abdomen above the navel
  - Often can be stopped through the use of comfort measures
- Cervix (by vaginal examination)
  - May be soft, but there is no significant change in effacement or dilation or evidence of bloody show
  - Is often in a posterior position
- Fetus
  - Presenting part is usually not engaged in the pelvis

---

not true contractions because they are not causing cervical dilation, or that they are still not strong or frequent enough for admission. During the third trimester of pregnancy, women should be instructed regarding the stages of labor and the signs indicating its onset. They should be informed of the possibility that they will not be admitted if they are 3 cm or less dilated. Later admission (i.e., during the active phase of labor at 4 cm or greater dilation) for low risk women has been associated with an increased rate of spontaneous vaginal birth and fewer obstetric interventions (Jackson, Lang, Ecker, Swartz, & Heeren, 2003).

If the woman lives near the hospital and has adequate support and transportation, she may be asked to stay home or return home to allow labor to progress (i.e., until the uterine contractions are more frequent and intense). The ideal setting for the low risk woman at this time is the familiar environment of her home. The nurse can use a telephone interview (Box 21-1) to assess the woman's status, to give instructions regarding the optimal time for admission, to reinforce teaching regarding the signs that require immediate notification of the primary health care provider, and to box 21-1 **Telephone Interview with Woman in Latent Phase of Labor**

ASSESSMENTS

- Gather data regarding the woman's status, including signs and symptoms indicative of true or false labor.
- Discuss instructions given by the woman's primary health care provider regarding when to come for admission.

INTERVENTIONS

- Decide whether the woman will come for labor assessment and admission or be encouraged to stay at home until contractions increase in duration, frequency, and intensity.
- Assure the woman that she is welcome to call the perinatal unit at any time to discuss her labor status.
- Answer questions the woman and her family may have regarding labor or provide instruction as needed (e.g., which entrance of the hospital to enter).
- Suggest a variety of positions she can assume to maximally enhance uteroplacental and renal blood flow (e.g., side-lying position) and enhance the progress of labor (e.g., upright positions and ambulation).
- Suggest diversional activities, such as walking, reading, watching television, talking to friends.
- Suggest measures to maintain comfort, such as a warm shower, or back or foot massage.
- Discuss the oral intake of foods and fluids appropriate for early labor (light foods or fluids or clear liquids depending on the preference of her primary health care provider).
- Instruct the woman to come in immediately if membranes rupture, bleeding occurs, or fetal movements change.

EVALUATION

- Evaluate whether instructions and information have been understood by the woman by asking her to verbalize her understanding.

The woman who lives at a considerable distance from the hospital or who lacks adequate support and transportation may be admitted in early labor. The same measures used by the woman at home should be offered to the hospitalized woman in early labor.

▬ Admission to Labor Unit

When the woman arrives at the perinatal unit, assessment is the top priority (Fig. 21-1). The nurse first performs a screening assessment by using the techniques of interview and physical assessment and reviews the laboratory and diagnostic test findings to determine the health status of the woman and her fetus and the progress of her labor. The primary health care provider is notified, and if the woman is admitted, a detailed systems assessment is done.

▬ LEGAL TIP Obstetric Triage and EMTALA

The Emergency Medical Treatment and Active Labor Act (EMTALA) is a federal regulation enacted to ensure that a woman gets emergency treatment or active labor care whenever such treatment is sought. According to the EMTALA, true labor is considered to be an emergency medical condition. Nurses working in labor and birth units must be familiar with their responsibilities according to the EMTALA regulations, which include providing services to pregnant women when they experience an urgent pregnancy problem (e.g., labor, decreased fetal movement, rupture of membranes, recent trauma) and fully documenting all relevant information (e.g., assessment findings, interventions implemented, client responses to care measures provided). A pregnant woman presenting in an obstetric triage is considered to be in "true" labor until a qualified health care provider certifies that she is not. Agencies need to have specific policies and procedures in place so that compliance with the EMTALA regulations is achieved while safe and efficient care is provided (Angelini & Mahlmeister, 2005; Caliendo, Millbauer, Moore, & Kitchen, 2004).

provide support and encouragement. Measures the woman and her significant others can use to enhance the progress of labor, reduce anxiety, and maintain comfort should be described. The woman should be informed that she can call back at any time to report concerns she may have or to ask questions. This is especially important for the primigravida who may be very anxious and lack confidence in her ability to cope with labor (Albers, 2003).

A warm shower can be relaxing for the woman in early labor; however, warm baths should be avoided until the cervix is approximately 5 cm dilated, because water immersion in early labor could prolong the labor process and increase the probability of oxytocin use to stimulate uterine contractions and epidural analgesia for pain reduction (Mackey, 2001). Soothing back, foot, and hand massage or a warm drink of preferred liquids such as tea or milk can help the woman to rest and even to sleep, especially if false or early labor is occurring at night. Diversional activities such as walking outdoors or in the house, reading, watching television, doing needlework, or talking with friends can reduce the perception of early discomfort, help the time pass, and reduce anxiety.

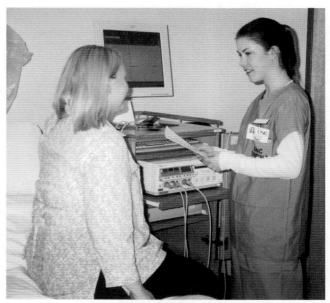

FIG. 21-1 Woman being assessed for admission to the labor and birth unit. (Courtesy Dee Lowdermilk, Chapel Hill, NC.)

When the woman is admitted, she usually is moved from an observation area to the labor room; the labor, delivery, and recovery (LDR) room; or the labor, delivery, recovery, and postpartum (LDRP) room. Because first impressions are important, the woman and her partner are welcomed by name and introduced to the staff members who will be involved in the woman's care. Women often express concern regarding the number of persons intruding on their labor experience, especially if the role of the person and purpose for his or her presence are not clearly identified (Hanson et al., 2001).

If the woman wishes, her partner is included in the assessment and admission process. Significant others not participating in this process may be directed to the appropriate waiting area, if that is the policy of the unit. Family-centered care is the trend in maternity today. This approach views labor as wellness and the woman and her support persons as active participants in the process of labor and birth. LDR or LDRP rooms are essential components of family-centered care, and the woman is encouraged to have anyone she wishes present for her support. After birth, the mother, baby, and support persons are permitted to stay together to celebrate the arrival of a new family member (Zwelling & Phillips, 2001).

The woman is asked to undress and put on her own gown or a hospital gown. An admissions band is placed on the woman's wrist and an allergy band (usually colored), if appropriate. Her personal belongings are put away safely or given to family members, according to agency policy. Often women who participate in expectant parents classes bring a birth bag or Lamaze bag with them. Tennis balls or rolling pins for counterpressure, a pillow for comfort and reminder of home, an object for a focal point (e.g., meaningful picture, stuffed animal), and rice bags for warm packs may be included in her bag. The woman and her partner are oriented to the layout and operation of the unit and room, including the use of the call light and telephone system, the location of personal storage areas in the bedside and over-the-bed tables, and how to adjust lighting in the room and the different positions of the bed.

The nurse reassures the woman and her partner that she is in competent, caring hands and that they can ask questions related to her care and her status and that of her fetus at any time during labor. The woman's anxiety can be minimized by explaining terms commonly used during labor. The woman's interest, response, and prior experience guide the depth of these explanations.

▪ Admission Data

Admission forms (Fig. 21-2) provide guidelines for the acquisition of important assessment information when a woman in labor is being evaluated or admitted. Additional sources of data include the prenatal record, the admission

FIG. 21-2 Obstetric admitting record. (Permission to use and/or reproduce this copyrighted material has been granted by the owner, Hollister, Inc., Libertyville, IL.)

interview, physical examination to determine baseline physiologic parameters (e.g., vital signs), laboratory and diagnostic test results, expressed psychosocial and cultural factors, and the clinical evaluation of labor status.

Prenatal Data. The nurse reviews the prenatal record to identify the woman's individual needs and risks. Complete information regarding a woman's prenatal health status is essential to ensure the quality and safety of the care provided to her and her fetus or newborn during labor and birth and in the postpartum period.

If the woman has not had any prenatal care or her prenatal record is unavailable, certain baseline information must be obtained. If the woman is having discomfort, the nurse should ask questions between contractions when the woman can concentrate more fully on her answers. At times the partner or support person(s) may need to be secondary sources of essential information.

It is important to know the woman's age so that the plan of care can be tailored to the needs of her age group. For example, a 14-year-old girl and a 40-year-old woman have different but specific needs, and their ages place them at risk for different problems. Height and weight relations are important to determine because a weight gain greater than that recommended may place the woman at a higher risk for cephalopelvic disproportion and cesarean birth. This is especially true for women who are petite and have gained 16 kg or more. Other factors to consider are the woman's general health status, current medical conditions or allergies, respiratory status, and previous surgical procedures.

Her obstetric and pregnancy history are carefully noted. These include gravidity, parity, and problems such as history of vaginal bleeding, gestational hypertension, anemia, pregestational or gestational diabetes, infections (e.g., bacterial or sexually transmitted), and immunodeficiency.

If this is not the woman's first labor and birth experience, it is important to note the characteristics of her previous experiences. This information includes the duration of previous labors, the type of anesthesia used, the kind of birth (e.g., spontaneous vaginal, forceps-assisted, vacuum-assisted, or cesarean birth) and the condition of the newborn. The woman's perception of her previous labor and birth experiences should be explored because it may influence her attitude toward her current experience. Women can retain long-term memories of their childbirth experiences. The memory of labor and birth events including her behavior and that of health care providers (e.g., physician, midwife, nurses, doula, partner) can affect a woman's postpartum emotional adjustment, self-esteem, and ability to parent effectively (Hanson et al., 2001).

It is important to confirm the expected date of birth (EDB). Other data in the prenatal record include patterns of maternal weight gain, physiologic measurements such as maternal vital signs (blood pressure, temperature, pulse, respirations); fundal height, baseline fetal heart rate (FHR), and laboratory and diagnostic test results. Laboratory tests include the woman's blood type and Rh factor, a complete or partial blood cell count (e.g., hemoglobin, hematocrit, white blood cell count, platelets), the 50-g blood glucose test, determination of the rubella titer, serologic tests (Venereal Disease Research Laboratories [VDRL] or rapid plasma reagin [RPR] test) for syphilis, hepatitis B surface antigen (HBsAg), culture for group B streptococcus, and urinalysis. Additional tests may include a tuberculosis screen with purified protein derivative (PPD), screening for the human immunodeficiency virus (HIV), and a screen for sickle cell trait or other genetic disorders (e.g., maternal serum alpha-fetoprotein). Diagnostic tests include amniocentesis, nonstress test (NST), contraction stress test (CST), biophysical profile (BPP), and ultrasound examination.

Interview. The woman's primary reason for coming to the hospital is determined in the interview. Her primary reason may be that her bag of waters (BOW, amniotic membranes) ruptured, with or without contractions. The woman may have come in for an obstetric check, which is a period of observation reserved for women who are unsure about the onset of their labor. This allows time on the unit for the diagnosis of labor without official admission and minimizes or avoids cost to the woman when used by the hospital and approved by her health insurance plan.

Even the experienced woman may have difficulty determining the onset of labor. The woman is asked to recall the events of the previous days and to describe the following:

- Time and onset of contractions and progress in terms of frequency, duration, and intensity
- Location and character of discomfort from contractions (e.g., back pain, suprapubic discomfort)
- Persistence of contractions despite changes in maternal position and activity (e.g., walking or lying down)
- Presence and character of vaginal discharge or show
- The status of amniotic membranes, such as a gush or seepage of fluid ([spontaneous] rupture of membranes [S][ROM]). If there has been a discharge that may be amniotic fluid, she is asked the date and time the fluid was first noted and the fluid's characteristics (e.g., amount, color, unusual odor). In many instances, a sterile speculum examination and a nitrazine (pH) or fern test can confirm that the membranes are ruptured (see Procedure box).

These descriptions help the nurse assess the degree of progress in the process of labor. Bloody or pink show is distinguished from bleeding by the fact that it is pink and feels sticky because of its mucoid nature. It is scant to begin with and increases with effacement and dilation of the cervix. A woman may report a scant brownish to bloody discharge that may be attributed to cervical trauma resulting from vaginal examination or coitus within the last 48 hours.

In case general anesthesia may be required in an emergency, it is important to assess the woman's respiratory status. The nurse determines this by asking the woman if she has a "cold" or related symptoms (e.g., "stuffy nose," sore throat, or cough). The status of allergies is

procedure

Tests for Rupture of Membranes

NITRAZINE TEST FOR pH

Explain procedure to woman/couple.

Procedure

- Wash hands.
- Use **nitrazine test** paper, a dye-impregnated test paper for determining pH (differentiates amniotic fluid, which is slightly alkaline, from urine and purulent material [pus], which are acidic).
- Wearing a sterile glove lubricated with water, place a piece of test paper at the cervical os.

OR

- Use a sterile, cotton-tipped applicator to dip deep into vagina to pick up fluid; touch applicator to test paper. (Procedure may be done during speculum examination.)

Read results:

- Membranes probably intact: identifies vaginal and most body fluids that are acidic:

Yellow	pH 5.0
Olive-yellow	pH 5.5
Olive-green	pH 6.0

- Membranes probably ruptured: identifies amniotic fluid that is alkaline:

Blue-green	pH 6.5
Blue-gray	pH 7.0
Deep blue	pH 7.5

- Realize that false test results are possible because of presence of bloody show, insufficient amniotic fluid, or semen.
- Provide pericare as needed.
- Remove gloves and wash hands.

Document Results

- Positive or negative

TEST FOR FERNING OR FERN PATTERN

- Explain procedure to woman/couple.
- Wash hands, apply sterile gloves, obtain specimen of fluid (usually during sterile speculum examination).
- Spread a drop of fluid from vagina on a clean glass slide with a sterile, cotton-tipped applicator.
- Allow fluid to dry.
- Examine slide under microscope: observe for appearance of **ferning** (a frondlike crystalline pattern) (do not confuse with cervical mucus test, when high levels of estrogen cause the ferning).
- Observe for absence of ferning (alerts staff to possibility that amount of specimen was inadequate or that specimen was urine, vaginal discharge, or blood).
- Provide pericare as needed.
- Remove gloves and wash hands.

Document Results

- Positive or negative

rechecked, including allergies to medications routinely used in obstetrics, such as opioids (e.g., hydromorphone [Dilaudid], butorphanol tartrate [Stadol], fentanyl [Sublimaze], nalbuphine [Nubain]), anesthetic agents (e.g., bupivacaine, lidocaine, ropivacaine), and antiseptics (Betadine). Some allergic responses cause swelling of the mucous membranes of the respiratory tract, which could interfere with breathing and the administration of inhalation anesthesia.

Because vomiting and subsequent aspiration into the respiratory tract can complicate an otherwise normal labor, the nurse records the time and type of the woman's most recent solid and liquid intake.

Any information not found in the prenatal record is obtained during the admission assessment. Pertinent data include the birth plan (Box 21-2), the choice of infant feeding method, the type of pain management preferred, and the name of the pediatric health care provider. A client profile is obtained that identifies the woman's preparation for childbirth, the support person or family members desired during childbirth and their availability, and ethnic or cultural expectations and needs. The woman's use of alcohol, drugs, and tobacco before or during pregnancy should be determined. Screening of the neonate for substances abused by the mother may be required. After birth, the nurse should assess the neonate for signs indicating maternal substance use during pregnancy (e.g., abstinence syndrome, size, and appearance).

The nurse reviews the birth plan; if no written plan has been prepared, the nurse helps the woman formulate

---

box 21-2 | The Birth Plan

The birth plan should include the woman's/couple's preferences related to the following:

- Presence of birth companions such as the partner, older children, parents, friends, or a doula, and the role each will play
- Presence of other persons such as students, male attendants, and interpreters
- Clothing to be worn
- Environmental modifications such as lighting, music, privacy, focal point, items from home such as pillows
- Labor activities such as preferred positions for labor and for birth, ambulation, birth balls, showers and whirlpool baths, and oral food and fluid intake
- Repertoire of comfort and relaxation measures
- Labor and birth medical interventions such as pharmacologic pain relief measures, intravenous therapy, electronic monitoring, induction or augmentation measures, and episiotomy
- Care and handling of the newborn immediately after birth such as cutting of the cord, eye care, and breastfeeding
- Cultural and religious requirements related to the care of the mother, newborn, and placenta

The childbirth.org website (**www.childbirth.org**) provides couples with an interactive birth plan along with examples of birth plans.

a birth plan by describing options available and finds out the woman's wishes and preferences. The nurse prepares the woman for the possibility that changes may be needed in her plan as labor progresses and assures her that information will be provided so that she can make informed decisions. The nurse uses the information in the birth plan to individualize the care given the woman during labor.

The nurse should discuss with the woman and her partner their plans for preserving childbirth memories by using photography and videotaping and provide information about the agency's policies regarding these practices and under what circumstances they are allowed. Protection of privacy and safety (e.g., flash photography in the presence of combustible gases) and infection control (e.g., where the person who is recording the event should stand) are major concerns for the parents-to-be and the agency. The woman's record should reflect that the childbirth was recorded.

Psychosocial Factors. The woman's general appearance and behavior (and that of her partner) provide valuable clues to the type of supportive care she will need. However, the nurse should keep in mind that general appearance and behavior may vary, depending on the stage and phase of labor (Table 21-1). Psychosocial factors to assess include the following:

Verbal interactions: Does the woman ask questions? Can she ask for what she needs? Does she talk to her support person(s)? Does she talk freely with the nurse or respond only to questions?

Body language: Is she relaxed or tense? What is her anxiety level? How does she react to being touched by the nurse or support person? Does she change positions or lie rigidly still? Does she avoid eye contact? Does she look tired? How much rest has she had during the past 24 hours?

Perceptual ability: Does she understand what the nurse says? Is there a language barrier? Are repeated explanations necessary because her anxiety level interferes with her ability to comprehend? Can she repeat what she has been told or demonstrate her understanding?

Discomfort level: To what degree does the woman describe what she is experiencing? How does she react to a contraction? Are any nonverbal pain messages seen? Does she complain to the nurse or her partner? Can she ask for comfort measures?

Women with a History of Sexual Abuse. Memories of sexual abuse can be triggered during labor by intrusive procedures such as vaginal examinations; loss of control; feeling helpless and isolated in a strange environment; being unable to move freely as a result of being confined to bed and "restrained" by monitors, intravenous (IV) lines, and epidurals; being watched by students; and having intense sensations in the uterus and genital area, especially at the time when she must push the baby out. Women who are abuse survivors may fight the labor process by reacting in panic or anger toward care providers, may take control of everyone and everything related to their childbirth, may surrender by being submissive and dependent, or may retreat by mentally dissociating themselves from the sensations of labor and birth (Hobbins, 2004; Simkin & Klaus, 2004).

The nurse can help these women to associate the sensations they are experiencing with the process of childbirth and not with their past abuse. The woman's sense of control should be maintained by explaining all procedures and why they are needed, validating her needs and paying close attention to her requests, proceeding at the woman's pace by waiting for her to give permission to touch her, accepting her often extreme reactions to labor, and protecting her privacy by limiting the amount of exposure of her body and the number of persons involved in her care. The nurse should avoid words and phrases that could cause the woman to recall the words of her abuser (e.g., "open your legs," "relax and it won't hurt so much"). The number of procedures that invade her body (e.g., vaginal examinations, urinary catheter, internal monitor, forceps or vacuum extractor) should be limited as much as possible. She should also be encouraged to choose a person (e.g., doula, friend, family member) to be with her during labor to provide continuous support and comfort and to act as her advocate. It is recommended that all laboring women be cared for in this manner, because it is not unusual for a woman to choose not to reveal a history of sexual abuse. These care measures can help a woman to perceive her childbirth experience in positive terms and to parent her new baby effectively (Hobbins, 2004; Simpkin & Klaus, 2004).

Stress in Labor. The way in which women and their support person or family members approach labor is related to the manner in which they have been socialized to the childbearing process. Their reactions reflect their life experiences regarding childbirth—physical, social, cultural, and religious. Society communicates its expectations regarding acceptable and unacceptable maternal behaviors during labor and birth. These expectations may be used by some women as the basis for evaluating their own actions during childbirth. An idealized perception of labor and birth may be a source of guilt and a sense of failure if the woman finds the process less than joyous, especially when the pregnancy is unplanned or is the product of a shaky or terminated relationship. Often women have heard horror stories or have seen friends or relatives going through labors that appear anything but easy. Multiparous women will often base their expectations of the present labor on their previous childbirth experiences.

Feelings a woman has about her pregnancy and fears regarding childbirth should be discussed. This is especially important if the woman is a primigravida who has not attended childbirth classes or is a multiparous woman who

table 21-1 Woman's Responses and Support Person's Actions During First Stage of Labor

WOMAN'S RESPONSES	NURSE OR SUPPORT PERSON'S ACTIONS*
DILATION OF CERVIX 0-3 CM (LATENT) (contractions 30-45 sec long, 5-30 min apart, mild to moderate)	
Mood: alert, happy, excited, mild anxiety	Provides encouragement, feedback for relaxation, companionship
Settles into labor room; selects focal point	Assists woman to cope with contractions
Rests or sleeps, if possible	Encourages use of focusing techniques
Uses breathing techniques	Helps to concentrate on breathing techniques
Uses effleurage, focusing, and relaxation techniques	Uses comfort measures
	Assists woman into comfortable position
	Informs woman of progress; explains procedures and routines
	Gives praise
	Offers fluids, food, ice chips as ordered
DILATION OF CERVIX 4-7 CM (ACTIVE) (contractions 40-70 sec long, 3-5 min apart, moderate to strong)	
Mood: seriously labor-oriented, concentration and energy needed for contractions, alert, more demanding	Acts as buffer; limits assessment techniques to between contractions
Continues relaxation, focusing techniques	Assists woman to cope with contractions
Uses breathing techniques	Encourages woman as needed to help her maintain breathing techniques
	Uses comfort measures
	Assists with frequent position changes, emphasizing side-lying and upright positions
	Encourages voluntary relaxation of muscles of back, buttocks, thighs, and perineum; performs effleurage
	Applies counterpressure to sacrococcygeal area
	Encourages and praises
	Keeps woman aware of progress
	Offers analgesics as ordered
	Checks bladder; encourages her to void
	Gives oral care; offers fluids, food, ice chips as ordered
DILATION OF CERVIX 8-10 CM (TRANSITION) (contractions 45-90 sec long, 2-3 min apart, strong)	
Mood: irritable, intense concentration, symptoms of transition (e.g., nausea, vomiting)	Stays with woman; provides constant support
Continues relaxation, needs greater concentration to do this	Assists woman to cope with contractions
Uses breathing techniques	Reminds, reassures, and encourages woman to reestablish breathing pattern and concentration as needed
If needed, changes to pattern-paced breathing (i.e., 4:1 breathing pattern) if using psychoprophylactic techniques	Alerts woman to begin breathing pattern before contraction becomes too intense
Uses panting to overcome urge to push if appropriate	Prompts panting respirations if woman begins to push prematurely
	Uses comfort measures
	Accepts woman's inability to comply with instructions
	Accepts irritable response to helping, such as counterpressure
	Supports woman who has nausea and vomiting; gives oral care as needed; gives reassurance regarding signs of end of first stage
	Uses relaxation techniques (effleurage and voluntary relaxation)
	Keeps woman aware of progress

*Provided by nurses and support persons in collaboration with the nurse.

has had a previous negative childbirth experience. Major fears and concerns relate to the process and effects of childbirth, maternal and fetal well-being, and the attitude and actions of the health care staff. Unresolved fears increase a woman's stress and can inhibit the process of labor as a result of the inhibiting effects of catecholamines associated with the stress response on uterine contractions (Melender, 2002).

Women in labor usually have a variety of concerns that they will voice if asked but rarely volunteer. It is important to ask the woman what she expects or to suggest that the woman ask her primary health care provider about an issue. The following are common concerns of women in labor: Will my baby be all right? Will I be able to stand labor? Will my labor be long? How will I act? Will I need medication? Will it work for me? Will my partner or someone be there to support me?

The nurse's responsibility to the woman in labor with regard to these concerns is to answer her questions or find out the answers, to provide support for her and her support person or family, to take care of her in partnership with those persons the woman wants as her support team, and to serve as their advocate. Women may equate emotional support with information giving. Nurses are perceived as supportive when they explain things in detail by using positive terms and provide accurate information and specific directions. Women feel empowered when they are given information they can understand and that shows support for their efforts. This feeling of empowerment gives women the sense that they have the freedom to participate fully in their labor and birth and fosters a positive perception of the experience. In contrast, a woman's level of anxiety and fear may increase when she does not understand what is being said. The woman who is unfamiliar with expressions such as "bloody show," "the membranes ruptured," "scalp electrode," and "baby's lying on the cord" could panic. Many such expressions sound violent and could conjure up thoughts of injury or pain.

The nurse communicates to the woman that she is not expected to act in any particular way and that the process will end in the birth of her baby, which is the only expectation she should have. Women need to be able to behave in a manner that is natural for them and be able to "let go." The woman's views and expectations regarding the nurse's role as caregiver should be determined. The nurse-client relationship will become increasingly important as labor progresses. Women need to trust in their own innate ability to give birth. Nurses need to support and protect the woman's efforts to achieve this outcome (Lothian, 2001).

Women prepare themselves for labor in a variety of ways. Some go to childbirth education classes, some read books and talk to friends and relatives about childbirth, and some prepare elaborate birth plans spelling out their wishes for labor and birth. The longer the list of "wishes," however, the greater the likelihood that expectations will not be met. It is the nurse's responsibility to integrate the woman's desires into the plan of care as much as possible. The nurse can help make sure various aspects of the birth plan are observed by reviewing the plan with the physician or midwife and telling the woman to remind her primary health provider in advance about what she wants.

The father, coach, or significant other(s) also experiences stress during labor. The nurse can assist and support these individuals by identifying their needs and expectations and by helping make sure these are met. The nurse can ascertain what role the support person intends to fulfill and whether he or she is prepared for that role by asking such questions as, "Has the couple attended childbirth classes?" "What role does this person expect to play?" and by making observations such as "Does he or she do all the talking?" "Is he or she nervous, anxious, aggressive, or hostile?" "Does he or she look hungry, tired, worried, or confused?" "Does he or she watch television, sleep, or stay out of the room instead of paying attention to the woman?" "Where does he or she sit?" "Does he or she touch the woman; what is the character of the touch?" Often the support this person is able to give the laboring woman is in direct proportion to the support he or she receives from the nurses and other health care providers.

Cultural Factors. As the population in the United States and Canada becomes more diverse, it is increasingly important to recognize a pregnant woman's ethnic (cultural) and religious values, beliefs, and practices in order to anticipate nursing interventions that should be included in a mutually acceptable plan of care that facilitates a feeling of safety and control. Nurses should be committed to providing culturally sensitive care and to developing an appreciation and respect for cultural diversity (Callister, 2005). The woman should be encouraged to request specific caregiving behaviors and practices that are important to her. If a special request contradicts usual practices in that setting, the woman or the nurse can ask the woman's primary health care provider to write an order to accommodate the special request. For example, in many cultures, it is unacceptable to have a male caregiver examine a pregnant woman. In some cultures, it is traditional to take the placenta home; in others, the woman is given only certain nourishments during labor. Some women believe that cutting her body, as with an episiotomy, allows her spirit to leave her body and that rupturing the membranes prolongs, not shortens, labor. It is important that the rationale for required care measures be carefully explained (Mattson, 2000) (see Cultural Considerations box).

cultural considerations

Birth Practices in Different Cultures

SOUTH KOREA
Stoic response to labor pain; fathers usually not present

JAPAN
Natural childbirth methods practiced; may labor silently; may eat during labor; father may be present

CHINA
Stoic response to pain; fathers usually not present; side-lying position preferred for labor and birth, because this position is thought to reduce infant trauma

INDIA
Natural childbirth methods preferred; father is usually not present; female relatives usually present

IRAN
Father not present; prefers female support and female caregivers

MEXICO
May be stoic about discomfort until second stage, then may request pain relief; fathers and female relatives may be present

LAOS
May use squatting position for birth; fathers may or may not be present; prefer female attendants

From D'Avanzo, C., & Geissler, E. (2003). *Pocket guide to cultural health assessment* (3rd ed.). St. Louis: Mosby.

Cultural beliefs and values can influence a woman's reliance on her primary health care provider during labor as well as her desire to participate in making decisions about the care she receives (Callister, 2005). It may be noted that a Japanese woman in labor may assume the traditional role of a "passive client" and may be reluctant to express her needs unless specifically asked to do so (Ito & Sharts-Hopko, 2002). Native American women, who view childbirth as a natural event, may find the high-technology environment of a hospital frightening and a disruption of the balance and harmony that are critical for a positive birth experience. They often prefer to be surrounded by a large number of family members, especially the grandparents, and become anxious in the presence of a large number of health care providers who come into the labor room and loudly discuss the progress of labor with each other (Molina, 2001). During contractions, a Navajo woman may wish to pull on a rope or sash belt that is suspended from the ceiling (Fig. 21-3). As the woman pulls on the rope, a caring person chosen by the woman (e.g., her husband, mother, or other female companion) sits, kneels, or stands behind her and holds her tight under her breasts and over her pregnant abdomen to support her in an upright position and to provide warmth against her back (Begay, 2004). Chinese women who believe in the balance of *yin-yang* view childbirth as a source of heat loss from the body. Providing hot fluids and a warm shower to these women during labor would be measures they would accept as a means of restoring the heat that is being lost (Cioffi, 2004).

In assessing a woman's cultural and religious preferences, Callister (1995) suggests that the nurse ask questions regarding the following:

• Value and meaning placed on the childbirth experience
• View of childbirth as a wellness or illness experience and as a private or social event
• Practices regarding diet, medications, activity, and emotional and physical support
• Appropriate maternal and paternal behaviors
• Birth companions—who they should be and what they should do
• Views regarding the newborn and the newborn's care immediately after birth

Within cultures, women may have the "right" way to behave in labor instilled in them and may react to the pain experienced in that way. These behaviors can range from total silence to moaning or screaming, but they are not in and of themselves a gauge of the degree of pain. A woman who moans with contractions may not be in as much physical pain as a woman who is silent but winces during contractions (Table 21-2). Chinese women, for example may be stoic and quiet during labor and may merely grimace during a contraction but not shout out. Rather than using pharmacologic measures for pain relief, they may prefer the support of family members and nonpharmacologic measures (Brathwaite & Williams, 2004; Cioffi, 2004). Some women feel it is shameful to scream or cry

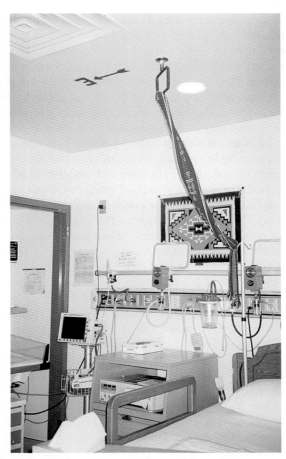

FIG. 21-3 Birthing room specific to a Native-American population. Note the arrow pointing east, the rug on the wall, and the rope or sash belt hanging from the ceiling. (Courtesy Patricia Hess, San Francisco, CA; Chinle Comprehensive Health Care Center, Chinle, AZ.)

out in pain if a man is present. If the woman's support person is her mother, she may perceive the need to "behave" more strongly than if her support person is the father of the baby. She will perceive herself as failing or succeeding on the basis of her ability to adhere to these "standards" of behavior. Conversely, a woman's behavior in response to pain may influence the support received from significant others. In some cultures, women who lose control and cry out in pain may be scolded, whereas in other cultures, support persons will become more helpful (D'Avanzo & Geissler, 2003).

Culture and Father Participation. A companion is an important source of support, encouragement, and comfort for women during childbirth. The nurse managing the care of pregnant women should help these women identify the person or persons they wish to be their supportive companions during childbirth. The choice of birth companion is influenced by the woman's cultural and religious background and by trends in the society in which she lives. For example, in Western societies, the father is viewed as the ideal birth companion. For European-

table 21-2 Sociocultural Basis of Pain Experience

WOMAN IN LABOR	NURSE
PERCEPTION OF MEANING	
Origin: Cultural concept of and personal experience with pain; for example: Pain in childbirth is inevitable, something to be endured. Pain in childbirth can be avoided completely. Pain in childbirth is punishment for sin. Pain in childbirth can be controlled.	Origin: Cultural concept of and personal experience with pain; in addition, nurse becomes accustomed to working with certain "expected" pain trajectories. For example, in obstetrics, pain is expected to increase as labor progresses, be intermittent, and have an end point; relief can be derived from medications once labor is well established and fetus or newborn can cope with amount and elimination of medications; relief can also come from woman's knowledge, attitude, and support from family or friends.
COPING MECHANISMS	
Woman may exhibit the following behaviors: Be traditionally vocal or nonvocal; crying out or groaning, or both, may be part of her ritual response to pain Use counterstimulation to minimize pain (e.g., rubbing, applying heat, or applying counterpressure) Use relaxation, distraction, or autosuggestion as pain-countering techniques Resist any use of "needles" as modes of administering pain-relief agents	Nurse may respond by: Using physical factors effectively (e.g., using tone of voice, closeness in space, and touch as media for conveying message of interest and caring) Using avoidance, belittling, or other distracting actions as protective device for self Offering comfort measures and other nonpharmacologic methods of pain relief Using pharmacologic resources at hand judiciously Assuming accountability for control and management of pain
EXPECTATIONS OF OTHERS	
Nurse may be seen as someone who will accept woman's statement of pain and act as her advocate. Medical personnel may be expected to relieve woman of all pain sensations. Nurse may be expected to be interested, gentle, kind, and accepting of behavior exhibited.	Only certain verbal or nonverbal responses to pain may be accepted as appropriate responses. Couple that is prepared for childbirth may be expected to refuse medication and to wish to "do everything on their own." Woman's definition of pain may not be accepted; that is, woman may wish to experience and participate in controlling pain or may not be able to accept any pain as reasonable.

American couples, attending childbirth classes together has become a traditional, expected activity. Laotian (Hmong) husbands traditionally participate actively in the labor process, often by supporting their wife's position, catching the baby as it emerges, cutting the cord, and burying the placenta. A Mormon woman expects her husband to be present during her labor and to lay his hands on her head in a blessing that imparts strength, comfort, and well-being for safe passage through childbirth (Callister, 1995). In some cultures, the father may be available, but his presence in the labor room with the mother may not be considered appropriate, or he may be present but resist active involvement in her care. Such behavior could be misconstrued by the nursing staff to represent a lack of concern, caring, or interest. Latina women expect their male partner to be present at their bedside during labor, to talk to them, keep them calm, and tell them everything is going to be okay and not to worry. The men are expected to show love and affection by telling the women they love them, by hugging them, and by holding their hands. However, Latino men do not become actively involved in giving their partners care during labor by performing such activities as backrubs

and helping with pushing (Khazoyan & Anderson, 1994). Mexican-American and Filipina women share an affectional bond with their female relatives when it comes to home-related activities such as childbearing. This also is true for the women of many other cultural groups. The presence of another woman or women is highly desired at such occasions. Women who come from some of these cultures and who give birth in the hospital like to have at least one woman present for assistance. Vietnamese, Chinese, Indian, Syrian, and Orthodox Jewish women prefer a female companion during childbirth and are very concerned about their modesty. In addition to feeling shy, they cite the belief that female caregivers are more respectful and would provide a higher degree of comfort and psychosocial support (Bashour & Abdulsalam, 2005; Choudhry, 1997; D'Avanzo & Geissler, 2003). Islamic women also are very modest (i.e., need to keep hair and body covered) and would not accept the presence of a man during childbirth, not even the father. The religious beliefs of some Orthodox Jews forbid the father to touch his wife during labor or to be present at the birth. Instead, while he prays, the female members of the laboring woman's family act as supportive childbirth companions.

If an unexpected intervention is required, the woman may need to wait to give consent until her husband consults with their rabbi (Callister, 1995; Semenic, Callister, & Feldman, 2004). In India, women are attended by other women, and in rural areas, by a local untrained midwife or *dai*. Men usually are not present and in some cases may not be allowed to see the face of their child until certain prayers are said or an astrologically appropriate time is reached (Choudhry, 1997). If couples from these cultures immigrate to the United States or Canada, their roles may change. The nurse will need to talk to the woman and her support persons to determine the roles they will assume.

The Non–English-Speaking Woman in Labor. A woman's level of anxiety in labor increases when she does not understand what is happening to her or what is being said. Some misunderstanding may occur with English-speaking women and cause some stress, but the effect of misunderstanding on non–English-speaking women is much more dramatic. These women often feel a complete loss of control over their situation if no health care provider is present who speaks their language. They can panic and withdraw or become physically abusive when someone tries to do something they perceive might harm them or their babies. Sometimes a support person is able to serve as an interpreter. However, this must be done with caution because the interpreter may not be able to convey exactly what the nurse or others are saying or what the woman is saying, which can increase the woman's stress level even more.

Ideally, a bilingual nurse will care for the woman. Alternatively, an employee or volunteer interpreter may be contacted for assistance (see Box 2-1). Preferably, the interpreter is from the woman's culture. For some women, a female interpreter may be more acceptable. If no one in the hospital is able to interpret, a service can be called so that interpretation can take place over the telephone. Another alternative is for the labor and birth unit staff to prepare a set of cards with graphic illustrations that depict common situations. These cards can be used to communicate with non–English-speaking women. Even when the nurse has limited ability to communicate verbally with the woman, in most instances, the nurse's efforts to communicate are meaningful and appreciated by the woman. Speaking slowly and avoiding complex words and medical terms can help a woman and her partner to understand (Mattson, 2000).

▬ Physical Examination

The initial physical examination includes a general systems assessment; performance of Leopold maneuvers to determine fetal presentation and position and the point of maximal intensity (PMI) for auscultating the FHR; assessment of fetal status; assessment of uterine contractions; and vaginal examination to assess the status of cervical effacement and dilation, fetal descent, and amniotic membranes and fluid. The findings of the admission physical examination serve as a baseline for assessing the woman's progress from that point.

It is important to obtain as many related pieces of information as possible before planning and implementing care. Women often focus on the nature of their contractions as the clearest indicator of how far advanced their labor is. However, the findings from the vaginal examination are more valid indicators of the phase of labor, especially for nulliparous women.

Expected maternal progress and minimal assessment guidelines during the first stage of labor are presented in Table 21-3 and the Care Path for the low risk woman in the first stage of labor.

The assessment procedures described in the following paragraphs can be used as a basis for teaching women and their significant others. The equipment needed, the nursing actions involved, and the rationale for each procedure should be discussed with the woman. Standard Precautions should guide all assessment and care measures (Box 21-3). Hand hygiene (e.g., washing hands with soap, application of an alcohol-based antiseptic rub) before and after

box 21-3 Standard Precautions During Childbirth

Birth is a time when nurses and other health care providers are exposed to a great deal of maternal and newborn blood and body fluids. Observation of Standard Precautions is necessary to prevent the transmission of infection. Perinatal infections most often are transmitted through contact with body fluids. The Standard Precautions applicable to childbirth include the following:

- Wash hands before and after putting on gloves and performing procedures.
- Wear gloves (clean or sterile, as appropriate) when performing procedures that require contact with the woman's genitalia and body fluids, including bloody show (e.g., during vaginal examination, amniotomy, hygienic care of the perineum, insertion of an internal scalp electrode and intrauterine pressure monitor, and catheterization).
- Wear a mask that has a shield or protective eyewear, and cover gown when assisting with the birth. Cap and shoe covers are worn for cesarean birth but are optional for vaginal birth in a birthing room. Gowns worn by the primary health care provider who is attending the birth should have a waterproof front and sleeves and should be sterile.
- Drape the woman with sterile towels and sheets as appropriate. Explain to the woman what can and cannot be touched.
- Help the woman's partner put on appropriate coverings for the type of birth, such as cap, mask, gown, and shoe covers. Show the partner where to stand and what can and cannot be touched.
- Wear gloves and gown when handling the newborn immediately after birth.
- Use an appropriate method to suction the newborn's airway, such as a bulb syringe, mechanical wall suction, or De Lee oral suction device that prevents the newborn's mucus from getting into the user's mouth or airway.

CD: Spanish Guidelines

table 21-3 **Expected Maternal Progress in First Stage of Labor**

	PHASES MARKED BY CERVICAL DILATION*		
CRITERION	**LATENT (0-3 CM)**	**ACTIVE (4-7 CM)**	**TRANSITION (8-10 CM)**
Duration†	About 6-8 hr	About 3-6 hr	About 20-40 min
Contractions			
Strength	Mild to moderate	Moderate to strong	Strong to very strong
Rhythm	Irregular	More regular	Regular
Frequency	5-30 min apart	3-5 min apart	2-3 min apart
Duration	30-45 sec	40-70 sec	45-90 sec
Descent			
Station of presenting part	Nulliparous: 0	Varies: +1 to +2 cm	Varies: +2 to +3 cm
Show	Multiparous: −2 cm to 0	Varies: +1 to +2 cm	Varies: +2 to +3 cm
Color	Brownish discharge, mucous plug, or pale pink mucus	Pink to bloody mucus	Bloody mucus
Amount	Scant	Scant to moderate	Copious
Behavior and appearance‡	Excited; thoughts center on self, labor, and baby; may be talkative or silent, calm or tense; some apprehension; pain controlled fairly well; alert, follows directions readily; open to instructions	Becomes more serious, doubtful of control of pain, more apprehensive; desires companionship and encouragement; attention more inwardly directed; fatigue evidenced; malar (cheeks) flush; has some difficulty following directions	Pain described as severe; backache common; frustration, fear of loss of control, and irritability may be voiced; vague in communications; amnesia between contractions; writhing with contractions; nausea and vomiting, especially if hyperventilating; hyperesthesia; circumoral pallor, perspiration of forehead and upper lips; shaking tremor of thighs; feeling of need to defecate, pressure on anus

*In the nullipara, effacement is often complete before dilation begins; in the multipara, it occurs simultaneously with dilation.
†Duration of each phase is influenced by such factors as parity, maternal emotions, position, level of activity, and fetal size, presentation, and position. For example, the labor of a nullipara tends to last longer, on average, than the labor of a multipara. Women who ambulate and assume upright positions or change positions frequently during labor tend to experience a shorter first stage. Descent is often prolonged in breech presentations and occiput posterior positions.
‡Women who have epidural analgesia for pain relief may not demonstrate some of these behaviors.

assessing the woman and providing care is a critical step in the prevention of infection transmission. The assessment findings are explained to the woman whenever possible. Throughout labor, accurate documentation, following agency policy, is done as soon as possible after a procedure has been performed (Fig. 21-4).

General Systems Assessment. A brief systems assessment is performed. This includes an assessment of the heart, lungs, and skin; an examination to determine the presence and extent of edema of the legs, the face, the hands, and the sacrum; and testing of deep tendon reflexes and for clonus.

Vital Signs. Vital signs (temperature, pulse, respirations, and blood pressure) are assessed on admission, and the initial values are used as the baseline for comparison with subsequent values. If the blood pressure is elevated, it should be reassessed 30 minutes later, between contractions, using a correct-size blood pressure cuff to obtain a reading after the woman has relaxed. To prevent supine

hypotension and fetal distress, the woman should be encouraged to lie on her side and not supine (Fig. 21-5). Her temperature is assessed so that signs of infection or a fluid deficit (e.g., dehydration associated with inadequate intake of fluids) can be identified. The woman's intake and output should be monitored. When appropriate, urinary protein and ketone levels may be determined by using a dipstick.

■ NURSE ALERT

During labor, blood pressures should be assessed using a sphygmomanometer and stethoscope for the most accurate results. Automatic devices that measure blood pressure have been found to overestimate the systolic pressure and underestimate the diastolic pressure. These devices further restrict freedom of movement and may also increase the discomfort of the woman as the cuff inflates and deflates on a regular basis. Maternal heart rate should be assessed by auscultation (i.e., apical rate) or by palpation (i.e., radial pulse rate) rather than using a pulse oximeter (Simpson, 2005).

care path ⟩	Low Risk Woman in First Stage of Labor		

	CERVICAL DILATION		
CARE MANAGEMENT	**0-3 CM (LATENT)**	**4-7 CM (ACTIVE)**	**8-10 CM (TRANSITION)**
I. ASSESSMENT MEASURES*	**Frequency**	**Frequency**	**Frequency**
• Blood pressure, pulse, respirations	Every 30-60 min	Every 30 min	Every 15-30 min
• Temperature†	Every 4 hr	Every 4 hr	Every 4 hr
• Uterine activity	Every 30-60 min	Every 15-30 min	Every 10-15 min
• Fetal heart rate (FHR)	Every 30-60 min	Every 15-30 min	Every 15-30 min
• Vaginal show	Every 30-60 min	Every 30 min	Every 15 min
• Behavior, appearance, mood, energy level of woman; condition of partner	Every 30 min	Every 15 min	Every 5 min
• Vaginal examination‡	As needed to identify progress	As needed to identify progress	As needed to identify progress
II. PHYSICAL CARE MEASURES§	Stay at home for as long as possible Relaxation measures; rest and sleep if at night Activity—ambulation; emphasize upright positions Diversional activities Nourishment—light foods and full liquids Encourage to void every 2 hr Perform basic hygiene measures	Coach breathing techniques Encourage effleurage Assist in using relaxation techniques between contractions Encourage ambulation, upright positions Assist with position changes Use comfort measures desired by woman: massage, hot or cold packs, touch, etc. Initiate hydrotherapy (shower, bath, Jacuzzi) Provide nourishment as desired Encourage voiding every 2 hr Assist with hygiene, perineal care Provide pharmacologic pain relief as requested by the woman and ordered by the primary health care provider Provide relief for partner	Coach breathing techniques Reduce touch if increased sensitivity is noted Help to relax between contractions Assist with position changes Use comfort measures according to acceptance level Continue hydrotherapy if effective Provide clear liquids: sips, ice chips Encourage voiding every 2 hr Provide hygiene measures, emphasizing mouth and perineal care Provide pharmacologic pain relief as requested by the woman and ordered by the primary health care provider Prepare for birth
III. EMOTIONAL SUPPORT	Review birth plan Review process of labor—what to expect, pain management techniques available Re-demonstrate breathing techniques Keep informed: progress, procedures	Provide feedback about performance Reduce distractions during contractions Role model comfort measures Reassure, encourage, praise Take charge, talk through contraction until control regained Continue to keep informed	Provide continuous support Reduce distractions Role model care measures to assist partner Continue reassurance, praise, and encouragement Keep informed Take charge as needed

*Full assessment using interview, physical examination, and laboratory testing is performed on admission. Subsequently, frequency of assessment is determined by the risk status of the maternal-fetal unit. More frequent assessment is required in high risk situations. Frequency of assessment and method of documentation are also determined by agency policy, which is usually based on the recommended care standards of medical and nursing organizations.

†If membranes have ruptured, the temperature should be assessed every 1 to 2 hr; assess orally or tympanically between contractions.

‡Perform vaginal examination at admission and thereafter only when signs indicate that progress has occurred (e.g., significant increase in frequency, duration, and intensity of contractions; rupture of membranes; perineal pressure); strict aseptic technique should be used. In the presence of vaginal bleeding, the primary health care provider performs the examination under a double setup in a delivery room, or an ultrasonography is performed to determine placental location.

§Physical care measures are performed by the nurse working together with the woman's partner and significant others. The woman is capable of greater independence in the latent phase but needs more assistance during the active and transition phases.

FIG. 21-4 Labor progress chart. (Permission to use and/or reproduce this copyrighted material has been granted by the owner, Hollister, Inc., Libertyville, IL.)

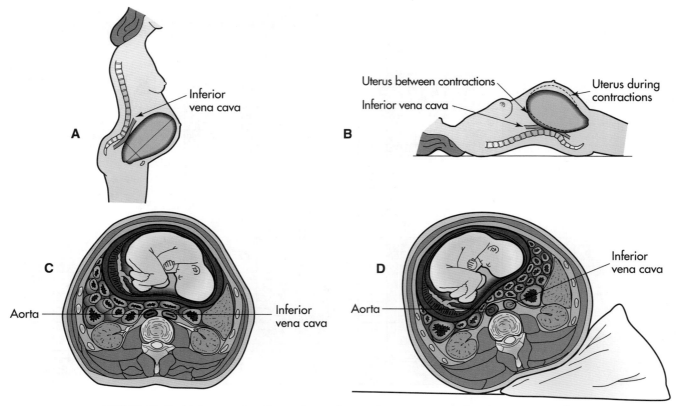

FIG. 21-5 Supine hypotension. Note relation of pregnant uterus to ascending vena cava in standing position **(A)**, and in the supine position **(B). C,** Compression of aorta and inferior vena cava with woman in supine position. **D,** Compression of these vessels is relieved by placement of a wedge pillow under the woman's right side.

CD: Assessment Video: Leopold Maneuvers

Leopold Maneuvers (Abdominal Palpation). Leopold maneuvers are performed with the woman briefly lying on her back (see Procedure box [Leopold maneuvers]). These maneuvers help identify the number of fetuses; the presenting part, fetal lie, and fetal attitude; the degree of the presenting part's descent into the pelvis; and the expected location of the point of maximum intensity (PMI) of the fetal heart rate (FHR) on the woman's abdomen.

Assessment of Fetal Heart Rate and Pattern. It is important for the nurse to understand the relation between the location of the PMI of the FHR and fetal presentation, lie, and position. A risk for childbirth complications may be revealed by variations in these findings. The PMI of the FHR is the location on the maternal abdomen where the FHR is heard the loudest (see Procedure Box [Finding PMI]). It is usually directly over the fetal back. The PMI also is an aid in determining the fetal presentation and position (Fig. 21-6). In a vertex presentation, the FHR is usually heard below the mother's umbilicus in either the right or left lower quadrant of the abdomen; in a breech presentation, the FHR is usually heard above the mother's umbilicus (Fig. 21-6, *A*, and Fig. 21-7, *C*). As the fetus descends and rotates internally, the FHR is heard lower and closer to the midline of the maternal abdomen. The PMI of the FHR of a fetus in the right occipitoanterior (ROA) position moves to the midline just over the symphysis pubis

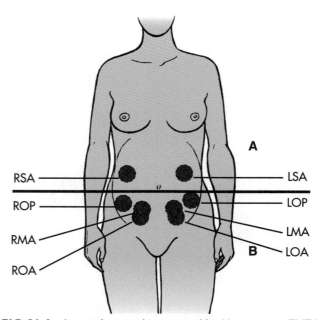

FIG. 21-6 Areas of maximal intensity of fetal heart tones (FHTs) for differing positions: *RSA,* right sacrum anterior; *ROP,* right occipitoposterior; *RMA,* right mentum anterior; *ROA,* right occipitoanterior; *LSA,* left sacrum anterior; *LOP,* left occipitoposterior; *LMA,* left mentum anterior; *LOA,* left occipitoanterior. **A,** Presentation is usually *breech* if FHTs are heard *above* umbilicus. **B,** Presentation is usually *vertex* if FHTs are heard *below* umbilicus.

procedure

Leopold Maneuvers

- Wash hands.
- Ask woman to empty bladder.
- Position woman supine with one pillow under her head and with her knees slightly flexed.
- Place small, rolled towel under woman's right or left hip to displace uterus off major blood vessels (prevents supine hypotensive syndrome; see Fig. 21-5, *D*).
- *If right-handed, stand on woman's right, facing her:*
  1. Identify fetal part that occupies the fundus. The head feels round, firm, freely movable, and palpable by ballottement; the breech feels less regular and softer. This maneuver identifies fetal lie (longitudinal or transverse) and presentation (cephalic or breech) **(Fig. A)**.
  2. Using palmar surface of one hand, locate and palpate the smooth convex contour of the fetal back and the irregularities that identify the small parts (feet, hands, elbows). This maneuver helps identify fetal presentation **(Fig. B)**.
  3. With right hand, determine which fetal part is presenting over the inlet to the true pelvis. Gently grasp the lower

pole of the uterus between the thumb and fingers, pressing in slightly **(Fig. C)**. If the head is presenting and not engaged, determine the attitude of the head (flexed or extended).
  4. Turn to face the woman's feet. Using both hands, outline the fetal head **(Fig. D)** with the palmar surface of the fingertips. When the presenting part has descended deeply, only a small portion of it may be outlined. Palpation of the cephalic prominence helps identify the attitude of the head. If the cephalic prominence is found on the same side as the small parts, this means that the head must be flexed and the vertex is presenting (see **Fig. D**). If the cephalic prominence is on the same side as the back, this indicates that the presenting head is extended and the face is presenting.
- Document fetal presentation, position, and lie and whether presenting part is flexed or extended, engaged, or free floating. Use agency's protocol for documentation (e.g., "Vtx, LOA, floating").

A   B   C   D

(Fig. 21-7, *A* and *B*). Just before birth, the fetal position is occipitoanterior (OA) and the fetal back is directly above the symphysis pubis. Assessments recommended for determining fetal status in the low risk woman during each stage of labor are summarized in the Care Paths. In addition to these scheduled assessments, the FHR and pattern also must be assessed immediately after ROM, because this is the most common time for the umbilical cord to prolapse; after any change in the contraction pattern or maternal status; and before and after the woman receives medications or a procedure is performed (Tucker, 2004).

Assessment of Uterine Contractions. A general characteristic of effective labor is regular uterine activity (i.e., contractions becoming more frequent and of increased duration), but uterine activity is not directly related to labor progress. Uterine contractions are the primary powers that act involuntarily to expel the fetus and the placenta from the uterus. Several methods are used to evaluate uterine contractions, including the woman's subjective description, palpation and timing of contractions by a health care provider, and internal electronic monitoring.

Each contraction exhibits a wavelike pattern. It begins with a slow increment (the "building up" of a contraction from its onset), gradually reaches an acme (intrauterine pressure less than 80 mm Hg), and then diminishes rapidly (decrement, the "letting down" of the contraction). An interval of rest (intrauterine pressure less than 20 mm Hg with a duration of at least 30 seconds) ends when the next contraction begins (Tucker, 2004). The outward appearance of the woman's abdomen during and between contractions and the pattern of a typical uterine contraction are shown in Fig. 21-8.

A uterine contraction is described in terms of the following characteristics:

- *Frequency:* How often uterine contractions occur; the time that elapses from the beginning of one contraction to the beginning of the next
- *Intensity:* The strength of a contraction at its peak
- *Duration:* The time that elapses between the onset and the end of a contraction
- *Resting tone:* The tension in the uterine muscle between contractions

Determination of Points of Maximal Intensity of the Fetal Heart Rate

- Wash hands.
- Perform Leopold maneuvers.
- Auscultate fetal heart rate (FHR) based on fetal presentation identified with Leopold maneuvers. The PMI is the location at which the FHR is the loudest, usually over the fetal back (see Fig. 21-6).
- Chart PMI of the FHR using a two-line figure to indicate the four quadrants of the maternal abdomen, as follows: right upper quadrant (RUQ), left upper quadrant (LUQ), left lower quadrant (LLQ), and right lower quadrant (RLQ):

RUQ	LUQ
RLQ	LLQ

- The umbilicus is the reference point for the quadrants (point at which the lines cross). The PMI of the FHR for the fetus in vertex presentation, in general flexion with the back on the mother's right side, commonly is found in the mother's right lower quadrant and is recorded with an "X" or with the FHR, as follows:

Uterine contractions are assessed by palpation or by an external or internal electronic monitor. Frequency and duration can be measured by all three methods of uterine activity monitoring. The accuracy of determining intensity varies by the method used. Palpation is subjective and is a less precise way of determining the intensity of uterine contractions. The following terms are used to describe what is felt on palpation:

- *Mild:* Slightly tense fundus that is easy to indent with fingertips (feels like touching finger to tip of nose)
- *Moderate:* Firm fundus that is difficult to indent with fingertips (feels like touching finger to chin)
- *Strong:* Rigid, boardlike fundus that is almost impossible to indent with fingertips (feels like touching finger to forehead)

Women in labor tend to describe the pain of contractions in terms of the sensations they are experiencing in the lower abdomen or back, which may be unrelated to the firmness of the uterine fundus. Thus their assessment of the strength of their contractions can be less valid than that of the health care provider, although the amount of discomfort reported is valid.

External electronic monitoring is not reliable for assessing intensity of uterine contractions. Internal electronic monitoring with an intrauterine pressure catheter is the most reliable way of assessing the intensity of uterine contractions.

On admission, a 20- to 30-minute baseline monitoring of uterine contractions and the fetal heart rate and pattern commonly is done. The minimal times for assessing

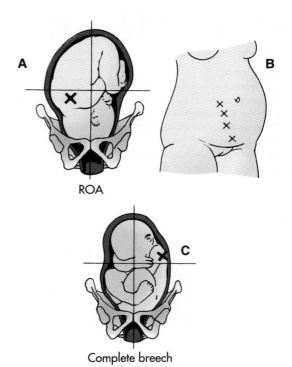

ROA

Complete breech

Lie: Vertical
Presentation: Breech (sacrum and feet presenting)
Reference point: Sacrum (with feet)
Attitude: General flexion

FIG. 21-7 Location of the fetal heart tones (FHTs). **A,** FHTs with fetus in right occipitoanterior (ROA) position. **B,** Changes in location of point of maximal intensity of FHTs as fetus undergoes internal rotation from ROA to OA and descent for birth. **C,** FHTs with fetus in left sacrum posterior position. (**A** and **C,** Courtesy Ross Laboratories, Columbus, OH.)

uterine activity during the various phases of labor are given in the Care Paths, and the findings expected as labor progresses are summarized in Tables 21-3 and 21-7.

The nurse's responsibility in the monitoring of uterine contractions is to ascertain whether they are powerful and frequent enough to accomplish the work of expelling the fetus and the placenta.

▬ NURSE ALERT

If the characteristics of contractions are found to be abnormal, either exceeding or falling below what is considered acceptable in terms of the standard characteristics, the nurse should report this finding to the primary health care provider.

Cervical Effacement and Dilation, Fetal Descent. Uterine activity must be considered in the context of its effect on cervical effacement and dilation and on the degree of descent of the presenting part (see Chapter 18). The effect on the fetus also must be considered. The progress of labor can be effectively verified through the use of graphic charts *(partograms)* on which cervical dilation and station (descent) are plotted. This type of graphic charting assists in early identification of deviations from expected labor patterns. Fig. 21-9 provides examples of partograms. Hospitals and

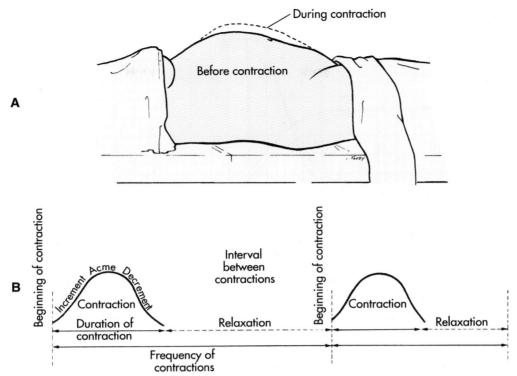

FIG. 21-8 Assessment of uterine contractions. **A,** Abdominal contour before and during uterine contraction. **B,** Wavelike pattern of contractile activity.

birthing centers may develop their own graphs for recording assessments. Such graphs may include not only data on dilation and descent but also data on maternal vital signs, FHR, and uterine activity.

▬ NURSE ALERT

It is important for the nurse to recognize that active labor can actually last longer than the expected labor patterns. This finding should not be a cause for concern unless the maternal-fetal unit exhibits signs of distress (e.g., nonreassuring fetal heart rate and patterns, maternal fever) (Cesario, 2004).

Vaginal Examination. The vaginal examination reveals whether the woman is in true labor and enables the examiner to determine whether the membranes have ruptured. Because this examination is often stressful and uncomfortable for the woman, it should be performed only when indicated by the status of the woman and her fetus. For example, a vaginal examination should be performed on admission, when significant change has occurred in uterine activity, on maternal perception of perineal pressure or the urge to bear down, when membranes rupture, or when variable decelerations of the FHR are noted. A full explanation of the examination and support of the woman are important factors in reducing the stress and discomfort associated with the examination. Chapter 5 describes a typical vaginal examination. Variations in the vaginal examinations of the woman in labor include the following:

1. Use a sterile glove and antiseptic solution or soluble gel; use water for lubrication during the initial examination if ROM is suspected and a nitrazine test is required.

2. Position the woman to prevent supine hypotension (see Fig. 21-5). Cleanse the perineum and vulva if needed.

3. Ask the woman for permission to touch her before proceeding and explain that she will feel insertion of the nurse's index and middle fingers into the vagina. Perform the examination gently, with concern for the woman's comfort. Acknowledge the woman's expressions of pain or discomfort and anxiety. Suggest she use slow breathing to help her relax.

4. Assess status of the following (Fig. 21-10):
   a. Dilation, effacement, and position (e.g., posterior, mid, anterior) of cervix
   b. Presenting part, position, station, and if vertex, any molding of the head
   c. Membranes—intact, bulging, or ruptured; amniotic fluid—color, clarity, and odor

5. Discuss the findings of the examination with the woman or couple.

6. Document the findings and report them to the primary health care provider.

▬ *Laboratory and Diagnostic Tests*

Analysis of Urine Specimen. A clean-catch urine specimen may be obtained to gather further data about the pregnant woman's health. It is a convenient and simple procedure that can provide information about her hydration status (e.g., specific gravity, color, amount), nutritional status (e.g., ketones), infection status (e.g., leukocytes), or the status of possible complications such as preeclampsia, shown by finding protein in the urine. The results can be

FIG. 21-9 Partograms for assessment of patterns of cervical dilation and descent. Individual woman's labor patterns *(colored)* are superimposed on prepared labor graph *(black)* for comparison. **A,** Labor of a nulliparous woman. **B,** Labor of a multiparous woman. The rate of cervical dilation is plotted with the circled plot points. A line drawn through these symbols depicts the slope of the curve. Station is plotted with Xs. A line drawn through the Xs reveals the pattern of descent.

obtained quickly and help the nurse determine appropriate interventions to implement.

Blood Tests. The blood tests performed vary with the hospital protocol and the woman's health status. An example of a minimal assessment is a hematocrit determination, in which the specimen is centrifuged in the perinatal unit. Blood can be obtained by a finger stick or from the hub of a catheter used to start an IV line. More comprehensive blood assessments such as white blood cell count, red blood cell count, the hemoglobin level, hematocrit, and platelet values are included in a complete blood count

(CBC). A CBC may be ordered for women with a history of infection, anemia, gestational hypertension, or other disorders.

If the woman's blood type has not been verified, blood is drawn for the purpose of determining the type and Rh factor. If blood typing has already been done, the primary health care provider may choose not to repeat the test. If obvious signs of immunocompromise or substance abuse are present, other blood tests may be ordered.

Assessment of Amniotic Membranes and Fluid. Labor is initiated at term by SROM in approximately

FIG. 21-10 Vaginal examination. **A,** Undilated, uneffaced cervix; membranes intact. **B,** Palpation of sagittal suture line. Cervix effaced and partially dilated.

table 21-4	Assessment of Amniotic Fluid Characteristics		
CHARACTERISTIC OF FLUID	**NORMAL FINDING**	**DEVIATION FROM NORMAL FINDING**	**CAUSE OF DEVIATION FROM NORMAL**
Color	Pale, straw-colored; may contain white flecks of vernix caseosa, lanugo, scalp hair	Greenish brown color	Hypoxic episode in fetus results in meconium passage into fluid May be normal finding in breech presentations related to pressure exerted on fetal abdominal wall during descent
		Yellow-stained fluid	Fetal hypoxia ≥36 hr before ROM; fetal hemolytic disease; intrauterine infection
		Port wine–colored	Bleeding associated with premature separation of the placenta (abruptio placentae)
Viscosity and odor	Watery; no strong odor	Thick, cloudy, foul-smelling	Intrauterine infection Large amount of meconium can make fluid thick
Amount (normally varies with gestational age)	400 ml (20 wk gestation)	≥2000 ml (32 to 36 wk gestation)	Hydramnios; associated with congenital anomalies of the fetus when fetus cannot drink or fluid is trapped in the body (e.g., fetal gastrointestinal obstruction or atresias); increased risk with maternal pregestational or gestational diabetes mellitus
	1000 ml (36 to 38 wk gestation)	≤500 ml (32 to 36 wk gestation)	Oligohydramnios; associated with incomplete or absent kidney; obstruction of urethra; fetus cannot secrete or excrete urine

ROM, Rupture of membranes.

25% of pregnant women. A lag period, rarely exceeding 24 hours, may precede the onset of labor. Membranes (the bag of waters) also can rupture spontaneously any time during labor, but most commonly in the transition phase of the first stage of labor.

▬ NURSE ALERT

The umbilical cord may prolapse when the membranes rupture. The fetal heart rate and pattern should be monitored closely for several minutes immediately after ROM to ascertain fetal well-being, and the findings should be documented.

The tests used to assess amniotic fluid are discussed in the Procedure box on p. 524 and the characteristics of the fluid are described in Table 21-4. Artificial rupture of membranes (AROM, ARM), or amniotomy, may be done to augment or induce labor or to facilitate placement of internal monitors when fetal status indicates the need for some form of direct assessment (e.g., insertion of a fetal scalp electrode or an intrauterine pressure catheter).

Infection. When membranes rupture, microorganisms from the vagina can then ascend into the amniotic sac, causing chorioamnionitis and placentitis to develop. For this reason, maternal temperature and vaginal discharge are assessed frequently (every 1 to 2 hours) so that an infection developing after ROM can be identified early. However, even when membranes are intact, microorganisms may ascend and cause infection that can lead to premature rupture of membranes (PROM). There is controversy regarding whether prophylactic antibiotic therapy can protect against infection (chorioamnionitis), which involves both the maternal and fetal sides of the membrane. Prophylactic antibiotics for prelabor ROM at term or preterm is a form of care of unknown effectiveness (Enkin et al., 2000).

Labor

- Intrauterine pressure of ≥80 mm Hg (determined by intrauterine pressure catheter monitoring) or resting tone of ≥20 mm Hg
- Contractions consistently lasting ≥90 sec
- Contractions consistently occurring ≤2 min apart
- Contraction interval <30 sec
- Fetal bradycardia, tachycardia, persistently decreased variability, or late or severe variable deceleration
- Irregular FHR; suspected fetal arrhythmias
- Appearance of meconium-stained or bloody fluid from the vagina
- Arrest in progress of cervical dilation or effacement, descent of the fetus, or both
- Maternal temperature of ≥38° C
- Foul-smelling vaginal discharge
- Persistent bright or dark red vaginal bleeding

The nurse's responsibility is to report findings promptly to the primary health care provider and to document findings in the labor record and on the monitor strip. If abnormal findings are noted, continuous electronic monitoring usually is implemented and maintained for the duration of labor. The presence of meconium-stained amniotic fluid alerts the nurse to the need to observe fetal status more closely. After birth, the newborn may be at risk for an alteration in respiratory status if meconium is aspirated into the lungs with the first breath.

Signs of Potential Problems. Although some problems of labor are anticipated, others may appear unexpectedly during the clinical course of labor (see Signs of Potential Complications box).

When establishing nursing diagnoses, the nurse should analyze the significance of findings ascertained during the assessment. Nursing diagnoses appropriate for the first stage of labor include the following:

- *Acute pain related to*
  –effects of uterine contractions and fetal descent
- *Anxiety related to*
  –negative experience with a previous childbirth
  –cultural differences
  –triggering of memories associated with history of sexual abuse
- *Impaired urinary elimination related to*
  –reduced intake of oral fluids
  –diminished sensations of bladder fullness associated with epidural anesthesia or analgesia
- *Impaired fetal gas exchange related to*
  –diminished placental perfusion associated with maternal hypertension or hypotension
    –maternal position
    –intense and frequent uterine contractions
  –compression of the umbilical cord

- *Situational low self-esteem (maternal) related to*
  –inability to meet self-expectations regarding performance during childbirth
  –loss of control during labor
- *Situational low self-esteem (father or partner) related to*
  –unrealistic expectations regarding role as labor coach
  –perceived ineffectiveness in meeting the needs of the laboring woman

▬ Expected Outcomes of Care

It is important for the nurse and woman to set priorities for expected outcomes that focus on the woman, the fetus, and the woman's significant others. Expected outcomes for the woman in the first stage of labor are that the woman will accomplish the following:

- Accept comfort and support measures from significant others and health care providers as needed.
- Actively participate in the labor process, with no evidence of injury to her or her fetus.
- Maintain adequate hydration status through oral or intravenous fluid intake.
- Void at least every 2 hours to prevent bladder distention.
- Verbalize discomfort and indicate the need for measures that help reduce discomfort and promote relaxation.
- Express satisfaction with her performance during labor.

▬ Plan of Care and Interventions
▬ *Standards of Care*

Standards of care guide the nurse in preparing for and implementing procedures with the expectant mother (Box 21-4). Protocols for care based on standards include the following tasks:

- Check the primary health care provider's orders.
- Review the primary health care provider's orders for completeness and correctness (e.g., the dose and route of the analgesic to be administered).
- Check labels on IV solutions, drugs, and other materials used for nursing care.
- Check the expiration date on any packs of supplies used for procedures.
- Ensure that information on the woman's identification band is accurate (e.g., the band is the appropriate color for allergies).
- Use an empathic approach when giving care:
  –Use words the woman can understand when explaining procedures; repeat as necessary.
  –Respect the woman's individual needs and behaviors.
  –Establish rapport with the woman and her significant others.
  –Be kind, caring, and competent when performing necessary procedures.
  –Be aware that pain and discomfort are as the woman describes them.
  –Carry out appropriate comfort measures such as mouth care and back care.

box 21-4 **Care Plan Using Protocols and Nursing Standards**

CARE PLAN FOR LABOR   **MARY J.**
                                                                     UNIT NO. 4587024

Date Initiated: _____   Time: _____   RN: _____

OUTCOME STANDARDS:
1. Client will demonstrate normal labor progress while the fetus tolerates the labor process without demonstrating nonreassuring signs. Date met: _____
2. Client will participate in decisions about her care. Date met: _____
3. Client and her partner will verbalize knowledge of labor process and their expectations for the birth experience. Date met: _____

INITIATED Date/RN	PROBLEM	NURSING INTERVENTIONS	DISCONTINUED Date/RN
	Impaired maternal/fetal gas exchange	Implement fetal monitoring per protocol or orders from health care provider	
	Risk related to labor progress:	Provide nursing care per hospital procedure manual	
	• Impaired urinary elimination	Implement labor care per protocol or care path	
	• Impaired tissue integrity related to birth	Notify primary health care provider of problems (see Signs of Potential Complications box)	
		Provide care for vaginal birth per hospital procedure manual	
		Provide immediate care for newborn per hospital procedure manual	
		Implement care for fourth stage of labor per protocol or care path	
	Anxiety related to maternal/fetal status	Encourage woman and her partner to express their concerns	
		Keep couple informed of labor progress	
		Involve woman in decision making regarding her care	
	Deficient knowledge about labor/procedures	Explain procedures in terms woman can understand	
	Acute pain related to process of labor	Promote use of relaxation techniques	
		Provide comfort measures	
		Offer pain medications as ordered	
		Evaluate response to pain relief measures	
	Other problems:		

–Include the support persons in the care as desired by the woman and the support persons.

–Recognize that a woman's current childbirth experience and the actions of nurses and other health care providers can have a positive or negative effect on the woman's future childbirth experiences.

• Use Standard Precautions, including precautions for invasive procedures (see Box 21-3).

• Document care according to hospital guidelines, and communicate information to the primary health care provider when indicated.

■ Physical Nursing Care During Labor

The physical nursing care rendered to the woman in labor is an essential component of her care. The current emphasis on evidence-based practice supports the management of care by using this approach to enhance the safety, effectiveness, and acceptability of the physical care measures chosen to support the woman during labor and birth (Enkin et al., 2000). The various physical needs, the requisite nursing actions, and the rationale for care are presented in Table 21-5, the Plan of Care, and the Care Paths on pp. 543 and 558.

General Hygiene. Women in labor should be offered the use of showers or warm water baths if they are available, to enhance the feeling of well-being and to minimize the discomfort of contractions (Benfield, 2002; Cluett, Nikodem, McCandlish, & Burns, 2002). Women also should be encouraged to wash their hands after voiding and to perform self-hygiene measures. Linen should be changed if it becomes wet or stained with blood, and linen savers (Chux) should be used and changed as needed.

Nutrient and Fluid Intake

Oral Intake. Traditionally the laboring woman has been offered only clear liquids or ice chips or given nothing by mouth during the active phase of labor to minimize the risk of anesthesia complications and their sequelae should general anesthesia be required in an emergency. These sequelae include the aspiration of gastric contents and resultant compromise in oxygen perfusion, which may endanger the lives of the mother and fetus. This practice is being challenged today because regional anesthesia is used more often than general anesthesia, even for emergency cesarean births. Women are awake during regional anesthesia and are able to participate in their own care and protect their airway.

(Text continued on p. 544.)

table 21-5 Physical Nursing Care During Labor

NEED	NURSING ACTIONS	RATIONALE
GENERAL HYGIENE		
Showers or bed baths, Jacuzzi bath	Assess for progress in labor	Determines appropriateness of the activity
	Supervise showers closely if woman is in true labor	Prevents injury from fall; labor may be accelerated
	Suggest allowing warm water to flow over back	Aids relaxation; increases comfort
Perineum	Cleanse frequently, especially after rupture of membranes and when show increases	Enhances comfort and reduces risk of infection
Oral hygiene	Offer toothbrush or mouthwash or wash the teeth with an ice-cold wet washcloth as needed	Refreshes mouth; helps counteract dry, thirsty feeling
Hair	Brush, braid per woman's wishes	Improves morale; increases comfort
Handwashing	Offer washcloths before and after voiding and as needed	Maintains cleanliness; prevents infection
Face	Offer cool washcloth	Provides relief from diaphoresis; cools and refreshes
Gowns and linens	Change as needed; fluff pillows	Improves comfort; enhances relaxation
NUTRIENT AND FLUID INTAKE		
Oral	Offer fluids and solid foods, following orders of primary health care provider and desires of laboring woman	Provides hydration and calories; enhances positive emotional experience and maternal control
Intravenous (IV)	Establish and maintain IV line as ordered	Maintains hydration; provides venous access for medications
ELIMINATION		
Voiding	Encourage voiding at least every 2 hr	A full bladder may impede descent of presenting part; overdistention may cause bladder atony and injury, as well as postpartum voiding difficulty
Ambulatory woman	Allow ambulation to bathroom according to orders of primary health care provider, if:	
	The presenting part is engaged	Reinforces normal process of urination
	The membranes are not ruptured	Precautionary measure to protect against prolapse of umbilical cord
	The woman is not medicated	Precautionary measure to protect against injury
Woman on bed rest	Offer bedpan	Prevents complications of bladder distention
	Allow tap water to run; pour warm water over the vulva; give positive suggestion	Encourages voiding
	Provide privacy	Shows respect for woman
	Put up side rails on bed	Prevents injury from fall
	Place call bell within reach	Reinforces safe care
	Offer washcloth for hands	Maintains cleanliness; prevents infection
	Wash vulvar area	Maintains cleanliness; enhances comfort; prevents infection
Catheterization	Catheterize according to orders of primary health care provider or hospital protocol if measures to facilitate voiding are ineffective	Prevents complications of bladder distention
	Insert catheter between contractions	Minimizes discomfort
	Avoid force if obstacle to insertion is noted	"Obstacle" may be caused by compression of urethra by presenting part
Bowel elimination—sensation of rectal pressure	Perform vaginal examination	Prevents misinterpretation of rectal pressure from the presenting part as the need to defecate
		Determine degree of descent of presenting part
	Help the woman ambulate to bathroom or offer bedpan if rectal pressure is not from presenting part	Reinforce normal process of bowel elimination and safe care
	Cleanse perineum immediately after passage of stool	Reduces risk of infection and sense of embarrassment

plan of care ❯ Labor and Birth

NURSING DIAGNOSIS Anxiety related to labor and the birthing process

Expected Outcome *Woman exhibits decreased signs of anxiety.*

Nursing Interventions/*Rationales*

- Orient woman and significant others to labor and birth unit and explain admission protocol *to allay initial feelings of anxiety.*
- Assess woman's knowledge, experience, and expectations of labor; note any signs or expressions of anxiety, nervousness, or fear *to establish a baseline for intervention.*
- Discuss the expected progression of labor and describe what to expect during the process *to allay anxiety associated with the unknown.*
- Actively involve woman in care decisions during labor, interpret sights and sounds of environment (monitor sights and sounds, unit activities), and share information on progression of labor (vital signs, FHR, dilation, effacement) *to increase her sense of control and allay fears.*

NURSING DIAGNOSIS Acute pain related to increasing frequency and intensity of contractions

Expected Outcome *Woman exhibits signs of ability to cope with discomfort.*

Nursing Interventions/*Rationales*

- Assess woman's level of pain and strategies that she has used to cope with pain *to establish a baseline for intervention.*
- Encourage significant other to remain as support person during labor process *to assist with support and comfort measures, because measures are often more effective when delivered by a familiar person.*
- Instruct woman and support person in use of specific techniques such as conscious relaxation, focused breathing, effleurage, massage, and application of sacral pressure *to increase relaxation, decrease intensity of contractions, and promote use of controlled thought and direction of energy.*
- Provide comfort measures such as frequent mouth care *to prevent dry mouth,* application of damp cloth to forehead, and changing of damp gown or bed covers *to relieve discomfort associated with diaphoresis;* positioning *to reduce stiffness.*
- Explain what analgesics and anesthesia are available for use during labor and birth *to provide knowledge to help woman make decisions about pain control.*

NURSING DIAGNOSIS Impaired urinary elimination related to sensory impairment secondary to labor

Expected Outcome *Woman does not show signs of bladder distention.*

Nursing Interventions/*Rationales*

- Palpate the bladder superior to the symphysis on a frequent basis *to detect a full bladder that occurs from increased fluid intake and inability to feel urge to void.*
- Encourage frequent voiding (at least every 2 hours) and catheterize if necessary *to avoid bladder distention, because it impedes progress of fetus down birth canal and may result in trauma to the bladder.*
- Assist woman to bathroom or commode to void, if appropriate, and provide privacy *to facilitate bladder emptying with an upright position (natural) and relaxation.*

NURSING DIAGNOSIS Ineffective coping related to birthing process

Expected Outcome *Woman actively participates in the birth process with no evidence of injury to her or her fetus.*

Nursing Interventions/*Rationales*

- Constantly monitor events of second-stage labor and birth, including physiologic responses of woman and fetus and emotional responses of woman and partner *to ensure maternal, partner, and fetal well-being.*
- Provide ongoing feedback to woman and partner *to allay anxiety and enhance participation.*
- Continue to provide comfort measures and minimizing distractions *to decrease discomfort and aid in focus on the birth process.*
- Encourage woman to experiment with various positions *to assist downward movement of fetus.*
- Ensure that woman takes deep cleansing breaths before and after each contraction *to enhance gas exchange and oxygen transport to the fetus.*
- Encourage woman to push spontaneously when urge to bear down is perceived during a contraction *to aid descent and rotation of fetus.*
- Encourage woman to exhale, holding breath for short periods while bearing down *to avoid holding breath and triggering a Valsalva maneuver and increasing intrathoracic and cardiovascular pressure and decreasing perfusion of placental oxygen, placing the fetus at risk.*
- Have woman take deep breaths and relax between contractions *to reduce fatigue and increase effectiveness of pushing efforts.*
- Have mother pant as fetal head crowns *to control birth of head.*
- Explain to woman and labor partner what is expected in the third stage of labor *to enlist cooperation.*
- Have woman maintain her position *to facilitate delivery of the placenta.*

NURSING DIAGNOSIS Fatigue related to energy expenditure required during labor and birth

Expected Outcome *Woman's energy levels are restored.*

Nursing Interventions/*Rationales*

- Educate woman and partner about need for rest and help them plan strategies (e.g., restricting visitors, increasing role of support systems performing functions associated with daily routines) that allow specific times for rest and sleep *to ensure that woman can restore depleted energy levels in preparation for caring for a new infant.*
- Monitor woman's fatigue level and the amount of rest received *to ensure restoration of energy.*

NURSING DIAGNOSIS Risk for deficient fluid volume related to decreased fluid intake and increased fluid loss during labor and birth

Expected Outcomes *Fluid balance is maintained, and the woman has no signs of dehydration.*

Nursing Interventions/*Rationales*

- Monitor fluid loss (i.e., blood, urine, perspiration) and vital signs; inspect skin turgor and mucous membranes for dryness *to evaluate hydration status.*
- Administer oral/parenteral fluid per physician/nurse-midwife orders *to maintain hydration.*
- Monitor the fundus for firmness after placental separation *to ensure adequate contraction and prevent further blood loss.*

CD: Plan of Care: Labor and Birth

Although gastric emptying is slowed as a result of labor, stress, and the use of opioids or sedatives, fasting does not cause gastric contents to be eliminated and may even cause them to become more acidic. In addition, fasting is identified by many laboring women as a stressor with which they must cope and a source of frustration and anxiety during labor related to a loss of control with regard to meeting their own nourishment needs. A woman's reaction to fasting may even result in activation of the stress response which is known to slow labor (Parsons, 2004).

An adequate intake of fluids and calories is required to meet the energy demands and fluid losses associated with childbirth. The progress of labor slows, and ketosis develops if these demands are not met and fat is metabolized. Reduced energy for bearing-down efforts (pushing) increases the risk for a forceps- or vacuum-assisted birth. This is most likely to occur in women who begin to labor early in the morning after a night without caloric intake. When women are permitted to consume fluids and food freely, they typically regulate their own oral intake, eating light foods (e.g., eggs, yogurt, ice cream, dry toast and jelly, fruit) and drinking fluids during early labor and tapering off to the intake of clear fluids and sips of water or ice chips as labor intensifies and the second stage approaches. Common practice is to allow clear liquids (e.g., water, tea, apple juice, clear sodas, gelatin, broth) during early labor, tapering off to ice chips and sips of water as labor progresses and becomes more active. Food and fluid consumed orally during labor can meet a laboring woman's hydration and energy demands more effectively and safely than fluid administered intravenously. In addition, the woman's sense of control and level of comfort are enhanced (Scheepers, Thans, deJong, Essed, LeCessie, & Kanhai, 2001). The CNM Data Group (1999) found that a woman's culture may influence what she will eat and drink during labor. In addition, women who used nonpharmacologic pain-relief measures and labored at home or in birthing centers were more likely to eat and drink during labor. The amount of solid and liquid carbohydrates to offer a woman in labor is still unclear. Though it is known that energy needs increase as labor becomes prolonged, there is limited evidence regarding the impact of oral carbohydrate intake in enhancing the progress of labor and reducing the risk for dystocia (Tranmer, Hodnett, Hannah, & Stevens, 2005).

Withholding food and fluids in labor is a form of care ❊ unlikely to be beneficial, and offering oral fluids is one that is demonstrably useful and should be encouraged (Enkin et al., 2000; Hofmeyr, 2005). Nurses should follow the orders of the woman's primary health care provider when offering the woman food or fluids during labor. As advocates, however, nurses can facilitate change by informing others of the current research findings that support the safety and effectiveness of the oral intake of food and fluid during labor and by initiating such research themselves.

Intravenous Intake. Fluids are administered intravenously to the laboring woman to maintain hydration, especially when a labor is long and the woman is unable to ingest a sufficient amount of fluid orally or if she is receiving epidural or intrathecal anesthesia. However, routine use of IV fluids during labor is a form of care that is ❊ unlikely to be beneficial and may be harmful (Enkin et al., 2000). In most cases, an electrolyte solution without glucose is adequate and does not introduce excess glucose into the bloodstream. The latter is important because an excessive maternal glucose level results in fetal hyperglycemia and fetal hyperinsulinism. After birth, the neonate's high levels of insulin will then deplete his or her glucose stores, and hypoglycemia will result. Infusions containing glucose can also reduce sodium levels in both the woman and the fetus, leading to transient neonatal tachypnea. If maternal ketosis occurs, the primary health care provider may order an IV solution containing a small amount of dextrose to provide the glucose needed to assist in fatty acid metabolism.

▬ NURSE ALERT

Nurses should carefully monitor the intake and output of laboring women receiving IV fluids because they also face an increased danger of hypervolemia as a result of the fluid retention that occurs during pregnancy.

Elimination

Voiding. Voiding every 2 hours should be encouraged. A distended bladder may impede descent of the presenting part, inhibit uterine contractions, and lead to decreased bladder tone or atony after birth. Women who receive epidural analgesia or anesthesia are especially at risk for the retention of urine, and the need to void should be assessed more frequently in them.

The woman should be assisted to the bathroom to void, unless the primary health care provider has ordered bed rest; the woman is receiving epidural analgesia or anesthesia; internal monitoring is being used; or, in the nurse's judgment, ambulation would compromise the status of the laboring woman, her fetus, or both. External monitoring can usually be interrupted for the woman to go to the bathroom.

Catheterization. If the woman is unable to void and her bladder is distended, she may need to be catheterized. Most hospitals have protocols that rely on the nurse's judgment concerning the need for catheterization. Before performing the catheterization, the nurse should clean the vulva and perineum, because vaginal show and amniotic fluid may be present. If there appears to be an obstacle that prevents advancement of the catheter, this is most likely the presenting part. If the catheter cannot be advanced, the nurse should stop the procedure and notify the primary health care provider of the difficulty.

Bowel Elimination. Most women do not have bowel movements during labor because of decreased intestinal motility. Stool that has formed in the large intestine often is moved downward toward the anorectal area by the pressure exerted by the fetal presenting part as it descends. This stool is often expelled during second-stage pushing and birth. However, the passage of stool with bearing-down efforts increases the risk of infection and may embarrass the woman, thereby reducing the effectiveness of these efforts. To prevent these problems, the nurse should immediately cleanse the perineal area to remove any stool, while reassuring the woman that the passage of stool at this time is a normal and expected event, because the same muscles used to expel the baby also expel stool. Routine use of an enema to empty the rectum is considered to be harmful or ineffective and should be eliminated (Enkin et al., 2000).

When the presenting part is deep in the pelvis, even in the absence of stool in the anorectal area, the woman may feel rectal pressure and think she needs to defecate. If the woman expresses the urge to defecate, the nurse should perform a vaginal examination to assess cervical dilation and station. When a multiparous woman experiences the urge to defecate, this often means birth will follow quickly.

Ambulation and Positioning. Freedom of maternal movement and choice of position throughout labor are forms of care likely to be beneficial for the laboring woman and should be encouraged (Enkin et al., 2000). The increased use of epidurals during childbirth accompanied by multiple medical interventions (e.g., monitors, intravenous infusions) and reduced motor control interfere with a woman's freedom of movement. In a national survey (Declercq, Sakala, Corry, Applebaum, & Risher, 2002), 71% of the participating women stated that they did not ambulate once labor became active because they were "hooked up" and could not walk.

The potential advantages of ambulation include enhanced uterine activity, distraction from labor's discomforts, enhanced maternal control, and an opportunity for close interaction with the woman's partner and care provider as they help her to walk. Ambulation is associated with a reduced rate of operative birth (i.e., cesarean birth, use of forceps, and vacuum extraction) and less frequent use of opioid analgesics (Albers et al., 1997).

Walking, sitting, or standing during labor is more comfortable than lying down and facilitates the progress of labor (Simkin & Ancheta, 2000). Ambulation should be encouraged if membranes are intact, if the fetal presenting part is engaged after ROM, and if the woman has not received medication for pain (Fig. 21-11). The woman also may find it comfortable to stand and lean forward on her partner, doula, or nurse for support at times during labor (Fig. 21-12, *A*). Ambulation may be contraindicated, however, because of maternal or fetal status.

When the woman lies in bed, she will usually change her position spontaneously as labor progresses (Albers

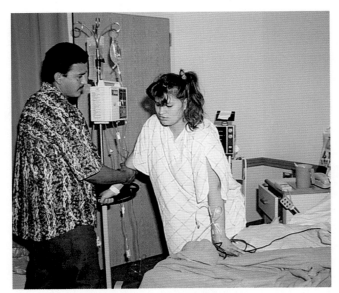

FIG. 21-11 Woman preparing to walk with partner. (Courtesy Marjorie Pyle, RNC, Lifecircle, Costa Mesa, CA.)

A

B

FIG. 21-12 **A,** Woman standing and leaning forward with support. **B,** Woman in hands-and-knees position. (Courtesy Marjorie Pyle, RNC, Lifecircle, Costa Mesa, CA.)

et al., 1997). If she does not change position every 30 to 60 minutes, she should be assisted to do so. The side-lying (lateral) position is preferred because it promotes optimal uteroplacental and renal blood flow and increases fetal oxygen saturation (Fig. 21-13, *B*). If the woman wants to lie supine, the nurse may place a pillow under one hip as a wedge to prevent the uterus from compressing the aorta and vena cava (see Fig. 21-5). Sitting is not contraindicated unless it adversely affects fetal status, which can be determined by checking the fetal heart rate and pattern. If the fetus is in the occiput posterior position, it may be helpful to encourage the woman to squat during contractions, because this position increases pelvic diameter, allowing the head to rotate to a more anterior position (see Fig. 21-13, *A*). A hands-and-knees position during contractions also is recommended to facilitate the rotation of the fetal occiput from a posterior to an anterior position, since gravity pulls the fetal back forward (see Fig. 21-12, *B*).

Much research continues to be directed toward acquiring a better understanding of the physiologic and psychologic effects of maternal position in labor. The variety of positions that are recommended for the laboring woman are described in Box 21-5.

A birth ball (gymnastic ball, physical therapy ball) can be used to support a woman's body as she assumes a variety of labor and birth positions (Fig. 21-14). The woman can sit on the ball while leaning over the bed, or she can lean over the ball to support her upper body and reduce stress on her arms and hands when she assumes a hands-and-knees position. The birth ball can encourage pelvic mobility and pelvic and perineal relaxation when the woman sits on the firm yet pliable ball and rocks in rhythmic movements. Warm compresses applied to the perineum and lower back can maximize this relaxation and comfort effect. The birth ball should be large enough so that when the woman sits, her knees are bent at a 90-degree angle and her feet are flat on the floor and approximately 2 feet apart (Perez, 2000).

▬ *Supportive Care During Labor and Birth*

Support during labor and birth involves emotional support, physical care and comfort measures, and provision of advice and information (Davies & Hodnett, 2002; Miltner, 2000). Effective support provided to women during labor can result in shorter labors; reduced rates of complications and surgical or obstetric interventions (e.g., cesarean births, labor augmentations and inductions, episiotomies, forceps- and vacuum-assisted births); and enhanced self-esteem and satisfaction (Hodnett, Lowe, Hannah, Willan, Stevens, & Weston, 2002; Miltner). Physical, emotional, and psychologic support of the woman during labor and birth is a beneficial form of care demonstrated by clear research evidence (Enkin et al., 2000; MacKinnon, McIntyre, & Quance, 2005).

Labor rooms should be airy, clean, and homelike. The laboring woman should feel safe in this environment and

FIG. 21-13 Maternal positions for labor. **A,** Squatting. **B,** Lateral position. Support person is applying sacral pressure while partner provides encouragement. (Courtesy Marjorie Pyle, RNC, Lifecircle, Costa Mesa, CA.)

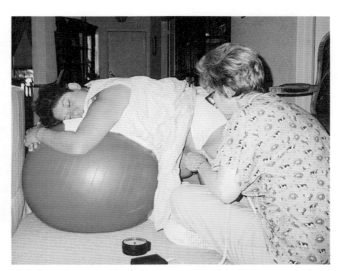

FIG 21-14 Woman laboring using birth ball. (Courtesy Polly Perez, Cutting Edge Press, Johnson, VT.)

| box 21-5 | Some Maternal Positions* During Labor and Birth |

SEMIRECUMBENT POSITION

With woman sitting with her upper body elevated to at least a 30-degree angle, place wedge or small pillow under hip to prevent vena cava compression and reduce likelihood of supine hypotension (see Fig. 21–16, A and Fig. 21-17, B).

- The greater the angle of elevation, the more gravity or pressure is exerted that promotes fetal descent, the progress of contractions, and the widening of pelvic dimensions.
- Convenient for rendering care measures and for external fetal monitoring.

LATERAL POSITION (SEE FIG. 21-13, B, AND 21-17, A)

Have woman alternate between left and right side-lying position, and provide abdominal and back support as needed for comfort.

- Removes pressure from the vena cava and back; enhances uteroplacental perfusion and relieves backache.
- Makes it easier to perform back massage or counterpressure.
- Associated with less frequent, but more intense, contractions.
- Obtaining good external fetal monitor tracings may be more difficult.
- May be used as a birthing position.
- Takes pressure off perineum, allowing it to stretch gradually.
- Reduces risk for perineal trauma.

UPRIGHT POSITION

The gravity effect enhances the contraction cycle and fetal descent: the weight of the fetus places increasing pressure on the cervix; the cervix is pulled upward, facilitating effacement and dilation; impulses from the cervix to the pituitary gland increase, causing more oxytocin to be secreted; and contractions are intensified, thereby applying more forceful downward pressure on the fetus, but they are less painful.

- Fetus is aligned with pelvis, and pelvic diameters are widened slightly.
- Effective upright positions include the following:
  - Ambulation (see Fig. 21-11)
  - Standing and leaning forward with support provided by coach (see Fig. 21-12, A), end of bed, back of chair, or birth ball (see Fig. 21-14); relieves backache and facilitates application of counterpressure or back massage
  - Sitting up in bed, chair, birthing chair, on toilet or bedside commode (see Fig. 21-16, B)
  - Squatting (see Fig. 21-13, A and Fig. 21-16, E)

HANDS-AND-KNEES POSITION—IDEAL POSITION FOR POSTERIOR POSITIONS OF THE PRESENTING PART (SEE FIG. 21-12, B)

Assume an "all fours" position in bed or on a covered floor; allows for pelvic rocking.

- Relieves backache characteristic of "back labor."
- Facilitates internal rotation of the fetus by increasing mobility of the coccyx, increasing the pelvic diameters, and using gravity to turn the fetal back and rotate the head.

*Assess the effect of each position on the laboring woman's comfort and anxiety level, progress of labor, and fetal heart rate (FHR) pattern. Alternate positions every 30 to 60 min, allowing woman to take control of her position changes.

---

free to be herself and to use the comfort and relaxation measures she prefers. To enhance relaxation, bright overhead lights should be turned off when not needed, and noise and intrusions should be kept to a minimum. The temperature is controlled to ensure the laboring woman's comfort. The room should be large enough to accommodate a comfortable chair for the woman's partner, the monitoring equipment, and hospital personnel. Couples may bring their own pillows to make the hospital surroundings more homelike and to facilitate position changes. This type of an environment can help women to view their childbirth experience as normal and not related to illness (Lowe, 2002). Environmental modifications should reflect the preferences of the woman, including the number of visitors and availability of a telephone, television, and music. Nurses should ensure that each woman labors in an optimal birth environment (Hanson et al., 2001).

Labor Support by the Nurse. The nurse can alleviate a woman's anxiety by communicating clearly, explaining unfamiliar terms, providing information and explanations without her having to ask and at a level she understands, and preparing her for sensations she will experience and procedures that will follow. By encouraging the woman or couple to ask questions and by providing honest, understandable answers, the nurse can play an important role in

helping the woman achieve a satisfying birth experience (Hodnett, Gates, Hofmeyr, & Sakala, 2003; Hodnett et al., 2002; Miltner, 2002; Sauls, 2002).

Supportive, empathetic nursing care for a woman in labor includes the following (MacKinnon et al., 2005; Matthews & Callister, 2004; Simkin, 2002; Sleutel, 2003):

- Helping the woman maintain control and participate to the extent she wishes in the birth of her infant
- Providing continuity of care that is nonjudgmental and respectful of her cultural and religious values and beliefs
- Meeting the woman's expected outcomes for her labor
- Listening to the woman's concerns and encouraging her to express her feelings
- Acting as the woman's advocate, supporting her decisions and respecting her choices as appropriate, and relating her wishes as needed to other health care providers
- Helping the woman conserve her energy and cope effectively with her pain and discomfort by using a variety of comfort measures that are acceptable to her
- Helping control the woman's discomfort
- Acknowledging the woman's efforts during labor including her strength and courage, as well as those of her partner, and providing positive reinforcement
- Protecting the woman's privacy, modesty, and dignity

EVIDENCE-BASED PRACTICE

Birthing Centers Say "There's No Place Like Home(like)"

BACKGROUND

- As the use of technology and interventions during labor and birth has become routine, there has been a paradoxical trend to create a nurturing, comforting homelike environment for birthing. Beyond just a redecorated room, this movement includes a model of care based on the philosophy that birth is normal. Birthing centers are typically staffed by nurse-midwives, who accept low risk clients for minimal intervention labor. Medical equipment is tucked away behind homelike, comfortable fixtures. Birthing centers are usually affiliated with conventional medical center for emergencies. Without continuous fetal monitoring, detection of emergent conditions and fetal distress may be delayed, and transport may delay emergency treatment.

OBJECTIVES

- The reviewers wished to compare the labor and birth outcomes of homelike birthing centers (but not home births) to conventional hospital maternity labor and birth settings. Their interests included staffing (shared or separate from the medical center), continuity of care (staff changing with shifts, versus staying throughout the birth), and physical proximity of the birthing center to the medical facility. Outcomes researched were medical interventions, complications, birth methods, perinatal mortality, neonatal health, breastfeeding, maternal satisfaction, and adjustment to mothering.

METHODS

Search Strategy

- The authors searched the Cochrane Pregnancy and Childbirth Group trials register, journals, and conference proceedings. They identified six randomized controlled trials, representing 8,677 women in Australia, Canada, Sweden, the United Kingdom, and the United States, dated 1986 to 2000.

Statistical Analyses

- Similar data were pooled. Reviewers calculated relative risk for dichotomous (categoric) data, such as type of birth, and weighted mean difference for continuous data, such as satisfaction. Differences between groups outside the 95% confidence interval were accepted as significant. All were analyzed in their original randomly assigned "intention to treat" categories, even if they changed their minds or were transported to hospital.

FINDINGS

- Birthing center care increased the likelihood of spontaneous vaginal birth, especially with separate staffing and continuity of care. Women at birthing centers gave birth without pain medication; they experienced both increased success initiating and sustaining breastfeeding, as well as increased maternal satisfaction. Perineal tears were more common to the birth center setting. There were fewer medical interventions, including detection of fetal heart rate abnormality; epidural analgesia, supine or semirecumbent position (see Evidence-Based Practice box in Chapter 1 about birth positions); episiotomy; labor augmentation; and instrumental or surgical births. Birthing centers did demonstrate a trend toward higher perinatal mortality over the conventional hospital setting.

LIMITATIONS

- Many (29% to 77%) of the women allocated to the homelike setting were transferred to the hospital for birth, which might alter risks and benefits for their original group, as well as maternal satisfaction scores. Reasons for transfer included failure to progress, fetal distress, and request for analgesia. There were differences between trials in the prenatal and postnatal care, time of enrollment, and "standard care" of the comparison group.

IMPLICATIONS FOR PRACTICE

- There are many benefits of a homelike birthing center for giving women the support, patience, and time to give birth without intervention. Women must weigh this against the earlier detection and treatment of problems in the hospital setting. Nurses can help support their clients' preferences for their ideal birth, while giving them a realistic idea of the transfer rate, and what to expect if they are transferred. This includes support for breastfeeding success in both settings.

IMPLICATIONS FOR FURTHER RESEARCH

- None of the trials examined free-standing birthing centers. There has to be more description of *standard care*, since it will vary across countries and time. Cost is an important driver for health care, and was not addressed. Staffing research needs to elucidate the effect of philosophy, and cross-staffing. The biggest confounder of these trials was the significant and varied transfer rate. A complete analysis of decision making and transfer experience on outcomes and satisfaction is needed.

Reference: Hodnett, E., Downe, S., Edwards, N., & Walsh, D. (2005). Home-like versus conventional institutional settings for birth. *The Cochrane Database of Systematic Reviews* 2006, Issue 3. Chichester, UK: John Wiley & Sons.

Couples who have attended childbirth education programs that teach the psychoprophylactic approach will know something about the labor process, coaching techniques, and comfort measures. The nurse should play a supportive role and keep such a couple informed of the progress. A review and repeated demonstration of methods learned in class and practiced in the familiar environment of their home without the pain and discomfort of labor and without the anxiety of being in an unfamiliar environment may be needed.

Even when expectant parents have not attended childbirth classes, the nurse can teach them simple breathing and relaxation techniques during the early phase of labor. In this case, the nurse may provide more of the coaching and supportive care until the support person feels ready to take on a more active coaching role. Comfort measures can be demonstrated by the nurse while encouraging the support person to assist and the laboring woman to express her needs and feelings. Observing the comforting approaches of the nurse can help the partner to learn effective comfort measures.

Comfort measures vary with the situation (Fig. 21-15). The nurse can draw on the couple's repertoire of comfort measures and relaxation techniques learned during the pregnancy and through life experiences (see Table 21-1 and Care Paths on pages 532 and 558). See Chapter 19 for a more detailed discussion of both pharmacologic and nonpharmacologic comfort measures.

Most women in labor respond positively to touch, but permission should be obtained before any measures involving touch. They appreciate gentle handling by staff members. Back rubs and counterpressure may be offered, especially if the woman is experiencing back labor. A support person may be taught to exert counterpressure against the woman's sacrum over the occiput of the head of a fetus in a posterior position (see Fig. 21-13, *B*). The back pain is caused by the occiput pressing on spinal nerves, and counterpressure lifts the occiput off these nerves, thereby providing some relief from pain. The partner will need to be relieved after a while, however, because exerting counterpressure is hard work. Hand and foot massage also can be soothing and relaxing (Simkin, Simkin & Ancheta, 2000; 2002).

The woman's perception of the soothing qualities of touch changes as labor progresses. Many women become more sensitive to touch (hyperesthesia) as labor progresses. This is a typical response during the transition phase (see Table 21-3). They may tell their coach to leave them alone or not to touch them. The partner who is unprepared for this normal response may feel rejected and may react by withdrawing active support. The nurse can reassure him or her that this response is a positive indication that the first stage is ending and the second stage is approaching. Women with increased sensitivity to touch may have a positive response when touched on surfaces of the body where hair does not grow, such as the forehead, the palms of the hands, and the soles of the feet.

Labor Support by the Father or Partner. Although another woman or a man other than the father may be the woman's partner, the father of the baby is usually the support person during labor. He often is able to provide the comfort measures and touch that the laboring woman needs. When the woman becomes focused on her pain, sometimes the partner can persuade her to try nonpharmacologic variations of comfort measures. In addition, he usually is able to interpret the woman's needs and desires for staff members.

Throughout the past 30 years, childbirth preparation education has been widely available. In the United States and Canada, the father's ideal role was thought to be that of labor coach, and he was expected to actively help the woman cope with labor. However, this expectation may be unrealistic, because some men have concerns about their labor-coaching abilities. Men can assume one of at least three different roles during labor and birth: coach, teammate, or witness (Chapman, 1992). As a *coach,* the father actively assists the woman during and after contractions. Men who are coaches express a strong need to be in control of themselves and of the labor experience. Women also express a great desire for the father to be physically involved in labor. The father who acts as the *teammate* assists the woman during labor and birth by responding to requests for physical or emotional support, or both. Teammates usually adopt the follower or helper role and look to the woman or nurse to tell them what to do. Women express a strong desire to have the father present and willing to help in any way. The father who acts as a *witness* acts as a companion, giving emotional and moral support. He watches the woman labor and give birth, but he often sleeps, watches television, or leaves the room for long periods. Witnesses believe that there is little they can do to help the woman physically and look to the nurses and health care providers to be in charge of the experience. Women do not expect more of this type of father than to just be present.

The degree of mutuality (level of interdependency and sharing) and understanding (the ability to know each other's needs) in a couple's relationship determines which role the father adopts. The coach and teammate roles are often assumed by men in couples with a high degree of mutuality. Men in couples in which mutuality is low tend to adopt the witness role. Because the father can participate in labor and birth in different ways, the nurse should encourage him to adopt the role most comfortable for him and for the woman, rather than to assume an unnatural role. Participation in the birth is ego building. The father can be of assistance; his presence is important.

The feelings of a first-time father change as labor progresses. Although he is often calm at the onset of labor, feelings of fear and helplessness begin to dominate as labor becomes more active and the father realizes that labor is more work than he anticipated. The first-time father may feel excluded as birth preparations begin during the transition phase. Once the second stage begins and birth nears, the father's focus changes from the woman to the baby who is about to be born. The father will be exposed to many sights and smells he may never before have experienced.

FIG. 21-15 Partner providing comfort measures. (Courtesy Marjorie Pyle, RNC, Lifecircle, Costa Mesa, CA.)

It is therefore important to tell him what to expect and to make him comfortable about leaving the room to regain his composure should something occur that surprises him. If he leaves the room, provision should be made for someone else to support the woman during his absence. Staff members should tell the father that his presence is helpful and encourage him to be involved in the care of the woman to the extent to which he is comfortable. Reassure him that he is not assuming the responsibility for observation and management of his partner's labor, but that his responsibility is to support her as the labor progresses. Suggest alternative comfort measures when those he is using are no longer helpful or are rejected by his partner.

Supporting both the father and the woman in labor elevates the nurse's role. It is another step forward for a nurse from merely providing custodial care to enacting a therapeutic role. Support of the father reflects the nurse's orientation and commitment to each person, the family, and the community. Therapeutic nursing actions convey several important concepts to the father: first, that the father is of value as a person; second, that he can learn to be a partner in the woman's care; and third, that childbearing is a partnership. Ways in which the nurse can support the father-partner are detailed in Box 21-6. A well-informed father can make an important contribution to the health and well-being of the mother and child, their family interrelationship, and his self-esteem.

Labor Support by Doulas. Continuity of care has been cited by women as a critical component of a satisfying childbirth experience. This need can be met by a spe-

cially trained, experienced female labor attendant called a doula. The doula provides a continuous, one-on-one caring presence throughout the labor and birth of the woman she is attending (Pascali-Bonaro & Kroeger, 2004). This is a beneficial form of care (Enkin et al., 2000).

The primary role of the doula is to focus on the laboring woman and provide physical and emotional support by using soft, reassuring words of praise and encouragement; touching, stroking, and hugging; administering nonpharmacologic comfort measures to reduce pain and enhance relaxation and coping; assisting the woman to move by walking with her, helping her to change positions, and encouraging her spontaneous, self-directed bearing-down efforts. Doulas provide information about labor progress and explain procedures and events. They advocate for the woman's right to participate actively in the management of her labor. These forms of caring help to reduce a woman's level of anxiety and fear, make her more confident and calm, and reduce the stress response that could inhibit the progress of labor (Kayne, Greulich, & Albers, 2001; Rosen, 2004; Trainor, 2002). Women participating in the Listening to Mother's Survey rated the doula highest among their caregivers during labor (Declercq et al., 2002).

The doula also supports the woman's partner, who often feels unqualified to be the sole labor support and may

---

box 21-6 Guidelines for Supporting the Father/Partner

- Orient to the labor room and the unit; explain location of the cafeteria, toilet, waiting room, and nursery; visiting hours; names and functions of personnel present.
- Inform him of sights and smells he can expect to encounter; encourage him to leave the room if necessary.
- Respect his or the couple's decision about the degree of his involvement. Offer them freedom to make decisions.
- Tell him when his presence has been helpful, and continue to reinforce this throughout labor.
- Offer to teach him comfort measures.
- Inform him frequently of the progress of the labor and the woman's needs. Keep him informed about procedures to be performed.
- Prepare him for changes in the woman's behavior and physical appearance.
- Remind him to eat; offer him snacks and fluids if possible.
- Relieve him of the job of support person as necessary. Offer him blankets if he is to sleep in a chair by the bedside.
- Acknowledge the stress experienced by each partner during labor and birth, and identify normal responses.
- Attempt to modify or eliminate unsettling stimuli, such as extra noise and extra light.

CRITICAL THINKING EXERCISE

Role of a Doula During Labor and Birth

Angela, a primigravida at 30 weeks of gestation, tells the nurse at a prenatal visit that she just read a magazine article about doulas and what they do to help women during labor. She says that when she asked her husband about hiring a doula for her labor he told her that he wanted to be her coach and felt they could work together without having to pay for someone to help them; in fact, they told the doctor they would probably opt for an epidural just like their friends. She asks the nurse if doulas are really all that helpful and worth their cost, especially since they heard that the nurses working on the labor unit where she will give birth are very good. How should the nurse respond to Angela's interest in doulas?

1. Evidence—Is there sufficient evidence to support the value of a doula as a caregiver for women in labor?
2. Assumptions—What assumptions can be made about the following issues related to the role of doulas in childbirth care?
   a. Benefits of having a doula as a caregiver during labor and birth
   b. Responsibilities of the doula during labor
   c. Role of the labor nurse as compared to that of the doula
3. How should the nurse address Angela's and her husband's belief that he can be an effective support for her and that the nurses on the floor are very good?
4. Does the evidence objectively support your response to Angela's belief?
5. Are there alternative perspectives to your conclusion?

find it difficult to watch the woman when she is experiencing pain. The doula can encourage and praise the partner's efforts, create a partnership as caregivers, and provide respite care. Doulas also facilitate communication between the laboring woman and her partner, as well as between the couple and the health care team (Pascali-Bonaro & Kroeger, 2004; Simkin & Young, 2005).

Continuous supportive care that begins early in labor significantly reduces the cesarean birth rate; duration of labor; use of oxytocin, analgesics, and forceps or vacuum extractor; and requests for epidural anesthesia. These reductions are greatest when the caregiver focuses solely on labor support and is not part of the staff of the labor unit (Hodnett et al., 2003; Rosen, 2004). Laboring women also reported a higher level of satisfaction with their childbirth experience and greater success with breastfeeding (Klaus, Kennell, & Klaus, 1993; Trainor, 2002). Long-term benefits of doula care are reflected in more positive maternal feelings regarding their parenting ability and lower rates of postpartum depression (Pascali-Bonaro & Kroeger, 2004; Rosen).

The role of the nurse and the doula are complementary. They should work together as a team, recognizing and respecting the role each plays in supporting and caring for the woman and her partner during the childbirth process. The doula provides supportive nonmedical care measures while the nurse focuses on monitoring the status of the maternal-fetal unit and implementing clinical care protocols, including pharmacologic interventions, and documenting assessment findings, actions, and responses (Adams & Bianchi, 2004; Simkin & Young, 2005).

Labor Support by Grandparents. When grandparents act as labor coaches, it is especially important to support and treat them with respect. They may have a way to relieve pain based on their experience. They should be encouraged to help as long as their actions do not compromise the status of the mother or the fetus. One example of an acceptable practice would be giving the woman herbal teas during labor. The nurse acts as a role model for parents by treating grandparents with dignity and respect, by acknowledging the value of the grandparents' contributions to parental support, and by recognizing the difficulty parents have in witnessing their child's discomfort or crisis, regardless of the age of the child. If they have never witnessed a birth, the nurse may need to provide explanations of what is happening. Many of the activities used to support fathers also are appropriate for grandparents.

When possible, the nurse offers the grandparents emotional support. A nurse can show such support by offering them liquid refreshment and by initiating discussion with open-ended questions or statements, such as, "It is sometimes hard to watch a daughter in labor." Nursing actions that provide support for the grandparents can have a therapeutic effect on all members of the family. In turn, a strong, supportive family unit is important for the optimal growth and development of its newest member.

Siblings During Labor and Birth. The preparation of siblings for acceptance of the new child helps promote the attachment process. Such preparation and participation during pregnancy and labor may help the older children accept this change. The older child or children who know themselves to be important to the family become active participants. Rehearsal for the event before labor is essential.

The age and developmental level of children influence their responses; therefore preparation for the children to be present during labor is adjusted to meet each child's needs. The child younger than 2 years shows little interest in pregnancy and labor; for the older child, such preparation may reduce fears and misconceptions. Parents need to be prepared for labor and birth themselves and feel comfortable about the process and the presence of their children. Most parents have a "feel" for their children's maturational level and their physical and emotional ability to observe and cope with the events of the labor and birth process. Preparation can include a description of the anticipated sights, events (e.g., ROM, monitors, IV infusions), smells, and sounds; a labor and birth demonstration; a tour of the birthing unit; and an opportunity to be around a real newborn. Children must learn that their mother will be working hard during labor and birth. She will not be able to talk to them during contractions. She may groan, scream, grunt, and pant at times as well as say things she would not say otherwise (e.g., "I can't take this anymore;" "Take this baby out of me;" or "This pain is killing me"). They can be told that labor is uncomfortable, but that their mother's body is made for the job. Storybooks about the birth process can be read to or by children to prepare them for the event. Films are available for preparing preschool and school-age children to participate in the labor and birth experience. Most agencies require that a specific person be designated to watch over the children who are participating in their mother's childbirth experience, to provide them with support, explanations, diversions, and comfort as needed. Health care providers involved in attending women during birth must be comfortable with the presence of children and the unpredictability of their questions, comments, and behaviors.

▅ Emergency Interventions

Emergency conditions that require immediate nursing intervention can arise with startling speed. Interventions for a nonreassuring FHR, inadequate uterine relaxation, vaginal bleeding, infection, and prolapse of the cord are detailed in the Emergency box.

▅ Evaluation

Evaluation of progress and outcomes is a continuous activity during the first stage of labor. The nurse must carefully evaluate each interaction with the mother-to-be and her family and critically appraise how well the expected outcomes of care are being met.

EMERGENCY

Interventions for Emergencies

SIGNS	INTERVENTIONS*
Nonreassuring FHR Pattern	
• Fetal bradycardia (FHR <110 beats/min for >10 min)†	Notify primary health care provider‡
• Fetal tachycardia (FHR >160 beats/min for >10 min in term pregnancy)§	Change maternal position
	Discontinue oxytocin (Pitocin) infusion, if being infused
• Irregular FHR, abnormal sinus rhythm shown by internal monitor	Increase IV fluid rate, if fluid being infused per protocol order
	Administer oxygen at 8 to 10 L/min by snug face mask
• Persistent decrease in baseline FHR variability without an identified cause	Check maternal temperature for elevation
	Start an IV line if one is not in place
• Late, severe variable, and prolonged deceleration patterns	Assist with amnioinfusion if ordered
• Absence of FHR	Stimulate fetal scalp or use sound stimulation
Inadequate Uterine Relaxation	
• Intrauterine pressure >75 mm Hg (shown by intrauterine pressure catheter monitoring)	Notify primary health care provider‡
	Discontinue oxytocin infusion, if being infused
• Contractions consistently lasting >90 sec	Change woman to side-lying position
• Contraction interval <2 min	Increase IV fluid rate, if fluid is being infused
	Administer oxygen at 8 to 10 L/min by snug face mask
	Start an IV line if one is not in place
	Palpate and evaluate contractions
	Give tocolytics (terbutaline), as ordered
Vaginal Bleeding	
• Vaginal bleeding (bright red, dark red, or in an amount in excess of that expected during normal cervical dilation)	Notify primary health care provider‡
	Anticipate emergency (stat) cesarean birth
• Continuous vaginal bleeding with FHR changes	*Do NOT perform a vaginal examination*
• Pain; may or may not be present	
Infection	
• Foul-smelling amniotic fluid	Notify primary health care provider‡
• Maternal temperature >38° C in presence of adequate hydration (straw-colored urine)	Institute cooling measures for laboring woman
	Start an IV line if one is not in place
• Fetal tachycardia >160 beats/min for >10 min	Assist with or perform collection of catheterized urine specimen and amniotic fluid sample and send to the laboratory for urinalysis and cultures
Prolapse of Cord	
• Fetal bradycardia with variable deceleration during uterine contraction	Call for assistance
	Have someone notify the primary health care provider immediately
• Woman reports feeling the cord after membranes rupture	
• Cord lies alongside or below the presenting part of the fetus; can be seen or felt in or protruding from the vagina	Glove the examining hand quickly and insert two fingers into the vagina to the cervix; with one finger on either side of the cord or both fingers to one side, exert upward pressure against the presenting part to relieve compression of the cord
• Major predisposing factors:	Place a rolled towel under the woman's hip
—Rupture of membranes with a gush	Place woman in extreme Trendelenburg or modified Sims position or knee-chest position
—Loose fit of presenting part in lower uterine segment	
—Presenting part not yet engaged	Wrap the cord loosely in a sterile towel saturated with warm, sterile normal saline if the cord is protruding from the vagina
—Breech presentation	Administer oxygen at 8 to 10 L/min by face mask until birth is accomplished
	Start IV fluids or increase existing drip rate
	Continue to monitor FHR by internal fetal scalp electrode, if possible
	Do not attempt to replace cord into cervix
	Prepare for immediate birth (vaginal or cesarean)

FHR, Fetal heart rate; *IV,* intravenous.

*Because emergency situations are often frightening events, it is important for the nurse to explain to the woman and her support person what is happening and how it is being managed.

†Practice is to intervene within 2 to 30 min of FHR of <110 beats/min.

‡In most emergency situations, nurses take immediate action, following a protocol and standards of nursing practice. Another person can notify the primary health care provider, or this can be done by the nurse as soon as possible.

§Nonreassuring sign when associated with late decelerations or absence of variability, especially of >180 beats/min.

■ SECOND STAGE OF LABOR

The second stage of labor is the stage in which the infant is born. This stage begins with full cervical dilation (10 cm) and complete effacement (100%) and ends with the baby's birth. The force exerted by uterine contractions, gravity, and maternal bearing-down efforts facilitates achievement of the expected outcome of a spontaneous, uncomplicated vaginal birth.

The second stage comprises three phases: the latent, descent, and transition phases. These phases are characterized by maternal verbal and nonverbal behaviors, uterine activity, the urge to bear down, and fetal descent.

The *latent phase* is a period of rest and relative calm (i.e., "laboring down"). During this early phase, the fetus continues to descend passively through the birth canal and rotate to an anterior position as a result of ongoing uterine contractions. The woman is quiet and often relaxes with her eyes closed between contractions. The urge to bear down is not well established and may not be experienced at all or only during the acme of a contraction. Allowing a woman to rest during this phase, and waiting until the urge to push intensifies, has been found to reduce maternal fatigue, conserve energy for bearing-down efforts, and provide optimal maternal and fetal outcomes (Minato, 2000; Simpson, 2005). Coaching a woman to push before her body signals readiness can result in a prolonged period of active pushing with limited to no progress. The woman may become dependent on her coach or nurses to tell her when and how to push (Roberts, 2002). However, women who have epidural analgesia may not feel the urge to bear down and will need coaching.

The *descent phase* or the phase of active pushing is characterized by strong urges to bear down as the reflex called the Ferguson reflex is activated; this is when the presenting part presses on the stretch receptors of the pelvic floor. At this point, the fetal station is usually +1, and the position is anterior. This stimulation causes the release of oxytocin from the posterior pituitary gland, which provokes stronger expulsive uterine contractions. The woman becomes more focused on bearing-down efforts, which become rhythmic. She changes positions frequently to find a more comfortable pushing position. The woman often announces the onset of contractions and becomes more vocal as she bears down. The urge to bear down intensifies as descent progresses.

In the *transition phase,* the presenting part is on the perineum, and bearing-down efforts are most effective for promoting birth. The woman may be more verbal about the pain she is experiencing; she may scream or swear and may act out of control (Roberts, 2002).

The nurse encourages the woman to "listen" to her body as she progresses through the phases of the second stage of labor. When a woman listens to her body to tell her when to bear down, she is using an internal locus of control and often feels more satisfied with her efforts to give birth to her baby. Her sense of self-esteem and accomplishment is enhanced, and her efforts become more effective. The

woman's trust in her own body and her ability to give birth to her baby should be fostered (Mayberry, Woods, Strange, Lee, Heisler, & Nielson-Smith, 2000).

If a woman is confined to bed, especially in a recumbent position, the rhythmic urge to bear down is delayed because gravity is not being used to press the presenting part against the pelvic floor. Being moved to another room and placed on a delivery table in the lithotomy position, as has been the custom in North America, also has an inhibiting effect on the urge to bear down. Today, Western societies have adopted the birthing practice of most non-Western societies in which labor and birth occur in the same room and women use various positions for bearing down, such as side-lying position, kneeling, squatting, sitting, or standing.

The duration of the second stage of labor is influenced by several factors, such as the effectiveness of the primary and secondary powers of labor; the type and amount of analgesia or anesthesia used; the physical and emotional condition, position, activity level, parity, and pelvic adequacy of the laboring woman; the size, presentation, and position of the fetus; and the nature and source of support the woman receives.

For many multiparous women, birth occurs within minutes of complete dilation, perhaps only one push later. Nulliparous women usually push for 1 to 2 hours before giving birth. If the woman has been given epidural analgesia, pushing can last more than 2 hours. Epidural analgesia blocks or reduces the urge to bear down and limits the woman's ability to attain an upright position to push. By adjusting dosages to the lowest effective level, allowing the epidural to wear off at full dilation or after 1 hour of pushing, or using mixtures containing an opioid agonist analgesic and a local anesthetic, the woman is better able to perceive the urge to bear down, to move more freely, and to attain an upright position with assistance as a result of increased strength and sensation in her legs. This approach can enhance the ability to bear down effectively and result in an uncomplicated vaginal birth (Mayberry et al., 2000). However, women also will have an increase in distress and the severity of pain. This results in an increase in sympathetic activity and the release of catecholamines. Catecholamines inhibit uterine contractions, potentially prolonging the second stage of labor. Allowing these women a "laboring down" period for fetal descent and rotation may result in a more positive outcome (Roberts, 2002).

Commonly, a second stage of more than 2 hours may be considered prolonged in women without regional analgesia and is reported to the primary health care provider. By using assessment findings such as the fetal heart rate and pattern, the descent of the presenting part, the quality of the uterine contractions, and the status of the woman, premature intervention with episiotomy or forceps- or vacuum-assisted birth can be avoided. If the status of the maternal-fetal unit is reassuring and progress is continuing, interventions to end the second stage of labor are unwarranted. Less emphasis should be placed on a definite time

Evolve/CD: Case Study: Second/Third Stages of Labor

limit for the second stage. The duration of active pushing has been found to be more relevant to the newborn's condition at birth than the duration of the second stage of labor itself (Cesario, 2004; Minato, 2000; Roberts, 2002).

▬ CARE MANAGEMENT

▬ Assessment and Nursing Diagnoses

The only certain objective sign that the second stage of labor has begun is the inability to feel the cervix during vaginal examination, indicating that the cervix is fully dilated and effaced. The precise moment that this occurs is not easily determined because it depends on when a vaginal examination is performed to validate full dilation and effacement. This makes timing of the actual duration of the second stage difficult (Roberts, 2002). Other signs that suggest the onset of the second stage include the following:

- Sudden appearance of sweat on upper lip
- An episode of vomiting
- Increased bloody show
- Shaking of extremities
- Increased restlessness; verbalization (e.g., "I can't go on")
- Involuntary bearing-down efforts

These signs commonly appear at the time the cervix reaches full dilation; however, women with an epidural block may not exhibit such signs. Other indicators for each phase of the second stage are given in Table 21-6.

Women can begin to experience an irresistible urge to bear down before full dilation. For some women, this occurs as early as 5 cm dilation. This is most often related to the station of the presenting part below the level of the ischial spines of the maternal pelvis. This occurrence creates a conflict between the woman, whose body is telling her to push, and her health care providers, who believe that pushing the fetal presenting part against an incompletely dilated cervix will result in cervical edema and lacerations, as well as a slowing down of labor progress. The premature urge to bear down must be evaluated as a phase of labor progress, possibly indicating the onset of the second stage

table 21-6 Expected Maternal Progress in Second Stage of Labor

CRITERION	LATENT PHASE (AVERAGE DURATION, 10-30 MIN)	DESCENT PHASE (AVERAGE DURATION VARIES)*	TRANSITION PHASE (AVERAGE DURATION 5-15 MIN)
Contractions Magnitude (intensity)	Period of physiologic lull for all criteria; period of peace and rest; "laboring down"	Significant increase	Overwhelmingly strong Expulsive
Frequency		2-2.5 min	1-2 min
Duration		90 sec	90 sec
Descent, station	0 to +2	Increases and Ferguson reflex† activated, +2 to +4	Rapid, +4 to birth Fetal head visible in introitus
Show: color and amount		Significant increase in dark red bloody show	Bloody show accompanies birth of head
Spontaneous bearing-down efforts	Slight to absent, except during acme of strongest contractions	Increased urge to bear down	Greatly increased
Vocalization	Quiet; concern over progress	Grunting sounds or expiratory vocalization; announces contractions	Grunting sounds and expiratory vocalizations continue; may scream or swear
Maternal behavior	Experiences sense of relief that transition to second stage is finished Feels fatigued and sleepy Feels a sense of accomplishment and optimism, because the "worst is over" Feels in control	Senses increased urge to push Alters respiratory pattern: has short 4- to 5-sec breath holds with regular breaths in between, 5 to 7 times per contraction Makes grunting sounds or expiratory vocalizations Frequent repositioning	Describes extreme pain Expresses feelings of powerlessness Shows decreased ability to listen or concentrate on anything but giving birth Describes *ring of fire* (burning sensation of acute pain as vagina stretches and fetal head crowns) Often shows excitement immediately after birth of head

Source: Roberts, J. (2002). The "push" for evidence: Management of the second stage. *Journal of Midwifery & Women's Health, 47*(1), 2-15; Simkin, P., & Ancheta, R. (2000). *The labor progress handbook*. Malden, MA: Blackwell Science.
*Duration of descent phase can vary depending on maternal parity, effectiveness of bearing-down effort, and presence of spinal anesthesia or epidural analgesia.
†Pressure of presenting part on stretch receptors of pelvic floor stimulates release of oxytocin from posterior pituitary, resulting in more intense uterine contractions.

of labor. The timing when a woman pushes in relation to whether or not her cervix is fully dilated should be based on research evidence rather than on tradition or routine practice. It may be safe and effective for a woman to push with the urge to bear down at the acme of a contraction if her cervix is soft, retracting, and 8 cm or more dilated and if the fetus is at a +1 station and rotating to an anterior position (Roberts, 2002).

Assessment is continuous during the second stage of labor. Professional standards and agency policy determine the specific type and timing of assessments, as well as the way in which findings are documented. The Care Path for the second and third stages of labor indicates typical assessments and the recommended frequency for their performance. Signs and symptoms of impending birth (see Table 21-6) may appear unexpectedly, requiring immediate action by the nurse (Box 21-7).

Nursing diagnoses that represent potential areas for concern during the second stage of labor include the following:

- *Risk for injury to mother and fetus related to*
  - persistent use of Valsalva maneuver during bearing-down efforts
- *Acute pain related to*
  - bearing-down efforts and distention of the perineum
- *Anxiety related to*
  - inability to control defecation during bearing-down efforts
  - deficient knowledge regarding perineal sensations associated with the urge to bear down
  - coaching that contradicts woman's physiologic urge to push
- *Risk for infection related to*
  - prolonged rupture of membranes
  - use of invasive measures (e.g., forceps, vacuum extraction) to facilitate birth
- *Situational low self-esteem (maternal) related to*
  - deficient knowledge of normal, beneficial effects of vocalization during bearing-down efforts
  - inability to carry out plan for birth

■ Expected Outcomes of Care

Planning for the second and third stages of labor is done during the first stage of labor. Previously determined expected outcomes may be modified as these stages progress. Expected outcomes for the woman in the second stage of labor are that the woman will accomplish the following:
- Actively participate in the process of giving birth.
- Sustain no injury to herself or her fetus during the birth process.
- Accept support measures from significant others and health care providers as needed during bearing-down efforts.

■ Plan of Care and Interventions

The nurse continues to monitor maternal-fetal status and events of the second stage and provide comfort measures for the mother, such as helping her to change positions; providing mouth care; maintaining clean, dry bedding; and keeping extraneous noise, conversation, and other distractions (e.g., laughing, talking of attending personnel in or outside the labor area) to a minimum. The woman is encouraged to indicate other support measures she would like (Table 21-7; Care Path for Low Risk Woman in Second and Third Stages of Labor; Plan of Care for Labor and Birth p. 543).

In the hospital, birth may occur in an LDR, LDRP, or delivery room. If the mother is to be transferred to the delivery room for birth, the nurse accomplishes the transfer early enough to avoid rushing the woman. The birth area also is readied for the birth.

Preparing for Birth

Maternal Position. There is no single position for childbirth. Labor is a dynamic, interactive process involving the woman's uterus, pelvis, and voluntary muscles. In addition, angles between the baby and the woman's pelvis constantly change as the infant turns and flexes down the birth canal. The woman may want to assume various positions for childbirth, and she should be encouraged and assisted in attaining and maintaining her position(s) of choice. Supine, semi-recumbent, or lithotomy positions are still widely used in Western societies despite evidence that women prefer upright positions for their bearing-down efforts and birth.

Birth attendants play a major role in influencing a woman's choice of positions for birth, with midwives tending to advocate the nonlithotomy positions for the second stage of labor. Upright positions for women with and without epidural anesthesia facilitate birth and fetal descent and reduce the duration of the second stage of labor and the need for episiotomy, forceps, or vacuum extractor in the following ways (Gupta & Hofmeyr, 2004):
- Straighten the longitudinal axis of the birth canal and improve the alignment of the fetus for passage through the pelvis
- Use gravity to direct the fetal head toward the pelvic inlet, thereby facilitating descent
- Enlarge pelvic dimensions and restrict the encroachment of the sacrum and coccyx into the pelvic outlet
- Increase uteroplacental circulation, resulting in more intense, efficient uterine contractions
- Enhance the woman's ability to bear down effectively, thereby minimizing maternal exhaustion

However, the upright positions may slightly increase the risk for second-degree lacerations and a blood loss greater than 500 ml. Further investigation is needed to determine the exact mechanism for these outcomes (Shorten, Donsante, & Shorten, 2002).

Squatting is highly effective in facilitating the descent and birth of the fetus. It is considered to be one of the best

CD: Critical Thinking Exercises: Positioning During Labor

| box 21-7 | Guidelines for Assistance at the Emergency Birth of a Fetus in the Vertex Presentation |

1. The woman usually assumes the position most comfortable for her. A lateral position is often recommended.
2. Reassure the woman that birth is usually uncomplicated and easy in these situations. Use eye-to-eye contact and a calm, relaxed manner. If there is someone else available, such as the partner, that person could help support the woman in the position, assist with coaching, and compliment her on her efforts.
3. Wash your hands and put on gloves, if available.
4. Place under woman's buttocks whatever clean material is available.
5. Avoid touching the vaginal area to decrease the possibility of infection.
6. As the head begins to crown, you should do the following:
   a. Tear the amniotic membrane if it is still intact.
   b. Instruct the woman to pant or pant-blow, thus minimizing the urge to push.
   c. Place the flat side of your hand on the exposed fetal head and apply gentle pressure toward the vagina to prevent the head from "popping out." The mother may participate by placing her hand under yours on the emerging head. NOTE: Rapid birth of the fetal head must be prevented because a rapid change of pressure within the molded fetal skull follows, which may result in dural or subdural tears and may cause vaginal or perineal lacerations.
7. After the birth of the head, check for the umbilical cord. If the cord is around the baby's neck, try to slip it over the baby's head or pull it *gently* to get some slack so that you can slip it over the shoulders.
8. Support the fetal head as restitution (external rotation) occurs. After restitution, with one hand on each side of the baby's head, exert *gentle* pressure downward so that the anterior shoulder emerges under the symphysis pubis and acts as a fulcrum; then, as *gentle* pressure is exerted in the opposite direction, the posterior shoulder, which has passed over the sacrum and coccyx, emerges.
9. Be alert! Hold the baby securely because the rest of the body may emerge quickly. The baby will be slippery!
10. Cradle the baby's head and back in one hand and the buttocks in the other. Keep the head down to drain away the mucus. Use a bulb syringe, if one is available, to remove mucus from the baby's mouth.
11. Dry the baby quickly to prevent rapid heat loss. Keep the baby at the same level as the mother's uterus until the end of the cord stops pulsating. NOTE: It is important to keep the baby at the same level as the mother's uterus to prevent the baby's blood from flowing to or from the placenta and the resultant hypovolemia or hypervolemia. Also, do not "milk" the cord.
12. Place the baby on the mother's abdomen, cover the baby (remember to keep the head warm, too) with the mother's clothing, and have her cuddle the baby. Compliment her (them) on a job well done, and on the baby, if appropriate.
13. Wait for the placenta to separate; *do not* tug on the cord. NOTE: Injudicious traction may tear the cord, separate the placenta, or invert the uterus. Signs of placental separation include a slight gush of dark blood from the introitus, lengthening of the cord, and change in the uterine contour from a discoid to globular shape.
14. Instruct the mother to push to deliver the separated placenta. Gently ease out the placental membranes using an up-and-down motion until the membranes are removed. If birth occurs outside a hospital setting, to minimize complications, do not cut the cord without proper clamps and a sterile cutting tool. Inspect the placenta for intactness. Place the baby on the placenta and wrap the two together for additional warmth.
15. Check the firmness of the uterus. Gently massage the fundus and demonstrate to the mother how she can massage her own fundus properly.
16. If supplies are available, clean the mother's perineal area and apply a peripad.
17. In addition to gentle massage of the fundus, the following measures can be taken to prevent or minimize hemorrhage:
    a. Put the baby to the mother's breast as soon as possible. Sucking or nuzzling and licking the nipple stimulates the release of oxytocin from the posterior pituitary. NOTE: If the baby does not or cannot nurse, manually stimulate the mother's nipples.
    b. Do not allow the mother's bladder to become distended. Assess the bladder for fullness and encourage her to void if fullness is found.
    c. Expel any clots from the mother's uterus.
18. Comfort or reassure the mother and her family or friends. Keep the mother and the baby warm. Give her fluids if available and tolerated.
19. If this is a multifetal birth, identify the infants in order of birth (using letters *A, B*, etc.).
20. Make notations regarding the following aspects of the birth:
    a. Fetal presentation and position
    b. Presence of cord around neck (nuchal cord) or other parts and number of times cord encircled part
    c. Color, character, and amount of amniotic fluid, if rupture of membranes occurs immediately before birth
    d. Time of birth
    e. Estimated time of determination of Apgar score (e.g., 1 and 5 min after birth), resuscitation efforts implemented, and ultimate condition of baby
    f. Sex of baby
    g. Time of placental expulsion, as well as the appearance and completeness of the placenta
    h. Maternal condition: affect, amount of bleeding, and status of uterine tonicity
    i. Any unusual occurrences during the birth (e.g., maternal or paternal response, verbalizations, or gestures in response to birth of baby)

and most natural positions for the second stage of labor (Mayberry et al., 2000; Roberts, 2002). Women should assume a modified, supported squat until the fetal head is engaged, at which time a deep squat can be used. A firm surface is required for this position, and the woman will need side support (see Fig. 21-13, *A*). In a birthing bed, a squat bar is available that she can use to help support herself (Fig. 21-16, *E*). A birth ball can also be used to help a woman maintain the squatting position. The fetus will be aligned with the birth canal, and pelvic and perineal

table. 21-7 Woman's Responses and Support Person's Actions During Second Stage of Labor	
WOMAN'S RESPONSES*	**NURSE OR SUPPORT PERSON'S ACTIONS†**
LATENT PHASE	
Experiences a short period of peace and rest:	Encourages woman to "listen" to her body
	Continues support measures allowing woman to rest
	Suggests an upright position to encourage progression of descent if descent phase does not begin after 20 min
DESCENT PHASE	
Senses increased urgency to bear down as Ferguson reflex is activated	Encourages respiratory pattern of short breath holds and open-glottis pushing
Notes increase in intensity of uterine contractions; alters respiratory pattern: short 4- to 5-sec breath holds, five to seven times per contraction	Stresses normality and benefits of grunting sounds and expiratory vocalizations
Makes grunting sounds or expiratory vocalizations	Encourages bearing-down efforts with urge to push
	Encourages or suggests maternal movement and position changes (upright, if descent is not occurring)
	Encourages woman to "listen" to her body regarding movement and position change if descent is occurring
	Discourages long breath holds (no longer than 5 to 7 sec)
	If birth is to occur in a delivery room, transfers woman to delivery room early to avoid rushing or, if permitted, offers her option of walking to delivery room
	Places woman in lateral recumbent position to slow descent if descent is too fast
TRANSITIONAL PHASE	
Behaves in manner similar to behavior during transition in first stage (8-10 cm)	Encourages slow, gentle pushing
Experiences a sense of severe pain and powerlessness	Explains that "blowing away the contraction" facilitates a slower birth of the head
Shows decreased ability to listen	Provides mirror to help woman see or touch the emerging fetal head (best to extend over two to three contractions) to help her understand the perineal sensations
Concentrates on birth of baby until head is born	
Experiences contractions as overwhelming in intensity	
Reports feeling ring of fire as head crowns	Coaches woman to relax mouth, throat, and neck to promote relaxation of pelvic floor
Maintains respiratory pattern of three to five 7-sec breath holds per contraction, followed by forced expiration	Applies warm compress to perineum to promote relaxation
Eases head out with short expirations	
Responds with excitement and relief after head is born	

*Woman's responses will be altered if epidural analgesia is being administered.
†Provided by nurses and support persons in collaboration with the nurse.

relaxation will be facilitated as she sits on the ball or holds it in front of her for support as she squats (see Fig. 21-14).

When a woman uses the supported standing position for bearing down, her weight is borne on both femoral heads, allowing the pressure in the acetabulum to cause the transverse diameter of the pelvic outlet to increase by up to 1 cm. This can be helpful if descent of the head is delayed because the occiput has not rotated from the lateral (transverse diameter of pelvis) to the anterior position. Birthing chairs or rocking chairs may be used to provide women with a good physiologic position to enhance her bearing-down efforts during childbirth, although some women feel restricted by a chair. The upright position also provides a potential psychologic advantage in that it allows the mother to see the birth as it occurs and to maintain eye contact with the attendant. Most birthing chairs are designed so that if an emergency occurs, the chair can be adjusted to the horizontal or the Trendelenburg position.

Oversized beanbag chairs and large floor pillows may be used for both labor and birth. They can mold around and support the mother in whatever position she selects. These chairs are of particular value for mothers who wish to be actively involved in the birth process. Birthing stools can be used to support the woman in an upright position similar to squatting. Women may want to sit on the toilet or commode during pushing because they are concerned about stool incontinence during this stage. These women must be closely monitored, however, and removed from the toilet before birth becomes imminent. Because sitting on chairs, stools, toilets, or commodes can increase perineal edema and blood loss, it is important to assist the woman to change her position frequently.

The side-lying position, with the upper part of the woman's leg held by the nurse or coach or placed on a pillow, is an effective position for the second stage of labor (Fig. 21-17, *A*). Women using the lateral position have more control over their bearing-down efforts. In addition,

care path ▷ Low Risk Woman in Second and Third Stages of Labor

CARE MANAGEMENT	SECOND STAGE OF LABOR	THIRD STAGE OF LABOR
I. ASSESSMENT MEASURES*	**Frequency**	**Frequency**
• Blood pressure, pulse, respirations	Every 5-30 min	Every 15 min
• Uterine activity	Assess every contraction	Assess for signs of placental separation
• Bearing-down effort	Assess each effort	
• Fetal heart rate (FHR)	Every 5-15 min	Assist with determination of Apgar score at 1 and 5 min
• Vaginal show	Every 15 min	Assess bleeding until placental expulsion
• Signs of fetal descent: urge to bear down, perineal bulging, crowning	Every 10-15 min	
• Behavior, appearance, mood, energy level of woman; condition of partner	Every 10-15 min	Assess response to completion of childbirth process, reaction to newborn
II. PHYSICAL CARE MEASURES†	**Latent Phase:**	
	Assist to rest in position of comfort	Assist to bear down to facilitate delivery of separated placenta
	Encourage relaxation to conserve energy	Administer oxytocic as ordered
	Promote urge to push; if delayed: ambulation, shower, pelvic rock, position changes	Provide pain relief as needed
		Provide hygiene and comfort measures as needed
	Descent Phase:	
	Assist to bear down effectively	
	Help to use recommended positions that facilitate descent	
	Encourage correct breathing during bearing-down efforts	
	Help to relax between contractions	
	Provide comfort measures as needed	
	Cleanse perineum immediately if fecal material is expelled	
	Transition Phase:	
	Assist to pant during contraction to avoid rapid birth of head	
	Coach to gently bear down between contractions	
III. EMOTIONAL SUPPORT	Keep informed of progress of fetal descent	Keep informed about progress of placental separation
	Provide feedback for bearing-down efforts	Explain purpose if medications given
	Explain purpose if medications given	Describe status of perineal tissue and inform if repair is needed
	Role model comfort measures	Introduce parents to their baby
	Provide continuous nursing presence	Assess and care for newborn within view of parents; delay eye prophylaxis to facilitate eye contact
	Create a quiet, calm environment	
	Reassure, encourage, praise	
	Take charge as needed, until woman regains confidence in ability to birth her baby	Provide private time for family to bond with their new baby and help them to create memories
	Offer mirror to watch birth	Encourage breastfeeding if desired

*Frequency of assessment is determined by the risk status of the maternal-fetal unit. More frequent assessment is required in high risk situations. Frequency of assessment and method of documentation are also determined by agency policy, which is usually based on the recommended care standards of medical and nursing organizations.
†Physical care measures are performed by the nurse working together with the woman's partner and significant others.

a slower, more controlled descent of the fetus results in a reduced risk of perineal trauma (Gupta & Hofmeyr, 2004). Some women prefer a semi-sitting (semi-recumbent) position. To maintain good uteroplacental circulation and to enhance the woman's bearing-down efforts in this position, the woman's back and shoulders should be elevated to at least a 30-degree angle, and a wedge should be placed under one hip (Fig. 21-17, *B*). The episiotomy rate for nulliparas has been found to be highest in this position (Shorten, Donsante, & Shorten, 2002).

FIG. 21-16 The versatility of today's birthing bed makes it practical in a variety of settings. NOTE: OB table used for lithotomy position. **A,** Labor bed. **B,** Birth chair. **C,** Birth bed. **D,** OB table. **E,** Squatting or birth bar. (Courtesy Julie Perry Nelson, Gilbert, AZ.)

The hands-and-knees position, along with pelvic rocking and abdominal stroking, is an effective position for birth because it enhances placental perfusion, helps rotate the fetus from a posterior to an anterior position, and may facilitate the birth of the shoulders, especially if the fetus is large. Perineal trauma also may be reduced (Simkin & Ancheta, 2000) (see Fig. 21-12, *B*).

The birthing bed is commonly used today and can be set for different positions according to the woman's needs (Figs. 21-16 and 21-18). The woman can squat, kneel, sit, recline, or lie on her side, choosing the position most comfortable for her for the birth. At the same time, there is excellent exposure for examinations, electrode placement, and birth. The bed also can be positioned for the administration of anesthesia and is ideal to help women receiving an epidural to assume different positions to facilitate birth. The bed can be used to transport the woman to the operating room if a cesarean birth is necessary. Squat bars, over-the-bed tables, birth balls, and pillows can be used for support.

Bearing-Down Efforts. As the fetal head reaches the pelvic floor, most women experience the urge to bear

CD: Animations

FIG. 21-18   Birth bed. (Courtesy Hill-Rom, Batesville, IN.)

FIG. 21-17   A, Pushing, side-lying position. Perineal bulging can be seen. **B,** Pushing, semi-sitting position. Midwife assists mother to feel top of fetal head. (**A,** Courtesy Michael S. Clement, MD, Mesa, AZ. **B,** Courtesy Roni Wernik, Palo Alto, CA.)

down. Reflexively the woman will begin to exert downward pressure by contracting her abdominal muscles while relaxing her pelvic floor. This bearing down is an involuntary response to the Ferguson reflex. A strong expiratory grunt or groan (vocalization) often accompanies pushing when the woman exhales as she pushes. This natural vocalization by women during open-glottis bearing-down efforts should not be discouraged by nurses.

When assisting a woman to push, the nurse should encourage her to push as she feels like pushing (instinctive, spontaneous pushing) rather than to give a prolonged push on command. A woman can become confused and anxious when she is being told to do something in conflict with what her body is telling her. Using phrases such as "you

CRITICAL THINKING EXERCISE

Spontaneous Versus Directed Bearing-Down Efforts

A controversy has arisen on the labor unit where you have your maternal-newborn clinical rotation. Some of the nurses and midwives and most of the obstetricians believe that women must be coached to begin pushing as soon as full dilation occurs to ensure that the second stage is not prolonged. The rest of the nurses and midwives and a few obstetricians believe that women know best when and how to push and encourage women in labor to follow what their bodies tell them. The nurse manager of the labor unit has encouraged those believing in spontaneous pushing to present a unit in-service to present evidence to show that spontaneous pushing enhances the well-being of the maternal-fetal unit without a significant effect on the progress of the second stage of labor. What should the proponents of spontaneous pushing present at the unit in-service?

1. Evidence—Is there evidence that will support the benefits of spontaneous pushing?
2. Assumptions—What assumptions can be made about the following issues related to spontaneous pushing during the second stage of labor?
   a. Benefits of spontaneous pushing
   b. Risks associated with directed pushing
   c. Impact of timing for the onset of pushing during the second stage of labor
3. What influence does a woman's position have on the effectiveness of the pushing technique she uses?
4. Does the evidence support a recommended position to enhance the woman's bearing-down efforts?
5. Are there alternative perspectives to your conclusion?

are doing so well," "you are moving the baby down," and "follow what your body is telling you" rather than "Push, push, push," encourages a woman to feel confident in her body and what she is feeling (Hansen, Clark, & Foster, 2002; Roberts, 2003; Sampselle, Miller, Luecha, Fischer, & Rosten, 2005).

Women will usually begin to push naturally as the contraction increases in intensity and the Ferguson reflex strengthens. The nurse should monitor the woman's breathing so that the woman does not hold her breath for more than 5 to 7 seconds at a time and should remind her to ventilate her lungs fully by taking deep cleansing breaths before and after each contraction. Bearing down while exhaling (open-glottis pushing) and taking breaths between bearing-down efforts helps maintain adequate oxygen levels for the mother and fetus, thereby enhancing fetal well-being. Approximately five pushes occur during a contraction, with each push lasting about 5 seconds (Mayberry et al., 2000). Maternal benefits associated with spontaneous pushing include less perineal trauma, less maternal fatigue, and fewer forceps- or vacuum-assisted births. In addition, evidence is indicating that the integrity of the pelvic floor is preserved reducing the risk for future incontinence and pelvic organ prolapse (Roberts, 2002; Sampselle et al., 2005; Simpson & James, 2005).

Prolonged breath-holding, or sustained, directed bearing down is still a common practice often beginning at 10 cm dilation and before the urge to bear down is perceived. The woman is coached to hold her breath, closing her glottis, and to push while the nurse or partner counts to 10. This method of bearing down triggers the Valsalva maneuver when the woman closes her glottis (closed-glottis pushing), thereby increasing intrathoracic and cardiovascular pressure, reducing cardiac output, and inhibiting perfusion of the uterus and the placenta. In addition, breath holding for more than 5 to 7 seconds causes the perfusion of oxygen across the placenta to be diminished, resulting in fetal hypoxia (Simpson, 2005). This approach to bearing down is harmful or ineffective and should be discouraged (Enkin et al., 2000).

A woman may reach the second stage of labor and then experience a lack of readiness to complete the process and give birth to her child. She may have doubts about her readiness to be a mother or may desire to wait for her support person or primary health care provider to arrive. Fear, anxiety, or embarrassment regarding unfamiliar or painful sensations and behaviors during pushing (e.g., sounds made, passage of stool) may be other inhibiting factors. Fear that the baby will be in danger once it emerges from the protective intrauterine environment also may be present.

By recognizing that a woman may experience a need to hold back the birth of her baby, the nurse can then address the woman's concerns and effectively coach the woman during this stage of labor.

To ensure the slow birth of the fetal head, the woman is encouraged to control the urge to bear down by coaching her to take panting breaths or to exhale slowly through pursed lips as the baby's head crowns. At this point, the woman needs simple, clear directions from one person.

Amnesia between contractions often is pronounced in the second stage, and the woman may have to be roused to get her to cooperate in the bearing-down process. Parents who have attended childbirth education classes may have devised a set of verbal cues for the laboring woman to follow. It is helpful for them to have these cues printed on a card that can be attached to the head of the bed so that the nurse can better substitute as coach if the partner has to leave.

Fetal Heart Rate and Pattern. As noted previously, the fetal heart rate must be checked. If the baseline rate begins to slow, if there is a loss of variability, or if deceleration patterns develop (e.g., late, variable), prompt treatment must be initiated. The woman can be turned on her side to reduce the pressure of the uterus against the ascending vena cava and descending aorta (see Fig. 21-5), and oxygen can be administered by mask at 8 to 10 L/min (Tucker, 2004). This is often all that is necessary to restore a reassuring pattern. If the FHR and pattern does not become reassuring immediately, medical intervention to hasten the birth may be indicated.

Support of the Father or Partner. During the second stage, the woman needs continuous support and coaching (see Table 21-7). Because the coaching process can be physically and emotionally tiring for support persons, the nurse offers them nourishment and fluids and encourages them to take short breaks. If birth occurs in an LDR or LDRP room, the partner may be allowed to wear street clothes or may be required to wear a clean scrub outfit, cap, and mask (for the birth). The support person who attends the birth in a delivery room is instructed to put on a cover gown or scrub clothes, mask, hat, and shoe covers, as required by agency policy. The nurse also specifies support measures that can be used for the laboring woman and points out areas of the room in which the partner can move freely.

Partners are encouraged to be present at the birth of their infants if this is in keeping with their cultural and personal expectations and beliefs. In this way the psychologic closeness of the family unit is maintained, and the partner can continue to provide supportive care during labor. The woman and her partner need to have an equal opportunity to initiate the attachment process with the baby.

▬ **LEGAL TIP** Documentation

Documentation of all observations (e.g., maternal vital signs, fetal heart rate and pattern, progress of labor) and nursing interventions, including client response, should be done concurrent with care. The course of labor and the maternal-fetal response may change without warning. It is important that all documentation be accurate, complete, timely, and according to agency policy.

Supplies, Instruments, and Equipment. To prepare for birth in any setting, the birthing table is usually set up during the transition phase for nulliparous women and during the active phase for multiparous women.

The birthing supples and instruments are arranged on a table or cart (Fig. 21-19). Standard procedures are followed for gloving, identifying and opening sterile packages, adding sterile supplies to the table, unwrapping sterile instruments, and handing them to the primary health care provider. The crib or radiant warmer and equipment are readied for the support and stabilization of the infant (Fig. 21-20).

The items used for birth may vary among different facilities; therefore each facility's procedure manual should

FIG. 21-19 Instrument table. (Courtesy Marjorie Pyle, RNC, Lifecircle, Costa Mesa, CA.)

FIG. 21-20 Radiant warmer for newborn. (Courtesy Dee Lowdermilk, Chapel Hill, NC.)

be consulted to determine the protocols specific to that facility.

The nurse estimates the time until the birth will occur and notifies the primary health care provider if he or she is not in the client's room. Even the most experienced nurse can miscalculate the time left before birth occurs; therefore every nurse who attends a woman in labor must be prepared to assist with an emergency birth if the primary health care provider is not present (see Box 21-7).

▬ *Birth in a Delivery Room or Birthing Room*

The woman will need assistance if she must move from the labor bed to the delivery table (Fig. 21-21). The various positions assumed for birth in a delivery room are the Sims or lateral position in which the attendant supports the upper part of the woman's leg, the dorsal position (supine position with one hip elevated), and the lithotomy position.

The lithotomy position has been the position most commonly used for birth in Western cultures, although this practice is slowly changing. The lithotomy position makes it more convenient for the primary health care provider to deal with complications that arise (see Fig. 21-16, *D*). To place the woman in this position, her buttocks are brought to the edge of the table and her legs are placed in stirrups. Care must be taken to pad the stirrups, to raise and place both legs simultaneously, and to adjust the shanks of the stirrups so that the calves of the legs are supported. There should be no pressure on the popliteal space. If the stirrups are not the same height, ligaments in the woman's back can be strained as she bears down, leading to considerable discomfort in the postpartum period. The lower portion of the table may be dropped down and rolled back under the table.

It should be noted that the routine use of a supine or lithotomy position for labor and birth has been identified ✳ as a clearly harmful or ineffective practice and should be discouraged (Enkin et al., 2000).

The maternal position for birth in a birthing room varies from a lithotomy position with the woman's legs in

CD:Video: Childbirth

FIG. 21-21 Delivery room. (Courtesy Michael S. Clement, MD, Mesa, AZ.)

stirrups, to one in which her feet rest on footrests while she holds onto a squat bar, to a side-lying position with the woman's upper leg supported by the coach, nurse, or squat bar. The foot of the bed can be removed so that the primary health care provider attending the birth can gain better perineal access for performing an episiotomy, delivering a large baby, using forceps or vacuum extractor, or getting access to the emerging head to facilitate suctioning. Otherwise the foot of the bed is left in place and lowered slightly to form a ledge that allows access for birth and that also serves as a place to lay the newborn (see Fig. 21-18).

Once the woman is positioned for birth either in a delivery room or birthing room, the vulva and perineum may be cleansed. Hospital protocols and the preferences of primary health care providers for cleansing may vary.

The labor nurse continues to coach and encourage the woman. The nurse auscultates the FHR or evaluates the monitor tracing every 5 to 15 minutes, depending on whether the woman is at low or high risk for problems or per protocol of the birthing facility, or continuously monitors the FHR with electronic monitoring. The primary health care provider is kept informed of the fetal heart rate and pattern (Tucker, 2004). An oxytocic medication such as oxytocin (Pitocin) may be prepared so that it is ready to be administered after expulsion of the placenta. Standard Precautions should always be followed as care is administered during the process of labor and birth (see Box 21-3).

In the delivery room, the primary health care provider puts on a cap, a mask that has a shield or protective eyewear, and shoe covers. Hands are scrubbed, a sterile gown (with waterproof front and sleeves) is donned, and gloves are put on. Nurses attending the birth also may need to wear caps, protective eyewear, masks, gowns, and gloves. The woman may then be draped with sterile drapes. In the birthing room, Standard Precautions are observed, but the amount and types of protective coverings worn by those in attendance may vary.

Nursing contact with the parents is maintained by touching, verbal comforting, explaining the reasons for care, and sharing in the parents' joy at the birth of their child.

■ Water Birth

There is evidence that immersion in water during first-stage labor can reduce the amount of pain and anxiety and does not appear to affect neonatal outcomes (Benfield, 2002; Cluett et al., 2002). However, the effects of immersion during birth and in the third stage have not been determined by randomized controlled trials that have a large enough sample to make a determination about maternal and neonatal outcomes.

If a woman wishes to have a water birth (Fig. 21-22) in the United States, the newborn will usually be removed from the water immediately after birth (Waterbirth International, 2005). The infant can be placed in the mother's arms until the cord is cut. The woman usually is assisted from the tub to the bed to deliver the placenta.

FIG. 21-22   Water birth. (Courtesy Global Maternal/Child Health Association, Inc., Wilsonville, OR.)

■ Mechanism of Birth: Vertex Presentation

The three phases of the spontaneous birth of a fetus in a vertex presentation are (1) birth of the head, (2) birth of the shoulders, and (3) birth of the body and extremities (see Chapter 18).

With voluntary bearing-down efforts, the head appears at the introitus (Fig. 21-23). Crowning occurs when the widest part of the head (the biparietal diameter) distends the vulva just before birth. The birth attendant may apply mineral oil to the perineum and stretch it as the head is crowning. Immediately before birth, the perineal musculature becomes greatly distended. If an episiotomy (incision into the perineum to enlarge vaginal outlet) is necessary, it is done at this time to minimize soft-tissue damage.

The physician or nurse-midwife may use a hands-on approach to control the birth of the head, believing that guarding the perineum results in a gradual birth that will prevent fetal intracranial injury, protect maternal tissues, and reduce postpartum perineal pain. This approach involves (1) applying pressure against the rectum, drawing it downward to aid in flexing the head as the back of the neck catches under the symphysis pubis; (2) then applying upward pressure from the coccygeal region (modified Ritgen maneuver) (Fig. 21-24) to extend the head during the actual birth, thereby protecting the musculature of the perineum; and (3) assisting the mother with voluntary control of the bearing-down efforts by coaching her to pant while letting uterine forces expel the fetus.

Some health care providers use a hands-poised (hands-off) approach when attending a birth. In this approach, hands are prepared to place light pressure on the fetal head to prevent rapid expulsion. Hands are not placed on the perineum or used to assist with birth of the shoulders and body.

The hands-on and hands-poised approaches have similar results in terms of perineal trauma and condition of the newborn. However, perineal pain is slightly less at

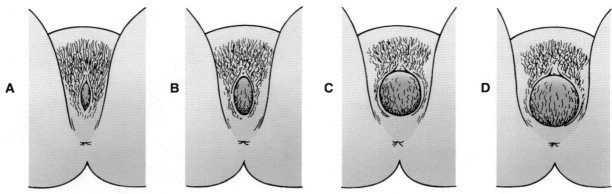

FIG. 21-23   Beginning birth with vertex presenting. **A,** Anteroposterior slit. **B,** Oval opening. **C,** Circular shape. **D,** Crowning.

FIG. 21-24   Birth of head with modified Ritgen maneuver. Note control to prevent too-rapid birth of head.

10 days postpartum when the hands-on approach is used (McCandlish, 2001). Guarding the perineum is a form of ❋ care likely to be beneficial (Enkin et al., 2000).

The umbilical cord often encircles the neck (nuchal cord) but rarely so tightly as to cause hypoxia. After the head is born, gentle palpation is used to feel for the cord. If present, the cord should be slipped gently over the head.

If the loop is tight or if there is a second loop, the cord is clamped twice, cut between the clamps, and unwound from around the neck before the birth is allowed to continue. Mucus, blood, or meconium in the nasal or oral passages may prevent the newborn from breathing. To eliminate this problem, moist gauze sponges are used to wipe the nose and mouth. A bulb syringe is first inserted into the mouth and oropharynx to aspirate contents, and then the nares are cleared in the same fashion while the head is supported.

Management of Infants Born in Meconium–Stained Fluid. The International Liaison Committee on Resuscitation (ILCOR) (2006) and the American Heart Association (2006) have published treatment recommendations for initial resuscitation of the newborn that include peripartum management of meconium. The widely used practice of routinely suctioning meconium from the infant's airway after the head is born but before the shoulders are born is no longer recommended. This recommendation is based on studies that have yielded conflicting results about the value of this practice and the results of a large multicenter randomized trial that found intrapartum suctioning of meconium does not decrease the incidence of meconium aspiration syndrome (Vain, Szyld, Prudent, Wiswell, Aguilar, & Vivas, 2004). ILCOR continues to recommended tra- ❋ cheal suctioning immediately after birth for meconium-stained depressed infants but not for meconium-stained infants who are at term gestation and vigorous.

▬ **NURSE ALERT**
Personnel skilled in neonatal resuscitation should be present for the birth of a meconium-stained infant (Miller, Fanaroff, & Martin, 2006).

Use of Fundal Pressure. Fundal pressure is the application of gentle, steady pressure against the fundus of the uterus to facilitate the vaginal birth. Historically it has been used when the administration of analgesia and anesthesia decreased the woman's ability to push during the birth, in cases of shoulder dystocia, and when second-stage fetal bradycardia or other nonreassuring FHR patterns were present. Use of fundal pressure by nurses is not advised because there is no standard technique available for this maneuver, and no current legal, professional, or regulatory standards exist for its use. (Simpson & Knox, 2001). In cases of shoulder dystocia, fundal pressure is not recommended: the all-fours position (Gaskin maneuver), suprapubic pressure, and maternal position changes are among the recommended interventions (Baxley & Gobbo, 2004) (see Chapter 36).

▬ Immediate Assessments and Care of the Newborn

The time of birth is the precise time when the entire body is out of the mother. This time must be recorded on the record. If the newborn's condition is not compromised, he or she may be placed on the mother's abdomen immediately after birth and covered with a warm, dry blanket. The cord may be clamped at this time, and the primary health care provider may ask if the woman's partner would like to cut the cord. If so, the partner is given a sterile pair of scissors and instructed to cut the cord 1 inch (2.5 cm) above the clamp.

The care given immediately after the birth focuses on assessing and stabilizing the newborn (see Chapter 26). The nurse's primary responsibility at this time is the infant, because the primary health care provider is involved with the delivery of the placenta and the care of the mother. The nurse must watch the infant for any signs of distress and initiate appropriate interventions should any appear.

A brief assessment of the newborn can be performed while the mother is holding the infant. This includes checking the infant's airway and Apgar score. Maintaining a patent airway, supporting respiratory effort, and preventing cold stress by drying the newborn and covering the newborn with a warmed blanket or placing him or her under a radiant warmer are the major priorities in terms of the newborn's immediate care. Further examination, identification procedures, and care can be postponed until later in the third stage of labor or early in the fourth stage.

▬ Perineal Trauma Related to Childbirth

Lacerations. Most acute injuries and lacerations of the perineum, the vagina, the uterus, and their support tissues occur during childbirth. Some injuries to the supporting tissues, whether they were acute or nonacute and whether they were repaired or not, may lead to genitourinary and sexual problems later in life (e.g., pelvic relaxation, fistulas, uterine prolapse, cystocele, rectocele, dyspareunia, urinary and bowel dysfunction).

Some damage occurs during every birth to the soft tissues of the birth canal and adjacent structures. The tendency to sustain lacerations varies with each woman; that is, the soft tissue in some women may be less distensible. Damage usually is more pronounced in nulliparous women because the tissues are firmer and more resistant than are those in multiparous women. Heredity also may be a factor. For example, the tissue of light-skinned women, especially those with reddish hair, is not so readily distensible as that of darker-skinned women, and healing may be less efficient. The perineal skin and vaginal mucosa may appear intact, but numerous small lacerations in underlying muscle and its fascia may be obscured. Damage to pelvic supports usually is readily apparent and is repaired after birth.

Immediate repair promotes healing, limits residual damage, and decreases the possibility of infection. Immediately after birth, the cervix, the vagina, and the perineum are inspected for damage. In addition, during the early postpartum period, the nurse and primary health care provider continue to inspect the perineum carefully and evaluate lochia and symptoms to identify any previously missed damage.

Perineal Lacerations. Perineal lacerations usually occur as the fetal head is being born. The extent of the laceration is defined in terms of its depth:

1. *First degree:* Laceration that extends through the skin and structures superficial to muscles
2. *Second degree:* Laceration that extends through muscles of the perineal body
3. *Third degree:* Laceration that continues through the anal sphincter muscle
4. *Fourth degree:* Laceration that also involves the anterior rectal wall

Perineal injury often is accompanied by small lacerations on the medial surfaces of the labia minora below the pubic rami and to the sides of the urethra (periurethral) and clitoris. Lacerations in this highly vascular area often result in profuse bleeding. Special attention must be paid to repair of third- and fourth-degree lacerations so that the woman retains fecal continence. Measures are taken to promote soft stools (e.g., roughage, fluid, activity, and stool softeners) to increase the woman's comfort and foster healing. Antimicrobial therapy may be instituted in some cases. Enemas and suppositories are contraindicated for these women. Simple perineal injuries usually heal without permanent disability, regardless of whether they were repaired. However, it is easier to repair a new perineal injury to prevent sequelae than it is to correct long-term damage.

Vaginal and Urethral Lacerations. Vaginal lacerations often occur in conjunction with perineal lacerations. Vaginal lacerations tend to extend up the lateral walls (sulci) and, if deep enough, involve the levator ani. Additional injury may occur high in the vaginal vault near the level of the ischial spines. Vaginal vault lacerations may be circular and may result from use of forceps to rotate the fetal head, rapid fetal descent, or precipitate birth.

Cervical Injuries. Cervical injuries occur when the cervix retracts over the advancing fetal head. These cervical lacerations occur at the lateral angles of the external os; most are shallow, and bleeding is minimal. More extensive lacerations may extend to the vaginal vault or beyond it into the lower uterine segment; serious bleeding may occur. Extensive lacerations may follow hasty attempts to enlarge the cervical opening artificially or to deliver the fetus before full cervical dilation is achieved. Injuries to the cervix can have adverse effects on future pregnancies and childbirths.

Episiotomy. An episiotomy is an incision made in the perineum to enlarge the vaginal outlet. It is performed more commonly in the United States and Canada than in Europe. The side-lying position for birth, used routinely in Europe, causes less tension on the perineum, making possible a gradual stretching of the perineum with fewer indications for episiotomies.

Clear evidence exists that routine performance of an episiotomy for birth is a form of care that is likely to be harmful or ineffective (Enkin et al., 2000; Hofmeyr, 2005). Routine performance of episiotomies has declined in the United States since the 1990s, most likely related to the clear evidence regarding the harmful effects of episiotomy in terms of increased postpartum pain, blood loss, risk for infection, and occurrence of third- and fourth-degree lacerations (Weeks & Kozak, 2001). The practice in many settings now is to support the perineum manually during birth and allow the perineum to tear rather than perform an episiotomy. Tears are often smaller than an episiotomy, are repaired easily or not at all, and heal quickly. The pain and discomfort resulting from episiotomies can interfere with mother-infant interaction, breastfeeding, reestablishment of the sexual relationship with partner, and even emotional recovery after birth.

When performed, the type of episiotomy is designated by the site and direction of the incision (Fig. 21-25). Midline (median) episiotomy is the most common type used in the United States. It is effective, easily repaired, and generally the least painful. However, midline episiotomies also are associated with a higher incidence of third- and fourth-degree lacerations. Sphincter tone is usually restored after primary healing and a good repair.

Mediolateral episiotomy is used in operative births when the need for posterior extension is likely. Although a fourth-degree laceration may be prevented, a third-degree laceration may occur. The blood loss also is greater and the repair more difficult and painful than with midline

episiotomies. It is also more painful in the postpartum period, and the pain lasts longer.

Risk factors associated with perineal trauma (e.g., episiotomy, lacerations) include nulliparity, maternal position, pelvic inadequacy (e.g., narrow subpubic arch with a constricted outlet), fetal malpresentation and position (e.g., breech, occiput posterior position), large (macrosomic) infants, use of instruments to facilitate birth, prolonged second stage of labor, fetal distress, and rapid labor in which there is insufficient time for the perineum to stretch. The rate of episiotomies also is higher when obstetricians rather than nurse midwives attend births (Shorten et al., 2002).

Factors found to reduce the risk of perineal trauma include avoiding episiotomies and using vacuum- rather than forceps-assisted vaginal birth if operative birth is required. Women should be assisted to avoid pushing when the perineum is tense and the fetal head is emerging. The primary health care provider should deliver the fetal head between contractions, while applying gentle pressure on the fetal head to prevent its rapid expulsion (Eason, Labrecque, Wells, & Feldman, 2000). Nurses acting as advocates can encourage women to use alternative birthing positions that reduce pressure on the perineum (e.g., lateral position) and to use spontaneous bearing-down efforts. In addition, nurses can educate other health care providers about measures to preserve perineal integrity and to be more flexible in defining the maximal limit for the duration of the second stage of labor as long as the maternal-fetal unit is stable.

Alternative measures for perineal management, such as warm compresses and massage with a lubricant (e.g., prenatal and intrapartum), have demonstrated limited effectiveness in reducing perineal trauma, though they may lessen the degree of perineal lacerations. Therefore, further research is recommended (Albers, Sedler, Bedrick, Teaf, & Peralta, 2005). Use of Kegel exercises in the prenatal and postpartum periods improves and restores the tone and strength of the perineal muscles. Health practices, including good nutrition and appropriate hygienic measures, help maintain the integrity and suppleness of the perineal tissue, enhance healing, and prevent infection.

■ *Emergency Childbirth*

Even under the best of circumstances, there probably will come a time when the perinatal nurse will be required to assist with the birth of an infant without medical assistance. Because it is neither possible nor desirable to prevent impending birth, the perinatal nurse must be able to function independently and be skilled in the safe birth of a vertex fetus (see Box 21-7).

A lateral Sims position may be the position of choice for birth when (1) the birth is progressing rapidly, and there is insufficient time for slow distention of the perineum; (2) the fetal head seems too large to pass through the introitus without laceration, and episiotomy is not possible; or (3) the apparent size of the fetus is consistent with possible shoulder dystocia. In the lateral Sims position, less

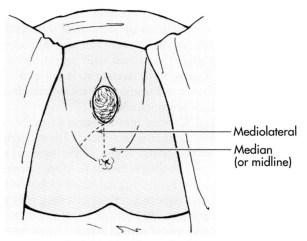

— Mediolateral
— Median (or midline)

FIG. 21-25 Types of episiotomies.

stress is placed on the perineum, and better visualization of the perineum is possible as the upper leg is supported by the woman's partner or the nurse (see Fig. 21-17, *A*). In the event of shoulder dystocia, the lateral Sims position increases the space needed for birth.

Evaluation

During the second stage of labor, the nurse evaluates the degree to which expected outcomes are being met, for example, the extent to which the woman has actively participated in the labor process, whether she or her fetus has sustained any injury during the labor process, the degree to which her birth plan has been fulfilled, and the extent to which she has been able to obtain comfort and support from her support person.

THIRD STAGE OF LABOR

The third stage of labor lasts from the birth of the baby until the placenta is expelled. The goal in the management of the third stage of labor is the prompt separation and expulsion of the placenta, achieved in the easiest, safest manner.

The placenta is attached to the decidual layer of the basal plate's thin endometrium by numerous fibrous an-

chor villi much in the same way as a postage stamp is attached to a sheet of postage stamps. After the birth of the fetus, strong uterine contractions cause the placental site to shrink markedly. This causes the anchor villi to break and the placenta to separate from its attachments. Normally the first few strong contractions that occur 5 to 7 minutes after the baby's birth cause the placenta to be sheared away from the basal plate. A placenta cannot detach itself from a flaccid (relaxed) uterus because the placental site is not reduced in size.

Placental Separation and Expulsion

Placental separation is indicated by the following signs (Fig. 21-26):
- A firmly contracting fundus
- A change in the uterus from a discoid to a globular shape as the placenta moves into the lower uterine segment
- A sudden gush of dark blood from the introitus
- Apparent lengthening of the umbilical cord as the placenta descends to the introitus
- The finding of vaginal fullness (the placenta) on vaginal or rectal examination or of fetal membranes at the introitus

Depending on the preferences of the primary health care provider, an expectant or active approach may be used

FIG. 21-26 Third stage of labor. **A,** Placenta begins to separate in central portion, accompanied by retroplacental bleeding. Uterus changes from discoid to globular shape. **B,** Placenta completes separation and enters lower uterine segment. Uterus has globular shape. **C,** Placenta enters vagina, cord is seen to lengthen, and there may be an increase in bleeding. **D,** Expulsion (delivery) of placenta and completion of third stage.

to manage the third stage of labor. Expectant management (watchful waiting) involves the natural, spontaneous separation and expulsion of the placenta by efforts of the mother with clamping and cutting of the cord after pulsation ceases. It may involve the use of gravity or nipple stimulation to facilitate separation and expulsion, but no oxytocic (uterotonic) medications are given. A quiet, relaxed environment that supports close skin-to-skin contact between mother and newborn also promotes the release of endogenous oxytocin.

Active management facilitates placenta separation and expulsion with administration of one or more oxytocic (uterotonic) medications after the birth of the anterior shoulder of the fetus, clamping and cutting of the umbilical cord immediately, and delivery of the placenta by application of controlled cord traction when signs of separation are noted. Research findings support the superiority of active management in terms of less blood loss and reduced risk of hemorrhage and other complications of the third stage of labor. However, active management is associated with nausea and vomiting and hypertension if the oxytocic used is ergometrine (Brucker, 2001; Prendiville, Elbourne, & McDonald, 2005). Active management of the third stage of labor is a beneficial form of care (Enkin et al., 2000).

To assist in the delivery of the placenta, the woman is instructed to push when signs of separation have occurred. If possible, the placenta should be expelled by maternal effort during a uterine contraction. Alternate compression and elevation of the fundus, plus minimal, controlled traction on the umbilical cord, may be used to facilitate delivery of the placenta and amniotic membranes. Oxytocics may be administered after the placenta is removed because they stimulate the uterus to contract, thereby helping to prevent hemorrhage.

Whether the placenta first appears by its shiny fetal surface (Schultze mechanism) or turns to show its dark roughened maternal surface first (Duncan mechanism) is of no clinical importance.

After the placenta and the amniotic membranes emerge, the primary health care provider examines them for intactness to ensure that no portion remains in the uterine cavity (i.e., no fragments of the placenta or membranes are retained) (Fig. 21-27).

Some women and their families may have culturally based beliefs regarding the care of the placenta and the manner of its disposal after birth, viewing the care and disposal of the placenta as a way of protecting the newborn from bad luck and illness. Requests by the woman to take the placenta home and dispose of it according to her customs may be at odds with health care agency policies, especially those related to infection control and the disposal of biologic wastes. Many cultures follow specific rules regarding the disposal of the placenta in terms of method (burning, drying, burying, eating), site for disposal (in or near the home), and timing of disposal (immediately after birth, time of day, astrologic signs). Disposal rituals may vary according to the gender of the child and the length of time before another child is desired. If eaten, the placenta can

FIG. 21-27 Examination of the placenta. (Courtesy Michael S. Clement, MD, Mesa, AZ.)

be a means of restoring a woman's well-being after birth or ensuring high-quality breast milk. Health care providers can provide culturally sensitive health care by encouraging women and their families to express their wishes regarding the care and disposal of the placenta and by establishing a policy to fulfill these requests (D'Avanzo & Geissler, 2003; Lemon, 2002; Molina, 2001).

▬ CARE MANAGEMENT

▬ Assessment and Nursing Diagnoses
▬ *Maternal Physical Status*

Physiologic changes after birth are profound. The cardiac output increases rapidly as maternal circulation to the placenta ceases and the pooled blood from the lower extremities is mobilized. The pulse rate slows in response to the change in cardiac output and tends to remain slightly slower than the prepregnancy rate for approximately 1 week.

Soon after the birth, the woman's blood pressure usually returns to prepregnancy levels. Several factors contribute to an elevated blood pressure at this time: the excitement of the second stage, certain medications, and the time of day (blood pressure is highest during the late afternoon). Analgesics and anesthetics may cause hypotension to develop in the hour after birth.

▬ *Signs of Potential Problems*

The major risk for women during the third stage of labor is postpartum hemorrhage. When the primary health care provider completes the delivery of the placenta, the nurse observes the mother for signs of excessive blood loss, including alteration in vital signs, pallor, light-headedness, restlessness, decreased urinary output, and alteration in level of consciousness and orientation (see Chapter 37).

Because of the rapid cardiovascular changes taking place (e.g., the increased intracranial pressure during pushing and the rapid increase in cardiac output), the risk of rupture of a preexisting cerebral aneurysm and the risk of formation of pulmonary emboli are greater than usual during this period. Another dangerous, unpredictable problem that may occur is the formation of an amniotic fluid embolism (see Chapter 36).

Women with a history of cardiac disorders are at increased risk for cardiac decompensation and pulmonary edema as a result of the circulatory changes associated with the birth of the fetus and expulsion of the placenta. The nurse should carefully assess the woman's respiratory pattern and effort, especially in the early postpartum period.

Nursing diagnoses that are relevant to the third stage of labor include the following:

- *Risk for deficient fluid volume related to*
  - blood loss occurring after placental separation and expulsion
  - ineffective contraction of the uterus
- *Risk for infection related to*
  - perineal trauma (e.g., laceration, episiotomy) associated with vaginal birth
- *Anxiety related to*
  - lack of knowledge regarding the separation and expulsion of the placenta
  - occurrence of perineal trauma and the need for repair
- *Fatigue related to*
  - energy expenditure associated with childbirth and the bearing-down efforts of the second stage of labor
- *Compromised family coping related to*
  - birth of infant whose gender was not preferred by the parents
  - unexpected birth of an infant with serious congenital anomalies
- *Situational low self-esteem (maternal and paternal) related to*
  - perceived inability to meet personal expectations regarding performance during childbirth

▬ Expected Outcomes of Care

As the woman progresses through the stages of labor, accomplishment of previously stated outcomes is determined. In addition, expected outcomes for the woman in the third stage of labor are that the woman will accomplish the following:

- Express satisfaction with her performance during labor and birth.
- Initiate, along with her partner and family, the process of bonding and attachment with the newborn.

▬ Plan of Care and Interventions
▬ *Care After Placental Delivery*

The woman may feel some discomfort when the placenta is delivered and while the primary health care provider carries out the postbirth vaginal examination. The nurse can assist the woman to use breathing and relaxation or distraction techniques to assist her in coping with the discomfort.

During the time the mother is being examined, the nurse has an opportunity to complete an assessment

of the newborn's physical condition. The baby can be weighed and measured, given a vitamin K injection, given an identification bracelet that corresponds to the mother's identification bracelet, wrapped in clean, warm blankets, and then given to the partner or back to the mother to hold when she is ready. In some agencies, the father of the baby (or another person designated by the mother) is also given a corresponding identification bracelet. Administration of eye prophylaxis can be delayed to promote parent-newborn attachment.

When the third stage is complete and any lacerations are repaired or an episiotomy is sutured, the vulvar area is gently cleansed with warm water or normal saline, and a perineal pad or an ice pack is applied to the perineum (some agencies or primary health care providers may require the use of sterile technique for perineal care immediately after birth). The birthing bed or table is repositioned, and the woman's legs are lowered simultaneously from the stirrups if she gave birth in the lithotomy position. Drapes are removed, and dry linen is placed under the woman's buttocks; she is provided with a clean gown and a blanket, which is warmed, if needed. She is assisted into her bed if she is to be transferred from the birthing area to the recovery area; assistance also is necessary to move the woman from the birthing table onto a bed if the woman has had anesthesia and does not have full use of her lower extremities. The side rails are raised during the transfer. She may be given the baby to hold during the transfer, or the father or partner may carry the baby or transport it in a crib, either to the nursery or to the recovery area. If the woman labors, gives birth, and recovers in the same bed and room, she is refreshed following the protocol already described. Maternal and neonatal assessments for the fourth stage of labor are instituted (see Chapter 23). When fourth-stage recovery is complete, the woman may be transferred via wheelchair to a room on the postpartum unit. Box 21-8 illustrates normal vaginal childbirth.

▬ *Care of the Family*

Most parents enjoy being able to handle, hold, explore, and examine the baby immediately after birth. Both parents can assist with the thorough drying of the infant. The infant may be wrapped in a receiving blanket and placed on the woman's abdomen. If skin-to-skin contact is desired, the unwrapped infant may be placed on the woman's abdomen and then covered with a warm blanket. Stockinette caps are often used to keep the newborn's head warm.

Many women may begin breastfeeding their newborns at this time to take advantage of the infant's alert state and to stimulate the production of oxytocin that promotes contraction of the uterus. Others prefer to wait until the fourth stage of labor.

▬ *Family-Newborn Relationships*

The woman's reaction to the sight of her newborn may range from excited outbursts of laughing, talking, and even crying to apparent apathy. A polite smile and nod may be her only acknowledgment of the comments of nurses and

box 21-8 Normal Vaginal Childbirth

FIRST STAGE

Anteroposterior slit. Vertex visible during contraction.

Oval opening. Vertex presenting. NOTE: nurse *(on left)* is wearing gloves, but support person *(on right)* is not.

SECOND STAGE

Crowning.

Nurse-midwife using Ritgen maneuver as head is born by extension.

After nurse-midwife checks for nuchal cord, she supports head during external rotation and restitution.

Use of bulb syringe to suction mucus.

Birth of posterior shoulder.

Birth of newborn by slow expulsion.

Second stage complete. Note that newborn is not yet completely pink.

Courtesy Michael S. Clement, MD, Mesa, AZ.

box 21-8 Normal Vaginal Childbirth—cont'd

THIRD STAGE

Newborn placed on mother's abdomen while cord is clamped and cut.

Note increased bleeding as placenta separates.

Expulsion of placenta.

Expulsion is complete, marking the end of the third stage.

THE NEWBORN

Newborn awaiting assessment. Note that color is almost completely pink.

Newborn assessment under radiant warmer.

Parents admiring their newborn.

the primary health care provider. Occasionally the reaction is one of anger or indifference; the woman turns away from the baby, concentrates on her own pain, and sometimes makes hostile comments. These varied reactions can arise from pleasure, exhaustion, or deep disappointment. When evaluating parent-newborn interactions after birth, the nurse also should consider the cultural characteristics of the woman and her family and the expected behaviors of that culture. In some cultures, the birth of a male child is preferred, and women may grieve when a female child is born (D'Avanzo & Geissler, 2003).

Whatever the reaction and its cause may be, the woman needs continuing acceptance and support from all staff. Notation regarding the parents' reaction to the newborn can be made in the recovery record. Nurses can assess this reaction by asking themselves such questions as, "How do the parents look?" "What do they say?" "What do they do?" Further assessment of the parent-newborn relationship can be conducted as care is given during the period of recovery. This is especially important if warning signs (e.g., passive or hostile reactions to the newborn, disappointment with gender or appearance of the newborn, absence of eye contact, or limited interaction of parents with each other) were noted immediately after birth. The nurse may find it helpful to discuss any warning signs that may have been noted with the woman's primary health care provider.

Siblings, who may have appeared only remotely interested in the final phases of the second stage, tend to experience renewed interest and excitement when the newborn appears. They can be encouraged to hold the baby (Fig. 21-28).

Parents usually respond to praise of their newborn. Many need to be reassured that the dusky appearance of their baby's extremities immediately after birth is normal until circulation is well established. If appropriate, the nurse should explain the reason for the molding of the newborn's head. Information about hospital routine can be communicated. It is important, however, for nurses to recognize that the cultural background of the parents may influence their expectations regarding the care and handling of their newborn immediately after birth. For example, some traditional Southeast Asians believe that the head should not be touched because it is the most sacred part of a person's body. They also believe that praise of the baby is dangerous because jealous spirits may then cause the baby harm or take it away (D'Avanzo & Geissler, 2003). Hospital staff members, by their interest and concern, can provide the environment for making this a satisfying experience for parents, family, and significant others.

▬ Evaluation

Determining a woman's satisfaction with and impressions of her childbirth experience is a critical component in the provision of high-quality maternal-newborn health care that meets the individual needs of women and families using these services. The woman may find it helpful to review her childbirth experience with a caring nurse who will listen, support, and provide explanations for events that occurred. This review process can help the woman to express her feelings about this significant event that will change her life forever (Semenic et al., 2004).

FIG. 21-28 Big brother becomes acquainted with new baby sister. (Courtesy Marjorie Pyle, RNC, Lifecircle, Costa Mesa, CA.)

---

community activity

1. Survey your community for doulas and complete the following activities:
   a. Create a list of the doulas that includes the following information:
      - Name of the doula and her credentials (e.g., education, certification)
      - Contact information: address, phone number, email
      - Cost and payment method
   b. Contact one of the doulas on your list and arrange to interview her. Write a description of this doula and her practice that includes the following information:
      - Her beliefs regarding the process of labor and her role in facilitating its progress
      - When she begins her contact with the women she will care for; what she does to assist these women before the onset of their labor
      - How she supports women in labor including physical comfort measures, emotional support, information giving, and advocacy
      - How she supports the woman's partner and support system
      - How she interacts with members of the labor and birth staff; how does she see her role different from theirs; has she encountered any difficulties and if so how did she handle the situation
      - Number of births she attends each year.
      - Length of contact including follow-up after discharge

key points

- The onset of labor may be difficult to determine for both nulliparous and multiparous women.
- The familiar environment of her home is most often the ideal place for a woman during the latent phase of the first stage of labor.
- The nurse assumes much of the responsibility for assessing the progress of labor and for keeping the primary health care provider informed about progress in labor and deviations from expected findings.
- The fetal heart rate and pattern reveal the fetal response to the stress of the labor process.
- Assessment of the laboring woman's urinary output and bladder is critical to ensure her progress and to prevent injury to the bladder.
- Regardless of the actual labor and birth experience, the woman's or couple's perception of the birth experience is most likely to be positive when events and performances are consistent with expectations, especially in terms of maintaining control and adequacy of pain relief.
- The woman's level of anxiety may increase when she does not understand what is being said to her about her labor because of the medical terminology used or because of a language barrier.
- Coaching, emotional support, and comfort measures assist the woman to use her energy constructively in relaxing and working with the contractions.
- The progress of labor is enhanced when a woman changes her position frequently during the first stage of labor.
- Doulas provide a continuous, supportive presence during labor that can have a positive effect on the process of childbirth and its outcome.
- The cultural beliefs and practices of a woman and her significant others, including her partner, can have a profound influence on their approach to labor and birth.
- The nurse who is aware of particular sociocultural aspects of helping and coping acts as an advocate or protective agent for the woman or couple during labor.
- The quality of the nurse-client relationship is a factor in the woman's ability to cope with the stressors of the labor process.
- Women with a history of sexual abuse often experience profound stress and anxiety during childbirth.
- Inability to palpate the cervix during vaginal examination indicates that complete effacement and full dilation have occurred and is the only certain, objective sign that the second stage has begun.
- Women may have an urge to bear down at various times during labor; for some it may be before the cervix is fully dilated and for others, it may not occur until the active phase of the second stage of labor.
- When allowed to respond to the rhythmic nature of the second stage of labor, the woman normally changes body positions, bears down spontaneously, and vocalizes (open-glottis pushing) when she perceives the urge to push (Ferguson reflex).
- Women should bear down several times during a contraction using the open-glottis pushing method; sustained closed-glottis pushing should be avoided because oxygen transport to the fetus will be inhibited.
- Nurses can use the role of advocate to prevent routine use of episiotomy and to reduce the incidence of lacerations by empowering women to take an active role in their birth and educating health care providers about approaches to managing childbirth that reduce the incidence of perineal trauma.
- Objective signs indicate that the placenta has separated and is ready to be expelled; excessive traction (pulling) on the umbilical cord, before the placenta has separated, can result in maternal injury.
- Siblings present for labor and birth need preparation and support for the event.
- Most parents/families enjoy being able to handle, hold, explore, and examine the baby immediately after the birth.
- Nurses should observe the progress in the development of parent-child relationships and be alert for warning signs that may appear during the immediate postpartum period.
- After an emergency childbirth out of the hospital, stimulation of the mother's nipple manually or by the infant's suckling stimulates the release of oxytocin from the maternal posterior pituitary gland; oxytocin stimulates the uterus to contract and thereby prevents hemorrhage.
- A woman benefits from reviewing her childbirth experience with the nurse who managed her care during the process of labor and birth.

REFERENCES

Adams, E., & Bianchi, A. (2004). Can a nurse and a doula exist in the same room? *International Journal of Childbirth Education, 19*(4), 12-15.

Albers, L. (2003). Commentary on "Impact of collaborative management and early admission in labor on method of delivery." *Journal of Obstetric, Gynecologic, and Neonatal Nursing, 32*(2), 158-160.

Albers, L., Anderson, D., Craigin, L., Daniels, S., Hunter, C, Sedler, K., et al. (1997). The relationship of ambulation in labor to operative delivery. *Journal of Nurse Midwifery, 42*(1), 4-8.

Albers, L., Sedler, K., Bedrick, E., Teaf, D., & Peralta, P. (2005). Midwifery care measures in the second stage of labor and reduction of genital tract trauma at birth: A randomized trial. *Journal of Midwifery & Women's Health, 50*(5), 365-372.

American Heart Association. (2006). 2005 American Heart Association (AHA) guidelines for cardiopulmonary resuscitation (CPR) and emergency cardiovascular care (ECC) of pediatric and neonatal patient: Pediatric basic life support. *Pediatrics, 117*(5), e989-e1004.

Angelini, D., & Mahlmeister, L. (2005). Liability in triage: Management of EMTALA regulations and common obstetric risks. *Journal of Midwifery & Women's Health, 50*(6), 472-478.

Bashour, H.,& Abdulsalam, A. (2005). Syrian women's preferences for birth attendant and birth place. *Birth, 32*(1), 20-25.

Baxley, E., & Gobbo, R. (2004). Shoulder dystocia. *American Family Physician, 69*(7), 1707-1714.

Begay, R. (2004). Changes in childbirth knowledge. *American Indian Quarterly, 28*(3 & 4), 550-565.

Benfield, R. (2002). Hydrotherapy in labor. *Journal of Nursing Scholarship, 34*(4), 347-352.

Brathwaite, A., & Williams, C. (2004). Childbirth experiences of professional Chinese Canadian women. *Journal of Obstetric, Gynecologic, and Neonatal Nursing, 33*(6), 748-755.

Brucker, M. (2001). Management of the third stage of labor: An evidence-based approach. *Journal of Midwifery & Women's Health, 46*(6), 381-392.

Caliendo, C., Millbauer, L., Moore, B., & Kitchen, E. (2004). Obstetric triage and EMTALA: Practice strategies for labor and delivery nursing units. *AWHONN Lifelines, 8*(5), 442-448.

Callister, L. (1995). Cultural meanings of childbirth. *Journal of Obstetric, Gynecologic, and Neonatal Nursing, 24*(4), 327-331.

Callister, L. (2005). What has the literature taught us about culturally competent care of women and children. *MCN American Journal of Maternal/Child Nursing, 30*(6), 380-388.

Cesario, S. (2004). Reevaluation of the Friedman labor cure: A pilot study. *Journal of Obstetric, Gynecologic, and Neonatal Nursing, 33*(6), 713-722.

Chapman, L. (1992). Expectant father's roles during labor and birth. *Journal of Obstetric, Gynecologic, and Neonatal Nursing, 21*(2), 114-120.

Choudhry, U. (1997). Traditional practices of women from India: Pregnancy, childbirth, and newborn care. *Journal of Obstetric, Gynecologic, and Neonatal Nursing, 26*(5), 533-539.

Cioffi, J. (2004). Caring for women from culturally diverse backgrounds: Midwives' experiences. *Journal of Midwifery & Women's Health, 49*(5), 437-442.

Cluett, E., Nikodem, V., McCandlish, R., and Burns, E. (2002). Immersion in water in pregnancy, labour, and birth. *The Cochrane Database of Systematic Reviews,* 2006, Issue 3. Chichester, UK: John Wiley & Sons.

CNM Data Group. (1999). Oral intake in labor: Trends in midwifery practice. The CNM Data Group, 1996. *Journal of Nurse Midwifery, 44*(2), 135-138.

D'Avanzo, C., & Geissler, E. (2003). *Pocket guide to cultural health assessment* (3rd ed.). St. Louis: Mosby.

Davies, B., & Hodnett, E. (2002). Labor support: Nurses' self-efficacy and views about factors influencing implementation. *Journal of Obstetric, Gynecologic, and Neonatal Nursing, 31*(1), 48-56.

Declercq, E., Sakala, C., Corry, M., Applebaum, S., & Risher, P. (2002). *Listening to mothers: Report of the first national U.S. survey of women's childbearing experiences.* New York: Maternity Center Association. Accessed www.maternitywise.org, October 25, 2005.

Eason, E., Labrecque, M., Wells, G., & Feldman, P. (2000). Preventing perineal trauma during childbirth: A systematic review. *Obstetrics and Gynecology, 95*(3), 464-471.

Enkin, M., Kierse, M., Neilson, J., Crowther, C., Duley, L., Hodnett, E., et al. (2000). *A guide to effective care in pregnancy and childbirth* (3rd ed.). Oxford, NY: Oxford University Press.

Goodman, P., Mackey, M., & Tavakoli, A. (2004). Factors related to childbirth satisfaction. *Journal of Advanced Nursing, 46*(2), 212-219.

Gross, M., Haunschild, T., Stoexen, T., Methner, V., & Guenter, H. (2003). Women's recognition of the spontaneous onset of labor. *Birth, 30*(4), 267-271.

Gupta, J., & Hofmeyr, G. (2004). Position in the second stage of labour for women without epidural anaesthesia. *The Cochrane Database of Systematic Reviews,* 2006, Issue 3. Chichester, UK: John Wiley & Sons.

Hansen, S., Clark, S., & Foster, J. (2002). Active pushing versus passive fetal descent in the second stage of labor: A randomized study. *Obstetrics and Gynecology, 99*(1), 29-34.

Hanson, L., VandeVusse, L., & Harrod, K. (2001). The theater of birth: Scenes from women's scripts. *Journal of Perinatal and Neonatal Nursing, 15*(2), 18-35.

Hobbins, D. (2004). Survivors of childhood sexual abuse: Implications for perinatal nursing. *Journal of Obstetric, Gynecologic, and Neonatal Nursing, 33*(4), 485-497.

Hodnett, E., Gates, S., Hofmeyr, G., & Sakala, C. (2003). Continuous support for women during childbirth. *The Cochrane Database of Systematic Reviews,* 2006, Issue 3. Chichester, UK: John Wiley & Sons.

Hodnett, E., Lowe, N., Hannah, M., Willan, A., Stevens, B., & Weston, J. (2002). Effectiveness of nurses as providers of birth support in North American hospitals. *Journal of the American Medical Association, 288*(11), 1373-1381.

Hofmeyr, G. (2005). Evidence-based intrapartum care. *Best Practices Research in Clinical Obstetrics and Gynaecology, 19*(1), 103-115.

(The) International Liaison Committee on Resuscitation (ILCOR). (2006). The International Liaison Committee on Resuscitation (ILCOR) consensus on science with treatment recommendations for pediatric and neonatal patients: Neonatal resuscitation. *Pediatrics, 117*(5), e978-e988.

Ito, M., & Sharts-Hopko, N. (2002). Japanese women's experience of childbirth in the United States. *Health Care for Women International, 23*(6-7), 666-677.

Jackson, D., Lang, J., Ecker, J., Swartz, W., & Heeren, T. (2003). Impact of collaborative management and early admission in labor on method of delivery. *Journal of Obstetric, Gynecologic, and Neonatal Nursing, 32*(2), 147-157.

Kayne, M., Greulich, M., & Albers, L. (2001). Doulas: An alternative yet complementary addition to care during childbirth. *Clinical Obstetrics and Gynecology, 44*(4), 692-703.

Khazoyan, C., & Anderson, N. (1994). Latina's expectations for their partners during childbirth. *MCN American Journal of Maternal/Child Nursing, 19*(4), 226-229.

Klaus, M., Kennell, J., & Klaus, P. (1993). *Mothering the mother.* Redwood City, CA: Addison-Wesley.

Lemon, B. (2002). Exploring Latino rituals in birthing. *AWHONN Lifelines, 6*(5), 443-445.

Lothian, J. (2001). Back to the future: Trusting birth. *Journal of Perinatal and Neonatal Nursing, 15*(3), 13-22.

Lowe, N. (2002). The nature of labor pain. *American Journal of Obstetrics and Gynecology, 186*(5), S16-S24.

Mackey, M. (2001). Use of water in labor and birth. *Clinical Obstetrics and Gynecology, 44*(4), 733-749.

MacKinnon, K., McIntyre, M., & Quance, M. (2005). The meaning of the nurse's presence during childbirth. *Journal of Obstetric, Gynecologic, and Neonatal Nursing, 34*(1), 28-36.

Matthews, R., & Callister, L. (2004). Childbearing women's perceptions of nursing care that promotes dignity. *Journal of Obstetric, Gynecologic, and Neonatal Nursing, 33*(4), 498-507.

Mattson, S. (2000). Working toward cultural competence: Making first steps through cultural assessment. *AWHONN Lifelines, 4*(4), 41-43.

Mayberry, L., Woods, S., Strange, L., Lee, L., Heisler, D., & Nielson-Smith, K. (2000). *Second stage labor management: Promotion of evidence-based practice and a collaborative approach to patient care.* Washington, DC: Association of Women's Health, Obstetric and Neonatal Nurses.

McCandlish, R. (2001). Perineal trauma: Prevention and treatment. *Journal of Midwifery & Women's Health, 46*(6), 396-401.

Melender, H. (2002). Experiences of fears associated with pregnancy and childbirth: A study of 329 pregnant women. *Birth, 29*(2), 101-111.

Miller, M., Fanaroff, A., & Martin, R. (2006). Respiratory disorders: Preterm and term infants. In R. Martin, A. Fanaroff, & M. Walsh (Eds). *Fanaroff and Martin's neonatal-perinatal medicine: Diseases of the fetus and infant* (8th ed). Philadelphia: Mosby

Miltner, R. (2000). Identifying labor support actions of intrapartum nurses. *Journal of Obstetric, Gynecologic, and Neonatal Nursing, 29*(5), 491-499.

Miltner, R. (2002). More than support: Nursing interventions provided to women in labor. *Journal of Obstetric, Gynecologic, and Neonatal Nursing, 31*(6), 753-761.

Minato, J. (2000). Is it time to push? Examining rest in second-stage labor. *AWHONN Lifelines, 4*(6), 20-23.

Molina, J. (2001). Traditional Native American practices in obstetrics. *Clinical Obstetrics and Gynecology, 44*(4), 661-670.

Parsons, M. (2004). Midwifery dilemma: To fast or feed the laboring woman. Part 2: The case supporting oral intake in labour. *Australian Midwifery Journal, 17*(1). 5-9.

Pascali-Bonaro, D., & Kroeger, M. (2004). Continuous female companionship during childbirth: A crucial resource in times of stress or calm. *Journal of Midwifery & Women's Health, 49*(4, Suppl.1), 19-27.

Perez, P. (2000). *Birth balls: The use of physical therapy balls in maternity care.* Johnson, VT: Cutting Edge Press.

Prendiville, W., Elbourne, D., & McDonald, S. (2005). Active versus expectant management in the third stage of labour. *The Cochrane Database of Systematic Reviews, 2006, Issue 3.* Chichester, UK: John Wiley & Sons.

Roberts, J. (2002). The "push" for evidence: Management of the second stage. *Journal of Midwifery & Women's Health, 47*(1), 2-15.

Roberts, J. (2003). A new understanding of the second stage of labor: Implications for care. *Journal of Obstetric, Gynecologic, and Neonatal Nursing, 32*(6), 794-801.

Rosen, P. (2004). Supporting women in labor: Analysis of different types of caregivers. *Journal of Midwifery & Women's Health, 49*(1), 24-31.

Sampselle, C., Miller, J., Luecha, Y., Fischer, K., & Rosten, L. (2005). Provider support of spontaneous pushing during the second stage of labor. *Journal of Obstetric, Gynecologic, and Neonatal Nursing, 34*(6), 695-702.

Sauls, D. (2002). Effects of labor support on mothers, babies, and birth outcomes. *Journal of Obstetric, Gynecologic, and Neonatal Nursing, 31*(6), 733-741.

Scheepers, H., Thans, H., deJong, P., Essed, G., LeCessie, S., & Kanhai, A. (2001). Eating and drinking in labor: The influence of caregiver advice on women's behavior. *Birth, 28*(2), 119-123.

Semenic, S., Callister, L., & Feldman, P. (2004). Giving birth: The voices of Orthodox Jewish women living in Canada. *Journal of Obstetric, Gynecologic, and Neonatal Nursing, 33*(1), 80-87.

Shorten, A., Donsante, J., & Shorten, B. (2002). Birth position, accoucheur, and perineal outcomes: Informing women about choices for vaginal birth. *Birth, 29*(1), 18-27.

Simkin, P. (2002). Supportive care during labor: A guide for busy nurses. *Journal of Obstetric, Gynecologic, and Neonatal Nursing, 31*(6), 721-732.

Simkin, P., & Ancheta, R. (2000). *The labor progress handbook.* Malden, MA: Blackwell Science.

Simkin, P., & Klaus, P. (2004). *When survivors give birth.* Seattle, WA: Classic Day.

Simkin, P., & Young, D. (2005). *Doulas of North America (DONA) International Position Paper: The birth doula's contribution to modern maternity care.* Accessed www.DONA.org, September 25, 2006.

Simpson, K. (2005). The context and clinical evidence for common nursing practices during labor. *MCN American Journal of Maternal/Child Nursing, 30*(6), 356-363.

Simpson, K., & James, D. (2005). Effects of immediate versus delayed pushing during second stage labor on fetal well-being: A randomized clinical trial. *Nursing Research, 54*(3), 149-157.

Simpson, K., & Knox, G. (2001). Fundal pressure during the second stage of labor: Clinical perspectives and risk management issues. *MCN American Journal of Maternal/Child Nursing, 26*(2), 64-71.

Sleutel, M. (2003). Intrapartum nursing: Integrating Rubin's framework with social support theory. *Journal of Obstetric, Gynecologic, and Neonatal Nursing, 32*(1), 76-82.

Trainor, C. (2002). Valuing labor support: A doula's perspective. *AWHONN Lifelines, 6*(5), 387-389.

Tranmer, J., Hodnett, E., Hannah, M., & Stevens, B. (2005). The effect of unrestricted oral carbohydrate intake on labor progress. *Journal of Obstetric, Gynecologic, and Neonatal Nursing, 34*(3), 319-328.

Tucker, S. (2004). *Pocket guide to fetal monitoring and assessment* (5th ed.). St. Louis: Mosby.

Tumblin, A., & Simkin, P. (2001). Pregnant women's perception of their nurse's role during labor and delivery. *Birth, 28*(1), 52-56.

Vain, N., Szyld, E., Prudent, L., Wiswell, T., Aguilar, A., & Vivas, N. (2004). Oropharyngeal and nasopharyngeal suctioning of meconium-stained neonates before delivery of their shoulders: Multicentre, randomized controlled trial. *Lancet, 364*(9434), 597-602.

Waterbirth International. (2005). *Frequently asked questions. How long is the baby in the water?* Accessed http://waterbirth.org, September 25, 2006.

Weeks, J., & Kozak, L. (2001). Trends in the use of episiotomy in the United States: 1980-1998. *Birth, 28*(3), 152-160.

Zwelling, E., & Phillips, C. (2001). Family-centered maternity care in the new millennium: Is it real or is it imagined? *Journal of Perinatal and Neonatal Nursing, 15*(3), 1-12.

Postpartum Physiology

learning objectives

- Describe the anatomic and physiologic changes that occur during the postpartum period.
- Identify characteristics of uterine involution and lochial flow and describe ways to measure them.

- List expected values for vital signs, deviations from normal findings, and probable causes of the deviations.

electronic resources

Additional information related to the content in Chapter 22 can be found on

the companion website at **evolve**
http://evolve.elsevier.com/Lowdermilk/MWHC/
- NCLEX Review Questions
- WebLinks

or on the interactive companion CD
- NCLEX Review Questions

THE postpartum period is the interval between the birth of the newborn and the return of the reproductive organs to their normal nonpregnant state. This period is sometimes referred to as the puerperium, or fourth trimester of pregnancy. Although the puerperium has traditionally been considered to last 6 weeks, this time frame varies among women. The distinct physiologic changes that occur as the processes of pregnancy are reversed are normal. To provide care during the recovery period that is beneficial to the mother, her infant, and her family, the nurse must synthesize knowledge of maternal anatomy and physiology, the newborn's physical and behavioral characteristics, infant care activities, and the family response to the birth of the child. This chapter focuses on anatomic and physiologic changes that occur in the woman during the postpartum period.

REPRODUCTIVE SYSTEM AND ASSOCIATED STRUCTURES

Uterus
Involution Process

The return of the uterus to a nonpregnant state after birth is known as involution. This process begins immediately after expulsion of the placenta with contraction of the uterine smooth muscle.

At the end of the third stage of labor, the uterus is in the midline, about 2 cm below the level of the umbilicus, with the fundus resting on the sacral promontory. At this time, the uterus weighs about 1000 g.

Within 12 hours, the fundus may be approximately 1 cm above the umbilicus (Fig. 22-1). By 24 hours postpartum, the uterus is about the same size it was at 20 weeks of gestation (Resnik, 2004). Involution progresses rapidly during the next few days. The fundus descends about 1 to 2 cm every 24 hours. By the sixth postpartum day, the fundus is normally located halfway between the umbilicus and the symphysis pubis. The uterus should not be palpable abdominally after 2 weeks (Resnik).

The uterus, which at full term is approximately 11 times its prepregnancy weight, involutes to about 500 g by 1 week after birth and 350 g by 2 weeks after birth. At 6 weeks postpartum, it weighs 50 to 60 g (see Fig. 22-1).

Increased estrogen and progesterone levels are responsible for stimulating the massive growth of the uterus during pregnancy. Prenatal uterine growth results from both hyperplasia, an increase in the number of muscle cells, and hypertrophy, enlargement of the existing cells. Postpartally the decrease in the secretion of these hormones causes autolysis, the self-destruction of excess hypertrophied tissue. The additional cells laid down during pregnancy remain, however, and account for the slight increase in uterine size after each pregnancy.

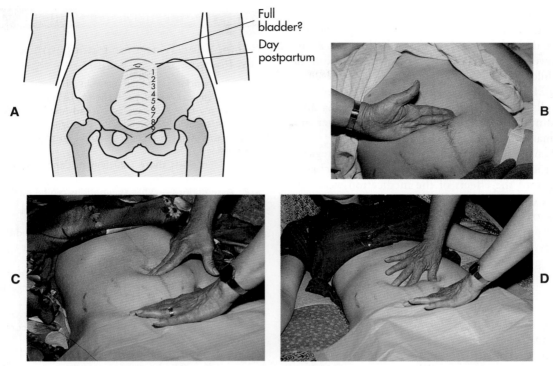

FIG. 22-1   Assessment of involution of uterus after childbirth. **A,** Normal progress, days 1 through 9. **B,** Size and position of uterus 2 hours after childbirth. **C,** Two days after childbirth. **D,** Four days after childbirth. (**B, C,** and **D** courtesy Marjorie Pyle, RNC, Lifecircle, Costa Mesa, CA.)

Subinvolution is the failure of the uterus to return to a nonpregnant state. The most common causes of subinvolution are retained placental fragments and infection (see Chapter 37).

Contractions

Postpartum hemostasis is achieved primarily by compression of intramyometrial blood vessels as the uterine muscle contracts, rather than by platelet aggregation and clot formation. The hormone oxytocin, released from the posterior pituitary gland, strengthens and coordinates these uterine contractions, which compress blood vessels and promote hemostasis. During the first 1 to 2 postpartum hours, uterine contractions may decrease in intensity and become uncoordinated. Because it is vital that the uterus remain firm and well contracted, exogenous oxytocin (Pitocin) is usually administered intravenously or intramuscularly immediately after expulsion of the placenta. Women who plan to breastfeed may also be encouraged to put the baby to breast immediately after birth, because suckling stimulates oxytocin release.

Afterpains

In first-time mothers, uterine tone is good, the fundus generally remains firm, and the woman usually perceives only mild uterine cramping. Periodic relaxation and vigorous contraction are more common in subsequent pregnancies and may cause uncomfortable cramping called afterpains (afterbirth pains) that persist throughout the early puerperium. Afterpains are more noticeable after births in which the uterus was overdistended (e.g., large baby, multifetal gestation, polyhydramnios). Breastfeeding and exogenous oxytocic medication usually intensify these afterpains, because both stimulate uterine contractions.

Placental Site

Immediately after the placenta and membranes are expelled, vascular constriction and thromboses reduce the placental site to an irregular nodular and elevated area. Upward growth of the endometrium causes sloughing of necrotic tissue and prevents the scar formation that is characteristic of normal wound healing. This unique healing process enables the endometrium to resume its usual cycle of changes and to permit implantation and placentation in future pregnancies. Endometrial regeneration is completed by postpartum day 16, except at the placental site (Resnik, 2004). Regeneration at the placental site usually is not complete until 6 weeks after birth.

Lochia

Postchildbirth uterine discharge, commonly called lochia, is initially bright red (lochia rubra) and may contain small clots. For the first 2 hours after birth the amount of uterine discharge should be approximately that of a heavy menstrual period. After that time, the lochial flow should steadily decrease.

Lochia rubra consists mainly of blood and decidual and trophoblastic debris. The flow pales, becoming pink or brown (lochia serosa) after 3 to 4 days. Lochia serosa consists of old blood, serum, leukocytes, and tissue debris. The median duration of lochia serosa discharge is 22 to 27 days (Bowes & Katz, 2002). In most women, about 10 days after childbirth the drainage becomes yellow to white (lochia alba). Lochia alba consists of leukocytes, decidua, epithelial cells, mucus, serum, and bacteria. Lochia alba usually continues for 10 to 14 days but may last longer and still be normal (Simpson & Creehan, 2001).

If the woman receives an oxytocic medication, regardless of the route of administration, the flow of lochia is often scant until the effects of the medication wear off. The amount of lochia is typically smaller after cesarean births. Flow of lochia usually increases with ambulation and breastfeeding. Lochia tends to pool in the vagina when the woman is lying in bed; upon standing, the woman may experience a gush of blood. This gush should not be confused with hemorrhage.

Persistence of lochia rubra early in the postpartum period suggests continued bleeding as a result of retained fragments of the placenta or membranes. Recurrence of bleeding approximately 7 to 14 days after birth is from the healing placental site. About 10% to 15% of women will still be experiencing normal lochia serosa discharge at their 6-week postpartum examination (Bowes & Katz, 2002). In the majority of women, however, a continued flow of lochia serosa or lochia alba by 3 to 4 weeks after birth may indicate endometritis, particularly if fever, pain, or abdominal tenderness is associated with the discharge. Lochia should smell like normal menstrual flow; an offensive odor usually indicates infection.

Not all postpartal vaginal bleeding is lochia; vaginal bleeding after birth may be a result of unrepaired vaginal or cervical lacerations. Table 22-1 distinguishes between lochial and nonlochial bleeding.

Cervix

The cervix is soft immediately after birth. Within 2 to 3 days postpartum it has shortened, become firm, and regained its form (Resnik, 2004). The cervix up to the lower uterine segment remains edematous, thin, and fragile for several days after birth. The ectocervix (portion of the cervix that protrudes into the vagina) appears bruised and has some small lacerations—optimal conditions for the development of infection. The cervical os, which dilated to 10 cm during

labor, closes gradually. Two fingers may still be introduced into the cervical os for the first 4 to 6 days postpartum; however, only the smallest curette can be introduced by the end of 2 weeks. The external cervical os never regains its prepregnancy appearance; it is no longer shaped like a circle but appears as a jagged slit often described as a "fish mouth" (see Fig. 14-2). Lactation delays the production of cervical and other estrogen-influenced mucus and mucosal characteristics.

Vagina and Perineum

Postpartum estrogen deprivation is responsible for the thinness of the vaginal mucosa and the absence of rugae. The greatly distended, smooth-walled vagina gradually returns to its prepregnancy size by 6 to 10 weeks after childbirth (Resnik, 2004). Rugae reappear within 3 weeks, but they are never as prominent as they are in the nulliparous woman. Most rugae are permanently flattened. The mucosa remains atrophic in the lactating woman, at least until menstruation resumes. Thickening of the vaginal mucosa occurs with the return of ovarian function.

CRITICAL THINKING EXERCISE

Telephone Triage for Management of Postpartum Bleeding

You are working as a staff nurse in a health department maternity clinic. One of your clients, LaToya, calls and states, "I had my baby 10 days ago. I had just about quit bleeding, but today I've noticed a lot of bright red blood. Do you think something is wrong? Should I go to the hospital right away?"

1. Evidence—Is there sufficient evidence to draw conclusions about LaToya's diagnosis and treatment?
2. Assumptions—What assumptions can be made about the following issues:
   a. Possible diagnoses for LaToya
   b. Assessment data which must be gathered during your phone conversation with LaToya in order to advise her properly
   c. Role of the staff nurse in telephone triage
3. What implications and priorities for nursing care can be made at this time?
4. Does the evidence objectively support your conclusion?
5. Are there alternative perspectives to your conclusion?

table 22-1 Lochial and Nonlochial Bleeding

LOCHIAL BLEEDING	NONLOCHIAL BLEEDING
Lochia usually trickles from the vaginal opening. The steady flow is greater as the uterus contracts. A gush of lochia may result as the uterus is massaged. If it is dark in color, it has been pooled in the relaxed vagina, and the amount soon lessens to a trickle of bright red lochia (in the early puerperium).	If the bloody discharge spurts from the vagina, there may be cervical or vaginal tears in addition to the normal lochia. If the amount of bleeding continues to be excessive and bright red, a tear may be the source.

Estrogen deficiency is also responsible for a decreased amount of vaginal lubrication. Localized dryness and coital discomfort (dyspareunia) may persist until ovarian function returns and menstruation resumes. The use of a water-soluble lubricant during sexual intercourse is usually recommended.

Initially the introitus is erythematous and edematous, especially in the area of the episiotomy or laceration repair. Afterward it is usually barely distinguishable from that of a nulliparous woman if lacerations and an episiotomy have been carefully repaired, hematomas are prevented or treated early, and the woman observes good hygiene during the first 2 weeks after birth.

Most episiotomies are visible only if the woman is lying on her side with her upper buttock raised or if she is placed in the lithotomy position. A good light source is essential for visualization of some episiotomies. Healing of an episiotomy is the same as any surgical incision. Signs of infection (pain, redness, warmth, swelling, or discharge) or the loss of approximation (separation of the incision edges) may occur. Healing should occur within 2 to 3 weeks.

Hemorrhoids (anal varicosities) are commonly seen (see Fig. 14-10). Internal hemorrhoids may evert while the woman is pushing during birth. Women often experience associated symptoms such as itching, discomfort, and bright red bleeding with defecation. Hemorrhoids usually decrease in size within 6 weeks of childbirth.

Pelvic Muscular Support

The supporting structure of the uterus and vagina may be injured during childbirth and may contribute to later gynecologic problems. Supportive tissues of the pelvic floor that are torn or stretched during childbirth may require up to 6 months to regain tone. Kegel exercises, which help to strengthen perineal muscles and encourage healing, are recommended after childbirth (see Teaching for Self-Care Box, Chapter 5, p. 120). Later in life, women can experience pelvic relaxation, the lengthening and weakening of the fascial supports of pelvic structures. These structures include the uterus, the upper posterior vaginal wall, the urethra, the bladder, and the rectum. Although pelvic relaxation can occur in any woman, it is usually a direct but delayed complication of childbirth (see Chapter 12).

ENDOCRINE SYSTEM

Placental Hormones

Significant hormonal changes occur during the postpartal period. Expulsion of the placenta results in dramatic decreases of the hormones produced by that organ. Decreases in human chorionic somatomammotropin, estrogens, cortisol, and the placental enzyme insulinase reverse the diabetogenic effects of pregnancy, resulting in significantly lower blood sugar levels in the immediate puerperium.

Mothers with type 1 diabetes will likely require much less insulin for several days after birth. Because these normal hormonal changes make the puerperium a transitional period for carbohydrate metabolism, it is more difficult to interpret glucose tolerance tests at this time.

Estrogen and progesterone levels decrease markedly after expulsion of the placenta, and reach their lowest levels 1 week postpartum. Decreased estrogen levels are associated with breast engorgement and with the diuresis of excess extracellular fluid accumulated during pregnancy. In nonlactating women, estrogen levels begin to rise by 2 weeks after birth and by postpartum day 17 are higher than in women who breastfeed (Bowes & Katz, 2002).

Human chorionic gonadotropin (hCG) disappears from maternal circulation in 14 days (Resnik, 2004).

Pituitary Hormones and Ovarian Function

Lactating and nonlactating women differ considerably in the time when the first ovulation occurs and when menstruation resumes. The persistence of elevated serum prolactin levels in breastfeeding women appears to be responsible for suppressing ovulation. Because levels of follicle-stimulating hormone (FSH) have been shown to be identical in lactating and nonlactating women, it is thought that ovulation is suppressed in lactating women because the ovary does not respond to FSH stimulation when increased prolactin levels are present (Resnik, 2004).

Prolactin levels in blood rise progressively throughout pregnancy. In women who breastfeed, prolactin levels remain elevated into the sixth week after birth (Lawrence & Lawrence, 2004). Serum prolactin levels are influenced by the frequency of breastfeeding, the duration of each feeding, and the degree to which supplementary feedings are used. Individual differences in the strength of an infant's sucking stimulus probably also affect prolactin levels. In nonlactating women, prolactin levels decline after birth and reach the prepregnant range by the third postpartum week (Bowes & Katz, 2002).

Ovulation occurs as early as 27 days after birth in nonlactating women, with a mean time of about 70 to 75 days (Bowes & Katz, 2002). Approximately 70% of nonbreastfeeding women resume menstruating by 3 months after birth (Lawrence & Lawrence, 2004). In women who breastfeed, the mean length of time to initial ovulation is 6 months (Bowes & Katz). In lactating women, both resumption of ovulation and return of menses are determined in large part by breastfeeding patterns (Resnik, 2004). Many women ovulate before their first postpartum menstrual period occurs; therefore there is need to discuss contraceptive options early in the puerperium (Lawrence & Lawrence).

The first menstrual flow after childbirth is usually heavier than normal. Within three to four cycles, the amount of menstrual flow returns to the woman's prepregnancy volume.

EVIDENCE-BASED PRACTICE

Kegel Exercises Prevent Incontinence

BACKGROUND

- Urinary incontinence affects more than half of all midlife women. Childbirth may stretch or damage the sling of muscles in the pelvic floor, causing inability to tightly close the urethral sphincter. Stress incontinence is the dribbling that occurs with increased intraabdominal pressure, such as with sneezing or laughter. Urge incontinence, caused by bladder fullness, is more profound, causing more loss of urine and decreased quality of life. Risk factors for urinary incontinence include current pregnancy, obesity, prolonged second-stage labor, instrumental birth, perineal tears, parity, and sizes of babies. In 1948, Kegel first described pelvic floor muscle exercises (PFME), now routinely taught to decrease incontinence by strengthening the perianal and perivaginal muscles.

OBJECTIVES

- The reviewers aimed to identify the efficacy of antenatal and postnatal PFME instruction on the outcomes of frequency and severity of incontinence. Other outcomes included pelvic floor strength and adherence to exercise program.

METHODS

Search Strategy

- The authors searched electronic databases, reference lists, and unpublished studies. Six randomized controlled trials met the criteria for comparing prenatal or postnatal PFME instruction to usual care. Seven randomized controlled trials and three nonrandomized controlled trials explored the efficacy of various instructional methods. Dates and countries of origin were not noted.

Statistical Analyses

- Similar data were pooled. Reviewers calculated weighted mean difference for continuous data, such as frequency of incontinence. Differences between groups outside the 95% confidence interval were accepted as significant.

FINDINGS

- *Antenatal:* Women began PFME at 20 weeks of gestation, and performed them at least 20 to 50 times daily. Two studies showed significant decrease in urinary incontinence in the PFME instruction group, when compared to usual care. A third trial showed improvement, but not to the level of significance.
- *Postnatal:* Instruction in PFME begun at 3 and 5 months postpartum was significantly beneficial, especially for women with preexisting incontinence.
- *Types of Instruction:* All comprehensive instruction methods, incorporating some combination of instruction sessions, home training, and written material resulted in significantly better adherence and increased reported number of daily exercises, for up to a year later.

LIMITATIONS

- Many postnatal subjects were lost to follow-up, limiting those conclusions. Some of the instruction efficacy trials were not randomized, which increases bias (the researchers may have chosen the more motivated women for the intervention). Multiple teaching interventions limit any conclusions about the efficacy of individual components (written, teaching session, home training). No study mentioned cost.

IMPLICATIONS FOR PRACTICE

- Nurses should advise all their prenatal and postnatal clients to practice PFME, to limit or resolve urinary incontinence. Benefits may be lifelong. The PFME program should be easy and realistic. Instruction which includes at least two sessions and written material appear effective. Nurses should be alert to scheduling an instruction session for early discharge postpartum clients.

IMPLICATIONS FOR FURTHER RESEARCH

- Research is needed to identify barriers to incorporating PFME into women's busy lives. Memory aids may be useful. Differences in sexual response and satisfaction may become apparent with PFME therapy. The cost of programs should be included. Investigators need to establish long-term benefits of PFME for preventing incontinence and the most efficacious interventions through randomized controlled studies.

Reference: Haddow, G., Watts, R., & Robertson, J. (2005). The effectiveness of a pelvic floor exercise program on urinary incontinence following childbirth. *International Journal of Evidence-Based Healthcare, 3*(5), 103-146.

▬ ABDOMEN

When the woman stands up during the first days after birth, her abdominal muscles protrude and give her a still-pregnant appearance. During the first 2 weeks after birth, the abdominal wall is relaxed. It takes approximately 6 weeks for the abdominal wall to return almost to its prepregnancy state (Fig. 22-2). The skin regains most of its previous elasticity, but some striae may persist. The return of muscle tone depends on previous tone, proper exercise, and the amount of adipose tissue. Occasionally, with or without overdistention because of a large fetus or multiple fetuses, the abdominal wall muscles separate, a condition termed diastasis recti abdominis (see Fig. 14-13).

Persistence of this defect may be disturbing to the woman, but surgical correction is rarely necessary. With time, the defect becomes less apparent.

▬ URINARY SYSTEM

The hormonal changes of pregnancy (i.e., high steroid levels) may be partly responsible for causing an increase in renal function; diminishing steroid levels after birth may partly explain the reduced renal function that occurs during the puerperium. Kidney function returns to normal within a month after birth. From 2 to 8 weeks is required for the pregnancy-induced hypotonia and dilation of

FIG. 22-2 Abdominal wall 6 weeks after vaginal birth is almost back to prepregnancy appearance. Note that the linea nigra is still visible. (Courtesy Jodi Brackett, Phoenix, AZ.)

the ureters and renal pelvis to return to the nonpregnant state (Cunningham, Leveno, Bloom, Hauth, Gilstrap, & Wenstrom, 2005). In a small percentage of women, dilation of the urinary tract may persist for 3 months, which increases the chance of developing a urinary tract infection.

Urine Components

The renal glycosuria induced by pregnancy disappears, but lactosuria may occur in lactating women. The blood urea nitrogen (BUN) level increases during the puerperium as autolysis of the involuting uterus occurs. This breakdown of excess protein in the uterine muscle cells also results in a mild (+1) proteinuria for 1 to 2 days after childbirth in 40% to 50% of women (Simpson & Creehan, 2001). Ketonuria may occur in women with an uncomplicated birth or after a prolonged labor with dehydration.

Postpartal Diuresis

Within 12 hours of birth, women begin to lose the excess tissue fluid accumulated during pregnancy. Profuse diaphoresis often occurs, especially at night, for the first 2 or 3 days after childbirth. Postpartal diuresis, caused by decreased estrogen levels, removal of increased venous pressure in the lower extremities, and loss of the remaining pregnancy-induced increase in blood volume, also aids the body in ridding itself of excess fluid. Fluid loss through perspiration and increased urinary output accounts for a weight loss of approximately 2.25 kg during the puerperium.

Urethra and Bladder

Birth-induced trauma, increased bladder capacity following childbirth, and the effects of conduction anesthesia combine to cause a decreased urge to void. In addition, pelvic soreness caused by the forces of labor, vaginal lacerations, or an episiotomy reduces or alters the voiding reflex.

Decreased voiding combined with postpartal diuresis, may result in bladder distention.

Immediately after birth, excessive bleeding can occur if the bladder becomes distended because it pushes the uterus up and to the side and prevents the uterus from contracting firmly. Later in the puerperium overdistention can make the bladder more susceptible to infection and impede the resumption of normal voiding (Cunningham et al., 2005). With adequate emptying of the bladder, bladder tone is usually restored 5 to 7 days after childbirth.

▬ GASTROINTESTINAL SYSTEM

Appetite

The mother is usually hungry shortly after giving birth and can tolerate a light diet. Most new mothers are very hungry after full recovery from analgesia, anesthesia, and fatigue. Requests for extra portions of food and frequent snacks are not uncommon.

Bowel Evacuation

A spontaneous bowel evacuation may not occur until 2 to 3 days after childbirth. This delay can be explained by decreased muscle tone in the intestines during labor and the immediate puerperium, prelabor diarrhea, lack of food, or dehydration. The mother often anticipates discomfort during the bowel movement because of perineal tenderness as a result of an episiotomy, lacerations, or hemorrhoids and resists the urge to defecate. Regular bowel habits should be reestablished when bowel tone returns.

Operative vaginal birth (forceps or vacuum use) and anal sphincter lacerations are associated with an increased risk of postpartum anal incontinence. If it occurs, anal incontinence is often temporary and may resolve within 6 months (Bowes & Katz, 2002). Women should be taught during pregnancy about episiotomy and its possible sequelae. Pelvic floor (Kegel) exercises should be encouraged.

▬ BREASTS

Promptly after birth, there is a decrease in the concentrations of hormones (i.e., estrogen, progesterone, hCG, prolactin, cortisol, and insulin) that stimulated breast development during pregnancy. The time it takes for these hormones to return to prepregnancy levels is determined in part by whether the mother breastfeeds her infant.

Breastfeeding Mothers

During the first 24 hours after birth, there is little, if any, change in the breast tissue. Colostrum, a clear, yellow fluid, may be expressed from the breasts. The breasts gradually become fuller and heavier as the colostrum transitions to milk by about 72 to 96 hours after birth; this is often referred to as the "milk coming in." The breasts may feel warm, firm, and somewhat tender. Bluish-white milk with a skim-milk appearance (true milk) can be expressed from the nipples. As milk glands and milk ducts fill with milk, breast tissue may feel somewhat nodular or lumpy. Unlike the lumps associated with fibrocystic breast disease or cancer (which may be palpated consistently in the same location), the nodularity associated with milk production tends to shift in position. Some women experience engorgement, but with frequent breastfeeding and proper care, this is a temporary condition that typically lasts only 24 to 48 hours (see Chapter 27).

Nonbreastfeeding Mothers

The breasts generally feel nodular in contrast to the granular feel of breasts in nonpregnant women. The nodularity is bilateral and diffuse. Prolactin levels drop rapidly. Colostrum is present for the first few days after childbirth. Palpation of the breasts on the second or third day, as milk production begins, may reveal tissue tenderness in some women. On the third or fourth postpartum day, engorgement may occur. The breasts are distended (swollen), firm, tender, and warm to the touch (because of vasocongestion). Breast distention is caused primarily by the temporary congestion of veins and lymphatics rather than by an accumulation of milk. Milk is present but should not be expressed. Axillary breast tissue (the tail of Spence) and any accessory breast or nipple tissue along the milk line may be involved. Engorgement resolves spontaneously, and discomfort usually decreases within 24 to 36 hours. A breast binder or well-fitted, supportive bra, ice packs, fresh cabbage leaves and/or mild analgesics may be used to relieve discomfort. Nipple stimulation is avoided. If suckling is never begun (or is discontinued), lactation ceases within a few days to a week.

■ CARDIOVASCULAR SYSTEM

Blood Volume

Changes in blood volume after birth depend on several factors, such as blood loss during childbirth and the amount of extravascular water (physiologic edema) mobilized and excreted. Blood lost at birth results in an immediate but limited decrease in total blood volume. Thereafter most of the blood volume increase during pregnancy (1000 to 1500 ml) is eliminated within the first 2 weeks after birth (Simpson & Creehan, 2001).

Pregnancy-induced hypervolemia (an increase in blood volume of at least 35% more than prepregnancy values near term) (Bowes & Katz, 2002) allows most women to tolerate considerable blood loss during childbirth. Many women lose approximately 500 ml of blood during vaginal birth of a single fetus and approximately twice this much during cesarean birth (Resnik, 2004).

Readjustments in the maternal vasculature after childbirth are dramatic and rapid. The woman's response to blood loss during the early puerperium differs from that in a nonpregnant woman. Three postpartum physiologic changes protect the woman by increasing the circulating blood volume: (1) elimination of uteroplacental circulation reduces the size of the maternal vascular bed by 10% to 15%, (2) loss of placental endocrine function removes the stimulus for vasodilation, and (3) mobilization of extravascular water stored during pregnancy occurs. Therefore hypovolemic shock usually does not occur in women who experience a normal blood loss.

Cardiac Output

Pulse rate, stroke volume, and cardiac output increase throughout pregnancy. Cardiac output remains increased for at least the first 48 hours postpartum because of an increase in stroke volume. This increased stroke volume is caused by the return of blood to the maternal systemic venous circulation, a result of rapid decrease in uterine blood flow and mobilization of extravascular fluid (Resnik, 2004). Cardiac output generally returns to normal by 6 weeks postpartum, but the rate of return appears to be variable (Resnik). Data suggest that stroke volume, cardiac output, and systemic vascular resistance remain elevated over nonpregnant values at least 12 weeks after birth (Resnik).

Vital Signs

Few alterations in vital signs are seen under normal circumstances. Heart rate and blood pressure return to nonpregnant levels within a few days (Resnik, 2004) (Table 22-2). Respiratory function returns to nonpregnant levels by 6 to 8 weeks after birth. After the uterus is emptied, the diaphragm descends, the normal cardiac axis is restored, and the point of maximal impulse (PMI) and the electrocardiogram (ECG) are normalized.

Blood Components
Hematocrit and Hemoglobin

During the first 72 hours after childbirth, there is a greater reduction of plasma volume than in the number of blood cells. This results in a rise in hematocrit and hemoglobin levels by the seventh day after the birth. There is no increased red blood cell (RBC) destruction during the puerperium, but any excess will disappear gradually in accordance with the life span of the RBC. The exact time at which RBC volume returns to nonpregnant values is not known, but it is within normal limits when measured 8 weeks after childbirth (Bowes & Katz, 2002).

White Blood Cell Count

Normal leukocytosis of pregnancy averages about 12,000/mm^3. During the first 10 to 12 days after childbirth values between 20,000 and 25,000/mm^3 are common. Neutrophils are the most numerous white blood cells. Leukocytosis, coupled with the normal increase in erythrocyte sedimentation rate, may obscure the diagnosis of acute infection at this time.

Coagulation Factors

Clotting factors and fibrinogen are normally increased during pregnancy and remain elevated in the immediate puerperium. When combined with vessel damage and immobility, this hypercoagulable state causes an increased risk of thromboembolism, especially after a cesarean birth.

table 22-2 Vital Signs After Childbirth

NORMAL FINDINGS	DEVIATIONS FROM NORMAL FINDINGS AND PROBABLE CAUSES
TEMPERATURE	
Temperature during first 24 hours may rise to 38° C as a result of dehydrating effects of labor. After 24 hours the woman should be afebrile.	A diagnosis of puerperal sepsis is suggested if a rise in maternal temperature to 38° C is noted after the first 24 hours after childbirth and recurs or persists for 2 days. Other possibilities are mastitis, endometritis, urinary tract infection, and other systemic infections.
PULSE	
Pulse returns to nonpregnant levels within a few days postpartum, although the rate of return varies among individual women.	A rapid pulse rate or one that is increasing may indicate hypovolemia as a result of hemorrhage.
RESPIRATIONS	
Respirations should decrease to within the woman's normal prepregnancy range by 6 to 8 weeks after birth.	Hypoventilation may follow an unusually high subarachnoid (spinal) block or epidural narcotic after a cesarean birth.
BLOOD PRESSURE	
Blood pressure is altered *slightly* if at all. Orthostatic hypotension, as indicated by feelings of faintness or dizziness immediately after standing up, can develop in the first 48 hours as a result of the splanchnic engorgement that may occur after birth.	A low or decreasing blood pressure may reflect hypovolemia secondary to hemorrhage. It is a late sign, however, and other symptoms of hemorrhage usually alert the staff. An increased reading may result from excessive use of vasopressor or oxytocic medications. Because gestational hypertension can persist into or occur first in the postpartum period, routine evaluation of blood pressure is needed. If a woman complains of headache, hypertension must be ruled out as a cause before analgesics are administered.

Fibrinolytic activity also increases during the first few days after childbirth (Bowes & Katz, 2002). Factors I, II, VII, VIII, IX, and X decrease to nonpregnant levels within a few days. Fibrin split products, probably released from the placental site, also can be found in maternal blood.

Varicosities

Varicosities (varices) of the legs (Fig. 22-3) and around the anus (hemorrhoids) are common during pregnancy. Surgical repair of varicosities is not considered during pregnancy. All varices, even the less common vulvar varices, begin to regress (empty) rapidly immediately after childbirth. Total or nearly total regression of varicosities is expected after childbirth.

▬ NEUROLOGIC SYSTEM

Neurologic changes during the puerperium are those that result from a reversal of maternal adaptations to pregnancy and those resulting from trauma during labor and childbirth.

Pregnancy-induced neurologic discomforts disappear after birth. The elimination of physiologic edema through the diuresis that occurs after childbirth relieves carpal tunnel syndrome by easing the compression of the median nerve. The periodic numbness and tingling of fingers that afflict 5% of pregnant women usually disappear after childbirth unless lifting and carrying the baby aggravates the condition. Headache requires careful assessment. Postpartum headaches may be caused by various conditions,

FIG. 22-3 Varicosities in legs. (Courtesy Bernadine Cunningham, Phoenix, AZ.)

including postpartum-onset preeclampsia, stress, and the leakage of cerebrospinal fluid into the extradural space during placement of the needle for administration of epidural or spinal anesthesia. Depending on the cause and effectiveness of the treatment, headaches last from 1 to 3 days to several weeks.

■ MUSCULOSKELETAL SYSTEM

Adaptations of the mother's musculoskeletal system that occur during pregnancy are reversed in the puerperium. These adaptations include the relaxation and subsequent hypermobility of the joints and the change in the mother's center of gravity in response to the enlarging uterus. The joints are completely stabilized by 6 to 8 weeks after birth. Although all other joints return to their normal prepregnancy state, those in the parous woman's feet do not. The new mother may notice a permanent increase in her shoe size.

■ INTEGUMENTARY SYSTEM

Chloasma of pregnancy usually disappears at the end of pregnancy. Hyperpigmentation of the areolae and linea nigra may not regress completely after childbirth. Some women will have permanent darker pigmentation of those areas. Striae gravidarum (stretch marks) on the breasts, the abdomen, the hips, and the thighs may fade but usually do not disappear.

Vascular abnormalities such as spider angiomas (nevi), palmar erythema, and epulis generally regress in response to the rapid decline in estrogens after the end of pregnancy. For some women, spider nevi persist indefinitely.

Hair growth slows during the postpartum period. Some women may actually experience hair loss, because the amount of hair lost is temporarily more than the amount regrown. The abundance of fine hair seen during pregnancy usually disappears after birth; however, any coarse or bristly hair that appears during pregnancy usually remains.

community activity

Perform an easy and fun experiment to assess the accuracy of subjective estimates of blood loss. Pour measured amounts of a red fluid (use expired blood from the blood bank, if available) on at least two brands of perineal pads and on plastic-backed underpads. Ask your classmates and instructors to make independent assessments of the volume. If possible, invite other health care professionals, including nursing or medical students, maternity nurses, obstetricians, nurse-midwives, anesthetists, and anesthesiologists to participate also. Calculate the percentage of correct responses among the total group and within each category of observer. Compare the results. Do profession, area of specialization, or years of experience correlate with more reliable estimates? Were people more likely to overestimate or underestimate the amount? Were the estimates for perineal pads or for underpads different? Were the errors in judgment large enough to raise concern about the accuracy of estimates of blood loss?

Fingernails return to their nonpregnant consistency and strength.

Profuse diaphoresis that occurs in the immediate postpartum period is the most noticeable change in the integumentary system.

■ IMMUNE SYSTEM

No significant changes in the maternal immune system occur during the postpartum period. The mother's need for a rubella vaccination or for prevention of Rh isoimmunization is determined.

key points

- The uterus involutes rapidly after birth and returns to the true pelvis within 2 weeks.
- The rapid drop in estrogen and progesterone levels after expulsion of the placenta is responsible for triggering many of the anatomic and physiologic changes in the puerperium.
- Assessment of lochia and fundal height is essential to monitor the progress of normal involution and to identify potential problems.
- The return of ovulation and menses is determined in part by whether the woman breastfeeds her infant.
- Under normal circumstances, few alterations in vital signs are seen after childbirth.
- Hypercoagulability, vessel damage, and immobility predispose the woman to thromboembolism.
- Marked diuresis, decreased bladder sensitivity, and overdistention of the bladder can lead to problems with urinary elimination.
- Pregnancy-induced hypervolemia, combined with several postpartum physiologic changes, allows the woman to tolerate considerable blood loss at birth.

REFERENCES

Bowes, W., & Katz, V. (2002). Postpartum care. In S. Gabbe, J. Niebyl, & J. Simpson (Eds.), *Obstetrics: Normal and problem pregnancies* (4th ed.). New York: Churchill Livingstone.

Cunningham, F., Leveno, K., Bloom, S., Hauth, J., Gilstrap, L., & Wenstrom, K. (2005). *Williams obstetrics* (22nd ed.). New York: McGraw-Hill.

Lawrence, R., & Lawrence, R. (2004). The breast and the physiology of lactation. In R. Creasy, R. Resnik, & J. Iams (Eds.), *Maternal-fetal medicine: Principles and practice* (5th ed.). Philadelphia: Saunders.

Resnik, R. (2004). The puerperium. In R. Creasy, R. Resnik, & J. Iams (Eds.), *Maternal-fetal medicine: Principles and practice* (5th ed.). Philadelphia: Saunders.

Simpson, K., & Creehan, P. (2001). *AWHONN's perinatal nursing* (2nd ed.). Philadelphia: Lippincott.

Nursing Care of the Postpartum Woman

learning objectives

- Identify the priorities of maternal care given during the fourth stage of labor.
- Identify common selection criteria for safe early postpartum discharge.
- Summarize nursing interventions to prevent infection and excessive bleeding, to promote normal bladder and bowel patterns, and to care for the breasts of women who are breastfeeding or bottle-feeding.

- Explain the influence of cultural expectations on postpartum adjustment.
- Identify psychosocial needs of the woman in the early postpartum period.
- Discuss discharge teaching and postpartum home care.

electronic resources

Additional information related to the content in Chapter 23 can be found on

the companion website at **evolve**
http://evolve.elsevier.com/Lowdermilk/MWHC/
- NCLEX Review Questions
- Case Study: Fourth Trimester
- WebLinks

or on the interactive companion CD
- NCLEX Review Questions
- Case Study: Fourth Trimester
- Critical Thinking Exercise: Postpartum Complications
- Critical Thinking Exercise: Priority Nursing Care—Postpartum Unit
- Plan of Care: Postpartum Care—Vaginal Birth

THE goal of nursing care in the immediate postpartum period is to assist women and their partners during their initial transition to parenting. The approach to the care of women after birth is wellness oriented. Consequently, in the United States most women remain hospitalized no more than 1 or 2 days after vaginal birth, and some for as few as 6 hours. Because there is so much important information to be shared with these women in a very short time, it is vital that their care be thoughtfully planned and provided. Care, which also includes other family members, is focused on the woman's physiologic recovery, her psychologic well-being, and her ability to care for herself and her new baby.

■ FOURTH STAGE OF LABOR

The first 1 to 2 hours after birth, sometimes called the fourth stage of labor, is a crucial time for mother and newborn. Both are not only recovering from the physical process of birth but are also becoming acquainted with each other and additional family members. During this time, maternal organs undergo their initial readjustment to

the nonpregnant state, and the functions of body systems begin to stabilize. Meanwhile, the newborn continues the transition from intrauterine to extrauterine existence.

Breastfeeding during the fourth stage of labor aids in the contraction of the uterus and the prevention of maternal hemorrhage. In most centers, the mother remains in the labor and birth area during this recovery time. In an institution where labor, delivery, and recovery (LDR) rooms are used, the woman stays in the same room where she gave birth. In traditional settings, women are taken from the delivery room to a separate recovery area for observation. Arrangements for care of the newborn vary during the fourth stage of labor. In many settings, the baby remains at the mother's bedside, and the labor or birth nurse cares for both of them. In other institutions, the baby is taken to the nursery for several hours of observation after an initial bonding period with the parents (Fig. 23-1).

Assessment

If the recovery nurse has not previously cared for the new mother, her assessment begins with an oral report from the nurse who attended the woman during labor and birth

Evolve/CD: Case Study: Fourth Trimester

FIG. 23-1 Mother, father, and sibling get acquainted with the newborn. (Courtesy Kim Molloy, Knoxville, IA.)

and a review of the prenatal, labor, and birth records. Of primary importance are conditions that could predispose the mother to hemorrhage, such as precipitous labor, a large baby, grand multiparity (i.e., having given birth to six or more viable infants), induced labor, or a magnesium

infusion during labor. For healthy women, hemorrhage is probably the most dangerous potential complication during the fourth stage of labor.

During the first hour in the recovery room, physical assessments of the mother are frequent. All factors except temperature are assessed every 15 minutes for 1 hour. Temperature is assessed at the beginning and end of the recovery period. After the fourth 15-minute assessment, if all parameters have stabilized within the normal range, the process is usually repeated once in the second hour. Box 23-1 and Fig. 23-2 describe the physical assessment of the mother during the fourth stage. Fig. 23-3 shows an easy-to-use flow sheet that combines the essential immediate postpartum and anesthesia recovery assessments. Within the past few years, many institutions have changed from paper to electronic charting, so that the same information is now recorded and stored on computer.

During the fourth stage of labor, intense tremors that resemble shivering from a chill are commonly seen; they are not related to infection. Several theories have been offered to explain these tremors or shivering, such as their being the result of a sudden release of pressure on pelvic nerves after birth, a response from a fetus-to-mother transfusion that occurred during placental separation, a reaction

---

box 23-1 **Assessment During Fourth Stage of Labor**

Before beginning the assessment, wash hands thoroughly, assemble necessary equipment, and explain the procedure to the client.

BLOOD PRESSURE
- Measure blood pressure per assessment schedule.

PULSE
- Assess rate and regularity.

TEMPERATURE
- Determine temperature.

FUNDUS
- Position woman with knees flexed and head flat.
- Just below umbilicus, cup hand and press firmly into abdomen. At the same time, stabilize the uterus at the symphysis with the opposite hand.
- If fundus is firm (and bladder is empty), with uterus in midline, measure its position relative to woman's umbilicus. Lay fingers flat on abdomen under umbilicus; measure how many fingerbreadths (fb) or centimeters (cm) fit between umbilicus and top of fundus. If the fundus is above the umbilicus, this is recorded as plus (+) fb or cm; if below, as minus (−) fb or cm.
- If fundus is not firm, massage it gently to contract and expel any clots before measuring distance from umbilicus.
- Place hands appropriately; massage gently only until firm.
- Expel clots while keeping hands placed as in Fig. 23-2. With upper hand, firmly apply pressure downward toward vagina; observe perineum for amount and size of expelled clots.

BLADDER
- Assess distention by noting location and firmness of uterine fundus and by observing and palpating bladder. A distended bladder is seen as a suprapubic rounded bulge that is dull to percussion and fluctuates like a water-filled balloon. When the bladder is distended, the uterus is usually boggy in consistency, well above the umbilicus, and to the woman's right side.
- Assist woman to void spontaneously. Measure amount of urine voided.
- Catheterize as necessary.
- Reassess after voiding or catheterization to make sure the bladder is not palpable and the fundus is firm and in the midline.

LOCHIA
- Put on clean examination gloves.
- Observe lochia on perineal pads and on linen under the mother's buttocks. Determine amount and color; note size and number of clots; note odor.
- Observe perineum for source of bleeding (e.g., episiotomy, lacerations).

PERINEUM
- Ask or assist woman to turn on her side and flex upper leg on hip.
- Lift upper buttock.
- Observe perineum in good lighting.
- Assess episiotomy site or laceration repair for intactness, hematoma, edema, bruising, redness, and drainage.
- Assess for presence of hemorrhoids.

FIG. 23-2 Palpating fundus of uterus during the fourth stage of labor. Note that upper hand is cupped over fundus; lower hand dips in above symphysis pubis and supports uterus while it is massaged gently.

to maternal adrenaline production during labor and birth, or a reaction to epidural anesthesia. Some useful interventions are warm blankets and reassurance that the chills or tremors are common, are self-limiting, and last only a short time.

The nutritional status of the woman is assessed. Restriction of food and fluid intake and the loss of fluids (blood, perspiration, or emesis) during labor cause many women to express a strong desire to eat or drink soon after birth. In the absence of complications, a woman who has given birth vaginally; has recovered from the effects of the anesthetic; and has stable vital signs, a firm uterus, and small to moderate lochial flow may have fluids and a regular diet as desired (American Academy of Pediatrics [AAP] & American College of Obstetricians and Gynecologists [ACOG], 2002). In the immediate postpartum period, women who give birth by cesarean are usually restricted to clear liquids and ice chips.

Postanesthesia Recovery

The woman who has given birth by cesarean or has received regional anesthesia for a vaginal birth requires special attention during the recovery period. Obstetric recovery areas are held to the same standard of care that would be expected of any other postanesthesia recovery (PAR) room (AAP & ACOG, 2002). A PAR score is determined for each client on arrival and is updated as part of every 15-minute assessment. Components of the PAR score include activity, respirations, blood pressure, level of consciousness, and color.

■ **NURSE ALERT**
Regardless of her obstetric status, no woman should be discharged from the recovery area until she has completely recovered from the effects of anesthesia.

If the woman received general anesthesia, she should be awake and alert and oriented to time, place, and person. Her respiratory rate should be within normal limits, and her oxygen saturation levels at least 95%, as measured by a pulse oximeter. If the woman received epidural or spinal anesthesia, she should be able to raise her legs, extended at the knees, off the bed, or to flex her knees, place her feet flat on the bed, and raise her buttocks well off the bed. The numb or tingling, prickly sensation should be entirely gone from her legs. Women vary greatly in regard to length of time required to recover from regional anesthesia. Often it takes several hours for these anesthetic effects to disappear.

Transfer from the Recovery Area

After the initial recovery period has been completed, the woman may be transferred to a postpartum room in the same or another nursing unit. In facilities with labor, delivery, recovery, postpartum (LDRP) rooms, the woman is not moved and the nurse who provides care during the recovery period usually continues caring for the woman. Women who have received general or regional anesthesia must be cleared for transfer from the recovery area by a member of the anesthesia care team.

In preparing the transfer report, the recovery nurse uses information from the records of admission, birth, and recovery. Information that must be communicated to the postpartum nurse includes identity of the health care provider; gravidity and parity; age; anesthetic used; any medications given; duration of labor and time of rupture of membranes; whether labor was induced or augmented; type of birth and repair; blood type and Rh status; group B streptococcus (GBS) status; status of rubella immunity; human immunodeficiency virus (HIV) and hepatitis B serology test results; other infections identified during pregnancy (e.g., syphilis, gonorrhea, chlamydia), and whether these were treated; intravenous infusion of any fluids; physiologic status since birth; description of fundus, lochia, bladder, and perineum; sex and weight of infant; time of birth; name of pediatric care provider; chosen method of feeding; any abnormalities noted; and assessment of initial parent-infant interaction.

Most of this information is also documented for the nursing staff in the newborn nursery if the infant is transferred to that unit. In addition, specific information should be provided regarding the infant's Apgar scores (see Chapter 26), weight, voiding, stooling, and whether fed since birth. Nursing interventions that have been completed (e.g., eye prophylaxis, vitamin K injection) as well as identification procedures done (e.g., footprints, arm bands) must also be recorded.

Table 23-1 gives examples for documenting this information before the transfer of the woman from the recovery area.

DIAGNOSIS:_____

PHYSICIAN:_____

ANESTHESIA:_____

ANESTHETIST:_____

ARMBANDS:_____mother _____infant

CLOTHING:_____c̄ family _____c̄ patient

ALLERGIES:_____

PAR SCORE: ADM:____ DC:____

ACTIVITY						
RESPIRATION						
BLOOD PRESSURE						
CONSCIOUS LEVEL						
COLOR						
TOTAL						

Activity
Able to move 4 extremities voluntarily or on command 2
Able to move 2 extremities voluntarily or on command 1
Able to move 0 extremities voluntarily or on command 0

Respiration
Able to deep breathe and cough freely 2
Dyspnea or limited breathing 1
Apneic 0

Blood Pressure
BP ± mm Hg of preanesthetic level 2
BP ± 25-50 mm Hg of preanesthetic level 1
BP ± Greater than 50 mm Hg of preanesthetic level 0

Conscious Level
Fully aware 2
Arousable on calling 1
Not responding 0

Color
Pink 2
Pale, dusky, blotchy, jaundiced, other 1
Cyanotic 0

Pain Scales
Wong Baker = WB
Numeric = N
Simple Descriptive = SD

Pain Characteristics
Location
Duration
Aggravating/Alleviating fx
Nature - dull, gnawing, hot, achy, sharp, burning, throbbing, shooting, stabbing

Observation Codes
A - Anxious D - Depressed H - Relaxed
B - Agitated, Restless E - Crying V - VS Change
C - Confused R - Restless W - Withdrawn
G - Grimace O - Other

Results Code
0 - No pain present
1 - Improved but still in pain
2 - No improvement

Pain Management Intervention
P - Pharmacological
NP - Non pharmacological

VITAL SIGNS:

	TIME								
	BP								
	PULSE								
	RESP / O₂ Sat								
	TEMP								
FUNDUS FB-FINGERBREADTH B-BOGGY FM-FIRM MD-MIDLINE	FUNDUS								
LOCHIA CL-CLOTS MOD-MODERATE SM-SMALL LG-LARGE	LOCHIA								
BLADDER D-DISTENDED F-FOLEY ND-NON-DISTENDED	BLADDER								
EPISIOTOMY/INCISION NL-NORMAL D-DRY ABNL-ABNORMAL I-INTACT	EPIS / INC								
CLEAR CL WHEEZING W DIMINISHED D	BREATH SOUNDS								
q 1° q / Shift	DTR / PROTEIN								
O₂ liters/min									
JP drain cc/hr									
INTAKE									
OUTPUT									
Pain Scale									
Observation Code									
Pain Management Intervention									
Results Code									
INITIALS									

DISCHARGE NOTE

PCA

PCA Medication, Concentration and Volume
_____

Loading Dose _____
Continuous Rate _____ 4 hour limit _____
Lockout Interval _____
RN _____ RN _____
____ / ____ / ____ ____:____ am / pm

Meds / IV / Rate	Time / Initial
	/
	/
	/
	/

INTAKE TOTAL Shift 7A 3P 11P

OUTPUT TOTAL Shift 7A 3P 11P

IV _____cc LTC @ D/C

Homans Sign Pos ☐ Neg ☐

BONDING
☐ appropriate
☐ inappropriate
☐ NA (explain)
_____

Social Services Notified
____ / ____ / ____
____:____ am/pm

TEACHING
☐ fundal massage
☐ TC & DB
☐ breastfeeding
☐ assistance on 1st ambulation
☐ Pain Scale
☐ PCA pump

Signatures/Initials
_____
_____

Report Called To:_____

ANESTHESIA D/C:_____
EPIDURAL CATHETER: IN OUT NA

Regional Medical Center at Memphis
MATERNITY RECOVERY ROOM RECORD
FORM NO. 68622 (10/01) White (Chart) Yellow (Pharmacy)

FIG. 23-3 An example of a maternity recovery room record. (Courtesy The Regional Medical Center at Memphis [The Med], Memphis, TN.)

table 23-1 Recovery Nurse's Report

ITEM	EXAMPLE OF DOCUMENTATION OF MOTHER	EXAMPLE OF DOCUMENTATION OF NEWBORN
Type of labor and birth: unusual observations, if any, of the placenta	Spontaneous or assisted (forceps) vaginal birth; vertex presentation	Spontaneous or assisted (forceps, vacuum extractor) vaginal birth in vertex presentation; time of ROM
Gravidity and parity, age	G1, P1, age 22 yr; 39 wk of gestation	G1, P1, age 22 yr; 39 wk of gestation
Anesthesia and analgesia used	None; epidural, low spinal, local	None; epidural, low spinal, or local
Condition of perineum	Episiotomy; repair of lacerations; intact	
Events since birth	Vital signs, BP, fundus, lochia, intake and output, medications (including dosage, time of administration, and results), response to newborn, observation of family interactions, including siblings, if present	Nursed at breast for _____ min. Voided × 1; meconium stool × 1 Eye prophylaxis given Vitamin K injection given Held by siblings who are happy (or have other response to newborn)
Condition and sex of newborn; other information	Time of birth; Apgar at 1 and 5 min; weight; whether breastfeeding or bottle-feeding; sex of baby	Time of birth: Apgar scores at 1 and 5 min Sex; weight; name of pediatrician; breastfeeding or bottle-feeding; mother's hepatitis B status and GBS status; whether or not mother received magnesium sulfate; time of last systemic analgesia
Relevant information from prenatal record	Need for rubella vaccination; presence of infections; hepatitis B status; HIV status; blood type; Rh status; GBS status and treatment if positive	Unremarkable pregnancy
Miscellaneous information: IV drip	If IV drip is infusing, rate of infusion, medication added (e.g., oxytocin [Pitocin]), whether to keep open or discontinue after completion of bag that is hung	
Social factors	If woman is releasing baby for adoption, whether or not she wants to see the baby, breastfeed, allow visitors, or other preferences she may have	Baby up for adoption; to stay in NBN until discharge

BP, Blood pressure; *GBS,* group B streptococcus; *HIV,* human immunodeficiency virus; *IV,* intravenous; *NBN,* newborn nursery; *ROM,* rupture of membranes.

Women who give birth in birthing centers may go home within a few hours, after the woman's and infant's conditions are stable.

▬ DISCHARGE: BEFORE 24 HOURS ▬ AND AFTER 48 HOURS

Early postpartum discharge, shortened hospital stay, and *1-day maternity stay* are all terms for the decreasing length of hospital stays of mothers and their babies after a low risk birth. The trend of shortened hospital stays is based largely on efforts to reduce health care costs coupled with consumer demands to have less medical intervention and more family-focused experiences (Meara, Kotagal, Atherton, & Lieu, 2004).

Laws Relating to Discharge

Health care providers have expressed concern with shortened stays because some medical problems do not show up in the first 24 hours after birth, and new mothers have not had sufficient time to learn how to care for their newborns and identify newborn health problems such as jaundice and dehydration related to breastfeeding difficulties (Meara et al., 2004).

The concern for the potential increase in adverse maternal-infant outcomes from hospital early-discharge practices led the American College of Obstetricians and Gynecologists (ACOG), the American Academy of Pediatrics (AAP), and other professional health care organizations to promote the enactment of federal and state maternity length-of-stay bills to ensure adequate care for both the mother and the newborn. The passage of the Newborns' and Mothers' Health Protection Act of 1996 provided minimum federal standards for health plan coverage for mothers and their newborns (AAP Committee on Fetus and Newborn, 2004). Under this Act, all health plans are required to allow the new mother and newborn to remain in the hospital for a minimum of 48 hours after a normal vaginal birth and for 96 hours after a cesarean birth unless the attending provider, in consultation with the mother, decides on early discharge.

Criteria for Discharge

Early discharge with postpartum home care can be a safe and satisfying option for women and their families when it is comprehensive and based on individual needs (AAP Committee on Fetus and Newborn, 2004). Hospital stays must be long enough to identify problems and to ensure that the woman is sufficiently recovered and is prepared to care for herself and the baby at home.

It is essential that nurses consider the medical needs of the woman and her baby and provide care that is coordinated to meet those needs in order to provide timely physiologic interventions and treatment to prevent morbidity and hospital readmission. With predetermined criteria for identifying low risk in the mothers and newborns (Box 23-2), the length of hospitalization can be based on medical need for care in an acute care setting or in consideration of the ongoing care needed in the home environment (AAP Committee on Fetus and Newborn, 2004). Early follow-up visits are key to reducing readmissions of newborns (Meara et al., 2004).

Care paths provide the nurse with an organized approach toward meeting essential maternal-newborn care and teaching goals within a limited time frame (see Care Path). Care paths can be developed for vaginal or cesarean births. Other methods such as postpartum order sets and maternal-newborn teaching checklists (Fig. 23-4) can be used to accomplish client care and educational outcomes.

Hospital-based maternity nurses continue to play invaluable roles as caregivers, teachers, and client and family advocates in developing and implementing effective home-care strategies. The nurse participates in the determination of whether the mother and newborn meet the criteria for early discharge.

▬ **LEGAL TIP** Early Discharge

Whether or not the woman and her family have chosen early discharge, the nurse and the primary health care provider are held responsible if the woman is discharged before her condition has stabilized within normal limits. If complications occur, the medical and nursing staff could be sued for abandonment.

▬ CARE MANAGEMENT—
▬ PHYSICAL NEEDS

▬ Assessment and Nursing Diagnoses

A complete physical assessment, including measurement of vital signs, is performed on admission to the postpartum unit. If the woman's vital signs are within normal limits, they are usually assessed every 4 to 8 hours for the remainder of her hospitalization. Other components of the initial assessment include the mother's emotional status, energy level, degree of physical discomfort, hunger, and thirst. Intake and output assessments should always be included if an intravenous infusion or a urinary catheter is in place. If the woman gave birth by cesarean, her incisional dressing should also be assessed. To some degree, her knowledge level concerning self-care and infant care also can be determined at this time.

▬ *Ongoing Physical Assessment*

The new mother should be evaluated thoroughly during each shift throughout hospitalization. Physical assessments include evaluation of the breasts, uterine fundus, lochia,

(Text continued on p. 594.)

---

box 23-2 | Criteria for Early Discharge

MOTHER
- Uncomplicated pregnancy, labor, vaginal birth, and postpartum course
- No evidence of premature rupture of membranes
- Blood pressure and temperature stable and within normal limits
- Ambulating unassisted
- Voiding adequate amounts without difficulty
- Hemoglobin >10 g
- No significant vaginal bleeding; perineum intact or no more than second-degree episiotomy or laceration repair; uterus is firm
- Received instructions on postpartum self-care

INFANT
- Term infant (38 to 42 weeks) with weight appropriate for gestational age
- Normal findings on physical assessment
- Temperature, respirations, and heart rate within normal limits and stable for the 12 hours preceding discharge
- At least two successful feedings completed (normal sucking and swallowing)
- Urination and stooling have occurred at least once

- No evidence of significant jaundice in the first 24 hours after the birth
- No excessive bleeding at the circumcision site for at least 2 hours
- Screening tests performed according to state regulations; tests to be repeated at follow-up visit if done before the infant is 24 hours old
- Initial hepatitis B vaccine given or scheduled for first follow-up visit
- Laboratory data reviewed: maternal syphilis and hepatitis B status; infant or cord blood type and Coombs' test results if indicated

GENERAL
- No social, family, or environmental risk factors identified
- Family or support person available to assist mother and infant at home
- Follow-up scheduled within 1 week if discharged before 48 hours after the birth
- Documentation of skill of mother in feeding (breastfeeding or bottle-feeding), cord care, skin care, perineal care, infant safety (use of car seat, sleeping positions), and recognizing signs of illness and common infant problems

Source: American Academy of Pediatrics (AAP) Committee on Fetus and Newborn. (2004). Hospital stay for healthy term infants. *Pediatrics, 113*(5), 1434-1436.

Abbott Northwestern Hospital
A HealthSpan™ Organization
SELF/FAMILY LEARNING CHECKLIST

Patient Name, Social Security #, Date of Birth

I learn best by: ☐ *Group classes*   ☐ *Individual instruction*   ☐ *Video instruction*   ☐ *Reading it myself*

Please indicate your desired learning needs by placing a check in one of the columns next to each topic.

KEY	1 = *Most important to learn before I go home* 2 = *I already know*

(Please DATE when learning need is met.)

CARING FOR YOURSELF	1	2	DATE	CARING FOR BABY	1	2	DATE
Episiotomy and perineal care				*Diapering*			
Vaginal discharge				*Baby bath, skin and cord care*			
Hemorrhoids/Constipation				*Circumcised/uncircumcised care*			
Breast care				*Burping*			
Nutrition				*Bowel movements/wet diapers*			
Activity				*Sleeping habits*			
Post partal exercises				*Newborn behavior*			
Return of menstruation				*Jaundice*			
Family planning				*Signs of illness*			
Blood clots				*Car seat safety*			
Post partum emotions				*General infant safety/poison control*			
Post partum warning signs				*Signs/symptoms of dehydration*			
				Bulb syringe			
Cesarean Birth							
Incisional care				**BREAST FEEDING**			
				Sore nipples			
				Positioning			
				Frequency of feedings			
AFTER DISCHARGE				*Expressing/storing milk*			
When to call health care provider				*Engorgement*			
				Feeding water			
				Nursing while working			
OTHER				*Weaning*			
Working mothers							
Day care				**BOTTLE FEEDING**			
Sibling adjustment				*Types of formula*			
Single parent support				*Preparing formula*			
Time out for parents				*Frequency of feedings*			
Infant safety and security							
Infant As A Person Class							
New Parent Connection							

MEDICATIONS AT HOME

MEDICATIONS	STRENGTH	DOSAGE	FREQUENCY	PURPOSE/SPECIAL INSTRUCTIONS
			times per day	
			times per day	
			times per day	

RESOURCES REFERRALS
☐ *Physician Discharge Instructions* _____
☐ *Home Care Agency* _____
☐ *Other Referrals* _____

VALUABLES: ☐ *Returned* ☐ *None*   **MEDICATIONS:** ☐ *Returned* ☐ *None*   ☐ *Room checked for belongings*
Patient verbalized understanding of discharge information received.

PATIENT OR
SUPPORT PERSON _____   NURSE'S
SIGNATURE _____   DATE _____

SELF/FAMILY LEARNING CHECKLIST (vertical, right margin)

SELF/FAMILY LEARNING CHECKLIST

FIG. 23-4   Self/family learning checklist. (Copyright Abbott Northwestern Hospital of Allina Health System, Minneapolis and St. Paul, MN.)

care path > **24-Hour Vaginal Birth Without Complications**

Date of Birth: _____
Hour of Birth: _____

The uncomplicated vaginal birth client's admission and discharge are based on a 24-hr length of stay after birth based on individual needs.

Time: _____

	RECOVERY	ADM. TO PP UNIT—8 HR	9-16 HR	17-24 HR—DISCHARGE
PRIMARY PHYSIOLOGIC FOCUS	Woman will have normal VS as documented on flow sheet.	Woman will have normal VS and moderate lochia rubra.	Woman will have normal VS and minimal lochia rubra.	Woman will have normal VS and minimal lochia rubra.
	NA MET VARIANCE	**NA MET VARIANCE**	**NA MET VARIANCE**	**NA MET VARIANCE**
	VS every 15 min ×1 hr, then every 4 hr. Assess perineum/episiotomy. Ice pack as needed (prn). Assess lochia.	VS every 4 hr. Assess perineum/episiotomy. Ice pack prn. Assess lochia.	VS every shift. Assess perineum/episiotomy. Ice pack prn. Assess lochia.	VS every shift. Assess perineum/episiotomy. Ice pack prn. Assess lochia.
	RECOVERY	**ADM. TO PP UNIT—8 HR**	**9-16 HR**	**17-24 HR—DISCHARGE**
IVs/LABWORK/ MEDICATIONS	Woman will have appropriate lab work done and medication given by time of transfer to mother/baby unit. IV may be infusing.	Woman will begin to verbalize understanding of hepatitis status and medication requirements. IV may be medlocked.	Woman will have appropriate lab work done by 16 hr PP. Medlock may be discontinued.	Woman will have appropriate lab work done and appropriate medications initiated.
	NA MET VARIANCE	**NA MET VARIANCE**	**NA MET VARIANCE**	**NA MET VARIANCE**
	CBC, if not done before birth. Urine drug screen if ordered. U/A–dipstick. (Send to lab, if abnormal.)	Review hepatitis B status. Medication regimen initiated.	CBC. Review rubella status. Review Hgb and Hct.	Iron tablet Prenatal vitamin. Rubella vaccine, if appropriate. Rh immune globulin, if indicated. Laxative prn.
	RECOVERY	**ADM. TO PP UNIT—8 HR**	**9-16 HR**	**17-24 HR—DISCHARGE**
NUTRITION/ ELIMINATION	Woman will be up to use bathroom before transfer.	Woman will resume normal nutritional status and bladder function.	Woman will resume normal nutritional status and bladder function.	Woman will have normal bowel and bladder function.
	NA MET VARIANCE	**NA MET VARIANCE**	**NA MET VARIANCE**	**NA MET VARIANCE**
	Assess bladder fullness. Assist to bathroom. Assess for tolerance of PO intake.	Encourage ambulation. Encourage PO fluids. Assist to bathroom as needed. Assess bladder function. Encourage PO intake.	Encourage ambulation. Encourage PO fluids. Assist to bathroom as needed. Assess bladder function. Encourage PO intake.	Encourage ambulation. Encourage PO fluids. Assist to bathroom as needed. Stool softener/ laxative PRN.
	RECOVERY	**ADM. TO PP UNIT—8 HR**	**9-16 HR**	**17-24 HR—DISCHARGE**
PSYCHOSOCIAL	Woman and family will begin attachment behaviors with newborn.	Woman and family will demonstrate appropriate attachment behaviors.	Family will verbalize comfort with new infant.	Family will verbalize comfort with new infant.
	NA MET VARIANCE	**NA MET VARIANCE**	**NA MET VARIANCE**	**NA MET VARIANCE**
	Encourage mother and family members to hold and touch infant. Provide skin-to-skin contact of mother and infant. Provide mother the opportunity to breastfeed, if applicable.	Offer flexible rooming-in with infant. Allow verbalization of woman's feelings. Assess discharge needs and need for social service consult.	Reinforce interventions.	Reinforce interventions. Complete birth certificate. Arrange for home visit if needed.

care path ▶ **24-Hour Vaginal Birth Without Complications—cont'd**

		RECOVERY	ADM. TO PP UNIT—8 HR	9-16 HR	17-24 HR—DISCHARGE
SELF-CARE ACTIVITY		Woman will begin self-care activities as tolerated.	Woman will be up to use bathroom or shower with assistance.	Woman will be up to use bathroom or shower independently.	Woman will be up to use bathroom or shower independently.
		NA MET VARIANCE	**NA MET VARIANCE**	**NA MET VARIANCE**	**NA MET VARIANCE**
		Instruct woman in pericare and pad changes and use of ice pack.	Reinforce proper pericare. Encourage woman to shower (if culturally appropriate).	Reinforce proper pericare. Instruct on use of sitz bath.	Reinforce proper pericare. Reinforce use of sitz bath.
TEACHING/DISCHARGE PLANNING		**RECOVERY**	**ADM. TO PP UNIT—8 HR**	**9-16 HR**	**17-24 HR—DISCHARGE**
		Woman will begin to verbalize and/or demonstrate self-care and infant-care activities.	Woman will begin to verbalize and/or demonstrate infant and self-care activities.	Woman and family will demonstrate appropriate infant-care activities.	Woman and family will demonstrate appropriate infant-care activities.
		NA MET VARIANCE	**NA MET VARIANCE**	**NA MET VARIANCE**	**NA MET VARIANCE**
		Date:			
		Initials:			
		Teaching to include following: Breastfeeding latch-on and positioning, if applicable. Appropriate handwashing techniques. Instruct in pain-relief techniques or medication.	Teaching to include following: Breastfeeding or formula initial feeding information. Breast care. Perineal care. Proper nutrition. Safety issues reviewed.	Teaching to include following: Attendance at mother/baby-care class or individual self/newborn care teaching. Breast care or formula information. Newborn channel. Lactation consult prn.	Teaching to include following: Reinforcement of self/newborn care teaching Plans for self/infant follow-up. Review IHSP.* Review Baby Net program. Telephone number for follow-up questions. Home-going meds and purposes.
		1.	1.	1.	1.
		2.	2.	2.	2.
		3.	3.	3.	3.
		4.	4.	4.	4.

Variance Documentation: _____

_____

_____

_____

_____

_____

CBC, Complete blood count; *Hct,* hematocrit; *Hgb,* hemoglobin; *PO,* oral (by mouth); *PP,* postpartum; *prn,* as needed; *U/A,* urinalysis; *VS,* vital signs.
*IHSP denotes a test done to determine whether follow-up is needed in the Infant Hearing Screening Program (IHSP).

perineum, bladder and bowel function, vital signs, and legs. If a woman has an intravenous line in place, her fluid and hematologic status should be evaluated before it is removed. Signs of potential problems that may be identified during the assessment process are listed in the Signs of Potential Complications box.

■ Routine Laboratory Tests

Several laboratory tests may be performed in the immediate postpartum period. Hemoglobin and hematocrit values are often evaluated on the first postpartum day to assess blood loss during childbirth, especially after cesarean birth. In some hospitals, a clean-catch or catheterized urine specimen may be obtained and sent for routine urinalysis or culture and sensitivity, especially if an indwelling urinary catheter was inserted during the intrapartum period. In addition, if the woman's rubella and Rh status are unknown, tests to determine her status and need for possible treatment should be performed at this time.

Nursing Diagnoses

Although all women experience similar physiologic changes during the postpartum period, certain factors act to make each woman's experience unique. From a physiologic standpoint, the length and difficulty of the labor, type of birth (i.e., vaginal or cesarean), presence of episiotomy or lacerations, and whether the mother plans to breastfeed or bottle-feed are factors to be considered with each woman. After analyzing the data obtained during the assessment process, the nurse establishes nursing diagnoses that will provide a guide for planning care. Examples of

nursing diagnoses commonly established for the postpartum woman include the following:

- *Risk for deficient fluid volume (hemorrhage) related to*
  –uterine atony after childbirth
- *Risk for constipation related to*
  –postchildbirth discomfort
  –childbirth trauma to tissues
  –decreased intake of solid food and/or fluids
- *Acute pain related to*
  –uterine involution
  –trauma to perineum, episiotomy
  –hemorrhoids
  –engorged breasts
- *Disturbed sleep patterns related to*
  –discomfort of postpartum period
  –long labor process
  –infant care and hospital routine
- *Ineffective breastfeeding related to*
  –maternal discomfort
  –infant positioning

■ Expected Outcomes of Care

The nursing plan of care includes both the postpartum woman and her infant, even if the nursery nurse retains primary responsibility for the infant. In many hospitals, couplet care (also called *mother-baby care* or *single-room maternity care*) is practiced. Nurses in these settings have been educated in both mother and infant care and function as the primary nurse for both mother and infant, even if the infant is kept in the nursery. This approach is a variation of

---

signs of potential complications

Physiologic Problems

TEMPERATURE
More than 38° C after the first 24 hr

PULSE
Tachycardia or marked bradycardia

BLOOD PRESSURE
Hypotension or hypertension

ENERGY LEVEL
Lethargy, extreme fatigue

UTERUS
Deviated from the midline, boggy consistency, remains above the umbilicus after 24 hr

LOCHIA
Heavy, foul odor, bright red bleeding that is not lochia

PERINEUM
Pronounced edema, not intact, signs of infection, marked discomfort

LEGS
Homans sign positive; painful, reddened area; warmth on posterior aspect of calf

BREASTS
Redness, heat, pain, cracked and fissured nipples, inverted nipples, palpable mass

APPETITE
Lack of appetite, nausea or vomiting

ELIMINATION
Urine: inability to void, urgency, frequency, dysuria
Bowel: constipation, diarrhea, gas pains

REST
Inability to rest or sleep

NEUROLOGIC
Headache, blurred vision

rooming-in, in which the mother and infant room together and mother and nurse share the care of the infant. The organization of the mother's care must take the newborn into consideration. The day actually revolves around the baby's feeding and care times.

Expected outcomes for the postpartum period are based on the nursing diagnoses identified for the individual woman. Examples of common expected outcomes for physiologic needs are that the woman will do the following:

- Demonstrate normal involution and lochial characteristics.
- Remain comfortable and injury free.
- Demonstrate normal bladder and bowel patterns.
- Demonstrate knowledge of breast care, whether breast-feeding or bottle-feeding.
- Integrate the newborn into the family.

▬ Plan of Care and Interventions

Once the nursing diagnoses are formulated, the nurse plans with the woman what nursing measures are appropriate and which are to be given priority. The nursing plan of care includes periodic assessments to detect deviations from normal physical changes, measures to relieve discomfort or pain, safety measures to prevent injury or infection, and teaching and counseling measures designed to promote the woman's feelings of competence in self-care and baby care. Family members are included in the teaching. The nurse evaluates continuously and is ready to change the plan if indicated. Almost all hospitals use standardized care plans or care paths as a basis for planning. The nurse's adaptation of the standardized plan to specific medical and nursing diagnoses results in individualized client care (Plan of Care).

Nurses assume many roles while implementing the nursing care plan. They provide direct physical care, teach mother-baby care, and provide anticipatory guidance and counseling. Perhaps most important of all, they nurture the woman by providing encouragement and support as she begins to assume the many tasks of motherhood. Nurses who take the time to "mother the mother" do much to increase feelings of self-confidence in new mothers.

The first step in providing individualized care is to confirm the woman's identity by checking her wristband. At the same time, the infant's identification number is matched with the corresponding band on the mother's wrist, and, in some instances, the father's wrist. The nurse determines how the mother wishes to be addressed and then notes her preference in her record and in her nursing care plan.

The woman and her family are oriented to their surroundings. Familiarity with the unit, routines, resources, and personnel reduces one potential source of anxiety—the unknown. The mother is reassured through knowing whom and how she can call for assistance and what she can expect in the way of supplies and services. If the woman's usual daily routine before admission differs from the facility's routine, the nurse works with the woman to develop a mutually acceptable routine.

Infant abduction from hospitals in the United States has increased over the past few years. The mother should be taught to check the identity of any person who comes to remove the baby from her room. Hospital personnel usually wear picture identification badges (see Fig. 26-14). On some units, all staff members wear matching scrubs or special badges. Other units use closed-circuit television, computer monitoring systems, or fingerprint identification pads. As a rule, the baby is never carried in a staff member's arms between the mother's room and the nursery but is always wheeled in a bassinet, which also contains baby care supplies. Clients and nurses must work together to ensure the safety of newborns in the hospital environment.

▬ *Prevention of Infection*

One important means of preventing infection is maintenance of a clean environment. Bed linens should be changed as needed. Disposable pads and draw sheets may have to be changed frequently. By not walking barefoot, women avoid contaminating the linens when they return to bed. A sitz bath or heat lamp used by multiple clients must be scrubbed after each woman's use. Personnel must be conscientious about their handwashing techniques to prevent cross-infection. Standard Precautions must be practiced. Staff members with colds, coughs, or skin infections (e.g., a cold sore on the lip [herpes simplex virus, type 1]) must follow hospital protocol when in contact with postpartum women. In many hospitals, staff members with open herpetic lesions, strep throat, conjunctivitis, upper respiratory infections, or diarrhea are encouraged to avoid contact with mothers and infants by staying home until the condition is no longer contagious.

Proper care of the episiotomy site and any perineal lacerations prevents infection in the genitourinary area and aids the healing process. Educating the woman to wipe from front to back (urethra to anus) after voiding or defecating is a simple first step. In many hospitals, a squeeze bottle filled with warm water or an antiseptic solution is used after each voiding to cleanse the perineal area. Heat lamps and sitz baths, once commonly used to promote healing, are now used much less frequently for this purpose (Box 23-3). The woman should change her perineal pad from front to back each time she voids or defecates and wash her hands thoroughly before and after doing so.

▬ *Prevention of Excessive Bleeding*

The most frequent cause of excessive bleeding after birth is uterine atony, failure of the uterine muscle to contract firmly. The two most important interventions for preventing excessive bleeding are maintaining good uterine tone and preventing bladder distention. If uterine atony occurs, the relaxed uterus distends with blood and clots, blood vessels in the placental site are not clamped off, and excessive bleeding results.

Excessive blood loss after childbirth also may be caused by vaginal or vulvar hematomas, unrepaired lacerations of the vagina or cervix, and retained placental fragments.

CD: Critical Thinking Exercise: Priority Nursing Care—Postpartum Unit

CD: Plan of Care: Postpartum Care—Vaginal Birth

NURSING DIAGNOSIS Risk for deficient fluid volume related to uterine atony and hemorrhage

Expected Outcomes *Fundus is firm, lochia is moderate, and there is no evidence of hemorrhage.*

Nursing Interventions/*Rationales*
- Monitor lochia (color, amount, consistency), and count and weigh sanitary pads if lochia is heavy *to evaluate amount of bleeding.*
- Monitor and palpate fundus for location and tone *to determine status of uterus and dictate further interventions because atonic uterus is most common cause of postpartum hemorrhage.*
- Monitor intake and output, assess for bladder fullness, and encourage voiding *because a full bladder interferes with involution of the uterus.*
- Monitor vital signs (increased pulse and respirations, decreased blood pressure) and skin temperature and color *to detect signs of hemorrhage or shock.*
- Monitor postpartum hematology studies *to assess effects of blood loss.*
- If fundus is boggy, apply gentle massage and assess tone response *to promote uterine contractions and increase uterine tone.* (Do not overstimulate because doing so can cause fundal relaxation.)
- Express uterine clots *to promote uterine contraction.*
- Explain to the woman the process of involution and teach her to assess and massage the fundus and to report any persistent bogginess *to involve her in self-care and increase sense of control.*
- Administer oxytocic agents per physician or nurse-midwife order and evaluate effectiveness *to promote continuing uterine contraction.*
- Administer fluids, blood, blood products, or plasma expanders as ordered *to replace lost fluid and lost blood volume.*

NURSING DIAGNOSIS Acute pain related to postpartum physiologic changes (hemorrhoids, episiotomy, breast engorgement, cracked and sore nipples)

Expected Outcome *Woman exhibits signs of decreased discomfort.*

Nursing Interventions/*Rationales*
- Assess location, type, and quality of pain *to direct intervention.*
- Explain to the woman the source and reasons for the pain, its expected duration, and treatments *to decrease anxiety and increase sense of control.*
- Administer prescribed pain medications *to provide pain relief.*
- If pain is perineal (episiotomy, hemorrhoids), apply ice packs in the first 24 hours *to reduce edema and vulvar irritation and reduce discomfort;* encourage sitz baths using cool water for first 24 hours *to reduce edema* and warm water thereafter *to promote circulation;* apply witch hazel compresses *to reduce edema;* teach woman to use prescribed perineal creams, sprays, or ointments *to depress response of peripheral nerves;* teach woman to tighten buttocks before sitting and to sit on flat, hard surfaces *to compress buttocks and reduce pressure on the perineum.* (Avoid donuts and soft pillows as they separate the buttocks and decrease venous blood flow, increasing pain.)
- If pain is from breasts and woman is breastfeeding, encourage use of a well-fitted, supportive bra *to increase comfort;* ascertain that infant has latched on correctly *to prevent sore nipples.*

- If breasts are engorged, have woman apply ice packs to breasts 15 minutes on, 45 minutes off or apply cabbage leaves in same manner *to relieve discomfort;* use warm compresses or take a warm shower before breastfeeding *to stimulate milk flow and relieve stasis;* hand-express milk or pump milk *to relieve discomfort if infant is unable to latch on and feed.*
- If nipples are sore, have woman rub breast milk into nipples after feeding and air-dry nipples; apply purified lanolin or other creams as prescribed; and wear breast shields in her bra *to minimize nipple irritation;* assist woman to correct latching-on problem *to prevent further nipple soreness.*
- If pain is from breast and woman is not breastfeeding, encourage use of a well-fitted, supportive bra or breast binder and application of ice packs and/or cabbage leaves *to suppress milk production and decrease discomfort.*

NURSING DIAGNOSIS Disturbed sleep patterns related to excitement, discomfort, and environmental interruptions

Expected Outcomes *Woman sleeps for uninterrupted periods of time and feels rested after waking.*

Nursing Interventions/*Rationales*
- Establish woman's routine sleep patterns and compare with current sleep patterns, exploring things that interfere with sleep, *to determine scope of problem and direct interventions.*
- Individualize nursing routines to fit woman's natural body rhythms (i.e., wake-sleep cycles), provide a sleep-promoting environment (i.e., darkness, quiet, adequate ventilation, appropriate room temperature), prepare for sleep using woman's usual routines (i.e., back rub, soothing music, warm milk), teach use of guided imagery and relaxation techniques *to promote optimum conditions for sleep.*
- Avoid things or routines (i.e., caffeine, foods that induce heartburn, fluids, strenuous mental or physical activity) *that may interfere with sleep.*
- Administer sedation or pain medication as prescribed *to enhance quality of sleep.*
- Advise woman or partner to limit visitors and activities *to avoid further fatigue.*
- Teach woman to use infant nap time as a time for her also *to nap and replenish energy and decrease fatigue.*

NURSING DIAGNOSIS Impaired urinary elimination related to perineal trauma and effects of anesthesia

Expected Outcomes *Woman will void within 6 to 8 hours after birth and will empty bladder completely.*

Nursing Interventions/*Rationales*
- Assess position and character of uterine fundus and bladder *to determine if any further interventions are indicated because of displacement of the fundus or distention of the bladder.*
- Measure intake and output *to assess for evidence of dehydration and subsequent anticipated decrease in urine output.*
- Encourage voiding by walking woman to bathroom, running water over perineum, running water in sink, and providing privacy *to encourage voiding.*
- Encourage oral intake *to replace fluids lost during birth and prevent dehydration.*
- Catheterize as necessary by indwelling or straight method *to ensure bladder emptying and allow uterine involution.*

| box 23-3 | **Self-Care Interventions for Episiotomy, Lacerations, and Hemorrhoids** |

Explain both procedure and rationale before implementation.

CLEANSING
- Wash hands before and after cleansing perineum and changing pads.
- Wash perineum with mild soap and warm water at least once daily.
- Cleanse from symphysis pubis to anal area.
- Apply peripad from front to back, protecting inner surface of pad from contamination.
- Wrap soiled pad and place in covered waste container.
- Change pad with each void or defecation or at least 4 times per day.
- Assess amount and character of lochia with each pad change.

ICE PACK
Apply a covered ice pack to perineum from front to back.
- During first 2 hours to decrease edema formation and increase comfort
- After the first 2 hours following the birth as needed to provide anesthetic effect

SQUEEZE BOTTLE
- Demonstrate for and assist woman; explain rationale.
- Fill bottle with tap water warmed to approximately 38° C (comfortably warm on the wrist).
- Instruct woman to position nozzle between her legs so that squirts of water reach perineum as she sits on toilet seat. Explain that it will take the whole bottle of water to cleanse perineum.
- Remind her to blot dry with toilet paper or clean wipes.
- Remind her to avoid contamination from anal area.
- Apply clean pad.

SITZ BATH
Built-in Type
- Prepare bath by thoroughly scrubbing with cleaning agent and rinsing.
- Pad with towel before filling.

- Fill one half to one third with water of correct temperature, 38° to 40.6° C. Some women prefer cool sitz baths. Ice is added to water to lower the temperature to the level comfortable for the woman.
- Encourage woman to use at least twice a day for 20 minutes.
- Place call light within easy reach.
- Teach woman to enter bath by tightening gluteal muscles and keeping them tightened and then relaxing them after she is in the bath.
- Place dry towels within reach.
- Ensure privacy.
- Check woman in 15 minutes; assess pulse as needed.

Disposable Type
- Clamp tubing and fill bag with warm water.
- Raise toilet seat, place bath in bowl with overflow opening directed toward back of toilet.
- Place container above toilet bowl.
- Attach tube into groove at front of bath.
- Loosen tube clamp to regulate rate of flow: fill bath to about one half full; continue as above for built-in sitz bath.

DRY HEAT
- Inspect lamp for defects.
- Cover lamp with towels.
- Position lamp 50 cm from perineum; use 3 times a day for 20-minute periods.
- Teach regarding use of 40-W bulb at home.
- Provide draping over woman.
- If same lamp is being used by several women, clean it carefully between uses.

TOPICAL APPLICATIONS
- Apply anesthetic cream or spray after cleansing perineal area: use sparingly 3 to 4 times per day.
- Offer witch hazel pads (Tucks) after voiding or defecating; woman pats perineum dry from front to back, then applies witch hazel pads.

▬ NURSE ALERT

A perineal pad saturated in 15 minutes or less and pooling of blood under the buttocks are indications of excessive blood loss, requiring immediate assessment, intervention, and notification of the physician or nurse-midwife.

Accurate visual estimation of blood loss is an important nursing responsibility. Blood loss is usually described subjectively as scant, light, moderate, or heavy (profuse). Figure 23-5 shows examples of perineal pad saturation corresponding to each of these descriptions.

Although postpartal blood loss may be estimated by observing the amount of staining on a perineal pad, it is difficult to judge the amount of lochial flow based only on observation of perineal pads. More objective estimates of blood loss include measuring serial hemoglobin or hematocrit values; weighing blood clots and items saturated

FIG. 23-5 Blood loss after birth is assessed by the extent of perineal pad saturation as (from left to right) scant (<2.5 cm), light (<10 cm), moderate (>10 cm), or heavy (one pad saturated within 2 hours).

with blood (1 mL equals 1 g); and establishing how many milliliters it takes to saturate perineal pads being used (Simpson & Creehan, 2001).

Any estimation of lochial flow is inaccurate and incomplete without consideration of the time factor. The woman who saturates a perineal pad in 1 hour or less is bleeding much more heavily than the woman who saturates one perineal pad in 8 hours.

Luegenbiehl (1997) found that nurses in general tend to overestimate, rather than underestimate, blood loss. Different brands of perineal pads vary in their saturation volume and soaking appearance. For example, blood placed on some brands tends to soak down into the pad, whereas on other brands it tends to spread outward. Nurses should determine saturation volume and soaking appearance for the brands used in their institution so that they may improve accuracy of blood loss estimation.

▬ NURSE ALERT

The nurse always checks under the mother's buttocks as well as on the perineal pad. Blood may flow between the buttocks onto the linens under the mother, although the amount on the perineal pad is slight; thus excessive bleeding may go undetected.

Blood pressure is not a reliable indicator of impending shock from early postpartum hemorrhage. More sensitive means of identifying shock are provided by respirations, pulse, skin condition, urinary output, and level of consciousness (Benedetti, 2002). The frequent physical assessments performed during the fourth stage of labor are designed to provide prompt identification of excessive bleeding (Emergency box).

Maintenance of Uterine Tone. A major intervention to restore good tone is stimulation by gently massaging the uterine fundus until it is firm (see Fig. 23-2). Fundal massage may cause a temporary increase in the amount of vaginal bleeding seen as pooled blood leaves the uterus. Clots also may be expelled. The uterus may remain boggy even after massage and expulsion of clots.

Fundal massage can be a very uncomfortable procedure. Understanding the causes and dangers of uterine atony and the purpose of fundal massage can help the woman to be more cooperative. Teaching the woman to massage her own fundus enables her to maintain some control and decreases her anxiety.

Additional interventions likely to be used are administration of intravenous fluids and oxytocic medications (drugs that stimulate contraction of the uterine smooth muscle). (See Table 37-1 for information about common oxytocic medications.)

▬ LEGAL TIP   Client Abandonment

In an emergency situation, the nurse must remain with the woman and call for help. Leaving the woman can lead to a charge of client abandonment.

Prevention of Bladder Distention. A full bladder causes the uterus to be displaced above the umbilicus and well to one side of midline in the abdomen. It also prevents

---

EMERGENCY

Hypovolemic Shock

SIGNS AND SYMPTOMS

- Persistent significant bleeding occurs—perineal pad is soaked within 15 minutes; may not be accompanied by a change in vital signs or maternal color or behavior.
- Woman states she feels weak, light-headed, "funny," or "sick to my stomach" or that she "sees stars."
- Woman begins to act anxious or exhibits air hunger.
- Woman's skin turns ashen or grayish.
- Skin feels cool and clammy.
- Pulse rate increases.
- Blood pressure decreases.

INTERVENTIONS

- Notify primary health care provider.
- If uterus is atonic, massage gently and expel clots to cause uterus to contract; compress uterus manually, as needed, using two hands. Add oxytocic agent to intravenous drip, as ordered.
- Give oxygen by face mask or nasal prongs at 8 to 10 L/min.
- Tilt the woman onto her side or elevate the right hip; elevate her legs to at least a 30-degree angle.
- Provide additional or maintain existing intravenous infusion of lactated Ringer's solution or normal saline solution to restore circulatory volume.
- Administer blood or blood products, as ordered.
- Monitor vital signs.
- Insert an indwelling urinary catheter to monitor perfusion of kidneys.
- Administer emergency drugs, as ordered.
- Prepare for possible surgery or other emergency treatments or procedures.
- Chart incident, medical and nursing interventions instituted, and results of treatments.

---

the uterus from contracting normally. Nursing interventions focus on helping the woman to empty her bladder spontaneously as soon as possible. The first priority is to assist the woman to the bathroom or onto a bedpan if she is unable to ambulate. Having the woman listen to running water, placing her hands in warm water, or pouring water from a squeeze bottle over her perineum may stimulate voiding. Other techniques include assisting the woman into the shower or sitz bath and encouraging her to void or placing oil of peppermint in a bedpan under the woman (the vapors may relax the urinary meatus and trigger spontaneous voiding). Administering analgesics, if ordered, may be indicated because some women may fear voiding because of anticipated pain. If these measures are unsuccessful, a sterile catheter may be inserted to drain the urine.

▬ Promotion of Comfort, Rest, Ambulation, and Exercise

Comfort. Most women experience some degree of discomfort during the postpartum period. Common causes of discomfort include afterbirth pains (afterpains), episiotomy or perineal lacerations, hemorrhoids, and breast engorgement. The woman's description of the type and severity of her pain is the best guide in choosing an appropriate intervention. To confirm the location and extent of discomfort, the nurse inspects and palpates areas of pain as appropriate for redness, swelling, discharge, and heat and observes for body tension, guarded movements, and facial tension. Blood pressure, pulse, and respirations may be elevated in response to acute pain. Diaphoresis may accompany severe pain. A lack of objective signs does not necessarily mean there is no pain, because there may also be a cultural component to the expression of pain. Nursing interventions are intended to eliminate the pain sensation entirely or reduce it to a tolerable level that allows the woman to care for herself and her baby. Nurses may use both nonpharmacologic and pharmacologic interventions to promote comfort. Pain relief is enhanced by using more than one method or route.

Nonpharmacologic Interventions. Warmth, distraction, imagery, therapeutic touch, relaxation, and interaction with the infant may decrease the discomfort associated with afterbirth pains. Simple interventions that can decrease the discomfort associated with an episiotomy or perineal lacerations include encouraging the woman to lie on her side whenever possible and to use a pillow when sitting. Other interventions include application of an ice pack; topical application (if ordered); dry heat; cleansing with a squeeze bottle; and a cleansing shower, tub bath, or sitz bath. Many of these interventions are also effective for hemorrhoids, especially ice packs, sitz baths, and topical applications (such as witch hazel pads). Box 23-3 gives more specific information about these interventions.

The discomfort associated with engorged breasts may be lessened by the application of ice, heat, or cabbage leaves to the breasts, and wearing a well-fitted support bra. Decisions about specific interventions for engorgement are based on whether the woman chooses breastfeeding or bottle-feeding (see Chapter 27).

Pharmacologic Interventions. Most health care providers routinely order a variety of analgesics to be administered as needed, including medications that are both narcotic and nonnarcotic (e.g., nonsteroidal antiinflammatory drugs [NSAIDs]), with their dosage and time frequency ranges. Topical application of antiseptic or anesthetic ointment or sprays is a common pharmacologic intervention for perineal pain. Patient-controlled analgesia (PCA) pumps and epidural analgesia are technologies commonly used to provide pain relief after cesarean birth.

■ NURSE ALERT
The nurse should carefully monitor all women receiving opioids because respiratory depression and decreased intestinal motility are side effects.

Many women want to participate in decisions about analgesia. Severe pain, however, may interfere with active participation in choosing pain relief measures. If an analgesic is to be given, the nurse must make a clinical judgment of the type, dosage, and frequency from the medications ordered.

The woman is informed of the prescribed analgesic and its common side effects; this teaching is documented.

Breastfeeding mothers often have concerns about the effects of an analgesic on the infant. Although nearly all drugs present in maternal circulation are also found in breast milk, many analgesics commonly used during the postpartum period are considered relatively safe for breastfeeding mothers. Often the timing of medications can be adjusted to minimize infant exposure. A mother may be given pain medication immediately after breastfeeding so that the interval between medication administration and the next nursing period is as long as possible. The decision to administer medications of any kind to a breastfeeding mother must always be made by carefully weighing the woman's need against actual or potential risks to the infant.

If acceptable pain relief has not been obtained in 1 hour and there has been no change in the initial assessment, the nurse may need to contact the primary care provider for additional pain relief orders or further directions. Unrelieved pain results in fatigue, anxiety, and a worsening perception of the pain. It might also indicate the presence of a previously unidentified or untreated problem.

Rest. The excitement and exhilaration experienced after the birth of the infant may make rest difficult. The new mother, who is often anxious about her ability to care for her infant or is uncomfortable, may also have difficulty sleeping. The demands of the infant, the hospital environment and routines, and the presence of frequent visitors contribute to alterations in her sleep pattern.

Fatigue. Fatigue is common in the postpartum period (Troy, 2003) and involves both physiologic components, associated with long labors, cesarean birth, anemia, and breastfeeding, and psychologic components, related to depression and anxiety. Infant behavior may also contribute to fatigue, particularly for mothers of more difficult infants.

Interventions must be planned to meet the woman's individual needs for sleep and rest. Backrubs, other comfort measures, and medication for sleep for the first few nights may be necessary. The side-lying position for breastfeeding minimizes fatigue in nursing mothers (Troy, 2003). Support and encouragement of mothering behaviors help reduce anxiety. Hospital and nursing routines may be adjusted to meet individual needs. In addition, the nurse can help the family limit visitors and provide a comfortable chair or bed for the partner.

Ambulation. Early ambulation is successful in reducing the incidence of thromboembolism and in promoting the woman's more rapid recovery of strength. Free movement is encouraged once anesthesia wears off unless an analgesic has been administered. After the initial recovery period is over, the mother is encouraged to ambulate frequently.

■ NURSE ALERT
Having a hospital staff or family member present the first time the woman gets out of bed after birth is wise because she may feel weak, dizzy, faint, or light-headed.

EVIDENCE-BASED PRACTICE

Treatment and Prevention of Nipple Pain

BACKGROUND

- New mothers typically experience some nipple pain during the first week of breastfeeding. When it is severe or persistent, it can discourage breastfeeding and inhibit the let-down reflex. Nipple lesions may manifest as chapped, cracked, bleeding, sore, erythematous, edematous, or blistered. Factors that may contribute to nipple pain include fair skin; estrogen or dietary deficiencies; improper infant feeding positioning; vigorous feeding; flat or retracted nipples; use of nipple shields or plastic breast pads; failure to break suction before detaching baby from the breast; and lack of nipple conditioning with sunlight, air, and friction. The use of soap, alcohol, petrolatum, or A&D preparations are not beneficial for nipple pain. Prenatal nipple conditioning may not be desirable, since it can cause uterine stimulation.

OBJECTIVES

- The goal of the review was to determine the efficacy of interventions for prevention and treatment of nipple pain.

METHODS

Search Strategy

- After extensive search of the literature databases and reference lists, the authors identified nine randomized controlled trials (RCTs) and three quasi-experimental (women served as their own controls—one breast experimental and one control) trials of nipple pain prevention interventions that met their criteria. The trials, dated 1986 to 2003, represented 1268 women. They also analyzed four RCTs and three quasi-experimental trials of nipple pain treatments. Countries of origin were not noted.

Statistical Analyses

- Similar data, where available, were pooled. Differences between groups outside the 95% confidence interval were accepted as significant. All were analyzed in their original randomly assigned "intention to treat" categories, even if they changed their minds.

FINDINGS

- Nipple pain was best prevented by keeping the nipples clean and dry. Warm water was superior to using breast milk, or teabag. Hydrogel was more preventive than lanolin. Chlorhexidine/alcohol spray before and after each feeding was more beneficial than distilled water spray. Groups that received postpartum education on breastfeeding, breast anatomy, attachment, and position reported less nipple pain than the control groups. Polyethylene film dressing decreased nipple pain, but caused discomfort when removed.
- Successful treatments for nipple pain included a combination of heat, positioning, and lanolin. Tea bags seemed to be effective. Air drying was superior to applying hydrogels while breasts were still moist, but both treatments reduced nipple pain. Use of soap increased nipple pain. Glycerin gel was more beneficial than breast shells or lanolin.

LIMITATIONS

- The trials were small, and mostly on Caucasian women. Bias from high attrition rates and inability to blind the subjects may have limited the generalizability. Women in the studies had various degrees of experience, commitment, cultural bias, and support.

IMPLICATIONS FOR PRACTICE

- Prevention of nipple soreness is much preferable to treatment after it has appeared. Comprehensive breastfeeding education, anticipatory guidance to prepare women for some discomfort during the first week, and proper positioning are first-line prevention practices. Nipple shields are potentially hazardous to the infant, and not recommended. Cleansing with warm water, applying breast milk, and air-drying are cost-free prevention and treatment. Lanolin or vitamin A ointments, plus heat, are effective. Breast shells may prevent friction pain. Occlusive dressings, such as glycerin gel and hydrogel, are soothing, but may foster infections.

IMPLICATIONS FOR FURTHER RESEARCH

- Well-designed RCTs of large, heterogeneous populations with excellent follow-up would yield more generalizable data. Research is needed on infant sucking strength and behaviors. Complementary and alternative therapies may prove beneficial and should be investigated.

Reference: Morland-Schultz, K., & Hill, P. (2004). Prevention of and therapies for nipple pain: A systematic review. *Journal of Obstetric, Gynecologic, and Neonatal Nursing, 34*(4), 428-437.

The rapid decrease in intraabdominal pressure after birth results in a dilation of blood vessels supplying the intestines (splanchnic engorgement) and causes blood to pool in the viscera. This condition contributes to the development of orthostatic hypotension when the woman who has recently given birth sits or stands up, first ambulates, or takes a warm shower or sitz bath. The nurse also needs to consider the baseline blood pressure; amount of blood loss; and type, amount, and timing of analgesic or anesthetic medications administered when assisting a woman to ambulate.

Prevention of clot formation is important. Women who must remain in bed after giving birth are at increased risk for the development of a thrombus. They may have antiembolic stockings (TED hose) and/or a sequential compression device (SCD boots) ordered prophylactically. If a woman remains in bed longer than 8 hours (e.g., because of postpartum magnesium sulfate therapy for preeclampsia), exercise to promote circulation in the legs is indicated, using the following routine:

- Alternate flexion and extension of feet.
- Rotate ankle in circular motion.

- Alternate flexion and extension of legs.
- Press back of knee to bed surface; relax.

If the woman is susceptible to thromboembolism, she is encouraged to walk about actively for true ambulation and is discouraged from sitting immobile in a chair.

Women with varicosities are encouraged to wear support hose. If a thrombus is suspected, as evidenced by complaint of pain in calf muscles or warmth, redness, or tenderness in the suspected leg (positive Homans sign [dorsiflexing the foot sharply with the knee flexed; may cause pain in the calf in the presence of deep vein thrombosis]), the primary health care provider should be notified immediately; meanwhile the woman should be confined to bed, with the affected limb elevated on pillows.

Exercise. Most women who have just given birth are extremely interested in regaining their nonpregnant figures. Postpartum exercise can begin soon after birth, although the woman should be encouraged to start with simple exercises and gradually progress to more strenuous ones. Figure 23-6 illustrates a number of exercises appropriate for the new mother. Abdominal exercises are postponed until approximately 4 weeks after cesarean birth.

Kegel exercises to strengthen muscle tone are extremely important, particularly after vaginal birth. Kegel exercises help women regain the muscle tone that is often lost as pelvic tissues are stretched and torn during pregnancy and birth. Women who maintain muscle strength may benefit years later by retaining urinary continence.

CRITICAL THINKING EXERCISE

Complications of Immobility After Cesarean Birth

Your client assignment today on the mother-baby unit includes LaTasha, who gave birth yesterday by cesarean. LaTasha has not yet gotten out of bed. She also refuses to turn herself in bed or perform deep breathing exercises because "both those things make me hurt." Based on your knowledge of postpartum physiology, you are concerned that LaTasha is at risk to develop a thromboembolism.

1. Evidence—Is there sufficient evidence to draw conclusions about risk factors for the development of a thromboembolism during the postpartum period in women who give birth by cesarean?
2. Assumptions—What assumptions can be made about the following issues:
   a. Differences in activity level between women who give birth vaginally and by cesarean during the immediate postpartum period
   b. The relationship between postoperative pain and the woman's activity level
   c. Cultural variations in reactions to pain and expression of pain
   d. Influence of supportive care by the nurse
3. What implications and priorities for nursing care can be made at this time?
4. Does the evidence objectively support your conclusion?
5. Are there alternative perspectives to your conclusion

It is essential that women learn to perform Kegel exercises correctly (see Teaching for Self-Care box p. 120. Approximately one fourth of all women who learn Kegel exercises do them incorrectly and may increase their risk of incontinence (Sampselle et al., 2000). This may occur when women inadvertently bear down on the pelvic floor muscles, thrusting the perineum outward. The woman's technique can be assessed during the pelvic examination at her checkup, by inserting two fingers intravaginally and checking whether the pelvic floor muscles correctly contract and relax.

▬ Promotion of Nutrition

During the hospital stay, most women display a good appetite and eat well; nutritious snacks are usually welcomed. Women may request that family members bring to the hospital favorite or culturally appropriate foods (Fig. 23-7). Cultural dietary preferences must be respected. This interest in food presents an ideal opportunity for nutritional counseling on dietary needs after pregnancy, such as for breastfeeding, preventing constipation and anemia, promoting weight loss, and promoting healing and well-being (see Chapter 15). Prenatal vitamins and iron supplements are often continued until 6 weeks postpartum or until the ordered supply has been used.

▬ Promotion of Normal Bladder and Bowel Patterns

Bladder Function. After giving birth the mother should void spontaneously within 6 to 8 hours. The first several voidings should be measured to document adequate emptying of the bladder. A volume of at least 150 ml is expected for each voiding. Some women experience difficulty in emptying the bladder, possibly as a result of diminished bladder tone, edema from trauma, or fear of discomfort. Nursing interventions for inability to void and bladder distention are discussed on p. 598.

Bowel Function. Nursing interventions to promote normal bowel elimination include educating the woman about measures to avoid constipation, such as ensuring adequate roughage and fluid intake and promoting exercise. Alerting the woman to side effects of medications such as narcotic analgesics (e.g., decreased gastrointestinal tract motility) may encourage her to implement measures to reduce the risk of constipation. Stool softeners or laxatives may be necessary during the early postpartum period. With early discharge, a new mother may be home before having a bowel movement. Some mothers experience gas pains. Antigas medications may be ordered. Ambulation or rocking in a rocking chair may stimulate passage of flatus and relief of discomfort.

▬ Breastfeeding Promotion and Lactation Suppression

Breastfeeding Promotion. The first 1 to 2 hours after birth is an excellent time to encourage the mother to breastfeed. The infant is typically in an alert state and will

Abdominal Breathing. Lie on back with knees bent. Inhale deeply through nose. Keep ribs stationary and allow abdomen to expand upward. Exhale slowly but forcefully while contracting the abdominal muscles; hold for 3 to 5 seconds while exhaling. Relax.

Reach for the Knees. Lie on back with knees bent. While inhaling, deeply lower chin onto chest. While exhaling, raise head and shoulders slowly and smoothly and reach for knees with arms outstretched. The body should only rise as far as the back will naturally bend while waist remains on floor or bed (about 6 to 8 inches). Slowly and smoothly lower head and shoulders back to starting position. Relax.

Double Knee Roll. Lie on back with knees bent. Keeping shoulders flat and feet stationary, slowly and smoothly roll knees over to the left to touch floor or bed. Maintaining a smooth motion, roll knees back over to the right until they touch floor or bed. Return to starting position and relax.

Leg Roll. Lie on back with legs straight. Keeping shoulders flat and legs straight, slowly and smoothly lift left leg and roll it over to touch the right side of floor or bed and return to starting position. Repeat, rolling right leg over to touch left side of floor or bed. Relax.

Combined Abdominal Breathing and Supine Pelvic Tilt (Pelvic Rock). Lie on back with knees bent. While inhaling deeply, roll pelvis back by flattening lower back on floor or bed. Exhale slowly but forcefully while contracting abdominal muscles and tightening buttocks. Hold for 3 to 5 seconds while exhaling. Relax.

Buttocks Lift. Lie on back with arms at sides, knees bent, and feet flat. Slowly raise buttocks and arch back. Return slowly to starting position.

Single Knee Roll. Lie on back with right leg straight and left leg bent at the knee. Keeping shoulders flat, slowly and smoothly roll left knee over to the right to touch floor or bed and then back to starting position. Reverse position of legs. Roll right knee over to the left to touch floor or bed and return to starting position. Relax.

Arm Raises. Lie on back with arms extended at 90 degree-angle from body. Raise arms so they are perpendicular and hands touch. Lower slowly.

FIG. 23-6 Postpartum exercise should begin as soon as possible. The woman should start with simple exercises and gradually progress to more strenuous ones.

FIG. 23-7 Special foods are considered essential for recovery in the Asian culture. (Courtesy Concept Media, Irvine, CA.)

suckle if put to the breast. This is an opportune time to instruct the mother in breastfeeding and to assess the physical appearance of the breasts and nipples. (See Chapter 27 for further information on assisting the breastfeeding woman.)

Lactation Suppression. Suppression of lactation is necessary when the woman has decided not to breastfeed or in the case of neonatal death. Wearing a well-fitted support bra or breast binder continuously for at least the first 72 hours after giving birth is important. Women should avoid breast stimulation, including running warm water over the breasts, newborn suckling, or pumping of the breasts. A few nonbreastfeeding mothers experience severe breast engorgement (swelling of breast tissue caused by increased blood and lymph supply to the breasts as the body produces milk, occurring at about 72 to 96 hours after birth). If breast engorgement occurs, it can usually be managed satisfactorily with nonpharmacologic interventions.

Ice packs to the breasts are helpful in decreasing the discomfort associated with engorgement. The woman should use a 15 minutes on, 45 minutes off schedule (to prevent the rebound swelling that can occur if ice is used continuously), or she can place fresh cabbage leaves inside her bra. Cabbage leaves have been used to treat swelling in other cultures for years (Ayers, 2000; Mass, 2004). The exact mechanism of action is not known, but it is thought that naturally occurring plant estrogens or salicylates may be responsible for the effects. The leaves are replaced each time they wilt. A mild analgesic also may be necessary to help the mother through this uncomfortable time. Medications that were once prescribed for lactation suppression (estrogen, estrogen and testosterone, and bromocriptine) are no longer used.

▬ Health Promotion for Future Pregnancies and Children

Rubella Vaccination. For women who have not had rubella (10% to 20% of all women) or women who are serologically not immune (titer of 1:8 or enzyme immunoassay level less than 0.8), a subcutaneous injection of rubella vaccine is recommended in the immediate postpartum period to prevent the possibility of contracting rubella in future pregnancies. Seroconversion occurs in approximately 90% of women vaccinated after birth. The live attenuated rubella virus is not communicable in breast milk; therefore breastfeeding mothers can be vaccinated. However, because the virus is shed in urine and other body fluids, the vaccine should not be given if the mother or other household members are immunocompromised. Rubella vaccine is made from duck eggs, so women who have allergies to these eggs may develop a hypersensitivity reaction to the vaccine, for which they will need adrenaline. A transient arthralgia or rash is common in vaccinated women but is benign. Because the vaccine may be teratogenic, women who receive the vaccine must be informed about this fact.

▬ LEGAL TIP   Rubella Vaccination

Informed consent for rubella vaccination in the postpartum period includes information about possible side effects and the risk of teratogenic effects. Women must understand that they must practice contraception to avoid pregnancy for 1 month after being vaccinated (ACOG, 2002).

Prevention of Rh Isoimmunization. Injection of Rh immune globulin (a solution of gamma globulin that contains Rh antibodies) within 72 hours after birth prevents sensitization in the Rh-negative woman who has had a fetomaternal transfusion of Rh-positive fetal red blood cells (RBCs) (see Medication Guide box). Rh immune globulin promotes lysis of fetal Rh-positive blood cells before the mother forms her own antibodies against them.

▬ NURSE ALERT

After birth, Rh immune globulin is administered to all Rh-negative, antibody (Coombs' test)–negative women who give birth to Rh-positive infants. Rh immune globulin is administered to the mother intramuscularly or intravenously. It should never be given to an infant.

The administration of 300 mcg (1 vial) of Rh immune globulin is usually sufficient to prevent maternal sensitization. If a large fetomaternal transfusion is suspected, however, the dosage needed should be determined by performing a Kleihauer-Betke test, which detects the amount of fetal blood in the maternal circulation. If more than 15 ml of fetal blood is present in maternal circulation, the dosage of Rh immune globulin must be increased.

A 1:1000 dilution of Rh immune globulin is crossmatched to the mother's RBCs to ensure compatibility. Because Rh immune globulin is usually considered a blood product, precautions similar to those used for transfusing blood are necessary when it is given. The identification number on the woman's hospital wristband should correspond to the identification number found on the laboratory slip. The nurse must also check to see that the lot number on the laboratory slip corresponds to the lot number on the vial. Finally, the expiration date on the vial should be checked to be certain of a usable product.

m e d i c a t i o n   g u i d e

Rh Immune Globulin, RhoGAM, Gamulin Rh, HypRho-D, Rhophylac

ACTION ■ Suppression of immune response in nonsensitized women with Rh-negative blood who receive Rh-positive blood cells because of fetomaternal hemorrhage, transfusion, or accident

INDICATIONS ■ Routine antepartum prevention at 20 to 30 weeks of gestation in women with Rh-negative blood; suppress antibody formation after birth, miscarriage, or pregnancy termination, abdominal trauma, ectopic pregnancy, amniocentesis, version, or chorionic villus sampling

DOSAGE AND ROUTE ■ Standard dose 1 vial (300 mcg) intramuscularly (IM) in deltoid or gluteal muscle; microdose 1 vial (50 mcg) IM in deltoid muscle; Rhophylac can be given IM or IV (available in prefilled syringes)

ADVERSE EFFECTS ■ Myalgia, lethargy, localized tenderness and stiffness at injection site, mild and transient fever, malaise, headache; rarely nausea, vomiting, hypotension, tachycardia, possible allergic response

NURSING CONSIDERATIONS ■ Give standard dose to mother at 28 weeks of gestation as prophylaxis, or after an incident or exposure risk that occurs after 28 weeks of gestation (e.g., amniocentesis, second-trimester miscarriage or abortion, after version) and within 72 hours after birth if baby is Rh positive.
■ Give microdose for first trimester miscarriage or abortion, ectopic pregnancy, chorionic villus sampling.
■ Verify that the woman is Rh negative and has not been sensitized, that Coombs' test is negative, and that baby is Rh positive. Provide explanation to the woman about procedure, including the purpose, possible side effects, and effect on future pregnancies. Have the woman sign a consent form if required by agency. Verify correct dosage and confirm lot number and woman's identity before giving injection (verify with another registered nurse or other procedure per agency policy); document administration per agency policy. Observe woman for allergic response for at least 20 minutes after administration.
■ The medication is made from human plasma (a consideration if woman is a Jehovah's Witness). The risk of transmitting infectious agents, including viruses, cannot be completely eliminated.

Rh immune globulin suppresses the immune response. Therefore the woman who receives both Rh immune globulin and rubella vaccine must be tested at 3 months to see if she has developed rubella immunity. If not, the woman will need another dose of rubella vaccine.

There is some disagreement about whether Rh immune globulin should be considered a blood product. Health care providers need to discuss the most current information about this issue with women whose religious beliefs conflict with having blood products administered to them.

■ Evaluation

The nurse can be reasonably assured that care was effective when the expected outcomes of care for physical needs have been achieved.

■ CARE MANAGEMENT— ■ PSYCHOSOCIAL NEEDS

Meeting the psychosocial needs of new mothers involves assessing the parents' reactions to the birth experience, feelings about themselves, and interactions with the new baby and other family members. Specific interventions are then planned to increase the parents' knowledge and self-confidence as they assume the care and responsibility of the new baby and integrate this new member into their existing family structure in a way that meets their cultural expectations (see Chapters 24 and 28).

■ Assessment and Nursing Diagnoses
■ *Impact of the Birth Experience*

Many women indicate a need to examine the birth process itself and look at their own intrapartal behavior in retrospect. Their partners may express similar desires. If their birth experience was different from their birth plan (e.g., induction, epidural anesthesia, cesarean birth), both partners may need to mourn the loss of their expectations before they can adjust to the reality of their actual birth experience. Inviting them to review the events and describe how they feel helps the nurse assess how well they understand what happened and how well they have been able to put their childbirth experience into perspective.

■ *Maternal Self-Image*

An important assessment concerns the woman's self-concept, body image, and sexuality. How this new mother feels about herself and her body during the puerperium may affect her behavior and adaptation to parenting. The woman's self-concept and body image also may affect her sexuality. Overweight women may experience symptoms of depression and anxiety up to 14 months postpartum (Carter, Baker, & Brownell, 2000).

Feelings related to sexual adjustment after childbirth are often a cause of concern for new parents. Women who have recently given birth may be reluctant to resume sexual intercourse for fear of pain or may worry that coitus could damage healing perineal tissue. Because many new parents are anxious for information but reluctant to bring up the subject, postpartum nurses should matter-of-factly include the topic of postpartum sexuality during their routine physical assessment. While examining the episiotomy site, for example, the nurse can say, "I know you're sore right now, but it probably won't be long until you (or you and your partner) are ready to make love again. Have you thought about what that might be like? Would you like to ask me questions?" This approach assures the woman and her partner that resuming sexual activity is a legitimate concern for new parents and indicates the nurse's willingness to answer questions and share information.

■ *Adaptation to Parenthood and Parent-Infant Interactions*

The psychosocial assessment also includes evaluating adaptation to parenthood, as evidenced by mother's and father's reactions to and interactions with the new baby.

FIG. 23-8 Bonding and attachment begun early after birth are fostered in the postpartum period. (Courtesy Wendy Larson-Harris, Roanoke, VA.)

FIG. 23-9 Active involvement of grandmother provides support for the mother and newborn. (Courtesy Nicole Larson, Eden Prairie, MN.)

Clues indicating successful adaptation begin to appear early in the postbirth period as parents react positively to the newborn infant and continue the process of establishing a relationship with their child (Fig. 23-8).

Parents are adapting well to their new roles when they exhibit a realistic perception and acceptance of their newborn's needs and his or her limited abilities, immature social responses, and helplessness. Examples of positive parent-infant interactions include taking pleasure in the infant and in the tasks done for and with him or her, understanding the infant's emotional states and providing comfort, and reading the infant's cues for new experiences and sensing his or her fatigue level (see Chapter 24).

Should these indicators be missing, the nurse must investigate further what is hindering the normal adaptation process. There are several questions that the nurse can ask, such as "Do you feel sad often?" or "Are there concerns that you have about being a good parent?" that will help to determine if the woman is experiencing the normal "baby blues" or if there is a more serious underlying condition (i.e., postpartum depression) (www.depressionafterdelivery.com) (Jesse & Graham, 2005). See Chapter 35 for further discussion of postpartum depression.

■ Family Structure and Functioning

A woman's adjustment to her role as mother is affected greatly by her relationships with her partner, her mother and other relatives, and any other children (Fig. 23-9). Nurses can help ease the new mother's return home by identifying possible conflicts among family members and helping the woman plan strategies for dealing with these problems before discharge. Such a conflict could arise when couples have very different ideas about parenting. Dealing with the stresses of sibling rivalry and unsolicited grandparent advice also can affect the woman's psychologic well-being. Only by asking about other nuclear and extended family members can the nurse discover potential problems in such relationships and help to plan workable solutions for them.

■ Impact of Cultural Diversity

The final component of a complete psychosocial assessment is the woman's cultural beliefs and values. Much of a woman's behavior during the postpartum period is strongly influenced by her cultural background. Nurses are likely to come in contact with women from many different countries and cultures. All cultures have developed safe and satisfying methods of caring for new mothers and babies. Only by understanding and respecting the values and beliefs of each woman can the nurse design a plan of care to meet the individual needs.

CRITICAL THINKING EXERCISE

Cultural Influences During the Postpartum Period

Kim, who is Asian, gave birth to her first child yesterday. This morning she refuses to eat her breakfast or take a shower, stating that to do either would cause an imbalance in her system. Although her chart indicates that she intends to breastfeed, she requests formula for her baby.

1. Evidence—Is there sufficient evidence to draw conclusions about the cultural beliefs of Asians as they relate to the postpartum period and breastfeeding?
2. Assumptions—What assumptions can be made about the following issues?
   a. Culturally appropriate diet, activity, and hygiene for the postpartum Asian woman
   b. Providing appropriate care for the newborn, including breastfeeding, in the Asian culture
   c. Role of other family members and friends in providing care to the postpartum woman and newborn
   d. Difficulty in establishing lactation if breastfeeding is not begun immediately
3. What implications and priorities for nursing care can be made at this time?
4. Does the evidence objectively support your conclusion?
5. Are there alternative perspectives to your conclusion?

Sometimes the psychosocial assessment indicates serious actual or potential problems that must be addressed. The Signs of Potential Complications box lists several psychosocial needs that, at a minimum, warrant ongoing evaluation following hospital discharge. Women exhibiting these needs should be referred to appropriate community resources for assessment and management.

After analyzing the data obtained during the assessment process, the nurse establishes nursing diagnoses to provide a guide for planning care. Nursing diagnoses related to psychosocial issues that are frequently established for the postpartum woman include the following:

- *Interrupted family processes related to*
  -unexpected birth of twins
- *Impaired verbal communication related to*
  -woman's hearing impairment
  -nurse's language being not the same as woman's
- *Impaired parenting related to*
  -long, difficult labor
  -unmet expectations of labor and birth
- *Anxiety related to*
  -newness of parenting role, sibling rivalry, or response of grandparent
- *Risk for situational low self-esteem related to*
  -body image changes

▬ Expected Outcomes of Care

Expected psychosocial outcomes during the postpartum period are based on the nursing diagnoses identified for the individual woman and her family. Examples of common expected outcomes include that the woman (family) will do the following:

- Identify measures that promote a healthy personal adjustment in the postpartum period.
- Maintain healthy family functioning based on cultural norms and personal expectations.

signs of potential complications

Psychosocial Needs

- Unable or unwilling to discuss labor and birth experience
- Refers to self as ugly and useless
- Excessively preoccupied with self (body image)
- Markedly depressed
- Lacks a support system
- Partner or other family members react negatively to the baby
- Refuses to interact with or care for baby; for example, does not name baby, does not want to hold or feed baby, is upset by vomiting and wet or dirty diapers (cultural appropriateness of actions must be considered)
- Expresses disappointment over baby's sex
- Sees baby as messy or unattractive
- Baby reminds mother of family member or friend she does not like
- Has difficulty sleeping
- Experiences loss of appetite

▬ Plan of Care and Interventions

The nurse functions in the roles of teacher, encourager, and supporter rather than doer while implementing the psychosocial plan of care for a postpartum woman. Implementation of the psychosocial plan of care involves carrying out specific activities to achieve the expected outcome of care planned for each individual woman. Topics that should be included in the psychosocial plan of care include promotion of parenting skills and family member adjustment to the newborn infant (see Chapter 24).

Cultural issues also must be considered when planning care. There are many traditional health beliefs and practices among the different cultures within the U.S. population. Traditional health practices that are used to maintain health or to avoid illnesses deal with the whole person (i.e., body, mind, and spirit) and tend to be culturally based.

Women from various cultures may view health as a balance between opposing forces (e.g., cold versus hot), being in harmony with nature, or just "feeling good." Traditional practices may include the observance of certain dietary restrictions, clothing, or taboos for balancing the body; participation in certain activities such as sports and art for maintaining mental health; and use of silence, prayer, or meditation for developing spiritually. Practices (e.g., using religious objects or eating garlic) are used to protect oneself from illness and may involve avoiding people who are believed to create hexes or spells or who have an "evil eye." Restoration of health may involve taking folk medicines (e.g., herbs, animal substances) or using a traditional healer.

Childbirth occurs within this sociocultural context. Rest, seclusion, dietary restraints, and ceremonies honoring the mother are all common traditional practices that are followed for the promotion of the health and well-being of the mother and baby.

There are several common traditional health practices used and beliefs held by women and their families during the postpartum period. In Asia, for example, pregnancy is considered to be a "hot" state, and childbirth results in a sudden loss of this state (Kim-Godwin, 2003). Therefore balance must be restored by facilitating the return of the hot state, which is present physically or symbolically in hot food, hot water, and warm air.

Another common belief is that the mother and baby remain in a weak and vulnerable state for a period of several weeks after birth. During this time, the mother may remain in a passive role, taking no baths or showers, and may stay in bed to prevent cold air from entering her body.

Women who have immigrated to the United States or other Western nations without their extended families may not have much help at home, making it difficult for them to observe these activity restrictions (Davis, 2001). The Cultural Considerations box lists some common cultural beliefs about the postpartum period and family planning.

It is important that nurses consider all cultural aspects when planning care and not use their own cultural beliefs as the framework for that care. Although the beliefs and

cultural considerations

Postpartum Period and Family Planning

POSTPARTUM CARE

- *Chinese, Mexican, Korean, and Southeast Asian women* may wish to eat only warm foods and drink hot drinks to replace blood loss and to restore the balance of hot and cold in their bodies. These women may also wish to stay warm and avoid bathing, exercises, and hair washing for 7 to 30 days after childbirth. Self-care may not be a priority; care by family members is preferred. The woman has respect for elders and authority. These women may wear abdominal binders. They may prefer not to give their babies colostrum.
- *Arabic women* eat special meals designed to restore their energy. They are expected to stay at home for 40 days after birth to avoid illness resulting from exposure to the outside air.
- *Haitian women* may request to take the placenta home to bury or burn.
- *Muslim women* follow strict religious laws on modesty and diet. A Muslim woman must keep her hair, body, arms to the wrist, and legs to the ankles covered at all times. She cannot be alone in the presence of a man other than her husband or a male relative. Observant Muslims will not eat pork or pork products and are obligated to eat meat slaughtered according to Islamic laws (halal meat). If halal meat is not available, kosher meat, seafood, or a vegetarian diet is usually accepted.

FAMILY PLANNING

- Birth control is government mandated in mainland *China*. Most *Chinese women* will have an intrauterine device (IUD) inserted after the birth of their first child. Women do not want hormonal methods of contraception because they fear putting these medications in their bodies.
- *Hispanic women* may choose the rhythm method or natural family planning because most are Catholic.
- *(East) Indian men* are encouraged to have voluntary sterilization by vasectomy.
- *Muslim couples* may practice contraception by mutual consent as long as its use is not harmful to the woman. Acceptable contraceptive methods include foam and condoms, the diaphragm, and natural family planning.
- *Hmong women* highly value and desire large families, which limits birth control practices.
- *Arabic women* value large families, and sons are especially prized.

behaviors of other cultures may seem different or strange, they should be encouraged as long as the mother wants to conform to them, and she and the baby suffer no ill effects. The nurse has to determine whether a woman is using any folk medicine during the postpartum period because active ingredients in folk medicine may have adverse physiologic effects when used in combination with prescribed medicines. The nurse should not assume that a mother desires to use traditional health practices that represent a particular cultural group merely because she is a member of that culture. Many young women who are

first- or second-generation Americans follow their cultural traditions only when older family members are present, or not at all.

■ Evaluation

The nurse can be reasonably assured that care was effective if expected outcomes of care for psychosocial needs have been met.

■ DISCHARGE TEACHING

Self-Care; Signs of Complications

Discharge planning begins at the time of admission to the unit and should be reflected in the plan of care developed for each individual woman. For example, a great deal of time during the hospital stay is usually spent in teaching about maternal and newborn care, because all women must be capable of providing basic care for themselves and their infants at the time of discharge. It is also crucial that every woman be taught to recognize physical signs and symptoms that might indicate problems and how to obtain advice and assistance quickly if these signs appear. The Signs of Potential Complications boxes on pp. 594 and 606 list several common indications of maternal physical and psychosocial problems in the postpartum period. (See Chapter 37 for more information on postpartum complications.) Before discharge, women also need basic instruction regarding the resumption of sexual intercourse, prescribed medications, routine mother-baby checkups, and contraception.

Just before the time of discharge, the nurse reviews the woman's chart to see that laboratory reports, medications, signatures, and so on are in order. Some hospitals have a checklist to use before the woman's discharge. The nurse verifies that medications, if ordered, have arrived on the unit; that any valuables kept secured during the woman's stay have been returned to her and that she has signed a receipt for them; and that the infant is ready to be discharged.

No medication that would make the mother sleepy should be administered if she is the one who will be holding the baby on the way out of the hospital. In most instances, the woman is seated in a wheelchair and is given the baby to hold. Some families leave unescorted and ambulatory, depending on hospital protocol. The woman's possessions are gathered and taken out with her and her family. The woman's and the baby's identification bands are carefully checked. The baby must be secured in a car seat for the drive home (see Fig. 28-2).

Sexual Activity and Contraception

Many couples resume sexual activity before the traditional postpartum checkup 6 weeks after childbirth. The risk of hemorrhage or infection is minimal by approximately 2 weeks postpartum. Couples may be anxious about the topic but uncomfortable and unwilling to bring it up. It is important that the nurse discuss the physical and

CD: Critical Thinking Exercise: Postpartum Complications

psychologic effects that giving birth can have on sexual activity (see Teaching for Self-Care box). Contraceptive options should also be discussed with women (and their partners, if present) before discharge so that they can make informed decisions about fertility management before resuming sexual activity. Waiting to discuss contraception at the 6-week checkup may be leaving it too late. It is possible, particularly in women who bottle-feed, for ovulation to occur as soon as 1 month after birth. A woman who engages in unprotected sex risks becoming pregnant. Current contraceptive options are discussed in detail in Chapter 9. Women who are undecided about contraception at the time of discharge need information about using condoms with foam or creams until the first postpartum checkup.

Prescribed Medications

Women routinely continue to take their prenatal vitamins and iron during the postpartum period. It is especially important that women who are breastfeeding or who are discharged with a lower than normal hematocrit take these medications as prescribed. Women with extensive episiotomies or vaginal lacerations (third or fourth degree) are

---

TEACHING FOR SELF-CARE

Resumption of Sexual Activity

- You can safely resume sexual activity by the second to fourth week after birth, when bleeding has stopped and the episiotomy/lacertion site has healed. For the first 6 weeks to 6 months, the vagina does not lubricate well.
- Your physical reactions to sexual stimulation for the first 3 months after birth will likely be slower and less intense. The strength of the orgasm may be reduced.
- A water-soluble gel, cocoa butter, or a contraceptive cream or jelly might be recommended for lubrication. If some vaginal tenderness is present, your partner can be instructed to insert one or more clean, lubricated fingers into the vagina and rotate them within the vagina to help relax it and to identify possible areas of discomfort. A position in which you have control of the depth of the insertion of the penis also is useful. The side-by-side or female-on-top position may be more comfortable.
- The presence of the baby influences postbirth lovemaking. Parents hear every sound made by the baby; conversely you may be concerned that the baby hears every sound you make. In either case, any phase of the sexual response cycle may be interrupted by hearing the baby cry or move, leaving both of you frustrated and unsatisfied. In addition, the amount of psychologic energy expended by you in child care activities may lead to fatigue. Newborns require a great deal of attention and time.
- Some women have reported feeling sexual stimulation and orgasms when breastfeeding their babies. Breastfeeding mothers often are interested in returning to sexual activity before nonbreastfeeding mothers.
- You should be instructed to correctly perform the Kegel exercises to strengthen your pubococcygeal muscle. This muscle is associated with bowel and bladder function and with vaginal feeling during intercourse.

---

usually prescribed stool softeners to take at home. Pain medications (analgesics or NSAIDs) may be prescribed, especially for women who had cesarean birth. The nurse should make certain that the woman knows the route, dosage, frequency, and common side effects of all ordered medications.

Routine Mother and Baby Checkups

Women who have experienced uncomplicated vaginal births are still commonly scheduled for the traditional 6-week postpartum examination. Women who have had a cesarean birth are often seen in the health care provider's office or clinic within 2 weeks after hospital discharge. The date and time for the follow-up appointment should be included in the discharge instructions. If an appointment has not been made before the woman leaves the hospital, she should be encouraged to call the health care provider's office or clinic and schedule an appointment.

Parents who have not already done so need to make plans for newborn follow-up at the time of discharge. Most offices and clinics like to see newborns for an initial examination within the first week or by 2 weeks of age. If an appointment for a specific date and time was not made for the infant before leaving the hospital, the parents should be encouraged to call the office or clinic right away.

Follow-Up After Discharge
Home Visits

Home visits to new mothers and babies within a few days of discharge can help bridge the gap between hospital care and routine visits to health care providers. Nurses are able to assess the mother, the infant, and the home environment; answer questions and provide education; and make referrals to community resources if necessary. Home visits have been shown to reduce the need for more expensive health care, such as emergency department visits and rehospitalization. They can also help to improve the overall quality of care provided to infants and their parents (Paul, Phillips, Widome, & Hollenbeak, 2004). Ideally, immediate follow-up contact and home visits are available 7 days a week.

Home nursing care may not be available, even if needed, because there are no agencies providing the service or there is no coverage for payment by third-party payers. If care is available, a referral form containing information about both mother and baby should be completed at hospital discharge and sent immediately to the home care agency. Figure 23-10 is an example of such a referral form.

The home visit is most commonly scheduled on the woman's second day home from the hospital, but it may be scheduled on any of the first 4 days at home, depending on the individual family's situation and needs. Additional visits are planned throughout the first week, as needed. The home visits may be extended beyond that time if the family's needs warrant it and if a home visit is the most appropriate option for carrying out the follow-up care required to meet the specific needs identified.

OB Homecare

Mother's Name: _____

Address/phone where mother will be staying:

Address: _____

City: _____

Phone #: _____

Language spoken: ☐ English   ☐ Other: _____

Understands English: ☐ Well   ☐ Poor

　　　　☐ Mother Needs Interpreter   ☐ Hearing Impaired

Who interpreted in hospital: _____

Mom agrees to this referral: ☐ Yes   ☐ No

Currently being seen by PHN: ☐ Yes   ☐ No

Mom's M.D./Midwife: _____

Phone #: _____

Next Appt: _____

MOTHER:

Gravida_____ T_____ P_____ A_____ L_____

Marital Status: S   M   W   D   Sep

Normal Maternal Exam: ☐ Yes   ☐ No (explain below)

Epis/Incision: _____

Hgb pp: _____

Meds: _____

Allergies: _____

OTHER ISSUES:

Diabetic: _____

Other: _____

Psycho/Social Issues:

☐ Parent/Child Interaction　　☐ Adolescent Mother

☐ Mental Health Status　　　　☐ Drug Use/Dependency

☐ Previous Losses　　　　　　☐ Hx of Family Abuse

☐ Developmentally Delayed Parents ☐ Limited Support System

☐ Other: _____

Husband/Significant Other: _____

Baby's Name: _____ ☐ M ☐ F

DOB/Time: _____

Mother's Discharge Date/Time: _____

Newborn Discharge Date:(if different from mother's) _____

Baby's M.D. (Full Name): _____

Phone #: _____

Next Appt: _____

BABY:

Gestation:_____Weeks   ☐ Fetal Loss

Birth Weight: _____ Discharge Weight: _____

Apgars: 1"_____   5"_____

Feeding Issues: _____

Feedings: Breast _____ Bottle _____

Normal Infant Exam: ☐ Yes   ☐ No (explain below)

Circumcised:　　　　　☐ Yes   ☐ No

Cord Clamp Off:　　　 ☐ Yes   ☐ No

Voidings:　　　　　　 ☐ Yes   ☐ No

Stooling:　　　　　　 ☐ Yes   ☐ No

☐ Newborn screen was done in hospital—after baby 24
　 hours of age.

☐ Newborn screen to be drawn at clinic.

☐ Newborn screen to be drawn at home.

　 ☐ Lab slip sent home with family.

ADDITIONAL COMMENTS or ABNORMAL FINDINGS FOR MOTHER OR BABY: _____

_____

_____

Faxed to Home Care　☐ *Facesheet*　☐ *Referral*　　*Referral Completed By:* _____

FIG. 23-10   Referral form. (Courtesy OB Homecare of Allina Hospitals and Clinics, Minneapolis, MN.)

During the home visit the nurse conducts a systematic assessment of mother and newborn to determine physiologic adjustment, identify any existing complications, and to answer any questions the mother has for herself as well as those the mother or family has about the newborn or newborn care. Conducting the assessment in a separate room provides private time for the mother to ask questions on topics such as breast care, family planning, and constipation. The assessment also focuses on the mother's emotional adjustment and her knowledge of self-care and infant care.

During the newborn assessment, the nurse can demonstrate and explain normal newborn behavior and capabilities and encourage the mother and family to ask questions or express concerns they may have. The home care nurse must verify if the newborn screen for phenylketonuria and other inborn errors of metabolism has been drawn. If the baby was discharged from the hospital before 24 hours of age, the newborn screen may be done by the home care nurse, or the family will need to take the infant to the clinic or physician's office.

Telephone Follow-Up

In addition to or instead of a home visit, many providers are adopting the practice of making one or more postpartum telephone follow-up calls to their clients for assessment, health teaching, and identification of complications to effect timely intervention and referrals. Telephone follow-up may be among the services offered by the hospital, the private physician or clinic, or a private agency; it may be either a separate service or combined with other strategies for extending postpartum care. Telephonic nursing assessments are frequently used after a postpartum home care visit to reassess a woman's knowledge about such things as signs of adequate intake by the breastfeeding infant or, after initiating home phototherapy, to assess the caregiver's knowledge regarding equipment complications.

The warm line is another type of telephone link between the new family and concerned caregivers or experienced parent volunteers. A warm line is a help line or consultation service, not a crisis intervention line. The warm line is appropriately used for dealing with less extreme concerns that may seem urgent at the time the call is placed but are not actual emergencies. Calls to warm lines commonly relate to infant feeding, prolonged crying, or sibling rivalry. Warm line services may extend beyond the fourth trimester. Families need to call when concerns arise and should be given phone numbers for easy access to answers to their questions.

Support Groups

A special group experience is sometimes sought by the woman adjusting to motherhood. On occasion, postpartum women who have met earlier in prenatal clinics or on the hospital unit may begin to associate for mutual support. Members of childbirth classes who attend a postpartum reunion may decide to extend their relationship during the fourth trimester.

A postpartum support group enables mothers and fathers to share with and support each other as they adjust to parenting. Many new parents find it reassuring to discover that they are not alone in their feelings of confusion and uncertainty. An experienced parent can often impart valuable concrete information to other group members. Inexperienced parents may find themselves imitating the behavior of others in the group whom they perceive as particularly capable.

Referral to Community Resources

To develop an effective referral system, it is important that the nurse have a clear understanding of the needs of the woman and family and of the organization and community resources available for meeting those needs. Locating and compiling information about available community services contributes to the development of a referral system. It is important for the nurse to develop his or her own resource file of local and national services that are frequently useful to postpartum families.

---

community activity

Interview a public health nurse from your local health department who provides maternal-child services. Ask the nurse to recommend resources available in your community to meet the needs of these mothers and newborns:
  a. Maria, age 18, an undocumented Hispanic woman who speaks no English. Maria just gave birth to her first child, a healthy boy born at term.
  b. Emily, a 25-year-old woman whose husband abused her throughout pregnancy. Emily is trying to breastfeed her new daughter but states, "I just don't think I can do this."
  c. Jasmine, who gave birth two weeks ago by cesarean to twin boys at 28 weeks of gestation. The babies are still in the neonatal intensive care unit. Jasmine has three other preschool-aged children at home.
In each situation, what additional information would the nurse need in order to make appropriate referrals?

---

key points

- Postpartum care is modeled on the concept of health.
- Cultural beliefs and practices affect the woman's response to the puerperium.
- The nursing care plan includes assessments to detect deviations from normal, comfort measures to relieve discomfort or pain, and safety measures to prevent injury or infection.
- Teaching and counseling measures are designed to promote the woman's feelings of competence in self-care and baby care.
- Common nursing interventions in the postpartum period include evaluating and treating the boggy uterus and the full urinary bladder; providing for nonpharmacologic and pharmacologic relief of pain and discomfort associated with the episiotomy, lacerations, or breastfeeding; and instituting measures to promote or suppress lactation.
- Administering rubella vaccine and Rh immune globulin if indicated helps to promote the health of the woman's future pregnancies and children.
- Meeting the psychosocial needs of new mothers involves planning care that takes into consideration the composition and functioning of the entire family.
- Early postpartum discharge will continue to be the trend as a result of consumer demand, medical necessity, discharge criteria for low risk childbirth, and cost-containment measures.
- Early discharge classes, telephone follow-up, home visits, warm lines, and support groups are effective means of facilitating physiologic and psychologic adjustments in the postpartum period.

REFERENCES

American Academy of Pediatrics (AAP) Committee on Fetus and Newborn. (2004). Hospital stay for healthy term infants. *Pediatrics, 113*(5), 1434-1436.

American Academy of Pediatrics (AAP) & American College of Obstetricians and Gynecologists (ACOG). (2002). *Guidelines for perinatal care* (5th ed.). Elk Grove Village, IL: AAP.

American College of Obstetricians and Gynecologists (ACOG). (2002). ACOG Committee Opinion #281. Rubella vaccine. *Obstetrics and Gynecology, 100*(6), 1417.

Ayers, J. (2000). The use of alternative therapies in the support of breastfeeding. *Journal of Human Lactation, 16*(1), 52-56.

Benedetti, T. (2002). Obstetric hemorrhage. In S. Gabbe, J. Niebyl, & J. Simpson (Eds.), *Obstetrics: Normal and problem pregnancies* (4th ed.). New York: Churchill Livingstone.

Carter, A., Baker, C., & Brownell, K. (2000). Body mass index, eating attitudes, and symptoms of depression and anxiety in pregnancy and the postpartum period. *Psychosomatic Medicine, 62*(2), 264-270.

Davis, R. (2001). The postpartum experience for Southeast Asian women in the United States. *MCN American Journal of Maternal/Child Nursing, 26*(4), 208-213.

Jesse, D., & Graham, M. (2005). Are you often sad and depressed? Brief measure to identify women at risk for depression in pregnancy. *MCN American Journal of Maternal/Child Nursing, 30*(1), 40-45.

Kim-Godwin, Y. (2003). Postpartum beliefs and practices among non-Western cultures. *MCN American Journal of Maternal/Child Nursing, 28*(2), 74-78.

Luegenbiehl, D. (1997). Improving visual estimation of blood volume on peripads. *MCN American Journal of Maternal/Child Nursing, 22*(6), 294-298.

Mass, S. (2004). Breast pain: Engorgement, nipple pain and mastitis. *Clinical Obstetrics and Gynecology, 47*(3), 676-682.

Meara, E., Kotagal, U., Atherton, H., & Lieu, T. (2004). Impact of early newborn discharge legislation and early follow-up visits on infant outcomes in a state Medicaid population. *Pediatrics, 113*(6), 1619-1627.

Paul, I., Phillips, T., Widome, M., & Hollenbeak, C. (2004). Cost-effectiveness of postnatal home nursing visits for prevention of hospital care for jaundice and dehydration. *Pediatrics, 114*(4), 1015-1022.

Sampselle, C., Wyman, J., Thomas, K., Newman, D., Gray, M., Dougherty, M., et al. (2000). Continence for women: A test of AWHONN's evidence-based protocol in clinical practice. *Journal of Obstetric, Gynecologic, and Neonatal Nursing, 29*(1), 18-26.

Simpson, K., & Creehan, P. (2001). *AWHONN's perinatal nursing* (2nd ed.). Philadelphia: Lippincott.

Troy, N. (2003). Is the significance of postpartum fatigue being overlooked in the lives of women? *MCN American Journal of Maternal/Child Nursing, 28*(4), 252-257.

Transition to Parenthood

learning objectives

- Identify parental and infant behaviors that facilitate and those that inhibit parent-infant attachment.
- Describe sensual responses that strengthen attachment.
- Examine the process of becoming a mother.
- Compare maternal adjustment and paternal adjustment to parenthood.
- Delineate ways to facilitate parent-infant adjustment.

- Examine the effects of the following on transition to parenting: parental age (adolescence and older than 35 years), social support, culture, socioeconomic conditions, personal aspirations, and sensory impairment.
- Describe sibling adjustment.
- Describe grandparent adaptation.

electronic resources

Additional information related to the content in Chapter 24 can be found on

the companion website at **evolve**
http://evolve.elsevier.com/Lowdermilk/MWHC/
- NCLEX Review Questions
- WebLinks

or on the interactive companion CD
- NCLEX Review Questions
- Critical Thinking Exercise: Postpartum Home Care
- Skill: Swaddling
- Plan of Care: The Multiparous Woman and Family

*B*ECOMING a parent creates a period of change and instability for all men and women who have children, whether they made a conscious decision to have children or the pregnancy was unplanned. This holds true whether parenthood is biologic or adoptive and whether the parents are married husband-wife couples, cohabiting couples, single mothers, single fathers, lesbian couples with one woman as biologic mother, or gay male couples who adopt a child. Parenting may be described as a process of role transition that begins during pregnancy or while awaiting adoption. The transition is an ongoing process as the parents and infant develop and change.

A thorough understanding of the process parents go through during their transition to parenthood guides the nurse in helping family members adapt. The parenting process requires cognitive and affective skills and knowledge as well as motor skills. The infant's well-being and development depend on these components. This chapter reviews the transition to parenthood, including the parenting process and the adjustment of parents, siblings, and grandparents.

■ PARENTAL ATTACHMENT, BONDING, AND ACQUAINTANCE

The process by which parents come to love and accept a child and a child comes to love and accept a parent is referred to as attachment (see Plan of Care). By using the terms attachment and bonding, Klaus and Kennell originally proposed that the period shortly after birth is important to mother-to-infant attachment (Klaus & Kennell, 1976). They defined the phenomenon of bonding as a sensitive period in the first minutes and hours after birth when mothers and fathers must have close contact with their infants for later optimal development (Klaus & Kennell). Klaus and Kennell (1982) later revised their theory of parent-infant bonding, modifying their claim of the critical nature of immediate contact with the infant after birth. They acknowledged the adaptability of human parents, stating that it took longer than minutes or hours for parents to form an emotional relationship with their infants. The terms attachment and bonding continue to be used interchangeably.

Attachment is developed and maintained by proximity and interaction with the infant, through which the parent becomes acquainted with the infant, identifies the infant as an individual, and claims the infant as a member of the family. Attachment is facilitated by positive feedback (i.e., social, verbal, and nonverbal responses, whether real or perceived, that indicate acceptance of one partner by the other). Attachment occurs through a mutually satisfying experience. A mother commented on her son's grasp reflex, "I put my finger in his hand, and he grabbed right on. It is just a reflex, I know, but it felt good anyway" (Fig. 24-1).

The concept of attachment has been extended to include mutuality; that is, the infant's behaviors and characteristics call forth a corresponding set of parental behaviors and characteristics. The infant displays signaling behaviors such as crying, smiling, and cooing that initiate the contact and bring the caregiver to the child. These behaviors are followed by executive behaviors such as rooting, grasping,

FIG. 24-1   Hands. (Courtesy Cheryl Briggs, RN, Annapolis, MD.)

and postural adjustments that maintain the contact. The caregiver is attracted to an alert, responsive, cuddly infant and repelled by an irritable, apparently disinterested infant. Attachment occurs more readily with the infant whose temperament, social capabilities, appearance, and sex fit the parent's expectations. If the child does not meet these expectations, resolution of the parent's disappointment can delay the attachment process. A list of infant behaviors affecting parental attachment that continues to be a classic comprehensive reference is presented in Table 24-1. A corresponding list of parental behaviors that affect infant attachment is presented in Table 24-2.

An important part of attachment is acquaintance. Parents use eye contact (Fig. 24-2), touching, talking, and exploring to become acquainted with their infant during the immediate postpartum period. Adoptive parents undergo the same process when they first meet their new child. During this period, families engage in the claiming process, which is the identification of the new baby (Fig. 24-3). The child is first identified in terms of "likeness" to other family members, then in terms of "differences," and finally in terms of "uniqueness." The unique newcomer is thus incorporated into the family. Mothers and fathers scrutinize their infant carefully and point out characteristics that the child shares with other family members and that are indicative of a relationship between them. The claiming process is revealed by maternal comments such as the following: "Matt held him close and said, 'She's the image of her father,' but I found one part like me—her toes are shaped like mine."

Conversely, some mothers react negatively. They "claim" the infant in terms of the discomfort or pain the baby causes. The mother interprets the infant's normal responses as being negative toward her and reacts to her child with dislike or indifference. She does not hold

table 24-1 **Infant Behaviors Affecting Parental Attachment**

FACILITATING BEHAVIORS	INHIBITING BEHAVIORS
Visually alert; eye-to-eye contact; tracking or following of parent's face	Sleepy; eyes closed most of the time; gaze averted
Appealing facial appearance; randomness of body movements reflecting helplessness	Resemblance to person parent dislikes; hyperirritability or jerky body movements when touched
Smiles	Bland facial expression; infrequent smiles
Vocalization; crying only when hungry or wet	Crying for hours on end; colicky
Grasp reflex	Exaggerated motor reflex
Anticipatory approach behaviors for feedings; sucks well; feeds easily	Feeds poorly; regurgitates; vomits often
Enjoys being cuddled, held	Resists holding and cuddling by crying, stiffening body
Easily consolable	Inconsolable; unresponsive to parenting, caretaking tasks
Activity and regularity somewhat predictable	Unpredictable feeding and sleeping schedule
Attention span sufficient to focus on parents	Inability to attend to parent's face or offered stimulation
Differential crying, smiling, and vocalizing; recognizes and prefers parents	Shows no preference for parents over others
Approaches through locomotion	Unresponsive to parent's approaches
Clings to parent; puts arms around parent's neck	Seeks attention from any adult in room
Lifts arms to parents in greeting	Ignores parents

From Gerson, E. (1973). *Infant behavior in the first year of life.* New York: Raven Press.

table 24-2 Parental Behaviors Affecting Infant Attachment

FACILITATING BEHAVIORS	INHIBITING BEHAVIORS
Looks; gazes; takes in physical characteristics of infant; assumes en face position; eye contact	Turns away from infant; ignores infant's presence
Hovers; maintains proximity; directs attention to, points to infant	Avoids infant; does not seek proximity; refuses to hold infant when given opportunity
Identifies infant as unique individual	Identifies infant with someone parent dislikes; fails to discern any of infant's unique features
Claims infant as family member; names infant	Fails to place infant in family context or identify infant with family member; has difficulty naming
Touches; progresses from fingertip to fingers to palms to encompassing contact	Fails to move from fingertip touch to palmar contact and holding
Smiles at infant	Maintains bland countenance or frowns at infant
Talks to, coos, or sings to infant	Wakes infant when infant is sleeping; handles roughly; hurries feeding by moving nipple continuously
Expresses pride in infant	Expresses disappointment, displeasure in infant
Relates infant's behavior to familiar events	Does not incorporate infant into life
Assigns meaning to infant's actions and sensitively interprets infant's needs	Makes no effort to interpret infant's actions or needs
Views infant's behaviors and appearance in positive light	Views infant's behavior as exploiting, deliberately uncooperative; views appearance as distasteful, ugly

From Mercer, R. (1983). Parent-infant attachment. In L. Sonstegard, K. Kowalski, & B. Jennings (Eds.), *Women's health* (Vol. 2), *Childbearing*. New York: Grune & Stratton.

FIG. 24-2 Mother interacts with newborn. (Courtesy Tricia Olson, North Ogden, UT.)

FIG. 24-3 Family members examine the new baby. They discuss how she resembles them and other family members. (Courtesy Marjorie Pyle, RNC, Lifecircle, Costa Mesa, CA.)

the child close or touch the child to be comforting; for example, "The nurse put the baby into Maggie's arms. She promptly laid him across her knees and glanced up at the television. 'Stay still until I finish watching—you've been enough trouble already.'"

Nursing interventions related to the promotion of parent-infant attachment are numerous and varied (Table 24-3). They can enhance positive parent-infant contacts by heightening parental awareness of an infant's responses and ability to communicate. As the parent attempts to become competent and loving in that role, nurses can bolster the parent's self-confidence and ego. Nurses are in

prime positions to identify actual and potential problems and collaborate with other health care professionals who will provide care for the parents after discharge.

Assessment of Attachment Behaviors

One of the most important areas of assessment is careful observation of those behaviors thought to indicate the formation of emotional bonds between the newborn and family, especially the mother. Unlike physical assessment of the neonate, which has concrete guidelines to follow, assessment of parent-infant attachment requires much more skill in observation and interviewing. Rooming-in of

table 24-3 Examples of Parent-Infant Attachment Interventions

INTERVENTION LABEL AND DEFINITION	ACTIVITIES
ATTACHMENT PROMOTION Facilitation of development of parent-infant relationship	Provide opportunity for parent(s) to see, hold, and examine newborn immediately after birth Encourage parent(s) to hold infant close to body Assist parent(s) to participate in infant care
ENVIRONMENTAL MANAGEMENT: ATTACHMENT PROCESS Manipulation of individuals' surroundings to facilitate development of parent-infant relationship	Provide rooming-in in hospital Create environment that fosters privacy Individualize daily routine to meet parents' needs Permit father or significant other to sleep in room with mother Develop policies that permit presence of significant others as much as desired
FAMILY INTEGRITY PROMOTION: CHILDBEARING FAMILY Facilitation of growth of individuals or families who are adding infant to family unit	Prepare parent(s) for expected role changes involved in becoming a parent Prepare parent(s) for responsibilities of parenthood Monitor effects of newborn on family structure Reinforce positive parenting behaviors
LACTATION COUNSELING Use of interactive helping process to assist in maintenance of successful breastfeeding	Correct misconceptions, misinformation, and inaccuracies about breastfeeding Evaluate parents' understanding of infant's feeding cues (e.g., rooting, sucking, alertness) Determine frequency of feedings in relation to infant's needs Demonstrate breast massage and discuss its advantages to increasing milk supply
PARENT EDUCATION: INFANT Instruction on nurturing and physical care needed during first year of life	Determine parents' knowledge, readiness, and ability to learn about infant care Provide anticipatory guidance about developmental changes during first year of life Teach parent(s) skills to care for newborn Demonstrate ways in which parent(s) can stimulate infant's development Discuss infant's capabilities for interaction Demonstrate quieting techniques
RISK IDENTIFICATION: CHILDBEARING FAMILY Identification of individual or family likely to experience difficulties in parenting and assigning priorities to strategies to prevent parenting problems	Determine developmental stage of parent(s) Review prenatal history for factors that predispose individuals or family to complications Ascertain understanding of English or other language used in community Monitor behavior that may indicate problem with attachment Plan for risk-reduction activities in collaboration with individual or family

Modified from Dochterman, J., & Bulechek, G. (2004). *Nursing interventions classification (NIC)* (4th ed.). St. Louis: Mosby.

mother and infant and liberal visiting privileges for father, siblings, and grandparents facilitate recognition of behaviors that demonstrate positive or negative attachment. An excellent opportunity exists during feeding. Guidelines for assessment of attachment behaviors are presented in Box 24-1.

During pregnancy, and often even before conception occurs, parents develop an image of the "ideal" or "fantasy" infant. At birth the fantasy infant becomes the real infant. How closely the dream child resembles the real child influences the bonding process. Assessing such expectations during pregnancy and at the time of

CD: Skill: Swaddling

box 24-1 Assessing Attachment Behavior

- When the infant is brought to the parents, do they reach out for the infant and call the infant by name? (Recognize that in some cultures, parents may not name the infant in the early newborn period.)
- Do the parents speak about the infant in terms of identification—whom the infant looks like; what appears special about their infant over other infants?
- When parents are holding the infant, what kind of body contact is there—do parents feel at ease in changing the infant's position; are fingertips or whole hands used; are there parts of the body they avoid touching or parts of the body they investigate and scrutinize?
- When the infant is awake, what kinds of stimulation do the parents provide—do they talk to the infant, to each other, or to no one; how do they look at the infant—direct visual contact, avoidance of eye contact, or looking at other people or objects?
- How comfortable do the parents appear in terms of caring for the infant? Do they express any concern regarding their ability or disgust for certain activities, such as changing diapers?
- What type of affection do they demonstrate to the newborn, such as smiling, stroking, kissing, or rocking?
- If the infant is fussy, what kinds of comforting techniques do the parents use, such as rocking, swaddling, talking, or stroking?

FIG. 24-4 Father interacts with his newborn son. (Courtesy Cheryl Briggs, RN, Annapolis, MD.)

the infant's birth allows identification of discrepancies between the parents' view of the fantasy child and the real child.

The labor process significantly affects the immediate attachment of mothers to their newborn infants. Factors such as a long labor, feeling tired or "drugged" after birth, and problems with breastfeeding can delay the development of initial positive feelings toward the newborn. Referral to groups such as La Leche League or Postpartum Support International (www.lalecheleague.org; www.chss.iup.edu/postpartum) can be useful.

▬ PARENT-INFANT CONTACT

Early Contact

Early close contact may facilitate the attachment process between parent and child. This does not mean that a delay will inhibit this process (humans are too resilient for that), but additional psychologic energy may be needed to achieve the same effect. No scientific evidence has demonstrated that immediate contact after birth is essential for the human parent-child relationship.

Parents who desire but are unable to have early contact with their newborn (for example, the infant was transferred to the neonatal intensive care nursery) can be reassured that such contact is not essential for optimal parent-infant interactions. Otherwise, adopted infants would not form affectional ties with their parents. Nor does the mode of infant-mother contact after birth (skin-to-skin versus wrapped) appear to have any important effect. Nurses need to stress that the parent-infant relationship is a process that occurs over time.

Extended Contact

The provision of rooming-in facilities for the mother and her baby is common in family-centered care. The infant is transferred to the area from the transitional nursery (if the facility uses one) after showing satisfactory extrauterine adjustment. The father is encouraged to participate in the care of the infant (Fig. 24-4), and siblings and grandparents also are encouraged to visit and become acquainted with the infant. Whether rooming-in or a family birth unit is the method of family-centered care, mothers and their partners are considered equal and integral parts of the developing family. Partners are encouraged to take as active a role as they wish.

Extended contact with the infant should be available for all parents but especially for those at risk for parenting inadequacies, such as adolescents and low-income women. Any activity that optimizes family-centered care is worthy of serious consideration by postpartum nurses.

▬ COMMUNICATION BETWEEN ▬ PARENT AND INFANT

The parent-infant relationship is strengthened through the use of sensual responses and abilities by both partners in the interaction. The nurse should keep in mind that there may be cultural variations in these interactive behaviors.

The Senses
Touch

Touch, or the tactile sense, is used extensively by parents and other caregivers as a means of becoming acquainted with the newborn. Many mothers reach out for their infants as soon as they are born and the cord is cut. Mothers lift their infants to their breasts, enfold them in their arms, and cradle them. Once the infant is close, they begin the exploration process with their fingertips, one of the most touch-sensitive areas of the body. Within a short time, the caregiver uses the palm to caress the baby's trunk and eventually enfolds the infant. Gentle stroking motions are used to soothe and quiet the infant; patting or gently rubbing the infant's back is a comfort after feedings. Infants also pat the mother's breast as they nurse. Both seem to enjoy sharing each other's body warmth. There is a desire in parents to touch, pick up, and hold the infant (Fig. 24-5). They comment on the softness of the baby's skin and are aware of milia and rashes. As parents become increasingly sensitive to the infant's like or dislike of different types of touch, they draw closer to their baby.

Variations in touching behaviors have been noted in mothers from different cultural groups (Galanti, 2003; Jiménez, 1995; Stewart & Jambunathan, 1996). For example, minimal touching and cuddling is a traditional Southeast Asian practice thought to protect the infant from evil spirits. Because of tradition and spiritual beliefs, women in India and Bali have practiced infant massage since ancient times (Miller, 2004; Zlotnick, 2000).

Eye Contact

Interest in having eye contact with the baby has been demonstrated repeatedly by parents. Some mothers remark that once their babies have looked at them, they feel much closer to them. Parents spend much time getting their babies to open their eyes and look at them. In the United States, eye contact appears to cement the development of a trusting relationship and is an important factor in human relationships at all ages. In other cultures, eye-to-eye contact may be perceived differently. For example, in Mexican culture, sustained direct eye contact is considered to be rude, immodest, and dangerous for some. This danger may arise from the *mal ojo* (evil eye), resulting from excessive admiration. Women and children are thought to be more susceptible to the *mal ojo* (D'Avanzo & Geissler, 2003).

FIG. 24-5 Father, mother, and newborn getting to know each other. (Courtesy Cheryl Briggs, RN, Annapolis, MD.)

As newborns become functionally able to sustain eye contact with their parents, time is spent in mutual gazing, often in the *en face* position. En face, "face-to-face," is a position in which the parent's face and the infant's face are approximately 8 inches apart and on the same plane (see Fig. 24-2).

Nursing and medical practices that encourage this interaction should be implemented. Immediately after birth, for example, the infant can be positioned on the mother's abdomen or breasts with the mother's and the infant's faces on the same plane so that they can easily make eye contact. Lights can be dimmed so that the infant's eyes will open. Instillation of prophylactic antibiotic ointment in the infant's eyes can be delayed until the infant and parents have had some time together in the first hour after birth.

Voice

The shared response of parents and infants to each other's voices also is remarkable. Parents wait tensely for the first cry. Once that cry has reassured them of the baby's health, they begin comforting behaviors. As the parents talk in high-pitched voices, the infant is alerted and turns toward them.

Infants respond to higher-pitched voices and can distinguish their mother's voice from others soon after birth. Infants use their cries to signal hunger, pain, boredom, and tiredness. With experience, parents learn to distinguish among such cries.

Odor

Another behavior shared by parents and infants is a response to each other's odor. Mothers comment on the smell of their babies when first born and have noted that each infant has a unique odor. Infants learn rapidly to distinguish the odor of their mother's breast milk.

Entrainment

Newborns move in time with the structure of adult speech, which is termed entrainment. They wave their arms, lift their heads, and kick their legs, seemingly "dancing in tune" to a parent's voice. Culturally determined rhythms of speech are ingrained in the infant long before spoken language is used to communicate. This shared rhythm also gives the parent positive feedback and establishes a positive setting for effective communication.

Biorhythmicity

The fetus is in tune with the mother's natural rhythms, such as heartbeats. After birth, a crying infant may be soothed by being held in a position where the mother's heartbeat can be heard or by hearing a recording of a heartbeat. One of the newborn's tasks is to establish a personal rhythm or to achieve biorhythmicity. Parents can help in this process by giving consistent loving care and using their infant's alert state to develop responsive behavior and thereby increase social interactions and opportunities for learning

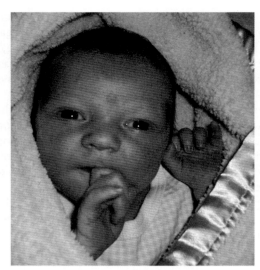

FIG. 24-6 Infant in alert state. (Courtesy Cheryl Briggs, RN, Annapolis, MD.)

FIG. 24-7 Sharing a smile: example of synchrony. (Courtesy Marjorie Pyle, RNC, Lifecircle, Costa Mesa, CA.)

(Fig. 24-6). The more quickly parents become competent in child care activities, the more quickly their psychologic energy can be directed toward observing the communication cues the infant gives them.

Reciprocity and Synchrony

Reciprocity is a type of body movement or behavior that provides the observer with cues. The observer or receiver interprets those cues and responds to them. Reciprocity often takes several weeks to develop with a new baby. For example, when the newborn fusses and cries, the mother responds by picking up and cradling the infant; the baby becomes quiet and alert and establishes eye contact; the mother verbalizes, sings, and coos while the baby maintains eye contact. The baby then averts the eyes and yawns; the mother decreases her active response. If the parent continues to stimulate the infant, the baby may become fussy.

Synchrony refers to the "fit" between the infant's cues and the parent's response. When parent and infant have a synchronous interaction, it is mutually rewarding (Fig. 24-7). Parents need time to interpret the infant's cues correctly. For example, after a certain time, the infant develops a specific cry in response to different situations such as boredom, loneliness, hunger, and discomfort. The parent may need assistance in deciphering these cries, along with trial-and-error interventions, before synchrony develops.

■ PARENTAL ROLE AFTER CHILDBIRTH

Adaptation involves a stabilizing of tasks, a coming to terms with commitments. Parents demonstrate growing competence in childcare activities and are more attuned to their infant's behavior. Typically, the period from the decision to conceive or to adopt through the first months of having a child is termed the transition to parenthood.

Transition to Parenthood

Historically the transition to parenthood was viewed as a crisis. The current perspective is that, for the majority of families, parenthood is a developmental transition rather than a major life crisis. The transition to parenthood is a time of disorder and disequilibrium, as well as satisfaction, for mothers and their partners. Usual methods of coping often seem ineffective. Some parents can be so distressed that they are unable to be supportive of each other. Because men typically identify their spouses as their primary or only source of support, the transition can be harder for the fathers, who feel deprived when the mothers, who are also experiencing stress, cannot provide their usual level of support. Strong emotions such as helplessness, inadequacy, and anger that arise when dealing with a crying infant catch many parents unprepared. On the other hand, parenthood allows adults to develop and display a selfless, warm, and caring side of themselves, which may not be expressed in other adult roles.

For the majority of mothers and their partners, the transition to parenthood is viewed as an opportunity rather than a time of danger. Parents are stimulated to try new coping strategies as they work to master their new roles and reach new developmental levels. As they work through the transition, personal strength and resourcefulness are revealed.

Parental Tasks and Responsibilities

Parents must reconcile the actual child with the fantasy and dream child. This means coming to terms with the infant's physical appearance, sex, innate temperament, and physical status. If the real child differs greatly from the fantasy child, parents may delay acceptance of the child. In some instances, they may never accept the child.

Some parents are startled by the normal appearance of the neonate—size, color, molding of the head, Mongolian spots, or bowed appearance of the legs. Many fathers have commented that they thought the odd shape of the infant's head (molding) meant the infant would be mentally retarded.

Parents may know the sex of the infant before birth because of the use of ultrasound assessments; for those who do not have this information, disappointment over the infant's sex can take time to resolve. The parents may provide adequate physical care but find it difficult to be sincerely involved with the infant until this internal conflict has been resolved. As one mother remarked,

> I really wanted a boy. I know it is silly and irrational, but when they said, "She's a lovely little girl," I was so disappointed and angry—yes, angry—I could hardly look at her. Oh, I looked after her okay, her feedings and baths and things, but I couldn't feel excited. To tell the truth, I felt like a monster not liking my child. Then one day she was lying there, and she turned her head and looked right at me. I felt a flooding of love for her come over me, and we looked at each other a long time. It's okay now. I wouldn't change her for all the boys in the world (Plan of Care).

Parents need to become adept in the care of the infant, including caregiving activities, noting the communication cues given by the infant to indicate needs and responding appropriately to the infant's needs. Self-esteem grows with competence. Breastfeeding makes mothers feel they are contributing in a unique way to the welfare of the infant. The infant's response to the parental care and attention may be interpreted by the parent as a comment on the quality of that care. Infant behaviors that are interpreted by parents as positive responses to their care include being consoled easily, enjoying being cuddled, and making eye contact. Spitting up frequently after feedings, crying, and being unpredictable may be perceived as negative responses to parental care. Continuation of these infant responses that are viewed as negative by the parent can result in alienation of parent and infant to the detriment of the infant.

Assistance, including advice by husbands, partners, wives, mothers, mothers-in-law, and professional workers, can be seen either as supportive or as an indication of how inept these people have judged the new parents to be. Criticism, real or imagined, of the new parents' ability to provide adequate physical care, nutrition, or social stimulation for the infant can prove to be devastating. By providing encouragement and praise for parenting efforts, nurses can bolster the new parents' confidence.

---

plan of care **The Multiparous Woman and Family**

NURSING DIAGNOSIS Risk for impaired maternal-infant attachment related to stress of birth of third baby boy when parents were hoping for a girl

Expected Outcome *Woman will demonstrate positive attachment toward the new infant.*

Nursing Interventions/Rationales
- Identify any negative maternal and paternal behaviors *to provide baseline for interventions.*
- Assist woman to identify positive coping methods *to provide ongoing support.*
- Interpret newborn's behaviors to mother *to facilitate positive response to infant.*
- Provide suggestions for introducing siblings to newborn *to minimize sibling rivalry.*
- Identify support systems and professional referrals *to promote expression of feelings and enhance maternal-infant attachment.*

NURSING DIAGNOSIS Ineffective family coping related to family disorganization

Expected Outcomes *Family will identify stressors and verbalize possible resources that will provide assistance during family role transition.*

Nursing Interventions/Rationales
- Assess for prominent stressors in family environment *to determine plan of care.*
- Assist family to identify positive coping strategies *to deal with family role transition.*
- Encourage family to identify appropriate resources *to decrease family stress.*

NURSING DIAGNOSIS Fatigue related to multiple role demands

Expected Outcome *Woman will report increased energy level.*

Nursing Interventions/Rationales
- Teach woman signs of fatigue *to recognize importance of immediate interventions.*
- Promote consumption of balanced diet with adequate vitamins and iron *to prevent nutritional deficiencies that may cause fatigue.*
- Assess availability of effective support systems *to provide meaningful assistance to the woman during this time of role transition.*
- Suggest modification of infant's behavioral cycle *to increase awake periods during the day and recommend sleeping when infant sleeps to prevent excessive fatigue.*

NURSING DIAGNOSIS Caregiver role strain related to demands of mothering four children

Expected Outcome *The caregiver will develop a plan to decrease role strain.*

Nursing Interventions/Rationales
- Discuss with woman and family a plan to provide infant care at home *to decrease role strain.*
- Allow time to discuss role transition for fourth child *to prepare for realistic role changes in the household.*
- Assist woman to develop time management plan for infant and self-care *to set realistic priorities.*
- List ways in which other members of the household can assist with infant care and household duties *to decrease demands on the woman.*
- Provide list of outside resources *to assist in decreasing caregiver role strain.*

CD: Plan of Care: The Multiparous Woman and Family

Parents must establish a place for the newborn within the family group. Whether the infant is the firstborn or the last born, all family members must adjust their roles to accommodate the newcomer. The firstborn child needs support to accept a rival for parental affections. An older child needs help dealing with losing a favored position in the family hierarchy. The parents are expected to negotiate these changes.

Becoming a Mother

Mercer (2004) has suggested that the concept of *maternal role attainment*, introduced by Rubin in 1967, be replaced with *becoming a mother* to signify the transformation and growth of the mother identity. Becoming a mother implies more than attaining a role. It includes learning new skills and increasing her confidence in herself as she meets new challenges in caring for her child(ren).

The transition to motherhood requires adjustment for the mother and her family. There is disruption inherent in that adjustment and some circumstances such as problems in postpartum recovery or giving birth to a high risk infant add to the disruption (Nelson, 2003). Martell (2001) described the postpartum period as "heading to a new normal."

Nelson (2003) identified two social processes in maternal transition. The primary process is engagement, that is, making a commitment to being a mother, actively caring for her child, and experiencing his/her presence. The secondary process is experiencing herself as a mother, which leads to growth and transformation. During this process, she must learn how to mother and adapt to a changed relationship with her partner and her family and friends; she must examine herself in relation to the past and her present, and come to view herself as a mother; and she must make decisions whether to and when to return to work.

The commitment to mothering is "world-defining" and results in a reorientation of the mother's life (Leonard, 1993). The mother is forever changed and commonly seeks new friends (those with children) and distances herself from those with no children.

Not all mothers experience the transition to motherhood in the same way. For some women, becoming a mother entails multiple losses. For example, for some single women, there may be a loss of the family of origin when they do not accept her decision to have the child, loss of a relationship with the father of the baby, with friends, and with their own sense of self. Women describe a loss of dreams including loss of job, financial security, and a future profession (Keating-Lefler & Wilson, 2004). Accompanying these losses is a loss of support.

Mercer (2004) provides new names for the stages in the process of establishing a maternal identity while becoming a mother. These include "(a) commitment, attachment, and preparation (pregnancy); (b) acquaintance, learning, and physical restoration (first 2 to 6 weeks following birth), (c) moving toward a new normal (2 weeks to 4 months); and (d) achievement of the maternal identity (around

4 months)." The time of achievement of the stages is variable and the stages may overlap. Achievement is influenced by mother and infant variables and the social environment (Mercer).

Nurses must individualize their assessments and interventions. More reality-based perinatal education programs are necessary to prepare mothers better and decrease their anxiety. Mothers need to know that it is common to feel overwhelmed, insecure, and to experience physical and mental fatigue in the first months of parenthood. They need to be assured that this situation is temporary and that it will take 3 to 6 months to become comfortable in caregiving and in being a mother (Nelson, 2003). Maternal support by professionals should not end with hospital discharge but extend over the next 4 to 6 months. Nurses can advocate for the extension of such support services well into the postpartum period.

Nurses can discuss, before and after birth, the usual postpartum concerns that mothers experience and can provide anticipatory guidance on coping strategies, such as resting when the infant sleeps and planning with an extended family member or friend to do the housework for the first week or two after the baby is born. Once a mother is home, periodic phone calls from a nurse who cared for her in the birth setting can provide the mother with an opportunity to vent her concerns and get support and advice from "her nurse." Nurses should plan additional supportive counseling for first-time mothers inexperienced in child care; women whose careers had provided outside stimulation; women who lack friends or family members with whom to share delights and concerns; and adolescent mothers. When possible, postpartum home visits are included in the plan of care.

Postpartum "Blues"

The "pink" period surrounding the first day or two after birth, characterized by heightened joy and feelings of well-being, is often followed by a "blue" period. Approximately 50% to 80% of women of all ethnic and racial groups experience the postpartum blues or "baby blues" (Beeber, 2002). When they have the blues, women are emotionally labile, often crying easily and for no apparent reason. This lability seems to peak around the fifth day and subside by the tenth day. Other symptoms of postpartum blues include depression, a let-down feeling, restlessness, fatigue, insomnia, headache, anxiety, sadness, and anger. Biochemical, psychologic, social, and cultural factors have been explored as possible causes of the postpartum depressive state; however, the etiology remains unknown.

Whatever the cause, the early postpartum period appears to be one of emotional and physical vulnerability for new mothers, who may be psychologically overwhelmed by the reality of parental responsibilities. The mother may feel deprived of the supportive care she received from family members and friends during pregnancy. Some mothers regret the loss of the mother–unborn child relationship and mourn its passing. Still others have a let-down feeling

EVIDENCE-BASED PRACTICE

Parenting Programs to Promote Mental Health

BACKGROUND

- Approximately one out of eight women has some mental health disorder. Some mental health issues that present around childbirth, such as depression, may mark the onset of chronicity. The mental health of the mother has a great impact on the short- and long-term well-being of the child. Parenting groups have become an accepted intervention, and have been shown to improve early childhood behavioral problems.

OBJECTIVES

- Having established in a similar review the children's outcomes of parenting programs, the review group wished to determine the benefits to the parents' psychosocial health. Of particular interest were maternal anxiety/stress, depression, self-esteem, attachment, marital adjustment, and social support.

METHODS

Search Strategy

- After thoroughly searching literature databases, reference lists, and consulting experts in the field, the reviewers identified 26 trials that met their criteria. The trials dated 1978 to 2001, and included 1717 women and families from Australia, Canada, Ireland, the United Kingdom, and the United States. There were five treatment categories, based on theoretical underpinnings: (1) behavioral, five studies that taught behavioral parenting strategies; (2) cognitive-behavioral, six studies that combined behavioral strategies with restructuring of parental thinking about themselves and their children; (3) multimodal, four studies that combined several approaches; (4) humanistic, six studies that relied on the Webster-Stratton series of role-modeling videotapes; and (5) rational-emotive, two studies that reduced stress by examining irrational fears.

Statistical Analyses

- Within the five theory categories, the treatment effect was standardized by finding the mean difference between intervention and control groups, and dividing by the pooled standard deviation. Five outcomes had enough data to justify metaanalysis: depression, anxiety, self-esteem, social support, and marital adjustment. Differences between groups outside the 95% confidence interval were accepted as significant.

FINDINGS

- Parenting groups reported significantly less depression, anxiety, and significantly better self-esteem and marital adjustment than the control group. Parenting groups showed a trend to improved social support, but not to the level of significance.

LIMITATIONS

- It is counter-intuitive that social support would be the weakest outcome, since parenting groups are social by their nature. However, the survey used creates skewed results, thus failing to capture the true differences between intervention and control. The small numbers in the samples led to large confidence intervals, thus making significance more difficult to achieve. Bias is a known hazard of mental health research. Blinding the subjects or the evaluators to treatment categories is impossible. None of the subjects were analyzed in their original randomly assigned "intention to treat" categories. Dropouts appear to have been higher risk parents. The severity of the children's problems at intake were not addressed. Fathers were not always tested. Most of the studies involved Caucasian families.

IMPLICATIONS FOR PRACTICE

- Parenting programs are beneficial for parents and therefore may benefit children. Groups provide a place for parents to identify their feelings as normal. Groups organized with a cognitive-behavioral or rational emotive approach strive to improve parental guilt and mood. Behavioral and multimodal approaches seek to improve parental competence and social support. Group leaders set the tone and model approaches, such as humor, warmth, and flexibility for the group.

IMPLICATIONS FOR FURTHER RESEARCH

- Further research is needed on drop-out parents, who may already be higher risk, and subsequently suffer guilt and lowered self-esteem. Research must account for the severity of the children's problems, since that adds stress and time constraints. As most of the studies were primarily looking for outcomes in children, more research needs to be designed to assess maternal and paternal outcomes. Therapist credentials and personality may cause greatly varied results. Measuring mental health by more objective means than self-report would decrease bias. Finally, larger and more diverse samples would increase generalizability of the findings.

Reference: Barlow, J., Coren, E., & Stewart-Brown, S. (2003). Parent-training programmes for improving maternal psychosocial healt. *The Cochrane Database of Systematic Reviews,* 2006, Issue 3. Chichester, UK: John Wiley & Sons.

when labor and birth are complete. Fatigue after childbirth is compounded by the around-the-clock demands of the new baby, and can accentuate the feelings of depression. To help mothers cope with postpartum blues, nurses can suggest various strategies (see Teaching for Self-Care box).

A few questions on a discharge checklist can help mothers to assess their level of "blues" and to decide when to seek advice from their nurse, nurse-midwife, or physician. Answering yes to any of these questions should alert

the woman to call her health care provider (Johnson & Johnson, 2006):

- Are you having trouble sleeping?
- Are you feeling isolated?
- Have you lost your appetite?
- Are you having thoughts about hurting yourself or your baby?

Home visits and telephone follow-up calls by the nurse are important to assess the mother's pattern of "blue" feelings and behavior over time.

TEACHING FOR SELF-CARE

Coping with Postpartum Blues

- Remember that the "blues" are normal.
- Get plenty of rest; nap when the baby does, if possible. Go to bed early, and let friends know when to visit.
- Use relaxation techniques learned in childbirth classes (or ask the nurse to teach you and your partner some techniques).
- Do something for yourself. Take advantage of the time your partner or family members care for the baby—soak in the tub or go for a walk.
- Plan a day out of the house—go to the mall with the baby, being sure to take a stroller or carriage, or go out to eat with friends without the baby. Many communities have churches or other agencies that provide child care programs such as Mothers' Morning Out.
- Talk to your partner about the way you feel—for example, about feeling tied down, how the birth met your expectations, and things that will help you.
- If you are breastfeeding, give yourself and your baby time to learn.
- Seek out and use community resources such as La Leche League or community mental health centers. One nationally recognized resource is:

  Postpartum Support International
  927 North Kellogg Avenue
  Santa Barbara, CA 93111
  805-967-7636
  www.chss.iup.edu/postpartum

Although the postpartum blues are usually mild and short lived, approximately half a million mothers in the United States each year experience a more severe syndrome termed postpartum depression (PPD) (Wisner, Parry, & Piontek, 2002). PPD symptoms can range from mild to severe, with women having "good days" and "bad days." Goodman (2004) noted that there is a high incidence of PPD in fathers (1% to 26%). Screening should be done in both the mother and father for PPD. PPD can go undetected because new parents generally do not voluntarily admit to this kind of emotional distress out of embarrassment, guilt, or fear. Nurses must include teaching about how to differentiate symptoms of the "blues" and PPD and urge parents to report depressive symptoms promptly if they occur.

Resuming Sexual Intimacy

The couple may begin to engage in sexual intercourse during the second to fourth week after the baby is born. Some couples begin earlier, as soon as it can be accomplished without discomfort, depending on factors such as timing, amount of vaginal dryness, and breastfeeding status. Sexual intimacy enhances the adult aspect of the family, and the adult pair shares a closeness denied to other family members. Changes in a woman's sexuality after childbirth are related to hormonal shifts, increased breast size, uneasiness with a body that has yet to return to a prepregnant

size, chronic fatigue related to sleep deprivation, and physical exhaustion (Bitzer & Alder, 2000). Many new fathers speak of the alienation experienced when they observe the intimate mother-infant relationship, and some are frank in expressing feelings of jealousy toward the infant. The resumption of sexual intimacy seems to bring the parents' relationship back into focus. Before and after birth, nurses should review with new parents their plans for other pregnancies and their preferences for contraception.

Postpartum Adjustment in the Lesbian Couple

Little is known about postpartum maternal adjustment in the lesbian couple. Relationship satisfaction in lesbian parent couples appears related to egalitarianism, commitment, sexual compatibility, and communication skills, as well as the birth mother's decision for insemination by an anonymous sperm donor (Osterwell, 1991; Reimann, 1999). Similar to heterosexual parent couples, most lesbian parent couples voice concern about less time and energy for their relationship after the arrival of the baby (Gartrell et al., 1996). Both partners consider themselves to be equal parents of the baby who share actively in childrearing (Brewaeys, Devroey, Helmerhorst, Van Hall, & Ponjaert, 1995). A primary concern of co-mothers is the legal vulnerability of lesbian families confounded by their social invisibility (Reimann, 1999).

Lesbian couples face strong social sanctions regarding pregnancy and parenting. Their families may not have resolved the initial dismay and guilt over learning of their daughters' homosexuality, or they may disagree with the lesbian couple's decision to conceive and be parents. Lesbian parents deal with public ignorance, social and legal invisibility, and the lack of biologic connection to the child by using a variety of techniques. These techniques include carefully planning and accomplishing their transition to parenthood, displaying public acts of equal mothering, sharing parenting at home, establishing a distinct parenting role within the family, and supporting each partner's sense of identity as a mother. In situations in which family support is limited or absent, the nurse can help lesbian couples locate more supportive social groups, lesbian or heterosexual.

Becoming a Father

Research on paternal adjustment to parenthood indicates that fathers go through predictable phases during their transition to becoming a father (Henderson & Brouse, 1991; St. John, Cameron, & McVeigh, 2005) (Table 24-4). During this period, fathers experience intense emotions. Many fathers acknowledge that their expectations were of limited value once they were immersed in the reality of parenthood. Feelings that often accompany this reality are sadness, ambivalence, jealousy, frustration at not being able to participate in breastfeeding, and an overwhelming desire to be more involved, most of which are different from the feelings mothers report. On the other hand, some fathers are pleasantly surprised at the ease and fun of parenting. In

table 24-4 Transition to Fatherhood: A Three-Stage Process

STAGES	CHARACTERISTICS
Stage 1: Expectations	Father has preconceptions about what life will be like after baby comes home

Stage 2: Reality	Father realizes that expectations are not always based on fact
	
	Common feelings experienced are as follows:
	    Sadness
	    Ambivalence
	    Jealousy
	    Frustration
	Overwhelming desire to be more involved
	Some fathers are pleasantly surprised at ease and fun of parenting

Stage 3: Transition to mastery	Father makes conscious decision to take control and become more actively involved with infant

FIG. 24-8 Engrossment: Father absorbed in looking at his son. (Courtesy Bill Olson, North Ogden, UT.)

their transition to mastery, fathers take control and become more actively involved in the infant's life.

First-time fathers perceive the first 4 to 10 weeks of parenthood in much the same way that mothers do, that is, as a period characterized by uncertainty, increased responsibility, disruption of sleep, and inability to control time needed to care for the infant and reestablish the marital dyad. Fathers express concerns about decreased attention from their partners relative to their personal relationship, the mother's lack of recognition of the father's desire to participate in decision making for the infant, and limited time available to establish a relationship with their infants (Steinberg, Kruckman, & Steinberg, 2000). These concerns can precipitate feelings of jealousy of the infant. The father should discuss his individual concerns/needs with the mother/partner, and become more involved with the infant. This can help alleviate feelings of jealousy in the father.

Father-Infant Relationship

In the U.S. culture, neonates have a powerful impact on their fathers, who become intensely involved with their babies (Fig. 24-8). The term used for the father's absorption, preoccupation, and interest in the infant is engrossment. Characteristics of engrossment include some of the sensual responses relating to touch and eye-to-eye contact discussed earlier and the father's keen awareness of features both unique and similar to himself that validate his claim to the infant. An outstanding response is one of strong attraction to the newborn. Fathers spend considerable time "communicating" with the infant and taking delight in the infant's response to them. A sense of increased self-esteem and a sense of being proud, bigger, more mature, and older are all experienced by fathers after seeing their baby for the first time (Table 24-5).

Fathers spend less time than mothers with infants, and fathers' interactions with infants tend to be characterized by stimulating social play rather than caretaking. The subtle and more open differences in stimulation from two

table 24-5 Development of a Father-Infant Relationship: Process Components

COMPONENT	CHARACTERISTICS
Making a commitment	Willingness to invest in and take responsibility for nurturing the relationship despite difficulties in parenting and other life demands Feeling the reality of commitment: at confirmation of pregnancy; during pregnancy and birth; when to provide infant care; when infant responds to them Helpless nature of infant causes a felt duty to nurture and protect Desire to get to know and be psychologically involved Rewarded by infant smile, increased self-esteem, gaining a new dimension in life, finding the child within self
Becoming connected	The basic psychologic process in the development of father-infant relationship First meeting with infant: feelings of joy, elation, awe, and wonderment Sense of a bond with the infant: may feel this at first meeting or when first touch/hold the infant or may develop gradually during the first 2 months Turning point: when perceives the infant as more responsive, predictable, and familiar
Making room for baby	Father makes changes in work and social/personal time, in relationship with wife/partner, and within self so more physically and emotionally available to infant

sources, mother and father, provide a wider social experience for the infant.

Fathers can benefit from nursing interventions during the postpartum period just as mothers can. Nurses can arrange to teach infant care when the father is present and provide anticipatory guidance for fathers about the transition to parenthood. Separate prenatal and parenting classes and parenting support groups for fathers can provide them with an opportunity to discuss their concerns and have some of their needs met. Postpartum phone calls and home visits by the nurse should include time for assessment of the father's adjustment and needs.

Infant-Parent Adjustment

It has long been recognized that newborns participate actively in shaping their parents' reaction to them. Behavioral characteristics of the infant influence parenting behaviors. The infant and the parent each have unique rhythms, behaviors, and response styles that are brought to every interaction. Infant-parent interactions can be facilitated in any of three ways: (1) modulation of rhythm, (2) modification of behavioral repertoires, and (3) mutual responsivity. Nurses can teach parents about these three aspects of infant-parent interaction through discussions, written materials, and videotapes on infant capabilities. A creative approach is to videotape the parent-infant pair during an interaction and then use the individualized tape to discuss the pair's rhythm, behavioral repertoire, and responsivity.

Rhythm

To modulate rhythm, both parent and infant must be able to interact. Therefore the infant must be in the alert state, one of the most difficult of the sleep-wake states to maintain. The alert state (see Fig. 24-6) occurs most often during a feeding or in face-to-face play. The parent must work hard to help the infant maintain the alert state long enough and often enough for interactions to take place. The *en face* position is usually assumed (Fig. 24-9, *D*). Multiparous mothers in particular are very sensitive and responsive to the infant's feeding rhythms. Mothers learn to reserve stimulation for pauses in sucking activity and not to talk or smile excessively while the infant is sucking because the infant will stop feeding to interact with her. With maturity the infant can sustain longer interactions by modulating activity rhythms, that is, limb movement, sucking, gaze alternation, and habituation. Meanwhile, the parent becomes more attuned to the infant's rhythms and learns to modulate the rhythms, facilitating a rhythmic turn-taking interaction.

Behavioral Repertoires

Both the infant and the parent have a repertoire of behaviors they can use to facilitate interactions. Fathers and mothers engage in these behaviors depending on the extent of contact and caregiving of the infant.

The infant's behavioral repertoire includes gazing, vocalizing, and facial expressions. The infant is able to focus and follow the human face from birth and also is able to alternate the gaze voluntarily, looking away from the parent's face when understimulated or overstimulated (Fig. 24-9, *F*). One of the key responses for the parents to learn is to be sensitive to the infant's capacity for attention and inattention. Developing this sensitivity is especially important when interacting with preterm infants.

Body gestures form a part of the infant's "early language." Babies greet parents with waving hands (Fig. 24-9, *E*) or a reaching out of hands. They can raise an eyebrow

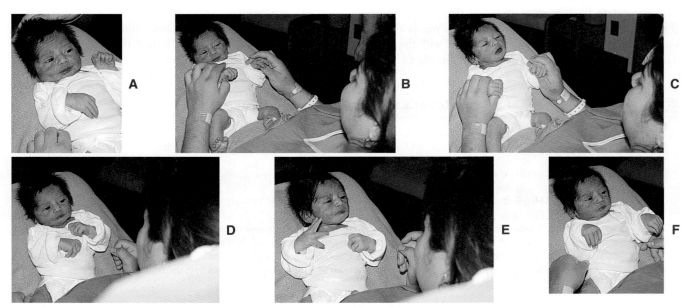

FIG. 24-9 Holding newborn in *en face* position, mother works to alert her daughter, 6 hours old. **A,** Infant is quiet and alert. **B,** Mother begins talking to daughter. **C,** Infant responds, opens mouth like her mother. **D,** Infant gazes at her mother. **E,** Infant waves hand. **F,** Infant glances away, resting. Hands relax. (Courtesy Marjorie Pyle, RNC, Lifecircle, Costa Mesa, CA.)

or soften their expression to elicit loving attention. Game playing can stimulate them to smile or laugh. Pouting or crying, arching of the back, and general squirming usually signal the end of an interaction.

The parents' repertoire includes various types of interactive behaviors such as constantly looking at the infant and noting the infant's response. New parents often remark that they are exhausted from looking at the baby and smiling. Adults also "infantilize" their speech to help the infant "listen." They do this by slowing the tempo, speaking loudly and rhythmically, and emphasizing key words. Phrases are repeated frequently. Infantilizing does not mean using "baby talk," which involves distortion of sounds.

To communicate emotions to the infant, parents often use facial expressions such as slow and exaggerated looks of surprise, happiness, and confusion. Games such as "peek-a-boo" and imitation of the infant's behaviors are other means of interaction. For example, if the baby smiles, so does the parent; if the baby frowns, the parent responds in kind.

Responsivity

Contingent responses (responsivity) are those that occur within a specific time and are similar in form to a stimulus behavior. The adult has the feeling of having an influence on the interaction. Infant behaviors such as smiling, cooing, and sustained eye contact, usually in *en face* position, are viewed as contingent responses. The infant's responses act as rewards to the initiator and encourage the adult to continue with the game when the infant responds positively. When the adult imitates the infant, the infant appears to enjoy it. A progression occurs in the types of behaviors that parents present for the baby to imitate; for example, in early interactions, the parent will grimace rather than laugh, which is in keeping with the infant's developmental level. Such "turnabout" behaviors sustain interactions and promote harmony in the relationship.

■ DIVERSITY IN TRANSITIONS ■ TO PARENTHOOD

How parents respond to the birth of their child is influenced by various factors including age, social networks, socioeconomic conditions, and personal aspirations for the future.

Age

Maternal age has a definite effect on the outcome of pregnancy. The mother and fetus are both at highest risk when the mother is an adolescent or is older than 35 years.

The Adolescent Mother

Although it is biologically possible for the adolescent female to become a parent, her egocentricity and concrete thinking interfere with her ability to parent effectively. The very young adolescent mother is inexperienced and unprepared to recognize the early signs of illness, potential danger, or household hazards. She may inadvertently neglect her child. The higher mortality rates among the infants of adolescent mothers are attributed to the inexperience, lack of knowledge, and immaturity of the mothers, which cause them to be unable to recognize a problem and obtain the necessary resources to rectify the situation. Nevertheless, in most instances, with adequate support and developmentally appropriate teaching, adolescents can learn effective parenting skills.

The transition to parenthood may be difficult for adolescent parents. Coping with the developmental tasks of parenthood is often complicated by the unmet developmental needs and tasks of adolescence. Some young parents may have difficulty accepting a changing self-image and adjusting to new roles related to the responsibilities of infant care. Other adolescent parents, however, may have higher self-concepts than their nonparenting peers (Dalla & Gamble, 2000).

As adolescent parents move through the transition to parenthood, they may feel "different" from their peers, excluded from "fun" activities, and prematurely forced to enter an adult social role. The conflict between their own desires and the infant's demands, in addition to the low tolerance for frustration that is typical of adolescence, further contribute to the normal psychosocial stress of childbirth.

Maintaining a relationship with the baby's father is beneficial for the teen mother and her infant. A close and satisfying relationship is positively correlated with maternal-fetal and maternal-infant attachment (Bloom, 1998). The involvement of the baby's father is related to appropriate maternal behaviors and positive mother-infant relationship (Diehl, 1997).

Adolescent mothers provide warm and attentive physical care; however, they use less verbal interaction than do older parents, tend to be less responsive, and interact less positively with their infants than do older mothers. Interventions emphasizing verbal and nonverbal communication skills between mother and infant are important. Such intervention strategies must be concrete and specific because of the cognitive level of adolescents. Although some observers suggest that some adolescents may use more aggressive behaviors, a higher incidence of child abuse has not been documented. In comparison with adult mothers, teenage mothers have a limited knowledge of child development. They tend to expect too much of their children too soon and often characterize their infants as being fussy. This limited knowledge may cause teenagers to respond to their infants inappropriately.

Many young mothers pattern their mothering behaviors on what they themselves experienced. Therefore nurses need to determine the kind of support that people close to the young mother are able and prepared to give, as well as the kinds of community aid available to supplement this support. Many teen mothers can identify a source of social support, with the predominant source being their own mothers.

The need for continued assessment of the new mother's parenting abilities during this postbirth period is essential. In addition, continued support should be provided by involving the grandparents and other family members, as well as home visits and group sessions for discussion of infant care and parenting problems. Outreach programs concerned with self-care, parent-child interactions, child injuries, and failure to thrive, in addition to programs that provide prompt and effective community intervention, prevent more serious problems from occurring. As the adolescent performs her mothering role within the framework of her family, she may need to address dependence versus independence issues. The adolescent's family members also may need help adapting to their new roles.

The Adolescent Father

The adolescent father and mother face immediate developmental crises, which include completing the developmental tasks of adolescence, making a transition to parenthood, and sometimes adapting to marriage. These transitions can be stressful. The nurse may initiate interaction with the adolescent father by asking him to be present when postpartum home visits are made and to accompany the mother and the baby to well-baby checks at the clinic or pediatrician's office. With the adolescent mother's agreement, the nurse may contact the father directly. Adolescent fathers need support to discuss their emotional responses to the pregnancy. The father's feelings of guilt, powerlessness, or bravado should be recognized because of their negative consequences for both the parents and the child. Counseling of adolescent fathers must be reality oriented. Topics such as finances, child care, parenting skills, and the father's role in the birth experience must be discussed. Teenage fathers also need to know about reproductive physiology and birth control options, as well as safer sex practices.

The adolescent father may continue to be involved in an ongoing relationship with the young mother and his baby. In many instances, he also plays an important role in the decisions about child care and raising the child. He may need help to develop realistic perceptions of his role as "father to a child." He is encouraged to use coping mechanisms that are not detrimental to his own, his partner's, or his child's well-being. The nurse enlists support systems, parents, and professional agencies on his behalf.

Maternal Age Greater Than 35 Years

Women older than 35 years have continued their childbearing either by choice or because of a lack or failure of contraception during the perimenopausal years. Added to this group are women who have postponed pregnancy because of careers or other reasons, as well as women of infertile couples who finally become pregnant with the aid of technologic advances.

Adjustment of older mothers to changes involved in becoming a parent and seeing themselves as competent is aided by support from their partners. Support from other family members and friends is also important for positive self-evaluation of parenting, a sense of well-being and satisfaction, and help in dealing with stress.

Changes in the sexual aspect of a relationship can be a stressor for new midlife parents. Mothers report that finding time and energy for a romantic rendezvous is more difficult. They attribute much of this to the reality of caring for an infant, but the decreasing libido that normally accompanies getting older also contributes.

Work and career issues are sources of conflict for older mothers. Conflicts emerge over being disinterested, worrying about giving enough attention to work with the distractions of a new baby, and anticipating what it will be like to return to work. Child care is a major factor causing stress about work.

Another major issue for older mothers with careers is the perception of loss of control. Mothers older than 35, when compared with younger mothers, are at a different stage in their careers, having attained high levels of education, career, and income. The loss of control experienced when going from the consistency of a work role to the inconsistency of the parent role comes as a surprise to many. Helping the older mother have realistic expectations of herself and of parenthood is essential.

New mothers who are also perimenopausal may find it hard to distinguish fatigue, loss of sleep, decreased libido, or other physiologic symptoms as the cause of the changes in their sex lives. Although many women view menopause as a natural stage of life, for midlife mothers this cessation of menstruation coincides with the state of parenthood. The changes of midlife and menopause can add more emotional and physical stress to older mothers' lives because of the time- and energy-consuming aspects of raising a young child.

Paternal Age Greater Than 35 Years

Older fathers describe their experience of midlife parenting as wonderful but not without drawbacks. What they see as positive aspects of parenthood in older years include increased love and commitment between the spouses, a reinforcement of why one married in the first place, a feeling of being complete, experiencing of "the child" again in oneself, more financial stability than in younger years, and more freedom to focus on parenting rather than on career. A common theme expressed is *sharing*: sharing joy, sharing in raising the child, sharing as a family. The main drawback of midlife parenting is the change that it makes in the relationships with their partners.

Social Support

Social support is strongly related to positive adaptation by new parents, including adolescent parents, during the transition to parenthood. Social support is multidimensional and includes the number of members in a person's social network, types of support, perceived general support, actual support received, and satisfaction with support available and received. The type and satisfaction of support seem to be more important than the total number of support network members.

Across cultural groups, families and friends of new parents form an important dimension of the parent's social network. Through seeking help within the social network, new mothers learn practices that are culturally valued and develop role competency.

Social networks provide a support system on which parents can rely for assistance, but they also can be a source of conflict. Sometimes a large network can cause problems because of the conflicting advice that comes from numerous people. Grandparents or in-laws are most appreciated when they assist with household responsibilities and do not intrude into the parents' privacy or judge them critically.

Because of the extent of restructuring and reorganization that occurs in a family with the birth of another child, the mother's moods and fatigue in the postpartum period can be helped more by situation-specific support from family and friends than by general support. General support addresses feeling loved, respected, and valued. Situation-specific support relates to practical concerns such as physical needs and child care.

Culture

Cultural beliefs and practices are important determinants of parenting behaviors. Culture defines what is socially acceptable in terms of eye contact, touch, and space. Culture influences the interactions with the baby as well as the parent's or family's caregiving style. For example, the provision for a period of rest and recuperation for the mother after birth is prominent in several cultures. Asian mothers must remain at home with the baby at least 30 days after birth and are not supposed to engage in household chores, including care of the baby. Many times the grandmother takes over the baby's care immediately, even before discharge from the hospital (D'Avanzo & Geissler, 2003; Kim-Goodwin, 2003). An example is the traditional Taiwanese ritual, *tso-yueh-tzu* (translated "doing, within the first month postpartum"). Jordanian mothers have a 40-day lying-in after birth during which their mothers or sisters care for the baby (D'Avanzo & Geissler). The Japanese tradition called *satogairi-bunben* requires a woman to return to her family of origin for rest during the last month of pregnancy and for the first 2 months after childbirth for recuperation. Hispanics practice an intergenerational family ritual, *la cuarentena*. For 40 days after birth, the mother is expected to recuperate and get acquainted with her infant. Traditionally this involves many restrictions concerning food (spicy or cold foods, fish, pork, and citrus are avoided; tortillas and chicken soup are encouraged), exercise, and activities, including sexual intercourse. Abdominal binding is a traditional practice, and many women avoid tub bathing and washing their hair. Traditional Hispanic husbands do not expect to see their wives or infants until both have been cleaned and dressed after birth. *La cuarentena* incorporates individuals into the family, instills parental responsibility, and integrates the family during a critical life event (D'Avanzo & Geissler).

Desire for and valuing of children is salient in all cultures. In Asian families, children are valued as a source of family strength and stability, are perceived as wealth, and are objects of parental love and affection. Infants almost always are given an affectionate "cradle" name that is used during the first years of life; for example, a Filipino girl might be called "Ling-Ling" and a boy "Bong-Bong." See Table 2-2 for examples of some traditional cultural beliefs that may be important to parents from African-American, Asian, and Hispanic cultures.

Knowledge of cultural beliefs can help the nurse make more accurate assessments and diagnoses of observed parenting behaviors. For example, nurses may become concerned when they observe cultural practices that appear to reflect poor maternal-infant bonding. Algerian mothers may not unwrap and explore their infants as part of the acquaintance process because in Algeria, babies are wrapped tightly in swaddling clothes to protect them physically and psychologically (D'Avanzo & Geissler, 2003). The nurse may observe a Vietnamese woman who gives minimal care to her infant but refuses to cuddle or further interact with her baby. This apparent lack of interest in the newborn is this cultural group's attempt to ward off "evil spirits" and actually reflects an intense love and concern for the infant (Galanti, 2003). An Asian mother might be criticized for almost immediately relinquishing the care of the infant to the grandmother and not even attempting to hold her baby when the infant is brought to her room. However, in Asian extended families, members show their support for a new mother's rest and recuperation by assisting with the care of the baby. Contrary to the guidance given to mothers in the United States about "nipple confusion," a mix of breastfeeding and bottle-feeding is standard practice for Japanese mothers. This is out of concern for the mother's rest during the first 2 to 3 months and does not lead to any problems with lactation; breastfeeding is widespread and successful among Japanese women.

Cultural beliefs and values give perspective to the meaning of childbirth for a new mother. Nurses can provide an opportunity for a new mother to talk about her perception of the meaning of childbearing. In helping new families adjust to parenthood, nurses must provide culturally sensitive care by following principles that enhance nursing practice within transcultural situations.

Socioeconomic Conditions

Socioeconomic conditions often determine access to available resources. Parents whose economic condition is made worse with the birth of each child and who are unable to use an effective method of fertility management may find childbirth complicated by concern for their own health and a sense of helplessness. Mothers who are single, separated, or divorced from their husbands or without a partner, family, and friends for whatever reason may view the birth of a child with dread. Serious financial problems may override any desire for mothering the infant.

Personal Aspirations

For some women, parenthood interferes with or blocks their plans for personal freedom or advancement in their careers. Resentment concerning this loss may not have been resolved during the prenatal period, and if it remains unresolved, it will spill over into caregiving activities. This may result in indifference and neglect of the infant, or in excessive concern and the setting of impossibly high standards by the mother for her own behavior or the child's performance.

Nursing intervention includes providing opportunities for mothers to express their feelings freely to an objective listener; to discuss measures to permit personal growth; and to learn about the care of their infant. Referring the woman to a support group of other mothers "in the same situation" may also be helpful.

Nurses also can be proactive in influencing changes in work policies related to maternity and paternity leaves, varying models of work sharing, and "family friendly" work environments. Some corporations already structure their work sites to support new mothers (e.g., by providing on-site daycare facilities and breastfeeding rooms).

▬ PARENTAL SENSORY IMPAIRMENT

In the early dialogue between the parent and child, each uses all senses—sight, hearing, touch, taste, and smell—to initiate and sustain the attachment process. A parent who has an impairment of one of the senses must maximize use of the remaining senses.

Visually Impaired Parent

Visual impairment alone does not seem to have a negative impact on mothers' early parenting experiences. These mothers, just as sighted mothers, express the wonders of parenthood and encourage other visually impaired persons to become parents. Mothers with disabilities tend to value the importance of performing parenting tasks in the perceived culturally usual way.

Although visually impaired mothers initially feel a pressure to conform to traditional, sighted ways of parenting, they soon adapt these ways and develop methods better suited to themselves. Examples of activities that visually impaired mothers do differently include preparation of the infant's nursery, clothes, and supplies. Mothers may put an entire clothing outfit together and hang it in the closet rather than keeping the items separately in drawers. They might develop a labeling system for the infant's clothing and put diapering, bathing, and other care supplies where these will be easy to locate with minimal searching. A strength that visually impaired parents have is a heightened sensitivity to other sensory outputs. A blind mother can tell when her infant is facing her because she can feel the baby's breath on her face.

One of the major difficulties that visually impaired parents experience is the skepticism, open or hidden, of health care professionals. Visually impaired people sense reluctance on the part of others to acknowledge that they have a right to be parents. All too often, nurses and doctors lack the experience to deal with the childbearing and child-rearing needs of visually impaired mothers, as well as mothers with other disabilities (such as hearing impaired, physically impaired, and mentally challenged). The best approach by the nurse is to assess the mother's capabilities. From that basis, the nurse can make plans to assist the woman, often in much the same way as for a mother with sight. Visually impaired mothers have made suggestions for providing care for women such as themselves during childbearing (Box 24-2). Such approaches by the nurse can help avoid a sense of increased vulnerability on the mother's part. Childbirth education and other materials are available in Braille (www.loc.gov/nls).

Eye contact is considered important in the U.S. culture. With a parent who is visually impaired, this critical factor in the parent-child attachment process is obviously missing. However, the visually-impaired parent, who may never have experienced this method of strengthening relationships, does not miss it. The infant will need other sensory input from that parent. An infant looking into the eyes of a mother who is visually impaired may not be aware that the eyes are unseeing. Other people in the newborn's environment can participate in active eye-to-eye contact to supply this need. A problem may arise, however, if the visually impaired parent has an impassive facial expression. Her infant, making repeated unsuccessful attempts to engage in face play with the mother, will abandon the behavior with her and intensify it with the father or other people in the household. Nurses can provide anticipatory guidance regarding this situation and help the mother learn to nod and smile while talking and cooing to the infant.

---

box 24-2 Nursing Approaches for Working with Visually Impaired Parents

- Parents who are visually impaired need oral teaching by health care providers because maternity information is not accessible to blind people.
- A visually impaired parent needs an orientation to the hospital room that allows the parent to move about the room independently. For example, "Go to the left of the bed and trail the wall until you feel the first door. That is the bathroom."
- Parents who are visually impaired need explanations of routines.
- Parents who are visually impaired need to feel devices (e.g., monitors, pelvic models) and to hear descriptions of the devices.
- Visually impaired parents need a chance to ask questions.
- Visually impaired parents need the opportunity to hold and touch the baby after birth.
- Nurses need to demonstrate baby care by touch and to follow with, "Now let me see you do it."
- Nurses need to give instructions such as, "I'm going to give you the baby. The head is to your left side."
- If parents read Braille, refer them to sources of materials printed in braille (www.loc.gov/nls).

Hearing-Impaired Parent

The parent who has a hearing impairment faces another set of problems, particularly if the deafness dates from birth or early childhood. The mother and her partner are likely to have established an independent household. A number of devices that transform sound into light flashes are now marketed and can be fitted into the infant's room to permit immediate detection of crying. Even if the parent is not speech trained, vocalizing can serve as both a stimulus and a response to the infant's early vocalizing. Deaf parents can provide additional vocal training by use of recordings and television so that from birth, the child is aware of the full range of the human voice. Young children acquire sign language readily, and the first sign used is as varied as the first word.

Section 504 of the Rehabilitation Act of 1973 requires that hospitals and other institutions receiving funds from the U.S. Department of Health and Human Services use various communication techniques and resources with the deaf, including having staff members or certified interpreters who are proficient in sign language. For example, provision of written materials with demonstrations and having nurses stand where the parent can read their lips (if the parent practices lip reading) can be used. A creative approach is for the nursing unit to develop videotapes in which information on postpartum care, infant care, and parenting issues is signed by an interpreter and spoken by a nurse. A videotape in which a nurse signs while speaking would be ideal. With the advent of the Internet, many resources are available to the deaf parent.

▬ SIBLING ADAPTATION

Because the family is an interactive, open unit, the addition of a new family member affects everyone in the family. Siblings have to assume new positions within the family hierarchy. The older child's goal is to maintain the lead position. Parents are faced with the task of caring for a new child while not neglecting the others. Parents must distribute their attention in an equitable manner.

Reactions of siblings may result from temporary separation from the mother or changes in the mother's or father's behavior. Positive behavioral changes include interest in and concern for the baby and increased independence. Regression in toileting and sleep habits, aggression toward the baby, and increased seeking of attention and whining are examples of negative behaviors.

The parents' attitudes toward the arrival of the baby can set the stage for the other children's reactions. Because the baby absorbs the time and attention of the important people in the other children's lives, jealousy (sibling rivalry) is to be expected once the initial excitement of having a new baby in the home is over. However, sibling rivalry, or negative behaviors in siblings, may have been overemphasized in the past. Developmentally appropriate behaviors in siblings are similar before and after the baby arrives. Firstborn children seem to continue their usual routines and are more pleased with the newborns and more understanding of the baby's need for care than the parents predict.

Parents, especially mothers, spend much time and energy promoting sibling acceptance of a new baby. Participating in sibling preparation classes makes a difference in the ability of mothers to cope with sibling behavior. Older children are actively involved in preparing for the infant, and this involvement intensifies after the birth of the child. Parents have to manage the feeling of guilt that the older children are being deprived of parental time and attention. They also have to monitor the behavior of older children toward the more vulnerable infant and to divert aggressive behavior. Strategies that parents have used to facilitate acceptance of a new baby by siblings are presented in Box 24-3.

Siblings demonstrate acquaintance behaviors with the newborn. The acquaintance process depends on the information given to the child before the baby is born and on the child's cognitive development level. The initial behaviors of siblings with the newborn include looking at the infant and touching the head (Fig. 24-10). The adjustment of older children to a newborn takes time, and children

---

CRITICAL THINKING EXERCISE

Hearing-Impaired Parents

You are assigned to care for Kathy, 22, and Ben, 23, who are first-time parents. Kathy gave birth to a daughter 6 hours ago. Both Kathy and Ben are deaf. Ben has been deaf since birth, and Kathy lost her hearing after having meningitis at age 8. Both Kathy and Ben read lips and sign; Kathy also has speech. Ben is a maintenance worker in a community college; Kathy is a teacher's assistant in a classroom for the hearing impaired. The infant, Angela, can hear. The parents plan to go home from the birth center tomorrow. They have done well in caring for the infant in the birth center but are concerned about how they will manage at home since they are unable to hear Angela when she cries. They have had many questions for the nurse about adaptations they can make at home to assure that Angela will be well cared for. How can the nurse help this couple?

1. Evidence—Is there sufficient evidence for the nurse to provide appropriate help for this couple?
2. Assumptions—What assumptions can be made about parenthood and child care by hearing-impaired parents?
   a. The nurse's approach to working with hearing-impaired parents
   b. Kathy and Ben's adjustment to parenthood
   c. The ability of these parents to safely care for their infant
   d. The infant's attachment to her parents
3. What implications and priorities for nursing can be made at this time?
4. Does the evidence objectively support your conclusion?
5. Are there alternative perspectives to your conclusion?

---

box 24-3 **Strategies for Facilitating Sibling Acceptance of a New Baby**

- Take your firstborn child on a tour of your hospital room and point out similarities to his or her birth. "This is like the room I was in with you, and the baby is in the same kind of bassinet that you were in."
- Have a small gift from the baby to give to your older child each day.
- Give the older child a T-shirt that says "I'm a big brother" (or "sister").
- Arrange for your children to be in the first group (grandparents, sister) to see the newborn. Let them hold the baby in the hospital. One mother and father arranged for their firstborn son to be present at the births of his three brothers and to be the first one to hold them.
- Plan time for both children. "When I get home, I'll arrange my day so that I can have the baby's care done in the morning while Sam (first child) is at school. Maybe the baby will

sleep part of the afternoon and I can spend some time with Sam."
- Fathers can spend time with the older sibling while mothers are taking care of the baby and vice versa. Siblings like to have time and attention from both parents.
- Give preschool and early school-age siblings a newborn doll as "their baby" to care for. Give sibling a photograph of the new baby to take to school to show off "his" or "her" baby. Older siblings may enjoy the responsibility of helping care for the newborn, such as learning how to give the baby a bottle or to change a diaper. One mother let her preschooler help burp the new baby by patting on the baby's back. She figured her son could pat the baby fairly firmly without harming him and at the same time get out some pent-up aggressive feelings.

FIG. 24-10 First meeting. Sister with mother during first meeting with new sibling. **A,** First tentative touch with fingertip. **B,** Relationship is more secure: it is now okay to touch with whole hand. **C,** Smiles indicate acceptance. (Courtesy Sara Kossuth, Los Angeles, CA.)

should be allowed to interact at their own pace rather than being forced to do so. To expect a young child to accept and love a rival for the parents' affection assumes an unrealistic level of maturity. Sibling love grows as does other love (i.e., by being with another person and sharing experiences). The relationship that develops between siblings has been conceptualized as sibling attachment. This bond between siblings involves a secure base in which one child provides support for the other, is missed when absent, and is looked to for comfort and security.

▬ GRANDPARENT ADAPTATION

Grandparents experience a transition to grandparenthood. Intergenerational relationships shift, and grandparents must deal with changes in practices and attitudes toward childbirth, childrearing, and men's and women's roles at home and in the workplace. The degree to which grandparents understand and accept current practices can influence how supportive they are perceived to be by their adult children.

While they are adjusting to grandparenthood, the majority of grandparents are experiencing normative middle- and old-age life transition issues, such as retirement and a move to smaller housing, and need support from their adult children. Some may feel regret about their limited involvement because of poor health or geographic distance. Maternal grandmothers, more than the other three grandparents, may have high expectations of themselves that cause them to be very self-critical.

The extent of involvement of grandparents in the care of the newborn depends on many factors, for example, the willingness of the grandparents to become involved, the proximity of the grandparents, and ethnic and cultural expectations of the grandparents' role. If the new parents live in the United States, Asian grandparents, for example, typically are asked to come to the United States to care for the baby and the mother after birth and to care for the children once the parents return to work. In the United States, paternal grandparents, in contrast to those in other cultures, frequently consider themselves secondary to the maternal grandparents. Less seems expected of them, and they are initially less involved. Nevertheless, these grandparents are eager to help and express great pleasure in their son's fatherhood and his involvement with the baby.

For first-time parents, pregnancy and parenthood can reawaken old issues related to dependence versus independence. Couples often do not plan on their parents' help immediately after the baby arrives. They may want time "to be a family," implying a couple-baby unit, not the intergenerational family network. Contrary to their expectations, many new parents do call on their parents for help, especially the maternal grandmother (Fig. 24-11). Many grandparents are aware of their adult children's wishes for autonomy, respect these wishes, and remain available to help when asked.

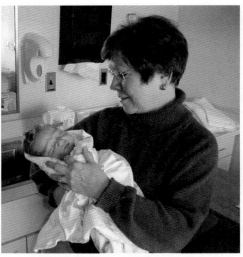

FIG. 24-11   Grandmother and new grandson get acquainted. (Courtesy Nicole Larson, Eden Prairie, MN.)

A simple technique to help people span the generation gap is through a printed "letter to new parents" (written from the grandparents' perspective), which can be included in prenatal kits distributed in childbirth preparation classes and made available to all family members on the postpartum unit. Grandparents' classes can be used to bridge the generation gap and help the grandparents understand their adult children's parenting concepts. The classes include information on up-to-date childbearing practices, family-centered care; infant care, feeding, and safety (car seats); as well as exploration of roles that grandparents play in the family unit.

The 2000 Census reported that 2.4 million grandparents had primary responsibility for grandchildren who lived with them. Of this number, 39% had cared for their grandchildren more than 5 years (Simmons & Dye, 2003). Increasing numbers of grandparents are providing permanent care to their grandchildren as a result of divorce, substance abuse, child abuse and/or neglect, abandonment, teenage pregnancy, death, human immunodeficiency virus (HIV) and acquired immunodeficiency syndrome (AIDS), unemployment, incarceration, and/or mental health problems. This emerging trend requires the nurse to evaluate the role of the grandparent in parenting the infant. Educational and financial considerations must be addressed and available support systems identified for these families.

community activity

Interview the health education teacher at a local high school. Are there resources at the school for adolescents who become pregnant? If yes, do these resources include the father of the baby? What are the resources available? If no, where are these adolescents referred? Are there community resources for pregnant and parenting teens?

key points

- The birth of a child necessitates changes in the existing inter-actional structure of a family.
- Becoming a mother or father signifies the transformation and growth of the mother or father identity.
- Attachment is the process by which the parent and infant come to love and accept each other.
- Both partners in the parent-infant interaction strengthen attachment through the use of sensual responses or interactions.
- The father is considered an equal and integral part of the developing family.

- Mothers may exhibit signs of postpartum blues (baby blues).
- Modulation of rhythm, modification of behavioral repertoires, and mutual responsivity facilitate infant-parent adjustment.
- Many factors influence adaptation to parenthood (e.g., age, culture, socioeconomic level, and expectations of what the child will be like).
- Parents face a number of tasks related to sibling adjustment that require creative parental interventions.
- Grandparents can be a source of knowledge and support and can have a positive influence on the postpartum family.

REFERENCES

Beeber, L. (2002). The pinks and the blues. *American Journal of Nursing, 102*(11), 91-98.

Bitzer, J., & Alder, J. (2000). Sexuality during pregnancy and the postpartum period. *Journal of Sex Education and Therapy, 25*(1), 49-58.

Bloom, K. (1998). Perceived relationship with the father of the baby and maternal attachment in adolescents. *Journal of Obstetric, Gynecologic, and Neonatal Nursing, 27*(4), 420-430.

Brewaeys, A., Devroey, P., Helmerhorst, F., Van Hall, E., & Ponjaert, I. (1995). Lesbian mothers who conceived after donor insemination: A follow-up study. *Human Reproduction, 10*(10), 2731-2735.

Dalla, R., & Gamble, E. (2000). Mother, daughter, teenager—who am I? Perceptions of adolescent maternity in a Navajo reservation community. *Journal of Family Issues, 21*(2), 225-245.

D'Avanzo, C., & Geissler, E. (2003). *Pocket guide to cultural health assessment* (3rd ed.). St. Louis: Mosby.

Diehl, K. (1997). Adolescent mothers: What produces positive mother-infant interaction? *MCN American Journal of Maternal/Child Nursing, 22*(2), 89-95.

Galanti, G. (2003). *Caring for patients from different cultures* (3rd ed.). Philadelphia: University of Pennsylvania Press.

Gartrell, N., Hamilton, J., Banks, A., Mosbacher, D., Reed, N., Sparks, C., et al. (1996). The National Lesbian Family Study: 1. Interviews with prospective mothers. *American Journal of Orthopsychiatry, 66*(2), 272-281.

Goodman, J. (2004). Paternal postpartum depression, its relationship to maternal postpartum depression, and implications for family health. *Journal of Advanced Nursing, 45*(1), 26-35

Henderson, A., & Brouse, A. (1991). The experiences of new fathers during the first three weeks of life. *Journal of Advanced Nursing, 16*(3), 293-298.

Jiménez, S. (1995). The Hispanic culture, folklore, and perinatal health. *Journal of Perinatal Education, 4*(1), 9-16.

Johnson & Johnson. (2006). *Compendium of postpartum care* (2nd ed.). Skillman, NJ: Johnson & Johnson Consumer Products.

Keating-Lefler, R., & Wilson, M. (2004). The experience of becoming a mother for single, unpartnered, Medicaid-eligible, first-time mothers. *Journal of Nursing Scholarship, 36*(1), 23-29.

Kim-Goodwin, Y. (2003). Beliefs and practices among non-Western cultures. *MCN American Journal of Maternal/Child Nursing, 28*(2), 74-78.

Klaus, M., & Kennell, J. (1976). *Maternal-infant bonding*. St. Louis: Mosby.

Klaus, M., & Kennell, J. (1982). *Parent-infant bonding* (2nd ed.). St. Louis: Mosby.

Leonard, V. (1993). Stress and coping in the transition to parenthood of first-time mothers with career commitments: An interpretive study. Doctoral dissertation, University of California, San Francisco, *Dissertation Abstracts International, 54*(08A), 3221.

Martell, L. (2001). Heading toward the new normal: A contemporary postpartum experience. *Journal of Obstetric, Gynecologic, and Neonatal Nursing, 30*(5), 496-506.

Mercer, R. (2004). Becoming a mother versus maternal role attainment. *Journal of Nursing Scholarship, 36*(3), 226-232.

Miller, E. (2004). Infant massage: A nurturing welcome to the world. *New Life Journal*, August-September.

Nelson, A. (2003). Transition to motherhood. *Journal of Obstetric, Gynecologic, and Neonatal Nursing, 32*(4), 465-477.

Osterwell, D. (1991). *Correlates of relationship satisfaction in lesbian couples who are parenting their first child together.* Doctoral dissertation, Berkeley, California School of Professional Psychology.

Reimann, R. (1999). *Becoming lesbian mothers: Lesbian couples' transition to parenthood.* 1999 ASA Conference proceedings. Washington, D.C.: American Sociological Association.

Rubin, R. (1967). Attainment of the maternal role. Part 1. Processes. *Nursing Research, 16*(4), 237-245.

Simmons, T., & Dye, J. (2003). Grandparents living with grandchildren. Internet document available at www.census.gov/prod/2003pubs/c2Kbr-31.pdf. Accessed October 5, 2006.

St. John, W., Cameron, C., & McVeigh, C. (2005). Meeting the challenges of new fatherhood during the early weeks. *Journal of Obstetric, Gynecologic, and Neonatal Nursing, 34*(2), 180-190.

Steinberg, S., Kruckman, L., & Steinberg, S. (2000). Reinventing fatherhood in Japan and Canada. *Social Science Medicine, 50*(9), 1257-1272.

Stewart, S., & Jambunathan, J. (1996). Hmong women and postpartum depression. *Health Care for Women International, 17*(4), 319-330.

Wisner, K., Parry, B., & Piontek, C. (2002). Clinical practice. Postpartum depression. *New England Journal of Medicine, 347*(3), 194-199.

Zlotnick, M. (2000). Infant massage: Building relationships through touch. *International Journal of Childbirth Education, 15*(1), 36-38.

Kathryn Rhodes Alden

Physiologic and Behavioral Adaptations of the Newborn

learning objectives

- Discuss the physiologic adaptations that the neonate must make during the period of transition from the intrauterine to the extrauterine environment.
- Describe the behavioral adaptations that are characteristic of the newborn during the transition period.
- Explain mechanisms of thermoregulation in the neonate and the potential consequences of hypothermia and hyperthermia.

- Recognize newborn reflexes and differentiate characteristic responses from abnormal responses.
- Discuss the sensory and perceptual functioning of the neonate.

electronic resources

Additional information related to the content in Chapter 25 can be found on

the companion website at **evolve**
http://evolve.elsevier.com/Lowdermilk/MWHC/
- NCLEX Review Questions
- Case Study: Newborn Health Problems
- WebLinks

or on the interactive companion CD
- NCLEX Review Questions
- Anatomy Review: Sutures and Fontanels
- Case Study: Newborn Health Problems
- Critical Thinking Exercise: Jaundice
- Skill: Thermoregulation
- Video: Crying female neonate, male breasts (supine position), cremasteric reflex, buttocks, neck (posterior), upper extremities, legs (symmetry, length), Moro reflex, plantar grasp, rooting and sucking

THE neonatal period includes the time from birth through day 28 of life. During this time the neonate must make many physiologic and behavioral adaptations to extrauterine life. Physiologic adjustment tasks are those that involve (1) establishing and maintaining respirations; (2) adjusting to circulatory changes; (3) regulating temperature; (4) ingesting, retaining, and digesting nutrients; (5) eliminating waste; and (6) regulating weight. Behavioral tasks include (1) establishing a regulated behavioral tempo independent of the mother, which involves self-regulation of arousal, self-monitoring of changes in state, and patterning of sleep; (2) processing, storing, and organizing multiple stimuli; and (3) establishing a relationship with caregivers and the environment. The term infant usually makes these adjustments with little or no difficulty.

■ TRANSITION TO EXTRAUTERINE LIFE

Newborn infants undergo a predictable series of events during the first 6 to 8 hours of life as they are transitioning from intrauterine to extrauterine existence. This transition period represents a time of vulnerability for the neonate and warrants careful observation by nurses. To detect disorders in adaptation soon after birth, nurses must be aware of normal features of the transition period. Labor and immediate neonatal events stimulate a sympathetic response reflected by changes in heart rate, color, respiration, motor activity, gastrointestinal function, and temperature of the infant. Behavioral characteristics also change during this transition period.

The first phase of the transition period lasts up to 30 minutes after birth and is called the *first period of reactivity.* The newborn's heart rate increases rapidly to 160 to

180 beats/min but gradually decreases after 30 minutes or so to a baseline rate of between 100 and 120 beats/min. Respirations are irregular for the first 15 minutes after birth, with a possible rate between 60 and 80 breaths/min. There may be pauses for up to 10 seconds between respirations. Crackles may be present on auscultation; audible grunting, nasal flaring, and retractions of the chest also may be noted. Coincident with these changes in heart rate and respiratory rate, the infant is alert. The infant's behavior is marked by spontaneous startle reactions, tremors, crying, and movement of the head from side to side. This characteristic exploratory behavior is accompanied by a decrease in body temperature and generalized increase in motor activity, with an increase in muscle tone. At this time, bowel sounds may be absent and there is minimal saliva (Hernandez, Fashaw, & Evans, 2005).

Between 30 minutes and 2 hours after birth, the neonate enters a *period of decreased responsiveness,* characterized by a marked decrease in motor activity and/or sleep. Respirations are rapid and shallow with a rate of up to 60 breaths per minute. The heart rate averages 100 to 120 beats/min. At this time the infant's color is pink. Bowel sounds are audible, and peristaltic waves may be noted over the abdomen. This period lasts for 60 to 100 minutes and is followed by a second period of reactivity (Hernandez et al., 2005).

The second period of reactivity occurs roughly between 2 and 8 hours after birth. This *second period of reactivity* lasts from 10 minutes to several hours. The infant becomes more responsive to all types of stimuli. Periods of tachycardia and tachypnea occur, associated with increased muscle tone, skin color, and mucus production. Meconium is commonly passed at this time. As this period diminishes, the infant is relatively stable (Hernandez et al., 2005).

All well newborns experience this transition, regardless of gestational age or type of birth. The length of time the periods last will vary depending on the amount and kind of stress experienced by the neonate before or after birth.

▬ PHYSIOLOGIC ADAPTATIONS

Respiratory System

As the infant emerges from the intrauterine environment and the umbilical cord is severed, profound adaptations are necessary for survival. The most critical of these adaptations is the establishment of effective respirations. Most newborns breathe spontaneously after birth and are able to maintain adequate oxygenation. Preterm infants often encounter respiratory difficulties related to immaturity of the lungs.

Initiation of Breathing

During intrauterine life, oxygenation of the fetus occurs through transplacental gas exchange. However, at birth the lungs must be established as the site of gas exchange. In utero, the fetus shunted blood away from the lungs, but when birth occurs, the pulmonary vasculature must be fully perfused for this purpose. Clamping of the umbilical cord causes a rise in blood pressure, which increases circulation and lung perfusion (Bloom, 2006).

It has been recognized that there is no one single trigger for newborn respiratory function. The initiation of respirations in the neonate is the result of a combination of chemical, mechanical, thermal, and sensory factors that stimulate the respiratory center in the medulla.

Chemical Factors. The activation of chemoreceptors in the carotid arteries and the aorta results from the relative state of hypoxia associated with labor. With each labor contraction, there is a temporary decrease in uterine blood flow and transplacental gas exchange resulting in transient fetal hypoxia and hypercarbia. While the fetus is able to recover between contractions, there appears to be a cumulative effect that results in progressive decline in Po_2, increased Pco_2, and lowered blood pH. Decreased levels of oxygen and increased levels of carbon dioxide seem to have a cumulative effect that is involved in the initiation of neonatal breathing. Another chemical factor may also play a role: it is thought that as a result of the clamping of the cord, there is a drop in levels of a prostaglandin that may inhibit respirations (Bloom, 2006; Hansen & Corbet, 2005).

Mechanical Factors. Respirations in the newborn may be stimulated by changes in intrathoracic pressure resulting from compression of the chest during vaginal birth. As the infant passes through the birth canal, the chest is compressed. With birth, this pressure on the chest is released and the negative intrathoracic pressure helps draw air into the lungs.

Thermal Factors. With birth, the newborn enters the extrauterine environment, in which the temperature is significantly lower. The profound change in environmental temperature stimulates receptors in the skin resulting in stimulation of the respiratory center in the medulla.

Sensory Factors. Sensory stimulation occurs in a variety of ways with birth. Some of these include handling of the infant by the physician or midwife, suctioning of the mouth and nose, and drying by the nurses. Pain associated with birth may also be a factor. The lights, sounds, and smells of the new environment may also be involved in stimulation of the respiratory center.

Breathing movements that began in utero as intermittent become continuous after birth, although the mechanism for this is not well understood. Respirations are often irregular, with short, periodic pauses. If the pause is longer than 20 seconds, it is known as apnea (Rigatto, 2004).

At term the lungs hold approximately 20 ml of fluid per kilogram. Air must be substituted for the fluid that filled the respiratory tract in utero. It has been traditionally thought that the thoracic squeeze occurring during normal vaginal birth resulted in significant clearance of lung fluid. However, it appears that this event has a minor role in the clearance of lung fluid. In the days preceding labor, there is a reduction in production of fetal lung fluid and a concomitant decrease in alveolar fluid volume. The process of labor provides a powerful stimulus for fluid clearance. The movement of lung fluid from the air spaces

EVIDENCE-BASED PRACTICE

Newborn Resuscitation: Room Air Versus Oxygen

BACKGROUND

- Most newborns transition from the uterus to breathing without help, but 5% to 10% do not breathe spontaneously and need resuscitation to avoid ischemic injury and death. Use of 100% oxygen has been conventional practice, but excess oxygen increases the work of breathing and releases free radicals, which can lead to retinopathy and bronchopulmonary dysplasia. Developing countries have the most birth asphyxia, yet have limited access to oxygen. Some animal studies have supported the efficacy of room air resuscitation.

OBJECTIVES

- The goal of the review was to compare the use of room air versus 100% oxygen during resuscitation of term newborns. The primary outcomes were death up to 5 years of age and neurologic disability, such as cerebral palsy or lower intelligence quotient (IQ). Secondary outcomes included Apgar scores, evidence of hypoxic ischemic encephalopathy, retinopathy, lung problems, vital signs, and blood gasses.

METHODS

Search Strategy

- The authors searched on-line databases, reference lists, and consulted experts in the field. They identified five randomized or quasi-randomized controlled trials, dated 1993 to 2003 and involving 1302 infants. Countries of origin were not noted, but the three largest studies, representing 1124 infants, were in developing countries.

Statistical Analyses

- Similar data were pooled. Reviewers calculated relative risk for dichotomous (categoric) data, such as presence of retinopathy, and weighted mean difference for continuous data, such as time to established respirations. Differences between groups outside the 95% confidence interval were accepted as significant. All were analyzed in their originally randomly assigned "intention to treat" categories, even though 26% of the room air group was given backup oxygen.

FINDINGS

- Although no individual study found significant differences in death rates, the pooled data allowed the statistical power

to determine that the death rate was significantly reduced for the room air group over the oxygen group. The air group demonstrated less time to established respirations and higher 5-minute Apgar scores. No differences were noted for neurologic outcomes at age 5 years, neurodevelopmental markers (cerebral palsy, time of developmental milestones, cranial ultrasound, electroencephalogram [EEG]), time to established heart rate over 100 beats/min, or results of arterial blood gas within 2 hours of birth. None of the studies reported lung or eye outcomes.

LIMITATIONS

- Generalizability and recommendations are limited by the small number of studies and the small samples. Oxygen use has been entrenched in medical practice for decades, making it difficult to compare to an alternative treatment. Its use for one quarter of the room air group limits interpretation of results. It is difficult to design a randomized controlled trial around an unpredictable, emergent condition. Limitations in randomization and blinding in some studies may have introduced bias. Follow-up was only at 28 days, or lost, bringing into question the true nature of neurodevelopmental outcomes. The preponderance of the trials occurred in developing countries, where care may be very different from developed countries.

IMPLICATIONS FOR PRACTICE

- Resuscitation with room air seems to be beneficial for term infants, causing fewer deaths than oxygen, and no evidence of harm. However, the authors do not yet recommend changing policies from oxygen to room air. Room air resuscitation shows promise as a choice in low-resource settings, with back up oxygen recommended.

IMPLICATIONS FOR FURTHER RESEARCH

- Larger trials are needed, from developed and developing countries. Randomization and blinding are necessary. Still unanswered is the question about long-term neurodevelopmental outcomes. The effect of oxygen versus room air for preterm infants on lung and eye outcomes needs investigation.

Reference: Tan, A., Schulze, A., O'Donnell, C., & Davis, P. (2005). Air versus oxygen for resuscitation of infants at birth. *The Cochrane Database of Systematic Reviews*, 2006, Issue 3. Chichester, UK: John Wiley & Sons.

occurs through active transport into the interstitium, with drainage occurring through the pulmonary circulation and lymphatic system. Retention of lung fluid may interfere with the infant's ability to maintain adequate oxygenation, especially if other factors (e.g., meconium aspiration, congenital diaphragmatic hernia, esophageal atresia with fistula, choanal atresia, congenital cardiac defect, immature alveoli) that compromise respirations are present. Infants born by cesarean in which labor did not occur prior to birth may experience some retention of lung fluid, although it typically clears without deleterious effects on the infant (Barker & Southern, 2004).

As the lungs expand after birth, surfactant release is stimulated. The alveoli of the term infant's lungs are lined with surfactant, a protein manufactured in type II cells of the lungs. Lung expansion is largely dependent on chest wall contraction and adequate secretion of surfactant. Surfactant reduces surface tension, therefore reducing the pressure required to keep the alveoli open with inspiration, and prevents total alveolar collapse on exhalation, thereby maintaining alveolar stability. The decreased surface tension results in increased lung compliance, helping to establish the functional residual capacity of the lungs (Bloom, 2006).

■ **NURSE ALERT**

Newborn infants are by preference nose breathers. The reflex response to nasal obstruction is to open the mouth to maintain an airway. This response is not present in most infants until 3 weeks after birth; therefore cyanosis or asphyxia may occur with nasal blockage.

Signs of Respiratory Distress

Certain respiratory patterns are characteristic of the normal term newborn. After respirations are established, breaths are shallow and irregular, ranging from 30 to 60 breaths/min, with short pauses of less than 15 seconds. These pauses in respirations occur most often during the active (rapid eye movement [REM]) sleep cycle and decrease in frequency and duration with age. Apneic episodes (longer than 20 seconds) should be evaluated.

Most term infants breathe spontaneously and continue to have normal respirations (Fig. 25-1, *A*). However, infants can manifest other problems through respiratory distress. Signs of respiratory distress may include nasal flaring, retractions (in-drawing of tissue between the ribs, below the rib cage, or above the sternum and clavicles), or grunting with expirations. Any increased use of the intercostal muscles may be a sign of distress. Seesaw respirations, instead of normal abdominal respirations, are not normal and should be reported (Fig. 25-1, *B*). Pallor or central cyanosis (seen as circumoral cyanosis) is often associated with respiratory difficulty. Within the first hour after birth the respiratory rate is between 40 and 60 breaths/min and should thereafter range from 30 to 60 breaths/min. A respiratory rate that is less than 30 or greater than 60 breaths/min with the infant at rest must be further evaluated. The respiratory rate of the infant may be slowed or depressed by the analgesics or anesthetics administered to the mother during labor and birth. Apneic episodes may be related to a number of events (rapid increase in body temperature; hypothermia, low blood glucose, and sepsis) that require careful evaluation. Tachypnea may result from inadequate clearance of lung

FIG. 25-1 Comparison of normal and seesaw respirations. **A,** Normal respiration. Chest and abdomen rise with inspiration. **B,** Seesaw respiration. Chest wall retracts and abdomen rises with inspiration. (Courtesy Mead Johnson & Co., Evansville, IN.)

fluid, or it may be an indication of newborn respiratory distress syndrome (RDS) (Bloom, 2006).

In the majority of newborn infants, auscultation of the chest reveals loud, clear breath sounds that seem very near, because little chest tissue intervenes. Breath sounds should be clear and equal bilaterally. The ribs of the infant articulate with the spine at a horizontal rather than a downward slope; consequently, the rib cage cannot expand with inspiration as readily as that of an adult. Because neonatal respiratory function is largely a matter of diaphragmatic contraction, abdominal breathing is characteristic of newborns. The newborn infant's chest and abdomen rise simultaneously with inspiration (see Fig. 25-1, *A*). Characteristics of the respiratory system of the neonate and the effects of these characteristics on respiratory function are listed in Table 25-1.

table 25-1	Characteristics of the Respiratory System of the Neonate
CHARACTERISTIC	**EFFECT ON FUNCTION**
Lung elastic tissue and recoil decreased	Lung compliance decreased; more work and higher pressure are required to expand; risk of atelectasis
Movement of diaphragm limited	Respiratory movement less effective; risk of atelectasis
By preference a nose breather; larynx and epiglottis high	Can breathe and swallow at the same time; risk of airway obstruction; difficulty intubating
Airway passages small and compliant; airway resistance high; cough reflex weak	Risk of obstruction of airway and apnea
Surfactant system altered in immature infants	Atelectatic areas; work of breathing increased; risk of respiratory distress syndrome (RDS)
Respiratory control immature	Respirations irregular; unable to increase rate and depth of respirations rapidly

From Blackburn, S. (1992). Alterations of the respiratory system in the neonate: Implications for clinical practice. *Journal of Perinatal and Neonatal Nursing, 6*(2), 46-58.

Cardiovascular System

The cardiovascular system changes markedly after birth. The infant's first breaths, combined with increased alveolar capillary distention, inflate the lungs and reduce pulmonary vascular resistance to the pulmonary blood flow from the pulmonary arteries. Pulmonary artery pressure drops, and pressure in the right atrium declines. Increased pulmonary blood flow from the left side of the heart increases pressure in the left atrium, which causes a functional closure of the foramen ovale. During the first few days of life, crying may reverse the flow through the foramen ovale temporarily and lead to mild cyanosis; conditions such as asphyxia may also cause the foramen to reopen. In most infants, it is permanently closed within a few months.

The ductus arteriosus begins to constrict as pulmonary circulation increases and arterial oxygen tension increases. In term infants the ductus arteriosus functionally closes within the first hours after birth hours; permanent closure usually occurs within 3 to 4 weeks. The ductus arteriosus may open in response to low oxygen levels in association with hypoxia, asphyxia, or prematurity. A patent ductus arteriosus may be detected with auscultation of the chest as a heart murmur (Clyman, 2004).

There is rapid constriction of the umbilical vein and arteries within the first 2 minutes after birth. It is thought that this is related to exposure of the cord to the cooler extrauterine environment and to increased oxygenation as the infant begins to breathe. With the clamping and severing of the cord, the umbilical arteries, the umbilical vein, and the ductus venosus are functionally closed; they are converted into ligaments within 2 to 3 months (Adamson, Myatt, & Byrne, 2004). Table 25-2 summarizes the cardiovascular changes at birth.

Heart Rate and Sounds

The term newborn has a resting heart rate between 100 and 160 beats/min, with brief fluctuations above and below these values, usually noted during sleeping and waking states. Shortly after the first cry the infant's heart rate may accelerate as high as 180 beats/min. The range of the heart

---

table 25-2 **Cardiovascular Changes at Birth**

PRENATAL STATUS	POSTBIRTH STATUS	ASSOCIATED FACTORS
PRIMARY CHANGES		
Pulmonary circulation: high pulmonary vascular resistance, increased pressure in right ventricle and pulmonary arteries	Low pulmonary vascular resistance; decreased pressure in right atrium, ventricle, and pulmonary arteries	Expansion of collapsed fetal lung with air
Systemic circulation: low pressures in left atrium, ventricle, and aorta	High systemic vascular resistance; increased pressure in left atrium, ventricle, and aorta	Loss of placental blood flow
SECONDARY CHANGES		
Umbilical arteries: patent, carrying blood from hypogastric arteries to placenta	Functionally closed at birth; obliteration by fibrous proliferation possibly taking 2-3 mo, distal portions becoming lateral ligaments, proximal portions remaining open as superior vesicle arteries	Closure preceding that of umbilical vein, probably accomplished by smooth muscle contraction in response to thermal and mechanical stimuli and alteration in oxygen tension, mechanically severed with cord at birth
Umbilical vein: patent, carrying blood from placenta to ductus venosus and liver	Closed, becoming ligament after obliteration	Closure shortly after umbilical arteries, hence blood from placenta possibly entering neonate for short period after birth, mechanically severed with cord at birth
Ductus venosus: patent, connection of umbilical vein to inferior vena cava	Closed, becoming ligament after obliteration	Loss of blood flow from umbilical vein
Ductus arteriosus: patent, shunting of blood from pulmonary artery to descending aorta	Functionally closed almost immediately after birth, anatomic obliteration of lumen by fibrous proliferation requiring 1-3 mo, becoming ligament	High systemic resistance increasing aortic pressure; low pulmonary resistance reducing pulmonary arterial pressure Increased oxygen content of blood in ductus arteriosus creating vasospasm of its muscular wall
Foramen ovale: formation of a valve opening that allows blood to flow directly to left atrium (shunting of blood from right to left atrium)	Functionally closed at birth, constant apposition gradually leading to fusion and permanent closure within a few months or years in majority of persons	Increased pressure in left atrium and decreased pressure in right atrium causing closure of valve over foramen

Modified from Wong, D. (1999). *Whaley and Wong's nursing care of infants and children* (6th ed.). St. Louis: Mosby.

rate in the term infant is about 85 to 100 beats/min during deep sleep and 120 to 160 beats/min while the infant is awake. A heart rate of 180 beats/min is not unusual when the infant cries. A heart rate that is either high (more than 160 beats/min) or low (fewer than 100 beats/min) should be reevaluated within 30 minutes to 1 hour or when the activity of the infant changes. Immediately after birth the heart rate can be palpated by grasping the base of the umbilical cord.

By term the infant's heart lies midway between the crown of the head and the buttocks, and the axis is more transverse than that in an adult (Fig. 25-2). The apical impulse (point of maximal impulse [PMI]) in the newborn is at the fourth intercostal space and to the left of the midclavicular line. The PMI is often visible because of the thin chest wall.

Apical pulse rates should be determined for all infants. Auscultation should be for a full minute, preferably when the infant is asleep. An irregular heart rate is not uncommon in the first few hours of life. After this time an irregular heart rate not attributed to changes in activity or respiratory pattern should be further evaluated.

Heart sounds during the neonatal period are of higher pitch, shorter duration, and greater intensity than those during adult life. The first sound is typically louder and duller than the second sound, which is sharp. Transient murmurs are common during the first few hours after birth. Most heart murmurs heard during the first few days of life have no pathologic significance; they usually result from a patent ductus arteriosus, tricuspid regurgitation, or the acute angle of the pulmonary artery bifurcation. If a murmur is present, it is important to note the presence of other signs of cardiovascular dysfunction such as tachypnea, tachycardia, pallor, cyanosis, absence of peripheral pulses, or poor perfusion (Miller & Newman, 2005).

FIG. 25-2 Differences in locations of apical pulse in newborn versus in adult. **A,** Neonate. **B,** Adult.

Blood Pressure

Although some institutions continue to assess blood pressure in newborn infants, the routine measurement of blood pressure in the screening of well neonates is no longer recommended by the American Academy of Pediatrics (AAP) and the American Academy of Obstetricians and Gynecologists (ACOG) (2002). A common practice is to obtain four-extremity blood pressures in the presence of any cardiovascular symptoms such as tachycardia, persistent murmur, abnormal pulses, poor perfusion, or abnormal precordial activity (Berryman & Glass, 2005).

Blood pressure varies according to weight and gestational age. The term newborn's average systolic blood pressure (BP) ranges from 60 to 80 mm Hg, and the average diastolic pressure is 40 to 50 mm Hg. A decrease in systolic BP of approximately 15 mm Hg during the first hour of life is common. Neonates are considered hypotensive if the mean BP is less than the gestational age. Hypertension is present if the mean pressure exceeds 50 to 70 mm Hg. Crying and movement result in changes in BP, especially in the systolic pressure. BP also is sensitive to the changes in blood volume that occur with the adaptations in circulation. The measurement of BP is best accomplished with a Doppler device and while the infant is at rest. A correctly sized BP cuff must be used for accurate measurement of an infant's BP (Sniderman & Taeusch, 2005).

Blood Volume

The blood volume of the newborn depends on the amount of blood transferred placentally. The blood volume of the term infant is approximately 85 ml/kg of body weight. Immediately after birth the total blood volume averages 300 ml, but this volume can increase by as much as 100 ml, depending on the length of time the infant is attached to the placenta. Early or late clamping of the umbilical cord changes circulatory dynamics of the newborn. Early clamping of the cord reduces the mean blood volume, whereas late clamping expands the blood volume from the so-called *placental transfusion*. This, in turn, causes an increase in heart size, higher systolic BP, and increased respiratory rate (Luchtman-Jones, Schwartz, & Wilson, 2006).

Signs of Risk for Cardiovascular Problems

Close monitoring of the infant's vital signs is important for early detection of impending problems. Persistent tachycardia (more than 160 beats/min) may be associated with anemia, hypovolemia, hyperthermia, or sepsis. Persistent bradycardia (less than 100 beats/min) may be a sign of a congenital heart block or hypoxemia. A significant difference between upper and lower extremity BPs may be an early sign of coarctation of the aorta (Berryman & Glass, 2005).

The newborn's skin color may be reflective of cardiovascular problems. Pallor in the immediate postpartum period is often symptomatic of underlying problems such as anemia or marked peripheral vasoconstriction as a result of intrapartum asphyxia or sepsis. Any prolonged cyanosis other than in the hands or feet may indicate respiratory and/or cardiac problems. The presence of jaundice may indicate ABO or Rh factor incompatibility problems (see Chapter 38).

Hematopoietic System

The hematopoietic system of the newborn exhibits certain variations from that of the adult. Levels of red blood cells (RBCs) and leukocytes differ, but platelet levels are relatively the same (see Table 25-3 for normal hematologic values in the newborn).

Red Blood Cells

Because fetal circulation is less efficient at oxygen exchange than the lungs, the fetus needs additional RBCs for transport of oxygen in utero. Therefore at birth the average levels of RBCs, hemoglobin, and hematocrit are higher than those in the adult; these levels fall slowly over the first month. At birth, the RBC count ranges from $4.8\text{-}7.1 \times 10^6/\text{mcl}$. The term newborn may have a hemoglobin concentration of 14 to 24 g/dl, decreasing gradually to 12 to 20 g/dl during the first 2 weeks. On the first day, the hematocrit ranges from 44% to 64% and by 8 weeks, it is between 39% and 59%. Polycythemia (central venous hematocrit >65%) may occur in term and preterm infants in relation to factors such as delayed cord clamping, maternal hypertension or diabetes, and intrauterine growth restriction (Pagana & Pagana, 2006).

In addition to delayed clamping of the cord, the source of the sample is another important factor because capillary blood yields higher values than venous blood. The time after birth when the blood sample is obtained also is significant; the slight increase in RBC numbers after birth is followed by a substantial decrease. At birth, 80% of the infant's blood contains fetal hemoglobin, but because of the shorter life span of the cells containing fetal hemoglobin, the percentage decreases to 55% by 5 weeks and to 5% by 20 weeks. Iron stores are generally sufficient to sustain normal RBC production for 5 months, and therefore mild, brief anemia is not serious.

Leukocytes

Leukocytosis, with a white blood cell (WBC) count of approximately $18,000/\text{mm}^3$ (range: 10,000 to $30,000/\text{mm}^3$), is normal at birth. The number of WBCs, predominantly

table 25-3	Normal Hematologic Values in Term Newborns
Hemoglobin	14-24 g/dl
Hematocrit	44%-64%
Red blood cell count	$4,800,000\text{-}7,100,000/\text{mm}^3$
Platelet count	$150,000\text{-}300,000/\text{mm}^3$
White blood cell count	$9,000\text{-}30,000/\text{mm}^3$

From Pagana, K., & Pagana, T. (2006). *Mosby's manual of diagnostic and laboratory tests* (3rd ed.). St. Louis: Mosby.

polymorphonuclear leukocytes, increases to approximately $22,000/\text{mm}^3$ the first day after birth. This early high WBC count of the newborn decreases rapidly, and a resting level of 11,000 to $12,000/\text{mm}^3$ is normally maintained during the neonatal period. Serious infection is not well tolerated by the newborn, and a marked increase in the WBC count is unlikely, even in critical sepsis (infection). In most instances, sepsis is accompanied by a decline in WBCs, particularly in neutrophils. The activity of the bone marrow is accurately reflected by the number of circulating cells, both RBCs and WBCs (Roberts, 2005).

Platelets

The platelet count ranges between 150,000 and $300,000/\text{mm}^3$ and is essentially the same in newborns as in adults. The levels of factors II, VII, IX, and X, found in the liver, are decreased during the first few days of life because the newborn cannot synthesize vitamin K. However, bleeding tendencies in the newborn are rare, and unless the vitamin K deficiency is great, clotting is sufficient to prevent hemorrhage (Pagana & Pagana, 2006).

Blood Groups

The infant's blood group is genetically determined and established early in fetal life. However, during the neonatal period, a gradual increase occurs in the strength of the agglutinogens present in the RBC membrane. Cord blood samples may be used to identify the infant's blood type and Rh status.

Thermogenic System

During the first 12 hours after birth the neonate attempts to achieve thermal balance in adjusting to extrauterine environmental temperature. Thermoregulation is the maintenance of balance between heat loss and heat production. The newborn must adjust to environmental temperatures at least $-6/6°$ C lower than inside the uterus. Rapid cooling occurs, requiring the infant to accelerate heat production. Newborns attempt to stabilize their internal body temperatures within a narrow range.

Anatomic and physiologic characteristics of neonates place them at risk for heat loss. Having less adipose tissue and subcutaneous fat, the newborn's thermal insulation is less than that of an adult. The blood vessels are closer to the surface of the skin. Changes in environmental temperature alter the temperature of the blood, thereby influencing temperature regulation centers in the hypothalamus. Newborns have larger body surface–to–body weight (mass) ratios than do children and adults (Sedin, 2006).

In an effort to conserve heat, term newborns assume a position of flexion that helps guard against heat loss because it diminishes the amount of body surface exposed to the environment. Infants also can reduce the loss of internal heat through the body surface by constricting peripheral blood vessels.

CD: Skill: Thermoregulation

Heat Loss

The body temperature of newborn infants is dependent on the heat transfer between the infant and the external environment. Factors that influence heat loss to the environment include the temperature and humidity of the air, the flow and velocity of the air, and the temperature of surfaces in contact with and around the infant. The goal of care is to maintain a neutral thermal environment for the neonate in which heat balance is maintained (Sedin, 2006).

Heat loss in the newborn occurs by four modes:

- *Convection* is the flow of heat from the body surface to cooler ambient air. Because of heat loss by convection, the ambient temperatures in the nursery are kept at approximately 24° C, and newborns are wrapped to protect them from the cold.
- *Radiation* is the loss of heat from the body surface to a cooler solid surface not in direct contact but in relative proximity. Nursery cribs and examining tables are placed away from outside windows to prevent this type of heat loss.
- *Evaporation* is the loss of heat that occurs when a liquid is converted to a vapor. In the newborn, heat loss by evaporation occurs as a result of vaporization of moisture from the skin. The process is invisible and is known as *insensible water loss (IWL)*. This heat loss can be intensified by failure to dry the newborn directly after birth or by too-slow drying of the infant after a bath.
- *Conduction* is the loss of heat from the body surface to cooler surfaces in direct contact. When admitted to the nursery, the newborn is placed in a warmed crib to minimize heat loss.

Loss of heat must be controlled to protect the infant. Control of such modes of heat loss is the basis of caregiving policies and techniques.

Thermogenesis

In response to cold, the neonate attempts to generate heat (thermogenesis) by increasing muscle activity. Cold infants may cry and appear restless. Because of vasoconstriction, the skin may feel cool to touch, and acrocyanosis may be present. There is an increase in cellular metabolic activity, primarily in the brain, heart, and liver; this also increases oxygen and glucose consumption.

While adults are able to produce heat through shivering, this shivering mechanism of heat production is insignificant in the newborn. The primary mechanism for heat production is nonshivering thermogenesis accomplished by metabolism of brown fat, a type of adipose tissue that is unique to the newborn. Brown fat is located in superficial deposits in the interscapular region and axillae, as well as in deep deposits at the thoracic inlet, along the vertebral column, and around the kidneys. Brown fat has a richer vascular and nerve supply than does ordinary fat. Heat produced by intense lipid metabolic activity in brown fat can warm the newborn by increasing heat production as much as 100%. Reserves of brown fat, usually present for several weeks after birth, are rapidly depleted with cold stress. The less mature the infant, the less reserve of this essential fat is available at birth (Rutter, 2005).

Cold Stress

Cold stress imposes metabolic and physiologic demands on all infants, regardless of gestational age and condition. The respiratory rate increases in response to the increased need for oxygen. In the cold-stressed infant, oxygen consumption and energy are diverted from maintaining normal brain and cardiac function and growth to thermogenesis for survival. If the infant cannot maintain an adequate oxygen tension, vasoconstriction jeopardizes pulmonary perfusion. As a consequence, the partial pressure of arterial oxygen (PO_2) is decreased, and the blood pH declines. These changes aggravate existing RDS. Moreover, decreased pulmonary perfusion and oxygen tension may maintain or reopen the right-to-left shunt across the patent ductus arteriosus.

The basal metabolic rate increases with cold stress (Fig. 25-3). If cold stress is protracted, anaerobic glycolysis occurs, resulting in increased production of acids. Metabolic acidosis develops, and if a defect in respiratory function is present, respiratory acidosis also develops. Excessive fatty acids displace the bilirubin from the albumin-binding sites. The resulting increased level of circulating unbound bilirubin heightens the risk of kernicterus even at serum bilirubin levels of 10 mg/dl or less (Rutter, 2005; Sedin, 2006).

Hyperthermia

Although occurring less frequently than hypothermia, hyperthermia can occur and must be corrected. A body temperature greater than 37.5° C is considered to be

FIG. 25-3 Effects of cold stress. When an infant is stressed by cold, oxygen consumption increases and pulmonary and peripheral vasoconstriction occur, thereby decreasing oxygen uptake by the lungs and oxygen delivery to the tissues; anaerobic glycolysis increases; and there is a decrease in PO_2 and pH, leading to metabolic acidosis.

abnormally high and is typically caused by excess heat production related to sepsis or to a decrease in heat loss. The clinical appearance of the infant who is hyperthermic often indicates the causative mechanism. Infants who are overheated due to environmental factors such as being swaddled in too many blankets, exhibit signs of heat-losing mechanisms: skin vessels dilate, skin appears flushed, hands and feet are warm to touch, and the infant assumes a posture of extension. The newborn who is hyperthermic because of sepsis will appear stressed: vessels in the skin are constricted, color is pale, and hands and feet are cool. Hyperthermia develops more rapidly in the newborn than in the adult because of the larger surface area of an infant. Sweat glands do not function well. Serious overheating of the newborn can cause cerebral damage from dehydration or even heat stroke and death (Sedin, 2006).

Renal System

At term gestation, the kidneys occupy a large portion of the posterior abdominal wall. The bladder lies close to the anterior abdominal wall and is an abdominal as well as a pelvic organ. In the newborn, almost all palpable masses in the abdomen are renal in origin.

A small quantity (approximately 40 ml) of urine is usually present at birth in the bladder of a term infant. Voiding at the time of birth often occurs. During the first 30 hours after birth, 98% of newborns will void. If a newborn has not voided within 48 hours, there may be renal impairment (Vogt, Dell, & Davis, 2006).

■ NURSE ALERT

Noting and recording the first voiding is important. An infant who has not voided by 24 hours should be assessed for adequacy of fluid intake, bladder distention, restlessness, and symptoms of pain. The pediatrician or neonatal nurse practitioner also should be notified.

The frequency of voiding varies according to the amount of fluid intake. It is expected that infants will void at least once during the first 24 hours, and that urination will increase as the infant takes in more fluid through breastfeeding or infant formula. Formula-fed infants may void more frequently; however, in breastfed infants, the urine output increases after the third or fourth day when the mother's milk has "come in." After the fourth day of life, all newborns should have at least six to eight voidings of straw-colored urine every 24 hours.

Normal urine during early infancy is usually straw colored and almost odorless. Sometimes pink-tinged stains (brick dust) appear on the diaper. These stains are caused by uric acid crystals and are normal during the first few days, but if seen later can be a sign of dehydration. Male infants may have some minimal bloody spotting from a circumcision. If there is no apparent cause of bleeding, the physician or neonatal nurse practitioner should be notified.

Fluid and Electrolyte Balance

In the term neonate, 75% of body weight consists of water. At birth, approximately 40% of the body weight is held within the extracellular fluid compartment. An abrupt reduction in extracellular fluid occurs soon after birth (Modi, 2005).

The daily fluid requirement for full-term neonates during the first 2 days of life is 40 to 60 ml/kg; this increases thereafter to 100 to 150 ml/kg/24 hrs (Tsang, DeMarini, & Rath, 2003). Loss of fluid through urine, feces, lungs, increased metabolic rate, and limited fluid intake usually results in a 5% to 10% loss of the birth weight (weight loss greater than 7% should be evaluated by the health care provider). This usually occurs during the first 3 to 5 days of life (Vogt et al., 2006). If the mother is breastfeeding and her milk supply has not come in yet (which happens on the third or fourth day after birth), the neonate is usually protected from dehydration by its increased extracellular fluid volume. The neonate should regain the birth weight within 14 days after birth.

Neonates have a limited ability to concentrate urine, which can increase the risk of dehydration. They are able to dilute urine similarly to adults; however, the kidneys do not manage well with large increases in fluid intake and increase the chance of fluid overload (Modi, 2005).

At birth, the glomerular filtration rate (GFR) of a newborn is approximately 30% to 50% that of the adult. This results in a decreased ability to remove nitrogenous and other waste products from the blood. The GFR rapidly increases during the first month of life as a result of postnatal physiologic changes including decreased renal vascular resistance, increased renal blood flow, and increased filtration pressure (Guignard, 2004).

Sodium reabsorption is decreased as a result of a reduced sodium- or potassium-activated adenosine triphosphatase (ATPase) activity. The decreased ability to excrete excessive sodium results in hypotonic urine compared with plasma, with a higher concentration of sodium, phosphates, chloride, and organic acids and a lower concentration of bicarbonate ions. The infant has a higher renal threshold for glucose.

Bicarbonate concentration and buffering capacity are decreased, which may lead to acidosis and electrolyte imbalance (Modi, 2005).

Signs of Risk for Renal System Problems

The renal system has a wide range of functions. Dysfunction resulting from physiologic abnormalities can range from the lack of a steady stream of urine to gross anomalies. Gross anomalies such as hypospadias and exstrophy of the bladder can be identified easily at birth. Enlarged or cystic kidneys may be identified as masses during abdominal palpation. Some kidney anomalies also can be detected by ultrasound examination during pregnancy.

Gastrointestinal System

The term newborn is capable of swallowing, digesting, metabolizing, and absorbing proteins and simple carbohydrates, and emulsifying fats. With the exception of pancreatic amylase, the characteristic enzymes and digestive juices are present even in low-birth-weight neonates.

Evolve/CD: Case Study: Newborn Health Problems

In the adequately hydrated infant the mucous membrane of the mouth is moist and pink. The hard and soft palates are intact. Retention cysts, small whitish areas (Epstein's pearls), may be found on the gum margins and at the juncture of the hard and soft palate. The cheeks are full because of well-developed sucking pads. These, like the labial tubercles (sucking calluses) on the upper lip, disappear when the sucking period is over, around the age of 12 months.

Coordinated sucking efforts are present in the fetus around 28 weeks of gestation. By 32 to 34 weeks of gestation, the fetus is capable of a mature sucking pattern that is effective in expressing milk from the breast or bottle. Neonatal sucking behavior is influenced by neuromuscular maturity, maternal medications and anesthetics received during labor and birth, and the type of initial feeding (Omari & Rudolph, 2004).

A special mechanism present in normal newborns coordinates the breathing, sucking, and swallowing reflexes necessary for oral feeding. Sucking in the newborn takes place in small bursts of three to eight sucks at a time. In the term newborn, longer and more efficient sucking attempts occur a few hours after birth. The infant is unable to move food from the lips to the pharynx; therefore placing the nipple (breast or bottle) well inside the baby's mouth is necessary. Peristaltic activity in the esophagus is uncoordinated in the first few days of life. It quickly becomes a coordinated pattern in normal infants, and they swallow easily (Omari & Rudolph, 2004).

Teeth begin developing in utero, with enamel formation continuing until about age 10 years. Tooth development is influenced by neonatal or infant illnesses, medications, and illnesses of or medications taken by the mother during pregnancy. The fluoride level in the water supply also influences tooth development. Occasionally an infant may be born with one or more teeth. Native American infants are commonly born with teeth.

Bacteria are not present in the infant's gastrointestinal tract at birth. Soon after birth, oral and anal orifices permit entry of bacteria and air. Generally the highest bacterial concentration is found in the lower portion of the intestine, particularly in the large intestine. Normal colonic bacteria are established within the first week after birth, and normal intestinal flora help synthesize vitamin K, folate, and biotin. Bowel sounds can usually be heard shortly after birth.

The capacity of the stomach varies from 30 to 90 ml, depending on the size of the infant. The emptying time for the stomach is highly variable. Several factors, such as time and volume of feedings or type and temperature of food, may affect the emptying time. The cardiac sphincter is immature, and nervous control of the stomach is not well established, so some regurgitation may occur. Regurgitation during the first day or two of life can be decreased by avoiding overfeeding, by burping the infant, and by positioning the infant with the head slightly elevated.

Digestion

The infant's ability to digest carbohydrates, fats, and proteins is regulated by the presence of certain enzymes. Most of these enzymes are functional at birth. One exception is amylase, produced by the salivary glands after about 3 months and by the pancreas at about 6 months of age. This enzyme is necessary to convert starch into maltose. The other exception is lipase, also secreted by the pancreas; it is necessary for the digestion of fat. Therefore the normal newborn is capable of digesting simple carbohydrates and proteins but has a limited ability to digest fats.

Further digestion and absorption of nutrients occur in the small intestine in the presence of pancreatic secretions, secretions from the liver through the common bile duct, and secretions from the duodenal portion of the small intestine.

Stools

At birth the lower intestine is filled with meconium. Meconium is formed during fetal life from the amniotic fluid and its constituents, intestinal secretions (including bilirubin), and cells (shed from the mucosa). Meconium is greenish black and viscous and contains occult blood. The first meconium passed is sterile, but within hours, all meconium passed contains bacteria. The majority of normal term infants pass meconium within the first 12 hours of life, and almost all do so by 24 hours. If no bowel movement has been passed by 72 hours, the infant may have an obstructive bowel problem (Miller & Newman, 2005). Stools change in color and consistency over the first 2 to 3 days as the infant feeds. Breast milk stools are generally more frequent and more liquid than formula stools. They contain small, yellow curds, whereas formula stools are more pasty in appearance, with larger, green-brown curds. Progressive changes in the appearance of stools and in the stooling pattern indicate a properly functioning gastrointestinal system (Box 25-1). Stooling also is an indicator of the adequacy of nutritional intake. For example, breastfed infants should have at least three stools per 24 hours after day 3 or 4 of life, when the mother's milk has increased in amount and has changed to mature milk. Formula-fed infants may stool less often, because formula tends to be more constipating than breast milk.

Feeding Behaviors

Variations occur among infants regarding interest in food, symptoms of hunger, and amount ingested at one time. The amount of food that the infant takes in at any feeding depends on the size, hunger level, and alertness of the infant. When put to breast, some infants feed immediately, whereas others require a longer learning period before breastfeeding is completely effective. Random hand-to-mouth movement and sucking of fingers are well developed at birth and intensify when the infant is hungry. Caregivers should be alert and responsive to these hunger cues (Lawrence & Lawrence, 2005).

| box 25-I | Bowel Elimination Pattern of Newborns |

MECONIUM

- First stool composed of amniotic fluid and its constituents, intestinal secretions, shed mucosal cells, and possibly blood (ingested maternal blood or minor bleeding of alimentary tract vessels).
- Passage of meconium should occur within first 24 to 48 hours. If no stool by 72 hours, there may be an obstructive problem.

TRANSITIONAL STOOLS

- Usually appear by third day after initiation of feeding; greenish brown to yellowish brown, thin, and less sticky than meconium; may contain some milk curds.

MILK STOOL

- Usually appears by fourth day.
- Breastfed infants: stools yellow to golden, pasty in consistency, may contain small, yellow curds, with an odor similar to that of sour milk. Expect 3 to 4 stools every 24 hours if infant receiving adequate feedings.
- Formula-fed infants: stools pale yellow to light brown, firmer in consistency, with a more offensive odor. Fewer stools than breastfed infants; one or two daily, or may have only one stool every 2 to 3 days.

Signs of Risk for Gastrointestinal Problems

The time, color, and character of the infant's first stool should be noted. A lack of passage of stool could indicate bowel obstruction related to conditions such as an inborn error of metabolism (e.g., cystic fibrosis) or a congenital disorder (e.g., Hirschsprung disease or an imperforate anus). An active rectal "wink" reflex (contraction of the anal sphincter muscle in response to touch) usually is a good sign of sphincter tone.

Fullness of the abdomen above the umbilicus may be due to problems such as hepatomegaly, duodenal atresia, or distention. Abdominal distention at birth usually indicates a serious disorder such as a ruptured viscus (from abdominal wall defects) or tumors. Distention that occurs later may be the result of overfeeding or may signal gastrointestinal disorders. A scaphoid (sunken) abdomen, with bowel sounds heard in the chest and signs of respiratory distress indicate a diaphragmatic hernia. Fullness below the umbilicus may indicate a distended bladder (Hernandez & Glass, 2005).

Some infants do not digest specific formulas well. If an infant is allergic to or unable to digest a formula, the stools may become very soft with a high water content that is signaled by a distinct water ring around the stool on the diaper. Forceful ejection of stool and a water ring around the stool are signs of diarrhea. Care must be taken to avoid misinterpreting transitional stools for diarrhea. The loss of fluid in diarrhea can rapidly lead to fluid and electrolyte imbalance. Passage of meconium from the vagina or urinary meatus is a sign of a possible fistulous tract from the rectum.

The amount and frequency of regurgitation ("spitting up") after feedings must be recorded. Color change, gagging, and projectile (very forceful) vomiting occur in association with esophageal and tracheoesophageal anomalies.

Hepatic System

The liver plays an important role in iron storage, carbohydrate metabolism, conjugation of bilirubin, and coagulation. In the newborn the liver can be palpated about 1 to 3.5 cm below the right costal margin in the midclavicular line. An enlarged liver (hepatomegaly) may be associated with congenital heart problems, hemolytic disease, or infection. The liver edge is normally sharp and soft, and the hepatic surface is smooth. If the liver edge is full or firm, this may indicate increased total blood volume, increased extramedullary hematopoiesis, or chronic infection (Hernandez & Glass, 2005).

Iron Storage

The infant's iron store in the liver is proportional to the body weight and, for the term infant, should be sufficient for the first 4 to 6 months. Preterm and small-for-date infants have lower iron stores, which are sufficient for only 2 to 3 months. Although both breast milk and cow's milk contain iron, the bioavailability of iron in breast milk is far superior. Full-term infants who are breastfed do not need supplemental iron for 6 months, whereas formula-fed infants should receive a formula that contains supplemental iron (Luchtman-Jones et al., 2006).

Carbohydrate Metabolism

At birth the newborn is cut off from its maternal glucose supply and, as a result, has an initial decrease in serum glucose, reaching its lowest level between 30 and 90 minutes after birth. In most healthy term newborns, blood glucose levels stabilize at 40 to 80 mg/dl during the first several hours after birth; by the end of the first week, blood glucose levels should be approximately 60 to 70 mg/dl. The initiation of feedings assists in the stabilization of the newborn's blood glucose levels. If the infant appears to be jittery or has tremors, the blood glucose level should be determined to rule out hypoglycemia. In general, blood glucose levels below 35 mg/dl are considered abnormal and warrant intervention. Hypoglycemia in the initial newborn period is most often transient and easily corrected through feeding. Persistent or recurrent hypoglycemia necessitates intravenous glucose therapy and may necessitate pharmacologic intervention (Kalhan & Parimi, 2006).

Conjugation of Bilirubin

Bilirubin is a yellow pigment derived from the hemoglobin released with the breakdown of RBCs and the myoglobin in muscle cells. The hemoglobin is phagocytized by the reticuloendothelial cells, converted to bilirubin, and released in an unconjugated form. Unconjugated bilirubin, termed

CD: Critical Thinking Exercise: Jaundice

indirect bilirubin, is relatively insoluble and almost entirely bound to circulating albumin, a plasma protein. The unbound bilirubin can leave the vascular system and permeate other extravascular tissues (e.g., the skin, sclera, and oral mucous membranes). The resultant yellow coloring is termed *jaundice* (Wong, DeSandre, Sibley, & Stevenson, 2006).

In the liver the unbound bilirubin is conjugated with glucuronide in the presence of the enzyme glucuronyl transferase. The conjugated form of bilirubin is excreted from liver cells as a constituent of bile. This form is termed *direct bilirubin* and is water soluble. Along with other components of bile, direct bilirubin is excreted into the biliary tract system, which carries the bile into the duodenum. Bilirubin is converted to urobilinogen and stercobilinogen within the duodenum by the action of the bacterial flora. Urobilinogen is excreted in urine and feces; stercobilinogen is excreted in the feces (Fig. 25-4). The total serum bilirubin level is the sum of the levels of both conjugated (direct) and unconjugated (indirect) bilirubin.

Adequate serum albumin–binding sites are available unless the infant has asphyxia neonatorum (respiratory failure in the newborn), cold stress, or hypoglycemia. A mother's prebirth ingestion of medications such as sulfa drugs and aspirin can reduce the amount of serum albumin–binding sites in the newborn. Although the neonate has the functional capacity to convert bilirubin, physiologic hyperbilirubinemia commonly occurs in infants (Wong et al., 2006).

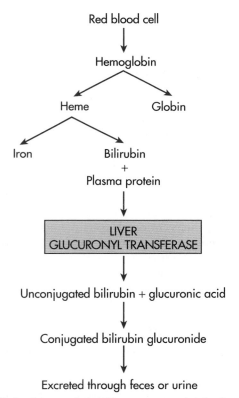

FIG. 25-4 Formation and excretion of bilirubin. (From Hockenberry, M. [2003]. *Wong's nursing care of infants and children* [7th ed.]. St. Louis: Mosby.)

Physiologic Jaundice

Physiologic jaundice or neonatal jaundice, or hyperbilirubinemia, occurs in as many as 60% of newborn infants but is more severe in preterm infants (Reiser, 2004). The incidence and severity of physiologic jaundice is increased in Asian and Native American infants. Although neonatal jaundice is considered benign, bilirubin may accumulate to hazardous levels and lead to a pathologic condition. Physiologic jaundice results from characteristics of normal newborn physiology, such as increased bilirubin production resulting from increased RBC mass, shortened life span of the fetal RBCs, and liver immaturity. Newborns also tend to resorb bilirubin from the small intestine.

The infant who is diagnosed with physiologic jaundice appears to be otherwise well and exhibits signs of jaundice after age 24 hours. Jaundice is clinically visible when bilirubin levels reach 5 to 7 mg/dl. Clinically the indirect bilirubin (unconjugated) is no more than 12 mg/dl by 3 days of age. In preterm infants the peak is higher (15 mg/dl) and tends to occur later. The peak indirect bilirubin level may be higher in breastfed infants (15 to 17 mg/dl). Jaundice is considered to be pathologic if it appears before 24 hours of age, increases more than 0.5 mg/dl/hr, peaks at greater than 13 mg/dl in a term infant, or is associated with anemia and hepatosplenomegaly. Jaundice that appears before 24 hours of age always warrants immediate attention. Pathologic jaundice is usually caused by blood group incompatibility or infection but may rarely be the result of RBC enzyme defects (glucose-6-phosphate dehydrogenase [G6PD], pyruvate kinase), RBC membrane disorders (spherocytosis, ovalocytosis), or hemoglobinopathy (thalassemia) (Frank & Frank, 2002).

CRITICAL THINKING EXERCISE

Jaundice in the Newborn

Margaret gave birth to a 6 lb baby boy 36 hours ago vaginally with the assistance of vacuum extraction. By dates and gestational assessment, the baby was estimated to be 38 weeks of gestation. As a result of the vacuum extraction, the baby's occiput is bruised and slightly edematous (caput succedeaneum). For the first 24 hours, he was very sleepy and difficult to arouse for feedings, but for the last 12 hours he has breastfed approximately every 3 hours for approximately 15 minutes. He has voided twice and passed only one small meconium stool since birth. The father was holding the baby this morning and stated, "Look at his handsome skin tones! Why, he looks like he has already been on vacation and started to get his suntan."

1. Evidence—Is there sufficient evidence to draw conclusions about the baby's skin color?
2. Assumptions—What assumptions can be made about the following?
   a. The baby's skin color
   b. Baby's intake and output since birth
   c. The parents' understanding of physiologic jaundice
3. What implications and priorities for nursing care can be made at this time?
4. Does the evidence objectively support your conclusion?
5. Are there alternative perspectives to your conclusion?

■ **NURSE ALERT**

At any serum bilirubin level, the appearance of jaundice during the first 24 hours of life or persistence beyond day 7 usually indicates a pathologic process.

Jaundice appears in a cephalocaudal manner. It is generally first noticed in the head, especially the sclera and mucous membranes, and then progresses gradually to the thorax, abdomen, and extremities. It dissipates in the reverse order.

Feeding practices may influence the appearance and degree of physiologic hyperbilirubinemia. Early (within the first hour) and frequent feeding tends to keep the serum bilirubin level low by stimulating intestinal activity (the gastrocolic reflex) and passage of meconium.

Cold stress of the newborn may result in acidosis and increase the level of free fatty acids. In the presence of acidosis, albumin binding of bilirubin is weakened, and bilirubin is freed.

Kernicterus, or acute bilirubin encephalopathy, is the most serious complication of neonatal hyperbilirubinemia. It occurs when bilirubin is deposited in the basal ganglia and brainstem, disrupting neuronal function and metabolism. Kernicterus usually occurs when bilirubin levels are higher than 25 mg/dl but may be noted with levels that are lower than 20 mg/dl in the presence of sepsis, meningitis, hypothermia, hypoglycemia, prematurity, and bilirubin-displacing drugs. In the acute stage of kernicterus, the infant is lethargic and hypotonic and has a poor suck. If untreated, the infant becomes hypertonic (with backward arching of the neck and trunk), has a high-pitched cry, and may develop fever. If an infant survives kernicterus, there may be residual cerebral palsy, epilepsy, and mental retardation. Although neonatal jaundice is common and kernicterus is rare, in recent years there has been a resurgence in the number of infants with kernicterus. This may be related to the shortened hospital stays after birth, an increase in the incidence of neonatal jaundice, and a lack of concern and attention to infants exhibiting signs of jaundice (Bhutani, Johnson, & Keren, 2005; Maisels, 2005a; Maisels, 2005b) (see Chapter 26). The Joint Commission on Accreditation of Healthcare Organizations (JCAHO) (2001) issued a sentinel event alert with guidelines for the prevention of neonatal kernicterus by health care workers and institutions.

Jaundice Associated with Breastfeeding

Breastfeeding is associated with an increased incidence of jaundice. Two types have been identified; however, nomenclature may vary among experts. Breastfeeding-associated jaundice (early-onset jaundice) begins at 2 to 4 days of age and occurs in approximately 10% to 25% of breastfed newborns. The jaundice is related to the process of breastfeeding and probably results from decreased caloric and fluid intake by breastfed infants before the milk supply is well established; this is related to decreased hepatic clearance of bilirubin. Breast milk jaundice (late-onset jaundice) has been defined as a progressive indirect hyperbilirubinemia beyond the first week of life; it typically occurs after 3 to 5 days of age and peaks by about 2 weeks. Despite high levels of bilirubin that may persist for 3 to 12 weeks, these infants are well. The jaundice may be caused by factors in the breast milk that either inhibit the conjugation or decrease the excretion of bilirubin. Less frequent stooling by breastfed infants in the first few days of life may allow for extended time for reabsorption of bilirubin from stools (Wong et al., 2006). (See Chapter 27 for a discussion of this topic.)

Coagulation

The liver plays an important role in blood coagulation. Coagulation factors, which are synthesized in the liver, are activated by vitamin K. The lack of intestinal bacteria needed to synthesize vitamin K results in a transient blood coagulation deficiency between days 2 and 5 of life. The levels of coagulation factors slowly increase to reach adult levels by age 9 months. An injection of vitamin K soon after birth helps prevent bleeding problems. Any bleeding problems noted in an infant should be reported immediately, and tests for clotting ordered (Luchtman-Jones et al., 2006).

Signs of Risk for Hepatic System Problems

Some problems such as kernicterus and hypoglycemia have already been discussed. The infant's hemoglobin levels must be assessed for anemia. Because infants may develop a coagulation deficiency, a male child who has been circumcised must be observed closely for signs of hemorrhage. Hemorrhage also could be caused by a clotting defect, indicating a serious problem such as hemophilia.

Immune System
Immunity

Beginning early in gestation, the immune system of the fetus is developing the capacity to respond to foreign antigens. The development of the immune system is necessary to equip the neonate to meet the numerous environmental challenges (microorganisms) associated with life in the extrauterine world.

At birth, most of the circulating antibodies in the newborn are immunoglobulin G (IgG) antibodies that were transported across the placenta from the maternal circulation. This transfer of antibodies from the mother begins as early as at 14 weeks of gestation and is greatest during the third trimester. By term, the IgG levels in the cord blood of the infant are higher than those in maternal blood. The passive immunity afforded the infant through the placental transfer of IgG usually provides sufficient antimicrobial protection during the first 3 months of life. Production of adult concentrations of IgG is reached by 4 to 6 years of age (Cant & Gennery, 2005; Kapur, Yoder, & Polin, 2006).

The fetus is capable of producing IgM by the eighth week of gestation, and low levels are present at term (<10% of adult levels). By the age of 2 years, IgM reaches adult levels. The production of IgA, IgD and IgE is much more gradual, and maximal levels are not attained until early childhood (Kapur et al., 2006).

Natural barrier mechanisms such as the acidity of the stomach and the production of pepsin and trypsin, which maintain sterility of the small intestine, are not fully developed until age 3 to 4 weeks.

The membrane-protective IgA is missing from the respiratory and urinary tracts, and unless the newborn is breast-fed, it also is absent from the gastrointestinal tract. Breast milk provides the newborn with important immunity. The secretory IgA in human milk acts locally in the intestines to neutralize bacterial and viral pathogens. It may also lessen the risk of allergy and food intolerance through modulation of exposure to foreign milk protein antigens (Cant & Gennery, 2005).

The newborn is capable of producing a protective immune response to vaccines, given as early as a few hours after birth. For example, when hepatitis B vaccine is administered at birth to the infant born to a mother with hepatitis B, there is an excellent immune response. This holds true even if the infant does not receive additional hepatitis B immunoglobulins.

The white blood cells of the newborn display a delayed response to invading bacteria. The influx of phagocytic cells to areas of inflammation is somewhat slowed, although the ability of these cells to attack and destroy bacteria is equivalent to that of adults (Kapur et al., 2006).

Risk for Infection

All newborns, and preterm newborns especially, are at high risk for infection during the first several months of life. During this period, infection is one of the leading causes of morbidity and mortality. The newborn cannot limit the invading pathogen to the portal of entry because of the generalized hypofunctioning of the inflammatory and immune mechanisms.

Early signs of infection must be recognized so that prompt diagnosis and treatment may ensue. Temperature instability or hypothermia may be symptomatic of serious infection; newborns do not typically exhibit fever, although hyperthermia can occur (temperature >38° C). Lethargy, irritability, poor feeding, vomiting or diarrhea, decreased reflexes, and pale or mottled skin color are some of the clinical signs that are suggestive of infection. Respiratory symptoms such as apnea, tachypnea, grunting, or retracting can be associated with infection such as pneumonia (Dear, 2005; Lott & Kenner, 2003).

Any unusual discharges from the infant's eyes, nose, mouth, or other orifice, must be investigated. If a rash appears, it must be evaluated closely; many normal rashes in the newborn are not associated with any infection. Infants must be protected from infections by the use of good handwashing techniques.

The greatest risk factor for neonatal infection is prematurity because of immaturity of the immune system. Other risk factors include premature rupture of membranes, maternal fever, antenatal or intrapartum asphyxia, invasive procedures, stress, and congenital anomalies (Dear, 2005; Lott & Kenner, 2003).

Integumentary System

All skin structures are present at birth. The epidermis and dermis are loosely bound and extremely thin. After 35 weeks of gestation, the skin is covered by vernix caseosa (a cheeselike, whitish substance) that is fused with the epidermis and serves as a protective covering. The amount of vernix decreases with age and is shed into the amniotic fluid. In the term newborn, vernix is present in the creases of the neck, the axilla, and the groin. Postterm infants have little vernix.

The term infant has an erythematous (red) skin for a few hours after birth, after which it fades to its normal color. The skin often appears blotchy or mottled, especially over the extremities. The hands and feet appear slightly cyanotic (acrocyanosis); this is caused by vasomotor instability, capillary stasis, and a high hemoglobin level. Acrocyanosis is normal and can appear intermittently over the first 7 to 10 days, especially with exposure to cold. Central cyanosis, seen as a bluish color of mucous membranes and periphery, suggests inadequate oxygenation and should be investigated. Jaundice that appears during the first 24 hours is considered abnormal (Hernandez & Glass, 2005).

The healthy term newborn appears plump. Subcutaneous fat accumulated during the last trimester acts as insulation. The newborn's skin may be slightly tight, suggesting fluid retention. Fine lanugo hair may be noted over the face, shoulders, and back. Actual edema of the face and ecchymosis (bruising) or petechiae may be present as a result of face presentation or forceps-assisted birth. Petechiae appearing on areas of the skin other than the face or neck can be associated with serious infection or hematologic problems (Lissauer, 2006; Rennie, 2005).

Creases can be found on the palms of the hands. The simian line, a single palmar crease, is often found in Asian infants or in infants with Down syndrome. The soles of the feet should be inspected for the number of creases. Premature newborns have few if any creases. Increasing numbers of creases correlate with a greater maturity rating (Lissauer, 2006).

Caput Succedaneum

Caput succedaneum is a generalized, easily identifiable edematous area of the scalp, most commonly found on the occiput (Fig. 25-5, A). With vertex presentation the sustained pressure of the occiput against the cervix results in compression of local vessels, thereby slowing venous return. The slower venous return causes an increase in tissue fluids within the skin of the scalp, and an edematous swelling develops, often accompanied by petechiae and ecchymosis. This boggy edematous swelling, present at birth, extends across suture lines of the fetal skull and disappears spontaneously within 3 to 4 days. Infants who are delivered with the assistance of vacuum extraction usually have a caput (and bruising) in the area where the cup was applied (Mangurten, 2006).

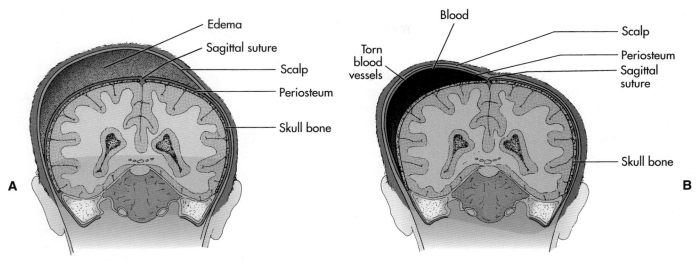

FIG. 25-5 Differences between caput succedaneum and cephalhematoma. **A,** Caput succedaneum: edema of scalp noted at birth; crosses suture lines. **B,** Cephalhematoma: bleeding between periosteum and skull bone appearing within first 2 days; does not cross suture lines.

Cephalhematoma

Cephalhematoma is a collection of blood between a skull bone and its periosteum; therefore a cephalhematoma does not cross a cranial suture line (Fig. 25-5, *B*). Caput succedaneum and cephalhematoma often occur simultaneously.

Bleeding resulting in cephalhematoma may occur with spontaneous birth from pressure against the maternal bony pelvis. Low forceps birth and difficult forceps rotation and extraction also may cause bleeding. This soft, fluctuating, irreducible fullness of cephalhematoma does not pulsate or bulge when the infant cries. The swelling may appear unilaterally or bilaterally, usually is minimal or absent at birth, increases over the first 3 days of life, and disappears gradually in 2 to 3 weeks. It may not become apparent until a caput succedaneum is absorbed. It is not aspirated because infection may develop if the skin is punctured. As the hematoma resolves, hemolysis of RBCs occurs, and jaundice may result. Hyperbilirubinemia may occur after the newborn is home (Mangurten, 2006). Less commonly the hematoma may calcify, causing a firm swelling that may persist for several months (Uhing, 2004).

Subgaleal Hemorrhage

Subgaleal hemorrhage is bleeding into the subgaleal compartment. The subgaleal compartment is a potential space that contains loosely arranged connective tissue; it is located beneath the galea aponeurosis, the tendinous sheath that connects the frontal and occipital muscles and forms the inner surface of the scalp. This space is potentially large, allowing a significant volume of blood to accumulate in an area bounded by the orbital ridges, the ears, and the occiput. The volume of blood loss can lead to hemorrhagic shock and anemia as well as hyperbilirubinemia. The injury occurs as a result of forces that compress and then drag the head through the pelvic outlet. Risk factors include forceps- and vacuum-assisted births, prolonged second stage of labor, fetal distress, macrosomia, and underlying coagulation disorders (Uchil & Arulkumaran, 2003; Uhing, 2004). Of these, a vacuum-assisted birth appears to have the highest association (Uchil & Arulkumaran). A subgaleal hemorrhage presents over the course of a few hours following birth as a soft, compressible mass that crosses suture lines. The bleeding extends beyond bone and continues after birth, with the potential for serious complications such as anemia or hypovolemic shock (Mangurten, 2006). Ongoing accumulation of blood may cause the ears to protrude and may extend down into the neck.

Early detection of the hemorrhage is vital; serial head circumference measurements and inspection of the back of the neck for increasing edema and a firm mass are essential. A boggy scalp, pallor, tachycardia, and increasing head circumference may also be early signs of a subgaleal hemorrhage. Computerized tomography or magnetic resonance imaging is useful in confirming the diagnosis. Replacement of lost blood and clotting factors is required in acute cases of hemorrhage (Uhing, 2004). The infant with a suspected subgaleal hemorrhage should have ongoing monitoring of vital signs including blood pressure and hemoglobin, hematocrit, and bilirubin levels, as well as coagulation studies. Monitoring the newborn for changes in level of consciousness and a decrease in the hematocrit are also key to early recognition and management. An increase in serum bilirubin levels may be seen as a result of the degrading blood cells within the hematoma (Mangurten, 2006).

Desquamation

Desquamation (peeling) of the skin of the term infant does not occur until a few days after birth. Its presence at birth is an indication of postmaturity.

Mongolian Spots

Mongolian spots, bluish-black areas of pigmentation, may appear over any part of the exterior surface of the body, including the extremities. They are more commonly noted on the back and buttocks (Fig. 25-6). These pigmented areas are most frequently noted in babies whose ethnic origins are in the Mediterranean area, Latin America, Asia, or Africa. They are more common in dark-skinned individuals, regardless of race. They fade gradually over months or years. Mongolian spots have no clinical significance but can be mistaken for bruises (Hernandez & Glass, 2005).

Nevi

Known as "stork bites" or "angel kisses," telangiectatic nevi are pink and easily blanched (Fig. 25-7, *A*). They may appear on the upper eyelids, the nose, the upper lip, the lower occipital area, and the nape of the neck. They have no clinical significance and fade by the second year of life (Lissauer, 2006).

The strawberry mark, or nevus vasculosus, is a common type of capillary hemangioma. It consists of dilated, newly formed capillaries occupying the entire dermal and subdermal layers, with associated connective tissue hypertrophy. The typical lesion is a raised, sharply demarcated, bright or dark red, rough-surfaced swelling that resembles a strawberry. Lesions usually are single but may be multiple, with the majority occurring on the head. These lesions can remain until the child is of school age or sometimes even longer (Narendran & Hoath, 2006).

A port-wine stain, or nevus flammeus, is usually observed at birth and is composed of a plexus of newly formed capillaries in the papillary layer of the corium. It is red to purple; varies in size, shape, and location; and is not elevated. True port-wine stains do not blanch on pressure or disappear. They are most frequently found on the face (Lissauer, 2006).

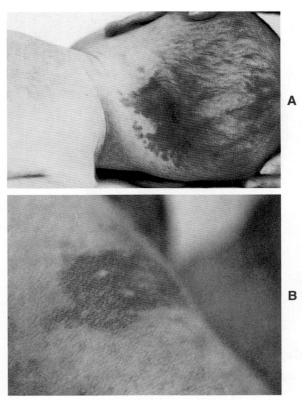

FIG. 25-7 **A,** Telangiectatic nevi (stork bite). **B,** Erythema toxicum (flea bite). (Courtesy Mead Johnson & Co., Evansville, IN.)

Erythema Toxicum

A transient rash, erythema toxicum, is also called *erythema neonatorum, newborn rash,* or *flea bite dermatitis.* It has lesions in different stages: erythematous macules, papules, and small vesicles (Fig. 25-7, *B*). The lesions may appear suddenly anywhere on the body. The rash is thought to be an inflammatory response. Eosinophils, which help decrease inflammation, are found in the vesicles. The rash is found in term neonates (gestational age of 36 weeks or more) during the first 3 weeks after birth. Although the appearance is alarming, the rash has no clinical significance and requires no treatment (Narendran & Hoath, 2006).

Signs of Risk for Integumentary Problems

Close observation of the newborn's skin color can lead to early detection of potential problems. Any pallor, plethora (deep purplish color from increased circulating RBCs), petechiae, central cyanosis, or jaundice should be noted and described. The skin should be examined for signs of birth injuries, such as forceps marks and lesions related to fetal monitoring. Bruises or petechiae may be present on the head, neck, and face of an infant born with a nuchal cord (cord around the neck) or in an infant who had a face presentation at birth. When bruises are present, the infant's bilirubin levels may be elevated. Petechiae may be present if increased pressure was applied to an area. Petechiae scattered over the infant's body should be reported

FIG. 25-6 Mongolian spot.

to the pediatrician because their presence may indicate underlying problems such as low platelet count or infection. Unilateral or bilateral periauricular papillomas (skin tags) occur fairly frequently. Their occurrence is usually a family trait and of no consequence.

Reproductive System
Female

At birth the ovaries contain thousands of primitive germ cells. These represent the full complement of potential ova; no oogonia form after birth in term infants. The ovarian cortex, which is made up primarily of primordial follicles, occupies a larger portion of the ovary in the female newborn than in the female adult. From birth to sexual maturity the number of ova decreases by approximately 90%.

An increase of estrogen during pregnancy followed by a decrease after birth results in a mucoid vaginal discharge and even some slight bloody spotting (pseudomenstruation). External genitals are usually edematous with increased pigmentation. In term newborn infants the labia majora and minora cover the vestibule (Fig. 25-8, *A*). In preterm infants, the clitoris is prominent, and the labia

FIG. 25-8 External genitalia. **A,** Genitals in female term infant. Note mucoid vaginal discharge. **B,** Genitals in male infant. Uncircumcised penis. Rugae cover scrotum, indicating term gestation. Cord has been swabbed with ethylene blue to prevent infection. (Courtesy Marjorie Pyle, RNC, Lifecircle, Costa Mesa, CA.)

majora are small and widely separated. Vaginal or hymenal tags are common findings and have no clinical significance. Vernix caseosa may be present between the labia (Rennie, 2005).

If the female was born in the breech position, the labia may be edematous and bruised. The edema and bruising resolve in a few days; no treatment is necessary.

Male

The foreskin completely covers the glans. The urethral opening may be completely covered by the prepuce, which is not retractable for 3 to 4 years. The position of the urethra should be at the tip of the penis. With hypospadias, the urethral opening is located in an abnormal position, on or adjacent to the glans, although it can be placed on the penile shaft or perineum. Small, white, firm lesions called *epithelial pearls* may be seen at the tip of the prepuce. By 28 to 36 weeks of gestation, the testes can be palpated in the inguinal canal, and a few rugae appear on the scrotum. At 36 to 40 weeks of gestation, the testes are palpable in the upper scrotum, and rugae appear on the anterior portion. After 40 weeks, the testes can be palpated in the scrotum, and rugae cover the scrotal sac. The postterm neonate has deep rugae and a pendulous scrotum. Hydroceles, caused by an accumulation of fluid around the testes, may be present. They can be easily transilluminated with a light and usually resolve without treatment (Rennie, 2005).

The scrotum is usually more deeply pigmented than the rest of the skin (Fig. 25-8, *B*), particularly in darker-skinned infants. A bluish discoloration of the scrotum suggests testicular torsion, which needs immediate attention. If the male infant was born in a breech presentation, the scrotum may appear very edematous and bruised. The swelling and discoloration resolve within a few days (Hernandez & Glass, 2005; Rennie, 2005).

Swelling of Breast Tissue

Swelling of the breast tissue in infants of both sexes is caused by the hyperestrogenism of pregnancy. In a few infants a thin discharge (witch's milk) can be seen. This condition has no clinical significance, requires no treatment, and subsides as the maternal hormones are eliminated from the infant's body within a few days (Lissauer, 2006).

The nipples should be symmetric on the chest. Breast tissue and areola size increase with gestation. The areola appears slightly elevated at 34 weeks of gestation. By 36 weeks, a breast bud of 1 to 2 mm is palpable; it increases to 12 mm by 42 weeks.

Signs of Risk for Reproductive System Problems

The infant must be closely inspected for ambiguous genitalia and other abnormalities. Normally in a female infant the urethral opening is located behind the clitoris. Any deviation from this may incorrectly suggest that the clitoris is a small penis, which can occur in conditions such as adrenal hyperplasia. Nearly all female infants are born with hymenal tags; absence of such tags could indicate vaginal agenesis. Fecal discharge from the vagina indicates a rectovaginal fistula. Any of these findings must be reported to the physician or neonatal nurse practitioner for further evaluation.

Hypospadias, undescended or maldescended testes, and other abnormalities of the male genitalia must be reported. Circumcision is contraindicated in the presence of hypospadias since the foreskin is used in repair of this anomaly (Hernandez & Glass, 2005).

Inguinal hernias may be present and become more obvious when the infant cries. They are common, especially in African-American neonates, and usually require no treatment since they resolve with time (Lissauer, 2006).

Skeletal System

The infant's skeletal system undergoes rapid development during the first year of life. At birth, more cartilage is present than ossified bone. Because of cephalocaudal (head-to-rump) development, the newborn looks somewhat out of proportion.

At term the head is one fourth the total body length. The arms are slightly longer than the legs. In the newborn, the legs are one third the total body length, but only 15% of the total body weight. As growth proceeds, the midpoint in head-to-toe measurements gradually descends from the level of the umbilicus at birth to the level of the symphysis pubis at maturity.

The face appears small in relation to the skull, which appears large and heavy. Cranial size and shape can be distorted by molding (the shaping of the fetal head by the overlapping of cranial bones to facilitate movement through the birth canal during labor) (Fig. 25-9).

The bones in the vertebral column of the newborn form two primary curvatures—one in the thoracic region and one in the sacral region (Fig. 25-10, *A*). Both are forward, concave curvatures. As the infant gains head control at approximately age 3 months, a secondary curvature appears in the cervical region (Fig. 25-10, *B*).

In some newborns, a significant separation of the knees occurs when the ankles are held together, resulting in an appearance of bowlegs (Fig. 25-11, *A*). If an infant was in the frank breech position in utero, the legs may be extended and remain in this position for several weeks. The newborn is also very flat footed because no clearly apparent arch to the foot is present (Fig. 25-11, *B*) (Lissauer, 2006).

The infant's extremities should be symmetric and of equal length. Fingers and toes should be equal in number and should have nails present. Digits may be missing (oligodactyly). Extra digits (polydactyly) are sometimes found on hands or feet. Fingers or toes may be fused (syndactyly) (Hernandez & Glass, 2005).

The infant is examined for developmental dysplasia of the hips (DDH). The hips are inspected for symmetry. Gluteal skin folds should be equal and symmetric, and legs should be of equal length. Hip integrity is assessed by

CD: Anatomy Review: Sutures and Fontanels

FIG. 25-9 Molding. **A,** Significant molding, soon after birth. **B,** Schematic of bones of skull when molding is present. (**A,** Courtesy Kim Molloy, Knoxville, IA.)

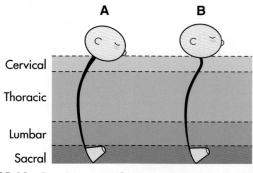

FIG. 25-10 Development of spinal curvatures. **A,** Newborn. **B,** Cervical secondary curvature. (From Wong, D. [1999]. *Whaley and Wong's nursing care of infants and children* [6th ed.]. St. Louis: Mosby.)

using the Barlow test and the Ortolani maneuver. For the Barlow test, the examiner places the middle finger over the greater trochanter and the thumb along the midthigh. The hip is flexed to 90 degrees and adducted followed by gentle downward pushing of the femoral head. If the hip can be dislocated with this maneuver, the femoral head moves out of the acetabulum and the examiner feels a "clunk." The hip is then checked to determine if the femoral head can be returned into the acetabulum using the Ortolani test. As the hip is abducted and upward leverage

FIG. 25-11   Extremities. **A,** Bowed appearance of legs. **B,** Normal absence of arch in newborn's foot. (Courtesy Marjorie Pyle, RNC, Lifecircle, Costa Mesa, CA.)

is applied, a dislocated hip will return to the acetabulum with a clunk. DDH occurs more often female infants, in breech presentations, and in infants with family history of DDH (Lissauer, 2006). These tests should be performed only by an expert examiner (Fig. 25-12).

The newborn's spine appears straight and can be easily flexed. The newborn can lift the head and turn it from side to side when prone. The vertebrae should appear straight and flat. If a pilonidal dimple is noted, further inspection is required to determine whether a sinus is present. A pilonidal dimple, especially with a sinus and nevus pilosis (hairy nevus), is significant because it can be associated with spina bifida (Hernandez & Glass, 2005).

Signs of Risk for Skeletal Problems

Skeletal deformities may be congenital or drug induced. Signs of congenital hip dislocation, additional digits or webbing of digits, and any other abnormality should be recorded and reported to the health care provider.

The feet may appear to be abnormally positioned. This may be indicative of congenital deformity or may be related to fetal positioning in the uterus. For example, clubfoot (talipes equinovarus), a deformity in which the foot turns inward and is fixed in a plantar-flexion position, is a congenital condition that warrants attention. If the foot is turned inward in the plantar-flexion position, but can be moved into the normal position, it is likely due to fetal positioning and should gradually resolve (Hernandez & Glass, 2005).

Neuromuscular System

Unlike the skeletal system, the neuromuscular system is almost completely developed at birth. The term newborn is a responsive and reactive being with remarkable sensory development and an amazing ability for self-organization and social interaction.

Growth of the brain after birth follows a predictable pattern of rapid growth during infancy and early childhood, more gradual growth during the remainder of the first decade, and minimal growth during adolescence. The

FIG. 25-12   Method of assessing for hip dysplasia or dislocation using the Ortolani maneuver. **A,** Examiner's middle fingers are placed over greater trochanter, and thumbs are placed over inner thigh opposite lesser trochanter. **B,** Gentle pressure is exerted to flex thigh on hip further, and thighs are rotated outward. If hip dysplasia is present, head of femur can be felt to slip forward in acetabulum and flip back when pressure is released and legs are returned to their original position. A "clunk" is sometimes heard (Ortolani sign). (Courtesy Marjorie Pyle, RNC, Lifecircle, Costa Mesa, CA.)

cerebellum ends its growth spurt, which began at about 30 weeks of gestation, by the end of the first year. This may be the reason the brain is vulnerable to nutritional deficiencies and trauma in early infancy.

The brain requires glucose as a source of energy and a relatively large supply of oxygen for adequate metabolism. Such requirements signal a need for careful assessment of the infant's respiratory status. The necessity for glucose requires attentiveness to those neonates who may have hypoglycemic episodes.

Spontaneous motor activity may be seen as transient tremors of the mouth and chin, especially during crying episodes, and of the extremities, notably the arms and hands. Transient tremors are normal and can be observed in nearly every newborn. These tremors should not be present when the infant is quiet and should not persist beyond 1 month of age. Persistent tremors or tremors involving the total body may indicate pathologic conditions. Marked tonicity, clonicity, and twitching of facial muscles are signs of seizure activity. Normal tremors, tremors of hypoglycemia, and central nervous system (CNS) disorders must be differentiated so that diagnostic workups and corrective care can be instituted as necessary (Lissauer, 2006).

The posture of the term newborn demonstrates flexion of the arms at the elbows and the legs at the knees. Hips are abducted and partially flexed. Intermittent fisting of the hands is common (Hernandez & Glass, 2005).

Muscle tone and strength are directly related. The infant with normal tone and strength exhibits some resistance to passive movement, such as when being pulled to sit, or when the arm or leg is extended by the examiner. The hypotonic neonate shows little resistance and may feel like a "rag doll." Hypertonia is evidenced by increased resistance to passive movement.

Although it is limited, some neuromuscular control is present in the newborn. If newborns are placed face down on a firm surface, they will turn their heads to the side to maintain an airway. They attempt to hold their heads in line with their bodies if they are raised by their arms (Hernandez & Glass, 2005; Lissauer, 2006).

Newborn Reflexes

The newborn has many primitive reflexes. The times at which these reflexes appear and disappear reflect the maturity and intactness of the developing nervous system. The most common reflexes found in the normal newborn are described in Table 25-4. The physical assessment includes a neurologic assessment of the newborn's reflexes. This provides useful information about the infant's nervous system and state of neurologic maturation. Many reflex behaviors are important for survival, for example, sucking and rooting. Other reflexes act as safety mechanisms, for instance, gagging, coughing, and sneezing. The assessment must be carried out as early as possible because abnormal signs present in the early neonatal period may disappear. They may reappear months or years later as abnormal functions (Rennie, 2005).

CD: Video: Newborn Assessment

Signs of Risk for Neuromuscular Problems

Any absence of a newborn reflex could indicate major neurologic problems. Birth trauma may cause nerve damage that results in facial asymmetry and paralysis. CNS depression resulting from maternal medications received during labor and birth also will influence neuromuscular functioning.

The cry of the term newborn is strong and "lusty." A weak cry is often associated with prematurity, neuromuscular disease, or sepsis. A high-pitched or shrill cry may suggest central nervous system abnormality. A low-pitched, husky cry may be related to hypothyroidism. Stridor with crying may indicate airway obstruction (Rennie, 2005).

Observation of the neonate for any abnormalities must be documented. A thorough physical examination of the newborn assists in detecting any potential complications (see Table 26-2).

▬ BEHAVIORAL CHARACTERISTICS

The healthy infant must achieve behavioral and biologic tasks to develop normally. Behavioral characteristics form the basis of the social capabilities of the infant. Normal newborns differ in their activity levels, feeding patterns, sleeping patterns, and responsiveness. Parents' reactions to their newborns often are determined by these differences. Showing parents the unique characteristics of their infant assists parents to develop a more positive perception of the infant with increased interaction between infant and parent.

Behavioral responses, as well as physical characteristics, change during the period of transition. The Brazelton Neonatal Behavioral Assessment Scale (BNBAS) can be used to assess the infant's behavior systematically (Brazelton, 1999; Brazelton & Nugent, 1996). The BNBAS is an interactive examination that assesses the infant's response to 28 areas organized according to the clusters in Box 25-2. It is generally used as a research or diagnostic tool, and its application requires special training.

Text continued on p. 657.

---

box 25-2 **Clusters of Neonatal Behaviors in the Brazelton Neonatal Behavioral Assessment Scale (BNBAS)**

Habituation—Ability to respond to and then inhibit responding to discrete stimuli (light, rattle, bell, pinprick) while asleep

Orientation—Quality of alert states and ability to attend to visual and auditory stimuli while alert

Motor performance—Quality of movement and tone

Range of state—Measure of general arousal level or arousability of infant

Regulation of state—How infant responds when aroused

Autonomic stability—Signs of stress (tremors, startles, skin color) related to homeostatic (self-regulator) adjustment of the nervous system

Reflexes—Assessment of several neonatal reflexes

From: Brazelton, T., & Nugent, K. (1996). *Neonatal behavioural assessment scale* (3rd ed.). London: MacKeith.

table 25-4 **Assessment of Newborn's Reflexes**

REFLEX	ELICITING THE REFLEX	CHARACTERISTIC RESPONSE	COMMENTS
Sucking and rooting	Touch infant's lip, cheek, or corner of mouth with nipple	Infant turns head toward stimulus, opens mouth, takes hold, and sucks	Response is difficult if not impossible to elicit after infant has been fed; if response weak or absent, consider prematurity or neurologic defect Parental guidance: Avoid trying to turn head toward breast or nipple, allow infant to root; response disappears after 3 to 4 mo* but may persist up to 1 yr
Swallowing	Feed infant; swallowing usually follows sucking and obtaining fluids	Swallowing is usually coordinated with sucking and usually occurs without gagging, coughing, or vomiting	If response is weak or absent, may indicate prematurity or neurologic defect Sucking and swallowing are often uncoordinated in preterm infant

Grasp
  Palmar
  Plantar
	Place finger in palm of hand
	Place finger at base of toes
		Infant's fingers curl around examiner's fingers, toes curl downward	Palmar response lessens by 3 to 4 mo; parents enjoy this contact with infant; plantar response lessens by 8 mo

Extrusion	Touch or depress tip of tongue	Newborn forces tongue outward	Response disappears about fourth month of life
Glabellar (Myerson's)	Tap over forehead, bridge of nose, or maxilla of newborn whose eyes are open	Newborn blinks for first four or five taps	Continued blinking with repeated taps is consistent with extrapyramidal disorder
Tonic neck or "fencing"	With infant falling asleep or sleeping, turn head quickly to one side	With infant facing left side, arm and leg on that side extend; opposite arm and leg flex (turn head to right, and extremities assume opposite postures)	Responses in leg are more consistent Complete response disappears by 3 to 4 mo, incomplete response may be seen until third or fourth year After 6 wk, persistent response is sign of possible cerebral palsy

Classic pose in spontaneous tonic neck reflex. (Courtesy Marjorie Pyle, RNC, Lifecircle, Costa Mesa, CA.)

*All durations for persistence of reflexes are based on time elapsed after 40 wk of gestation, that is, if this newborn was born at 36 wk of gestation, add 1 mo to all time limits given.

Continued

table 25-4 **Assessment of Newborn's Reflexes—cont'd**

REFLEX	ELICITING THE REFLEX	CHARACTERISTIC RESPONSE	COMMENTS
Moro	Hold infant in semi-sitting position, allow head and trunk to fall backward to an angle of at least 30 degrees Place infant on flat surface, strike surface to startle infant	Symmetric abduction and extension of arms are seen; fingers fan out and form a C with thumb and forefinger; slight tremor may be noted; arms are adducted in embracing motion and return to relaxed flexion and movement Legs may follow similar pattern of response Preterm infant does not complete "embrace"; instead, arms fall backward because of weakness	Response is present at birth; complete response may be seen until 8 wk; body jerk is seen only between 8 and 18 wk; response is absent by 6 mo if neurologic maturation is not delayed; response may be incomplete if infant is deeply asleep; give parental guidance about normal response Asymmetric response may connote injury to brachial plexus, clavicle, or humerus Persistent response after 6 mo indicates possible brain damage

Moro reflex. (From Dickason, E., Silverman, B., & Kaplan, J. [1998]. *Maternal-infant nursing care* [3rd ed.]. St. Louis: Mosby.)

REFLEX	ELICITING THE REFLEX	CHARACTERISTIC RESPONSE	COMMENTS
Stepping or "walking"	Hold infant vertically, allowing one foot to touch table surface	Infant will simulate walking, alternating flexion and extension of feet; term infants walk on soles of their feet, and preterm infants walk on their toes	Response is normally present for 3 to 4 wk

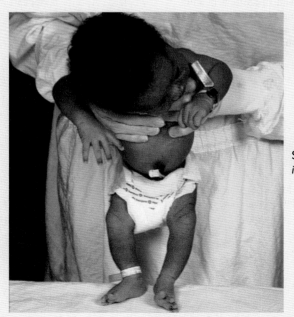

Stepping reflex. (From Dickason, E., Silverman, B., & Kaplan, J. [1998]. *Maternal-infant nursing care* [3rd ed.]. St. Louis: Mosby.)

REFLEX	ELICITING THE REFLEX	CHARACTERISTIC RESPONSE	COMMENTS
Crawling	Place newborn on abdomen	Newborn makes crawling movements with arms and legs	Response should disappear about 6 wk of age

table 25-4 **Assessment of Newborn's Reflexes—cont'd**

REFLEX	ELICITING THE REFLEX	CHARACTERISTIC RESPONSE	COMMENTS
Deep tendon	Use finger instead of percussion hammer to elicit patellar, or knee jerk, reflex; newborn must be relaxed	Reflex jerk is present; even with newborn relaxed, nonselective overall reaction may occur	This reflex should be present during newborn period.
Crossed extension	Infant should be supine; extend one leg, press knee downward, stimulate bottom of foot; observe opposite leg	Opposite leg flexes, adducts, and then extends	

Crossed extension reflex. (Courtesy Marjorie Pyle, RNC, Lifecircle, Costa Mesa, CA.)

Babinski reflex (plantar)	On sole of foot, beginning at heel, stroke upward along lateral aspect of sole, then move finger across ball of foot	All toes hyperextend, with dorsiflexion of big toe; recorded as a positive sign	Absence requires neurologic evaluation, should disappear after 1 yr of age

Babinski reflex. (From Hockenberry, M. [2003]. *Wong's nursing care of infants and children* [7th ed.]. St. Louis: Mosby.)

Pull-to-sit (traction)	Pull infant up by wrists from supine position with head in midline	Head will lag until infant is in upright position, then head will be held in same plane with chest and shoulder momentarily before falling forward; infant will attempt to right head	Response depends on general muscle tone and maturity and condition of infant

Continued

table 25-4 Assessment of Newborn's Reflexes—cont'd

REFLEX	ELICITING THE REFLEX	CHARACTERISTIC RESPONSE	COMMENTS
Trunk incurvation (Galant)	Place infant prone on flat surface, run finger down back about 4 to 5 cm lateral to spine, first on one side and then down other	Trunk is flexed, and pelvis is swung toward stimulated side With transverse lesions of cord, no response below the level of the lesion is present.	Response disappears by fourth week Absence suggests general depression of nervous system Response may vary but should be obtainable in all infants, including preterm ones.

Trunk incurvation reflex. (Courtesy Marjorie Pyle, RNC, Lifecircle, Costa

Magnet	Place infant in supine position, partially flex both lower extremities and apply pressure to soles of feet **(A)**	Both lower limbs should extend against examiner's pressure **(B)**	Absence suggests damage to spinal cord or malformation Reflex may be weak or exaggerated after breech birth

A

B

Magnet reflex. (Courtesy Michael S. Clement, MD, Mesa, AZ.)

Additional newborn responses: yawn, stretch, burp, hiccup, sneeze	These are spontaneous behaviors	May be slightly depressed temporarily because of maternal analgesia or anesthesia, fetal hypoxia, or infection	Parental guidance: Most of these behaviors are pleasurable to parents Parents need to be assured that behaviors are normal Sneeze is usually response to lint, etc., in nose and not an indicator of a cold No treatment is needed for hiccups; sucking may help

In addition to use as initial and ongoing tools to assess neurologic and behavioral responses, the scales can be used to assess initial parent-infant relationships and as a guide for parents to help them focus on their infant's individuality and to develop a deeper attachment to their child. See Chapter 24 for further discussion of attachment.

Sleep-Wake States

Variations in the state of consciousness of infants are called sleep-wake states (Brazelton, 1999). The six states form a continuum from deep sleep to extreme irritability (Fig. 25-13): two sleep states (deep sleep and light sleep) and four wake states (drowsy, quiet alert, active alert, and crying). Each state has specific characteristics and state-related behaviors. The optimal state of arousal is the quiet alert state. During this state, infants smile, vocalize, move in synchrony with speech, watch their parents' faces, and respond to people talking to them. The infants' reactions to internal and external stimuli and ability to control their responses while in these sleep-wake states reflect their ability to organize behavior.

Infants use purposeful behavior to maintain the optimal arousal state (the quiet alert state): (1) actively withdrawing by increasing physical distance, (2) rejecting by pushing away with hands and feet, (3) decreasing sensitivity by falling asleep or breaking eye contact by turning head, or (4) using signaling behaviors, such as fussing and crying. These behaviors permit infants to quiet themselves and reinstate readiness to interact.

The first 6 weeks of life involve a steady decrease in the proportion of active REM sleep to total sleep. A steady increase in the proportion of quiet sleep to total sleep also occurs. Periods of wakefulness increase. For the first few weeks the wakeful periods seem dictated by hunger, but soon a need for socializing appears as well. The newborn sleeps approximately 17 hours a day, with periods of wakefulness gradually increasing. By the fourth week of life, some infants stay awake from one feeding to the next.

Other Factors Influencing Newborn Behavior
Gestational Age

The gestational age of the infant and level of CNS maturity affect the observed behavior. In an infant with an immature CNS, the entire body responds to a pinprick of the foot. The mature infant withdraws only the foot. CNS immaturity is reflected in reflex development and sleep-wake cycles. Preterm infants have brief periods of alertness but have difficulty maintaining this state. Premature or sick infants show fatigue or stress sooner than term healthy infants.

Time

The time elapsed since birth affects the behavior of infants as they attempt to become organized initially. Time elapsed since the previous feeding and time of day also may influence infants' responses.

FIG. 25-13 Summary of newborn sleep-wake states. States of consciousness: **A,** Deep sleep. **B,** Light sleep. **C,** Drowsy. **D,** Quiet alert. **E,** Active alert. **F,** Crying. (Courtesy Marjorie Pyle, RNC, Lifecircle, Costa Mesa, CA.)

Stimuli

Environmental events and stimuli affect the behavioral responses of infants. The newborn responds differently to animate and inanimate stimuli. Nurses in intensive care nurseries observe that infants respond to loud noises, bright lights, monitor alarms, and tension in the unit. If a mother is tense and has a fast heartbeat while feeding an infant, the infant will have an increase in heart rate that is similar to the mother's.

Medication

Analgesic and anesthetic medications administered to the mother during labor may affect the newborn's neurologic status and behavior temporarily. Narcotics are likely to cause CNS depression and hypotonia and may even cause apnea. These medications also can affect the infant's sucking ability, at the breast or from a bottle.

Sensory Behaviors

From birth, infants possess sensory capabilities that indicate a state of readiness for social interaction. Infants effectively use behavioral responses in establishing their first dialogues. These responses, coupled with the newborns' "baby appearance" (e.g., facial proportions of forehead and eyes larger than the lower portion of the face) and their small size and helplessness, arouse feelings of wanting to hold, protect, and interact with them.

Vision

Compared with other sensory systems, the visual system is the least mature at term gestation. Development of the visual system parallels brain growth, progressing rapidly over the first 6 months, with visual acuity reaching adult levels by 4 to 5 years of age.

The neonate's pupils react to light, the blink reflex is easily stimulated, and the corneal reflex is activated by light touch. Infants are sensitive to light, preferring low illumination. If the room is darkened, they will open their eyes wide and look about. Newborns respond to a flash of bright light by frowning, blinking, and withdrawing the head by arching the entire body. Reflex tearing in response to irritants is present at birth. Emotional tearing begins at about 3 weeks of age and is fully developed by 3 months (Gupta, Hamming, & Miller, 2006).

Newborns have a limited ability to fixate at birth. Their eyes will follow a visual stimulus for short periods. By 3 months of age, infants can fixate and track a high-contrast object horizontally and vertically. They display preference for black-and-white objects. Infants seem attentive to the human face and track their parents' eyes (Gupta et al., 2006).

Visual acuity is difficult to determine, although it appears that the clearest visual distance for the newborn is approximately 19 cm, which is about the distance the infant's face is from the mother's face as she breastfeeds or cuddles. Newborns prefer to look at patterns rather than plain surfaces, even if the latter are brightly colored, and they prefer more complex patterns to simple ones (Brazelton, 1999).

Hearing

As soon as the amniotic fluid drains from the ear, the infant's hearing is similar to that of an adult. This may occur as early as 1 minute after birth. Loud sounds of about 90 decibels cause the infant to respond with a startle reflex. The newborn responds to low-frequency sounds such as a heartbeat or lullaby by decreasing motor activity or stopping crying. High-frequency sound elicits an alerting reaction.

The infant responds readily to the mother's voice. Studies indicate a selective listening to maternal voice sounds and rhythms during intrauterine life that prepares newborns for recognition and interaction with their primary caregivers—their mothers. Newborns are accustomed in the uterus to hearing the regular rhythm of the mother's heartbeat. As a result, they respond by relaxing and ceasing to fuss and cry if a regular heartbeat simulator is placed in their cribs.

The internal and middle portions of the ear are larger at birth, but the external canal is small. The mastoid process and bony parts of the external canal have not developed; therefore the tympanic membrane and facial nerve are very close to the surface and can be easily damaged. Hearing loss is common at birth; 1 in 1000 newborn infants is afflicted with a sensorineural hearing loss significant enough to affect speech and language development. Approximately half of those are due to hereditary loss and the other half are due to an acquired loss. The most common cause of acquired hearing loss is infection that is transmitted from the mother to the fetus transplacentally (Arnold & Sprecher, 2006).

Smell

Newborns have a highly developed sense of smell and can detect and discriminate distinct odors. It has been shown that preterm infants as early as 28 weeks are capable of reacting to odors. By 29 to 32 weeks, preterm infants respond to odors similarly to term newborns (Philbin, White, Schaal, & Hoath, 2006). Newborns react to strong odors such as alcohol or vinegar by turning their heads away, but are attracted to sweet smells. By the fifth day of life, newborn infants can recognize their mother's smell (Brazelton, 1999). Breastfed infants are able to smell breast milk and can differentiate their mothers from other lactating women (Lawrence & Lawrence, 2005).

Taste

As early as 25 weeks of gestation, the fetus is capable of detecting and discriminating sweet, bitter, acid, and salty tastes. It is thought that the components of amniotic fluid stimulate taste receptors in utero. The newborn can distinguish among tastes, and various types of solutions elicit differing facial expressions. A tasteless solution produces no response; a sweet solution elicits eager sucking. A sour solution causes a puckering of the lips, and a bitter liquid produces a grimace. Newborns prefer glucose water to plain water (Philbin et al., 2006).

Young infants are particularly oriented toward the use of their mouths, both for meeting their nutritional needs for rapid growth and for releasing tension through sucking. The early development of circumoral sensation, muscle activity, and taste would seem to be preparation for survival in the extrauterine environment.

Touch

The infant is responsive to touch on all parts of the body. The face (especially the mouth), the hands, and the soles of the feet appear to be the most sensitive. Reflexes can be elicited by stroking the infant. The newborn's responses to touch suggest that this sensory system is well prepared to receive and process tactile messages. Touch and motion are essential to normal growth and development; however, each infant is unique, and variations can be seen in newborns' responses to touch. Birth trauma or stress and depressant drugs taken by the mother decrease the infant's sensitivity to touch or painful stimuli.

Response to Environmental Stimuli
Temperament

Classic studies identified individual variations in the primary reaction pattern of newborns and described them as temperament. Their style of behavioral response to stimuli is guided by the temperament affecting the newborn's sensory threshold, ability to habituate, and response to maternal behaviors. The newborn possesses individual characteristics that affect selective responses to various stimuli present in the internal and external environments.

Habituation

Habituation is a protective mechanism that allows the infant to become accustomed to environmental stimuli. Habituation is a psychologic and physiologic phenomenon whereby the response to a constant or repetitive stimulus is decreased. In the term newborn this can be demonstrated in several ways. Shining a bright light into a newborn's eyes will cause a startle or squinting the first 2 or 3 times. The third or fourth flash will elicit a diminished response, and by the fifth or sixth flash, the infant ceases to respond (Brazelton, 1999). The same response pattern holds true for the sounds of a rattle or a pinprick to the heel. A newborn presented with new stimuli becomes wide eyed and alters his or her gaze for a time but will eventually show a diminished interest.

The ability to habituate also allows the newborn to select stimuli that promote continued learning about the social world, thereby avoiding overload. The intrauterine experience seems to have programmed the newborn to be especially responsive to human voices, soft lights, soft sounds, and sweet tastes.

The newborn quickly learns the sounds in a newborn nursery and the home and is able to sleep in their midst. The selective responses of the newborn indicate cerebral organization capable of remembering and making choices. The ability to habituate depends on state of consciousness, hunger, fatigue, and temperament. These factors also affect consolability, cuddliness, irritability, and crying.

Consolability

Newborns vary in their ability to console themselves or to be consoled. In the crying state, most newborns initiate one of several methods for reducing their distress. Hand-to-mouth movements are common, with or without sucking, as well as alerting to voices, noises, or visual stimuli.

Cuddliness

Cuddliness is especially important to parents because they often gauge their ability to care for the child by the child's responses to their actions. There is variability in the degree to which newborns will mold into the contours of the persons holding them. Babies are soothed and become alert with the vestibular stimulation of being picked up and moved.

Irritability

Some newborns cry longer and harder than others. For some the sensory threshold seems low. They are readily upset by unusual noises, hunger, wetness, or new experiences, and therefore respond intensely. Others with a high sensory threshold require a great deal more stimulation and variation to reach the active, alert state.

Crying

Crying in an infant may signal hunger, pain, desire for attention, or fussiness. Most mothers learn to distinguish among the cries. The duration of crying is highly variable in each infant; newborns may cry for as little as 5 minutes or as much as 2 hours or more per day. The amount of crying peaks in the second month and then decreases. The diurnal rhythm of crying typically includes more crying in the evening hours. Crying does not seem to differ with different caregivers.

---

community activity

Determine whether newborn classes are available in your community. Are there classes available in languages other than English? Interview the instructor to determine what is included in the class content. Is there attention to normal physical characteristics of the neonate? What information do parents receive related to newborn behaviors? What suggestions would you make for additional content related to physiologic and behavioral adaptations of the newborn? What is the value of providing expectant parents with this information?

key points

- By term the infant's various anatomic and physiologic systems have reached a level of development and functioning that permits a physical existence apart from the mother.
- The infant has sensory capabilities that indicate a state of readiness for social interaction.
- Several significant differences exist between the respiratory, renal, and thermogenic systems of the newborn and those of an adult.
- At any serum bilirubin level, the appearance of jaundice during the first 24 hours of life or persistence of jaundice for more than 7 days usually indicates a pathologic process in term infants.

- Loss of heat in a newborn, even a healthy newborn, may result in acidosis and increase the level of free fatty acids, leading to cold stress.
- Many reflex behaviors are important for the newborn's survival.
- Individual personalities and behavioral characteristics of infants play major roles in their relationships with their parents.
- Sleep-wake states and other factors influence the newborn's behavior.
- Each newborn has a predisposed capacity to handle the multitude of stimuli in the external world.

REFERENCES

Adamson, S., Myatt, L., & Byrne, B. (2004). Regulation of umbilical blood flow. In R. Polin, W. Fox, & S. Abman (Eds.), *Fetal and neonatal physiology.* (3rd ed.). Philadelphia: Saunders.

American Academy of Pediatrics (AAP) & American College of Obstetricians and Gynecology (ACOG). (2002). *Guidelines for perinatal care* (5th ed). Elk Grove, IL: (AAP).

Arnold, J., & Sprecher, J. (2006). Hearing loss in the newborn. In R. Martin, A. Fanaroff, & M. Walsh (Eds.), *Fanaroff and Martin's neonatal-perinatal medicine: Diseases of the fetus and infant* (8th ed.). Philadelphia: Mosby.

Barker, P., & Southern, K. (2004). Regulation of liquid secretion and absorption by the fetal and neonatal lung. In R. Polin, W. Fox, & S. Abman (Eds.), *Fetal and neonatal physiology* (3rd ed.). Philadelphia: Saunders.

Berryman, R., & Glass, S. (2005). Routine care. In P. Thureen, J. Deacon, J. Hernandez, & D. Hall (Eds.), *Assessment and care of the well newborn* (2nd ed.). St. Louis: Saunders.

Bhutani, V., Johnson, L., & Keren, R. (2005). Treating acute bilirubin encephalopathy—before it's too late. *Contemporary Pediatrics, 22*(5), 57-70.

Bloom, R. (2006). Delivery room resuscitation of the newborn: Part 1 Overview and initial management. In R. Martin, A. Fanaroff, & M. Walsh (Eds.), *Fanaroff and Martin's neonatal-perinatal medicine: Diseases of the fetus and infant* (8th ed.). Philadelphia: Mosby.

Brazelton, T. (1999). Behavioral competence. In G. Avery, M. Fletcher, & M. MacDonald (Eds.), *Neonatology: Pathophysiology and management of the newborn* (5th ed.). Philadelphia: Lippincott Williams & Wilkins.

Brazelton, T., & Nugent, K. (1996). *Neonatal behavioural assessment scale* (3rd ed.). London: MacKeith.

Cant, A., & Gennery, A. (2005). Neonatal infection. In J. Rennie (Ed.), *Robertson's textbook of neonatology* (4th ed.). Philadelphia: Churchill Livingstone.

Clyman, R. (2004). Mechanisms regulating closure of the ductus arteriosus. In R. Polin, W. Fox, & S. Abman (Eds.), *Fetal and neonatal physiology* (3rd ed.). Philadelphia: Saunders.

Dear, P. (2005). Infection in the newborn. In J. Rennie (Ed.), *Robertson's textbook of neonatology* (4th ed.). Philadelphia: Churchill Livingstone.

Frank, C., & Frank, P. (2006). Jaundice. In G. Merenstein, & S. Gardner (Eds.), *Handbook of neonatal intensive care* (5th ed.). St. Louis: Mosby.

Guignard, J. (2004). Postnatal development of glomerular filtration rate in neonates. In R. Polin, W. Fox, & S. Abman (Eds.), *Fetal and neonatal physiology* (3rd ed.). Philadelphia: Saunders.

Gupta, B., Hamming, N., & Miller, M. (2006). The eye: Diagnosis and evaluation. In R. Martin, A. Fanaroff, & M. Walsh (Eds.), *Fanaroff and Martin's neonatal-perinatal medicine: Diseases of the fetus and infant* (8th ed.). Philadelphia: Mosby.

Hansen, T., & Corbet, A. (2005). Control of breathing. In H. Taeusch, R. Ballard, & C. Gleason (Eds.), *Avery's diseases of the newborn* (8th ed.). Philadelphia: Saunders.

Hernandez, J., Fashaw, L., & Evans, R. (2005). Adaptation to extrauterine life and management during normal and abnormal transition. In P. Thureen, J. Deacon, J. Hernandez, & D. Hall (Eds.), *Assessment and care of the well newborn* (2nd ed.). St. Louis: Saunders.

Hernandez, J., & Glass, S. (2005). Physical assessment of the newborn. In P. Thureen, J. Deacon, J. Hernandez, & D. Hall (Eds.), *Assessment and care of the well newborn* (2nd ed.). St. Louis: Saunders.

Joint Commission on Accreditation of Healthcare Organizations (JCAHO). (2001). *Sentinel event alert: Kernicterus threatens healthy newborns,* Issue 18, April. Accessed www.jcaho.org/edu_pub/sealert/sea18.html, October 5, 2006.

Kalhan, S., & Parimi, P. (2006). Metabolic and endocrine disorders. In R. Martin, A. Fanaroff, & M. Walsh (Eds.), *Fanaroff and Martin's neonatal-perinatal medicine: Diseases of the fetus and infant* (8th ed.). Philadelphia: Mosby.

Kapur, R., Yoder, M., & Polin, R. (2006). Developmental immunology. In R. Martin, A. Fanaroff, & M. Walsh (Eds.), *Fanaroff and Martin's neonatal-perinatal medicine: Diseases of the fetus and infant* (8th ed.). Philadelphia: Mosby.

Lawrence, R., & Lawrence R. (2005). *Breastfeeding: A guide for the medical profession* (6th ed.). St. Louis: Mosby.

Lissauer, T. (2006). Physical examination of the newborn. In R. Martin, A. Fanaroff, & M. Walsh (Eds.), *Fanaroff and Martin's neonatal-perinatal medicine: Diseases of the fetus and infant* (8th ed.). Philadelphia: Mosby.

Lott, J., & Kenner, C. (2003). Assessment and management of the immune system. In C. Kenner, & J. Lott (Eds.), *Comprehensive neonatal nursing: A physiologic perspective* (3rd ed.). Philadelphia: Saunders.

Luchtman-Jones, L., Schwartz, A., & Wilson, D. (2006). Hematologic problems in the fetus and neonate. In R. Martin, A. Fanaroff, & M. Walsh (Eds.), *Fanaroff and Martin's neonatal-perinatal medicine: Diseases of the fetus and infant* (8th ed.). Philadelphia: Mosby.

Mangurten, H. (2006). Birth injuries. In R. Martin, A. Fanaroff, & M. Walsh (Eds.), *Fanaroff and Martin's neonatal-perinatal medicine: Diseases of the fetus and infant* (8th ed.). Philadelphia: Mosby.

Maisels, M. (2005a). Jaundice in a newborn: Answers to questions about a common clinical problem. *Contemporary Pediatrics, 22*(5), 34-41.

Maisels, M. (2005b). Jaundice in a newborn: How to head off an urgent situation. *Contemporary Pediatrics, 22*(5), 41-50.

Miller, C., & Newman, T. (2005). Routine newborn care. In H. Taeusch, R. Ballard, & C. Gleason (Eds.), *Avery's diseases of the newborn* (8th ed.). Philadelphia: Saunders.

Modi, N. (2005). Fluid and electrolyte balance. In J. Rennie (Ed.), *Robertson's textbook of neonatology* (4th ed.). Philadelphia: Churchill Livingstone.

Narendran, V., & Hoath, S. (2006). The skin. In R. Martin, A. Fanaroff, & M. Walsh (Eds.), *Fanaroff and Martin's neonatal-perinatal medicine: Diseases of the fetus and infant* (8th ed.). Philadelphia: Mosby.

Omari, R., & Rudolph, C. (2004). Gastrointestinal motility. In R. Polin, W. Fox, & S. Abman (Eds.), *Fetal and neonatal physiology* (3rd ed.). Philadelphia: Saunders.

Pagana, K., & Pagana, T. (2006). *Mosby's manual of diagnostic and laboratory tests* (3rd ed.). St. Louis: Mosby.

Philbin, M., White, R., Schaal, B., & Hoath, S. (2006). The sensory environment of the intensive care nursery. In R. Martin, A. Fanaroff, & M. Walsh (Eds.), *Fanaroff and Martin's neonatal-perinatal medicine: Diseases of the fetus and infant* (8th ed.). Philadelphia: Mosby.

Reiser, D. (2004). Neonatal jaundice: Physiologic variation or pathologic process. *Critical Care Clinics of North America, 16*(2), 257-269.

Rennie, J. (2005). Examination of the newborn. In J. Rennie (Ed.), *Robertson's textbook of neonatology* (4th ed.). Philadelphia: Churchill Livingstone.

Rigatto, H. (2004). Control of breathing in fetal life and onset and control of breathing in the neonate. In R. Polin, W. Fox, & S. Abman (Eds.), *Fetal and neonatal physiology* (3rd ed.). Philadelphia: Saunders.

Roberts, I. (2005). Haematological values in the newborn. In J. Rennie (Ed.), *Robertson's textbook of neonatology* (4th ed.). Philadelphia: Churchill Livingstone.

Roberts, I., & Murray, N. (2005). Haematology. In J. Rennie (Ed.), *Robertson's textbook of neonatology* (4th ed.). Philadelphia: Churchill Livingstone.

Rutter, N. (2005). Temperature control and disorders. In J. Rennie (Ed.), *Robertson's textbook of neonatology* (4th ed.). Philadelphia: Churchill Livingstone.

Sedin, G. (2006). Physical environment: Part 1 The thermal environment of the newborn infant. In R. Martin, A. Fanaroff, & M. Walsh (Eds.), *Fanaroff and Martin's neonatal-perinatal medicine: Diseases of the fetus and infant* (8th ed.). Philadelphia: Mosby.

Sniderman, S., & Taeusch, H. (2005). Initial evaluation: History and physical examination of the newborn. In H. Taeusch, R. Ballard, & C. Gleason (Eds.), *Avery's diseases of the newborn* (8th ed.). Philadelphia: Saunders.

Tsang, R., Demarini, S., Rath, L. (2003). Fluids, electrolytes, vitamins, and trace minerals. In C. Kenner, & J. Lott (Eds.), *Comprehensive neonatal nursing: A physiologic perspective* (3rd ed.). Philadelphia: Saunders.

Uchil, D., & Arulkumaran, S. (2003). Neonatal subgaleal hemorrhage and its relationship to delivery by vacuum extraction. *Obstetrical and Gynecological Survey, 58*(1), 687-693.

Uhing, M. (2004). Management of birth injuries. *Pediatric Clinics of North America, 51*(4), 1169-86, xii.

Vogt, B., Dell, K., & Davis, I. (2006). The kidney and urinary tract. In R. Martin, A. Fanaroff, & M. Walsh (Eds.), *Fanaroff and Martin's neonatal-perinatal medicine: Diseases of the fetus and infant* (8th ed.). Philadelphia: Mosby.

Wong, R., DeSandre, G., Sibley, E., & Stevenson, D. (2006). Neonatal jaundice and liver disease. In R. Martin, A. Fanaroff, & M. Walsh (Eds.), *Fanaroff and Martin's neonatal-perinatal medicine: Diseases of the fetus and infant* (8th ed.). Philadelphia: Mosby.

CHAPTER 26

Kathryn Rhodes Alden

Nursing Care of the Newborn

learning objectives

- Describe the purpose and components of the Apgar score.
- Describe the method for estimating the gestational age of a newborn.
- Explain the procedure for assessment of the newborn.
- Describe common deviations from normal physiologic findings during physical examination of the newborn.
- Discuss the nursing care needed during the newborn's transition to extrauterine life.
- Explain what is meant by a protective environment.

- Discuss phototherapy and the guidelines for teaching parents about this treatment.
- Explain purposes for and methods of circumcision, the postoperative care of the circumcised infant, and parent teaching regarding circumcision.
- Describe procedures for doing a heel stick, collecting urine specimens, assisting with venipuncture, and restraining the newborn.
- Describe evaluation and management of pain in the newborn.

electronic resources

Additional information related to the content in Chapter 26 can be found on

the companion website at *evolve*
http://evolve.elsevier.com/Lowdermilk/MWHC/
- NCLEX Review Questions
- Case Study: The Normal Newborn
- WebLinks

or on the interactive companion CD
- NCLEX Review Questions
- Case Study: The Normal Newborn
- Critical Thinking Exercise: Circumcision
- Plan of Care: The Normal Newborn
- Skill: Pain Assessment
- Video: Circumcision

THE numerous biologic changes the neonate makes during the transition to extrauterine life are discussed in the preceding chapter. The first 24 hours are critical because respiratory distress and circulatory failure can occur rapidly and with little warning. Although most infants make the necessary biopsychosocial adjustment to extrauterine existence without undue difficulty, their well-being depends on the care they receive from others. This chapter describes assessment and care of the infant immediately after birth until discharge, as well as important parent education related to ongoing infant care. A discussion of pain in the neonate and its management is included.

■ CARE MANAGEMENT: FROM BIRTH THROUGH THE FIRST 2 HOURS

Care begins immediately after birth and focuses on assessing and stabilizing the newborn's condition. The nurse has primary responsibility for the infant during this period,

because the physician or midwife is involved with delivery of the placenta and caring for the mother. The nurse must be alert for any signs of distress and must initiate appropriate interventions.

With the possibility of transmission of viruses such as hepatitis B virus (HBV) and human immunodeficiency virus (HIV) via maternal blood and blood-stained amniotic fluid, the newborn must be considered a potential contamination source until proved otherwise. In keeping with Standard Precautions, nurses should wear gloves when handling the newborn until blood and amniotic fluid are removed by bathing.

■ Assessment and Nursing Diagnoses

The initial assessment of the neonate is done at birth by using the Apgar score (Table 26-1) and a brief physical examination (Box 26-1). A gestational age assessment is done within 2 hours of birth (Fig. 26-1). A more comprehensive physical assessment is completed within 24 hours of birth (Table 26-2).

table 26-1 Apgar Score

SIGN	SCORE		
	0	**1**	**2**
Heart rate	Absent	Slow (<100)	>100
Respiratory rate	Absent	Slow, weak cry	Good cry
Muscle tone	Flaccid	Some flexion of extremities	Well flexed
Reflex irritability	No response	Grimace	Cry
Color	Blue, pale	Body pink, extremities blue	Completely pink

---

box 26-1 Initial Physical Assessment by Body System

CNS	[ ]	moves extremities, muscle tone good
	[ ]	symmetric features, movement
	[ ]	suck, rooting, Moro response, grasp reflexes good
	[ ]	anterior fontanel soft and flat
CV	[ ]	heart rate strong and regular
	[ ]	no murmurs heard
	[ ]	pulses strong and equal bilaterally
RESP	[ ]	lungs clear to auscultation bilaterally
	[ ]	no retractions or nasal flaring
	[ ]	respiratory rate, 30-60 breaths/min
	[ ]	chest expansion symmetric
	[ ]	no upper airway congestion
GU	[ ]	male: urethral opening at tip of penis; testes descended bilaterally
	[ ]	female: vaginal opening apparent
GI	[ ]	abdomen soft, no distention
	[ ]	cord attached and clamped
	[ ]	anus appears patent
ENT	[ ]	eyes clear
	[ ]	palates intact
	[ ]	nares patent
SKIN	Color	[ ] pink [ ] acrocyanotic
	[ ]	no lesions or abrasions
	[ ]	no peeling
	[ ]	birthmarks _____
	[ ]	caput and molding
	[ ]	vacuum "cap"
	[ ]	forceps marks
	[ ]	other

Comments: _____

_____

_____

_____

CNS, Central nervous system; *CV*, cardiovascular; *ENT*, ear, nose, and throat; *GI*, gastrointestinal; *GU*, genitourinary; *RESP*, respiratory.

▬ Apgar Score

The Apgar score permits a rapid assessment of the need for resuscitation based on five signs that indicate the physiologic state of the neonate: (1) heart rate, based on auscultation with a stethoscope; (2) respiratory rate, based on observed movement of the chest wall; (3) muscle tone, based on degree of flexion and movement of the extremities; (4) reflex irritability, based on response to gentle slaps on the soles of the feet; and (5) generalized skin color,

---

box 26-2 Significance of the Apgar Score

The Apgar score was developed to provide a systematic method of assessing an infant's condition at birth. Researchers have tried to correlate Apgar scores with various outcomes such as development, intelligence, and neurologic development. In some instances, researchers have attempted to attribute causality to the Apgar score, that is, to suggest that the low Apgar score caused or predicted later problems. This is an inappropriate use of the Apgar score. Instead the score should be used to ensure that infants are systematically observed at birth to ascertain the need for immediate care. Either a physician or a nurse may assign the score; however, to avoid the real or perceived appearance of bias, the person assisting with the birth should not assign the score. Lack of consistency in the assigned scores limits studies of the Apgar's long-term predictive value. Prospective parents and the public need education on the significance of the Apgar score, as well as its limits. Because infants often do not receive the maximum score of 10, parents need to know that scores of 7 to 10 are within normal limits. Attorneys involved in litigation related to injury of an infant at birth or negative outcomes, either short-term or long-term, also need education about the Apgar score, its significance, and its limits. This useful tool needs to be used appropriately; health care providers, parents, and the public may need education to ensure appropriate use of the score.

Data from Montgomery, K. (2000). Apgar scores: Examining the long-term significance. *Journal of Perinatal Education, 9*(3), 5-9.

described as pallid, cyanotic, or pink. Each item is scored as a 0, 1, or 2. Evaluations are made 1 and 5 minutes after birth. Scores of 0 to 3 indicate severe distress; scores of 4 to 6 indicate moderate difficulty in adjusting to extrauterine life; and scores of 7 to 10 indicate that the infant is having no difficulty adjusting to extrauterine life. Apgar scores do not predict future neurologic outcome but are useful for describing the newborn's transition to the extrauterine environment (Box 26-2). Should resuscitation be required, it should be initiated before the 1-minute Apgar score (American Academy of Pediatrics [AAP] and American College of Obstetricians and Gynecologists [ACOG], 2002).

▬ Initial Physical Assessment

The initial physical assessment includes a brief review of systems (see Box 26-1):

1. *External:* Note skin color, general activity, position; assess nasal patency by covering one nostril at a time

NEUROMUSCULAR MATURITY

	−1	0	1	2	3	4	5
Posture							
Square Window (wrist)	> 90°	90°	60°	45°	30°	0°	
Arm Recoil		180°	140° - 180°	110° 140°	90° - 110°	< 90°	
Popliteal Angle	180°	160°	140°	120°	100°	90°	< 90°
Scarf Sign							
Heel to Ear							

A PHYSICAL MATURITY

Skin	sticky friable transparent	gelatinous red, translucent	smooth pink, visible veins	superficial peeling or rash, few veins	cracking pale areas rare veins	parchment deep cracking no vessels	leathery cracked wrinkled
Lanugo	none	sparse	abundant	thinning	bald areas	mostly bald	
Plantar Surface	heel-toe 40-50 mm: -1 <40 mm: -2	>50 mm no crease	faint red marks	anterior transverse crease only	creases ant. 2/3	creases over entire sole	
Breast	imperceptible	barely perceptible	flat areola no bud	stippled areola 1-2 mm bud	raised areola 3-4 mm bud	full areola 5-10 mm bud	
Eye/Ear	lids fused loosely: -1 tightly: -2	lids open pinna flat stays folded	sl. curved pinna; soft; slow recoil	well-curved pinna; soft but ready recoil	formed & firm instant recoil	thick cartilage ear stiff	
Genitals (male)	scrotum flat, smooth	scrotum empty faint rugae	testes in upper canal rare rugae	testes descending few rugae	testes down good rugae	testes pendulous deep rugae	
Genitals (female)	clitoris prominent labia flat	prominent clitoris small labia minora	prominent clitoris enlarging minora	majora & minora equally prominent	majora large minora small	majora cover clitoris & minora	

MATURITY RATING

score	weeks
-10	20
-5	22
0	24
5	26
10	28
15	30
20	32
25	34
30	36
35	38
40	40
45	42
50	44

FIG. 26-1 Estimation of gestational age. **A,** New Ballard Scale for newborn maturity rating. Expanded scale includes extremely premature infants and has been refined to improve accuracy in more mature infants. (From Ballard, J., Khoury, J., Wedig, K., Wang, L., Eilers-Walsman, B., & Lipp, R. [1991]. New Ballard Score, expanded to include extremely premature infants. *Journal of Pediatrics, 119*[3], 417-423).

while observing respirations; skin: peeling, or lack of subcutaneous fat (dysmaturity or postterm); note meconium staining of cord, skin, fingernails, or amniotic fluid (staining may indicate fetal release of meconium, often related to hypoxia; offensive odor may indicate intrauterine infection); note length of nails and creases on soles of feet.

2. *Chest:* Auscultate apical heart for rate and rhythm, heart tones and presence of abnormal sounds; note character of respirations and presence of crackles or other adventitious sounds; note equality of breath sounds by auscultation.

3. *Abdomen:* Observe characteristics of abdomen (rounded, flat, concave) and absence of anomalies; note number of vessels in cord.

4. *Neurologic:* Check muscle tone; assess Moro and suck reflexes; palpate anterior fontanel; note by palpation the presence and size of the fontanels and sutures.

5. *Genitourinary:* Note external sex characteristics and any abnormality of genitalia; check anal patency (by appearance), presence of meconium; note passage of urine.

6. *Other observations:* Note gross structural malformations obvious at birth that may require immediate medical attention.

Text continued on p. 678.

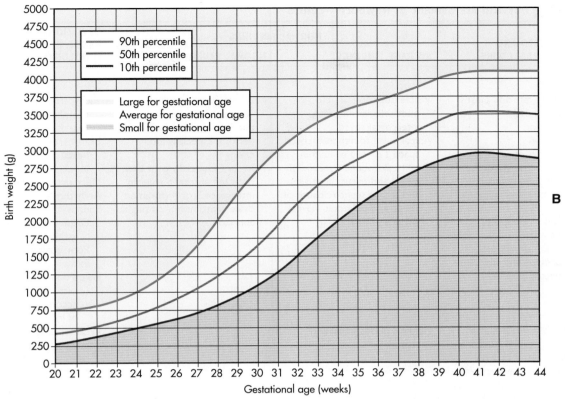

FIG. 26-1, cont'd Estimation of gestational age. **B,** Intrauterine growth: birth weight percentiles based on live single births at gestational ages 20 to 44 weeks. (Data from Alexander, G., Himes, J., Kaufman, R., Mor, J., & Kogan M. [1996]. A United States national reference for fetal growth. *Obstetrics and Gynecology, 87*[2], 163-168.)

table 26-2 Physical Assessment of Newborn

AREA ASSESSED AND APPRAISAL PROCEDURE	NORMAL FINDINGS		DEVIATIONS FROM NORMAL RANGE: POSSIBLE PROBLEMS (ETIOLOGY)
	AVERAGE FINDINGS	**NORMAL VARIATIONS**	
POSTURE			
Inspect newborn before disturbing for assessment	Vertex: arms, legs in moderate flexion; fists clenched	Frank breech: legs straighter and stiff, newborn assuming intrauterine position in repose for a few days	Hypotonia, relaxed posture while awake (prematurity or hypoxia in utero, maternal medications)
Refer to maternal chart for fetal presentation, position, and type of birth (vaginal, surgical), because newborn readily assumes prenatal position	Resistance to having extremities extended for examination or measurement, crying possible when attempted	Prenatal pressure on limb or shoulder possibly causing temporary facial asymmetry or resistance to extension of extremities	Hypertonia (drug dependence, central nervous system [CNS] disorder)
	Cessation of crying when allowed to resume curled-up fetal position		Opisthotonos (CNS disturbance)
	Normal spontaneous movement bilaterally asynchronous (legs moving in bicycle fashion) but equal extension in all extremities		Limitation of motion in any of extremities (see pp. 676-677)

Continued

table 26-2 Physical Assessment of Newborn—cont'd

AREA ASSESSED AND APPRAISAL PROCEDURE	NORMAL FINDINGS		DEVIATIONS FROM NORMAL RANGE: POSSIBLE PROBLEMS (ETIOLOGY)
	AVERAGE FINDINGS	NORMAL VARIATIONS	
VITAL SIGNS			
Check heart rate and pulses: Thorax (chest) Inspection Palpation Auscultation Apex: mitral valve Second interspace, left of sternum: pulmonic valve Second interspace, right of sternum: aortic valve Junction of xiphoid process and sternum: tricuspid valve	Visible pulsations in left midclavicular line, fifth intercostal space Apical pulse, fourth intercostal space 120-160 beats/min Quality: *first sound* (closure of mitral and tricuspid valves) and *second sound* (closure of aortic and pulmonic valves) sharp and clear	100 beats/min (sleeping) to 180 beats/min (crying); possibly irregular for brief periods, especially after crying Murmurs, especially over base or at left sternal border in interspace 3 or 4 (foramen ovale anatomically closing at approximately 1 yr)	Tachycardia: persistent, ≥160 beats/min (respiratory distress syndrome [RDS]) Bradycardia: persistent, ≤120 beats/min (congenital heart block) Murmurs (possibly functional) Arrhythmias: irregular rate Sounds Distant (pneumomediastinum) Poor quality Extra Heart on right side of chest: (dextrocardia, often accompanied by reversal of intestines)
For femoral pulse palpation, place fingers along inguinal ligament about midway between symphysis pubis and iliac crest; feel bilaterally and simultaneously	Femoral pulses equal and strong		Weak or absent femoral pulses (hip dysplasia, coarctation of aorta, thrombus)
Obtain temperature: Axillary: method of choice until age 6 yr Electronic: thermistor probe (avoid taping over bony area)	Axillary: 37° C Temperature stabilized by 8-10 hr of age Undeveloped shivering mechanism	36.5° C to 37.2° C Heat loss: 200 kcal/kg/ min from evaporation, conduction, convection, radiation	Subnormal (prematurity, infection, low environmental temperature, inadequate clothing, dehydration) Increased (infection, high environmental temperature, excessive clothing, proximity to heating unit or in direct sunshine, drug addiction, diarrhea and dehydration) Temperature not stabilized by 10 hr after birth (if mother received magnesium sulfate, newborn less able to conserve heat by vasoconstriction; maternal analgesics possibly reducing thermal stability in newborn)
Check respiratory rate and effort: Observe respirations when infant is at rest Count respirations for full minute Check apnea monitor Listen for sounds audible without stethoscope Observe respiratory effort	40 breaths/min Tendency to be shallow and irregular in rate, rhythm, and depth when infant is awake No sounds audible on inspiration or expiration Breath sounds: bronchial; loud, clear, near	30-50 breaths/min Possibly appearing to be Cheyne-Stokes with short periods of apnea and no evidence of respiratory distress First period (reactivity): 50-60/min Second period: 50-70/min Stabilization (1-2 days): 30-40/min	Apneic episodes: >15 sec (preterm infant: "periodic breathing," rapid warming or cooling of infant) Bradypnea: <25/min (maternal narcosis from analgesics or anesthetics, birth trauma) Tachypnea: >60/min (RDS, aspiration syndrome, diaphragmatic hernia)

table 26-2 Physical Assessment of Newborn—cont'd

AREA ASSESSED AND APPRAISAL PROCEDURE	NORMAL FINDINGS		DEVIATIONS FROM NORMAL RANGE: POSSIBLE PROBLEMS (ETIOLOGY)
	AVERAGE FINDINGS	NORMAL VARIATIONS	
VITAL SIGNS—cont'd			

			Sounds
			    Crackles, rhonchi, wheezes (fluid in lungs)
			    Expiratory grunt (narrowing of bronchi)
			    Distress evidenced by nasal flaring, retractions, chin tug, labored breathing (RDS, fluid in lungs)

Measure blood pressure (BP) (usually assessed only if a problem is suspected)
Check electronic monitor
    BP cuff: BP cuff width affects readings, use cuff 2.5 cm wide and palpate radial pulse
	80s-90s/40s-50s (approximately)
	At birth
	    Systolic: 60-80 mm Hg
	    Diastolic: 40-50 mm Hg
	At 10 days
	    Systolic: 95-100 mm Hg
	    Diastolic: slight increase
		Variation with change in activity level: awake, crying, sleeping	Difference between upper and lower extremity pressures (coarctation of aorta)
			Hypotension (sepsis, hypovolemia)
			Hypertension (coarctation of aorta)

WEIGHT* Put protective liner cloth or paper in place and adjust scale to 0 Weigh at same time each day Protect newborn from heat loss	Female, 3400 g Male, 3500 g Birth weight regained within first 2 weeks	2500-4000 g Acceptable weight loss: ≤10% Second baby weighs more than first	Weight ≤2500 g (prematurity, small for gestational age, rubella syndrome) Weight ≥4000 g (large for gestational age, maternal diabetes, heredity—normal for these parents) Weight loss >10% (dehydration)
LENGTH Measure length from top of head to heel; measuring is difficult in term infant because of presence of molding, incomplete extension of knees	50 cm	45-55 cm	<45 cm or >55 cm (chromosomal aberration, heredity—normal for these parents)

Weighing the infant. The scale is covered to protect against cross-infection. The nurse never leaves the infant alone on the scale. (Courtesy Wendy and Marwood Larson-Harris, Roanoke, VA.)

Length, crown to rump. To determine total length, include length of legs. If measurements are taken before the infant's initial bath, wear gloves. (Courtesy Marjorie Pyle, RNC, Lifecircle, Costa Mesa, CA.)

*NOTE: Weight, length, and head circumference all should be close to the same percentile for any newborn.

Continued

table 26-2 Physical Assessment of Newborn—cont'd

AREA ASSESSED AND APPRAISAL PROCEDURE	NORMAL FINDINGS		DEVIATIONS FROM NORMAL RANGE: POSSIBLE PROBLEMS (ETIOLOGY)
	AVERAGE FINDINGS	NORMAL VARIATIONS	
HEAD CIRCUMFERENCE Measure head at greatest diameter: occipitofrontal circumference May need to remeasure on second or third day after resolution of molding and caput succedaneum	33-35 cm Circumference of head and chest approximately the same for first 1 or 2 days after birth	32-36.8 cm	Small head ≤32 cm: microcephaly (rubella, toxoplasmosis, cytomegalic inclusion disease) Hydrocephaly: sutures widely separated, circumference 4 cm more than chest circumference (mal-development, infection) Increased intracranial pressure (hemorrhage, space-occupying lesion)
CHEST CIRCUMFERENCE Measure at nipple line	2-3 cm less than head circumference, averages between 30 and 33 cm		≤30 cm (prematurity)

Circumference of head. (Courtesy Marjorie Pyle, RNC, Lifecircle, Costa Mesa, CA.)

Circumference of chest. (Courtesy Marjorie Pyle, RNC, Lifecircle, Costa Mesa, CA.)

ABDOMINAL CIRCUMFERENCE Not usually measured unless specific indication	Abdomen enlargement after feeding because of lax abdominal muscles Same size as chest		Enlarging abdomen between feedings (abdominal mass or blockage in intestinal tract)

Abdominal circumference. (Courtesy Marjorie Pyle, RNC, Lifecircle, Costa Mesa, CA.)

table 26-2 Physical Assessment of Newborn—cont'd

AREA ASSESSED AND APPRAISAL PROCEDURE	NORMAL FINDINGS		DEVIATIONS FROM NORMAL RANGE: POSSIBLE PROBLEMS (ETIOLOGY)
	AVERAGE FINDINGS	NORMAL VARIATIONS	
SKIN			
Check color:			
Inspect and palpate	Generally pink	Mottling	Dark red (prematurity,
Inspect naked newborn in well-lit, warm area without drafts; natural daylight provides best lighting	Varying with ethnic origin, skin pigmentation beginning to deepen right after birth in basal layer of epidermis	Harlequin sign Plethora Telangiectases ("stork bites" or capillary hemangiomas) (see Fig. 25-7, A)	polycythemia) Pallor (cardiovascular problem, CNS damage, blood dyscrasia, blood loss, twin-to-twin transfusion,
Inspect newborn when quiet and when active	Acrocyanosis, especially if chilled	Erythema toxicum or neonatorum ("newborn rash") (see Fig. 25-7, B) Milia	nosocomial infection) Cyanosis (hypothermia, infection, hypoglycemia, cardiopulmonary diseases, cardiac, neurologic, or respiratory malformations)
		Petechiae over presenting part	Petechiae over any other area (clotting factor deficiency, infection)
		Ecchymoses from forceps in vertex births or over buttocks, genitalia, and legs in breech births	Ecchymoses in any other area (hemorrhagic disease, traumatic birth) Gray (hypotension, poor perfusion)
Check for jaundice	None at birth	Physiologic jaundice in 50% of term infants after first 24 hr	Jaundice within first 24 hr (Rh isoimmunization, ABO incompatibility, increased hemolysis)
Check birthmarks:			
Inspect and palpate for location, size, distribution, characteristics, color	Transient hyperpigmentation Areolae Genitals Linea nigra	Mongolian spotting (see Fig. 25-6) Infants of African- American, Asian, and Native American origin: 70%–85% Infants of Caucasian origin: (5%–13%)	Hemangiomas Nevus flammeus: port-wine stain Nevus vasculosus: strawberry mark Cavernous hemangiomas
Check condition:			
Inspect and palpate for intactness, smoothness, texture, edema	No skin edema Opacity: few large blood vessels visible indistinctly over abdomen	Slightly thick; superficial cracking, peeling, especially of hands, feet No visible blood vessels, a few large vessels clearly visible over abdomen Some fingernail scratches	Edema on hands, feet; pitting over tibia (overhydration) Texture thin, smooth, or of medium thickness; rash or superficial peeling visible (prematurity) Numerous vessels very visible over abdomen (prematurity) Texture thick, parchment-like; cracking, peeling (postmaturity) Skin tags, webbing Papules, pustules, vesicles, ulcers, maceration (impetigo, candidiasis, herpes, diaper rash)
Assess hydration and consistency			
Weigh infant routinely Inspect and palpate Gently pinch skin between thumb and forefinger over abdomen and inner thigh to check for turgor	Dehydration: loss of weight best indicator After pinch released, skin returns to original state immediately	Normal weight loss after birth: ≤10% of birth weight Possibly puffy Variation in amount of subcutaneous fat	Loose, wrinkled skin (prematurity, postmaturity, dehydration: fold of skin persisting after release of pinch) Tense, tight, shiny skin (edema, extreme cold, shock, infection)

Continued

table 26-2 Physical Assessment of Newborn—cont'd

AREA ASSESSED AND APPRAISAL PROCEDURE	NORMAL FINDINGS		DEVIATIONS FROM NORMAL RANGE: POSSIBLE PROBLEMS (ETIOLOGY)
	AVERAGE FINDINGS	NORMAL VARIATIONS	
SKIN—cont'd			
Check subcutaneous fat deposits (adipose pads) over cheeks, buttocks			Lack of subcutaneous fat, prominence of clavicle or ribs (prematurity, malnutrition)
Check vernix caseosa:			
Observe amount		Variation in amount; usually more found in creases, folds	Absent or minimal (postmaturity) Excessive (prematurity)
Observe its color and odor before bath or wiping	Whitish, cheesy, odorless		Yellow color (possible fetal anoxia >36 hr before birth, Rh or ABO incompatibility) Green color (possible in utero release of meconium or presence of bilirubin) Odor (possible intrauterine infection)
Assess lanugo			
Inspect for this fine, downy hair, including its amount, distribution	Over shoulders, pinnas of ears, forehead	Variation in amount	Absent (postmaturity) Excessive (prematurity, especially if lanugo abundant and long and thick over back)
HEAD			
Palpate skin	See "Skin"	Caput succedaneum, possibly showing some ecchymosis (see Fig. 25-5, A)	Cephalhematoma (birth trauma) (see Fig. 25-5, B)
Inspect shape, size	Making up one fourth of body length Molding (see Fig. 25-9)	Slight asymmetry from intrauterine position Lack of molding (prematurity, breech presentation, cesarean birth)	Molding Severe molding (birth trauma) Indentation (fracture from trauma)
Palpate, inspect, measure fontanels	Anterior fontanel 5 cm diamond, increasing as molding resolves Posterior fontanel triangle, smaller than anterior	Variation in fontanel size with degree of molding Difficulty in feeling fontanels possible because of molding	Fontanels Full, bulging (tumor, hemorrhage, infection) Large, flat, soft (malnutrition, hydrocephaly, retarded bone age, hypothyroidism) Depressed (dehydration)
Palpate sutures	Palpable and unjoined sutures	Possible overlap of sutures with molding	Sutures Widely spaced (hydrocephaly) Premature closure
Inspect pattern, distribution, amount of hair; feel texture	Silky, single strands lying flat; growth pattern toward face and neck	Variation in amount	Fine, woolly (prematurity) Unusual swirls, patterns, hairline or coarse, brittle (endocrine or genetic disorders)

table 26-2 Physical Assessment of Newborn—cont'd

AREA ASSESSED AND APPRAISAL PROCEDURE	NORMAL FINDINGS		DEVIATIONS FROM NORMAL RANGE: POSSIBLE PROBLEMS (ETIOLOGY)
	AVERAGE FINDINGS	NORMAL VARIATIONS	
EYES			
Check placement on face	Eyes and space between eyes each one third the distance from outer-to-outer canthus	Epicanthal folds: normal racial characteristic	Epicanthal folds when present with other signs (chromosomal disorders such as Down, *cri-du-chat* syndromes)
Check for symmetry in size, shape	Symmetric in size, shape		
Check eyelids for size, movements, blink	Blink reflex	Edema if silver nitrate instilled; also may occur with instillation of erythromycin and tetracycline	
Assess for discharge	None	Some discharge if silver nitrate used	
Evaluate eyeballs for size, shape	No tears	Occasional presence of some tears	Discharge: purulent (infection)
	Both present and of equal size, both round, firm	Subconjunctival hemorrhage	Agenesis or absence of one or both eyeballs
			Small eyeball (rubella syndrome)
			Lens opacity or absence of red reflex (congenital cataracts, possibly from rubella)
			Lesions: coloboma, absence of part of iris (congenital)
			Pink color of iris (albinism)
			Jaundiced sclera (hyperbilirubinemia)
Check pupils	Present, equal in size, reactive to light		Pupils: unequal, constricted, dilated, fixed (intracranial pressure, medications, tumors)
Evaluate eyeball movement	Random, jerky, uneven, focus possible briefly, following to midline	Transient strabismus or nystagmus until third or fourth month	Persistent strabismus
			Doll's eyes (increased intracranial pressure)
			Sunset (increased intracranial pressure)
Assess eyebrows: amount of hair, pattern	Distinct (not connected in midline)		Connection in midline (Cornelia de Lange syndrome)

Eyes. In pseudostrabismus, inner epicanthal folds cause the eyes to appear misaligned; however, corneal light reflexes are perfectly symmetric. Eyes are symmetric in size and shape and are well placed.

Continued

table 26-2 Physical Assessment of Newborn—cont'd

AREA ASSESSED AND APPRAISAL PROCEDURE	NORMAL FINDINGS		DEVIATIONS FROM NORMAL RANGE: POSSIBLE PROBLEMS (ETIOLOGY)
	AVERAGE FINDINGS	**NORMAL VARIATIONS**	
NOSE Observe shape, placement, patency, configuration of bridge of nose	Midline Apparent lack of bridge, flat, broad Some mucus but no drainage Preferential nose breather Sneezing to clear nose	Slight deformity from passage through birth canal	Copious drainage, with or without regular periods of cyanosis at rest and return of pink color with crying (choanal atresia, congenital syphilis) Malformed (congenital syphilis, chromosomal disorder) Flaring of nares (respiratory distress)
EARS Observe size, placement on head, amount of cartilage, open auditory canal	Correct placement: line drawn through inner and outer canthi of eyes reaching to top notch of ears (at junction with scalp) Well-formed, firm cartilage	Size: small, large, floppy Darwin's tubercle (nodule on posterior helix)	Agenesis Lack of cartilage (prematurity) Low placement (chromosomal disorder, mental retardation, kidney disorder) Preauricular tags Size: possibly overly prominent or protruding ears
Assess hearing	Responses to voice and other sounds	State (e.g., alert, asleep) influencing response	Deaf: no response to sound

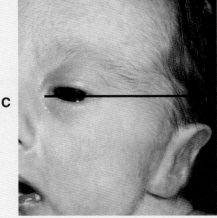

Placement of ears on the head in relation to a line drawn from the inner to the outer canthus of the eye. **A,** Normal position. **B,** Abnormally angled ear. **C,** True low-set ear. (Courtesy Mead Johnson Nutritionals, Evansville, IN.)

table 26-2 Physical Assessment of Newborn—cont'd

AREA ASSESSED AND APPRAISAL PROCEDURE	NORMAL FINDINGS		DEVIATIONS FROM NORMAL RANGE: POSSIBLE PROBLEMS (ETIOLOGY)
	AVERAGE FINDINGS	NORMAL VARIATIONS	
FACIES			
Observe overall appearance of face	"Normal" appearance, well-placed, proportionate, symmetric features	Positional deformities	Infant appearance "odd" or "funny" Usually accompanied by other features such as low-set ears, other structural disorders (hereditary, chromosomal aberration)
MOUTH			
Inspect and palpate Check placement on face Assess lips for color, configuration, movement	Symmetry of lip movement	Transient circumoral cyanosis	Gross anomalies in placement, size, shape (cleft lip and/or palate, gums) Cyanosis, circumoral pallor (respiratory distress, hypothermia) Asymmetry in movement of lips (cranial nerve VII paralysis)
Check gums	Pink gums	Inclusion cysts (Epstein pearls—Bohn nodules, whitish, hard nodules on gums or roof of mouth)	Teeth: predeciduous or deciduous (hereditary)
Assess tongue for attachment, mobility, movement, size	Tongue not protruding, freely movable, symmetric in shape, movement	Short frenulum	Macroglossia (prematurity, chromosomal disorder)
Evaluate cheeks	Sucking pads inside cheeks		Thrush: white plaques on cheeks or tongue that bleed if touched (*Candida albicans*)
Assess palate (soft, hard): Arch Uvula	Soft and hard palates intact Uvula in midline	Anatomic groove in palate to accommodate nipple, disappearance by 3 to 4 yr of age Epstein pearls	Cleft hard or soft palate
Assess chin	Distinct chin		Micrognathia (Pierre Robin or other syndrome)
Evaluate saliva for amount, character	Mouth moist		Excessive saliva (esophageal atresia, tracheoesophageal fistula)
Check reflexes: Rooting Sucking Extrusion	Reflexes present	Reflex response dependent on state of wakefulness and hunger	Absent (prematurity)
NECK			
Inspect and palpate length	Short, thick, surrounded by skin folds; no webbing		Webbing (Turner syndrome)
Check sternocleidomastoid muscles, movement and position of head	Head held in midline (sternocleidomastoid muscles equal), no masses Freedom of movement from side to side and flexion and extension, no movement of chin past shoulder	Transient positional deformity apparent when newborn is at rest: passive movement of head possible	Restricted movement, holding of head at angle (torticollis [wryneck], opisthotonos) Absence of head control (prematurity, Down syndrome)
Assess trachea for position and thyroid gland	Thyroid not palpable		Masses (enlarged thyroid) Distended veins (cardiopulmonary disorder)

Continued

table 26-2 Physical Assessment of Newborn—cont'd

AREA ASSESSED AND APPRAISAL PROCEDURE	NORMAL FINDINGS		DEVIATIONS FROM NORMAL RANGE: POSSIBLE PROBLEMS (ETIOLOGY)
	AVERAGE FINDINGS	NORMAL VARIATIONS	
CHEST			
Inspect and palpate Observe shape	Almost circular, barrel shaped	Tip of sternum possibly prominent	Bulging of chest, unequal movement (pneumothorax, pneumomediastinum) Malformation (funnel chest— pectus excavatum)
Check respiratory movements	Symmetric chest movements, chest and abdominal movements synchronized during respirations	Occasional retractions, especially when crying	Retractions with or without respiratory distress (prematurity, RDS)
Evaluate clavicles	Clavicles intact		Fracture of clavicle (trauma); crepitus (see Fig. 38-4)
Assess ribs	Rib cage symmetric, intact; moves with respirations		Poor development of rib cage and musculature (prematurity)
Assess nipples for size, placement, number	Nipples prominent, well formed; symmetrically placed		Nipples Supernumerary, along nipple line Malpositioned or widely spaced
Check breast tissue	Breast nodule: approximately 6 mm in term infant	Breast nodule: 3-10 mm Secretion of witch's milk caused by pregnancy hormones	Lack of breast tissue (prematurity)
Auscultate: Heart sounds and rate and breath sounds (see "Vital Signs")			Sounds: bowel sounds (see "Abdomen")
ABDOMEN			
Inspect, palpate, and smell umbilical cord	Two arteries, one vein Whitish gray Definite demarcation between cord and skin, no intestinal structures within cord Dry around base, drying Odorless		One artery (renal anomalies) Meconium stained (intrauterine distress) Bleeding or oozing around cord (hemorrhagic disease) Redness or drainage around cord (infection, possible persistence of urachus)
	Cord clamp in place for 24 hr	Reducible umbilical herniation	Hernia: herniation of abdominal contents into area of cord (e.g., omphalocele); defect covered with thin, friable membrane, possibly extensive
Inspect size of abdomen and palpate contour	Rounded, prominent, dome-shaped because abdominal musculature not fully developed Liver possibly palpable 1-2 cm below right costal margin No other masses palpable No distention	Some diastasis of abdominal musculature	Gastroschisis: fissure of abdominal cavity Distention at birth (ruptured viscus, genitourinary masses or malformations: hydronephrosis, teratomas, abdominal tumors) Mild (overfeeding, high gastrointestinal tract obstruction) Marked (lower gastrointestinal tract obstruction, imperforate anus) Intermittent or transient (overfeeding)

table 26-2 Physical Assessment of Newborn—cont'd

AREA ASSESSED AND APPRAISAL PROCEDURE	NORMAL FINDINGS		DEVIATIONS FROM NORMAL RANGE: POSSIBLE PROBLEMS (ETIOLOGY)
	AVERAGE FINDINGS	NORMAL VARIATIONS	
ABDOMEN—cont'd			
			Partial intestinal obstruction (stenosis of bowel)
			Visible peristalsis (obstruction)
			Malrotation of bowel or adhesions
			Sepsis (infection)
Auscultate bowel sounds and note number, amount, and character of stools; note behavior—crying, fussiness—before or during elimination	Sounds present within 1-2 hr after birth Meconium stool passing within 24-48 hr after birth		Scaphoid, with bowel sounds in chest and respiratory distress (diaphragmatic hernia)
Assess color		Linea nigra possibly apparent and caused by hormone influence during pregnancy	
Check movement with respiration	Respirations primarily diaphragmatic, abdominal and chest movement synchronous		Decreased abdominal breathing (intrathoracic disease, diaphragmatic hernia) "Seesaw" (respiratory distress)
GENITALIA			
Female (see Fig. 25-8, A)			
Inspect and palpate			
General appearance	Female genitals	Increased pigmentation caused by pregnancy hormones	Ambiguous genitals—enlarged clitoris with urinary meatus on tip, fused labia (chromosomal disorder, maternal drug ingestion)
Clitoris	Usually edematous		
Labia majora	Usually edematous, covering labia minora in term newborns	Edema and ecchymosis after breech birth	
Labia minora	Possible protrusion over labia majora	Blood-tinged discharge from pseudomenstruation caused by pregnancy hormones	
Discharge	Smegma		
Vagina	Open orifice Mucoid discharge Hymenal or vaginal tag	Some vernix caseosa between labia possible	Labia majora widely separated and labia minora prominent (prematurity) Absence of vaginal orifice or imperforate hymen Fecal discharge (fistula) Stenosed meatus
Urinary meatus	Beneath clitoris, difficult to see (to watch for voiding)		
Check urination	Voiding within 24 hours	Rust-stained urine (uric acid crystals)*	
Male (see Fig. 25-8, B)			
Inspect and palpate			
General appearance			
Penis	Male genitals	Increased size and pigmentation caused by pregnancy hormones	Ambiguous genitals
Urinary meatus as slit	Meatus at tip of penis		Urinary meatus not on tip of glans penis (hypospadias, epispadias)
Prepuce	Prepuce (foreskin) covering glans penis and not retractable	Prepuce removed if circumcised Wide variation in size of genitals	Round meatal opening

*To determine whether rust color is caused by uric acid or blood, rinse diaper under running warm tap water; uric acid washes out, blood does not.

Continued

table 26-2 Physical Assessment of Newborn—cont'd

AREA ASSESSED AND APPRAISAL PROCEDURE	NORMAL FINDINGS		DEVIATIONS FROM NORMAL RANGE: POSSIBLE PROBLEMS (ETIOLOGY)
	AVERAGE FINDINGS	**NORMAL VARIATIONS**	
GENITALIA—cont'd			
Male—cont'd			
Scrotum	Large, edematous, pendulous	Scrotal edema and ecchymosis	Scrotum smooth and testes
Rugae (wrinkles)	in term infant; covered with	if breech birth	undescended (prematurity,
	rugae	Hydrocele, small,	cryptorchidism)
		noncommunicating	Hydrocele
			Inguinal hernia
Testes	Palpable on each side	Bulge palpable in inguinal canal	Undescended (prematurity)
Check urination	Voiding within 24 hr, stream	Rust-stained urine (uric acid	
	adequate, amount adequate	crystals)*	
Check reflexes:			
Cremasteric	Testes retracted, especially		
	when newborn is chilled		
EXTREMITIES			
Make a general check:			
Inspect and palpate	Assuming of position	Transient (positional)	Limited motion
Degree of flexion	maintained in utero	deformities	(malformations)
Range of motion	Attitude of general flexion		Poor muscle tone
Symmetry of motion	Full range of motion,		(prematurity, maternal
Muscle tone	spontaneous movements		medications, CNS
			anomalies)
Check arms and hands:			
Inspect and palpate	Longer than legs in newborn	Slight tremors sometimes	Asymmetry of movement
Color	period	apparent	(fracture or crepitus,
Intactness	Contours and movement	Some acrocyanosis, especially	brachial nerve trauma,
Appropriate placement	symmetric	when chilled	malformations)
			Asymmetry of contour
			(malformations, fracture)
			Amelia or phocomelia
			(teratogens)
			Palmar creases
			Simian line with short,
			incurved little fingers
			(Down syndrome)
Check number of fingers	Five on each hand		Webbing of fingers: syndactyly
	Fist often clenched with		Absence or excess of fingers
	thumb under fingers		Strong, rigid flexion; persistent
			fists; positioning of fists in
			front of mouth constantly
			(CNS disorder)
Palpate humerus	Intact		Fractured humerus
Evaluate joints	Full range of motion,		Increased tonicity, clonicity,
Shoulder	symmetric contour		prolonged tremors (CNS
Elbow			disorder)
Wrist			
Fingers			
Check reflex: grasp			
Check legs and feet:			
Inspect and palpate	Appearance of bowing	Feet appearing to turn in	Amelia (absence of limbs),
Color	because lateral muscles	but can be easily rotated	phocomelia (shortened
Intactness	more developed than	externally, positional defects	limbs) (chromosomal defect,
Length in relation to	medial muscles	tending to correct while	teratogenic effect)
arms and body and to		infant is crying	
each other			

*To determine whether rust color is caused by uric acid or blood, rinse diaper under running warm tap water; uric acid washes out, blood does not.

table 26-2 **Physical Assessment of Newborn—cont'd**

AREA ASSESSED AND APPRAISAL PROCEDURE	NORMAL FINDINGS		DEVIATIONS FROM NORMAL RANGE: POSSIBLE PROBLEMS (ETIOLOGY)
	AVERAGE FINDINGS	NORMAL VARIATIONS	
EXTREMITIES—cont'd			
Number of toes	Five on each foot	Acrocyanosis	Webbing, syndactyly (chromosomal defect)
			Absence or excess of digits (chromosomal defect, familial trait)
Femur	Intact femur		Femoral fracture (difficult breech birth)
Head of femur as legs are flexed and abducted, placement in acetabulum (see Fig. 25-12)	No click heard, femoral head not overriding acetabulum		Congenital hip dysplasia or dislocation
Major gluteal folds	Major gluteal folds even		
Soles of feet	Soles well lined (or wrinkled) over two thirds of foot in term infants		Soles of feet Few lines (prematurity) Covered with lines (postmaturity)
	Plantar fat pad giving flat-footed effect		Congenital clubfoot Hypermobility of joints (Down syndrome)
Evaluate joints: Hip Knee Ankle Toes	Full range of motion, symmetric contour		Temperature of one leg differing from that of the other (circulatory deficiency, CNS disorder)
Check reflexes (see Table 25-3)			Asymmetric movement (trauma, CNS disorder)
BACK			
Assess anatomy:			
Inspect and palpate Spine Shoulders Scapulae Iliac crests Base of spine—pilonidal area	Spine straight and easily flexed Infant able to raise and support head momentarily when prone Shoulders, scapulae, and iliac crests lining up in same plane	Temporary minor positional deformities, correction with passive manipulation	Limitation of movement (fusion or deformity of vertebra) Pigmented nevus with tuft of hair, location anywhere along the spine, often associated with spina bifida occulta Spina bifida cystica (meningocele, myelomeningocele)
Check reflexes (spinal-related) Test trunk incurvation reflex	Trunk flexed and pelvis swings to stimulated side	May not be apparent in first few days but is usually present in 5-6 days	If transverse lesion is present, no response below lesion; absence of response: nervous system abnormality or general depression
Test magnet reflex	Lower limbs extend as pressure applied to feet with legs in semiflexed position	Weak or exaggerated response with breech presentation	Absence: suggestive of spinal cord damage or malformation
ANUS			
Inspect and palpate Placement Number Patency	One anus with good sphincter tone Passage of meconium within 24 hr after birth	Passage of meconium within 48 hr of birth	Low obstruction: anal membrane High obstruction: anal or rectal atresia

Continued

table 26-2 Physical Assessment of Newborn—cont'd

AREA ASSESSED AND APPRAISAL PROCEDURE	NORMAL FINDINGS		DEVIATIONS FROM NORMAL RANGE: POSSIBLE PROBLEMS (ETIOLOGY)
	AVERAGE FINDINGS	NORMAL VARIATIONS	
ANUS—cont'd Test for sphincter response (active "wink" reflex) Observe for following: Abdominal distention Passage of meconium Passage of fecal drainage from surrounding orifices	Good "wink" reflex of anal sphincter		Drainage of fecal material from vagina in female or urinary meatus in male (rectal fistula)
STOOLS Observe frequency, color, consistency	Meconium followed by transitional and soft yellow stools		No stool (obstruction) Frequent watery stools (infection, phototherapy)

The nurse responsible for the care of the newborn immediately after birth verifies that respirations have been established, dries the infant, assesses temperature, and places identical identification bracelets on the infant and the mother. In some settings, the father or partner also wears an identification bracelet. Information on the identification bracelets should include name, sex, date and time of birth, and identification number, according to hospital protocol. Infants also are footprinted using a form that includes the mother's fingerprints, name, and date and time of birth. These identification procedures must be performed before the mother and infant are separated after birth. The infant may be wrapped in a warm blanket and placed in the arms of the mother, given to the partner to hold, or kept partially undressed under a radiant warmer. In some settings, immediately after birth the infant is placed on the mother's abdomen to allow skin-to-skin contact. This contributes to maintenance of the infant's optimum temperature and parental bonding. The infant may be admitted to a nursery or may remain with the parents throughout the hospital stay.

The initial examination of the newborn can occur while the nurse is drying and wrapping the infant, or observations can be made while the infant is lying on the mother's abdomen or in her arms immediately after birth. Efforts should be directed to minimizing interference in the initial parent-infant acquaintance process. If the infant is breathing effectively, is pink in color, and has no apparent life-threatening anomalies or risk factors requiring immediate attention (e.g., infant of a diabetic mother), further examination can be delayed until after the parents have had an opportunity to interact with the infant. Routine procedures and the admission process may be carried out in the mother's room or in a separate nursery. Box 26-3 shows an example of newborn routine orders.

Nursing diagnoses are established after analysis of the findings of the physical assessment and may include the following:

- *Ineffective airway clearance related to*
  –airway obstruction with mucus, blood, and amniotic fluid
- *Impaired gas exchange related to*
  –airway obstruction
  –hypothermia
- *Ineffective thermoregulation related to*
  –excess heat loss

box 26-3 Routine Admission Orders

- Vital signs on admission and q30min × 2, q1hr × 2, then q8hr
- Weight, length, and head and chest circumferences on admission; then weigh daily
- Tetracycline or erythromycin ophthalmic ointment 5 mg 1 to 2 cm line in lower conjunctiva of each eye after initial parent-infant contact (but within 2 hr of birth)
- Vitamin K 0.5 to 1 mg intramuscularly
- Breastfeeding on demand may be initiated immediately after birth
- If formula feeding, give formula of mother's choice q3-4 hr on demand
- Allow rooming-in as desired and infant's condition permits
- Newborn screening panel per state health department protocol (phenylketonuria [PKU], thyroxine [T_4], and galactosemia or other newborn screening tests as ordered at least 24 hr after first feeding)
- Perform hearing screening and document results before discharge
- Serum bilirubin measurement if clinical jaundice evident
- Hepatitis B injection if indicated

• *Risk for infection related to*
  –intrauterine or extrauterine exposure to virulent virus or bacteria
  –multiple sites for opportunistic bacterial and viral entry (e.g., umbilical cord, lesions from fetal scalp electrode or vacuum extraction)

■ Expected Outcomes of Care

The expected outcomes for the newborn during the immediate recovery period include that the infant will achieve the following:
• Maintain effective breathing patterns.
• Maintain effective thermoregulation.
• Remain free from infection.
• Receive necessary nutrition for growth.

■ Plan of Care and Interventions

Changes can occur rapidly in newborns immediately after birth. Assessment must be followed quickly by the implementation of appropriate care.

■ *Stabilization*

Generally, the normal term infant born vaginally has little difficulty clearing the airway. Most secretions are moved by gravity and brought to the oropharynx by the cough reflex. The infant is often maintained in a side-lying position (head stabilized, not in Trendelenburg) with a rolled blanket at the back to facilitate drainage.

If the infant has excess mucus in the respiratory tract, the mouth and nasal passages may be suctioned with the bulb syringe (Procedure box and Fig. 26-2). The nurse may perform gentle percussion over the chest wall using a soft circular mask or a percussion cup to aid in loosening secretions before suctioning (Fig. 26-3). Routine chest percussion is avoided, especially in preterm newborns, because this may cause more harm than good; the head should be kept steady during the procedure and the infant's tolerance

FIG. 26-2 Bulb syringe. Bulb must be compressed before insertion. (Courtesy Cheryl Briggs, RN, Annapolis, MD.)

FIG. 26-3 Chest percussion. Nurse performs gentle percussion over the chest wall by using a percussion cup to aid in loosening secretions before suctioning. (Courtesy Shannon Perry, Phoenix, AZ.)

of the procedure carefully evaluated (Hagedorn, Gardner, Dickey, & Abman, 2006). The infant who is choking on secretions should be supported with the head to the side.

■ *Use of Nasopharyngeal Catheter with Mechanical Suction Apparatus*

Deeper suctioning may be needed to remove mucus from the newborn's nasopharynx or posterior oropharynx. Proper tube insertion and suctioning for 5 seconds or less per tube insertion helps prevent vagal stimulation and hypoxia (Niermeyer, 2005) (Procedure box).

■ *Relieving Airway Obstruction*

A choking infant needs immediate attention. Often, simply repositioning the infant and suctioning the mouth and nose with the bulb syringe eliminates the problem. The infant should be positioned to facilitate gravity drainage. The

---

procedure

Suctioning with a Bulb Syringe

• The mouth is suctioned first to prevent the infant from inhaling pharyngeal secretions by gasping as the nares are touched.
• The bulb is compressed (see Fig. 26-2) and inserted into one side of the mouth. The center of the infant's mouth is avoided because this could stimulate the gag reflex.
• The nasal passages are suctioned one nostril at a time.
• When the infant's cry does not sound as though it is through mucus or a bubble, suctioning can be stopped. The bulb syringe should always be kept in the infant's crib.
• The parents should be given demonstrations on how to use the bulb syringe and asked to perform a return demonstration.

procedure

Suctioning with a Nasopharyngeal Catheter with Mechanical Suction Apparatus

To remove excessive or tenacious mucus from the infant's nasopharynx:

- If wall suction is used, adjust the pressure to <80 mm Hg. Proper tube insertion and suctioning for 5 sec per tube insertion helps prevent laryngospasms and oxygen depletion.
- Lubricate the catheter in sterile water and then insert either orally along the base of the tongue or up and back into the nares.
- After the catheter is properly placed, create suction by placing your thumb over the control as the catheter is carefully rotated and gently withdrawn.
- Repeat the procedure until the infant's cry sounds clear and air entry into the lungs is heard by stethoscope.

nurse also should listen to the infant's respiration and lung sounds with a stethoscope to determine whether there are crackles, rhonchi, or inspiratory stridor. Fine crackles may be auscultated for several hours after birth. If air movement is adequate, the bulb syringe may be used to clear the mouth and nose. If the bulb syringe does not clear mucus interfering with respiratory effort, mechanical suction can be used.

If the newborn has an obstruction that is not cleared with suctioning, further investigation must be performed to determine if there is a mechanical defect (e.g., tracheo-esophageal fistula, choanal atresia) causing the obstruction (see Emergency: Relieving Airway Obstruction, p. 752). All personnel working with infants must have current infant cardiopulmonary resuscitation (CPR) certification. Many institutions offer infant CPR courses to new parents before discharge. Such instruction is especially important for parents whose infants were preterm or had cardiac or respiratory problems. Babysitters also should learn CPR.

▬ LEGAL TIP Neonatal Resusitation

It is the nurse's responsibility to ensure that the area for neonatal resuscitation is equipped and functional.

▬ *Maintaining an Adequate Oxygen Supply*

Four conditions are essential for maintaining an adequate oxygen supply:

- A clear airway
- Effective respiratory efforts
- Adequate circulation, adequate perfusion, and effective cardiac function
- Adequate thermoregulation (exposure to cold stress increases oxygen and glucose needs)

Signs of potential complications related to abnormal breathing are listed in the Signs of Potential Complications box.

signs of potential complications

Abnormal Newborn Breathing

- Bradypnea: respirations (≤25/min)
- Tachypnea: respirations (≥60/min)
- Abnormal breath sounds: crackles, rhonchi, wheezes, expiratory grunt
- Respiratory distress: nasal flaring, retractions, chin tug, labored breathing

▬ *Maintenance of Body Temperature*

Effective neonatal care includes maintenance of an optimal thermal environment. Cold stress increases the need for oxygen and may deplete glucose stores. The infant may react to exposure to cold by increasing the respiratory rate and may become cyanotic. Ways to stabilize the newborn's body temperature include placing the infant directly on the mother's abdomen and covering with a warm blanket (skin-to-skin contact); drying and wrapping the newborn in warmed blankets immediately after birth; keeping the head well covered; and keeping the ambient temperature of the nursery or mother's room at 23.8° to 26.1° C (AAP & ACOG, 2002).

If the infant does not remain with the mother during the first 1 to 2 hours after birth, the nurse places the thoroughly dried infant under a radiant warmer until the body temperature stabilizes. The infant's skin temperature is used as the point of control in a warmer with a servocontrolled mechanism. The control panel usually is maintained between 36° and 37° C. This setting should maintain the healthy newborn's skin temperature at approximately 36.5° to 37° C. A thermistor probe (automatic sensor) is taped to the right upper quadrant of the abdomen immediately below the right intercostal margin (never over a bone). A reflector adhesive patch may be used over the probe to provide adequate warming. This will ensure detection of minor changes resulting from external environmental factors or neonatal factors (peripheral vasoconstriction, vasodilation, or increased metabolism) before a dramatic change in core body temperature develops. The servocontroller adjusts the temperature of the warmer to maintain the infant's skin temperature within the present range. The sensor must be checked periodically to make sure it is securely attached to the infant's skin. The axillary temperature of the newborn is checked every hour (or more often as needed) until the newborn's temperature stabilizes. The time to stabilize and maintain body temperature varies; each newborn should therefore be allowed to achieve thermal regulation as necessary, and care should be individualized.

During all procedures, heat loss must be avoided or minimized for the newborn; therefore examinations and activities are performed with the newborn under a heat panel. The initial bath is postponed until the newborn's skin temperature is stable and can adjust to heat loss from a bath. The exact and optimal timing of the bath for each newborn remains unknown.

Even a normal term infant in good health can become hypothermic. Birth in a car on the way to the hospital, a cold birthing room, or inadequate drying and wrapping immediately after birth may cause the newborn's temperature to fall below the normal range (hypothermia). Warming the hypothermic infant is accomplished with care. Rapid warming may cause apneic spells and acidosis in an infant. The warming process is monitored to progress slowly over a period of 2 to 4 hours.

▬ Therapeutic Interventions

It is the nurse's responsibility to perform certain interventions immediately after birth to provide for the safety and well-being of the newborn.

Eye Prophylaxis. The instillation of a prophylactic agent in the eyes of all neonates is mandatory in the United States as a precaution against ophthalmia neonatorum (Fig. 26-4). This is an inflammation of the eyes resulting from gonorrheal or chlamydial infection contracted by the newborn during passage through the mother's birth canal. The agent used for prophylaxis varies according to hospital protocols, but the usual agent is erythromycin, tetracycline, or silver nitrate. Canadian hospitals have not recommended the use of silver nitrate since 1986. Its use in the United States is minimal because silver nitrate does not protect against chlamydial infection and can cause chemical conjunctivitis. In some institutions, eye prophylaxis is delayed until an hour or so (up to 2 hours) after birth so that eye contact and parent-infant attachment and bonding are facilitated. The Centers for Disease Control and Prevention specifies that it should be given as soon as possible after birth; if instillation is delayed, there should be a monitoring process in place to ensure that all newborns are treated (Centers for Disease Control and Prevention,

FIG. 26-4 Instillation of medication into eye of newborn. Thumb and forefinger are used to open the eye; medication is placed in the lower conjunctiva from the inner to the outer canthus. (Courtesy Marjorie Pyle, RNC, Lifecircle, Costa Mesa, CA.)

---

medication guide

Eye Prophylaxis: Erythromycin Ophthalmic Ointment, 0.5%, and Tetracycline Ophthalmic Ointment, 1%

ACTION ▬ These antibiotic ointments are both bacteriostatic and bactericidal. They provide prophylaxis against *Neisseria gonorrhoeae* and *Chlamydia trachomatis*.

INDICATION ▬ These medications are applied to prevent ophthalmia neonatorum in newborns of mothers who are infected with gonorrhea, conjunctivitis, or chlamydia.

NEONATAL DOSAGE AND ROUTE ▬ Apply a 1- to 2-cm ribbon of ointment to the lower conjunctival sac of each eye; also may be used in drop form.

ADVERSE EFFECTS ▬ May cause chemical conjunctivitis that lasts 24 to 48 hours; vision may be blurred temporarily.

NURSING CONSIDERATIONS ▬ Administer within 1 to 2 hr of birth. Wear gloves. Cleanse eyes if necessary before administration. Open eyes by putting a thumb and finger at the corner of each lid and gently pressing on the periorbital ridges. Squeeze the tube and spread the ointment from the inner canthus of the eye to the outer canthus. Do not touch the tube to the eye. After 1 min, excess ointment may be wiped off. Observe eyes for irritation. Explain treatment to parents. ▬ Eye prophylaxis for ophthalmia neonatorum is required by law in all states of the United States.

Workowski & Berman, 2006) (Medication Guide). In the United States, if parents object to eye prophylaxis, they may be asked to sign an informed refusal form, and their refusal will be noted in the infant's record.

Topical antibiotics such as tetracycline and erythromycin, silver nitrate, and a 2.5% povidone-iodine solution (currently unavailable in commercial form in the United States) have not proved to be effective in the treatment of chlamydial conjunctivitis. A 14-day course of oral erythromycin or an oral sulfonamide may be given for chlamydial conjunctivitis (AAP & ACOG, 2002).

Vitamin K Administration. Administering vitamin K intramuscularly is routine in the newborn period in the United States. A single injection of 0.5 to 1 mg of vitamin K is given soon after birth to prevent hemorrhagic disease of the newborn. Vitamin K is produced in the gastrointestinal tract by bacteria starting soon after microorganisms are introduced. By day 8, normal newborns are able to produce their own vitamin K (Medication Guide).

▬ NURSE ALERT

Vitamin K is never administered via the intravenous route for prevention of hemorrhagic disease of the newborn except in some cases of a preterm infant who has no muscle mass. In such cases, the medication should be diluted and given over 10 to 15 minutes, with the infant being closely monitored (cardiorespiratory monitor). Rapid bolus administration of vitamin K may cause cardiac arrest.

Umbilical Cord Care. The cord is clamped immediately after birth. The care of the umbilical cord is an important aspect of nursing care and parent teaching. The goal of care is prevention and early detection of hemorrhage

medication guide

Vitamin K: Phytonadione (AquaMEPHYTON, Konakion)

ACTION ■ This intervention provides vitamin K, necessary because the newborn does not have the intestinal flora to produce this vitamin in the first week after birth. It also promotes formation of clotting factors (II, VII, IX, X) in the liver.
INDICATION ■ Vitamin K is used for prevention and treatment of hemorrhagic disease in the newborn.
NEONATAL DOSAGE ■ Administer a 0.5- to 1-mg (0.25- to 0.5-ml) dose intramuscularly within 2 hr of birth; may be repeated if newborn shows bleeding tendencies.
ADVERSE REACTIONS ■ Edema, erythema, and pain at injection site may occur rarely; hemolysis, jaundice, and hyperbilirubinemia have been reported, particularly in preterm infants.
NURSING CONSIDERATIONS ■ Wear gloves. Administer in the middle third of the vastus lateralis muscle using a 25-gauge, ⅝-inch needle. Inject into skin that has been cleaned, or allow alcohol to dry on puncture site for 1 min to remove organisms and prevent infection. Stabilize leg firmly, and grasp muscle between the thumb and fingers. Insert the needle at a 90-degree angle; aspirate, and inject medication slowly if there is no blood return. Massage the site with a dry gauze square after removing needle to increase absorption. Observe for signs of bleeding from the site.

FIG. 26-5 With special scissors, remove clamp after cord dries (about 24 hours). (Courtesy Cheryl Briggs, RN, Annapolis, MD.)

or infection. The umbilical cord stump is an excellent medium for bacterial growth and can easily become infected (Miller & Newman, 2005).

Hospital protocol directs the technique for routine cord care. Many hospitals have subscribed to the practice of "dry care" consisting of cleaning the periumbilical area with soap and water and wiping it dry. Others apply an antiseptic solution such as triple dye or alcohol to the cord (Janssen, Selwood, Dobson, Peacock, & Thiessen, 2003). Current recommendations for cord care by the Association of Women's Health, Obstetric and Neonatal Nurses (AWHONN) include cleaning the cord with sterile water or a neutral pH cleanser. Subsequent care entails cleansing the cord with water (AWHONN, 2001). The stump and base of the cord should be assessed for edema, erythema, and drainage with each diaper change. The stump deteriorates through the process of dry gangrene; therefore odor alone is not a positive indicator of omphalitis (infection of the umbilical cord). Cord separation time is influenced by a number of factors, including type of cord care, type of birth, and other perinatal events. The average cord separation time is 10 to 14 days.

The cord clamp is removed once the stump has started drying and is no longer bleeding, typically in 24 hours (Fig. 26-5).

■ *Promoting Parent-Infant Interaction*

Today's childbirth practices strive to promote the family as the focus of care. Parents generally desire to share in the birth process and have early contact with their infants. Early contact between mother and newborn can be important in developing future relationships. It also has a positive effect on the duration of breastfeeding. The physiologic benefits of early mother-infant contact include increased oxytocin and prolactin levels in the mother and activation of sucking reflexes in the infant. The infant can be put to breast soon after birth. The process of developing active immunity begins as the infant ingests flora from the mother's colostrum.

■ Evaluation

Evaluation of the effectiveness of immediate care of the newborn is based on the previously stated outcomes.

■ CARE MANAGEMENT: FROM 2 HOURS AFTER BIRTH UNTIL DISCHARGE

The infant's admission to the nursery may be delayed, or may never occur. Depending on the routine of the hospital, the infant frequently remains in the labor area and is then transferred to either the nursery or the postpartum unit with the mother. With the emphasis on family-centered maternity care, efforts are made to keep the mother and newborn together from birth. Many hospitals have adopted variations of single-room maternity care (SRMC) or mother-baby care in which one nurse provides care for the mother and newborn. SRMC allows the infant to remain with the parents after the birth.

Many of the procedures, such as assessment of weight and measurement (i.e., circumference of head and chest, length), instillation of eye medications, intramuscular administration of vitamin K, and physical assessment, may be carried out in the labor and birth unit. Nurses who work in an SRMC unit; labor, delivery, and recovery (LDR) room; or labor, delivery, recovery, and postpartum (LDRP) room must be knowledgeable and competent in intrapartal, neonatal, and postpartum nursing care. If an infant is transferred to the nursery, the infant's identification is verified by the nurse receiving the infant, who places the baby in a warm environment and begins the admission process.

Regardless of the physical organization for care, many hospitals have a small holding nursery, which is available for procedures or on the request of the mother who wishes her infant to be placed there. This arrangement promotes parent-infant bonding while still allowing the new parents some time to be alone.

▬ Assessment and Nursing Diagnoses
▬ Baseline Measurements of Physical Growth

The examiner records baseline measurements to help assess the progress of the neonate and to determine the neonate's growth patterns. These may be recorded on growth charts. The following measurements are made.

Weight. The newborn is usually weighed shortly after birth. This may be done in the labor and birthing area, the mother's room, or on admission to the nursery. The totally unclothed neonate is placed in the center of the scale, which is usually covered with a disposable pad or diaper to prevent heat loss from conduction and infection (see p. 667). The nurse should remain in close proximity to prevent the infant from falling off the scales. The infant is commonly weighed at the same time every day during the hospital stay. Birth weight of a term infant ranges from 2500 to 4000 g.

Circumferences and Length. The head is measured at the widest part, which is the occipitofrontal diameter (see p. 668). The tape measure is placed around the head just above the infant's eyebrows.

The chest circumference usually measures about 2 cm less than the head circumference. Frequently the chest is the same size as the head but should not exceed it. The tape is placed around the infant's chest at the nipple line (see p. 668).

Abdominal circumference is measured by placing the tape around the abdomen (see p. 668). Measurements vary with the size of the infant. The abdomen should be cylindrical and protrude slightly. Abdominal measurements are not always taken but should be made when abdominal distention is suspected.

The length may be difficult to measure because of the flexed posture of the newborn (see p. 667). The examiner places the newborn on a flat surface and extends the leg until the knee is flat against the surface. Placing the head against a perpendicular surface and extending the leg may assist with this measurement. In the term infant, head-to-heel length ranges from 45 to 55 cm.

▬ Gestational Age Assessment

Assessment of gestational age is an important criterion because perinatal morbidity and mortality rates are related to gestational age and birth weight. The simplified Assessment of Gestational Age (Ballard, Novak, & Driver, 1979) is commonly used to assess gestational age of infants between 35 and 42 weeks. It assesses six external physical and six neuromuscular signs. Each sign has a number score, and the cumulative score correlates with a maturity rating of 26 to 44 weeks of gestation. The score is accurate to plus or minus 2 weeks and is accurate for infants of all races.

The New Ballard Score, a revision of the original scale, can be used with newborns as young as 20 weeks of gestation. The tool has the same physical and neuromuscular sections but includes −1 to −2 scores that reflect signs of extreme prematurity, such as fused eyelids; imperceptible breast tissue; sticky, friable, transparent skin; no lanugo; and square-window (flexion of wrist) angle greater than 90 degrees (see Fig. 26-1, A). The examination of infants with a gestational age of 26 weeks or less should be performed at a postnatal age of less than 12 hours. For infants with a gestational age of at least 26 weeks, the examination can be performed up to 96 hours after birth. To ensure accuracy, it is recommended that the initial examination be performed within the first 48 hours of life. Neuromuscular adjustments after birth in extremely immature neonates require that a follow-up examination be performed to further validate neuromuscular criteria. The scale overestimates gestational age by 2 to 4 days in infants younger than 37 weeks of gestation, especially at gestational ages of 32 to 37 weeks (Ballard, Khoury, Wedig, Wang, Eilers-Walsman, & Lipp, 1991).

▬ Classification of Newborns by Gestational Age and Birth Weight

Classification of infants at birth by both birth weight and gestational age provides a more satisfactory method for predicting mortality risks and providing guidelines for management of the neonate than estimating by gestational age or birth weight alone. The infant's birth weight, length, and head circumference are plotted on standardized graphs that identify normal values for gestational age. A normal range of birth weights exists for each gestational week (see Fig. 26-1, B), but the birth weights of preterm, term, postterm, or postmature newborns also may be outside these normal ranges. Birth weights are classified in the following ways:

- *Large for gestational age (LGA):* Weight is above the 90th percentile (or two or more standard deviations above the norm) at any week.
- *Appropriate for gestational age (AGA):* Weight falls between the 10th and 90th percentiles for infant's age.
- *Small for gestational age (SGA):* Weight is below the 10th percentile (or two or more standard deviations below the norm) at any week.
- *Low birth weight (LBW):* Weight of 2500 g or less at birth. These newborns have had either less than the expected rate of intrauterine growth or a shortened gestation period. Preterm birth and LBW commonly occur together (e.g., less than 32 weeks of gestation and birth weight of less than 1200 g).
- *Very low birth weight (VLBW):* Weight of 1500 g or less at birth.
- *Intrauterine growth restriction (IUGR):* Term applied to the fetus whose rate of growth does not meet expected norms.

Newborns are classified according to their gestational ages in the following ways:

- *Preterm or premature:* Born before completion of 37 weeks of gestation, regardless of birth weight
- *Late preterm or near term:* Born between 34 and 37 weeks of gestation
- *Term:* Born between the beginning of week 38 and the end of week 42 of gestation
- *Postterm (postdate):* Born after completion of week 42 of gestation
- *Postmature:* Born after completion of week 42 of gestation and showing the effects of progressive placental insufficiency

Maternal Effects on Gestational Age Assessment and Birth Weight. Some maternal conditions can affect the results of the gestational assessment. For instance, any infant who has had oxygen deprivation during labor will show poor muscle tone. Infants in respiratory distress tend to be flaccid and assume a "frog-leg" posture. Even though an infant may look large, such as the infant of a diabetic mother, it may respond more like a premature infant. The infant of a mother who has been receiving magnesium sulfate will tend to be somewhat lethargic.

▬ Physical Assessment

Although the initial assessment following birth may reveal significant anomalies, birth injuries, and cardiopulmonary problems that have immediate implications, a more detailed, thorough physical examination should follow within 12 to 18 hours after birth (see Table 26-2; Box 26-4).

---

box 26-4 Nursing Considerations in Examining the Newborn

- Before the assessment, review the maternal history and prenatal and intrapartal records to provide a background for the recognition of any potential problems.
- Check that equipment and supplies are working properly and are accessible.
- Provide a normothermic and nonstimulating examination area.
- Undress only the body area to be examined to prevent heat loss. Examine under a radiant warmer if available.
- Proceed in an orderly sequence (usually head to toe) with the following exceptions:
  - Perform all procedures that require quiet first, such as auscultating the lungs, heart, and abdomen.
  - Perform disturbing procedures, such as testing reflexes, last.
  - Measure head, chest, and length at the same time to compare results.
- Comfort the infant during and after examination; involve parents in the following:
  - Talking softly
  - Holding the infant's hands against chest
  - Swaddling and holding
  - After obtaining parental consent, giving pacifier or gloved finger to suck

---

The parents' presence during this and other examinations encourages discussion of parental concerns and actively involves the parents in the health care of their infant from birth. It also affords the nurse an opportunity to observe parental interactions with the infant. The findings provide a database for implementing the nursing process with newborns and providing anticipatory guidance for the parents. Ongoing assessments are made throughout the hospital stay; another detailed physical examination is performed before discharge.

An assessment of the newborn's reflexes (see Table 25-4) provides useful information about the infant's nervous system and state of neurologic maturation. The assessment must be carried out as early as possible because abnormal signs present in the early neonatal period may disappear. They may reappear months or years later as abnormal functions.

▬ Common Problems in the Newborn

Physical Injuries. Birth trauma includes any physical injury sustained by a newborn during labor and birth. Although most injuries are minor and resolve during the neonatal period without treatment, some types of trauma require intervention. A few are serious enough to be fatal.

Factors that may predispose the neonate to birth trauma include prolonged or precipitous labor, preterm labor, fetal macrosomia, cephalopelvic disproportion, abnormal presentation, and congenital anomalies. Injury can be the result of obstetric birth techniques such as forceps-assisted birth, vacuum extraction, version and extraction, and cesarean birth (Efird & Hernandez, 2005).

Soft-Tissue Injuries. Cephalhematoma is the most common type of cranial injury in newborns and can be associated with an underlying skull fracture. Caput succedaneum is diffuse swelling of the soft tissues of the scalp and is a result of pressure of the uterus or vaginal wall on the fetal head (Efird & Hernandez, 2005). Caput succedaneum and cephalhematoma are described in Chapter 25 (see Fig. 25-5).

Subconjunctival and retinal hemorrhages result from rupture of capillaries caused by increased pressure during birth (see Chapter 38). These hemorrhages usually clear within 5 days after birth and present no further problems. Parents need explanation and reassurance that these injuries will resolve without sequelae.

Erythema, ecchymoses, petechiae, abrasions, lacerations, or edema of buttocks and extremities may be present. Localized discoloration may appear over presenting parts and may result from the application of forceps or the vacuum extractor. Ecchymoses and edema may appear anywhere on the body. The specific location of these injuries should be documented.

Bruises over the face may be the result of face presentation (see Fig. 38-1). In a breech presentation, bruising and swelling may be seen over the buttocks or genitalia (see Fig. 38-2). The skin over the entire head may be ecchymotic and covered with petechiae caused by a tight nuchal cord. Petechiae (pinpoint hemorrhagic areas) acquired during birth may extend over the upper trunk and face. These lesions are benign if they disappear within 2 or 3 days of birth and no new lesions appear. Ecchymoses and petechiae may be signs of a more serious disorder, such as thrombocytopenic purpura.

■ **NURSE ALERT**
To differentiate hemorrhagic areas from skin rashes and discolorations, try to blanch the skin with two fingers. Petechiae and ecchymoses do not blanch because extravasated blood remains within the tissues, whereas skin rashes and discolorations do.

Trauma resulting from dystocia occurs to the presenting fetal part. Forceps injury and bruising from the vacuum extractor cup occur at the site where the instruments were applied. In a forceps injury, commonly a linear mark appears across both sides of the face in the shape of the forceps blades. The affected areas are kept clean to minimize the risk of infection. If the skin is abraded, an antibiotic ointment may be ordered. With the increased use of the vacuum extractor and the use of padded forceps blades, the incidence of these lesions may be significantly reduced (Mangurten, 2006).

Accidental lacerations may be inflicted with a scalpel during a cesarean birth. These cuts may occur on any part of the body but are most often found on the face, scalp, buttocks, and thighs. Usually they are superficial and only need to be kept clean. Liquid skin adhesive or butterfly adhesive strips can hold together the edges of more serious lacerations. Rarely are sutures needed.

Skeletal Injuries. Fracture of the clavicle (collarbone) is the most common birth injury. This injury is often associated with macrosomia and is a result of compression of the shoulder or manipulation of the affected arm during delivery. A fractured clavicle usually heals without treatment, although the arm and shoulder may be immobilized for comfort (Efird & Hernandez, 2005).

Fractures of the humerus and femur may occur during a difficult birth, but such fractures in newborns generally heal rapidly. Immobilization is accomplished with slings, splints, swaddling, and other devices.

The infant's immature, flexible skull can withstand a great deal of molding before fracture results. Fractures may occur during difficult births and result from the head pressing on the bony pelvis or from the injudicious application of forceps. The location of a skull fracture determines whether it is insignificant or fatal. Spontaneous or nonsurgical elevation of the indentation using a hand breast pump or vacuum extractor has been reported.

Nerve injuries may result in temporary or permanent paralysis. Brachial plexus injuries can affect movement of the shoulder, arm, wrist, or hand. Phrenic nerve palsy can occur because of hyperextension of the neck during difficult delivery and can cause respiratory distress. Facial palsy affects one side of the face and is usually self-limiting (Efird & Hernandez, 2005).

Parents need emotional support when it comes to handling a newborn with birth injuries because they are often fearful of hurting their newborn. Parents are encouraged to practice handling, changing, and feeding the injured newborn under the guidance of the nursing staff. This increases the parents' knowledge and confidence, in addition to facilitating attachment. A plan for follow-up therapy is developed with the parents so that the times and arrangements for therapy are convenient for them.

Physiologic Problems
Physiologic Jaundice. The infant who is diagnosed with physiologic jaundice appears to be otherwise well and exhibits signs of jaundice after age 24 hours. Jaundice is clinically visible when bilirubin levels reach 5 to 7 mg/dl. Clinically the indirect-reacting bilirubin (unconjugated) is no more than 12 mg/dl by 3 days of age. In preterm infants the peak is higher (15 mg/dl) and tends to occur later. The peak indirect bilirubin level may be higher in breast-fed infants (15 to 17 mg/dl). Jaundice is considered to be pathologic if it appears before 24 hours of age, increases more than 0.5 mg/dl/hr, peaks at greater than 13 mg/dl in a term infant, or is associated with anemia and hepatosplenomegaly. Jaundice that appears before 24 hours of age always warrants immediate attention. Pathologic jaundice is usually caused by blood group incompatibility or infection but may rarely be the result of RBC enzyme defects (glucose-6-phosphate dehydrogenase [G6PD], pyruvate kinase), RBC membrane disorders (spherocytosis, ovalocytosis), or hemoglobinopathy (thalassemia) (Frank & Frank, 2006) (see Chapter 39).

■ **NURSE ALERT**
At any serum bilirubin level, the appearance of jaundice during the first 24 hours of life or persistence beyond day 7 usually indicates a pathologic process.

Every newborn is assessed for jaundice. The blanch test helps differentiate cutaneous jaundice from skin color. To do the test, apply pressure with a finger over a bony area (e.g., the nose, forehead, sternum) for several seconds to empty all the capillaries in that spot. If jaundice is present, the blanched area will look yellow before the capillaries refill. The conjunctival sacs and buccal mucosa also are assessed, especially in darker-skinned infants. It is better to assess for jaundice in daylight, because artificial lighting and reflection from nursery walls can distort the actual skin color.

Jaundice appears in a cephalocaudal manner. It is generally first noticed in the head, especially the sclera and mucous membranes, and then progresses gradually to the thorax, abdomen, and extremities. It dissipates in the reverse order.

Feeding practices may influence the appearance and degree of physiologic hyperbilirubinemia. Early (within the first hour) and frequent feeding tends to keep the serum bilirubin level low by stimulating intestinal activity (the gastrocolic reflex) and passage of meconium.

Cold stress of the newborn may result in acidosis and increase the level of free fatty acids. In the presence of acidosis, albumin binding of bilirubin is weakened, and bilirubin is freed.

Noninvasive monitoring of bilirubin via cutaneous reflectance measurements (transcutaneous bilirubinometry [TcB]) allows for repetitive estimations of bilirubin levels (Fig. 26-6). These devices work well on dark- and light-skinned infants and correlate fairly well with serum measurements of bilirubin levels in term infants. With shorter maternity stays, the transcutaneous bilirubin measurement can be valuable as an assessment tool for home care follow-up. It is important to note that the intensity of jaundice is not always related to the degree of hyperbilirubinemia. Transcutaneous bilirubin meters have been significantly improved in the last 2 decades and may reduce or obviate the need for blood sampling in certain healthy neonates. The new TcB monitors provide accurate measurements within 2 to 3 mg/dl in most neonatal populations at serum levels less than 15 mg/dl (American Academy of Pediatrics [AAP], 2004).

■ **NURSE ALERT**

After phototherapy has been initiated, TcB is no longer useful as a screening tool.

A newer method to screen healthy infants in need of close follow-up is the end-tidal carbon monoxide (CO) levels in the breath corrected for inhaled CO (ETCOc). CO binds to hemoglobin and is eliminated from the body by the lungs through exhalation (Juretschke, 2005).

The use of hour-specific serum bilirubin levels to predict newborns at risk for rapidly rising levels has now become an official recommendation of the AAP Subcommittee on Hyperbilirubinemia (2004), for the monitoring of healthy neonates at 35 weeks of gestation or greater before discharge from the hospital. Using a nomogram with three levels (high, intermediate, or low risk) of rising total serum bilirubin may be done at the same time as the routine newborn profile (phenylketonuria [PKU], galactosemia, and others) (Fig. 26-7).

In many institutions the hour-specific bilirubin risk nomogram is used to determine the infant's risk for development of hyperbilirubinemia requiring medical treatment or closer screening. Risk factors recognized to place infants in the high risk category include gestational age less than 38 weeks, breastfeeding, previous sibling with significant jaundice, and jaundice appearing before discharge (AAP Subcommittee on Hyperbilirubinemia, 2004; Maisels, 2005).

It is recommended that healthy infants (35 weeks or greater) receive follow-up care and assessment of bilirubin within 3 days of discharge if discharged at less than 24 hours as well as a risk assessment with tools such as the hour-specific nomogram. Newborns discharged at 24 to 47.9 hours should receive follow-up evaluation within 4 days (96 hours), and those discharged between 48 and 72 hours should receive follow-up within 5 days (AAP Subcommittee on Hyperbilirubinemia, 2004).

■ **NURSE ALERT**

In cases in which the infant is discharged from the hospital before 48 hours after birth or the infant is born at home, a professional attendant may not be available to assess pathologic increases in circulating unbound bilirubin. Therefore all parents need instruction in how to assess jaundice and when to call the health care provider.

The overall goal is to prevent neonatal bilirubin levels from increasing to levels that place the infant at risk for acute bilirubin encephalopathy or kernicterus (Bhutani, Johnson, & Keren, 2005) (see Chapter 39). The parent should notify the health care provider if the jaundice appears to be increasing, that is, extending to the abdomen, arms, or legs; if the sclera appear yellow; or if the newborn is difficult to awaken, is fussy, or not nursing or taking formula well. Placing the baby in sunlight is not recommended because it is effective only if the infant is completely undressed. This presents danger in terms of hypothermia and the risk of sunburn (AAP, 2004). (Jaundice associated with breastfeeding is discussed in Chapter 27.)

Hypoglycemia. Hypoglycemia during the early newborn period of a term infant is defined as a blood glucose concentration of less than 35 mg/dl or a plasma concentration of less than 40 mg/dl. When the neonate is born and abruptly disconnected from the continuous supply of maternal glucose, there is a period of adjustment as the newborn begins to regulate blood glucose concentration in accordance with intermittent feedings. Hypoglycemia can result if this metabolic adaptation is delayed, if early feedings result in limited intake, or if the neonate is stressed. The glucose level normally declines during the first hours after birth. Not all newborns are routinely screened for hypoglycemia. Instead, those who are symptomatic and those considered to be at risk for hypoglycemia are tested. Risk factors for hypoglycemia include birth weight less than 2500 g or greater than 4000 g, gestational age less than 37 weeks or greater than 42 weeks,

FIG. 26-6 Trancutaneous monitoring of bilirubin with a TcB monitor. (Courtesy Cheryl Briggs, RN, Annapolis, MD.)

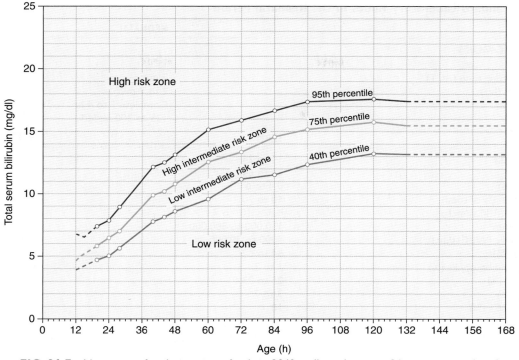

FIG. 26-7 Nomogram for designation of risk in 2840 well newborns at 36 or more weeks of gestational age with birth weight of 2000 g or more or 35 or more weeks of gestational age and birth weight of 2500 g or more based on the hour-specific serum bilirubin values. (This nomogram should not be used to represent the natural history of neonatal hyperbilirubinemia.) (From Bhutani, V., Johnson, L., & Sivieri, E. [1999]. Predictive ability of a predischarge hour-specific serum bilirubin for subsequent significant hyperbilirubinemia in healthy term and near-term newborns. *Pediatrics, 103*[1], 6-14.)

LGA infant, SGA infant, maternal diabetes, and 5-minute APGAR of 5 or less. Blood glucose levels should be checked initially between 30 minutes and 2 hours of life, and repeated every 30 minutes to 1 hour until the levels are consistently within normal limits. Glucose levels may continue to be measured every 4 hours until the risk period has passed (Townsend, 2005).

Signs of hypoglycemia include jitteriness; an irregular respiratory effort; cyanosis; apnea; a weak, high-pitched cry; feeding difficulty; hunger; lethargy; twitching; eye rolling; and seizures. The signs may be transient and recurrent.

Hypoglycemia in the low risk term infant is usually eliminated by feeding the infant. Occasionally the intravenous administration of glucose is required for newborns with persistently high insulin levels or those with depleted glycogen stores.

Hypocalcemia. Hypocalcemia (serum calcium levels of less than 7.8 to 8 mg/dl in term infants and 7 mg/dl in preterm infants) may occur in newborns of diabetic mothers or in those who had perinatal asphyxia or trauma, and in LBW and preterm infants. Early-onset hypocalcemia occurs within the first 72 hours after birth. Signs of hypocalcemia include jitteriness, high-pitched cry, irritability, apnea, intermittent cyanosis, abdominal distention, and laryngospasm, although some hypocalcemic infants are asymptomatic (Blackburn, 2003).

In most instances, early-onset hypocalcemia is self-limiting and resolves within 1 to 3 days. Treatment includes early feeding and, occasionally, the administration of calcium supplements. Preterm or asphyxiated infants may require intravenous elemental calcium.

Jitteriness is a symptom of both hypoglycemia and hypocalcemia; therefore hypocalcemia must be considered if the therapy for hypoglycemia proves ineffective. In many newborns, jitteriness remains despite therapy and cannot be explained by hypoglycemia or hypocalcemia (Rigo & De Curtis, 2006).

▬ *Laboratory and Diagnostic Tests*

Because newborns experience many transitional events in the first 28 days of life, laboratory samples are often gathered to determine adequate physiologic adaptation and to identify disorders that may adversely affect the child's life beyond the neonatal period. Tests that are commonly performed include blood glucose levels, bilirubin levels, complete blood count (CBC), newborn screening tests, and toxicology screening. Standard laboratory values for a term newborn are given in Table 26-3.

Newborn Genetic Screening. Before hospital discharge, a heel-stick blood sample is obtained to detect a variety of congenital conditions. Mandated by U.S. law, newborn genetic screening is an important public health

table 26-3 Standard Laboratory Values in the Neonatal Period

NEONATAL

1. HEMATOLOGIC VALUES

Clotting factors

Activated clotting time (ACT)	2 min
Bleeding time (Ivy)	2 to 7 min
Clot retraction	Complete 1 to 4 hr
Fibrinogen	125 to 300 mg/dl*

	TERM	PRETERM
Hemoglobin (g/dl)	14 to 24	15 to 17
Hematocrit (%)	44 to 64	45 to 55
Reticulocytes (%)	0.4 to 6	Up to 10
Fetal hemoglobin (% of total)	40 to 70	80 to 90
Red blood cells (RBCs)/mcl	4.8×10^6 to 7.1×10^6	
Platelet count/mm³	150,000 to 300,000	120,000 to 180,000
White blood cells (WBCs)/mcl	9000 to 30,000	10,000 to 20,000
Neutrophils (%)	54 to 62	47
Eosinophils and basophils (%)	1 to 3	
Lymphocytes (%)	25 to 33	33
Monocytes (%)	3 to 7	4
Immature WBCs (%)	10	16

*dl refers to deciliter (1 dl = 100 ml); this conforms to the SI system (standardized international measurements).
†mcl refers to microliter.

NEONATAL

2. BIOCHEMICAL VALUES

Bilirubin, direct			0 to 1 mg/dl
Bilirubin, total	Cord:		<2 mg/dl
	Peripheral blood:	0 to 1 day	6 mg/dl
		1 to 2 days	8 mg/dl
		2 to 5 days	12 mg/dl
Blood gases		Arterial:	pH 7.31 to 7.49
			Pco_2 26 to 41 mm Hg
			Po_2 60 to 70 mm Hg
		Venous:	pH 7.31 to 7.41
			Pco_2 40 to 50 mm Hg
			Po_2 40 to 50 mm Hg
Serum glucose			40 to 60 mg/dl

NEONATAL

3. URINALYSIS

Color	Clear, straw
Specific gravity	1.001 to 1.020
pH	5 to 7
Protein	Negative
Glucose	Negative
Ketones	Negative
RBCs	0 to 2
WBCs	0 to 4
Casts	None

Volume: 24 to 72 ml/kg excreted daily in the first few days; by week 1, 24-hr urine volume close to 200 ml.
Protein: may be present in first 2 to 4 days.
Osmolarity (mOsm/L): 100 to 600.

Some data from Hockenberry, M. (2003). Wong's nursing care of infants and children (7th ed.). St. Louis: Mosby; Pagana, K., & Pagana, T. (2006). Mosby's manual of diagnostic and laboratory tests (3rd ed.). St. Louis: Mosby.

program that is aimed at early detection of genetic diseases that result in severe health problems if not treated early. Newborn screening is regulated by the states and there is marked variation in the types of disorders included in routine screening tests. All states in the U.S. and provinces in Canada screen for PKU and hypothyroidism, but each state and province determine whether other tests are performed. Other genetic defects that are included in some screening programs include galactosemia, cystic fibrosis, maple syrup urine disease, and sickle cell disease. It is recommended that the screening test be repeated at age 1 to 2 weeks if the initial specimen was obtained when the infant was younger than 24 hours (Albers & Levy, 2005; Zinn, 2006).

Newborn Hearing Screening. Hearing loss is one of the most frequently occurring problems present at birth, occurring in 3 in 1000 infants. During the first 2 years of life, a child learns speech and language. When hearing loss is identified early, interventions can help prevent early developmental delays (Newborn hearing screening devices, 2005). To address this problem, 38 states have enacted legislation mandating universal hearing screening (www.newborn-hearing-screening.org/about_screening.htm), and it is performed routinely in other states. Infants in the neonatal intensive care unit (NICU) and those with other risk factors are screened in many settings where universal screening is not routinely done. The majority (90%) of newborns are screened for hearing loss in the United States. before leaving the nursery (Johnson et al., 2005).

Screening involves an ABR (auditory brainstem response), an OAE (otoacoustic emissions testing), or a combination of the two. Infants are usually screened at birth with an OAE (Fig. 26-8, *A*). If the infant fails the OAE, he or she is next screened with the ABR. Infants who fail the ABR are referred for diagnostic testing (Johnson et al., 2005). Neither test is definitive in diagnosis of hearing loss; they are used to determine whether further, more accurate hearing testing is needed.

In the OAE, a soft rubber earpiece which makes a soft clicking noise is placed in the baby's outer ear (Fig. 26-8, *B*). A healthy ear will "echo" the click sound back to a microphone inside the earpiece that is in the baby's ear. The ABR is performed by attaching sensors to the baby's forehead and behind each ear. An earphone is placed in the baby's outer ear and sends a series of quiet sounds into the sleeping baby's ear (Fig. 26-8,*C*). The sensors measure the responses of the baby's acoustic nerve. The responses are recorded and stored in a computer.

The AAP recommends routine hearing screening for all newborns before hospital discharge through early hearing detection and intervention programs (EHDI). Using

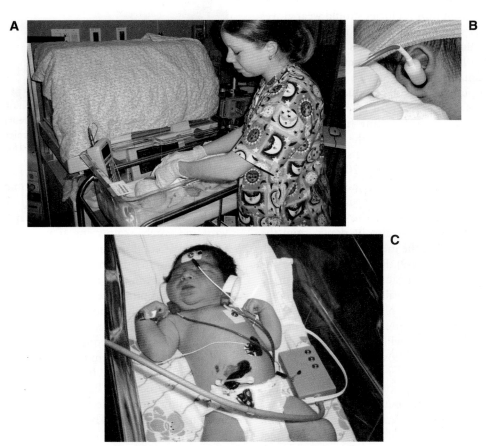

FIG. 26-8   Hearing screening in a newborn nursery. **A,** OAE (otoacoustic emissions testing). **B,** Earpiece in place for OAE, **C,** ABR (auditory brainstem response) testing. (**A** and **B,** Courtesy Cheryl Briggs, RN, Annapolis, MD; **C,** Courtesy Dee Lowdermilk, Chapel Hill, NC.)

noninvasive technology, newborn hearing screening provides information about the pathways from the external ear to the cerebral cortex. Newborns who do not pass the initial screening test should be followed and evaluated within 3 months. Regardless of the outcome of hearing testing, any infant with risk factors for hearing loss should have ongoing audiologic and medical follow-up for 3 years so that any hearing loss may be promptly identified and treated (Joint Committee on Infant Hearing, 2000).

▬ Collection of Specimens

Ongoing evaluation of a newborn often requires obtaining blood by the heel-stick or venipuncture method or the collection of a urine specimen.

Heel Stick. Most blood specimens are drawn by laboratory technicians. Nurses, however, may be required to perform heel sticks to obtain blood for glucose monitoring and to measure hematocrit levels. The same technique is needed to obtain a blood sample for newborn genetic screening tests.

It may be helpful to warm the heel before the sample is taken, because the application of heat for 5 to 10 minutes helps dilate the vessels in the area. A cloth soaked with warm water and wrapped loosely around the foot can effectively warm the foot. Disposable heel warmers also are available from a variety of companies but should be used with care to prevent burns. Nurses should wear gloves when collecting any specimen. The nurse first cleanses the area with alcohol, allows it to dry, restrains the infant's foot with his or her free hand, and then punctures the site. A spring-loaded automatic puncture device causes less pain and requires fewer punctures than a manual lance blade.

The most serious complication of an infant heel stick is necrotizing osteochondritis resulting from lancet penetration of the bone. To prevent this, the stick should be made at the outer aspect of the heel and should penetrate no deeper than 2.4 mm (Hockenberry, 2003). To identify the appropriate puncture site, the nurse should draw an imaginary line from between the fourth and fifth toes that runs parallel to the lateral aspect of the heel, where the stick should be made; a line can also be drawn from the great toe that runs parallel to the medial aspect of the heel, another site for a stick (Fig. 26-9). Repeated trauma to the walking surface of the heel can cause fibrosis and scarring that may lead to problems with walking later in life.

After the specimen has been collected, pressure should be applied with a dry gauze square, but no further alcohol should be applied because this will cause the site to continue to bleed. The site is then covered with an adhesive bandage. The nurse ensures proper disposal of equipment used, reviews the laboratory slip for correct identification, and checks the specimen for accurate labeling and routing.

A heel stick is traumatic for the infant and causes pain. After several heel sticks, infants often withdraw their feet when they are touched. To reassure the infant and promote feelings of safety, the neonate should be cuddled and comforted when the procedure is complete and appropriate pain management measures taken to minimize the pain.

FIG. 26-9 A, Heel stick sites (*shaded areas*) on infant's foot for obtaining samples of capillary blood. **B,** Venipuncture using a butterfly needle. (**B,** Courtesy Cheryl Briggs, RN, Annapolis, MD.).

Venipuncture. A venipuncture may be less painful than a heel stick for blood sampling. Venous blood samples can be drawn from antecubital, saphenous, superficial wrist and, rarely, scalp veins. If an intravenous site is used to obtain a blood specimen, it is important to consider the type of infusion fluid, because mixing of the blood sample with the fluid can alter the results.

When venipuncture is required, positioning of the needle is extremely important. Although regular venipuncture needles may be used, some prefer butterfly needles. A 25-gauge needle is adequate for blood sampling in neonates, with minimal hemolysis occurring when the proper procedure is followed. It is necessary to be very patient during the procedure, because the blood return in small veins is slow, and consequently the small needle must remain in place longer. The mummy restraint commonly is used to help secure the infant (Fig. 26-10).

For external jugular venipuncture, "mummy" the infant as necessary, and then lower the infant's head over a rolled towel, the edge of a table, or your knee, and stabilize. For femoral venipuncture, place your hands over the infant's

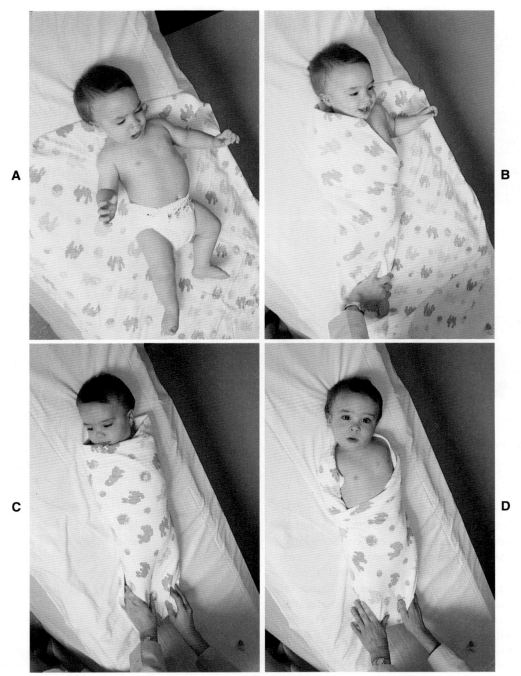

FIG. 26-10 Application of mummy restraint. **A,** Infant is placed on folded corner of blanket. **B,** One corner of blanket is brought across body and secured beneath the body. **C,** Second corner is brought across body and secured, and lower corner is folded and tucked or pinned in place. **D,** Modified mummy restraint with chest uncovered. (From Hockenberry, M. [2003]. *Wong's nursing care of infants and children* [7th ed.]. St. Louis: Mosby.)

knees, but avoid pressing your fingers over the inner aspect of the thigh (Fig. 26-11, *A*). Both of these positions ensure the safety of the infant and exposure of the puncture sites. If the radial vein is used, the infant's arm is exposed and held securely in place.

If venipuncture or arterial puncture is being performed for blood gas studies, crying, fear, and agitation will affect the values; therefore every effort must be made to keep the infant quiet during the procedure. For blood gas studies,

the blood sample tubes are packed in ice (to reduce blood cell metabolism) and are taken immediately to the laboratory for analysis.

Pressure must be maintained over an arterial or femoral vein puncture with a dry gauze square for at least 3 to 5 minutes to prevent bleeding from the site. For an hour after any venipuncture, the nurse should then observe the infant frequently for evidence of bleeding or hematoma formation at the puncture site. The infant's tolerance of the

FIG. 26-11 A, Restraining infant for femoral vein puncture. **B,** Modified side-lying position for lumbar puncture. (From Hockenberry, M. [2003]. *Wong's nursing care of infants and children* [7th ed.]. St. Louis: Mosby.)

procedure also should be recorded. The infant should be cuddled and comforted when the procedure is completed.

Obtaining a Urine Specimen. Examination of urine is a valuable laboratory tool for infant assessment; the way in which the urine specimen is collected may influence the results. The urine sample should be fresh and analyzed within 1 hour of collection.

A variety of urine collection bags are available, including the Hollister U-Bag (Fig. 26-12). These are clear plastic, single-use bags with an adhesive material around the opening at the point of attachment.

To prepare the infant, the nurse removes the diaper and places the infant in a supine position. The genitalia, perineum, and surrounding skin are washed and thoroughly dried because the adhesive on the bag will not stick to moist, powdered, or oily skin surfaces. The protective paper is removed to expose the adhesive (Fig. 26-12, *A*). In female infants, the perineum is first stretched to flatten skin folds, and then the adhesive area on the bag is pressed firmly onto the skin all around the urinary meatus and vagina. (*NOTE:* Start with the narrow portion of the butterfly-shaped adhesive patch.) Starting the application at the bridge of skin separating the rectum from the vagina and working upward is most effective (Fig. 26-12, *B*). In male infants, the penis and scrotum are tucked through the opening into the collection bag before the protective paper is removed from the adhesive and it is pressed firmly onto the perineum, making sure the entire adhesive is firmly attached to skin and the edges of the opening do not pucker (Fig. 26-12, *C*). This helps ensure a leakproof seal and decreases the chance of contamination from stool. Cutting a slit in the diaper and pulling the bag through the slit also may help prevent leaking.

The diaper is carefully replaced, and the bag is checked frequently. When a sufficient amount of urine (this amount varies according to the test done) appears, the bag is removed. The infant's skin is observed for signs of irritation while the bag is in place. The specimen can be aspirated with a syringe or drained directly from the bag.

Collection of a 24-hour specimen can be a challenge; the infant may need to be restrained. The 24-hour urine bag is applied in the manner just described, and the urine is drained into a receptacle. During the collection, the infant's skin is observed closely for signs of irritation and for lack of a proper seal.

For some types of urine tests, urine can be aspirated directly from the diaper by means of a syringe without a needle. If the diaper has absorbent gelling material that traps urine, a small gauze dressing or some cotton balls can be placed inside the diaper and the urine aspirated from them (Hockenberry, 2003).

▬ Restraining the Infant

Infants may need to be restrained to (1) protect the infant from injury, (2) facilitate examinations, and (3) limit discomfort during tests, procedures, and specimen collections

FIG. 26-12 Collection of urine specimen. **A,** Protective paper is removed from the adhesive surface. **B,** Applied to girls. **C,** Applied to boys. (Permission to use and/or reproduce this copyrighted material has been granted by the owner, Hollister Incorporated, Libertyville, IL.)

(see Figs. 26-10 and 26-11). The following special considerations must be kept in mind when restraining an infant:

- Apply restraints and check them to make sure they are not irritating the skin or impairing circulation.
- Maintain proper body alignment.
- Apply restraints without using knots or pins if possible. If knots are necessary, make the kind that can be released quickly. Use pins with care so that there is no danger of their puncturing or pressing against the infant's skin.
- Check the infant hourly, or more frequently if indicated.

Restraint Without Appliance. The nurse may restrain the infant by using the hands and body. Figure 26-10, illustrates ways to restrain an infant in this manner.

Possible nursing diagnoses for the newborn from 2 hours after birth until discharge include the following:

- *Ineffective breathing pattern related to*
  - –obstructed airway
- *Impaired gas exchange related to*
  - –ineffective breathing pattern
- *Ineffective thermoregulation related to*
  - –excess heat loss to the environment
- *Acute pain related to*
  - –circumcision
  - –heel stick, venipuncture

Possible nursing diagnoses for the parents are as follows:

- *Readiness for enhanced family coping related to*
  - –knowledge of newborn's social capabilities
  - –knowledge of newborn's dependency needs
  - –knowledge of biologic characteristics of the newborn
- *Situational low self-esteem related to*
  - –misinterpretation of newborn's behavioral cues

Examples of nursing diagnoses derived from specific assessment findings are listed in the Plan of Care.

▬ Expected Outcomes of Care

The expected outcomes for newborn care relate to the infant and parents. The outcomes for the infant are that the infant will do the following:

- Continue to maintain an effective breathing pattern.
- Continue to maintain effective thermoregulation.
- Remain free from infection.
- Establish adequate feeding and elimination patterns.
- Experience minimal pain.

For the parents, expected outcomes include the following:

- Attain knowledge, skill, and confidence relevant to infant care activities.
- State understanding of biologic and behavioral characteristics of their newborn.
- Have opportunities to intensify their relationship with the infant.
- Integrate the infant into the family.

▬ Plan of Care and Interventions

In the inpatient setting, priorities of care must be established and a systematic teaching plan devised for infant care. One way to accomplish this is to use critical path case management. A care path may be developed to cover the changes expected in the infant during the first several days of life (Care Path). When variations from the care path occur, further assessment and intervention may be necessary.

▬ *Protective Environment*

The provision of a protective environment is basic to the care of the newborn. The construction, maintenance, and operation of nurseries in accredited hospitals are monitored by national professional organizations such as the AAP, Joint Commission on Accreditation of Healthcare Organizations (JCAHO), Occupational Safety and Health Administration (OSHA), and local or state governing bodies. In addition, hospital personnel develop their own policies and procedures for protecting the newborns under their care. Prescribed standards cover areas such as the following:

- *Environmental factors:* Provision of adequate lighting, elimination of potential fire hazards, safety of electrical appliances, adequate ventilation, and controlled temperature (i.e., warm and free of drafts) and humidity (lower than 50%).
- *Infection control factors:* Adequate floor space to permit the positioning of bassinets at least 3 feet apart in all directions, handwashing facilities, and areas for cleaning and storing equipment and supplies.
  - –Only those personnel directly involved in the care of mothers and infants are allowed in these areas, thereby reducing the opportunities for the transmission of pathogenic organisms.

▬ NURSE ALERT

Personnel are instructed to use good handwashing techniques. Handwashing before and after each infant handling is the single most important measure in the prevention of neonatal infection. An alternative to handwashing may be the use of an approved antimicrobial hand cleanser. Before caring for any newborn, the nurse must cleanse her hands according to the policy of the particular institution.

- –Health care personnel must wear gloves when handling the infant until blood and amniotic fluid have been removed from the infant's skin, when drawing blood (e.g., heel stick), when caring for a fresh wound (e.g., circumcision), and during diaper changes.
- –Visitors and health care providers such as nurses, physicians, parents, brothers and sisters, department supervisors, electricians, and housekeepers are expected to wash their hands before having contact with infants or equipment. Cover gowns are not necessary.
- –Individuals with infectious conditions are excluded from contact with newborns or must take special precautions when working with infants. This includes persons with upper respiratory tract infections, gastrointestinal tract infections, and infectious skin

CD: Plan of Care: The Normal Newborn

plan of care ▶   The Normal Newborn

NURSING DIAGNOSIS Risk for ineffective airway clearance related to excess mucus production or improper positioning

Expected Outcomes *Neonate's airway remains patent, breath sounds are clear, and no respiratory distress is evident.*

Nursing Interventions/Rationales
- Teach parents that gagging, coughing, and sneezing are normal neonatal responses *that assist the neonate in clearing airways.*
- Teach parents feeding techniques that prevent overfeeding and distention of the abdomen and to burp neonate frequently *to prevent regurgitation and aspiration.*
- Position neonate on back when sleeping *to prevent suffocation.*
- Suction mouth and nasopharynx with bulb syringe as needed; clean nares of crusted secretions *to clear airway and prevent aspiration and airway obstruction.*

NURSING DIAGNOSIS Risk for imbalanced body temperature related to larger body surfaces in relationship to mass

Expected Outcome *Neonate temperature remains in range of 36.5° C to 37.2° C.*

Nursing Interventions/Rationales
- Maintain neutral thermal environment *to identify any changes in neonate's temperature that may be related to other causes.*
- Monitor neonate's temperature frequently *to identify any changes promptly and ensure early interventions.*
- Bathe neonate efficiently when temperature is stable, using warm water, drying carefully, and avoiding exposing neonate to drafts *to avoid heat losses from evaporation and convection.*
- Report any alterations in temperature findings promptly *to assess and treat for possible infection.*

NURSING DIAGNOSIS Risk for infection related to immature immunologic defenses and environmental exposure

Expected Outcome *The neonate will be free from signs of infection.*

Nursing Interventions/Rationales
- Review maternal record for evidence of any risk factors *to ascertain whether the neonate may be predisposed to infection.*
- Provide prescribed eye prophylaxis *to prevent infection.*
- Monitor vital signs *to identify early possible evidence of infection, especially temperature instability.*
- Have all care providers, including parents, practice good handwashing techniques before handling newborn *to prevent spread of infection.*

- Keep genital area clean and dry using proper cleansing techniques *to prevent skin irritation, cross-contamination, and infection.*
- Keep umbilical stump clean and dry and keep exposed to air *to allow to dry and minimize chance of infection.*
- If infant is circumcised, keep site clean and apply diaper loosely *to prevent trauma and infection.*
- Teach parents to keep neonate away from crowds and environmental irritants *to reduce potential sources of infection.*

NURSING DIAGNOSIS Risk for injury related to sole dependence on caregiver

Expected Outcome *Neonate remains free of injury.*

Nursing Interventions/Rationales
- Monitor environment for hazards such as sharp objects, long fingernails of caretaker and neonate, and jewelry of caretaker that may be sharp *to prevent injury.*
- Handle neonate gently and support head; place infant on back to sleep; ensure correct use of car seat by parents; teach parents never to place neonate on high surface unsupervised, and to supervise pet and sibling interactions *to prevent injury.*
- Assess neonate frequently for any evidence of jaundice *to identify rising bilirubin levels, treat promptly, and prevent kernicterus.*

NURSING DIAGNOSIS Readiness for enhanced family coping related to anticipatory guidance regarding responses to neonate's crying

Expected Outcomes *Parents will verbalize understanding of methods of coping with neonate's crying and describe increased success in interpreting neonate's cries.*

Nursing Interventions/Rationales
- Alert parents to crying as neonate's form of communication and that cries can be differentiated to indicate hunger, wetness, pain, and loneliness *to provide reassurance that crying is not indicative of neonate's rejection of parents and that parents will soon be able to interpret the different cries of their child.*
- Differentiate self-consoling behaviors from fussing or crying *to give parents concrete examples of interventions.*
- Discuss methods of consoling a neonate who has been crying, such as checking and changing diapers, talking softly to neonate, holding neonate's arms close to body, swaddling, picking neonate up, rocking, using a pacifier, feeding, or burping *to provide anticipatory guidance.*

---

conditions. Most agencies have now coupled this day-to-day self-screening of personnel with yearly health examinations.

- *Safety factors:* Health care institutions must be proactive in protecting newborns from abductions. Examples of measures taken to this end include placing identification bracelets on infants and their parents, using identification bands with radiofrequency transmitters that set off an alarm if the bracelet is removed or if a certain threshold is crossed (e.g., doorway to exit unit or building) (Fig. 26-13), and footprinting

or taking identification pictures immediately after birth, before the infant leaves the mother's side. Personnel wear picture identification badges or other badges that identify them as newborn unit personnel (Fig. 26-14). Mother-baby units may have infant tracking systems that will set off an alarm if a baby is left alone or is with unauthorized personnel. Mothers are instructed to be certain they know the identity of anyone who cares for the infant and never to release the infant to anyone who is not wearing the appropriate identification.

FIG. 26-13   Neonatal safety device. (Courtesy Shannon Perry, Phoenix, AZ.)

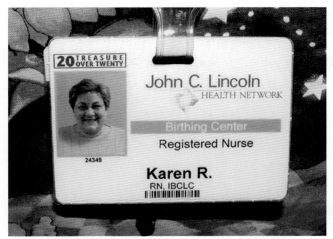

FIG. 26-14   Photo ID for personnel working in maternity settings. (Courtesy Shannon Perry, Phoenix, AZ.)

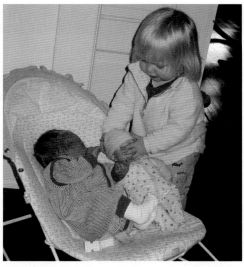

FIG. 26-15   Older sibling sharing her "baby" with brother. (Courtesy Wendy and Marwood Larson-Harris, Roanoke, VA.)

cultural considerations

Cultural Beliefs and Practices

Nurses working with childbearing families from other cultures and ethnic groups must be aware of cultural beliefs and practices that are important to individual families. People with a strong sense of heritage may hold on to traditional health beliefs long after adopting other U.S. lifestyle practices. These health beliefs may involve practices regarding the newborn. For example, some Asians, Hispanics, eastern Europeans, and Native Americans delay breastfeeding because they believe that colostrum is "bad." Some Hispanics and African-Americans place a belly band over the infant's navel. The birth of a male child is generally preferred by Asians and Indians, and some Asians and Haitians delay naming their infants.*

* D'Avanzo, C., & Geissler, E. (2003). *Pocket guide to cultural health assessment* (3rd ed.). St. Louis: Mosby.

▬ Supporting Parents in the Care of Their Infant

The sensitivity of the caregiver to the social responses of the infant is basic to the development of a mutually satisfying parent-child relationship. Sensitivity increases over time as parents become more aware of their infant's social capabilities (Cultural Considerations box).

Social Interaction. The activities of daily care during the neonatal period are the best times for infant and family interactions. While caring for their baby, the mother and father can talk to the infant, play baby games, caress and cuddle the child, and perhaps use infant massage. Too much stimulation should be avoided after feeding and before a sleep period. Older children's contact with a newborn is encouraged and supervised based on the developmental level of the child (Fig. 26-15).

Infant Feeding. The infant is put to breast as soon as possible after birth or at least within 4 hours. Thereafter, the mother should attempt to breastfeed at least every 3 hours in the day and at least once during the night, such that the infant is feeding 8 to 12 times in 24 hours. If the infant is to be bottle-fed, a nurse may first offer a few sips of sterile water to make certain the sucking and swallowing reflexes are intact and that there are no anomalies such as a tracheoesophageal fistula. Formula-fed infants need to be fed approximately every 3 to 4 hours. For a thorough discussion of infant feeding, see Chapter 27.

▬ Therapeutic and Surgical Procedures

Intramuscular Injection. As discussed previously, it is routine to administer a single dose of 0.5 to 1 mg of vitamin K intramuscularly to an infant soon after birth (see Medication Guide box on p. 682).

Hepatitis B (Hep B) vaccination is recommended for all infants. Infants at highest risk for contracting hepatitis B are those born to women who come from Asia, Africa, South America, the South Pacific, or southern or eastern Europe (Medication Guide). If the infant is born to an infected mother or to a mother who is a chronic carrier, hepatitis vaccine and hepatitis B immune globulin (HBIG)

Text continued on p. 700.

care path >	**Healthy Term Newborn**		
CARE ASPECTS	**FIRST HOUR**	**2-3 HR**	**6 HR**
Safety	ID band on and verified to match parents'; bulb syringe (for suction) at bedside; newborn (NB) safety alarm system activated*	ID band on Parent teaching regarding bulb syringe; NB alarm system active	ID band on Bulb syringe in crib; NB alarm system active
Temperature (axillary)	36.5°-37.2° C	36.5°-37.2° C	36.5°-37.2° C
Vital signs	Blood pressure on admission per protocol (not usual unless indicated)		
Heart rate	100-180 beats/min	80-180 beats/min	120-140 beats/min
Respiratory rate	30-60 breaths/min (may be less if asleep)	30-60 breaths/min	30-60 breaths/min
Feeding			
Breast	Initiated—latch-on		1 latch-on‡
Formula		Sips to verify suck, swallow, and breathing	Sips to verify suck, swallow, and breathing
Elimination			
Voiding		Check for urine	Check for urine
Stooling	Verify anal patency	Check for stool	Check for stool

Prepared by David Wilson, MS, RNC.
DPNB, Dorsal penile nerve block; *HBsAg,* hepatitis B surface antigen; *hr,* hour(s); *ID,* identification; *PKU,* phenylketonuria; *VS,* vital signs.
*NB alarm system is the hospital protocol designed to protect infant from abduction.
†If still in hospital.
‡Minimum observed and documented.

care path >	Healthy Term Newborn—cont'd		
12 HR	**18 HR**	**24 HR**	**36-48 HR TO DISCHARGE**
ID band on	ID band on	ID band on	ID band on†
Bulb syringe in crib; NB alarm system active	Bulb syringe in crib; NB alarm system active	Bulb syringe in crib; NB alarm system active	Remove at discharge only
			Parents verbalize appropriate car seat in place
			Discuss and reinforce home safety, including abduction prevention, infection prevention, car seat safety, and falls prevention
			Reinforce teaching for use of bulb syringe
			Discuss sleep position—on back, always; sleep environment (mattress, crib rails)
			Reinforce smoke-free environment around infant
			Deactivate NB alarm system at discharge
36.5°-37.2° C	36.5°-37.2° C	36.5°-37.2° C	36.5°-37.2° C
			Reinforce teaching for taking axillary temperature and when to take
			Thermometer type
			Normal ranges
			Discuss home environment temperature
120-140 beats/min	VS stable	VS stable: 120-140 beats/min	VS stable and documented
			If murmur present, document
			Monitor blood pressure per protocol
30-60 breaths/min		30-60 breaths/min	
1 latch-on‡	2 latch-ons verified	3-4 successful latch-ons verified‡	Feeding successfully 8-10 times/day; discuss and reinforce feeding cues and associated behaviors
2 feedings—15-25 ml each	3 successful feedings verified—15-30 ml each	4-5 feedings verified; adequate suck, swallow, and breathing coordination	Feeding successfully 5-6 times/day; discuss and reinforce feeding cues and associated behaviors
1 void		Minimum of 3 voids/24 hr in first few days	2-3 voids minimum; or number of voids = number of days old
Check for stool		1 meconium documented	Reinforce teaching and care—minimum of 5 to 6 voids/day
			1 meconium documented
			Reinforce teaching and care—approximately 1-2 stools/72-96 hr after first week of life depending on feeding method; more if breastfeeding

Continued

CARE ASPECTS	FIRST HOUR	2-3 HR	6 HR
Parent interaction	Initiated eye contact and verbalization	Ongoing contact	Exhibit newborn care interest and involvement
Cord care	Cord clamped	Cord care per institutional protocol	
Circumcision			
Bilirubin	<5-6 mg/dl		
	No visible jaundice; pink	No visible jaundice; pink	
Newborn screening			
Medications		Eye prophylaxis Vitamin K Maternal HBsAg status verified and documented	Hepatitis B vaccine within 12 hr of birth if mother positive; document
Activity	Active, flexed, primitive reflexes present (Moro, suck, tonic neck, Babinski)	May be drowsy but arousable	Active and alert Flexed, strong suck reflex

12 HR	18 HR	24 HR	36-48 HR TO DISCHARGE
Involvement in newborn care		Continued involvement in newborn care	Demonstrates interest in newborn care; participates in newborn care; asks appropriate questions regarding home care; follow-up time and location provided
Clamped; no drainage		Cord drying; no drainage	Cord drying; care reinforced to parents; clamp removed before discharge
	Pain management—recommend topical anesthesia with DPNB or regional and oral sucrose; verify after procedure	Pain management—recommend topical anesthesia with DPNB or regional and oral sucrose; verify after procedure	Continued evaluation for absence of bleeding and presence of voiding
			Dressing and Vaseline applied with each diaper change depending on method (Gomco and Mogen clamp)
			Ring intact if PlastiBell
			Reinforce teaching on care of circumcision at home; pain management care
<5-6 mg/dl		≤5-6 mg/dl; color pink; note if jaundice present and documented; transcutaneous bilirubin check per protocol	Note skin color; transcutaneous jaundice meter reading per protocol AND check serum bilirubin at 24-36 hr: <7 mg/dl—low risk 7 to 11 mg/dl—low-intermediate risk 11-13 mg/dl—high-intermediate risk >13 mg/dl—high risk
No visible jaundice; pink		Check for jaundice	Note color—document
			Provide parent instruction regarding jaundice and follow-up visit with primary care practitioner within 3-4 days
Hearing screening completed and documented		Newborn screening completed after 24 hr—document time and method	Verify newborn screening completed, including PKU after 24 hr of oral intake—reschedule if needed
		Check eye status; verify free of drainage	Reinforce hepatitis B vaccination at follow-up if not given in birth hospital
	Active and alert Sleep periods noted Reflexes present Neurologic status intact		Discuss and reinforce sleep-wake patterns with parents; reinforce cues to active engagement with infant (eye contact, socialization); potential signs of danger (decreased activity; not arousable for feedings; color changes [not acrocyanosis], central cyanosis, apnea)

Hepatitis B Vaccine (Recombivax HB, Engerix-B)

ACTION ▪ Hepatitis B vaccine induces protective antihepatitis B antibodies in 95% to 99% of healthy infants who receive the recommended three doses. The duration of protection of the vaccine is unknown.

INDICATION ▪ Hepatitis B vaccine is for immunization against infection caused by all known subtypes of hepatitis B virus (HBV).

NEONATAL DOSAGE AND ROUTE ▪ The usual dosage is Recombivax HB, 5 mcg/0.5 ml, or Engerix-B, 10 mcg/0.5 ml, at 0, 1, and 6 mo. An alternate dosing schedule is at 0, 1, 2, and 12 mo and is usually for newborns whose mothers were positive for hepatitis B surface antigen (HBsAg).

ADVERSE EFFECTS ▪ Common adverse reactions are rash, fever, erythema, swelling, and pain at injection site.

NURSING CONSIDERATIONS ▪ Parental consent must be obtained before administration. Wear gloves. Administer in the middle third of the vastus lateralis muscle by using a 25-gauge, ⅝-inch needle. Inject into skin that has been cleaned, or allow alcohol to dry on puncture site for 1 min to remove organisms and prevent infection. Stabilize leg firmly and grasp muscle between the thumb and fingers. Insert the needle at a 90-degree angle; aspirate, and inject medication slowly if there is no blood return. Massage the site with a dry gauze square after removing needle to increase absorption. If the infant was born to HBsAg-positive mother, hepatitis B immune globulin (HBIG) should be given within 12 hr of birth in addition to the HB vaccine. Separate sites must be used.

Hepatitis B Immune Globulin

ACTION ▪ Hepatitis B immune globulin (HBIG) provides a high titer of antibody to hepatitis B surface antigen (HBsAg).

INDICATION ▪ The HBIG vaccine provides prophylaxis against infection in infants born of HBsAg-positive mothers.

NEONATAL DOSAGE AND ROUTE ▪ Administer one 0.5-ml dose intramuscularly within 12 hr of birth.

ADVERSE EFFECTS ▪ Hypersensitivity may occur.

NURSING CONSIDERATIONS ▪ Must be given within 12 hr of birth. Wear gloves. Administer in the middle third of the vastus lateralis muscle by using a 25-gauge, ⅝-inch needle. Inject into skin that has been cleaned, or allow alcohol to dry on puncture site for 1 min to remove organisms and prevent infection. Stabilize leg firmly, and grasp muscle between the thumb and fingers. Insert the needle at a 90-degree angle; aspirate, and inject medication slowly if there is no blood return. Massage the site with a dry gauze square after removing needle to increase absorption. May be given at same time as hepatitis B vaccine but at a different site.

should be administered within 12 hours of birth (Medication Guide). The hepatitis vaccine is given in one site and the HBIG in another. For infants born to healthy women, the first dose of the vaccine may be given at birth or at age 1 or 2 months. Parental consent should be obtained before these vaccines are administered.

In most cases, a 25-gauge, ⅝-inch needle should be used for the vitamin K and hepatitis vaccine injections. A 22-gauge needle may be necessary if thicker medications such as some penicillins are to be given.

Selection of the site for injection is important. Injections must be given in muscles large enough to accommodate the medication, and major nerves and blood vessels must be avoided. The muscles of newborns may not tolerate more than a 0.5 ml per intramuscular injection. The injection site for newborns is the vastus lateralis (Fig. 26-16). The dorsogluteal muscle is very small, poorly developed, and dangerously close to the sciatic nerve, which occupies a larger area in infants compared with older children. Therefore it is not recommended that it be used as an injection site until the child has been walking for at least

FIG. 26-16 Intramuscular injection. **A,** Acceptable intramuscular injection site for newborn infant. *X,* Injection site. **B,** Infant's leg stabilized for intramuscular injection. Nurse is wearing gloves to give injection. (**B,** Courtesy Marjorie Pyle, RNC, Lifecircle, Costa Mesa, CA.)

1 year. The newborn's deltoid muscle has an inadequate amount of muscle for intramuscular injection.

Gloves should be worn by the person giving the injection. In preparing to administer the injection, the neonate's leg is stabilized. The nurse cleanses the injection site with an appropriate skin antiseptic (e.g., alcohol), then pinches up the infant's muscle between the thumb and forefinger. The needle is inserted into the vastus lateralis at a 90-degree angle. The muscle is released and the plunger of the syringe gently withdrawn. If no blood is aspirated, the medication is injected. If blood is aspirated, the needle is withdrawn and the injection is given in another site. After the injection has been given, the needle is withdrawn quickly and the site massaged with a gauze square to hasten absorption, unless contraindicated. A small amount of bleeding at the injection site is not uncommon, but it is not necessary to cover the site with an adhesive bandage. Pressure should be applied until bleeding stops.

The nurse should always remember to comfort the infant after an injection and to discard equipment properly. It is important to record the name of the medication, date and time of administration, amount, route, and site of injection on the newborn's chart.

Therapy for Hyperbilirubinemia. The best therapy for hyperbilirubinemia is prevention. Because bilirubin is excreted primarily through stooling, prevention can be facilitated by early feeding, which stimulates the passage of meconium. However, despite early passage of meconium, the newborn may have trouble conjugating the increased amount of bilirubin derived from disintegrating fetal red blood cells, especially if the infant was born at less than 38 weeks of gestation or has excessive bruising from traumatic birth. As a result, the serum levels of unconjugated bilirubin may increase beyond normal limits, causing hyperbilirubinemia (see Chapter 25). The goal of treatment for hyperbilirubinemia is to help reduce the newborn's serum levels of unconjugated bilirubin. The two principal ways of doing this are phototherapy and, rarely, exchange blood transfusion. Exchange transfusion treats those infants whose increased levels of bilirubin cannot be controlled by phototherapy (Ip et al., 2004). The use of intravenous immunoglobulin (IVIG) may preclude the need for exchange transfusion (Mundy, 2005).

Phototherapy. During phototherapy the unclothed infant is placed beneath a bank of lights. The distance may vary based on unit protocol and the type of light used. There should always be a Plexiglas panel or shield between the lights and the infant when conventional lighting is used. The most effective therapy is achieved with lights at 400 to 500 nanometers, and blue light spectrum is the most efficient. The lamp energy should be monitored routinely during treatment with a photometer to ensure efficacy of therapy. Phototherapy is carried out until the infant's serum bilirubin level decreases to within an acceptable range. The decision to discontinue therapy is based on the observation of a definite downward trend in the bilirubin values. After therapy has been terminated, the infant

may have a rebound in bilirubin levels, which is usually harmless (Kliegman, 2002).

Several precautions must be taken while the infant is undergoing phototherapy. The infant's eyes must be protected by an opaque mask to prevent overexposure to the light. The eye shield should cover the eyes completely but not occlude the nares (Fig. 26-17). Before the mask is applied, the infant's eyes should be closed gently to prevent excoriation of the corneas. The mask should be removed during infant feedings so that the eyes can be checked and the parents can have visual contact with the infant.

To promote optimal skin exposure during phototherapy, the diaper may be left off, or a "string bikini" made from a disposable face mask may be used to cover the infant's genital area. Before placing the mask on the infant, the metal strip must be removed from the face mask to prevent burning the infant. Lotions and ointments should not be used during phototherapy because they absorb heat, and this can cause burns.

Phototherapy may cause changes in the infant's temperature, depending partially on the bed used: bassinet, isolette, or radiant warmer. The infant's temperature is closely monitored. Phototherapy lights may increase insensible water loss, placing the infant at risk for fluid loss and dehydration; therefore it is important that the infant be adequately hydrated. Hydration maintenance in the healthy newborn is accomplished with human milk or infant formula; there is no reason to administer glucose water or plain water because these do not promote excretion of bilirubin in the stools and may actually perpetuate enterohepatic circulation, thus delaying bilirubin excretion. Urine output may be decreased or unaltered; the urine may have a brown or gold appearance. All aspects of the

FIG. 26-17 Eye patches for newborns receiving phototherapy. **A,** Small Velcro patch stuck to both sides of head. **B,** Eye cover sticks to Velcro patch, which reduces movement of eye cover and facilitates removal for feedings.

phototherapy treatment should be accurately recorded in the infant's chart.

The number and consistency of stools are monitored. Bilirubin breakdown increases gastric motility, which results in the formation of loose stools that can cause skin excoriation and breakdown. The infant's buttocks are cleaned after each stool to help maintain skin integrity. A fine maculopapular rash may appear during phototherapy, but this is transient. Because visualization of the infant's skin color is difficult with blue light, appropriate cardiorespiratory monitoring should be implemented based on the infant's overall condition.

An alternative device for phototherapy that is safe and effective is a fiberoptic panel attached to an illuminator. This fiberoptic blanket may be wrapped around the newborn's torso or placed flat in the bed, thus delivering continuous phototherapy. Although the fiberoptic lights do not produce heat as do conventional lights, staff should ensure that there is a covering pad between the infant's skin and the fiberoptic device. This helps to prevent burns, especially in preterm infants. During treatment with the fiberoptic blanket the newborn can remain in the mother's room in an open crib or in her arms; follow unit protocol for the use of eye patches. The blanket also may be used for home care (see Chapter 28 for a discussion of home phototherapy). In certain instances the infant's bilirubin levels may be increasing rapidly and intensive phototherapy is required; this involves the use of a combination of conventional lights and fiberoptic blankets.

See Chapter 39 for a discussion of exchange transfusion.

Circumcision. Neonatal circumcision, removal of the foreskin of the penis, is commonly performed in the United States, although there is ongoing controversy over its value. The AAP Task Force on Circumcision (1999) noted that, although there is scientific evidence of potential medical benefits of circumcision, the data are not sufficient to recommend routine circumcision.

Circumcision is a matter of personal parental choice. Parents usually decide to have their newborn circumcised for one or more of the following reasons: hygiene, religious conviction, tradition, culture, or social norms. Regardless of the reason for the decision, parents should be given unbiased information and the opportunity to discuss the benefits and risks of the procedure (Ressler-Maerlender & Sorensen, 2005). Suggested medical benefits of circumcision for the infant include decreased incidence of urinary tract infection and decreased risk for sexually transmitted infection, penile cancer, and human papilloma virus (HPV) infection. There may be a lower risk of cervical cancer among female partners of circumcised men (Alanis & Lucidi, 2004). Risks and potential complications associated with circumcision include hemorrhage, infection, and penile injury (removal of excessive skin, damage to the meatus or glans) (Alanis & Lucidi).

The incidence of newborn circumcision is declining as parents are more educated about the risks and benefits. In addition, many third party payers including Medicaid do

CD: Critical Thinking Exercise: Circumcision

CD: Video: Circumcision

CRITICAL THINKING EXERCISE

Sudden Infant Death Syndrome and Infant Sleep Position

- Carly gave birth to a full-term male infant; she and her son, Daniel, are being discharged today. The nurse has given her instructions about placing the baby on his back for sleep. Carly said that she had noticed that the nurses placed Daniel on his side in the nursery and wondered why they did that when she was instructed to place Daniel on his back.
- Michelle gave birth to Michael at 32 weeks. During the stay in the neonatal intensive care unit (NICU) the nurses placed Michael on his abdomen to sleep. At discharge, Michelle was instructed to place Michael on his back to sleep. Michelle asked why she had to place Michael on his back to sleep when he was used to sleeping on his abdomen.

How should the nurses respond to the concerns of these mothers?

1. Evidence—Is there sufficient evidence to draw conclusions about the safety and efficacy of the supine position for sleep in reducing the incidence of sudden infant death syndrome (SIDS)?
2. Assumptions—What assumptions can be made about the following factors related to infant positioning?
   a. Role modeling by nurses
   b. Sleep position in the nursery versus sleep position at home
   c. Sleep position for preterm versus term infants
   d. Nurses' knowledge and use of research evidence
3. What implications and priorities for nursing care can be made at this time?
4. Does the evidence objectively support your conclusion?
5. Are there alternative perspectives to your conclusion?

not provide coverage/reimbursement for the procedure. Parents should be encouraged to explore financial implications as they consider circumcision.

Expectant parents should begin learning about circumcision during the prenatal period, but circumcision often is not discussed with the parents before labor. In many instances, it is only when the mother is being admitted to the hospital or birth unit that parents are first confronted with the decision regarding circumcision. Because the stress of the intrapartal period makes this a difficult time for parental decision making, this is not an ideal time to broach the topic of circumcision and expect a well-thought-out decision.

Newborn circumcision requires written informed parental consent. This should be obtained on admission (if the fetus is known to be a male) or within a few hours after birth.

Procedure. Circumcision involves removing the prepuce (foreskin) of the glans. The procedure is usually not done immediately after birth because of the danger of cold stress, but is performed in the hospital before the infant's discharge. The circumcision of a Jewish male is commonly performed on the eighth day after birth and is done at home, in a ceremony called a *bris*. This timing is logical from a physiologic standpoint because clotting factors decrease somewhat immediately after birth and do not return to prebirth levels until the end of the first week.

Formula feedings are usually withheld up to 4 hours before the circumcision to prevent vomiting and aspiration. Breastfed infants may be allowed to nurse up until the procedure is done; this varies with unit protocol.

Prior to circumcision, the infant is properly identified. To prepare the infant for the circumcision, he is positioned on a plastic restraint form (Fig. 26-18), and his penis is cleansed with soap and water or a preparatory solution such as povidone-iodine. The infant is draped to provide warmth and a sterile field, and the sterile equipment is readied for use.

Although some circumcision procedures require no special equipment or appliances, newborn circumcision is often done with the use of a surgical device: the Gomco or Yellen clamp, the PlastiBell device, or the Mogen clamp (www.cirp.org/library/procedure/). Use of the Gomco or Mogen clamp (Fig. 26-19) may make this an almost bloodless operation because hemostasis occurs due to pressure

from the device (www.circumcisionquotes.com/metods. html). After it is completed, a small petrolatum gauze dressing or a generous amount of petrolatum may be applied for the first day or two to prevent the diaper from adhering to the site.

A PlastiBell also may be used for the circumcision. With this technique, the PlastiBell device is fitted over the glans; excess foreskin is pulled over the plastic ring. A suture tied around the rim applies pressure to blood vessels as the excess foreskin is removed (Fig. 26-20).

Discomfort. Circumcision is painful, and the pain is manifested by both physiologic and behavioral changes in the infant. The AAP recommends the use of environmental, nonpharmacologic, and pharmacologic pain interventions to prevent, decrease, or alleviate pain during neonatal circumcision (AAP Task Force on Circumcision, 1999). Use of a padded restraint board, use of only lower limb restraints, and application of warm blankets to the upper body increase infant comfort during the procedure (Glass, 2005).

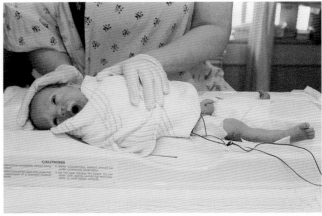

FIG. 26-18 Proper positioning of infant in Circumstraint. (Photo by Paul Vincent Kuntz, Texas Children's Hospital, Houston, TX.)

FIG. 26-19 Circumcision with Gomco clamp. Prepuce is drawn over cone and the clamp applied, hemostasis occurs, and then prepuce (over cone) is cut away. (Courtesy Cheryl Briggs, RN, Annapolis, MD.)

FIG. 26-20 Circumcision by using Hollister PlastiBell. **A,** Suture around rim of PlastiBell controls bleeding. **B,** Plastic rim and suture drop off in 7 to 10 days. (Permission to use and/or reproduce this copyrighted material has been granted by the owner, Hollister Incorporated, Libertyville, IL.)

EVIDENCE-BASED PRACTICE

Circumcision Pain Relief

BACKGROUND

- Although the American Academy of Pediatrics does not recommend it, over a million newborn boys are circumcised every year in the United States. Most circumcisions are performed without anesthesia, despite growing evidence that neonates experience pain intensely. Physicians report little training about neonatal pain management in medical school, concerns about adverse effects of medications, technical difficulties, and "wait time" with administering medication, and the belief that anesthesia is not necessary for circumcision. Babies who experience painful procedures, such as circumcision, show increased sensitivity to pain at 6 months of age. Pain levels of newborns must be inferred from their limited responses: facial grimacing, crying, increased heart rate and blood pressure, decreased oxygen saturation, vomiting, and cyanosis. Pain relief measures include dorsal penile nerve block (DPNB), topical eutectic mixture of local anesthesia (EMLA), oral sucrose, nonnutritive sucking, acetaminophen, touch, and music.

OBJECTIVES

- The reviewers sought to compare the safety and efficacy of pain-relief interventions for circumcision. Primary outcomes were vital signs and cortisol levels, cry variables, and validated neonatal pain scales. Secondary outcomes were methemoglobinemia (a rare but serious side effect from the prilocaine in EMLA), local skin damage, bleeding, and behavioral responses (choking, vomiting, or withdrawal).

METHODS

Search Strategy

- After a thorough search of research databases, reference lists, and conference proceedings, the authors identified 35 randomized controlled trials, dated 1983 to 2002, representing 1,984 newborns. Countries of origin were not noted.

Statistical Analyses

- Similar data were pooled. Reviewers calculated weighted mean difference for continuous data, such as pain scale. For dissimilar data, the treatment effect was standardized by finding the mean difference between intervention and control groups, and dividing by the pooled standard deviation. Differences between groups outside the 95% confidence interval were accepted as significant.

FINDINGS

- No intervention completely relieved circumcision pain response. Penile blocks and topical anesthesia decreased many pain responses, when compared to placebo. The penile blocks were significantly superior to EMLA in relieving pain. Side effects of both were minor and transient. No increase in methemoglobinemia was found with EMLA. Sucrose results varied. Nonnutritive sucking (pacifier), acetaminophen, touch, and music did not differ significantly from placebo in relieving pain.

LIMITATIONS

- Conclusions were limited by small sample sizes. Two studies included preterm infants in a neonatal intensive care unit (NICU), who have immature nervous systems and undergo other painful experiences. Procedures for pain relief and circumcision varied, as did operator technique and expertise. Some trials used subjective and unvalidated measures for pain. No distinction was made between pain and distress, such as being restrained instead of swaddled. Preoperative fasting varied. Some intervention protocols did not account for concurrent use of pacifiers, which may provide relief from pain by calming or distraction. Administration of local anesthetic requires skill to apply, has a 60-minute "wait time," and must be reapplied if the infant voids. Sucrose doses and delivery varied.

IMPLICATIONS FOR PRACTICE

- Circumcision is an entrenched cultural and medical practice. Nurses should advocate vigorously for anesthesia for their tiniest clients, who may feel pain even more intensely than older children and adults. Penile blocks are more effective than topical anesthesia against circumcision pain, but nothing relieves it completely. There is not enough evidence that oral sucrose, acetaminophen, touch, or music are beneficial for circumcision pain.

IMPLICATIONS FOR FURTHER RESEARCH

- It is no longer acceptable to have a placebo/no treatment group. Future studies should compare promising interventions with each other. Larger studies are needed to increase the power to draw conclusions. Interventions with shorter "wait times" are needed, as are optimal combination therapies, such as the additive effect of pacifiers or doses of oral sucrose with other therapies. Evidence for neonatal circumcision pain relief may be generalizable to other painful procedures in the NICU.

Reference: Brady-Fryer, B., Wiebe, N., & Lander, J. (2004). Pain relief for neonatal circumcision. *The Cochrane Database of Systematic Reviews*, 2006, Issue 3. Chichester, UK: John Wiley & Sons.

Three types of anesthesia and analgesia are used in newborns that undergo circumcisions. These include (from most effective to less effective) ring block, dorsal penile nerve block (DPNB), and topical anesthetic (AAP Task Force on Circumcision, 1999). Nonpharmacologic methods such as nonnutritive sucking, containment, and swaddling may be used in addition to pharmacologic use of oral acetaminophen and a concentrated oral glucose solution. A combination of ring block or DPNB, topical anesthetic, nonnutritive sucking, oral acetaminophen, concentrated oral sucrose solution (2 ml of a 24% concentration given during the procedure on a pacifier, with a syringe or nipple), and swaddling has been shown to be the most effective means of decreasing the pain associated with circumcision (Anand, Johnston, Oberlander, Taddio, Lehr, & Walco, 2005).

A ring block is the injection of buffered lidocaine administered subcutaneously on each side of the penile shaft. A DPNB includes subcutaneous injections of buffered lidocaine at the 2 o'clock and 10 o'clock positions at the base of the penis. The circumcision should not be done for 3 to 5 minutes after these injections.

A topical cream containing prilocaine-lidocaine such as EMLA has been shown to be effective in preventing pain from circumcision (Weise & Nahata, 2005). This cream can be applied to the base of the penis at least 1 hour before the circumcision. The area where the prepuce attaches to the glans is well coated with 1 g of the cream and then covered with a transparent occlusive dressing or finger cot. Just before the procedure, the cream is removed. Blanching or redness of the skin may occur.

After the circumcision, the infant is comforted until he is quieted. If the parents were not present during the procedure, the infant is returned to them. The infant may be fussy for several hours, or he may be sleepy and difficult to awaken for feedings. Oral acetaminophen may be administered after the procedure every 4 hours (as ordered by the practitioner) for a maximum of five doses in 24 hours or a maximum of 75 mg/kg/day (Alanis & Lucidi, 2004).

Nurses are instrumental in implementing changes in health care practices to effectively manage the pain of neonatal circumcision (Razmus, Dalton, & Wilson, 2004).

Care of the Newly Circumcised Infant. Bleeding is the most common complication of circumcision. The nurse checks the infant hourly for the 12 hours after the procedure to make sure no bleeding is occurring and that voiding is normal. If bleeding is noted from the circumcision, the nurse applies gentle pressure to the site of bleeding with a folded sterile gauze square; absorbable gelatin sponge (Gelfoam) powder or sponge may be applied to stop bleeding. If bleeding is not easily controlled, a blood vessel may require ligation. In this event, one nurse notifies the physician and prepares the necessary equipment (circumcision tray and suture material), while another nurse maintains intermittent pressure until the physician arrives. If the parents take the baby home before the end of the 12-hour observation period, they must be instructed about postcircumcision care and when to notify the physician. Before the infant is discharged, the nurse checks to see that the parents have the physician's telephone number.

If the PlastiBell technique was used, the parents are instructed to observe the position of the plastic ring on the glans; it should remain on the glans (not on the shaft of the penis) for a minimum of 24 to 48 hours and should routinely fall off within 5 to 7 days. No petrolatum is used in caring for the penis circumcised with the PlastiBell technique (Glass, 2005). Otherwise, care is the same as for the other types of circumcision.

■ Evaluation

Evaluation is based on the expected outcomes of care. The plan is revised as needed, based on the evaluation findings.

■ NEONATAL PAIN

Until recent years, pain in the neonate was unrecognized and untreated. A common myth was that because newborns are developmentally immature, they neither experience pain, nor do they recall having felt pain. Care providers now acknowledge that newborns actually do feel pain, and also remember pain. Much attention has been drawn to assessment of neonatal pain as well as to interventions that alleviate discomfort and return the newborn to a state of equilibrium (Clifford, Stringer, Christensen, & Mountain, 2004).

Pain has physiologic and psychologic components. The psychologic component of pain and the diffuse total body response to pain exhibited by the neonate led many health care providers to believe that infants, especially preterm infants, do not experience pain. The central nervous system is well developed, however, as early as 24 weeks of gestation. The peripheral and spinal structures that transmit pain information are present and become functional between the first and second trimesters. The pituitary-adrenal axis also is well developed at this time, and a fight-or-flight reaction is observed in response to the catecholamines released in response to stress (AAP & Canadian Paediatric Society, 2000; Walden & Franck, 2003).

The physiologic response to pain in neonates can be life threatening. Pain response can decrease tidal volume, increase demands on the cardiovascular system, increase metabolism, and cause neuroendocrine imbalance. The hormonal-metabolic response to pain in a term infant has greater magnitude and shorter duration than that in adults. The newborn's sympathetic response to pain is less mature and therefore less predictable than an adult's.

Assessment

Pain can be assessed in behavioral, physiologic or autonomic, and metabolic categories (Walden & Franck, 2003).

Behavioral Responses

The most common behavioral sign of pain is a vocalization or crying, ranging from a whimper to a distinctive high pitched, shrill cry. Facial expressions of pain include grimacing, eye squeeze, brow contraction, deepened nasolabial furrows, a taut and quivering tongue, and open mouth (Fig. 26-21). The infant will flex and adduct the upper body

FIG. 26-21 The face of pain after heel stick. Note eye squeeze, brow bulge, nasolabial furrow, and wide-spread mouth. (Photo by Paul Vincent Kuntz, Texas Children's Hospital, Houston, TX.)

CD: Skill: Pain Assessment

and lower limbs in an attempt to withdraw from the painful stimulus (Clifford et al., 2004).

Physiologic or Autonomic Responses. The neonate may respond to pain by exhibiting a variety of physical changes. These include increased heart rate, increased respiratory rate, shallow respirations, blood pressure alterations (increases or decreases), pallor, flushing, diaphoresis, and dilated pupils (Walden & Franck, 2003).

Metabolic Responses

In response to pain, infants release epinephrine, norepinephrine, glucagon, corticosterone, cortisol, 11-deoxycorticosterone, lactate, pyruvate, and glucose (Walden & Franck, 2003).

In assessing pain, the care provider needs to consider the health of the neonate, the type and duration of the painful stimulus, environmental factors, and the infant's state of alertness. For example, severely compromised neonates may be unable to generate a pain response, although

they are, in fact, experiencing pain. In addition, every neonate should have an initial pain assessment as well as a pain management plan. Pain should be assessed and documented on a regular basis.

Several pain assessment tools have been developed for use with neonates. A combination of behavioral and physiologic indicators of pain are used to diagnose and differentiate infant pain levels. Tools that have been shown to have validity and reliability include the Neonatal Infant Pain Scale (NIPS) (Lawrence, Alcock, McGrath, Kay, MacMurray, & Dulberg, 1993) and the Premature Infant Pain Profile (PIPP) (Stevens, Johnston, Petryshen, & Taddio, 1996). One pain assessment tool used by nurses in the NICU is the CRIES (Krechel & Bildner, 1995) (Table 26-4). This tool was developed for use by nurses who work with preterm and term infants. CRIES is an acronym for the physiologic and behavioral indicators of pain used in the tool: *c*rying, *r*equiring increased oxygen, *i*ncreased vital signs, *e*xpression, and *s*leeplessness. Each indicator is

---

table 26-4 CRIES Neonatal Postoperative Pain Scale

	0	1	2
Crying	No	High pitched	Inconsolable
Requires O$_2$ for saturation >95%	No	<30%	>30%
Increased vital signs	Heart rate and blood pressure equal to or less than preoperative state	Heart rate and blood pressure <20% of preoperative state	Heart rate and blood pressure >20% of preoperative state
Expression	None	Grimace	Grimace and grunt
Sleepless	No	Wakes at frequent intervals	Constantly awake

CODING TIPS FOR USING CRIES

Crying	The characteristic cry of pain is high pitched.
	If no cry or cry that is not high pitched, score 0.
	If cry is high pitched but infant is easily consoled, score 1.
	If cry is high pitched and infant is inconsolable, score 2.
Requires O$_2$ for saturation >95%	Look for changes in oxygenation. Infants experiencing pain manifest decreases in oxygenation as measured by oxygen saturation. (Consider other causes of changes in oxygenation, such as atelectasis, pneumothorax, oversedation.)
	If no oxygen is required, score 0.
	If <30% O$_2$ is required, score 1.
	If >30% O$_2$ is required, score 2.
Increased vital signs	NOTE: Measure blood pressure last because this may wake child, causing difficulty with other assessments. Use baseline preoperative parameters from a nonstressed period.
	Multiply baseline heart rate (HR) × 0.2, then add this to baseline HR to determine the HR that is 20% over baseline. Do likewise for blood pressure (BP). Use mean BP.
	If HR and BP are both unchanged or less than baseline, score 0.
	If HR or BP is increased but increase is <20% of baseline, score 1.
	If either one is increased >20% over baseline, score 2.
Expression	The facial expression most often associated with pain is a grimace. This may be characterized by brow lowering, eyes squeezed shut, deepening of the nasolabial furrow, open lips and mouth.
	If no grimace is present, score 0.
	If grimace alone is present, score 1.
	If grimace and noncry vocalization grunt is present, score 2.
Sleepless	This is scored based on the infant's state during the hour preceding this recorded score.
	If the child has been continuously asleep, score 0.
	If he or she has awakened at frequent intervals, score 1.
	If he or she has been awake constantly, score 2.

Neonatal pain assessment tool developed at the University of Missouri–Columbia. From Krechel, S., & Bildner, J. (1995). CRIES: A new neonatal postoperative pain measurement score: Initial testing of validity and reliability. *Pediatric Anaesthesia, 5*(1), 53-61.

scored from 0 to 2. The total possible pain score, which represents the worst pain, is 10. A pain score greater than 4 should be considered significant. This tool can be used on infants between ages 32 weeks of gestation and 20 weeks after birth (Pasero, 2002).

Management of Neonatal Pain

The anticipation and prevention of pain are essential to newborn care (Saniski, 2005). In treating neonatal pain, the goals are to (1) minimize the intensity, duration, and physiologic cost of the pain; and (2) maximize the neonate's ability to cope with and recover from the pain (Walden & Franck, 2003). Nonpharmacologic and pharmacologic strategies are used to achieve these goals (Walden, 2001).

Nonpharmacologic Management

Containment, also known as *swaddling*, is effective in reducing excessive immature motor responses. This may provide comfort through other senses, such as thermal, tactile, and proprioceptive senses. Nonnutritive sucking on a pacifier, with or without sucrose, is a common comfort measure used with newborns. Sucrose solution, ranging from 12% to 24%, can be very useful for pain control in newborns. It seems to have a twofold effect, first calming the infant and later producing an endogenous opioid effect. The standard dosage is 1 to 2 ml (Saniski, 2005). Skin-to-skin contact with the mother during a painful procedure can help to reduce pain. Combining these nonpharmacologic methods results in greater pain reduction. Distraction with visual, oral, auditory, or tactile stimulation may be helpful in term or older infants (Clifford et al., 2004; Walden & Franck, 2003).

Pharmacologic Management

Pharmacologic agents are used to alleviate pain in neonates related to procedures. Local anesthesia has become routine during procedures such as circumcision. Topical anesthesia has been used for circumcision, lumbar puncture, venipuncture, and heel sticks. Nonopioid analgesia (acetaminophen) is effective for mild to moderate pain from inflammatory conditions. Morphine and fentanyl are the most widely used opioid analgesics for pharmacologic management of neonatal pain. Continuous or bolus intravenous infusion of opioids provides effective and safe pain control. Acetaminophen is often used for control of postoperative pain following circumcision (AAP & Canadian Paediatric Society, 2000; Anand et al., 2005).

---

community activity

Investigate infant car seat safety laws in your state. Find out age and weight guidelines for the various types of safety seats. Where can parents go to have their infant car seats checked for proper installation? Are there programs in your community to provide car seats for low income families? What are hospitals in your area doing to promote infant safety?

---

key points

- Assessment of the newborn requires data from the prenatal, intrapartal, and postnatal periods.
- The newborn assessment should proceed systematically so that each system is thoroughly evaluated.
- Gestational assessment should be completed within 12 hours of birth for infants with less than 26 weeks of gestation and within 48 hours of birth for infants with at least 26 weeks of gestation.
- The immediate nursing assessment of the newborn includes Apgar scoring and a general evaluation of physical status.
- Nursing care of the newborn immediately after birth includes maintaining a patent airway, preventing heat loss, stabilizing the infant, and promoting parent-infant interaction.
- Nursing care of the newborn may include diagnostic and therapeutic procedures.
- Providing a protective environment is a key responsibility of the nurse and includes such measures as careful identification procedures, support of physiologic functions, measures to prevent infection, and restraining techniques.
- Circumcision is an elective surgical procedure.
- Pain in neonates must be assessed and managed.

REFERENCES

Alanis, M., & Lucidi, R. (2004). Neonatal circumcision: A review of the world's oldest and most controversial operation. *Obstetrical and Gynecological Survey, 59*(5), 379-395.

Albers, S., & Levy, H. (2005). Newborn screening. In H. Taeusch, R. Ballard, & C. Gleason (Eds.), *Avery's diseases of the newborn* (8th ed.). Philadelphia: Saunders.

American Academy of Pediatrics. (2004). *Questions and answers: Jaundice and your newborn.* Accessed www.aap.org/family/, April 23, 2006.

American Academy of Pediatrics Subcommittee on Hyperbilirubinemia. (2004). Management of hyperbilirubinemia in the newborn infant 35 or more weeks of gestation. *Pediatrics, 114*(1), 297-316.

American Academy of Pediatrics (AAP) Task Force on Circumcision. (1999). Circumcision policy statement. *Pediatrics, 103*(3), 686-693.

American Academy of Pediatrics (AAP) and American College of Obstetricians and Gynecologists (ACOG). (2002). *Guidelines for perinatal care* (5th ed.). Elk Grove Village, IL: AAP.

American Academy of Pediatrics (AAP) & Canadian Paediatric Society. (2000). Prevention and management of pain and stress in the neonate. *Pediatrics, 105*(2), 454-461.

Anand, K., Johnston, C., Oberlander, R., Taddio, A., Lehr, V., & Walco, G. (2005). Analgesia and local anesthesia during invasive procedures in the neonate. *Clinical Therapeutics, 27*(6), 844-876.

Association of Women's Health, Obstetric and Neonatal Nurses (AWHONN). (2001). *Evidence-based clinical practice guideline: Neonatal skin care.* Washington, DC: Author.

Ballard, J., Khoury, J., Wedig, K., Wang, L., Eilers-Walsman, B., & Lipp, R. (1991). New Ballard score, expanded to include extremely premature infants. *Journal of Pediatrics, 119*(3), 417-423.

Ballard, J., Novak, K., & Driver, M. (1979). A simplified score for assessment of fetal maturation of newly born infants. *Journal of Pediatrics, 95*(5 Pt 1), 769-774.

Bhutani, V., Johnson, L., & Keren, R. (2005). Treating acute bilirubin encephalopathy—before it's too late. *Contemporary Pediatrics, 22*(5), 57-70.

Blackburn, S. (2003). *Maternal, fetal, and neonatal physiology: A clinical perspective* (2nd ed.). St. Louis: Saunders.

Centers for Disease Control and Prevention, Workowski K., & Berman, S. (2006). Sexually transmitted disease treatment guidelines, 2006. *MMWR Morbidity and Mortality Weekly Report.* 55(RR-11), 1-94.

Clifford, P., Stringer, M., Christensen, H., & Mountain, D. (2004). Pain assessment and intervention for term newborns. *Journal of Midwifery & Women's Health, 49*(6), 514-519.

Efird, M., & Hernandez, J. (2005). Birth injuries. In P. Thureen, J. Deacon, J. Hernandez, & D. Hall, (Eds.), *Assessment and care of the well newborn* (2nd ed.). St. Louis: Saunders.

Frank, C., & Frank, P. (2006). Jaundice. In G. Merenstein, & S. Gardner (Eds.), *Handbook of neonatal intensive care* (6th ed.). St. Louis: Mosby.

Glass, S. (2005). Circumcision. In P. Thureen, J. Deacon, J. Hernandez, & D. Hall (Eds.), *Assessment and care of the well newborn* (2nd ed.). St. Louis: Saunders.

Hagedorn, M., Gardner, S., & Dickey, L. (2006). Respiratory diseases. In G. Merenstein & S. Gardner (Eds.), *Handbook of neonatal intensive care* (6th ed.). St. Louis: Mosby.

Hockenberry, M. (2003). *Wong's nursing care of infants and children* (7th ed.). St. Louis: Mosby.

Ip, S., Chung, M., Kulig, J., O'Brien, R., Sege, R., Glicken, S., et al. (2004). An evidence-based review of important issues concerning neonatal hyperbilirubinemia. *Pediatrics, 114*(1), e130-e153.

Janssen, P., Selwood, B., Dobson, S., Peacock, D., & Thiessen, P. (2003). To dye or not to dye: A randomized, clinical trial of a triple dye/alcohol regime versus dry cord care. *Pediatrics, 111*(1), 15-20.

Johnson, J., White, K., Widen, J., Gravel, J., James, M. Kennalley, T. et al. (2005). A multicenter evaluation of how many infants with permanent hearing loss pass a two-stage otoacoustic emissions/automated auditory brainstem response newborn hearing screening protocol. *Pediatrics, 116*(3), 663-672.

Joint Committee on Infant Hearing, American Academy of Audiology, American Academy of Pediatrics, American Speech-Language-Hearing Association, and Directors of Speech and Hearing Programs in State Health and Welfare Agencies. (2000). Year 2000 Position statement: Principles and guidelines for early hearing detection and intervention programs *Pediatrics,* 106(4), 798-817.

Juretschke, L. (2005). Kernicterus: Still a concern. *Neonatal Network,* 24(2), 7-19.

Kliegman, R. (2002). Fetal and neonatal medicine. In R. Behrman & R. Kliegman (Eds.), *Nelson essentials of pediatrics* (4th ed.). Philadelphia: Saunders.

Krechel, S., & Bildner, J. (1995). CRIES: A new neonatal postoperative pain measurement score—Initial testing of validity and reliability. *Pediatric Anaesthesia, 5*(1), 53-61.

Lawrence, J., Alcock, D., McGrath, P., Kay, J., MacMurray, S., & Dulberg, C. (1993). The development of a tool to assess neonatal pain. *Neonatal Network, 12*(6), 59-66.

Maisels, M. (2005). Jaundice in a newborn: How to head off an urgent situation. *Contemporary Pediatrics, 22*(5), 41-50.

Mangurten, H. (2006). Birth injuries. In R. Martin, A. Fanaroff, & M. Walsh (Eds.), *Fanaroff and Martin's neonatal-perinatal medicine: Diseases of the fetus and infant* (8th ed.). Philadelphia: Mosby.

Miller, C., & Newman, T. (2005). Routine newborn care. In H. Taeusch, R. Ballard, & C. Gleason, (Eds.), *Avery's diseases of the newborn* (8th ed.). Philadelphia: Saunders.

Mundy, C. (2005). Intravenous immunoglobulin in the management of hemolytic disease of the newborn. *Neonatal Network, 24*(6), 17-24.

Newborn hearing screening devices: Sound advice on choosing the right technology. (2005). *Health Devices, 34*(10), 350-356.

Niermeyer, S. (2005). Resuscitation of the newborn. In H. Taeusch, R. Ballard, & C. Gleason (Eds.), *Avery's diseases of the newborn* (8th ed.). Philadelphia: Saunders.

Pasero, C. (2002). Pain assessment in infants and young children: Neonates. *American Journal of Nursing, 102*(8), 61, 63, 65.

Razmus, I., Dalton, M., & Wilson, D. (2004). Pain management for newborn circumcision. *Pediatric Nursing, 30*(5), 414-417, 427.

Ressler-Maerlender, J., & Sorensen, R. (2005). Circumcision: An informed choice. *AWHONN Lifelines, 9*(2),146-150.

Rigo, J., & De Curtis, M. (2006). Disorders of calcium, phosphorus, and magnesium metabolism. In R. Martin, A. Fanaroff, & M. Walsh (Eds.), *Fanaroff and Martin's neonatal-perinatal medicine: Diseases of the fetus and infant* (8th ed.). Philadelphia: Mosby.

Saniski, D. (2005). Neonatal pain relief protocols in their infancy. *Nurse Week News.* Accessed www.nurseweek.com/news/features/05-02/Clinical_BabyPain, November 3, 2005.

Stevens, B., Johnston, C., Petryshen, P., & Taddio, A. (1996). Premature infant pain profile: Development and initial validation. *Clinical Journal of Pain, 12*(1), 13-22.

Townsend, S. (2005). Approach to the infant at risk for hypoglycemia. In P. Thureen, J. Deacon, J. Hernandez, & D. Hall (Eds.), *Assessment and care of the well newborn* (2nd ed.). St. Louis: Saunders.

Walden, M. (2001). *Pain assessment and management: Guidelines for practice.* Glenview, IL: NANN.

Walden, M., & Franck, L. (2003). Identification, management, and prevention of newborn/infant pain. In C. Kenner, & J. Lott (Eds.), *Comprehensive neonatal nursing: A physiologic perspective* (3rd ed.). St. Louis: Saunders.

Weise, K., & Nahata, M. (2005). EMLA for painful procedures in infants. *Journal of Pediatric Health Care, 19*(1), 42-47.

Zinn, A. (2006). Inborn errors of metabolism. In R. Martin, A. Fanaroff, & M. Walsh (Eds.), *Fanaroff and Martin's neonatal-perinatal medicine: Diseases of the fetus and infant* (8th ed.). Philadelphia: Mosby.

Kathryn Rhodes Alden

Newborn Nutrition and Feeding

learning objectives

- Describe current recommendations for infant feeding.
- Explain the nurse's role in helping families to choose an infant feeding method.
- Describe nutritional needs of infants.
- Recognize newborn feeding-readiness cues.
- Explain maternal and infant indicators of effective breastfeeding.
- Discuss benefits of breastfeeding for infants, mothers, families, and society.

- Describe the anatomy and physiology of breastfeeding.
- Examine nursing interventions to facilitate and promote successful breastfeeding.
- Analyze common problems associated with breastfeeding and nursing interventions to help resolve them.
- Compare powdered, concentrated, and ready-to-use forms of commercial infant formula.
- Develop a teaching plan for parents of a formula-fed infant.

electronic resources

Additional information related to the content in Chapter 27 can be found on

the companion website at *evolve*
http://evolve.elsevier.com/Lowdermilk/MWHC/
- NCLEX Review Questions
- Case Study: Breastfeeding
- WebLinks

or on the interactive companion CD
- NCLEX Review Questions
- Case Study: Breastfeeding
- Critical Thinking Exercise: Breastfeeding
- Critical Thinking Exercise: Formula Preparation
- Plan of Care: Breastfeeding and Infant Nutrition
- Skill: Infant Feeding

GOOD nutrition in infancy fosters optimal growth and development. Infant feeding is more than the provision of nutrition; it is an opportunity for social, psychologic, and even educational interaction between parent and infant. It also can establish a basis for developing good eating habits that last a lifetime. Health supervision of infants requires knowledge of their nutritional needs.

Through preconception and prenatal education and counseling, nurses play an instrumental role in assisting parents with the selection of an infant feeding method, which ideally will be breastfeeding or at least the provision of expressed breast milk fed with bottles. Regardless of the chosen method of infant feeding, nurses provide support and ongoing education to enable parents to safely and effectively provide nutrition to their infants. Education of parents is necessarily based on current research findings and standards of practice.

This chapter focuses on meeting nutritional needs for normal growth and development from birth to age 6 months, with emphasis on the neonatal period, when feeding practices and patterns are being established. Both breastfeeding and formula feeding are addressed.

■ RECOMMENDED INFANT NUTRITION

The American Academy of Pediatrics (AAP) recommends exclusive breastfeeding or human milk feeding for the first 6 months of life and that breastfeeding or human milk feeding continue as the sole source of milk for the next 6 months. During the second 6 months of life, appropriate complementary foods (solids) are added to the infant diet. If infants are weaned from breast milk before 12 months of age, they should receive iron-fortified infant formula, not cow's milk (Gartner et al., 2005).

Exclusive breastfeeding for the first six months of life is also recommended by other health organizations such as the American Academy of Family Physicians (AAFP, 2001) and the World Health Organization (WHO, 2001). Other health care organizations that promote and support breastfeeding include the Academy of Breastfeeding Medicine (2006), the American College of Obstetricians and Gynecologists (2000), the American Dietetic Association (2003), and the Association of Women's Health, Obstetric and Neonatal Nurses (1999).

■ BREASTFEEDING RATES

Breastfeeding rates in the United States have risen steadily over the past decade, reaching record levels with 70.1% of mothers initiating breastfeeding in the hospital. When their babies are 6 months old, 33.2% of mothers are still breastfeeding (Abbott Laboratories, 2003). If breastfeeding rates continue to rise at their current rate, it is likely that the breastfeeding goals of *Healthy People 2010* will be attained; the goals are for breastfeeding initiation rates to reach 75%, continuance rates at 6 months to reach 50%, and that at least 25% of infants will still be breastfeeding at 1 year of age (U.S. Department of Health and Human Services, 2000).

Although breastfeeding rates have increased in recent years across all demographic groups, certain trends still remain. Women least likely to breastfeed typically are younger than 25 years of age, have a lower income, are African-American, are primiparas, have a high-school education or less, are employed full time outside the home, and participate in the Special Supplemental Nutrition Program for Women, Infants, and Children (WIC) (Abbott Laboratories, 2003; Ryan, Wenjun, & Acosta, 2002).

■ BENEFITS OF BREASTFEEDING

The AAP states that "human milk is species-specific, and all substitute feeding preparations differ markedly from it, making human milk uniquely superior for infant feeding" (Gartner et al., 2005).

Human milk is bacteriologically safe and always fresh. The nutrients in breast milk are ideally balanced and more easily absorbed than are those in formula. The composition of breast milk changes over time to meet changing needs as infants grow.

Numerous research studies have identified the beneficial effects of human milk for infants during the first year of life. The greatest benefits are associated with exclusive breastfeeding for the first 6 months. Long-term epidemiologic studies have shown that these benefits do not cease when the infant is weaned, but instead extend into childhood and beyond. Breastfeeding has many advantages for mothers, for families, and for society in general. In discussing the benefits of breastfeeding with parents, it is critical that nurses and other health care professionals have a thorough understanding of these benefits from both a physiologic and a psychosocial perspective. Benefits for the infant include the following:

- Breast milk enhances maturation of the gastrointestinal (GI) tract and contains immune factors that contribute to a lower incidence and severity of diarrheal illness, necrotizing enterocolitis, Crohn's disease, and celiac disease (Bhandari et al., 2003; Gianino et al., 2002; Morrow et al., 2004).
- Breastfed infants receive specific antibodies and cell-mediated immunologic factors that help decrease the incidence and severity of otitis media, respiratory illnesses such as respiratory syncytial virus (RSV) and pneumonia, urinary tract infections, bacteremia, and bacterial meningitis (Bachrach, Schwarz, & Bachrach, 2003; Bulkow, Singleton, Karron, Harrison, & Alaska RSV Study Group, 2002; Hanson & Korotkova, 2002; Oddy, 2004; Oddy et al., 2003b).
- Breastfeeding seems to protect against the development of atopic disease such as eczema; the effect appears to be stronger in children with a family history of atopic disease. Asthma, which is often of an allergic nature, is less frequent among children who were breastfed (Chan-Yeung, Manfreda, Dimich-Ward, Ferguson, Watson, & Becker, 2000; Chulada, Arbes, Dunson, & Zeldin, 2003; Dell & To, 2001; Gdalevich, Mimouni, David, & Mimouni, 2001; Oddy, 2004; Oddy et al., 2004; Van Odijk et al., 2003).
- Breast milk may have a protective effect against certain childhood cancers such as lymphoma and leukemia (Bener, Denic, & Galadari, 2001; Kwan, Buffler, Abrams, & Kiley, 2004).
- Children who are breastfed are less likely to develop insulin-dependent (type 1) diabetes (Sadauskaite-Kuehne, Ludvigsson, Padaiga, Jasinskiene, & Samuelsson, 2004).
- Breast milk and breastfeeding may enhance cognitive development (Feldman & Eidelman, 2003; Horwood & Fergusson, 1998; Mortensen, Michaelsen, Sanders, & Reinisch, 2002; Oddy et al., 2003a).
- Breastfeeding enhances jaw development, decreasing problems with malocclusions and malalignment of teeth (Page, 2001).
- Breastfeeding decreases the risk of childhood obesity (Arenz, Ruckerl, Koletzko, & von Kries, 2004; Gillman et al., 2001; Grummer-Strawn & Mei, 2004).
- Breastfeeding appears to have an analgesic effect for infants undergoing painful procedures such as venipuncture (Carbajal, Veerapen, Couderc, Jugie, & Ville, 2003; Gray, Miller, Philipp, & Blass, 2002).

Maternal benefits include the following:

- Women who breastfeed have a decreased risk of breast cancer (Collaborative Group on Hormonal Factors in Breast Cancer, 2002; Ursin et al., 2004) and ovarian cancer (Riman, Nilsson, & Persson, 2004).
- Breastfeeding initiates the release of oxytocin into the circulation, causing uterine contractions. This helps to expel the placenta in the immediate postpartum period, promotes uterine involution, and reduces the risk of postpartum hemorrhage (Lawrence & Lawrence, 2005).
- Mothers who breastfeed experience lactational amenorrhea (LAM). Return of menses is usually delayed with

(left margin, vertical text) CD: Critical Thinking Exercise: Breastfeeding   Evolve/CD: Case Study: Breastfeeding

increased frequency and exclusivity of breastfeeding. Breastfeeding also delays the return of fertility but is not considered to be an effective method of birth control (Lawrence & Lawrence, 2005).

• Breastfeeding may enhance postpartum weight loss (King, 2000).

• Breastfeeding increases bone density, thereby providing some protection against the development of osteoporosis (Grimes & Wimalawansa, 2003; Paton et al., 2003).

• Breastfeeding provides a unique bonding experience that is important in the development of a strong and healthy relationship between mother and infant; it also increases maternal role attainment (Lawrence & Lawrence, 2005).

Benefits to families and society include the following:

• Breastfeeding is convenient; breast milk does not need to be warmed and does not require a clean water supply or a clean serving container. No bottles or other necessary equipment must be purchased or cleaned. When traveling, fewer supplies must be taken along.

• Breastfeeding saves money. The cost of formula far exceeds the cost of extra food for the lactating mother. Because breastfed infants have a lower incidence of illness and infection, health care costs are lower for families and federal, state, and local governments. Breastfeeding represents cost savings to employers: less time is lost from work by parents who must stay home with sick infants. Breastfeeding families who are eligible for WIC represent a cost savings to the government (Weimer, 2001).

• Intangible benefits for families and society include better quality of life because of psychologic benefits for mothers and infants, increased mothering behaviors, and more free time for interaction with family and friends.

• Breastfeeding benefits the environment. It is a natural resource that is renewable with each pregnancy. It requires no fossil fuels, and no advertising, shipping, or disposal is needed.

▬ CHOOSING AN INFANT ▬ FEEDING METHOD

Breastfeeding is a natural extension of pregnancy and childbirth; it is much more than simply a means of supplying nutrition for infants. Women who elect to breastfeed their babies most often do so because they are aware of the benefits to the infant. Many are seeking the unique bonding experience between mother and infant that is characteristic of breastfeeding. The support of the partner and family is a major factor in the mother's decision to breastfeed and in her ability to do so successfully. Prenatal preparation ideally includes the father of the baby, giving him information about benefits of breastfeeding and how he can participate in infant care and nurturing (Pollock, Bustamante-Forest, & Giarrantano, 2002).

Parents who choose to formula-feed often make this decision without complete information and understanding of the benefits of breastfeeding and the potential hazards of formula feeding. Even women who are educated about the advantages of breastfeeding may still decide to formula-feed. Cultural beliefs, as well as myths and misconceptions about breastfeeding, influence women's decision making. Many women see bottle-feeding as more convenient or less embarrassing than breastfeeding. Formula feeding is often viewed as a way to ensure that the father, other family members, and day care providers can feed the baby. Some women lack confidence in their ability to produce breast milk of an adequate quantity or quality. Women who have had previous unsuccessful breastfeeding experiences may choose to formula feed subsequent infants. Breastfeeding is seen by some women as incompatible with an active social life, or they think that it will prevent them from going back to work. Modesty issues and societal barriers exist against breastfeeding in public. A major barrier for many women is the influence of family and friends; this is especially true for lower-income mothers.

There are situations in which breastfeeding is contraindicated. Newborns who have galactosemia should not be breastfed. Mothers with active tuberculosis or human immunodeficiency virus (HIV) infection and those who are positive for human T-cell lymphotropic virus type I or type II should not breastfeed. Breastfeeding is not recommended when mothers have active herpes lesions on their breasts. It is contraindicated if the mother is receiving chemotherapy or radioactive isotopes (e.g., with diagnostic

---

CRITICAL THINKING EXERCISE

Painful Breastfeeding

Mary was discharged from the birthing center at 48 hours postpartum with her newborn son, Matthew. He is now 4 days old, and she has brought him to the clinic for a follow-up visit. She states that her milk came in yesterday, and her breasts have been hard and painful ever since. It has been difficult to latch the baby on. She reports that breastfeeding is very painful and that her nipples are cracked and so sore she "can hardly stand to feed the baby." Matthew has had only one wet diaper and no bowel movements in the last 24 hours. He is crying most of the time and never seems to settle down to sleep for very long. Mary states, "I am ready to give up on this breastfeeding thing and just switch to formula."

1. Evidence—Is there sufficient evidence to draw conclusions about the feeding difficulties experienced by this mother and infant?
2. Assumptions—What assumptions can be made about the following issues?
   a. Mary's milk supply
   b. Mary's sore nipples
   c. Matthew's urinary output and bowel elimination pattern
   d. Mary's commitment to breastfeeding
3. What implications and priorities for nursing care can be made at this time?
4. Does the evidence objectively support your conclusion?
5. Are there alternative perspectives to your conclusion?

procedures). Maternal use of drugs of abuse ("street drugs") is incompatible with breastfeeding (Gartner et al., 2005; Kline et al., 2003).

To make an informed decision about an infant feeding method, parents must be presented with factual information about the nutritional and immunologic needs of the infant that are met by human milk, the potential benefits to the infant and the mother, and the inherent risks associated with infant formulas. The nurse must provide this information to parents in a nonjudgmental manner and respect their decision. Some health care professionals may attempt to avoid this responsibility with the rationalization that they do not want parents to feel guilty if they choose not to breastfeed. However, the nurse should give complete information about infant feeding to parents and to document having done so.

The key to encouraging mothers to breastfeed is education, beginning as early as possible during pregnancy and even before pregnancy.

Prenatal breastfeeding classes are an excellent vehicle to relay important information to expectant parents. Each encounter with an expectant mother is an opportunity to educate, dispel myths, clarify misinformation, and address personal concerns. It may be helpful to connect expectant

---

EVIDENCE-BASED PRACTICE

Encouraging Breastfeeding

BACKGROUND

- Breastfeeding is beneficial for infant and mother, less expensive, and requires less effort. Well-documented benefits include significantly reduced mortality in preterm infants, less gastrointestinal, respiratory, urinary tract and middle ear infections, and less atopic illness. Breastfed infants demonstrate significantly higher cognitive abilities. Long-term, breastfeeding provides important public health benefits, such as less diabetes. Yet breastfeeding initiation remains discouraging low, possibly due to cultural attitudes, employment barriers, and the availability of subsidized formula. Breastfeeding rates are highest in eastern Europe, Scandinavia, and Japan and considerably lower in the United States and the United Kingdom. The higher the income and education level, the more likely a woman is to breastfeed.

OBJECTIVES

- The reviewers' task was to identify and compare effective interventions that promote breastfeeding. Secondary outcomes included duration of breastfeeding and cultural and community support for breastfeeding.

METHODS

Search Strategy

- The authors thoroughly searched the Cochrane Pregnancy and Childbirth Group's trial registry, reference lists, and conference proceedings. They identified seven randomized controlled trials, dated 1987 to 2004, representing 1388 women from Nicaragua and the United States.

Statistical Analyses

- Similar data, where available, were pooled. Reviewers calculated relative risk for dichotomous (categoric) data, such as initiation of breastfeeding, and weighted mean difference for continuous data, such as length of breastfeeding. Differences between groups outside the 95% confidence interval were accepted as significant. All were analyzed in their original randomly assigned "intention to treat" categories, even if they changed their minds.

FINDINGS

- The interventions varied, but all forms of health education significantly increased breastfeeding initiation by low-income women, when compared to usual care. Prenatal education, postnatal support, and education of the professional staff increased this beneficial effect, and prolonged the duration of breastfeeding. No differences in breastfeeding initiation rates were noted in a single trial between high-income women who were given a breastfeeding promotion pack and those that received a commercial formula pack. The trial conducted in Nicaragua, which has much higher breastfeeding rates than the United States, showed that early mother-baby contact, followed by separation for the rest of the hospital stay did not promote breastfeeding more than the usual care of complete separation during hospitalization (normally 12 to 24 hours).

LIMITATIONS

- The health education trials were of low-income, American women, and were small, which limited generalizability. Women receiving promotional packs reported they received formula samples and promotion elsewhere. Bias may have occurred through lack of blinding and attrition in these studies. The credentials of the educator and the personality and demographic characteristics may have influenced women's decisions to breastfeed. The Nicaraguan study was small, its population young (mean age 20 years), and standard care was counter to the World Health Organization recommendation that mothers and babies be together.

IMPLICATIONS FOR PRACTICE

- Lactation consultants, usually nurses, are the gold standard educators used by hospitals for health education. Health education that begins prenatally and continues with follow-up support promotes breastfeeding initiation and duration. Early and ongoing contact between mother and baby promote bonding and breastfeeding.

IMPLICATIONS FOR FURTHER RESEARCH

- Further research is needed in various settings with larger numbers to determine which health education intervention combinations are most effective for promoting breastfeeding: prenatal, hospital stay, or postpartum support, especially for vulnerable populations. The training of the most effective educators needs to be determined. Broader interventions in the community may help shift a cultural bias, including family support and employment barriers to breastfeeding.

Reference: Dyson, L., McCormick, F., & Renfrew, M. (2005). Interventions for promoting the initiation of breastfeeding. *The Cochrane Database of Systematic Reviews*, 2006, Issue 3. Chichester, UK: John Wiley & Sons.

mothers with women from similar backgrounds who are breastfeeding or have successfully breastfed. Peer counseling programs, such as those instituted by WIC programs, are beneficial, particularly in lower socioeconomic groups, in which bottle-feeding is the norm (Chapman, Damio, Young, & Perez-Escamilla, 2004; Dennis, Hodnett, Gallop, & Chalmers, 2002).

The postnatal period is not too late to educate parents about the benefits of breastfeeding. For those women with limited access to health care, the postpartum period may provide the first opportunity for education about breastfeeding. Even women who have indicated the desire to bottle-feed may benefit from information about the differences in formula and breast milk for their infants. Offering these women the chance to try breastfeeding with the assistance of a nurse may influence a change in infant feeding practices.

It is the responsibility of the nurse and other health care professionals to promote feelings of competence and confidence in the breastfeeding mother and to reinforce the unequaled contribution she is making toward the health and well-being of her infant. The role of the nurse in promotion of successful breastfeeding is emphasized by AWHONN (1999) (Box 27-1).

| box 27-1 | **AWHONN Clinical Position Statement: The Role of the Nurse in the Promotion of Breastfeeding** |

The nurse plays a key role in providing education aimed at successful initiation and maintenance of breastfeeding. AWHONN believes that nurses who care for women and infants in the prenatal and postpartum periods should foster an environment supportive of breastfeeding. Responsibilities of the nurse include:

- Pursue professional basic and continuing education regarding the benefits of breastfeeding, the anatomy and physiology of lactation, initiation of lactation, and management of common concerns and problems.
- Promote nonseparation of mother-baby in postpartum period.
- As part of preconception counseling, counsel on the benefits of breastfeeding.
- Provide breastfeeding education to all women during the prenatal period and explore concerns, fears, and myths that may inhibit successful breastfeeding.
- Work in collaboration with lactation specialists and/or other health care providers to optimize the breastfeeding experience for the mother and infant.
- Integrate culturally appropriate and sensitive information into all breastfeeding education.
- Ensure breastfeeding initiation in the immediate postpartum period, barring maternal or neonatal complications.
- Provide information about breastfeeding resources in all discharge planning.
- Utilize and conduct research related to breastfeeding.

Adapted from Association of Women's Health, Obstetric and Neonatal Nurses (AWHONN). (1999). *Clinical position statement: The role of the nurse in the promotion of breastfeeding.* Washington, DC: Author.

■ CULTURAL INFLUENCES ■ ON INFANT FEEDING

Cultural beliefs and practices are significant influences on infant feeding methods. Although recognized cultural norms exist, one cannot assume that generalized observations about any cultural group hold true for all members of that group. Within the United States, many regional and ethnic cultures are found. Dealing effectively with these groups requires that the nurse be knowledgeable about and sensitive to the cultural factors influencing infant feeding practices.

In nonindustrialized societies throughout the world that continue to practice ancient traditions of childrearing, breastfeeding is common, with the duration extending well beyond 1 year (Lawrence & Lawrence, 2005). Persons who have immigrated to the United States from poorer countries often stray from their traditional cultural practices, choosing to formula feed their infants because they believe it is a better, more "modern" method or because they want to adapt to U.S. culture and perceive that it is the custom to formula feed. In addition, many have relocated to the United States and have left extended family behind, which often means a lack of family support for breastfeeding and loss of breastfeeding role models.

Among some cultural groups within the United States, breastfeeding rates have declined. As increasing numbers of families leave Native-American reservations to reside in urban areas, the traditional practice of breastfeeding often shifts to formula feeding. The separation from female relatives who lend childbirth and lactation support may be a factor in the change in feeding practices (Houghton, 2001).

The onset of breastfeeding varies among cultures. Because of beliefs about the harmful nature of colostrum, there may be restrictions on breastfeeding for a period of days after birth; this is true for many cultures in Southern Asia, the Pacific islands, and parts of sub-Saharan Africa (Holman & Grimes, 2003; Morse, Jehle, & Gamble, 1990). Before the mother's milk is deemed to be "in," babies are fed prelacteal food (Lefeber & Voorhoeve, 1999) (Table 27-1). Latinos may think that colostrum is insufficient and offer supplements before the milk comes in. Other cultures begin breastfeeding immediately and offer the breast each time the infant cries. Cultural attitudes regarding modesty and breastfeeding are important considerations.

Some cultures have specific beliefs and practices related to the mother's intake of foods that foster milk production. Korean mothers often eat seaweed soup and rice to enhance milk production. Hmong women believe that boiled chicken, rice, and hot water are the only appropriate nourishments during the first postpartum month. The balance between energy forces, hot and cold, or *yin* and *yang* is integral to the diet of the lactating mother. Hispanics, Vietnamese, Chinese, East Indians, and Arabs often use this belief in choosing foods. "Hot" foods are considered best for new mothers; this does not necessarily relate to the temperature or spiciness of foods. For example, chicken

table 27-1	Advised First Food for Newborns in Countries of Africa, Asia, and Latin America			
	COUNTRY	**PEOPLE**	**FIRST FOOD**	**RATIONALE**
Africa	Ghana	Asante	Gin, rum, lime-juice	To clear the infant's throat
	Nigeria	Yoruba	Palm wine	
	South Africa	Pedi, Zulu, Sotho	Watery porridge, cow's milk, water dextrose/water mixture	To clear the infant's throat
	Zambia	Lozi, Mbunda	Light beer (mahel)	To clear the infant's bowel of meconium
Asia	Bangladesh		Mustard oil	To clean intestine of meconium
			Honey, sugar (gur or talmisri) Sugar water	For ritual and/or medicinal purpose
	India		Honey, water	To clean and purify the body
			Castor oil, herbs	To remove the fluids of the womb ingested by the newborn during birth
	Thailand	Karen	Rice	To learn the taste
	Indonesia	Minangkabau	Honey, coconut water	
			Rice water	To learn the taste
	Iran Jaya			
	Lowland		Sago, sago-porridge	To learn the taste
	Highland		Taro (yam), pork fat	To learn the taste
Latin America	Jamaica		Mint tea, castor oil	To cough up mucus
	Haiti		Castor oil	To clear the infant's bowel of meconium
	Guatemala	Maya, Ladinos	Tea, boiled with anise, sugar, onion stalk, garlic, salt, tea of chicoria	
	Bolivia		Wine, cow's milk, water with herbs or salt, coffee	

From Lefeber, Y., & Voorhoeve, H. (1999). Indigenous first feeding practices in newborn babies. *Midwifery, 15*(2), 97-100.

and broccoli are considered "hot," whereas many fresh fruits and vegetables are considered "cold." Families often bring desired foods into the health care setting.

■ NUTRIENT NEEDS

Fluids

The fluid requirement for normal infants is 100 to 140 ml of water per kilogram of body weight per 24 hours; however, during the first 24 hours after birth, most infants need only 60 to 80 ml/kg/24 hours (Kliegman, 2002). In general, neither breastfed nor formula-fed infants need to be fed water, not even those living in very hot climates. Breast milk contains 87% water, which easily meets fluid requirements. Feeding water to infants may only decrease caloric consumption at a time when infants are growing rapidly.

Infants have room for little fluctuation in fluid balance and should be monitored closely for fluid intake and water loss. Infants lose water through excretion of urine and insensibly through respiration. Under normal circumstances, infants are born with some fluid reserve, and some of the weight loss during the first few days is related to fluid loss. In some cases, however, infants do not have this fluid reserve, possibly because of inadequate maternal hydration during labor or birth.

Energy

Infants require adequate caloric intake to provide energy for growth, digestion, physical activity, and maintenance of organ metabolic function. For the first 3 months, the infant needs 110 kcal/kg/day. From 3 months to 6 months, the requirement is 100 kcal/kg/day. This decreases slightly to 95 kcal/kg/day from 6 to 9 months and increases to 100 kcal/kg/day from 9 months to 1 year (AAP, 2003).

Human milk provides 67 kcal/100 ml or 20 kcal/oz; the greatest amount of energy is provided by the fat content of breast milk. Infant formulas are made to simulate the caloric content of human milk; standard formulas contain 20 kcal/oz, with differences in composition varying among brands.

During the first 3 months, formula-fed infants consume more energy than breastfed infants and therefore tend to grow more rapidly (Ziegler, Fomon, & Carlson, 2003).

Carbohydrate

The average daily intake of carbohydrates for infants is 10 to 30 g/kg. Because newborns have only small hepatic glycogen stores, carbohydrates should provide at least 40% to 50% of the total calories in the diet. Moreover, newborns may have a limited ability to carry out gluconeogenesis (the formation of glucose from amino acids and other substrates) and ketogenesis (the formation of ketone bodies from fat), the mechanisms that provide alternative sources of energy.

As the primary carbohydrate in human milk and cow's-milk formula, lactose is the most abundant carbohydrate in the diet of infants up to age 6 months. Lactose provides calories in an easily available form. Its slow breakdown and absorption also increase calcium absorption. Corn syrup solids or glucose polymers are added to infant formulas to supplement the lactose in the cow's milk and thereby provide sufficient carbohydrates.

Oligosaccharides, another form of carbohydrates found in breast milk, are important in the development of microflora in the intestinal tract of the newborn. These prebiotics promote an acidic environment in the intestines, preventing the growth of gram-negative and other pathogenic bacteria, thus increasing the breastfed infant's resistance to GI illness (Uauy & Araya, 2004; Ziegler et al., 2003).

Fat

The daily fat intake for infants should be approximately 5 to 7 g/kg/day. For infants to acquire adequate calories from human milk or formula, at least 15% of the calories provided must come from fat (triglycerides). This fat must therefore be easily digestible. The fat in human milk is easier to digest and absorb than that in cow's milk because of the arrangement of the fatty acids on the glycerol molecule. Fat absorption also is related to the natural lipase activity present in human milk.

Cow's milk is used in most infant formulas, but the milk fat is removed, and another fat source such as corn oil, which can be digested and absorbed by the infant, is added in its place. If whole milk or evaporated milk without added carbohydrate is fed to infants, the resulting fecal loss of fat (and therefore loss of energy) may be excessive, because the milk moves through the infant's intestines too quickly for adequate absorption to take place. This can lead to poor weight gain.

Human milk contains the essential fatty acids (EFAs), linoleic acid and linolenic acid, as well as the long chain polyunsaturated fatty acids arachidonic acid (ARA) and docosahexaenoic acid (DHA). Fatty acids are important in the development of cellular membranes and are particularly important in eye and brain development. Cow's milk contains fewer of the EFAs and no polyunsaturated fatty acids. Most formula companies add DHA and ARA to their products (Preedy, Grimble, & Watson, 2001).

Protein

The protein requirement per unit of body weight is greater in the newborn than at any other time of life. The recommended daily allowance (RDA) for protein during the first 6 months is 2.25 to 4 g/kg.

The protein content of human milk, which is lower than that of unmodified cow's milk, is ideal for the newborn. The primary protein in human milk is whey, mainly consisting of lactoalbumin, lactoferrin, secretory immunoglobulin A (IgA), and enzymes (e.g., lysozyme and lipase).

The immunologic properties of IgA provide protective effects against diarrhea and other infectious illnesses. The major protein in cow's milk is casein, which is more difficult to digest. Lactoglobulins in cow's milk are responsible for much of the widely recognized intolerance to cow's milk protein (Preedy et al., 2001).

Vitamins

Human milk contains all of the vitamins required for infant nutrition, with individual variations based on maternal diet and genetic differences. Vitamins are added to cow's-milk formulas to resemble levels found in breast milk. Although cow's milk contains adequate amounts of vitamin A and vitamin B complex, vitamin C (ascorbic acid), vitamin E, and vitamin D must be added. Infants of mothers who are strict vegans also should receive vitamin B_{12} supplements (Terschakovec & Stallings, 2002).

Human milk contains small amounts of vitamin D, and therefore it is recommended that breastfeeding infants receive 200 international units of oral vitamin D drops daily starting during the first 2 months and continuing until the infant is consuming at least 500 ml per day of vitamin D–fortified formula or milk (Gartner et al., 2005; Henderson, 2005). Vitamin K, required for blood coagulation, is produced by intestinal bacteria. However, the gut is sterile at birth, and a few days are needed for intestinal flora to become established and produce vitamin K. To prevent hemorrhagic problems in the newborn, an injection of vitamin K is given at birth to all newborns, regardless of feeding method (Gartner et al.).

Minerals

The mineral content of commercial infant formula is designed to reflect that of breast milk. Minerals are typically highest in human milk during the first few days after birth and decrease slightly throughout lactation. Unmodified cow's milk is much higher in mineral content than is human milk, which makes it unsuitable for infants during the first year of life.

The ratio of calcium to phosphorus in human milk is 2:1, a proportion optimal for bone mineralization. Although cow's milk is high in calcium, the calcium-to-phosphorus ratio is low, resulting in decreased calcium absorption. Consequently, young infants fed unmodified cow's milk are at risk for hypocalcemia, seizures, and tetany. The calcium-to-phosphorus ratio in commercial infant formula is between that of human milk and cow's milk.

Iron levels are low in all types of milk; however, iron from human milk is better absorbed (50%) than that from cow's milk, iron-fortified formula, or infant cereals. Breastfed infants draw on iron reserves deposited in utero and benefit from the high lactose and vitamin C levels in human milk that facilitate iron absorption. The infant who is entirely breastfed normally maintains adequate hemoglobin levels for the first 6 months. After that time, iron-fortified cereals and other iron-rich foods are added to the diet. Infants who are weaned from the breast before 6 months of age and all formula-fed infants should receive an iron-fortified commercial infant formula until 12 months of age.

Fluoride levels in human milk and commercial formulas are low. This mineral, which is important in the prevention of dental caries, may cause spotting of the permanent teeth (fluorosis) in excess amounts. It is recommended that no fluoride supplements be given to infants under 6 months of age. From 6 months to 3 years, fluoride supplements are based on the concentration of fluoride in the water supply (Gartner et al., 2005).

▬ ANATOMY AND PHYSIOLOGY
▬ OF LACTATION

Breast Development

Each female breast is composed of approximately 15 to 25 segments (lobes) embedded in fat and connective tissues and well supplied with blood vessels, lymphatic vessels, and nerves (Fig. 27-1). Within each lobe are alveoli, the milk-producing cells, surrounded by myoepithelial cells, which contract to send the milk forward into the ductules. Each ductule enlarges into lactiferous ducts and sinuses where milk collects just behind the nipple. Each nipple has 15 to 20 pores through which milk is transferred to the suckling infant.

The size of the breast is not an accurate indicator of its ability to produce milk. Although nearly every woman can lactate, a small number have insufficient mammary gland development to breastfeed their infants exclusively. Typically, these women experience few breast changes during puberty or early pregnancy. In some cases, women may still be able to breastfeed and offer supplemental nutrition to support optimal infant growth. Devices are available to allow mothers to offer supplements while the baby is nursing at the breast (Fig. 27-2).

Early in pregnancy the breasts are preparing for lactation. Because of the effects of estrogen and progesterone during pregnancy, the lobular components of the breast enlarge while the ductal system proliferates and differentiates. The nipples become more erect, and pigmentation of the areola increases. Nipples and areola may enlarge. The breasts increase in size and sensitivity and exhibit more prominent veins. Around week 16 of gestation, the alveoli begin producing colostrum (early milk) in response to human placental lactogen.

Lactogenesis

After the mother gives birth, a precipitate decrease in estrogen and progesterone levels triggers the release of prolactin from the anterior pituitary gland. During pregnancy, prolactin prepares the breasts to secrete milk and, during lactation, to synthesize and secrete milk. Prolactin levels are highest during the first 10 days after birth, gradually declining over time, but remaining above baseline levels for the duration of lactation. Prolactin is produced in response to infant suckling and emptying of the breasts (lactating breasts are never completely empty; milk is constantly being

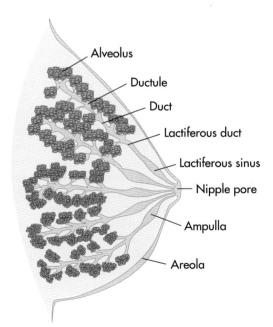

FIG. 27-1 Detailed structural features of human mammary gland.

Alveolus
Ductule
Duct
Lactiferous duct
Lactiferous sinus
Nipple pore
Ampulla
Areola

FIG. 27-2 Supplemental nursing system. (Courtesy Medela, Inc., McHenry, IL.)

produced by the alveoli as the infant feeds) (Fig. 27-3, *A*). Milk production is a supply-meets-demand system; that is, as milk is removed from the breast, more is produced. Incomplete emptying of the breasts with feedings can lead to a decreased milk supply.

Oxytocin is the other hormone essential to lactation. As the nipple is stimulated by the suckling infant, the posterior pituitary is prompted by the hypothalamus to produce oxytocin. This hormone is responsible for the milk ejection reflex (MER), or let-down reflex (Fig. 27-3, *B*). The myoepithelial cells surrounding the alveoli respond to oxytocin by contracting and sending the milk forward through the ducts to the nipple. Many "let-downs" can occur with each feeding session. The MER can be triggered

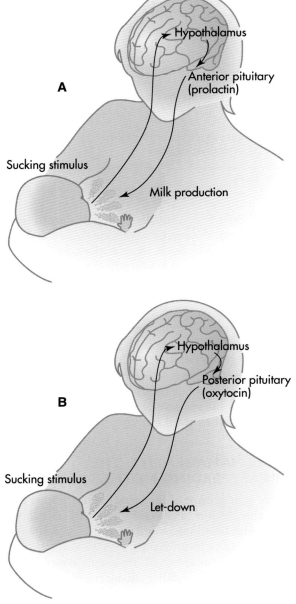

FIG. 27-3   Maternal breastfeeding reflexes. **A,** Milk production. **B,** Let-down.

by thoughts, sights, sounds, or odors that the mother associates with her baby (or other babies), such as hearing the baby cry. Let-down may occur during sexual activity, because oxytocin is released during orgasm.

Oxytocin is the same hormone that stimulates uterine contractions during labor. Consequently, the laboring woman can experience let-downs that may be evidenced by leakage of colostrum. This readies the breast for immediate feeding by the infant after birth. Oxytocin has the important function of contracting the mother's uterus after birth to control postpartum bleeding and promote uterine involution. Thus mothers who breastfeed are at decreased risk for postpartum hemorrhage. These uterine contractions or "afterpains" that occur with breastfeeding can be painful during and after feeding for the first 3 to 5 days, particularly in multiparas.

Prolactin and oxytocin have been referred to as the "mothering hormones," because they are known to affect the postpartum woman's emotions, as well as her physical state. Many women report feeling thirsty or very relaxed during breastfeeding, probably as a result of these hormones.

The nipple-erection reflex is an integral part of lactation. When the infant cries, suckles, or rubs against the breast, the nipple becomes erect. This assists in the propulsion of milk through the lactiferous sinuses to the nipple pores. Nipple sizes, shapes, and ability to become erect vary with individuals. Some women have flat or inverted nipples that do not become erect with stimulation. Babies are usually able to learn to breastfeed successfully with any nipple. It is important that these infants not be offered bottles or pacifiers until breastfeeding is well established.

Uniqueness of Human Milk

Human milk is a highly complex, species-specific fluid containing more than 200 constituents, which meets the needs of the human infant. It is a dynamic substance whose composition changes to meet the changing nutritional and immunologic needs of the infant as growth and development ensue. Breast milk is specific to the needs of each newborn; for example, the milk of preterm mothers differs in composition from that of mothers who give birth at term.

Human milk contains antimicrobial factors (antibodies) that provide some protection against a broad spectrum of bacterial, viral, and protozoan infections. Secretory immunoglobulin A (IgA) is the major antibody in human milk. Other factors in human milk that help protect against infection include lactoferrin, the bifidus factor, oligosaccharides, milk lipids, and milk leukocytes. Antiinflammatory agents, growth factors, hormones, and enzymes are found in human milk, many of which contribute to the maturation of the infant's intestine. Immunomodulating agents found in human milk are instrumental in preventing disease after infancy (Table 27-2).

Human milk composition and volumes vary according to the stage of lactation. In lactogenesis stage I, beginning at approximately the 16th week of pregnancy, the breasts prepare for milk production. Colostrum is present in the

table 27-2 Summary of Immune Properties of Breast Milk

COMPONENT	ACTION
WHITE BLOOD CELLS	
B lymphocytes	Give rise to antibodies targeted against specific microbes
Macrophages	Kill microbes outright in baby's gut, produce lysozyme, and activate other components of the immune system
Neutrophils	May act as phagocytes, ingesting bacteria in baby's digestive system
T lymphocytes	Kill infected cells directly or send out chemical messages to mobilize other defenses
	Proliferate in the presence of organisms that cause serious illness in infants
	Manufacture compounds that can strengthen an infant's own immune response
MOLECULES	
Antibodies of secretory immunoglobulin A (IgA) class	Bind to microbes in infant's digestive tract and thereby prevent them from passing through walls of the gut into body tissues
B_{12}-binding protein	Reduces amount of vitamin B_{12}, which bacteria need to grow
Bifidus factor	Promotes growth of *Lactobacillus bifidus*, a harmless bacterium, in infant's gut. Growth of such nonpathogenic bacteria helps crowd out dangerous varieties
Fatty acids	Disrupt membranes surrounding certain viruses and destroy them
Fibronectin	Increases antimicrobial activity of macrophages; helps repair tissues that have been damaged by immune reactions in infant's gut
Interferon-gamma	Enhances antimicrobial activity of immune cells
Hormones and growth factors	Stimulate infant's digestive tract to mature more quickly. Once the initially "leaky" membranes lining the gut mature, infants become less vulnerable to microorganisms
Lactoferrin	Binds to iron, a mineral many bacteria need to survive. By reducing the available amount of iron, lactoferrin thwarts growth of pathogenic bacteria
Lysozyme	Kills bacteria by disrupting their cell walls
Mucins	Adhere to bacteria viruses, thus keeping such microorganisms from attaching to mucosal surfaces
Oligosaccharides	Bind to microorganisms and bar them from attaching to mucosal surfaces

From Newman, J. (1995). How breast milk protects newborn. *Scientific American, 273*(6), 76-79.

breasts at this time. Colostrum, a clear yellowish fluid, is more concentrated than mature milk and is extremely rich in immunoglobulins. It has higher concentrations of protein and minerals but less fat than mature milk. The high protein level of colostrum facilitates binding of bilirubin, and the laxative action of colostrum promotes early passage of meconium.

Lactogenesis stage II begins at birth with the drop in progesterone levels. Over the next few days, colostrum gradually changes to mature milk; this is referred to as "the milk coming in." By day 3 to 5 after birth, most women have experienced this onset of copious milk secretion. Breast milk continues to change to mature milk for approximately 10 days and continues to change over the months of breastfeeding (Lawrence & Lawrence, 2005).

The onset of lactogenesis may be delayed in women who are diabetic, those who experienced a stressful birth, and in those who experience a retained placenta. In the absence of signs of lactogenesis during the first 72 hours postbirth, further assessment and intervention may be indicated (Lawrence & Lawrence, 2005).

Composition of mature milk changes during each feeding. As the infant nurses, the fat content of breast milk increases. Initially, a bluish-white foremilk is released that is part skim milk (about 60% of the volume) and part whole milk (about 35% of the volume). It provides primarily lactose, protein, and water-soluble vitamins. The hindmilk, or cream (about 5%), is usually let down 10 to 20 minutes into the feeding, although it may occur sooner. It contains the denser calories from fat necessary for ensuring optimal growth and contentment between feedings. Because of this changing composition of human milk during each feeding, it is important to breastfeed the infant long enough to supply a balanced feeding.

According to the supply-meets-demand principle, milk production increases as the baby grows. Babies have fairly predictable growth spurts (at about 10 days, 3 weeks, 6 weeks, 3 months, and 4 to 6 months), when more frequent feedings stimulate increased milk production. These growth spurts usually last 24 to 48 hours, and then the infants resume their usual feeding pattern.

▬ CARE MANAGEMENT: THE BREASTFEEDING MOTHER AND INFANT

Effective management of the breastfeeding mother and infant requires that the caregivers be knowledgeable about the benefits of breastfeeding, as well as about basic anatomy and the physiology of breastfeeding, how to assist the mother with feeding, and interventions for common problems. Ongoing support of the mother enhances her self-confidence and promotes a satisfying and successful breastfeeding experience. Planning care for the breastfeeding couplet is based on thorough assessment of both the mother and infant.

■ Assessment and Nursing Diagnoses
■ *Infant*

Before the initiation of breastfeeding, the nurse must consider the following in preparing to assist the breastfeeding infant effectively:

- Maturity level: gestational age, term or preterm, birth weight (small for gestational age [SGA], large for gestational age [LGA])
- Labor and birth: length of labor, maternal medications (narcotics, magnesium sulfate); type of birth: vaginal (with or without use of vacuum extraction or forceps) or cesarean; type of anesthesia
- Birth trauma: fractured clavicle, bruising of face or head
- Maternal risk factors: diabetes, preeclampsia, infection, HIV, herpes, hepatitis B
- Congenital defects: cleft lip or palate, cardiac anomalies, Down syndrome or other genetic anomalies
- Physical stability: vital signs within normal limits, unlabored respirations, bowel sounds present
- State of alertness: awake, sleepy, crying

Feeding Readiness. Term neonates are born with reflexes that facilitate feeding: rooting, sucking, and swallowing. However, coordination of sucking, swallowing, and breathing in order to feed requires adaptation by the infant. Although the majority of newborns experience minimal hunger or thirst in the first hours after birth, they will suckle when given the opportunity.

Physical assessment of the newborn reveals signs that the baby is physiologically ready to begin feeding:
- Vital signs within normal limits
- Unlabored respirations; nares patent; no cyanosis
- Active bowel sounds
- No abdominal distention

When newborns feel hunger, they usually cry vigorously until their needs are met. Some infants, however, will withdraw into sleep because of discomfort associated with hunger. Babies exhibit feeding-readiness cues that can be recognized by a knowledgeable caregiver. Instead of waiting to feed until the infant is crying in a distraught manner or withdrawing into sleep, it is better to begin a feeding when the baby exhibits some of these cues (even during light sleep):
- Hand-to-mouth or hand-to-hand movements
- Sucking motions
- Rooting
- Mouthing

Babies normally consume small amounts of milk during the first 3 days of life. The breastfed infant receives colostrum, a very concentrated, high-protein fluid containing enzymes, antiinfective agents, hormones, and growth factors. Similarly, bottle-fed infants initially require small feedings. However, as the baby adjusts to extrauterine life and the digestive tract is cleared of meconium, milk intake increases from 15 to 30 ml per feeding in the first 24 hours to 60 to 90 ml by the end of the first week.

At birth and for several months thereafter, all of the secretions of the infant's digestive tract contain enzymes especially suited to the digestion of human milk. The ability to digest foods other than milk depends on the physiologic development of the infant. The capacities for salivary, gastric, pancreatic, and intestinal digestion increase with age, indicating that the natural time for introduction of solid foods may be around 6 months of age.

Babies are born with a tongue extrusion reflex that causes them to push out of the mouth anything placed on the tongue. This reflex disappears by 6 months—another indication of physiologic readiness for solids.

Early introduction of solids may make the infant more prone to food allergies. Regular feeding of solids can lead to decreased intake of breast milk or formula and may be associated with early cessation of breastfeeding.

Assessment During Feeding. The infant is assessed for the following by direct observation while breastfeeding:
- Latch-on (attachment of the infant to the breast for feeding)
- Position, alignment
- Sucking and swallowing

Assessment of the Infant
- Behavior after and between feedings: contented, sleepy
- Elimination patterns: within 24 hours after birth, at least one wet diaper and one stool; by day 3, three to four wet diapers and three to four stools that are beginning to change from meconium to yellowish; after day 4 (and mother's milk has "come in"), six to eight wet diapers and three to six stools per day
- General assessment: presence of jaundice; weight loss of less than 10% during the first week; regaining of birth weight by age 10 to 14 days; consistent gain of 140 to 200 g per week

■ *Mother*

Before breastfeeding is begun, it is important that the nurse carefully assess the mother's knowledge of breastfeeding, as well as her physical and psychologic readiness to breastfeed. This assessment can be accomplished through interviews, discussion, and direct observation. Factors to consider include the following:
- Previous experience with breastfeeding: first baby; successful or unsuccessful breastfeeding with previous infants
- Knowledge about breastfeeding: prenatal classes, support groups, books and pamphlets, videos, friends or relatives who breastfed; knowledge about positioning, latch-on, frequency and duration of feedings, and so forth
- Cultural factors: cultural beliefs, modesty issues, language barrier
- Feelings about breastfeeding: anxiety, fear of failure; confidence, expectation of success
- Physical features: development of breast tissue, symmetry of breasts, protractility of nipples (flat or inverted), previous breast surgery (reduction or mammoplasty), chronic illness, carpal tunnel syndrome, visual or hearing impairment, physical limitations

- Physical and psychologic readiness: risk factors, time since giving birth, type of birth, complications, perineal discomfort, level of pain, medications, mood (eager, cheerful), energy level (tired, exhausted)
- Support: father of baby, family members, or friends and their knowledge about breastfeeding

As breastfeeding is becoming established, the nurse performs ongoing assessment of the mother and infant to determine appropriate interventions. During the time in the hospital, the nurse can help the mother to view each breastfeeding session as a "feeding lesson" or "practice session" that will foster maternal confidence and a satisfying breastfeeding experience for mother and baby. Items that should be assessed are the following:

- Condition of nipples: during feeding; mother should feel a "tugging" sensation, but no pain after the initial latch-on; check for presence of soreness, redness, cracking, bleeding
- Transition to mature milk: milk should be "in" by day 3 to 5 (by which time she may be home)
- Consistency of breasts: breasts feel softer or lighter after feeding
- How mother is feeling during feeding: may feel relaxed or sleepy
- Presence of uterine cramping and/or increased lochia flow during or after feeding
- Comfort with breastfeeding techniques, including positioning and latch-on

Nursing diagnoses for the breastfeeding woman include the following:

- *Effective breastfeeding related to*
  -mother's knowledge of breastfeeding techniques
  -mother's appropriate response to infant's feeding-readiness cues
  -mother's ability to facilitate efficient breastfeeding
  -mother's adequate fluid and caloric intake for breastfeeding
- *Ineffective breastfeeding related to:*
  -insufficient knowledge regarding newborn's reflexes and breastfeeding techniques
  -lack of support from father of baby, family, friends
  -lack of maternal self-confidence; anxiety, fear of failure
  -poor infant sucking reflex
  -difficulty waking sleepy baby

▬ Expected Outcomes of Care

In planning care, the nurse discusses the desired outcomes with the parents. The expected outcomes include that the infant will do the following:

- Latch on and feed effectively 8 to 12 times per day.
- Gain weight appropriately.
- Remain well hydrated (have six to eight wet diapers and three to six bowel movements every 24 hours after day 4).
- Sleep or seem contented between feedings.

Examples of expected outcomes for the mother include that she will do the following:

- Verbalize or demonstrate understanding of breastfeeding techniques, including positioning and latch-on, signs of adequate feeding, self-care.
- Report no nipple discomfort with breastfeeding.
- Express satisfaction with the breastfeeding experience.
- Consume a nutritionally balanced diet with appropriate caloric and fluid intake to support breastfeeding.

▬ Plan of Care and Interventions

Interventions are based on the expected outcomes and are influenced by the resources and time available to achieve the desired goals. In the early days after birth, interventions focus on helping the mother and the newborn initiate breastfeeding and achieve some degree of success and satisfaction before discharge from the hospital or birthing center. Interventions to promote successful breastfeeding include basics such as latch-on and positioning, signs of adequate feeding, and self-care measures such as prevention of engorgement. An important intervention is to provide the parents with a list of resources that they may contact after discharge from the hospital.

The ideal time to begin breastfeeding is immediately after birth. Newborns without complications should be allowed to remain in direct skin-to-skin contact with the mother until the baby is able to breastfeed for the first time (Gartner et al., 2005). Each mother should receive instruction, assistance, and support in positioning and latching on until she is able to do so independently.

▬ *Positioning*

The four basic positions for breastfeeding are the football hold, cradle, modified cradle or across-the-lap, and side-lying position (Fig. 27-4). Initially it is advantageous to use the position that most easily facilitates latch-on while allowing maximal comfort for the mother. The football hold is often recommended for early feedings because the mother can easily see the baby's mouth as she guides the infant onto the nipple. The football hold is usually preferred by mothers who gave birth by cesarean. The modified cradle or across-the-lap hold also works well for early feedings, especially with smaller babies. The side-lying position allows the mother to rest while breastfeeding and is often preferred by women with perineal pain and swelling. Cradling is the most common breastfeeding position for infants who have learned to latch on easily and feed effectively. Before discharge from the hospital, the mother can be assisted to try all of the positions so that she will feel confident in her ability to vary positions at home.

Whichever position is used, the mother should be comfortable. The infant is placed at the level of the breast, supported by pillows or folded blankets, turned completely on his or her side, and facing the mother so that the infant is "belly to belly," with the arms "hugging" the breast. The baby's mouth is directly in front of the nipple. It is important that the mother support the baby's neck and shoulders with her hand and not push on the occiput.

FIG. 27-4 Three breastfeeding positions. **A,** Football hold. **B,** Cradling. **C,** Lying down. (**B** and **C** Courtesy Marjorie Pyle, RNC, Lifecircle, Costa Mesa, CA.)

Pushing on the back of the head may cause the newborn to bite, hyperextend the neck, or develop an aversion to being brought near the breast. The baby's body is held in correct alignment (ears, shoulders, and hips are in a straight line) during latch-on and feeding.

▬ Latch-on

In preparation for latch-on, it may be helpful for the mother to manually express a few drops of colostrum or milk and spread it over the nipple. This lubricates the nipple and may entice the baby to open the mouth as the milk is tasted.

To facilitate latch-on, the mother supports her breast in one hand with the thumb on top and four fingers underneath at the back edge of the areola. The breast is compressed slightly, as one might compress a large sandwich in preparing to take a bite, so that an adequate amount of breast tissue is taken into the mouth with latch-on (Weissinger, 1998). Most mothers need to support the breast during feeding for at least the first days until the infant is adept at feeding.

With the baby held close to the breast with the mouth directly in front of the nipple, the mother tickles the baby's lower lip with the tip of her nipple, stimulating the mouth to open. When the mouth is open wide and the tongue is down, the mother quickly pulls the baby onto the nipple. She brings the baby to the breast, not the breast to the baby. If the breast is pushed into the baby's mouth, the typical response is for the baby to close the mouth too soon, which precludes correct latch-on (Fig. 27-5).

The amount of areola in the baby's mouth with correct latch-on depends on the size of the baby's mouth and the size of the areola and the nipple. In general, the baby's mouth should cover the nipple and an areolar radius of approximately 2 to 3 cm all around the nipple. (It is incorrect to tell all mothers that the baby should take the entire areola into the mouth with latch-on because areolae vary in size from very small to the size of a saucer.)

When the baby is latched on correctly, the tip of the nose, cheeks, and chin should all be touching the breast (Fig. 27-6). It is important for the mother not to pull the nipple out of the mouth when trying to create a breathing space for the baby's nose. Depressing the breast tissue around the baby's nose is not necessary. If she is worried about the baby's breathing, the mother can raise the baby's hips slightly to change the angle of the baby's head at the breast. The nurse should reassure the mother that if the baby cannot breathe, innate reflexes will prompt the baby to move the head and pull back to breathe.

When the baby is latched on correctly and sucking appropriately, (1) the mother reports a firm tugging sensation on her nipples, but no pinching or pain; (2) the baby sucks with cheeks rounded, not dimpled; (3) the baby's jaw glides smoothly with sucking; and (4) swallowing is audible. Sucking creates a vacuum in the intraoral cavity as the breast is compressed between the tongue and the palate. If the mother feels pinching or pain after the initial sucks or does not feel a strong tugging sensation on the nipple, the latch-on and positioning should be evaluated. If each suck is painful, the baby may be having difficulty keeping the tongue out over the lower gum ridge. Clicking or smacking may be audible when this occurs. The nurse can place a finger on the side of the baby's lower jaw, pulling down gently but firmly as the baby sucks, to help stabilize the jaw so that the tongue stays in place.

Any time the signs of adequate latch-on and sucking are not present, the baby should be taken off the breast and latch-on attempted again. To prevent nipple trauma as the baby is taken off the breast, the mother is instructed to break the suction by inserting a finger in the side of the baby's

FIG. 27-5 Latching on. **A,** Tickle baby's lower lip with your nipple until he or she opens wide. **B,** Once baby's mouth is opened wide, quickly pull baby onto breast. **C,** Baby should have as much areola (dark area around nipple) in his or her mouth as possible, not just the nipple. (Courtesy Medela, Inc., McHenry, IL.)

mouth between the gums and leaving it there until the nipple is completely out of the baby's mouth (Fig. 27-7).

▬ Milk Ejection or Let-Down

As the baby begins sucking on the nipple, the let-down, or milk ejection, reflex is stimulated (see Fig. 27-3, *B*). The following signs indicate that let-down has occurred:

- The mother may feel a tingling sensation in the nipples, although many women never feel their milk let down.

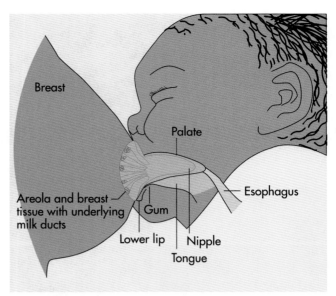

FIG. 27-6 Correct attachment (latch-on) of infant at breast.

FIG. 27-7 Removing infant from the breast. (Courtesy Marjorie Pyle, RNC, Lifecircle, Costa Mesa, CA.)

- The baby's suck changes from quick, shallow sucks to a slower, more drawing, sucking pattern.
- Swallowing is heard as the baby sucks.
- The mother feels uterine cramping and may have increased lochia during and after feedings.
- The mother feels relaxed, even sleepy, during feedings.
- The opposite breast may leak.

▬ Frequency of Feedings

Newborns need to breastfeed 8 to 12 times in a 24-hour period. Feeding patterns are variable because every baby is unique. Some infants will breastfeed every 2 to 3 hours throughout a 24-hour period. Others may cluster-feed, breastfeeding every hour or so for three to five feedings and then sleeping for 3 to 4 hours between clusters. During the first 24 to 48 hours after birth, most babies do not awaken this often to feed. It is important that parents understand that they should awaken the baby to feed at least every 3 hours during the day and at least every 4 hours at night. (Feeding frequency is determined by counting from the beginning of one feeding to the beginning of the next.) Once the infant is feeding well and gaining weight adequately, it is more appropriate to go to demand feeding, in which the infant determines the frequency of feedings. (With demand feeding, the infant should still receive at least eight feedings in 24 hours.) Parents should be cautioned about attempting to place newborn infants on strict feeding schedules.

Infants should be fed whenever they exhibit feeding cues such as hand-to-mouth movements and mouth and tongue movements.

▬ Duration of Feedings

The duration of breastfeeding sessions is highly variable because the timing of milk transfer differs for each mother-baby pair. The average time for feeding is 30 to 40 minutes, or approximately 15 to 20 minutes per breast. Some mothers do one-sided nursing, in which the baby nurses on only one breast at each feeding. The first breast offered should be alternated at each feeding to ensure that each breast receives equal stimulation and emptying. In reality, instructing mothers to feed for a set number of minutes is inappropriate. It is better to teach mothers how to determine when a baby has finished a feeding: the baby's suck and swallow pattern has slowed, the breast is softened, and the baby appears content and may fall asleep or release the nipple.

If a baby seems to be feeding effectively and the urine output is adequate but the weight gain is not satisfactory, the mother may be switching to the second breast too soon. The high-lactose, low-fat foremilk may cause the baby to have explosive stools, gas pains, and inconsolable crying. Feeding on the first breast until it softens ensures that the baby will receive the hindmilk, which usually results in increased weight gain.

▬ Indicators of Effective Breastfeeding

In the newborn period, when breastfeeding is becoming established, it is important to teach parents the signs that breastfeeding is going well (Box 27-2). When they understand these signs, they will be more likely to recognize when problems arise and know when to seek assistance.

During the time in the hospital and in the first weeks at home, parents should be encouraged to record the time and duration of each breastfeeding session, along with the infant's urine output and bowel movements. This helps to provide them and their health care provider with evidence of adequate feeding (Gartner et al., 2005).

▬ Supplements, Bottles, and Pacifiers

The AAP recommends that, unless a medical indication exists, no supplements should be given to breastfeeding infants. With sound breastfeeding knowledge and practice, supplements rarely are needed (Gartner et al., 2005).

---

box 27-2 **Indicators of Effective Breastfeeding During the First Week**

INFANT

Physical Assessment

- The baby is alert when awake and appears well hydrated, with normal skin turgor and moist mucous membranes. The fontanels are soft and flat, and the baby demonstrates a strong and coordinated suck. Periods of wakefulness and hunger alternate with periods of contentment or sleeping. Weight loss is less than 7% by day 3 after birth, and the infant gains 20 to 28 g/day after milk is "in." Birth weight should be regained by 10 to 14 days.

Feeding Frequency

- The infant should breastfeed 8 to 12 times in 24 hours.

Feeding Behavior

- Baby latches on easily and sucks with gliding jaw movements in bursts of 10 to 12 sucks and swallows at beginning of feeding, slowing to bursts of 2 to 3 sucks and swallows at end of feeding. Swallowing is audible. Baby appears relaxed during feeding and contented when finished.

Output

- In the first 3 days of life, a newborn should have at least one wet diaper and one stool for each day of life. After day 4, when milk has come in, the baby should have 6 to 8 wet diapers every 24 hours. The baby may stool with every feeding, but should minimally have 3 bowel movements every 24 hours. Stools transition from meconium to milk stools, becoming lighter in color by day 3, and by day 5, appearing mustard-yellow in color.

MOTHER

Physical Assessment

- Nipples are intact (no redness, cracking, scabs, or bleeding), and nipple tenderness is minimal. Breasts are full, soft, and without engorgement, with no redness and minimal tenderness to palpation. The mother should have no fever.

Breastfeeding Behavior

- Milk is "in" by the third or fourth day. Breasts are full at beginning of feeding and soften as baby breastfeeds. Baby softens at least one breast per feeding. There should be no pinching or nipple pain with sucking, and the mother should feel a strong tugging sensation as the baby sucks.
- Mother easily positions and latches baby on and experiences let-down with feeding. She may have a tingling sensation in the nipples as the milk lets down. During the first 4 or 5 days after birth, she may feel uterine cramping and have increased lochia. As she breastfeeds, the mother may be thirsty and experience leaking from the opposite breast. She should feel relaxed during feeding.

Supplementary feeding may become necessary in situations such as babies with low birth weight, hypoglycemia, dehydration, or inborn errors of metabolism. Mothers may be unable to breastfeed because of severe illness or complications of birth, or they may be taking medications incompatible with breastfeeding.

Offering formula to a baby after breastfeeding just to "make sure the baby is getting enough" is normally unnecessary and should be avoided. This can contribute to low milk supply because the baby becomes overly full and does not breastfeed often enough. Supplementation interferes with the supply-meets-demand system of milk production. The parents may interpret the baby's willingness to take a bottle to mean that the mother's milk supply is inadequate. They need to know that a baby will automatically suck from a bottle, as the easy flow of milk from the nipple triggers the suck and swallow reflex.

Babies who receive supplementary feedings may develop nipple confusion (i.e., difficulty knowing how to latch on to the breast). This is because breastfeeding and bottle feeding require different skills. The way babies use their tongues, cheeks, and lips, as well as the sucking and swallowing patterns, are very different. Some babies can transition easily between breast and bottle, but some have considerable difficulty. It is impossible to predict which babies will adapt well and which ones will not; therefore it is best to avoid bottles until breastfeeding is well established, usually after 3 to 4 weeks. If parents choose to use bottles, a slow-flow nipple is recommended. Although some parents combine breastfeeding and bottle feeding, many babies never take a bottle and go directly from the breast to a cup as they grow.

Pacifiers are not recommended until breastfeeding is well established (Gartner et al., 2005). Their use has been associated with shorter duration of breastfeeding, sore nipples, and insufficient milk supply (Howard et al., 2003; Kloeblen-Tarver, 2001). Newborns need to learn the association between sucking and satiation. Although some infants have nonnutritive sucking needs between feedings, it is best to wait to introduce a pacifier until the infant is proficient at breastfeeding.

■ Special Considerations

Sleepy Baby. During the first few days of life, some babies need to be awakened for feedings. Parents are instructed to be alert for behavioral signs or feeding cues such as rapid eye movements under the eyelids, sucking movements, or hand-to-mouth motions. When these signs are present, it is a good time to attempt breastfeeding. If the infant is awakened from a sound sleep, attempts at feeding are more likely to be unsuccessful. Unwrapping the baby, changing the diaper, sitting the baby upright, talking to the baby with variable pitch, gently massaging the baby's chest or back, and stroking the palms or soles may bring the baby to an alert state (Box 27-3).

Fussy Baby. Babies sometimes awaken from sleep crying frantically. Although they may be hungry, they cannot

---

box 27-3 Waking the Sleepy Newborn

- Lay the baby down and unwrap.
- Change the diaper.
- Hold the baby upright, turn from side to side.
- Talk to the baby.
- Gently, but firmly, massage the chest and back.
- Rub the baby's hands and feet.
- Do baby "sit-ups." Gently rock the baby from a lying to sitting position and back again until the eyes open.
- Adjust lighting up for stimulation or down to encourage the baby to open the eyes.
- Apply cool cloth to face.

---

box 27-4 Calming the Fussy Baby

- Swaddle the baby.
- Hold closely.
- Move or rock gently.
- Talk soothingly.
- Reduce environmental stimuli.
- Allow baby to suck on adult finger.
- Place baby skin-to-skin with mother.

---

focus on feeding until they are calmed. The nurse can encourage parents to swaddle the baby, hold the baby close, talk soothingly, and allow the baby to suck on a clean finger until calm enough to latch on to the breast (Box 27-4).

Babies sometimes cry as soon as they are positioned for feeding. The infant may be experiencing physical discomfort related to bruising or birth injury such as a previously undetected fractured clavicle. This problem may be alleviated by assisting the mother to change the feeding position.

Infants who were suctioned extensively or intubated at birth may demonstrate an aversion to oral stimulation. The baby may scream and stiffen if anything approaches the mouth. Parents may need to spend time holding and cuddling the baby before attempting to breastfeed.

An infant may become fussy and appear discontented when sucking if the nipple does not extend far enough into the mouth. The feeding may begin with well-organized sucks and swallows, but the infant soon begins to pull off the breast and cry. It may be helpful for the mother to support her breast throughout the feeding so that the nipple stays in the same position as the feeding proceeds and the breast softens.

Fussiness may be related to GI distress (i.e., cramping and gas pains). This may occur in response to an occasional feeding of infant formula, or it may be related to something the mother has ingested. Although most mothers can consume their normal diet without affecting the baby, foods such as broccoli, cabbage, or onions may irritate some babies. Others may react to cow's-milk protein ingested by the mother. If gas is a problem, the physician may suggest giving the baby liquid simethicone drops before feeding.

Parents should be taught that persistent crying or refusing to breastfeed can indicate illness, and the health care provider should be notified. Ear infections, sore throat, or oral thrush may cause the infant to be fussy and not breastfeed well.

Slow Weight Gain. Newborn infants typically lose about 5% of body weight before they begin to show weight gain. Weight loss of 7% in a breastfeeding infant during the first 3 days of life should be investigated (Gartner et al., 2005; Lawrence & Lawrence, 2005). Neonates should not lose more than 10% of birth weight during the first week. Thereafter they should begin to show a weight gain of 140 to 200 g/week or 20 to 28 g/day for the first 3 months. (Breastfed infants usually do not gain weight as quickly as formula-fed infants.) The infant who continues to lose weight after 5 days, who does not regain birth weight by 14 days, or whose weight is below the 10th percentile by 1 month should be evaluated and closely monitored by a health care provider.

Most often, slow weight gain is related to inadequate breastfeeding. Feedings may be short or infrequent, or the infant may be latching on incorrectly or sucking ineffectively or inefficiently. Other possibilities are illness or infection, malabsorption, or circumstances that increase the baby's energy needs such as congenital heart disease, cystic fibrosis, or simply being SGA.

Maternal factors may be the cause of slow weight gain. There may be a problem with inadequate emptying of the breasts, pain with feeding, or inappropriate timing of feedings. Inadequate glandular breast tissue or previous breast surgery may affect milk supply. Maternal diabetes, severe intrapartum or postpartum hemorrhage, illness, or medications may decrease milk supply. Stress and fatigue also may negatively affect milk production.

Usually the solution to slow weight gain is to improve the feeding technique. Positioning and latch-on are evaluated, and adjustments made. It may help to add a feeding or two in a 24-hour period. If the problem is a sleepy baby, parents are taught waking techniques.

Using alternate breast massage during feedings may help increase the amount of milk going to the infant. With this technique, the mother massages her breast from the chest wall to the nipple whenever the baby has sucking pauses. Some think this technique also may increase the fat content of the milk, which aids in weight gain.

When babies are calorie deprived and need supplementation, expressed breast milk or formula can be given with a nursing supplementer (see Fig. 27-2), cup, syringe, or bottle. In most cases, supplementation is needed only for a short time until the baby gains weight and is feeding adequately.

Jaundice. Jaundice (hyperbilirubinemia) in the newborn is discussed in detail in Chapter 25. Physiologic jaundice usually occurs after age 24 hours and peaks by the third day. When jaundice occurs before 24 hours of age, it is considered abnormal and warrants intervention.

Two clinical conditions are recognized that associate breastfeeding with jaundice: early breast milk jaundice and breast milk jaundice. The first is a common condition that occurs in healthy newborns, whereas the latter is a rare condition.

Early breast milk jaundice or *jaundice while breastfeeding* may be associated with insufficient breastfeeding and infrequent stooling. Colostrum has a natural laxative effect and promotes early passage of meconium. Bilirubin is excreted from the body primarily through the intestines. Infrequent stooling allows bilirubin in the stool to be reabsorbed into the infant's system, thus promoting hyperbilirubinemia.

The American Academy of Pediatrics recommends that when jaundice occurs in the healthy breastfeeding infant, breastfeeding should not be interrupted. Instead, the infant should be fed frequently (at least 8 to 12 times in 24 hours) (Gartner et al., 2005). Breastfeeding is evaluated in terms of frequency and length of feedings, positioning and latch-on, and the infant's ability to empty the breast. Factors such as a sleepy or lethargic baby or breast engorgement may interfere with effective breastfeeding and should be corrected. If supplementation is needed, the infant should be fed expressed breast milk or formula through a supplemental feeding device. A supplemental feeding device may be used to deliver additional breast milk or formula while the infant is nursing. Hyperbilirubinemia may reach levels that require treatment with phototherapy administered with a light or a fiberoptic blanket (see Chapter 26).

Late-onset jaundice or *breast milk jaundice* affects a few breastfed infants and develops in the second week of life, peaking at about age 10 days. Affected infants are typically thriving, gaining weight, and stooling normally; all pathologic causes of jaundice have been ruled out. It was once postulated that an enzyme in the milk of some mothers caused the bilirubin level to increase. It now appears that a factor in human milk increases the intestinal absorption of bilirubin. In most cases, no intervention is necessary, although some experts recommend temporary interruption of breastfeeding for 12 to 24 hours to allow bilirubin levels to decrease. During this time, the mother pumps her breasts, and the baby is offered alternative nutrition, usually formula (Lawrence & Lawrence, 2005).

Preterm Infants. Human milk is the ideal food for preterm infants, with unique benefits over and above those received by term, healthy infants. Breast milk enhances retinal maturation in the preterm infant and improves neurocognitive outcome. It also decreases the risk of necrotizing enterocolitis. Greater physiologic stability occurs with breastfeeding as compared with bottle feeding (Lawrence & Lawrence, 2005).

Depending on gestational age and physical condition, many preterm infants are capable of breastfeeding for at least some feedings each day. Mothers of preterm infants who are not able to breastfeed their infants should begin pumping their breasts as soon as possible after birth with a hospital-grade electric pump (Fig. 27-8). To establish an optimal milk supply, the mother should use a dual collection kit and pump 8 to 10 times daily for 10 to 15 minutes

FIG. 27-8 Hospital-grade electric breast pump.

FIG. 27-9 Breastfeeding twins. (Courtesy Marjorie Pyle, RNC, Lifecircle, Costa Mesa, CA.)

and/or until the milk flow has ceased for a few minutes. These women are taught proper handling and storage of breast milk to minimize bacterial contamination and growth (Riordan, 2005).

There are numerous benefits and challenges for mothers who are providing breast milk for their infants. The mothers of preterm infants often receive specific emotional benefits in breastfeeding or providing breast milk for their babies. They find rewards in knowing they can provide the healthiest nutrition for the infant and believe that breastfeeding enhances feelings of closeness to the infant. Challenges often come in being separated from the infant who must remain in the hospital, establishing and maintaining milk supply, and transitioning from gavage feeding to breastfeeding (Callen & Pinelli, 2005).

Breastfeeding Multiple Infants. Breastfeeding is especially beneficial to twins, triplets, and other higher-order multiples because of the immunologic and nutritional advantages, as well as the opportunity for the mother to interact with each baby frequently. Most mothers are capable of producing an adequate milk supply for multiple infants. Parenting multiples may be overwhelming and mothers, as well as fathers, need extra support and assistance learning how to manage feedings.

Twins are the most common type of multiple birth. In the hospital, a mother usually learns to feed each baby separately, and as her comfort level increases, she may begin to feed both babies at once. Each baby feeds from one breast per feeding, usually for about 20 to 30 minutes. Some mothers assign each baby a breast; others switch babies from one breast to the other, either on a schedule or randomly. If one twin nurses more vigorously than the other, the more vigorous baby should be alternated between breasts to equalize breast stimulation. The mother may find it easiest to use a modified demand feeding schedule. This involves feeding the first baby who wakes and then waking the second baby for feeding.

If the mother wants to feed the babies simultaneously, she may wish to experiment with positions. The easiest position to feed both babies is the football hold (Fig. 27-9). Alternatively, one baby could be held in the football hold and the other in the cradle hold, or the babies could each be held in a cradling position.

It is possible to breastfeed triplets and higher-order multiples. For example, with triplets, one baby alternately receives expressed breast milk or formula from a bottle at each feeding while the other two are breastfeeding. Obviously, this requires that the mother has someone to assist with feedings.

▬ *Expressing and Storing Breast Milk*

In some situations, expression of breast milk is necessary or desirable, such as when engorgement occurs, the mother and baby are separated (e.g., preterm or sick infant), the mother is employed outside the home and needs to maintain her milk supply, the nipples are severely sore or damaged, or the mother is leaving the infant with a caregiver and will not be present for feeding.

Because pumping and hand expression are rarely as efficient as a baby in removing milk from the breast, the milk supply should never be judged based on the volume expressed.

Hand Expression. After her hands are thoroughly washed, the mother places one hand on her breast at the edge of the areola. With her thumb above and fingers below, she presses in toward her chest wall and gently compresses the breast while rolling her thumb and fingers forward toward the nipple. These motions are repeated rhythmically until the milk begins to flow. The mother simply maintains steady, light pressure while the milk is flowing easily. The thumb and fingers should not pinch the breast or slip down to the nipple, and the mother should rotate her hand to reach all sections of the breast. After expressing milk from the second breast, she should return and express milk from the first breast, and then repeat with the second breast until all readily available milk is expressed.

Pumping. For most women, it is advisable to initiate pumping only after the milk supply is well established and the infant is latching on and breastfeeding well. However, when breastfeeding is delayed after birth, pumping is started as soon as possible and continued regularly until the infant is able to breastfeed effectively.

Numerous ways exist to approach pumping. Some women pump on awakening in the morning, or when the baby has fed but did not completely empty the breast. Others choose to pump after feedings or may pump one breast while the baby is feeding from the other. Double pumping (pumping both breasts at the same time) saves time and may stimulate the milk supply more effectively than single pumping (Fig. 27-10).

The amount of milk obtained when pumping depends on the type of pump being used, the time of day, how long it has been since the baby breastfed, the mother's milk supply, how practiced she is at pumping, and her comfort level (pumping is uncomfortable for some women). Breast milk may vary in color and consistency, depending on the time of day, the age of the baby, and foods the mother has eaten.

Types of Pumps. Many types of breast pumps are available, varying in price and effectiveness. Before purchasing or renting a breast pump, the mother would benefit from counseling by a nurse or lactation consultant to determine which pump best suits her needs.

Manual or hand pumps are least expensive and may be the most appropriate where portability and quietness of operation are important. These are most often used by mothers who are pumping for an occasional bottle (Fig. 27-11).

Full-service electric pumps, or hospital-grade pumps (see Fig. 27-8) most closely duplicate the sucking action and pressure of the breastfeeding infant. When breastfeeding is delayed after birth (e.g., preterm or ill newborn), or when mother and baby are separated for lengthy periods, these pumps are most appropriate. Because hospital-grade breast pumps are very heavy and expensive, portable versions of these pumps can be rented for home use.

Electric, self-cycling double pumps are efficient and easy to use. These pumps were designed for working mothers. Some of these pumps come with carry bags containing coolers to store pumped milk.

FIG. 27-11   Manual breast pumps. (Courtesy Marjorie Pyle, RNC, Lifecircle, Costa Mesa, CA.)

Smaller electric or battery-operated pumps also are available. Some have automatic suck/release cycling, and others require use of a finger to regulate strength and speed of suction. These are typically used when pumping is done occasionally, but some models are satisfactory for working mothers or others who pump on a regular basis.

Storage of Breast Milk. Breast milk can be safely stored in any clean glass or plastic container. Plastic bags especially designed for freezing breast milk can be purchased. Plastic ice cube trays can also be used to freeze breast milk. For full-term, healthy infants, freshly expressed breast milk can be stored at room temperature for up to 8 hours and can be refrigerated safely for 5 days. Milk can be frozen for 3 to 6 months in the freezer section of a refrigerator with a separate door, and for 6 to 12 months in a deep freeze (0° C). When breast milk is stored, the container should be dated, and the oldest milk should be used first (Eglash, Chantry, & Howard, 2004).

Frozen milk is thawed by placing the container in the refrigerator for gradual thawing or in warm water for faster thawing. It must not be refrozen and should be used within 24 hours. After thawing, the container should be shaken to mix the layers that have separated (Teaching for Self-Care box).

■ **NURSE ALERT**

Frozen milk is never thawed or heated in a microwave oven. Microwaving does not heat evenly and can cause encapsulated boiling bubbles to form in the center of the liquid. This may not be detected when drops of milk are checked for temperature. Babies have sustained severe burns to the mouth, throat, and upper GI tract as a result of microwaved milk (Lawrence & Lawrence, 2005).

■ *Being Away from the Baby*

Many women are able to combine breastfeeding successfully with employment, attending school, or other commitments. If feedings are missed, the milk supply may be affected. Some women's bodies adjust the milk supply to the times she is with the baby for feedings, whereas other

FIG. 27-10   Bilateral breast pumping. (Courtesy Medela, Inc., McHenry, IL.)

TEACHING FOR SELF-CARE

Breast Milk Storage Guidelines for Home Use

- Before expressing breast milk, wash your hands.
- Containers for storing milk should be washed in hot, soapy water and rinsed thoroughly; they can also be washed in a dishwasher. Plastic bags designed specifically for breast milk storage can be used.
- Write the date of expression on the container before storing the milk.
- It is acceptable to store breast milk in the refrigerator or freezer with other food items.
- When storing milk in a refrigerator or freezer, place the containers in the middle or back of the freezer, not on the door.
- Freeze milk in serving sizes of 2 to 4 ounces to avoid waste.
- When filling a storage container that will be frozen, allow space at the top of the container for expansion.
- To thaw frozen breast milk, place the container in the refrigerator for gradual thawing, or place the container under warm, running water for quicker thawing. Never boil or microwave.
- Milk thawed in the refrigerator can be stored for 24 hours. Milk thawed in warm water can be refrigerated for use within 4 hours.
- Thawed breast milk should never be refrozen.
- Shake the milk container before feeding baby, and test the temperature of the milk on the inner aspect of your wrist.
- Any unused milk left in the bottle after feeding must be discarded.
- Freshly expressed breast milk can be stored at room temperature (less than 78° F [25.6° C]) for up to 8 hours.
- Breast milk can be stored in the refrigerator for 3 to 5 days.
- Frozen breast milk can be stored for 2 weeks in a freezer compartment within a refrigerator.
- Frozen breast milk can be stored for up to 3 to 6 months in a freezer section with a separate door.
- Frozen breast milk can be stored for 6 to 12 months in a deep freeze (32° F [0° C] or lower)

From Lawrence, R., & Lawrence, R. (2005). *Breastfeeding: A guide for the medical profession* (6th ed.). Philadelphia: Mosby.

FIG. 27-12 Lactation room. Note the breast pump, rocking chair and nursing foot stool, changing table, books, and supplies. (Courtesy Cheryl Briggs, RN, Annapolis, MD.)

women find they must pump or the supply diminishes quickly. Nurses and other health care providers can provide useful information for mothers about continuing to breastfeed once they return to the workforce or to school (Tully, 2005). Employers are becoming increasingly more aware of the importance of supporting breastfeeding mothers who return to work; some businesses provide rooms where mothers can nurse their infants or use breast pumps (Fig. 27-12).

▬ Weaning

Weaning is initiated when babies are introduced to foods other than breast milk and concludes with the last breastfeeding. Gradual weaning, over a period of weeks or months, is easier for mothers and infants. Abrupt weaning is likely to be distressing for both mother and baby, as well as physically uncomfortable for the mother.

Infant-led weaning means that the infant moves at his or her own pace in omitting feedings. Drinking from a cup and increasing the amount of solid foods substitute for breastfeeding and allow a gradual decrease in the mother's milk supply.

Mother-led weaning means that the mother decides which feedings to drop. This is most easily done by omitting the feeding of least interest to the baby or the one the infant is most likely to sleep through. It also can be the feeding most convenient for the mother to omit. After a week or more, another feeding is dropped, and so on, until the infant is weaned from the breast. Allowing time for the milk supply to adjust before omitting another feeding prevents discomfort for the mother as her supply gradually decreases.

Infants can be weaned directly from the breast to a cup. Bottles are usually offered to infants younger than 6 months. If the infant is weaned before age 1 year, formula should be fed to the infant instead of cow's milk.

If abrupt weaning is necessary, breast engorgement often occurs. The mother is instructed to take mild analgesics, wear a supportive bra, apply ice packs or cabbage leaves to the breasts, and pump small amounts if needed to increase comfort. It is best to avoid pumping because the breasts should remain full enough to promote a decrease in the milk supply.

Weaning can be a very emotional time for mothers. Many women feel that weaning is the end to a special, satisfying relationship with the infant and benefit from time to adapt to the changes. Sudden weaning may evoke feelings of guilt and disappointment; some women go through a grieving period after weaning. The nurse can assist the mother by discussing other ways to continue this nurturing relationship with the infant, such as skin-to-skin contact while bottle feeding, or holding and cuddling the baby. Support from the father of the baby and other family members is essential at this time.

■ Milk Banking

For those infants who cannot be breastfed but cannot survive except on human milk, banked donor milk is critically important. Because of the antiinfective and growth-promoting properties of human milk, as well as its superior nutrition, donor milk is used in many neonatal intensive care units for preterm or sick infants when the mother's own milk is not available. Donor milk also is used therapeutically for a variety of medical conditions, such as in transplant recipients who are immunocompromised, chronic renal failure, leukemia, intractable pneumonia, and HIV.

The Human Milk Banking Association of North America (HMBANA) has established annually reviewed guidelines for the operation of donor human milk banks. Donor milk banks collect, screen, process, and distribute the milk donated by breastfeeding mothers who are feeding their own infants and pumping a few ounces extra each day for the milk bank. All donors are screened both by interview and serologically for communicable diseases. Donor milk is stored frozen until it is heat processed to kill potential pathogens; then it is refrozen for storage until it is dispensed for use. The heat processing adds a level of protection for the recipient that is not possible with any other donor tissue or organ. Banked milk is dispensed only by prescription. A per-ounce fee is charged by the bank to pay for the processing costs, but the HMBANA guidelines prohibit payment to donors (HMBANA, 2003).

■ Care of the Mother

Diet. Women who generally consume a nutritious diet will produce healthy breast milk for their infants. Chronically undernourished mothers whose dietary intake of vitamins and minerals is limited and who have low body stores may produce milk that is lacking in vitamins such as A, D, B_6, or B_{12}. Women who are breastfeeding should consume about 2700 calories per day (equal to 500 calories more than a nonpregnant, nonnursing woman). In dietary teaching, it is important to consider the mother's family situation, cultural beliefs, socioeconomic status, and individual energy and nutrient needs.

No specific foods or drinks need be either consumed or avoided. Lactating mothers should ideally consume a balanced diet of nutrient-dense foods. Adequate amounts of calcium, minerals, and fat-soluble vitamins are important. Breastfeeding mothers are encouraged to continue taking their prenatal vitamins until the baby is weaned.

If the breastfeeding mother is drinking enough fluids to quench her thirst, she is likely drinking enough to support lactation. Typically, women find that they are drinking as much as 2 to 3 quarts of fluid each day, with the choice

of fluid depending on the mother's preference. Because of her increased need for fluids, the breastfeeding mother may wish to keep a drink within reach during feedings. An indicator of adequate fluid intake is the color of the mother's urine. If she is drinking enough fluids, her urine should be clear to light yellow throughout the day.

Weight Loss. Because it takes energy to produce milk, many mothers have a gradual weight loss while breastfeeding, as fat stores deposited during pregnancy are used (Dewey, 2004). For overweight women, this can be an added incentive for breastfeeding. However, the mother who wants to diet while lactating should avoid losing large amounts of weight quickly because fat-soluble environmental contaminants to which she has been exposed are stored in her body's fat reserves, and these may be released into her milk. In addition, some mothers find that their milk supply decreases when their caloric intake is severely restricted. Most mothers find that they can lose about 1 kg per week without affecting their milk supply (King, 2000).

Exercise. Exercising in moderation is healthy for the breastfeeding mother and is not likely to affect her milk supply. Exercising to exhaustion may cause increased lactic acid levels in the breast milk, and subsequently the infant may refuse the breast (Larson-Meyer, 2002). For comfort, mothers may find it beneficial to engage in exercise soon after breastfeeding, when their breasts are as empty as possible. Wearing a well-designed, supportive bra also may be helpful. Hydration is important for the breastfeeding woman, therefore, the nursing mother who is exercising needs to consume adequate amounts of fluid to maintain good hydration status.

Rest. It is important for the breastfeeding mother to rest as much as possible, especially in the first 1 or 2 weeks after birth. Fatigue, stress, and worry can negatively affect milk production and let-down. The nurse can encourage the mother to sleep when the baby sleeps. Breastfeeding in a side-lying position promotes rest for the mother. Assistance with household chores and caring for other children can be done by the father, grandparents or other relatives, and friends.

Breast Care. The breastfeeding mother's normal routine bathing is all that is necessary to keep her breasts clean. Soap can have a drying effect on nipples, so she should be instructed to avoid washing the nipples with soap.

Breast creams should not be used routinely because they may block the natural oil secreted by the Montgomery glands on the areola. Some breast creams contain alcohol, which may dry the nipples. Vitamin E oil or cream is not recommended for use on nipples because it is a fat-soluble vitamin, and a breastfeeding infant might consume enough vitamin E from the nipple to reach toxic levels. In addition, some people are allergic to vitamin E oil.

The mother with flat or inverted nipples will likely benefit from wearing breast shells in her bra (see Fig. 16-10). Breast shells also are useful for sore nipples to keep the

FIG. 27-13 Breast shells.

mother's bra or clothing from touching the nipples (Fig. 27-13).

If a mother needs breast support, she will likely be uncomfortable unless she wears a bra, because the ligament that supports the breast (Cooper's ligament) will otherwise stretch and be painful. If she is comfortable without a bra, there is no reason for her to wear one. If a woman prefers to wear a bra, it should fit well, offer nonbinding support, and feel comfortable. Underwire bras or improperly fitting bras may contribute to clogged milk ducts. Mothers should be encouraged to breastfeed at least once daily without a bra on so that all milk ducts can empty well.

Leakage of milk between feedings is a problem for some women. Using breast pads (disposable or washable) inside a bra and wearing layered or printed tops can help camouflage the leakage. Plastic-lined breast pads are not recommended because they trap moisture and may contribute to sore nipples. To stop leakage, the mother can be alert to any sensation, such as tingling, that her milk is letting down. If this happens, she can usually stop the let-down by pressing straight back on her nipples. In public, she can fold her arms across her chest to apply pressure unobtrusively.

Although few cases of breast cancer are diagnosed during pregnancy or lactation, the breastfeeding woman should perform monthly breast self-examination (BSE). The woman who is not menstruating should choose a convenient date on which to do her BSE each month. She needs to become familiar with the normal nodularity of her lactating breasts so that she can detect anything unusual on examination. Nodules that match in location in both breasts are likely breast tissue. Nodules that increase and decrease in size are probably milk glands or ducts. Because lactating breasts are very dense, mammography is of limited diagnostic value. Should a suggestive nodule be discovered, a biopsy can usually be done without interrupting breastfeeding.

Effect of Menstruation. The return of menstrual periods varies among lactating women. The majority will resume menstruation by 6 months postpartum. Menstruation has no effect on breastfeeding. There are no hormonal effects on the infant, although some babies may seem fussy for the first day. The quality of the milk is not affected (Lawrence & Lawrence, 2005).

Sexual Sensations. Some women experience rhythmic uterine contractions during breastfeeding. Such sensations are not unusual because uterine contractions and milk ejection are both triggered by oxytocin. Occasionally, these uterine contractions may provoke sensations resembling an orgasmic response, which is disturbing to some mothers.

Breastfeeding and Contraception. Although breastfeeding confers a period of infertility, it is not considered an effective method of contraception. Breastfeeding delays the return of ovulation and menstruation; however, ovulation may occur even before the first menstrual period after birth. The breastfeeding woman who is relying on the lactational amenorrhea (LAM) method of birth control needs to be knowledgeable about ways to determine when ovulation occurs (i.e., basal body temperature, consistency of cervical mucus, and cervical position). Hormonal contraceptives, including pills, injectables, and implants, may cause a decrease in the milk supply and are best avoided during the first 6 weeks after birth. Oral contraceptives containing estrogen are not recommended for breastfeeding mothers. Progestin-only birth control pills are less likely to interfere with the milk supply. Some women find that the progestin-only injection (Depo-Provera) interferes with milk production, although others notice no alteration in the milk supply. Nonhormonal contraceptive methods (e.g., foam, condoms, nonhormonal intrauterine device [IUD], natural family planning, sterilization) are less likely to have a detrimental effect on breastfeeding (Lawrence & Lawrence, 2005) (see Chapter 9).

Breastfeeding During Pregnancy. It is possible for a breastfeeding woman to conceive and continue breastfeeding throughout the pregnancy if there are no medical contraindications (e.g., risk of preterm labor). When the baby is born, colostrum is produced. The practice of breastfeeding a newborn and an older child is called *tandem nursing.* The nurse should remind the mother always to feed the infant first to ensure that the newborn is receiving adequate nutrition. The supply-meets-demand principle works in this situation, just as with breastfeeding multiples.

The Mother with Diabetes. The mother with diabetes is encouraged to breastfeed. In addition to benefits for the infant, as well as maternal satisfaction, breastfeeding has an antidiabetogenic effect. Blood glucose levels and insulin requirements are lower because of the carbohydrate used in milk production. During lactation, the woman may be able to eat more food and still take less insulin. However, insulin dosage must be adjusted as the baby is weaned. Some women with diabetes are at increased risk for sore nipples caused by monilial infections and may have an increased risk for mastitis.

Medications and Breastfeeding. Although there is much concern about the compatibility of drugs and breastfeeding, few drugs are absolutely contraindicated during lactation. However, there is concern that the relative number of medications taken by mothers is rising.

In addition to the commonly prescribed analgesics, sedatives, methylergonovine, and antihypertensives, there has been an increase in the use of antibiotics, antidepressants, antipsychotics, steroids, and antiepileptics (Hale, 2004). In evaluating the safety of a specific medication during breastfeeding, the health care provider considers the pharmacokinetics of the drug in the maternal system, as well as the absorption, metabolism, distribution, storage, and excretion in the infant. The gestational and chronologic age of the infant, body weight, and breastfeeding pattern also are considered. Breastfeeding mothers should be cautioned about taking any medications except those that are deemed essential; they should be advised to check with their physician before taking any medication. If a breastfeeding mother is taking a medication that has questionable effect on the infant, she can be advised to take the medication just after nursing the baby or just before the infant is expected to sleep for a long time. References are available with specific information about medications and breastfeeding (AAP Committee on Drugs, 2001; Hale, 2004; Hale & Berens, 2002).

Smoking may impair milk production; it also exposes infants to the effects of second-hand smoke. Mothers should be encouraged to stop smoking, however, those who continue to smoke tobacco when lactating should be advised not to smoke within 2 hours before breastfeeding and never to smoke in the same room with the infant (AAP Committee on Drugs, 2001).

Breastfeeding mothers should not consume alcoholic beverages, because alcohol is concentrated in the milk and is passed on to the infant. Alcohol can also inhibit milk production and let-down. If a mother chooses to consume alcohol, she should be advised to minimize its effects by having only one occasional drink, and not to breastfeed for 2 hours after the drink (Gartner et al., 2005). The mother who is pumping for a sick or preterm infant should avoid alcohol entirely until her infant is healthy (Lawrence & Lawrence, 2005).

Caffeine intake by breastfeeding mothers is typically not problematic provided the mother is not consuming excessive amounts. Although only 1% of the caffeine ingested by the mother is passed into her breast milk, the infant's immature system limits the ability to excrete the caffeine. Caffeine accumulates in the infant's system and can cause irritability and poor sleeping patterns. Mothers need to be aware that caffeine is found in many sources including coffee, tea, some soft drinks, as well as in some pain relievers and cold medications. Theobromine, found in chocolate and cocoa, can have similar effects on the infant (Lawrence & Lawrence, 2005).

Herbs and herbal teas are becoming more widely used during lactation. Because herbal preparations are not regulated by the Food and Drug Administration (FDA), there is concern about their components. Although some are considered safe, others contain pharmacologically active compounds that may have detrimental effects. A thorough maternal history should include the use of any herbal remedies. Each remedy should then be evaluated for its compatibility with breastfeeding. The regional poison control center may provide information on the active properties of herbs. If herbal preparations are used, pure forms are recommended over mixtures of unknown herbals and standard recommended doses should not be exceeded (Hale, 2004).

Environmental Contaminants. Except under unusual circumstances, breastfeeding is not contraindicated because of exposure to environmental contaminants such as DDT (an insecticide) and tetrachloroethylene (used in dry cleaning plants) (Lawrence & Lawrence, 2005).

■ Special Considerations

The breastfeeding mother may have some common problems. In the majority of cases, these complications are preventable if the mother receives appropriate education about breastfeeding. Early recognition and resolution of these problems is important to prevent interruption of breastfeeding and to promote the mother's comfort and sense of well-being. The nurse or lactation consultant is likely to be the first contact the mother makes when these problems arise. By using astute interview and assessment skills, the nurse can gather essential data related to these problems, make necessary referrals to the physician or nurse practitioner, and assist the mother in initiating the appropriate treatment plan. Emotional support provided by the nurse or lactation consultant is essential to help allay the mother's frustration and anxiety and to prevent early cessation of breastfeeding.

Engorgement. Breast fullness is a normal phenomenon of lactogenesis that is noticed by most mothers about 36 hours after birth, gradually increasing until about the third to fifth day. Breasts may feel heavy and full, but soft and without pain. Engorgement, characterized by painful overfilling of the breasts, can occur as a result of infrequent or ineffective emptying of the breasts. It typically occurs 3 to 5 days after birth when the milk "comes in" and lasts about 24 hours. It is a common response of the breasts to the sudden change in hormones and the presence of an increased volume of milk. There is vascular congestion and increased vascularity, accumulation of milk in the breast tissue, and edema due to swelling and obstruction of lymphatic drainage (Mass, 2004). The breasts are firm, tender, and hot and may appear shiny and taut. The areolae are firm, and the nipples may flatten. The unyielding areolae make it difficult for the infant to latch on. Because back pressure on full milk glands inhibits milk production, if milk is not removed from the breasts, the milk supply may diminish.

Preparing the mother for what to expect when the milk comes in may help prevent engorgement or minimize its severity. Breastfeeding the baby frequently, at least every 2 to 3 hours, as the milk is coming in may help prevent engorgement. The baby should be encouraged to feed at least 15 to 20 minutes on each breast or until one breast softens per feeding.

When engorgement occurs, the nurse should reassure the mother that this a temporary condition usually resolved within 24 hours. The mother is instructed to feed every 2 hours, massaging the breasts as the baby is feeding. The baby should feed on the first breast until it softens before switching to the other side. If the infant does not soften the second breast, the mother may use a breast pump to empty the breast. Pumping during engorgement will not cause a problematic increase in milk supply. A warm shower just before feeding or pumping can aid in relaxation and let-down.

Because of the swelling of breast tissue surrounding the milk glands and milk ducts, cold compresses (ice packs) may reduce swelling, vascularity, and pain. Cold compresses are usually applied after feeding or pumping. Raw cabbage leaves placed over the breasts between feedings may help reduce the swelling. The mother washes the cabbage leaves and places them in her refrigerator until they are cool. She then crushes the leaves and places them over the breasts for 15 to 20 minutes. This can be repeated for two or three sessions; frequent application of cabbage leaves can decrease milk supply. (They are often very effective for formula-feeding mothers who want their milk to "dry up"). Cabbage leaves should not be used if the mother is allergic to cabbage or sulfa drugs or develops a skin rash (Lactation Education Resources, 2004).

Antiinflammatory medications, such as ibuprofen, may help reduce the pain and swelling associated with engorgement. Mothers often have a low-grade fever with engorgement and experience aching in their breasts, which ibuprofen can help remedy.

Sore Nipples. Mild nipple discomfort at the beginning of feedings or mild nipple tenderness during the first few days of breastfeeding is not abnormal. Severe soreness and abraded, cracked, or bleeding nipples are not normal and most often result from poor positioning, incorrect latch-on, improper suck, or a monilial infection. Many women expect breastfeeding to be painful, based on stories they have heard from family and friends. The nurse or lactation consultant must emphasize that breastfeeding should not be a painful experience; infant suckling should feel like a strong tugging sensation, but without pain or pinching. Limiting the time at the breast will not prevent sore nipples; the key to preventing sore nipples is correct breastfeeding technique (see Critical Thinking Exercise on p. 711).

For the first few days after birth, the mother may have some tenderness with the infant's initial sucks at the beginning of a feeding. This should quickly dissipate as the colostrum or milk begins to flow. To make the initial sucks less painful, the mother can express a few drops of colostrum or milk to moisten the nipple and areola before latch-on.

If the mother continues to experience nipple pain or discomfort after the first few sucks, it is necessary to help the mother evaluate the latch-on and baby's position at the breast.

If the mother reports a pinching sensation on the nipple as the baby sucks, it may be helpful to pull down on the side of the baby's jaw gently during sucking to increase the amount of breast tissue in the baby's mouth. If the nipple pain continues, the mother needs to remove the baby from the breast, breaking suction with her finger in the baby's mouth. She then proceeds to attempt latch-on again, making sure the baby's mouth is open wide before the baby is pulled quickly to the breast (see Fig. 27-5). Often sore nipples are the result of the mother latching the baby onto the breast before the mouth is open wide.

The infant's suck can be assessed by the nurse or lactation consultant simply by inserting a clean gloved finger into the baby's mouth and stimulating the baby to suck. If the baby is not extruding the tongue over the lower gum, and the mother reports pain or pinching with sucking, the baby may have ankyloglossia. With ankyloglossia (commonly referred to as "tongue-tie"), the sublingual frenulum inhibits the tongue from extending and elevating with sucking, which interferes with effective milk transfer and may result in nipple trauma. Sometimes this is corrected surgically to free the tongue for less painful, more effective breastfeeding (Griffiths, 2004; Lawrence & Lawrence, 2005).

The treatment for sore nipples is first to correct the cause. Once the problem is identified and corrected, sore nipples should heal within a few days, even though the baby continues to breastfeed regularly.

When sore nipples occur, it is more comfortable to start the feeding on the least sore nipple. Applying ice to the nipple for 2 to 3 minutes provides a numbing effect that increases comfort with latch-on. After feeding, the nipples are wiped with water to remove the baby's saliva. A few drops of milk can be expressed, rubbed into the nipple, and allowed to air dry.

Rapid healing of sore nipples is critical to relieve the mother's discomfort, maintain breastfeeding, and prevent mastitis. Although numerous creams, ointments, and gels have been used to treat sore nipples, no one topical agent has shown better results than others in relief of nipple discomfort (Morland-Schultz & Hill, 2005). Purified lanolin ointment and hydrogel are commonly used treatments for sore nipples. Purified lanolin helps sore nipples by retaining the skin's natural moisture and protecting the nipple from further abrasion. It is applied to nipples after feeding and need not be removed for the next feeding. (Mothers with history of wool allergy should not use lanolin until a skin test is done). A more recent technique for treating sore nipples is the use of hydrogel dressings. These create a soothing, moist healing environment by using a glycerin-based gel or saline-based hydrophilic polymer to provide a healing environment and bacterial barrier. Hydrogel pads are applied to the sore nipples after feeding, pumping, or bathing; they will not wipe off onto clothing or stick to sore nipples. They can be rinsed and reused for several days. Hydrogel also is available in a cream. An antibiotic ointment may be recommended if nipples are cracked, abraded, or bleeding; this must be washed off before the feeding.

If nipples are extremely sore or damaged, and the mother cannot tolerate breastfeeding, she may be advised to use an electric breast pump for 24 to 48 hours to allow the nipples to begin healing before resuming breastfeeding. It is important that the mother use a pump that will effectively empty the breasts; a rental pump is likely the best choice (see Fig. 27-10).

Sore nipples should be open to air as much as possible. Breast shells worn inside the bra allow air to circulate while keeping clothing off sore nipples (see Fig. 27-13).

Modern silicone nipple shields have been marketed as a treatment for sore nipples; however, they do not protect the nipple and can actually chafe the nipple as the baby sucks. The danger of the baby not receiving adequate milk flow through the shield exists because it is difficult for most infants to get far enough back on the breast to compress the lactiferous sinuses adequately and get the milk to flow. In special situations, nipple shields are useful; however, they should be used only by trained lactation consultants who closely monitor the infant's intake of milk and growth (Riordan, 2005).

Nipple Infections. Painful lesions on the nipples can be caused by bacterial *(staphyloccus)* or viral (herpes virus) infection. Such lesions are cultured and appropriate medications prescribed. If the mother has an active herpes lesion on her nipple or breast, the infant should not be allowed to breastfeed until healing occurs. The mother will need to pump her breasts to maintain milk supply and decrease discomfort from engorgement.

Nipple soreness may be caused by a monilial (yeast) infection. Sore nipples that occur after the newborn period are often the result of a yeast infection. The mother usually reports sudden onset of severe nipple pain and tenderness, burning, or stinging and may have sharp, shooting, burning pains into the breasts during and after feedings. The nipples appear somewhat pink and shiny or may be scaly or flaky; there may be a visible rash, small blisters, or thrush. Most often, the pain is out of proportion to the appearance of the nipple. Yeast infections of the nipples and breasts can be excruciatingly painful and can lead to early cessation of breastfeeding if not recognized and treated promptly (Hoover, 2001).

Babies may or may not exhibit symptoms of monilial infection. Oral thrush and a red, raised diaper rash are common indications of a yeast infection. An affected infant is often very fussy and gassy. When feeding, the baby is likely to pull off the breast soon after starting to feed, crying with apparent pain. The infant may be biting or gumming at the breast.

The most common predisposing factors for yeast infection of the breast include previous antibiotic use, vaginal yeast infections, and nipple damage.

Mothers and babies must be treated simultaneously, even if the infant has no visible signs of infection. Treatment for the mother is typically an antifungal cream applied to the nipples after feedings. Most pediatricians prescribe an oral antifungal medication, such as Nystatin, for infants. If maternal symptoms do not respond to topical treatment, oral antifungal medications may be needed. Treatment of mother and baby should continue for at least 7 days after symptoms begin to improve. Careful hand-

washing is essential to prevent the spread of yeast. Family members may have symptoms of yeast infections and should receive appropriate treatment. Jock itch and finger or toenail fungus are types of yeast infections. Other children in the family may have diaper rash because of yeast (Hoover, 2001).

Eczema. Red, scaly, cracked nipples may be a result of eczema, a type of dermatitis; this is usually treated with a topical steroid cream. It is important that this is not confused with Paget's disease, a rare type of breast cancer that often presents with itching, burning, scaling, and redness of the nipple (Lawrence & Lawrence, 2005).

Raynaud's Phenomenon. Extreme nipple pain during and after feedings may be related to vasospasm, or Raynaud's phenomenon. The nipple appears blanched after feeding and may turn red or blue before returning to the normal color. Nifedipine may be prescribed; mothers may find some comfort in taking an antiinflammatory such as ibuprofen and applying warmth to the breasts (Anderson, Held, & Wright, 2004; Riordan, 2005).

Plugged Milk Ducts. A milk duct may become plugged or clogged, causing a red, tender area or small lump in the breast, which may or may not be tender. This area typically does not empty or soften with feeding or pumping. A small white blister or "pearl" may be seen on the tip of the nipple; this is the curd of milk blocking the flow. The mother is afebrile and has no generalized symptoms.

Plugged milk ducts are most often the result of inadequate emptying of the breast. This may be occur because of poor breastfeeding, delayed or missed feedings, always using the same position for feeding, clothing that is too tight, or a poorly fitting or underwire bra.

Application of warm compresses to the affected area and to the nipple before feeding helps promote emptying of the breast and release of the plug. (A disposable diaper filled with warm water makes an easy compress.) Soaking in a warm bath before feeding may be helpful.

Frequent feeding is recommended, with the baby beginning the feeding on the affected side to foster more complete emptying. The mother is advised to massage the affected area while the baby nurses or while she is pumping. Varying feeding positions and feeding without wearing a bra may be useful in resolving a plugged duct.

If the mother develops fever or flulike symptoms, she may have mastitis and should notify her health care provider. Plugged milk ducts do not necessarily cause mastitis, but milk stasis may increase the susceptibility to a breast infection. Women with recurrent plugged milk ducts may find that taking oral lecithin capsules is helpful.

Mastitis. A breast infection, or mastitis, is characterized by the sudden onset of flulike symptoms such as fever, chills, body aches, and headache. (Flulike symptoms in a breastfeeding mother should be considered indicative of mastitis, until proven otherwise.) Localized breast pain and tenderness usually is accompanied by a warm, reddened area on the breast, often resembling the shape of a pie wedge. Mastitis most commonly occurs in the upper outer quadrant of the breast; it may affect one or both breasts.

Certain factors may predispose a woman to mastitis. Inadequate emptying of the breasts is common, related to engorgement, plugged ducts, a sudden decrease in the number of feedings, abrupt weaning, or wearing underwire bras. Sore, cracked nipples may lead to mastitis by providing a portal of entry for causative organisms (*Staphylococcus, Streptococcus,* and *Escherichia coli* are most common). Stress and fatigue, ill family members, breast trauma, and poor maternal nutrition also are predisposing factors for mastitis (Mass, 2004).

Breastfeeding mothers should be taught the signs of mastitis before they are discharged from the hospital after birth, and they need to know to call the health care provider promptly if the symptoms occur. Treatment includes antibiotics such as cephalexin or dicloxacillin for 10 to 14 days, and analgesic and antipyretic medications such as ibuprofen. The mother is advised to rest as much as possible, and she should feed the baby or pump frequently, striving to empty the affected side adequately. Warm compresses to the breast before feeding or pumping may be useful. Adequate fluid intake and a balanced diet are important for the mother with mastitis (Hale & Berens, 2002).

Complications of mastitis include breast abscess, chronic mastitis, or fungal infections of the breast. Most complications can be prevented by early recognition and treatment (Mass, 2004).

Breast Surgery. Previous breast surgery may impact the mother's ability to breastfeed successfully. Surgical procedures can damage nerves and interrupt milk ducts. Women who have had augmentation mammoplasty (breast implants) should be able to breastfeed successfully, particularly if the implants are placed underneath the chest wall muscle. Reduction mammoplasty is more likely to cause problems with the ability to successfully lactate due to interference with milk ducts, removal of glandular tissue, and nerve damage. Even so, many women are still able to breastfeed completely or partially. Mothers with a history of previous breast surgery are instructed to carefully monitor their infants for signs of adequate feeding. Before undergoing breast surgery, all women should discuss their lactation potential with their surgeon (Riordan, 2005).

▬ Role of the Nurse in Promoting Successful Lactation

Providing a birth environment in which breastfeeding is initiated and supported is an important nursing responsibility. The optimal environment in which to promote breastfeeding is a "Baby Friendly" hospital that promotes a family-centered approach and facilitates breastfeeding. The Baby Friendly Hospital Initiative (BFHI), sponsored by the WHO and United Nations Children's Fund (UNICEF), was founded in 1991 to encourage institutions to offer optimal levels of care for lactating mothers. When a hospital achieves the "Ten Steps to Successful Breastfeeding for Hospitals," it is recognized as a Baby Friendly Hospital (see Box 27-5) (BFHI USA, 2004).

Nurses working in a variety of perinatal settings can play a major role in breastfeeding education and support for new parents. In prenatal settings, nurses are often the first to inquire about the mother's plans regarding infant feeding. Nurses can educate the mother and her partner about the advantages of breastfeeding and explore reasons that they may prefer formula feeding. Current reading materials and information about prenatal classes are made available to expectant parents. At each encounter, the nurse offers to answer questions and provide additional information as needed. Assessment of the mother's breasts and nipples during pregnancy is important. The nurse should inquire about previous breast surgery and breast changes during pregnancy, such as enlargement of the breasts. Flat or inverted nipples are identified, and the mother is offered breast shells (see Fig. 27-13) to wear during the last month of pregnancy to encourage eversion of the nipples.

Prenatal education of the mother who plans to breastfeed includes information about breast and nipple care. It is not necessary to prepare nipples for breastfeeding; this is accomplished through normal physiologic changes of pregnancy.

Parents often expect that because breastfeeding is "natural," it comes naturally for both mother and baby. This misconception should be clarified early so that parents may view breastfeeding as a learning process. Then they are able to give themselves and their baby permission to learn, without unrealistic expectations. Nurses, physicians, and other health care providers who are knowledgeable about breastfeeding can offer needed support and encouragement to parents, helping to instill a sense of confidence.

---

box 27-5 Baby-Friendly Hospital Initiative: Ten Steps to Successful Breastfeeding

1. Have a written breastfeeding policy that is routinely communicated to all health care staff.
2. Train all health care staff in skills necessary to implement this policy.
3. Inform all pregnant women about the benefits and management of breastfeeding.
4. Help mothers initiate breastfeeding within 1 half hour of birth.
5. Show mothers how to breastfeed and maintain lactation, even if they should be separated from their infants.
6. Give newborn infants no food or drink other than breast milk, unless medically indicated.
7. Practice rooming-in—that is, allow mothers and infants to remain together 24 hours a day.
8. Encourage breastfeeding on demand.
9. Give no artificial teats or pacifiers (also called dummies or soothers) to breastfeeding infants.
10. Foster the establishment of breastfeeding support groups and refer mothers to them on discharge from the hospital or clinic.

From BFHI USA: *Implementing the UNICEF/WHO Baby-Friendly Hospital Initiative in the United States.* (2004). Accessed www.babyfriendlyusa.org, April 25, 2006.

Nurses often work in collaboration with lactation consultants in hospitals, physician offices, or community settings. Although the vast majority are registered nurses, lactation consultants come from a variety of backgrounds such as nutrition, physical or occupational therapy, home economics, psychology, social work, education, or the basic sciences. Lactation consultants have had specialized education, training, and clinical experience related to breastfeeding. Most lactation consultants are certified by the International Board of Lactation Consultant Examiners, having met specific criteria for academic and clinical experience and having passed the certifying examination. The professional organization for lactation consultants is the International Lactation Consultant Association (ILCA) (www.ilca.org) and is open to anyone interested in breastfeeding. The organization publishes the *Journal of Human Lactation,* which includes research and clinical articles related to breastfeeding.

■ Follow-up After Hospital Discharge

Problems with sore nipples, engorgement, and jaundice are likely to occur after discharge. It is the role of the nurse to educate and prepare the mother for problems she may encounter once she is home. It is important that the mother be given a list of resources for help with breastfeeding concerns and that she realizes when to call for assistance. Community resources for breastfeeding mothers include lactation consultants in hospitals, physician offices, or in private practice; nurses in pediatric or obstetric offices; support groups such as La Leche League (www.laleche.org); and peer counseling programs (e.g., those offered through WIC).

Telephone follow-up by hospital, birth center, or office nurses within the first day or two after discharge can provide a means to identify problems and offer needed advice and support. The AAP recommends that breastfeeding infants should be seen by a health care provider at 3 to 5 days of age and again at 2 to 3 weeks to assess weight gain and offer encouragement and support to the mother (Gartner et al., 2005).

■ Evaluation

Evaluation is based on the expected outcomes, and the plan of care is revised as needed based on the evaluation (Plan of Care).

---

plan of care ▶ Breastfeeding and Infant Nutrition

NURSING DIAGNOSIS Ineffective breastfeeding related to knowledge deficit of mother as evidenced by ongoing incorrect latch-on technique

Expected Outcomes *Mother will demonstrate correct latch-on technique. Infant will latch on and suck with gliding jaw movements and audible swallowing. Mother will report no nipple pain with infant suckling.*

Nursing Interventions/Rationales
- Assess mother's knowledge and motivation for breastfeeding *to acknowledge woman's desire for effective outcome and provide starting point for teaching.*
- Observe a breastfeeding session *to provide database for positive reinforcement and problem identification.*
- Describe and demonstrate ways to stimulate the sucking reflex, various positions for breastfeeding, and the use of pillows during a session *to promote maternal and neonatal comfort and effective latch-on.*
- Monitor neonatal position of mouth on areola and position of head and body *to give positive reinforcement for correct latch-on position or to correct poor latch-on position.*
- Teach woman ways to stimulate neonate to maintain an awake state by diapering, unwrapping, massaging, or burping *to complete a breastfeeding thoroughly and satisfactorily.*
- Give woman information regarding lactation diet, expression of milk by hand or pump, and storage of expressed breast milk *to provide basic information.*
- Make sure woman has written information on all aspects of breastfeeding *to reinforce verbal instructions and demonstrations.*
- Refer to support groups and lactation consultant if needed *to provide further information and group support.*

NURSING DIAGNOSIS Ineffective infant feeding pattern related to inability to coordinate sucking and swallowing

Expected Outcome *Neonate will coordinate sucking and swallowing in order to accomplish an effective feeding pattern.*

Nursing Interventions/Rationales
- Assess for factors that may contribute to ineffective sucking and swallowing *to provide a basis for plan of care.*
- Teach mother to observe feeding readiness cues *to enhance effective feeding.*
- Modify feeding methods as needed *to maintain hydration status and nutritional requirements.*
- Promote a calm, relaxed atmosphere *to provide a pleasant breastfeeding experience for woman and neonate.*
- Refer to lactation consultant *to provide specialized support.*

NURSING DIAGNOSIS Anxiety related to ineffective infant feeding pattern

Expected Outcomes *Woman will report a decrease in anxiety level and will express confidence in ability to provide adequate nutrition to her infant.*

Nursing Interventions/Rationales
- Monitor anxiety level during feeding sessions *to provide a basis for care planning.*
- Provide positive reinforcement for feeding pattern improvement *to decrease anxiety.*
- Monitor weight, intake, and output *to provide information regarding effective feeding.*
- Enlist assistance of support persons *to provide positive feedback for increasing skill.*
- Provide information for lactation support *to decrease anxiety after discharge.*

CD: Plan of Care: Breastfeeding and Infant Nutrition

▬ FORMULA FEEDING

The vast majority of infants in the United States receive infant formula at some point during their first year of life (Ryan et al., 2002). Although some parents may choose to exclusively formula feed, formula also may be used to supplement breastfeeding if the mother's milk supply appears to be inadequate, or it may be fed to the baby when the mother will be away and wishes to leave a bottle of formula instead of expressed breast milk.

Parent Education

Mothers and fathers who are formula feeding their infants need teaching, counseling, and support, particularly if they are first-time parents or if they have never formula fed. Parents are likely to have questions related to feeding frequency, the appropriate amount of formula to give the infant at each feeding, formula intolerance, weight gain, and "spitting up" (Borghese-Lang, Morrison, Ogle, & Wright, 2003). They may need assistance with the feeding process and with any problems they may have. Emphasis on the beneficial use of feeding times for close contact and socializing with the infant can help promote bonding and infant interaction.

The alarming increase in childhood and adolescent obesity in the United States is prevalent among low-income populations and minorities who receive WIC benefits. Many of these mothers believe that heavier infants are healthier and thus an indication of successful parenting. Solids are introduced earlier and the feeding environment promotes parental control over infant intake. Parents who choose formula feeding are more likely to feed on a regular schedule, without attending to infant feeding readiness cues (Birch & Davison, 2001; Borghese-Lang et al., 2003; Gillman et al., 2001). Teaching parents to observe for signs that the infant is hungry and how to tell if the baby is full can help decrease the likelihood of overfeeding.

Readiness for Feeding

The first feeding of formula is ideally given after the initial transition to extrauterine life is made. Feeding-readiness cues include such things as stability of vital signs, presence of bowel sounds, an active sucking reflex, and those described earlier for breastfed infants. The type of formula is usually determined by the pediatrician. Parents are advised to avoid switching formulas unless instructed to do so by the physician.

Before the first formula feeding, some institutions have the policy of offering sips of sterile water to the newborn to assess patency of the GI tract and absence of tracheoesophageal fistula. If the infant sucks and swallows the water without difficulty, formula is then offered.

Feeding Patterns

Typically, a newborn will drink 15 to 30 ml of formula per feeding during the first 24 hours, with the intake gradually increasing during the first week of life. Most newborn infants should be fed every 3 to 4 hours, even if that requires waking the baby for the feedings. The infant showing an adequate weight gain can be allowed to sleep at night and fed only on awakening. Most newborns need six to eight feedings in 24 hours, and the number of feedings decreases as the infant matures. Usually by 3 to 4 weeks after birth, a fairly predictable feeding pattern has developed. Scheduling feedings arbitrarily at predetermined intervals may not meet a baby's needs, but initiating feedings at convenient times often moves the baby's feedings to times that work for the family.

Mothers will usually notice increases in the infant's appetite at 7 to 10 days, 3 weeks, 6 weeks, 3 months, and 6 months. These appetite spurts correspond to growth spurts. The amount of formula per feeding should be increased by about 30 ml to meet the baby's needs at these times.

Feeding Technique

Parents who choose formula feeding often need education regarding feeding techniques. Babies should be held for all feedings. During feedings, parents are encouraged to sit comfortably, holding the infant closely in a semiupright position with good head support. Feedings provide opportunities to bond with the baby through touching, talking, singing, or reading to the infant. Parents should consider feedings as a time of peaceful relaxation with the baby (Fig. 27-14).

A bottle should never be propped with a pillow or other inanimate object and left with the infant. This practice may result in choking, and it deprives the infant of important interaction during feeding. Moreover, propping the bottle has been implicated in causing nursing bottle caries,

FIG. 27-14 Father bottle feeding infant son. Note the angled bottle that ensures that milk covers nipple area. (Courtesy Eugene Doerr, Leitchfield, KY.)

CD: Skill: Infant Feeding

or decay of the first teeth resulting from continuous bathing of the teeth with carbohydrate-containing fluid as the infant sporadically sucks the nipple.

The bottle should be held so that fluid fills the nipple and none of the air in the bottle is allowed to enter the nipple (see Fig. 27-14). When the infant falls asleep, turns aside the head, or ceases to suck, it is usually an indication that enough formula has been taken to satisfy the baby. Parents should be taught to look for these cues and avoid overfeeding, which can contribute to obesity.

Most infants swallow air when fed from a bottle and should be given a chance to burp several times during a feeding (Fig. 27-15).

Spitting up. Parents need to know what to do if the infant is spitting up. They may need to decrease the amount of feeding, or feed smaller amounts more frequently. Burping the infant several times during a feeding, such as when the infant's sucking slows down or stops, may decrease spitting. It may help to hold the baby upright for 30 minutes after feeding, and to avoid bouncing or placing the infant on the abdomen soon after the feeding is finished. Spitting may be a result of overfeeding or may be symptomatic of gastroesophageal reflux. Vomiting one third or more of the feeding at most feeding sessions or projectile vomiting should be reported to the health care provider.

Bottles and Nipples

Various brands and styles of bottles and nipples are available to parents. Most babies will feed well with any bottle and nipple. It is important that the bottles and nipples be washed in warm soapy water, using a bottle and nipple brush to facilitate thorough cleansing. Careful rinsing is necessary. Boiling of bottles and nipples is not needed unless there is some question about the safety of the water supply.

Infant Formulas

Commercial Formulas. Human milk is used as the "gold standard" on which all infant formulas are based. Commercial infant formulas are designed to resemble human milk as closely as possible, although none has ever duplicated it. The exact composition of infant formula varies with the manufacturer, but all must meet specific standards.

In an effort to make formula as similar to breast milk as possible, formula manufacturers have added a variety of ingredients including iron and nucleotides. Recently, manufacturers have added long-chain polyunsaturated fatty acids (LCPUFAs), consisting of arachidonic acid and docosahexaenoic acid, to enhance brain growth and retinal development. Research is ongoing to determine if, in fact, this is true (Morin, 2004). Other possible additives are currently under consideration such as probiotics to promote the development of fecal flora and enhance the intestinal immune response (Agostoni & Haschke, 2003; Institute of Medicine, 2004).

Infants who are not breastfed should be given commercial formulas for the first year of life (Gartner et al., 2005). If this is too expensive, the family would likely be eligible for services through the WIC program, which provides iron-fortified commercial infant formula. Cow's milk is the basis for most infant formulas, although soy-based and other specialized formulas are available for the infant who cannot tolerate cow's milk. Parents should be encouraged to use infant formulas that are fortified with iron.

Commercial formulas are available in three forms: powder, concentrate, and ready-to-feed. All are equivalent in terms of nutritional content, but they vary considerably in cost:

- Powdered formula is the least expensive type. It is easily mixed by using one scoop for every 60 ml of water. One feeding at a time should be prepared; unused formula in the bottle should be discarded.

FIG. 27-15 Positions for burping an infant. **A,** Sitting. **B,** On the shoulder. **C,** Across the lap. (Courtesy Julie Perry Nelson, Gilbert, AZ.)

- Concentrated formula is more expensive than powder. It is diluted with equal parts of water and can be stored in the refrigerator for 48 hours after opening.
- Ready-to-feed formula is the most expensive but easiest to use. The desired amount is poured into the bottle. The opened can is safely refrigerated for 48 hours. This type of formula can be purchased in individual disposable bottles for the most convenient feeding.

Special Formulas. Some infants have an allergic reaction to cow's-milk formula. They may have diarrhea, rash, colic, or vomiting, and, in extreme cases, failure to thrive. Some of these infants may better tolerate a soy-milk formula; however, some may be allergic to soy protein. If hypersensitivity to cow's-milk protein is suspected, a hydrolyzed casein formula may be recommended; however, special formulas are very expensive. Some women may be able to begin breastfeeding or, in life-threatening cases, obtain human milk through a milk bank, at least temporarily. Other special formulas are available for infants with a variety of disorders such as protein allergy, malabsorption syndromes, and inborn errors of metabolism.

Formulas for preterm infants contain higher calorie concentration (22 to 24 cal/oz) and higher concentrations of some nutrients such as protein, vitamin A, folic acid, and zinc (Morrow, 2004).

Evaporated Milk. Although evaporated milk is concentrated and less expensive than commercial formula, the mixing of evaporated milk and water to feed a baby is no longer recommended because evaporated milk does not provide adequate nutrition for an infant.

Unmodified Cow's Milk. Unmodified cow's milk is not suited to the nutritional needs of the human infant in the first year of life. Specific concerns include the excessive amounts of calcium, phosphorus, and other minerals it contains; an imbalance of calcium and phosphorus; its excessive protein content; the poor absorption of the fat it contains; and its low iron concentration. In addition, its use in infants is apt to cause microscopic hemorrhages that lead to GI blood loss. This blood loss, as well as the low levels of iron in the milk, increases the likelihood of iron-deficiency anemia.

Formula Preparation

The commercial infant formula must include directions for preparation and use with pictures and symbols for the benefit of persons who cannot read. Some manufacturers are translating the directions into various languages, such as Spanish, French, Vietnamese, Chinese, and Arabic to prevent misunderstanding and errors in formula preparation.

Although manufacturers of commercial formula include directions for preparing their products, the nurse should review formula preparation with the parents. It is especially important that formula be mixed properly. The newborn's kidneys are immature, and giving the infant overly concentrated formula may provide protein and minerals in amounts that exceed the kidney's excretory ability. In contrast, if the formula is diluted too much (sometimes done

CD: Critical Thinking Exercise: Formula Preparation

in an effort to save money), the infant does not consume enough calories and does not grow well (Renfrew, Ansell, & Macleod, 2003).

▬ NURSE ALERT

It is important to impress on families that the proportions must not be altered—neither diluted to expand the amount of formula nor concentrated to provide more calories.

Sterilization of formula rarely is recommended for those families with access to a safe public water supply. Instead, the formula is prepared with attention to cleanliness. When water from a private well is used, parents should be advised to contact the health department to have a chemical and bacteriologic analysis of the water done before using the water in formula preparation. The presence of nitrates, excess fluoride, or bacteria may be harmful to the infant.

If the sanitary conditions in the home appear unsafe, it would be better to recommend the use of ready-to-feed formula or to teach the mother to sterilize the formula. The two traditional methods for sterilization are terminal heating and the aseptic method. In the terminal-heating method, the prepared formula is placed in the bottles, which are topped with the nipples placed upside down and covered with the caps, and then sealed loosely with the rings. The bottles are then boiled together in a water bath for 25 minutes. In the aseptic method, the bottles, rings, caps, nipples, and any other necessary equipment, such as a funnel, are boiled separately, after which the formula is poured into the bottles. Any formula left in the bottle after the feeding should be discarded because the baby's saliva has mixed with it. Instructions for formula preparation and feeding are provided in the Teaching for Self-Care box.

Vitamin and Mineral Supplementation

Commercial iron-fortified formula has all of the nutrients the infant needs for the first 6 months of life. After 6 months, the only mineral supplementation required is fluoride if the local water supply is not fluoridated.

Weaning

The bottle-fed infant will gradually learn to use a cup, and the parents will find that they are preparing fewer bottles. Often the bottle feeding before bedtime is the last one to remain. Babies have a strong need to suck, and the baby who has the bottle taken away too early or abruptly will compensate with nonnutritive sucking on his or her fingers, thumb, a pacifier, or even his or her own tongue. Weaning from a bottle should therefore be done gradually, because the baby has learned to rely on the comfort that sucking provides.

Introducing Solid Foods

The infant receives the right balance of nutrients from breast milk or formula during the first 4 to 6 months. It is not true that the feeding of solids will help the infant sleep through the night. Cereal should not be put into

TEACHING FOR SELF-CARE

Formula Preparation and Feeding

FORMULA PREPARATION

- Wash your hands and clean the bottle, nipple, and can opener carefully before preparing formula.
- If new nipples seem too firm or stiff, they can be softened by boiling them in water for 5 minutes before use.
- Read the label on the container of formula and mix it exactly according to the directions.
- Use tap water to mix concentrated or powdered formula unless directed otherwise by your baby's physician or nurse.
- Test the size of the nipple hole by holding a prepared bottle upside down. The formula should drip from the nipple. If it runs in a stream, the hole is too big and should not be used. If it has to be shaken for the formula to come out, the hole is too small. You can either buy a new nipple or enlarge the hole by boiling the nipple for 5 minutes with a sewing needle inserted in the hole.
- If a nipple collapses when your baby sucks, loosen the nipple ring a little to let in air.
- Opened cans of ready-to-feed or concentrated formula should be covered and refrigerated. Any unused portions must be discarded after 48 hours. Record on the can the date and time the can was opened.
- Bottles or cans of unopened formula can be stored at room temperature.
- If the formula is refrigerated, warm it by placing the bottle in a pan of hot water. Never use a microwave to warm any food to be given to a baby. Test the temperature of the formula by letting a few drops fall on the inside of your wrist. If the formula feels comfortably warm to you, it is the correct temperature.

FEEDING TECHNIQUES AND TIPS

- Newborns should be fed at least every 3 to 4 hours and should never go longer than 4 hours without feeding until a satisfactory pattern of weight gain is established. This may take 2 weeks. If a baby cries or fusses between feedings, check to see if the diaper should be changed, and if the baby needs to be picked up and cuddled. If the baby continues to cry and acts hungry, go ahead and feed. Babies do not get hungry on a regular schedule.
- Babies gradually increase the amount of milk they drink with each feeding. The first day or so, most newborns consume

15 to 30 ml (½ to 1 ounce) with each feeding. This amount increases as the infant grows. If any formula remains in the bottle as the feeding ends, that milk must be thrown away, because saliva from the baby's mouth can cause the formula to spoil.

- It is a good idea to keep a feeding diary, writing down the amount of formula the baby drinks with each feeding for the first week or so. Also record the wet diapers and bowel movements the baby is having. Take this "diary" with you when you take the baby for the first pediatrician visit.
- For feeding, hold the baby close in a semi-reclining position. Talk to the baby during the feeding. This is a great time for social interaction and cuddling.
- Place the nipple in the baby's mouth on the tongue. It should touch the roof of the mouth to stimulate the baby's sucking reflex. Hold the bottle like a pencil. Keep the bottle tipped so that the nipple stays filled with milk and the baby does not suck in air.
- It is normal for babies to take a few sucks and then pause briefly before continuing to suck again. Some newborns take longer to feed than others. Be patient. It may be necessary to keep the baby awake and to encourage sucking. Moving the nipple gently in the baby's mouth may stimulate sucking.
- Newborns are apt to swallow air when sucking. Give the baby opportunities to burp several times during a feeding. As the baby gets older, you will know better when it is necessary to stop for burping.
- After the first 2 or 3 days, the stools of a formula-fed infant are yellow and soft, but formed. The baby may have a stool with each feeding in the first 2 weeks, although this may decrease to one or two stools each day.

SAFETY TIPS

- Babies should be held and never left alone while feeding. Never prop the bottle. The baby might inhale formula or choke on any that was spit up. Babies who fall asleep with a propped bottle of milk or juice may be prone to cavities when the first teeth come in.
- Know how to use the bulb syringe and how to help a baby who is choking (see Chapter 26).

---

the infant's bottle. Introduction of solid foods before the infant is 4 to 6 months of age may result in overfeeding and decreased intake of formula. The infant cannot communicate feeling full as can an older child, who is able to turn the head away. The proper balance of carbohydrate, protein, and fat for an infant to grow properly is in the breast milk or formula.

The infant's individual growth pattern should help determine the right time to start solids. The primary health care provider will advise when to introduce solid foods. The schedule for introducing solid foods and the types of foods to serve will be discussed during well-baby supervision visits with the pediatrician or pediatric nurse practitioner.

community activity

Explore the resources in your community for breastfeeding mothers after they are discharged from the hospital. Find out if there are lactation consultants in hospitals, pediatricians' offices, or health departments, or in private practice, who are accessible to mothers. What services are provided (e.g., phone consultations, one-on-one consultations)? Is there a charge to the client for these services? Are there peer counselors for nursing mothers through the local WIC program? Are there nursing support groups in the community, such as La Leche League, where mothers can attend meetings to gain information and support?

key points

- Human breast milk is species-specific and is the recommended form of infant nutrition. It provides immunologic protection against many infections and diseases.
- Breast milk changes in composition with each stage of lactation, during each feeding, and as the infant grows.
- During the prenatal period, parents should be informed of the benefits of breastfeeding for infants, mothers, families, and society.
- Infants should be breastfed as soon as possible after birth and at least 8 to 12 times per day thereafter.
- Specific, measurable indicators show that the infant is breastfeeding effectively.

- Breast milk production is based on a supply-meets-demand principle: the more the infant nurses, the greater the milk supply.
- Commercial infant formulas provide satisfactory nutrition for most infants.
- All infants should be held for feedings.
- Parents should be instructed about the types of commercial infant formulas, proper preparation for feeding, and correct feeding technique.
- Solid foods should be started after age 4 to 6 months.
- Nurses must be knowledgeable about feeding methods and provide education and support for families.

REFERENCES

Abbott Laboratories. (2003). *New data show U.S. breastfeeding rates at all-time recorded high.* News release, 11/25/2003. Abbott Park, IL: Ross Products Division.

Academy of Breastfeeding Medicine. (2006). *Breastfeedng a top priority in addressing infant growth and nutrition, accoding to Academy of Breastfeeding Medicine and UNICEF.* Internet document accessed at www.bfmed.org August 16, 2006.

Agostoni, C., & Haschke, F. (2003). Infant formulas: Recent developments and new issues. *Minerva Pediatrics, 55*(3), 181-194.

American Academy of Family Physicians (AAFP). (2001). *AAFP Policy Statement on Breastfeeding.* Leawood, KS: Author.

American Academy of Pediatrics (AAP). (2003). *Pediatric nutrition handbook* (5th ed.). Elk Grove Village, IL: Author.

American Academy of Pediatrics (AAP) Committee on Drugs. (2001). The transfer of drugs and other chemicals into human milk. *Pediatrics, 108*(3), 776-789.

American College of Obstetricians and Gynecologists (ACOG). (2000). Breastfeeding: Maternal and infant aspects. *ACOG Educational Bulletin No. 258.* Washington, DC: Author.

American Dietetic Association (ADA). (2003). *Promoting and supporting breastfeeding.* Accessed www.eatright.org, April 25, 2006.

Anderson, J., Held, N., & Wright, K. (2004). Raynaud's phenomenon of the nipple: A treatable cause of painful breastfeeding. *Pediatrics, 13*(4), e360-e364.

Arenz, S., Ruckerl, R., Koletzko, B., & von Kries, R. (2004). Breastfeeding and childhood obesity—a systematic review. *International Journal of Obesity and Related Metabolic Disorders, 28*(10), 1247-1256.

Association of Women's Health, Obstetric and Neonatal Nurses (AWHONN). (1999). *Clinical position statement: The role of the nurse in the promotion of breastfeeding.* Washington, DC: Author.

Bachrach, V., Schwarz, E., & Bachrach, L. (2003). Breastfeeding and the risk of hospitalization for respiratory disease in infancy. *Archives of Pediatric and Adolescent Medicine, 157*(3), 237-243.

Bener, A., Denic, S., & Galadari, S. (2001). Longer breastfeeding and protection against childhood leukemia and lymphomas. *European Journal of Cancer, 37*(2), 234-238.

BFHI USA: *Implementing the UNICEF/WHO Baby-Friendly Hospital Initiative in the United States.* (2004). Accessed www.babyfriendlyusa. org, April 25, 2006.

Bhandari, N., Bahl, R., Mazumdar, S., Martines, J., Black, R., Bhan, M., et al. (2003). Effect of community-based promotion of exclusive breastfeeding on diarrhoeal illness and growth: A cluster randomized controlled trial. Infant Feeding Study Group. *Lancet, 361*(9367), 1418-1423.

Birch, L., & Davison, K. (2001). Family environmental factors influencing the developing behavioral controls of food intake and childhood overweight. *Pediatric Clinics of North America, 48*(4), 893-907.

Borghese-Lang, T., Morrison, L., Ogle, A., & Wright, A. (2003). Successful bottle feeding of the young infant. *Journal of Pediatric Health Care, 17*(2), 94-101.

Bulkow, L., Singleton, R., Karron, R., Harrison, L., & Alaska RSV Study Group. (2002). Risk factors for severe respiratory syncytial virus infection among Alaska native children. *Pediatrics, 109*(2), 210-216.

Callen, J., & Pinelli, J. (2005). A review of the literature examining the benefits and challenges, incidence and duration, and barriers to breastfeeding in preterm infants. *Advances in Neonatal Care, 5*(2), 72-88.

Carbajal, R., Veerapen, S., Couderc, S., Jugie, M., & Ville, Y. (2003). Analgesic effect of breastfeeding in term neonates: Randomized controlled trial. *BMJ, 326*(7379), 13.

Chan-Yeung, M., Manfreda, J., Dimich-Ward, H., Ferguson, A., Watson, W., & Becker, A. (2000). A randomized controlled study of the effectiveness of a multifaceted intervention program in the primary prevention of asthma in high risk infants. *Archives of Pediatrics and Adolescent Medicine, 154*(7), 657-663.

Chapman, D., Damio, G., Young, S., & Perez-Escamilla, R. (2004). Effectiveness of breastfeeding peer counseling in a low-income, predominantly Latina population: A randomized controlled trial. *Archives of Pediatric and Adolescent Medicine, 158*(9), 897-902.

Chulada, P., Arbes, S. Jr., Dunson, D., & Zeldin, D. (2003). Breastfeeding and the prevalence of asthma and wheeze in children: Analyses from the Third National Health and Nutrition Examination Survey, 1988-1994. *Journal of Allergy and Clinical Immunology, 111*(2), 328-336.

Collaborative Group on Hormonal Factors in Breast Cancer. (2002). Breast cancer and breastfeeding: Collaborative reanalysis of individual data from 47 epidemiological studies in 30 countries, including 50302 women with breast cancer and 96,973 women without the disease. *Lancet, 360*(9328), 187-195.

Dell, S., & To, T. (2001). Breastfeeding and asthma in young children: Findings from a population-based study. *Archives of Pediatric and Adolescent Medicine, 155*(11), 1261-1265.

Dennis, C., Hodnett, E., Gallop, R., & Chalmers, B. (2002). The effect of peer support on breastfeeding duration among primiparous women: A randomized controlled trial. *Canadian Medical Association Journal, 166*(1), 21-28.

Dewey, K. (2004). Impact of breastfeeding on maternal nutritional status. *Advances in Experimental Medical Biology, 554,* 91-100.

Eglash, A., Chantry, C., & Howard, C. (2004). Protocol #8: Human milk storage information for home use for healthy term infants. *The Academy of Breastfeeding Medicine.* Accessed www.bfmed.org, April 25, 2006.

Feldman, R., & Eidelman, A. (2003). Direct and indirect effects of breast milk on the neurobehavioral and cognitive development of premature infants. *Developmental Psychobiology, 43*(2), 109-119.

Gartner, L., Morton, J., Lawrence, R., Naylor, A., O'Hare, D., Schanler, R., et al. (2005). Breastfeeding and the use of human milk. *Pediatrics, 115*(2), 496-506.

Gdalevich, M., Mimouni, D., David, M., & Mimouni, M. (2001). Breastfeeding and the onset of atopic dermatitis in childhood: A systematic review and meta-analysis of prospective studies. *Journal of the American Academy of Dermatology, 45*(4), 520-527.

Gianino, P., Mastretta, A., Longo, P., Laccisaglia, A., Sartore, M., Russo, R., et al. (2002). Incidence of nosocomial rotavirus infections, symptomatic and asymptomatic, in breastfed and non-breastfed infants. *Journal of Hospital Infection, 50*(1), 13-17.

Gillman, M., Rifas-Shiman, S., Camargo, C., Berkey, S., Frazier, L., Rockett, H., et al. (2001). Risk of overweight among adolescents who were breastfed as infants. *Journal of the American Medical Association, 285*(19), 2461-2467.

Gray, L., Miller, L., Philipp, B., & Blass, E. (2002). Breastfeeding is analgesic in healthy newborns. *Pediatrics, 109*(4), 590-593.

Griffiths, D. (2004). Do tongue ties affect breastfeeding? *Journal of Human Lactation, 20*(4), 409-414.

Grimes, J., & Wimalawansa, S. (2003). Breastfeeding and post-menopausal osteoporosis. *Current Women's Health Reports, 3*(3), 193-198.

Grummer-Strawn, L., & Mei, Z. (2004). Does breastfeeding protect against pediatric overweight? Analysis of longitudinal data from the Centers for Disease Control and Prevention Pediatric Nutrition Surveillance System [Electronic version]. *Pediatrics, 113*(2). Accessed www.pediatrics.org/cgi/content/full/113/2/e81, March 31, 2005.

Hale, T. (2004). Maternal medications during breastfeeding. *Clinical Obstetrics and Gynecology, 47*(3), 696-711.

Hale, T., & Berens, P. (2002). *Clinical therapy in breastfeeding patients.* Amarillo, TX: Pharmasoft.

Hanson, L., & Korotkova, M. (2002). The role of breastfeeding in prevention of neonatal infection. *Seminars in Perinatology, 7*(4), 275-281.

Henderson, A. (2005). Vitamin D and the breastfed infant. *Journal of Obstetric, Gynecologic, and Neonatal Nursing, 34*(3), 367-372.

Holman, D., & Grimes, M. (2003). Patterns for the initiation of breastfeeding in humans. *American Journal of Human Biology, 15*(6), 765-780.

Horwood, L., & Fergusson, D. (1998). Breastfeeding and later cognitive academic outcomes. *Pediatrics, 101*(1), e9. Accessed http://pediatrics.aappublications.org/cgi/content/101/1/e9, August 17, 2006.

Hoover, K. (2001). Yeast infections of the nipples and breasts. *Medela Messenger, 18*(3), 11-12.

Houghton, M. (2001). Breastfeeding practices of Native-American mothers participating in WIC. *Journal of the American Dietetic Association, 101*(2), 245-247.

Howard, C., Howard, F., Lanphear, B., Eberly, S., deBlieck, E., Oakes, D., et al. (2003). Randomized clinical trial of pacifier use and bottle-feeding or cupfeeding and their effect on breastfeeding. *Pediatrics, 111*(3), 511-518.

Human Milk Banking Association of North America (HMBANA). (2003). *Human milk banking: General information.* Accessed www.hmbana.org, April 25, 2006.

Institute of Medicine. (2004). *Infant formula: Evaluating the safety of new ingredients.* Washington, DC: National Academies Press.

King, D. (2000). Statistics: Weight loss and lactation. *International Journal of Childbirth Education, 15*(3), 44.

Kliegman, R. (2002). Fetal and neonatal medicine. In R. Behrman, & R. Kliegman (Eds.), *Nelson essentials of pediatrics* (4th ed.). Philadelphia: Saunders.

Kline, M., Boyle, R., Futterman, D., Havens, P., Henry-Reid, L., King, S., et al. (2003). Human milk, breastfeeding, and transmission of human immunodeficiency virus type 1 in the United States. *Pediatrics, 112*(5), 1196-1205.

Kloeblen-Tarver, A. (2001). Pacifier use is associated with shorter breastfeeding duration among low-income women. *Pediatrics, 108*(2), 526.

Kwan, M., Buffler, P., Abrams, B., & Kiley, V. (2004). Breastfeeding and the risk of childhood leukemia: A metanalysis. *Public Health Reports, 119*(6), 521-535.

Lactation Education Resources. (2004). *Breast engorgement.* Internet document Accessed August 17, 2006. www.leron-line.com/handouts/Breast_Engorgement.htm.

Larson-Meyer, D. (2002). Effect of postpartum exercise on mothers and their offspring: A review of the literature. *Obstetric Research, 10*(8), 841-853.

Lawrence, R., & Lawrence, R. (2005). *Breastfeeding: A guide for the medical profession* (6th ed.). Philadelphia: Mosby.

Lefeber, Y., & Voorhoeve, H. (1999). Indigenous first feeding practices in newborn babies. *Midwifery, 15*(2), 97-100.

Mass, S. (2004). Breast pain: Engorgement, nipple pain, and mastitis. *Clinical Obstetrics and Gynecology, 47*(3), 676-682.

Morin, K. (2004). Current thoughts on healthy term infant nutrition: The first twelve months. *MCN American Journal of Maternal/Child Nursing, 29*(5), 312-317.

Morland-Schultz, K., & Hill, P. (2005). Prevention of and therapies for nipple pain: A systematic review. *Journal of Obstetric, Gynecologic, and Neonatal Nursing, 34*(3), 428-437.

Morrow, A. (2004). Choosing an infant or pediatric formula. *Journal of Pediatric Health Care, 18*(1), 49-52.

Morrow, A., Ruiz-Palacios, G., Altaye, M., Jiang, X., Guerrero, M., Meinzen-Derr, J., et al. (2004). Human milk oligosaccharides are associated with protection against diarrhea in breast-fed infants. *Journal of Pediatrics, 145*(3), 297-303.

Morse, J., Jehle, C., & Gamble, D. (1990). Initiating breastfeeding: A world survey of the timing of postpartum breastfeeding. *International Journal of Nursing Studies, 27*(3), 303-313.

Mortensen, E., Michaelsen, K., Sanders, S., & Reinisch, J. (2002). The association between duration of breastfeeding and adult intelligence. *Journal of the American Medical Association, 287*(18), 2365-2371.

Oddy, W. (2004). A review of the effects of breastfeeding on respiratory infections, atopy, and childhood asthma. *Journal of Asthma, 41*(6), 605-621.

Oddy, W., Kendall, G., Blair, E., de Klerk, N., Stanley, F., Landau, L., et al. (2003a). Breastfeeding and cognitive development in childhood: A prospective birth cohort study. *Paediatric and Perinatal Epidemiology, 17*(1), 81-90.

Oddy, W., Sheriff, J., de Klerk, N., Kendall, G., Sly, P., Beilin, L., et al. (2004). The relation of breastfeeding and body mass index to asthma and atopy in children: A prospective cohort study to age 6 years. *American Journal of Public Health, 94*(9), 1531-1537.

Oddy, W., Sly, P., de Klerk, N., Landau, L., Kendall, G., Holt, P., et al. (2003b). Breastfeeding and respiratory morbidity in infancy: A birth cohort study. *Archives of Diseases in Childhood, 88*(3), 224-228.

Page, D. (2001). Breastfeeding is early functional jaw orthopedics (an introduction). *Functional Orthodontics, 18*(3), 24-27.

Paton, L., Alexander, J., Nowson, C., Margerison, C., Frame, M., Kaymakci, B., et al. (2003). Pregnancy and lactation have no long-term deleterious effect on measures of bone mineral in healthy women: A twin study. *American Journal of Clinical Nutrition, 77*(3), 707-714.

Pollock, C., Bustamante-Forest, R., & Giarrantano, G. (2002). Men of diverse cultures: Knowledge and attitudes about breastfeeding. *Journal of Obstetric, Gynecologic, and Neonatal Nursing, 31*(6), 673-679.

Preedy, V., Grimble, G., & Watson, R. (2001). *Nutrition in the infant.* London: Greenwich Medical Media.

Renfrew, M., Ansell, P., & Macleod, K. (2003). Formula feed preparation: Helping reduce the risks: A systematic review. *Archives of Diseases in Childhood, 88*(10), 855-858.

Riman, T., Nilsson, S., & Persson, I. (2004). Review of epidemiological evidence for reproductive and hormonal factors in relation to the risk of epithelial ovarian malignancies. *Acta Obstetricia et Gynecologica Scandinavica, 83*(9), 783-795.

Riordan, J. (2005). *Breastfeeding and human lactation* (3rd ed.). Boston: Jones & Bartlett.

Ryan, A., Wenjun, Z., & Acosta, A. (2002). Breastfeeding continues to increase into the new millennium. *Pediatrics, 110*(6), 1103-1109.

Sadauskaite-Kuehne, V., Ludvigsson, J., Padaiga, Z., Jasinskiene, E., & Samuelsson, U. (2004). Longer breastfeeding is an independent protective factor against development of type one diabetes mellitus in childhood. *Diabetes and Metabolic Research Review, 20*(2), 150-157.

Terschakovec, A., & Stallings, V. (2002). Pediatric nutrition and nutritional disorders. In R. Behrman, & R. Kliegman (Eds.), *Nelson essentials of pediatrics* (4th ed.). Philadelphia: Saunders.

Tully, M. (2005). Working and breastfeeding. *AWHONN Lifelines, 9*(3), 198-203.

Uauy, R., & Araya, M. (2004). Novel oligosaccharides in human milk: Understanding mechanisms may lead to better prevention of enteric and other infections. *Journal of Pediatrics, 145*(3), 283-285.

Ursin, G., Bernstein, L., Wang, Y., Lord, S., Deapen, D., Liff, J. et al. (2004). Reproductive factors and risk of breast carcinoma in a study of white and African-American women. *Cancer, 101*(2), 353-362.

U.S. Department of Health and Human Services. (2000). *Healthy People 2010.* (Conference edition) (Vol. 2). Washington, DC: Author. Accessed www.health.gov/healthypeople/document/default.htm, April 25, 2006.

Van Odijk, J., Kull, I., Borres, M., Brandtzaeg, P., Edberg, U., Hanson, L., et al. (2003). Breastfeeding and allergic disease: A multidisciplinary review of the literature (1966-2001) on the mode of early feeding in infancy and its impact on later atopic manifestations. *Allergy, 58*(9), 833-843.

Weimer, J. (2001). *The economic benefits of breastfeeding: A review and analysis. Food Assistance and Nutrition Research Report No. 18.* Washington, DC: Food and Rural Economics Division, Economic Research Service, U.S. Department of Agriculture.

Weissinger, D. (1998). A breastfeeding teaching tool using a sandwich analogy for latch-on. *Journal of Human Lactation, 14*(1), 51-56.

World Health Organization (WHO) Fifty-fourth Annual Assembly. (2001). *Global strategy for infant and young child feeding. The optimal duration of exclusive breastfeeding.* Geneva, Switzerland: Author.

Ziegler, E., Fomon, S., & Carlson, S. (2003). The term infant. In W. Walker, J. Watkins, & C. Duggan (Eds.), *Nutrition in pediatrics* (3rd ed.). London: BC Decker.

Shannon E. Perry

Care of the Newborn at Home

learning objectives

- Discuss nursing care management for assisting parents in the care of the infant during the first weeks at home.
- Explain continuing care of the infant who was circumcised.
- Review the anticipatory guidance nurses provide parents before discharge.

- Describe infant cardiopulmonary resuscitation (CPR).
- Discuss home phototherapy and the guidelines for teaching parents about this treatment.
- Review developmental milestones with parents to help them have realistic expectations of their infant.

electronic resources

Additional information related to the content in Chapter 28 can be found on

the companion website at *evolve*
http://evolve.elsevier.com/Lowdermilk/MWHC/
- NCLEX Review Questions
- WebLinks

or on the interactive companion CD
- NCLEX Review Questions
- Plan of Care: Home Care Follow-Up: Transition to Parenthood
- Skill: Changing a Diaper
- Skill: Infant Bathing

MOTHERS and infants are ordinarily discharged from the place of birth (hospital, birthing center) between 6 and 48 hours after birth. The time of discharge depends on the condition of the mother and infant, whether breastfeeding is established, preferences of the parents, and insurance coverage.

Before discharge, the nurse provides anticipatory guidance related to feeding, elimination, care of the circumcised infant, crying, behavior, sleeping, signs of illness, and community resources, including support groups. Many hospitals have 24-hour in-house television channels where infant care topics can be viewed. When the opportunity presents, a bath demonstration may be provided. A sample Infant Teaching/Discharge Record is in Fig. 23-4. Note that the parents can check the information that is most important to them, enabling the nurse to focus her teaching. This chapter addresses the care of the infant in the first 6 weeks after birth.

THE TRIP HOME

The optimal time for the baby to travel is after a feeding. A satisfied infant will usually sleep during the ride and the couple will have adequate time to get home and relatively settled before the next feeding. If the trip is lengthy, providing bottles of formula for the formula-fed infant will reduce anxiety during the trip and prevent the rushed preparation of formula. The breastfeeding mother will be able to nurse the infant immediately.

The infant must be secured in a car seat for the trip home (see later discussion of car seat safety). Although the nurse is not responsible for securing the infant in the car seat, she should query the parents about whether the car seat is present and properly installed. If parents do not have a car seat, the nurse should be able to provide information about resources in the hospital or community where they may borrow or be given a car seat.

It is usually best if siblings remain at home when the mother and baby are discharged so that the parents can concentrate on the mother and the care and safety of the newborn during the trip home. When the mother arrives home, the father can carry the baby into the house while the mother greets the siblings. Siblings need some undivided attention on this first day as well as every day. This often provides the father an opportunity to spend time with the children that he otherwise might not have.

■ PROTECTIVE ENVIRONMENT

The provision of a protective environment is basic to the care of the infant. The bassinet or crib should be placed on an inner wall to prevent cold stress by radiation. For the first few weeks at home, the bassinet is commonly placed in the parents' bedroom so that they can easily hear the infant. Proximity of the infant also facilitates breastfeeding. As the parents become more secure, the bassinet may be moved to the infant's own room or to one shared with a sibling.

All visitors should wash their hands before touching the infant. Persons with infectious conditions including upper respiratory infections, gastrointestinal (GI) tract infections, and infectious skin conditions should be excluded from contact with the newborn. Some health care providers recommend that infants not be taken out in crowds, particularly when there is an increased risk for being exposed to communicable diseases such as the flu or colds.

■ KNOWLEDGE OF AND SKILL ■ IN CHILD CARE ACTIVITIES

Parents must learn skills such as feeding, holding, clothing, and bathing the infant and protecting the baby from harm. The ability to perform these task-oriented activities competently and confidently does not appear automatically with the birth of a child. Many parents must learn to do these tasks, and this learning process can be difficult. However, almost all parents become adept in caregiving activities when they have the desire to learn and the support of others.

Nurses can help inexperienced parents feel confident and competent in their new roles. They can provide opportunities for parents to practice child care tasks in the hospital, birth setting, or in the home, where assistance and feedback are available. Nursing approaches and strategies can enhance parents' self-concept by helping them feel more comfortable and confident in their parenting skills.

CARE MANAGEMENT: PRACTICAL ■ SUGGESTIONS FOR THE ■ FIRST WEEKS AT HOME

Numerous changes occur during the first weeks of parenthood. Care management should be directed toward helping parents cope with infant care, role changes, altered lifestyle, and changes in family structure resulting from the addition of a new baby. Parents may have inadequate or incorrect understanding of what to expect in the early postpartum weeks. Developing skill and confidence in caring for an infant can be especially anxiety provoking.

Nurses, especially those making postpartum visits to parents' homes, are in a prime position to help new families. The nurse's role becomes primarily one of teacher-supporter, focusing on enabling new parents to become capable of self-care and infant care and of meeting the needs of the family unit.

■ Assessment and Nursing Diagnoses

Assessment should include a psychosocial assessment focusing on parent-infant attachment, adjustment to the parental role, sibling adjustment, social support, and education needs, as well as mother's and baby's physical adaptation (see Chapter 24). Early home visits are an excellent opportunity for the nurse to assess beginnings of successful or harmful parenting behaviors (see Table 24-2). Parents who demonstrate loving and nurturing behaviors with their infant need to be given positive reinforcement. Parents who interact in inappropriate or abusive ways with their infant should be monitored more closely, instructed in positive ways to interact, and an appropriate mental health practitioner or professional social worker should be notified.

Home visits often offer an opportunity to involve all family members. The mother, father, siblings, and even grandparents may ask questions and express concerns. The nurse can share her assessments and observations, role model appropriate care, and develop a plan of care collaboratively with the family. Nursing diagnoses pertinent to the period of transition to parenthood include the following:

- *Readiness for enhanced family coping related to*
  –Positive attitude and realistic expectations for the newborn and adapting to parenthood
  –Verbalizing positive factors in lifestyle change
- *Risk for impaired parenting related to*
  –Lack of knowledge of infant care
  –Feelings of incompetence or lack of confidence
  –Unrealistic expectations of infant
  –Fatigue from interrupted sleep
- *Parental role conflict related to*
  –Role transition and role attainment
  –Unwanted pregnancy
  –Lack of resources to support parenting (e.g., no paid leave)
- *Risk for impaired parent-infant attachment related to*
  –Postpartum complications
  –Neonatal complications/anomalies

■ Expected Outcomes of Care

A plan of care is formulated in collaboration with the family, incorporating their priorities and preferences, to meet their specific needs. Expected outcomes for effective transition to parenthood include that the parents will do the following:

- Interact with the infant in a loving and nurturing way.
- Incorporate the infant into the family.
- Promote acceptance of the infant by siblings.
- Demonstrate behaviors that reflect appreciation of sensory and behavioral capacities of the infant.
- Respond appropriately to infant cues.
- Verbalize increasing confidence and competence in feeding, diapering, dressing, and sensory stimulation of the infant.

- Identify deviations from normal in the infant that should be brought to the immediate attention of the primary health care provider.
- Describe or demonstrate emergency procedures and verbalize ways of getting emergency help.

■ Plan of Care and Interventions
■ *Instructions for the First Days at Home*

Parents, especially first-time parents, must be helped to anticipate what the transition from hospital to home will be like. Anticipatory guidance can help prevent a shock of reality that might negate the parents' joy or cause them undue stress. Even the simplest strategies can provide enormous support (see Teaching for Self-Care box).

- Classes in the prenatal period or during the postpartum stay are helpful.
- Written information reinforcing education topics is helpful to provide to parents, as is a list of available community resources, both local and national.

TEACHING FOR SELF-CARE

Newborn Home Care: Expected Findings After Early Discharge*

- Interactions with infant are loving and caring.
- Breastfeeding: successful latch-on and feeding 8 to 12 times per 24 hours
- Formula-feeding: taking approximately 2 to 3 ounces every 3 to 4 hours
- Wet diapers: at least 6 to 8 per day after 4 days of age
- Stools: at least one every 48 hours (bottle feeding) or at least three per day (breastfeeding) after 4 days
- Circumcision: wash with warm water only; petroleum jelly to glans if Yellen or Gomco clamp technique; yellow exudate forming, no bleeding, no signs of infection; PlastiBell intact for at least 48 hours
- Color: pink to ruddy when crying; pink centrally when at rest or asleep
- Activity: has four or five wakeful periods per day and alerts to environmental sounds and voices
- Jaundice: physiologic jaundice (appearing after 24 to 36 hours of age), feeding, voiding, and stooling as noted above, or practitioner notification for suspicion of pathologic jaundice (appears within 24 hours of birth, ABO/Rh problem suspected; hemolysis); decreased activity; poor feeding; dark orange skin color persisting beyond fifth day in light-skinned newborn
- Cord: kept above diaper line; drying; periumbilical area skin pink (erythematous circle at umbilical site may be sign of omphalitis); no drainage or odor
- Vital signs: heart rate 110 to 140 beats/min at rest; respiratory rate 30 to 60 breaths/min at rest without evidence of retractions, grunting, or nasal flaring; temperature 36.5° to 37.2° C axillary
- Position of sleep: back

Adapted from Hockenberry, M. (2003). *Wong's nursing care of infants and children.* (7th ed.). St. Louis: Mosby.
*Any deviation from the above or suspicion of poor newborn adaptation should be reported to the practitioner at once.

- An excellent resource for the nurse is the *Compendium of Postpartum Care,* developed by Johnson & Johnson Products, Inc., (2006) in association with the Association of Women's Health, Obstetric, and Neonatal Nurses (AWHONN). Postpartum nurses will find the "Patient Handouts" section especially useful. It includes handouts on topics such as rest and exercise, emotional well-being during adaptation to parenthood, understanding the blues, and what to expect and do regarding the infant's health.

Instructions for the first days at home should minimally include activities of daily living, dealing with visitors, and activity and rest.

Activities of Daily Living. Given the demands of a newborn, the mother's discomfort or fatigue associated with giving birth, and a busy homecoming day, even small details of daily life can become stressful. Such things as using disposable diapers or having a diaper service for the first week or so, preparing frozen and/or microwavable dinners, or getting takeout meals can decrease stress by eliminating at least one or two parental responsibilities during the first few days at home.

Visitors. New parents are often inadequately prepared for the reality of bringing a new infant home because they romanticize the homecoming. One mother stated,

> By the time we drove an hour through traffic, my stitches were hurting, and all I wanted was a warm sitz bath and some private time with Bill and the baby, in that order. Instead, a carload of visitors pulled into the driveway as we were unbuckling the baby from his car seat. I thought I would surely cry.

The nurse can help parents explore ways, in advance, to assert their need to limit visitors. When family and friends ask what they can do to help, new parents can suggest they prepare and bring them a meal or pick up items at the store. Parents can work out a signal for alerting the partner that the mother is becoming tired or uncomfortable and needs the partner to invite the visitors to another room or to leave. Some mothers find that wearing a robe and not appearing ready for company leads visitors to stay a shorter time. A sign on the front door saying, "Mother and baby resting.... Please do not disturb" may be useful.

Activity and Rest. Because mothers have reported fatigue as a major problem during the first few weeks after giving birth, mothers should be encouraged to limit their activities and be realistic about their level of fatigue. Activities should not be sustained for long periods. Family, friends, and neighbors can be solicited for support and help with meals, housecleaning, picking up other children, and so forth. Rest periods throughout the day are important. Mothers can nap when their baby sleeps. Adequate nutrition also is important for postpartum recovery and for dealing with fatigue. Because many women are anemic or have a low normal hemoglobin and hematocrit, providing a list of foods high in iron may be useful. Increasing fiber and fluid intake helps reestablish bowel function.

▬ *Physical Care and Safety*

Providing practical suggestions for infant care can help parents adjust to parenthood. Mothers and fathers want to feel capable and confident in the physical care of their infant (Fig. 28-1). The nurse should assess each parent's need for instruction on care, such as care of the circumcised infant, bathing, clothing, and safety.

Umbilical Cord Care. The cord should be kept clean and dry by folding the diaper below the cord to allow drying. The cord clamp is removed when the cord is dry, usually about 24 hours after birth before the infant is discharged. The recommendation of AWHONN (2001) for cord care is to cleanse the cord with water. The stump and base of the cord should be assessed for edema, redness, and purulent drainage with each diaper change. The cord usually falls off in 10 to 14 days. Cord separation time is influenced by a number of factors, including type of cord care, type of birth, and other perinatal events.

Care of the Circumcised Infant Male. The infant is often circumcised the day of discharge. The infant is observed to assure that excessive bleeding does not occur and that the infant voids at least once before discharge (see Teaching for Self-Care box). Petroleum jelly is applied to the penis with each diaper change for at least the first 24 hours after circumcision to prevent the diaper from adhering to the penis. If the PlastiBell technique was used, no petrolatum is necessary. The penis is kept clean with gentle cleansing with warm water. The diaper is applied loosely. A yellow exudate covers the glans within 24 hours. This is normal and will persist for 2 to 3 days. No attempt should be made to remove it.

Circumcision is painful; the infant may be fussy and should be comforted. A prescription for oral acetaminophen may be written and the medication given as needed if the infant is not consoled by other means.

Infant Bathing. Bathing serves a number of purposes. It provides opportunities for (1) completely cleansing the infant, (2) observing the infant's condition, (3) promoting comfort, and (4) parent-child-family interaction. Some fathers consider this their own special time with their babies. While bathing their baby, parents can talk to and caress and cuddle the infant, and engage in arousal and imitation of facial expressions and smiling.

Sponge baths are usually used until the infant's umbilical cord falls off and the umbilicus is healed (see Teaching for Self-Care box). Bathing the newborn by immersion has been found to allow less heat loss and stimulate less crying; however, tub bathing is usually delayed until the umbilical cord falls off, which occurs at about 10 to 14 days after birth (Box 28-1). A daily bath is not necessary for achieving cleanliness and may do harm by disrupting the integrity of the newborn's skin and the acid mantle. Cleansing the perineum after a soiled diaper and daily cleansing of the face and creases may suffice. Parents can pick a time for the bath that is easy for them and when the baby is awake, usually before a feeding. Other suggestions include:

(Side margin, rotated text) CD: Skill: Infant Bathing

FIG. 28-1 Father participates in care of his newborn son. (Courtesy Wendy and Marwood Larson-Harris, Roanoke, VA.)

TEACHING FOR SELF-CARE

Care of the Circumcised Newborn at Home

- Wash hands before touching the newly circumcised penis.

CHECK FOR BLEEDING
- Check circumcision for bleeding with each diaper change.
- If bleeding occurs, apply gentle pressure with a folded sterile gauze square. If bleeding does not stop with pressure, notify primary health care provider.

OBSERVE FOR URINATION
- Check to see that the infant urinates after being circumcised.
- Infant should have a wet diaper 6 to 8 times per 24 hours.

KEEP AREA CLEAN
- Change diaper and inspect circumcision at least every 4 hours.
- Wash penis gently with warm water to remove urine and feces. Apply petrolatum to the glans with each diaper change (omit petrolatum if PlastiBell was used).
- Use soap only after circumcision is healed (5 to 6 days).
- Fanfold diaper to prevent pressure on the circumcised area.

CHECK FOR INFECTION
- Glans penis is dark red after circumcision, then becomes covered with yellow exudates in 24 hours. This is normal and will persist for 2 to 3 days. Do not attempt to remove it.
- Redness, swelling, or discharge indicates infection. Notify primary health care provider if you think the circumcision area is infected.

PROVIDE COMFORT
- Circumcision is painful. Handle the area gently.
- Provide extra holding, feeding, and opportunities for nonnutritive sucking for a day or two.

EVIDENCE-BASED PRACTICE

Cord Care

BACKGROUND

- After being the lifeline for the growing fetus, the umbilical cord is cut after birth. A layer of polymorphonuclear leukocytes lines the separation site for the stump, which dries up and falls off in 5 to 15 days after birth. Most of the newborn skin is colonized by nonpathogenic bacteria from the mother, especially when mother and baby room-in. However, the open wound of the umbilicus can colonize streptococci and coliform bacteria, such as *Escherichia Coli*. Under-resourced countries may use unclean implements to cut the cords and various household or farm substances to dry the cord. A common result is neonatal tetanus. Other infections can manifest as local inflammation and odor, and subtle systemic signs of infant septicemia. To prevent infection in modern settings, caregivers use clean cutting technique, and cord care with antiseptics (alcohol, silver sulfadiazine, iodine, chlorhexadine, gentian violet, triple dye) or antibiotics (bacitracin, nitrofurazone, tetracycline) or drying powders.

OBJECTIVES

- The reviewers sought to determine good umbilical cord care practice in both high and low resource settings for the prevention of neonatal infection and death. Outcomes included clinical infections, bacterial colonization, and time to cord separation.

METHODS

Search Strategy

- After searching the Cochrane Pregnancy and Childbirth Group trials register, reference lists, and conference proceedings, the authors identified 21 randomized controlled trials on the subject, published 1977 to 2003. The trials represented 8959 infants from Canada, Israel, Italy, Norway, Spain, Taiwan, Thailand, the United Kingdom, and the United States. Two studies were comprised of preterm infants.

Statistical Analyses

- Similar data were pooled. Reviewers calculated relative risk for dichotomous (categoric) data, such as type of birth, and weighted mean difference for continuous data, such as pain scale. Differences between groups outside the 95% confidence interval were accepted as significant.

FINDINGS

- Antiseptic versus dry cord care: Bacterial colonization, including *Staphylococcus* and *E. coli*, was significantly reduced with the use of alcohol, silver sulfadiazine, and triple dye. However, there were no differences in clinical cord infection symptoms: redness, swelling, or odor. Triple dye was the superior antiseptic.
- Antibiotics versus antiseptics: There were no clinical infections and no differences in colonization in trials comparing triple dye, silver sulfadiazine, or povidone-iodine to neomycin or bacitracin.
- Studies of time to cord separation showed the shortest times with powders and no treatment and the longest times with use of triple dye and silver sulfadiazine.
- Preterm infants were more at risk for nosocomial infections, and had a longer time to cord separation.

LIMITATIONS

- Most of these trials were from high-resource areas, which have lower risk for neonatal tetanus. Wealthier countries are shifting to rooming-in care, which reduces infections. Follow-up in these trials ended at cord separation, and subsequent infections were not addressed. Time to cord separation is of unknown clinical value. Skin colonization does not always lead to clinical infection.

IMPLICATIONS FOR PRACTICE

- In developed countries, umbilical cord infections are rare. The authors recommended clean technique at birth, followed by keeping the cord clean and dry. There was insufficient evidence to recommend antiseptics or antibiotics for cord care, except with infants with higher risk for nosocomial infections, such as those born preterm. Antiseptics are cheaper. Rooming-in of mothers and breastfeeding infants continues to be the gold standard for preventing infections.

IMPLICATIONS FOR FURTHER RESEARCH

- More research could illuminate the clinical variations in cord separation. Measures of longer-term outcomes, including maternal satisfaction, are needed, including absorption of topical treatments and subsequent immune status and infections. Much more research is needed in low-resource countries for cord interventions that are affordable and accessible, such as application of colostrum.

Reference: Zupan, J., Garner, P., & Omari, A. (2004). Topical umbilical cord care at birth. *The Cochrane Database of Systematic Reviews*, 2006, Issue 3. Chichester, UK: John Wiley & Sons.

- Alkaline soaps (such as Ivory), oils, powders, and many lotions should not be used since they alter the acid mantle and provide a medium for bacterial growth.
- Use of commercial diaper wipes should be discouraged because they can alter the acid mantle (AWHONN, 2001).
- Powders are not recommended, because the infant can inhale powder and experience respiratory distress. If parents use powder, it should be shaken onto the parent's hand and smoothed onto the skin of the infant.

Diaper Rash. To maintain optimal skin condition in the diaper region, diapers should be changed frequently. Disposable diapers made with absorbent gel materials may be advantageous for promoting skin integrity. Washing and drying the wet and soiled area and changing the diaper immediately after voiding or stooling will prevent and help treat diaper rash. Parents can be taught to expose the buttocks to air to help dry up diaper rash. Because bacteria thrive in moist dark areas, exposing the skin to dry air decreases bacterial proliferation. Plastic pants should be

Skill: Changing a Diaper

left off until the diaper area heals. A skin barrier ointment such as zinc oxide may be effective in preventing further excoriation, especially in the presence of loose stools or systemic gastrointestinal candidiasis; the latter will require treatment with a systemic antifungal drug.

The warm, moist atmosphere in the diaper area provides an optimal environment for *Candida albicans* growth; dermatitis appears in the perianal area, inguinal folds, and lower abdomen. The affected area is intensely erythematous with a sharply demarcated, scalloped edge, often with

---

box 28-1 Tub Bathing

- See guidelines for sponge bathing (Teaching for Self-Care box).
- Place liner on bottom of tub to prevent infant from slipping.
- Add up to 5 inches of comfortably warm water (36.6° C to 37.2° C—pleasantly warm to your inner wrist) or water deep enough to cover the shoulders to prevent heat loss from evaporation.
- Undress baby. Lower infant slowly into water.
- Hold baby safely with fingers under the baby's armpit, with your thumb around the shoulder. Use the other hand to support the baby's bottom and legs.
- Wash face and shampoo hair as for sponge bath.

- Wash the front of the baby.
- Go from front to back between the legs. Rinse with a wet washcloth.
- Wash the baby's back with your free hand lathered with soap.
- Rinse well with the wet washcloth.
- Remove infant from the water, and gently pat dry. Wrap in a warm blanket and leave wrapped for up to 10 minutes before dressing. Dressing immediately if the baby is still damp will get clothes wet and cause heat loss. After dressing, wrap in a warm blanket.

TEACHING FOR SELF-CARE

Sponge Bathing

FITTING BATHS INTO FAMILY'S SCHEDULE

- Give a bath at any time convenient to you but not immediately after a feeding period because the increased handling may cause regurgitation.

PREVENTING HEAT LOSS

- The temperature of the room should be 24° C (75° F), and the bathing area should be free of drafts.
- Control heat loss during the bath to conserve the infant's energy. Bathing the infant quickly, exposing only a portion of the body at a time, and thorough drying are all parts of the bathing technique.

GATHERING SUPPLIES AND CLOTHING BEFORE STARTING

- Clothing suitable for wearing indoors: diaper, shirt; stretch suit or nightgown optional
- Unscented, mild soap
- Pins, if needed for diaper, closed and placed well out of baby's reach
- Cotton balls
- Towels for drying infant and a clean washcloth
- Receiving blanket
- Tub for water

BATHING THE BABY

- Bring infant to bathing area when all supplies are ready.
- *Never leave the infant alone* on bath table or in bath water, not even for a second! If you have to leave, take the infant with you or put back into crib.
- Test temperature of the water. It should feel pleasantly warm to the inner wrist 36.6° to 37.2° C (98° to 99° F).
- Do not hold infant under running water—water temperature may change, and infant may be scalded or chilled rapidly.
- Undress the baby and wrap in a towel with the head exposed. Uncover the parts of the body you are washing, taking care to keep the rest of the baby covered as much as possible to prevent heat loss.

Wash hair with baby wrapped to limit heat loss. (Courtesy Marjorie Pyle, RNC, Lifecircle, Costa Mesa, CA.)

- Begin by washing the face with water; do not use soap on the face. Cleanse the eyes from the inner canthus outward, using separate parts of a clean washcloth for each eye. For the first 2 to 3 days, a discharge may result from the reaction of the conjunctiva to the substance (erythromycin) used as a prophylactic measure against infection. Any discharge should be considered abnormal and reported to the health care provider.
- If the hair is to be washed, begin by wrapping the infant in a towel with the head exposed. Hold the infant in a football position with one hand, using the other hand to wash the hair (see figure). Wash the scalp with water and mild soap and a soft brush; rinse well and dry thoroughly. Scalp desquamation, called *cradle cap,* often can be prevented by removing any scales with a fine-toothed comb or brush after washing. If condition persists, the health care provider may prescribe an ointment to massage into the scalp. A blow dryer is never used on an infant because the temperature is too hot for a baby's skin.

numerous satellite lesions that extend beyond the larger lesion. The usual source of infection is from handling by persons who do not practice adequate handwashing. It may also appear 2 to 3 days after an oral infection (thrush).

Therapy consists of applications of an anticandidal ointment, such as clotrimazole or miconazole, with each diaper change. Sometimes the infant also is given an oral antifungal preparation such as nystatin or fluconazole to eliminate any gastrointestinal source of infection.

Other Rashes. A rash on the cheeks may result from the infant's scratching with long unclipped fingernails or from rubbing the face against the crib sheets, particularly if regurgitated stomach contents are not washed off promptly. The newborn's skin begins a natural process of peeling and sloughing after birth. Dry skin may be treated with a neutral pH lotion, with approval of the health care provider, but this should be used sparingly. Newborn rash, erythema toxicum, and newborn "acne" are common findings (see Chapter 25) and should resolve with no treatment.

Nail Care. Fingernails and toenails should not be cut immediately after birth, but should be allowed to grow out far enough to avoid cutting the attached skin. If needed, the infant's hands can be covered with loose-fitting mittens to prevent scratching the face. However, this should be avoided if possible, because mittens inhibit the infant from sucking on fingers for self-consolation (see Teaching for Self Care box on sponge bathing).

Infant Clothing. Parents commonly ask how warmly they should dress their infant. A simple rule of thumb is to dress the child as the parents dress themselves, adding or subtracting clothes and wraps for the infant as necessary. A cotton shirt and diaper may be sufficient clothing for the young infant. A cap or bonnet is needed to protect the scalp and to minimize heat loss if it is cool or to protect against

TEACHING FOR SELF-CARE

Sponge Bathing—cont'd

BATHING THE BABY—cont'd

- Creases under the chin and arms and in the groin may need daily cleansing. The crease under the chin may be exposed by elevating the infant's shoulders 5 cm and letting the head drop back.
- Cleanse ears and nose with twists of moistened cotton or a corner of the washcloth. Do not use cotton-tipped swabs because they may cause injury.
- Undress baby and wash body and arms and legs. Pat dry gently. Baby may be tub bathed after the cord drops off and umbilicus and circumcised penis are completely healed.

CARE OF THE CORD

- Cleanse around base of the cord where it joins the skin with water. If the use of alcohol on the cord is suggested, use cotton-tipped swabs dipped in alcohol to cleanse the cord at the base where the cord meets the skin; this should be done with each diaper change. Notify the health care provider of any odor, discharge, or skin inflammation around the cord. The clamp is removed when the cord is dry (approximately 24 hr). The diaper should not cover the cord because a wet or soiled diaper will slow or prevent drying of the cord and foster infection. When the cord drops off, usually in 10 to 14 days, small drops of blood may be seen when the baby cries. This will heal by itself. It is not dangerous.

CARE OF HANDS AND FEET

- Wash and dry between the fingers and toes when bathing the infant.
- When the nails have grown, the fingernails and toenails can be cut more easily with manicure scissors (preferably scissors with rounded tips) or clippers; nails should be cut straight across. The ideal time to do this is when the infant is asleep. Soft emery boards may be used to file the nails. Nails should be kept short.

CLEANSING GENITALS

- Cleanse the genitals of infants daily and after voiding or defecating. For girls, the genitals may be cleansed by separating the labia and gently washing from the pubic area to the anus.

For uncircumcised boys, gently pull back on the foreskin. Stop when resistance is felt. Wash and rinse the tip (glans) with soap and warm water, and replace the foreskin. The foreskin must be returned to its original position to prevent constriction and swelling. Once healed, the circumcised penis does not require any special care other than cleansing with diaper changes. In most newborns, the inner layer of the foreskin adheres to the glans and the foreskin cannot be retracted. By 3 years of age in 90% of boys, the foreskin can be retracted easily without causing pain or trauma. For others, the foreskin is not retractable until adolescence. As soon as the foreskin is partly retractable and the child is old enough, he can be taught self-care.

SKIN CARE

- The skin of a newborn is sensitive and should be cleaned only with water between baths. Soap is drying and its use is limited to bathing. Routine use of creams, lotions, ointments, or powders are not recommended. If the skin seems excessively dry during the first 2 to 3 weeks after birth, an unscented, non–alcohol-based lotion may be used; it is best to check with the health care provider for suggestions on skin care products.
- The fragile skin can be injured by too vigorous cleansing. If stool or other debris has dried and caked on the skin, soak the area to remove it. Do not attempt to rub it off, because abrasion may result. Gentleness, patting dry rather than rubbing, and use of a mild soap without perfumes or coloring are recommended. Chemicals in the coloring and perfume can cause rashes on sensitive skin.
- Babies are very prone to sunburn and should be kept out of direct sunlight. Use of sunscreens should be discussed with the health care provider.
- Babies often develop rashes that are normal. Neonatal acne resembles pimples and may appear at 2 to 4 weeks of age, resolving without treatment by 6 to 8 months. Heat rash is common in warm weather; this appears as a fine red rash around creases or folds where the baby sweats.

sunburn and to shade the eyes if it is sunny and hot. Wrapping the infant snugly in a blanket maintains body temperature and promotes a feeling of security. Overdressing in warm temperatures can cause discomfort, as can underdressing in cold weather. Parents are encouraged to dress the infant at all times in flame-retardant clothing. Infant sunglasses are available to protect the infant's eyes when outdoors.

Infants have sensitive skin; therefore new clothes should be washed before putting them on the infant. Baby clothes should be washed separately with a mild detergent and hot water. A double rinse usually removes traces of the potentially irritating cleansing agent or acid residue from urine or stool. If possible, the clothing and bed linens are dried in the sun to neutralize residue.

Bedding requires frequent changing. The top of a plastic-coated mattress should be washed frequently, and the crib or bassinet should be dusted with a damp cloth. The infant's toilet articles may be kept convenient for use in a box, basket, or plastic carrier.

Infant Safety. Providing for the safety of an infant is not a matter of just using common sense. New parents may not be aware of many potential dangers to their infant (e.g., window blind cords near the crib or a parent throwing an infant in the air during play). Nurses should provide parents with concrete instructions on infant safety (Box 28-2).

Sleeping. In 2005, the American Academy of Pediatrics (AAP) released revised recommendations regarding sudden infant death syndrome (SIDS) prevention in which the back sleep position is recommended during every sleep period. Side-sleeping is no longer recognized as an acceptable alternative to the fully supine position (AAP Task Force on Sudden Infant Death Syndrome, 2005).

Positional plagiocephaly, flattening of the head, has increased since the back sleep position has been used. Turning the infant's head from side to side during sleep and encouraging "tummy time" while awake may be useful to prevent the flattening.

Infants should sleep on a firm surface: specifically, on a firm crib mattress covered by a sheet. Soft materials such as comforters, quilts, pillows, or sheepskins should not be placed under the sleeping infant. These same objects should be kept out of the infant's sleeping environment. Loose bedding such as sheets and blankets may be dangerous and if used, should be tucked securely around the crib mattress to prevent the infant's face from being covered by the bedding. Sleep clothing such as infant sleep sacks are useful to keep the infant covered without the danger of covering the head (AAP, 2005).

It is important to avoid overheating the infant during sleep. Overbundling is to be avoided; the baby should not feel hot to the touch. (AAP, 2005).

Bed sharing is not recommended during infant sleep. Infants may be brought into the parent's bed for comforting or for breastfeeding, but should be returned to the crib or bassinet before the parent goes to sleep. Room sharing (infant sleeping in the parent's room) is associated with a decreased risk of SIDS (AAP, 2005).

Use of Car Seat. Infants should travel only in federally approved, rear-facing safety seats that meet Federal Motor Vehicle Safety Standard (FMVSS) 213 and that are secured in the rear seat (www.nhtsa.dot.gov) (Fig. 28-2). Parents should bring the car seat to the hospital before discharge for training on positioning and securing the infant as well as proper installation of the car seat. Many hospitals have staff who are specially trained and certified in car seat safety; parents can also check with local fire, police, or highway patrol agencies for assistance with proper installation of car seats (AAP Committee on Injury and Poison Prevention, 2002).

---

box 28-2 **Tips for Keeping Your Baby Safe**

- Never leave your baby alone on a bed, couch, or table. Even newborns can move enough to reach the edge eventually and fall off.
- Never put your baby on a cushion, pillow, beanbag, or waterbed to sleep. Your baby may suffocate. Do not keep pillows, large floppy toys, or loose plastic sheeting in the crib.
- Do not place your infant on his or her stomach to sleep. The back-lying position is recommended.
- When using an infant carrier, stay within arm's reach when the carrier is on a high place, such as a table, sofa, or store counter. If at all possible, place the carrier on the floor near you.
- Infant carriers do not keep your baby safe in a car. Always place your baby in an approved car safety seat in the back seat (see Fig. 28-2) when traveling in a motor vehicle (car, truck, bus, or van). Car safety seats are recommended for travel on trains and airplanes as well.
- When bathing your baby, never leave him or her alone. Newborns and infants can drown in 1 to 2 inches of water.
- Be sure that your hot water heater is set at 49° C or less. Always check bath water temperature with your elbow before putting your baby in the bath.

- Do not tie anything around your baby's neck. Pacifiers tied around the neck with a ribbon or string may strangle your baby.
- Check your baby's crib for safety. Slats should be no more than 2.5 inches apart. The space between the mattress and sides should be less than 2 finger widths. There should be no decorative knobs on the bedposts.
- Keep crib or playpen away from window blind and drapery cords; your baby could strangle on them.
- Keep crib and playpen well away from radiators, heat vents, and portable heaters. Linens in crib or playpen could catch fire if in contact with these heat sources.
- Install smoke detectors on every floor of your home. Check them once a month to be sure they work. Change batteries at least once a year.
- Avoid exposing your baby to cigarette or cigar smoke in your home or other places. Passive exposure to tobacco smoke greatly increases the likelihood that your infant will have respiratory symptoms and illnesses.
- Be gentle with your baby. Do not pick your baby up or swing your baby by the arms or throw him or her up in the air.

FIG. 28-2 Rear-facing infant seat in rear seat of car. (Courtesy Brian and Mayannyn Sallee, Las Vegas, NV.)

The safest area of the car is in the back seat. A car seat that faces the rear gives the best protection for the disproportionately weak neck and heavy head of an infant. In this position, the force of a frontal crash is spread over the head, neck, and back; the back of the car seat supports the spine.

▬ NURSE ALERT

Infants should use a rear-facing car seat from birth to 20 pounds *and* to 1 year of age. If the infant reaches the weight limit before the first birthday, the rear-facing position should still be used. In cars equipped with air bags, rear-facing infant seats must not be placed in the front seat. Serious injury can occur if the air bag inflates because these types of infant seats fit close to the dashboard (AAP, 2002).

The car seat is secured by using the vehicle seat belts; the infant is secured using the harness system in the car seat. If the infant must ride in the front seat, the air bag must be turned off to prevent injury from the air bag (AAP, 2002).

To secure the infant in the rear-facing car safety seat, shoulder harnesses are placed in the slots at or below the level of the infant's shoulders. The harness is snug, and the retainer clip is placed at the level of the infant's armpits as opposed to on the abdomen or neck area (AAP, 2002).

Infants are positioned at a 45 degree angle in a car seat to prevent slumping and subsequent airway obstruction. Many seats allow for adjustment of the seat angle. For seats that are not adjustable, a tightly rolled newspaper, a solid-core Styrofoam roll, or a firm roll of fabric can be placed under the car safety seat to place the infant at a 45 degree angle (AAP, 2002).

Infants born at less than 37 weeks of gestation and with birth weight less than 2500 g should be observed in a car seat for a period of time (equal to the length of the car ride home) before discharge. The infant is monitored for apnea, bradycardia, and a decrease in oxygen saturation. It may be necessary to place blanket rolls on either side of the infant for support of the head and trunk. To prevent slumping,

the back-to-crotch strap distance should be 14 cm (AAP, 2002).

If the parents do not have a car safety seat, arrangements should be made to make an appropriate seat available for purchase, loan, or donation. Parents need to be cautioned about purchasing second-hand car safety seats, due to the possibility that the seat may be been involved in an auto accident and may no longer be considered reliable.

Cardiopulmonary Resuscitation. Parents should receive instruction in relieving airway obstruction (see Emergency box) and CPR (see Emergency box). Often classes are offered in hospitals and clinics during the prenatal period or to parents of newborns. Such instruction is especially important for parents whose infants were preterm or had cardiac or respiratory problems. Babysitters also should learn CPR.

▬ *Nonnutritive Sucking*

Sucking is the infant's chief pleasure. However, sucking may not be satisfied by breastfeeding or bottle feeding alone. Sucking is such a strong need that infants who are deprived of sucking, such as those with a cleft lip, will suck on their tongues. Some newborns are born with sucking pads on their fingers that developed during in utero sucking. Several benefits of nonnutritive sucking have been demonstrated, such as an increased weight gain in preterm infants, increased ability to maintain an organized state, and decreased crying.

Problems arise when parents are concerned about the sucking of fingers, thumb, or pacifier and try to restrain this natural tendency. Before giving advice, nurses should investigate the parents' feelings and base the guidance they give on the information elicited. For example, some parents may see no problem with the use of a finger but may find the use of a pacifier objectionable. In general, there is no need to restrain either practice, unless thumb sucking persists past 4 years of age or past the time when the permanent teeth erupt. Parents are advised to consult with their pediatrician or pediatric nurse practitioner about this topic.

A parent's excessive use of the pacifier to calm the child should be explored. It is not unusual for parents to place a pacifier in their infant's mouth as soon as the infant begins to cry, thus reinforcing a pattern of distress-relief.

The AAP (2005) has recognized an association between pacifier use and reduced risk of SIDS. Therefore, they suggest pacifier use during the first year of life with specific guidelines: The infant is given the pacifier when placed down for sleep, but it is not to be reinserted once the baby is asleep; pacifiers are not to be coated with sweet solutions; regular cleaning and replacement of pacifiers is needed; and pacifier use in breastfeeding infants should be delayed until 1 month of age to allow for establishment of breastfeeding.

If parents choose to let their infant use a pacifier, they must be aware of certain safety considerations before purchasing one. A homemade or poorly designed pacifier

Relieving Airway Obstruction in an Infant

Back blow and chest thrusts are used to clear an airway obstructed by a foreign body.

BACK BLOWS

- Position the infant prone over forearm with the head down and the infant's jaw firmly supported.
- Rest the supporting arm on the thigh.
- Deliver five back blows forcefully between the infant's shoulder blades with the heel of the free hand.

TURN INFANT

- Place the free hand on the infant's back to sandwich the baby between both hands; one hand supports the neck, jaw, and chest, while the other supports the back.
- Turn the infant over, and place the head lower than the chest, supporting the head and neck.
- Alternative position: Place the infant face down on your lap with the head lower than the trunk; firmly support the head. Apply back blows, and then turn the infant as a unit.

CHEST THRUSTS

- Provide five downward chest thrusts on the lower third of the sternum.
- Perform finger sweeps to remove foreign body only if it is visible.

OPEN AIRWAY

- Open airway with the head tilt–chin lift maneuver, and attempt to ventilate.
- Repeat the sequence of back blows, turning, and chest thrusts.
- Continue these emergency procedures until signs of recovery occur:
  —Palpable peripheral pulses return.
  —The pupils become normal in size and are responsive to light.
  —Mottling and cyanosis disappear.
- Record the time and duration of the procedure and the effects of this intervention.

Back blows and chest thrust in infant to clear airway obstruction. **A,** Back blow. **B,** Chest thrust.

can be dangerous because the entire object may be aspirated if it is small, or a portion may become lodged in the pharynx. Improvised pacifiers, such as those commonly made in hospitals from a padded nipple, also pose dangers because the nipple may separate from the plastic collar and be aspirated. Safe pacifiers are made of one piece that includes a shield or flange that is large enough to prevent entry into the mouth and a handle that can be grasped (Fig. 28-3).

▬ *Anticipatory Guidance Regarding Infant Development*

Anticipatory guidance helps prepare new parents for what to expect as their newborn grows and develops. Parents with realistic expectations of infant needs and behavior are prepared better to adjust to the demands of a new baby and to parenthood itself.

FIG. 28-3 Safe pacifiers for term and preterm infants. Note one-piece construction, easily grasped handle, and large shield with ventilation holes. (Courtesy Julie Perry Nelson, Gilbert, AZ.)

EMERGENCY

Cardiopulmonary Resuscitation (CPR) for Infants

- Wash hands before and after touching infant and equipment. Wear gloves, if possible.

ASSESS RESPONSIVENESS
- Observe color; tap or gently shake shoulders.
- Yell for help; if alone, perform cardiopulmonary resuscitation (CPR) for 1 min before calling for help again.

POSITION INFANT
- Turn the infant onto back, supporting the head and neck.
- Place the infant on firm, flat surface.

AIRWAY
- Open the airway with the head tilt–chin lift method.
- Place one hand on the infant's forehead, and tilt the head back.
- Place the fingers of other hand under the bone of the lower jaw at the chin.

BREATHING
- Assess for evidence of breathing:
  - Observe for chest movement.
  - Listen for exhaled air.
  - Feel for exhaled air flow.
- To breathe for infant:
  - Take a breath.
  - Place mouth over the infant's nose and mouth to create a seal.
- NOTE: When available, a mask with a one-way valve should be used.
- Give two slow breaths (1 to 1.5 sec/breath), pausing to inhale between breaths.
- NOTE: Gently puff the volume of air in your cheeks into infant. Do not force air.
- The infant's chest should rise slightly with each puff; keep fingers on the chest wall to sense air entry.
- The rescue breathing rate is 40 to 60 breaths per minute.

CIRCULATION
- Assess circulation:
  - Check pulse of the brachial or femoral artery while maintaining the head tilt.
  - If the pulse is present, initiate rescue breathing. Continue doing once every 3 sec or 12-20 times/min until spontaneous breathing resumes.
  - If the pulse is absent, initiate chest compressions and coordinate them with breathing.
- Chest compression

There are two systems of chest compression. Nurses should know both methods.

- Maintain the head tilt and
  1. Place thumbs side by side in the middle third of the sternum with fingers around the chest and supporting the back.
     - Compress the sternum to one third the depth of the chest.
  2. Place index finger of hand just under an imaginary line drawn between the nipples. Place the middle and ring fingers on the sternum adjacent to the index finger.
     - Using the middle and ring fingers, compress the sternum to one third the depth of the chest.
- Avoid compressing the xiphoid process.
- Release the pressure without moving the thumbs/fingers from the chest.
- Use a 30:2 compression-ventilation ratio for all 1-rescuer and a 15:2 compression-ventilation ratio for 2-rescuer CPR.
- Repeat at least 100 times/min, doing five compressions in 3 sec or less.
- Perform 10 cycles of five compressions and one ventilation.
- Avoid giving compressions and ventilations simultaneously.
- After the cycles, check the brachial artery to determine whether there is a pulse.
- Discontinue compressions when the infant's spontaneous heart rate reaches or exceeds 80 beats/min.
- Record the time and duration of the procedure and the effects of intervention.

A, Opening airway with head tilt–chin lift method. **B,** Checking pulse of brachial artery. **C,** Side-by-side thumb placement for chest compressions in newborn.

Source: American Heart Association. (2005). American Heart Association guidelines for cardiopulmonary resuscitation and emergency cardiovascular care. *Circulation, 112,* IV-12–IV-18. Accessed www.circulationaha.org, August 19, 2006.

New parents can be overwhelmed by a large volume of information and may become anxious. Anticipatory guidance should include the following: newborn sleep-wake cycles, interpretation of crying and quieting techniques, infant developmental milestones, sensory enrichment/ infant stimulation, recognizing signs of illness, and well-baby follow-up and immunizations. Printed materials and audiotapes or videotapes for parents to take home are helpful. These resources (1) reinforce content discussed in the hospital, (2) allow parents another chance to review the material in private and at their own pace, and (3) provide new information not covered in the hospital. For visually impaired parents, free Talking Books about childbirth are available. To locate a library that participates in this program, access the following website: www. loc.gov/nls.

Development of Day-Night Routines. Nurses can help prepare new parents for the fact that most newborns cannot tell the difference between night and day and must learn the rhythm of day-night routines. Nurses should provide basic suggestions for settling a newborn and for helping him or her develop a predictable routine. Examples of such suggestions include

- In the late afternoon, bring the baby out to the center of family activity. Keep the baby there for the rest of the evening. If the baby falls asleep, let the baby do so in the infant seat or in someone's arms. Save the crib or bassinet for nighttime sleep.
- Give the baby a bath right before bedtime. This soothes the baby and helps him or her expend energy.
- Give the baby the last evening feeding around 11 PM and put him or her to bed in the crib or bassinet.
- For nighttime feedings and diaper changes, keep a small night-light on to avoid turning on bright lights. Talk in soft whispers (if at all) and handle the baby gently and only as absolutely necessary to feed and diaper. Nighttime feedings should be all business and no play. Babies usually go back to sleep if the room is quiet and dark.

A predictable, stable routine gradually develops for most babies; however, some babies never develop one. New parents will find it easier if they are willing to be flexible and to give up some control during those early weeks.

Interpretation of Crying and Quieting Techniques. Crying is an infant's first social communication. Some babies cry more than others, but all babies cry. They cry to communicate that they are hungry, uncomfortable, wet, ill, or bored, and sometimes for no apparent reason at all. Crying increases to about 2.5 hours per day, peaks in the second month of life, and decreases after that time. Infants with high responsivity cry more than other infants (St. James-Roberts, Goodwin, Peter, Adams, & Hunt, 2003). However, caretaking behaviors of mothers of children who cry more are not different from behaviors of mothers whose infants cry less.

The longer parents are around their infants, the easier it becomes to interpret what a cry means. Many infants,

CRITICAL THINKING EXERCISE

Infant Crying

Marta, an 18-year-old primiparous single mother of a 3-week-old baby, called her pediatric nurse practitioner (PNP). She was distraught and crying, stating, "My baby is crying all the time, and I don't know what to do. I fed him and changed him and he just keeps crying. What is the matter with him? I can't stand his crying anymore." What should the nurse's initial response be? What are some causes of infant crying? What questions should the nurse ask? To what risks is the infant exposed? To what resources can Marta be referred? Make a handout listing ways to soothe infants that could be distributed to parents.

1. Evidence—Is there sufficient evidence to draw conclusions about what information and advice the PNP should provide Marta?
2. Assumptions—What assumptions can be made about the following factors:
   a. The frequency and amount of normal infant crying
   b. Mother's tolerance of infant crying
   c. Relationship between crying and abuse
   d. Marta's single status and tolerance of infant crying
3. What implications and priorities for nursing care can be made at this time?
4. Does the evidence objectively support your conclusion?
5. Are there alternative perspectives to your conclusion?

especially between ages 3 and 12 weeks, have a fussy period during the day, often in the late afternoon or early evening when everyone is naturally tired. Environmental tension adds to the length and intensity of crying spells. Babies also have periods of vigorous crying that no comforting helps. These periods of crying may last for long stretches until the infants seem to cry themselves to sleep. Possibly the infants are trying to discharge enough energy so that they can settle themselves down. Time and infant maturation will take care of these types of cries.

Crying because of colic is a common concern of new parents. Babies with colic cry inconsolably for several hours, pull their legs up to their stomach, and pass large amounts of gas. No one really knows what colic is or why babies have it. Parents can be encouraged to contact their nurse practitioner or pediatrician if they are concerned that their baby has colic.

Certain types of sensory stimulation can calm and quiet infants and help them get to sleep. Important characteristics of this sensory stimulation—whether tactile, vestibular, auditory, or visual—appear to be that the stimulation is mild, slow, rhythmic, and consistently and regularly presented. Tactile stimulation can include warmth, patting, back rubbing, and covering the skin with textured cloth. Swaddling to keep arms and legs close to the body (as in utero) provides widespread and constant tactile stimulation and a sense of security. Vestibular stimulation is especially effective and can be accomplished by mild rhythmic movement such as rocking or by holding the infant upright, as on the parent's shoulder.

The health care provider should ask about infant crying during well-child visits. The nurse can teach parents a number of strategies that help quiet a fussy baby, prevent crying, and induce quiet attention or sleep (Boxes 28-3 and 28-4). Excessive crying is not caused by inadequate parental caregiving (St. James-Roberts et al., 2003). Unemployment and maternal smoking are risk factors for excessive crying (Reijneveld, Brugman, & Hiarsing, 2002). If excessive crying is reported, the nurse can suggest that the parents keep a crying diary to document the amount and type of crying. Additional support services and follow-up should be provided for those parents who appear unable to cope with the crying; mothers should be encouraged to stop smoking. Parents report smothering, slapping, and shaking babies who will not stop crying (Reijneveld, van der Wal, Brugman, Sing, & Verloove-Vanharick, 2004). Health care providers should be aware that inconsolable infant crying sometimes provokes abuse by parents that is sometimes fatal. Referrals to community support groups is appropriate.

Developmental Milestones. Knowledge of infant growth and development helps parents have realistic

expectations of what an infant can do. When parents understand and appreciate the limitations and developing abilities of their infant, adjustment to parenthood can go more smoothly. Emphasizing the individuality of the infant enhances the capacity of the family to offer their infant an optimally nurturing environment.

Brazelton (1995) suggested the concept of "touchpoints" for intervention, that is, points at which a change in the system (baby, parent, and family) is brought about by the baby's spurts in development (cognitive, motor, or emotional) (www.touchpoints.org). Immediately before each spurt in development, there is a predictable short period of disorganization in the baby. Parents are likely to feel disorganized and stressed as well. Because these periods of disorganization are predictable, nurses can offer parents anticipatory guidance to help them understand what happens with infant development and to prepare them for the subsequent spurts in development.

Two touch-points occur during the early postpartum-newborn period: one soon after birth and another at 2 to 3 weeks (Brazelton, 1995). In the hospital or at a home visit during the first week, the nurse can use the Newborn Behavioral Observations (NBO) system to demonstrate to parents their baby's amazing repertoire of abilities. In this way, parents begin to appreciate their baby's individuality and become more sensitive to their baby's behavioral cues (www.brazelton.institute@childrens.harvard.edu).

It also is helpful for nurses to provide parents with information on month-by-month infant growth and development. Written information that parents can refer to later is especially helpful. See Table 28-1 for a summary of infant growth and development during the first 2 to 3 months.

Infant Stimulation. Interacting with their parents is an important way in which infants learn about themselves and

---

box 28-3 How to Swaddle an Infant (see Fig. 26-10)*

1. Fold down the top corner of the blanket. Position the infant on the blanket, with the infant's neck near the fold.
2. Bring the blanket around the infant's right side and across the infant, tucking the corner under the left side.
3. Bring the bottom of the blanket up to the infant's chest.
4. Bring the remaining corner of the blanket across the infant, tucking the corner under the infant's right side. The infant should be wrapped securely but not tightly; some room should be left for the infant to move.

*Swaddling uses the same techniques as the morning restraint.

---

box 28-4 Infant Quieting Techniques

- Many newborns feel insecure in the center of a large crib. They prefer a small, warm, soft space that reminds them of intrauterine life. Try a smaller bed, such as a bassinet, portable crib, buggy, or cradle, or use a rolled-up blanket to turn a corner of the big crib into a smaller place.
- Carry your baby in a frontpack or backpack.
- Swaddle your newborn snugly in a receiving blanket. Swaddling keeps your newborn's arms and legs close to his or her body, similar to the intrauterine position. It makes the newborn feel more secure.
- Prewarm the crib sheets with a hot water bottle or heating pad that you remove before putting your baby to bed. Some babies startle when placed on a cold sheet.
- Some newborns need extra sucking to soothe themselves to sleep. Breastfeeding mothers may prefer to let their infant suckle at the breast as a soothing technique. Other mothers choose to use a pacifier. Around age 3 months, infants become able to find and suck their thumbs consistently as a way of self-consoling.
- A rhythmic, monotonous noise simulating the intrauterine sounds of your heartbeat and blood flow may help your infant

settle down. Some parents have found that putting the baby in a portable crib beside the dishwasher or washing machine helps settle a fussy baby.
- Movement often helps quiet a baby. Take your baby for a ride in the car, or take your baby for an outing in a stroller or carriage. Rock your baby in a rocking chair or cradle.
- Place your baby on his or her stomach across your lap; pat and rub his or her back while gently bouncing your legs or swaying them from left to right.
- Babies enjoy close skin-to-skin contact. A combination of this and warm water often helps soothe a fussy baby. Fill your tub with warm water. Get in and let the baby lie on your chest so that the baby is immersed in the water up to his or her neck. Cuddle the baby close.
- Let your baby see your face. Talk to your baby in a soothing voice.
- Your baby may simply be bored. Bring him or her into the room where you and the rest of the family are.
- Change your baby's position; many babies like to be upright, such as being held up on your shoulder.

table 28-1 Growth and Development During Infancy

	1 MONTH	2 MONTHS	3 MONTHS

PHYSICAL

1 MONTH	2 MONTHS	3 MONTHS
Weight gain of 5 to 7.5 oz (150 to 210 g) weekly for first 6 mo Height gain of 1 in (2.5 cm) monthly for first 6 mo Head circumference increases by 0.6 in (1.5 cm) monthly for first 6 mo Primitive reflexes present and strong Doll's eye reflex and dance reflex fading Preferential nose breathing (most infants)	Posterior fontanel closed Crawling reflex disappears	Primitive reflexes fading

GROSS MOTOR

1 MONTH	2 MONTHS	3 MONTHS
Assumes flexed position with pelvis high but knees not under abdomen when prone (at birth, knees flexed under abdomen)† Can turn head from side to side when prone, lifts head momentarily from bed† Has marked head lag, especially when pulled from lying to sitting position Holds head momentarily parallel and in midline when suspended in prone position Assumes asymmetric tonic neck reflex position when supine When held in standing position, body limp at knees and hips In sitting position, back is uniformly rounded; absence of head control	Assumes less flexed position when prone—hips flat, legs extended, arms flexed, head to side† Less head lag when pulled to sitting position Can maintain head in same plane as rest of body when held in ventral suspension When prone, can lift head almost 45 degrees off table When held in sitting position, head is held up but bobs forward Assumes asymmetric tonic neck reflex position intermittently	Able to hold head more erect when sitting, but still bobs forward Has only slight head lag when pulled to sitting position Assumes symmetric body positioning Able to raise head and shoulders from prone position to a 45-to 90-degree angle from table; bears weight on forearms When held in standing position, able to bear slight fraction of weight on legs Regards own hand

FINE MOTOR

1 MONTH	2 MONTHS	3 MONTHS
Hands predominantly closed Grasp reflex strong Hand clenches on contact with rattle	Hands often open Grasp reflex fading	Actively holds rattle but will not reach for it† Grasp reflex absent Hands kept loosely open Clutches own hand; pulls at blanket and clothes

SENSORY

1 MONTH	2 MONTHS	3 MONTHS
Able to fixate on moving object in range of 45 degrees when held at a distance of 8 to 10 in. Visual acuity approaches 20/100* Follows light to midline Quiets when hears a voice	Binocular fixation and convergence to near objects beginning When supine, follows dangling toy from side to point beyond midline Visually searches to locate sounds Turns head to side when sound is made at level of ear	Follows object to periphery (180 degrees)† Locates sound by turning head to side and looking in same direction† Begins to have ability to coordinate stimuli from various sense organs

VOCALIZATION

1 MONTH	2 MONTHS	3 MONTHS
Cries to express displeasure Makes small throaty sounds Makes comfort sounds during feeding	Vocalizes, distinct from crying† Crying becomes differentiated Coos Vocalizes to familiar voice	Squeals aloud to show pleasure† Coos, babbles, chuckles Vocalizes when smiling "Talks" a great deal when spoken to Less crying during periods of wakefulness

SOCIALIZATION AND COGNITION

1 MONTH	2 MONTHS	3 MONTHS
Is in sensorimotor phase—stage I, use of reflexes (birth-1 mo), and stage II, primary circular reactions (1-4 mo) Watches parent's face intently as she or he talks to infant	Demonstrates social smile in response to various stimuli†	Displays considerable interest in surroundings Ceases crying when parent enters room Can recognize familiar faces and objects, such as feeding bottle Shows awareness of strange situations

From Hockenberry, M. (2003). *Wong's nursing care of infants and children* (7th ed.). St. Louis: Mosby.
† Milestones that represent essential integrative aspects of development that lay the foundation for the achievement of more advanced skills.
*Degree of visual acuity varies according to vision measurement procedure used.

their environment. Nurses can teach parents a variety of ways to stimulate their infant's development and to enrich the infant's learning environment. Home health nurses are in a prime position to evaluate the home environment and to make suggestions to parents for promotion of their baby's physical, cognitive, and emotional development. Suggestions for teaching infants during the first few months are presented in Boxes 28-5 and 28-6. Table 28-2 presents suggestions for visual, auditory, tactile, and kinetic stimulation.

Another method of sensory enrichment that parents can learn to use is infant massage. This type of nurturing touch can help create a loving bond between the infant and parent and has been shown to contribute to the physical and emotional well-being of both massage giver and receiver (Box 28-7). Infant massage is not manipulative, but a gentle, warm communication done with the infant, not to the infant. The focus is on reciprocal interaction between infant and parent; the parent talks to the infant, asks permission to start the massage, questions the infant, and facilitates dialogue (www.infantmassageusa.org).

One of the most important skills for the parents is the improved ability to read their infant's cues. Positive cues include eye contact, smiling, looking at the parent's face, babbling or cooing, and smooth movements of arms and legs. Negative cues from the infant include pulling away, frowning, grimacing, turning the head away, arching the back, crying, squirming, and flailing the arms and legs. Increased ability to read their infant's cues can increase parental confidence and self-esteem, thereby assisting adaptation to parenthood (see Chapter 24).

Well-Baby Follow-Up and Immunizations

Parents should plan for their infant's health follow-up care at the following ages: within 3 days if early discharge to check for status of jaundice, feeding, and elimination; 2 to 4 weeks, and then every 2 months until 6 to 7 months; then every 3 months until 18 months, at 2 years, at 3 years, at preschool, and every 2 years thereafter. These well-baby follow-up visits with a nurse practitioner or pediatrician are important for the parents, as well as for the infant. They provide a time for parents to have questions answered, to receive reassurance about their adaptation to parenthood, and to receive anticipatory guidance for the ensuing weeks before the next well-baby visit.

Immunizations. The schedule for immunizations should be reviewed with parents (Table 28-3). An infant's

---

box 28-5 | Teaching Your Newborn

- Newborns learn things every day. You can teach your newborn by playing with him or her and giving your newborn toys that help him or her to learn.
- Talk to your baby a lot. Tell your baby what is going on in the room ("Listen to the dog barking."). Label objects that you see or use ("Here's the washcloth.") and describe things you are doing ("Let's put the shirt over Kerry's head!").
- Look at your baby's face and make eye contact. Play face-making games: smile, stick out your tongue, open your eyes wide. As your baby gets older, he or she will try to imitate these facial expressions.
- Babies like music and rhythmic movement. Rock or swing your baby as you sing to him or her in a gentle voice.

- Acknowledge your baby's attempts to "answer" your talking and singing. He or she will respond to you by looking in your direction, making eye contact, moving his or her arms and legs, and/or making sounds.
- Babies like bright colors and vivid contrasts. Show your baby pictures and objects that are black and white, bright primary colors (red, blue, yellow, green), and/or large patterns. Keep colorful mobiles and toys where your baby can see them.
- Babies like to be held upright. Holding your newborn on your shoulder lets your baby look around his or her world and provides vestibular stimulation. Let your baby lift his or her head for a few seconds. Keep your hand ready to support your baby's head.

---

box 28-6 | Teaching Your 1- to 2-Month-Old Infant

At age 1 to 2 months, your infant is gaining more control of his or her movements: more head control, even holding an object briefly in his or her hand. Your baby also is becoming more social. He or she demonstrates behaviors to engage you in interaction: smiling, cooing, making longer eye contact, and following you with his or her eyes.

During these months you can help your baby learn if you do the following:
- Put your baby on his or her abdomen on a blanket on the floor. Lie on your abdomen facing your baby. Talk to your baby to get him or her to raise his or her head to see you.
- Roll your baby onto his or her back and play with your baby's legs. Move the legs in a bicycle-riding motion. Try to get your baby to kick his or her legs.
- Play hand games, such as pat-a-cake, with your baby; kiss your baby's fingers; place your baby's hands on your face. Bring

your baby's hands in front of his or her eyes as you play; get your baby to look at his or her hands.
- Encourage your baby to watch and follow things with his or her eyes. Use a noise-making toy, such as a rattle or a chime, or a brightly colored object about 12 inches from his or her eyes; move it slowly to one side and then the other. Objects hanging from a play frame are good for your baby to watch while he or she is on his or her back or sitting in an infant seat.
- Continue to talk and sing a lot to your baby. Continue to tell your baby what you are doing with him or her and what is going on in the immediate environment.
- Keep your baby near you during times when the family usually is together, such as at mealtimes. Infant seats, especially ones that bounce or rock, and infant swings are good to use at these times.

table 28-2 Play During Infancy: Suggested Activities for Birth Through 3 Months				
AGE (MONTHS)	**VISUAL STIMULATION**	**AUDITORY STIMULATION**	**TACTILE STIMULATION**	**KINETIC STIMULATION**
Birth-1	Look at infant at close range Hang bright, shiny object within 9 to 10 inches of infant's face and in midline Hang mobiles with black-and-white contrast designs	Talk to infant, sing in soft voice Play music box, radio, television Have ticking clock or metronome nearby	Hold, caress, cuddle Keep infant warm Infant may like to be swaddled	Rock infant, place in cradle Use carriage for walks
2–3	Provide bright objects Make room bright with pictures or mirrors on walls Take infant to various rooms while doing chores Place infant in infant seat for vertical view of environment	Talk to infant Include in family gatherings Expose to various environmental noises other than those of home Use rattles, wind chimes	Caress infant while bathing, at diaper change Comb hair with a soft brush	Use infant swing Take in car for rides Exercise body by moving extremities in swimming motion Use cradle gym

From Hockenberry, M. (2003). *Wong's nursing care of infants and children* (7th ed.). St. Louis: Mosby.

box 28-7 Benefits of Infant Massage

BENEFITS TO BABY RECEIVING MASSAGE

- Relaxes child and helps to decrease stress for you and your baby.
- Relieves discomfort from constipation, gas, and colic.
- Helps normalize muscle tone and improve blood circulation.
- Helps baby sleep better (and, therefore, parents sleep better!).
- Stimulates brain development and improves sensory awareness.
- Babies cry less, as the parent is more responsive to babies' cues.
- Promotes bonding and attachment.

BENEFITS TO THE PARENT OF GIVING MASSAGE

- Caregivers report feeling more comfortable and confident in their ability to care for baby.
- Parents learn to understand and respond to baby's cues.
- Parents learn techniques to soothe and comfort their babies.
- Provides an additional avenue for close and nurturing contact.
- Provides special baby-focused time for mothers, fathers, and caregivers.

From Infant Massage USA. *About Infant Massage.* Accessed www.infantmassageusa.org, March 16, 2006.

table 28-3 Recommended Childhood Immunization Schedule Birth to 18 Mo—United States, 2006

VACCINES	AGE (THROUGH 18 MO)
Hep B (Hepatitis B)	Birth, 1-4 mo, 6-18 mo
HBIG (Hepatitis immune globulin)	Within 12 hours of birth if mother is HbsAg positive
DTaP (diphteria, tetanus, pertussis)	2, 4, 6, 15-18 mo
Haemophilus influenzae type b	2, 4, 6, 12-15 mo
IPV (inactivated polio)	2, 4, 6-18 mo
MMR (measles, mumps, rubella)	12-15 mo
Varicella	12-18 mo
PCV (Pneumococcal)	2, 4, 6, 12-15 mo
Influenza	Yearly starting at 6-18 mo

For additional information, see the National Immunization Program Website at www.cdc.gov/nip or call the National Immunization Hotline at 800-232-2522 (English) or 800-232-0233 (Spanish).

Parents can print an individualized immunization schedule for their child(ren) from this site.

ability to protect himself or herself against antigens by the formation of antibodies develops sequentially; therefore the infant must be developmentally capable of responding to these antibodies.

A form of passive immunity is already present in colostrum and breast milk. These antibodies are specific for microbes present in the mother's GI tract and protect against overgrowth as fresh colonization occurs in the term newborn.

The active ingredients in immunizations for diphtheria-pertussis-tetanus (DPT), hepatitis B, rubella, measles, and mumps, as well as the oral poliovirus vaccine (OPV), are not altered by breast milk and should be given according to the regular recommended schedule (Lawrence & Lawrence, 2005).

Recognizing Signs of Illness. As well as explaining the need for well-baby follow-up visits, the nurse should discuss with parents the signs of illness in newborns (Box 28-8). Parents should be advised to call their nurse practitioner or pediatrician immediately if they notice such signs and to ask about over-the-counter medications, such as acetaminophen for infants, to keep at home (see Plan of Care).

box 28-8 **Signs of Illness to Report Immediately**

- Fever: temperature above 100.4° F axillary (under arm); also, a continual increase in temperature
- Hypothermia: temperature below 97.8° F axillary
- Poor feeding or little interest in food: refusal to eat for two feedings in a row
- Vomiting: more than one episode of forceful vomiting or frequent vomiting (over a 6-hr period)
- Diarrhea: two consecutive green, watery stools (NOTE: Stools of breastfed infants are normally looser than stools of formula-fed infants. Diarrhea will leave a water ring around the stool, whereas breastfed stools will not.)
- Decreased bowel movements: less than two soiled diapers per day after 48 hr or fewer than three soiled diapers per day by day 5 of life
- Decreased urination: no wet diapers for 18 to 24 hr or fewer than six to eight wet diapers per day
- Breathing difficulties: labored breathing with flared nostrils or absence of breathing for more than 15 sec (NOTE: A newborn's breathing is normally irregular and between 30 to 40 breaths/min. Count the breaths for a full minute.)
- Cyanosis, whether accompanying a feeding or not
- Lethargy: sleepiness, difficulty waking, or periods of sleep longer than 6 hr (Most newborns sleep for short periods, usually from 1 to 4 hr, and wake to be fed.)
- Inconsolable crying (attempts to quiet not effective) or continuous high-pitched cry
- Bleeding or purulent drainage from umbilical cord or circumcision
- Drainage developing in the eyes

▬ Home Phototherapy

Healthy term infants may at times be discharged home and need phototherapy for hyperbilirubinemia (see Fig. 26-16). Candidates for home phototherapy include those infants who are healthy and active with no signs and symptoms of other complications; the parents or other caregivers must be willing and able to assume responsibility for therapy maintenance and monitoring, and the home environment should be adequate with a telephone, heat, and electricity. Client considerations for administering home phototherapy are included in Box 28-9. Home health care nurses are usually responsible for assessing the parents' or other caregivers' willingness to use the equipment and monitor the infant (Box 28-10) and making home visits to assess the infant's response to therapy, including obtaining blood specimens for measuring bilirubin levels. The company that provides the home therapy equipment is responsible for setting up the phototherapy unit and teaching the parents/caregivers how to use the equipment. The home care nurse schedules home visits to assess the infant's response to therapy including weight, feeding, output, and temperature stability. Additional education of parents may be necessary; their understanding of the therapy and their responsibilities is assessed. Blood may be drawn for laboratory work, and results reported to the primary health care provider. When therapy is discontinued, follow-up visits for monitoring may be ordered. The equipment company is called to arrange for pick-up of the phototherapy unit.

box 28-9 **Considerations for Selecting Infant Home Phototherapy Over Hospital Therapy**

Infant >36 weeks of gestation
Infant age >24 hr
Birthweight >2300 g
Breast or bottle feeding well
Weight loss <10% of birth weight
Stooling and voiding by 24 hr of age; continued adequate amount
Not at risk for sepsis
Blood work results:
- Coombs <1+
- ABO compatible or evidence of resolving initial hyperbilirubinemia
- Central hematocrit <65%
- Direct bilirubin <1.5 mg/100 ml
- If bilirubin history is known
  - <10 mg/100 ml at 24 hr
  - <15 mg/100 ml at 48 hr
  - <20 mg/100 ml at 72 hr

From University of California San Francisco Home Health Care. (2001). *Guidelines for home therapy*. San Francisco: University of California.

box 28-10 **Parent Information for Home Phototherapy Using a Biliblanket**

Information for parents:
- As much of the infant's skin as possible should be in direct contact with the lighted section of the pad. The infant's back or chest should be placed directly on the pad, with the tip of the pad at the shoulder and the cable at the feet.
- Follow the equipment supplier's instructions regarding safety and use of the phototherapy unit.
- Phototherapy can be discontinued for brief periods without harming your baby.
- Temperature instability may occur when starting and stopping phototherapy and when collecting laboratory specimens.
- Effects of phototherapy may include changes in frequency and color of the infant's stools and rash due to an increase in the number of loose stools.

Notify your child's health care provider if
- A notable change is seen in activity level
- The infant's temperature is not maintained at 97° F or 100° F
- The infant is feeding poorly
- The infant is not voiding 6 times per day or does not void within a 6-hr period
- Infant vomits two or more feedings

Notify your home care agency if
- Phototherapy is discontinued
- An equipment malfunction occurs

From University of California San Francisco Home Health Care. (2001). *Guidelines for home therapy*. San Francisco: University of California.

▬ Evaluation

Evaluation is based on the expected outcomes of care. The plan is revised as needed, based on the evaluation findings.

NURSING DIAGNOSIS Deficient knowledge of infant care related to lack of experience/lack of support

Expected Outcomes *Infant care routines are adequate, and infant appears healthy.*

Nursing Interventions/Rationales
- Observe infant care routines (bathing, diapering, feeding, play) *to evaluate parental ease with care and adequacy of techniques.*
- Observe infant appearance (height-weight ratio, head circumference, fontanels, skin tone and turgor); assess infant's vital signs, overall tone, reflexes, and age-appropriate developmental skills *to evaluate for signs indicative of inadequate care.*
- Explore available support systems for infant care *to determine adequacy of existing system.*
- Demonstrate care routines that are troublesome to parents and have involved family members return demonstration *to facilitate improvements in care.*
- Provide ongoing follow-up as needed *to remediate identified potential and actual care deficits.*

NURSING DIAGNOSIS Disturbed maternal sleep pattern related to infant demands and environmental interruptions

Expected Outcomes *Mother sleeps for uninterrupted periods and feels rested on waking.*

Nursing Interventions/Rationales
- Discuss woman's routine and specify things that interfere with sleep *to determine scope of problem and direct interventions.*
- Explore ways woman and significant others can make environment more conducive to sleep (e.g., privacy, darkness, quiet, back rubs, soothing music, warm milk); teach use of guided imagery and relaxation techniques *to promote optimal conditions for sleep.*
- Eliminate things or routines (e.g., caffeine, foods that induce heartburn, strenuous mental/physical activity) *that may interfere with sleep.*
- Advise family to limit visitors and activities *to avoid further taxation and fatigue.*
- Have family plan specific times to care for the newborn *to allow mother time to sleep;* have mother learn to use infant nap time as a time for her to nap as well *to replenish energy and decrease fatigue.*

NURSING DIAGNOSIS Impaired home maintenance related to addition of new family member/inadequate resources/inadequate support systems

Expected Outcome *Home exhibits signs of safe and functional environment.*

Nursing Interventions/Rationales
- Observe the home environment (e.g., available living space and sleeping arrangements; adequacy of facilities for food preparation and storage, hygiene and toileting; overall state of repair; cleanliness; presence of safety hazards) *to determine adequacy and effective use of resources.*
- Observe arrangements for the newborn, such as sleeping space, care equipment, and supplies (bathing, changing, feeding, transportation) *to determine adequacy of resources.*
- Explore who is responsible for cooking, cleaning, child care, and newborn care and determine whether the mother seems adequately rested *to determine adequacy of support systems.*
- Identify and arrange referrals to needed social agencies (e.g., Aid to Families with Dependent Children [AFDC], Women, Infants, and Children [WIC] program, food pantries) *to address resource deficits (finances, supplies, equipment).*

NURSING DIAGNOSIS Interrupted family processes related to inclusion of new family member

Expected Outcome *Infant is successfully assimilated into family structure.*

Nursing Interventions/Rationales
- Explore with family the ways that the birth and neonate have changed family structure and function *to evaluate functional and role adjustment.*
- Observe family interaction with the newborn and note degree of bonding, evidence of sibling rivalry, and involvement in newborn care *to evaluate acceptance of newest family member.*
- Clarify identified misinformation and misperceptions *to promote clear communication.*
- Assist family to explore options for solutions to identified problems *to promote effective problem resolution.*
- Support family efforts as they move toward adjusting and incorporating the new member *to reinforce new functions and roles.*
- If needed, make referrals to appropriate social services or community agencies *to ensure ongoing support and care.*

community activity

Go to a local toy or department store and examine toys for infants from birth to 3 months of age. Are there toys labeled as educational or to provide stimulation? What types of stimulation do the toys provide? What kind of education do the toys provide? Do the toys have information about safety in the use of the toys? Are the toys easy to clean? What is the range of price for the toys? Are some of the toys in a price range that would make them available for parents with a limited income? How can you use this information in your contact with parents?

key points
- Anticipatory guidance helps prepare new parents for what to expect.
- Topics to include in parent teaching include feeding, elimination, care of the circumcised infant, crying, behavior, developmental milestones, sleeping, signs of illness, and community resources including support groups.
- Parents may need assistance in providing a protective environment for the infant.
- Nurses are responsible for teaching parents about home phototherapy when it is ordered and for monitoring the infant's response to therapy.

REFERENCES

American Academy of Pediatrics (AAP) Committee on Injury and Poison Prevention. (2002). Selecting and using the most appropriate care safety seats for growing children: Guidelines for counseling parents. *Pediatrics, 109*(3), 550-553.

American Academy of Pediatrics (AAP) Task Force on Sudden Infant Death Syndrome. (2005). The changing concept of sudden infant death syndrome: Diagnostic coding shifts, controversies regarding the sleeping environment, and new variables to consider in reducing risk. *Pediatrics, 116*(5), 1245-1255.

Association of Women's Health, Obstetric, and Neonatal Nurses (AWHONN). (2001). *Neonatal skin care: Evidence-based clinical practice guideline.* Washington, DC: Author.

Brazelton, T. (1995). Working with families: Opportunities for early intervention. *Pediatric Clinics of North America, 42*(1), 1-9.

Johnson & Johnson. (2006). *Compendium of postpartum care* (2nd ed.). Skillman, NJ: Johnson & Johnson Consumer Products.

Lawrence, R., & Lawrence, R. (2005). *Breastfeeding: A guide for the medical profession* (6th ed.). Philadelphia: Mosby.

Reijneveld, S., Brugman, E., & Hirasing, R. (2002). Excessive infant crying: Definitions determine risk groups. *Archives of Disease in Childhood, 87*(1), 43-44.

Reijneveld, S., van der Wal, M., Brugman, E., Sing, R., & Verloove-Vanharick, S. (2004). Infant crying and abuse. *Lancet, 364*(9442), 1340-1342.

St. James-Roberts, I., Goodwin, J., Peter, B., Adams, D., & Hunt, S. (2003). Individual differences in responsivity to a neurobehavioural examination predict crying patterns of 1-week-old infants at home. *Developmental Medicine & Child Neurology, 45*(6), 400-407.

Cynthia Garrett

Assessment for Risk Factors

learning objectives

- Explore physiologic and psychologic aspects of high risk pregnancy.
- Discuss regionalization of health care services.
- Examine risk factors identified through history, physical examination, and diagnostic techniques.

- Differentiate among diagnostic techniques, including when they are used in pregnancy and for what purposes.
- Develop a teaching plan to explain diagnostic techniques and implications of findings to women and their families.

electronic resources

Additional information related to the content in Chapter 29 can be found on

the companion website at **evolve**
http://evolve.elsevier.com/Lowdermilk/MWHC/
- NCLEX Review Questions
- WebLinks

or on the interactive companion CD
- NCLEX Review Questions

PPROXIMATELY 500,000 of the 4 million births that occur in the United States each year will be categorized as high risk because of maternal or fetal complications. Identification of the risks, together with appropriate and timely intervention during the perinatal period, can prevent morbidity and mortality among mothers and infants.

With the changing demographics in the United States, more women and families can be identified as at risk because of factors other than biophysical criteria. The increasing numbers of homeless, single, or uninsured pregnant women who have no access to prenatal care during any stage of pregnancy and the behaviors and lifestyles that pose a risk to the health of the mother and fetus contribute to the problem (U.S. Department of Health and Human Services [USDHHS], 2000).

Care of these high risk clients requires the unified efforts of medical and nursing personnel. The high risk woman and the factors associated with a diagnosis of high risk are identified in this chapter; diagnostic techniques used to monitor the maternal-fetal unit are emphasized.

DEFINITION AND SCOPE OF THE PROBLEM

A high risk pregnancy is one in which the life or health of the mother or fetus is jeopardized by a disorder coincidental

with or unique to pregnancy. For the mother, the high risk status arbitrarily extends through the puerperium (4 to 6 weeks after childbirth). Postbirth maternal complications are usually resolved within 1 month of birth, but perinatal morbidity may continue for months or years.

High risk pregnancy is a critical problem for modern medical and nursing care. The new social emphasis on the quality of life and the wanted child has resulted in a reduction of family size and the number of unwanted pregnancies. At the same time, technologic advances have facilitated pregnancies in previously infertile couples. As a consequence, emphasis is on the safe birth of normal infants who can develop to their potential. Scientific and technologic advances have allowed perinatal health care in developed countries to reach a level far beyond that previously available.

The diagnosis of high risk imposes a situational crisis on the family (e.g., loss of pregnancy before the anticipated date, development of gestational diabetes mellitus with its potential complications, or birth of a neonate who does not meet cultural, societal, or familial norms and expectations).

Maternal Health Problems

The leading causes of maternal death attributable to pregnancy differ over the world. In general, three major causes have persisted for the last 50 years: hypertensive disorders, infection, and hemorrhage. The three leading causes of maternal mortality in the United States today are gestational hypertension, pulmonary embolism, and hemorrhage. Factors that are strongly related to maternal death include age (younger than 20 years and 35 years or older), lack of prenatal care, low educational attainment, unmarried status, and nonwhite race. African-American maternal mortality rates are more than 3 times higher than those for Caucasian women (Hoyert, Heron, Murphy, & Kung, 2006). Reaching the goal set by *Healthy People 2010* of no more than 3.3 maternal deaths per 100,000 live births (USDHHS, 2000) presents a significant challenge.

Although the overall number of maternal deaths is small, maternal mortality remains a significant problem because a high proportion of deaths are preventable, primarily through improving the access to and use of prenatal care services. Nurses can be instrumental in educating the public about the importance of obtaining early and regular care during pregnancy.

Fetal and Neonatal Health Problems

The leading cause of death in the neonatal period is congenital anomalies (Hoyert et al., 2006). Other causes of neonatal death include disorders related to short gestation and low birth weight, sudden infant death, respiratory distress syndrome, and the effects of maternal complications. Racial differences in the infant mortality rates continue to challenge public health experts. Increased rates of survival during the neonatal period have resulted largely from high quality prenatal care and the improvement in perinatal services, including technologic advances in neonatal intensive care and obstetrics.

What can be done to prevent antepartum fetal deaths? Some factors are presumed avoidable, such as failure to respond appropriately to abnormalities of pregnancy and labor. Such abnormalities may include results of fetal growth or fetal well-being assessments, significant maternal weight loss, or decreased fetal movements (Druzin, Gabbe, & Reed, 2002). In addition, commitment at national, state, and local levels is required to reduce the infant mortality rate. More research is needed to identify the extent to which financial, educational, sociocultural, and behavioral factors individually and collectively affect perinatal morbidity and mortality. Barriers to care must be removed and perinatal services modified to meet contemporary health care needs.

Regionalization of Health Care Services

Early and ongoing risk assessment is a crucial component of perinatal care. Conditions associated with perinatal morbidity and mortality can be prevented, treated, or referred to more skilled health care providers. Factors to consider when determining a client's risk status include resources available locally to treat the condition, availability of appropriate facilities for transport if needed, and determination of the best match for the client's needs.

Not all facilities develop and maintain the full spectrum of services required for high risk perinatal clients. As a consequence, regionalization of hospital-based perinatal health care services emerged. This system of coordinated care, in which facilities within a geographic region are organized to provide different levels of care, was also applied to preconception and ambulatory prenatal care services.

Guidelines have been established regarding the level of care that could be expected at any given facility. In ambulatory settings, providers must distinguish themselves by the level of care they provide. *Basic care* is provided by obstetricians, family physicians, certified nurse-midwives, and other advanced practice clinicians approved by local governance. Routine risk-oriented prenatal care, education, and support is provided. Providers offering *specialty care* are obstetricians who must provide fetal diagnostic testing and management of obstetric and medical complications in addition to basic care. *Subspecialty care* is provided by maternal-fetal medicine specialists and includes the aforementioned in addition to genetic testing, advanced fetal therapies, and management of severe maternal and fetal complications (American Academy of Pediatrics [AAP] & American College of Obstetricians and Gynecologists [ACOG], 2002).

In hospital settings, perinatal services also are designated as basic, specialty, or subspecialty. Criteria for basic perinatal services include care of all clients admitted to the service, with an established triage system for high risk clients who should be transferred to a higher level of care; ability to perform a cesarean birth within 30 minutes of a decision to do so; availability of blood and blood products; availability of radiology, anesthesia, and laboratory services on a 24 hour basis; presence of newborn and postpartum care; resuscitation and stabilization of all neonates born in the hospital; availability of transport for all sick neonates; family visitation; and data collection and retrieval (AAP & ACOG, 2002).

Specialty hospital care includes these requirements in addition to care of high risk mothers and fetuses, stabilization of ill neonates before transfer, and care of preterm infants with a birth weight of 1500 g or more. Women in preterm labor or those with impending births at 32 weeks of gestation or less should be transferred for subspecialty care. Additional criteria for subspecialty care include provision of comprehensive perinatal care for women and infants of all risk categories, evaluation and use of new high risk technologies and therapies, and data collection and retrieval. Collaboration among providers to meet the client's needs is the key in reducing perinatal morbidity and mortality (AAP & ACOG, 2002).

Assessment of Risk Factors

Pregnancies can be designated as high risk for any of several undesirable outcomes. Those considered to be at risk for uteroplacental insufficiency (UPI; the gradual decline in delivery of needed substances by the placenta to the fetus) carry a serious threat for fetal growth restriction, intrauterine fetal death, intrapartum death, intrapartum fetal distress, and various types of neonatal morbidity.

In the past, risk factors were evaluated only from a medical viewpoint; therefore only adverse medical, obstetric, or physiologic conditions were considered to place the woman at risk. Today, a more comprehensive approach to high risk pregnancy is used, and the factors associated with high risk childbearing are grouped into broad categories based on threats to health and pregnancy outcome. Categories of risk are biophysical, psychosocial, sociodemographic, and environmental (Gilbert & Harmon, 2003) (Box 29-1).

Biophysical risks include factors that originate within the mother or fetus and affect the development or functioning of either one or both. Examples include genetic disorders, nutritional and general health status, and medical or obstetric-related illnesses.

Psychosocial risks consist of maternal behaviors and adverse lifestyles that have a negative effect on the health of the mother or fetus. These risks may include emotional distress and disturbed interpersonal relationships, as well as inadequate social support and unsafe cultural practices.

---

box 29-1 Categories of High Risk Factors

BIOPHYSICAL FACTORS

- *Genetic considerations.* Genetic factors may interfere with normal fetal or neonatal development, result in congenital anomalies, or create difficulties for the mother. These factors include defective genes, transmissible inherited disorders and chromosome anomalies, multiple pregnancy, large fetal size, and ABO incompatibility.
- *Nutritional status.* Adequate nutrition, without which fetal growth and development cannot proceed normally, is one of the most important determinants of pregnancy outcome. Conditions that influence nutritional status include the following: Young age; three pregnancies in the previous 2 years; tobacco, alcohol, or drug use; inadequate dietary intake because of chronic illness or food fads; inadequate or excessive weight gain; and hematocrit value less than 33%.
- *Medical and obstetric disorders.* Complications of current and past pregnancies, obstetric-related illnesses, and pregnancy losses put the woman at risk (see Box 29-2).

PSYCHOSOCIAL FACTORS

- *Smoking.* A strong, consistent, causal relation has been established between maternal smoking and reduced birth weight. Risks include low-birth-weight infants, higher neonatal mortality rates, increased miscarriages, and increased incidence of premature rupture of membranes. These risks are aggravated by low socioeconomic status, poor nutritional status, and concurrent use of alcohol.
- *Caffeine.* Birth defects in humans have not been related to caffeine consumption. High intake (three or more cups of coffee per day) has been related to a slight decrease in birth weight.
- *Alcohol.* Although its exact effects in pregnancy have not been quantified and its mode of action is largely unexplained, alcohol exerts adverse effects on the fetus, resulting in fetal alcohol syndrome, fetal alcohol effects, learning disabilities, and hyperactivity.
- *Drugs.* The developing fetus may be adversely affected by drugs through several mechanisms. They can be teratogenic, cause metabolic disturbances, produce chemical effects, or cause depression or alteration of central nervous system function. This category includes medications prescribed by a health care provider or bought over the counter, as well as commonly abused drugs such as heroin, cocaine, and marijuana. (See Chapter 35 for more information about drug and alcohol abuse.)
- *Psychologic status.* Childbearing triggers profound and complex physiologic, psychologic, and social changes, with evidence to suggest a relation between emotional distress and birth complications. This risk factor includes conditions such as specific intrapsychic disturbances and addictive lifestyles; a history of child or spouse abuse; inadequate support systems; family disruption or dissolution; maternal role changes or conflicts; noncompliance with cultural norms; unsafe cultural, ethnic, or religious practices; and situational crises.

SOCIODEMOGRAPHIC FACTORS

- *Low income.* Poverty underlies many other risk factors and leads to inadequate financial resources for food and prenatal care, poor general health, increased risk of medical complications of pregnancy, and greater prevalence of adverse environmental influences.
- *Lack of prenatal care.* Failure to diagnose and treat complications early is a major risk factor arising from financial barriers or lack of access to care; depersonalization of the system resulting in long waits, routine visits, variability in health care personnel, and unpleasant physical surroundings; lack of understanding of the need for early and continued care or cultural beliefs that do not support the need; and fear of the health care system and its providers.
- *Age.* Women at both ends of the childbearing age spectrum have a higher incidence of poor outcomes; however, age may not be a risk factor in all cases. Both physiologic and psychologic risks should be evaluated.
  - *Adolescents.* More complications are seen in young mothers (younger than 15 years), who have a 60% higher mortality rate than those older than 20 years, and in pregnancies occurring less than 6 years after menarche. Complications include anemia, preeclampsia, prolonged labor, and contracted pelvis and cephalopelvic disproportion. Long-term social implications of early motherhood are lower educational status, lower income, increased dependence on government support programs, higher divorce rates, and higher parity.
  - *Mature mothers.* The risks to older mothers are not from age alone but from other considerations such as number and spacing of previous pregnancies; genetic disposition of the parents; and medical history, lifestyle, nutrition, and prenatal care. The increased likelihood of chronic diseases and complications that arises from more invasive medical management of a pregnancy and labor combined with demographic characteristics put an older woman at risk. Medical conditions more likely to be experienced by mature women include hypertension and preeclampsia, diabetes, prolonged labor, cesarean birth, placenta previa, abruptio placentae, and mortality. The fetus is at greater risk for low birth weight and macrosomia, chromosomal abnormalities, congenital malformations, and neonatal mortality.
- *Parity.* The number of previous pregnancies is a risk factor associated with age and includes all first pregnancies, especially a first pregnancy at either end of the childbearing age continuum. The incidence of preeclampsia and dystocia is higher with a first birth.

---

box 29-1 | **Categories of High Risk Factors—cont'd**

SOCIODEMOGRAPHIC FACTORS—cont'd

- *Marital status.* The increased mortality and morbidity rates for unmarried women, including a greater risk for preeclampsia, are often related to inadequate prenatal care and a younger childbearing age.
- *Residence.* The availability and quality of prenatal care varies widely with geographic residence. Women in metropolitan areas have more prenatal visits than do those in rural areas, who have fewer opportunities for specialized care and consequently a higher incidence of maternal mortality. Health care in the inner city, where residents are usually poorer and begin childbearing earlier and continue for longer, may be of lower quality than in a more affluent neighborhood.
- *Ethnicity.* Although ethnicity by itself is not a major risk, race is an indicator of other sociodemographic risk factors. Nonwhite

women are more than 3 times as likely as Caucasian women to die of pregnancy-related causes. African-American babies have the highest rates of prematurity and low birth weight, with the infant mortality rate among African-Americans being more than double that among Caucasians.

ENVIRONMENTAL FACTORS

- Various environmental substances can affect fertility and fetal development, the chance of a live birth, and the child's subsequent mental and physical development. Environmental influences include infections, radiation, chemicals such as pesticides, therapeutic drugs, illicit drugs, industrial pollutants, cigarette smoke, stress, and diet. Paternal exposure to mutagenic agents in the workplace has been associated with an increased risk of miscarriage.

---

box 29-2 | **Specific Pregnancy Problems and Related Risk Factors**

PRETERM LABOR

- Age younger than 16 or older than 35 years
- Low socioeconomic status
- Maternal weight below 50 kg
- Poor nutrition
- Previous preterm birth
- Incompetent cervix
- Uterine anomalies
- Smoking
- Drug addiction and alcohol abuse
- Pyelonephritis, pneumonia
- Multiple gestation
- Anemia
- Abnormal fetal presentation
- Preterm rupture of membranes
- Placental abnormalities
- Infection
- Abdominal surgery in current pregnancy
- History of cervical surgery

POLYHYDRAMNIOS

- Diabetes mellitus
- Multiple gestation
- Fetal congenital anomalies
- Isoimmunization (Rh or ABO)
- Nonimmune hydrops
- Abnormal fetal presentation

INTRAUTERINE GROWTH RESTRICTION (IUGR)

- Multiple gestation
- Poor nutrition

- Maternal cyanotic heart disease
- Prior pregnancy with IUGR
- Maternal collagen diseases
- Chronic hypertension
- Preeclampsia
- Recurrent antepartum hemorrhage
- Smoking
- Maternal diabetes with vascular problems
- Fetal infections
- Fetal cardiovascular anomalies
- Drug addiction and alcohol abuse
- Fetal congenital anomalies
- Hemoglobinopathies

OLIGOHYDRAMNIOS

- Renal agenesis (Potter's syndrome)
- Prolonged rupture of membranes
- IUGR
- Intrauterine fetal death

POSTTERM PREGNANCY

- Anencephaly
- Placental sulfatase deficiency
- Perinatal hypoxia, acidosis
- Placental insufficiency

CHROMOSOMAL ABNORMALITIES

- Maternal age 35 years or older
- Balanced translocation (maternal and paternal)

Reference: Gillem-Goldstein, J., et al. (2003). Methods of assessment for pregnancy at risk. In A. DeCherney, & L. Nathan (Eds.), *Current obstetric and gynecologic diagnosis and treatment* (9th ed.). New York: Lange Medical Books/McGraw-Hill.

Sociodemographic risks arise from the mother and her family. These risks may place the mother and fetus at risk. Examples include lack of prenatal care, low income, marital status, and ethnicity (see Box 29-1).

Environmental factors include hazards in the workplace and the woman's general environment and may include environmental chemicals (e.g., pesticides, lead and mercury), radiation, and pollutants (Silbergeld & Patrick, 2005).

Risk factors are interrelated and cumulative in their effects. Box 29-2 lists specific pregnancy problems and risk factors. Risk factors for the postpartum woman and the newborn are shown in Box 29-3.

The development of a comprehensive database for pregnancy risk assessment will help generate appropriate nursing diagnoses. For example, use of functional health patterns can be the basis for an assessment tool (Box 29-4).

---

box 29-3 Factors That Place the Postpartum Woman and Neonate at High Risk

MOTHER
- Hemorrhage
- Infection
- Abnormal vital signs
- Traumatic labor or birth
- Psychosocial factors

INFANT (FOR ADMISSION TO NICU)
High Risk
- Infants who continue with or develop signs of RDS or other respiratory distress
- Asphyxiated infants (Apgar score less than 6 at 5 min), resuscitation required at birth
- Preterm infants, dysmature infants
- Infants with cyanosis or suspected cardiovascular disease, persistent cyanosis
- Infants with major congenital malformations requiring surgery, chromosomal anomalies
- Infants with convulsions, sepsis, hemorrhagic diathesis, or shock
- Meconium aspiration syndrome
- CNS depression for more than 24 hr
- Hypoglycemia
- Hypocalcemia
- Hyperbilirubinemia

Moderate Risk
- Dysmaturity
- Prematurity (weight between 2000 and 2500 g)
- Apgar score less than 5 at 1 min
- Feeding problems
- Multifetal birth
- Transient tachypnea
- Hypomagnesemia or hypermagnesemia
- Hypoparathyroidism
- Failure to gain weight
- Jitteriness or hyperactivity
- Cardiac anomalies not requiring immediate catheterization
- Heart murmur
- Anemia
- CNS depression for less than 24 hr

CNS, Central nervous system; *NICU,* neonatal intensive care unit; *RDS,* respiratory distress syndrome.

---

box 29-4 Assessment for High Risk Pregnancy with Functional Health Patterns

For each of the following functional health patterns, the nurse includes questions that will provide data about the woman, her family, her community, and her cultural practices and beliefs:

- *Health perception or health management pattern.* Current health, medical history, family medical history, environmental or chemical exposure, family decision making about health, community resources, beliefs about health care during pregnancy
- *Nutritional-metabolic pattern.* Nutritional status, knowledge of pregnancy needs, pregnancy discomforts, community resources (e.g., WIC), cultural eating practices
- *Elimination pattern.* Urinary and bowel patterns, family or cultural practices (e.g., laxatives), community waste and sanitation services
- *Activity-exercise pattern.* Usual exercise, recreation, community resources, cultural practices or taboos for activities during pregnancy
- *Sleep-rest pattern.* Usual sleep patterns, use of remedies, family sleep arrangements, cultural beliefs about sleep and rest in pregnancy
- *Cognitive-perceptual pattern.* Communication problems, knowledge deficits about pregnancy and birth (individual and family), community resources for support for high risk pregnant clients, cultural beliefs about pain and its management
- *Self-perception or self-concept pattern.* Body image, responses of family to high risk pregnancy, housing conditions, cultural practices about parenting
- *Role-relationship pattern.* Feelings of security, occupation, hobbies, family living arrangements, community resources
- *Sexuality-reproductive pattern.* Sexual activities, problems, restrictions, obstetric history, current obstetric status, cultural beliefs about sexual practices during pregnancy
- *Coping-stress pattern.* Life stressors, losses experienced, coping mechanisms, support systems, community resources, spiritual or religious practices or beliefs that are important

References: Gilbert, E., & Harmon, J. (2003). *Manual of high risk pregnancy & delivery* (3rd ed.). St. Louis: Mosby; Gordon, M. (2002). *Manual of nursing diagnosis* (10th ed.). St. Louis: Mosby.
WIC, Special Supplemental Nutrition Program for Women, Infants, and Children.

▬ ANTEPARTUM TESTING: ▬ BIOPHYSICAL ASSESSMENT

The major expected outcome of all antepartum testing is the detection of potential fetal compromise. Ideally the technique used identifies fetal compromise before intrauterine asphyxia of the fetus, so that the health care provider can take measures to prevent or minimize adverse perinatal outcomes. No single test can provide this information. Assessment tests should be selected based on their effectiveness, and the results must be interpreted in light of the complete clinical picture. The most reliable evidence for effectiveness is provided by randomized controlled trials. Nurses can be informed about the most recent research on fetal assessment by using an up-to-date systematic review such as the Cochrane Database of Systematic Reviews (Enkin et al., 2001). Table 29-1 lists the evidence for recommending care for fetal assessment screening based on this database.

Daily Fetal Movement Count

Assessment of fetal activity by the mother is a simple yet valuable method for monitoring the condition of the fetus. The daily fetal movement count (DFMC) (also called "kick counts") can be done at home, is noninvasive, is simple to understand, and usually does not interfere with a daily routine. The DFMC is frequently used to monitor the fetus in pregnancies complicated by conditions that

table 29-1 Fetal Assessment Screening: Recommendations for Care

FETAL ASSESSMENT TEST	RECOMMENDATION OR CONCLUSION
• Doppler ultrasound use in pregnancy at high risk for fetal compromise	Beneficial effects
• Ultrasound use to estimate gestational age in first and early second trimesters • Ultrasound use to confirm suspected multiple pregnancy • Ultrasound use for placental location in suspected placenta previa • Ultrasound use to assess amniotic fluid volume • Early second trimester amniocentesis for identification of chromosomal abnormalities • Transabdominal instead of transvaginal chorionic villus sampling (CVS)	Effects likely to be beneficial
• Formal systems of risk scoring • Routine use of early ultrasound • CVS versus amniocentesis for diagnosing chromosomal abnormalities • Serum alpha-fetoprotein screening for neural tube defects • Triple screen test for Down syndrome and neural tube defects	Trade-off between beneficial and adverse effects
• Placental grading by ultrasound to improve perinatal outcome • Biophysical profile for fetal surveillance • Routine fetal movement counts to improve perinatal outcome	Unknown effectiveness
• Routine use of ultrasound for fetal anthropometry (body measurements) in late pregnancy • Use of Doppler ultrasound screening in all pregnancies • Measurement of placental hormones (estriol and human placental lactogen)	Unlikely to be beneficial
• Nipple stimulation test to improve perinatal outcome • Nonselective nonstress test to improve perinatal outcome • Contraction stress test to improve perinatal outcome	Likely to be ineffective or harmful

Source: Enkin, M., Keirse, M., Neilson, J., Crowther, C., Duley, L., Hodnett, E., et al. (2001). Effective care in pregnancy and childbirth: A synopsis. *Birth, 28*(1), 41-51.

may affect fetal oxygenation. These conditions include but are not limited to gestational hypertension or chronic hypertension and diabetes. The presence of movements is generally a reassuring sign of fetal health.

Several methods are used for counting. One recommendation is to count all fetal movements in a 12-hour period each day until a minimum of 10 movements are counted. Another common recommendation is that mothers count fetal activity 2 or 3 times daily (e.g., after meals or before bedtime) for 2 hours until 10 movements are counted (Armour, 2004). Except for establishing a very low number of daily fetal movements or a trend toward decreased motion, the clinical value of the absolute number of fetal movements has not been established, except in the situation in which fetal movements cease entirely for 12 hours (the so-called *fetal alarm signal*). If less than 10 movements are felt within the specified time or movement is perceived to be less than the previous day, the woman should notify her health care provider for further evaluation (Armour).

Women should be taught the significance of the presence and/or absence of fetal movements, the procedure for counting that is to be used, how to record findings on a DFMC record, and when to notify the health care provider.

■ **NURSE ALERT**

In assessing fetal movements, it is important to remember that they are usually not present during the fetal sleep cycle; they may be temporarily reduced if the woman is taking depressant medications, drinking alcohol, or smoking a cigarette. They do not decrease as the woman nears term. Obesity decreases the ability of the mother to assess fetal movement.

Ultrasonography

Sound is a form of wave energy that causes small particles in a medium to oscillate. The frequency of sound, which refers to the number of peaks or waves that move over a given point per unit of time, is expressed in hertz (Hz). Sound with a frequency of 1 cycle, or one peak per second, has a frequency of 1 Hz. When directional beams of sound strike an object, an echo is returned. The time delay between the emission of the sound and the return of the echo and the direction of the echo are noted. From these data, the distance and location of an object can be calculated. Ultrasound is sound frequency higher than that detectable by humans (greater than 20,000 Hz). Diagnostic ultrasound instruments operate within a frequency range of 2 to 10 million Hz (or 2 to 10 MHz), which is below the range used by sonar and radar equipment. Ultrasound images are a reflection of the strength of the sending beam, the strength of the returning echo, and the density of the medium (e.g., muscle [uterus], bone, tissue [placenta], fluid, or blood) through which the beam is sent and returned (Chervenak & Gabbe, 2002).

Diagnostic ultrasonography is an important, safe technique in antepartum fetal surveillance. It provides critical information to health care providers regarding fetal activity and gestational age, normal versus abnormal fetal growth curves, visual assistance with which invasive tests may be performed more safely, fetal and placental anatomy, and fetal well-being (Chervenak & Gabbe, 2002). Ultrasound examination can be done abdominally or transvaginally during pregnancy. Both produce a three-dimensional view from which a pictorial image is obtained. Abdominal ultrasonography is more useful after the first trimester when the pregnant uterus becomes an abdominal organ. For the procedure, the woman usually should have a full bladder to displace the uterus upward to get a better image of the fetus. Transmission gel or paste is applied to the woman's abdomen before a transducer is moved over the skin to enhance transmission and reception of the sound waves. She is positioned with small pillows under her head and knees. The display panel is positioned so that the woman and/or her partner can observe the images on the screen if they desire.

Transvaginal ultrasonography, in which the probe is inserted into the vagina, allows pelvic anatomy to be evaluated in greater detail and intrauterine pregnancy to be diagnosed earlier (Manning, 2004). A transvaginal ultrasound examination is well tolerated by most clients because it alleviates the need for a full bladder. It is especially useful in obese women whose thick abdominal layers cannot be penetrated adequately with an abdominal approach. A transvaginal ultrasound may be performed with the woman in a lithotomy position or with her pelvis elevated by towels, cushions, or a folded pillow. This pelvis tilt is optimal to image the pelvic structures. A protective cover such as a condom, the finger of a clean rubber surgical glove, or a special probe cover provided by the manufacturer is used to cover the transducer probe. The probe is lubricated with a water-soluble gel and placed in the vagina either by the examiner or by the woman herself. During the examination, the position of the probe or the tilt of the examining table may be changed so that the complete pelvis is in view. The procedure is not physically painful, although the woman will feel pressure as the probe is moved. Transvaginal ultrasonography is optimally used in the first trimester to detect ectopic pregnancies, monitor the developing embryo, help identify abnormalities, and help establish gestational age. In some instances it may be used as an adjunct to abdominal scanning to evaluate preterm labor in second- and third-trimester pregnancies.

Levels of Ultrasonography

The American College of Obstetricians and Gynecologists (ACOG, 2004) describes three levels of ultrasonography. The *standard* examination is used most frequently and can be performed by ultrasonographers or other health care professionals, including nurses, who have had special training. Indications for standard ultrasonography are described in detail in the next section; its primary use is to detect fetal viability, determine the presentation of the fetus, assess gestational age, locate the placenta, examine the fetal anatomy for malformations, and determine amniotic fluid volume (AFV). *Limited* examinations are performed for specific indications such as identifying fetal presentation during labor or evaluating fetal heart activity when it is not detected by other methods (ACOG). *Specialized* or targeted examinations are performed if a woman is suspected of carrying an anatomically or a physiologically abnormal fetus. Indications for this comprehensive examination include abnormal findings on clinical examination, especially with polyhydramnios or oligohydramnios, elevated alphafetoprotein (AFP) levels, and a history of offspring with anomalies that can be detected by ultrasound examination. Specialized ultrasonography is performed by highly trained and experienced personnel (ACOG).

Indications for Use

Major indications for obstetric sonography are shown by trimester in Table 29-2. During the first trimester, ultrasound examination is performed to obtain information regarding (1) number, size, and location of gestational sacs; (2) presence or absence of fetal cardiac and body movements; (3) presence or absence of uterine abnormalities (e.g., bicornuate uterus or fibroids) or adnexal masses (e.g., ovarian cysts or an ectopic pregnancy); (4) determination of gestational age (by measuring the crown-rump length); and (5) presence and location of an intrauterine contraceptive device.

During the second and third trimesters, information regarding the following conditions is sought: (1) fetal

table 29-2 **Major Uses of Ultrasonography During Pregnancy**

FIRST TRIMESTER	SECOND TRIMESTER	THIRD TRIMESTER
Confirm pregnancy	Establish or confirm dates	Confirm gestational age
Confirm viability	Confirm viability	Confirm viability
Determine gestational age	Detect polyhydramnios, oligohydramnios	Detect macrosomia
Rule out ectopic pregnancy	Detect congenital anomalies	Detect congenital anomalies
Detect multiple gestation	Detect intrauterine growth restriction (IUGR)	Detect IUGR
Use for visualization during chorionic villus sampling	Confirm placenta placement	Determine fetal position
Detect maternal abnormalities such as bicornuate uterus, ovarian cysts, fibroids	Use for visualization during amniocentesis	Detect placenta previa or abruptio placentae
		Use for visualization during amniocentesis, external version
		Biophysical profile
		Amniotic fluid volume assessment
		Doppler flow studies
		Detect placental maturity

viability, number, position, gestational age, growth pattern, and anomalies; (2) AFV; (3) placental location and maturity; (4) uterine fibroids and anomalies; (5) adnexal masses; and (6) cervical length.

Ultrasonography provides earlier diagnoses, allowing therapy to be instituted early in the pregnancy, thereby decreasing the severity and duration of morbidity, both physical and emotional, for the family. For instance, early diagnosis of a fetal anomaly gives the family choices such as (1) intrauterine surgery or other therapy for the fetus, (2) termination of the pregnancy, or (3) preparation for the care of an infant with a disorder.

Fetal Heart Activity. Fetal heart activity can be demonstrated as early as 6 to 7 weeks by real-time echo scanners and at 10 to 12 weeks by Doppler mode. By 9 to 10 weeks, gestational trophoblastic disease can be diagnosed. Fetal death can be confirmed by lack of heart motion, the presence of fetal scalp edema, and maceration and overlap of the cranial bones.

Gestational Age. Gestational dating by ultrasonography is indicated for conditions and situations such as (1) uncertain dates for the last normal menstrual period, (2) recent discontinuation of oral contraceptives, (3) bleeding episode during the first trimester, (4) uterine size that does not agree with dates, and (5) other high risk conditions.

During the first 20 weeks of gestation, ultrasonography provides an accurate assessment of gestational age because most normal fetuses grow at the same rate. Accuracy is increased as the fetus ages because more than one variable is measured. The four methods of fetal age estimation used include (1) determination of gestational sac dimensions (at about 8 weeks), (2) measurement of crown-rump length (between 7 and 12 weeks), (3) measurement of the biparietal diameter (BPD) (after 12 weeks), and (4) measurement of femur length (after 12 weeks). Fetal BPD at 36 weeks should be approximately 8.7 cm. Term pregnancy and fetal maturity can be diagnosed with some confidence if the biparietal measurement by ultrasound examination is greater than 9.8 cm, especially when this is combined with appropriate femur length measurement.

In later gestational periods, serial measurements can provide a more accurate determination of fetal age. Two and preferably three composite measurements are recommended, at least 2 weeks apart, and these are plotted against standard fetal growth curves. This method, when applied between 24 and 32 weeks of gestation, yields an estimation error of 10 days more or less than the actual age (Manning, 2004).

Fetal Growth. Fetal growth is determined by both intrinsic growth potential and environmental factors. Conditions that require ultrasound assessment of fetal growth include (1) poor maternal weight gain or pattern of weight gain, (2) previous pregnancy with intrauterine growth restriction (IUGR), (3) chronic infections, (4) ingestion of drugs (tobacco, alcohol, and over-the-counter and street drugs), (5) maternal diabetes mellitus, (6) hypertension,

(7) multifetal pregnancy, and (8) other medical or surgical complications.

Serial evaluations of BPD, limb length, and abdominal circumference can allow differentiation among size discrepancy resulting from inaccurate dates, true IUGR, and macrosomia. IUGR may be symmetric (the fetus is small in all parameters) or asymmetric (head and body growth vary). Symmetric IUGR reflects a chronic or long-standing insult and may be caused by low genetic growth potential, intrauterine infection, undernutrition, heavy smoking, or chromosomal aberration. Asymmetric growth suggests an acute or late-occurring deprivation, such as placental insufficiency resulting from hypertension, renal disease, or cardiovascular disease. Reduced fetal growth is still one of the most frequent conditions associated with stillbirth.

Macrosomic infants (those weighing 4000 g or more) are at increased risk for dystocia, traumatic injury, and asphyxia during birth. In addition, fetal macrosomia associated with maternal glucose intolerance or diabetes carries an increased risk of intrauterine fetal death. Macrosomia in the infant of a diabetic mother is asymmetric and characterized by increases in fat and muscle in the abdomen and shoulders, while head circumference remains normal. Macrosomia in an infant whose mother is obese without glucose intolerance results in symmetric changes—excessive growth of abdominal and head circumferences (Chervenak & Gabbe, 2002).

Fetal Anatomy. Anatomic structures that can be identified by ultrasonography (depending on the gestational age) include the following: head (including ventricles and blood vessels) (Fig. 29-1), neck, spine, heart, stomach, small bowel, liver, kidneys, bladder, and limbs. Ultrasonography permits the confirmation of normal anatomy, as well as the detection of major fetal malformations. The presence of an anomaly may influence the location of birth (e.g., a

CRITICAL THINKING EXERCISE

Fetal Growth Assessment

Jenna and Cody, both 23, are expecting their first baby. Jenna is 15 weeks pregnant and has insulin-dependent diabetes mellitus. She tells the nurse that she is relieved to be having an ultrasound done today because the procedure will show whether or not the baby is growing properly and whether she will need to have any more tests. What response to Jenna's statement by the nurse would be appropriate?

1. Evidence—Is there sufficient evidence to draw conclusions about what response the nurse should give?
2. Assumptions—Describe underlying assumptions about the following issues:
   a. Maternal diabetes and potential risks to the fetus
   b. Ultrasound use by trimester
   c. Suggested prenatal follow-up
3. What implications and priorities for nursing care can be made at this time?
4. Does the evidence objectively support your conclusion?
5. Are there alternative perspectives to your conclusion?

FIG. 29-1 Two views of the fetus during ultrasonography. **A,** Fetal face (20 weeks). **B,** Umbilical cord (26 weeks). (Courtesy Advanced Technology Laboratories, Bothell, WA.)

it is seen to be low lying, its relation to the internal cervical os can sometimes be dramatically altered by varying the fullness of the maternal bladder. In approximately 15% to 20% of all pregnancies in which ultrasound scanning is performed during the second trimester, the placenta seems to be overlying the os, but the incidence of placenta previa at term is only 0.5%. Therefore the diagnosis of placenta previa can seldom be confirmed before 27 weeks, primarily because of the elongation of the lower uterine segment as pregnancy advances.

Another use for ultrasonography is grading of placental maturation. Calcium deposits are of significance in postterm pregnancies because as they increase, the available surface area that can be adequately bathed by maternal blood decreases. The point at which this results in fetal

FIG. 29-2 Fetal nuchal translucency. **A,** Nuchal lucency (calipers) and nasal bone (*arrow*) in 12-week fetus. **B,** Increased nuchal translucency. Transvaginal ultrasound performed at 12 weeks demonstrates a sonolucent area (*asterisk*) over the posterior neck and upper thorax. (From Martin, R., Fanaroff, A., & Walsh, M. (2006). *Fanaroff and Martin's neonatal-perinatal medicine: Diseases of the fetus and infant* (8th ed.). Philadelphia: Mosby.)

delivery room versus a labor, delivery, recovery room, or a subspecialty center versus a basic care center) and the method of birth to optimize neonatal outcomes.

The number of fetuses and their presentations also may be assessed by ultrasonography, allowing plans for therapy and mode of birth to be made in advance.

Fetal Genetic Disorders and Physical Anomalies. A prenatal screening technique called *fetal nuchal translucency* (FNT) screening uses ultrasound measurement of fluid in the nape of the fetal neck between 10 and 14 weeks of gestation to identify possible fetal abnormalities (Fig. 29-2). A finding of abnormal fluid collection that is greater than 2.5 mm is considered abnormal, whereas a measurement of 3 mm or greater is highly indicative of genetic disorders and/or physical anomalies. If the FNT is abnormal, diagnostic genetic testing is recommended (ACOG, 2004).

Placental Position and Function. The pattern of uterine and placental growth and the fullness of the maternal bladder influence the apparent location of the placenta by ultrasonography. During the first trimester, differentiation between the endometrium and small placenta is difficult. By 14 to 16 weeks, the placenta is clearly defined, but if wastage and hypoxia cannot be determined precisely; however, the effects are usually observable by 42 weeks and are progressive (Gilbert & Harmon, 2003).

Adjunct to Other Invasive Tests. The safety of amniocentesis is increased when the positions of the fetus, placenta, and pockets of amniotic fluid can be identified accurately. Ultrasound scanning has reduced risks previously associated with amniocentesis, such as fetomaternal hemorrhage from a pierced placenta. Percutaneous umbilical blood sampling (PUBS) and chorionic villus sampling also are guided by ultrasonography to identify the cord and chorion frondosum accurately (see Fig. 29-1, *B*).

Fetal Well-Being

Physiologic parameters of the fetus that can be assessed with ultrasound scanning include amniotic fluid volume, vascular waveforms from the fetal circulation, heart motion, fetal breathing movements (FBMs), fetal urine production, and fetal limb and head movements. Assessment of these parameters, singly or in combination, yields a fairly reliable picture of fetal well-being. The significance of these findings is discussed in the following sections.

Doppler Blood Flow Analysis. One of the major advances in perinatal medicine is the ability to study blood flow noninvasively in the fetus and placenta with ultrasound. Doppler blood flow analysis is a helpful adjunct in the management of pregnancies at risk because of hypertension, IUGR, diabetes mellitus, multiple fetuses, or preterm labor.

When a sound wave is reflected from a moving target, there is a change in frequency of the reflected wave relative to the transmitted wave. This is called the *Doppler effect*. An ultrasound beam scattered by a group of red blood cells (RBCs) is an example of this effect. The velocity of the RBCs can be determined by measuring the change in the frequency of the sound wave reflected off the cells.

The shifted frequencies can be displayed as a plot of velocity versus time, and the shape of these waveforms can be analyzed to give information about blood flow and resistance in a given circulation. Velocity waveforms from umbilical and uterine arteries, reported as systolic/diastolic (S/D) ratios, can be first detected at 15 weeks of pregnancy. Because of the progressive decline in resistance in both the umbilical and uterine arteries, this ratio decreases as pregnancy advances. Most fetuses will achieve an S/D ratio of 3 or less by 30 weeks. Persistent elevation of S/D ratios after 30 weeks is associated with IUGR, usually resulting from UPI (Druzin et al., 2002). In postterm pregnancies evaluated by Doppler umbilical flow studies, an elevated S/D ratio indicates a poorly perfused placenta. Abnormal results also are seen with certain chromosome abnormalities (trisomy 13 and 18) in the fetus and with lupus erythematosus in the mother. Exposure to nicotine from maternal smoking also has been reported to increase the S/D (Fig. 29-3).

Amniotic Fluid Volume. Abnormalities in amniotic fluid volume (AFV) are frequently associated with fetal disorders. Subjective determinants of oligohydramnios (decreased fluid) include the absence of fluid pockets in the uterine cavity and the impression of crowding of small fetal parts. An objective criterion of decreased AFV is met if the largest pocket of fluid measured in two perpendicular planes is less than 2 cm (Manning, 2004). In polyhydramnios (increased fluid), subjective criteria include multiple large pockets of fluid, the impression of a floating fetus, and free movement of fetal limbs. The diagnosis may be made when the largest pocket of fluid exceeds 8 cm in two perpendicular planes (Chervenak & Gabbe, 2002).

FIG. 29-3   Umbilical artery velocity waveform. (From Callen, P. [2000]. *Ultrasonography in obstetrics and gynecology* [4th ed.]. Philadelphia: Saunders.)

The total AFV can be evaluated by a method in which the depths (in centimeters) of the amniotic fluid in all four quadrants surrounding the maternal umbilicus are totaled, providing an amniotic fluid index (AFI). An AFI less than 5 cm indicates oligohydramnios; 5 to 19 cm is considered a normal measurement; and a measurement greater than 20 cm reflects polyhydramnios (Chervenak & Gabbe, 2002). Oligohydramnios is associated with congenital anomalies (such as renal agenesis), growth restriction, and fetal distress during labor. Polyhydramnios is associated with neural tube defects (NTDs), obstruction of the fetal gastrointestinal tract, multiple fetuses, and fetal hydrops.

Biophysical Profile. Real-time ultrasound permits detailed assessment of the physical and physiologic characteristics of the developing fetus and cataloging of normal and abnormal biophysical responses to stimuli. The biophysical profile (BPP) is a noninvasive dynamic assessment of a fetus that is based on acute and chronic markers of fetal disease. The BPP includes AFV, FBMs, fetal movements, and fetal tone determined by ultrasound and fetal heart rate (FHR) and patterns determined by means of a nonstress test (NST). The BPP may therefore be considered a physical examination of the fetus, including determination of vital signs. The fetal response to central hypoxia is alteration in movement, muscle tone, breathing, and heart rate patterns. The presence of normal fetal biophysical activities indicates that the central nervous system (CNS) is functional, and the fetus therefore is not hypoxemic (Harman, 2004). BPP variables and scoring are detailed in Table 29-3.

The BPP is an accurate indicator of impending fetal death. Fetal acidosis can be diagnosed early with a nonreactive NST and absent FBMs. An abnormal BPP score and oligohydramnios are indications that labor should be induced (Harman, 2004). Fetal infection in women whose membranes rupture prematurely (at less than 37 weeks of gestation) can be diagnosed early by changes in biophysical activity that precede the clinical signs of infection and indicate the necessity for immediate birth. When the BPP score is normal and the risk of fetal death low, intervention is indicated only for obstetric or maternal factors.

Nursing Role

Although a growing number of nurses perform ultrasound scans and BPPs in certain centers, the main role of nurses is in counseling and educating women about the procedure (Garcia et al., 2002). Providing accurate information regarding the procedure is imperative to allay the mother's anxiety. Although ultrasound scanning has become a widely used diagnostic tool, recommendations for the procedure are based on expectations of a fetal problem and therefore may cause concern. Women should be provided ample opportunity to ask questions and be reassured that the procedure is safe. In the 30 years that diagnostic ultrasonography has been used, no conclusive evidence of any harmful effects on humans has emerged. Although the possibility of unidentified biologic effects exists, the benefits to the woman of prudent use of diagnostic ultrasonography appear to outweigh any possible risk (Chervenak & Gabbe, 2002).

■ **LEGAL TIP** Performance of Limited Ultrasound Examinations

Nurses who have the training and competence may perform limited ultrasound examinations if it is within the scope of practice in their state or area and consistent with regulations of the agencies in which they practice (Menihan, 2000). Limited ultrasound examinations include identification of fetal number, fetal presentation, fetal cardiac activity, location of the placenta,

table 29-3	Biophysical Profile	
VARIABLES	**NORMAL (SCORE = 2)**	**ABNORMAL (SCORE = 0)**
Fetal breathing movements	One or more episodes in 30 min, each lasting ≥30 sec	Episodes absent or no episode ≥30 sec in 30 min
Gross body movements	Three or more discrete body or limb movements in 30 min (episodes of active continuous movement are considered as a single movement)	Less than three episodes of body or limb movements in 30 min
Fetal tone	One or more episodes of active extension with return to flexion of fetal limb(s) or trunk; opening and closing of hand is considered normal tone	Slow extension with return to flexion, movement of limb in full extension, or fetal movement absent
Reactive fetal heart rate	Two or more episodes of acceleration (≥15 beats/min) in 20 min, each lasting ≥15 sec and associated with fetal movement	Less than two episodes of acceleration or acceleration of <15 beats/min in 20 min
Qualitative amniotic fluid volume	One or more pockets of fluid measuring ≥1 cm in two perpendicular planes	Pockets absent or pocket <1 cm in two perpendicular planes
SCORE		
Normal	8-10 (if amniotic fluid index is adequate)	
Equivocal	6	
Abnormal	<4	

Reference: Harman, C. (2004). Assessment of fetal health. In R. Creasy, R. Resnik, & J. Iams (Eds.), *Maternal-fetal medicine: Principles and practice* (5th ed.). Philadelphia: Saunders.

and BPP, including AFV assessment. Women should be informed about the limited information provided by these examinations. They are not meant to evaluate or identify fetal anomalies, assess fetal age, or estimate fetal weight (Stringer, Miesnik, Brown, Menei, & Macones, 2003). The obstetric health care provider is responsible for obtaining a more comprehensive ultrasound examination when complete client assessment is necessary (Association of Women's Health, Obstetric and Neonatal Nurses [AWHONN], 1998).

Magnetic Resonance Imaging

Magnetic resonance imaging (MRI) is a noninvasive radiologic technique used for obstetric and gynecologic diagnosis. Like computed tomography (CT), MRI provides excellent pictures of soft tissue. Unlike CT, ionizing radiation is not used; therefore vascular structures within the body can be visualized and evaluated without injection of an iodinated contrast medium, thus eliminating any known biologic risk. Like sonography, MRI is noninvasive and can provide images in multiple planes, but there is no interference from skeletal, fatty, or gas-filled structures, and imaging of deep pelvic structures does not require a full bladder.

With MRI, the examiner can evaluate (1) fetal structure (CNS, thorax, abdomen, genitourinary tract, musculoskeletal system) and overall growth; (2) placenta (position, density, and presence of gestational trophoblastic disease); (3) quantity of amniotic fluid; (4) maternal structures (uterus, cervix, adnexa, and pelvis); (5) biochemical status (pH, adenosine triphosphate content) of tissues and organs; and (6) soft-tissue, metabolic, or functional anomalies.

The woman is placed on a table in the supine position and slid into the bore of the main magnet, which is similar in appearance to a CT scanner. Depending on the reason for the study, the procedure may take from 20 to 60 minutes, during which time the woman must be perfectly still except for short respites. Because of the long time needed to produce MRIs, the fetus will probably move, which will obscure anatomic details. The only way to ensure that this does not occur is to administer a sedative to the mother, but this approach should be reserved for selected cases in which visualization of fetal detail is critical.

MRI has little effect on the fetus; concerns that the FHR or fetal movement would decrease have not been supported.

■ BIOCHEMICAL ASSESSMENT

Biochemical assessment involves biologic examination (e.g., chromosomes in exfoliated cells) and chemical determinations (e.g., lecithin/sphingomyelin [L/S] ratio and bilirubin level) (Table 29-4). Procedures used to obtain the needed specimens include amniocentesis, PUBS, chorionic villus sampling, and maternal sampling (Box 29-5).

box 29-5 Fetal Rights

Amniocentesis, percutaneous umbilical blood sampling (PUBS), and chorionic villus sampling (CVS) are prenatal tests used for diagnosing fetal defects in pregnancy. They are invasive and carry risks to the mother and fetus. A consideration of elective abortion is linked to the performance of these tests because there is no treatment for genetically affected fetuses; therefore, the issue of fetal rights is a key ethical concern in prenatal testing for fetal defects.

table 29-4 Summary of Biochemical Monitoring Techniques

TEST	POSSIBLE FINDINGS	CLINICAL SIGNIFICANCE
MATERNAL BLOOD		
Coombs' test	Titer of 1:8 and increasing	Significant Rh incompatibility
Alpha-fetoprotein (AFP)	See below	See below
AMNIOTIC FLUID ANALYSIS		
Color	Meconium	Possible hypoxia or asphyxia
Lung profile		Fetal lung maturity
L/S ratio	>2:1	
Phosphatidylglycerol	Present	
Creatinine	>2 mg/dl	Gestational age >36 weeks
Bilirubin (ΔOD, 450/nm)	<0.015	Gestational age >36 weeks, normal pregnancy
	High levels	Fetal hemolytic disease in Rh-isoimmunized pregnancies
Lipid cells	>10%	Gestational age >35 weeks
AFP	High levels after 15 week gestation	Open neural tube or other defect
Osmolality	Decline after 20-week gestation	Advancing nonspecific gestational age
Genetic disorders	Dependent on cultured cells for karyotype and enzymatic activity	Counseling possibly required
Sex-linked		
Chromosomal		
Metabolic		

AFP, Alpha-fetoprotein; *L/S,* lecithin-sphingomyelin; *ΔOD,* delta optical density.

Amniocentesis

Amniocentesis is performed to obtain amniotic fluid, which contains fetal cells. Under direct ultrasonographic visualization, a needle is inserted transabdominally into the uterus, amniotic fluid is withdrawn into a syringe, and the various assessments are performed (Fig. 29-4). Amniocentesis is possible after week 14 of pregnancy, when the uterus becomes an abdominal organ, and sufficient amniotic fluid is available for testing. Indications for the procedure include prenatal diagnosis of genetic disorders or congenital anomalies (NTDs in particular), assessment of pulmonary maturity, and diagnosis of fetal hemolytic disease.

Complications in the mother and fetus occur in fewer than 1% of the cases and include the following:
- *Maternal:* Hemorrhage, fetomaternal hemorrhage with possible maternal Rh isoimmunization, infection, labor, abruptio placentae, inadvertent damage to the intestines or bladder, and amniotic fluid embolism. Because of the possibility of fetomaternal hemorrhage, it is standard practice after an amniocentesis to administer Rh$_o$D immune globulin to the woman who is Rh negative.
- *Fetal:* Death, hemorrhage, infection (amnionitis), direct injury from the needle, miscarriage or preterm labor, and leakage of amniotic fluid.

Many of the complications have been minimized or eliminated by using ultrasonography to direct the procedure.

Indications for Use

Genetic Concerns. Prenatal assessment of genetic disorders is indicated in women older than 35 years (Box 29-6), with a previous child with a chromosomal abnormality, or with a family history of chromosomal anomalies. Inherited inborn errors of metabolism (such as Tay-Sachs disease, hemophilia, and thalassemia) and other disorders for which marker genes are known also may be detected. Fetal cells are cultured for karyotyping of chromosomes (see Chapter 3). Karyotyping also permits determination of fetal sex, which is important if an X-linked disorder (occurring almost always in a male fetus) is suspected.

Biochemical analysis of enzymes in amniotic fluid can detect inborn errors of metabolism. For example, alpha-fetoprotein (AFP) levels in amniotic fluid are assessed as a follow-up for elevated levels in maternal serum. High AFP levels in amniotic fluid help confirm the diagnosis of an NTD such as spina bifida or anencephaly or an abdominal wall defect such as omphalocele. The elevation results from the increased leakage of cerebrospinal fluid into the amniotic fluid through the closure defect. AFP levels may also be elevated in a normal multifetal pregnancy and

---

box 29-6 Elimination of Maternal Age as an Indication for Invasive Prenatal Diagnosis

Maternal age of 35 years and older has been a standard indication for invasive prenatal testing since 1979 despite a sensitivity of only 30%. The importance of age as a single indication for testing is being reevaluated, as serum screening has evolved. The most effective use of resources involves screening the whole population of pregnant women. At present many centers offer the option of serum screening before invasive testing for women over 35 years of age.

Reference: Jenkins, T., & Wapner, R. (2004). Prenatal diagnosis of congenital disorders. In R. Creasy, R. Resnik, & J. Iams (Eds.), *Maternal-fetal medicine: Principles and practice* (5th ed.). Philadelphia: Saunders.

FIG. 29-4 **A,** Amniocentesis and laboratory use of amniotic fluid aspirant. **B,** Transabdominal amniocentesis. (**B,** Courtesy Marjorie Pyle, RNC, Lifecircle, Costa Mesa, CA.)

with intestinal atresia, presumably caused by lack of fetal swallowing.

A concurrent test that finds the presence of acetylcholinesterase almost always indicates a fetal defect (Jenkins & Wapner, 2004). In such instances, follow-up ultrasound examination is recommended.

Fetal Maturity. Accurate assessment of fetal maturity is possible through examination of amniotic fluid or its exfoliated cellular contents. The laboratory tests described are determinants of term pregnancy and fetal maturity (see Table 21-4). A quick means of determining an approximate L/S ratio is the *shake test,* foam test, or bubble stability test. Serial dilutions of fresh amniotic fluid are mixed with ethanol and shaken. After 15 minutes, the amount of bubbles present at different dilutions indicates the presence of surfactant.

Fetal Hemolytic Disease. Another indication for amniocentesis is the identification and follow-up of fetal hemolytic disease in cases of isoimmunization. The procedure is usually not done until the mother's antibody titer reaches 1:8 and is increasing. Currently PUBS is the procedure of choice to evaluate and treat fetal hemolytic disease.

EVIDENCE-BASED PRACTICE

Postmaturity of Pregnancy

BACKGROUND
- In the United States, 7% of all pregnancies extend beyond 42 weeks. Prolonged pregnancy may cause the fetus to outgrow the blood supply provided by the aging placenta. Uteroplacental insufficiency may lead to stillbirth, meconium aspiration, growth restriction, and intrapartal asphyxia. Macrosomia may lead to labor abnormalities and trauma. Nonstress and contraction stress tests, biophysical profile, and Doppler blood flow tests are used frequently to monitor fetal well-being of the postmature pregnancy. The Bishop score and fibronectin tests help determine cervical readiness for labor. Interventions are labor induction or cesarean birth.

OBJECTIVES
- The task of the reviewers was to examine risks, benefits, and costs of prenatal testing and management of postmature pregnancy. Specifically, they wanted to know the safety and benefits of fetal well-being tests and labor induction methods. Clinically relevant outcomes included cervical changes, perinatal and maternal mortality, fetal distress, type of birth, labor augmentation, complications, and costs.

METHODS
Search Strategy
- The authors searched research databases and reference lists, and consulted experts for studies dated 1980 to 2001. They identified randomized controlled trials, cohort studies, and large case studies. Number of trials, subjects, and countries of origin were not noted. To enhance the epidemiologic and demographic picture, data was included from the Nationwide Inpatient Sample, a databank from over 1000 hospitals in 22 states, representing 20% of all U.S. hospitals.

Statistical Analyses
- Similar data were pooled. Reviewers calculated relative risk for dichotomous (categoric) data, such as type of birth, and weighted mean difference for continuous data, such as gestational age. Differences between groups outside the 95% confidence interval were accepted as significant.

FINDINGS
- Stillbirth increases with postmaturity. No evidence links postmaturity fetal well-being testing to better outcomes. Testing that combined fetal heart rate and amniotic fluid index was the most sensitive. Testing becomes less sensitive as gestational age advances. Planned induction was safer and less expensive than waiting beyond 41 weeks. Cervical examination, while predictive for labor induction success, was still subject to clinician skill.
- Labor induction was accomplished best by misoprostol, then by prostaglandins, oxytocin, manual nipple stimulation, sweeping membranes, and castor oil. Any intervention which shortened labor tended to increase the risk for uterine hyperstimulation and fetal compromise. Mifepristone (RU-486) was effective at reducing time to birth, but was associated with fetal compromise and lower Apgar scores.
- There were no ethnic differences for incidence of postmaturity, but African-American women with prolonged pregnancies were more likely to have intrauterine growth restriction and oligohydramnios.

LIMITATIONS
- Not all the included data comes from randomized controlled trials, the gold standard for minimizing bias. The available report is a summary, with no information about the trials selected. Costs were rarely mentioned.

IMPLICATIONS FOR PRACTICE
- Decision making for postmaturity involves weighing risks and benefits of intervention versus expectant management. After the clinician makes the judgment call, it typically falls to the nurse to answer the questions of worried parents. It appears that induction is preferable to waiting after 41 weeks. There was not enough evidence to recommend a particular induction intervention.

IMPLICATIONS FOR FURTHER RESEARCH
- Much research is needed about postmaturity management for ethnic and socioeconomic groups. Factors such as nutrition and stress may be factors in prolonged pregnancy. Low-technology interventions which can be easily reversed will be best suited for low-resource countries. Researchers can determine safety, specific timing, dosing, and costs of intervention for induction.

Reference: Myers, E., Blumrick, R., Christian, A., Datta, S., Gray, R., Kolimaga, J., et al. (2002). *Management of prolonged pregnancy (AHRQ Publication No. 02-E018)*. Rockville, MD: Agency for Healthcare Research and Quality.

Meconium. The presence of meconium in the amniotic fluid is usually determined by visual inspection of the sample. The significance of meconium in the fluid varies depending on when it is found.

Antepartal Period. Meconium in the amniotic fluid before the beginning of labor is not usually associated with an adverse fetal outcome. The finding may be the result of acute and subsequently corrected fetal stress, chronic continuing stress, or simply the physiologic passage of meconium. Because there has been some association between meconium in amniotic fluid in the third trimester and hypertensive disorders and postmaturity, the fetus should undergo further antepartum evaluation if the birth is not imminent (Glantz & Woods, 2004).

Intrapartal Period. Intrapartal meconium-stained amniotic fluid is an indication for more careful evaluation by electronic fetal monitoring (EFM) and perhaps fetal scalp blood sampling. The presence of meconium, however, should not be the sole indicator for intervention.

Three possible reasons for the passage of meconium during the intrapartal period are as follows: (1) it is a normal physiologic function that occurs with maturity (meconium passage being infrequent before weeks 23 or 24, with an increased incidence after 38 weeks) or with a breech presentation; (2) it is the result of hypoxia-induced peristalsis and sphincter relaxation; and (3) it may be a sequel to umbilical cord compression–induced vagal stimulation in mature fetuses. Thick, fresh meconium passed for the first time in late labor and in association with nonremediable severe variable or late FHR decelerations is an ominous sign.

It is a common practice for the birth team to suction the nasopharynx or oropharynx of infants born in the presence of meconium-stained amniotic fluid at the time of birth, usually before the first breath is taken, to reduce the incidence and severity of meconium aspiration. However, this practice is no longer recommended. Research does not support the efficacy of routine intrapartum suctioning to prevent meconium aspiration syndrome (Vain, Szyld, Prudent, Wiswell, Aguilar, & Vivas, 2004).

Chorionic Villus Sampling

The combined advantages of earlier diagnosis and rapid results have made chorionic villus sampling (CVS) a popular technique for genetic studies, although some risks to the fetus exist. Although indications for CVS are similar to those for amniocentesis, second-trimester amniocentesis appears to be safer than CVS (Alfirevic, Sundberg, & Brigham, 2003). The benefits of earlier diagnosis must be weighed against the increased risk of pregnancy loss and risk of anomalies.

The procedure is performed between 10 and 12 weeks of gestation and involves the removal of a small tissue specimen from the fetal portion of the placenta (Fig. 29-5). Because chorionic villi originate in the zygote, this tissue reflects the genetic makeup of the fetus.

CVS procedures can be accomplished either transcervically or transabdominally. In transcervical sampling, a sterile catheter is introduced into the cervix under continuous ultrasonographic guidance, and a small portion of the chorionic villi is aspirated with a syringe. The aspiration cannula and obturator must be placed at a suitable site, and rupture of the amniotic sac must be avoided.

If the abdominal approach is used, an 18 gauge spinal needle with stylet is inserted under sterile conditions

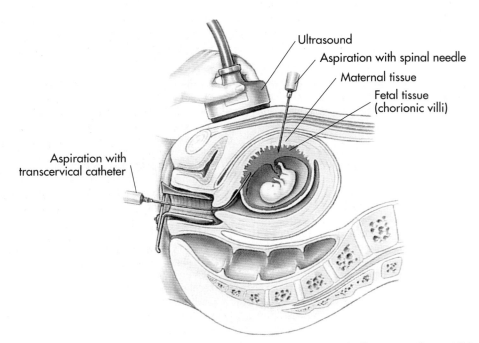

Ultrasound
Aspiration with spinal needle
Maternal tissue
Fetal tissue (chorionic villi)
Aspiration with transcervical catheter

FIG. 29-5 Chorionic villus sampling. (Courtesy Medical and Scientific Illustration, Crozet, VA.)

through the abdominal wall into the chorion frondosum under ultrasound guidance. The stylet is then withdrawn, and the chorionic tissue is aspirated into a syringe (see Fig. 29-5).

Complications of the procedure include vaginal spotting or bleeding immediately afterward, miscarriage (in 0.3% of cases), rupture of membranes (in 0.1% of cases), and chorioamnionitis (in 0.5% of cases). Because of the possibility of fetomaternal hemorrhage, women who are Rh negative should receive immune globulin to avoid isoimmunization (Gilbert & Harmon, 2003). An increased risk of limb anomalies (transverse digital anomalies) has been noted when CVS is done before 10 weeks of gestation (Wilson, 2000).

Use of amniocentesis and CVS is declining because of advances in noninvasive screening techniques. These techniques include measurement of nuchal translucency, maternal serum screening tests in the first and second trimesters, and ultrasonography in the second trimester (Benn, Egan, Fang, & Smith-Bindman, 2004).

Percutaneous Umbilical Blood Sampling

Direct access to the fetal circulation during the second and third trimesters is possible through percutaneous umbilical sampling (PUBS), or cordocentesis, which is the most widely used method for fetal blood sampling and transfusion. PUBS involves the insertion of a needle directly into a fetal umbilical vessel under ultrasound guidance. Ideally, the umbilical cord is punctured 1 to 2 cm from its insertion into the placenta (Fig. 29-6) (Simpson, 2002). At this point the cord is well anchored and will not move, and the risk of maternal blood contamination (from the placenta) is slight. Generally, 1 to 4 ml of blood is removed and tested immediately by the Kleihauer-Betke procedure to ensure that it is fetal in origin. Indications for use of PUBS include prenatal diagnosis of inherited blood disorders, karyotyping of malformed fetuses, detection of fetal infection, determination of the acid-base status of fetuses with IUGR, and assessment and treatment of isoimmunization and thrombocytopenia in the fetus (Jenkins & Wapner, 2004). Complications that can occur include leaking of blood from the puncture site, cord laceration, thromboembolism, preterm labor, premature rupture of membranes, and infection (Simpson).

In fetuses at risk for isoimmune hemolytic anemia, PUBS permits precise identification of fetal blood type and RBC count and may prevent the need for further intervention. If the fetus is positive for the presence of maternal antibodies, a direct blood test can confirm the degree of anemia resulting from hemolysis. Intrauterine transfusion of severely anemic fetuses can be done 4 to 5 weeks earlier than through the intraperitoneal route.

Follow-up includes continuous FHR monitoring for several minutes to 1 hour and a repeated ultrasound examination 1 hour later to ensure that no further bleeding or hematoma formation has occurred.

FIG. 29-6 Technique for percutaneous umbilical blood sampling guided by ultrasound.

Maternal Assays
Alpha-Fetoprotein

Maternal serum alpha-fetoprotein (MSAFP) levels have been used as a screening tool for NTDs in pregnancy. Through this technique, approximately 80% to 85% of all open NTDs and open abdominal wall defects can be detected early in pregnancy. Screening is recommended for all pregnant women.

The cause of NTDs is not well understood, but 95% of all affected infants are born to women with no family history of similar anomalies (Jenkins & Wapner, 2004). The defect occurs in 1 to 2 per 1000 births in most parts of the United States. The birth of one affected child increases the risk of NTD recurrence in future pregnancies to 1% to 5% (Fanaroff, Martin, & Rodriguez, 2004).

AFP is produced by the fetal liver, and increasing levels are detectable in the serum of pregnant women from 14 to 34 weeks. Although amniotic fluid AFP is diagnostic for NTD, MSAFP is a screening tool only and identifies candidates for the more definitive procedures of amniocentesis and ultrasound examination. MSAFP screening can be done with reasonable reliability any time between 15 and 22 weeks of gestation (16 to 18 weeks being ideal) (Jenkins & Wapner, 2004).

Once the maternal level of AFP is determined, it is compared with normal values for each week of gestation. Values also should be correlated with maternal age, weight, race, and whether the woman has insulin-dependent diabetes. If findings are abnormal, follow-up procedures include genetic counseling for families with a history of NTD, repeated AFP, ultrasound examination and, possibly, amniocentesis.

Down syndrome and probably other autosomal trisomies are associated with lower-than-normal levels of MSAFP and amniotic fluid AFP. The *triple-marker test* also is performed at 16 to 18 weeks of gestation and uses the levels of three maternal serum markers, MSAFP, unconjugated estriol, and human chorionic gonadotropin (hCG), in combination with maternal age, to calculate a new risk level. In the presence of a fetus with Down syndrome, the MSAFP and unconjugated estriol levels are low, whereas the hCG level is elevated. With these two additional screening tests, approximately 60% of cases of Down syndrome can be identified. Other maternal markers are being investigated as predictors of fetal abnormalities as well. Serum pregnancy-associated placental protein A (PAPP-A) is low in Down syndrome, whereas another substance, inhibin-A, is elevated in Down syndrome and other trisomies (Simpson, 2002).

As with MSAFP, these tests are screening procedures only and are not diagnostic. A definitive examination of amniotic fluid for AFP and chromosomal analysis combined with ultrasound visualization of the fetus is necessary for diagnosis.

Coombs' Test

The indirect Coombs' test is a screening for Rh incompatibility. If the maternal titer for Rh antibodies is greater than 1:8, amniocentesis for determination of bilirubin in amniotic fluid is indicated to establish the severity of fetal hemolytic anemia. Coombs' test also can detect other antibodies that may place the fetus at risk for incompatibility with maternal antigens.

▬ ANTEPARTAL ASSESSMENT USING ▬ ELECTRONIC FETAL MONITORING

Indications

First- and second-trimester antepartal assessment is directed primarily at the diagnosis of fetal anomalies. The goal of third-trimester testing is to determine whether the intrauterine environment continues to be supportive to the fetus. The testing is often used to determine the timing of childbirth for women at risk for UPI. Gradual loss of placental function results first in inadequate nutrient delivery to the fetus, leading to IUGR. Subsequently, respiratory function also is compromised, resulting in fetal hypoxia. Common indications for both the nonstress test (NST) and the contraction stress test (CST) are listed in Box 29-7.

---

box 29-7 Indications for Electronic Fetal Monitoring Assessment Using NST and CST

- Maternal diabetes mellitus
- Chronic hypertension
- Hypertensive disorders in pregnancy
- Intrauterine growth restriction
- Sickle cell disease
- Maternal cyanotic heart disease
- Postmaturity
- History of previous stillbirth
- Decreased fetal movement
- Isoimmunization
- Meconium-stained amniotic fluid at third-trimester amniocentesis
- Hyperthyroidism
- Collagen disease
- Older pregnant woman
- Chronic renal disease

CST, Contraction stress test; *NST,* nonstress test.

No clinical contraindications exist for the NST, but results may not be conclusive if gestation is 26 weeks or less. Absolute contraindications for the CST are the following: rupture of membranes, previous classic incision for cesarean birth, preterm labor, placenta previa, and abruptio placentae. Other conditions in which the CST may be contraindicated are multifetal pregnancy, previous preterm labor, hydramnios, more than 36 weeks of gestation, and incompetent cervix. As a rule, reactive patterns with the NST or negative results with the CST are associated with favorable outcomes.

Fetal Responses to Hypoxia and Asphyxia

Observable fetal responses to hypoxia or asphyxia are the clinical basis for testing with EFM. Hypoxia or asphyxia elicits a number of responses in the fetus. Blood flow is redistributed to certain vital organs. This series of responses (redistribution of blood flow favoring vital organs, decrease in total oxygen consumption, and switch to anaerobic glycolysis) is a temporary mechanism that enables the fetus to survive up to 30 minutes of limited oxygen supply without decompensation of vital organs. However, during more severe asphyxia or sustained hypoxemia, these compensatory responses are no longer maintained, and a decrease in the cardiac output, arterial blood pressure, and blood flow to the brain and heart occurs (Parer & Nageotte, 2004), with characteristic FHR patterns reflecting these changes.

Variability

Considerable evidence supports the clinical belief that FHR variability indicates an intact nervous pathway through the cerebral cortex, midbrain, vagus nerve, and cardiac conduction system. With 98% accuracy in predicting fetal well-being, the presence of normal FHR variability is a reassuring indicator. Inputs from various areas of the brain decrease after cerebral asphyxia, leading to a decrease in variability after failure of the fetal hemodynamic compensatory mechanisms to maintain cerebral oxygenation (Parer & Nageotte, 2004).

Nonstress Test

The NST is the most widely applied technique for antepartum evaluation of the fetus. It is an ideal screening test and is the primary method of antepartum fetal assessment at most sites. The basis for the NST is the principle that the normal fetus will produce characteristic HR patterns in response to fetal movement. In the healthy fetus with an intact CNS, 90% of gross fetal body movements are associated with accelerations of the FHR. The acceleration with movement response may be blunted by hypoxia, acidosis, drugs (analgesics, barbiturates, and beta-blockers), fetal sleep, and some congenital anomalies (Tucker, 2004). The NST can be performed easily and quickly in an outpatient setting because it is noninvasive, is relatively inexpensive, and has no known contraindications. Disadvantages center around the high rate of false-positive results for non-reactivity as a result of fetal sleep cycles, chronic tobacco smoking, medications, and fetal immaturity. The test also is slightly less sensitive in detecting fetal compromise than are the CST or BPP.

Procedure

The woman is seated in a reclining chair (or in semi-Fowler position) with a slight left or right tilt to optimize uterine perfusion and avoid supine hypotension. The FHR is recorded with a Doppler transducer, and a to-codynamometer is applied to detect uterine contractions or fetal movements. The tracing is observed for signs of fetal activity and a concurrent acceleration of FHR. If evidence of fetal movement is not apparent on the tracing, the woman may be asked to depress a button on a hand-held event marker connected to the monitor when she feels fetal movement. The movement is then noted on the tracing. Because almost all accelerations are accompanied by fetal movement, the movements need not be recorded for the test to be considered reactive. The test is usually completed within 20 to 30 minutes, but it may take longer if the fetus must be awakened from a sleep state.

It has been suggested that the woman drink orange juice or be given glucose to increase her blood sugar level and thereby stimulate fetal movements. This practice is common; however, research has not proven it to be effective (Tan & Sabapathy, 2004). Some sources suggest that fetal movements increase when maternal glucose levels are low. Other methods that have been used to stimulate fetal activity, such as manipulating the woman's abdomen or using a transvaginal light, have not been very effective either. Only vibroacoustic stimulation has had some impact (Tan & Smyth, 2004).

Interpretation

Generally accepted criteria for a reactive tracing are as follows:
- Two or more accelerations of 15 beats/min lasting for 15 seconds over a 20 minute period
- Normal baseline rate
- Moderate variability

If the test does not meet the criteria after 40 minutes, it is considered nonreactive (Fig. 29-7 and Table 29-5), in which case further assessments are needed with a CST or BPP. The current recommendation is that the NST be performed twice weekly (after 28 weeks of gestation) with women who have diabetes or are at risk for having a fetal death (Druzin et al., 2002).

Vibroacoustic Stimulation

Vibroacoustic stimulation (also called *fetal acoustic stimulation test*) is another method of testing antepartum FHR response and is sometimes used in conjunction with the NST. The test takes approximately 15 minutes to complete, with the fetus monitored for 5 to 10 minutes before stimulation to obtain a baseline FHR. If the fetal baseline pattern is nonreactive, the sound source (usually a laryngeal stimulator) is then activated for 3 seconds on the maternal abdomen over the fetal head. Monitoring continues for another 5 minutes, after which the monitor tracing is assessed. A test is considered reactive if there is an immediate and sustained increase in long-term variability and HR accelerations. The accelerations produced may have a significant increase in duration. The test may be repeated at 1-minute intervals up to 3 times when there is no response. Further evaluation is needed with BPP or CST if the pattern is still nonreactive (Druzin et al., 2002).

Contraction Stress Test

The CST is one of the first electronic methods to be developed for assessment of fetal health. It was devised as a graded stress test of the fetus, and its purpose was to identify the jeopardized fetus that was stable at rest but showed evidence of compromise after stress. Uterine contractions decrease uterine blood flow and placental perfusion. If this decrease is sufficient to produce hypoxia in the fetus,

FIG. 29-7 Reactive nonstress test (fetal heart rate acceleration with movement). (From Tucker, S. [2004]. *Pocket guide to fetal monitoring and assessment* [5th ed.]. St. Louis: Mosby.)

table 29-5	Interpretation of the Nonstress Test	
RESULT	**INTERPRETATION**	**CLINICAL SIGNIFICANCE**
Reactive	Two or more accelerations of FHR of 15 beats/min lasting ≥15 sec, associated with each fetal movement in 20 min period (see Fig. 29-7)	As long as twice-weekly NSTs remain reactive, most high risk pregnancies are allowed to continue
Nonreactive	Any tracing with either no FHR accelerations or accelerations <15 beats/min or lasting <15 sec throughout any fetal movement during testing period	Further indirect monitoring may be attempted with abdominal fetal electrocardiography in effort to clarify FHR pattern and quantify variability; external monitoring should continue, and CST or BPP should be done
Unsatisfactory	Quality of FHR recording not adequate for interpretation	Test is repeated in 24 hr or CST is done, depending on clinical situation

Reference: Tucker, S. (2004). *Pocket guide to fetal monitoring and assessment* (5th ed.). St. Louis: Mosby.
BPP, Biophysical profile; *CST*, contraction stress test; *FHR*, fetal heart rate; *NST*, nonstress test.

a deceleration in FHR will result, beginning at the peak of the contraction and persisting after its conclusion (late deceleration).

▬ NURSE ALERT

In a healthy fetoplacental unit, uterine contractions usually do not produce late decelerations, whereas if there is underlying uteroplacental insufficiency, contractions will produce late decelerations.

The CST provides an earlier warning of fetal compromise than the NST and with fewer false-positive results. In addition to the contraindications described earlier, the CST is more time consuming and expensive than the NST. It also is an invasive procedure if oxytocin stimulation is required. The CST is infrequently used.

Procedure

The woman is placed in semi-Fowler position or sits in a reclining chair with a slight left or right tilt to optimize uterine perfusion and avoid supine hypotension. She is monitored electronically with the fetal ultrasound transducer and uterine tocodynamometer. The tracing is observed for 10 to 20 minutes for baseline rate, moderate variability, and the possible occurrence of spontaneous contractions. The two methods of CST are the nipple-stimulated contraction test and the oxytocin-stimulated contraction test.

Nipple-Stimulated Contraction Test. Several methods of nipple stimulation have been described. In one approach the woman applies warm, moist washcloths to both breasts for several minutes. The woman is then asked to massage one nipple for 10 minutes. Massaging the nipples causes a release of oxytocin from the posterior pituitary. An alternative approach is for her to massage the nipple for 2 minutes, rest for 5 minutes, and repeat the cycles of massage and rest as necessary to achieve adequate uterine activity. When adequate contractions or hyperstimulation (defined as uterine contractions lasting more than 90 seconds or five or more contractions in 10 minutes) occurs, stimulation should be stopped (Druzin et al., 2002).

Oxytocin-Stimulated Contraction Test. Exogenous oxytocin also can be used to stimulate uterine contrac-

tions. An intravenous (IV) infusion is begun with a scalp needle. The oxytocin is diluted in an IV solution (e.g., 10 units in 1000 ml of fluid), infused into the tubing of the main IV device through a piggyback port, and delivered by an infusion pump to ensure accurate dosage. One method of oxytocin infusion is to begin at 0.5 milliunits/min and increase the dose by 0.5 milliunits/min at 15- to 30-minute intervals until three uterine contractions of good quality are observed within a 10-minute period. A rate of 10 milliunits/min is usually adequate to elicit uterine contractions (Druzin et al., 2002).

Interpretation

If no late decelerations are observed with the contractions, the findings are considered negative (Fig. 29-8, *A*). Repetitive late decelerations render the test results positive (Fig. 29-8, *B*, and Table 29-6).

FIG. 29-8 Contraction stress test (CST). **A,** Negative CST. **B,** Positive CST. (From Tucker, S. [2004]. *Pocket guide to fetal monitoring and assessment* [5th ed.]. St. Louis: Mosby.)

table 29-6	Guide for Interpretation of the Contraction Stress Test
INTERPRETATION	**CLINICAL SIGNIFICANCE**
NEGATIVE No late decelerations, with minimum of three uterine contractions lasting 40 to 60 sec within 10 min period (see Fig. 29-8, A)	Reassurance that the fetus is likely to survive labor should it occur within 1 wk; more frequent testing may be indicated by clinical situation
POSITIVE Persistent and consistent late decelerations occurring with more than half of contractions (see Fig. 29-8, B)	Management decision lies between use of other tools of fetal assessment such as BPP and termination of pregnancy; a positive test result indicates that fetus is at increased risk for perinatal morbidity and mortality; physician may perform expeditious vaginal birth after successful induction or may proceed directly to cesarean birth; decision to intervene is determined by fetal monitoring and presence of FHR reactivity
SUSPICIOUS Late decelerations occurring in less than half of uterine contractions once adequate contraction pattern established	NST and CST should be repeated within 24 hr; if interpretable data cannot be achieved, other methods of fetal assessment must be used*
HYPERSTIMULATION Late decelerations occurring with excessive uterine activity (contractions more often than every 2 min or lasting >90 sec) or persistent increase in uterine tone	
UNSATISFACTORY Inadequate uterine contraction pattern, or tracing too poor to interpret	

Reference: Tucker, S. (2004). *Pocket guide to fetal monitoring and assessment* (5th ed.). St. Louis: Mosby.
BPP, Biophysical profile; *CST,* contraction stress test; *FHR,* fetal heart rate; *NST,* nonstress test.
*Applies to results noted as suspicious, hyperstimulation, or unsatisfactory.

After interpretation of the FHR pattern, the oxytocin infusion is halted, and the maintenance IV solution infused until uterine activity has returned to the prestimulation level. If the CST is negative, the IV device is removed, and the fetal monitor disconnected. If the CST is positive, continued monitoring and further evaluation of fetal well-being are indicated.

▬ NURSING ROLE IN ANTEPARTAL ▬ ASSESSMENT FOR RISK

The nurse's role is that of educator and support person when the woman is undergoing such examinations as ultrasonography, MRI, CVS, PUBS, and amniocentesis. In some instances, the nurse may assist the physician with the procedure. In many settings, nurses perform NSTs, CSTs, and BPPs; conduct an initial assessment; and begin necessary interventions for nonreassuring patterns. These nursing procedures are accomplished after additional education and training, under guidance of established protocols, and in collaboration with obstetrics providers (Menihan, 2000; Stringer et al., 2003). Client teaching, which is an integral component of this role, involves preparing the woman for the procedure, interpreting the findings, and providing psychosocial support when needed.

Psychologic Considerations

All women who undergo antepartal assessments are at risk for real and potential problems and may be in an anxious frame of mind. In most instances, the tests are ordered because of suspected fetal compromise, deterioration of a maternal condition, or both. In the third trimester, pregnant women are most concerned about protecting themselves and their fetuses and consider themselves most vulnerable to outside influences. The label of high risk will increase this sense of vulnerability.

When a woman is diagnosed with a high risk pregnancy, she and her family will likely experience stress related to the diagnosis. The woman may exhibit various psychologic responses including anxiety, low self-esteem, guilt, frustration, and inability to function. The development of a high risk pregnancy also can affect parental attachment, accomplishment of the tasks of pregnancy, and family adaptation to the pregnancy (Ramer & Frank, 2001).

Women with complicated pregnancies perceive their risks as higher than do women with uncomplicated pregnancies (Gupton, Heaman, & Cheung, 2001). If the mother has to be placed on bed rest for pregnancy complications, separation from family, finances, and worry about children and home create further stress (Maloni, Brezinski-Tomasi, & Johnson, 2001).

If the woman is fearful for her own well-being, she may continue to feel ambivalence about the pregnancy or may not accept the reality of the pregnancy. She may not be able to complete preparations for the baby or go to childbirth classes if she is on bed rest or hospitalized. The family may become frustrated because they cannot engage in these activities that prepare them for parenthood.

Antepartal hospitalization is an added stressor for the high risk pregnant woman and her family. The woman may be lonely because she is separated from her home and family. She may feel powerless and unable to make decisions for herself because her care is out of her control. Likewise, preparation for the birth process may be out of control of the woman and her family. Unexpected procedures and care for the woman or fetus may take priority over the usual birth plan and may not allow choices that would have been selected if the pregnancy had been normal.

Attachment to the newborn can be affected if the mother or newborn is ill after the birth. Early contact may not be possible. Time, support, and intervention by the health care team may be necessary to help the family begin the attachment process.

The nurse can help the woman and her family regain control and balance in their lives by providing support and encouragement, providing information about the pregnancy problem and its management, and providing opportunities to make as many choices as possible about the woman's care (Coffman & Ray, 2002).

The impact of the effects of a specific pregnancy complication and its management is discussed in the following chapters in this unit.

community activity

Contact the nearest March of Dimes office to assess the resources available for parents (e.g., pamphlets, websites for high risk pregnancies) and what screening is recommended during pregnancy to identify problems. How can pregnant women get access to the March of Dimes information? What information or resources are available in your community for the problems identified?

key points

- A high risk pregnancy is one in which the life or well-being of the mother or infant is jeopardized by a biophysical or psychosocial disorder coincidental with or unique to pregnancy.
- Biophysical, sociodemographic, psychosocial, and environmental factors place the pregnancy and fetus or neonate at risk.
- Psychosocial perinatal warning indicators include characteristics of the parents, the child, their support systems, and family circumstances.
- Maternal and perinatal mortality rates for Caucasians are considerably lower than for other ethnic groups in the United States.

- Mortality rate decreases when risk is identified early and intensive care is applied.
- Biophysical assessment techniques include fetal movement counts, ultrasonography, and MRI.
- Biochemical monitoring techniques include amniocentesis, PUBS, CVS, and MSAFP.
- Reactive NSTs and negative CSTs suggest fetal well-being.
- Most assessment tests have some degree of risk for the mother and fetus and usually cause some anxiety for the woman and her family.

REFERENCES

Alfirevic, Z., Sundberg, K., & Brigham, S. (2003). Amniocentesis and chorionic villi sampling for prenatal diagnosis. In *The Cochrane Database of Systematic Reviews*, 2006, Issue 3. Chichester, UK: John Wiley & Sons.

American Academy of Pediatrics (AAP) & American College of Obstetricians and Gynecologists (ACOG). (2002). *Guidelines for perinatal care* (5th ed.). Elk Grove Village, IL: Authors.

American College of Obstetricians and Gynecologists (ACOG). (2004). Ultrasonography in pregnancy. Practice Bulletin Number 58. *Obstetrics and Gynecology 104*(6), 1149-1158.

Armour, K. (2004). Antepartum maternal-fetal assessment. Using surveillance to improve maternal and fetal outcomes. *AWHONN Lifelines, 8*(3), 232-240.

Association of Women's Health, Obstetric and Neonatal Nurses (AWHONN). (1998). *Nursing practice competencies and educational guidelines for limited ultrasound examination in obstetric and gynecology/infertility settings* (2nd ed.). Washington, DC: Author.

Benn, P., Egan, J., Fang, M., & Smith-Bindman, R. (2004). Changes in utilization of prenatal diagnosis. *Obstetrics and Gynecology, 103*(6), 1255-1260.

Chervenak, F., & Gabbe, S. (2002). Obstetric ultrasound: Assessment of fetal growth and anatomy. In S. Gabbe, J. Niebyl, & J. Simpson (Eds.), *Obstetrics: Normal and problem pregnancies* (4th ed.). New York: Churchill Livingstone.

Coffman, S., & Ray, M. (2002). African American women describe support processes during high-risk pregnancy and postpartum. *Journal of Obstetric, Gynecologic, and Neonatal Nursing, 31*(5), 536-544.

Druzin, M., Gabbe, S., & Reed, K. (2002). Antepartum fetal evaluation. In S. Gabbe, J. Niebyl, & J. Simpson (Eds.), *Obstetrics: Normal and problem pregnancies* (4th ed.). New York: Churchill Livingstone.

Enkin, M., Keirse, M., Neilson, J., Crowther, C., Duley, L., Hodnett, E., et al. (2001). Effective care in pregnancy and childbirth: A synopsis. *Birth, 28*(1), 41-51.

Fanaroff, A., Martin, J., & Rodriguez, R. (2004). Identification and management of problems in the high-risk neonate. In R. Creasy, R. Resnik, & J. Iams (Eds.), *Maternal-fetal medicine: Principles and practice* (5th ed.). Philadelphia: Saunders.

Garcia, J., Bricker, L., Henderson, J., Martin, M., Mugford, M., Neilson, J., et al. (2002). Women's views of pregnancy ultrasound: A systematic review. *Birth, 29*(4), 225-247.

Gilbert, E., & Harmon, J. (2003). *Manual of high risk pregnancy and delivery* (3rd ed.). St. Louis: Mosby.

Glantz, J., & Woods, J. (2004). Significance of amniotic fluid meconium. In R. Creasy, R. Resnik, & J. Iams (Eds.), *Maternal-fetal medicine: Principles and practice* (5th ed.). Philadelphia: Saunders.

Gupton, A., Heaman, M., & Cheung, L. (2001). Complicated and uncomplicated pregnancies: Women's perception of risk. *Journal of Obstetric, Gynecologic, and Neonatal Nursing, 30*(2), 192-201.

Harman, C. (2004). Assessment of fetal health. In R. Creasy, R. Resnik, & J. Iams (Eds.), *Maternal-fetal medicine: Principles and practice* (5th ed.). Philadelphia: Saunders.

Hoyert, D., Heron, M., Murphy, S., & Kung, H. (2006). Deaths: Final data for 2003. *Health E-Stats.* Released January 19, 2006. Hyattsville, MD: National Center for Health Statistics.

Jenkins, T., & Wapner, R. (2004). Prenatal diagnosis of congenital disorders. In R. Creasy, R. Resnik, & J. Iams (Eds.), *Maternal-fetal medicine: Principles and practice* (5th ed.). Philadelphia: Saunders.

Maloni, J., Brezinski-Tomasi, J., & Johnson, L. (2001). Antepartum bed rest: Effect upon the family. *Journal of Obstetric, Gynecologic, and Neonatal Nursing, 30*(2), 67-77.

Manning, F. (2004). General principles and applications of ultrasound. In R. Creasy, R. Resnik, & J. Iams (Eds.), *Maternal-fetal medicine: Principles and practice* (5th ed.). Philadelphia: Saunders.

Menihan, C. (2000). Limited ultrasound in nursing practice. *Journal of Obstetric, Gynecologic, and Neonatal Nursing, 29*(3), 325-330.

Parer, J., & Nageotte, M. (2004). Intrapartum fetal surveillance. In R. Creasy, R. Resnik, & J. Iams (Eds.), *Maternal-fetal medicine: Principles and practice* (5th ed.). Philadelphia: Saunders.

Ramer, L., & Frank, B. (2001). *Pregnancy: Psychosocial perspectives* (3rd ed.). White Plains, NY: March of Dimes Birth Defects Foundation.

Silbergeld, E., & Patrick, T. (2005). Environmental exposures, toxicologic mechanisms, and adverse pregnancy outcomes. *American Journal of Obstetrics and Gynecology, 192*(5), S11-121.

Simpson, J. (2002). Genetic counseling and prenatal diagnosis. In S. Gabbe, J. Niebyl, & J. Simpson (Eds.), *Obstetrics: Normal and problem pregnancies* (4th ed.). New York: Churchill Livingstone.

Stringer, M., Miesnik, S., Brown, L., Menei, L., & Macones, G. (2003). Limited obstetric ultrasound examinations: Competency and cost. *Journal of Obstetric, Gynecologic, and Neonatal Nursing, 32*(3), 307-312.

Tan, K., & Sabapathy, A. (2004). Maternal glucose administration for facilitating tests of fetal wellbeing. In *The Cochrane Database of Systematic Reviews,* 2006, Issue 3. Chichester, UK: John Wiley & Sons.

Tan, K., & Smyth, R. (2004). Fetal vibroacoustic stimulation for facilitation of tests of fetal wellbeing. In *The Cochrane Database of Systematic Reviews,* 2006, Issue 3. Chichester, UK: John Wiley & Sons.

Tucker, S. (2004). *Pocket guide to fetal monitoring and assessment* (5th ed.). St. Louis: Mosby.

U.S. Department of Health and Human Services (USDHHS). (2000). *Healthy People 2010.* (Conference Edition) (Vols. 1-2). Washington, DC: U.S. Government Printing Office.

Vain, N., Szyld, E., Prudent, L., Wiswell, T., Aguilar, A., & Vivas, N. (2004). Oropharyngeal and nasopharyngeal suctioning of meconium-stained neonates before delivery of their shoulders: Multicentre, randomized, controlled trial. *Lancet, 364*(9434), 597-602.

Wilson, R. (2000). Amniocentesis and chorionic villus sampling. *Current Opinion in Obstetrics and Gynecology, 12*(2), 81-86.

Hypertensive Disorders in Pregnancy

learning objectives

- Differentiate the defining characteristics of gestational hypertension, preeclampsia and eclampsia, and chronic hypertension.
- Review risk factors for developing preeclampsia.
- Describe the pathophysiology of preeclampsia.
- Evaluate maternal, fetal, and newborn morbidity and mortality attributable to the hypertensive disorders of pregnancy.
- Identify assessment techniques for preeclampsia.

- Differentiate between the management of the woman with mild versus severe preeclampsia.
- Describe HELLP syndrome, including appropriate nursing actions.
- Identify the priorities for management of eclamptic seizures.
- Evaluate the use of anticonvulsant and antihypertensive medications.

electronic resources

Additional information related to the content in Chapter 30 can be found on

the companion website at *evolve*
http://evolve.elsevier.com/Lowdermilk/MWHC/
- NCLEX Review Questions
- Case Study: Preeclampsia
- WebLinks

or on the interactive companion CD
- NCLEX Review Questions
- Case Study: Preeclampsia
- Critical Thinking Exercise: Preeclampsia
- Plan of Care: Mild Preeclampsia: Home Care
- Plan of Care: Severe Preeclampsia: Hospital Care

THIS chapter focuses on the classification, pathophysiology and management of hypertensive disorders of pregnancy. Hypertensive disorders of pregnancy contribute significantly to maternal and perinatal morbidity and mortality. Blood pressure elevations in pregnancy may be related to preeclampsia, eclampsia, gestational hypertension, or chronic hypertension. Preeclampsia and eclampsia are the primary focus of the chapter. Nurses working in a variety of clinical settings can use this information to expand their knowledge base so that they can identify pregnant women with hypertensive disorders who then can be treated appropriately.

■ SIGNIFICANCE AND INCIDENCE

Hypertensive disorders complicate 6% to 8% of all pregnancies, and are the most common medical complication reported during pregnancy (Martin, Hamilton, Sutton, Ventura, Menacker, & Munson, 2005; Peters & Flack, 2004). Preeclampsia complicates approximately 4.5% to 11% of all pregnancies (Longo, Dola, & Pridjian, 2003). The rate of pregnancy-related hypertension has risen steadily, by about

30% to 40%, since 1990 for all ages, races, and ethnic groups to the current rate of 37.8 per 1000 live births. Rates for chronic hypertension have increased moderately (8.4 per 1000), whereas the rate for preeclampsia has declined (4 per 1000 live births). Maternal race also influences the rate of pregnancy-related hypertension, with the highest rates seen in Native American (46.5 per 1000) and African-American (41.5 per 1000) women. Hispanic women have an intermediate rate (25.9 per 1000) (Martin et al.). Hispanic women, when compared to non-Hispanic Caucasian women with pregnancy-related hypertension, were more than three times as likely to develop preeclampsia (Wolf, Shah, Jimenez-Kimble, Sauk, Ecker, & Thadhani, 2004). Asian or Pacific Islander women have the lowest rate for pregnancy-related hypertension (19.6 per 1000) (Martin et al.).

■ MORBIDITY AND MORTALITY

In the United States, hypertension in pregnancy is the second leading cause of maternal and perinatal morbidity and mortality (Longo et al., 2003; Peters & Flack, 2004). Hypertensive disorders predispose the woman to serious complications, including abruptio placentae (also called placental abruption), thrombocytopenia, disseminated intravascular coagulation (DIC), acute renal failure, hepatic failure, pulmonary edema, adult respiratory distress syndrome, aspiration pneumonia, and cerebral hemorrhage (American College of Obstetricians and Gynecologists [ACOG], 2002; Peters & Flack; Zhang, Meikle & Trumble, 2003). Women younger than 20 or older than 35, have significantly higher morbidity rates. Hypertension in pregnancy also increases the woman's risk for a cesarean birth (Martin et al., 2005; Zhang et al., 2003).

Hypertensive disorders constitute almost 15% of pregnancy-related deaths (Longo et al., 2003). The overall rate of reported maternal death from preeclampsia-eclampsia was 1.8 per 100,000. African-American women experienced the most severe complications and had higher mortality rates than other races (Kochanek, Murphy, Anderson, & Scott, 2004; Zhang et al., 2003). Maternal mortality from preeclampsia is primarily a result of complications from abruptio placentae, eclampsia, and liver rupture (Longo et al.).

Preeclampsia occurs primarily after the second trimester of pregnancy and represents a great danger to the fetus and neonate. If the preeclampsia is severe, the fetus most likely will be born preterm. An infant born at 24 to 28 weeks of gestation is at risk for respiratory distress syndrome, chronic lung disease, intraventricular hemorrhage, sepsis, necrotizing enterocolitis, and failure to thrive (Bashiri, Zmora, Sheiner, Hershkovitz, Shoham-Vardi, & Mazor, 2003; Longo et al., 2003). Prematurity and low birth weight are the leading causes of neonatal mortality. Premature infants can face neurologic disabilities such as cerebral palsy, asthma, vision and hearing loss, and behavior problems, attention deficit hyperactivity disorders, and lower levels of academic achievement when older (Wener & Lavigne, 2004). Neonatal death rates were highest when the women had HELLP syndrome (defined and discussed later in this chapter), a variant of severe preeclampsia (Aslan, Gul, & Cebeci, 2004).

■ CLASSIFICATION

The classification system used in the United States today is based on reports from the American College of Obstetricians and Gynecologists (ACOG) (2002) and the National High Blood Pressure Education Program (NHBPEP) Working Group on High Blood Pressure in Pregnancy (2000). This classification system is summarized in Table 30-1.

Gestational Hypertension

Gestational hypertension is the onset of hypertension, without proteinuria, after 20 weeks of pregnancy, which may be transient or chronic in nature. Transient hypertension occurs when the blood pressure elevations return to normal by 12 weeks after the birth. If the hypertension does not resolve by 12 weeks postpartum, then the diagnosis of chronic hypertension is made. Gestational hypertension is considered a benign diagnosis with good pregnancy outcomes (Longo et al., 2003; Peters & Flack, 2004).

Preeclampsia

Preeclampsia, a pregnancy-specific syndrome in which hypertension develops after 20 weeks of gestation in a previously normotensive woman, is characterized by the presence of hypertension and proteinuria. Preeclampsia is a vasospastic, systemic disorder with a clinical continuum from mild to severe (Table 30-2). With mild preeclampsia, hypertension and proteinuria are present, and there is no evidence of organ dysfunction (ACOG, 2002; Longo et al., 2003).

Hypertension, whether gestational or chronic, is defined as a systolic blood pressure (BP) greater than 140 mm Hg, or a diastolic BP greater than 90 mm Hg, or a mean arterial pressure (MAP) greater than 105 mm Hg, recorded on

Evolve/CD: Case Study: Preeclampsia

table 30-1 Classification of Hypertensive States of Pregnancy

TYPE	DESCRIPTION
Gestational hypertension	Blood pressure elevation detected first time after midpregnancy (20 wks) without proteinuria
Transient hypertension	Gestational hypertension with no signs of preeclampsia present at the time of birth, and hypertension resolves by 12 weeks postpartum. This is a retrospective diagnosis
Preeclampsia	Pregnancy-specific syndrome that usually occurs after 20 weeks of gestation and is determined by gestational hypertension plus proteinuria
Eclampsia	The occurrence of seizures in a woman with preeclampsia that cannot be attributed to other causes
Chronic hypertension	Hypertension that is present and observable before pregnancy or that is diagnosed before week 20 of gestation
Preeclampsia superimposed on chronic hypertension	Chronic hypertension with new proteinuria or an exacerbation of hypertension (previously well controlled) or increased proteinuria, thrombocytopenia, or increases in hepatic enzymes (alanine aminotransferase [ALT] or aspartate aminotransferase [AST]

Adapted from: American College of Obstetricians and Gynecologists. (2002). *Diagnosis and management of preeclampsia and eclampsia.* ACOG Practice Bulletin Number 33. Washington, DC: ACOG; Blackburn, S. (2003). *Maternal, fetal, & neonatal physiology: A clinical perspective* (2nd ed.). St. Louis: Saunders; and National High Blood Pressure Education Program (NHBPEP) Working Group on High Blood Pressure in Pregnancy. (2000). Report of the National High Blood Pressure Education Program Working Group on High Blood Pressure in Pregnancy. *American Journal of Obstetrics and Gynecology, 183*(1),S1-S22.

table 30-2 Differentiation Between Mild and Severe Preeclampsia

	MILD PREECLAMPSIA	SEVERE PREECLAMPSIA
MATERNAL EFFECTS		
Blood pressure	BP reading of >140/90 mm Hg × 2, 4-6 hr apart, no more than 1 wk apart	Rise to ≥160/110 mm Hg on two separate occasions
Mean arterial pressure (MAP)	>105 mm Hg	>105 mm Hg
Proteinuria		
Quantitative 24 hr analysis	Proteinuria of ≥0.3 g in a 24 hr specimen	Proteinuria of ≥2 g in a 24 hr specimen
Qualitative dipstick	≥30 mg/dl (≥ 1+) on dipstick	2+ to 3+ protein on dipstick
Reflexes	May be normal	Hyperreflexia ≥3+, possible ankle clonus
Urine output	Output matching intake, ≤30 ml/hr or <650 ml/24 hr	<20 ml/hr or <400 ml to 500 ml/24 hr
Headache	Absent/transient	Persistent or severe
Visual problems	Absent	Blurred, photophobia, blind spots on funduscopy
Irritability/changes in affect	Transient	Severe
Epigastric pain	Absent	Present
Serum creatinine	Normal	Elevated >1.2 mg/dl
Thrombocytopenia	Absent	Present <100,000/mm³
AST elevation	Normal or minimal	Marked
FETAL EFFECTS		
Placental perfusion	Reduced	Decreased perfusion expressing as IUGR in fetus; FHR: late decelerations
Premature placental aging	Not apparent	At birth, placenta appearing smaller than normal for duration of pregnancy, premature aging apparent with numerous areas of broken syncytia, ischemic necroses (white infarcts) numerous, intervillous fibrin deposition (red infarcts)

Sources: American College of Obstetricians and Gynecologists. (2002). *Diagnosis and management of preeclampsia and eclampsia.* ACOG Practice Bulletin Number 33. Washington, DC: Author; and National High Blood Pressure Education Program (NHBPEP) Working Group on High Blood Pressure in Pregnancy. (2000). Report of the National High Blood Pressure Education Program Working Group on High Blood Pressure in Pregnancy. *American Journal of Obstetrics and Gynecology, 183*(1)S1-S22.
AST, Aspartate aminotransferase; *BP,* blood pressure; *FHR,* fetal heart rate; *IUGR,* intrauterine growth restriction.

two separate occasions at least 4 to 6 hours apart (ACOG, 2002; Longo et al., 2003). Elevations over prepregnancy values are no longer considered diagnostic for preeclampsia. However, women who demonstrate an increase of 30 mm Hg systolic or 15 mm Hg diastolic warrant closer observation if the BP elevation occurs with proteinuria and hyperuricemia (uric acid of 6 mg/dl or more) (ACOG).

Proteinuria is defined as a concentration of ≥30 mg/dl (≥1+ on dipstick measurement) or more in at least two random urine specimens collected at least 6 hours apart with no evidence of urinary tract infection. In a 24 hour specimen, *proteinuria* is defined as a concentration of ≥300 mg/24 hours. Because of the discrepancy between random protein determinations, the diagnosis of proteinuria should be based on a 24 hour urine collection if possible, or a timed collection corrected for creatinine excretion if a 24 hour specimen is not feasible (ACOG, 2002; Longo et al., 2003).

Severe Preeclampsia

Severe preeclampsia is the presence of a systolic BP greater than 160 mm Hg or a diastolic BP greater than 110 mm Hg and proteinuria ≥2 g/24 hr specimen or ≥2+ on dipstick. Other signs and symptoms associated with severe

preeclampsia include the following: oliguria; cerebral disturbances such as altered level of consciousness, confusion, or headache; visual disturbances such as scotoma, or blurred vision; hepatic involvement, including epigastric pain, right upper quadrant pain, impaired liver function or elevated liver enzymes; thrombocytopenia with a platelet count less than 100,000/mm³; hemolytic anemia; pulmonary edema; and fetal intrauterine growth restriction (ACOG, 2002; Longo et al., 2003).

Eclampsia

Eclampsia is the onset of seizure activity or coma in the woman diagnosed with preeclampsia, with no history of preexisting pathology that can result in seizure activity (ACOG, 2002). The initial presentation of eclampsia varies, with one third of the women developing eclampsia during the pregnancy, one third during labor, and one third within 72 hours postpartum (Emery, 2005).

Chronic Hypertension

Chronic hypertension is defined as hypertension present before the pregnancy or diagnosed before 20 weeks of gestation. Most women will experience uncomplicated pregnancies; however, there is an increased risk of poor

CRITICAL THINKING EXERCISE

Severe Preeclampsia

Kathy is a 28-year-old primigravida who arrives at the obstetrics (OB) clinic for her routine prenatal visit at 30 weeks of gestation. She is accompanied by her husband. During the interview, Kathy reports that she has been very tired, and she complains of occasional headaches, nausea, mild cramping, and seeing "shooting stars." Her OB history is negative for chronic diseases such as hypertension and diabetes. Kathy has gained 8 pounds the last month and has significant ankle edema. Her urine specimen shows 4+ protein and her blood pressure (BP) is 200/115. Kathy rests on her left side for 15 minutes and her BP is 190/110. The physician examines Kathy and decides to admit her to the labor and birth unit immediately. Kathy and her husband are frightened at the suddenness of the decision and are concerned about their baby.

1. Evidence—Is there sufficient evidence to draw conclusions about her diagnosis and preferred treatment?
2. Assumptions—What assumptions can be made about the following items?
   a. Possible diagnosis
   b. Physical assessment, laboratory tests, and diagnostic procedures that will be done to make a diagnosis
   c. Factors contributing to the diagnosis
3. What implications and priorities for nursing care can be made at this time?
4. Does the evidence objectively support your conclusion?
5. Are there alternative perspectives to your conclusion?

fetal growth and fetal demise. Preconception counseling is recommended for women with chronic hypertension (ACOG, 2002; Longo et al., 2003).

Chronic Hypertension with Superimposed Preeclampsia

Approximately 25% of women with chronic hypertension may develop preeclampsia or eclampsia. This disorder is associated with severe maternal and fetal complications. Chronic hypertension with superimposed preeclampsia is defined with the following findings:

- In women with hypertension before 20 weeks of gestation, with new-onset proteinuria
- In women with both hypertension and proteinuria before 20 weeks of gestation
- Sudden increase in proteinuria
- A sudden increase in BP in a woman whose hypertension has previously been well controlled
- Thrombocytopenia
- Elevated liver enzymes (ACOG, 2002; Longo et al., 2003; Peters & Flack, 2004)

■ PREECLAMPSIA

Etiology

Preeclampsia is a condition unique to human pregnancy; signs and symptoms develop only during pregnancy and disappear quickly after birth of the fetus and placenta. The ultimate cause remains unknown. Preeclampsia is seen more frequently in primigravidas. Age distribution remains U-shaped,

with women younger than 20 years and older than 40 years having the highest rates of occurrence. Certain risk factors are associated with development of the condition, such as multiple gestation, hydatiform moles and chronic medical disorders (Box 30-1) (Duckitt & Harrington, 2005; Longo et al., 2003; Peters & Flack, 2004). Some studies have shown an increased risk for preeclampsia in multiparous women with new partners for subsequent pregnancies (Longo et al.). Other studies found that a change of partner did not increase the recurrence rate of preeclampsia (Hjartardottir, Leifsson, Geirsson, & Steinthorsdottir, 2004).

The etiology of preeclampsia is theorized to include various possibilities: abnormal prostaglandin action, endothelial cell dysfunction, coagulation abnormalities, vasoconstrictor tone, and dietary deficiencies or excesses. Immunologic factors and genetic disposition may also play an important role (Sibai, 2002b). Animal studies have suggested that abnormalities of the placenta are the cause of preeclampsia. The trophoblast cells of the placenta usually alter the spiral arteries in the uterus to accommodate increased blood flow. Instead, the vessels seen in preeclampsia are abnormally thick-walled and muscular and have higher resistance. The condition also results in a distinctive lesion called acute atherosis, and there are increased numbers of placental infarcts. Placental perfusion is decreased, resulting in hypoxia; this causes several pathophysiologic abnormalities, especially, endothelial damage. Thus, many of the pathophysiologic changes of preeclampsia occur before clinical symptoms develop (Longo et al., 2003; Peters & Flack, 2004).

Pathophysiology

The pathophysiology of preeclampsia reflects alterations in the normal adaptations of pregnancy. Normal physiologic adaptations to pregnancy include increased blood

CD: Critical Thinking Exercise: Preeclampsia

---

box 30-1 Risk Factors Associated with the Development of Preeclampsia

- Chronic renal disease
- Chronic hypertension
- Family history of preeclampsia
- Multifetal gestation
- Primigravidity or multiparous woman with new partner for current pregnancy
- Extremes of maternal age: <20 years or >40 years
- Diabetes
- Rh incompatibility
- Obesity
- African-American ethnicity
- Insulin resistance
- Limited sperm exposure with same partner
- Preeclampsia in a previous pregnancy
- Pregnancies after donor insemination, oocyte donation, embryo donation
- Maternal infections

Data from American College of Obstetricians and Gynecologists (ACOG). (2002). *Diagnosis and management of preeclampsia and eclampsia.* ACOG Practice Bulletin Number 33. Washington, DC: Author; Gilbert, E., & Harmon, J. (2003). *Manual of high risk pregnancy and delivery* (3rd ed.). St. Louis: Mosby; and Sibai, B., Dekker, G., & Kupferminic, M. (2005). Preeclampsia. *Lancet, 365*(9461), 785-799.

plasma volume, vasodilation, decreased systemic vascular resistance, elevated cardiac output, and decreased colloid osmotic pressure (Box 30-2). With preeclampsia, the main pathogenic factor is not an increase in BP but poor perfusion as a result of vasospasm and reduced plasma volume. Arteriolar vasospasm diminishes the diameter of blood vessels, which impedes blood flow to all organs and increases BP (Longo et al., 2003; Peters & Flack, 2004; Roberts, Pearson, Cutler, Lindheimer, & NHLBI Working Group on Research on Hypertension during Pregnancy, 2003). Function in organs such as the placenta, kidneys, liver, and brain is depressed by as much as 40% to 60%. The pathophysiologic sequelae are shown in Fig. 30-1.

Reduced kidney perfusion decreases the glomerular filtration rate and leads to degenerative glomerular changes and possibly oliguria. Pathologic changes in the endothelial cells of the glomeruli (glomerular endotheliosis) are uniquely characteristic of preeclampsia. Protein, primarily albumin, is lost in the urine. Uric acid clearance is decreased; however, blood urea nitrogen (BUN), serum creatinine, and serum uric acid levels increase. Sodium and water are retained (Longo et al., 2003; Peters & Flack, 2004).

Plasma colloid osmotic pressure decreases as serum albumin levels decrease. Intravascular volume is reduced as fluid moves out of the intravascular compartment, resulting in hemoconcentration, increased blood viscosity, and tissue

box 30-2 Normal Physiologic Adaptations to Pregnancy

CARDIOVASCULAR
- ↑ Blood volume; plasma volume expansion greater than red cell mass expansion, leading to physiologic anemia of pregnancy
- ↓ Total peripheral resistance, decreases in blood pressure readings and MAP
- ↑ Cardiac output resulting from increased blood volume, slight increase in heart rate to compensate for peripheral relaxation
- ↑ Oxygen consumption
- Physiologic edema related to ↓ plasma colloid osmotic pressure and ↑ venous capillary hydrostatic pressure

HEMATOLOGIC
- ↑ Clotting factors, predisposing to DIC and clotting
- ↓ Serum albumin resulting in decreases in colloid osmotic pressure, predisposing to pulmonary edema

RENAL
- ↑ Renal plasma flow and glomerular filtration rate

ENDOCRINE
- ↑ Estrogen production resulting in ↑ renin–angiotensin II–aldosterone secretion
- ↑ Progesterone production blocking aldosterone effect (slight ↓ Na)
- ↑ Vasodilator prostaglandins resulting in resistance to angiotensin II (slight ↓ blood pressure)

DIC, disseminated intravascular coagulation; *MAP,* Mean arterial pressure.

edema. The hematocrit value increases as fluid leaves the intravascular space. In severe preeclampsia, blood volume may decrease to or below nonpregnancy levels; severe edema develops, and rapid weight gain is seen. Arteriolar vasospasm can cause endothelial damage and contribute to an increased capillary permeability. This increases edema and further decreases intravascular volume, predisposing the woman with preeclampsia to pulmonary edema (Fig. 30-2) (Longo et al., 2003; Peters & Flack, 2004; Roberts et al., 2003).

Decreased liver perfusion results in impaired liver function. Liver enzyme levels increase in the wake of liver damage. If hepatic edema and subcapsular hemorrhage develop, the women may complain of epigastric or right upper quadrant pain. Rupture of a subcapsular hematoma is a life-threatening complication and a surgical emergency (Longo et al., 2003; Peters & Flack, 2004).

Arteriolar vasospasms and decreased blood flow to the retina lead to visual symptoms such as scotomata (blind spots) and blurring. Neurologic complications associated with preeclampsia include cerebral edema and hemorrhages and increased central nervous system (CNS) irritability, which manifests as headache, hyperreflexia, positive ankle clonus, and seizures (Longo et al., 2003) (see Fig. 30-2).

Preeclampsia contributes significantly to restrictions of fetal growth and incidence of placental abruption. Impaired placental perfusion leads to early degenerative aging of the placenta. The rate of fetal complications is directly related to the severity of the disease (Longo et al., 2003).

HELLP Syndrome

HELLP syndrome is a laboratory diagnosis for a variant of severe preeclampsia that involves hepatic dysfunction; it is characterized by hemolysis (H), elevated liver enzymes (EL), and low platelets (LP). A woman's platelet count must be less than $100,000/mm^3$, and her liver enzyme levels (aspartate aminotransferase [AST] and alanine aminotransferase [ALT]) must be elevated. A unique form of coagulopathy (not DIC) occurs with HELLP syndrome. The platelet count is low, but coagulation factor assays, prothrombin time (PT), partial thromboplastin time (PTT), and bleeding time remain normal. In some instances hemolysis does not occur and the condition is called ELLP (Sibai, Dekker, & Kupferminic, 2005).

HELLP syndrome appears in approximately 20% of women with severe preeclampsia (ACOG, 2002; Emery, 2005). Most commonly, HELLP syndrome is seen in older Caucasian, multiparous women. About 90% of women report a history of malaise for several days. Epigastric or right upper quadrant abdominal pain (possibly related to hepatic ischemia) is noted by 65% of women with the syndrome, and 50% complain of nausea and vomiting. Many women with HELLP syndrome may not have signs or symptoms of severe preeclampsia or may have only slight elevations in BP. As a result, women with HELLP syndrome are often misdiagnosed as having a variety of other medical or surgical disorders (Sibai et al., 2005).

Recognition of the clinical and laboratory findings associated with HELLP syndrome is important if early, aggressive therapy is to be initiated to prevent maternal and neonatal mortality. Complications reported with HELLP syndrome include renal failure, pulmonary edema, ruptured liver hematoma, DIC, placental abruption, and preterm birth (Sibai et al., 2005). Perinatal mortality rates range from 7.7% to 60%, and maternal mortality ranges from 0% to 24% (Moldenhauer & Sibai, 2002; Sibai et al., 2005).

■ CARE MANAGEMENT

■ Identifying and Preventing Preeclampsia

There have been numerous clinical trials studying various methods for preventing preeclampsia. These interventions included the use of low-dose aspirin, antioxidants, calcium, magnesium, and zinc, and restricted sodium intake and fish oil supplementation. None of the interventions demonstrated

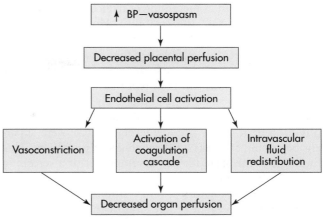

FIG. 30-1   Etiology of preeclampsia: Endothelial cell dysfunction.

FIG. 30-2   Pathophysiology of preeclampsia. (Modified from Gilbert, E., & Harmon, J. [2003]. *Manual of high risk pregnancy & delivery* [3rd ed.]. St. Louis: Mosby.)

❊ a significant benefit in preventing or reducing the severity of preeclampsia (ACOG, 2002; Atallah, Hofmeyr, & Duley, 2002; Peters & Flack, 2004; Zhang et al., 2002).

There has been no reliable test that could be used as a routine screening tool for predicting preeclampsia (Peters & Flack, 2004). Research findings reported by Cockey (2005) suggested that women were more likely to develop preeclampsia if they had low levels of placental growth factor (PlGF) in their urine. The low levels of PlGF were apparent beginning at weeks 25 through 28 of pregnancy. This finding sets the stage for the development of a screening tool for women that are at high risk for preeclampsia. Once these women are identified, future studies could target effective ways to prevent progression of the disease and to prevent dangerous complications from occurring (Cockey). Nurses should be aware of what strategies are being studied and use the most reliable evidence about the results so that they can counsel pregnant women about interventions that are likely to be beneficial. One excellent resource for evidence-based care is the Cochrane Pregnancy and Childbirth Database (www.cochrane.org).

▪ Assessment and Nursing Diagnoses

Hypertensive disorders of pregnancy can occur without warning or with the gradual development of symptoms. The best prevention methods include early prenatal care for identification of women at risk and early detection of preeclampsia. The woman is assessed for risk factors at her first prenatal visit (see Box 30-1).

▪ *Interview*

Medical history is reviewed, especially the presence of diabetes mellitus, renal disease, and hypertension. Family history is explored for hypertensive disorders, diabetes mellitus, and other chronic conditions. The social history provides information about the woman's marital status, nutritional status, cultural beliefs, activity level, and lifestyle behaviors such as smoking and alcohol and drug use.

A review of systems adds to the database for detecting BP changes from baseline, abnormal weight gain, and the presence of edema. During each subsequent visit, the woman is assessed for signs and symptoms of preeclampsia.

▪ *Physical Examination*

Accurate and consistent BP assessment is important for establishing a baseline and monitoring subtle changes throughout the pregnancy. BP readings are affected by maternal position and measurement techniques. Consistency must be ensured in that proper equipment and cuff size are used, and the woman is seated with her arm at heart level. Diastolic pressure should be recorded at Korotkoff phase V (disappearance of sound) not Korotkoff phase IV (muffling sound). If the initial measurement is elevated, the woman should be allowed to relax and have a repeated measurement. Normally, the diastolic blood pressure drops an average of 10 mm Hg below nonpregnant values by midgestation and then slowly reaches nonpregnant levels in the third trimester. Evaluation of BP focuses on trends, not on a single reading (ACOG,

2002; Peters & Flack, 2004). Box 30-3 presents recommendations for standardizing this procedure.

Observation of edema in addition to hypertension warrants additional investigation. Edema is assessed for distribution, degree, and pitting. Edema may be described as dependent or pitting.

Dependent edema is edema of the lowest or most dependent parts of the body, where hydrostatic pressure is greatest. If a pregnant woman is ambulatory, this edema may first be evident in the feet and ankles. If the pregnant woman is confined to bed, the edema is more likely to occur in the sacral region.

Pitting edema is edema that leaves a small depression or pit after finger pressure is applied to the swollen area. The pit, which is caused by movement of fluid to adjacent tissue away from the point of pressure, normally disappears within 10 to 30 seconds. Although the amount of edema is difficult to quantify, the method described in Fig. 30-3 may be used to record relative degrees of edema formation.

Although it is not a routine assessment during the prenatal period, evaluation of the fundus of the eye yields valuable data. An initial baseline finding of normal eye grounds assists in differentiating preexisting disease from a new disease process (Fig. 30-4).

Deep tendon reflexes (DTRs) are evaluated as a baseline and to detect any changes. The biceps and patellar reflexes and ankle clonus are assessed and the findings recorded (Fig. 30-5; Table 30-3). To elicit the biceps reflex, the examiner strikes a downward blow over the thumb, which is situated over the biceps tendon (see Fig. 30-5, *A*). Normal response is flexion of the arm at the elbow, described

---

box 30-3 Blood Pressure Measurement

- Measure blood pressure with the woman seated (ambulatory) or in the left lateral recumbent position with the arm at heart level.
- After positioning, allow the woman at least 10 minutes of quiet rest before blood pressure measurement, to encourage relaxation.
- No tobacco or caffeine use 30 minutes before blood pressure measurement.
- Use the same arm each time for blood pressure measurement.
- Hold the arm in a roughly horizontal position at heart level.
- Use the proper-sized cuff (cuff should cover approximately 80% of the upper arm or be 1.5 times the length of the upper arm).
- Maintain a slow, steady deflation rate.
- Take the average of two readings at least 4 to 6 hours apart to minimize recorded blood pressure variations across time.
- Use Korotkoff phase V (disappearance of sound) for recording the diastolic value (some sources recommend recording both phase IV [the muffled sound] and phase V).
- Use accurate equipment. The manual sphygmomanometer is the most accurate device.
- If interchanging manual and electronic devices, use caution in interpreting different blood pressure values.

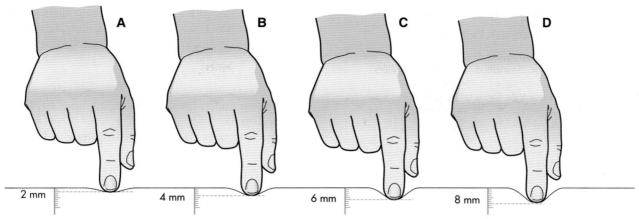

FIG. 30-3 Assessment of pitting edema of lower extremities. **A,** 1+. **B,** 2+. **C,** 3+. **D,** 4+.

FIG. 30-4 Funduscopic evidence of severe preeclampsia: arteriospasm, edema, hemorrhage, arteriovenous nicking, and exudates.

FIG. 30-5 **A,** Biceps reflex. **B,** Patellar reflex with woman's legs hanging freely over end of examining table. **C,** Test for ankle clonus. (Courtesy Shannon Perry, Phoenix, AZ.)

as a 2+ response. The patellar reflex is elicited with the woman's legs hanging freely over the end of the examining table or with the woman lying on her side with the knee slightly flexed (see Fig. 30-5, *B*). A blow with a percussion hammer is dealt directly to the patellar tendon, inferior to the patella. Normal response is the extension or kicking out of the leg. To assess for hyperactive reflexes (clonus) at the ankle joint, the examiner supports the leg with the knee flexed (see Fig. 30-5, *C*). With one hand, the examiner sharply dorsiflexes the foot, maintains the position for a moment, and then releases the foot. Normal *(negative clonus)* response is elicited when no rhythmic oscillations (jerks) are felt while the foot is held in dorsiflexion. When the foot is released, no oscillations are seen as the foot drops to the plantar-flexed position. Abnormal *(positive clonus)* response is recognized by rhythmic oscillations of one or more "beats" felt when the foot is in dorsiflexion and seen as the foot drops to the plantar-flexed position.

During the physical examination, the pregnant woman is examined for signs and symptoms of progression of mild preeclampsia to severe preeclampsia, such as headaches, epigastric pain, and visual disturbances. The signs of mild versus severe preeclampsia are summarized in Table 30-2.

table 30-3 Assessing Deep Tendon Reflexes

GRADE	DEEP TENDON REFLEX RESPONSE
0	No response
1+	Sluggish or diminished
2+	Active or expected response
3+	More brisk than expected, slightly hyperactive
4+	Brisk, hyperactive, with intermittent or transient clonus

From Seidel, H., Ball, J., Dains, J., & Benedict, G. (2006). *Mosby's guide to physical examination* (6th ed.). St. Louis: Mosby.

Uteroplacental perfusion is decreased in women with preeclampsia. Biophysical monitoring, such as nonstress testing, biophysical profile, and serial ultrasonography, are used to assess fetal status. The fetal heart rate (FHR) is assessed for baseline rate, variability, and presence of accelerations. Abnormal baseline rate, decreased or absent variability, and late or variable decelerations are indications of fetal intolerance to the intrauterine environment. Since the woman with preeclampsia is at risk for abruptio placentae, it is important to assess uterine tone and tenderness and the presence of vaginal bleeding. Doppler flow velocimetry studies may also be used to evaluate uteroplacental perfusion (see Chapter 29).

■ NURSE ALERT

Uterine tenderness in the presence of increasing tone may be the earliest finding of an abruption. Idiopathic preterm contractions also may be an early sign.

■ *Laboratory Tests*

Blood and urine specimens are collected to aid in the diagnosis and treatment of preeclampsia, HELLP syndrome, and chronic hypertension. Baseline laboratory test information is useful in cases of early diagnosis of preeclampsia, because it can be compared with later results to evaluate

progression and severity of disease (Table 30-4). An initial blood specimen is obtained for the following tests to assess the disease process and its effect on renal and hepatic functioning:

- Complete blood count (CBC) (including a platelet count)
- Clotting studies (including bleeding time, PT, PTT, and fibrinogen)
- Liver enzymes (lactate dehydrogenase [LDH], AST, ALT)
- Chemistry panel (BUN, creatinine, glucose, uric acid)
- Type and screen, possible crossmatch

The hematocrit, hemoglobin, and platelet levels are monitored closely for changes indicating a worsening of preeclampsia. Because hepatic involvement is a possible complication, serum glucose levels are monitored if liver function tests indicate elevated liver enzymes. Once the platelet count decreases below 100,000/mm^3, coagulation profiles are needed to identify developing DIC (Sibai, 2002b).

Urine output is assessed for volume of at least 30 ml/hr or 120 ml/4 hr. Proteinuria is determined from dipstick testing of a clean catch or catheterized urine specimen. A reading of 2+ or 3+ on two or more occasions, at least 6 hours apart, should be followed by a 24 hour urine collection. A 24 hour collection to test for protein and creatinine clearance is more reflective of true renal status. Renal laboratory assessments include monitoring trends in serum creatinine and BUN levels. As renal function becomes compromised, renal excretion of creatinine and other waste products, including magnesium sulfate, decreases. As renal excretion decreases, serum levels of creatinine, BUN, uric acid, and magnesium increase. Proteinuria is usually a late sign in the course of preeclampsia (ACOG, 2002; Longo et al., 2003).

table 30-4 Common Laboratory Changes in Preeclampsia

	NORMAL (NONPREGNANT)	PREECLAMPSIA	HELLP
Hemoglobin/hematocrit	12 to 16 g/dl/37% to 47%	May ↑	↓
Platelets	150,000 to 400,000/mm^3	Unchanged or <100,000/mm^3	<100,000/mm^3
Prothrombin time (PT)/partial thromboplastin time (PTT)	12 to 14 sec/60 to 70 sec	Unchanged	Unchanged
Fibrinogen	200 to 400 mg/dl	300 to 600 mg/dl	↓
Fibrin split products (FSPs)	Absent	Absent/Present	Present
Blood urea nitrogen (BUN)	10 to 20 mg/dl	↑	↑
Creatinine	0.5 to 1.1 mg/dl	>1.2 mg/dl	↑
Lactate dehydrogenase (LDH)*	45 to 90 units/L	↑	↑ (>600 units/L)
Aspartate aminotransferase (AST)	4 to 20 units/L	Unchanged to minimal ↑	↑ (>70 units/L)
Alanine aminotransferase (ALT)	3 to 21 units/L	Unchanged to minimal ↑	↑
Creatinine clearance	80 to 125 ml/min	130 to 180 ml/min	↓
Burr cells or schistocytes	Absent	Absent	Present
Uric acid	2 to 6.6 mg/dl	>5.9 mg/dl	>10 mg/dl
Bilirubin (total)	0.1 to 1 mg/dl	<1.2 mg/dl	↑ (>1.2 mg/dl)

Sources: Cunningham, F., Leveno, K., Bloom, S., Hauth, J., Gilstrap, L., & Wenstrom, K. (2005). *Williams obstetrics* (22nd ed.). New York: McGraw-Hill; Dildy, G. (2004). Complications of preeclampsia. In G. Dildy, M. Belfort, G. Saade, J. Phelan, G. Hankins, & S. Clark (Eds.), *Critical care obstetrics* (4th ed). Malden, MA: Blackwell Science; Roberts, J. (2004). Pregnancy-related hypertension. In R. Creasy, R. Resnik, & J. Iams (Eds.), *Maternal-fetal medicine: Principles and practice* (5th ed.). Philadelphia: Saunders.
*LDH values differ according to the test/assays being done

Protein readings are designated as follows:

0	negative
Trace	trace
1+	30 mg/dl (equivalent to 0.3 g/L)
2+	100 mg/dl
3+	300 mg/dl
4+	1000 mg (1 g)/dl

Renal laboratory assessments include monitoring trends in serum creatinine and BUN levels. As renal function becomes compromised, renal excretion of creatinine and other waste products decreases, and serum levels for creatinine, BUN, and uric acid increase.

■ Nursing Diagnoses

Nursing diagnoses for the woman with hypertensive disorders in pregnancy may include the following:

- *Anxiety related to*
  –preeclampsia and its effect on woman and infant
- *Deficient knowledge related to*
  –management of preeclampsia (diet, medications, activity restrictions)
- *Ineffective family coping related to*
  –restricted activity and concern over a complicated pregnancy
  –financial concerns
  –transfer of the woman to a tertiary center for more intensive management
- *Powerlessness related to*
  –inability to prevent or control condition and outcomes
- *Ineffective tissue perfusion related to*
  –hypertension
  –cyclic vasospasms
  –cerebral edema
  –hemorrhage
- *Risk for injury to fetus related to*
  –uteroplacental insufficiency
  –preterm birth
  –abruptio placentae
- *Risk for injury to mother related to*
  –CNS irritability secondary to cerebral edema, vasospasm, decreased renal perfusion
  –magnesium sulfate and antihypertensive therapies

■ Expected Outcomes of Care

Expected outcomes for care of women with hypertensive disorders of pregnancy include that the woman will do the following:
- Recognize and immediately report signs and symptoms indicative of worsening condition.
- Adhere to the medical regimen to minimize risk to herself and her fetus.
- Identify and use available support systems.

- Verbalize her fears and concerns to cope with the condition and situation.
- Develop no signs of eclampsia and its complications.
- Give birth to a healthy infant.
- Develop no sequelae to preeclampsia, or its management.

■ Plan of Care and Interventions

The treatment and management of preeclampsia varies according to the severity of the disease and the gestational age at diagnosis. The only cure for preeclampsia is the birth of the fetus; however, immediate birth may not be in the best interest of the fetus. Women suspected of preeclampsia should be hospitalized for a thorough evaluation of both the maternal and the fetal condition. To determine the severity of the disease, laboratory studies should be obtained. When mild preeclampsia is diagnosed in a preterm pregnancy (less than 37 weeks of gestation), bed rest with close maternal and fetal surveillance (expectant management) until the birth is recommended (Longo et al., 2003).

A multidisciplinary plan of care is developed, together with the woman and her family. The diagnosis of a high risk pregnancy and the associated restrictions can be very stressful for the woman and her family. Emotional support is essential to assist them with coping with the impact of a high risk pregnancy. The family will need to use coping mechanisms and support systems to help them through this crisis.

■ Mild Preeclampsia and Home Care

If the woman has mild preeclampsia (BP is stable, urine protein is less than 300 mg in a 24 hour collection, and no subjective complaints), she may be managed at home. The maternal-fetal condition should be assessed 2 to 3 times per week. Many agencies are available to provide this assessment in the home. Arrangements for this service may be made, depending on the woman's insurance coverage. If home nursing care is not possible, the woman may be asked to perform self-assessment daily, including weight, urine dipstick protein determinations, BP measurement, and fetal movement counting. She will be instructed to report the development of any subjective symptoms immediately to her health care provider (see Teaching for Self-Care box) and to return to the physician's office or high risk clinic for all appointments as scheduled.

The fetal condition also is closely monitored to allow additional time for fetal growth and maturation. An evaluation of fetal growth by ultrasound should be obtained every 3 weeks. Fetal movement is counted daily. Other fetal assessment tests include a nonstress test (NST), once or twice a week, and a biophysical profile (BPP) as needed. Fetal jeopardy as evidenced by inappropriate growth or abnormal test results necessitates immediate intervention (ACOG, 2002; Sibai, 2002b).

Activity Restriction. Bed rest in the lateral recumbent position is a standard therapy for preeclampsia and may improve uteroplacental blood flow. Complete bed

TEACHING FOR SELF-CARE

Assessing and Reporting Clinical Signs of Preeclampsia

- *Report immediately any increase in your blood pressure, protein in urine, weight gain, decreased fetal movement.**
- *Take your blood pressure on the same arm in a sitting position each time for consistent and accurate readings. Support arm on a table in a horizontal position at heart level.*
- *Use the same scale, wearing the same clothes, at the same time each day,* after voiding, before breakfast, for reliable daily weights.
- *Dipstick test your clean-catch urine sample to assess proteinuria; report frequency or burning on urination and decreased urine output.*
- *Assess your baby's activity daily.* Decreased activity (e.g., three or fewer movements per hour) may indicate fetal compromise.
- *It is important to keep your scheduled prenatal appointments* so that any changes in your or your baby's condition can be detected immediately.
- *Keep a daily log or diary* of your assessments for your home health care nurse, or bring it with you to your next prenatal visit.

*Thresholds for blood pressure, weight gain, fetal movement counts, and proteinuria are set by the physician or institutional protocol.

rest has been shown to be beneficial in decreasing blood pressure and promoting diuresis. Adverse physiologic outcomes related to bed rest include cardiovascular deconditioning; diuresis with accompanying fluid, electrolyte, and weight loss; muscle atrophy; and psychologic stress. These changes begin on the first day of bed rest and continue for the duration of therapy. Thus, modified bed rest with bathroom privileges may be ordered to help decrease negative effects (Maloni, Alexander, Schluchter, Shah, & Park, 2004; Sibai, 2002b).

TEACHING FOR SELF-CARE

Coping with Bed Rest

- *In bed, lie on your side.* This allows more blood to get to your uterus (womb) and the baby. The bed or sofa should be near a window and a bathroom.
- *Increase your fluid intake* to 8 glasses/day and add roughage (bran, fruits, leafy vegetables) to your diet to decrease constipation. Keep a bowl of fruit and a large container full of water close by.
- *Include diversionary activities,* such as puzzles, reading, and crafts, to reduce boredom. Place a box or table within reach to store magazines, books, telephone, and so forth.
- *Do gentle exercises,* such as circling your hands and feet or gently tensing and relaxing arm and leg muscles. This improves muscle tone, circulation, and sense of well-being.
- *Encourage family participation* in your care.
- *Have significant others assist you* with care of the house, children, and so forth.
- *Use relaxation to help cope with stress.* Relax your body one muscle at a time, or imagine some pleasant scene, word, or image. Soothing music can also help you relax.

Women with mild preeclampsia feel reasonably well; boredom from activity restriction is therefore common. Diversionary activities, visits from friends, telephone conversations, and creation of a comfortable and convenient environment are ways to cope with the boredom (see Teaching for Self-Care box). Gentle exercise (e.g., range of motion, stretching, Kegel exercises, pelvic tilts) is important in maintaining muscle tone, blood flow, regularity of bowel function, and a sense of well-being. Relaxation techniques can help reduce the stress associated with a high risk pregnancy and prepare the woman for labor and birth.

Diet. Diet and fluid recommendations are much the same as for healthy pregnant women. Diets high in protein and low in salt have been suggested to prevent preeclampsia; however, the efficacy of these diets has not been proven (Sibai, 2002b). The exception may be the woman with chronic hypertension that was successfully controlled with a low salt diet before the pregnancy. Adequate fluid intake helps maintain optimum fluid volume and aids in renal perfusion and bowel function (see Teaching for Self-Care box).

Successful home care requires the woman to be well educated about preeclampsia and highly motivated to follow the plan of care. All teaching should include the woman and her family, and time must be allowed for assimilation of information, questions, and concerns. The woman's knowledge base is directly associated with her compliance with the prescribed treatment program. Methods for enhancing learning include visual aids, videotapes, handouts, and demonstrations with return demonstrations. Furthermore, the effects of illness, language, age, culture, beliefs, and support systems must be considered (see Plan of Care).

▬ *Severe Preeclampsia and HELLP Syndrome*

Hospital Care. The women with severe preeclampsia or HELLP syndrome should receive appropriate management in a tertiary care center. The woman may be admitted to an antepartum or a labor and birth unit, depending on the hospital. If the woman's condition is severe, she may be placed in an obstetric critical care unit or a medical intensive care unit for hemodynamic monitoring. If severe preeclampsia is diagnosed at less than 32 weeks, an initial

TEACHING FOR SELF-CARE

Nutrition

- Eat a nutritious, balanced diet (60 to 70 g protein; 1200 mg calcium; and adequate zinc, magnesium, and vitamins). Consult with registered dietitian on the diet best suited for you as an individual.
- There is no sodium restriction; however, consider limiting excessively salty foods (luncheon meats, pretzels, potato chips, pickles, sauerkraut).
- Eat foods with roughage (whole grains, raw fruits, and vegetables).
- Drink six to eight 8-oz glasses of water per day.
- Avoid alcohol, and limit caffeine intake.

EVIDENCE-BASED PRACTICE

Treatments for Preeclampsia

BACKGROUND

- Preeclampsia is a common complication of pregnancy associated with endothelial inflammation leading to high blood pressure and proteinuria. When severe, it can affect the maternal liver, kidneys, clotting factors, and brain. Uteroplacental hypoperfusion can compromise fetal growth and lead to hypoxia and early delivery. For unknown reasons, preeclampsia can lead to eclampsia, seizures that can be life threatening for mother and fetus. Clinicians use anticonvulsants such as diazepam and phenytoin, but the most accepted treatment worldwide is magnesium sulfate, a central nervous system depressant and smooth muscle relaxer. Side effects include hypotension, nausea, flushing, and muscle weakness. Adverse effects include respiratory depression in mother and newborn, possibly increased cesarean births due to its tocolytic effects, and postpartum hemorrhage and retained placenta due to decreased muscle tone of uterus.

OBJECTIVES

- The reviewers' goal was to assess efficacy and risks of treatments for preeclampsia. They sought evidence about various therapies, and their use with varying degrees of disease severity. Outcomes for women included eclampsia and complications, hospital stay, induction of labor, type of birth, hemorrhage, retained placenta, and death. Outcomes for the baby included Apgar scores, hemorrhage, development, admission to special care nursery, hospital stay, and death.

METHODS

Search Strategy

- The authors searched the Cochrane Pregnancy and Childbirth Group trials register. They identified 13 studies of 15,588 women from Denmark, Malaysia, Mexico, South Africa, Taiwan, and the United States, dated 1992 to 2003.

Statistical Analyses

- Similar data were pooled. The largest pool was 11,444 women in six trials comparing magnesium sulfate to placebo/no treatment. Reviewers calculated relative risk for dichotomous (categoric) data, such as type of birth. From that, they calculated the "number needed to treat" (NNT) in order to prevent one incidence of harm, such as one case of eclampsia. Differences between groups outside the 95% confidence interval were accepted as significant.

FINDINGS

- Magnesium sulfate cut the risk of eclampsia by half and greatly decreased the chance of dying, when compared to placebo/no treatment, and was also superior to other anticonvulsants. The NNT to prevent one case of eclampsia was 100. In severe disease, the NNT was 50. The most common side effect was flushing. The only sign of toxicity that reached significance was respiratory depression. Where intramuscular injection was the route, there were problems at the injection site. Magnesium sulfate groups had less chance of placental abruption, but a slightly increased chance of cesarean birth than placebo. There was no increased need for induction, or increased postpartum hemorrhage, retained placenta, stillbirth, or admission to the special care nursery, when compared to placebo.

LIMITATIONS

- Even in reviews representing thousands of women, some adverse effects, such as placental abruption, are rare enough that trials do not detect a treatment effect. The trials varied as to criteria for preeclampsia, and some only admitted women with moderate or severe disease. This means the NNT might be higher for mild disease. Intramuscular injections do not provide the consistent systemic dosing, nor the reversibility of intravenous dosing. Most of the studies had little blinding.

IMPLICATIONS FOR PRACTICE

- Magnesium sulfate is the anticonvulsant of choice. The reviewers recommend treatment not exceed 24 hours and or 1 g/hour. This is less than typically used in many U.S. hospitals, where serum levels can be monitored. Nurses need to monitor the respirations, reflexes, and urine output during intravenous administration. Low drug cost and absence of need to monitor serum level at the recommended doses make it suitable for low-resource countries.

IMPLICATIONS FOR FURTHER RESEARCH

- The reviewers already plan a future review about the optimal dosing and administration of magnesium sulfate. Much more information is needed to determine the long-range consequences for mother and development of the child, and long-range cost-effectiveness. Accumulating more data may give a better picture of treatment effect on rare events, such as abruption.

Reference: Duley, L., Gulmezoglu, A., & Henderson-Smart, D. (2003). Magnesium sulphate and other anticonvulsants for women with pre-eclampsia. In *The Cochrane Database of Systematic Reviews*, 2006, Issue 3. Chichester, UK: John Wiley & Sons.

■ **NURSE ALERT**

The woman's BP, pulse, and respiratory status should be monitored closely while the loading dose is being administered IV, and every 15 to 30 minutes at other times, depending on the stability of the woman's condition.

Magnesium sulfate is rarely given IM because the absorption rate cannot be controlled, injections are painful, and tissue necrosis may occur. However, the IM route may be used with some women who are being transported to a tertiary care center. The IM dose is 4 to 5 g given in each buttock, a total of 10 g (with 1% procaine possibly being added to the solution to reduce injection pain), and can be repeated at 4 hour intervals. Z-track technique should be used for the deep IM injection, followed by gentle massage at the site.

Magnesium sulfate interferes with the release of acetylcholine at the synapses, decreasing neuromuscular irritability, depressing cardiac conduction, and decreasing CNS irritability. Because magnesium circulates free and unbound to protein and is excreted in the urine, accurate recordings of maternal urine output must be obtained. Since magnesium sulfate is a CNS depressant, the nurse

| box 30-5 | **Protocol for Care of Women with Preeclampsia Receiving Magnesium Sulfate** |

MAGNESIUM SULFATE ADMINISTRATION

Client and Family Teaching
Explain technique, rationale, and reactions to expect
- Route and rate
- Purpose of "piggyback"
Reasons for use
- Tailor information to woman's readiness to learn
- Explain that it is to prevent disease progression
- Explain that it is to prevent seizures
Reactions to expect from medication
- Initially woman will feel flushed, hot, and sedated, especially during the bolus
- Sedation will continue
Monitoring to anticipate
- Maternal: blood pressure, pulse, DTRs, level of consciousness, urine output (indwelling catheter likely), presence of headache, visual disturbances, epigastric pain
- Fetal: FHR and activity

Administration
- Verify physician order
- Position woman in side-lying position
- Prepare solution and administer with an infusion control device (pump)
- Piggyback a solution of 40 g magnesium sulfate in 1000 ml of lactated Ringer's solution with an infusion control device at the ordered rates: loading dose: initial bolus of 4-6 g over 15 to 30 min; maintenance dose: 1-3 g/hr

Maternal and Fetal Assessments
- Monitor blood pressure, pulse, respiratory rate, FHR, and contractions every 15-30 min, depending on client condition
- Monitor intake and output, proteinuria, DTRs, presence of headache, visual disturbances, and epigastric pain at least hourly
- Restrict hourly fluid intake to a total of 100 to 125 ml/hr; urinary output should be ≥30 ml/hr

Reportable Conditions
- Blood pressure: systolic, ≥160 mm Hg; diastolic, ≥110 mm Hg, or both
- Respiratory rate: ≤12 breaths/min
- Urinary output <30 ml/hr
- Presence of headache, visual disturbances, or epigastric pain
- Increasing severity or loss of DTRs, increasing edema, proteinuria
- Any abnormal laboratory values (magnesium levels, platelet count, creatinine clearance, levels of uric acid, AST, ALT, prothrombin time, partial thromboplastin time, fibrinogen, fibrin split products)
- Any other significant change in maternal or fetal status

Emergency Measures
- Keep emergency drug tray at bedside with calcium gluconate and intubation equipment
- Keep side rails up
- Keep lights dimmed, and maintain a quiet environment

Documentation
- All of the above

ALT, alanine aminotransferase; *AST,* aspartate aminotransferase; *DTR,* Deep tendon reflex; *FHR,* fetal heart rate.

assesses for signs and symptoms of magnesium toxicity. Early symptoms of toxicity include nausea, a feeling of warmth, flushing, muscle weakness, decreased reflexes, and slurred speech (see Box 30-5). Serum magnesium levels are obtained per hospital protocol or if any signs of toxicity are present (Cunningham et al., 2005; Sibai, 2002b).

▬ NURSE ALERT

Loss of patellar reflexes, respiratory depression, oliguria, and decreased level of consciousness are signs of magnesium toxicity. Action must be taken to prevent respiratory or cardiac arrest. If magnesium toxicity is suspected, the infusion should be discontinued immediately. Calcium gluconate, the antidote for magnesium sulfate, also may be ordered (10 ml of a 10% solution, or 1 g) and given by slow IV push (usually by the physician) over at least a 3 minute period to avoid undesirable reactions such as arrhythmias, bradycardia, and ventricular fibrillation (Cunningham et al., 2005; Nick, 2004; Sibai, 2002b).

Magnesium sulfate does not seem to affect the FHR in a healthy, term fetus. Neonatal serum magnesium levels approximate those levels of the mother. Doses of magnesium sulfate that prevent maternal seizures have been determined to be safe for the fetus. Toxic levels in the newborn can cause depressed respirations and hyporeflexia at birth (Cunningham et al., 2005). It is important that the neonatal team attend the birth in order to provide resuscitation measures as needed. The long-term effects of magnesium administration on mothers and infants is under investigation (Magpie Trial Follow-Up Study Management Group, 2004).

▬ NURSE ALERT

Because magnesium sulfate also is a tocolytic agent, its use may increase the duration of labor. A preeclamptic woman receiving magnesium sulfate may need augmentation with oxytocin during labor. The amount of oxytocin needed to stimulate labor may be more than that needed for a woman who is not receiving magnesium sulfate.

Control of Blood Pressure. Antihypertensive medications may be ordered to lower the diastolic blood pressure. Initiation of antihypertensive therapy reduces maternal morbidity and mortality rates associated with left ventricular failure and cerebral hemorrhage. Because a degree of maternal hypertension is necessary to maintain uteroplacental perfusion, antihypertensive therapy must not decrease the arterial pressure too much or too rapidly. The target range for the diastolic pressure is therefore less than 110 mm Hg and the systolic pressure less than 160 mm Hg (ACOG, 2002; Cunningham et al., 2005).

IV hydralazine remains the antihypertensive agent of choice for the treatment of hypertension in severe preeclampsia. Labetalol hydrochloride, nifedipine, verapamil, and oral methyldopa are also used (ACOG, 2002; Chan & Winkle, 2006; Cunningham et al., 2005; Peters & Flack, 2004). The choice of agent used depends on the woman's response and physician preference. Table 30-5 compares antihypertensive agents used to treat hypertension in pregnancy.

■ NURSE ALERT

When administering antihypertensive therapy, the nurse must remember that the drug effects are dependent on intravascular volume. Because preeclampsia is associated with contracted intravascular volume, initial doses should be given with caution, and maternal response monitored closely.

■ *Eclampsia*

Eclampsia is usually preceded by various premonitory symptoms and signs, including headache, severe epigastric pain, and hyperreflexia. However, convulsions can appear suddenly and without warning in a seemingly stable woman with only minimum blood pressure elevations (Longo et al., 2003; Sibai, 2004). The convulsions that occur in eclampsia are frightening to observe. Increased hypertension and tonic contraction of all body muscles (seen as arms flexed, hands clenched, legs inverted) precede the tonic-clonic convulsions (Fig. 30-6). During this stage, muscles alternately relax and contract. Respirations are halted and then begin again with long, deep, stertorous inhalations. Hypotension follows, and coma ensues. Nystagmus and muscular twitching persist for a time. Disorientation and amnesia cloud the immediate recovery. Seizures may recur within minutes of the first convulsion, or the woman may never have another. During the convulsion the pregnant woman and fetus are not receiving oxygen, so eclamptic seizures produce a marked metabolic insult to both the woman and the fetus (Cunningham et al., 2005).

Immediate Care. The immediate goal of care during a convulsion is to ensure a patent airway (see Emergency box). When convulsions occur, turn the woman onto her side to prevent aspiration of vomitus and supine hypotension syndrome. Note the time and the duration of the convulsion. After the convulsion ceases, suction food and fluids from the glottis, and administer 10 L of oxygen by a facemask. If an IV infusion is not in place, insert one with an 18 gauge needle. Magnesium sulfate 2 to 4 g is given by IV push, and repeated every 15 minutes with a maximum of 6 g. If eclampsia develops after the initiation of magnesium sulfate therapy, additional magnesium sulfate or another anticonvulsant (e.g., diazepam) may be

FIG. 30-6 Eclampsia (convulsions or seizures).

EMERGENCY

Eclampsia
TONIC-CLONIC CONVULSION SIGNS
- Stage of invasion: 2-3 sec, eyes are fixed, twitching of facial muscles occurs
- Stage of contraction: 15-20 sec, eyes protrude and are bloodshot, all body muscles are in tonic contraction
- Stage of convulsion: Muscles relax and contract alternately (clonic); respirations are halted and then begin again with long, deep, stertorous inhalation; coma ensues

INTERVENTION
- Keep airway patent: Turn head to one side, place pillow under one shoulder or back if possible
- Call for assistance
- Protect with side rails up
- Observe and record convulsion activity

AFTER CONVULSION OR SEIZURE
- Do not leave unattended until fully alert
- Observe for postconvulsion coma, incontinence
- Use suction as needed
- Administer oxygen via face mask at 10 L/min
- Start intravenous fluids and monitor for potential fluid overload
- Give magnesium sulfate or anticonvulsant drug as ordered
- Insert indwelling urinary catheter
- Monitor blood pressure
- Monitor fetal and uterine status
- Expedite laboratory work as ordered to monitor kidney function, liver function, coagulation system, and drug levels
- Provide hygiene and a quiet environment
- Support woman and family and keep them informed
- Be prepared to assist with birth when woman is in stable condition

administered (ACOG, 2002; Sibai et al., 2005). Fetal and neonatal effects of diazepam include decreased FHR variability, neonatal hyotonia, decreased respirations, and depressed sucking reflex. With adequate blood magnesium levels, the eclamptic woman will rarely continue to have seizures (Chan & Winkle, 2006; Cunningham et al., 2005; Roberts, 2004).

Aspiration is a leading cause of maternal morbidity and mortality after eclamptic seizure. After initial stabilization and airway management, the nurse should anticipate orders for a chest radiograph and possibly arterial blood gases to rule out the possibility of aspiration.

A rapid assessment of uterine activity, cervical status, and fetal status is performed after a convulsion. During the convulsion, membranes may have ruptured; the cervix may have dilated, because the uterus becomes hypercontractile and hypertonic; and birth may be imminent. If not, once a woman's seizure activity and BP are controlled, a decision should be made regarding whether birth should take place. The target levels for blood pressure management are a systolic blood pressure between 140 and 160 mm Hg and a diastolic pressure between 90 and 110 mm Hg. Blood

table 30-5 Pharmacologic Control of Hypertension in Pregnancy

ACTION AND DOSAGE	TARGET TISSUE	MATERNAL EFFECTS	FETAL EFFECTS	NURSING ACTIONS
HYDRALAZINE (APRESOLINE, NEOPRESOL)*				
Arteriolar vasodilator; usually administered intravenously (IV) or intramuscularly (IM). Start with 5 mg IV or 10 mg IM; may be repeated at 20-min intervals (5 to 10 mg depending on response). Once BP is controlled, repeat as needed (usually every 3 hours). If no success after 20 mg IV or 30 mg IM total dose, consider another drug	Peripheral arterioles: to decrease muscle tone, decrease peripheral resistance; hypothalamus and medullary vasomotor center for minor decrease in sympathetic tone	Headache, flushing, palpitation, tachycardia, some decrease in uteroplacental blood flow, increase in heart rate and cardiac output, increase in oxygen consumption, nausea and vomiting	Tachycardia; late decelerations and bradycardia if maternal diastolic pressure <90 mm Hg	Assess for effects of medications, alert mother (family) to expected effects of medications, assess blood pressure frequently because precipitate decrease can lead to shock and perhaps abruptio placentae; assess urinary output; maintain bed rest in a lateral position with side rails up; use with caution in presence of maternal tachycardia
LABETALOL HYDROCHLORIDE (NORMODYNE)*				
Beta-blocking agent causing vasodilation without significant change in cardiac output; usually administered intravenously. Start with 20 mg IV as a bolus; if effect is suboptimal, give 40 mg 10 min later and 80 mg every 10 min for 2 more doses (to a maximum dose of 220 mg). If BP control not achieved, switch to another drug	Peripheral arterioles (see hydralazine)	Minimal: flushing, tremulousness; minimal change in pulse rate	Minimal, if any	See hydralazine; less likely to cause excessive hypotension and tachycardia; less rebound hypertension than hydralazine
NIFEDIPINE (PROCARDIA)*				
Calcium channel blocker; usually administered orally. Start with 10 mg orally and repeat in 30 min if necessary	Arterioles: to reduce systemic vascular resistance by relaxation of arterial smooth muscle	Headache, flushing; possible potentiation of effects on CNS if administered concurrently with magnesium sulfate, may interfere with labor	Minimal	See hydralazine; use caution if woman also getting magnesium sulfate
METHYLDOPA (ALDOMET)†				
Alpha$_2$-receptor agonist; usually administered orally. Dose ranges from 250 mg to 500 mg orally every 8 hr.	Postganglionic nerve endings: interferes with chemical neurotransmission to reduce peripheral vascular resistance, causes CNS sedation	Sleepiness, postural hypotension, constipation; rare: drug-induced fever in 1% of women and positive Coombs' test result in 20%	After 4 mo maternal therapy, positive Coombs' test result in infant after birth	See hydralazine

CNS, Central nervous system.
*For acute severe hypertension—blood pressure ≥160 mmHg systoloc, ≥105 mmHg diastolic, or both if sustained.
†Maintenance therapy if needed.

pressure may be managed with hydralazine (10 mg doses) or labetalol (20 to 40 mg intravenously) every 15 minutes (Sibai et al., 2005). The more serious the condition of the woman, the greater the need to proceed to birth. The route of birth—induction of labor versus cesarean birth—depends on maternal and fetal condition, fetal gestational age, presence of labor, and the cervical Bishop score (Sibai et al.). In pregnancies of less than 34 weeks of gestation, antenatal corticosteroids may be given to promote fetal lung maturation. If the birth can be delayed for 48 hours, steroids such as betamethasone (12 mg IM 24 hours apart) may be given to the woman (Cunningham et al., 2005; Sibai et al.). General anesthesia is usually not recommended since there is an increased risk of aspiration, but maternal pain can be controlled with epidural anesthesia or systemic opioids. Regional anesthesia is not recommended for eclamptic women with coagulopathy or a platelet count less than 50,000/mm^3 (Sibai et al.).

The woman may have been incontinent of urine and stool during the convulsion; she will need assistance with hygiene and a change of gown.

▬ NURSE ALERT

Immediately after a seizure, the woman may be very confused and can be combative. Pad the side rails to prevent injury, and maintain a quiet, darkened environment. It may take several hours for the woman to regain her usual level of mental functioning. The woman should not be left alone. Provide emotional support to the family and discuss with them the management and its rationale and the woman's progress.

Laboratory tests are ordered to assess for HELLP syndrome. Blood is typed and crossmatched in the event of an emergency transfusion. Whole blood or packed red blood cells may be infused in the event of hemorrhage or shock, since the eclamptic women is high risk for abruptio placentae. Other tests include determination of electrolyte levels, liver function, and a CBC and a clotting profile, including platelet count and fibrin split product levels (to assess for DIC). Since aspiration is a leading cause of maternal morbidity and mortality after a seizure, a chest radiograph or arterial blood gases may also be ordered.

▬ *Postpartum Nursing Care*

After birth, the symptoms of preeclampsia or eclampsia resolve quickly, usually within 48 hours. Resolution of the disease process is manifested by diuresis, which usually occurs within 24 hours after the birth (Longo et al., 2003). The hematopoietic and hepatic complications of HELLP syndrome may persist longer. Usually an abrupt decrease in platelet count occurs, with a concomitant increase in LDH and AST levels, after a trend toward normalization of values has begun. Generally the laboratory abnormalities seen with HELLP syndrome resolve in 72 to 96 hours.

The nursing care of the woman with hypertensive disease differs from that required in the usual postpartum period in a number of respects. The following material describes variations in the nursing process.

The woman will need careful assessment of her vital signs, intake and output, DTRs, level of consciousness, uterine tone, and lochia flow throughout the postpartum period. The magnesium sulfate infusion is continued for 12 to 24 hours for seizure prophylaxis. Since magnesium sulfate potentiates the action of narcotics, CNS depressants, and calcium channel blockers, these drugs must be administered with caution. Even if no convulsions occurred before the birth, they may occur during the postpartum period. The nurse should also assess the woman for any symptoms of preeclampsia such as headaches, visual disturbances, or epigastric pain.

Later postpartum eclampsia is eclampsia occurring after 48 hours but before 4 postpartal weeks. These women may present with clinical manifestations of preeclampsia intrapartally or during the immediate postpartum, although other women present with the initial symptoms and convulsions after 48 hours postpartum (Sibai et al., 2005).

▬ NURSE ALERT

The woman is at risk for a boggy uterus and a large lochia flow as a result of the magnesium sulfate therapy. Uterine tone and lochia flow should be assessed frequently.

The preeclamptic woman is unable to tolerate excessive postpartum blood loss because of hemoconcentration. Oxytocin or prostaglandin products are used to control bleeding. Ergot products (e.g., Ergotrate and Methergine) are contraindicated, because they increase blood pressure.

Postpartum recovery may be prolonged as a result of the physiologic consequences of prolonged bed rest. The nurse should accompany the woman when she ambulates after prolonged bed rest and assess for weakness, dizziness, and shortness of breath and muscle soreness. Also, the woman will need reassurance that the physiologic effects of bed rest will reverse over time, when she resumes normal activity (Simpson & James, 2005).

It is important to provide emotional support to the woman and her family during this stressful period. Coping mechanisms should be assessed and appropriate referrals initiated. If the preeclampsia was severe, the infant may be premature and in a special care nursery. The woman and her family may be worried about their infant's survival, and the day-to-day fluctuations in the infant's status can be emotionally draining (Simpson & James, 2005). Emotional stress can also decrease the woman's ability to process information. Thus, the nurse should include the family during all discharge teaching and provide them with written information. The woman and her family should also be informed that there is a sevenfold increase in the chance of developing preeclampsia or eclampsia in a future pregnancy, and that comprehensive prenatal care is essential for assessment and early intervention (Duckitt & Harrington, 2005).

▬ Evaluation

Evaluation of the effectiveness of care of the woman with preeclampsia is based on the expected outcomes.

▪ CHRONIC HYPERTENSION

Chronic hypertension affects 5% of pregnant women. Of these women, 95% to 98% have essential hypertension, and 2% have secondary hypertension as a result of a medical condition such as renal disease or Cushing's syndrome (Longo et al., 2003). Chronic hypertension in pregnancy is associated with an increased incidence of abruptio placentae, superimposed preeclampsia, and increased perinatal mortality (three- or fourfold). Fetal effects include fetal growth restriction and small-for-gestational-age infants (Cunningham et al., 2005).

Ideally, the management of chronic hypertension in pregnancy begins before conception. Many women with chronic hypertension are treated with an antihypertensive medication when they become pregnant. It is important for women to discontinue any antihypertensive medications known to be embryotoxic. Because of the antihypertensive effects of pregnancy, the antihypertensive medication may be discontinued or changed to another medication. Antihypertensive medications are reinstituted when the blood pressure increases with gestational age, especially after 28 weeks (Longo et al., 2003; Peters & Flack, 2004).

Based upon the history and physical findings, women with chronic hypertension are identified as being at either high or low risk for pregnancy complications (Sibai, 2002a). Women who are at high risk are managed with antihypertensive medication and frequent assessments of maternal and fetal well-being. The goal of treatment is to maintain a blood pressure below 150 to 160 mm Hg systolic and 100 to 110 mm Hg diastolic. Methyldopa (Aldomet) is the drug of choice for treating chronic hypertension in pregnancy. If methyldopa is ineffective in reducing blood pressure, then hydralazine, beta-blockers, or calcium channel blockers may be used (Chan & Winkle, 2006; Cunningham et al., 2005: Longo et al., 2003; Peters & Flack, 2004). The treatment of low risk women is controversial. Evidence has not shown improvement in maternal or fetal outcome or a decreased risk of developing superimposed preeclampsia with treatment (Abalos, Duley, Steyn, & Henderson-Smart, 2001; Longo et al.; Peters & Flack).

It is important to counsel the woman and her family about lifestyle changes to help minimize the risks associated with chronic hypertension in pregnancy. These changes include limiting sodium intake, exercise as appropriate, consuming a well-balanced diet, limiting caffeine intake, avoidance of alcohol and tobacco use, and losing weight in the preconception period if overweight. Also, they should be taught how to perform blood pressure monitoring and fetal movement counting and the importance of maintaining bed rest (Gilbert & Harmon, 2003; Longo et al., 2003; Peters & Flack, 2004).

The time of birth is individualized, but a woman at low risk can usually wait until her cervix is favorable for induction at 37 weeks (Gregg, 2004). However, women at high risk are followed closely, and the method and timing of the birth is dependent upon the maternal and fetal status. After giving birth, the woman should be monitored closely for complications such as pulmonary edema, renal failure, heart failure, and encephalopathy (Sibai, 2002a). Since all antihypertensive medications are found in breast milk, the drug of choice for women who breastfeed is methyldopa or hydralazine. Short-term studies have not found any adverse effects on infants, but no long-term human studies have examined the drug effects on infants (Peters & Flack, 2004).

community activity

Contact the nearest Health Department Prenatal Clinic or private OB office. Assess the educational resources and recommended screening tools available for women with hypertensive disorders of pregnancy in these agencies. Are these available in languages other than English? How can these resources be made available to pregnant women in the community?

key points

- Hypertensive disorders during pregnancy are a leading cause of worldwide infant and maternal morbidity and mortality.
- The cause of preeclampsia is unknown, and there are no known reliable tests for predicting which women are at risk for preeclampsia.
- Preeclampsia is a multisystem disease rather than only an increase in BP.
- Failure of trophoblastic invasion of spiral arterioles is proposed as the triggering mechanism that eventually leads to vasospasm and organ ischemia; the cure is birth of the fetus and delivery of the placenta.
- The pathologic changes of preeclampsia, involving every organ system in the body, are present long before clinical manifestations are evident.
- Historic risk factors (e.g., first pregnancy or pregnancy of new genetic makeup, history of vascular disease, and multiple gestation) are associated with a higher incidence of preeclampsia.
- Progression of hypertensive disorders during pregnancy is unpredictable; mild hypertension must therefore be taken seriously and managed as for preeclampsia.
- Once preeclampsia becomes clinically evident, therapeutic intervention is palliative (bed rest, diet); this may slow the progression of the disease and allow the pregnancy to continue.
- Home care management is an option only for women whose condition is stable and who are able to comply with the medical regimen, reliably perform self-monitoring, and immediately recognize and report abnormal signs and symptoms.
- HELLP syndrome can occur in women with severe preeclampsia and is considered life threatening.
- Magnesium sulfate, the anticonvulsive agent of choice for preventing eclampsia, requires careful monitoring of reflexes, respirations, and urinary output; its antidote, calcium gluconate, should be available at the bedside.

Continued

key points—cont'd

- The intent of emergency interventions for eclampsia is to prevent self-injury, ensure adequate oxygenation, reduce aspiration risk, establish seizure control with magnesium sulfate, and correct maternal acidemia.
- Chronic hypertension in pregnancy is associated with abruptio placentae and superimposed preeclampsia.

REFERENCES

Abalos, E., Duley, L., Steyn, N., & Henderson-Smart, D. (2001). Antihypertensive drug treatment for mild to moderate hypertension in pregnancy. *The Cochrane Database of Systematic Reviews, 2006*, Issue 3. Chichester, UK: John Wiley & Sons.

American College of Obstetricians and Gynecologists (ACOG). (2002). *Diagnosis and management of preeclampsia and eclampsia.* ACOG Practice Bulletin Number 33. Washington, DC: Author.

Aslan, H., Gul, A., & Cebeci, A. (2004). Neonatal outcome in pregnancies after preterm delivery for HELLP syndrome. *Gynecologic and Obstetric Investigation, 58*(2), 96-99.

Atallah, A., Hofmeyr, G., & Duley, L. (2002). Calcium supplementation during pregnancy for preventing hypertensive disorders and related problems. *The Cochrane Database of Systematic Reviews,* 2006, Issue 3. Chichester, UK: John Wiley & Sons.

Bashiri, A., Zmora, E., Sheiner, E., Hershkovitz, R., Shoham-Vardi, I., & Mazor, M. (2003). Maternal hypertensive disorders are an independent risk factor for the development of necrotizing enterocolitis in very low birth weight infants. *Fetal Diagnosis and Therapy, 18*(6), 404-407.

Chan, P., & Winkle, C. (2006). *Gynecology and obstetrics: Current clinical strategies.* Laguna Hills, CA: CCS Publishing.

Cockey, C. (2005). Predicting preeclampsia. *AWHONN Lifelines, 9*(1), 25-26.

Cunningham, F., Leveno, K., Bloom, S., Hauth, J., Gilstrap, L., & Wenstrom, K. (2005). *Williams obstetrics* (22nd ed.). New York: McGraw-Hill.

Duckitt, R., & Harrington, D. (2005). Risk factors for pre-eclampsia at antenatal booking: Systematic review of controlled studies. *BMJ, 333*(7491), 565.

Emery, S. (2005). Hypertensive disorders of pregnancy: Overdiagnosis is appropriate. *Cleveland Clinic Journal of Medicine, 72*(4), 345-352.

Gilbert, E., & Harmon, J. (2003). *Manual of high risk pregnancy & delivery* (3rd ed.). St. Louis: Mosby.

Gregg, A. (2004). Hypertension in pregnancy. *Obstetric and Gynecologic Clinics of North America, 31*(2), 223-241.

Hjartardottir, S., Leifsson, B., Geirsson, R. & Steinthorsdottir, V. (2004). Paternity change and the recurrence risk in familial hypertensive disorders in pregnancy. *Hypertension in Pregnancy, 23*(2), 219-225.

Kochanek, K., Murphy, S., Anderson, R., & Scott, C. (2004). Deaths: Final data for 2002. *National Vital Statistics Report, 53*(5), 1-115.

Longo, S., Dola, C., & Pridjian, G. (2003). Preeclampsia and eclampsia revisited. *Southern Medical Journal, 96*(9), 891-898.

Magpie Trial Follow-Up Study Management Group. (2004).The Magpie trial follow-up study: Outcome after discharge from hospital for women and children recruited to a trial comparing magnesium sulfate with placebo for pre-eclampsia. *BMC Pregnancy and Childbirth 4*(1), 5.

Maloni, J., Alexander, G., Schluchter, M., Shah, D., & Park, S. (2004). Antepartum bed rest: Maternal weight gain change and infant birth weight. *Biological Research for Nursing, 5*(3), 177-186.

Martin, J., Hamilton, B., Sutton, P., Ventura, S., Menacker, F., & Munson, M. (2005). Births: Final data for 2003. *National Vital Statistics Reports, 54*(2), 1-116.

Moldenhauer, J., & Sibai, B. (2002). HELLP syndrome: Pinpointing the diagnosis. *Women's Health Gynecologic Edition, 2*(3), 139-150.

National High Blood Pressure Education Program (NHBPEP) Working Group on High Blood Pressure in Pregnancy. (2000). Report of the National High Blood Pressure Education Program Working Group on High Blood Pressure in Pregnancy. *American Journal of Obstetrics and Gynecology, 183*(1)S1-S22.

Nick, J. (2004). Deep tendon reflexes, magnesium, and calcium: Assessments and implications. *Journal of Obstetric, Gynecologic, and Neonatal Nursing 33*(2), 221-230.

Peters, R., & Flack, J. (2004). Hypertensive disorders of pregnancy. *Journal of Obstetric, Gynecologic, and Neonatal Nursing, 33*(2), 209-219.

Roberts, J. (2004). Pregnancy-related hypertension. In R. Creasy, R. Resnik, & J. Iams (Eds.), *Maternal-fetal medicine: Principles and practice* (5th ed.). Philadelphia: Saunders.

Roberts, J., Pearson, G., Cutler, J., Lindheimer, M., & NHLBI Working Group on Research on Hypertension During Pregnancy. (2003). Summary of the NHLBI working group on research on hypertension during pregnancy. *Hypertension, 41*(3), 437-445.

Sibai, B. (2002a). Chronic hypertension in pregnancy. *Obstetrics and Gynecology, 100*(2), 369-377.

Sibai, B. (2002b). Hypertension in pregnancy. In S. Gabbe, J. Niebyl, & J. Simpson (Eds.), *Obstetrics: Normal and problem pregnancies* (4th ed.). New York: Churchill Livingstone.

Sibai, B. (2004). Diagnosis, controversies, and management of the syndrome of hemolysis, elevated liver enzymes, and low platelet count. *Obstetrics and Gynecology, 103*(5 Part 1), 981-991.

Sibai, B., Dekker, G., Kupferminic, M. (2005). Pre-eclampsia. *Lancet, 365*(9461), 785-799.

Simpson, K., & James, D. (2005). *Postpartum care.* White Plains, NY: March of Dimes.

Wener, M., & Lavigne, S. (2004). Can periodontal disease lead to premature delivery? *AWHONN Lifelines, 8*(5), 424-430.

Wolf, M., Shah, A., Jimenez-Kimble, R., Sauk, J., Ecker, J., & Thadhani, R. (2004). Differential risk of hypertensive disorders of pregnancy among Hispanic women. *Journal of the American Society of Nephrology, 15*(5), 1330-1338.

Zhang, J., Meikle S., & Trumble, A. (2003). Severe maternal morbidity associated with hypertensive disorders in pregnancy in the United States. *Hypertension in Pregnancy, 22*(2), 203-212.

Zhang, C., Williams, M., Sorensen, T., King, I., Kestin, M., Thompson, M., et al. (2002). Vitamin C and the risk of preeclampsia: Results from dietary questionnaire and plasma assay. *Epidemiology, 13*(4), 409-416.

Antepartal Hemorrhagic Disorders

learning objectives

- Differentiate among causes, signs and symptoms, possible complications, and management of miscarriage, ectopic pregnancy, incompetent cervix, and hydatidiform mole.
- Compare and contrast abruptio placentae and placenta previa in relation to signs and symptoms, complications, and management.
- Discuss clotting disorders in pregnancy, with emphasis on disseminated intravascular coagulation.

- Revise plans of care for the woman with an unruptured ectopic pregnancy versus the one with a ruptured ectopic pregnancy.
- Review the physiology of a hydatidiform mole and the risk factors for the woman's immediate health future.
- Examine the role of the nurse in the health care team approach to the treatment of bleeding disorders.

electronic resources

Additional information related to the content in Chapter 31 can be found on

the companion website at **evolve**
http://evolve.elsevier.com/Lowdermilk/MWHC/
- NCLEX Review Questions
- WebLinks

or on the interactive companion CD
- NCLEX Review Questions
- Plan of Care: Placenta Previa

A maternal hypervolemic state is the result of adaptations in the hematologic and cardiovascular systems of the woman during pregnancy. Systemic and pulmonary vascular resistance also increase. Plasma volume and red blood cell mass increases occur as early as 4 to 8 weeks of gestation and serve to (1) meet the metabolic demands of the mother and fetus, (2) protect against the potentially deleterious impairment in venous return caused by the pressure of an enlarging uterus, and (3) safeguard the mother against the effects of blood loss at birth. Any bleeding in pregnancy may therefore jeopardize both maternal and fetal well-being. Maternal blood loss decreases oxygen-carrying capacity, which predisposes the woman to increased risk for hypovolemia, anemia, infection, and preterm labor and adversely affects oxygen delivery to the fetus. Fetal risks from maternal hemorrhage include blood loss or anemia, hypoxemia, hypoxia, anoxia, and preterm birth. If the bleeding involves fetal blood loss, the effects are exponential because of the smaller fetal blood volume.

Hemorrhagic disorders in pregnancy are medical emergencies; the incidence and type of bleeding vary by trimester. Antepartal hemorrhage is a leading cause of maternal death. Ruptured ectopic pregnancy and abruptio placentae

have the highest incidence of maternal mortality. Prompt assessment and intervention by the health care team is essential to save the life of the woman and fetus.

■ EARLY PREGNANCY BLEEDING

Bleeding during early pregnancy is alarming to the woman and of concern to health care providers. The common bleeding disorders of early pregnancy include miscarriage (spontaneous abortion), incompetent cervix, ectopic pregnancy, and hydatidiform mole (molar pregnancy). Women with advanced maternal age, smoking exposure, and prior preterm birth are more likely to experience intense vaginal bleeding during pregnancy (Yang et al., 2005).

Miscarriage (Spontaneous Abortion)

A pregnancy that ends as a result of natural causes before 20 weeks of gestation is defined as a spontaneous abortion. This 20 week marker is considered to be the point of viability, when a fetus may survive in an extrauterine environment. A fetal weight less than 500 g also may be used to define an abortion (Cunningham, Leveno, Bloom, Hauth, Gilstrap, & Wenstrom, 2005).

The term miscarriage is used throughout this discussion as it is a more appropriate term to use with clients; *abortion* has been perceived as an insensitive term to use with families who are grieving a pregnancy loss. Therapeutic or elective induced abortion is discussed in Chapter 9.

Incidence and Etiology

Approximately 10% to 20% of all confirmed pregnancies in the United States end in miscarriage (White & Bouvier, 2005). An early miscarriage is one that occurs before 12 weeks of gestation. At least 50% of all clinically recognized pregnancy losses result from chromosomal abnormalities (Griebel, Halvorsen, Goleman, & Day, 2005; Simpson, 2002). The majority (more than 90%) of miscarriages occur early, before 8 weeks of gestation (Simpson). Possible causes include endocrine imbalance (as in women who have luteal phase defects or insulin-dependent diabetes mellitus with high blood glucose levels in the first trimester), immunologic factors (e.g., antiphospholipid antibodies), infections (e.g., bacteriuria and *Chlamydia trachomatis*), systemic disorders (e.g., lupus erythematosus), and genetic factors (Cunningham et al., 2005; Gilbert & Harmon, 2003).

A late miscarriage occurs between 12 and 20 weeks of gestation. It usually results from maternal causes, such as

EVIDENCE-BASED PRACTICE

Vitamins to Prevent Miscarriage

BACKGROUND

- Approximately 1 out of 7 pregnancies ends in miscarriage (pregnancy loss before 20 weeks of gestation). Most losses in the first trimester are thought to be due to chromosomal abnormalities, and the majority in the second trimester may be due to structural abnormalities of the uterus or cervix. Other causes include autoimmunity, or vascular pathology such as preeclampsia or blood clotting problems. Miscarriages can cause hemorrhage, infection, stress, and grief. Poor diet and oxidative stress are thought to be risk factors for miscarriage. Dietary and supplemental nutrients, including vitamins, may help prevent miscarriages, but excessive fat-soluble vitamins A, D, E, and K may accumulate in the body and become toxic.

OBJECTIVES

- The authors set out to assess the efficacy and safety of any vitamin supplementation from preconception through 20 weeks of gestation. Fetal outcomes included fetal loss, prematurity, birth weight, congenital abnormalities (excluding neural tube defect, covered in another review), Apgar scores, hospitalization, and long-term development. Maternal outcomes included multiple pregnancies, preeclampsia, placental abnormalities, anemia, breastfeeding, and subsequent pregnancies.

METHODS

Search Strategy

- After a thorough search of the Cochrane Pregnancy and Childbirth Group's trial register, the authors qualified 17 randomized or quasi-randomized controlled trials representing 35,812 women during 37,353 pregnancies. The earliest trial was The People's League Study, an extraordinary example of dedication to research. It was a quasi-randomized study, representing 5515 pregnant women, seen 1938 to 1939, of whom 494 were lost to follow-up when they were evacuated from London during World War II. The study was completed and published in 1942. Other selected trials dated 1968 to 2003 and originated from Hungary, India, Indonesia, Ireland, Japan, Malawi, Nigeria, Portugal, Tanzania, the United Kingdom, and the United States.

Statistical Analyses

- Similar data were pooled. Reviewers calculated relative risk for dichotomous (categoric) data, such as type of birth, and weighted mean difference for continuous data, such as pain scale. Differences between groups outside the 95% confidence interval were accepted as significant.

FINDINGS

- No vitamins, single or combined, prevented miscarriage or stillbirth. Multivitamins and vitamins C and E were associated with significantly less preeclampsia. The vitamin C groups had a greater risk of preterm birth. Vitamin A and multivitamins were associated with increased multiple births. One suggested reason for this is an increase in multiple conceptions, rather than just improved survival of twins.

LIMITATIONS

- Some trials included pregnancy loss through 26 or 28 weeks of gestation, or did not define miscarriage. Blinding of participants and evaluators was unclear in most trials. Placebos varied—some had trace elements or vitamins in them. Two trials had no placebos. Trials that spanned decades and wars and availability of resources made an enriched but heterogenous mix of data, challenging to metaanalyze. Some of the women were randomized, but never became pregnant during the trial period, yet were counted as not having miscarried, skewing the results.

IMPLICATIONS FOR PRACTICE

- Vitamins do not prevent miscarriages, but multivitamins and vitamins C and E may reduce the incidence of preeclampsia. This may be offset, somewhat, by an increase in the incidence of multiple pregnancies, which carry risks. The advantages of folic acid in preventing neural tube defects are well established (see Evidence-Based Practice box for Chapter 13). Vitamins seem safe, at recommended doses.

IMPLICATIONS FOR FURTHER RESEARCH

- Multiple pregnancies are higher risk for adverse outcomes, and much more research is needed to clarify whether multivitamins, now so commonly recommended in industrialized countries, are beneficial. Well-designed randomized, placebo-controlled trials can establish the doses and combinations needed for safety and beneficial outcomes.

Reference: Rumbold, A., Middleton, P., & Crowther, C. (2005). Vitamin supplementation for preventing miscarriage. *The Cochrane Database of Systematic Reviews,* 2006, Issue 3. Chichester, UK: John Wiley & Sons.

advancing maternal age and parity, chronic infections, premature dilation of the cervix and other anomalies of the reproductive tract, chronic debilitating diseases, inadequate nutrition, and recreational drug use (Cunningham et al., 2005). Little can be done to avoid genetically caused pregnancy loss, but correction of maternal disorders, immunization against infectious diseases, adequate early prenatal care, and treatment of pregnancy complications can do much to prevent other causes of miscarriage.

Types

The types of miscarriage include threatened, inevitable, incomplete, complete, and missed. All types of miscarriage can recur in subsequent pregnancies; all types except the threatened miscarriage can lead to infection (Fig. 31-1).

Clinical Manifestations

Signs and symptoms of miscarriage depend on the duration of pregnancy. The presence of uterine bleeding, uterine contractions, or uterine pain is an ominous sign during early pregnancy and must be considered a threatened miscarriage until proven otherwise.

If miscarriage occurs before the sixth week of pregnancy, the woman may report a heavy menstrual flow. Miscarriage that occurs between weeks 6 and 12 of pregnancy causes moderate discomfort and blood loss. After week 12, miscarriage is typified by more severe pain, similar to that of labor, because the fetus must be expelled. Diagnosis of the type of miscarriage is based on the signs and symptoms present (Table 31-1).

Symptoms of a *threatened* miscarriage (see Fig. 31-1, *A*) include spotting of blood but with the cervical os closed. Mild uterine cramping may be present.

Inevitable (see Fig. 31-1, *B*) and *incomplete* (see Fig. 31-1, *C*) miscarriages involve a moderate to heavy amount of bleeding with an open cervical os. Tissue may be present with the bleeding. Mild to severe uterine cramping may be present. An inevitable miscarriage is often accompanied by rupture of membranes (ROM) and cervical dilation; passage of the products of conception will occur. An incomplete miscarriage involves the expulsion of the fetus with retention of the placenta (Cunningham et al., 2005).

In a *complete* miscarriage (see Fig. 31-1, *D*), all fetal tissue is passed, the cervix is closed, and there may be slight bleeding. Mild uterine cramping may be present.

The term *missed* miscarriage (see Fig. 31-1, *E*) refers to a pregnancy in which the fetus has died, but the products of

FIG. 31-1   Miscarriage. **A,** Threatened. **B,** Inevitable. **C,** Incomplete. **D,** Complete. **E,** Missed.

table 31-1 Assessing Miscarriage and the Usual Management

TYPE OF MISCARRIAGE	AMOUNT OF BLEEDING	UTERINE CRAMPING	PASSAGE OF TISSUE	CERVICAL DILATION	MANAGEMENT
Threatened	Slight, spotting	Mild	No	No	Bed rest (controversial), sedation, and avoidance of stress, sexual stimulation, and orgasm usually recommended. Acetaminophen-based analgesics may be given. Further treatment depends on woman's response to treatment.
Inevitable	Moderate	Mild to severe	No	Yes	Bed rest if no pain, fever, or bleeding. If pain, rupture of membranes (ROM), bleeding, or fever is present, then prompt termination of pregnancy is accomplished, usually by dilation and curettage.
Incomplete	Heavy, profuse	Severe	Yes	Yes, with tissue in cervix	May or may not require additional cervical dilation before curettage. Suction curettage may be done.
Complete	Slight	Mild	Yes	No	No further intervention may be needed if uterine contractions are adequate to prevent hemorrhage and there is no infection. Suction or curettage may be performed to ensure no fetal or maternal tissue is retained.
Missed	None, spotting	None	No	No	If spontaneous evacuation of the uterus does not occur within 1 month, pregnancy is terminated by method appropriate to duration of pregnancy. Blood clotting factors are monitored until uterus is empty. Disseminated intravascular coagulation (DIC) and incoagulability of blood with uncontrolled hemorrhage may develop in cases of fetal death after the twelfth week, if products of conception are retained for longer than 5 weeks.
Septic	Varies, usually malodorous	Varies	Varies	Yes, usually	Immediate termination of pregnancy by method appropriate to duration of pregnancy. Cervical culture and sensitivity studies are done, and broad-spectrum antibiotic therapy (e.g., ampicillin) is started. Treatment for septic shock is initiated if necessary.
Recurrent (generally defined as 3 or more consecutive abortions)	Varies	Varies	Yes	Yes, usually	Varies, depends on type. Prophylactic cerclage may be done if premature cervical dilation is the cause. Tests of value include parental cytogenetic analysis and lupus, anticoagulant, and anticardiolipin antibodies assays.

From Cunningham, F., Leveno, K., Bloom, S., Hauth, J., Gilstrap, L., & Wenstrom, K. (2005). *Williams obstetrics* (22nd ed.). New York: McGraw-Hill; Gilbert, E., & Harmon, J. (2003). *Manual of high risk pregnancy and delivery* (3rd ed.). St. Louis: Mosby.

conception are retained in utero for up to several weeks. It may be diagnosed by ultrasonic examination after the uterus stops increasing in size or even decreases in size. No bleeding or cramping may be present, and the cervical os remains closed.

Habitual miscarriage or recurrent spontaneous abortion (RSA) is three or more consecutive pregnancy losses before 20 weeks of gestation. The etiology is often unclear but is thought to be multifactorial in nature (Pandey, Rani & Agrawal, 2005). Anticardiolipin antibodies are also being investigated for their impact on pregnancy and as an indicator for RSA (Velayuthaprabhu & Archunan, 2005). Women with a history of habitual miscarriage are at increased risk for preterm birth, placenta previa, and fetal anomalies in subsequent pregnancies (Cunningham et al., 2005). Miscarriage can become septic, although this is not a common occurrence. Symptoms of a septic miscarriage include fever and abdominal tenderness. Vaginal bleeding, which may be slight to heavy, is usually malodorous. Surgical evacuation is required at this point (Butler, Kelsberg, St. Anna, & Crawford, 2005).

▬ CARE MANAGEMENT

▬ Assessment and Nursing Diagnoses

Whenever a woman has vaginal bleeding early in pregnancy, a thorough assessment should be performed (Box 31-1). The data to be collected include pain, bleeding, and date of last menstrual period (LMP) to determine the approximate duration of gestation. The initial database includes vital signs (a temperature higher than 38° C may indicate infection), previous pregnancies, previous pregnancy losses, type and location of pain, quantity and nature of bleeding, allergies, and emotional status (see Box 31-1). The woman may be anxious and fearful regarding what may happen to her and to her pregnancy.

Various laboratory findings are characteristic of miscarriage. Evaluation of human chorionic gonadotropin (hCG), a placental hormone, is used in the diagnosis of pregnancy and pregnancy loss. Human chorionic gonadotropin is produced by the syncytiotrophoblast, and the beta subunit of hCG (β-hCG) can be detected in maternal plasma and urine 8 to 9 days after ovulation if the woman is pregnant. In early pregnancy, the concentration of β-hCG should double every 1.4 to 2.0 days until about 60 or 70 days of gestation (Cunningham et al., 2005). Before 8 weeks of gestation, if miscarriage is suspected, measurement of two serum quantitative β-hCG levels is performed 48 hours apart. If a normal pregnancy is present, the β-hCG level doubles in this time. Ultrasonography can then be used to determine the presence of a viable gestational sac. With considerable or persistent blood loss, anemia is likely (hemoglobin level less than 11 g/dl). If infection is present, the white blood cell count (WBC) is greater than 12,000/mm^3. Sedimentation rate is not helpful for differential diagnostic purposes because an increased sedimentation rate occurs with pregnancy, anemia, and infection.

---

box 31-1 **Assessment of Bleeding in Pregnancy**

INITIAL DATABASE
- Chief complaint
- Vital signs
- Gravidity, parity
- Date of last menstrual period and estimated date of birth
- Pregnancy history (previous and current)
- Allergies
- Nausea and vomiting
- Pain (onset, quality, precipitating event, location)
- Bleeding or coagulation problems
- Level of consciousness
- Emotional status

EARLY PREGNANCY
- Confirmation of pregnancy
- Bleeding (bright or dark, intermittent or continuous)
- Pain (type, intensity, persistence)
- Vaginal discharge

LATE PREGNANCY
- Estimated date of birth
- Bleeding (quantity, associated pain)
- Vaginal discharge
- Amniotic membrane status
- Uterine activity
- Abdominal pain
- Fetal status/viability

The following nursing diagnoses are appropriate for the woman experiencing a miscarriage:

- *Anxiety/fear related to*
  - unknown outcome and unfamiliarity with medical procedures
- *Deficient fluid volume related to*
  - excessive bleeding secondary to miscarriage
- *Acute pain related to*
  - uterine contractions
- *Anticipatory grieving related to*
  - unexpected pregnancy outcome
- *Situational low self-esteem related to*
  - inability to carry a pregnancy successfully to term gestation
- *Risk for infection related to*
  - surgical treatment
  - dilated cervix

▬ Expected Outcomes of Care

Expected outcomes of care for the woman experiencing miscarriage may include that the woman will do the following:
- Discuss the impact of the loss on her and her family.
- Identify and use available support systems.
- Display no signs or symptoms of physiologic or psychologic complications (e.g., hemorrhage, infection, depression).

- Identify health promotion measures that decrease her risk of miscarriage, and state understanding of reasons for diagnostic and genetic follow-up if needed.
- Report relief from pain.

■ Plan of Care and Interventions
■ *Medical/Surgical Management*

Medical management (see Table 31-1) depends on the classification of the miscarriage and on signs and symptoms. Traditionally, threatened miscarriages have been managed with bed rest and supportive care. Follow-up treatment depends on whether the threatened miscarriage progresses to actual miscarriage, or symptoms subside and the pregnancy remains intact. Dilation and curettage (D&C) is a surgical procedure in which the cervix is dilated and a curette is inserted to scrape the uterine walls and remove uterine contents. A D&C is commonly performed to treat inevitable and incomplete miscarriage. The nurse reinforces explanations, answers any questions or concerns, and prepares the woman for surgery.

Dilation and evacuation, performed after 16 weeks of gestation, consists of wide cervical dilation followed by instrumental removal of the uterine contents.

Before either surgical procedure is performed, a full history should be obtained, and general and pelvic examinations should be performed. General preoperative and postoperative care is appropriate for the woman requiring surgical intervention. Analgesics and anesthesia appropriate to the procedure are used.

Outpatient management of first-trimester pregnancy loss may be accomplished with the use of misoprostol intravaginally for up to 2 days (Moodliar, Bagratee, & Moodley, 2005; Zhang et al., 2005). There has been no difference in short-term psychologic outcomes between expectant and surgical management. If evidence of infection, unstable vital signs, or uncontrollable bleeding exist, a surgical evacuation is performed (Butler et al., 2005).

For late incomplete, inevitable, or missed miscarriages (16 to 20 weeks), prostaglandins may be administered into the amniotic sac or by vaginal suppository to induce or augment labor and cause the products of conception to be expelled. Intravenous (IV) oxytocin also may be used.

■ *Nursing Care*

Immediate nursing care focuses on physiologic stabilization. Typical orders to be followed are initiation of an IV line, request for blood testing of hemoglobin and hematocrit, blood type and Rh status determination, and indirect Coombs' screen. An ultrasound examination is ordered for diagnostic confirmation.

Nursing care is similar to care for any woman whose labor is being induced (see Chapter 36). Special care may be needed for management of side effects of prostaglandin such as nausea, vomiting, and diarrhea. If the products of conception are not passed in entirety, the woman may be prepared for manual or surgical evacuation of the uterus.

After evacuation of the uterus, 10 to 20 units of oxytocin in 1000 ml of fluids may be given to prevent hemorrhage.

For excessive bleeding, ergot products such as ergonovine or a prostaglandin derivative such as carboprost tromethamine may be given to contract the uterus. Three or four doses of ergonovine, 0.2 mg orally or intramuscularly (IM) every 4 hours, may be given if the woman is normotensive. A 25 mg dose of carboprost may be given IM every 15 to 90 minutes for as many as eight doses (Cunningham et al., 2005). Antibiotics are given as necessary. Analgesics, such as antiprostaglandin agents, may decrease discomfort from cramping. Transfusion therapy may be required for shock or anemia. The woman who is Rh negative and is not isoimmunized is given an IM injection of $Rh_o(D)$ immune globulin within 72 hours of the miscarriage.

Psychosocial aspects of care focus on what the pregnancy loss means to the woman and her family. Grief from perinatal loss is complex and unique to each individual (Hutti, 2005). Explanations are provided regarding the nature of the miscarriage, expected procedures, and possible implications for future childbearing.

As with other fetal or neonatal losses, the woman should be offered the option of seeing the products of conception. She also may want to know what the hospital does with the products of conception or whether she needs to make a decision about final disposition of fetal remains.

■ NURSE ALERT
Procedures for disposition of the fetal remains vary from hospital to hospital and state to state. The nurse should know what the usual procedures are in his or her setting.

■ *Home Care*

The woman will likely be discharged home within a few hours after a D&C or as soon as vital signs are stable, vaginal bleeding remains minimal, and she has recovered from anesthesia. Discharge teaching emphasizes the need for rest. If significant blood loss has occurred, iron supplementation may be ordered. Teaching includes information about normal physical findings such as cramping, type and amount of bleeding, resumption of sexual activity, and family planning (see Teaching for Self-Care box). Follow-up care should assess the woman's physical and emotional recovery. Referrals to local support groups should be provided as needed.

Follow-up phone calls after a loss are important. The woman may appreciate a phone call on what would have been her due date. These calls provide opportunities for the woman to ask questions, seek advice, and receive information to help process her grief.

■ Evaluation

The expected outcomes of care are used to evaluate the care of the woman who experienced a miscarriage.

Incompetent Cervix (Recurrent Premature Dilation of the Cervix)

Another cause of late miscarriage is incompetent cervix (recurrent premature dilation of the cervix), which has traditionally been defined as passive and painless dilation of the cervix during the second trimester. This definition

TEACHING FOR SELF-CARE

Discharge Teaching for the Woman After Early Miscarriage

- Advise the woman to report any heavy, profuse, or bright red bleeding to health care provider.
- Reassure the woman that a scant, dark discharge may persist for 1 to 2 weeks.
- To reduce the risk of infection, remind the woman not to put anything into the vagina for 2 weeks or until bleeding has stopped (e.g., no tampons, no vaginal intercourse). She should take antibiotics as prescribed.
- Advise the woman to eat foods high in iron and protein.
- Acknowledge that the woman has experienced a loss and that time is required for recovery. She may have mood swings and depression.
- Refer the woman to support groups, clergy, or professional counseling as needed.
- Advise the woman that attempts at pregnancy should be postponed for at least 2 months to allow her body to recover.

From Gilbert, E., & Harmon, J. (2003). *Manual of high risk pregnancy and delivery* (3rd ed.). St. Louis: Mosby.

assumes an "all-or-nothing" role for the cervix; it is either "competent" or "incompetent." Current research contends that cervical competence is variable and exists as a continuum that is determined in part by cervical length. Other factors include composition of the cervical tissue and the individual circumstances associated with the pregnancy in terms of maternal stress and lifestyle. Iams (2002) referred to this condition as abnormal or reduced cervical competence.

Etiology

Etiologic factors include a history of previous cervical lacerations during childbirth, excessive cervical dilation for curettage or biopsy, or the woman's mother's ingestion of diethylstilbestrol during pregnancy with the woman. Multiple gestation may provide an additional stress on the cervix but alone does not produce cervical incompetency or justify prophylactic cervical cerclage (Parilla, Haney, & MacGregor, 2003). Other instances may result from a congenitally short cervix or cervical or uterine anomalies. Reduced cervical competence is a clinical diagnosis, based on history. Short labors and recurring loss of the pregnancy at progressively earlier gestational ages are characteristics of reduced cervical competence. Ultrasound examination is used to diagnose this condition objectively. A short cervix (less than 25 mm in length) is indicative of reduced cervical competence. Often, but not always, the short cervix is accompanied by cervical funneling (beaking), or effacement of the internal cervical os (Iams, 2002; Rust, Atlas, Kimmel, Roberts, & Hess, 2005).

Collaborative Care

Medical-Surgical Management. Conservative management consists of bed rest, hydration, and tocolysis (inhibition of uterine contractions). A cervical cerclage may

be performed. During gestation, a McDonald cerclage, a band of homologous fascia or nonabsorbable ribbon (Mersilene), may be placed around the cervix beneath the mucosa to constrict the internal os of the cervix (Fig. 31-2). A cerclage procedure can be classified according to time, or whether it is elective (prophylactic), urgent, or emergent (Rust & Roberts, 2005).

Prophylactic cerclage is placed at 10 to 14 weeks of gestation, after which the woman is told to refrain from intercourse, prolonged (more than 90 minute) standing, and heavy lifting. She is monitored during the course of her pregnancy with ultrasound scans to assess for cervical shortening and funneling. The cerclage is electively removed (usually an office or a clinic procedure) when the woman reaches 37 weeks of gestation, or it may be left in place and a cesarean birth performed. Approximately 80% to 90% of pregnancies treated with cerclage result in live, viable births (Iams, 2002). If removed, the cerclage must be replaced with each successive pregnancy.

A woman whose reduced cervical competence is diagnosed during the current pregnancy may undergo emergency cerclage placement. Under ideal circumstances emergency cerclage can significantly prolong pregnancy and increase the chance of a viable pregnancy outcome (Cockwell & Smith, 2005). Risks of the procedure include premature ROM, preterm labor, and chorioamnionitis. Because of these risks, and because bed rest and tocolytic therapy can be used to prolong the pregnancy, cerclage is rarely performed after 25 weeks of gestation (Iams, 2002).

FIG. 31-2 **A,** Cerclage correction of premature dilation of the cervical os. **B,** Cross-sectional view of closed internal os.

Nursing Care. The nurse assesses the woman's feelings about her pregnancy and her understanding of reduced cervical competence. It also is important to evaluate the woman's support systems. Because the diagnosis of reduced cervical competence is usually not made until the woman has lost one or two pregnancies, she may feel guilty or to blame for this impending loss. It is therefore important to assess for previous reactions to stresses and appropriateness of coping responses. The woman needs the support of her health care providers, as well as that of her family.

If a cervical cerclage is performed, the nurse monitors the woman postoperatively for contractions, ROM, and signs of infection. Discharge teaching focuses on continued monitoring of these aspects at home. Home uterine monitoring may be indicated with follow-up from a home health agency.

Home Care. The woman must understand the importance of activity restriction at home and the need for close observation and supervision. She must be instructed on the importance of taking oral tocolytic medication if prescribed, the expected response, and possible side effects. Tocolytics may be given prophylactically to prevent uterine contractions and further dilation of the cervix. If home uterine monitoring is implemented, the woman is taught how to apply a uterine contraction monitor and transmit the monitor tracing by telephone to the monitoring center. Nurses at the monitoring center assess the tracing for contractions, answer questions, provide emotional support and education, and report information to the woman's physician or nurse-midwife. The woman must be aware that strong contractions less than 5 minutes apart, ROM, severe perineal pressure, and an urge to push will warrant immediate transfer to the hospital setting. If management is unsuccessful and the fetus is born before viability, appropriate grief support should be provided. If the fetus is born prematurely, appropriate anticipatory guidance and support will be necessary.

Ectopic Pregnancy

Incidence and Etiology

Ectopic pregnancy is one in which the gestational sac is implanted outside the uterine cavity (Fig. 31-3). The incidence of ectopic pregnancy in the general population is 2%. The frequency is consistent across maternal age ranges and ethnic origins (Murray, Baakdah, Bardell, & Tulandi, 2005).

Approximately 95% of ectopic pregnancies occur in the uterine (fallopian) tube, with most located on the ampullar or largest portion of the tube. Other sites include the abdominal cavity (3% to 4%), the ovary (1%), and the cervix (1%).

Ectopic pregnancy is responsible for 10% of all maternal mortality, and it is the leading pregnancy-related cause of first trimester maternal mortality (Simpson, 2002). Moreover, ectopic pregnancy is a leading cause of infertility. Women have increased difficulty conceiving after an ectopic pregnancy and are at an increased risk of developing a subsequent ectopic pregnancy.

The reported incidence of ectopic pregnancy is increasing as a result of improved diagnostic techniques, such as

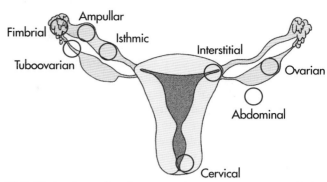

FIG. 31-3 Sites of implantation of ectopic pregnancies. Order of frequency of occurrence is ampulla, isthmus, interstitium, fimbria, tuboovarian ligament, ovary, abdominal cavity, and cervix (external os).

more sensitive β-hCG assays and the availability of transvaginal ultrasound. An increased incidence of sexually transmitted infections, better treatment of pelvic inflammatory disease (which formerly would have caused sterility), increased numbers of tubal sterilizations, and surgical reversal of tubal sterilizations also have resulted in more ectopic pregnancies (Simpson, 2002).

Ectopic pregnancy is classified according to site of implantation (e.g., tubal or ovarian). The uterus is the only organ capable of containing and sustaining a term pregnancy. However, abdominal pregnancy with birth by laparotomy may result in a living infant in 5% to 25% of such pregnancies (Fig. 31-4); the risk of deformity is as high as 40% (Gilbert & Harmon, 2003).

Clinical Manifestations

A missed period, adnexal fullness, and tenderness may suggest an unruptured tubal pregnancy. The tenderness can progress from a dull pain to a colicky pain when the tube stretches. Pain may be unilateral, bilateral, or diffuse over

FIG. 31-4 Ectopic pregnancy, abdominal.

the abdomen. Dark red or brown abnormal vaginal bleeding occurs in 50% to 80% of women. If the ectopic pregnancy ruptures, pain increases. This pain may be generalized, unilateral, or acute deep lower quadrant pain caused by blood irritating the peritoneum. Referred shoulder pain can occur as a result of diaphragmatic irritation caused by blood in the peritoneal cavity. The woman may exhibit signs of shock related to the amount of bleeding in the abdominal cavity and not necessarily related to obvious vaginal bleeding. An ecchymotic blueness around the umbilicus (Cullen's sign), indicating hematoperitoneum, may develop in an undiagnosed ruptured intraabdominal ectopic pregnancy.

Collaborative Care

The differential diagnosis of ectopic pregnancy involves consideration of numerous disorders that share many signs and symptoms. Many of these women present to the emergency room experiencing first-trimester bleeding or pain. The physician, nurse-midwife, or nurse practitioner must consider miscarriage, ruptured corpus luteum cyst, appendicitis, salpingitis, ovarian cysts, torsion of the ovary, and urinary tract infection (Table 31-2). The key to early detection of ectopic pregnancy is having a high index of suspicion for this condition. Any woman with complaints of abdominal pain, vaginal spotting or bleeding, and a positive pregnancy test should undergo screening for ectopic

table 31-2 Differential Diagnosis of Ectopic Pregnancy

	ECTOPIC PREGNANCY	APPENDICITIS	SALPINGITIS	RUPTURED OVARIAN CYST	MISCARRIAGE
Pain	Unilateral cramps and tenderness before rupture May be colicky after rupture Sudden sharp abdominal pelvic pain Abdominal tenderness	Epigastric, periumbilical, then right lower quadrant pain, tenderness localizing at McBurney's point, rebound tenderness	Usually in both lower quadrants with or without rebound Mild to severe pelvic pressure	Unilateral, becoming general with progressive bleeding, dull cramping	Mild uterine cramps to severe uterine pain
Nausea and vomiting	Occasionally before, frequently after rupture	Usual, precedes shift of pain to right lower quadrant	Infrequent	Rare	Almost never
Menstruation	Some aberration, missed period, spotting	Unrelated to menses	Hypermenorrhea, metrorrhagia, or both	Period delayed, then bleeding, often with pain	Amenorrhea then spotting, then brisk bleeding
Temperature, pulse, and blood pressure (BP)	37.2°-37.8° C, pulse variable, normal before and rapid after rupture, ↓ BP after rupture	37.2°-37.8° C, pulse rapid	37.2°-40° C, pulse elevated in proportion to fever	Not over 37.2° C, pulse normal unless blood loss marked, then rapid	To 37.2° C Signs of shock related to obvious bleeding
Pelvic examination	Unilateral tenderness, especially on movement of cervix, crepitant mass on one side or in cul-de-sac; dark red or brown vaginal discharge	No masses, rectal tenderness high on right side No vaginal discharge	Bilateral tenderness on movement of cervix Purulent discharge	Tenderness over affected ovary, no masses	Cervix open or closed, uterus slightly enlarged, irregularly softened, tender with infection, vaginal bleeding
Laboratory findings	WBC normal to 15,000/mm³ Pregnancy test result is positive Ultrasound to rule out pregnancy after 6 weeks	WBC 10,000-18,000/mm³ (rarely normal) Pregnancy test result is negative	WBC 15,000-30,000/mm³ Pregnancy test result is negative	WBC normal to 10,000/mm³ Pregnancy test is negative unless also pregnant Ultrasound will show ovarian cyst	WBC normal Pregnancy test result is positive

Modified from Gilbert, E., & Harmon, J. (2003). *Manual of high risk pregnancy and delivery* (3ʳᵈ ed.). St. Louis: Mosby.
WBC, White blood cell.

pregnancy. Laboratory screening includes determination of serum progesterone and quantitative β-hCG levels. If either of these values is lower than would be expected for a normal pregnancy, the woman is asked to return within 48 hours for serial measurements. Transvaginal ultrasonography is done to confirm intrauterine or tubal pregnancy (Farquhar, 2005). Ultrasonographic identification of an intrauterine pregnancy (gestational sac plus yolk sac) rules out ectopic pregnancy in most women (Murray et al., 2005).

The woman also should be assessed for the presence of active bleeding, which is associated with tubal rupture. If internal bleeding is present, assessment may reveal vertigo, shoulder pain, hypotension, and tachycardia. A vaginal examination should be performed only once, and then with great caution. Approximately half of the women who have a tubal pregnancy have a palpable mass on examination. It is possible to rupture the mass during a bimanual examination, so gentleness is critical (Simpson, 2002).

Removal of the ectopic pregnancy by salpingostomy is possible before rupture. Residual tissue is dissolved with a dose of methotrexate postoperatively. Methotrexate is a folic acid analog that destroys the rapidly dividing cells. It may be used IM in a single-dose injection to treat unruptured pregnancies (Takacs, Chakhtoura, DeSantis, & Verma, 2005). It has been shown to produce results similar to those of surgical therapy, in terms of high success rate, low complication rate, and good reproductive potential (Simpson, 2002).

Advanced ectopic abdominal pregnancy requires laparotomy as soon as the woman has been stabilized for operation. If the placenta of a second- or third-trimester abdominal pregnancy is attached to a vital organ, such as the liver, separation is usually not attempted because of the risk of hemorrhage. The cord is cut flush with the placenta, and the abdomen is closed, with the placenta left in place. Degeneration and absorption of the placenta usually occur without complication, although infection and intestinal obstruction may occur. Methotrexate may be given to dissolve the residual tissue (Cunningham et al., 2005).

Hospital Care. If surgery is planned for the woman with an ectopic pregnancy, general preoperative and postoperative care is appropriate. Vital signs (pulse, respirations, and blood pressure) are assessed preoperatively every 15 minutes or as needed, according to severity of the bleeding and the woman's condition. Preoperative laboratory tests include determination of blood type and Rh factor, complete blood count (CBC), and serum quantitative β-hCG assay. Ultrasonography is used to confirm an extrauterine pregnancy. Blood replacement may be necessary. The nurse verifies the woman's Rh and antibody status and administers $Rh_o(D)$ immune globulin if appropriate. The woman should be encouraged to verbalize her feelings related to the loss. Referral to community resources may be appropriate.

Home Care. Some women can be treated on an outpatient basis if they meet certain criteria. Hemodynamically stable women with ectopic pregnancies are eligible for methotrexate therapy if the mass is unruptured and measures less than 4 cm in diameter by ultrasonography (Simpson, 2002), if there is no fetal cardiac activity noted on ultrasound, if the serum β-hCG level is less than 5000 international units/L, and if the woman is willing to comply with posttreatment monitoring (Murray et al., 2005). Methotrexate therapy avoids surgery and is a safe, effective, and cost-conscious way of managing many cases of tubal pregnancy. The woman is informed how the medication works, what adverse effects are possible, whom to call if she has concerns or if problems develop, and the importance of follow-up care (Box 31-2).

■ **NURSE ALERT**

The woman receiving methotrexate therapy who drinks alcohol and takes vitamins containing folic acid (e.g., prenatal vitamins) increases her risk of having side effects of the drug or exacerbating the ectopic rupture.

---

box 31-2 **Nursing Considerations for Clients Undergoing Methotrexate Treatment for Ectopic Pregnancy**

ADMINISTRATION
- Check to make sure laboratory and diagnostic tests have been completed
  - Complete blood count and blood type and Rh-antibody status
  - Liver and renal function tests
  - Serum β-hCG levels <5000 international units/L
  - Transvaginal ultrasound confirming size of mass and absence of fetal cardiac activity
- Administer methotrexate 50 mg/m² intramuscularly (IM)
- Administer $Rh_O(D)$ immune globulin (50 mcg to 300 mcg IM as ordered if woman has Rh-negative blood)

CLIENT AND FAMILY TEACHING
- Review how methotrexate works
- Advise woman to discontinue folic acid supplements
- Advise woman to avoid sun exposure since the drug will make her more photosensitive

- Advise woman to refrain from strenuous activities
- Advise woman not to put anything in her vagina—no tampons, douches, or vaginal intercourse
- Inform woman of possible side effects—stomatitis and conjunctivitis are common; rare effects include pleuritis, gastritis, dermatitis, alopecia, enteritis, increased liver enzymes, and bone marrow suppression
- Advise woman to report to her health care provider immediately if she has severe abdominal pain that may be a sign of impending or actual rupture

FOLLOW-UP
- Inform woman to return to clinic/office in 1 week for measurement of β-hCG and vaginal ultrasound and possible second methotrexate injection
- Advise woman that she will need to return to the clinic/office for weekly measurements of β-hCG until level is <15 international units/L

Reference: Murray, H., Baakdah, H., Bardell, T., Tulandi, T., et al. (2005). Diagnosis and treatment of ectopic pregnancy. *Canadian Medical Association Journal, 173*(8), 905-912.

Future fertility should be discussed. Any woman who has been diagnosed with an ectopic pregnancy should be told to contact her health care provider as soon as she suspects that she might be pregnant, because of the increased risk for recurrent ectopic pregnancy. These women may need referral to grief or infertility support groups such as SHARE: Pregnancy and Infant Loss Support Inc. (www. nationalshareoffice.com). In addition to the loss of the current pregnancy, they are faced with the possibility of future pregnancy losses and infertility.

Hydatidiform Mole (Molar Pregnancy)

Hydatidiform mole (molar pregnancy) is a gestational trophoblastic disease. Gestational trophoblastic disease (GTD) includes disorders that arise from the placental trophoblast. It includes hydatidiform mole and gestational trophoblastic neoplasia (GTN). A hydatiform mole may be further categorized as a complete or partial mole. GTN refers to persistent trophoblastic tissue that is presumed to be malignant (Berman, DiSaia, & Tewari, 2004; Gilbert & Harmon, 2003). Metastatic trophoblastic neoplasia is commonly staged as low risk, intermediate risk, and high risk GTN (American College of Obstetricians and Gynecologists [ACOG], 2004). Once almost invariably fatal, because of early diagnosis and treatment, GTN is now the most curable gynecologic malignancy (Berman et al.) (see discussion in Chapter 12).

Incidence and Etiology

Hydatidiform mole occurs in 1 in 1200 pregnancies in the United States, but a higher incidence has been reported in Asian countries (Berman et al., 2004). The etiology is unknown, although there may be an ovular defect or nutritional deficiency. Women at higher risk for hydatidiform mole formation are those who have undergone ovulation stimulation with clomiphene (Clomid) and those who are in their early teens or older than 40 years. The risk of a second mole is 1% to 2%. Other risk factors include history of miscarriage and nutritional factors (e.g., deficient intake of carotene and animal fats) (Bess & Wood, 2006).

Types

The complete mole results from fertilization of an egg with a lost or inactivated nucleus (Fig. 31-5, *A*). The nucleus of a sperm (23,X) duplicates itself (resulting in the diploid number, 46,XX) because the ovum has no genetic material or the material is inactive. The mole resembles a bunch of white grapes (Fig. 31-5, *B*). The hydropic (fluid-filled) vesicles grow rapidly, causing the uterus to be larger than expected given the duration of the pregnancy. Usually the complete mole contains no fetus, placenta, amniotic membranes, or fluid. Maternal blood has no placenta to receive it; therefore hemorrhage into the uterine cavity and vaginal bleeding occur. In about 20% of cases of complete mole, progression toward choriocarcinoma occurs.

For a partial mole, chromosomal studies often show a karyotype of 69,XXY; 69,XXX; or 69,XYY. This occurs as a

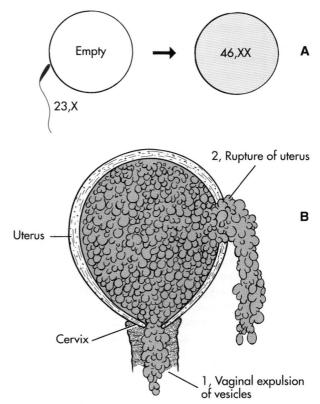

FIG. 31-5 A, Chromosomal origin of complete mole. Single sperm *(color)* fertilizes an "empty" ovum. Reduplication of sperm's 23, X set gives completely homozygous diploid 46, XX. Similar process follows fertilization of empty ovum by two sperm with two independently drawn sets of 23, X or 23, Y; both karyotypes of 46, XX and 46, XY can therefore result. **B,** Uterine rupture with hydatidiform mole. *1,* Vaginal expulsion of mole through cervix. *2,* Rupture of uterus and spillage of mole into peritoneal cavity (rare).

result of two sperm fertilizing an apparently normal ovum (Fig. 31-6). Partial moles often have embryonic or fetal parts and an amniotic sac. Congenital anomalies are usually present. The potential for malignant transformation is less than 6% (Copeland & Landon, 2002).

Clinical Manifestations

The clinical manifestations of a complete hydatidiform mole in the early stages cannot be distinguished from those of normal pregnancy. Vaginal bleeding occurs later in almost 95% of cases. The vaginal discharge may be dark brown (resembling prune juice) or bright red and either scant or profuse, and may continue for only a few days or intermittently for weeks. Early in pregnancy, the uterus in about half of affected women is significantly larger than expected from menstrual dates. The percentage of women with an excessively enlarged uterus increases as length of time since LMP increases. Approximately 25% of affected women have a uterus smaller than would be expected from menstrual dates.

Anemia from blood loss, excessive nausea and vomiting (hyperemesis gravidarum), and abdominal cramps

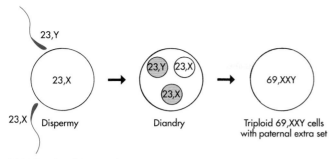

FIG. 31-6 Chromosomal origin of triploid partial mole. Normal ovum with 23,X haploid set is fertilized by two sperms to give total of 69 chromosomes. Sex configuration of XXY, XXX, or XYY is possible.

caused by uterine distention are relatively common findings. Preeclampsia occurs in about 15% of cases, usually between 9 and 12 weeks of gestation, but any symptoms of gestational hypertension before 24 weeks of gestation may suggest hydatidiform mole. Hyperthyroidism and pulmonary embolization of trophoblastic elements occur less commonly but are serious complications of hydatidiform mole. Partial moles cause few of these symptoms and may be mistaken for an incomplete or missed miscarriage.

▬ Collaborative Care

Medical-Surgical Management. Although most moles abort spontaneously, suction curettage offers a safe, rapid, and effective method of evacuation of hydatidiform mole if necessary (Gilbert & Harmon, 2003). Induction of labor with oxytocic agents or prostaglandins is not recommended because of the increased risk of embolization of trophoblastic tissue (Copeland & Landon, 2002). Administration of $Rh_o(D)$ immune globulin to women who are Rh negative is necessary to prevent isoimmunization.

Nursing Care. Nursing assessments during prenatal visits should include observation for signs of molar pregnancy during the first 24 weeks. If hydatidiform mole is suspected, ultrasonography and serial β-hCG immunoassays will be used to confirm the diagnosis. The sonographic pattern of a molar pregnancy is characterized by a diffuse "snowstorm" pattern. A β-hCG titer will remain high or increase above the normal peak after the time at which it normally decreases (70 to 100 days) (Cunningham et al., 2005).

The nurse provides the woman and her family with information about the disease process, the necessity for a long course of follow-up, and the possible consequences of the disease. The nurse helps the woman understand and cope with pregnancy loss and recognize that the pregnancy was abnormal. The woman and her family are encouraged to express their feelings, and information is provided about support groups or counseling resources if needed. Explanations about the importance of the need to postpone a subsequent pregnancy and contraceptive counseling are provided to emphasize the importance of consistent and reliable use of the method chosen.

▬ NURSE ALERT

To avoid confusion with signs of pregnancy, pregnancy should be avoided for 6 months to 1 year. Any contraceptive method except an intrauterine device is acceptable. Oral contraceptives are preferred as they are highly effective.

Home Care. Follow-up management includes frequent physical and pelvic examinations along with biweekly measurements of β-hCG level until the level decreases to normal and remains normal for 3 weeks. Monthly measurements are taken for 6 months and then every 2 months for a total of 1 year. A rising titer and an enlarging uterus may indicate choriocarcinoma (see Chapter 12). Women with a complete hydatidiform molar pregnancy are at a 15% to 28% risk of requiring further management with chemotherapy for persistent trophoblastic disease (Wolfberg, Berkowitz, Goldstein, Feltmate, & Lieberman, 2005). Referral to community support resources may be needed. Internet resources such as Share: Pregnancy and Infant Loss Support Inc., and International Society for the Study of Trophoblastic Disease at www. isstd.org may also be useful.

▬ LATE PREGNANCY BLEEDING

Late pregnancy bleeding disorders include placenta previa, premature separation of placenta (abruptio placentae), and variations in the cord insertion and the placenta. Expedient assessment for and diagnosis of the cause of bleeding are essential to reduce maternal and perinatal morbidity and mortality (Fig. 31-7).

Placenta Previa

In placenta previa, the placenta is implanted in the lower uterine segment near or over the internal cervical os. Historically, the degree to which the internal cervical os is covered by the placenta has been used to classify four types of placenta previa; total, partial, marginal, and low-lying (Fig. 31-8). The categorization of placenta previa may change in relationship to the dilation of the cervix. With a total previa the internal os is entirely covered by the placenta. Partial placenta previa implies incomplete coverage of the internal os. Marginal placenta previa indicates that only an edge of the placenta extends to the margin of the internal os. The term low-lying placenta is used when the placenta is implanted in the lower uterine segment but does not reach the os. Clark (2004) suggests that this classification has become obsolete, in part as a result of better ultrasound diagnosis of placenta previa. Clark offers a more descriptive classification that includes placenta previa (in the third trimester, the placenta covers the internal os) and marginal placenta previa (the distance of the placenta is 2 to 3 cm from the internal os and does not cover it). When the exact relationship of the os to the placenta has not been determined or in the case of apparent placenta previa in the second trimester, the term low-lying placenta is used (Clark).

A *vasa previa* occurs when unprotected fetal vessels pass across the cervical os in front of the presenting part of the

FIG. 31-7 Assessment and management of bleeding during late pregnancy. *CBC*, Complete blood count; *DIC*, disseminated intravascular coagulation; *IV*, intravenous.

fetus. The vessels are surrounded only by the amnion and are not covered with Wharton's jelly. Vasa previa is usually seen with a velamentous insertion of the umbilical cord (see later discussion). Vasa previa should be suspected when identification of the presenting part is difficult. The examiner may be able to feel the pulsation of the umbilical cord, however, this is not always the case. The umbilical blood vessels are at risk for laceration at any time, most frequently occurring during ROM (Clark, 2004). The sudden appearance of bright red blood at the time of ROM (spontaneous or artificial) and a sudden change in the fetal heart rate without other known risk factors should immediately alert the nurse to the possibility of vasa previa.

Although it occurs rarely, vasa previa is associated with high incidence of fetal morbidity and mortality because of the potential for fetal exsanguination (Benedetti, 2002). Diagnosis before birth is unusual, although examiners have

reported palpating a pulsing vessel, and ultrasound antenatal diagnosis is possible. There is a higher incidence of this condition with in vitro fertilization conceptions (Bhide & Thilaganathan, 2004). Best outcomes occur with early prenatal diagnosis and cesarean birth at 35 weeks or earlier (Oyelese et al., 2004).

Incidence and Etiology

The incidence of placenta previa is approximately 0.5% of births (Francois, Johnson, & Harris, 2003). The risk of placenta previa increases with previous history of placenta previa, previous cesarean birth or endometrial scarring, multiple gestation (because of the larger placental area), closely spaced pregnancies, maternal age older than 35 years, African or Asian ethnicity, smoking, and cocaine use (Ananth, Demissie, Smulian & Vintzileos, 2003; Clark, 2004).

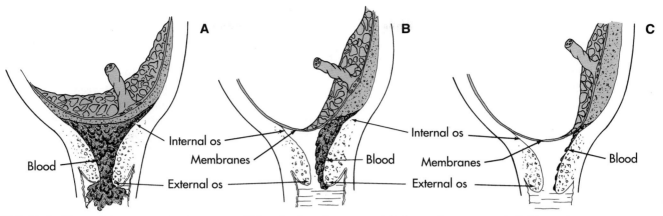

FIG. 31-8   Types of placenta previa after onset of labor. **A,** Complete, or total. **B,** Incomplete, or partial. **C,** Marginal.

Clinical Manifestations

Approximately 70% of women with placenta previa have painless vaginal bleeding; 20% have vaginal bleeding associated with uterine activity. Placenta previa should be suspected whenever vaginal bleeding occurs after 24 weeks of gestation. This bleeding is associated with the stretching and thinning of the lower uterine segment that occurs during the third trimester. Placental attachment is gradually disrupted, and bleeding occurs when the uterus is not able to contract adequately and stop blood flow from open vessels (Benedetti, 2002). The initial bleeding is usually a small amount and stops as clots form; however, it can recur at any time (Table 31-3). It is bright red.

Vital signs may be normal, even with heavy blood loss, because a pregnant woman can lose up to 40% of blood volume without showing signs of shock. Clinical presentation and decreasing urinary output may be better indicators of

table 31-3 Summary of Findings: Abruptio Placentae and Placenta Previa

	Abruptio Placentae			
	GRADE 1 MILD SEPARATION (10% TO 20%)	**GRADE 2 MODERATE SEPARATION (20% TO 50%)**	**GRADE 3 SEVERE SEPARATION (>50%)**	**PLACENTA PREVIA**
Bleeding, external, vaginal	Minimal	Absent to moderate	Absent to moderate	Minimal to severe and life threatening
Total amount of blood loss	<500 ml	1000-1500 ml	>1500 ml	Varies
Color of blood	Dark red	Dark red	Dark red	Bright red
Shock	Rare; none	Mild shock	Common, often sudden, profound	Uncommon
Coagulopathy	Rare, none	Occasional DIC	Frequent DIC	None
Uterine tonicity	Normal	Increased, may be localized to one region or diffuse over uterus, uterus fails to relax between contractions	Tetanic, persistent uterine contraction, boardlike uterus	Normal
Tenderness (pain)	Usually absent	Present	Agonizing, unremitting uterine pain	Absent
Ultrasonographic findings				
Location of placenta	Normal, upper uterine segment	Normal, upper uterine segment	Normal, upper uterine segment	Abnormal, lower uterine segment
Station of presenting part	Variable to engaged	Variable to engaged	Variable to engaged	High, not engaged
Fetal position	Usual distribution*	Usual distribution*	Usual distribution*	Commonly transverse, breech, or oblique
Gestational or chronic hypertension	Usual distribution*	Commonly present	Commonly present	Usual distribution*
Fetal effects	Normal fetal heart rate pattern	Nonreassuring fetal heart rate pattern	Nonreassuring fetal heart rate pattern, death can occur	Normal fetal heart rate pattern

DIC, Disseminated intravascular coagulation.
*Usual distribution refers to the usual variations of incidence seen when there is no concurrent problem.

acute blood loss than are vital signs alone. The fetal heart rate will be reassuring unless there is a major detachment of the placenta (Gilbert & Harmon, 2003).

Abdominal examination usually reveals a soft, relaxed, nontender uterus with normal tone. If the fetus is lying longitudinally, the fundal height is usually greater than expected for gestational age because the low placenta hinders descent of the presenting fetal part. Leopold maneuvers may reveal a fetus in an oblique or breech position or lying transverse because of the abnormal site of placental implantation.

Maternal and Fetal Outcome

Maternal morbidity is about 5%, and mortality is less than 1% with placenta previa (Clark, 2004). Complications associated with placenta previa include preterm ROM, preterm labor and birth, surgery-related trauma to structures adjacent to the uterus, anesthesia complications, blood transfusion reactions, overinfusion of fluids, abnormal placental attachments, postpartum hemorrhage, anemia, thrombophlebitis, and infection (Cunningham et al., 2005). Women with complete placenta previa have poorer pregnancy outcome. They are at a higher risk of giving birth prematurely and requiring a hysterectomy at the time of cesarean birth (Dola, Garite, Dowling, Friend, Ahdoot, & Asrat, 2003).

The greatest risk of fetal mortality is caused by preterm birth. Other fetal risks include malpresentation and congenital anomalies (Gilbert & Harmon, 2003). Infants who are small for gestational age or have intrauterine growth restriction also have been associated with placenta previa. This is thought to be a result of poor placental exchange or hypovolemia resulting from maternal blood loss and maternal anemia.

▪ CARE MANAGEMENT

▪ Assessment and Nursing Diagnoses

A woman with third-trimester vaginal bleeding requires immediate evaluation. Necessary history data include gravidity, parity, estimated date of birth, general status, bleeding (quantity, precipitating event, associated pain), vital signs, and fetal status (see Box 31-1). Abdominal assessment reveals a soft, relaxed, nontender uterus with normal tone. Laboratory studies include a CBC, determination of blood type and Rh factor, coagulation profile, and possible type and crossmatch.

The standard for diagnosis of placenta previa is a transabdominal ultrasonographic examination. This study is accurate 93% to 97% of the time, with false-negative and false-positive results occurring as a result of factors such as an engaged cephalic presentation, a posteriorly implanted placenta, maternal obesity, and compression of the lower uterine segment by an overdistended bladder. At term, women with a placental edge located within 2 cm of the internal cervical os require a cesarean birth (Bhide & Thilaganathan, 2004). If ultrasonographic scanning reveals a normally implanted placenta, a speculum examination is performed to rule out local causes of bleeding (e.g., cervicitis, polyps, or

carcinoma of the cervix), and a coagulation profile is obtained to rule out other causes of bleeding. If expectant management is to be implemented, a vaginal speculum examination by the health care provider is postponed until fetal viability has been reached (preferably after 34 weeks of gestation). If a pelvic examination is needed before that time, anticipate the possibility that an immediate cesarean birth may be required. The woman is taken to a delivery or operating room set up for cesarean birth because profound hemorrhage can occur during the examination. This type of vaginal examination, known as the *double-setup procedure,* is not done often.

Potential nursing diagnoses for the woman with a placenta previa include the following:

- *Decreased cardiac output related to*
  –excessive blood loss secondary to placenta previa
- *Deficient fluid volume related to*
  –excessive blood loss secondary to placenta previa
- *Excess fluid volume related to*
  –fluid resuscitation
- *Ineffective peripheral tissue perfusion related to*
  –hypovolemia and shunting of blood to central circulation
- *Risk for injury to fetus related to*
  –decreased placental perfusion secondary to placenta previa
- *Anxiety/fear related to*
  –maternal condition and pregnancy outcome
- *Deficient knowledge related to*
  –hospitalization and treatment regimens
- *Interrupted family processes related to*
  –mother's condition and hospitalization
- *Anticipatory grieving related to*
  –actual/perceived threat to self, pregnancy, or infant
- *Risk for infection related to*
  –anemia, hemorrhage, placenta previa, and transfusions
- *Risk for injury to mother related to*
  –invasive monitoring procedures and treatment

▪ Expected Outcomes of Care

Expected outcomes for the woman with placenta previa may include that the woman will do the following:

- Verbalize understanding of her condition and its management.
- Identify and use available support systems.
- Demonstrate compliance with prescribed activity limitations.
- Develop no complications related to bleeding.
- Give birth to a healthy infant at or near term.

▪ Plan of Care and Interventions
▪ Hospital Care

Active Management. Once placenta previa has been diagnosed, a management plan is developed based on gestational age, amount of bleeding, and fetal condition. If the woman is at term (longer than or equal to 37 weeks of gestation) and in labor or bleeding persistently, immediate birth by cesarean is almost always indicated. In women with partial or marginal placenta previa who have minimal bleeding, vaginal birth may be attempted. Vaginal birth also may be indicated for previable gestations or births involving intrauterine fetal demise (Benedetti, 2002).

If cesarean birth is undertaken, the nurse continuously assesses maternal and fetal status while preparing the woman for surgery. Maternal vital signs are assessed frequently for decreasing blood pressure, increasing pulse rate, changes in level of consciousness (LOC), and oliguria. Fetal assessment is maintained by continuous electronic fetal monitoring to assess for signs of hypoxia.

Blood loss may not cease with the birth of the infant. The large vascular channels in the lower uterine segment may continue to bleed because of that segment's diminished muscle content. The natural mechanism to control bleeding so characteristic of the upper part of the uterus—the interlacing muscle bundles, the "living ligature" contracting around open vessels—is absent in the lower part of the uterus. Postpartum hemorrhage may therefore occur even if the fundus is contracted firmly.

Emotional support for the woman and her family is extremely important. The actively bleeding woman is concerned not only for her own well-being but for the well-being of her fetus. All procedures should be explained, and a support person should be present. The woman should be encouraged to express her concerns and feelings. If the woman and her support person or family desire pastoral support, the nurse can notify the hospital chaplaincy service or provide information about other supportive resources.

Expectant Management. If the woman is at less than 36 weeks of gestation, not in labor, and the bleeding is mild or has stopped, expectant management is generally the treatment of choice to give the fetus time to mature in utero. Expectant management consists of rest and close observation. The woman is usually placed on bed rest, although she may be allowed bathroom privileges and limited activity (up in a wheelchair for an hour or so daily). Bleeding is assessed by checking the amount of bleeding on perineal pads, bed pads, and linens. Weighing pads, although not a method often used, is one way to assess blood loss accurately: 1 g represents 1 ml of blood.

Ultrasonographic examinations may be done every 2 to 3 weeks. Fetal surveillance may include nonstress testing (NST) or biophysical profiles once or twice weekly. Serial laboratory values are evaluated for decreasing hemoglobin and hematocrit levels and changes in coagulation values. Venous access with an IV infusion or medication lock may be placed, in case blood or blood component therapy should be needed. Antepartum steroids (betamethasone) may be ordered to promote fetal lung maturity if the woman is at less than 34 weeks of gestation. No vaginal or rectal examinations are performed, and the woman is placed on pelvic rest (nothing in the vagina). Once she reaches 37 weeks of gestation, and fetal lung maturity is documented, cesarean birth can be scheduled.

During her hospitalization, the woman with placenta previa should always be considered a potential emergency because massive blood loss with resulting hypovolemic shock can occur quickly if bleeding resumes. The possibility always exists that she may require an emergency cesarean for birth. Placenta previa in a preterm gestation may be an indication for transfer to a tertiary perinatal center, because many community hospitals are not equipped to perform emergency cesarean births 24 hours per day, 7 days per week.

Home Care. Criteria for home care management vary among primary perinatal providers and home care agencies and are usually determined on a case-by-case basis. To be considered for home care referral, the woman must be in stable condition with no evidence of active bleeding and must have resources to be able to return to the hospital immediately if active bleeding resumes.

She must have close supervision by family or friends in the home. The woman should be taught how to assess fetal and uterine activity and bleeding and told to avoid intercourse, douching, and enemas. She should limit her activities according to the advice of her physician, and be advised to keep all appointments for fetal testing, laboratory assessments, and prenatal care. Follow-up home care visits by a perinatal nurse may be arranged.

If hospitalization or home care with activity restriction is prolonged, the woman may have concerns about her work- or family-related responsibilities or may become bored with inactivity. She should be encouraged to participate in her own care and decisions about care as much as possible. Provision of diversionary activities or encouragement to participate in activities she enjoys and can do during bed rest is needed (see Teaching for Self-Care activities in Chapter 30, p. 794).

■ Evaluation

The expected outcomes of care are used to evaluate the care for the woman with placenta previa (see Plan of Care).

Premature Separation of Placenta

Premature separation of the placenta, also termed abruptio placentae, is the detachment of part or all of the placenta from its implantation site (Fig. 31-9). Separation occurs in the area of the decidua basalis after 20 weeks of pregnancy and before the birth of the baby.

Incidence and Etiology

Premature separation of the placenta is a serious event that accounts for significant maternal and fetal morbidity and mortality. Maternal hypertension is probably the most consistently identified risk factor for abruption (Benedetti, 2002). Cocaine use is also a risk factor because of the hypertensive state it can cause. Blunt external abdominal trauma, most often the result of motor vehicle accidents or maternal battering, is an increasingly significant cause of placental abruption (Benedetti, 2002). In the past, maternal age older than 35 years and parity, short umbilical cord, and folic acid deficiency were all thought to increase

| plan of care ▶ | **Placenta Previa** |

NURSING DIAGNOSIS Decreased cardiac output related to bleeding secondary to placenta previa

Expected Outcome *Woman will exhibit signs of increased blood volume and restoration of cardiac output (i.e., normal pulse and blood pressure; normal heart and breath sounds; normal skin color, tone, and turgor; normal capillary refill).*

Nursing Interventions/Rationales

• Palpate uterus for tenderness and tone; assess bleeding rate, amount, color, degree of bleeding, CBC values, and coagulation profile *to determine severity of situation.* Do not perform vaginal examination *because it may stimulate further bleeding.*

• Establish baseline data for cardiac output (vital signs; heart and breath sounds; skin color, tone, turgor; capillary refill; level of consciousness; urinary output; pulse oximetry) *to use as basis for evaluating effectiveness of treatment.*

• Initiate intravenous therapy or blood transfusions and medications per physician order *to restore blood volume and prevent organ compromise to mother and fetus.*

• Place woman on bed rest *to decrease oxygen demands.*

• Monitor vital signs, intake and output, hemodynamic status, and laboratory values *to evaluate treatment response.*

• Provide emotional support to woman and her family (e.g., explain procedures and their rationale; explain what is happening and what to expect; keep support person present) *to allay fears and provide the family with some sense of control.*

• After stabilization, teach woman home management, including bed rest, watching for spotting/bleeding, close follow-up with her health care provider, and preparation for immediate return to hospital if needed *to prevent or stem further complications.*

NURSING DIAGNOSIS Risk for injury to the fetus related to decreased uterine/placental perfusion secondary to bleeding

Expected Outcome *Ongoing signs of fetal well-being will be exhibited (i.e., adequate fetal movement, normal fetal heart rate, reactive NST, normal BPP).*

Nursing Interventions/Rationales

• Monitor fetus daily for signs of tachycardia, decreased movement, and loss of reactivity on NST *to identify and treat changes in fetal status early.*

• Obtain BPP per physician order *to assess for signs of chronic asphyxia.*

• Maintain maternal side-lying position *to prevent compression of aorta and vena cava.*

NURSING DIAGNOSIS Risk for infection related to anemia and bleeding secondary to placenta previa

Expected Outcome *Woman will show no signs of intrauterine infection.*

Nursing Interventions/Rationales

• Monitor vital signs for elevated temperature, pulse, and blood pressure; monitor laboratory results for elevated white blood cell count and differential shift; check for uterine tenderness and malodorous vaginal discharge *to detect early signs of infection resulting from exposure of placental tissue.*

• Provide/teach perineal hygiene *to decrease the risk of ascending infection.*

BPP, Biophysical profile; *CBC,* complete blood count; *NST,* nonstress test.

---

risk; however, more recent research has failed to confirm this (Benedetti, 2002). As gestational plurality increases from one to three, the risk of placental abruption rises, but the risk for related perinatal mortality decreases (Salihu, Bekan, Aliyu, Rouse, Kirby, & Alexander, 2005).There is a significant (5% to 17%) recurrence risk for placental abruption (Ananth, Oyelese, Yeo, Pradhan, & Vintzileos, 2005). A woman who has had two previous premature separations has a 25% recurrence risk in the next pregnancy (Benedetti, 2002).

Classification Systems

The most common classification of placental abruption is according to type and severity. This classification system is summarized in Table 31-3.

Clinical Manifestations

The separation may be partial or complete, or only the margin of the placenta may be involved. Bleeding from the placental site may dissect (separate) the membranes from the decidua basalis and flow out through the vagina; it may remain concealed (retroplacental hemorrhage); or it may

do both (Fig. 31-9). Clinical symptoms vary with degree of separation (see Table 31-3).

Classic symptoms of abruptio placentae include vaginal bleeding, abdominal pain, and uterine tenderness and contractions. Vaginal bleeding is present in as many as 70% to 80% of women with abruption (Clark, 2004). Although abdominal pain and uterine tenderness are characteristic for this complication, either finding may be absent in the presence of a silent abruption (Cunningham et al., 2005). Bleeding may result in maternal hypovolemia (shock, oliguria, anuria) and coagulopathy. Mild to severe uterine hypertonicity is present. Pain is mild to severe and localized over one region of the uterus or diffuse over the uterus with a boardlike abdomen.

Extensive myometrial bleeding damages the uterine muscle. If blood accumulates between the separated placenta and the uterine wall, it may produce a Couvelaire uterus. The uterus appears purplish and copper colored, it is ecchymotic, and contractility is lost. Shock may occur and is out of proportion to apparent blood loss. Laboratory findings include a positive *Apt test* result (blood in amniotic fluid); a decrease in hemoglobin and hematocrit

Partial separation
(concealed hemorrhage)

Partial separation
(apparent hemorrhage)

Complete separation
(concealed hemorrhage)

FIG. 31-9 Abruptio placentae. Premature separation of normally implanted placenta.

levels (which may appear later); and a decrease in coagulation factor levels. Clotting defects (e.g., disseminated intravascular coagulation [DIC]) develop in 10% to 30% of clients (most within 8 hours of hospital admission). A *Kleihauer-Betke test* may be ordered to determine the presence of fetal-to-maternal bleeding (transplacental hemorrhage). A positive Kleihauer-Betke test predicts increased risk of preterm labor after maternal trauma (Dhanraj & Lambers, 2004; Muench et al., 2004).

Maternal, Fetal, and Neonatal Outcomes

The maternal mortality rate approaches 1% for abruptio placentae; this condition remains a leading cause of maternal death. The mother's prognosis depends on the extent of placental detachment, overall blood loss, degree of DIC, and time between placental detachment and birth.

Maternal complications are associated with the abruption or its treatment. Hemorrhage, hypovolemic shock, hypofibrinogenemia, and thrombocytopenia are associated with severe abruption. Couvelaire uterus, DIC, and infection may occur. Renal failure and pituitary necrosis (Sheehan's syndrome) may result from ischemia. In rare cases, women who are Rh negative can become sensitized if fetal-to-maternal hemorrhage occurs and the fetal blood type is Rh positive.

Perinatal mortality rates range from 15% to 30%. Mortality occurs as a result of fetal hypoxia, preterm birth, and status as small for gestational age. Risks of neurologic defects are increased (Cunningham et al., 2005).

Collaborative Care

Abruptio placentae should be strongly suspected in the woman who has a sudden onset of intense, usually localized, uterine pain, with or without vaginal bleeding. Initial assessment is much the same as that for placenta previa. Physical examination usually reveals abdominal pain, uterine tenderness, and contractions. The fundal height may be measured over time, because increasing fundal height indicates concealed bleeding. Vaginal bleeding is present in about 80% of cases (Benedetti, 2002). Approximately 60% of live fetuses exhibit nonreassuring signs on the electronic fetal heart monitor, such as loss of variability and late decelerations; uterine hyperstimulation and increased resting tone may also be noted on the monitor tracing (Benedetti). Many women demonstrate coagulopathy, as evidenced by abnormal clotting studies (fibrinogen, platelet count, prothrombin time [PT], partial thromboplastin time [PTT], fibrin split products). Sonographic examination is used to rule out placenta previa; however, it is not always diagnostic for abruption. A retroplacental mass may be detected with ultrasonographic examination, but negative findings do not rule out a life-threatening abruption (Clark, 2004; Cunningham et al., 2005). However, better imaging

CRITICAL THINKING EXERCISE

Abruptio Placentae

Summer is a 25-year-old woman who has just been admitted to the emergency room after an automobile accident. She has intermittent states of consciousness, but states she is pregnant. Her admitting vital signs are the following: temperature, 36.8; pulse, 112; respirations, 18; and blood pressure 102/74. She has a 3-inch laceration above her left eye with a dressing applied. Her abdomen is distended. Fetal heart rate ausculated at 112 in the righ lower quadrant of the abdomen. She has no vaginal bleeding. A Foley catheter is inserted; 300 ml of pink-tinged urine return. An open fracture to the right lower leg is present.

1. Evidence—Is there sufficient evidence to draw conclusions about her diagnosis and preferred treatment?
2. Assumptions—What assumptions can be made about the following items?
   a. Possible diagnosis for Summer
   b. Physical assessment, laboratory tests, and diagnostic procedures that will be done to make a diagnosis
   c. The circumstances under which antepartal treatment will become immediate
3. What implications and priorities for nursing care can be made at this time?
4. Does the evidence objectively support the conclusion?
5. Are there alternative perspectives to your conclusion?

technology has made it possible to demonstrate ultrasonographic evidence of hemorrhage in more than 50% of cases of confirmed placental abruption (Benedetti).

Nursing diagnoses and expected outcomes of care are similar to those described for placenta previa.

Hospital Care. Treatment depends on the severity of blood loss and fetal maturity and status. If the abruption is mild and the fetus is less than 36 weeks of gestation and not in distress, expectant management may be implemented. The woman is hospitalized and observed closely for signs of bleeding and labor. The fetal status also is monitored with intermittent fetal heart rate monitoring and NST or biophysical profiles until fetal maturity is determined, or until the woman's condition deteriorates and immediate birth is indicated. Use of corticosteroids to accelerate fetal lung maturity is appropriately included in the plan of care for expectant management (National Institutes of Health Consensus Development Conference, 2000). Women who are Rh negative may be given Rh₀(D) immune globulin if fetal-to-maternal hemorrhage occurs and the fetal blood is Rh positive.

Delivery is the treatment of choice if the fetus is at term gestation or if the bleeding is moderate to severe and mother or fetus is in jeopardy. At least one large-bore (16 gauge) IV line should be started. Maternal vital signs are monitored frequently to observe for signs of declining hemodynamic status, such as increasing pulse rate and decreasing blood pressure. Serial laboratory studies include hematocrit or hemoglobin determinations and clotting studies. Continuous electronic fetal monitoring is mandatory. An indwelling Foley catheter is inserted for continuous assessment of urine output, an excellent indirect measure of maternal organ perfusion (Benedetti, 2002).

Blood and fluid volume replacement will most likely be ordered, with a goal of maintaining the urine output at 30 ml/hr or more, and the hematocrit at 30% or more. If this goal is not reached despite vigorous attempts at replacement, hemodynamic monitoring may be necessary (Benedetti, 2002). Fresh frozen plasma or cryoprecipitate may be given to maintain the fibrinogen level at a minimum of 100 to 150 mg/dl.

Vaginal birth is usually feasible and is desirable especially in cases of fetal death. Cesarean birth should be reserved for cases of fetal distress or other obstetric indications. Cesarean birth should not be attempted when the woman has severe and uncorrected coagulopathy, because it may result in surgically uncontrollable bleeding (Benedetti, 2002).

Nursing care of women experiencing moderate to severe abruption is demanding, because it requires meticulous assessment of maternal and fetal condition, as described previously. Information about abruptio placentae, including cause, treatment, and expected outcome, is given to the woman and her family. Emotional support also is extremely important because the woman and her family may be experiencing fetal loss in addition to the woman's critical illness.

Home Care. Women with abruptio placentae are usually not managed out of the hospital because the placenta can separate further at any time, and immediate intervention may be necessary.

■ Cord Insertion and Placental Variations

Velamentous insertion of the cord is a rare placental anomaly associated with placenta previa and multiple gestation. The cord vessels begin to branch at the membranes and then course onto the placenta (Fig. 31-10, *A*). ROM or traction on the cord may tear one or more of the fetal vessels. As a result, the fetus may rapidly bleed to death. Battledore (marginal) insertion of the cord (Fig. 31-10, *B*) increases the risk of fetal hemorrhage, especially after marginal separation of the placenta.

Rarely the placenta may be divided into two or more separate lobes, resulting in succenturiate placenta (Fig. 31-10, *C*). Each lobe has a distinct circulation; the vessels collect at the periphery, and the main trunks eventually unite to form the vessels of the cord. Blood vessels joining the lobes may be supported only by the fetal membranes and are therefore in danger of tearing during labor, birth, or expulsion of the placenta. During recovery of the placenta, one or more of the separate lobes may remain attached

FIG. 31-10 Cord insertion and placental variations. **A,** Velamentous insertion of cord. **B,** Battledore placenta. **C,** Placenta succenturiate.

to the decidua basalis, preventing uterine contraction and increasing the risk of postpartum hemorrhage.

■ CLOTTING DISORDERS IN PREGNANCY

Normal Clotting

Normally a delicate balance (homeostasis) exists between the opposing hemostatic and fibrinolytic systems. The hemostatic system is involved in the life-saving process. This system stops the flow of blood from injured vessels, in part through the formation of insoluble fibrin, which acts as a hemostatic platelet plug. The phases of the coagulation process involve an interaction of the coagulation factors in which each factor sequentially activates the factor next in line, the "cascade effect" sequence. The fibrinolytic system is the process through which the fibrin is split into fibrinolytic degradation products and circulation is restored.

Clotting Problems

A history of abnormal bleeding, inheritance of unusual bleeding tendencies, and a report of significant aberrations of laboratory findings indicate a bleeding or clotting problem. For the pregnant woman, bleeding disorders are suspected if the woman has gestational hypertension, HELLP syndrome (involving *h*emolysis, *e*levated *l*iver *e*nzymes, and *low p*latelets; see Chapter 30), retained dead fetus syndrome, amniotic fluid embolism, sepsis, or hemorrhage. Determination of hemostasis is made by testing the usual mechanisms for the control of bleeding, the function of platelets, and the necessary clotting factors. Most clotting disorders are more a concern in the immediate postpartum period. Recognition in the antepartum period may decrease hemorrhagic problems (see Chapter 37).

Disseminated Intravascular Coagulation

Disseminated intravascular coagulation (DIC) or consumptive coagulopathy is a pathologic form of clotting that is diffuse and consumes large amounts of clotting factors, causing widespread external bleeding, internal bleeding, or both, and clotting (Cunningham et al., 2005). DIC is most often triggered by the release of large amounts of tissue thromboplastin. This occurs in abruptio placentae and in retained dead fetus and amniotic fluid embolus syndromes. Severe preeclampsia, HELLP syndrome, and gram-negative sepsis are examples of conditions that can trigger DIC because of widespread damage to vascular integrity (Cunningham et al., 2005; Kilpatrick & Laros, 2004). DIC is an overactivation of the clotting cascade and the fibrinolytic system, resulting in depletion of platelets and clotting factors. This results in the formation of multiple fibrin clots throughout the body's vasculature, even in the microcirculation. Blood cells are destroyed as they pass through these fibrin-choked vessels. Thus DIC results in a clinical picture of clotting, bleeding, and ischemia (Cunningham et al., 2005; Labelle & Kitchens, 2005). DIC is always a secondary diagnosis. Clinical manifestations and laboratory tests are discussed in Box 31-3.

---

box 31-3 **Antepartal Clinical Manifestations and Laboratory Screening Results for Pregnant Patients with Disseminated Intravascular Coagulation**

POSSIBLE PHYSICAL EXAMINATION FINDINGS
- Spontaneous bleeding from gums, nose
- Oozing, excessive bleeding from venipuncture site, intravenous access site, or site of insertion of urinary catheter
- Petechiae, for example on the arm where blood pressure cuff was placed
- Other signs of bruising
- Hematuria
- Gastrointestinal bleeding
- Tachycardia
- Diaphoresis

LABORATORY COAGULATION SCREENING TEST RESULTS
- Platelets—decreased
- Fibrinogen—decreased
- Factor V (proaccelerin)—decreased
- Factor VIII (antihemolytic factor)—decreased
- Prothrombin time—prolonged
- Partial prothrombin time—prolonged
- Fibrin degradation products—increased
- D-dimer test (specific fibrin degradation fragment)—increased
- Red blood smear—fragmented red blood cells

Sources: Cunningham, F., Leveno, K., Bloom, S., Hauth, J., Gilstrap, L., & Wenstrom, K. (2005). *Williams obstetrics* (22nd ed.). New York: McGraw-Hill; Kilpatrick, S., & Laros, R. (2004). Maternal hematologic disorders. In R. Creasy, R. Resnik, & J. Iams (Eds.), *Maternal-fetal medicine: Principles and practice* (5th ed.). Philadelphia: Saunders; Labelle, C., & Kitchens, C. (2005). Disseminated intravascular coagulation: Treat the cause, not the lab values. *Cleveland Clinic Journal of Medicine, 72*(5), 377-397.

Collaborative Care. Medical management during pregnancy includes correcting the underlying cause and replacement of essential factors and fluid volume (see Chapter 37 for further discussion).

The nurse caring for the pregnant woman at risk for DIC must be aware of risk factors. Careful and thorough assessment is required, with particular attention to signs of bleeding (petechiae, oozing from injection sites, and hematuria). Because renal failure is one consequence of DIC, urinary output is carefully monitored by using an indwelling Foley catheter. Vital signs are assessed frequently.

Supportive measures include keeping the pregnant woman in a side-lying tilt to maximize blood flow to the uterus. Oxygen may be administered through a tight-fitting, rebreathing mask at 8 to 10 L/min, or per hospital protocol or physician order. Blood and blood products must be administered safely. Fetal assessments are done to monitor fetal well-being (Labelle & Kitchens, 2005). DIC usually is "cured" with the birth and as coagulation abnormalities resolve.

The educational and emotional needs of the woman and her family must be recognized and supported. They need information about her condition and explanations of procedures and will most likely be very anxious about the health of mother and baby.

community activity

Identify perinatal loss support groups in your community (frequently listed in the newspaper and phone book). Attend two different support meetings from an observational perspective. Obtain a March of Dimes (MOD) bereavement kit (from the website or your local community MOD). Compare and contrast the different support modalities. When would you refer a client to these programs? Would the programs be appropriate for both parents? What is the nurse's role in supporting these families?

key points

- Blood loss during pregnancy should always be regarded as a warning sign until the cause is determined.
- Some miscarriages occur for unknown reasons, but fetal or placental maldevelopment and maternal factors account for many others.
- The type of miscarriage directs care management.
- Ectopic pregnancy is a significant cause of maternal morbidity and mortality, even in developed countries.
- The two distinctive types of hydatidiform mole are complete and partial.
- Premature separation of the placenta and placenta previa are differentiated by type of bleeding, uterine tonicity, and presence or absence of pain.
- Clotting disorders are associated with many obstetric complications.
- Management of late-pregnancy bleeding requires immediate evaluation; care is based on gestational age, amount of bleeding, and fetal condition.

REFERENCES

American College of Obstetricians and Gynecologists. (2004). Diagnosis and treatment of gestational trophoblastic disease. ACOG Practice Bulletin Number 53. *Obstetrics and Gynecology, 103*(6), 1365-1377.

Ananth, C., Demissie, K., Smulian, J., & Vintzileos, A. (2003). Placenta previa in singleton and twin births in the United States, 1989 through 1998: A comparison of risk factor profiles and associated conditions. *American Journal of Obstetrics and Gynecology, 188*(1), 275-282.

Ananth, C., Oyelese, Y., Yeo, L., Pradhan, A., & Vintzileos, A. (2005). Placental abruption in the United States, 1979 through 2001: Temporal trends and potential determinants. *American Journal of Obstetrics and Gynecology, 192*(1), 191-198.

Benedetti, T. (2002). Obstetric hemorrhage. In S. Gabbe, J. Niebyl, & J. Simpson (Eds.), *Obstetrics: Normal and problem pregnancies* (4th ed.). New York: Churchill Livingstone.

Berman, M., DiSaia, P., & Tewari, K. (2004). Pelvic malignancy, gestational trophoblastic neoplasm, and nonpelvic malignancies. In R. Creasy, R. Resnik, & J. Iams (Eds.), *Maternal-fetal medicine: Principles and practice* (5th ed.). Philadelphia: Saunders.

Bess, K., & Wood, T. (2006). Understanding gestational trophoblastic disease: How nurses can help those dealing with a diagnosis. *AWHONN Lifelines, 10*(4), 320-326.

Bhide, A., & Thilaganathan, B. (2004). Recent advances in the management of placenta previa. *Current Opinion in Obstetrics & Gynecology, 16*(6), 447-451.

Butler, C., Kelsberg, G., St. Anna, L., & Crawford, P. (2005). How long is expectant management safe in first-trimester miscarriage? *Journal of Family Practice, 54*(10), 889-890.

Clark, S. (2004). Placenta previa and abruptio placentae. In R. Creasy, R. Resnik, & J. Iams (Eds.), *Maternal-fetal medicine: Principles and practice* (5th ed.). Philadelphia: Saunders.

Cockwell, H., & Smith, G. (2005). Cervical incompetence and the role of emergency cerclage. *Journal of Obstetrics and Gynaecology Canada, 27*(2), 123-129.

Copeland, L., & Landon, M. (2002). Malignant diseases and pregnancy. In S. Gabbe, J. Niebyl, & J. Simpson (Eds.), *Obstetrics: Normal and problem pregnancies* (4th ed.). New York: Churchill Livingstone.

Cunningham, F., Leveno, K., Bloom, S., Hauth, J., Gilstrap, L., & Wenstrom, K. (2005). *Williams obstetrics* (22nd ed.). New York: McGraw-Hill.

Dhanraj, D., & Lambers, D. (2004). The incidences of positive Kleihauer-Betke test in low-risk pregnancies and maternal trauma patients. *American Journal of Obstetrics and Gynecology, 190*(5), 1461-1463.

Dola, C., Garite, T., Dowling, D., Friend, D., Ahdoot, D., & Asrat, T. (2003). Placenta previa: Does its type affect pregnancy outcome? *American Journal of Perinatology, 20*(7), 353-360.

Farquhar, C. (2005). Ectopic pregnancy. *Lancet, 366*(9485), 583-591.

Francois, K., Johnson, J., & Harris, C. (2003). Is placenta previa more common in multiple gestations? *American Journal of Obstetrics and Gynecology, 188*(5), 1226-1228.

Gilbert, E., & Harmon, J. (2003). *Manual of high risk pregnancy and delivery* (3rd ed.). St. Louis: Mosby.

Griebel, C., Halvorsen, J., Golemon, T., & Day, A. (2005). Management of spontaneous abortion. *American Family Physician, 72*(7), 1243-1250.

Hutti, M. (2005). Social and professional support needs of families after perinatal loss. *Journal of Obstetric, Gynecologic, and Neonatal Nursing, 34*(5), 630-638.

Iams, J. (2002). Preterm birth. In S. Gabbe, J. Niebyl, & J. Simpson (Eds.), *Obstetrics: Normal and problem pregnancies* (4th ed.). New York: Churchill Livingstone.

Kilpatrick, S., & Laros, R. (2004). Maternal hematologic disorders. In R. Creasy, R. Resnik, & J. Iams (Eds.), *Maternal-fetal medicine: Principles and practice* (5th ed.). Philadelphia: Saunders.

Labelle, C., & Kitchens, C. (2005). Disseminated intravascular coagulation: Treat the cause, not the lab values. *Cleveland Clinic Journal of Medicine, 72*(5), 377-397.

Moodliar, S., Bagratee, J., & Moodley, J. (2005). Medical versus surgical evacuation of first-trimester spontaneous abortion. *International Journal of Gynecology and Obstetrics, 91*(1), 21-26.

Muench, M., Baschat, A., Reddy, U., Mighty, H., Weiner, C., Scalea, T., et al. (2004). Kleihauer-Betke testing is important in all cases of maternal trauma. *Journal of Trauma, 57*(5), 1094-1098.

Murray, H., Baakdah, H., Bardell, T., & Tulandi, T. (2005). Diagnosis and treatment of ectopic pregnancy. *Canadian Medical Association Journal, 173*(8), 905-912.

National Institutes of Health Consensus Development Conference. (2000). *Statement on repeated courses of corticosteroids, August 17-18, 2000,* Bethesda, MD. Accessed August 10, 2006, consensus.nih.gov.

Oyelese, Y., Catanzarite, V., Prefumo, F., Lashley, S., Schachter, M., Tovbin, Y., et al. (2004). Vasa previa: The impact of prenatal diagnosis on outcomes. *Obstetrics and Gynecology, 103*(5), 937-942.

Pandey, M., Rani, R., & Agrawal, S. (2005). An update in recurrent spontaneous abortion. *Archives of Gynecology and Obstetrics, 272*(2), 95-108.

Parilla, B., Haney, E., & MacGregor, S. (2003). The prevalence and timing of cervical cerclage placement in multiple gestations. *International Journal of Gynecology and Obstetrics, 80*(2), 123-128.

Rust, O., & Roberts, W. (2005). Does cerclage prevent preterm birth? *Obstetrics and Gynecology Clinics of North America, 32*(3), 441-456.

Rust, O., Atlas, R., Kimmel, S., Roberts, W., & Hess, L. (2005). Does the presence of a funnel increase the risk of adverse perinatal outcome in a patient with a short cervix? *American Journal of Obstetrics and Gynecology, 192*(4), 1060-1066.

Salihu, H., Bekan, B., Aliyu, M., Rouse, D., Kirby, R., & Alexander, G. (2005). Perinatal mortality associated with abruption placenta in singletons and multiples. *American Journal of Obstetrics and Gynecology, 193*(1), 198-203.

Simpson, J. (2002). Fetal wastage. In S. Gabbe, J. Niebyl, & J. Simpson (Eds.), *Obstetrics: Normal and problem pregnancies* (4th ed.). New York: Churchill Livingstone.

Takacs, P., Chakhtoura, N., DeSantis, T., & Verma, U. (2005). Evaluation of the relationship between endometrial thickness and failure of single-dose methotrexate in ectopic pregnancy. *Archives of Gynecology and Obstetrics, 272*(4), 269-272.

Velayuthaprabhu, S., & Archunan, G. (2005). Evaluation of anticardiolipin antibodies and antiphosphatidylserine antibodies in women with recurrent abortion. *Indian Journal of Medical Science, 59*(8), 347-352.

White, H., & Bouvier, D. (2005). Caring for a patient having a miscarriage. *Nursing 2005, 35*(7), 18-19.

Wolfberg, A., Berkowitz, R., Goldstein, D., Feltmate, C., & Lieberman, E. (2005). Postevacuation hCG levels and risk of gestational trophoblastic neoplasia in women with complete molar pregnancy. *Obstetrics and Gynecology, 106*(3), 548-552.

Yang, J., Savitz, D., Dole, N., Hartmann, K., Herring, A., Olshan, A., et al. (2005). Predictors of vaginal bleeding during the first two trimesters of pregnancy. *Paediatric and Perinatal Epidemiology, 19*(4), 276-283.

Zhang, J., Gilles, J., Barnhart, K., Creinin, M., Westhoff, C., Frederick, M., et al. (2005). A comparison of medical management with misoprostol and surgical management for early pregnancy failure. *New England Journal of Medicine, 353*(8), 761-769.

CHAPTER *32*

Kitty Cashion

Endocrine and Metabolic Disorders

learning objectives

- Differentiate the types of diabetes mellitus and their respective risk factors in pregnancy.
- Compare insulin requirements during pregnancy, post-partum, and with lactation.
- Identify maternal and fetal risks or complications associated with diabetes in pregnancy.
- Develop a plan of care for the pregnant woman with pregestational or gestational diabetes.
- Explain the effects of hyperemesis gravidarum on maternal and fetal well-being.

- Discuss the management of the woman with hyperemesis gravidarum in the hospital and at home.
- Explain the effects of thyroid disorders on pregnancy.
- Compare the management of a pregnant woman with hyperthyroidism with one who has hypothyroidism.
- Examine the effects of maternal phenylketonuria on pregnancy outcome.
- Discuss care management for the woman with phenylketonuria during the perinatal period.

electronic resources

Additional information related to the content in Chapter 32 can be found on

the companion website at **evolve**
http://evolve.elsevier.com/Lowdermilk/MWHC/
- NCLEX Review Questions
- Case Study: Pregestational Diabetes
- WebLinks

or on the interactive companion CD
- NCLEX Review Questions
- Case Study: Pregestational Diabetes
- Critical Thinking Exercise: Gestational Diabetes
- Plan of Care: Hyperemesis Gravidarum
- Plan of Care: Pregnancy Complicated by Pregestational Diabetes

$\mathcal{E}$NDOCRINE and metabolic disorders, which often complicate pregnancy, require careful management to promote maternal and fetal well-being and a positive pregnancy outcome. Diabetes mellitus is the most common endocrine disorder associated with pregnancy. Hyperemesis gravidarum and disorders of the thyroid, although encountered less often, also require careful planning for care. Phenylketonuria, an inborn error of metabolism, is a relatively new disorder of women of reproductive age, and it has significant implications for pregnancy outcome.

Providing safe and effective care for women with these endocrine and metabolic disorders and their fetuses can be a challenge. Although there are unique needs related to these conditions, pregnant women with endocrine and metabolic disorders also experience the feelings, needs, and concerns associated with a normal pregnancy. The primary objective of nursing care is to achieve optimal outcomes for both the pregnant woman and the fetus.

■ DIABETES MELLITUS

The perinatal mortality rate for well-managed diabetic pregnancies, excluding major congenital malformations, is about the same as that for any other pregnancy (Landon, Catalano, & Gabbe, 2002; Moore, 2004). The key to an optimal pregnancy outcome is strict maternal glucose control before conception, as well as throughout the gestational period. Consequently, for women with diabetes much emphasis is placed on preconception counseling.

Pregnancy complicated by diabetes is still considered high risk. It is most successfully managed by a multidisciplinary approach involving the obstetrician, internist or diabetologist, ophthalmologist, nephrologist, neonatologist, nurse, nutritionist or dietitian, and social worker, as needed. A favorable outcome requires commitment and active participation by the pregnant woman and her family. It is preferable to plan the pregnancy, working before conception with the woman and her family (Slocum et al., 2004).

826

Pathogenesis

Diabetes mellitus refers to a group of metabolic diseases characterized by hyperglycemia resulting from defects in insulin secretion, insulin action, or both (Expert Committee on the Diagnosis and Classification of Diabetes Mellitus [ECDCDM], 2003). Insulin, produced by the beta cells in the islets of Langerhans in the pancreas, regulates blood glucose levels by enabling glucose to enter adipose and muscle cells, where it is used for energy. When insulin is insufficient or ineffective in promoting glucose uptake by the muscle and adipose cells, glucose accumulates in the bloodstream, and hyperglycemia results. Hyperglycemia causes hyperosmolarity of the blood, which attracts intracellular fluid into the vascular system, resulting in cellular dehydration and expanded blood volume. Consequently, the kidneys function to excrete large volumes of urine (polyuria) in an attempt to regulate excess vascular volume and to excrete the unusable glucose (glycosuria). Polyuria, along with cellular dehydration, causes excessive thirst (polydipsia).

The body compensates for its inability to convert carbohydrate (glucose) into energy by burning proteins (muscle) and fats. However, the end products of this metabolism are ketones and fatty acids which, in excess quantities, produce ketoacidosis and acetonuria. Weight loss occurs as a result of the breakdown of fat and muscle tissue. This tissue breakdown causes a state of starvation that compels the individual to eat excessive amounts of food (polyphagia).

Over time, diabetes causes significant changes in both the microvascular and macrovascular circulations. These structural changes affect a variety of organ systems, particularly the heart, the eyes, the kidneys, and the nerves. Complications resulting from diabetes include premature atherosclerosis, retinopathy, nephropathy, and neuropathy.

Diabetes may be caused by either impaired insulin secretion, when the beta cells of the pancreas are destroyed by an autoimmune process, or by inadequate insulin action in target tissues at one or more points along the metabolic pathway. Both of these conditions are commonly present in the same person, and it is unclear which, if either, abnormality is the primary cause of the disease (ECDCDM, 2003).

Classification

The current classification system includes four groups: type 1 diabetes also called insulin-dependent diabetes; type 2 diabetes, also called insulin-resistant diabetes, other specific types (e.g., diabetes caused by infection or drug-induced diabetes); and gestational diabetes mellitus (GDM). Approximately 8.7% of women older than 20 years have diabetes mellitus (Bernasko, 2004), with approximately 4% to 7% of those women developing gestational diabetes or diabetes in pregnancy (American Diabetes Association [ADA], 2006; ADA, 2004a). Of the women with pregestational diabetes, the majority (65%) have type 2 diabetes (Chan & Winkle, 2006).

Type 1 diabetes includes those cases that are primarily caused by pancreatic islet beta cell destruction and that are prone to ketoacidosis. People with type 1 diabetes usually have an absolute insulin deficiency. Type 1 diabetes includes cases currently thought to be caused by an autoimmune process, as well as those for which the cause is unknown (ECDCDM, 2003).

Type 2 diabetes is the most prevalent form of the disease and includes individuals who have insulin resistance and usually relative (rather than absolute) insulin deficiency. Specific causes of type 2 diabetes are unknown at this time. Type 2 diabetes often goes undiagnosed for years, because hyperglycemia develops gradually and often is not severe enough for the person to recognize the classic signs of polyuria, polydipsia, and polyphagia. Many people who develop type 2 diabetes are obese or have an increased amount of body fat distributed primarily in the abdominal area. Other risk factors for the development of type 2 diabetes include aging, a sedentary lifestyle, hypertension, and prior gestational diabetes. Type 2 diabetes often has a strong genetic predisposition (ECDCDM, 2003).

Pregestational diabetes mellitus is the label sometimes given to type 1 or type 2 diabetes that existed before pregnancy.

Gestational diabetes mellitus (GDM) is any degree of glucose intolerance with the onset or first recognition occurring during pregnancy. This definition is appropriate whether or not insulin is used for treatment or the diabetes persists after pregnancy. It does not exclude the possibility that the glucose intolerance preceded the pregnancy. Women experiencing gestational diabetes should be reclassified 6 weeks or more after the pregnancy ends (ECDCDM, 2003).

Metabolic Changes Associated with Pregnancy

Normal pregnancy is characterized by complex alterations in maternal glucose metabolism, insulin production, and metabolic homeostasis. During normal pregnancy, adjustments in maternal metabolism allow for adequate nutrition for both the mother and the developing fetus. Glucose, the primary fuel used by the fetus, is transported across the placenta through the process of carrier-mediated facilitated diffusion. This means that the glucose levels in the fetus are directly proportional to maternal levels. Although glucose crosses the placenta, insulin does not. Around the tenth week of gestation, the fetus begins to secrete its own insulin at levels adequate to use the glucose obtained from the mother. Therefore, as maternal glucose levels rise, fetal glucose levels are increased, resulting in increased fetal insulin secretion.

During the first trimester of pregnancy, the pregnant woman's metabolic status is significantly influenced by the rising levels of estrogen and progesterone. These hormones stimulate the beta cells in the pancreas to increase insulin production, which promotes increased peripheral use of glucose and decreased blood glucose, with fasting levels being reduced by approximately 10% (Fig. 32-1, *A*). A concomitant increase in tissue glycogen stores and a decrease

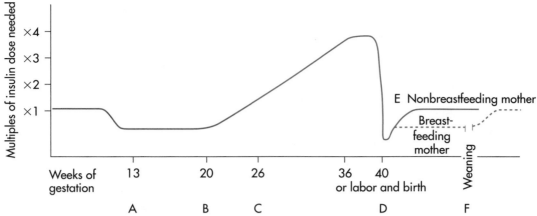

FIG. 32-1 Changing insulin needs during pregnancy. **A,** First trimester: Insulin need is reduced because of increased insulin production by pancreas and increased peripheral sensitivity to insulin; nausea, vomiting, and decreased food intake by mother and glucose transfer to embryo or fetus contribute to hypoglycemia. **B,** Second trimester: Insulin needs begin to increase as placental hormones, cortisol, and insulinase act as insulin antagonists, decreasing insulin's effectiveness. **C,** Third trimester: Insulin needs may double or even quadruple but usually level off after 36 weeks of gestation. **D,** Day of birth: Maternal insulin requirements decrease drastically to approach prepregnancy levels. **E,** Breastfeeding mother maintains lower insulin requirements, as much as 25% less than those of prepregnancy; insulin needs of nonbreastfeeding mother return to prepregnancy levels in 7 to 10 days. **F,** Weaning of breastfeeding infant causes mother's insulin needs to return to prepregnancy levels.

in hepatic glucose production occur, which further encourage lower fasting glucose levels. As a result of these normal metabolic changes of pregnancy, women with insulin-dependent diabetes are prone to hypoglycemia during the first trimester.

During the second and third trimesters, pregnancy exerts a "diabetogenic" effect on the maternal metabolic status. Because of the major hormonal changes, there is decreased tolerance to glucose, increased insulin resistance, decreased hepatic glycogen stores, and increased hepatic production of glucose. Increasing levels of human chorionic somatomammotropin, estrogen, progesterone, prolactin, cortisol, and insulinase increase insulin resistance through their actions as insulin antagonists. Insulin resistance is a glucose-sparing mechanism that ensures an abundant supply of glucose for the fetus. Maternal insulin requirements gradually increase from about 18 to 24 weeks of gestation to about 36 weeks of gestation. Maternal insulin requirements may double or quadruple by the end of the pregnancy (Fig. 32-1, *B* and *C*).

At birth, expulsion of the placenta prompts an abrupt decrease in levels of circulating placental hormones, cortisol, and insulinase (Fig. 32-1, *D*). Maternal tissues quickly regain their prepregnancy sensitivity to insulin. For the nonbreastfeeding mother, the prepregnancy insulin-carbohydrate balance usually returns in about 7 to 10 days (Fig. 32-1, *E*). Lactation uses maternal glucose; therefore the breastfeeding mother's insulin requirements will remain low during lactation. On completion of weaning, the mother's prepregnancy insulin requirement is reestablished (Fig. 32-1, *F*).

Pregestational Diabetes Mellitus

Approximately 2 per 1000 pregnancies are complicated by preexisting diabetes. Women who have pregestational diabetes may have either type 1 or type 2 diabetes, which may

or may not be complicated by vascular disease, retinopathy, nephropathy, or other diabetic sequelae. Type 2 is the more common diagnosis. Almost all women with pregestational diabetes are insulin dependent during pregnancy.

The diabetogenic state of pregnancy imposed on the compromised metabolic system of the woman with pregestational diabetes has significant implications. The normal hormonal adaptations of pregnancy affect glycemic control, and pregnancy may accelerate the progress of vascular complications.

During the first trimester, when maternal blood glucose levels are normally reduced and the insulin response to glucose is enhanced, glycemic control is improved. The insulin dosage for the woman with well-controlled diabetes may have to be reduced to avoid hypoglycemia. Nausea, vomiting, and cravings typical of early pregnancy result in dietary fluctuations that influence maternal glucose levels and may also necessitate a reduction in insulin dosage.

Because insulin requirements steadily increase after the first trimester, insulin dosage must be adjusted accordingly to prevent hyperglycemia. Insulin resistance begins as early as 14 to 16 weeks of gestation, and continues to rise until it stabilizes during the last few weeks of pregnancy.

Preconception Counseling

Preconception counseling is recommended for all women of reproductive age who have diabetes, because it is associated with an improved pregnancy outcome (Moore, 2004). Under ideal circumstances, women with pregestational diabetes are counseled before the time of conception to plan the optimal time for pregnancy, establish glycemic control before conception, and diagnose any vascular complications of diabetes. However, it has been estimated that fewer than 20% of women with diabetes in the United States

Evolve/CD: Case Study: Pregestational Diabetes

participate in preconception counseling (Landon et al., 2002).

The woman's partner should be included in the counseling to assess the couple's level of understanding related to the effects of pregnancy on the diabetic condition and of the potential complications of pregnancy as a result of diabetes. The couple should also be informed of the anticipated alterations in diabetic management during pregnancy and the need for a multidisciplinary team approach to health care. Financial implications of diabetic pregnancy and other demands related to frequent maternal and fetal surveillance should be discussed. Contraception is another important aspect of preconception counseling to assist the couple in planning effectively for pregnancy. The American Diabetes Association website, www.diabetes.org, is an excellent resource for information about pregnancy and diabetes.

Maternal Risks and Complications

Although maternal morbidity and mortality rates have improved significantly, the pregnant woman with diabetes remains at risk for the development of significant complications during pregnancy. Poor glycemic control around the time of conception and in the early weeks of pregnancy is associated with an increased incidence of miscarriage. Women with good glycemic control before conception and in the first trimester are no more likely to miscarry than women who do not have diabetes (Moore, 2004).

Poor glycemic control later in pregnancy, particularly in women without vascular disease, increases the rate of fetal macrosomia. Macrosomia occurs in 20% to 25% of diabetic pregnancies. Macrosomic infants tend to have a disproportionate increase in shoulder and trunk size. Because of this, the risk of shoulder dystocia is greater in these babies than in other macrosomic infants. Women with diabetes therefore face an increased likelihood of cesarean birth because of failure of fetal descent or labor progress, or of operative vaginal birth (birth involving the use of episiotomy, forceps, or vacuum extractor) (Moore, 2004).

Preeclampsia and eclampsia occur more frequently in diabetic pregnancies. The highest incidence occurs in women with preexisting vascular changes related to diabetes (Moore, 2004). Diabetic nephropathy has more impact on perinatal outcome than any other vascular complication. Increased risks of preterm labor, intrauterine growth restriction (IUGR), fetal distress, stillbirth, and neonatal death are associated with this condition (Moore).

Hydramnios (polyhydramnios) occurs approximately 10 times more often in diabetic than in nondiabetic pregnancies. Hydramnios (amniotic fluid in excess of 2000 ml) is associated with premature rupture of membranes (PROM), onset of preterm labor, and postpartum hemorrhage (Cunningham, Leveno, Bloom, Hauth, Gilstrap, & Wenstrom, 2005).

Infections are more common and more serious in pregnant women with diabetes. Disorders of carbohydrate metabolism alter the body's normal resistance to infection. The inflammatory response, leukocyte function, and vaginal pH are all affected. Vaginal infections, particularly monilial vaginitis, are more common. Urinary tract infections (UTIs) are also more prevalent. Infection is serious because it causes increased insulin resistance and may result in ketoacidosis. Postpartum infection is more common among women who are insulin dependent.

Ketoacidosis (accumulation of ketones in the blood resulting from hyperglycemia and leading to metabolic acidosis) occurs most often during the second and third trimesters, when the diabetogenic effect of pregnancy is the greatest. When the maternal metabolism is stressed by illness or infection, the woman is at increased risk for diabetic ketoacidosis (DKA). The use of tocolytic drugs such as terbutaline (Brethine) to treat preterm labor may also contribute to the risk for hyperglycemia and subsequent DKA (Cunningham et al., 2005; Iams & Creasy, 2004). DKA may also occur because of the woman's failure to take insulin appropriately. The onset of previously undiagnosed diabetes during pregnancy is another cause of DKA. DKA may occur with blood glucose levels barely exceeding 200 mg/dl, compared with 300 to 350 mg/dl in the nonpregnant state. In response to stress factors such as infection or illness, hyperglycemia (excess glucose in the blood) occurs as a result of increased hepatic glucose production and decreased peripheral glucose use. Stress hormones, which act to impair insulin action and further contribute to insulin deficiency, are released. Fatty acids are mobilized from fat stores to enter into the circulation. As they are oxidized, ketone bodies are released into the peripheral circulation.

CRITICAL THINKING EXERCISE

Hyperglycemia in a Woman with GDM

Cindy, who was diagnosed with gestational diabetes mellitus (GDM) 3 weeks ago, comes to the clinic for a routine prenatal visit. Although Cindy was placed on a 2000 calorie American Diabetes Association diet at diagnosis, her blood sugar record from home reveals that her fasting and postprandial values are too high. When you talk with Cindy about her hyperglycemia she states, "I don't see how my blood sugar could possibly be too high. I'm not eating ANY sweets!" Cindy also declares, "I don't want to take insulin shots!"

1. Evidence—Is there sufficient evidence to draw conclusions about why Cindy continues to have hyperglycemia?
2. Assumptions—What assumptions can be made about the following issues?
   a. Common diet-related reasons for hyperglycemia in women with GDM
   b. The relationship between advancing gestational age and increasing levels of hyperglycemia
   c. The importance of blood glucose control during pregnancy
   d. Influence of education and emotional support by the nurse
3. What implications and priorities for nursing care can be made at this time?
4. Does the evidence objectively support your conclusion?
5. Are there alternative perspectives to your conclusion?

The woman's buffering system is unable to compensate, and metabolic acidosis develops. The excessive blood glucose and ketone bodies result in osmotic diuresis with subsequent loss of fluid and electrolytes, volume depletion, and cellular dehydration. Prompt treatment of DKA is necessary to avoid maternal coma or death. Ketoacidosis occurring at any time during pregnancy can lead to intrauterine fetal death. It is also a cause of preterm labor. The risk of fetal demise is approximately 10% with maternal ketoacidosis (Moore, 2004) (Table 32-1).

The risk of hypoglycemia (a less than normal amount of glucose in the blood) is also increased. Early in pregnancy, when hepatic production of glucose is diminished and peripheral use of glucose is enhanced, hypoglycemia occurs frequently, often during sleep. Later in pregnancy, hypoglycemia may also result as insulin doses are adjusted to maintain euglycemia (a normal blood glucose level). Women with a prepregnancy history of severe hypoglycemia are at increased risk for severe hypoglycemia during gestation. Mild to moderate hypoglycemic episodes do not appear to have significant deleterious effects on fetal well-being (see Table 32-1).

Fetal and Neonatal Risks and Complications

From the moment of conception, the infant of a woman with diabetes faces an increased risk of complications that may occur during the antepartum, intrapartum, or neonatal periods. Infant morbidity and mortality rates associated

table 32-1 Differentiation of Hypoglycemia (Insulin Shock) and Hyperglycemia (Diabetic Ketoacidosis)

CAUSES	ONSET	SYMPTOMS	INTERVENTIONS
HYPOGLYCEMIA (INSULIN SHOCK)			
Excess insulin	Rapid (regular insulin)	Irritability	Check blood glucose level
Insufficient food	Gradual (modified insulin or	Hunger	when symptoms first
(delayed or missed meals)	oral hypoglycemic agents)	Sweating	appear
Excessive exercise or work		Nervousness	Eat or drink 10 to 15 g
Indigestion, diarrhea, vomiting		Personality change	simple carbohydrate
		Weakness	immediately
		Fatigue	Recheck blood glucose level
		Blurred or double vision	in 15 min and eat or drink
		Dizziness	another 10 to 15 g simple
		Headache	carbohydrate if glucose
		Pallor; clammy skin	remains low
		Shallow respirations	Recheck blood glucose level
		Rapid pulse	in 15 min
		Laboratory values	Notify primary health care
		Urine: negative for sugar and	provider if no change in
		acetone	glucose level
		Blood glucose: ≤60 mg/dl	If woman is unconscious,
			administer 50% dextrose
			by IV push, 5% to 10%
			dextrose in water IV drip,
			or glucagon
			Obtain blood and urine
			specimens for laboratory
			testing
HYPERGLYCEMIA (DKA)			
Insufficient insulin	Slow (hours to days)	Thirst	Notify primary health care
Excess or wrong kind of food		Nausea or vomiting	provider
Infection, injuries, illness		Abdominal pain	Administer insulin in
Emotional stress		Constipation	accordance with blood
Insufficient exercise		Drowsiness	glucose levels
		Dim vision	Give IV fluids such as normal
		Increased urination	saline solution or one half
		Headache	normal saline solution;
		Flushed, dry skin	potassium when urinary
		Rapid breathing	output is adequate;
		Weak, rapid pulse	bicarbonate for pH <7
		Acetone (fruity) breath odor	Monitor laboratory testing of
		Laboratory values	blood and urine
		Urine: positive for sugar	
		and acetone	
		Blood glucose: ≥200 mg/dl	

DKA, Diabetic ketoacidosis; *IV,* intravenous.

with diabetic pregnancy are significantly reduced with strict control of maternal glucose levels before and during pregnancy.

Despite the improvements in care of pregnant women with diabetes, sudden and unexplained stillbirth (birth of a dead fetus) is still a major concern. Typically, this is observed in pregnancies after 36 weeks of gestation in women with vascular disease or poor glycemic control. It may also be associated with DKA, preeclampsia, hydramnios, or macrosomia. Although the exact cause of stillbirth is unknown, it may be related to chronic intrauterine hypoxia.

The most important cause of perinatal loss in pregestational diabetic pregnancy is congenital malformations, accounting for 30% to 50% of all perinatal loss (Lindsay, 2006). The incidence of congenital malformations is related to the severity and duration of the diabetes. Anomalies commonly seen in infants primarily affect the cardiovascular system, the central nervous system (CNS), and the skeletal system (Cunningham et al., 2005; Moore, 2004) (see Chapter 38).

The fetal pancreas begins to secrete insulin at 10 to 14 weeks of gestation. The fetus responds to maternal hyperglycemia by secreting large amounts of insulin (hyperinsulinism). Insulin acts as a growth hormone, causing the fetus to produce excess stores of glycogen, protein, and adipose tissue, leading to increased fetal size or macrosomia. Macrosomia is often defined as a weight of greater than 4500 g (American College of Obstetricians and Gynecologists [ACOG], 2000). During birth the macrosomic infant is at risk for a fractured clavicle, liver or spleen laceration, brachial plexus injury, facial palsy, phrenic nerve injury, or subdural hemorrhage (Moore, 2004) (for further discussion, see Chapter 38).

Infants of mothers with diabetes are also at increased risk for respiratory distress syndrome. Hyperglycemia and hyperinsulinemia may be instrumental in delaying pulmonary maturation in the fetus (Moore, 2004).

For infants born to diabetic women the transition to extrauterine life is often associated with metabolic abnormalities. Within the first 30 to 60 minutes after birth, neonatal hypoglycemia often occurs. This is caused by the interruption of the glucose supply with the cutting of the umbilical cord, the effects of fetal hyperinsulinism, and the rapid use of glucose after birth. Hypocalcemia, hypomagnesemia, hyperbilirubinemia, and polycythemia also occur more frequently (Cunningham et al., 2005; Landon et al., 2002; Moore, 2004).

■ CARE MANAGEMENT

■ Assessment and Nursing Diagnoses
■ Interview

When a pregnant woman with diabetes initiates prenatal care, a thorough evaluation of her health status is completed. In addition to the routine prenatal assessment, a detailed history regarding the onset and course of the diabetes and its management and the degree of glycemic

control before pregnancy is obtained. Effective management of the diabetic pregnancy depends on the woman's adherence to a plan of care. At the initial prenatal visit, the woman's knowledge regarding diabetes and pregnancy, potential maternal and fetal complications, and the plan of care are also assessed. With subsequent visits, follow-up assessments are completed. Data from these assessments are used to identify the woman's specific learning needs.

The woman's emotional status is assessed to determine how she is coping with pregnancy superimposed on preexisting diabetes. Although normal pregnancy typically evokes some degree of stress and anxiety, pregnancy designated as "high risk" serves to compound anxiety and stress levels. Fear of maternal and fetal complications is a major concern. Strict adherence to the plan of care may necessitate alterations in patterns of daily living and may be an additional source of stress.

The woman's support system is assessed to identify those people significant to her and their roles in her life. It is important to assess reactions of the family and significant other to the pregnancy and to the strict management plan, and their involvement in the treatment regimen.

■ Physical Examination

At the initial visit, a thorough physical examination is performed to assess the woman's current health status. In addition to the routine prenatal examination, efforts are made to assess the effects of the diabetes, specifically diabetic retinopathy, nephropathy, autonomic neuropathy, and coronary artery disease (ADA, 2004c). A baseline electrocardiogram (ECG) may be done to assess cardiovascular status. Evaluation for retinopathy is done, with follow-up by an ophthalmologist each trimester and more frequently if retinopathy is diagnosed. Blood pressure is monitored carefully throughout pregnancy because of the increased risk for preeclampsia. The woman's weight gain also is monitored at each visit. Fundal height is measured, noting any abnormal increase in size for dates, which may indicate hydramnios or fetal macrosomia.

■ Laboratory Tests

Routine prenatal laboratory examinations are performed. In addition, baseline renal function may be assessed with a 24 hour urine collection for total protein excretion and creatinine clearance. Urinalysis and culture are performed on the initial prenatal visit and as needed throughout the pregnancy to assess for the presence of UTI, which is common in diabetic pregnancy. At each visit, urine is tested for the presence of glucose and ketones. Because of the risk of coexisting thyroid disease, thyroid function tests may also be performed (see later discussion of thyroid disorders).

For the woman with pregestational type 1 or type 2 diabetes, laboratory tests may be done to assess past glycemic control. At the initial prenatal visit, the glycosylated hemoglobin A_{1C} level may be measured. With prolonged hyperglycemia, some of the hemoglobin remains saturated with glucose for the life of the red blood cell (RBC). Therefore a test for glycosylated hemoglobin provides a measure of glycemic control over time, specifically over the previous 4 to 6 weeks. Regular measurements of glycosylated hemoglobin provide data for altering the treatment plan and lead to improvement of glycemic control. Values for the measurement of hemoglobin A_{1C}, the most commonly used index of glycosylated hemoglobin, are as follows (Pagana & Pagana, 2003):

- Adult or elderly without diabetes: 2.2% to 4.8%
- Good diabetic control: 2.5% to 5.9%
- Fair diabetic control: 6% to 8%
- Poor diabetic control: Greater than 8%

Fasting blood glucose and/or random (1 to 2 hours after eating) glucose levels may be assessed during antepartum visits (Fig. 32-2). Blood glucose self-monitoring records may also be reviewed.

Nursing diagnoses for the woman with pregestational diabetes include the following:

- *Deficient knowledge related to*
  - –diabetic pregnancy, management, and potential effects on pregnant woman and fetus
  - –insulin administration and its effects
  - –hypoglycemia and hyperglycemia
  - –diabetic diet
- *Anxiety, fear, dysfunctional grieving, powerlessness, disturbed body image, situational low self-esteem, spiritual distress, ineffective role performance, interrupted family processes related to*
  - –stigma of being labeled "diabetic"
  - –effects of diabetes and its potential sequelae on the pregnant woman and the fetus
- *Noncompliance related to*
  - –lack of understanding of diabetes and pregnancy and requirements of treatment plan
  - –lack of financial resources to purchase blood glucose monitoring supplies or insulin and necessary supplies
  - –insufficient funds or lack of transportation to grocery store to follow dietary regimen
- *Risk for injury to fetus related to*
  - –uteroplacental insufficiency
  - –birth trauma
- *Risk for injury to mother related to*
  - –improper insulin administration
  - –hypoglycemia and hyperglycemia
  - –cesarean or operative vaginal birth
  - –postpartum infection

■ Expected Outcomes of Care

Expected outcomes of management for the pregnant woman with pregestational diabetes include that she will do the following:

- Demonstrate or verbalize understanding of diabetic pregnancy, the plan of care, and the importance of glycemic control.
- Achieve and maintain glycemic control.

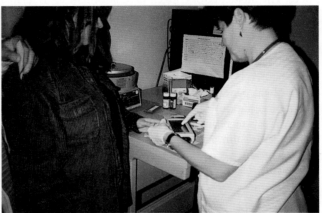

FIG. 32-2 A, Clinic nurse collects blood to determine glucose level. **B,** Nurse interprets glucose value displayed by monitor. (Courtesy Dee Lowdermilk, UNC Ambulatory Care Clinics, Chapel Hill, NC.)

- Demonstrate effective coping.
- Give birth to a healthy infant at term.

■ Plan of Care and Interventions
■ *Antepartum*

Because of her high risk status, a woman with diabetes is monitored much more frequently and thoroughly than are other pregnant women. During the first and second trimesters of pregnancy, her routine prenatal care visits may be scheduled every 1 to 2 weeks. In the last trimester, she will likely be seen 1 to 2 times each week. In the past, routine hospitalization for management of the diabetes, such as insulin dose changes, was common. With the availability of better home glucose monitoring and the growing reluctance of third-party payers to reimburse for hospitalization, pregnant women with diabetes are now generally managed as outpatients. Some client and family education and maternal and fetal assessment may be done in the home, depending on the woman's insurance coverage and care provider preference.

Achieving and maintaining constant euglycemia, with blood glucose levels in the range of 65 to 105 mg/dl preprandially (Table 32-2), is the primary goal of medical ther-

table 32-2	Target Blood Glucose Levels During Pregnancy

TIME OF DAY	TARGET PLASMA GLUCOSE LEVEL (mg/dl)
Premeal	>65 but <105
Postmeal (1 hr)	<155
Postmeal (2 hr)	<130

Sources: American Diabetes Association (ADA). (2004a). Gestational diabetes mellitus. *Diabetes Care, 27*(Suppl 1), S88-S90; Moore, T. (2004). Diabetes in pregnancy. In R. Creasy, R. Resnik, & J. Iams (Eds.), *Maternalfetal medicine: Principles and practice* (5th ed.). Philadelphia: Saunders.

apy (ADA, 2004a; Moore, 2004). Euglycemia is achieved through a combination of diet, insulin, and exercise. Providing the woman with the knowledge, skill, and motivation she needs to achieve and maintain excellent blood glucose control is the primary nursing goal.

Achieving euglycemia requires commitment on the part of the woman and her family to make the necessary lifestyle changes, which can sometimes seem overwhelming. Maintaining tight blood glucose control necessitates that the woman follow a consistent daily schedule. She must get up and go to bed, eat, exercise, and take insulin at the same time each day. Blood glucose measurements are done frequently to determine how well the major components of therapy (diet, insulin, and exercise) are working together to control blood glucose levels. The pregnant woman with diabetes should wear a medical identification bracelet at all times and carry insulin, syringes, and "glucose boosters" with her whenever she is away from home.

Because the woman with diabetes is at increased risk for infections, eye problems, and neurologic changes, foot care and general skin care are important. A daily bath that includes good perineal care and foot care is important. For dry skin, lotions, creams, or oils can be applied. Tight clothing should be avoided. Shoes or slippers should be worn at all times, should fit properly, and are best worn with socks or stockings. Feet should be inspected regularly; toenails should be cut straight across, and professional help should be sought for any foot problems. Extremes of temperature should be avoided.

Diet. The woman with pregestational diabetes has usually had nutritional counseling regarding management of her diabetes. However, because pregnancy precipitates special nutritional concerns and needs, the woman must be educated to incorporate these changes into dietary planning. For the woman who has "controlled" her diabetes for a number of years, the changes in her insulin and dietary needs mandated by pregnancy may be difficult. Nutritional counseling usually is provided by a registered dietitian.

Dietary management during diabetic pregnancy must be based on blood (not urine) glucose levels. The diet is individualized to allow for increased fetal and metabolic requirements, with consideration of such factors as prepregnancy weight and dietary habits, overall health, ethnic background, lifestyle, stage of pregnancy, knowledge of nutrition, and insulin therapy. The dietary goals are to

provide weight gain consistent with a normal pregnancy, to prevent ketoacidosis, and to minimize wide fluctuation of blood glucose levels.

For nonobese women, dietary counseling based on preconceptional body mass index (BMI) is 30 kcal/kg/day (Cunningham et al., 2005). In contrast, for obese women with a BMI greater than 30, it is recommended that the caloric intake total 25 kcal/kg/day (Moore, 2004). The average diet includes 2200 calories (first trimester) to 2500 calories (second and third trimesters). Total calories may be distributed among three meals and one evening snack or, more commonly, three meals and at least two snacks. Meals should be eaten on time and never skipped. Snacks must be carefully planned in accordance with insulin therapy to avoid fluctuations in blood glucose levels. A large bedtime snack of at least 25 g of carbohydrate with some protein is recommended to help prevent hypoglycemia and starvation ketosis during the night.

Attention to the ratio of carbohydrate, protein, and fat or the carbohydrate-to-insulin ratio (C:I ratio) is important to meet the metabolic needs of the woman and the fetus (Bernasko, 2004). Approximately 40% to 50% of the total calories should be carbohydrates, with 30% to 40% fats and proteins providing the remainder of the caloric intake (ADA, 2004b; Bernasko) (see Teaching for Self-Care box). Simple carbohydrates are limited; complex carbohydrates that are high in fiber content are recommended because the starch and protein in such foods help regulate the blood glucose level by more sustained glucose release. Weight gain for women with a normal BMI (19.8 to 26) should be approximately 12 kg during the pregnancy (Gilbert & Harmon, 2003).

Exercise. Although it has been shown that exercise enhances the use of glucose and decreases insulin need in nondiabetic women, there are limited data regarding exercise in women with pregestational diabetes. Any prescription of exercise during pregnancy for women with diabetes should be done by the primary health care provider and should be closely monitored to prevent complications,

TEACHING FOR SELF-CARE

Dietary Management of Diabetic Pregnancy

- Follow the prescribed diet plan.
- Eat a well-balanced diet, including daily food requirements for a normal pregnancy.
- Divide daily food intake between three meals and two to four snacks, depending on individual needs.
- Eat a substantial bedtime snack to prevent a severe drop in blood glucose level during the night.
- Limit the intake of fats if weight gain occurs too rapidly.
- Take daily vitamins and iron as prescribed by the health care provider.
- Avoid foods high in refined sugar.
- Eat consistently each day; never skip meals or snacks.
- Reduce the intake of saturated fat and cholesterol.
- Eat foods high in dietary fiber.
- Avoid alcohol and caffeine.

especially for women with vasculopathy. Women with vasculopathy usually depend completely on exogenous insulin and are at greater risk for wide fluctuations in blood glucose levels and ketoacidosis, which can be made worse by exercise.

When exercise is prescribed by the health care provider as part of the treatment plan, careful instructions are given to the woman. Exercise need not be vigorous to be beneficial: 15 to 30 minutes of walking 4 to 6 times a week is satisfactory for most pregnant women. Other exercises that may be recommended are non–weight-bearing activities such as arm exercises or use of a recumbent bicycle. The best time for exercise is after meals, when the blood glucose level is rising. To monitor the effect of insulin on blood glucose levels, the woman can measure blood glucose before, during, and after exercise.

■ **NURSE ALERT**

Uterine contractions may occur during exercise; the woman should stop exercising immediately if they are detected.

Insulin Therapy. Adequate insulin is the primary factor in the maintenance of euglycemia during pregnancy, thus ensuring proper glucose metabolism of the woman and fetus. Insulin requirements during pregnancy change dramatically as the pregnancy progresses, necessitating frequent adjustments in insulin dosage. In the first trimester, from weeks 3 to 7 of gestation there is an increase in insulin requirement, followed by a decrease between weeks 7 and 15 of gestation. However, insulin dosage may have to be decreased because of hypoglycemia. The commonly prescribed insulin dosage is 0.7 units/kg in the first trimester for women with type 1 diabetes (Moore, 2004). During the second and third trimesters, because of insulin resistance, dosage must be increased to maintain target glucose levels. As insulin needs rise, women with type 1 diabetes require a dosage increase to 0.8 units/kg during gestational weeks 18 to 26, 0.9 units/kg during gestational weeks 27 to 36, and 1 unit/kg from 37 gestational weeks until labor (Bloomgarden, 2004; Moore).

For the woman with type 1 pregestational diabetes who has typically been accustomed to one injection per day of intermediate-acting insulin, multiple daily injections of mixed insulin are a new experience. The woman with type 2 diabetes previously treated with oral hypoglycemics is faced with the task of learning to self-administer injections of insulin. The nurse is instrumental in education and support of pregestational diabetic women with regard to insulin administration and adjustment of insulin dosage to maintain euglycemia (see Teaching for Self-Care box).

Since 1982, most insulin preparations have been produced by inserting portions of DNA ("recombinant DNA") into special lab-cultivated bacteria or yeast cells. The cells then produce complete human insulin, which is less likely to cause antibody formation than animal-derived (beef or pork) insulin. More recently, insulin products called "insulin analogs," in which the structure differs slightly from human insulin, have been produced. This small alteration in

TEACHING FOR SELF-CARE

Administration of Insulin

PROCEDURE FOR MIXING INTERMEDIATE-ACTING (N) AND SHORT-ACTING (R) INSULIN
- Wash hands thoroughly and gather supplies. Be sure the insulin syringe corresponds to the concentration of insulin you are using.
- Check insulin bottle to be certain it is the appropriate type and check the expiration date.
- Gently rotate (do not shake) the insulin vial to mix the insulin.
- Wipe off rubber stopper of each vial with alcohol.
- Draw into syringe the amount of air equal to total dose.
- Inject air equal to intermediate-acting dose into N vial. Remove syringe from vial.
- Inject air equal to regular insulin dose into R insulin vial.
- Invert regular insulin bottle and withdraw regular insulin dose.
- Without adding more air to N vial, carefully withdraw intermediate-acting dose.

PROCEDURE FOR SELF-INJECTION OF INSULIN
- Select proper injection site (remember to rotate sites).
- Injection site should be clean. Use of alcohol is not necessary. If alcohol is used, let it dry before injecting.
- Pinch the skin up to form a subcutaneous pocket and, holding the syringe like a pencil, puncture the skin at a 45- to 90-degree angle. If there is a great deal of fatty tissue at the site, spread the skin taut and inject the syringe at a 90-degree angle.
- Slowly inject the insulin.
- As you withdraw the needle, cover the injection site with sterile gauze and apply gentle pressure to prevent bleeding.
- Record insulin dosage and time of injection.

insulin structure results in changes in the onset and peak of action of the medication. Currently, the most commonly used insulin preparations include rapid-acting (lispro or aspart), short-acting (regular), intermediate-acting (N), and long-acting (glargine) (Lewis, 2002). (Table 32-3). Mixtures of short- and intermediate-acting insulins in several proportions are also available (Lewis).

Lispro (Humalog), is a commonly prescribed rapid-acting insulin with a shorter duration of action than regular insulin. Advantages of rapid-acting insulin, such as lispro, include convenience, because it is injected immediately before mealtime; less hyperglycemia after meals; and fewer hypoglycemic episodes in some people. Because its effects last only 3 to 5 hours, most clients require a longer-acting insulin in addition to maintain optimal blood glucose levels (Landon et al., 2002; Lewis, 2002; Moore, 2004).

Glargine (Lantus) is a long-acting insulin lasting approximately 16 to 24 hours. Glargine is categorized as a pregnancy category C drug by the U.S. Food and Drug Administration (FDA) (Aventis Pharmaceuticals, 2004). Small

table 32-3 Common Insulin Preparations

TYPE OF INSULIN	EXAMPLES GENERIC (TRADE) NAME	ONSET OF ACTION	PEAK OF ACTION	DURATION OF ACTION
Rapid-acting	Lispro (Humalog) Aspart (NovoLog)	15 minutes	30-90 minutes	3-5 hours
Short-acting (Regular)	Humulin R or Novolin R	30-60 minutes	50-120 minutes	5-8 hours
	Humulin N or Novolin N	1-3 hours	8 hours	20 hours
Intermediate-acting (NPH)	Humulin L or Novolin L	1-2.5 hours	7-15 hours	20 hours
Long-acting	Ultralente			
	Humulin U	4-8 hours	8-12 hours	36 hours
	Glargine (Lantus)	1 hour	none	24 hours

From: Lewis, C. (2002). Diabetes: A growing public health concern. U.S. Food and Drug Administration. *FDA Consumer, 36*(1). Accessed http://www.fda.gov/fdac/features/2002/102_diab.html#insulin, August 14, 2006.

amounts of glargine insulin are slowly released, with no pronounced peak. This insulin preparation is most often used with women who have insulin-resistant diabetes (type 2) requiring high doses of long-acting insulin. Glargine insulin is combined with a rapid-acting insulin to prevent hypoglycemia. Major concerns with this medication include the need for monitoring for nocturnal hypoglycemia (Moore, 2004) and not mixing with other insulins or solutions (Aventis Pharmaceuticals). Glargine insulin provides a more stable basal blood glucose with less risk of nocturnal hypoglycemia than intermediate-acting insulin (Cianni et al., 2005).

Most women with insulin-dependent diabetes are managed with two to three injections per day, also known as multiple injection therapy (MIT) (Bernasko, 2004). Usually, two thirds of the daily insulin dose, with longer-acting (i.e., intermediate and rapid- or short-acting (lispro or regular) insulin combined in a 2:1 ratio, is given before breakfast. The remaining one third, again a combination of longer- and short-acting insulin, is administered in the evening before dinner. To reduce the risk of hypoglycemia during the night, separate injections are often administered, with short-acting insulin given before dinner, followed by longer-acting insulin at bedtime. Another alternative insulin regimen that works well for some women is to administer short-acting insulin before each meal and longer-acting insulin at bedtime (Moore, 2004).

Continuous subcutaneous insulin infusion (CSII) systems are increasingly used during pregnancy. The insulin pump is designed to mimic more closely the function of the pancreas in secreting insulin (Fig. 32-3). This portable, battery-powered device is worn, like a pager, during most daily activities. The pump infuses regular insulin at a set basal rate and has the capacity to deliver up to four different basal rates in 24 hours. It also delivers bolus doses of insulin before meals to control postprandial blood glucose levels. A fine-gauge plastic catheter is inserted into subcutaneous tissue, usually in the abdomen, and attached to the pump syringe by connecting tubing. The subcutaneous catheter and connecting tubing are changed every 2 to 3 days, although the infusion tubing can be left in place for

FIG. 32-3 Insulin pump shows basal rate for pregnant women with diabetes. (Courtesy MiniMed, Inc., Sylmar, CA.)

several weeks without local complications. Although the insulin pump is convenient and generally provides good glycemic control, complications such as DKA, infection, or hypoglycemic coma can still develop (Moore, 2004). Use of the insulin pump requires a knowledgeable, motivated client, skilled health care providers, and an alternative mode of insulin delivery in case of pump failure (Bernasko, 2004; Moore).

Monitoring Blood Glucose Levels. Blood glucose testing at home with a glucose reflectance meter or biosensor monitor is the commonly accepted method for monitoring blood glucose levels and the most important tool available to the woman to assess her degree of glycemic control.

To perform blood glucose monitoring, an individual obtains a drop of blood by means of a finger stick and places it on a test strip. After a specified amount of time, the glucose level can be read by the meter (see Teaching for Self-Care box Testing Blood Glucose Level). Blood glucose levels are routinely measured at various times throughout the day, such as before breakfast, lunch, and dinner; 2 hours after each meal; at bedtime; and in the middle of the night. When there is any readjustment in insulin

TEACHING FOR SELF-CARE

Testing Blood Glucose Level

- Gather supplies, check expiration date, and read instructions on testing materials. Prepare glucose reflectance meter for use according to manufacturer's directions.
- Wash hands in warm water (warmth increases circulation).
- Select site on side of any finger (all fingers should be used in rotation).
- Pierce site with lancet (may use automatic, spring-loaded puncturing device). Cleaning the site with alcohol is not necessary.
- Drop hand down to side; with other hand gently squeeze finger from hand to fingertip.
- Allow blood to drop onto testing strip. Be sure to cover entire reagent area.
- Determine blood glucose value using the glucose reflectance meter, following manufacturer's instructions.
- Record results.
- Repeat daily as instructed by health care provider and as needed for signs of hypoglycemia or hyperglycemia.

Source: American Diabetes Association. (2000). *Medical management of pregnancy complicated by diabetes* (3rd ed.). Alexandria, VA: The Association.

TEACHING FOR SELF-CARE

Treatment for Hypoglycemia

- Be familiar with signs and symptoms of hypoglycemia (nervousness, headache, shaking, irritability, personality change, hunger, blurred vision, sweaty skin, tingling of mouth or extremities).
- Check blood glucose level immediately when hypoglycemic symptoms occur.
- If blood glucose is <60 mg/dl, immediately eat or drink something that contains 10 to 15 g of simple carbohydrate. Examples:
  - ½ cup (4 ounces) unsweetened fruit juice
  - ½ cup (4 ounces) regular (not diet) soda
  - 5 to 6 Life Savers candies
  - 1 tablespoon honey or corn (Karo) syrup
  - 1 cup (8 ounces) milk
  - 2 to 3 glucose tablets
- Rest for 15 min, then recheck blood glucose.
- If glucose level is still <60 mg/dl, eat or drink another serving of one of the "glucose boosters" listed above.
- Wait 15 min, then recheck blood glucose. If it is still <60 mg/dl, notify health care provider immediately.

Source: American Diabetes Association. (2000). *Medical management of pregnancy complicated by diabetes* (3rd ed.). Alexandria, VA: Author; Becton Dickinson & Co. (1997). *Controlling low blood sugar reactions.* Franklin Lakes, NJ: Author.

dosage or diet, more frequent measurement of blood glucose is warranted. If nausea, vomiting, or diarrhea occurs, or if any infection is present, the woman will be asked to monitor her blood glucose levels more closely.

▬ NURSE ALERT

Hyperglycemia will most likely be identified in 2 hour postprandial values, because blood glucose levels peak about 2 hours after a meal.

Target levels of blood glucose during pregnancy are lower than nonpregnant values. Acceptable fasting levels are generally between 60 and 105 mg/dl, and 2 hour postprandial levels should be less than 130 mg/dl (ADA, 2004a; Moore, 2004) (see Table 32-2). The woman should be told to immediately report episodes of hypoglycemia (less than 60 mg/dl) and hyperglycemia (more than 200 mg/dl) to her health care provider so that adjustments in diet or insulin therapy can be made.

Pregnant women with diabetes are much more likely to develop hypoglycemia than hyperglycemia. Most episodes of mild or moderate hypoglycemia can be treated with oral intake of 10 to 15 g of simple carbohydrate (see Teaching for Self-Care box Treatment for Hypoglycemia). If severe hypoglycemia occurs, in which the woman experiences a decrease in or loss of consciousness or an inability to swallow, she will require a parenteral injection of glucagon or intravenous (IV) glucose. Because hypoglycemia can develop rapidly and because impaired judgment can be associated with even moderate episodes, it is vital that family members, friends, and work colleagues be able to quickly recognize signs and symptoms and initiate proper treatment if necessary.

Hyperglycemia is less likely to occur, but it can rapidly progress to DKA, which is associated with an increased risk of fetal death (Cunningham et al., 2005; Moore, 2004). Maternal hyperglycemia is predictive of macrosomia (Bloomgarden, 2004). Women and family members should be particularly alert for signs and symptoms of hyperglycemia, especially when infections or other illnesses occur (see Table 32-1 and Teaching for Self-Care box on p. 837).

Urine Testing. Although urine testing for glucose is not beneficial during pregnancy, urine testing for ketones continues to have a place in diabetic management (ADA, 2004a). Monitoring for urine ketones may detect inadequate caloric or carbohydrate intake (ADA). Women may be taught to perform urine testing daily with the first morning urine. Testing may also be done if a meal is missed or delayed, when illness occurs, or when the blood glucose level is greater than 200 mg/dl.

Complications Requiring Hospitalization. Occasionally hospitalization is necessary to regulate insulin therapy and stabilize glucose levels. Infection, which can lead to hyperglycemia and DKA, is an indication for hospitalization, regardless of gestational age. Hospitalization during the third trimester for closer maternal and fetal observation may be indicated for women whose diabetes is poorly controlled. In addition, women with diabetes are 20% to 30% more likely to also have preexisting hypertension (Moore, 2004), or develop preeclampsia or eclampsia, which may necessitate hospitalization.

Fetal Surveillance. Diagnostic techniques for fetal surveillance are often performed to assess fetal growth and

TEACHING FOR SELF-CARE

What to Do When Illness Occurs

- Be sure to take insulin even though appetite and food intake may be less than normal. (Insulin needs are increased with illness or infection.)
- Call the health care provider and relay the following information:
  - Symptoms of illness (e.g., nausea, vomiting, diarrhea)
  - Fever
  - Most recent blood glucose level
  - Urine ketones
  - Time and amount of last insulin dose
- Increase oral intake of fluids to prevent dehydration.
- Rest as much as possible.
- If unable to reach health care provider and blood glucose exceeds 200 mg/dl with urine ketones present, seek emergency treatment at the nearest health care facility. Do not attempt to self-treat for this.

well-being. The goals of fetal surveillance are to detect fetal compromise as early as possible and to prevent intrauterine fetal death or unnecessary preterm birth.

Early in pregnancy, the estimated date of birth (EDB) is determined. A baseline sonogram is done during the first trimester to assess gestational age. Follow-up ultrasound examinations are usually performed during the pregnancy (as often as every 4 to 6 weeks) to monitor fetal growth; estimate fetal weight; and detect hydramnios, macrosomia, and congenital anomalies.

Because the fetus of a diabetic woman is at greater risk for neural tube defects (e.g., spina bifida, anencephaly, microcephaly), measurement of maternal serum alpha-fetoprotein is performed between 16 and 20 weeks of gestation (Cunningham et al., 2005). This is often done in conjunction with a detailed ultrasound study to examine the fetus for neural tube defects.

Fetal echocardiography may be performed between 20 and 22 weeks of gestation to detect cardiac anomalies (Moore, 2004). Some practitioners repeat this fetal surveillance test at 34 weeks of gestation. Doppler studies of the umbilical artery may be performed in women with vascular disease to detect placental compromise.

The majority of fetal surveillance measures are concentrated in the third trimester, when the risk of fetal compromise is greatest. Pregnant women should be taught how to do daily fetal movement counts, beginning at 28 weeks of gestation (see Chapter 29) (Moore, 2004).

The nonstress test (NST), done weekly or twice weekly, to evaluate fetal well-being is typically begun around 28 weeks of gestation (Moore, 2004) (see Chapter 29). For the woman with vascular disease, testing may begin earlier and continue more frequently. In the presence of a nonreactive nonstress test, a contraction stress test (CST) or fetal biophysical profile (BPP) may be used to evaluate fetal well-being (Landon et al., 2002; Moore).

Determination of Birth Date and Mode of Birth. Today, most diabetic pregnancies are allowed to progress to 38.5 to 40 weeks of gestation as long as good metabolic control is maintained and all parameters of antepartum fetal surveillance remain within normal limits. Reasons to proceed with birth before term include poor metabolic control, worsening hypertensive disorders, fetal macrosomia, or fetal growth restriction (Cunningham et al., 2005; Moore, 2004).

Many practitioners plan for elective labor induction between 38 and 40 weeks of gestation. To confirm fetal lung maturity before birth, an amniocentesis should be performed in pregnancies between 37 and 38.5 weeks of gestation (Moore, 2004). For the pregnancy complicated by diabetes, fetal lung maturation is better predicted by the amniotic fluid phosphatidylglycerol (>3%) (Moore) than by the lecithin/sphingomyelin ratio. If the fetal lungs are still immature, birth should be postponed as long as the results of fetal assessment remain reassuring. Amniocentesis may be repeated to monitor lung maturity (Landon et al., 2002). Birth, despite poor fetal lung maturity, may be necessary when testing suggests fetal compromise, worsening maternal renal function or vision, or preeclampsia.

Although vaginal birth is expected for most women with pregestational diabetes, the cesarean rate for these women ranges from 30% to 80% (Cunningham et al., 2005; Moore, 2004). Cesarean birth is often performed when antepartum testing suggests fetal distress or the estimated fetal weight is greater than 4500 g (Moore). Also, cesarean birth is necessary when the cervix fails to dilate completely during induction of labor (Moore).

■ *Intrapartum*

During the intrapartum period, the woman with pregestational diabetes must be monitored closely to prevent complications related to dehydration, hypoglycemia, and hyperglycemia. Most women use large amounts of energy (calories) to accomplish the work and manage the stress of labor and birth. However, this calorie expenditure varies with the individual. Blood glucose levels and hydration must be carefully controlled during labor. An IV line is inserted for infusion of a maintenance fluid, such as lactated Ringer's solution, 5% dextrose in lactated Ringer's solution, or 10% dextrose (Bloomgarden, 2004). Most commonly, insulin is administered by continuous infusion. Only regular insulin may be administered intravenously. Determinations of blood glucose levels are made every hour, and fluids and insulin are adjusted to maintain blood glucose levels between 80 and 120 mg/dl (Balsells, Corcoy, Adelantado, & Garcia-Patterson, Altirriba, & de Leiva, 2000; Bernasko, 2004). It is essential that these target glucose levels be maintained because hyperglycemia during labor can precipitate metabolic problems, particularly hypoglycemia, in the neonate.

During labor, continuous fetal heart monitoring is necessary. The woman should assume an upright or side-lying position during bed rest in labor to prevent supine hypotension because of a large fetus or polyhydramnios. Labor is allowed to progress, provided normal rates of cervical dilation, fetal descent, and fetal well-being are maintained. Failure to progress may indicate a macrosomic infant and cephalopelvic disproportion, necessitating a cesarean birth. The woman is observed and treated during labor for diabetic complications such as hyperglycemia, ketosis, ketoacidosis, and glycosuria. During second-stage labor, shoulder dystocia may occur during vaginal birth of a macrosomic infant (see Chapter 36). A neonatologist, pediatrician, or neonatal nurse practitioner may be present at the birth to initiate assessment and neonatal care.

If a cesarean birth is planned, it should be scheduled in the early morning to facilitate glycemic control. Dependent upon the provider, no morning insulin may be given or the bedtime dose of intermediate-acting insulin may be given in the morning and every 8 hours until surgery (Chan & Winkle, 2006). The woman is given nothing by mouth. Epidural anesthesia is recommended because hypoglycemia can be detected earlier if the woman is awake. After surgery, glucose levels should be monitored at least every 2 hours if an IV solution containing 5% dextrose is being infused. Target plasma glucose levels are between 80 and 160 mg/dl (Moore, 2004).

▬ Postpartum

During the first 24 hours postpartum, insulin requirements decrease substantially because the major source of insulin resistance, the placenta, has been removed. Women with type 1 diabetes may require only one fourth to one third of the prenatal insulin dose on the first postpartum day, provided that they are eating a full diet (Bernasko, 2004). In women with type 1 diabetes who give birth by cesarean, an intravenous infusion of glucose and insulin may be required for the first 2 to 3 postpartum days (Moore, 2004). It takes several days after birth to reestablish carbohydrate homeostasis (see Figure 32-1, *D* and *E*). Since insulin needs decrease significantly following birth, some women may not require insulin for 24 to 72 hours postpartum (Chan & Winkle, 2006). Blood glucose levels are monitored in the postpartum period, and insulin dosage is adjusted, often using a sliding scale. The woman who has insulin-dependent diabetes must realize the importance of eating on time, even if the baby needs feeding or other pressing demands exist. Women with type 2 diabetes often require only 40% to 50% of their prebirth insulin doses in the postpartum period and are soon able to maintain euglycemia through diet alone or with oral hypoglycemics (Moore).

Possible postpartum complications include preeclampsia and/or eclampsia, hemorrhage, and infection. Hemorrhage is a possibility if the mother's uterus was overdistended (hydramnios, macrosomic fetus) or overstimulated (oxytocin induction). Postpartum infections such as endometritis are more likely to occur in a woman with diabetes.

Mothers are encouraged to breastfeed. In addition to the advantages of maternal satisfaction and pleasure, breastfeeding has an antidiabetogenic effect for the children of women with diabetes and for women with gestational diabetes (Lindsay, 2006; Moore, 2004). Insulin requirements may be half of prepregnancy levels because of the carbohydrate used in human milk production. Because glucose levels are lower, breastfeeding women are at increased risk for hypoglycemia, especially in the early postpartum period and after breastfeeding sessions, particularly after late-night feedings (Moore). Breastfeeding mothers with diabetes may be at increased risk for mastitis and yeast infections of the breast. Insulin dosage, which is decreased during lactation, must be recalculated at weaning (Landon et al., 2002; Lawrence & Lawrence, 2005) (see Fig. 32-1, *F*).

The mother may have early breastfeeding difficulties. Poor metabolic control may delay lactogenesis and contribute to decreased milk production (Moore, 2004). Initial contact and opportunity to breastfeed the infant may be delayed for mothers who had cesarean birth or if infants are placed in neonatal intensive care units or special care nurseries for observation during the first hours after birth. Support and assistance from nursing staff and lactation specialists can facilitate the mother's early experience with breastfeeding and encourage her to continue.

The new mother needs information about family planning and contraception. Although family planning is important for all women, it is essential for the woman with diabetes to safeguard her own health and to promote optimal outcomes in future pregnancies. The woman and her partner should be informed that the risks associated with pregnancy increase with the duration and severity of the diabetic condition and that pregnancy may contribute to vascular changes associated with diabetes.

The risks and benefits of contraceptive methods should be discussed with the mother and her partner before discharge from the hospital. Barrier methods are often recommended as safe, inexpensive options that have no inherent risks for women with diabetes (Landon et al., 2002). However, barrier methods such as the diaphragm or condom and spermicide are not as effective as some other forms of contraception, and inconsistent use often leads to unplanned pregnancy (Landon et al.).

Use of oral contraceptives by diabetic women is controversial because of the risk of thromboembolic and vascular complications and the effect on carbohydrate metabolism. In women without vascular disease or other risk factors, combination low-dose oral contraceptives may be prescribed. Progestin-only oral contraceptives also may be used because they minimally affect carbohydrate metabolism (Cunningham et al., 2005; Landon et al., 2002). Close monitoring of blood pressure and lipid levels is necessary to detect complications (Landon et al.).

Some health care providers are reluctant to use intrauterine contraceptive devices (IUDs) in women with diabetes because of concerns about infection. However, this method has been used successfully by women with diabetes, though an increased incidence of pelvic infections has been reported in this population (Cunningham et al., 2005).

Opinion is divided about the use of long-acting parenteral progestins, such as Depo-Provera. Some health care providers recommend their use, especially in women who may not be compliant with daily dosing for oral contraceptives. In contrast, other health care providers believe this method may adversely affect diabetic control. Transdermal (patch) and transvaginal (vaginal ring) administration are newer contraceptive options, particularly effective in women who prefer weekly or every-third-week dosing, respectively. For women weighing more than 90 kg (198 pounds) there is a higher contraceptive failure rate with transdermal administration (Cunningham et al., 2005). Therefore use of the patch would not be recommended for these women. Limited data are available regarding patch and vaginal ring use in women with diabetes.

The risks associated with pregnancy increase with the duration and severity of diabetes, and vascular changes may worsen. This information must be thoroughly discussed with the woman and her partner. Sterilization is often recommended for the woman who has completed her family, who has poor metabolic control, or who has significant vascular problems.

▬ Evaluation

Evaluation of the care of the pregnant woman with pregestational diabetes is based on the previously stated expected outcomes of care and is closely associated with the degree of maternal metabolic control during pregnancy (see Plan of Care).

Gestational Diabetes Mellitus (GDM)

GDM complicates approximately 4% to 7% of all pregnancies in the United States (ADA, 2006; ADA, 2004a) and accounts for over 75% of all cases of diabetic pregnancy (Chan & Winkle, 2006). Prevalence varies (1% to 14%) by racial and ethnic groups (ADA, 2006). GDM is more likely to occur among Hispanic, Native-American, Asian, and African-American populations than in Caucasians (ADA, 2006; Moore, 2004). GDM is likely to recur in future pregnancies, and there is an increased risk for development of overt diabetes in later life (Moore). This is especially true for women whose GDM is diagnosed early in pregnancy or who are obese (Landon et al., 2002). Classic risk factors for GDM include maternal age over 25 years; obesity; family history of type 2 diabetes; and an obstetric history of an infant weighing more than 4500 g, hydramnios, unexplained stillbirth, miscarriage, or an infant with congenital anomalies (Moore). Women at high risk for GDM are often screened at their initial prenatal visit and then are rescreened later (at 24 to 28 weeks of gestation) if the initial screen is negative.

GDM is usually diagnosed during the second half of pregnancy. As fetal nutrient demands rise during the late second and the third trimesters, maternal nutrient ingestion induces greater and more sustained levels of blood glucose. At the same time, maternal insulin resistance is also increasing because of the insulin-antagonistic effects of the placental hormones, cortisol, and insulinase. Consequently, maternal insulin demands rise as much as threefold. Most pregnant women are capable of increasing insulin production to compensate for insulin resistance and to maintain euglycemia. When the pancreas is unable to produce sufficient insulin or the insulin is not used effectively, however, gestational diabetes can result.

Maternal-Fetal Risks

Women with GDM have an increased risk (10% to 40%) of developing hypertensive disorders compared with normal pregnant women (ADA, 2004a; Moore, 2004). They also have increased risk for fetal macrosomia, which can lead to increased rates of perineal lacerations, episiotomy, and cesarean birth (ADA). In addition, fetal macrosomia may be associated with shoulder dystocia and birth trauma. GDM also places the neonate at increased risk for hypoglycemia, hypocalcemia, hyperbilirubinemia, thrombocytopenia, polycythemia, and respiratory distress syndrome (Moore).

The overall incidence of congenital anomalies among infants of women with gestational diabetes approaches that of the general population because gestational diabetes usually develops after the critical period of organogenesis (first trimester) has passed. However, Anderson, Waller, Canfield, Shaw, Watkins, and Werler (2005) found that women who were obese before conception (BMI >30 kg/m²) and developed gestational diabetes were at greater risk to give birth to infants with CNS defects.

Collaborative Care

Screening for Gestational Diabetes Mellitus. ACOG recommends that all pregnant women be screened for GDM, either by history, clinical risk factors, or laboratory screening of blood glucose levels (ACOG, 2001). Based on history and clinical risk factors, some women are at such low risk for the development of GDM that glucose testing is not cost-effective (ECDCDM, 2003). This group includes normal-weight women younger than 25 years of age who have no family history of diabetes, are not members of an ethnic or a racial group known to have a high prevalence of the disease, and have no previous history of abnormal glucose tolerance or adverse obstetric outcomes usually associated with GDM (ACOG; ADA, 2006; ADA, 2004a; ECDCDM).

Women at high risk for GDM should be screened at their initial prenatal visit and then rescreened later (at 24 to 28 weeks of gestation) in pregnancy if the initial screen is negative (ADA, 2006; ADA, 2004a). The screening test (glucola screening) most often used consists of a 50-g oral glucose load, followed by a plasma glucose determination 1 hour later. It is not necessary that the woman be fasting. A glucose value of 140 mg/dl or greater is considered a positive screen and should be followed by a 2-hour (75-g) or 3-hour

CD: Critical Thinking Exercise: Gestational Diabetes

plan of care	Pregnancy Complicated by Pregestational Diabetes

CD: Plan of Care: Pregestational Diabetes

NURSING DIAGNOSIS Deficient knowledge related to lack of recall of information as evidenced by woman's questions and concerns

Expected Outcome *Woman will be able to verbalize important information regarding diabetes, its management, and potential effects on the pregnant woman and fetus.*

Nursing Interventions/*Rationales*
- Assess woman's current knowledge base regarding disease process, management, effects on pregnancy and fetus, and potential complications *to provide database for further teaching.*
- Review the pathophysiology of diabetes, effects on pregnancy and fetus, and potential complications *to promote recall of information and compliance with treatment plan.*
- Review procedure for insulin administration, demonstrate procedure for blood glucose monitoring and insulin measurement and administration, and obtain return demonstration *to establish woman's comfort and competence with procedures.*
- Discuss diet and exercise as prescribed by diabetologist *to promote self-care.*
- Review signs and symptoms of complications of hypoglycemia and hyperglycemia and appropriate interventions *to promote prompt recognition of complications and self-care.*
- Provide contact numbers for health care team for prompt interventions and answers to questions on an ongoing basis *to promote collaboration between woman and health care team.*

NURSING DIAGNOSIS Risk for fetal injury related to elevated maternal glucose levels

Expected Outcomes *Fetus will remain free of injury and be born at term in a healthy state.*

Nursing Interventions/*Rationales*
- Assess woman's current diabetic control *to identify risk for fetal mortality and congenital anomalies.*
- Monitor fundal height during each prenatal visit *to identify appropriate fetal growth.*
- Monitor for signs and symptoms of preeclampsia *to identify early manifestations because pregnant women with diabetes are more at risk.*
- Assess fetal movement and heart rate during each prenatal visit, and perform weekly nonstress tests during the last 4 weeks of pregnancy *to assess fetal well-being.*
- Review procedure for blood glucose testing and insulin administration *to promote self-care.*

NURSING DIGANOSIS Anxiety related to threat to maternal and fetal well-being as evidenced by woman's verbal expressions of concern

Expected Outcomes *Woman will identify sources of anxiety and report feeling less anxious.*

Nursing Interventions/*Rationales*
- Through therapeutic communication, promote an open relationship with woman *to promote trust.*
- Listen to woman's feelings and concerns *to assess for any misconception or misinformation that may be contributing to anxiety.*
- Review potential dangers by providing factual information *to correct any misconceptions or misinformation.*
- Encourage woman to share concerns with her health care team *to promote collaboration in her care.*

NURSING DIAGNOSIS Risk for imbalanced nutrition: less than body requirements related to inability to ingest nutrients that are needed for pregnancy complicated by diabetes

Expected Outcomes *Woman will verbalize understanding of dietary needs during pregnancy, will gain weight that is consistent with a normal pregnancy, and will maintain blood sugar levels between 65 and 130 mg/dl.*

Nursing Interventions/*Rationales*
- Assess caloric intake and dietary pattern using 24 hour recall *to evaluate woman's understanding and/or adherence to dietary regimen.*
- Review importance of regularity of meals and snacks *to promote compliance with treatment plan.*
- Review blood glucose monitoring *to determine if woman is competent with procedure.*
- Weigh woman at each prenatal visit *to assess appropriate weight gain.*
- Refer to dietitian for individualized counseling if needed *to plan diet that assists the woman to maintain euglycemia and to gain the appropriate amount of weight.*
- Instruct woman to do daily fetal movement counts *to assess well-being of fetus.*
- Encourage woman to join a support group or use online support website *to decrease anxiety and to share findings and concerns.*

(100-g) oral glucose tolerance test (OGTT) (ADA, 2006; ADA, 2004a; Cunningham et al., 2005; Moore, 2004). The OGTT is administered after an overnight fast and at least 3 days of unrestricted diet (at least 150 g of carbohydrate) and physical activity. The woman is instructed to avoid caffeine because it will increase glucose levels and to abstain from smoking for 12 hours before and during the test. The 3-hour OGTT, the gold standard test, requires a fasting blood glucose level, which is drawn before giving a 100-g glucose load. Blood glucose levels are then drawn 1, 2, and 3 hours later. The woman is diagnosed with gestational diabetes if two or more values are met or exceeded (ADA, 2006; ADA, 2004a; Moore) (Fig. 32-4).

Nursing diagnoses and expected outcomes of care for women with GDM are basically the same as those for women with pregestational diabetes, except that the time frame for planning may be shortened with GDM because the diagnosis is usually made later in pregnancy.

Antepartum Care. When the diagnosis of gestational diabetes is made, treatment begins immediately, allowing little or no time for the woman and her family to adjust to the diagnosis before they are expected to participate in the treatment plan. With each step of the treatment plan, the nurse and other health care providers should educate the woman and her family, providing detailed and comprehensive explanations to ensure understanding, participation, and

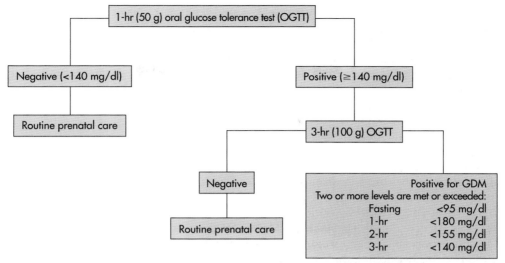

FIG. 32-4 Screening and diagnosis for gestational diabetes. (From American Diabetes Association. [2004a]. Position statement: Gestational diabetes mellitus. *Diabetes Care* 27[Suppl 1], S88-S90.)

adherence to the necessary interventions. Potential complications should be discussed, and the need for maintenance of euglycemia throughout the remainder of the pregnancy reinforced. It may be reassuring for the woman and her family to know that gestational diabetes typically disappears when the pregnancy is over.

As with pregestational diabetes, the aim of therapy in women with GDM is strict blood glucose control. Fasting blood glucose levels should range between 65 and 105 mg/dl, and 2-hour postprandial blood levels should be less than 130 mg/dl (ADA, 2004a; Moore, 2004).

Diet. Dietary modification is the mainstay of treatment for GDM. The woman with GDM is placed on a standard diabetic diet. The usual prescription is for 30 kcal/kg/day based on a normal preconceptional weight. For obese women, the usual prescription is up to 25 kcal/kg/day, which translates into 1500 to 2000 kcal/day for most women (ADA, 2004a; Chan & Winkle, 2006). Carbohydrate intake is restricted to approximately 35% to 40% of caloric intake (ADA). Dietary counseling by a nutritionist is recommended.

Exercise. Exercise in women with GDM helps lower blood glucose levels and may be instrumental in decreasing the need for insulin (ADA, 2004a). Women with GDM who already have an active lifestyle should be encouraged to continue an exercise program.

Monitoring Blood Glucose Levels. Blood glucose monitoring is necessary to determine whether euglycemia can be maintained by diet and exercise. Women are encouraged to monitor their blood sugar daily. At a minimum, fasting and postprandial glucose levels should be monitored at least weekly (ACOG, 2001). However, the optimal frequency and timing of blood glucose monitoring has not been established (ACOG). Women with GDM may perform self-monitoring at home, or monitoring may be done at the clinic or office visit.

Insulin Therapy. Up to 20% of women with GDM will require insulin during the pregnancy to maintain adequate blood glucose levels, despite compliance with the prescribed diet. In contrast to women with pregestational diabetes, women with gestational diabetes are initially managed with diet and exercise alone. If fasting glucose levels are greater than 105 mg/dl, then insulin therapy is begun (ADA, 2004a). Either lower or higher thresholds for initiating insulin may be used (Landon et al., 2002). One oral hypoglycemic agent, glyburide, is being used experimentally during pregnancy in women with diabetes. Although limited data exist, minimal placental transfer occurs, and maternal and fetal complications are comparable with those of maternal insulin administration (Cianni et al., 2005). Women with diabetes who are unable or unwilling to take insulin injections or are cognitively impaired may be candidates for glyburide use.

Fetal Surveillance. There is no standard recommendation for fetal surveillance in pregnancies complicated by GDM. Women whose blood glucose levels are well controlled by diet are at low risk for fetal complications. Limited antepartum fetal testing is done in women with gestational diabetes as long as their fasting and 2-hour postprandial blood glucose levels remain within normal limits and they have no other risk factors. Daily fetal movement counts are done beginning at 28 weeks of gestation and nonstress tests may be done twice weekly beginning at 36 weeks of gestation (Moore, 2004). Usually these women progress to term and spontaneous labor without intervention.

Women with GDM whose blood glucose levels are poorly controlled or who require insulin therapy, have hypertension, or have a history of previous stillbirth generally receive more intensive fetal biophysical monitoring. NSTs and BPPs are often performed weekly, beginning anywhere from 28 to 36 weeks of gestation (Bernasko, 2004; Moore, 2004).

Intrapartum Care. During the labor and birth process, blood glucose levels are monitored at least every 2 hours to maintain levels at 80 to 120 mg/dl (Bernasko, 2004; Moore, 2004). Glucose levels within this range will decrease the incidence of neonatal hypoglycemia. It may be necessary to infuse regular insulin intravenously during labor in order to maintain blood glucose levels within this range. IV fluids containing glucose are not commonly given during labor. Although gestational diabetes is not an indication for cesarean birth, it may be necessary in the presence of problems such as preeclampsia or macrosomia. Women with gestational diabetes are encouraged to breastfeed.

Postpartum Care. Most women with GDM will return to normal glucose levels after childbirth. However, GDM is likely to recur in future pregnancies, and women with GDM are at significant risk for developing glucose intolerance later in life. Assessment for carbohydrate intolerance with a 75 g oral glucose tolerance test should be done at 6 to 12 weeks postpartum or after breastfeeding has stopped (ADA, 2004a). Obesity is a major risk factor for the later development of diabetes. Women with a history of GDM, particularly those who are overweight, should be encouraged to make lifestyle changes that include weight loss and exercise to reduce this risk (ADA). The risk of developing GDM in subsequent pregnancies is 50% or higher. Infants born to women with GDM are at increased risk to develop type 2 diabetes or impaired glucose tolerance. Infants are also at risk for becoming obese in childhood or adolescence (Lindsay, 2006).

▬ HYPEREMESIS GRAVIDARUM

Nausea and vomiting complicate approximately 70% of all pregnancies beginning typically at 4 to 6 weeks of gestation and are usually confined to the first trimester or the first 16 to 20 weeks of gestation, peaking from 8 to 12 weeks of gestation (Cunningham et al., 2005; Scott & Abu-Hamda, 2004). Although these manifestations are distressing, they are typically benign, with no significant metabolic alterations or risks to the mother or fetus. Theories include increasing levels of estrogens, human chorionic gonadotropin, transient maternal hyperthyroidism, and stress and interrelated psychosocial components (Davis, 2004; Meighan & Wood, 2004; Scott & Abu-Hamda).

When vomiting during pregnancy becomes excessive enough to cause weight loss of at least 5% of prepregnancy weight and is accompanied by dehydration, electrolyte imbalance, ketosis, and acetonuria, the disorder is termed hyperemesis gravidarum. The estimated incidence varies from 3.3 to 10 per 1000 births (Scott & Abu-Hamda, 2004). Approximately 1% of women with this disorder require hospitalization. Hyperemesis gravidarum usually begins during the first 10 weeks of pregnancy. It has been associated with women who are nulliparous, have increased body weight, have a history of migraines, are pregnant with twins (Davis, 2004; Scott & Abu-Hamda) or hydatidiform mole (Berman, DiSaia, & Tewari, 2004). In addition, an interrelated psychologic component has been associated with hyperemesis and must be assessed (Cunningham et al., 2005; Scott & Abu-Hamda). The effects of hyperemesis gravidarum on perinatal outcome vary with the severity of the disorder. Women with hyperemesis gravidarum have a decreased risk of spontaneous abortion (Scott & Abu-Hamda).

Etiology

The etiology of hyperemesis gravidarum remains obscure. Several theories have been proposed as to the cause, although none of them adequately explains the disorder. Hyperemesis gravidarum may be related to high levels of estrogen or human chorionic gonadotropin (hCG) and may be associated with transient hyperthyroidism during pregnancy. Some research has found that a woman who has severe nausea and vomiting has a 1.5-fold increased chance of carrying a female infant, supporting the association between increased estrogen exposure and hyperemesis gravidarum (Cunningham et al., 2005; Davis, 2004). Esophageal reflux, reduced gastric motility, and decreased secretion of free hydrochloric acid may contribute to the disorder.

Psychosocial factors also may play a part in the development of hyperemesis gravidarum for some women. Ambivalence toward the pregnancy and increased stress may be associated with this condition (Cunningham et al., 2005; Davis, 2004; Scott & Abu-Hamda, 2004). Conflicting feelings regarding prospective motherhood, body changes, and lifestyle alterations may contribute to episodes of vomiting, particularly if these feelings are excessive or unresolved.

Clinical Manifestations

The woman with hyperemesis gravidarum usually has significant weight loss and dehydration. She may have a decreased blood pressure, increased pulse rate, and poor skin turgor (Scott & Abu-Hamda, 2004). She is frequently unable to keep down even clear liquids taken by mouth. Laboratory tests may reveal electrolyte imbalances.

Collaborative Care

Whenever a pregnant woman has nausea and vomiting, the first priority is a thorough assessment to determine the severity of the problem. In most cases the woman should be told to come immediately to the health care provider's office or to the emergency department, because the severity of the illness is often difficult to determine by phone conversation.

The assessment should include frequency, severity, and duration of episodes of nausea and vomiting. If the woman reports vomiting, then the assessment should also include the approximate amount and color of the vomitus. Other symptoms such as diarrhea, indigestion, and abdominal pain or distention also are identified. The woman is asked to report any precipitating factors relating to the onset of her symptoms. Any pharmacologic or nonpharmacologic treatment measures used should be recorded. Prepregnancy weight and documented weight gain or loss during pregnancy are important to note.

The woman's weight and vital signs are measured, and a complete physical examination is performed, with attention to signs of fluid and electrolyte imbalance and nutritional status. The most important initial laboratory test to be obtained is a dipstick determination of ketonuria. Other laboratory tests that may be ordered are a urinalysis, a complete blood count (CBC), electrolytes, liver enzymes, and bilirubin levels. These tests help rule out the presence of underlying diseases such as gastroenteritis, pyelonephritis, pancreatitis, cholecystitis, and hepatitis (Cunningham et al., 2005). Because of the recognized association between hyperemesis gravidarum and hyperthyroidism, thyroid levels may also be measured (Scott & Abu-Hamda, 2004).

Psychosocial assessment includes asking the woman about anxiety, fears, and concerns related to her own health and the effects on pregnancy outcome. Family members should be assessed both for anxiety and in regard to their role in providing support for the woman.

Initial Care

Initially the woman who is unable to keep down clear liquids by mouth will require IV therapy for correction of fluid and electrolyte imbalances. She should be kept on nothing-by-mouth (NPO) status until dehydration has been resolved and for at least 48 hours after vomiting has stopped to prevent rapid recurrence of the problem (Gordon, 2002). In the past, women requiring IV therapy were admitted to the hospital. Today, however, they may be, and often are, successfully managed at home, even if on enteral therapy. Medications may be used if nausea and vomiting are uncontrolled. The most frequently prescribed drugs include pyridoxine (vitamin B_6) 25 mg to 75 mg daily, alone or in combination with doxylamine (Unisom) 25 mg, promethazine (Phenergan), and metoclopramide (Reglan) (ACOG, 2004; Cunningham et al., 2005; Weiner & Buhimschi, 2004). Other less commonly used medications include meclizine (Antivert), dimenhydrinate (Dramamine), diphenhydramine (Benadryl), prochlorperazine (Compazine), and ondansetron (Zofran) (Cunningham et al.). Corticosteroids (methylprednisolone [Medrol]) may also be used to treat refractory hyperemesis gravidarum (Cunningham et al.). Lastly, enteral or parenteral nutrition may be used for women nonresponsive to other medical therapies (Cunningham et al.). In addition to medical management, some women can also benefit from psychotherapy or stress reduction techniques (Scott & Abu-Hamda, 2004). Once the vomiting has stopped, feedings are started in small amounts at frequent intervals, and the diet is slowly advanced as tolerated.

Nursing care of the woman with hyperemesis gravidarum involves implementing the medical plan of care, whether this care be given in the hospital or home setting. Interventions may include initiating and monitoring IV therapy, administering drugs and nutritional supplements, and monitoring the woman's response to interventions. The nurse observes the woman for any signs of complications such as metabolic acidosis (secondary to starvation), jaundice, or hemorrhage and alerts the physician should these occur. Monitoring includes assessment of the woman's nausea, retching without vomiting, and vomiting, since the two symptoms, although related, are separate. A standardized assessment tool such as the PUQE (Pregnancy-Unique Quantification of Emesis) allows quantification of the presence and severity of the nausea and vomiting and promotes accurate monitoring (Davis, 2004).

Accurate measurement of intake and output, including the amount of emesis, is an important aspect of care. Oral hygiene while the woman is receiving nothing by mouth, and after episodes of vomiting, helps allay associated discomforts. Assistance with positioning and providing a quiet, restful environment that is free from odors may increase the woman's comfort. When the woman begins responding to therapy, limited amounts of oral fluids and bland foods such as crackers, toast, or baked chicken are begun. The diet is progressed slowly as tolerated by the woman until she is able to consume a nutritionally sound diet. Because sleep disturbances may accompany hyperemesis gravidarum, promoting adequate rest is important. The nurse can assist in coordinating treatment measures and periods of visitation to provide opportunity for rest periods (see Plan of Care).

Follow-Up Care

Most women are able to take nourishment by mouth after several days of treatment. Women should be encouraged to eat small, frequent meals consisting of low-fat, high-protein foods; to avoid greasy and highly seasoned foods; and to increase dietary intake of potassium and magnesium. Herbal teas such as ginger, chamomile, or raspberry leaf may decrease nausea (Jewell & Young, 2003; Nursing, 2006; Smith, Crowther, Willson, Hotham, & McMillian, 2004; Tiran & Mack, 2000). Many pregnant women find exposure to cooking odors nauseating. Having other family members cook may lessen the woman's nausea and vomiting, even if only temporarily. Dietary instructions include ingestion of dry, bland foods, high protein foods, small, frequent meals, cold foods, a snack before bedtime, drinking liquids from a cup with a lid, drinking tea or water with lemon slices, and avoidance of high-fat or spicy foods (Davis, 2004). The woman is counseled to contact her health care provider immediately if the nausea and vomiting recur. Complications accompanying severe hyperemesis gravidarum include esophageal rupture and deficiencies of vitamin K and thiamine with resulting Wernicke encephalopathy (CNS involvement) (Cunningham et al., 2005).

A few women will continue to experience intractable nausea and vomiting throughout pregnancy. Rarely, it may be necessary to maintain a woman on enteral, parenteral, or total parenteral nutrition to ensure adequate nutrition for the mother and fetus (Cunningham et al., 2005). Many home health agencies are able to provide these services,

EVIDENCE-BASED PRACTICE

Ginger for Nausea and Vomiting of Pregnancy

BACKGROUND

- Nausea is commonly estimated to affect about three out of four women in the first trimester of pregnancy, with half of all pregnant women experiencing vomiting. "Morning sickness," so-called because queasiness is more likely when fasting, can last all day. In its most severe form, hyperemesis gravidarum, the pregnant woman can take nothing by mouth and may require parenteral fluids and nutrition. Concerns of teratogenic effects from conventional medications have led to increased interest in complementary and alternative therapies, such as vitamin B_6 (pyridoxine); herbs such as ginger, chamomile, peppermint, and raspberry leaf; homeopathic therapies; and acupressure and acupuncture. Ginger is widely used and accepted in the United States and Europe as an aid for digestion and nausea.

OBJECTIVES

- Assessment of the efficacy and safety of ginger as a therapy for the nausea and vomiting of pregnancy was the reviewers' goal.

METHODS

Search Strategy

- The authors searched the international literature and identified six randomized controlled trials that met the predetermined criteria for inclusion. The studies represented 675 women, from Australia, Canada, Denmark, and Thailand. Bias was lowered by the studies being double-blinded, meaning neither the subjects nor their clinicians knew what therapy they were taking.

Statistical Analyses

- Meaningful pooling of the data was not possible because of differences in measures and different control groups.

FINDINGS

- Four studies compared ginger to placebo. Ginger preparation varied; the doses ranged from 125 to 250 mg, taken up to 4 times a day. Outcomes were results of several scales of nausea and retching, as well as episodes of vomiting. Ginger was significantly beneficial for nausea and vomiting in all four trials. The effect began to show up after several days of use.

- Two trials compared ginger to vitamin B_6, given 3 times a day. In both trials, nausea and vomiting were significantly reduced from baseline after several days. Ginger was found to be as effective as vitamin B_6.
- Adverse effects in four out of six trials included headache, diarrhea, drowsiness, and reflux. There were no adverse pregnancy outcomes.

LIMITATIONS

- Metaanalysis was not possible because of differences in nausea measures and doses. The two studies comparing ginger to vitamin B_6 had no placebo, whereas the trials with placebos all showed some placebo effects. Ginger was found equivalent to vitamin B_6, but evidence for B_6 has not been "compelling." Some trials allowed subjects to take other antiemetics. Ginger root was prepared in several different ways: ground fresh and dried to powder, or as a syrup; the preparation may affect the efficacy, and the taste may have unblinded the subjects.

IMPLICATIONS FOR PRACTICE

- The authors suggest ginger as a safe and effective therapy for the nausea and vomiting of pregnancy. Ginger is readily available as tea, capsules, syrup, and in ginger ale, and it is not expensive. It may provide some relief alone or in combination with other complementary and alternative therapies such as acupressure, another evidence-based recommendation for pregnancy nausea.

IMPLICATIONS FOR FURTHER RESEARCH

- Future trials should control for the placebo effect, which is impressive in these trials. More data about vitamin B_6, chamomile, raspberry leaf and peppermint may determine effectiveness and safety of these popularly accepted therapies for use during pregnancy. Other evidence-based complementary and alternative therapies such as hypnosis may benefit pregnant women.

Reference: Borelli, F., Capasso, R., Aviello, G., Pittler, M., & Izzo, A. (2005). Effectiveness and safety of ginger in the treatment of pregnancy-induced nausea and vomiting. *Obstetrics and Gynecology, 105*(4), 849-856.

and arrangements for service may be made depending on the woman's insurance coverage.

The woman with hyperemesis gravidarum needs calm, compassionate, and sympathetic care, with recognition that the manifestations of hyperemesis can be physically and emotionally debilitating to the woman and stressful for her family. Irritability, tearfulness, and mood changes are often consistent with this disorder. Fetal well-being is a primary concern of the woman. The nurse can provide an environment conducive to discussion of concerns and assist the woman in identifying and mobilizing sources of support. The family should be included in the plan of care whenever possible. Their participation may help alleviate some of the emotional stress associated with this disorder.

▬ THYROID DISORDERS

Hyperthyroidism

Hyperthyroidism in pregnancy is rare, occurring in approximately 1 or 2 of every 1000 pregnancies (Cunningham et al., 2005; Nader, 2004b). In 90% to 95% of pregnant women, it is caused by Graves' disease (Nader). Clinical manifestations of hyperthyroidism include tachycardia, fatigue, heat intolerance, emotional lability, weight loss, and severe nausea and vomiting. Exophthalmos and enlargement of the thyroid gland (goiter) may also occur. Many of these symptoms also occur with pregnancy, so the disorder can be difficult to diagnose. Signs that may help differentiate hyperthyroidism from normal pregnancy changes include weight loss, goiter, and a pulse rate greater

plan of care ▸ Hyperemesis Gravidarum

NURSING DIAGNOSIS Deficient fluid volume related to excessive vomiting as evidenced by fluid and electrolyte imbalance

Expected Outcome *Woman's fluid and electrolyte balance will be restored.*

Nursing Interventions/Rationales
- Assess and document skin turgor, condition of mucous membranes, vital signs, and urine specific gravity *to provide database for planning care.*
- Obtain daily weight *to provide ongoing evaluation of care.*
- Monitor laboratory values and report deviations from normal *to prevent complications.*
- Maintain accurate intake and output record *to assess for evidence of fluid deficit.*
- Initiate and maintain intravenous (IV) therapy carefully *to maintain fluid balance.*
- Administer antiemetics as prescribed *to inhibit nausea and vomiting.*
- Begin oral fluids slowly and carefully *to slowly increase tolerance and restore fluid balance.*

NURSING DIAGNOSIS Imbalanced nutrition: less than body requirements, related to nausea and persistent vomiting as evidenced by weight decrease as compared with prepregnant weight

Expected Outcomes *Woman will exhibit no further weight losses, and weight will stabilize. Woman will tolerate regular diet with adequate nutrients for pregnancy with no further nausea and vomiting.*

Nursing Interventions/Rationales
- Ascertain woman's prepregnant weight, and monitor current weight and intake and output *to provide a database for care planning.*
- Resume oral diet as tolerated and prescribed by caregiver *to provide oral nutrition at optimal time.*

- Provide small, frequent, bland meals as woman tolerates *to assess her response to limited oral intake.*
- Administer antiemetic medications as prescribed *to decrease or eliminate episodes of vomiting.*
- Provide a quiet, restful environment *to decrease associated discomforts.*
- Teach woman the importance of a low-fat, high-protein diet with fluids between meals *to provide optimal nutrition for fetal growth and keep nausea to a minimum.*
- Refer to dietitian to develop optimal diet plan individualized to woman's current preferences, culture, and lifestyle *to encourage ongoing compliance.*
- Discuss with woman the importance of contacting health care provider if intractable nausea and vomiting recur *to provide prompt treatment and avoid complications.*

NURSING DIAGNOSIS Anxiety related to effects of hyperemesis on fetal well-being as evidenced by woman's statements of concern

Expected Outcome *Woman will exhibit decreased incidence of anxiety.*

Nursing Interventions/Rationales
- Use therapeutic communication to listen to woman's concerns *to maintain a relationship and feeling of trust.*
- Provide information regarding any potential risks to the fetus *to alleviate anxiety.*
- Assist woman to identify personal strengths and previous coping mechanisms *to reinforce to woman those strengths and coping mechanisms that may be of assistance during this illness.*
- Help woman identify sources of support and mobilize support person or group of her choice *to provide support as needed.*
- Refer for psychological assessment if needed *for ongoing evaluation and assistance.*

CD: Plan of Care: Hyperemesis Gravidarum

---

than 100 beats/min (Nader). Laboratory findings include elevated free thyroxine (T_4) and triiodothyronine (T_3) levels and suppressed thyroid-stimulating hormone (TSH) levels (Cunningham et al.; Nader). Moderate and severe hyperthyroidism must be treated during pregnancy; untreated or inadequately treated women have an increased risk of preterm birth, and giving birth to stillborn infants and infants with goiter, and hypothyroidism or hyperthyroidism (Cunningham et al.). Women with hyperthyroidism are also at increased risk to develop severe preeclampsia (Nader). Women with hyperemesis gravidarum often present with elevated thyroid hormone levels because of high levels of human chorionic gonadotropin (Cunningham et al.).

The primary treatment of hyperthyroidism during pregnancy is drug therapy; the medication of choice is propylthiouracil (PTU). The usual starting dose is 100 to 150 mg every 8 hours, with higher doses required for some women (Nader, 2004b). Women generally show clinical improvement within 2 weeks of beginning therapy, but the medication requires 6 to 8 weeks to reach full effectiveness. During

therapy, the woman's free T_4 levels are measured monthly and the results used to taper the drug to the smallest effective dosage to prevent unnecessary fetal hypothyroidism (Nader). PTU is well tolerated by most women. Rare side effects include pruritus, skin rash, fever, a metallic taste, nausea, bronchospasm, oral ulcerations, hepatitis, and a lupus-like syndrome (Nader; Weiner & Buhimschi, 2004). The most severe side effect is agranulocytosis, which occurs very rarely and usually develops only in women over 40 years of age and in those taking high doses of PTU (Nader). Symptoms of agranulocytosis are fever and sore throat; these symptoms should be reported immediately to the health care provider, and the woman should stop taking the PTU. Leukopenia of a transient and benign nature may occur as a result of PTU therapy. PTU readily crosses the placenta and may induce fetal hypothyroidism and goiter (Mestman, 2002; Nader).

Beta-adrenergic blockers such as propranolol may be used in severe hyperthyroidism to control maternal symptoms, especially maternal heart rate. Long-term use of these medications is not recommended because of the potential for IUGR and altered response to anoxic stress, postnatal bradycardia, and hypoglycemia.

Radioactive iodine must not be used in diagnosis or treatment of hyperthyroidism in pregnancy because it may compromise the fetal thyroid. Mothers choosing to breastfeed who are also taking hyperthyroid medication should be informed that, although small amounts of the drug are excreted in breast milk, PTU has not been found to adversely affect the neonate's thyroid function (Weiner & Buhimschi, 2004).

In severe cases, surgical treatment of hyperthyroidism, subtotal thyroidectomy, may be performed during the second or third trimester. Because of the increased risk of miscarriage and preterm labor associated with major surgery, this treatment is usually reserved for women with severe disease, those for whom drug therapy proves toxic, and those who are unable to adhere to the prescribed medical regimen.

■ **NURSE ALERT**
A serious but uncommon complication of undiagnosed or partially treated hyperthyroidism is thyroid storm, which may occur in response to stress such as infection, birth, or surgery. A woman with this emergency disorder may have fever, restlessness, tachycardia, vomiting, hypotension, or stupor. Prompt treatment is essential; IV fluids and oxygen are administered along with high doses of PTU. After administration of PTU, iodide is given. Other medications include antipyretics, dexamethasone, and beta-blockers (Cunningham et al., 2005; Nader, 2004b).

Hypothyroidism

Hypothyroidism during pregnancy is less common (1.3 per 1000) than is hyperthyroidism. Hypothyroidism is often associated with menstrual and fertility problems, including an increased risk of miscarriage (Cunningham et al., 2005). Hypothyroidism is usually caused by glandular destruction by autoantibodies, most commonly because of Hashimoto's thyroiditis. Characteristic symptoms of hypothyroidism include weight gain; fatigue; cold intolerance; constipation; cool, dry skin; coarsened hair; and muscle weakness. Laboratory values in pregnancy include low or low-normal T_3 and T_4 levels and elevated levels of TSH (Cunningham et al.; Nader, 2004b).

Pregnant women with untreated hypothyroidism are at risk for preeclampsia, placental abruption, and stillbirth (Cunningham et al., 2005). Infants born to mothers with hypothyroidism may be of low birth weight. For the most part, however, if such women are treated before conception or early in the pregnancy, their infants are healthy and without evidence of thyroid dysfunction (Nader, 2004b).

Thyroid hormone supplements are used to treat hypothyroidism. Levothyroxine (e.g., l-thyroxine [Synthroid]) is most often prescribed during pregnancy. The usual beginning dosage is 0.1 to 0.15 mg per day with adjustment by 25 to 50 mcg every 4 to 6 weeks as necessary based on the maternal TSH level (Cunningham et al., 2005; Nader, 2004b). The aim of drug therapy is to maintain the woman's TSH level at the lower end of the normal range for pregnant women. In contrast, women on thyroid replacement therapy before conception usually will have a dose increase of 25% to 50% during the pregnancy (DiPiro, Talbert, Yee, Matzke, Wells, & Posey, 2005).

■ **NURSE ALERT**
If taking iron supplementation, pregnant women should be told to take l-thyroxine 2 hours before or after iron tablets, because ferrous sulfate decreases absorption of T_4 (Spratto & Woods, 2004).

The fetus depends on maternal thyroid hormones until 12 weeks of gestation, when fetal production begins (Blackburn, 2003). Decreased levels of T_4 in the second trimester have been associated with permanent neonatal neurologic deficits (Cunningham et al., 2005; Nader, 2004b). Careful monitoring of the neonate's thyroid status to detect any abnormalities is important.

Nursing Care

Education of the pregnant woman with thyroid dysfunction is essential to promote compliance with the plan of treatment. It is important to discuss with the woman and her family the disorder and its potential impact on her, her family, and her fetus; the medication regimen and possible side effects; the need for continuing medical supervision; and the importance of compliance.

The woman often needs assistance from the nurse in coping with the discomforts and frustrations associated with symptoms of the disorder. For example, the woman with hyperthyroidism who has nervousness and hyperactivity concomitant with weakness and fatigue may benefit from suggestions to channel excess energies into quiet diversional activities such as reading or crafts. Discomfort associated with hypersensitivity to heat (hyperthyroidism) or cold intolerance (hypothyroidism) can be minimized by appropriate clothing and regulation of environmental temperatures, and by avoidance of temperature extremes.

Nutritional counseling with a registered dietitian may provide guidance in selecting a well-balanced diet. The woman with hyperthyroidism who has increased appetite and poor weight gain and the hypothyroid woman who has anorexia and lethargy need counseling to ensure adequate intake of nutritionally sound foods to meet both maternal and fetal needs.

▬ MATERNAL PHENYLKETONURIA

Phenylketonuria (PKU), a recognized cause of mental retardation, is an inborn error of metabolism caused by an autosomal recessive trait that creates a deficiency in the enzyme phenylalanine hydrolase. Absence of this enzyme impairs the body's ability to metabolize the amino acid phenylalanine, found in all protein foods. Consequently, there is toxic accumulation of phenylalanine in the blood, which interferes with brain development and function.

PKU affects 1 in every 15,000 live births in the United States (Cunningham et al., 2005).

PKU was the first inborn error of metabolism to be universally screened for in the United States. Since 1961, all newborns have been tested soon after birth for this disorder. Prompt diagnosis and therapy with a phenylalanine-restricted diet significantly decreases the incidence of mental retardation. It is recommended that dietary therapy for PKU be continued throughout life (Blackburn, 2003; Brown et al., 2002). Some people discontinue the restricted diet because of the difficulty in adhering to the specially prepared foods (Blackburn; Brown et al.). Women who discontinue the phenylalanine-restricted diet may demonstrate a decline in intellectual function (Cunningham et al., 2005).

The keys to prevention of fetal anomalies caused by PKU are the identification of women in their reproductive years who have the disorder and dietary compliance for those women diagnosed. Screening for undiagnosed homozygous maternal PKU at the first prenatal visit may be warranted, especially in individuals with a family history of the disorder, with low intelligence of uncertain etiology, or who have given birth to microcephalic infants. Women with PKU should continue the low-protein diet during pregnancy. Nutritional phenylalanine intake and phenylalanine levels must be monitored. It is recommended that maternal phenylalanine levels range between 2 and 6 mg/dl. These levels are associated with a decrease in fetal sequelae (Cunningham et al., 2005). High maternal phenylalanine levels are associated with microcephaly with mental retardation and congenital heart defects (Cunningham et al.; Landon et al., 2002). Ultrasound examinations are used for fetal surveillance beginning in the first trimester. A spontaneous vaginal birth is anticipated.

Women with PKU may breastfeed, but their maternal blood levels are followed closely (Lawrence & Lawrence, 2005; Riordan, 2005) because their milk contains high levels of phenylalanine (Nader, 2004a). Mothers who choose to breastfeed must still supplement the infant's diet with a special milk preparation, phenylalanine (PHE)-free formula that contains little or no phenylalanine (Riordan).

community activity

Stroll through your local pharmacy and examine the diabetic equipment and supplies you find there. Locate glucose meters, urine test strips, insulin syringes, and insulin pens. How expensive are each of these items? Check to see what costs are covered by most types of insurance and Medicaid. Read the directions for use of each item. How easily could you follow the directions? Could a woman who has low literacy skills read and understand them? Do the directions contain pictures? Are they written in more than one language (for example, in Spanish or French) in addition to English?

CRITICAL THINKING EXERCISE

Preconception Counseling for the Woman with PKU

Toni, who has just gotten married, comes in for her yearly well-woman exam. She and her husband are anxious to start a family right away. Toni tells you that she has phenylketonuria (PKU) but has not followed a special diet since she was "just a little girl."

1. Evidence—Is there sufficient evidence to draw conclusions about the damaging effects of untreated PKU on children born with this disorder?
2. Assumptions—What assumptions can be made about the following issues?
   a. Risk that the baby will inherit this disorder
   b. Relationship between excessive levels of maternal phenylalanine and the development of fetal anomalies
   c. Effectiveness of dietary management of PKU
   d. Importance of education and support by the nurse
3. What implications and priorities for nursing care can be made at this time?
4. Does the evidence objectively support your conclusion?
5. Are there alternative perspectives to your conclusion?

key points

- In pregnant women with diabetes, lack of glycemic control before conception and in the first trimester of pregnancy may be responsible for fetal congenital malformations.
- For pregnant women who have diabetes and are insulin dependent, insulin requirements increase as the pregnancy progresses and may quadruple by term as a result of insulin resistance created by placental hormones, insulinase, and cortisol. After birth, levels decrease dramatically; breastfeeding will affect insulin needs.
- Poor glycemic control before and during pregnancy in women who have diabetes can lead to maternal complications such as miscarriage, infection, and dystocia (difficult labor) caused by fetal macrosomia.
- Careful glucose monitoring, insulin administration when necessary, and dietary counseling are used to create a normal intrauterine environment for fetal growth and development in the pregnancy complicated by diabetes mellitus.
- Because GDM is usually asymptomatic, most women undergo routine screening during pregnancy.
- The woman with hyperemesis gravidarum may have significant weight loss and dehydration; management focuses on restoring fluid and electrolyte balance and preventing recurrence of nausea and vomiting.
- Thyroid dysfunction during pregnancy requires close monitoring of thyroid hormone levels to regulate therapy and prevent fetal insult.
- High levels of PKU in the maternal bloodstream cross the placenta and are teratogenic to the developing fetus. Damage can be prevented or minimized by dietary restriction of phenylalanine before and during pregnancy.

REFERENCES

American College of Obstetricians and Gynecologists (ACOG). (2000). Fetal macrosomia. *ACOG Practice Bulletin No. 22.* Washington, DC: Author.

American College of Obstetricians and Gynecologists (ACOG). (2001). Gestational diabetes. *ACOG Practice Bulletin No. 30.* Washington, DC: Author.

American College of Obstetricians and Gynecologists (ACOG). (2004). Nausea and vomiting of pregnancy. *ACOG Practice Bulletin No. 52.* Washington, DC: Author.

American Diabetes Association (ADA). (2006). Diagnosis and classification of diabetes mellitus. *Diabetes Care, 29*(Suppl), S543-S548.

American Diabetes Association (ADA). (2004a). Gestational diabetes mellitus. *Diabetes Care, 27*(Suppl 1), S88-S90.

American Diabetes Association (ADA). (2004b). Nutrition principles and recommendations in diabetes. *Diabetes Care, 27*(Suppl 1), S36-S46.

American Diabetes Association (ADA). (2004c). Preconception care of women with diabetes. *Diabetes Care, 27*(Suppl 1), S76-S78.

Anderson, J., Waller, D., Canfield, M., Shaw, G., Watkins, M., & Werler, M. (2005). Maternal obesity, gestational diabetes, and central nervous system birth defects. *Epidemiology, 16*(1), 87-92.

Aventis Pharmaceuticals. (2004). *Lantus prescribing information.* Kansas City, MO: Author.

Balsells, M., Corcoy, R., Adelantado, J., Garcia-Patterson, A., Altirriba, O., & de Leiva, A. (2000). Gestational diabetes mellitus: Metabolic control during labour. *Diabetes, Nutrition, & Metabolism, 13*(5), 257-262.

Berman, M., DiSaia, P., & Tewari, K. (2004). Pelvic malignancies, gestational trophoblastic neoplasia, and nonpelvic malignancies. In R. Creasy, R. Resnik, & J. Iams (Eds.), *Maternal-fetal medicine: Principles and practice* (5th ed.). Philadelphia: Saunders.

Bernasko, J. (2004). Contemporary management of type 1 diabetes mellitus in pregnancy. *Obstetrical and Gynecological Survey, 59*(8), 628-636.

Blackburn, S. (2003). *Maternal, fetal, and neonatal physiology: A clinical perspective* (2nd ed.). St. Louis: Saunders.

Bloomgarden, Z. (2004). Inpatient diabetes control: *Rationale. Diabetes Care, 27*(8), 2074-2080.

Brown, A., Fernhoff, P., Waisbren, S., Frazier, D., Singh, R., Rohr, F., et al. (2002). Barriers to successful dietary control among pregnant women with phenylketonuria. *Genetics in Medicine, 4*(2), 84-89.

Chan, P., & Winkle, C. (2006). *Gynecology and obstetrics: Current clinical strategies.* Laguna Hills, CA: CCS Publishing.

Cianni, G., Volpe, L., Lencioni, C., Chatzianagnostou, K., Cuccuru, J., Ghio, A., et al. (2005). Use of insulin glargine during the first weeks of pregnancy in five type 1 diabetic women. *Diabetes Care, 28*(4), 982-983.

Cunningham, F., Leveno, K., Bloom, S., Hauth, J., Gilstrap, L., & Wenstrom, K. (Eds.). (2005). *Williams obstetrics* (22nd ed.). New York: McGraw-Hill.

Davis, M. (2004). Nausea and vomiting of pregnancy: An evidence-based review. *Journal of Perinatal and Neonatal Nursing, 18*(4), 312-328.

DiPiro, J., Talbert, R., Yee, G., Matzke, G., Wells, B., & Posey, L. (2005). *Pharmacotherapy: A pathophysiologic approach* (6th ed.). New York: McGraw-Hill.

Expert Committee on the Diagnosis and Classification of Diabetes Mellitus (ECDCDM). (2003). Follow-up report on the diagnosis of diabetes mellitus. *Diabetes Care, 26*(11), 3160-3167.

Gilbert, E., & Harmon, J. (2003). *Manual of high risk pregnancy and delivery* (3rd ed.). St. Louis: Mosby.

Gordon, M. (2002). Maternal physiology in pregnancy. In S. Gabbe, J. Niebyl, & J. Simpson (Eds.), *Obstetrics: Normal and problem pregnancies* (4th ed.). New York: Churchill Livingstone.

Iams, J., & Creasy, R. (2004). Preterm labor and delivery. In R. Creasy, R. Resnik, & J. Iams, (Eds.), *Maternal-fetal medicine: Principles and practice* (5th ed.). Philadelphia: Saunders.

Jewell, D., & Young, G. (2003). Interventions for nausea and vomiting in early pregnancy. *The Cochrane Database of Systematic Reviews,* 2006, Issue 3. Chichester, UK: John Wiley & Sons.

Landon, M., Catalano, P., & Gabbe, S. (2002). Diabetes mellitus. In S. Gabbe, J. Niebyl, & J. Simpson (Eds.), *Obstetrics: Normal and problem pregnancies* (4th ed.). New York: Churchill Livingstone.

Lawrence, R., & Lawrence, R. (2005). *Breastfeeding: A guide for the medical profession* (6th ed.). Philadelphia: Mosby.

Lewis, C. (2002). Diabetes: A growing public health concern. U.S. Food and Drug Administration. *FDA Consumer 36*(1). Accessed http://www.fda.gov/features/2002/102_diab.html, March 15, 2006.

Lindsay, C. (2006). Pregnancy complicated by diabetes mellitus. In R. Martin, A. Fanaroff, & M. Walsh (Eds.), *Fanaroff and Martin's neonatal-perinatal medicine: Diseases of the fetus and infant* (8th ed.). Philadelphia: Mosby.

Meighan, M., & Wood, A. (2004). The impact of hyperemesis gravidarum on maternal role assumption. *Journal of Obstetric, Gynecologic, and Neonatal Nursing, 34*(2), 172-179.

Mestman, J. (2002). Endocrine diseases in pregnancy. In S. Gabbe, J. Niebyl, & J. Simpson (Eds.), *Obstetrics: Normal and problem pregnancies* (4th ed.). New York: Churchill Livingstone.

Moore, T. (2004). Diabetes in pregnancy. In R. Creasy, R. Resnik, & J. Iams, (Eds.), *Maternal-fetal medicine: Principles and practice* (5th ed.). Philadelphia: Saunders.

Nader, S. (2004a). Other endocrine disorders of pregnancy. In R. Creasy, R. Resnik, & J. Iams, (Eds.), *Maternal-fetal medicine: Principles and practice* (5th ed.). Philadelphia: Saunders.

Nader, S. (2004b). Thyroid disease and pregnancy. In R. Creasy, R. Resnik, & J. Iams, (Eds.), *Maternal-fetal medicine: Principles and practice* (5th ed.). Philadelphia: Saunders.

Nursing 2006. (2006). *Nursing 2006 drug handbook* (26th ed.). Philadelphia: Lippincott Williams & Wilkins.

Pagana, K., & Pagana, T. (2003). *Mosby's diagnostic and laboratory test reference* (6th ed.). St. Louis: Mosby.

Riordan, J. (2005). *Breastfeeding and human lactation* (3rd ed.). Boston: Jones & Bartlett.

Scott, L., & Abu-Hamda, E. (2004). Gastrointestinal disease in pregnancy. In R. Creasy, R. Resnik, & J. Iams, (Eds.), *Maternal-fetal medicine: Principles and practice* (5th ed.). Philadelphia: Saunders.

Slocum, J., Barcio, L., Darany, J., Friedley, K., Homko, C., Jennings-Mills, J., et al. (2004). Preconception to postpartum: Management of pregnancy complicated by diabetes. *Today's Educator, 30*(5), 740-753.

Smith, C., Crowther, C., Willson, K., Hotham, N., & McMillian, V. (2004). A randomized controlled trial of ginger to treat nausea and vomiting in pregnancy. *Obstetrics and Gynecology, 103*(4), 639-645.

Spratto, G., & Woods, A. (2004). *PDR: Nurses' drug handbook.* Clifton Park, NY: Delmar.

Tiran, D., & Mack, E. (Eds). (2000). *Complementary therapies for pregnancy and childbirth* (2nd ed.). Edinburgh: Bailliere Tindall.

Weiner, C., & Buhimschi, C. (2004). *Drugs for pregnant and lactating women.* New York: Churchill Livingstone.

Medical-Surgical Problems in Pregnancy

learning objectives

- Describe the management of cardiovascular disorders in pregnant women.
- Identify nursing interventions for the pregnant woman with a cardiovascular disorder.
- Discuss anemia during pregnancy.
- Explain the care of pregnant women with pulmonary disorders.
- Examine the effect of a gastrointestinal disorder on gastrointestinal function during pregnancy.

- Identify the effects of neurologic disorders on pregnancy.
- Describe the care of women whose pregnancies are complicated by autoimmune disorders.
- Delineate the basic principles of care for a pregnant woman having surgery.

electronic resources

Additional information related to the content in Chapter 33 can be found on

the companion website at *evolve*
http://evolve.elsevier.com/Lowdermilk/MWHC/
- NCLEX Review Questions
- Case Study: Class III Cardiac Disorder
- WebLinks

or on the interactive companion CD
- NCLEX Review Questions
- Case Study: Class III Cardiac Disorder
- Plan of Care: The Pregnant Woman with Heart Disease

THE effects of selected preexisting medical disorders on pregnancy and the nursing care that can lead to their effective management are presented in this chapter. These disorders, including cardiovascular, respiratory, gastrointestinal (GI), integumentary, and central nervous system (CNS) disorders, are sometimes first diagnosed during pregnancy. Abdominal surgery and the related nursing roles also are discussed.

■ CARDIOVASCULAR DISORDERS

During a normal pregnancy, the maternal cardiovascular system undergoes many changes that put a physiologic strain on the heart. The major cardiovascular changes that occur during a normal pregnancy and that affect the woman with cardiac disease are increased intravascular volume, decreased systemic vascular resistance, cardiac output changes occurring during labor and birth, and the intravascular volume changes that occur just after childbirth. The strain is present during pregnancy and continues for a few weeks after birth. The normal heart can compensate for the increased workload so that pregnancy, labor, and birth are generally well tolerated, but the diseased heart is hemodynamically challenged.

If the cardiovascular changes are not well tolerated, cardiac failure can develop during pregnancy, labor, or the postpartum period. In addition, if myocardial disease develops, valvular disease exists, or a congenital heart defect is present, **cardiac decompensation** (inability of the heart to maintain a sufficient cardiac output) is anticipated.

About 1% to 4% of pregnancies are complicated by heart disease (Foley, 2004), accounting for about 10% to 25% of maternal mortality. Congenital diseases and mitral valve disease are increasing in incidence in women of childbearing age while the incidence of rheumatic fever, is diminishing. Other cardiac diseases are uncommon (Gilbert & Harmon, 2003). Maternal mortality rates range from negligible to 25% depending on the cardiac defect (Foley). A perinatal mortality of up to 50% is anticipated with persistent cardiac decompensation. See Box 33-1 for maternal cardiac disease risk groups.

The degree of disability experienced by the woman with cardiac disease is often more important in the treatment and prognosis of cardiac disease complicating pregnancy

| box 33-1 | Maternal Cardiac Disease Risk Groups |

GROUP I (MORTALITY 1%)
- Corrected tetralogy of Fallot
- Pulmonic/tricuspid disease
- Mitral stenosis (Classes I, II)
- Patent ductus arteriosus
- Ventricular septal defect
- Atrial septal defect
- Porcine valve

GROUP II (MORTALITY 5%-15%)
- Mitral stenosis with atrial fibrillation
- Artificial heart valves
- Mitral stenosis (Classes III, IV)
- Uncorrected tetralogy of Fallot
- Aortic coarctation (uncomplicated)
- Aortic stenosis
- Marfan syndrome with normal aorta

GROUP III (MORTALITY 25%-50%)
- Aortic coarctation (complicated)
- Myocardial infarction (previous)
- Marfan syndrome with aortic involvement
- Pulmonary hypertension

From Gilbert, E., & Harmon, J. (2003). *Manual of high risk pregnancy and delivery* (3rd ed.). St. Louis: Mosby

Evolve/CD: Case Study: Class III Cardiac Disorder

than is the diagnosis of cardiovascular disease. The New York Heart Association's (NYHA) functional classification of organic heart disease is a widely accepted standard (American Heart Association Science Advisory, 2000):
- Class I: asymptomatic without limitation of physical activity
- Class II: symptomatic with slight limitation of activity
- Class III: symptomatic with marked limitation of activity
- Class IV: symptomatic with inability to carry on any physical activity without discomfort

No classification of heart disease can be considered rigid or absolute, but the NYHA classification offers a basic practical guide for treatment, assuming that frequent prenatal visits, good client cooperation, and appropriate obstetric care occur. Medical therapy is conducted by a team approach and includes the cardiologist, the obstetrician, and nurses. The functional classification may change for the pregnant woman because of the hemodynamic changes that occur in the cardiovascular system. A 30% to 50% increase in cardiac output occurs compared with nonpregnancy resting values, with most of the increase in the first trimester and the peak at 20 to 26 weeks of gestation (Blanchard & Shabetai, 2004). The functional classification of the disease is determined at 3 months and again at 7 or 8 months of gestation. Pregnant women may progress from class I or II to III or IV during the pregnancy. Women with cyanotic congenital heart disease do not fit into the

NYHA classification because their exercise-induced symptoms have causes not related to heart failure. An Ability Index was developed for assessment of these clients (Gei & Hankins, 2001).

Contraindications to pregnancy in women with heart disease are listed in Box 33-2. The incidence of miscarriage is increased, and preterm labor and birth are more prevalent in the pregnant woman with cardiac problems. In addition, *intrauterine growth restriction (IUGR)* (impeded or delayed development of the fetus) is common, probably because of low oxygen pressure (PO_2) in the mother.

The incidence (5% to 10%) of a fetus being affected by congenital heart disease exists, depending on the defect (Setaro & Caulin-Glaser, 2004). Preconception and genetic counseling are essential components of care.

A diagnosis of cardiac disease depends on the history, physical examination, radiographic findings, electrocardiogram (ECG), Holter monitoring, echocardiography and, if indicated, ultrasonogram results. The differential diagnosis of heart disease also involves ruling out respiratory problems and other potential causes of chest pain.

Maternal mortality rate in women with cardiac events is higher than that for abortion, genital sepsis, and hemorrhage (Setaro & Caulin-Glaser, 2004). The highest risk of complications or death occurs in women with pulmonary hypertension, complicated coarctation of the aorta, and Marfan syndrome with aortic involvement (Foley, 2004).

▬ ASSOCIATED CARDIOVASCULAR ▬ DISORDERS

Nursing care of the woman with a cardiovascular disorder combines routine peripartum care with care specific for the cardiac diagnosis. Cardiac diseases vary in their impact on pregnancy according to their acuteness or chronicity. The following discussion focuses first on congenital cardiac diseases such as septal defects, patent ductus arteriosus, and cyanotic and acyanotic lesions. The second group of cardiac diseases are acquired diseases, specifically mitral stenosis, aortic stenosis, ischemic heart disease, and other cardiac diseases (pulmonary hypertension, Marfan syndrome, peripartum cardiomyopathy, and presence of artificial valves). A review of the care of the pregnant woman who has had a heart transplant concludes the discussion.

| box 33-2 | Contraindications to Pregnancy in a Woman with Heart Disease |

- Pulmonary hypertension
- Shunt lesions associated with Eisenmenger syndrome
- Complex cyanotic congenital heart disease
- Aortic coarctation complicated by aortic dissection
- Poor ventricular function
- Marfan syndrome with marked aortic dilation

Adapted from Mendelson, M. (1997). Congenital cardiac disease and pregnancy. *Clinical Perinatology, 24*(2), 467-482.

Congenital Cardiac Disease
Septal Defects

Atrial septal defect (ASD) (an abnormal opening between the atria), one of the causes of a left-to-right shunt, is the most common congenital defect seen during pregnancy. This defect may go undetected because the woman usually is asymptomatic. The pregnant woman with an ASD will most likely have an uncomplicated pregnancy. Some women may have right-sided heart failure or arrhythmias as the pregnancy progresses as a result of increased plasma volume.

Ventricular septal defect (VSD) (an abnormal opening between the right and left ventricles), another cause of a left-to-right shunt, is usually diagnosed and corrected during infancy or childhood. As a result, a VSD is not very common in pregnancy. Women with a small, uncomplicated VSD usually do not have pregnancy complications. For women with a large VSD, there is a higher risk for arrhythmias, heart failure, and pulmonary hypertension. Medical management includes rest and decrease of physical activity, as well as administration of anticoagulants.

Patent ductus arteriosus (PDA) is another cause of a left-to-right shunt that is usually diagnosed and corrected during infancy. Possible complications of a PDA include those of VSD as well as endocarditis and pulmonary emboli. Medical management is the same as for VSD.

Mortality rates for women with shunt defects are less than 1% (Foley, 2004).

Acyanotic Lesions

Coarctation of the aorta (localized narrowing of the aorta near the insertion of the ductus) is an example of an acyanotic congenital heart lesion. Pregnancy is usually relatively safe for the woman with uncomplicated, uncorrected, coarctation. Maternal mortality is about 4% (Blanchard & Shabetai, 2004). Complications that can occur include hypertension, congestive heart failure, aortic dissection, aneurysm, and rupture. The mainstays of treatment for uncorrected coarctation of the aorta during pregnancy are rest and antihypertensive medications, preferably beta-adrenergic blocking agents. Vaginal birth is possible with epidural anesthesia and shortening of the second stage with vacuum extraction or use of forceps, if necessary. Beta-blockers should be continued throughout labor. Because of the risk of endocarditis, antibiotic prophylaxis is recommended at birth (see later discussion). The rate of fetal loss is about 10% (Setaro & Caulin-Glaser, 2004).

Cyanotic Lesions

Tetralogy of Fallot is the most common cyanotic heart disease present during pregnancy, accounting for 5% to 6% of congenital heart malformations (Veldtman, Connolly, Grogan, Ammash, & Warnes, 2004). Components of tetralogy of Fallot include a VSD, pulmonary stenosis, overriding aorta, and right ventricular hypertrophy, leading to a right-to-left shunt. Women with corrected tetralogy of Fallot have less than 1% mortality; however, women with uncorrected tetralogy of Fallot have a 5% to 15% mortality rate (Foley, 2004). Medical management for women with uncorrected tetralogy of Fallot includes anticoagulant therapy, high-concentration oxygen administration, and hemodynamic monitoring during labor and birth.

Acquired Cardiac Disease
Mitral Valve Stenosis

Mitral valve stenosis (narrowing of the opening of the mitral valve caused by stiffening of valve leaflets, which obstructs blood flow from the atrium to the ventricles) is the characteristic lesion resulting from rheumatic heart disease (RHD) (Setaro & Caulin-Glaser, 2004). Even though a history of rheumatic fever may be absent, it remains the most likely cause of mitral stenosis. As the mitral valve narrows, dyspnea worsens, occurring first on exertion and eventually at rest. A tight stenosis plus the increase in blood volume and cardiac output of normal pregnancy may cause ventricular failure, pulmonary edema, and atrial arrhythmias (Klein & Galan, 2004). Maternal mortality rate in classes III and IV can be as high as 5% to 7%, with perinatal mortality rates of 12% to 31% (Klein & Galan).

Atrial fibrillation can precipitate a decrease in the cardiac output. Pharmacologic treatment for women with a history of rheumatic heart disease includes daily prophylactic penicillin, diuretics to prevent pulmonary edema, and beta-blockers or calcium channel blockers to prevent tachycardia (Klein & Galan, 2004). A combination of drugs will most likely be needed. Cardioversion may be needed for new-onset atrial fibrillation. Women who have chronic atrial fibrillation may need digoxin or beta-blockers to control the heart rate. In addition, anticoagulant therapy may be needed to prevent embolism. About 25% of women with mitral valve stenosis may become symptomatic for the first time during pregnancy (Setaro & Caulin-Glaser, 2004). The care of the woman with mitral stenosis typically is managed by reducing her activity, restricting dietary sodium, and increasing bed rest. The pregnant woman with mitral stenosis should be monitored clinically for symptoms and with echocardiograms to monitor the atrial and ventricular size, as well as heart valve function. Prophylaxis for intrapartum endocarditis and pulmonary infections may be provided for women at high risk (Easterling & Otto, 2002) (Box 33-3).

During labor, adequate pain control is required to prevent tachycardia. Epidural analgesia for labor is preferred (Easterling & Otto, 2002). Shortening the second stage of labor is also important to decrease the cardiac workload. Even with close monitoring, the woman with moderate to severe mitral stenosis is at risk for pulmonary edema, right-sided heart failure, and hypotension. Intensive invasive pulmonary artery catheter monitoring should continue through labor, birth, and the postpartum period because fluid shifts can place the woman at risk for pulmonary edema (Easterling & Otto).

box 33-3 **Prophylaxis for Bacterial Endocarditis During Labor and Birth**

HIGH RISK CLIENTS

In active labor: ampicillin 2 g IV or IM plus gentamicin 1.5 mg/kg (not to exceed 120 mg)
6 hours later: ampicillin 1 g IV or IM or amoxicillin 1 g PO

Penicillin-Allergic Clients

In active labor: vancomycin 1 g IV over 1-2 hr plus gentamicin as above

MODERATE RISK CLIENTS

In active labor: amoxicillin 2 g PO or ampicillin 2 g IV or IM

Penicillin-Allergic Clients

In active labor: vancomycin 1 g IV over 1-2 hr

Sources: Easterling, T., & Otto, C. (2002). Heart disease. In S. Gabbe, J. Niebyl, & J. Simpson (Eds.), *Obstetrics: Normal and problem pregnancies* (4th ed.). New York: Churchill Livingstone.
IM, Intramuscular route; *IV*, intravenous route; *PO*, by mouth.

For women with NYHA class III or IV cardiac disease, percutaneous balloon mitral valvuloplasty can be performed. This procedure should be considered only when symptoms cannot be controlled by standard means. Mitral balloon valvuloplasty is optimally performed after the first trimester to decrease radiation risks to the fetus. This relatively safe nonsurgical procedure is being performed more frequently.

Mitral Valve Prolapse

Mitral valve prolapse (MVP) is a common, usually benign, condition occurring in 2% to 3% of women of reproductive age (Cunningham, Leveno, Bloom, Hauth, Gilstrap, & Wenstrom, 2005). The mitral valve leaflets prolapse into the left atrium during ventricular systole, allowing some backflow of blood. Midsystolic click and late systolic murmur are hallmarks of this syndrome. Most cases are asymptomatic. A few women have atypical chest pain (sharp and located in the left side of the chest) that occurs at rest and does not respond to nitrates. They may also have anxiety, palpitations, dyspnea on exertion, and syncope. Specific treatment usually is not necessary except for symptomatic tachyarrhythmias and rarely, heart failure. Women usually are treated with beta-blockers such as propranolol (Inderal) or beta-adrenergic blockers such as atenolol (Tenormin) (Blanchard & Shabetai, 2004; Cunningham et al.). Pregnancy and its associated hemodynamic changes may change or alleviate the murmur and click of MVP, as well as symptoms. Pregnancy usually is well tolerated unless bacterial endocarditis occurs. As with RHD, antibiotic prophylaxis is given before invasive procedures for women with mitral regurgitation, thickened mitral valves, and complicated vaginal births to prevent bacterial endocarditis (Blanchard & Shabetai; Cunningham et al.).

Aortic Stenosis

Aortic stenosis (narrowing of the opening of the aortic valve leading to an obstruction to left ventricular ejection) is rarely encountered as a complication of pregnancy. The reported maternal mortality rate is 17% (Sataro & Caulin-Glaser, 2004). Medical management is similar to that for mitral stenosis.

Ischemic Heart Disease

Myocardial infarction (MI) (an acute ischemic event) is a rare event in women of childbearing age; it is estimated to occur in only 1 in 10,000 women during pregnancy (Klein & Galan, 2004). It is anticipated that the occurrence will increase, considering the increase in the age of childbearing women and of other risk factors such as stress, smoking, and cocaine use. Other risk factors for coronary artery disease that may affect childbearing women are familial hyperlipidemia, diabetes mellitus, family history of coronary artery disease, hypertension, multiple gestation, sickle cell anemia, and the use of oral contraceptives (Easterling & Otto, 2002). Finally, the cardiac changes that normally occur in a pregnant woman may provoke symptoms for the first time.

MI occurs most frequently in the last trimester and in women older than 33 years. Maternal mortality rates from MIs during pregnancy range from 19% to 35% (Foley, 2004). Women who have MIs during pregnancy or the postpartum period should be assessed for thrombophilias (deficiency of proteins involved in coagulation inhibition), such as antiphospholipid antibody.

Medical management for pregnant women with MI is the same as for nonpregnant women and includes the administration of oxygen, aspirin, beta-blockers, nitrates, and heparin. Women who have had symptomatic cardiac disease during the pregnancy should continue cardiac medications and receive oxygen during labor. Because pain can lead to tachycardia and increased cardiac demands, pain control during labor is crucial. The side-lying position is preferred to avoid pressure on the vena cava. Vaginal birth is preferable, with avoidance of maternal pushing and a vacuum- or forceps-assisted birth. Postpartum diuretics usually are given (Easterling & Otto, 2002).

Other Cardiac Diseases and Conditions
Pulmonary Hypertension

Women with primary pulmonary hypertension (PPH) have constriction of the arteriolar vessels in the lungs, leading to an increase in the pulmonary artery pressure. As a result of this pathology, there is right ventricular hypertension, right ventricular hypertrophy and dilation, and finally, right ventricular failure with tricuspid regurgitation and systemic congestion.

Woman with PPH are usually young and have an increased incidence of Raynaud's phenomenon. A connection may be found with recurrent pulmonary embolism, appetite suppressants, and cocaine use (Easterling & Otto, 2002). The woman may have dyspnea, occasional chest pain, fatigue, edema, and ascites. Congestive heart failure may be evidenced by jugular vein distention, hepatomegaly, ascites, and edema.

Diagnostic tests performed are chest x-ray, electrocardiogram, echocardiogram, Doppler studies, and Swan-Ganz catheterization. Mortality rates reported during pregnancy are as high as 50%, with half of these deaths occurring during the early postpartum period (Esterling & Otto, 2002). These women should be strongly discouraged from getting pregnant.

Medical management of pregnant women with PPH includes antepartal therapy with oral nifedipine or intravenous (IV) prostacyclin for pulmonary vasodilation; intrapartal intensive hemodynamic monitoring, use of anti-embolic stockings, side-lying position, the administration of oxygen, and the use of epidural analgesia to promote hemodynamic stability. Anticoagulant therapy also is indicated to prevent pulmonary embolus. Women with PPH are considered candidates for heart-lung transplants.

Marfan Syndrome

Marfan syndrome is an autosomal dominant genetic disorder characterized by generalized weakness of the connective tissue, resulting in joint deformities, ocular lens dislocation, and weakness of the aortic wall and root (Foley, 2004). Associated cardiovascular changes include mitral valve prolapse, mitral regurgitation, aortic regurgitation, aortic root dilatation, and possible dissection or rupture of the aortic root (Klein & Galan, 2004). Excruciating chest pain is the most common symptom of aortic dissection. Aortic dissection most often occurs in the third trimester or postpartally. Marfan syndrome also may be responsible for cervical incompetence, placenta previa, and postpartum hemorrhage. Preconception genetic counseling is recommended to make women aware of the risks of pregnancy with this condition, with a 50% risk of inheritance of the syndrome (Klein & Galan, 2004). Baseline data should be gathered about the aortic root before pregnancy or at the first prenatal visit by noninvasive imaging with transesophageal echocardiography, computed tomography, or magnetic resonance imaging (MRI).

Management during pregnancy includes restricted activity and use of beta-blockers; surgery may be indicated in some women. Antibiotic prophylaxis is suggested for labor; regional analgesia is well tolerated. Mortality rates may be as high as 50% in women who have severe cardiac disease (Easterling & Otto, 2002).

Infective Endocarditis

Infective endocarditis (inflammation of the innermost lining—endocardium—of the heart caused by invasion of microorganisms) is an uncommon disorder during pregnancy (Mendelson & Lang, 2000). It may be seen in women taking IV street drugs. Bacterial endocarditis, leading to incompetence of heart valves and thus congestive heart failure and cerebral emboli, can result in death. Treatment is with antibiotics.

Eisenmenger Syndrome

Eisenmenger syndrome is a right-to-left or bidirectional shunting that can be at the atrial or ventricular level and is combined with elevated pulmonary vascular resistance (Blanchard & Shabetai, 2004). The syndrome is associated with high mortality (50% in mothers and 50% in fetuses), and thus pregnancy is contraindicated (Blanchard & Shabetai). Contraception is essential, and tubal ligation should be considered because oral contraceptives and intrauterine devices carry considerable risk (Mendelson & Lang, 2000). If pregnancy occurs, termination may be recommended if the woman has significant pulmonary hypertension (Easterling & Otto, 2002).

In women who continue pregnancy despite the risks, physical activity is strictly limited. Hospitalization may be necessary to provide optimal care, including the administration of oxygen in order to maintain the maternal PaO_2 at 70% or higher (Foley, 2004). During labor and birth, intrathecal or epidural morphine sulfate is recommended (Foley). Pulse oximetry is a useful assessment tool to guide the treatment plan during labor and birth.

Peripartum Cardiomyopathy

The classic criteria for the diagnosis of peripartum cardiomyopathy (PPCM) include development of congestive heart failure in the last month of pregnancy or within the first 5 postpartum months, lack of another cause for heart failure, and absence of heart disease before the last month of pregnancy (Blanchard & Shabetai, 2004). Incidence ranges from 1 in 1300 to 1 in 1500 pregnancies (Setaro & Caulin-Glaser, 2004). The etiology of the disease is unknown; theories suggest genetic predisposition, auto-immunity, and viral infections.

Associated risk factors include maternal age older than 35 years, multifetal gestation, preeclampsia, gestational hypertension, multiparity, African descent, and prolonged tocolytic therapy (Klein & Galan, 2004). Maternal mortality has been estimated in the range of 25% to 50% (Setaro & Caulin-Glaser, 2004). Clinical findings are those of congestive heart failure (left ventricular failure). Clinical manifestations include dyspnea, fatigue, and edema, as well as radiologic findings of cardiomegaly (Fig. 33-1). The prognosis is good if left ventricular dysfunction resolves before 6 months postpartum. There is no agreement on recommendations for future pregnancies; however, the mortality and morbidity rate is greatly increased for women who have persistent left ventricular dysfunction (Setaro & Caulin-Glaser). PPCM tends to recur in subsequent pregnancies, even if cardiac function stabilizes. Women whose hearts remain enlarged at or beyond 6 months postpartum will have PPCM in future pregnancies.

Medical management of cardiomyopathy during pregnancy includes a regimen used for congestive heart failure: diuretics, sodium and fluid restriction, afterload-reducing agents, and digoxin (Klein & Galan, 2004). Angiotensin-converting enzyme inhibitors can be used only in the postpartum period, because they are associated with fetal renal

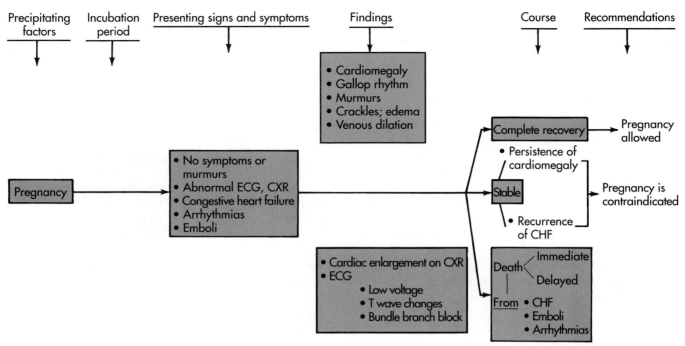

FIG. 33-1 Summary of course of peripartum cardiomyopathy. *CHF,* Congestive heart failure; *CXR,* chest x-ray; *ECG,* electrocardiogram.

dysfunction. The nursing care of women with peripartum cardiomyopathy is essentially the same as for those with other types of cardiac problems.

Valve Replacement

Pregnant women with mechanical or tissue prosthetic heart valves require specialized care for this high risk situation. Maternal risks include death, heart failure, thromboemboli, hemorrhage, arrhythmias, and bacterial endocarditis (Setaro & Caulin-Glaser, 2004). The primary medical management through the use of anticoagulants is controversial and complicated. A high risk for thromboembolism is present because of the hypercoagulability of pregnancy. In addition, the use of anticoagulants during pregnancy presents the possibility of maternal and fetal hemorrhage. Some oral anticoagulants pose a significant risk to the fetus, such as fetal abnormalities and fetal intracranial hemorrhage. Prosthetic heart valve thrombosis is a life-threatening emergency during pregnancy. This situation requires clot removal surgery, which has a high mortality rate. The use of recombinant tissue-type plasminogen activator (rtPA) has been described as a treatment for thrombosis in pregnancy (Mendelson & Lang, 2000). Women with porcine heterograft valves usually do not require anticoagulation during pregnancy. This type of valve is an ideal replacement for women of childbearing age. A disadvantage of this type of valve is premature valve failure, which may be exacerbated by pregnancy.

The current recommendations for pregnant women with mechanical prosthetic valves who need anticoagulation therapy involve several different treatment regimens. Because the most effective and safest management has not been determined through controlled trials, the decision on the choice of therapy should be made between the physician and the woman, who should be fully informed about the potential risks of the various options to her and her unborn child (Danik & Fuster, 2004). One option is to use subcutaneous heparin (either unfractionated or low-molecular-weight) for the first 12 weeks of gestation. Warfarin (Coumadin) then is used to week 35 of gestation, followed by a return to heparin (intravenous) until after the birth. If prothrombin time results are reported in the international normalized ratio (INR) values, the goal is 3. A second option is to use warfarin for the entire pregnancy up to 35 weeks of gestation and then to use intravenous heparin. With both of these options, low-dose aspirin (80 to 100 mg/day) is recommended to maximize the antithrombotic effect of the therapy (Eklayam, Singh, Irani, & Akhter, 2004). Another option is to use subcutaneous unfractionated or low-molecular-weight heparin throughout pregnancy (Elkayam et al.). Anticoagulation therapy should be discontinued at the time of active labor and reactivated within 6 hours of vaginal birth or 12 to 24 hours after cesarean birth. Because of the possibility of epidural hematoma, regional analgesia/anesthesia is not recommended.

Nursing care of the pregnant woman with a valve replacement is similar to care for any woman with a cardiac disorder. Emphasis should be placed on teaching the woman how to administer subcutaneous injections (if that option of anticoagulation is used), how to recognize preterm labor, and how to monitor for adverse effects of anticoagulant therapy, primarily bleeding.

Heart Transplantation

Increasing numbers of heart recipients are successfully completing pregnancies. Before conception, the woman should be assessed for quality of ventricular function and potential rejection of transplant. The woman should be considered to be stabilized on the immunosuppressant regimen. Women who have no evidence of rejection and have normal cardiac function at the beginning of the pregnancy appear to do well during pregnancy, labor, and birth. Risks to the woman include gestational hypertension, preterm birth, and low-birth-weight neonates (Foley, 2004).

■ CARE MANAGEMENT

The presence of cardiac disease makes the decision to become pregnant more difficult (see Box 33-2). Planned pregnancy requires that the woman understand the peripartum risks. If the pregnancy is unplanned, the nurse should explore the woman's desire to continue the pregnancy after examining the risks in relation to the status of her cardiac condition. The nurse should review with the woman options for pregnancy termination if her cardiac status is tenuous and abortion is an acceptable alternative. The woman's significant other and family should be included in the discussion. Teaching sessions for the woman and her support persons should be offered as indicated by their learning needs.

Care of these women at high risk requires a multidisciplinary approach. The multidisciplinary team includes a cardiologist who is familiar with expected cardiovascular changes in pregnancy; a perinatologist; an anesthesiologist, and nurses skilled in advanced hemodynamic monitoring.

■ Assessment and Nursing Diagnoses

The pregnant woman with cardiac disease requires detailed assessment throughout the peripartum period to determine the potential for optimal maternal health and a viable fetus. If she chooses to continue the pregnancy, the high risk pregnant woman's condition may be assessed as often as weekly.

■ *Interview*

The nurse solicits information from the woman regarding her personal medical history and that of her family. Special notation is made of diseases of cardiovascular significance, including congenital heart disease, streptococcal infections, rheumatic fever, valvular disease, endocarditis, congestive heart failure, angina, or MI.

The nurse assesses for factors that would increase stress on the heart, such as anemia (discussed later in this chapter), infection, and edema. In reviewing for symptoms, the nurse should assess how the woman is adapting to the physiologic changes of pregnancy.

In assessing the pregnant woman with a cardiovascular disorder, special attention is given to the review of the cardiovascular and pulmonary systems. The nurse should determine whether the woman has had chest pain at rest or on exertion; edema of the face, hands, or feet; hypertension; heart murmurs; palpitations; paroxysmal nocturnal dyspnea; diaphoresis; pallor; or syncope. Pulmonary symptoms such as cough, hemoptysis, shortness of breath, and orthopnea also can be signs of cardiac dis-

table 33-1 Cardiovascular Signs and Symptoms During Pregnancy

NORMAL	ABNORMAL
SIGNS	
Neck vein pulsation	Neck vein distention
Diffuse or displaced apical pulse	Cardiomegaly; heave
Split S_1, accentuated S_2	Loud P_2; wide split of S_2
Third heart sound—loud	Summation gallop
Systolic murmur (1-2/6) (92%-95%)	Loud systolic murmur (4-6/6)
Venous hum	Diastolic murmur
Sinus arrhythmia	Sustained arrhythmia
Peripheral edema, particularly lower extremities	Clubbing or cyanosis
SYMPTOMS	
Fatigue	Symptoms at rest
Chest pain	Exertional chest pain
Dyspnea	Exertional severe dyspnea
Orthopnea	Orthopnea (progressive)
Hyperpnea	Paroxysmal nocturnal dyspnea
Palpitations	Tachycardia (>120 beats/min); irregular pulse
Syncope (vasovagal)	Exertional syncope

Adapted from Blackburn, S. (2003). *Maternal, fetal, and neonatal physiology: A clinical perspective* (2nd ed.). St. Louis: Saunders.

ease. See Table 33-1 for normal and abnormal cardiovascular signs and symptoms during pregnancy.

The nurse documents all medications taken by the woman—including over-the-counter (OTC) medications such as supplemental iron—and is alert to their potential side effects and interactions. The woman also is assessed for undue emotional stress that might further compromise cardiac status. Examples of emotional stress are depression, anxiety or fear of morbidity or mortality for herself and the fetus, financial concerns related to extended hospitalization, anger because of impaired social interaction, and feelings of inadequacy regarding her inability to meet family and household demands. Women and their families may have a number of problems associated with the prescription of antepartum bed rest. Reported difficulties include anxiety over not being able to assume role functions, emotional stress for family and children, and financial difficulties (Maloni, Brezinski-Tomasi, & Johnson, 2001).

The woman's cultural background may affect the amount of support she is able to receive from significant others. Family size (number of children and extended family members in the home) as well as role expectations within the family may be dictated by cultural norms. For the woman with cardiac impairment, family expectations may be a cause of major stress if she is unable to bear the expected number of children or if it is unacceptable to receive help with domestic chores. The nurse should be aware of the cultural customs of the pregnant woman and her family.

■ *Physical Examination*

Routine assessments continue during the prenatal period, including monitoring the amount and pattern of edema, vital signs, oxygen saturation level, discomforts of pregnancy, and amount and pattern of weight gain. The woman is observed for signs of cardiac decompensation, that is, progressive generalized edema, crackles at the base of the lungs, or pulse irregularity (see Signs of Potential Complications box). Symptoms of cardiac decompensation may appear abruptly or gradually. Medical intervention must be instituted immediately to maintain optimal cardiac status. Dyspnea, palpitations, syncope, and edema may occur in pregnant women and can mask the symptoms of a developing or worsening cardiovascular disorder. A woman's sudden inability to perform activities that she previously was comfortable doing may indicate cardiovascular decompensation.

■ *Laboratory and Diagnostic Tests*

Routine urinalysis and blood work (complete blood cell count and blood chemistry) are completed during the initial visit. The woman with cardiac impairment requires a baseline 12-lead ECG at the beginning of her pregnancy, if not before pregnancy, which permits vital diagnostic comparisons of subsequent ECGs. Echocardiograms and pulse oximetry studies may be performed as indicated. Chest films may be necessary during late pregnancy, provided the abdomen is carefully shielded. In addition, fetal ultrasound, fetal movement studies, or fetal nonstress tests (NSTs) may be used to determine fetal well-being.

The following lists nursing diagnoses that may be formulated. As always, individualization of diagnoses is vital.

- *Fear related to*
  - increased peripartum risk
- *Risk for ineffective individual/family coping related to*
  - woman's cardiac condition
  - changes in role performance
- *Iineffective tissue perfusion related to*
  - hypotensive syndrome
- *Activity intolerance related to*
  - cardiac condition
- *Deficient knowledge related to*
  - cardiac condition
  - pregnancy and how it affects cardiac condition
  - medication: dosages and possible side effects
  - requirements to alter self-care activities
- *Self-care deficit (bathing, grooming, dressing) related to*
  - fatigue or activity intolerance
  - need for bed rest
- *Impaired home maintenance related to*
  - woman's confinement to bed and/or limited activity level

■ **Expected Outcomes of Care**

The pregnant woman with cardiovascular problems faces curtailment of her activities. Bed rest during pregnancy affects all of the organ systems, but especially the cardio-

---

signs of potential complications

Cardiac Decompensation

PREGNANT WOMAN: SUBJECTIVE SYMPTOMS

- Increasing fatigue or difficulty breathing, or both, with usual activities
- Feeling of smothering
- Frequent cough
- Palpitations; feeling that her heart is racing
- Swelling of face, feet, legs, fingers (e.g., rings do not fit anymore)

NURSE: OBJECTIVE SIGNS

- Irregular weak, rapid pulse (≥100 beats/min)
- Progressive, generalized edema
- Crackles at base of lungs after two inspirations and exhalations
- Orthopnea; increasing dyspnea
- Rapid respirations (≥25 breaths/min)
- Moist, frequent cough
- Increasing fatigue
- Cyanosis of lips and nail beds

---

vascular and the musculoskeletal systems. In addition, psychologic side effects can be debilitating, especially stress (Cunningham et al., 2005; Maloni et al., 2001). The community health nurse, the social worker, and the physical or occupational therapist are resource persons whose services may be incorporated into the plan of care. Expected outcomes that might be appropriate include that the pregnant woman (and family, if appropriate) will do the following:

- Verbalize understanding of the disorder, its management, and its probable outcome.
- Describe her role in management, including when and how to take medication, adjust diet, and prepare for and participate in treatment.
- Cope with emotional reactions to pregnancy and infant at risk.
- Adapt to the physiologic stressors of pregnancy and labor and birth.
- Identify and use support systems.
- Carry her fetus to viability or to term.
- Develop no complications in the postpartum period.

■ **Plan of Care and Interventions**
■ *Antepartum Care*

Therapy for the pregnant woman with heart disease is focused on minimizing stress on the heart, which is greatest between 28 and 32 weeks of gestation as the hemodynamic changes reach their maximum. Factors that increase the risk of cardiac decompensation are avoided. The workload of the cardiovascular system is reduced by appropriate treatment of any coexisting emotional stress, hypertension, anemia, hyperthyroidism, or obesity.

Signs and symptoms of cardiac decompensation are reviewed during the prenatal period. The woman with class I or II heart disease requires 8 to 10 hours of sleep every day and should take 30-minute naps after eating. Her activities are restricted, with housework, shopping, and exercise limited to the amount allowed for the functional classification of her heart disease. Information on how to cope with activity limitations is important in meeting the emotional needs of the woman. Referral to a support group may help the woman and her family to handle stress.

The pregnant woman with class II cardiac disease should avoid heavy exertion and should stop any activity that causes even minor signs and symptoms of cardiac decompensation. She should also be admitted to the hospital near term (earlier if signs of cardiac overload or arrhythmia develop) for evaluation and treatment.

Bed rest for much of each day is necessary for pregnant women with class III cardiac disease. About 30% of these women have cardiac decompensation during pregnancy. With this possibility, a woman may require hospitalization for the remainder of the pregnancy. Because decompensation occurs even at rest in persons with class IV cardiac disease, a major initial effort must be made to improve the cardiac status of the pregnant woman in this category who chooses to continue her pregnancy (Box 33-4).

Infections are treated promptly because respiratory, urinary, or GI tract infections can complicate the condition by accelerating the heart rate and by direct spread of organisms

box 33-4 The Pregnant Woman at Risk for Cardiac Decompensation

- Assess lifestyle patterns, emotional status, and environment of woman.
- Arrange for consultations as needed (i.e., dietitian, home care, child care, social work).
- Determine woman's and her family's understanding of her heart disease and how the disease affects her pregnancy.
- Determine stressors in the woman's life. Assist woman in identifying effective coping strategies.
- Instruct woman to report signs of cardiac decompensation or congestive heart failure: generalized edema, distention of neck veins, dyspnea, pulmonary crackles, cough, palpitations, sudden weight gain.
- Instruct woman to be watchful for signs of thromboembolism, such as redness, tenderness, pain, or swelling of the legs. Instruct woman to seek medical help immediately if such symptoms occur.
- Instruct woman to avoid constipation and thus straining with bowel movements (Valsalva maneuver) by taking in adequate fluids and fiber. A stool softener may be ordered.
- Explore with woman ways to obtain the needed rest throughout the day. Depending on the level of her cardiac disease, she may need to sleep 10 hr per night and rest 30 min after meals (class I or II) or rest for most of the day (class III or IV).
- Help woman make use of community resources, including support groups, as indicated.
- Emphasize the importance of keeping her prenatal appointments.

From Gilbert, E., & Harmon, J. (2003). *Manual of high risk pregnancy & delivery* (3rd ed.). St. Louis: Mosby; Health Care Resources. (1997). *Handbook of high risk perinatal home care.* St. Louis: Mosby; Lowdermilk, D., & Grohar, J. (1998). *High risk antepartal home care.* White Plains, NY: March of Dimes.

(e.g., streptococci) to the heart structure. The woman should notify her physician at the first sign of infection or exposure to an infection. Vaccination against influenza and pneumococcus may be given. Prophylactic antibiotics against bacterial endocarditis during pregnancy are not recommended by the American Heart Association but may be needed by women with valvular disorders (Easterling & Otto, 2002).

Nutrition counseling is necessary, optimally with the woman's family present. The pregnant woman needs a well-balanced diet with iron and folic acid supplementation, high protein, and adequate calories to gain weight. Iron supplements tend to cause constipation. The pregnant woman should increase her intake of fluids and fiber. A stool softener may be prescribed. It is important that the woman with a cardiac disorder avoid straining during defecation, thus causing the Valsalva maneuver (forced expiration against a closed airway, which when released, causes blood to rush to the heart and overload the cardiac system). If sodium restriction is necessary, the amount should not be less than 2.5 g/day (Gilbert & Harmon, 2003). The woman's intake of potassium is monitored to prevent hypokalemia, especially if she is taking diuretics. A referral to a registered dietitian may be necessary.

Cardiac medications are prescribed as needed for the pregnant woman, with attention to fetal well-being. The physiologic changes that occur during pregnancy, labor, and the postpartum period can significantly alter how drugs are used and excreted by the body. Monitoring of the drug levels during the pregnancy is crucial to maintain effective therapy for the woman while minimizing risk to the fetus. The nurse should review current pharmacologic literature, especially when administering any medication to a pregnant woman (Table 33-2).

Anticoagulant therapy may be needed during pregnancy in various situations, such as recurrent vein thrombosis, pulmonary embolus, rheumatic heart disease, prosthetic valves, or cyanotic congenital heart defects.

If anticoagulant therapy is required during pregnancy a number of various regimens may be recommended. See the section on valve disorders for more discussion of anticoagulant therapy. The nurse should be aware of the goals of therapy and monitor the prothrombin time (e.g., PT, INR) accordingly. The woman may need to learn to self-administer injectable agents such as heparin or low-molecular-weight heparin. She also requires specific nutritional teaching to avoid foods high in vitamin K, such as raw, dark green, and leafy vegetables, which counteract the effects of heparin. In addition, she will require a folic acid supplement.

Tests for fetal maturity and well-being and placental sufficiency may be necessary. Other therapy is directly related to the functional classification of heart disease. The nurse must reinforce the need for close medical supervision.

Heart Surgery During Pregnancy. The ideal scenario is for a woman to have surgical correction of the cardiac lesion before pregnancy; in some women, however, cardiac disease is diagnosed for the first time during pregnancy. When medical therapy for a pregnant woman fails, cardiac

table 33-2 Selected Drugs Used in Treatment of Cardiac Disorders in the Pregnant Woman

DRUG	CROSSES PLACENTA	CONSIDERATIONS
Digoxin	Yes	Can cause maternal arrhythmias and fetal low birth weight
		Possible need to increase maternal dose because of increased blood volume while keeping in therapeutic range
Procainamide	Yes	No known teratogenic effects
		Caution needed with use
Verapamil	Yes	Considered safe for use in pregnancy but can produce maternal hypotension with decreased uterine blood flow
		No controlled human studies on fetal effects
Propranolol	Yes	Considered safe for use in pregnancy
		No known teratogenic effects
		Associated with fetal bradycardia, diminished uterine blood flow, IUGR, increased uterine irritability, and premature labor, hypoglycemia, maternal bradycardia, hypotension
Heparin	No	If anticoagulant therapy needed, heparin usually used (see discussion of use in pregnant women with valve replacement on p. 854)
		Risk of maternal hemorrhage, preterm birth, stillbirth, fetal hemorrhage
Warfarin	Yes	Warfarin embryopathy, fetal hemorrhage, CNS abnormalities
		Maternal hemorrhage
		Contraindicated in first trimester and at term
Furosemide	Yes	Fetal levels estimated to be equal to maternal levels
		No known teratogenic effects
		Limit use in first trimester
		Necessary to monitor for decreased plasma volume, which could lead to decreased placental perfusion
Thiazides	Yes	Neonatal jaundice, thrombocytopenia, hemolytic anemia, hypoglycemia, maternal electrolyte imbalances
Lidocaine	Yes	Safe as long as toxic levels avoided
		Toxic dose—fetal CNS depression
		Can cause maternal arrhythmia
Quinidine	Yes	Toxic dose may induce preterm labor and cause damage to the fetal 8th cranial nerve
		Neonatal thrombocytopenia reported
		Fetal distress due to maternal hypotension
Nifedipine	Yes	Maternal orthostatic hypotension, headache, tachycardia; potential for fetal toxicity needs to be determined
		May inhibit labor; may be synergistic with magnesium
Diazoxide	Yes	Fetal and maternal hyperglycemia possible
		Reserved for severe hypertension unresponsive to other medications
		Potent relaxant of uterine smooth muscle
Sodium nitroprusside	Yes	Low dose does not appear to cause toxic cyanide levels (fetal cyanide toxicity possibly occurring with higher doses)

References: Blanchard, D., & Shabetai, R. (2004). *Cardiac diseases* In R. Creasy, R. Resnik. (J. Iams (Eds.), *Maternal-fetal medicine: Principles and practice* (5th ed.). Philadelphia: Saunders; Klein, L., & Galan, H. (2004). Cardiac disease in pregnancy. *Obstetrics and Gynecology Clinics of North America, 31*(2), 429-459.
CNS, Central nervous system; *IUGR,* intrauterine growth restriction.

surgery may be performed. Ideally, surgery should be performed early in the third trimester in order to decrease the risks to the fetus (Blanchard & Shabetai, 2004). The woman, the fetus, and uterine activity must be monitored carefully during surgery. Electrocardiography monitoring and intraarterial and Swan-Ganz catheters are recommended for intraoperative and postoperative assessment. In some cases, transesophageal echocardiography may be required (Blanchard & Shabetai). Closed cardiac surgery, such as release of a stenotic mitral orifice, can be accomplished with little risk to mother or fetus. Open heart surgery requires extracorporeal circulation, and under these circumstances, fetal bradycardia may occur as a result of low blood-flow rates. Periods of hypoxemia for the fetus can lead to various kinds of neurologic insults. Increase in flow rates on

cardiopulmonary bypass as well as intravenous nitroprusside may correct fetal bradycardia. Preterm labor occurs more frequently in women having cardiac surgery.

■ *Intrapartum Care*

For all pregnant women, the intrapartum period is the one that evokes the most apprehension in clients and caregivers. The woman with impaired cardiac function has additional reasons to be anxious, because labor and giving birth place an additional burden on her already compromised cardiovascular system.

Assessments include the routine assessments for all laboring women, as well as assessments for cardiac decompensation. In addition, arterial blood gases (ABGs) may be needed to assess for adequate oxygenation. A Swan-Ganz catheter may be inserted to monitor hemodynamic status accurately during labor and birth (see Chapter 34). ECG monitoring and continuous monitoring of blood pressure and pulse oximetry are usually instituted for the woman, and continuous fetal monitoring is used to monitor the fetus.

▪ NURSE ALERT

A pulse rate of 100 beats/min or greater or respirations 25 breaths/min or greater are a concern. Respiratory status is checked frequently for developing dyspnea, coughing, or crackles at the base of the lungs. The color and temperature of the skin are noted. Pale, cool, clammy skin may indicate cardiac shock.

Nursing care during labor and birth focuses on the promotion of cardiac function. Anxiety is minimized by maintaining a calm atmosphere in the labor and birth rooms. The nurse provides anticipatory guidance by keeping the woman and her family informed of labor progress and events that will probably occur, as well as answering any questions they have. The woman's childbirth preparation method should be supported to the degree it is feasible for her cardiac condition. Nursing techniques that promote comfort, such as back massage, are used.

Cardiac function is supported by keeping the woman's head and shoulders elevated and body parts resting on pillows. The side-lying position usually facilitates positive hemodynamics during labor. Discomfort is relieved with medication and supportive care. Epidural regional analgesia provides better pain relief than narcotics and causes fewer alterations in hemodynamics (Easterling & Otto, 2002).

▪ LEGAL TIP Cardiac and Metabolic Emergencies

The management of emergencies such as maternal cardiopulmonary distress or arrest or maternal metabolic crisis should be documented in policies, procedures, and protocols. Any independent nursing actions appropriate to the emergency should be clearly identified.

Beta-adrenergic agents such as terbutaline are associated with various side effects, including tachycardia, irregular pulse, myocardial ischemia, and pulmonary edema. A synthetic oxytocin (Syntocinon) can be used for induction of labor. This drug does not appear to cause significant coronary artery constriction in doses prescribed for labor induction or control of postpartum uterine atony. Cervical ripening agents containing prostaglandin are usually tolerated well, but should be used cautiously.

If there are no obstetric problems, vaginal birth is recommended and may be accomplished with the woman in the side-lying position to facilitate uterine perfusion. If the supine position is used, a pad is positioned under the hip to displace the uterus laterally and to minimize the danger of supine hypotension. The knees are flexed, and the feet are flat on the bed. To prevent compression of popliteal veins and an increase in blood volume in the chest and trunk as a result of the effects of gravity, stirrups are not used. Open-glottis pushing is recommended, and the Valsalva maneuver must be avoided during pushing in the second stage of labor because it reduces diastolic ventricular filling and obstructs left ventricular outflow. Mask oxygen is important. Episiotomy and vacuum extraction or outlet forceps may be used because these procedures decrease the length of the second stage of labor and decrease the workload of the heart in second-stage labor. Cesarean birth is not routinely recommended for women who have cardiovascular disease because there are risks of dramatic fluid shifts, sustained hemodynamic changes, and increased blood loss.

Penicillin prophylaxis may be ordered for nonallergic pregnant women with class II or higher cardiac disease to protect against bacterial endocarditis in labor and during the early puerperium (see Box 33-3). Dilute IV oxytocin immediately after birth of the placenta may be given to prevent postbirth hemorrhage. Ergot products should not be used, because they increase blood pressure. Fluid balance should be maintained and blood loss replaced. If tubal sterilization is desired, surgery is delayed at least several days to ensure homeostasis.

▪ Postpartum Care

Monitoring for cardiac decompensation in the postpartum period is essential. The first 24 to 48 postpartum hours are the most hemodynamically difficult for the woman. Hemorrhage or infection, or both, may worsen the cardiac condition. The woman with a cardiac disorder may continue to require a Swan-Ganz catheter and ABG monitoring.

▪ NURSE ALERT

The immediate postbirth period is hazardous for a woman whose heart function is compromised. Cardiac output increases rapidly as extravascular fluid is remobilized into the vascular compartment. At the moment of birth, intraabdominal pressure is reduced drastically; pressure on veins is removed, the splanchnic vessels engorge, and blood flow to the heart is increased. When blood flow increases to the heart, a **reflex bradycardia** (slowing of the heart in response to the increased blood flow) may result.

Nursing diagnoses appropriate for the postpartum period include the following:

- *Anxiety related to*
  - –fear for infant's safety
- *Fear of dying related to*
  - –perceived physiologic inability to cope with stress of labor
- *Risk for impaired gas exchange related to*
  - –cardiac condition
- *Excess fluid volume related to*
  - –extravascular fluid shifts
- *Situational low self-esteem related to*
  - –restriction placed on involvement in care of infant
  - –ineffective (compromised) family coping
- *Ineffective breastfeeding related to*
  - –fatigue from cardiac condition
- *Risk for impaired mother/infant attachment related to*
  - –separation due to prematurity
  - –fatigue from cardiac condition

Care in the postpartum period is tailored to the woman's functional capacity. Postpartum assessment of the woman with cardiac disease includes vital signs, oxygen saturation levels, lung and heart auscultation, edema, amount and character of bleeding, uterine tone and fundal height, urinary output, pain (especially chest pain), the activity-rest pattern, dietary intake, mother-infant interactions, and emotional state. The head of the bed is elevated, and the woman is encouraged to lie on her side. Bed rest may be ordered, with or without bathroom privileges. Progressive ambulation may be permitted as tolerated. The nurse may help the woman meet her grooming and hygiene needs and other activities. Bowel movements without stress or strain for the woman are promoted with stool softeners, diet, and fluids.

The woman may need a family member to help in the care of the infant. Breastfeeding is not contraindicated, but not all women with heart disease (particularly those with life-threatening disease) will be able to do it. The woman who chooses to breastfeed will need the support of her family and the nursing staff to be successful. For example, the woman may need assistance in positioning herself and/or the infant for feeding. Further to conserve the woman's energy, the infant may be brought to the mother and taken from her after the feeding. Women who breastfeed may need less medication for their cardiac condition, especially diuretics. Because diuretics can cause neonatal diuresis that can lead to dehydration, lactating women must be monitored closely to determine if medication doses can be reduced and still be effective.

If the woman is unable to breastfeed and her energies do not allow her to bottle feed the infant, the baby can be kept at the bedside so she can look at and touch her baby to establish an emotional bond with her baby with a low expenditure of energy. The infant should be held at the mother's eye level and near her lips and brought to her fingers. At the same time, involving the mother passively in her infant's care helps the mother feel vitally important—as she is—to the infant's well-being (e.g., "You can offer something no one else can: provide your baby with your sounds, touch, and rhythms that are so comforting"). Perhaps the woman can be encouraged to make a tape recording of her talking, singing, or whispering, which can be played for the baby in the nursery to help the infant feel her presence and be in contact with her voice. This also enhances maternal-infant bonding.

Preparation for discharge is carefully planned with the woman and family. Provision of help for the woman in the home by relatives, friends, and others must be addressed. If necessary, the nurse refers the family to community resources (e.g., for homemaking services). Rest and sleep periods, activity, and diet must be planned. The couple may need information about reestablishing sexual relations and contraception or sterilization. Oral contraception, particularly combined estrogen-progestin pills, are usually avoided because of the risk for thrombophlebitis. Sterilization may be a risk for women with class III or IV heart disease. Intrauterine devices (IUDs) may put the woman at risk for infection, especially if she has a valve replacement. Injectable progestins are effective and safe (Easterling & Otto, 2002).

Monitoring for cardiac decompensation continues through the first few weeks after birth because of hormonal shifts that affect hemodynamics. Maternal cardiac output is usually stabilized by 2 weeks postpartum (Easterling & Otto, 2002).

■ Cardiopulmonary Resuscitation of the Pregnant Woman

Trauma, pulmonary embolism, preeclampsia, anesthesia complications, drug overdose, hemorrhage, sepsis, or amniotic fluid embolism may result in cardiac arrest. Preexisting congenital or acquired heart disease also increases the risk of cardiac arrest. The incidence of cardiac arrest in pregnancy is estimated to be about 1 in 30,000 pregnancies (Mallampalli, Powner, & Gardner, 2004).

Various protocols exist for cardiopulmonary resuscitation (CPR) during pregnancy. If birth is accomplished within 5 minutes of the time of maternal cardiac arrest, intact neurologic neonatal survival is likely. Beyond 15 minutes, neonatal impairment or death is likely (Hueppchen & Satin, 2004). The primary and secondary surveys include the standard *A* for airway, *B* for breathing, *C* for circulation, and *D* for defibrillation. No matter what protocol is used, nurses and other health care providers must be prepared if CPR is to be successful.

In the event of cardiac arrest, standard resuscitative efforts with a few modifications are implemented. To prevent supine hypotension, the pregnant woman is placed on a firm surface with the uterus displaced laterally either manually or with a wedge or rolled blanket or towel under one hip (Mallampalli et al., 2004; Morris & Stacey, 2005). If defibrillation is needed, the paddles need to be placed one rib interspace higher than usual because the heart is displaced slightly by the enlarged uterus. If possible, the fetus should be monitored during the cardiac arrest (see Emergency box).

Complications may be associated with CPR on a pregnant woman. These complications may include laceration of the liver, rupture of the spleen or uterus, hemothorax, hemopericardium, or fracture of ribs or the sternum. Fetal complications also may occur. These include cardiac arrhythmia or asystole related to maternal defibrillation and medications, and CNS depression related to antiarrhythmic drugs and inadequate uteroplacental perfusion, with possible fetal hypoxemia and acidemia (Hueppchen & Satin, 2004).

If there is successful resuscitation, the woman and her fetus must receive careful monitoring. The woman remains at increased risk for recurrent cardiac arrest and arrhythmias (ventricular tachycardia, supraventricular tachycardia, bradycardia). Therefore her cardiovascular, pulmonary, and neurologic status should be assessed continuously. Uterine activity and resting tone must be monitored. Fetal status and gestational age should be determined and used in decision making regarding the continuation of the pregnancy or the timing and route of birth.

EMERGENCY

Cardiopulmonary Resuscitation (CPR) for the Pregnant Woman

AIRWAY

- Determine unresponsiveness.
- Activate emergency medical system and get the automated external defibrillator (AED) if available.
- Position woman on flat, firm surface with uterus displaced laterally with a wedge (e.g., a rolled towel placed under her hip) or manually, or place her in a lateral position.
- Open airway with head tilt–chin lift maneuver.

BREATHING

- Determine breathlessness (look, listen, feel).
- If the woman is not breathing, give two breaths, 1 second each.

CIRCULATION

- Determine pulselessness by feeling carotid pulse.
- If there is no pulse, begin chest compressions at rate of 100 per minute. Chest compressions may be performed slightly higher on the sternum if the uterus is enlarged enough to displace the diaphragm into a higher position.
- After five cycles of 30 compressions and two breaths (or about 2 minutes), check her pulse. If pulse is not present, continue CPR.

DEFIBRILLATION

- Use an AED according to standard protocol to analyze heart rhythm and deliver shock if indicated.

RELIEF OF FOREIGN BODY AIRWAY OBSTRUCTION

- If the pregnant woman is unable to speak or cough, perform chest thrusts. Stand behind the woman and place your arms under her armpits to encircle her chest. Press backward with quick thrusts until the foreign body is expelled (Fig. 33-2). If the woman becomes unresponsive, follow the steps for victims who become unresponsive, but use chest thrusts instead of abdominal thrusts.

From American Heart Association (AHA). (2005). American Heart Association guidelines for cardiopulmonary resuscitation and emergency cardiovascular care, Part 10.8: Cardiac arrest associated with pregnancy. *Circulation, 112*(24 Suppl), IV-150–IV-153.

FIG. 33-2 Heimlich maneuver. Clearing airway obstruction in woman in late stage of pregnancy (can also be used in markedly obese victim). **A,** Standing behind victim, place your arms under woman's armpits and across chest. Place thumb side of your clenched fist against middle of sternum, and place other hand over fist. **B,** Perform backward chest thrusts until foreign body is expelled or woman becomes unconscious. If pregnant woman becomes unconscious because of foreign-body airway obstruction, place her on her back and kneel close to the victim's side. (Be sure uterus is displaced laterally by using, for example, a rolled blanket under her hip.) Open mouth with tongue-jaw lift, perform finger sweep, and attempt rescue breathing. If unable to ventilate, position hands as for chest compression. Deliver five chest thrusts firmly to remove obstruction. Repeat this sequence of Heimlich maneuver, finger sweep, and attempt to ventilate. Continue sequence until pregnant woman's airway is clear of obstruction or help has arrived to relieve you. If woman is unconscious, give chest compressions as for woman without pulse.* (American Heart Association [AHA]. (2005). American Heart Association guidelines for cardiopulmonary resuscitation and emergency cardiovascular care, Part 10.8: *Circulation 112*[24 Suppl], IV-150–IV-153.)

Clearing an airway obstruction in a woman in the second or third trimester of pregnancy also requires a modification of the Heimlich maneuver (Fig. 33-2) (Hueppchen & Satin, 2004).

▬ Evaluation

The nurse uses the previously stated expected outcomes as criteria to evaluate the care of the woman with cardiac disease (see Plan of Care).

▬ OTHER MEDICAL DISORDERS ▬ IN PREGNANCY

Anemia

Anemia is the most common medical disorder of pregnancy, affecting at least 20% of pregnant women.

Anemia results in reduction of the oxygen-carrying capacity of the blood, and the heart tries to compensate by increasing the cardiac output. This effort increases the workload of the heart and stresses ventricular function.

CD: Plan of Care: The Pregnant Woman with Heart Disease

plan of care ▶ The Pregnant Woman with Heart Disease

NURSING DIAGNOSIS Activity intolerance related to effects of pregnancy on the woman with rheumatic heart disease with mitral valve stenosis

Expected Outcome *Woman will verbalize a plan to change lifestyle throughout pregnancy in order to avoid risk of cardiac decompensation.*

Nursing Interventions/Rationales
- Assist woman to identify factors that decrease activity tolerance and explore extent of limitations *to establish a baseline for evaluation.*
- Help woman to develop an individualized program of activity and rest, taking into account the living and working environment as well as support of family and friends *to maintain sufficient cardiac output.*
- Teach woman to monitor physiologic response to activity (i.e., pulse rate, respiratory rate) and reduce activity that causes fatigue or pain *to maintain sufficient cardiac output and prevent potential injury to fetus.*
- Enlist family and friends to assist woman in pacing activities and to provide support in performing role functions and self-care activities that are too strenuous *to increase chances of compliance with activity restrictions.*
- Suggest that woman maintain an activity log that records activities, time, duration, intensity, and physiologic response *to evaluate effectiveness of and adherence to activity program.*
- Discuss various quiet diversional activities that could be done by the woman *to decrease the potential for boredom during rest periods.*

NURSING DIAGNOSIS Ineffective therapeutic regimen management related to woman's first pregnancy and perceived sense of wellness

Expected Outcome *Woman will participate in an effective therapeutic regimen for pregnancy complicated by heart disease.*

Nursing Interventions/Rationales
- Identify factors, such as insufficient knowledge about the effect of cardiac disease on pregnancy that could inhibit the woman from participating in a therapeutic regimen *to promote early interventions, such as teaching about the importance of rest.*
- Teach woman and family about factors such as lack of rest or not taking prescribed medications that could adversely affect the pregnancy *to provide information and promote empowerment over the situation.*
- Encourage expression of feelings about the disease and its potential effect on the pregnancy *to promote a sense of trust.*

- Identify resources in the community *to provide a shared sense of common experiences.*
- Encourage woman to verbalize her plan for carrying out the regimen of care *to evaluate the effects of teaching.*

NURSING DIAGNOSIS Decreased cardiac output related to increased circulatory volume secondary to pregnancy and cardiac disease

Expected Outcome *The woman will exhibit signs of adequate cardiac output (i.e., normal pulse and blood pressure; normal heart and breath sounds; normal skin color, tone, and turgor; normal capillary refill; normal urine output; and no evidence of edema).*

Nursing Interventions/Rationales
- Reinforce the importance of activity/rest cycles *to prevent cardiac complications.*
- Plan with woman a frequent visit schedule to caregiver *to provide adequate surveillance of high risk pregnancy.*
- Teach woman to lie in lateral position *to increase uteroplacental blood flow* and to elevate legs while sitting *to promote venous return.*
- Monitor intake and output and check for edema *to assess for renal complications or venous return problems.*
- Monitor FHR and fetal activity, and perform NST as indicated *to assess fetal status and detect uteroplacental insufficiency.*

NURSING DIAGNOSIS Ineffective tissue perfusion related to cardiac condition secondary to increased circulatory needs during pregnancy

Expected Outcomes *The woman will exhibit signs of hemodynamic stability (i.e., blood pressure, pulse, ABGs, and WBC counts are within normal limits). The fetus will exhibit signs of well-being (i.e., fetal activity and FHR are within normal limits).*

Nursing Interventions/Rationales
- Monitor heart rate and rhythm, blood pressure, skin color and temperature, WBCs, hemoglobin and hematocrit, and ABGs *to detect early signs of cardiac failure/hypoxia.*
- Monitor fetal activity and FHR, and perform nonstress testing as indicated *to assess fetal status and detect uteroplacental insufficiency.*
- Teach woman how to detect and report early signs of cardiac decompensation *to prevent maternal/fetal complications.*

ABGs, Arterial blood gases; *FHR*, fetal heart rate; *NST*, nonstress test; *WBCs*, white blood cells.

Therefore anemia that occurs with any other complication (e.g., preeclampsia) may result in congestive heart failure.

An indirect index of the oxygen-carrying capacity is the packed red blood cell (RBC) volume, or hematocrit level. The normal hematocrit range in nonpregnant women is 37% to 47%. However, normal values for pregnant women with adequate iron stores may range from 33% to 44%. This has been explained by hydremia (dilution of blood), or the physiologic anemia of pregnancy.

According to the Centers for Disease Control and Prevention (CDC), anemia in pregnancy is defined as hemoglobin less than 11 g/dl in the first and third trimesters and 10.5 g/dl in the second trimester (Kilpatrick & Laros, 2004).

When a woman has anemia during pregnancy, the loss of blood at birth, even if minimal, is not well tolerated. She is at an increased risk for requiring blood transfusions. Women with anemia have a higher incidence of puerperal complications, such as infection, than pregnant women with normal hematologic values.

Nursing care of the anemic pregnant woman requires that the nurse be able to distinguish between the normal physiologic anemia of pregnancy and the disease states. The most common cases of anemia in pregnancy are of the iron deficiency type. The other types embrace a considerable variety of acquired and hereditary anemias, including folic acid deficiency, sickle cell anemia, and thalassemia.

During prenatal visits, the nurse should take a diet history and provide dietary teaching as appropriate. Pregnancy may cause increased fatigue, stress, and financial difficulties for a woman with anemia as she copes with her activities of daily living. The nurse should assess the woman's needs and provide her with appropriate resources or referral.

Iron Deficiency Anemia

Pathologic anemia of pregnancy is primarily caused by *iron deficiency*. Without iron therapy, even pregnant women who have excellent nutrition will end pregnancy with an iron deficit. Iron is actively transported across the placenta for fetal erythropoiesis. Diet alone cannot replace gestational iron losses. Inadequate nutrition without therapy will certainly mean iron deficiency anemia during late pregnancy and the puerperium. Successful iron therapy during pregnancy can be carried out in most cases with oral iron supplements (e.g., elemental iron of 60 to 80 mg/day). It is important to teach the woman the significance of the iron therapy (see Teaching for Self-Care box in Chapter 15, p. 363). In addition, the woman should be instructed in dietary ways to decrease the GI side effects of iron therapy. Some pregnant women cannot tolerate the prescribed oral iron because of nausea and vomiting. In such cases, the woman should receive parenteral iron such as an iron-dextran complex (Imferon).

Folic Acid Deficiency Anemia

Folic acid deficiency during conception and early pregnancy is associated with an increased incidence of neural tube defects, cleft lip, and cleft palate. Even in well-nourished women, it is common to have a folate deficiency. Poor diet, cooking with large volumes of water, or home canning of food (especially vegetables) may lead to folate deficiency. Malabsorption may play a part in the development of anemia caused by a lack of folic acid. Folic acid deficiency anemia is common in multiple gestations. During pregnancy the recommended daily intake is 600 mcg of folic acid per day; women who have a deficiency may need a supplement.

Sickle Cell Hemoglobinopathy

Sickle cell hemoglobinopathy is a disease caused by the presence of abnormal hemoglobin in the blood. *Sickle cell trait* (SA hemoglobin pattern), sickling of the RBCs but with a normal RBC life span, usually causes only mild clinical symptoms. *Sickle cell anemia* (sickle cell disease) is a recessive, hereditary, familial hemolytic anemia that affects those of African-American or Mediterranean ancestry. These individuals usually have abnormal hemoglobin types (SS or SC). People with sickle cell anemia have recurrent attacks (crises)

of fever and pain in the abdomen or extremities. These attacks are attributed to vascular occlusion (from abnormal cells), tissue hypoxia, edema, and RBC destruction. Crises are associated with normochromic anemia, jaundice, reticulocytosis, a positive sickle cell test, and the demonstration of abnormal hemoglobin (usually SS or SC).

Almost 10% of African-Americans in North America have the sickle cell trait, but fewer than 1% have sickle cell anemia. The anemia is often complicated by iron and folic acid deficiency.

Women with sickle cell trait usually do well in pregnancy, although they are at increased risk for urinary tract infections (UTIs) and may be deficient in iron (Kilpatrick & Laros, 2004). If the woman has sickle cell anemia, the anemia that occurs in normal pregnancies may aggravate the condition and bring on more crises. Fetal complications include preterm birth and IUGR. Pregnant women with sickle cell anemia are prone to pyelonephritis, bone abnormalities, strokes, cardiomyopathy, congestive heart failure, and preeclampsia (Cunningham et al., 2005; Moore & Martin, 2004). An aplastic crisis may follow serious infection, for example, with the parvovirus B19. Transfusions of the woman have been the usual treatment for symptomatic clients who have not responded to conservative management. Prophylactic transfusions are controversial and not usually recommended during pregnancy, unless the client has very severe symptoms (Rappaport, Velazquez, & Williams, 2004). Vaginal birth is preferred. Cesarean birth is warranted only for obstetric indications.

Table 33-3 identifies some considerations for management of the woman with sickle cell disease during pregnancy and childbirth.

Thalassemia

Thalassemia (Mediterranean or Cooley's anemia) is a relatively common anemia in which an insufficient amount of hemoglobin is produced to fill the RBCs. The condition eventually manifests itself in severe bone deformities caused by massive marrow tissue expansion. Thalassemia is a hereditary disorder that involves the abnormal synthesis of the alpha or beta chains of hemoglobin. Beta thalassemia is the more common variety in the United States and often is diagnosed in persons of Italian, Greek, southern Chinese, Mediterranean, North African, African- American, Middle Eastern, southern Asian, or Indo-Pakistani descent (Kilpatrick & Laros, 2004). The unbalanced synthesis of hemoglobin leads to premature RBC death, resulting in severe anemia. *Thalassemia major* is the homozygous form of this disorder; *thalassemia minor* is the heterozygous form. Couples with the thalassemia trait should seek genetic counseling. Women with the thalassemia trait usually have an uncomplicated pregnancy.

Women with thalassemia major or minor have infertility problems, so few pregnancies will occur. As many as 50% of these pregnancies are complicated by stillbirth, IUGR, preeclampsia, and preterm birth. Medical management

Trial of Labor Versus Elective Repeat Cesarean Birth

BACKGROUND

- Although cesarean births now account for more than one birth out of four, subsequent births do not necessarily mean repeat cesarean birth. A trial of labor (TOL) for vaginal birth after cesarean (VBAC) became more accepted in the early 1990s, until concerns about uterine rupture and fetal outcomes caused some decline in its popularity. Some researchers suggested that use of labor augmentation may increase the risk for uterine rupture. The alternative is the elective repeat cesarean birth (ERCB), available to women who had a low, transverse scar. Cesarean birth carries surgical risks and costs, and may contribute to newborn respiratory problems.

OBJECTIVES

- The reviewers' goal was to compare the maternal and fetal outcomes of TOL versus ERCB for women giving birth after cesarean, and the rate of successful VBAC. Information relevant to clinical decision making included useful predictive tools; maternal and fetal outcomes, particularly uterine rupture; client preferences and satisfaction; cost; individual risk factors; and administrative influences such as legal, hospital, and insurance practices.

METHODS

Search Strategy

- After a thorough search of the literature, the authors identified 180 relevant studies, which included randomized controlled trials, cohort studies, case-controlled studies, cross-sectional studies, large case studies, and decision models. The studies, published 1982 to 2001, were from Australia, Canada, France, Hong Kong, Ireland, Israel, the Netherlands, Singapore, Sweden, Switzerland, the United Kingdom, and the United States. The numbers of subjects varied with each question studied.

Statistical Analyses

- Similar data of good quality were pooled. Reviewers calculated relative risk for dichotomous (categoric) data, such as type of birth, and weighted mean difference for continuous data, such as length of labor. Differences between groups outside the 95% confidence interval were accepted as significant. All were analyzed in their original randomly assigned "intention to treat" categories, even if they changed their minds.

FINDINGS

- Success rates for VBAC ranged from 60% to 82%, with a rate of 75.9% at tertiary and university settings. Vaginal birth was 10% less likely with oxytocin use. Radiologic pelvimetry did not predict route of birth. There were no differences in maternal deaths between TOL and ERCB groups, but cesarean births were associated with increased infection, especially if TOL was attempted first. The evidence was insufficient to assess risk to infants for lower Apgar scores, respiratory disease, or infection. Most studies showed varying degrees of increased perinatal death with TOL versus ERCB. Symptomatic uterine rupture was significantly more likely with TOL, and led to infant death and/or hysterectomy. Fetal bradycardia frequently accompanied uterine rupture. Women who chose TOL were more likely to have a history of vaginal birth, white race, desire for easy recovery, and lower anxiety. Successful VBAC was more likely for women under 40 with prior vaginal birth, favorable cervix, and history of nonrecurrent indication for cesarean (such as breech). Risk factors for failed VBAC were increasing number of previous cesarean births, gestation over 40 weeks, birth weight greater than 4000 g, and augmentation of labor. Rates of VBAC were higher in teaching hospitals and in states where standardized VBAC guidelines were issued to obstetric providers. VBACs are cost-effective if the success rate is 76% or higher.

LIMITATIONS

- The studies varied in definitions and measures, making comparisons difficult. Benefits and harm had to be abstracted indirectly. There was no way to determine that the TOL group was comparable to the ERCB group, which would have decreased the confounders. Practice and attitudes varied enormously across regions and time. Use of oxytocin did not necessarily cause cesarean birth; rather, both may have resulted from inefficient labor. All the studies were conducted in developed countries, limiting its generalizability to low-resource areas.

IMPLICATIONS FOR PRACTICE

- Cesarean birth is one of the most common surgeries performed on women, yet the literature is unclear on its benefits and risks. Low risk women have a good chance of successful VBAC, which will decrease their surgical risks, recovery time, and costs, and increases their chance of successful future VBAC. Providers are influenced by hospital and regional guidelines.

IMPLICATIONS FOR FURTHER RESEARCH

- Future researchers need to insure that groups are identical in every way except route of birth. More information will determine the role that augmentation plays in VBAC success. More precision in definitions of important outcomes such as mortality, hemorrhage, and infection will give much clearer information for clinical decision making.

Reference: Guise, J., McDonagh, M., Hashima, J., Kraemer, D., Eden, K., Berlin, M., et al. (2003). *Vaginal birth after cesarean (VBAC)*. AHRQ Publications No 03-E018. Rockville, MD: Agency for Healthcare Research and Quality.

consists of ongoing monitoring, aggressive transfusion, and iron chelation therapy. Treatment has improved life expectancy and fertility and enabled women with thalassemia major to accomplish successful pregnancies (Rappaport et al., 2004).

Women with thalassemia minor have a mild, persistent anemia, but the RBC level may be normal or even elevated. However, no systemic problems are caused by the anemia. Thalassemia minor must be distinguished from iron deficiency anemia.

Pregnancy will neither worsen thalassemia minor nor be compromised by the disease. Iron therapy should only be prescribed for women with iron deficiency. Folic acid supplementation is recommended. People with thalassemia minor should have a normal life span despite a moderately reduced hemoglobin level.

table 33-3 Sickle Cell Anemia: Considerations for Pregnancy and Childbirth

FIRST TRIMESTER	SECOND TRIMESTER	THIRD TRIMESTER	LABOR AND BIRTH
Genetic counseling if desired to identify parents as having the disease or as a carrier	Genetic testing if desired and counseling about results and options	Urine cultures, checking hemoglobin and hematocrit levels, and treatment for crisis as described in first trimester	Expect spontaneous labor and vaginal birth; consider induction of labor or cesarean birth for fetal compromise
Nutritional counseling	Alpha fetoprotein testing if desired	Assess for preeclampsia, signs of preterm labor or other complications (e.g., thromboembolism or congestive heart failure	Have typed and crossmatched blood available; assist with transfusion if needed
Folic acid 1 mg/day orally supplementation for all of pregnancy	Urine cultures, checking hemoglobin and hematocrit levels, and treatment for crisis as described in first trimester	Weekly serial ultrasound examination for fetal growth and amniotic fluid volume	Administer oxygen by face mask continuously during labor
Urine cultures and treat urinary tract infection if present	Ultrasound for fetal growth and to identify anomalies if present		Use lateral position for labor
Assess for respiratory infection and treat with antibiotics as ordered			Coach for relaxation and to lessen anxiety
Determine hemoglobin (Hb) and hematocrit (Hct) to maintain Hb at ≥8g and Hct at ≥20%			Maintain adequate hydration; observe for signs of fluid overload
Ultrasound to determine fetal gestational age			Consider epidural analgesia
If in crisis, treat with analgesia, adequate hydration and oxygen; transfusion if needed			Monitor fetal status with continuous electronic fetal monitoring

Sources: Cunningham, G., Leveno, K., Bloom, S., Hauth, J., Gilstrap, L., & Wenstrom, K. (Eds.). (2005). *Williams obstetrics* (22nd ed.). New York: McGraw-Hill; Kilpatrick, S., & Laros, R. (2004). Maternal hematologic disorders. In R. Creasy, R. Resnik, & J. Iams (Eds.), *Maternal-fetal medicine: Principles and practice* (5th ed.). Philadelphia: Saunders; Samuels, P. (2002). Hematologic complications of pregnancy. In S. Gabbe, J. Niebyl, & J. Simpson (Eds.), *Obstetrics: Normal and problem pregnancies* (4th ed.). New York: Churchill Livingstone.

Women with thalassemia syndromes require intense maternal and fetal surveillance throughout the pregnancy. Women need to be monitored for anemia and the fetus assessed with ultrasound testing, NSTs, biophysical profiles (BPPs), Doppler flow studies, and fetal lung maturity studies (Poole, 2003).

Pulmonary Disorders

As pregnancy advances and the uterus impinges on the thoracic cavity, any pregnant woman may have increased respiratory difficulty. This difficulty will be compounded by pulmonary disease. A pulmonary disorder in pregnancy requires assessment, planning, and interventions specific to the disease process, in addition to routine peripartum care. The nurse also must be alert to pulmonary complications precipitated by pregnancy.

Asthma

Bronchial asthma is an acute respiratory illness caused by allergens, marked change in ambient temperature, or emotional tension. In many cases the actual cause may be unknown. A family history of allergy is common in people with asthma. In response to stimuli, there is widespread but reversible narrowing of the hyperreactive airways, making it difficult to breathe. The clinical manifestations are expiratory wheezing, productive cough, thick sputum, and/or dyspnea.

From 0.5% to 8% of pregnant women have asthma (Gardner & Doyle, 2004), one of the most common complications of pregnancy. The effect of pregnancy on asthma is unpredictable. In one study, about 50% of the asthma conditions remained the same, 30% improved, and 20% worsened (Gardner & Doyle). Physiologic alterations induced by pregnancy do not make the pregnant woman more prone to asthmatic attacks. Women often have few symptoms of asthma in the first trimester and in the last 4 weeks of pregnancy. The severity of symptoms usually peaks between 24 and 36 weeks of gestation (Gardner & Doyle).

Risks to pregnancies complicated by asthma include hyperemesis gravidarum, preterm birth, preeclampsia, gestational diabetes, IUGR, and neonatal mortality. The more severe the asthma, the more likely that risks will occur for the woman and fetus (Conversations with Colleagues, 2005).

Therapy for asthma has four major goals: (1) optimal control of asthma symptoms, (2) attainment of normal pulmonary function, (3) prevention and reversal of asthma attacks, and (4) prevention of maternal and fetal complications (Guy, Kirumaki, & Hanania, 2004). These goals can be achieved in pregnancy by assessment and monitoring of maternal lung function and fetal well-being, avoidance or elimination of environmental triggers (e.g., dust mites, animal dander, pollen, wood smoke), drug therapy (e.g., bronchodilators and antiinflammatory agents), and client education (Guy et al.). Respiratory infections should be treated, and mist or steam inhalation used to aid expectoration of mucus. Acute episodes may require β-agonists such as albuterol, steroids, aminophylline, and oxygen. Almost all asthma medications are considered safe in pregnancy (Gluck & Gluck, 2005; Murdock, 2002) (Table 33-4).

Asthma attacks can occur in labor; thus medications for asthma are continued in labor and the postpartum period. Pulse oximetry should be instituted during labor. Epidurals are recommended for pain relief. Morphine and meperidine are histamine-releasing narcotics and should be avoided (Guy et al., 2004).

During the postpartum period, women who have asthma are at increased risk for hemorrhage. If excessive bleeding occurs, oxytocin is the recommended drug. Asthma medications are usually safe for administration during the postpartum period and lactation. The woman usually returns to her prepregnancy asthma status within 3 months after giving birth.

Cystic Fibrosis

Cystic fibrosis is a common autosomal recessive genetic disorder in which the exocrine glands produce excessive viscous secretions, which causes problems with both respiratory and digestive functions. There is an increase in pulmonary capillary permeability, decrease of lung volume, and shunting, which results in arterial hypoxemia. Respiratory failure and early death may occur.

Since the gene for cystic fibrosis was identified in 1989, data can be collected for the purposes of genetic counseling for couples regarding carrier status. About 4% of the Caucasian population in the United States are heterozygous carriers. Cystic fibrosis occurs in about 1 in 3000 Caucasian live births (Whitty & Dombrowski, 2004). Improvements in diagnosis and treatment have allowed an increasing number of women with cystic fibrosis to sur-

vive to adulthood. The median age of survival for clients is 40 years (Cohen, Talwar, & Efferen, 2004). Preconception counseling is essential for women with cystic fibrosis. Fewer than one in five women are able to become pregnant, as a result of very thick cervical mucus (Whitty & Dombrowski). Women should be advised of the risks of pregnancy, depending on their status. If possible, women should be 90% of their ideal body weight before conception (Whitty & Dombrowski).

In women who do not have severe disease, pregnancy is usually tolerated well. Lung function seems to be associated with the ability to carry the pregnancy to term (Cohen et al., 2004).

In those with severe disease, the pregnancy is often complicated by chronic hypoxia and frequent pulmonary infections. Women with cystic fibrosis show a decrease in their residual volume during pregnancy, as do normal pregnant women, and are unable to maintain vital capacity. Presumably the pulmonary vasculature cannot accommodate the increased cardiac output of pregnancy. The results are decreased oxygen to the myocardium, decreased cardiac output, and increased hypoxemia. A pregnant woman with less than 50% of expected vital capacity usually has a difficult pregnancy. Increased maternal and perinatal mortality is related to severe pulmonary infection. There is an increased incidence of preterm births, IUGR, and neonatal deaths in clients with severe cystic fibrosis. Predictors of adverse affects to the fetus and neonate are inadequate weight gain, dyspnea, and cyanosis.

In addition to the respiratory implications, women with cystic fibrosis may develop gestational diabetes and liver disease. Pancreatic insufficiency may put the woman at risk for malnutrition, because she cannot meet the increased nutritional requirements of pregnancy. Fat-soluble vitamins may not be absorbed as well, resulting in deficiency in those nutrients.

There are no national guidelines regarding the management of pregnant clients with cystic fibrosis.

table 33-4 Medications Used in Pregnancy in Clients with Asthma

STAGE/CONDITION OF PREGNANCY	PREFERRED MEDICATION	MEDICATION(S) TO AVOID (RATIONALE)
Labor	Continue asthma medications	
Induction	Prostaglandin E_2 and E_1 may be used for cervical ripening Oxytocin	15-methyl prostaglandin $F_{2\alpha}$ (may cause bronchoconstriction or bronchospasm)
Pain relief	Fentanyl Epidural anesthesia	Morphine and meperidine (Demerol) (release histamine)
Preterm labor	Magnesium sulfate	β-agonist (e.g., terbutaline) if client is already taking one for her asthma (may cause respiratory distress) Indomethacin may cause brochospasm NSAIDs (may exacerbate asthma)
Postpartum hemorrhage	Oxytocin	Methylergonovine and 15-methyl prostaglandin $F_{2\alpha}$ (may worsen asthma)

Data from Whitty, J., & Dombrowski, M. (2004). Respiratory diseases in pregnancy. In R. Creasy, R. Resnik, & J. Iams. (Eds.), *Maternal-fetal medicine: Principles and practice.* (5th ed.). Philadelphia: Saunders.
NSAIDs, Nonsteroidal antiinflammatory drugs.

Throughout pregnancy, frequent monitoring of the woman's weight, blood glucose, hemoglobin, total protein, serum albumin, prothrombin time, and fat-soluble vitamins A and E are suggested. Baseline pulmonary function tests should be ideally completed before pregnancy and continued as needed during pregnancy. Early detection and treatment of infection is essential throughout pregnancy. Antibiotic regimens should be appropriate for the organism and blood levels monitored. Chest physiotherapy and drainage is an important component of care. Fetal assessment is essential, since the fetus can be at risk from uteroplacental insufficiency. Fundal height, amniotic fluid index, daily fetal movement counts, NSTs, and BPPs provide important data for decision making regarding birth. Women with severe pancreatic insufficiency may require enteral tube feedings or total parenteral nutrition.

During labor, monitoring for fluid and electrolyte balance is required. Increase in cardiac output could lead to cardiopulmonary failure. The amount of sodium lost through sweat can be significant, and hypovolemia can occur. Conversely, if any degree of cor pulmonale is present, fluid overload is a concern. Oxygen is given by face mask during labor, and monitoring by pulse oximetry is recommended. Diuretics may be prescribed for fluid overload. Epidural or local analgesia is the preferred analgesic for birth.

Breastfeeding appears to be safe as long as the sodium content of the milk is not abnormal (Lawrence & Lawrence, 2005). Pumping and discarding the milk is done until the sodium content has been determined. Milk samples should be tested periodically for sodium, chloride, and total fat, and the infant's growth pattern should be monitored.

Adult Respiratory Distress Syndrome

Adult respiratory distress syndrome (ARDS), or shock lung, occurs when the lungs are unable to maintain levels of oxygen and carbon dioxide within normal limits. Severe hypoxemia, in spite of high levels of inspired oxygen, is accompanied by an increase in pulmonary capillary permeability, a decrease in lung volume, and shunting of blood.

ARDS is not specific to pregnancy; it also can result from trauma, pneumonia, sepsis, aspiration of gastric contents, fat emboli, acute pancreatitis, and drug overdose. When ARDS is associated with pregnancy, the precipitating factors may be inhalation of gastric contents during anesthesia, disseminated intravascular coagulation (DIC), preeclampsia, eclampsia, abruptio placentae, dead fetus syndrome, amniotic fluid embolism, hemorrhage, or chorioamnionitis (Bandi, Munnar, & Matthay, 2004). An initial intervention is to find and correct the underlying cause, if possible. To provide the best fetal environment, early intubation and mechanical ventilation is recommended. With severe lung injury, positive end-expiratory pressure (PEEP) may be necessary (Bandi et al.). Sedatives may be prescribed for intubation and ventilation. The administration of vasoactive agents, inotropic agents, and corticosteroids may be necessary. Maintaining fluid balance is a challenge and a key component of management. For the woman who is hypovolemic, administration of blood may help to increase cardiac output. For the woman who is hypervolemic, diuretics may be necessary to maintain adequate cardiac output. The optimum treatment for women with ARDS after 28 weeks of gestation is birth (induction of labor and vaginal birth or scheduled cesarean).

The postpartum incidence of ARDS is affected not by the method of birth but by the amount of trauma occurring during pregnancy and birth. It also may occur after miscarriage or therapeutic abortion.

Laboratory reports are important in identifying the origin of acute pulmonary problems. Chest radiographs can indicate the presence of infiltrates in the lungs, and ABGs identify the status of acid-base balance. The priority assessments to note are vital signs, oxygen saturation, signs of thrombophlebitis, and hemorrhage. During the postpartum period, apprehension, distended neck veins, cyanosis, diaphoresis, or pallor may indicate hypoxemia. Mental confusion or disorientation also may be noted.

The pulse rate increases to compensate for respiratory insufficiency of any origin. The severity of the pulmonary problem increases as the pulse rate increases. An initial increase in blood pressure occurs as cardiac output increases in an attempt to supply the tissue with oxygen. When lung damage is severe, blood pressure decreases.

Respiratory changes are the most important indicators of ARDS. The rate and depth of respirations, respiratory pattern, symmetry of chest movement, and use of accessory muscles should be noted; therefore observation of respiratory characteristics after activity is important.

■ NURSE ALERT

If there is any indication of abnormality, respirations are counted for a full minute; an error in rate of plus or minus four respirations per minute may be highly significant.

On auscultation, crackles, rhonchi, wheezes, or a pleural friction rub should be reported, especially when they occur after an earlier assessment with normal findings. The pregnant woman should be positioned for breathing comfort. Oxygen and emergency equipment should be available. The woman should be reassured and coached in relaxation techniques to lessen her anxiety.

This syndrome has a high mortality rate. The prognosis is good if the woman is otherwise healthy and if ventilatory support can be maintained until the underlying disease can be treated (Cunningham et al., 2005).

Integumentary Disorders

The skin surface may exhibit many physiologic conditions during pregnancy. Dermatologic disorders induced by pregnancy include melasma (chloasma), vascular "spiders," palmar erythema, and striae gravidarum. Skin problems generally aggravated by pregnancy are acne vulgaris (in the first trimester), erythema multiforme, herpetiform dermatitis (fever blisters and genital herpes), granuloma inguinale (Donovan bodies), condylomata acuminata (genital warts), neurofibromatosis (von Recklinghausen disease), and pemphigus. Dermatologic disorders usually improved by pregnancy include acne vulgaris (in the third trimester), seborrheic dermatitis (dandruff), and psoriasis (Cunningham et al., 2005). An unpredictable course during pregnancy may be expected in atopic dermatitis, lupus erythematosus, and herpes simplex. Disease processes during and soon after pregnancy may be extremely difficult to diagnose and treat.

Pruritus is a common symptom in pregnancy-specific inflammatory skin diseases. The most common pregnancy-specific causes of pruritus are polymorphic eruption of pregnancy (also known as *pruritic urticarial papules and plaques of pregnancy [PUPPP]*) (Fig. 33-3), prurigo gestationis, and cholestasis of pregnancy. Symptoms usually appear in the third trimester and usually subside in the postpartum period. The abdomen is usually affected, but lesions can spread to the arms, the thighs, the back, and the buttocks. Topical steroid therapy usually provides relief, but some women may require systemic steroid therapy for severe symptoms (Stambuk & Colvin, 2002).

Pemphigoid gestationis and impetigo herpetiformis are rare complications that can cause fetal morbidity. Antepartal fetal assessments are recommended (Stambuk & Colvin, 2002).

▬ NURSE ALERT
Isotretinoin (Accutane), commonly prescribed for cystic acne, is highly teratogenic. There is a risk for craniofacial, cardiac, and CNS malformations in exposed fetuses. This drug should not be taken during pregnancy.

Explanation, reassurance, and commonsense measures should suffice for normal skin changes. In contrast, disease processes during and soon after pregnancy may be extremely difficult to diagnose and treat.

Neurologic Disorders

The pregnant woman with a neurologic disorder must deal with potential teratogenic effects of prescribed medications, changes of mobility during pregnancy, and ability to

FIG. 33-3 Woman with pruritic urticarial papules and plaques of pregnancy. Lesions also are present on her arms, back, abdomen, and buttocks. (Courtesy Shannon Perry, Phoenix, AZ.)

care for the baby. The nurse should be aware of all drugs the woman is taking and the associated potential for producing congenital anomalies. As the pregnancy progresses, the woman's center of gravity shifts and causes balance and gait changes. The nurse should advise the woman of these expected changes and suggest safety measures as appropriate. Family and community resources should be identified to provide infant care for the neurologically impaired woman.

Epilepsy

Epilepsy is a disorder of the brain causing recurrent seizures; it is the most common neurologic disorder accompanying pregnancy (Constantino & Varner, 2004). Epilepsy may result from developmental abnormalities or injury, or may have no known cause. Convulsive seizures may be more frequent or severe during complications of pregnancy, such as edema, alkalosis, fluid-electrolyte imbalance, cerebral hypoxia, hypoglycemia, and hypocalcemia. They also may be related to hormonal changes, fatigue, or sleep deprivation. However, the effects of pregnancy on epilepsy are unpredictable: some women have no change or even a decrease in seizure frequency (Constantino & Varner).

The differential diagnosis between epilepsy and eclampsia may pose a problem. Epilepsy and eclampsia can coexist. However, a history of seizures and a normal plasma uric acid level, as well as the absence of hypertension, generalized edema, or proteinuria, point to epilepsy.

During pregnancy, the risk of vaginal bleeding is doubled, and there is a threefold risk of abruptio placentae (Donaldson & Duffy, 2004). Abnormal presentations are more common in labor and birth, and there is an increased possibility that the fetus will experience seizures in utero (Aminoff, 2004).

Metabolic changes in pregnancy usually alter pharmacokinetics. In addition, nausea and vomiting may interfere with ingestion and absorption of medication. Failure to take medications is a common factor leading to worsening of seizure activity during pregnancy, particularly during the first trimester (Constantino & Varner, 2004). This is largely because of the message that drugs for epilepsy are harmful to the fetus. Teratogenicity of antiepileptic drugs (AEDs) is well documented. Therefore, monotherapy and the use of the smallest dose possible to control seizures during pregnancy is recommended (Aminoff, 2004; Constantino & Varner; Shehata & Okosun, 2004). Congenital anomalies that can occur with AEDs include cleft lip or palate, congenital heart disease, urogenital defects, and neural tube defects (Weiner & Buhimschi, 2004). AEDs prescribed in pregnancy should also be administered with folic acid. Daily folic acid supplementation is important because of the depletion that occurs when anticonvulsants are taken (Shehata & Okosun).

Vaginal birth is preferred. The risk of seizures during labor exists; approximately 1% to 2% of women have a tonic-clonic seizure, and another 1% to 2% have a seizure within 24 hours postpartum (Shehata & Okosun, 2004). Prolonged labor may be problematic, since the effectiveness of oral AEDs may diminish over time. If the women is taking phenytoin or phenobarbital, these drugs may be administered parenterally. Fetal monitoring is essential, because seizures can precipitate fetal bradycardia.

During the neonatal period, infants can have a hemorrhagic disorder associated with AED-induced vitamin K deficiency. Prophylaxis consists of administering vitamin K, 20 mg orally, daily during the last month of pregnancy and administering 1 mg intramuscularly (IM) to the newborn at birth (Pschirrer, 2004). Breastfeeding is safe with many of the antiepilepsy drugs. More data are needed on the effects of some of the newer antiepilepsy drugs. Neonatal sedation may be a side effect of carbamazepine, phenobarbital, and primidone. Neonatal drug levels should be monitored if the mother is taking phenobarbital, gabapentin, lamotrigine, or oxcarbazepine (Pschirrer).

Multiple Sclerosis

Multiple sclerosis (MS), a patchy demyelinization of the spinal cord and CNS, may be a viral disorder. MS has a greater prevalence in female subjects and is more common during the childbearing years, with onset between the ages of 20 and 40 years (Shehata & Okosun, 2004). Infertility, miscarriage, stillbirth, and fetal anomalies do not appear to be increased in women with MS.

MS may occasionally complicate pregnancy, but exacerbations and remissions are unrelated to the pregnant state. Some women have flare-up in the third trimester and the postpartum period, whereas others have fewer symptoms. Bowel and bladder problems, increased difficulty in walking, and fatigue may be more pronounced in women with MS. Medications such as Avonex (interferon beta-1a), Betaseron (interferon beta-1b), and Copaxone (glatiramer acetate) that are given to reduce the frequency and intensity of attacks and slow the progression of disease should not be taken during pregnancy (Donaldson & Duffy, 2004). Nursing care of the pregnant woman with MS is similar

---

CRITICAL THINKING EXERCISE

Epilepsy

Sarah, 24, is a gravida 1, para 0 at 12 weeks of gestation who is being evaluated at the prenatal clinic. She asks you, the registered nurse, about the risks of her epilepsy to the fetus and the pregnancy.
1. Evidence—Are her questions and concerns valid?
2. Assumptions—What assumptions can be made about the following?
   a. Risks of antiepileptic medications on fetal development
   b. Effects of epilepsy on pregnancy and vice versa
   c. Importance of folic acid supplementation
   d. Safety of antiepileptic medications on breastfeeding
3. What implications and priorities for nursing care can be made at this time?
4. Does the evidence objectively support your conclusion?
5. Are there alternative perspectives to your conclusion?

---

to the care of the normal pregnant woman. Breastfeeding is permitted.

Bell's Palsy

An association between Bell's palsy (idiopathic facial paralysis) and pregnancy was first cited by Bell in 1830. The incidence of Bell's palsy in pregnancy is about 3 times higher than in nonpregnant women of the same age (Donaldson & Duffy, 2004). The clinical manifestations include the sudden development of a unilateral facial weakness, often discovered first thing in the morning. In addition, taste on the anterior two thirds of the tongue may be lost, depending on the location of the lesion. Pain may occur in and around the ear. The incidence usually peaks during the third trimester and the puerperium. A relationship with the hypertensive disorders of pregnancy may be present. Women with Bell's palsy occurring during pregnancy should be monitored for preeclampsia or hypertension (Donaldson & Duffy).

No effects of maternal Bell's palsy have been observed in infants. Maternal outcome is generally good unless there is a complete block in nerve conduction. Steroid therapy is the only medical treatment prescribed. Supportive care includes prevention of injury to the exposed cornea, facial muscle massage, careful chewing and manual removal of food from inside the affected cheek, and reassurance that return of total neurologic function is likely in about 85% of women affected (Shehata & Okosun, 2004).

Autoimmune Disorders

Autoimmune disorders make up a large group of diseases that disrupt the function of the immune system of the body. In these types of disorders, the body develops antibodies that attack its normally present antigens, causing tissue damage. Autoimmune disorders have a predilection for women in their reproductive years; therefore associations with pregnancy are not uncommon (Warren & Silver, 2004). Pregnancy may affect the disease process. Some disorders adversely affect the course of pregnancy or are detrimental to the fetus. Autoimmune disorders of concern in pregnancy include systemic lupus erythematosus (SLE) and myasthenia gravis (MG).

Systemic Lupus Erythematosus

One of the most common serious disorders of childbearing age, systemic lupus erythematosus (SLE) is a chronic, multisystem inflammatory disease characterized by autoimmune antibody production that affects the skin, the joints, the kidneys, the lungs, the CNS, the liver, and other body organs (Warren & Silver, 2004). The exact cause is unknown, but viral infection and hormonal and genetic factors may be related.

Early symptoms such as fatigue, weight loss, skin rashes, and arthralgias may be overlooked. Pericarditis is often the presenting symptom. Eventually all organs become involved. The condition is characterized by a series of exacerbations and remissions.

If the diagnosis has been established and the woman desires a child, she is advised to wait until she has been in remission for at least 6 months before attempting to become pregnant (Gilbert & Harmon, 2003). An exacerbation of SLE during pregnancy or postpartum occurs in 50% of women.

SLE during pregnancy is associated with increased rates of preeclampsia, fetal loss, IUGR, and preterm birth (Hankins & Suarez, 2004; Warren & Silver, 2004).

Medical therapy is kept to a minimum in women who are in remission or who have a mild form of SLE. Nonsteroidal antiinflammatory drugs (NSAIDs) and aspirin are ordinarily the most commonly used antiinflammatory drugs, but are not recommended in pregnancy. Steroids such as hydrocortisone, prednisone, or prednisolone may be used because they pose minimal risk to the fetus. Other immunosuppressive drugs are not recommended during pregnancy. Nursing care focuses on early recognition of signs of SLE exacerbation and pregnancy complications, education and support of the woman and her family, and assessment of fetal well-being.

Vaginal birth is preferred. Corticosteroid therapy should be administered to women who are currently receiving steroids. During labor, efforts are aimed at reducing the risk of infection, which is the leading cause of death in women with SLE.

During the postpartum period, the mother should rest as much as possible to prevent an exacerbation of SLE. Breastfeeding is encouraged unless the mother is taking immunosuppressive agents. Family planning is important. Oral contraceptives are used with caution because vascular disease commonly accompanies SLE. Intrauterine devices may increase the risk of infection. Barrier methods such as the diaphragm, the condom, and spermicides should be considered (Laskin, 2004).

Myasthenia Gravis

Myasthenia gravis (MG), an autoimmune motor (muscle) end-plate disorder that involves acetylcholine use, affects the motor function at the myoneural junction. Muscle weakness results, particularly of the eyes, the face, the tongue, the neck, the limbs, and the respiratory muscles. In addition, women may experience ptosis, diplopia, and dysphagia. Women are affected twice as often as men, with incidence peaking between the ages of 20 and 30 years (Samuels, 2002a). The response of women with MG to pregnancy is unpredictable; remission, exacerbation, or continued stability during pregnancy may occur.

Treatment is the same as for a nonpregnant woman. Usual medications include immunosuppressive medications and acetylcholinesterase inhibitors. Monitoring blood glucose values is important because hyperglycemia may be the result of corticosteroid therapy. Thymectomy may result in remission of the disease but is best performed before or after pregnancy, if at all possible. For severe weakness, plasmapheresis or IV immunoglobulin therapy may be needed.

Women with MG usually tolerate labor well, but vacuum or forceps assistance for birth may be required because of muscle weakness. Oxytocin may be given, but magnesium sulfate is contraindicated because it inhibits the release of acetylcholine. Narcotic analgesia may be used with careful monitoring. Regional analgesia is preferred. After birth, women must be carefully supervised because relapses often occur during the puerperium.

In approximately 10% to 25% of neonates, neonatal myasthenia develops, with symptoms of feeble cry, poor sucking, and rarely respiratory distress. With proper management, complete recovery of the neonate should occur within 3 to 15 weeks.

Gastrointestinal Disorders

Compromise of GI function during pregnancy is a concern. Obvious physiologic alterations, such as the greatly enlarged uterus, and less apparent changes, such as hormonal differences and *hypochlorhydria* (deficiency of hydrochloric acid in the stomach's gastric juice), require understanding for proper diagnosis and treatment. Gallbladder disease is an example of a GI disorder that may occur during pregnancy.

Cholelithiasis and Cholecystitis

Women are twice as likely to have cholelithiasis (presence of gallstones in the gallbladder) as are men, and pregnancy seems to make the woman more vulnerable to gallstone formation (Blackburn, 2003), with 1 in 1000 pregnant women developing cholelithiasis (Cunningham et al., 2005). Decreased muscle tone allows gallbladder distention, thickening of the bile, and prolonged emptying time. Increased progesterone levels result in a slight hypercholesterolemia.

Cholecystitis (inflammation of the gallbladder) also is more common in pregnancy, probably because pressure of the enlarged uterus interferes with the normal circulation and drainage of the gallbladder. The incidence of acute cholecystitis is about 0.02% to 0.16%, most often seen in multiparous women who have a history of previous attacks. Gallbladder disease is the second most common indication for nonobstetric surgical intervention in pregnancy (Angelini, 2002).

Women with acute cholecystitis usually have fatty food intolerance along with colicky abdominal pain radiating to the back or shoulder, nausea, and vomiting (see Teaching for Self-Care box). Fever and an increased leukocyte count also may be present. Ultrasound is often used to detect the presence of stones or dilation of the common bile duct (Samuels, 2002b). Obese multiparous women are usually without symptoms.

Generally, gallbladder surgery should be postponed until the puerperium. Usually the woman can be treated with medical therapy, consisting of antibiotics, analgesics, intravenous fluids, bowel rest, and nasogastric suctioning. Total parenteral nutrition (TPN) can be used in some cases as an alternative to surgery. Morphine should

---

TEACHING FOR SELF-CARE

Nutritional Counseling for the Pregnant Woman with Cholecystitis or Cholelithiasis

- Assess your diet for foods that cause discomfort and flatulence, and omit foods that trigger episodes.
- Reduce dietary fat intake to 40 to 50 g/day.
- Limit protein to 10% to 12% of total calories.
- Choose foods so that most of the calories come from carbohydrates.
- Prepare food without adding fats or oils as much as possible.
- Avoid fried foods.

not be used as an analgesic because it may cause ductal spasm. The woman's condition should improve significantly within 48 hours of beginning treatment. Surgery may be necessary if the woman has repeated attacks of biliary colic, acute cholecystitis, obstructive jaundice, peritonitis, or pancreatitis. Laparoscopic cholecystectomy performed in the second trimester or even third semester increasingly appears to be safe (Samuels, 2002b). Other procedures performed may be endoscopic retrograde cholangiopancreatography (ERCP) or open cholecystectomy (Angelini, 2002).

Inflammatory Bowel Disease

The incidence of inflammatory bowel disease, particularly Crohn's disease and ulcerative colitis, is not increased in pregnancy (Cunningham et al., 2005). Active disease at conception may continue during pregnancy and worsen, with an increased risk of poor maternal-fetal outcomes (Cunningham et al.; Scott & Abu-Hamda, 2004). Treatment of inflammatory bowel disease is the same for the pregnant woman as it is for the nonpregnant woman. Medicines include prednisone and sulfasalazine. Fat-soluble vitamin and folic acid supplementation is especially important because of problems with intestinal malabsorption. With complications, such as hemorrhage, or if there is no response to medical therapy, surgery may be indicated (Cunningham et al.). Effects of inflammatory bowel disease on pregnancy are usually minimal; however, if the woman is severely debilitated, preterm birth, low birth weight, or fetal death can occur (Scott & Abu-Hamda).

Surgery During Pregnancy

The incidence of surgery requiring anesthesia during pregnancy ranges from 0.2% to 2.2% (Ludmir & Stubblefield, 2002). The need for abdominal surgery occurs as frequently among pregnant women as among nonpregnant women of comparable age. However, pregnancy may make the diagnosis more difficult. An enlarged uterus and displaced internal organs may make abdominal palpation more difficult, alter the position of an affected organ, and/or change the usual signs and symptoms associated with a particular disorder. The most common condition necessitating abdominal surgery during pregnancy is appendicitis.

Appendicitis

Appendicitis occurs approximately once in 2000 pregnancies. This condition occurs in approximately the same frequency during each trimester of pregnancy and the postpartum period (Ludmir & Stubblefield, 2002). The diagnosis of appendicitis is often delayed because the usual signs and symptoms mimic some normal changes of pregnancy such as nausea and vomiting and increased white blood cell (WBC) count. As pregnancy progresses, the appendix is pushed upward and to the right from its usual anatomic location (see Fig. 14-14). Because of these changes, appendiceal rupture and peritonitis occur 2 to 3 times more often in pregnant women than in nonpregnant women.

Most commonly the woman with appendicitis is first seen with right lower quadrant abdominal pain, nausea and vomiting, and loss of appetite. Approximately half of these affected women have muscle guarding. Moving the uterus tends to increase the pain. Temperature may be normal or mildly increased (to 38.3° C). Because of the physiologic increase in WBCs that occurs in pregnancy, laboratory findings are not helpful in the diagnosis (Scott & Abu-Hamda, 2004).

The diagnosis of appendicitis requires a high level of suspicion because the typical signs and symptoms are similar to those found in many other conditions, including pyelonephritis, round ligament pain, placental abruption, torsion of an ovarian cyst, cholecystitis, and preterm labor (Ludmir & Stubblefield, 2002) (see Table 31-2).

Appendectomy before rupture usually does not require either antibiotic or tocolytic therapy. If surgery is delayed until after rupture, multiple antibiotics are ordered. Rupture is likely to result in preterm labor, perhaps necessitating the use of tocolytic agents.

Collaborative Care

Initial assessment of the pregnant woman requiring surgery focuses on her presenting signs and symptoms. A thorough history and physical examination are performed. Laboratory testing includes, at a minimum, a complete blood count with differential and a urinalysis. Additional laboratory and other diagnostic tests may well be necessary to reach a diagnosis. In addition, fetal heart rate (FHR) and activity, along with uterine activity, should be monitored, and constant vigilance for symptoms of impending obstetric complications maintained. The extent of presurgery assessment is determined by the immediacy of surgical intervention and the specific disorder that requires surgery.

Hospital Care. When surgery becomes necessary during pregnancy, the woman and her family are concerned about the effects of the procedure and medication on fetal well-being and the course of pregnancy. An important part of preoperative nursing care is encouraging the woman to express her fears, concerns, and questions.

Preoperative care for a pregnant woman differs from that for a nonpregnant woman in one significant aspect: the presence of at least one other person, the fetus. Continuous FHR and uterine contraction monitoring should be performed if the fetus is considered viable. Procedures such as preparation of the operative site and time of insertion of IV lines and urinary retention catheters vary with the physician and the facility. However, in every instance, there is a total restriction of solid foods and liquids or a clear specification of the type, amount, and time at which clear liquids may be taken before surgery. Some bowel preparation such as clear liquids and laxatives may be required before surgery. Food by mouth is restricted for several hours before a scheduled procedure. Even if she has had nothing by mouth—but more important, if surgery is unexpected—the woman is in danger of vomiting and aspirating, and special precautions are taken before anesthetic is administered (e.g., administering an antacid).

Intraoperatively, perinatal nurses may collaborate with the surgical staff to increase their knowledge about the special needs of pregnant women undergoing surgery. One intervention to improve fetal oxygenation is positioning the woman on the operating table with a lateral tilt to avoid maternal venacaval compression. Continuous fetal and uterine monitoring during the procedure is recommended because of the risk for preterm labor. Monitoring may be accomplished by using sterile aquasonic gel and a sterile sleeve for the transducer. During abdominal surgery, uterine contractions may be manually palpated.

In the immediate recovery period, general observations and care pertinent to postoperative recovery are initiated. Frequent assessments are carried out for several hours after surgery. Whether the woman is cared for in the surgical postanesthesia recovery area or in a labor and birth unit, continuous fetal and uterine monitoring will likely be initiated or resumed because of the increased risk of preterm labor. Tocolysis may be necessary if preterm labor occurs (see Chapter 36).

Home Care. Plans for the woman's return home and for convalescent care should be completed as early as possible before discharge. Depending on her insurance coverage, nursing care may be provided through a home health agency. If not, the woman and other support persons must be taught necessary skills and procedures, such as wound care. Ideally, the woman and other caregivers should have opportunities for supervised practice before discharge so that they can feel comfortable with their knowledge and ability before being totally responsible for providing care. Box 33-5 lists information that should be included in discharge teaching for the postoperative client. The woman also may need referrals to various community agencies for evaluation of the home situation, child care, home health care, and financial or other assistance.

---

box 33-5 | Discharge Teaching for Home Care

- Care of incision site
- Diet and elimination related to gastrointestinal (GI) function
- Signs and symptoms of developing complications: wound infection, thrombophlebitis, pneumonia
- Equipment needed and technique for assessing temperature
- Recommended schedule for resumption of activities of daily living
- Treatments and medications ordered
- List of resource persons and their telephone numbers
- Schedule of follow-up visits

If birth has not occurred:
- Assessment of fetal activity (daily fetal movement count)
- Signs of preterm labor

---

community activity

Contact the local chapter of the American Heart Association to collect data on what information is available for women who have heart defects and are considering pregnancy. What resources are available for preconception counseling for women of childbearing age who are concerned about the effect of a cardiac defect on a potential pregnancy? How can women access this information?

---

key points

- The stress of the normal maternal adaptations to pregnancy on a heart whose function is already taxed may cause cardiac decompensation.
- In the case of a cardiac arrest in a pregnant woman, the standard advanced cardiac life support guidelines should be implemented with a few slight modifications: the uterus must be displaced laterally, and the defibrillation paddles should be placed one rib interspace higher.
- Maternal morbidity and mortality is a significant risk in a pregnancy complicated by mitral stenosis.
- The normal hemodynamic values are significantly altered as a result of pregnancy.
- Anemia, the most common medical disorder of pregnancy, affects at least 20% of pregnant women.
- Asthma is the most common respiratory crisis complicating pregnancy.
- Pruritus is a common symptom in pregnancy-specific inflammatory skin diseases.
- Epilepsy is the most common neurologic disorder of pregnancy and can be confused with eclampsia; however, a history of seizures and no signs of preeclampsia point to epilepsy.
- Cholecystitis and cholelithiasis are common gastrointestinal problems in pregnancy.
- Autoimmune disorders (e.g., SLE, MG) show a predilection for women in their reproductive years; therefore associations with pregnancy are not uncommon.
- In the pregnant woman, an enlarged uterus, displaced internal organs, and altered laboratory values may confound differential diagnosis when the need for immediate abdominal surgery occurs.
- Preoperative care for a pregnant woman differs from that for a nonpregnant woman in one significant aspect: the presence of at least one other person, the fetus.

REFERENCES

American Heart Association Science Advisory. (2000). Assessment of functional capacity in clinical and research applications. *Circulation, 102*(13), 1591-1597.

American Heart Association (AHA). (2005). American Heart Association guidelines for cardiopulmonary resuscitation and emergency cardiovascular care, Part 10.8: Cardiac arrest associated with pregnancy. *Circulation, 112*(24 Suppl), IV-150-IV-153.

Aminoff, M. (2004). Neurologic disorders. In R. Creasy, R. Resnik & J. Iams (Eds.), *Maternal-fetal medicine: Principles and practice* (5th ed.). Philadelphia: Saunders.

Angelini, D. (2002). Gallbladder and pancreatic disease during pregnancy. *Journal of Perinatal and Neonatal Nursing, 15*(4), 1-12.

Bandi, V., Munnar, V., & Matthay, M. (2004). Acute lung injury and acute respiratory distress syndrome in pregnancy. *Critical Care Clinics, 20*(4), 577-607.

Blackburn, S. (2003). *Maternal, fetal, and neonatal physiology: A clinical perspective* (2nd ed.). St. Louis: Saunders.

Blanchard, D., & Shabetai, R. (2004). Cardiac diseases. In R. Creasy, R. Resnik, & J. Iams (Eds.), *Maternal-fetal medicine: Principles and practice* (5th ed.), Philadelphia: Saunders.

Cohen, R., Talwar, A., & Efferen, L. (2004). Exacerbation of underlying pulmonary disease in pregnancy. *Critical Care Clinics, 20*(4), 713-730.

Constantino, T., & Varner, M. (2004). Seizures and status epilepticus. In G. Dildy, M. Belfort, G. Saade, J. Phelan, G. Hankins, & S. Clark, (Eds.), *Critical care obstetrics* (4th ed.). Malden, MA: Blackwell Science.

Conversation with Colleagues. (2005). Treating asthma in pregnant women. *AWHONN Lifelines, 9*(2), 123-124.

Cunningham, G., Leveno, K., Bloom, S., Hauth, J., Gilstrap, L., & Wenstrom, K. (Eds.). (2005). *Williams obstetrics* (22nd ed.). New York: McGraw-Hill.

Danik, S., & Fuster, V. (2004). Anticoagulation in pregnant women with prosthetic heart valves. *The Mount Sinai Journal of Medicine, 7*(15), 322-329.

Donaldson, J., & Duffy, T. (2004). Neurologic complications. In G. Burrow, T. Duffy, and J. Copel (Eds.), *Medical complications during pregnancy* (6th ed.). Philadelphia: Saunders.

Easterling, T., & Otto, C. (2002). Heart disease. In S. Gabbe, J. Niebyl, & J. Simpson (Eds.), *Obstetrics: Normal and problem pregnancies* (4th ed.). New York: Churchill Livingstone.

Eklayam, U., Singh, H., Irani, A., Akhter, M. (2004). Anticoagulation in pregnant women with prosthetic heart valves. *Journal of Cardiovascular Pharmacology and Therapeutics, 9*(2), 107-115.

Foley, M. (2004). Cardiac disease. In G. Dildy, M. Belfort, G. Saade, J. Phelan, G. Hankins, & S. Clark (Eds.), *Critical care obstetrics* (4th ed.). Malden, MA: Blackwell Science.

Gardner, M., & Doyle, N. (2004). Asthma in pregnancy. *Obstetrics and Gynecology Clinics of North America, 31*(2), 385-413.

Gei, A., & Hankins, G. (2001). Cardiac disease and pregnancy. *Obstetrics and Gynecology Clinics of North America, 28*(3), 465-512.

Gilbert, E., & Harmon, J. (2003). *Manual of high risk pregnancy & delivery* (3rd ed.). St. Louis: Mosby.

Gluck, J., & Gluck, P. (2005). Asthma controller therapy during pregnancy. *American Journal of Obstetrics and Gynecology, 192*(2), 369-380.

Guy, E., Kirumaki, A., & Hanania, N. (2004). Acute asthma in pregnancy. *Critical Care Clinics, 20*(4), 731-745.

Hankins, G., & Suarez, V. (2004). Rheumatologic and connective tissue disorders. In R. Creasy, R. Resnik, & J. Iams (Eds.), *Maternal-fetal medicine: Principles and practice* (5th ed.). Philadelphia: Saunders.

Hueppchen, N., & Satin, A. (2004). Cardiopulmonary resuscitation. In G. Dildy, M. Belfort, G. Saade, J. Phelan, G. Hankins, & S. Clark, (Eds.), *Critical care obstetrics* (4th ed.). Malden, MA: Blackwell Science.

Kilpatrick. S., & Laros, R. (2004). Maternal hematologic disorders. In R. Creasy, R. Resnik, & J. Iams (Eds.), *Maternal-fetal medicine: Principles and practice* (5th ed.). Philadelphia: Saunders.

Klein, L., & Galan, H. (2004). Cardiac disease in pregnancy. *Obstetrics and Gynecology Clinics of North America, 31*(2), 429-459.

Laskin, C. (2004). Pregnancy and the rheumatic diseases. In G. Burrow, T. Duffy, & J. Copel (Eds.), *Medical complications during pregnancy* (6th ed.). Philadelphia: Saunders.

Lawrence, R., & Lawrence, R. (2005). *Breastfeeding: A guide for the medical profession* (6th ed.). Philadelphia: Mosby.

Ludmir, J. & Stubblefield, P. (2002). Surgical procedures in pregnancy. In S. Gabbe, J. Niebyl, & J. Simpson (Eds.), *Obstetrics: Normal and problem pregnancies* (4th ed.). New York: Churchill Livingstone.

Mallampalli, A., Powner, D., & Gardner, M. (2004). Cardiopulmonary resuscitation and somatic support of the pregnant patient. *Critical Care Clinics, 20*(4), 747-761.

Maloni, J., Brezinski-Tomasi, J., & Johnson, L. (2001). Antepartum bed rest: Effect upon the family. *Journal of Obstetric, Gynecologic, and Neonatal Nursing, 30*(2), 67-77.

Mendelson, M., & Lang, R. (2000). Pregnancy and cardiovascular disease. In W. Barron & M. Lindheimer (Eds.), *Medical disorders during pregnancy* (3rd ed.). Philadelphia: Mosby.

Moore, L., & Martin, J. (2004). Sickle-cell crisis. In G. Dildy, M. Belfort, G. Saade, J. Phelan, G. Hankins, & S. Clark (Eds.), *Critical care obstetrics* (4th ed.). Malden, MA: Blackwell Science.

Morris, S., & Stacey, M. (2005). Resuscitation in pregnancy. *BMJ, 327* (7426), 1277-1279.

Murdock, M. (2002). Asthma in pregnancy. *Journal of Perinatal and Neonatal Nursing, 15*(4), 27-36.

Poole, J. (2003). Thalassemia and pregnancy. *Journal of Perinatal and Neonatal Nursing, 17*(3), 196-208.

Pschirrer, E. (2004). Seizure disorders in pregnancy. *Obstetrics and Gynecology Clinics of North America, 31*(2), 373-384.

Rappaport, V., Velazquez, M., & Williams, K. (2004). Hemoglobinopathies in pregnancy. *Obstetrics and Gynecology Clinics of North America, 31*(2), 287-317.

Samuels, P. (2002a). Collagen vascular diseases. In S. Gabbe, J. Niebyl, & J. Simpson (Eds.), *Obstetrics: Normal and problem pregnancies* (4th ed.). New York: Churchill Livingstone.

Samuels, P. (2002b). Hepatic disease. In S. Gabbe, J. Niebyl & J. Simpson (Eds.), *Obstetrics: Normal and problem pregnancies* (4th ed.). New York: Churchill Livingstone.

Scott, L., & Abu-Hamda, E. (2004). Gastrointestinal disease in pregnancy. In R. Creasy, R. Resnik, & J. Iams (Eds.), *Maternal-fetal medicine: Principles and practice* (5th ed.). Philadelphia: Saunders.

Setaro, J., & Caulin-Glaser, T. (2004). Pregnancy and cardiovascular disease. In G. Burrow, T. Duffy, & J. Copel (Eds.), *Medical complications during pregnancy* (6th ed.). Philadelphia: Saunders.

Shehata, H., & Okosun, H. (2004). Neurologic disorders in pregnancy. *Current Opinion in Obstetrics and Gynecology, 16*(2), 117-122.

Stambuk, R., & Colvin, R. (2002). Dermatologic disorders. In S. Gabbe, J. Niebyl, & J. Simpson (Eds.), *Obstetrics: Normal and problem pregnancies* (4th ed.). New York: Churchill Livingstone.

Veldtman, G., Connolly, H., Grogan, M., Ammash, N., & Warnes, C. (2004). Outcomes of pregnancy in women with Tetralogy of Fallot. *Journal of the American College of Cardiology, 44*(1), 174-180.

Warren, J., & Silver, R. (2004). Autoimmune disease in pregnancy: Systemic lupus erythematosus and antiphospholipid syndrome. *Obstetrics and Gynecology Clinics of North America, 31*(2), 345-372.

Weiner, C., & Buhimschi, C. (2004). *Drugs for pregnant and lactating women.* New York: Churchill Livingstone.

Whitty, J., & Dombrowski, M. (2004). Respiratory diseases in pregnancy. In R. Creasy, R. Resnik, & J. Iams (Eds.), *Maternal-fetal medicine: Principles and practice* (5th ed.). Philadelphia: Saunders.

Obstetric Critical Care

learning objectives

- Discuss factors that have contributed to the development of the specialty of critical care obstetrics.
- Describe conditions that may place a pregnant woman in a critically ill state.
- Examine factors that affect the provision of obstetric critical care when a pregnant woman becomes critically ill.
- Describe significant cardiovascular, pulmonary, and hematologic alterations during pregnancy that affect critical care for the pregnant woman.
- Describe the parameters measured and normal values for pulmonary artery and arterial pressure monitoring.
- Identify treatment strategies based on interpretation of hemodynamic profiles.
- Identify physiologic alterations of pregnancy that affect stabilization and treatment of the pregnant woman who has undergone trauma.
- Describe immediate assessment and stabilization measures for the pregnant victim of trauma.
- Compare components of the primary and secondary surveys for the pregnant woman who has undergone trauma.
- Discuss inclusion of the components of family-centered maternity care for the critically ill pregnant woman.
- Examine the impact of maternal death on families and nursing staff members who cared for the woman.

electronic resources

Additional information related to the content in Chapter 34 can be found on

the companion website at **evolve**
http://evolve.elsevier.com/Lowdermilk/MWHC/
- NCLEX Review Questions
- WebLinks

or on the interactive companion CD
- NCLEX Review Questions

*O*BSTETRIC and critical care units are equally challenged whenever presented with the multiple, complex needs of a critically ill pregnant woman and her fetus. Optimal outcome for mother and fetus depends on (1) swift recognition of severe complications and (2) delivery of critical care therapies adjusted for the physiologic alterations of pregnancy. Fetal effects of therapies also must be considered. Management of the critically ill pregnant woman includes measures to assess both maternal and fetal status continually, selection of therapeutic interventions appropriate for both mother and fetus, and careful management for the timing of birth.

The provision of critical care and hemodynamic monitoring for the seriously ill pregnant woman has developed slowly in many institutions. This seems to have been the result of two factors: (1) obstetric nurses and physicians, expert in the care of pregnant women, feel threatened by pressure transducers, alarms, hemodynamic monitoring,

and ventilators; and (2) critical care nurses and physicians, expert in hemodynamic monitoring and mechanical ventilation, feel threatened by the pregnant uterus, labor, birth, the fetus, and fetal monitoring. The result is that few institutions have been able to provide optimal care whenever a sudden, acute, life-threatening complication has occurred in a pregnant woman.

■ OBSTETRIC INTENSIVE CARE UNIT

Critical care obstetrics evolved as a subspecialty of perinatal medicine in response to the need for optimal care for the critically ill pregnant woman and her fetus. This subspecialty prepares the obstetric team, which has in-depth knowledge of pregnancy, to use critical care techniques in the management of the critically ill pregnant woman and her fetus. Obstetric intensive care units (OBICUs) have been developed in some centers so that expensive, specific equipment and individuals with special training and expertise in obstetric care and critical care are available to provide this care.

Complications may develop during pregnancy that are so severe and life threatening that optimal maternal and fetal outcome, and many times survival, depend on the woman receiving critical care that meets her specific needs. Maternal adaptations that are normal for the pregnancy state alter physiologic status and make the pregnant woman hemodynamically different from the nonpregnant woman.

Before the development of OBICUs, care for the critically ill pregnant woman was usually provided in an ICU for adults, where management modalities were based on hemodynamic values that are normal for the nonpregnant individual but resulted in less than desirable outcomes for pregnant women. Research in some of the first OBICUs reported on physical and hemodynamic differences during the pregnant state. Normal hemodynamic values for pregnancy were identified. Maternal and fetal outcomes improved when management of care was based on the enhanced hemodynamic state that accompanies normal pregnancy and care was provided in the specialized units (Mabie & Sibai, 1990).

▬ PROVISION OF OBSTETRIC ▬ CRITICAL CARE

Anyone providing care for pregnant women may encounter the pregnant woman with a life-threatening complication and be challenged to recognize the need for immediate, critical care and to provide such care. This care may be delivered in a variety of ways. Problems can be decreased by development of a viable plan to provide care for the critically ill pregnant woman; adequate education of nursing, medical, and ancillary staff; provision of necessary equipment at the bedside; and liberal consultation between the obstetric and critical care units.

The most practical, efficient, and economic method to provide care for the critically ill obstetric client who requires invasive hemodynamic monitoring, mechanical ventilation, or both depends primarily on the numbers of pregnant women cared for annually and the referral patterns in a specific facility. The ideal method to provide care for the pregnancy would be a specially trained team of obstetricians and obstetric nurses in an OBICU, augmented by anesthesiologists, pulmonologists, cardiologists, and intensivists as needed. The larger tertiary center is more likely to have this type of unit because the census of pregnant women cared for annually in the referral center would support development of the service. OBICUs are often small and may consist of one bed. Admissions may be limited only to the very sickest women and may not include all women eligible for a bed in the OBICU.

However, even in many large, tertiary centers, the number of truly critically ill pregnant women is not enough to warrant such an investment in equipment and training of medical staff. In these centers, collaborative practice between obstetrics and intensive care has been successful in providing the best care for these women (Zeeman, Wendel, & Cunningham, 2003). If the woman remains pregnant, the optimal place for her is the labor and birth suite, with a critical care nurse in attendance. However, the ICU is the most usual site for this collaborative care. In this instance, obstetric practitioners serve a vital role in monitoring the woman as well as assessing the fetus. The institution must develop policies and procedures so that care is provided where it is most advantageous to the pregnant woman. Some institutions provide dual training for selected nurses (i.e., an ICU nurse receives advanced education in obstetrics or an obstetric nurse receives advanced education in intensive care nursing).

▬ LEGAL TIP   Nursing Assignments

Continuous assignment of an obstetric and an intensive care nurse, or one nurse experienced in both specialties, is required in the care of the critically ill woman with a viable pregnancy.

In still other institutions, an obstetric service may be established to provide care during the low risk pregnancy. The plan for the smaller unit or the low risk unit may be for the nursing and medical team to recognize the critical illness immediately, stabilize the woman, and initiate measures for transport to the tertiary center and/or the OBICU. *Standards and Guidelines for Professional Nursing Practice in the Care of Women and Newborns* (Association of Women's Health, Obstetric and Neonatal Nurses [AWHONN], 2003) includes guidelines for the care of the pregnant woman requiring critical care.

▬ LEGAL TIP   Client Care Standards

Client care standards established for both obstetric care and intensive care must be met within the plan developed by an institution to provide complex, critical care for the critically ill pregnant woman. Standards of care from both specialties must be followed.

Obstetric clients requiring critical care are at risk for undesirable outcomes of the pregnancy because of the severity of complications, including decreased oxygen transport and multiple system organ failure and the possibility of long-term residual physical effects of the illness.

▬ LEGAL TIP   Legal Review

Because an optimal outcome is uncertain when the pregnant woman is critically ill, the medical records, with documentation of the medical and nursing care that mother, fetus, and neonate received, are more likely to be subjected to legal review than are medical records of other clients.

▬ EQUIPMENT AND EXPERTISE

The usual equipment for a labor, birth, and recovery suite is mandatory for an ICU or surgical suite where this woman may be admitted for care. Staff and equipment for neonatal resuscitation must also be available. The usual equipment for intensive care, including hemodynamic monitoring and mechanical ventilation, is equally necessary whenever the critically ill client is in the labor and birth unit.

Obstetric critical care may be delivered according to individual plans developed by individual institutions on the basis of a needs assessment. However, it is imperative that all institutions providing care for pregnant women have a plan and staff educated to care for the occasional woman who has a life-threatening complication during pregnancy. Pregnant women with a critical complication must receive the care needed; critical care must not be denied to pregnant women. Pregnancy is not a contraindication for invasive hemodynamic monitoring.

INDICATIONS FOR OBSTETRIC CRITICAL CARE

A severe complication of pregnancy may prompt the need for obstetric critical care with hemodynamic monitoring or mechanical ventilation. See Box 34-1 for a list of complications that indicate a need for critical care.

The number of pregnant women who need obstetric critical care has increased in recent years. This apparently is the result of women surviving childhood illnesses because of advances in pediatric care. These include the development of pediatric ICUs; improved surgical procedures for infants with congenital defects, such as cardiac lesions; and advanced knowledge in pediatric care for children with chronic health problems, including diabetes, cystic fibrosis, and pulmonary disorders. The wish to become a parent is not eliminated by a chronic health problem, and many women each year risk their lives to have a baby. Women have had successful pregnancies after kidney transplants (Hou, 2003; Sgro et al., 2002), after heart transplants (Cowan et al., 2002), and after liver transplants (Miller, Mastrobattista, & Katz, 2000). More pregnant women with chronic health problems are predicted as graduates of neonatal ICUs reach adulthood.

Other pregnant women need critical care because of trauma resulting from automobile crashes or violence and battering. These causes account for most of the traumatic injuries during pregnancy.

The most common diagnosis for admission to an OBICU is severe preeclampsia with complications including refractory pulmonary edema, refractory oliguria, hypertensive crisis, severe hemorrhage or disseminated intravascular coagulation (DIC), and renal failure. Massive hemorrhage or DIC is reported as the second most common reason for admission (Zeeman et al., 2003). Conditions that classify the parturient as critically ill and indicate the need for a pulmonary artery catheter include the following (American College of Obstetricians and Gynecologists [ACOG], 1992):

- Sepsis with refractory hypotension or oliguria
- Unexplained or refractory pulmonary edema, congestive heart failure, or oliguria
- Severe preeclampsia with pulmonary edema or refractory oliguria
- Intraoperative or intrapartum cardiovascular decompensation
- Massive blood loss or volume replacement needs
- Adult respiratory distress syndrome
- Shock of undefined source
- Chronic disease, particularly when associated with labor or major surgery

The identification of women needing OBICU services merits careful consideration. It is important not to visualize just the "sickest client scenario"—that dramatic case, never to be forgotten. Instead, the typical picture of a critically ill pregnant woman is one with severe preeclampsia, whose condition has worsened and today has headache, high blood pressure (BP), oliguria, and low platelets. Or, the woman may be sent in for referral from the level I center with a preexisting cardiac lesion exacerbated by pregnancy that has gradually deteriorated from class I to class III cardiac disease. Her presenting complaint may be "feeling extremely tired."

CARDIORESPIRATORY CHANGES OF PREGNANCY

The normal physiologic adaptations that accompany pregnancy and produce profound hemodynamic changes are the primary factors that make the pregnant woman a different type of critical care client and merit a separate critical care facility. Knowledge of the effects of the physiologic alterations during pregnancy is essential for optimal critical care management. Normal maternal alterations during pregnancy affect the major systems: the cardiovascular, pulmonary, renal, and hematologic systems (Norwitz, Robinson, & Malone, 2004).

---

box 34-1 | **Complications of Pregnancy That Indicate the Need for Critical Care**

- Severe preeclampsia or eclampsia with complications
  - Refractory pulmonary edema
  - Refractory oliguria
  - Hypertensive crisis
  - Severe hemorrhage or disseminated intravascular coagulation (DIC)
  - Renal failure
- Hemorrhage or DIC that requires multiple transfusions
- Cardiac problems

- Chronic health problems
  - Systemic lupus erythematosus
  - Diabetic ketoacidosis
  - Sickle cell disease
  - Diabetes complicated by vascular changes
  - Others
- Trauma victim
  - Motor vehicle crash
  - Violence, battering

EVIDENCE-BASED PRACTICE

Can Aspirin Prevent Preeclampsia?

BACKGROUND

- Preeclampsia is a significant problem, particularly in vulnerable populations and developing countries. Deficient placental implantation probably leads to poor perfusion and ischemia, resulting in a generalized inflammatory response and platelet activation. The inflammation causes endothelial damage, narrowing of the arteries, and subsequent hypertension, greater than 170 mm Hg systolic or 110 mm Hg diastolic. Preeclampsia can affect the liver, the kidneys, the brain, and the clotting systems in the mother, and cause low birth weight and prematurity in the infant. Late symptoms include headache, epigastric pain, visual changes, and feeling unwell. Severe preeclampsia can lead to seizures, and even maternal and perinatal death.

- Interest in antiplatelet therapy, especially low-dose aspirin, followed some small, successful trials. Several systemic reviews established the safety of low-dose aspirin, but efficacy and dosing are still controversial, as is which clients benefit the most. Several other therapies in use, including calcium, protein, magnesium sulfate (see the Evidence-Based Practice box in Chapter 30), nutritional advice, fish oil, and antioxidants (see the Evidence-Based Practice box in Chapter 15) are promising, but not proven.

OBJECTIVES

- The authors sought to examine the risks and benefits of antiplatelet therapy (aspirin) for prevention of preeclampsia. Their interest was to establish the benefits of treatment of high risk (previous severe preeclampsia, diabetes, chronic hypertension, or autoimmune disease) versus moderate risk women, onset of therapy, and dosing. They planned a separate review of treatment for preeclampsia.

METHODS

Search Strategy

- The authors searched the Cochrane Pregnancy and Childbirth Group trials register and conference proceedings. They identified 51 randomized controlled trials representing 36,500 women from 24 countries on every major continent, mostly Europe and North America.

Statistical Analyses

- Similar data were pooled. Reviewers calculated relative risk for dichotomous (categoric) data, such as type of birth, and weighted mean difference for continuous data, such as weeks

of gestation. Differences between groups outside the 95% confidence interval were accepted as significant. All were analyzed in their original randomly assigned "intention to treat" categories, even if they changed their minds.

FINDINGS

- Low-dose aspirin did not prevent gestational hypertension, except for high risk women. It did, however, reduce preeclampsia by 19% overall. Aspirin doses of greater than 75 mg were more beneficial than lower doses. There was a 7% reduction in preterm birth, an 8% reduction in small-for-gestational-age births, and 16% fewer perinatal deaths with aspirin therapy over placebo. There was no difference noted for eclampsia, placental abruption, maternal deaths, cesarean births, induction, neonatal intensive care unit admission, or neonatal bleeding.

LIMITATIONS

- Small trials showing negative effects of aspirin may have gone against the general moral, intellectual, and cultural climate of the 1980s and 1990s, and so may not have been published, and may be missing from this review. The onset of aspirin therapy may have to be during the first half of pregnancy to show certain threshold benefits. Doses varied, so the division of greater than or less than 75 mg may not have shown true benefits for certain women. The definition of high risk varied among countries and across decades.

IMPLICATIONS FOR PRACTICE

- Women may worry about taking aspirin during pregnancy, against conventional wisdom, but the nurse can reassure women that aspirin has been shown to safely prevent preeclampsia and its adverse outcomes, especially in high risk women. The woman should be instructed to not exceed the dosage, and to take acetaminophen, not more aspirin, if she requires pain relief. Aspirin is a cost-efficient and available intervention, suitable for low-resource areas.

IMPLICATIONS FOR FURTHER RESEARCH

- Since aspirin is anticlotting, more information is needed on the outcome of aspirin therapy on maternal hemorrhage. More studies of early intervention (before 12 weeks of gestation) and with higher doses are needed to establish safety and efficacy for low and high risk women.

Reference: Duley, L., Henderson-Smart, D., Knight, M., & King, J. (2003). Antiplatelet agents for preventing pre-eclampsia and its complications. *The Cochrane Database for Systematic Reviews*, 2006, Issue 3. Chichester, UK: John Wiley & Sons.

Cardiovascular Changes

The cardiovascular system changes dramatically during pregnancy. Pregnancy is a state of high flow and low resistance, so that pregnancy is hemodynamically similar to early sepsis. Hypervolemia is the result of the influence of estrogen and progesterone on aldosterone, which produces an increase in circulating blood volume. The increase in maternal blood volume begins with a 22% increase by 8 weeks of gestation. Total expansion increases progressively to a maximum of

45% by 32 to 34 weeks of gestation. This represents an increase of approximately 1570 ml for the singleton gestation. This includes a 40% to 50% increase in plasma volume and a 20% to 30% increase in red blood cell mass, a disproportional increase that results in a state of hemodilution. An increase in total body water of 6 to 8 L in the extravascular compartment, accompanied by an accumulation of 500 to 900 mEq of sodium, also occurs during pregnancy. Heart rate (HR) increases 20% (10 to 15 beats/min) with the major

table 34-1 Cardiovascular Changes During Pregnancy

PARAMETER	CHANGE
Blood volume	40%-50% increase
Plasma volume	40%-50% increase (1200-1300 ml)
Red blood cell mass	20%-30% increase (250-450 ml)
Heart	Displaced to the left and upward
Point of maximal intensity (PMI)	Fourth intercostal space and lateral
Rate	20% increase (10-15 beats/min)
Sounds	Exaggerated splitting first sound
	Systolic murmur usually present
	Third sound present
Stroke volume	32% increase by 20-24 wk
Cardiac output	Increases by 30%-50%
	22% increase by 28 wk
	43% increase by term
	Increases during labor
	≤3 cm, 17% increase
	4-7 cm, 23% increase
	≥8 cm, 34% increase

Source: Norwitz E., Robinson, J., & Malone, F. (2004). Pregnancy-induced physiologic alterations. In G. Dildy, M. Belfort, G. Saade, J. Phelan, G. Hankins, & S. Clark (Eds.). *Critical care obstetrics* (4th ed.). Malden, MA: Blackwell Science.

increase in the third trimester, and stroke volume increases to accommodate the increased circulating volume. See Table 34-1 for a summary of cardiovascular adaptations.

Colloid Osmotic Pressure

Colloid osmotic pressure (COP) is the gradient controlling whether fluid remains inside the capillary or moves into the interstitial space. The force to keep the fluid inside the vessel is the pulling pressure of the colloids, or proteins, present in the plasma. The most important plasma proteins are albumin, globulin, and fibrinogen. Pregnancy produces a decrease in COP values resulting from the hemodilution state that reduces the concentration of plasma proteins. Severe preeclampsia usually produces renal damage, with a subsequent loss of proteins in the urine, further reducing the COP. The force exerted to push fluids through the membrane is the capillary hydrostatic pressure and is measured as the pulmonary capillary wedge pressure (PCWP). COP is measured with an oncometer. Colloid osmotic (oncotic) values in pregnancy are shown in Table 34-2. This measurement is not available in many institu-

table 34-2 Colloid Osmotic (Oncotic) Pressure Values

Nonpregnant	25.4 ± 2.3 mm Hg
Pregnant, antepartum	22.4 ± 0.54 mm Hg
Pregnant, postpartum	15.4 ± 2.1 mm Hg
Preeclampsia, antepartum	17.9 ± 0.68 mm Hg
Preeclampsia, postpartum	13.7 ± 0.46 mm Hg

tions; however, knowledge of this key concept is helpful in understanding one of the basic differences between pregnant and nonpregnant women. Pulmonary edema tends to develop in pregnant women at a lower PCWP than in those who are not pregnant and have a normal COP.

The lower the COP and the higher the PCWP, the more likely pulmonary edema is to develop, as reflected by a lower COP-PCWP gradient. COP-PCWP gradient values are as follows: nonpregnant, 14.5 ± 2.5; pregnant, 10.5 ± 2.7.

Pulmonary edema is more likely to develop in pregnancy. For example, the normal PCWP is 6 to 10 mm Hg during pregnancy and 4 to 9 mm Hg in the nonpregnant state (Clark et al., 1989). With a PCWP of 8, calculations of the COP-PCWP gradient show:
- Nonpregnant woman: COP of 25 − PCWP of 8 = 17 mm Hg
- Pregnant woman with severe preeclampsia: COP of 13 − PCWP of 8 = 5 mm Hg

Lower COP-PCWP gradients during pregnancy are usually caused by lower COP values occurring during pregnancy.

Respiratory Changes

Anatomic and physiologic alterations during pregnancy are necessary to supply adequate oxygenation to mother and fetus. A relative hyperventilation of pregnancy begins in the first trimester and increases 42% by term. Respiratory rate increases only slightly. Tidal volume and minute ventilations increase about 50% by term to meet increased oxygen consumption needs. The enlarging uterus pushes the diaphragm upward approximately 4 to 7 cm, reducing lung volume. Compensation is necessary to meet increased ventilatory demands, and the transverse diameter of the thorax increases 2 to 4 cm as the rib cage flares out. The functional residual capacity decreases 25% since more of the inhaled air is used, resulting in decreased reserve. These women become short of breath easily, as seen in walking or even light exercise. This can become critical if the oxygen demands of the pregnant woman increase. The hyperventilation of pregnancy is associated with a resting arterial carbon dioxide tension less than 30 mm Hg. Maternal alkalosis is prevented by the compensatory decrease in serum bicarbonate of about 4 mEq/L, from 26 to 22 mEq. During gestation, respiratory acidosis and metabolic acidosis develop more rapidly than in the nonpregnant state.

Normal arterial blood gas (ABG) values for pregnancy reflect a chronic state of compensated respiratory alkalosis, represented by a right shift in the oxyhemoglobin dissociation curve caused by the increased levels of 2,3-diphosphoglycerate from the high progesterone and estrogen levels present. Normal pregnancy values in comparison with those in the nonpregnant state are listed in Table 34-3.

Hematologic Changes

Pregnancy is a hypercoagulable state, as preparation is made for blood loss that accompanies childbirth. Table 34-4 gives a summary of alterations that enhance coagulation.

table 34-3 Arterial Blood Gas (ABG) Values

ABGS	NONPREGNANT	PREGNANT
pH	7.35-7.45	7.40-7.45
Po_2 (mm Hg)	80-100	104-108
Pco_2 (mm Hg)	35-42	27-32
Bicarbonate (HCO_3) (mEq/L)	26	18-31

table 34-4 Gestational Changes That Enhance Coagulation

Fibrinogen	Increased 30%-50% (from 300 to 480 mg/dl)
Coagulation factors VII-X	Increased
Fibrinolysis	Depressed

Bleeding and clotting times remain unchanged even when hypervolemia and hemodilution are present. The critically ill pregnant woman is at increased risk for thrombus formation whenever hemoconcentration develops, as occurs with severe preeclampsia or dehydration.

Systemic Vascular Resistance

Systemic vascular resistance (SVR) is a measure of the tension required for the ejection of blood into the circulation (afterload). To describe the physiologic relations between pressure and flow, measurements are made by the following formula as a ratio of pressure to flow:

$$SVR = \frac{[(MAP - CVP) \times 80]}{CO}$$

where MAP is mean arterial pressure (in millimeters of mercury), CVP is central venous pressure (in millimeters of mercury), and CO is cardiac output (in liters per minute).

Vasodilation of arterial vessels, a result of hormonal influences, and development of the uteroplacental circulation result in a decrease in SVR of 20% to 25% and a decrease in pulmonary vascular resistance of 40% during pregnancy. Systolic and diastolic blood pressures decrease during pregnancy, reaching the nadir at midtrimester, with a gradual return to prepregnancy values by term.

▬ HEMODYNAMIC MONITORING

Anatomic and Physiologic Characteristics of Circulation

An in-depth knowledge of normal functioning and hemodynamics of the cardiovascular system is the basis for understanding hemodynamic monitoring; therefore a review of these functions is included. The purpose of the cardiopulmonary system is to deliver oxygenated blood to the tissues throughout the body and to remove waste products through the dynamics of normal circulation as follows (Fig. 34-1).

Deoxygenated blood flows from the capillaries into the veins and the right side of the heart through the superior vena cava, draining the upper part of the body, and from

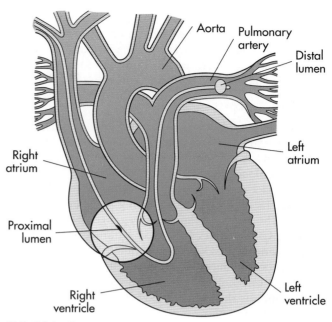

FIG. 34-1 Diagram of heart with position of pulmonary artery catheter.

the inferior vena cava, draining the lower part of the body. Venous blood flows into the right atrium, a holding chamber for the right side of the heart. When the atrium is filled, the tricuspid valve opens, and blood flows through this valve into the right ventricle.

When the right ventricle is filled, its muscles (myocardium) contract, and blood is ejected through the pulmonic valve into the pulmonary artery. Blood is pushed through the pulmonary artery and its branches to the capillary beds (pulmonary beds) in both lungs. Gas exchange occurs in the capillary beds as carbon dioxide is released and oxygen enters the circulation across the alveolar membrane.

Oxygenated blood drains from the pulmonary beds into the pulmonary veins, two from each lung, into the left atrium, the holding chamber for the left side of the heart. When the left atrium is filled, the mitral valve opens, and blood flows through this valve into the left ventricle. After the left ventricle is filled, the muscles of the left ventricle contract, and the oxygenated blood is ejected through the aortic valve into the aorta and then pumped throughout the systemic arterial system so that oxygen is supplied to the organs and tissues of the body.

Synchronization by the electrical conduction system of the myocardium causes the right and left atrial and ventricular contractions to occur simultaneously. The period of the cardiac cycle when both ventricles are relaxed and filling is termed *diastole,* and the period of the cardiac cycle when both ventricles contract is termed *systole.*

Left ventricle contractions must generate enough force to pump blood throughout the systemic circulation. Force required for right ventricular work is less because the right ventricle has to exert only enough force for blood to flow through the pulmonary circulation. Therefore the left ventricle is referred to as the *hemodynamic ventricle,* and the left side of the heart is referred to as the *hemodynamic heart.* Hemodynamic monitoring with a pulmonary artery catheter (PAC) provides left heart values, and during a critical illness, values of left heart function are more significant than are values of right heart function.

Cardiac Output

Cardiac output (CO) is the volume of blood ejected from the left ventricle in 1 minute; it is measured in liters per minute. CO is the product of stroke volume (SV), the volume of blood ejected from the left ventricle during one cardiac cycle, and heart rate (HR); thus CO = HR × SV. Because HR and SV increase during pregnancy, CO increases. The normal prepregnancy range of CO is 3 to 5 L/min. CO increases 40% to 50% during pregnancy, to produce a normal CO in the last trimester of 6 to 7 L/min at rest. Labor produces an additional 40% increase in CO because of catecholamine release in response to pain perception and the shunting of blood from the placental-fetal unit with uterine contractions, for a CO range during labor of 8 to 10 L/min. CO increases further after birth because of significant hemodynamic fluctuations that reflect the net effect of blood loss at birth and the autotransfusion with approximately 1000 ml of blood that occurs after the uterus is emptied. Soon after birth, the accumulated 6 to 8 L of extravascular fluid is mobilized into the intravascular compartment. The large increase in CO remains for 7 to 10 days after birth in the healthy woman but will continue longer if the usual diuresis fails to occur because of a complication.

Positional Changes

Maternal CO in the last trimester is position dependent. Clark and colleagues (1991) showed the effect of maternal position on CO output (Table 34-5).

The right or left lateral recumbent position provides optimal CO for the critically ill pregnant woman. Any time maternal CO is decreased, compensatory mechanisms are initiated. The first compensatory response is to shunt blood away from the peripheral circulation to the central circulation, to save the heart and brain. Peripheral circulation includes circulation to the skin, the renal system, the gastrointestinal system, the lung beds, and the reproductive system. Enhancing maternal CO enhances fetal perfusion.

table 34-5 Effect of Maternal Position on Cardiac Output	
Knee-chest	6.9 (±2.1)
Right lateral	6.8 (±1.3)
Left lateral	6.6 (±1.4)
Sitting	6.2 (±2.0)
Supine	6.0 (±1.4)
Standing	5.4 (±2.0)

▬ NURSE ALERT

During the last trimester, CO decreases so significantly when the woman is supine that a hip wedge under one hip or manual displacement of the uterus to one side is necessary to prevent a sudden decrease in CO and a subsequent decrease in fetal perfusion.

Cardiac Output Determinants

The four determinants of CO are reflected in the calculation for cardiac output (CO = HR × SV) because SV is the result of preload, afterload, and contractility.

Preload is defined as the volume of blood in the ventricles at the end of diastole; preload is determined by intraventricular pressure and volume. Right preload is assessed by right atrial or CVP, and left preload is assessed by PCWP. The volume of blood in the ventricles stretches the myocardial muscle fibers and produces the intraventricular pressure. Measurements are made at end diastole, the time immediately preceding systole when the ventricles reach maximal stretch because of the extra amount of blood delivered into the ventricles when the tricuspid and mitral valves snap closed.

Right preload reflects the blood circulating through the right side of the heart, and left preload reflects the amount of blood circulating in the left side of the heart. The two sides of the heart are not equal when cardiac or pulmonary complications are present; therefore they are measured separately.

Preload must be adequate to maintain CO, and plotting of CO against preload gives a cardiac function curve (Fig. 34-2). As preload increases, CO increases up to the point of failure. The cardiac function curve shows that a heart in failure will require a higher preload than the healthy heart to produce the same CO. Bedside manipulations of preload are possible with continuous hemodynamic monitoring to determine effects on CO. A low preload can be increased by the administration of fluids, including crystalloid, colloid, or blood, and by positioning with legs

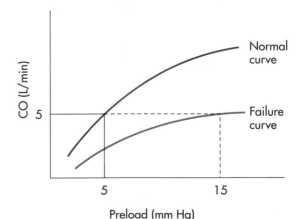

FIG. 34-2 Relation of preload to cardiac output. Ventricular function (Starling) curve for heart, showing both normal function and during failure.

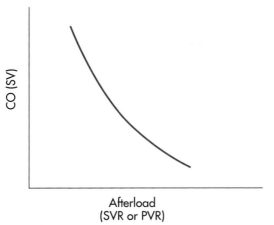

FIG. 34-3 Relation of afterload to cardiac output when preload is maintained constant. As afterload increases, cardiac output decreases.

elevated. A high preload can be decreased by the administration of a vasodilator or diuretic or by phlebotomy and positioning in an upright position.

Afterload is defined as the ventricular wall tension during systole, or the resistance the blood meets as blood is ejected from the ventricles. Afterload is dependent on the end-diastolic radius of the ventricle, the aortic pressure, and the thickness of the ventricle wall. As afterload increases, CO decreases, and bedside manipulation of afterload is possible to achieve optimal cardiac output (Fig. 34-3). Right afterload is assessed by the pulmonary vascular resistance (PVR), and left afterload is assessed by the SVR. Arterial BP measurement does not give as accurate an indication of left ventricular work as the SVR but is used clinically as reflecting left afterload. Therefore control of the woman's blood pressure is used to control left afterload.

Afterload must be adequate for circulation and CO; extremes of afterload may decrease CO. Increased left afterload occurs with hypertensive disease caused by the systemic arterial vasoconstriction. Increased right afterload occurs with pulmonary hypertension resulting from vasoconstriction in the pulmonary circulation.

Increased afterload can be corrected by the administration of vasodilator drugs. Hydralazine is commonly used as the first-line drug for hypertension. It is an arterial vasodilator that is usually effective, safe for mother and fetus, and has as an added bonus that the majority of obstetric personnel are comfortable in its use. However, many believe that the calcium channel blockers (such as nifedipine, orally) and the beta-blockers (such as labetalol) cause less hypotension (Roberts, 2004) (see Table 30-5). Sodium nitroprusside has the potential to produce such immediate changes in SVR that continuous intraarterial BP monitoring is required. Sodium nitroprusside produces cyanide as a metabolite; fetal cyanide toxicity must be a concern if this drug is administered during pregnancy. Of paramount importance is the correction of hypovolemia before ad-

ministration of any antihypertensive to prevent acute hypotension (National Institutes of Health & National Heart, Lung, and Blood Institute, 2000).

■ **NURSE ALERT**
Sodium nitroprusside by continuous intravenous infusion is the vasodilator drug used most commonly in the adult intensive care setting, but it is saved for emergency use for pregnant women.

Severe vasodilation and loss of arterial resistance with a decreased afterload impedes venous return of blood to the right side of the heart and decreases CO. This situation is seen with septic shock. Decreased afterload can be corrected by fluid administration to fill the vascular space or by the administration of alpha-adrenergic drugs such as phenylephrine (Gonik & Foley, 2004). Contractility (inotropic state of the heart) is defined as the force and velocity of ventricular contractions when preload and afterload are held constant. Contractility is governed by the Frank-Starling law, which states that the greater the length of the muscle fibers before contraction, the greater will be the contraction of the fibers, up to the point of failure. Fiber length is related to the maximal stretch of preload, because as more blood volume enters the ventricles, the more the fibers in the myocardium stretch to accommodate the increased volume.

Decreased contractility results in decreased CO. The first response to correct this problem is bedside manipulation to optimize both preload and afterload. If this fails to increase CO to the desired level, medications to increase myocardial contractility are indicated. Inotropic drugs such as dopamine hydrochloride or dobutamine are administered. Digitalis therapy also may be necessary.

Heart rate is the fourth determinant of cardiac output. The rate at which the ventricles fill and contract affects CO. Extremes of HR may decrease CO.

Sustained tachycardia can decrease CO as a result of myocardial ischemia or the decreased time for adequate filling of the ventricles during diastole and shortened systolic ejection times. The cause, such as fever, hypoxia, pain, hypovolemia, or hyperthyroidism, should be determined and treated. Drugs to correct tachycardia are seldom necessary for obstetric clients. However, propranolol, digoxin, or calcium channel blockers such as verapamil are effective agents to decrease HR if needed.

Bradycardia can compromise CO when the number of ventricular contractions per minute that occur are inadequate to deliver the circulating volume needed to perfuse and oxygenate the body. If treatment is necessary for this problem, atropine or cardiac pacing is used.

Invasive Hemodynamic Monitoring

Invasive hemodynamic monitoring provides continuous measurements of preload, afterload, myocardial contractility, and HR in the critically ill pregnant woman so that therapeutic manipulations may be made quickly at the bedside in response to changes in client status. Monitoring may be done by use of a pulmonary artery catheter (PAC) (a balloon-tipped, multilumen catheter) or by CVP.

Although few adequate clinical studies at this time demonstrate the benefit of pulmonary artery catheterization for the critically ill client, most critical care bedside clinicians use the PAC to direct their therapy modalities.They believe that use of the PAC does improve outcomes in selected critically ill clients (Fujitani & Baldisseri, 2005).

Use of a PAC allows the management of care to be based on immediate recognition of changes in hemodynamic values from the left ventricle. Immediate information is obtained, calculations are made, and management is adjusted quickly as needed. Results of therapeutic strategies can be calculated and evaluated (ACOG, 1992). The continuous hemodynamic measurements obtained will reinforce therapies in use or show that therapy should be changed. Use of a PAC or Swan-Ganz catheter in combination with an arterial pressure catheter and a pulse oximeter provides adequate data to assess cardiac, fluid, and pulmonary status of the client continuously. Indications for the use of invasive hemodynamic monitoring are the same in obstetrics as in any other area of medicine.

It is essential to evaluate risks and benefits of any procedure before use, especially because there are risks associated with invasive techniques. The information obtained from hemodynamic monitoring is essential for management of critical, complex cases and is unavailable by other means; thus the benefits outweigh the risks in most cases. The overall complication rate in the obstetric population is low, approximately 1%. This low rate of complications is related to three factors: (1) the pregnant woman usually needs the device because of an acute event, (2) the duration of use is usually short, and (3) the majority of pregnant women requiring its use are young and healthy before the acute event.

It is essential that meticulous attention be paid to each step and detail of all procedures to decrease problems with the technique itself. The complications seen with invasive monitoring seem to be most closely correlated with the technical skill and experience of the clinician (Gonik & Foley, 2004).

Pulmonary Artery Catheter

A PAC, commonly called the Swan-Ganz catheter, provides continuous measurements of pulmonary artery pressure (PAP) and right atrial pressure (RAP) or CVP.

Intermittent measurements of PCWP and CO also are possible. The standard flow-directed thermodilution PAC has three lumina and a thermistor connector (Fig. 34-4). The distal lumen or port is located in the pulmonary artery after insertion. It is connected to a transducer with a heparinized pressure line to measure a continuous PAP when the balloon is deflated and intermittent PCWP when the balloon is inflated. A continuous flush of 3 ml per hour of heparinized solution maintains patency of the lumen.

The proximal lumen or port exits approximately 30 cm from the tip of the catheter and is located in the right atrium after insertion. This port also is connected to a transducer with a heparinized line, and it can be used to measure continuous RAP, which is comparable to the CVP, or to administer fluid or drugs. Both the proximal and distal lumina of the catheter can be used to withdraw blood samples for laboratory studies.

The balloon lumen ends in a small latex balloon, located 0.5 inch from the tip of the PAC. Inflation of the balloon is used to assist in the insertion of the catheter and to obtain PCWP readings.

The thermodilution port is connected to a thermistor, a temperature sensor, located 5 cm proximal to the tip of the PAC. The thermistor continuously measures the temperature of the blood in the pulmonary artery.

Other types of PACs are available in addition to the standard PAC. Some have an extra right atrial port for intracardiac infusions. The small size of the ports makes them more effective for the administration of vasopressors or drugs such as antibiotics, rather than for the use of rapid administration of large volumes of blood or fluids. A fiberoptic PAC includes a sensor that can continuously measure the hemoglobin saturation of mixed venous blood, the SvO_2, in the pulmonary artery and is useful in cases of decreased oxygen transport, such as with preeclampsia and eclampsia. Another type for selected cases is a modified PAC with a heated filament to provide continuous CO values (Leather et al., 2004).

Venous Access. The internal or external jugular vein or the subclavian vein is most commonly used for venous access for invasive hemodynamic monitoring during pregnancy. Access with femoral or antecubital veins is not used so frequently for pregnant women because of the greater difficulty in positioning the catheter when this route is accessed. Furthermore, with use of a vein in the inguinal area,

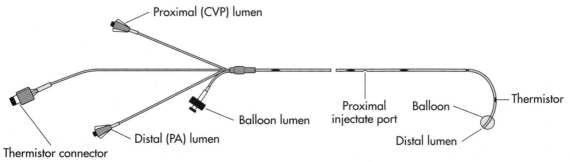

FIG. 34-4 Standard triple-lumen flow-directed pulmonary artery catheter.

CRITICAL THINKING EXERCISE

Nursing Care of the Critically Ill Pregnant Woman

Janna, a 32-year-old gravida 2, para 0, is brought to the hospital by ambulance with complaints of a severe epigastric pain that she had when she awoke that morning. She is at 29 weeks of gestation. Her blood pressure (BP) is 170/112 mm Hg. An intravenous (IV) line is started and blood drawn to rule out preeclampsia. Urine dipstick shows 4+ proteinuria, and magnesium sulfate is started for seizure prophylaxis. A Foley catheter is inserted to assess urine output. The laboratory results are indicative of severe preeclampsia with elevated liver enzymes. Induction of labor is started with oxytocin. She has been on oxytocin for 4 hours. Her last hourly urine output was 20 ml. The physician orders a fluid challenge of 1000 ml lactated Ringer's solution (LR). In 1 hour, her urine output is 22 ml. A pulmonary artery catheter is inserted to determine volume status and the cause of oliguria.

Her hemodynamic profile is as follows:

CVP	2 mm Hg
PAP	13/4 mm Hg
PCWP	34 mm Hg
CO	6 L/min

1. Evidence—Is there sufficient information to determine what action is needed?
2. Assumptions—What assumptions can be made about the following?
   a. Fluid challenge as treatment for hypovolemia
   b. Hemodynamic values in pregnancy
3. What implications and priorities for nursing care can be made at this time?
4. Does the evidence objectively support your conclusion?
5. Are there alternative perspectives to your conclusion?

procedure

How to Set Up, Calibrate, and Zero-Reference Pressure Lines

1. Connect pressure tubing to sterile disposable pressure transducer.
2. Check all connections for a tight fit to prevent leakage.
3. Heparinize flush solution of normal saline solution. Heparin is necessary for the pregnant client to prevent thrombus formation.
4. Connect the pressure tubing to the intravenous bag of heparinized solution.
5. Gently flush both pressure tubing and transducer to remove all air. Cap stopcocks with nonvented covers.
6. Connect transducer to hemodynamic monitor.
7. Place a pressure bag on the heparinized solution. Inflate to 300 mm Hg of pressure. (This allows a continuous rate of 3 ml/hr of heparinized solution to flow as a flush solution.) The heparinized solution and continuous flow of fluid prevent clot formation on the tip of the catheter.
8. Calibrate the pressure transducer by zeroing the line.
9. Zero-reference the transducer by positioning the woman supine with a hip wedge under the right hip, locating the phlebostatic axis at the fourth intercostal space at the midaxillary line, and marking on the chest wall.
10. Open stopcock to air. Push zero button on the monitor to identify zero. The transducer negates atmospheric pressure and establishes a baseline for subsequent readings. Close the stopcock to air.

NOTE: The phlebostatic axis is the physiologic reference point used when measuring pulmonary and arterial line pressures (see Fig. 34-7 for an illustration of this procedure).

birth of the infant at a critical time can limit access to and manipulation of the catheter. With certain disorders, such as a coagulopathy, antecubital access may be preferred to decrease the possibility of intrathoracic bleeding (Gonik & Foley, 2004).

The flow-directed PAC is usually inserted at the bedside after preparations are complete. Meticulous attention to detail is critical when the equipment is prepared. Flushing the pressure tubing to eliminate any air, establishing a zero reference point, and both zeroing and calibrating the pressure transducer are done carefully before insertion. The Procedure box explains how to set up a pressure line and how to zero-reference and calibrate a pressure transducer. Box 34-2 describes nursing care during insertion and continuing care for a PAC.

Hemodynamic monitoring systems have three major components: (1) a pressure transducer that converts physiologic pressures into electrical energy, (2) an amplifier to magnify the volume of the signal being measured, and (3) a monitor screen to display in digital and graphic form the converted physiologic signal (Fig. 34-5).

Waveforms and Pressure Readings. The basis of interpretation of assessments obtained by hemodynamic

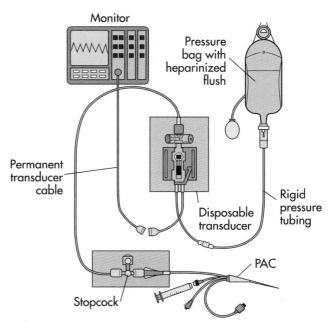

FIG. 34-5 Components of hemodynamic monitoring system: pressurized tubing, pressure transducer, and hemodynamic monitor.

box 34-2 **Pulmonary Artery Catheter (PAC) Protocol**

SETUP
- Prepare two pressure lines for the distal and proximal ports as described in the Procedure box on p. 883 how to set up, calibrate, and zero-reference pressure lines.
- Connect an intravenous line of normal saline solution, per infusion pump, to the introducer.
- Check PAC balloon for symmetric inflation, absence of air leak, and ease of spontaneous deflation.

CLIENT PREPARATION FOR INSERTION
- Assess woman's knowledge level and explain procedure to ensure her understanding, cooperation, and acceptance of the procedure.
- Confirm that informed consent form is signed and attached to chart.
- Provide support and encouragement throughout the procedure.
- Initiate electrocardiographic (ECG) monitoring. Obtain baseline ECG pattern.

NURSING MANAGEMENT DURING INSERTION
- Monitor ECG continuously as catheter passes through right ventricle to recognize any ventricular ectopy (premature beats) present.
- Use a slight Trendelenburg position with a hip wedge. This position engorges the neck veins and facilitates placement of the catheter. When the internal jugular approach is used, tilt head to the side away from the site of cannulation.
- Be available to provide assistance to the operator throughout the procedure.
- Adjust intravenous line connected to the introducer to maintain patency.
- Observe waveform patterns on the monitor screen and record pressures as the catheter advances through the chambers in the heart.
- Have lidocaine hydrochloride available for arrhythmias.
- Ensure that balloon is deflated. Deflate balloon passively.
- Anticipate orders for chest radiograph film to verify catheter placement.
- Apply dressing after physician secures introducer.
- Observe monitor screen for continuous tracing of pulmonary artery pressures.

NURSING ASSESSMENTS
- Verify that alarms are set at all times.
- Observe monitor screen closely for pressures and waveforms that denote placement of catheter. Be prepared to intervene when necessary (see Box 34-3).

- Record hemodynamic parameters according to client status and unit care protocols. Follow the procedure for obtaining a pulmonary capillary wedge pressure reading (see Procedure box).
- Inspect all connection sites every 2 hr and entire monitor system for presence of air or blood clots.
- Examine insertion site frequently for bleeding or signs of infection. Perform site care every shift or daily, as indicated by unit infection control policy.
- Change pressure and intravenous lines every 24 to 48 hr, as indicated by unit infection control policy.
- Monitor heparinized pressure flush for continuous correct pressure (300 mm Hg).
- Rezero and calibrate transducer every shift and as necessary.

NURSING MANAGEMENT FOR CATHETER REMOVAL
- Document vital signs and ECG pattern.
- Monitor for ECG arrhythmias during removal.
- After catheter removal, pressure to site must be applied for 5 min. Anticipate that physician may request application of pressure. Ensure that bleeding has stopped completely before pressure is removed.
- Apply pressure dressing to site, per unit protocol. Keep pressure dressing in place for 8 hr.

DOCUMENTATION
- Presence of signed informed consent form on chart
- Date, time, site of insertion, type of introducer, and name of operator who performed procedure
- Type of pulmonary catheter, number of attempts, confirmation of placement by x-ray studies, and any ventricular ectopy
- Woman's tolerance of procedure
- Zeroing and calibration of transducers and verification of alarm settings
- Hemodynamic parameters obtained according to client status
- Pertinent nursing assessments and medical and nursing care
- Site assessments and care
- Changes of pressure and intravenous lines
- Date and time of removal of intact catheter, date and removal of introducer
- Nursing care and assessments after catheter removal

monitoring is to understand the relation to cardiovascular status of the waveforms observed on the monitor screen and the pressure readings obtained.

Specific chambers in the heart have different pressures that are reflected by changing waveform patterns, and placement of the PAC is evaluated through the pressure and waveform changes that appear on the monitor screen to reflect the position of the catheter. Fig. 34-6 displays pressure waveforms in different chambers of the heart.

Because the right atrium is a holding chamber with relatively small muscle mass, the waveform pattern for this chamber has a low amplitude. Right atrium pressures reflect intravascular volume and compliance of the right ventricle. Mean right atrium pressures in pregnancy are relatively low, 0 to 7 mm Hg.

When the catheter is inserted into the right ventricle, pressures change, and a distinct spiking waveform appears. The low-amplitude waveform of the right atrium converts

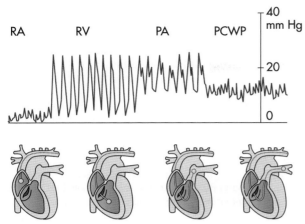

FIG 34-6 Pressure waveform in relation to catheter position from right atrium *(RA)*, to right ventricle *(RV)*, to pulmonary artery *(PA)*, to pulmonary capillary wedge pressure *(PCWP)*.

procedure

Obtaining a Pulmonary Capillary Wedge Pressure Reading

1. Inflate balloon slowly while observing waveform on monitor screen. Stop inflation as soon as pulmonary artery waveform changes to pulmonary capillary wedge pressure waveform.
2. Note amount of air necessary to achieve wedge waveform. Do NOT inflate balloon further than necessary to obtain wedge waveform.
3. Keep balloon inflated only long enough to obtain pressure reading, about 5 sec. Complications associated with sustained wedging (>10 sec) are pulmonary infarction and pulmonary rupture.
4. Release syringe and allow balloon to deflate passively. Do NOT aspirate air from syringe. (Passive deflation of the balloon correlates with an intact balloon.)
5. Note return of pulmonary artery waveform after deflation of balloon.
6. Document assessments made.

to a high-amplitude waveform with distinct systolic and diastolic components in the right ventricle, with a baseline pressure of 0 mm Hg. Right ventricular pressures are measured as systolic and diastolic. Normal right ventricle systolic pressure is 18 to 30 mm Hg, and the normal diastolic pressure is 0 to 7 mm Hg.

The catheter is then advanced into the pulmonary artery. This is reflected by a different spiking waveform with baseline pressures greater than 0 mm Hg. Pulmonary artery systolic pressures are equal to the systolic pressures in the right ventricle, but pulmonary artery diastolic pressures abruptly increase to the range of 6 to 10 mm Hg.

The catheter advances through the pulmonary artery as far as possible and becomes "wedged" in the vessel. This wedging is reflected by a distinct waveform of a dampened tracing with respiratory variation. This relatively low amplitude reflects the low pressures in the capillary beds of the lungs.

The PCWP is obtained when the balloon is inflated, with all pressures from the right side of the heart ob-structed, so that the distal port now reads pressures from the left side of the heart across the lungs, because there are no valves in the pulmonary circulation. The PCWP measures left atrial filling pressures or left-sided preload. During right ventricular diastole, the pulmonic valve is closed, with the mitral valve open; the diastolic PAP is measured. In the absence of a problem, such as mitral valve disease or pulmonary edema, PAP diastolic readings reflect PCWP or left ventricular preload. The diastolic PAP is therefore used clinically to reflect left preload (Darovic, 2002). See the Procedure box for obtaining a PCWP reading.

The normal PCWP during pregnancy is 6 to 10 mm Hg. Pressures higher than 20 mm Hg are usually caused by abnormal left ventricular performance, such as left ventricular failure, mitral valve stenosis, or fluid volume overload. Lower-than-normal readings are seen usually with hypovolemia (see Fig. 34-6).

Box 34-3 describes nursing measures for managing selected problems that may arise with a PAC.

Arterial Pressure Catheter

Percutaneous arterial catheterization, in which a Teflon intravenous catheter, usually 20 gauge, is placed in an artery and connected to a hemodynamic monitor by a pressure line, provides continuous measurements of the systolic, diastolic, and mean arterial blood pressures. The arterial pressure catheter produces a waveform and also provides access for ABG sampling and analysis.

Indications for use of this type of hemodynamic monitoring include situations in which frequent and accurate BP measurements are needed, such as the administration of potent drugs (e.g., dopamine to treat septic shock or nitroprusside to treat severe hypertensive disease), or when frequent ABG determinations are needed. Characteristics of desirable arteries for an arterial line are (1) a vessel that

FIG. 34-7 Location of phlebostatic axis and zeroing.

box 34-3 **Trouble-Shooting Pulmonary Artery Catheter Problems**

SPONTANEOUS WEDGING: PCWP WAVEFORM APPEARS ON MONITOR SCREEN

- Assess syringe. Determine if balloon is inflated or deflated.
- Have woman turn her head, cough deeply 2 to 3 times, and then take a few deep breaths while observing monitor screen for return of pulmonary artery waveform.
- If wedge form continues, call physician immediately to the bedside to reposition catheter. (Catheter will need to be pulled back into larger-diameter vessel.)
- Monitor screen for return of pulmonary artery waveform.

MIGRATION OF CATHETER BACKWARD: RIGHT VENTRICULAR WAVEFORM ON SCREEN

- Call physician immediately to bedside to reposition catheter. (Balloon must be reinflated for catheter to flow back into the pulmonary artery.)
- Monitor ECG pattern for ventricle ectopy, especially premature ventricle contractions if catheter tip irritates wall of right ventricle.
- Have lidocaine hydrochloride available.

SUSPECTED BALLOON RUPTURE: ABSENCE OF RESISTANCE FELT WHEN INFLATING BALLOON OR INABILITY TO OBTAIN PCWP READING

- Confirm tight attachment of syringe. Do NOT inject air. Slowly withdraw plunger.
- Rupture may be assumed if unable to aspirate blood or fluid because of absence of resistance in syringe. Do NOT inject any air. Tape closed and label balloon inflation port, "balloon rupture."
- Notify physician.
- Usually does not necessitate change of catheter, especially if diastolic PAP and PCWP readings have been similar. Diastolic PAP will be monitored to reflect left preload values.

ECG, Electrocardiogram; *PAP,* pulmonary artery pressure; *PCWP,* pulmonary capillary wedge pressure.

has a diameter large enough for accurate measurement of pressure without occlusion of the artery by the catheter, (2) adequate collateral circulation, (3) ease of access to the site for care, and (4) a site not prone to infection. The most common vessels used in the pregnant woman are the radial, axillary, and pedal arteries, in that order.

In preparation for insertion of the arterial line into the radial artery, the procedure should be explained to the woman in simple terms, informed consent obtained, and Allen's test performed to validate collateral circulation into the hand by demonstrating a patent ulnar artery. Box 34-4 describes the steps to perform Allen's test.

The most common risk associated with an intraarterial line is infection. More serious, but less common risks include hemorrhage, thrombus formation, and embolization. The heparinized continuous flush solution of the pressure line helps prevent thrombus formation. Once the line is in place, a transparent occlusive dressing is applied. The transducer is then rezeroed, and an arm board is used to prevent movement of the wrist.

box 34-4 **Allen's Test Procedure**

1. Determine the woman's dominant hand. Use opposite extremity.
2. Elevate woman's hand and occlude both radial and ulnar arteries.
3. Have woman clench and unclench fist to facilitate venous drainage.
4. Observe that palm is blanched.
5. Release pressure on the ulnar artery only. Radial artery remains occluded.
6. Observe and time the palm for capillary refill (normal time is ≤5 sec).
7. If it takes >5 sec, collateral circulation may be impaired.

The hemodynamic monitor displays an arterial waveform and the systolic, diastolic, and MAPs for the health care team to interpret. Normal versus abnormal waveforms must be recognized at the bedside, and immediate intervention must be available as needed. The normal waveform should include the following (Fig. 34-8):

- Rapid upstroke to systole
- Clear dicrotic notch, which denotes closure of the aortic valve
- Definite end-diastolic wave

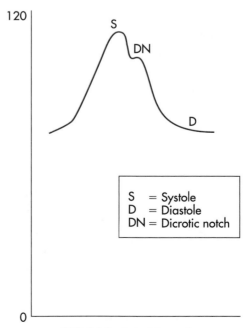

FIG. 34-8 Arterial waveform.

A blood pressure taken with a sphygmomanometer should be ascertained periodically to verify accuracy of the hemodynamic monitor.

Continuing assessments and documentation include the following:

- Systolic and diastolic arterial pressures
- Cuff pressure readings
- Intraarterial strip recording
- Site care
- Dressing and line changes
- Transducer zeroing and calibration
- Description of the circulation in the extremity

Pressure Lines

All pressure lines use a specialized high-pressure tubing to transmit the physiologic signal to the transducer and monitor. The pressure tubing is rigid to prevent the dampening or absorption of pressure itself, so that the physiologic pressures are transmitted directly from the catheter tip to the transducer through the fluid that fills the length of the tubing. The line includes a continuous flushing mechanism to ensure patency (see Fig. 34-5).

Data Collection

Continuous measurements of the CVP and PAPs and intermittent PCWPs are obtained from the PAC. CO is also calculated intermittently by the use of a PAC with the thermodilution technique. Electrocardiographic (ECG) monitoring permits continuous evaluation of HR and rhythm. Newer ECG monitors with sensitive leads connected to the chest wall also monitor respiratory rate. Systemic arterial BP can be evaluated by a manual or an automatic sphygmomanometer or by an arterial pressure line. Placement of an arterial pressure line also permits ready access for frequent arterial blood sampling and analysis, especially for ABGs.

Mean pressure values are used to evaluate client status. They can be determined for the pulmonary arterial and systemic circulations by electronic dampening of the respective tracing or by use of the following calculation formula (Gonik & Foley, 2004):

$$\text{MAP} = \frac{\text{systolic pressure} + 2(\text{diastolic pressure})}{3}$$

The PCWP is reported as a mean value, determined by the average of its maximal and minimal deflections on the monitor screen or oscilloscope. Reading values from the oscilloscope is usually adequate for clinical management at the bedside; however, for complex cases, strip chart recordings are recommended. See the Procedure box for making and recording hemodynamic assessments.

When the thermodilution procedure to calculate CO in a pregnant woman is performed, the injectate should be chilled to obtain an accurate reading because of the high COs normal for pregnancy (Wallace & Winslow, 1993). The thermistor at the tip of the PAC measures the speed with which the blood temperature cools and returns to nor-

procedure

Making and Recording Hemodynamic Assessments

1. Position woman in supine position with a hip wedge.
2. Rezero all pressure transducers.
3. Print a strip recording of the PAC and arterial line blood pressures. Observe oscilloscope for mean values.
4. Record findings of the PAP, central venous pressure, and arterial BP.
5. Calibrate PCWP according to the Procedure box for obtaining a PCWP reading. Record the mean determination.
6. Calibrate cardiac output (CO) according to the Procedure box outlining the thermodilution procedure for measuring CO.
7. Document all findings and woman's tolerance of procedures.

mal after the chilled fluid is injected. The time required for the temperature changes is computed, and a CO readout is given. The Procedure box describes the thermodilution procedure for measuring CO.

Oxygenation

Oxygen delivery to and use by the peripheral tissues must be adequate. Determination of oxygen transport is essential in the care of the critically ill pregnant woman. Oxygen delivery is directly proportional to CO; if CO decreases 50%, oxygen delivery decreases 50%. Conversely, increasing CO 50% doubles oxygen delivery. Oxygen delivery also can be improved by improving the hemoglobin value, which can be accomplished by the administration of red blood cells.

SaO_2 Monitoring. Oxygen is transported to the tissues in two ways: dissolved in plasma and bound to hemoglobin. The oxygen dissolved in plasma (PaO_2) makes up only 1% to 2% of the total oxygen content, whereas the oxygen bound to hemoglobin (SaO_2) makes up 98% to 99%

procedure

Thermodilution Procedure for Measuring Cardiac Output

1. Enter the cardiac output (CO) coefficient into the computer.
2. Chill injectate in ice bath.
3. Use insulated syringe.
4. Flush coiled tubing with injectate solution to remove all air.
5. Connect syringe to three-way stopcock at the proximal port.
6. Draw injectate (5 or 10 ml per unit protocol) into insulated syringe.
7. Depress the CO control on the computer.
8. Inject the injectate as rapidly as possible with both hands. Observe oscilloscope for a smooth curve.
9. Repeat the procedure twice. Calculate results. If readings are within 15% of each other, average the three to determine CO. If not, omit the highest and lowest.

of the total oxygen content. Results of arterial blood gas determination reflect the dissolved oxygen according to the PaO$_2$ value. The PaO$_2$ reflects the partial pressure that oxygen exerts when it is dissolved in blood; it is measured in millimeters of mercury. The normal PaO$_2$ for the pregnant state is 100 to 106 mm Hg. The adequacy of maternal oxygenation for delivery to the fetus can be evaluated by the usual methods of fetal well-being assessment such as electronic fetal monitoring or biophysical profile. The partial pressure of the oxygen tension is important because circulation transports the higher PaO$_2$ blood to organs with a lower PaO$_2$, and gas exchange occurs as gases move from the higher concentration to the lower concentration. The higher tension (PaO$_2$) pushes the oxygen molecule off the hemoglobin molecule through the cell membrane so that tissues receive a supply of oxygen.

The oxygen that cells can use is the oxygen molecules bound to hemoglobin (SaO$_2$). Each molecule of hemoglobin has four binding sites for oxygen; when all four sites are bound, an oxyhemoglobin molecule results. The saturation of hemoglobin with oxygen (SaO$_2$) is evaluated with the pulse oximeter (SaO$_2$ monitoring). The normal range for SaO$_2$ is 95% to 100%, and normal SaO$_2$ values for pregnancy are 97% to 100%. Critically ill pregnant women benefit from continuous SaO$_2$ monitoring.

SvO$_2$ Monitoring. The percentage of saturation of hemoglobin with oxygen in mixed venous and arterial blood is reflected as an SvO$_2$ value. SvO$_2$ monitoring involves insertion of a fiberoptic PAC that is connected to a bedside microprocessor to give a continuous SvO$_2$ value. Mixed venous blood saturation reflects the balance between oxygen delivery and oxygen use. It reflects tissue perfusion, the variation in oxygen requirements for different organs, and the affinity of hemoglobin to accept and then release oxygen. The normal value of SvO$_2$ is 60% to 80%; values less than 60% are interpreted as abnormally low.

Fiberoptic PACs and bedside microprocessors provide the technology to plot the mixed venous blood oxygen saturation continuously. Plotting of mixed venous oxygen content is used as an early warning system, because values may decrease before any other evidence of hemodynamic instability is seen (Fujitani & Baldisseri, 2005).

Use of pulse oximetry permits evaluation of the SaO$_2$, arterial blood saturation. Arterial blood usually has a saturation of 90% or greater. Because of the shape of the oxyhemoglobin dissociation curve, fluctuations at the high levels of oxygen tension, 90% and higher, are reflected by a small change in arterial oxygen saturation (SaO$_2$). However, the lower levels of oxygen tension in mixed venous blood (40% or less) produce a linear relation between saturation and tension, resulting in the SvO$_2$ becoming a sensitive alarm to detect physiologic instability.

Arterial blood analysis evaluates pulmonary oxygen exchange and ventilation but does not evaluate overall adequacy of oxygen delivery to the peripheral tissues. However, mixed venous blood analysis (SvO$_2$) reflects the end product of supply and demand and is used to evaluate overall adequacy of oxygen delivery to the peripheral tissues. This technique provides additional data and can be especially useful to support or change management strategies when used in conjunction with thermodilution CO calculations.

▬ NURSE ALERT

Stable CO measurements in conjunction with an improvement in SvO$_2$ readings are associated with clinical improvement and are a good prognostic sign. The same improved SvO$_2$ readings in conjunction with a 100% increase in CO are a common first sign of the development of sepsis.

Continuous monitoring of SvO$_2$ is recommended for titration of vasoactive or inotropic drugs; during adjustments of positive end-expiratory pressure, evaluation of fluid administration, and routine care of critically ill pregnant women.

Central Venous Pressure Lines

Before the development of the flow-directed PAC in the early 1970s, CVP lines were used for the critically ill. Two primary problems with the use of CVP lines became apparent. First, CVP monitoring provides right-sided heart information only, the right preload. When a cardiac or pulmonary complication is present, right- and left-sided values are not equal. CVP monitoring gives no information about left ventricular function. Second, changes in CVP values occur much later with left ventricular dysfunction. This type of monitoring does not permit rapid calculation of the effects of treatment modalities. Additionally, several studies reported disparities in the relationship between CVP and PCWP in preeclampsia (Gonik & Foley, 2004). Considering that the risks for insertions are similar, when invasive hemodynamic monitoring is required, use of the PAC is preferred.

Interpretation of Hemodynamic Data

Data obtained with hemodynamic monitoring techniques include values that reflect blood volume in the pulmonary and systemic circulations, which profoundly affect cardiac performance, in the following ways:

- Right atrial pressure or CVP indicates right end-diastolic pressure and reflects right preload.
- PAP: Pulmonary vascular resistance (PVR) is the calculation for right afterload. Clinically, mean PAP reflects right afterload.
- Diastolic PAP approximates PCWP and reflects left preload.
- PCWP indicates left end-diastolic pressure and reflects left preload.
- CO refers to the volume of blood ejected from the left ventricle in liters per minute.
- SVR is the calculation for left afterload; arterial BP reflects left afterload.

Hemodynamic profiles provide valuable data for evaluating status of the client and changing treatment strategies as needed. Normal hemodynamic values in pregnancy for calculation in the cases described in the following material

table 34-6 Normal Hemodynamic Values in Pregnancy

Right atrial pressure (RAP) or central venous pressure (CVP)	0-7 mm Hg
Pulmonary artery pressure (PAP)	18-30 mm Hg (systolic) 6-10 mm Hg (diastolic)
Pulmonary capillary wedge pressure (PCWP)	6-10 mm Hg
Cardiac output (CO)	6-7 L/min
Systemic vascular resistance (SVR)	1210 ± 266
Pulmonary vascular resistance (PVR)	78 ± 22

are shown in Table 34-6. Table 34-7 compares normal non-pregnant hemodynamic values with normal values during pregnancy.

Oliguria is diagnosed if urine output is less than 25 to 30 ml for 2 consecutive hours. It may indicate severe renal dysfunction (Roberts, 2004). If oliguria is not corrected with fluid challenge, the woman is diagnosed as having oliguria refractory to conservative therapy.

Refractory oliguria caused by preeclampsia may be associated with three different hemodynamic subsets: hypovolemia, hypervolemia, and renal artery spasm. Treatment strategies for correction of oliguria are different for each hemodynamic subset. Noninvasive assessments do not differentiate the type of treatment that would be appropriate for the pregnant woman. Recognition of which hemodynamic subset has produced the refractory oliguria is obtained only by the use of a PAC. Failure to use PAC when refractory oliguria is present can result in inappropriate treatment.

Examples of three different pregnant women with preeclampsia complicated by refractory oliguria are included in Box 34-5 to demonstrate how useful hemodynamic monitoring is to determine the appropriate care for the individual woman with this complication. These three women, all with severe preeclampsia with similar noninvasive assessment findings, illustrate the need for use of a PAC when the pregnant woman with hypertensive disease and oliguria fails a fluid challenge test. Noninvasive parameters do not reflect volume status. Completely different treatment modalities to correct oliguria are indicated for each of these three women.

table 34-7 Central Hemodynamic Normal Values

PARAMETER	NONPREGNANT	PREGNANT
CO (L/min)	4.3 ± 0.9	6.2 ± 1
HR (beats/min)	71 ± 10	83 ± 10
SVR (dynes/cm/sec^{-5})	1530 ± 520	1210 ± 266
PVR (dynes/cm/sec^{-5})	119 ± 47	78 ± 22
PCWP (mm Hg)	6.3 ± 2.1	7.5 ± 1.8
CVP (mm Hg)	3.7 ± 2.6	3.6 ± 2.5
Left ventricular work index	41 ± 8	48 ± 6

Reference: Clark, S., et al. (1989). Central hemodynamic assessment of normal term pregnancy. *American Journal of Obstetrics and Gynecology, 16*(6), 1439-1442.

Pulmonary Edema

One of the most common uses of the PAC during pregnancy is the differentiation of cardiogenic (heart failure or hydrostatic) pulmonary edema from noncardiogenic (permeability or lung failure) pulmonary edema (Mabie, 2004). Optimal therapies for the two types of pulmonary edema are dramatically different; however, the correct diagnosis can be determined only by evaluation of the hemodynamic profile.

Cardiogenic or heart failure pulmonary edema develops as a result of left ventricular failure or acute fluid overload. The PCWP is elevated because of the increased volume of fluid in the pulmonary circulation. Therapy is focused on improvement of myocardial contractility with an inotropic drug, decreasing left afterload, if elevated, with an arterial vasodilator and reducing preload with a diuretic drug to a normal range. This type of pulmonary edema usually responds to therapy within a few hours, and a normal PCWP is restored.

Pulmonary edema also may result from damage to the pulmonary alveolar capillary membrane by numerous factors, the most common being sepsis. Disturbance of membrane permeability results in the leakage of both protein and fluid into the pulmonary interstitium and alveoli, in the presence of normal cardiac function and ventricular filling pressures (Mabie, 2004). The PCWP is normal. Alveolar membranes require days to heal, and adult respiratory distress disease may develop if the source of injury is not found and eradicated. The focus of therapy is to maintain the PCWP in the low-normal range to minimize transudation of protein and fluid into the lung and to eliminate the source of injury.

When radiography reveals pulmonary edema, evaluation of the hemodynamic profile is the only way to diagnose correctly the type of pulmonary edema present, as illustrated in the following two hemodynamic profiles (refer to Table 34-6 for the normal values):

Case I

CVP	4 mm Hg
PAP	44/21 mm Hg
PCWP	20 mm Hg
CO	6.1 L/min

The high wedge pressure reflects a high left preload and correlates with cardiogenic pulmonary edema. Treatment would include an inotropic drug such as dobutamine, a vasodilator such as hydralazine if hypertension is present, and a diuretic such as furosemide (Lasix) because CO is adequate.

Case II

CVP	2 mm Hg
PAP	23/8 mm Hg
PCWP	7 mm Hg
CO	7.1 L/min

All readings are in the normal range, although pulmonary edema is present. This correlates with noncardiogenic pulmonary edema. A diuretic should not be administered. Preload is in the low-normal range. Reducing the preload with a diuretic drug could decrease CO and jeopardize

box 34-5 Case Studies

CASE 1

Jessie is a 24-year-old woman, gravida 4, para 2, at 35 weeks of gestation, diagnosed with severe preeclampsia. She is scheduled for labor induction today because of the increasing severity of the disease.

Everything went well for the first 5 hr after admission. However, this hour's urine output is only 22 ml. The physician orders a fluid challenge of 1000 ml of LR; one hr after this fluid infusion is completed, urine output is 24 ml.

This is a failed fluid challenge. A Swan-Ganz catheter (PAC) is inserted to determine volume status and to help determine why the kidneys are not excreting urine. The woman's hemodynamic profile was determined to be the following:

CVP	2 mm Hg
PAP	15/5 mm Hg
PCWP	4 mm Hg
CO	6.1 L/min

Evaluation

Evaluation of this profile shows a low PCWP of 4 mm Hg, which denotes decreased left preload and reflects hypovolemia. The low PAP reflects the decreased pulmonary circulating volume. CO is low for a laboring woman, probably as a result of the decreased preload. Her CO at 6.1 L/min is probably being maintained by her elevated HR; however, she is not in danger of dying with a CO of 6 L/min. This hemodynamic profile correlates with hypovolemia as the reason for oliguria. Urine is not being produced because the renal system is not adequately perfused. Additional fluids are needed rapidly. The oliguria is due to compensatory mechanisms that shunt the blood from the peripheral circulation to the central circulation in response to the extremely low preload. The 1000 ml of fluid given in the fluid challenge was not adequate to correct the hypovolemia. Additional fluid should be administered until left preload is adequate.

CASE 2

Shavone is an 18-year-old primigravid woman at 34 weeks of gestation with a diagnosis of severe preeclampsia. She is scheduled for induction of labor today because of increasing severity of the disease.

Everything went well for the first 5 hr after admission. However, this hour's urine output is only 23 ml. The physician orders a fluid challenge of 1000 ml of LR. One hour after this fluid is infused, urine output is 24 ml.

This is a failed fluid challenge. A Swan-Ganz catheter is inserted to determine volume status and to help determine the cause of the oliguria. The hemodynamic profile is determined to be the following:

CVP	2 mm Hg
PAP	22/9 mm Hg
PCWP	8 mm Hg
CO	7.8 L/min

Evaluation

Evaluation of this profile shows a normal PCWP of 8 mm Hg, a normal PAP, and a CO of 7.8 L/min. A normal hemodynamic profile in conjunction with refractory oliguria is associated with renal artery spasm that decreases perfusion and oxygenation to the kidneys and results in decreased urine output. Renal dose (low-dose) dopamine is used as the first-line management strategy to correct this type of oliguria. An arterial pressure line will be used during administration of the drug to monitor BP closely. Relaxation of the renal artery will improve renal system perfusion and correct the oliguria.

CASE 3

Bonnie is a 32-year-old woman, gravida 5, para 4, at 36 weeks of gestation with a diagnosis of severe preeclampsia. She is scheduled for labor induction today because of increasing severity of the disease.

Everything went well for the first 5 hr after admission. However, this hour's urine output is only 20 ml. The physician orders a fluid challenge of 1000 ml of LR. One hour after this fluid infusion is completed, urine output is 22 ml.

This is a failed fluid challenge. A Swan-Ganz catheter is inserted to determine volume status and to help determine the cause of the oliguria. Hemodynamic profile is determined to be the following:

CVP	2 mm Hg
PAP	44/20 mm Hg
PCWP	18 mm Hg
CO	6.6 L/min

Evaluation

Evaluation of this profile shows a high PCWP of 18 mm Hg, which denotes an increased left preload. CO is adequate. This profile correlates with oliguria in the hypervolemic pregnant woman. Lack of urine excretion is probably due to renal damage from the ischemia accompanying the severe hypertensive disease. Intravenous fluids should be restricted to 50 ml/hr. The high wedge pressure correlates with pulmonary edema during pregnancy. With such severe preeclampsia, pulmonary edema is usually a combined cardiogenic and noncardiogenic type. Cardiogenic pulmonary edema is a result of the increased SVR, which increased the resistance that the left ventricle must overcome to eject blood. This can lead to congestive heart failure. The noncardiogenic pulmonary edema is a result of an extremely low COP, a result of renal disease and protein excretion. Reduction of left afterload with hydralazine is the initial management strategy to correct the pulmonary edema. CO is adequate, probably because of the increased HR and circulating volume. The high PAP reflects the increased pressures in the pulmonary circulation because of the excessive fluid that is present, produced by the increased left afterload. Immediate delivery by cesarean birth will permit further renal studies to evaluate renal function. Dialysis may be indicated.

BP, Blood pressure; *CO*, cardiac output; *COP*, colloid osmotic pressure; *CVP*, central venous pressure; *LR*, lactated Ringer's solution; *PAC*, pulmonary artery catheter; *PAP*, pulmonary artery pressure; *PCWP*, pulmonary capillary wedge pressure; *SVR*, systemic vascular resistance.

the client's status. Instead, sepsis should be suspected, and treatment should focus on antibiotic therapy and elimination of foci of infection, continuing assessments, and support of vital systems while lung membranes heal.

▬ TRAUMA DURING PREGNANCY

Trauma continues to be a common complication during pregnancy because of the continuation of usual activities by the majority of pregnant women in the United States.

Significance

Approximately 8% of pregnancies have been reported to be complicated by physical trauma (Van Hook, Gei, & Pacheco, 2004). As pregnancy progresses, the risk of trauma seems to increase because more cases of trauma are reported in the third trimester than earlier in gestation. Most maternal injuries are a result of motor vehicle accidents; however falls, assaults, and burns are other major sources (Mattox & Goetzl, 2005).

Acts of violence are a significant health problem in the United States. Unfortunately, in 1999, homicide was the third highest cause of injury-related death for women of childbearing age, and second among African-American women (Chang et al., 2003). The risk of trauma caused by battering and abuse is increased during pregnancy, and rates of recurrence are high. The reported incidence of physical abuse during pregnancy ranges from 4% to 30% (El Kady, Gilbert, Xing, & Smith, 2005). Up to 45% of women subject to intimate partner violence before pregnancy continue to be abused during the pregnancy. Abuse also may have its onset with the pregnant state. An even more frightening statistic is that women who are abused during pregnancy have a threefold risk of being murdered compared with their nonpregnant abused controls (McFarlane, Campbell, Sharps, & Watson, 2002). The report goes on to say that African-American women have a threefold higher risk than Caucasian women in the same pregnancy group (McFarlane et al.).

Trauma occurs in 5% of all pregnancies but is the leading nonobstetric cause of maternal mortality (Weinberg, Steele, Pugh, Higgins, Herbert, & Story, 2005). Motor vehicle accidents account for more than 50% of maternal trauma incidents. About 50% of fetal deaths are associated with maternal trauma, and most of these are due to motor vehicle accidents (Mattox & Goetzl, 2005). Maternal death caused by trauma is usually the result of head injury or hemorrhagic shock. Fetal death usually occurs as a sequela to maternal death or as a result of placental abruption.

Fortunately, the majority of trauma injuries during pregnancy are minor and have no impact on pregnancy outcome. However, each case of trauma during pregnancy must be evaluated carefully, because pregnancy can mask signs of severe injury. Research has not yet revealed an accurate "trauma score" to predict risk of adverse pregnancy outcome from the initial physical assessment. The incidence of fetal loss is increased with a high injury severity score, elevated base deficit, or abnormal uterine activity (Mattox & Goetzl, 2005). However, prolonged assessments are usually completed before discharge from the unit even in seemingly "mild" cases of trauma.

Multisystem trauma during pregnancy is usually the result of a serious motor vehicle crash, especially if the woman is not wearing a seat belt with a shoulder harness and is ejected from the vehicle. To improve chances of survival for both mother and fetus, ACOG (1998) recommends that pregnant women wear properly positioned restraints at all times when in a motor vehicle (see Fig. 16-17). Failure to wear restraining devices occurred in 66% of cases in one study (Ikossi, Lazar, Morabito, Fildes, & Knudson, 2005). Another study found 95% of pregnant women surveyed either maintained or increased their seat belt use during pregnancy, and a large majority (73%) demonstrated correct usage. The perception that wearing a seat belt would protect them and their baby positively influenced their decision to wear a seat belt, though only 37% of these women reported being given seat belt information during their pregnancy (McGwin, Russell, Rux, Leath, Valent, & Rue, 2004).

Trauma increases the incidence of miscarriage, preterm labor, abruptio placentae, and stillbirth (Mattox & Goetzl, 2005). The effect of trauma on pregnancy is influenced by the length of gestation, type and severity of the trauma, and degree of disruption of uterine and fetal physiologic features. Fetal death as a result of trauma is more common than the occurrence of both maternal and fetal death (Shah & Kilcline, 2003). Less serious trauma is associated with numerous complications for pregnancy, including fetomaternal hemorrhage, abruptio placentae, intrauterine fetal death, and preterm labor and birth (Gilbert & Harmon, 2003). Careful evaluation of mother and fetus after all types of trauma is imperative (American Academy of Pediatrics [AAP] & ACOG, 2002).

Special considerations for mother and fetus are necessary when trauma occurs during pregnancy because of the physiologic alterations that accompany pregnancy and because of the presence of the fetus. Fetal survival depends on maternal survival; therefore the pregnant woman must receive immediate stabilization and appropriate care for optimal fetal outcome.

Maternal Physiologic Characteristics

Optimal care for the pregnant woman after trauma is dependent on understanding the physiologic state of pregnancy and its effects on trauma. The pregnant woman's body will exhibit responses different from those of a nonpregnant person to the same traumatic insults. Because of the different responses to injury during pregnancy, management strategies must be adapted for appropriate resuscitation, fluid therapy, positioning, assessments, and most other interventions. Significant maternal adaptations and the relation to trauma are summarized in Table 34-8.

The uterus and bladder are confined to the bony pelvis during the first trimester of pregnancy and are at reduced risk for injury in cases of abdominal trauma. After pregnancy progresses beyond the fourteenth week, the uterus becomes an abdominal organ, and the risk for injury in cases of abdominal trauma increases. During the second and third trimesters, the distended bladder becomes an abdominal organ and is at increased risk for injury and rupture. Bowel injuries occur less often during pregnancy because of the protection provided by the enlarged uterus.

The elevated levels of progesterone that accompany pregnancy relax smooth muscle and profoundly affect the gastrointestinal tract. Gastrointestinal motility decreases,

table 34-8 **Maternal Adaptations During Pregnancy and Relation to Trauma**

SYSTEM	ALTERATION	CLINICAL RESPONSES
Respiratory	↑ Oxygen consumption	↑ Risk of acidosis
	↑ Tidal volume	↑ Risk of respiratory mismanagement
	↓ Functional residual capacity	
	Chronic compensated alkalosis	↓ Blood-buffering capacity
	↓ PaCO₂	
	↓ Serum bicarbonate	
Cardiovascular	↑ Circulating volume, 1600 ml	Can lose 1000 ml blood
	↑ CO	No signs of shock until blood loss >30% total blood volume
	↑ Heart rate	↓ Placental perfusion in supine position
	↓ SVR	
	↓ Arterial blood pressure	Point of maximal impulse, fourth intercostal space
	Heart displaced upward to left	
Renal	↑ Renal plasma flow	
	Dilation of ureters and urethra	↑ Risk of stasis, infection
	Bladder displaced forward	↑ Risk of bladder trauma
Gastrointestinal	↓ Gastric motility	↑ Risk of aspiration
	↑ Hydrochloric acid production	
	↓ Competency of gastroesophageal sphincter	Passive regurgitation of stomach acids if head lower than stomach
Reproductive	↑ Blood flow to organs	Source of ↑ blood loss
	Uterine enlargement	Vena caval compression in supine position
Musculoskeletal	Displacement of abdominal viscera	↑ Risk of injury, altered rebound response
	Pelvic venous congestion	Altered pain referral
	Cartilage softened	↑ Risk of pelvic fracture
		Center of gravity changed
	Fetal head in pelvis	↑ Risk of fetal injury
Hematologic	↑ Clotting factors	↑ Risk of thrombus formation
	↓ Fibrinolytic activity	

with a resultant increased time required for gastric emptying, whereas the production of hydrochloric acid increases in the last trimester, and the gastroesophageal sphincter relaxes (Norwitz et al., 2004). Airway management of the unconscious pregnant woman is of critical importance.

■ **NURSE ALERT**
The unconscious pregnant woman is at increased risk for regurgitation of gastric contents and aspiration whenever her head is positioned lower than her stomach or if abdominal pressure is applied.

A pregnant woman has decreased tolerance for hypoxia and apnea because of her decreased functional residual capacity and increased renal loss of bicarbonate. Acidosis develops more quickly in the pregnant than in the nonpregnant state.

CO increases 44% to 50% over prepregnancy values and is position dependent in the third trimester. Because of compression of the inferior vena cava and descending aorta by the pregnant uterus, CO will decrease dramatically if the woman is placed in the supine position. The supine position must be avoided, even in women with cervical spine injuries. It is a primary priority that lateral uterine displacement be accomplished without any head movement. As soon as the neck is immobilized, the stretcher should be tilted laterally.

Circulating blood volume increases 50% during gestation, and pregnant women can tolerate a 1000 ml blood loss readily without demonstrating clinical signs. Hemodynamic instability that indicates the need for transfusion may not be apparent until blood loss nears 1500 to 2000 ml (Gonik & Foley, 2004). Clinical signs of hemorrhage do not appear until after a 30% loss of circulating volume occurs. Although HR increases with pregnancy, a maternal HR greater than 100 beats/min should be considered abnormal.

Fetal Physiologic Characteristics

Perfusion of the uterine arteries, which provide the primary blood supply to the uteroplacental unit, depends on adequate maternal arterial pressure, because these vessels lack autoregulation. Therefore maternal hypotension decreases uterine and fetal perfusion. Maternal shock results in splanchnic and uterine artery vasoconstriction, which decreases blood flow and oxygen transport to the fetus. Electronic fetal monitoring (EFM) tracings can assist in the evaluation of maternal status after trauma. EFM tracings reflect fetal cardiac responses to hypoxia and hypoperfusion, including tachycardia or bradycardia, decreased or absent baseline variability, and late decelerations.

Careful monitoring of fetal status assists greatly in maternal assessment, because the fetal monitor tracing works as an "oximeter" of internal maternal well-being. Hypoperfusion may be present in the pregnant woman before the onset of clinical signs of shock. The EFM tracings show the first signs of maternal compromise, such as when maternal

HR, BP, and color appear normal, yet the EFM printout shows signs of fetal hypoxia (Murray, 1997).

Mechanisms of Trauma
Blunt Abdominal Trauma

Blunt abdominal trauma is most commonly the result of motor vehicle crashes but also may be the result of battering or falls. Maternal and fetal mortality and morbidity rates are directly correlated with whether the mother remains inside the vehicle or is ejected. Maternal death is usually the result of a head injury or exsanguination from a major vessel rupture. Serious retroperitoneal hemorrhage after lower abdominal and pelvic trauma is reported more frequently during pregnancy. Serious maternal abdominal injuries are usually the result of splenic rupture or liver or renal injury.

When maternal survival of trauma occurs, fetal death is usually the result of abruptio placentae occurring within 48 hours of the accident (Shah & Kilcline, 2003). Placental separation is thought to be a result of deformation of the elastic myometrium around the relatively inelastic placenta. Shearing of the placental edge from the underlying decidua basalis results and is worsened by the increased intrauterine pressure resulting from the impact. It is critical that all pregnant victims be carefully evaluated for signs and symptoms of abruptio placentae after even minor blunt abdominal trauma.

■ NURSE ALERT

Signs and symptoms of abruptio placentae include uterine tenderness or pain, uterine irritability, uterine contractions, vaginal bleeding, leaking of amniotic fluid, or a change in FHR characteristics.

Pelvic fracture may result from severe injury and may produce bladder trauma or retroperitoneal bleeding with the two-point displacement of pelvic bones that usually occurs. One point of displacement is commonly at the symphysis pubis, and the second point is posterior, because of the structure of the pelvis. Careful evaluation for clinical signs of internal hemorrhage is indicated.

Direct fetal injury as a complication of trauma during pregnancy most often involves the fetal skull and brain (Gilbert & Harmon, 2003). Most commonly this injury accompanies maternal pelvic fracture in late gestation, after the fetal head becomes engaged. When the force of the impact is great enough to fracture the maternal pelvis, the fetus will often sustain a skull fracture. Evaluation for fetal skull fracture or intracranial hemorrhage is indicated.

Uterine rupture as a result of trauma is rare, occurring in only 0.6% of all reported cases of trauma during pregnancy. Uterine rupture depends on numerous factors, including gestational age, the intensity of the impact, and the presence of a predisposing factor such as a distended uterus caused by polyhydramnios or multiple gestation or the presence of a uterine scar resulting from previous uterine surgery (Cunningham, Leveno, Bloom, Hauth, Gilstrap, & Wenstrom, 2005). When uterine rupture occurs, the force responsible is usually a direct, high-energy blow. Fetal death is common with traumatic uterine rupture. However, maternal death occurs less than 10% of the time, and when it occurs, it is usually the result of massive injuries sustained from an impact severe enough to rupture the uterus.

Penetrating Abdominal Trauma

Bullet wounds are the most frequent cause of penetrating abdominal injury, followed by stab wounds. Penetrating abdominal wounds have disparate prognoses for mother and fetus in almost 66% of cases; that is, the woman survives, but the fetus does not. The enlarged uterus may protect other maternal organs, but the fetus is more vulnerable (Cunningham et al., 2005).

Numerous factors determine the extent and severity of maternal and fetal injury from a bullet wound, including size and velocity of the bullet, anatomic region penetrated, angle of entry, path of the bullet, organs damaged, gestational age, and exit wound. Once the bullet enters the body, it may ricochet several times as it encounters organs or bone, or it may sever a large blood vessel. During the second half of pregnancy, the fetus usually sustains a direct injury from the bullet. Gunshot wounds require surgical exploration to determine the extent of injury and repair damage as needed.

Stab wounds are limited by the length and width of the penetrating object and are usually confined to the pathway of the weapon. Maternal and fetal injury are less if the stab wound is located in the upper abdomen and from movement of the penetrating object from above the head downward toward the abdomen than from movement of the penetrating object from the ground upward toward the lower abdomen. Stab wounds usually require surgical exploration to clean out debris, determine extent of injury, and repair damage.

Thoracic Trauma

Thoracic trauma is reported to produce 25% of all trauma deaths. Pulmonary contusion results from nearly 75% of blunt thoracic trauma and is a potentially life-threatening condition. Pulmonary contusion can be difficult to recognize, especially if flail chest also is present or if there is no evidence of thoracic injury. Pulmonary contusion should be suspected in cases of thoracic injury, especially after blunt acceleration or deceleration trauma, such as that occurring when a rapidly moving vehicle crashes into an immovable object.

Penetrating wounds into the chest can result in pneumothorax or hemothorax. This type of injury is usually caused by a vehicular crash that results in impalement by the steering column or a loose article in the vehicle that became a projectile with the force of impact. Stab wounds into the chest also may occur as a result of violence.

Immediate Stabilization

Immediate priorities for stabilization of the pregnant woman after trauma should be identical to those of the nonpregnant trauma client. Pregnancy should not result in any restriction of the usual diagnostic, pharmacologic, or resuscitative procedures or maneuvers (ACOG, 1998). The initial response of many trauma team members when caring for the pregnant woman is to assess fetal status first because of the concern for a healthy neonate. Instead, the trauma team should follow a methodical evaluation of maternal status to ensure complete assessment and stabilization of the mother. Fetal survival depends on maternal survival, and stabilization of the mother improves fetal chance of survival.

▬ NURSE ALERT

Priorities of care for the pregnant woman after trauma must be to resuscitate the woman and stabilize her condition first, and then consider fetal needs.

Primary Survey

The systematic evaluation begins with a primary survey and the initial *ABCs* of resuscitation: establishment of and maintaining an *airway,* ensuring adequate *breathing,* and maintenance of an adequate *circulatory volume.*

Increased oxygen needs during gestation necessitate a rapid response. The presence of a cervical spine injury is always assumed.

▬ NURSE ALERT

Hyperextension of the neck is avoided; instead jaw thrust is used to establish an airway for the trauma victim.

Once an airway is established, assessment should focus on adequacy of oxygenation. The chest wall is observed for movement. If breathing is absent, ventilations and endotracheal intubation are initiated. Supplemental oxygen should be administered with a tight-fitting, nonrebreathing face mask at 10 to 12 L per minute to maintain adequate oxygen availability to the fetus. The chest wall is assessed for penetrating chest wound or flail chest. Breathing with a flail chest will be rapid and labored; chest wall movements will be uncoordinated and asymmetric; crepitus from bony fragments may be palpated.

Rapid placement of two large-bore (14 to 16 gauge) intravenous lines is necessary in the majority of seriously injured clients. It is important to place the lines while veins are still distended. Cardiac arrest during the immediate stabilization period is usually the result of profound hypovolemia, necessitating massive fluid resuscitation. Infusion of crystalloids such as Ringer's solution or normal saline solution should be given as a 3:1 ratio; that is, 3 ml of crystalloid replacement to 1 ml of the estimated blood loss is given over the first 30 to 60 minutes of acute resuscitation (ACOG, 1998). Because of the 50% increase in blood volume during pregnancy, published formulas for nonpregnant adults used for estimating crystalloid and blood replacement to counter blood loss must be adjusted upward for pregnancy.

Replacement of red blood cells and other blood components is anticipated, and blood is drawn for type, crossmatch, complete blood cell count, and platelet count (Van

Hook et al., 2004). Infusion of type-specific whole blood or packed red blood cells is usually necessary to improve fetal oxygenation status and to replace blood loss. During an extreme emergency, type O Rh-negative blood may be administered without matching.

Vasopressor drugs to restore maternal arterial BP should be avoided, if possible, until volume replacement is administered. Although vasopressor agents result in decreased perfusion to the uterus, they should be given, and not withheld, if needed for successful resuscitation of the mother (ACOG, 1998).

After 20 weeks of gestation, venous return to the heart is best accomplished by positioning the uterus to one side to eliminate the weight of the uterus compressing the inferior vena cava or the descending aorta. This facilitates efforts to establish the forward flow of blood through resuscitation and stabilization. If a lateral position is not possible because of resuscitative efforts or cervical spine immobilization, the uterus can be manually deflected to the left, or a wedge should be inserted underneath the right side of the backboard or stretcher.

Signs of bleeding may be more difficult to recognize in the pregnant woman because a 30% to 35% loss of maternal blood volume may produce only a minimal change in maternal MAP. Hypovolemia can be detrimental for the fetus because the vascular bed of the uterus is a low-resistance system that depends on adequate maternal arterial pressure to maintain uterine and fetal perfusion. Maternal hypovolemia can be fatal for the fetus (Friese & Wojciehoski, 2005).

Establishing a baseline neurologic status (level of consciousness, pupil size and reactivity) is essential. The Glasgow Coma Scale is commonly used at the scene of the accident to help determine the extent of the head injury. The scale is simple and easy to use (Box 34-6).

Secondary Survey

After immediate resuscitation and successful stabilization measures, a more detailed secondary survey of the mother and fetus should be accomplished. A complete physical assessment including all body systems is performed.

The maternal abdomen should be evaluated carefully, because a large percentage of serious injuries involve the uterus, intraperitoneal structures, and the retroperitoneum. The pregnant woman's stomach is assumed to be full. A nasogastric tube can be used to empty the stomach to help prevent acid aspiration syndrome. An empty stomach facilitates respiratory efforts. The uterus should be evaluated for evidence of gross deformity, tenderness, irritability, or contractions (ACOG, 1998).

The greatest clinical concern after vehicular crashes is abruptio placentae, since up to 40% of these women will have an abruption (Mattox & Goetzl, 2005). Assessments should focus on recognition of this complication, with careful evaluation of fetal monitor tracings, uterine tenderness, labor, or vaginal bleeding. Ultrasound examination may be performed to determine gestational age, viability of

box 34-6	Glasgow Coma Scale			
Eyes	Open	Spontaneously	4
		To verbal command	3
		To pain	2
		No response	1
Best motor response	To verbal command	Obeys	6
	To painful stimulus	Localizes pain	5
		Flexion-withdrawal	4
		Flexion-abnormal (decorticate rigidity)	3
		Extension (decerebrate rigidity)	2
		No response	1
Best verbal response		Oriented and converses	5
		Disoriented and converses	4
		Inappropriate words	3
		Incomprehensible sounds	2
		No response	1
Total			3-15

fetus, and placental location. However, ultrasound studies cannot exclude abruptio placentae.

Peritoneal lavage for the pregnant woman after blunt abdominal trauma has proved to be a safe procedure and can be helpful in the early diagnosis of intraperitoneal injury or hemorrhage. Under direct visualization, the peritoneum is incised, and a peritoneal dialysis catheter is positioned. If aspiration yields free-flowing blood, the test is considered positive, and a laparotomy should be performed. This procedure is not necessary before laparotomy if intraperitoneal bleeding is clinically apparent. Indications for peritoneal lavage include abdominal symptoms or signs suggestive of intraperitoneal bleeding, alteration in mental status, unexplained shock, and severe multiple injuries (Cunningham et al., 2005).

If trauma is the result of a penetrating wound, the woman should be completely undressed and carefully examined for all entrance and exit wounds. A bullet may be located on x-ray films. Exploratory laparotomy is necessary after a gunshot wound to explore the abdominal cavity for organ damage and to repair any damage present, with careful examination of all organs, the entire bowel, and posterior vessels. If uterine injury is determined, a careful evaluation of the risks and benefits of cesarean birth is quickly accomplished. A cesarean birth is desirable if the fetus is alive and near term and may be necessary for the preterm fetus because of the high incidence of fetal injury in these cases. The fetus usually tolerates surgery and anesthesia if adequate uterine perfusion and oxygenation are maintained. Tetanus prophylaxis guidelines are not changed by pregnancy.

Trauma may affect numerous systems in the maternal body and may affect more than the pregnancy. External signs of maternal trauma should suggest the possibility of internal trauma. Back and neck pain suggest spine injury, abrasions on the chest suggest chest injury, and limb pain and malposition suggest limb fractures. If head injury results in nonresponsiveness, suspect spinal, thoracic, and abdominal injuries. Hypovolemic shock can occur with internal hemorrhage, fracture of long bones, ruptured liver or spleen, hemothorax, or arterial dissection.

Once immediate stabilization is achieved, obstetric clients with severe trauma and massive blood loss that merits vigorous fluid resuscitation will usually benefit from the use of hemodynamic monitoring with a fiberoptic pulmonary catheter to determine cardiac and pulmonary function more precisely and to calculate volume and oxygen needs. The hemodynamic profile permits precise fluid resuscitation volumes. Oxygenation status calculations, including oxygen content, delivery, and consumption, will demonstrate which fluids are needed to enhance oxygen transport. Precise determinations can help prevent the potential sequelae of too little or too much fluid administration. With massive trauma, this care may be best provided in a regional trauma center with the obstetric team working closely with the trauma team, the obstetric team providing the obstetric care while the trauma team provides the trauma care.

All female trauma victims of childbearing age should be considered pregnant until proven otherwise. Determination of the health history and a history of the events preceding the trauma are important components of care. If the pregnant woman was involved in a vehicular crash, it should be determined whether she was the driver or a passenger and if she was ejected from the vehicle or used a restraining device and remained within the vehicle.

The physical examination should be performed in a systematic manner (Box 34-7).

Electronic Fetal Monitoring

Use of EFM may be predictive of abruptio placentae in pregnant trauma victims beyond week 20 of gestation (ACOG, 1998). Continuous EFM may show early signs of abruptio placentae, including a change in baseline rate, loss of accelerations, or the presence of late decelerations. Fetal monitoring should be initiated soon after the woman is stable, because abruptio placentae usually becomes apparent shortly after the injury. Fetal monitoring should be continued and further evaluation initiated if any of the

box 34-7 Physical Examination of the Pregnant Trauma Victim

HEAD

- Check scalp for signs of cuts, bruises, or edema. Examine skull for deformities, depressions, or lumps. Examine eyes and eyelids. Evaluate pupils for size, equality, and reaction to light. If contact lenses are present, remove them. Examine nose and ears, and observe for serous or bloody fluid. Open the mouth and look for blood, vomitus, loose teeth, and dentures.
- Neurologic function should be evaluated frequently, because the most frequent cause of death in women not using seat belts is head trauma (ACOG, 1998). If neurologic checks show a possible head trauma, a complete neurologic consultation and examination should be obtained quickly, including skull films and computed tomographic examination.

NECK

- Palpate for tenderness over the cervical spine area. Immobilize with a cervical collar and backboard if complaints of tenderness are present or any injury is suspected. Tilt backboard to side as soon as the pregnant woman is placed on backboard.

CHEST

- Observe for lacerations, contusions, wounds, or impaled objects. Observe chest wall movement for symmetry and equal expansion. Assess breath sounds and quality and rate of respirations. Observe for deviated trachea, sounds of sucking wounds, and flail chest. Palpate ribs, sternum, and clavicle.

ABDOMEN

- Observe for lacerations, contusions, wounds, or impaled objects. Perform light and then deep palpation. Apply electronic fetal monitoring (EFM) devices, both the ultrasound Doppler device and tocodynamometer. Palpate for intensity of uterine contractions and determine uterine resting tone. Observe fetal heart rate tracing for signs of fetal reassurance or compromise.

LOWER BACK

- Palpate for tenderness. Observe for contusions, deformities, or other signs of injury.

EXTREMITIES

- Examine for deformities, edema, dislocation, bleeding, contusions, and fractures. Palpate for tenderness. Assess radial and pedal pulses. Request pregnant woman to move extremities; observe response.

VAGINA

- Use digital examination for term gestation without vaginal bleeding; use sterile speculum examination for preterm gestation or if vaginal bleeding is present. Assess for signs of labor, injuries to tissues, or evidence of ruptured membranes.

URINARY TRACT

- Observe for the presence of blood in the urine. Trauma to the lower urinary tract is usually accompanied by a fractured pelvis, requiring use of a Foley catheter. Rupture of the bladder may occur in late pregnancy without a pelvic fracture because the full bladder becomes an abdominal organ. Maintain accurate intake and output and observe color of urine.

---

aforementioned signs occur. The external device to monitor uterine activity, the tocodynamometer, is unable to measure pressures, and the pattern made with this device shows the frequency and duration of contractions only. Palpation is required to evaluate the intensity of contractions and the uterine resting tone. It is important to palpate between contractions to verify that the uterus is well relaxed. If the uterus does not relax between contractions, abruptio placentae could be present.

Abruptio placentae occurring after trauma may be delayed up to 48 hours after the incident. EFM periods of 2 to 6 hours after minor trauma are adequate if there are no uterine contractions, uterine tenderness, or bleeding (ACOG, 1998). However, fetal reassurance must be established after minor trauma before fetal monitoring is discontinued and the woman is discharged.

■ LEGAL TIP Care of the Pregnant Woman Involved in a Minor Trauma Situation

After minor trauma, the pregnant woman may be discharged after an adequate period of EFM that demonstrates fetal reassurance and absence of uterine contractions. However, clear instructions must be given for immediate return if vaginal bleeding, leaking of amniotic fluid, decreased fetal movement, or abdominal pain occurs (ACOG, 1998).

Fetal-Maternal Hemorrhage

The potential for fetal-maternal hemorrhage exists after trauma; hemorrhage can lead to fetal anemia, distress, or even death. If the pregnant trauma victim is Rh negative, fetal-maternal hemorrhage can result in sensitization and hemolytic disease of the neonate. The routine use of the Kleihauer-Betke assay in women with blunt abdominal trauma or multiple trauma helps identify cases with a hemorrhage of more than 30 ml (ACOG, 1998). Because most cases have less than 30 ml of hemorrhage, the routine administration of 300 mg (one ampule) of $Rh_o(D)$ immunoglobulin is appropriate, because this practice would protect almost all pregnant trauma clients negative for $Rh_o(D)$ from isoimmunization (ACOG, 1998).

Ultrasound

Ultrasonography after trauma is not as sensitive as EFM for diagnosing abruptio placentae. Ultrasound may be useful to help establish gestational age, locate the placenta, evaluate cardiac activity (to determine whether the fetus is alive), and determine amniotic fluid volume (ACOG, 1998). Ultrasound may also be used to evaluate the presence of intraabdominal fluid that would suggest the presence of intraabdominal hemorrhage.

Radiation Exposure

If the pregnant woman has sustained serious injuries, any necessary radiographic examination should be performed, regardless of fetal exposure. If radiographic examination would be performed for the nonpregnant trauma victim, it also should be performed for the pregnant woman. Special efforts can minimize the dose to the lower abdomen. Shielding the uterus during irradiation procedures and eliminating duplicate films usually exposes the fetus to a radiation dose of less than 1 rad (ACOG, 1998).

In some victims with blunt abdominal trauma, abdominal-pelvic computed tomography (CT) is preferred to visualize extraperitoneal and retroperitoneal structures and the genitourinary tract. This procedure, in general, exposes the fetus to 5 to 10 rad and should not be withheld for the pregnant woman.

Blunt head trauma and loss of consciousness necessitate skull films and CT assessment with neurosurgical consultation. Magnetic resonance imaging also may be used to assess injuries (ACOG, 1998).

Perimortem Cesarean Delivery

In the presence of multisystem trauma, perimortem cesarean delivery may be indicated. Removal of the stressor of pregnancy early in the process of resuscitation may increase the chance for maternal survival. Fetal survival is unlikely if cesarean delivery is accomplished more than 20 minutes after maternal death. Therefore, to facilitate resuscitative efforts, consideration may be given to cesarean delivery for maternal benefit after 5 minutes of resuscitative efforts that produce no response in the mother (Gonik & Foley, 2004). It should be emphasized that this procedure is rarely successful.

▬ FAMILY-CENTERED OBSTETRIC
▬ CRITICAL CARE

Obstetric critical care should include the components of family-centered maternity care because this critically ill woman also is experiencing pregnancy and birth.

Components of family-centered critical care include the following elements:
- Open visitation so that spouse, significant other, or family members are present and provide support during labor, birth, and the postpartum period.
- Facilitation of parent-infant contact and attachment. The neonate should be brought to the bedside frequently if the condition permits. When the infant's condition does not permit leaving the neonatal intensive care unit (NICU), pictures of the infant should be placed within focus of the mother's eyes. Staff and family can talk about the infant and keep her updated on the infant's condition.
- Sibling visitation, reassuring the mother that the older child is included in the experience.
- Family visitation as the mother desires. This can be arranged around necessary care procedures. The critically ill mother needs this care, perhaps even more than the healthy mother does.

Obstetric nurses have become accustomed to family-centered maternity care. When the critically ill mother receives care in an OBICU, there seem to be fewer problems for inclusion of the components of family-centered care than when the mother has to be transported to the adult ICU, probably because the obstetric staff is accustomed to this care and the nursery is more readily available to the labor suite than to the ICU. Obstetric and critical care nurses can work together to include the components of family-centered care. Many ICUs are adopting the family-centered care philosophy, which ranges from open visitation to more inclusion of the family in the woman's care—depending mainly on her condition (Henneman & Cardin, 2002).

Never assume that the mother is too ill to see and hold her infant. Encourage this and observe her body language to determine how much contact with the infant she desires. If perinatal loss occurs as a result of severe illness, provide grief support. Initiate all the components of grief support as usual for the institution. Burial plans can be delayed until the mother's condition improves so that her concerns are addressed (see Chapter 41).

Maternal Death

It is extremely rare for a woman to die in childbirth, but it does happen. The yearly occurrence of maternal deaths in the United States is 11.8 per 100,000 live births (Chang et al., 2003). The leading causes of maternal death are embolism and preeclampsia. Older women ($\geq$35) and those without prenatal care are at greatest risk. A higher mortality ratio exists in African American women compared to Caucasian women. The father and extended family who are faced with mourning not only the death of a wife and mother but also the death of the baby have a particularly difficult time. Conversely, the father may be faced with parenting a baby without a surviving mother. Death of a mother disrupts the family structure and leaves the father with the care of a baby when he is greatly distressed. Thus the father and extended family, especially other children and grandparents, need supportive grief counseling at the time of death and after discharge for them to heal after such a devastating loss.

The nursing care of families at this time is similar to that described in Chapter 41. Options need to be offered, memories made, and mementos obtained and held for the family until they are ready for them. These families are at risk for complicated bereavement and altered parenting of the surviving baby and other children in the family. Referral to social services to help the family mobilize support systems and for counseling can help combat potential problems before they develop. Such a referral may be beneficial not only at the time of the loss but also in the future.

The emotional toll that a maternal death can take on the nursing and medical staff also must be addressed. Guilt, anger, fear, sadness, and depression are all common responses to a maternal death. The staff may want to review the situation surrounding the events, the chart, and their responses in the forum of a mortality-morbidity review and a critical incident debriefing to help in coping with the feelings and emotions that result after a maternal death. Attending memorial or funeral services may benefit staff and family.

community activity

Investigate the hospitals in your community to determine where and how OB critical care clients are treated. If women need to be transferred to another hospital, what is the procedure and how is the woman's family included?

key points

- The numbers of critically ill pregnant women are increasing, paralleling improvements in pediatric and neonatal care. Any nurse providing care for pregnant women may encounter the critically ill pregnant woman and must be able to initiate appropriate care.
- Nurses must recognize early signs of severe complications and expedite the institution's plan for the critically ill pregnant woman to receive necessary complex care.
- The institutional plan may consist of actual implementation of critical care procedures in a labor and birth unit, stabilization, and preparation for transport to a tertiary center or adult ICU, with obstetric consultation after transport.
- Normal physiologic alterations during pregnancy produce profound hemodynamic changes. The critical care team should base care on knowledge of normal hemodynamic values for the pregnant state.
- Pregnancy is not a contraindication for hemodynamic monitoring.
- Invasive hemodynamic monitoring is associated with potential complications. However, the benefits usually outweigh the risks when the woman is critically ill.
- Pulmonary artery catheterization provides continuous information about left ventricle function; this information is not available from any other method.
- Use of a PAC in combination with an arterial pressure catheter and pulse oximeter provides adequate data to assess continuously both cardiac and pulmonary status.

- The fiberoptic PAC provides a continuous SvO_2, which is a sensitive marker of physiologic instability because it reflects overall adequacy of oxygen delivery to the tissues.
- The active roles assumed by most pregnant women today place them at risk for vehicular crashes, falls, violence, and other injuries.
- Intimate partner violence and battering increase during pregnancy.
- Pregnancy does not limit or restrict resuscitative, diagnostic, or pharmacologic treatment after trauma.
- Fetal survival depends on maternal survival. After trauma the first priority, before consideration of fetal concerns, is resuscitation and stabilization of the mother.
- Optimal care for the pregnant victim of trauma depends on knowledge of the physiologic state of pregnancy.
- Minor trauma is associated with major complications for the pregnancy, including abruptio placentae, fetomaternal hemorrhage, preterm labor and birth, and fetal death.
- Trauma from accidents is the most common cause of death in women of childbearing age.
- Care of the critically ill pregnant woman should include the components of family-centered childbirth.
- Death of a woman in childbirth is rare; it disrupts family structure, and the family needs supportive grief counseling.

REFERENCES

American Academy of Pediatrics (AAP) & American College of Obstetricians and Gynecologists (ACOG). (2002). *Guidelines for perinatal care* (5th ed.). Elk Grove Village, IL: Authors.

American College of Obstetricians and Gynecologists (ACOG). (1992). *Invasive hemodynamic monitoring in obstetrics and gynecology.* ACOG Technical Bulletin No. 175. Washington, DC: Author.

American College of Obstetricians and Gynecologists (ACOG). (1998). *Trauma during pregnancy.* ACOG Education Bulletin No. 251. Washington, DC: Author.

Association of Women's Health, Obstetric and Neonatal Nurses (AWHONN). (2003). *Standards and guidelines for professional nursing practice in the care of women, and newborns* (6th ed.). Washington, DC: Author.

Berg, C., Chang, J., Callaghan, W., & Whitehead, S. (2003). Pregnancy-related mortality in the United States, 1991-1997. *Obstetrics and Gynecology, 101*(2), 289-296.

Chang, J., Elam-Evans, L., Berg, C., Herndon, J., Flowers, L., Seed, K., et al. (2003). Pregnancy-related mortality surveillance—United

States, 1991-1999. *MMWR Morbidity and Mortality Weekly Report, 52*(SS02), 1-8.

Clark, S., Cotton, D., Lee, W., Bishop, C., Hill, T., Southick, J., et al. (1989). Central hemodynamic assessment of normal term pregnancy. *American Journal of Obstetrics and Gynecology, 161*(6), 1439-1442.

Clark, S., Cotton, D., Pivarnik, J., Lee, W., Hankins, G., Benedett, T., et al. (1991). Position change and central hemodynamic profile during normal third-trimester pregnancy and postpartum. *American Journal of Obstetrics and Gynecology, 164*(3), 883-887.

Cowan, S., Coscia, L., Philips, L., Wagoner, L., Mannion, J., Moritz, M., et al. (2002) Pregnancy outcomes in female heart and heart-lung transplant recipients. *Transplantation Proceedings, 34*(2), 1855-1856.

Cunningham, G., Leveno, K., Bloom, S., Hauth, J., Gilstrap, L., & Wenstrom, K. (Eds.). (2005). *Williams obstetrics* (22nd ed.). New York: McGraw-Hill.

Darovic, G. (2002). *Hemodynamic monitoring: Invasive and noninvasive clinical application.* Philadelphia: Saunders.

El Kady, D., Gilbert, W., Xing, G., & Smith, L. (2005). Maternal and neonatal outcomes of assaults during pregnancy. *Obstetrics and Gynecology, 105*(2), 357-363.

Friese, G., & Wojciehoski, R. (2005). Fetal trauma from motor vehicle collisions. *Journal of Emergency Medical Services, 30*(5), 110-127.

Fujitani, S., & Baldisseri, M. (2005). Hemodynamic assessment in a pregnant and peripartum patient. *Critical Care Medicine, 33*(Suppl), S354–S361.

Gilbert, E., & Harmon, J. (2003). *Manual of high risk pregnancy & delivery* (3rd ed.). St. Louis: Mosby.

Gonik, B., & Foley, M. (2004). Intensive care monitoring of the critically ill pregnant patient. In R. Creasy, R. Resnik, & J. Iams (Eds.). *Maternal-fetal medicine: Principles and practice* (5th ed.). Philadelphia: Saunders.

Henneman, E., & Cardin, S. (2002). Family-centered critical care: A practical approach to making it happen. *Critical Care Nursing, 22*(6), 12-19.

Hou, S. (2003). Pregnancy in renal transplant recipients. *Advances in Renal Replacement Therapy, 10*(1), 40-47.

Ikossi, D., Lazar, A., Morabito, D., Fildes, J., & Knudson, M. (2005). Profile of mothers at risk: An analysis of injury and pregnancy loss in 1,195 trauma patients. *Journal of the American College of Surgeons, 200*(1), 49-56.

Leather, H., Vuylsteke, A., Bert, C., M'Fam, W., Segers, P., Sergeant, P., et al. (2004). Evaluation of a new continuous cardiac output monitor in off-pump coronary artery surgery. *Anaesthesia, 59*(4), 385-389.

Mabie, W. (2004). Pulmonary edema. In G. Dildy, M. Belfort, G. Saade, J. Phelan, G. Hankins, & S. Clark (Eds.), *Critical care obstetrics* (4th ed.). Malden, MA: Blackwell Science.

Mabie, W., & Sibai, B. (1990). Treatment in an obstetric intensive care unit. *American Journal of Obstetrics and Gynecology, 162*(1), 1-4.

Mattox, K., & Goetzl, L. (2005). Trauma in pregnancy. *Critical Care Medicine, 33*(10S), S385-S389.

McFarlane, J., Campbell, J., Sharps, P., & Watson, K. (2002). Abuse during pregnancy and femicide: Urgent implications for women's health. *Obstetrics and Gynecology, 100*(1), 27-36.

McGwin, G., Russell, S., Rux, R., Leath, C., Valent, F., & Rue, L. (2004). Knowledge, beliefs, and practices concerning seat belt use, during pregnancy. *Journal of Trauma, 56*(3), 670-675.

Miller, J., Mastrobattista, J., & Katz, A. (2000). Obstetrical and neonatal outcome in pregnancies after liver transplantation. *American Journal of Perinatology, 17*(6), 299-302.

Murray, M. (1997). *Antepartal and intrapartal fetal monitoring* (2nd ed.). Albuquerque, NM: Learning Resources International.

National Institutes of Health & National Heart, Lung, and Blood Institute. (2000). *Classification of the hypertensive disorders of pregnancy. Working report on hypertension in pregnancy*. Bethesda, MD: NIH.

Norwitz, E., Robinson, J., & Malone, F. (2004). Pregnancy-induced physiologic alterations. In G. Dildy, M. Belfort, G. Saade, J. Phelan, G. Hankins, & S. Clark (Eds.), *Critical care obstetrics* (4th ed.). Malden, MA: Blackwell Science.

Roberts, J. (2004). Pregnancy-related hypertension. In R. Creasy, R. Resnik, & J. Iams (Eds.), *Maternal-fetal medicine: Principles and practice* (5th ed.), Philadelphia: Saunders.

Shah, A., & Kilcline, B. (2003). Trauma in pregnancy. *Emergency Medicine Clinics of North America, 21*(3), 615-629.

Sgro, M., Barozzino, T., Mirghani, H., Sermer, M., Moscato, L., Akoury, H., et al. (2002). Pregnancy outcome post renal transplantation. *Teratology, 65*(1), 5-9.

Van Hook, J., Gei, A., & Pacheco, L. (2004). Trauma in pregnancy. In G. Dildy, M. Belfort, G. Saade, J. Phelan, G. Hankins, & S. Clark (Eds.), *Critical care obstetrics* (4th ed.). Malden, MA: Blackwell Science.

Wallace, D., & Winslow, E. (1993). Effects of iced and room temperature injectate on cardiac output measurements in critically ill patients with low and high cardiac outputs. *Heart and Lung, 32*(1), 2-12.

Weinberg, L., Steele, R., Pugh, R., Higgins, S., Herbert, M., & Story, D. (2005). The pregnant trauma patient. *Anaesthesia and Intensive Care, 33*(2), 167-180.

Zeeman, G., Wendel, G., & Cunningham, F. (2003). A blueprint for obstetric critical care. *American Journal of Obstetrics and Gynecology, 188*(2), 532-536.

CHAPTER 35

Anne Hopkins Fishel

Mental Health Disorders and Substance Abuse

learning objectives

- Delineate emotional complications during pregnancy, including management of anxiety disorders and mood disorders.
- Examine substance abuse during pregnancy, including dual diagnosis, prevalence, risk factors, legal considerations, treatment programs, barriers to treatment, and care management.

- Identify postpartum emotional complications, including incidence, risk factors, signs and symptoms, and management.
- Evaluate the role of the nurse in assessing and managing care of women with emotional complications during pregnancy and postpartum.

electronic resources

Additional information related to the content in Chapter 35 can be found on

the companion website at **evolve**
http://evolve.elsevier.com/Lowdermilk/MWHC/
- NCLEX Review Questions
- WebLinks

or on the interactive companion CD
- NCLEX Review Questions
- Critical Thinking Exercise: Postpartum Depression
- Plan of Care: Postpartum Depression
- Plan of Care: Substance Abuse During Pregnancy

*M*ANAGEMENT of mental health disorders takes place primarily in community settings. Women who have serious mental disorders may be engaging in sexual activities that can result in pregnancy. Mental health disorders have implications for the pregnant woman, the fetus, the newborn, and the entire family. Between 10% and 20% of women have these disorders (Lehmann, 2004). The symptoms and treatment can complicate pregnancy, childbirth, and the postpartum period (Goodman, 2005).

■ MENTAL HEALTH DISORDERS ■ DURING PREGNANCY

The pregnant woman may have a history of mood disorder, anxiety disorder, substance use disorder, schizophrenia, personality disorder, or developmental disorder. If she is currently not in treatment, assessment throughout pregnancy and the postpartum period is critical to the mother's and the baby's health. With a history of mental illness, referral to a mental health specialist for evaluation is recommended. Some psychiatric disorders, such as panic disorder, may improve or abate during pregnancy; in contrast, obsessive-compulsive disorder (OCD) appears to be more

prevalent during pregnancy, with one study citing that more than 25% of women with OCD reported symptom onset during pregnancy (Schatzberg, & Nemeroff, 2004). Psychiatric disorders with a psychotic component, such as schizophrenia, generally worsen during pregnancy.

Mood Disorders

Women who are being treated for depression may become pregnant, either intentionally or accidentally. In a review of 21 research articles, the prevalence of depression during pregnancy was cited as being 7.4% during the first trimester, 12.8% during the second trimester, and 12% during the third trimester (Bennett, Einarson, Toddio, Koren, & Einarson, 2004). Of all pregnant women treated for depression, approximately one third of them have a first occurrence during their pregnancy (Pigarelli, Kraus, & Potter, 2005). These findings dispel the myth that pregnancy is a "pleasant and happy event" for all women.

Mood disorders are defined as disorders that have as their dominant feature a disturbance in the prevailing emotional state. To be diagnosed with major depression, at least five of the following signs or symptoms must be present nearly every day: depressed mood, often with spontaneous crying; markedly diminished interest in all activities;

insomnia or hypersomnia; weight changes (increases and decreases); psychomotor retardation or agitation; fatigue or loss of energy; feelings of worthlessness or inappropriate guilt; diminished ability to concentrate; and suicidal ideation with or without a suicidal plan (American Psychiatric Association [APA], 2000).

■ **NURSE ALERT**

Diagnostic assessment for depression in pregnant women is difficult because many of the symptoms of pregnancy mimic depression. Critical cues are the presence of psychologic symptoms, a suicide plan, and major disruptions in sleep pattern. Risk factors for developing depression in pregnancy include a prior history in self or family, a lack of social support, stressful life events, partner discord, and history of premenstrual syndrome (PMS).

Collaborative Care

Medical management of depression is usually a combination of antidepressants and cognitive-behavioral or interpersonal psychotherapy. Self-help strategies such as exercise, respite from caregiving, self-help groups, and making time for one's self can be helpful (Fishel, 1999). Nursing strategies include educating the woman about depression as an illness, about treatment success, and about antidepressant medications. For the woman who refuses medications during pregnancy, the nurse should discuss alternative treatments and respect her choice. The nurse also can be effective by maintaining a caring relationship, which includes being hopeful. The nurse can ask about a time when the woman was coping well and how she was able to combat the depression then.

If a woman becomes psychotic during pregnancy, usually because she has quit taking mood stabilizers or antipsychotics, or because she has a history of schizophrenia, this is a medical emergency. To treat a psychotic state, antipsychotic medication or electroconvulsive therapy (ECT) is preferable to lithium or anticonvulsant medications (Kaplan & Sadock, 2005). However, lithium is currently considered the first-line medication for the treatment of bipolar disorder during pregnancy (Pigarelli et al., 2005).

Antidepressant Medications. No consensus exists about safety in the use of antidepressant medications with pregnant women. To date, the U.S. Food and Drug Administration (FDA) has not approved any psychotropic medication for use during pregnancy. None of these medications is rated as an FDA category A drug (controlled studies show no risk to the fetus) (see Table 35-1 for FDA pregnancy risk category of most common antidepressant medications). Amitriptyline, imipramine, and nortriptyline, along with the monoamine oxidase inhibitors (MAOIs) are the most risky. Because the majority of women are not aware of their pregnancy until at least 6 weeks of gestation, psychotropic medications may not be discontinued until after the period of greatest potential risk to the fetus has passed (Stowe, Strader, & Nemeroff, 2005). For women with severe depression who would be at risk of suicide without medication, clinical judgment usually dictates continued use of antidepressants. In one study, 75% of women who had discontinued antidepressant medications relapsed during pregnancy; the majority occurred in the first trimester, and relapse was more prevalent in women with histories of more chronic depression (Cohen et al., 2004). The commonly used antidepressant drugs are often divided into four groups: selective serotonin reuptake inhibitors (SSRIs), serotonin/norepinephrine reuptake inhibitors (SNRIs), tricyclic antidepressants (TCAs), and MAOIs (Kando, Wells, & Hayes, 2005).

Many scientists are reluctant to do research on the effects of psychotropic medications on fetuses. Concerns about safety of antidepressants are common; however, untreated depression may have adverse effects on the developing fetus, including preterm birth, small head circumference, and low Apgar scores (Pigarelli et al., 2005). In a landmark study, Nulman and colleagues (1997) reported that in utero exposure to fluoxetine or TCAs did not affect either neurodevelopment or behavior in preschool-age children. However, some studies have reported higher rates of perinatal complications (low maternal weight gain, premature birth, and delayed fetal growth rate) associated with third-trimester use of fluoxetine (Hendrick & Altshuler, 2002). In a study comparing 17 SSRI-exposed and 17 nonexposed newborns, the women who used SSRIs during pregnancy had healthy infants; however, the infants also showed disruptions in a wide range of neurobehavioral outcomes (Zeskind & Stephens, 2004). In reviewing 93 cases of SSRI-induced neonatal withdrawal syndrome, paroxetine caused the most cases (64 babies), followed by fluoxetine (14), Zoloft (9), and Celexa (7) (Sanz, 2005).

Although less information is known about SSRIs (than TCAs) during pregnancy, they are emerging as first-line agents in treatment (Pigarelli et al., 2005). They are relatively safe and carry fewer side effects than the TCAs. However, if an SSRI is taken with dextromethorphan, an agent found in cough syrup, the combination could trigger the serotonin syndrome (mental status changes, agitation, hyperreflexia, shivering, diarrhea, etc.). The most frequent side effects with the SSRIs are gastrointestinal (GI) disturbances (nausea, diarrhea), headache, and insomnia. In about one third of clients, the SSRIs reduce libido, arousal, or orgasmic function (Kando et al., 2005). SSRIs also can inhibit specific P-450 isoenzymes, resulting in marked elevations in drug concentrations and reduction in drug clearance.

The TCAs cause many central nervous system (CNS) and peripheral nervous system (PNS) side effects. Although some are simply annoying, others are significant or even dangerous (Kando et al., 2005). In overdose, these medications can cause death. A common CNS effect is sedation, and this could easily interfere with mothers caring for their babies. A mother could doze off while holding the baby and drop him or her, or she could have trouble becoming fully awake during the night to care for the baby. Other side effects include weight gain, tremors, grand mal seizures, nightmares, agitation or mania, and extrapyramidal side effects. Anticholinergic side effects include dry

table 35-1 **Antidepressant Medications**	PREGNANCY RISK CATEGORY*	LACTATION RISK CATEGORY*
SELECTIVE SEROTONIN REUPTAKE INHIBITORS		
Citalopram (Celexa)	C	L3
Escitalopram (Lexapro)	C	L3 in older infants
Fluoxetine (Prozac)	C	L2 in older infants; L3 in neonates
Fluvoxamine (Luvox)	C	L2
Paroxetine (Paxil)	B	L2
Sertraline (Zoloft)	B	L2
SEROTONIN/NOREPINEPHRINE REUPTAKE INHIBITORS		
Bupropion (Wellbutrin) IR & SR	B	L3
Maprotiline (Ludiomil)	B	L3
Mirtazapine (Remeron)	C	L3
Trazodone (Desyrel)	C	L2
Venlafaxine (Effexor)	C	L3
TRICYCLICS		
Amitriptyline (Elavil)	D	L2
Amoxapine (Asendin)	C	L2
Clomipramine (Anafranil)	C	L2
Desipramine (Norpramin)	C	L2
Doxepin (Sinequan)	C	L5
Imipramine (Tofranil)	D	L2
Nortriptyline (Pamelor)	D	L2
MONOAMINE OXIDASE INHIBITORS		
Phenelzine (Nardil)	unknown	unknown
Tranylcypromine (Parnate)	unknown	unknown

*Source: Hale, T. (2004). *Medications and mother's milk* (11th ed.). Amarillo, TX: Pharmasoft.
IR, Intermediate release; *SR*, sustained release.
B = Animal studies haven't shown fetal risk, but no controlled studies in pregnant women OR animal studies showed adverse effect that was not confirmed in controlled studies in women in first trimester—no risk in later trimesters.
C = Animal studies show adverse effects on fetus and no controlled studies in pregnant women OR no studies available
D = Positive evidence of human fetal risk
L2 = Drug studied in limited number of breastfeeding women with no adverse effects in infant OR evidence is remote
L3 = No controlled studies OR studies show minimal nonthreatening effects
L5 = Contraindicated because studies have shown significant and documented risk to infant

mouth, blurred vision (usually temporary), difficulty voiding, constipation, sweating, and orgasm difficulty (Kando et al.). The lack of research data on the use of MAOIs during pregnancy along with the dietary constraints and potential for hypertensive crisis generally discourage their use during pregnancy.

Anxiety Disorders

Anxiety disorders are the most common mental disorder. They include phobias (irrational fears that lead a person to avoid common objects, events, or situations), panic disorder (repeated, unprovoked episodes of intense fear, which develop without warning and are not related to any specific event), generalized anxiety disorder (constant worry unrelated to any event), obsessive compulsive disorder (OCD), and posttraumatic stress disorder (PTSD) (APA, 2000).

OCD symptoms include recurrent, persistent, and intrusive thoughts that cause anxiety, which a person tries to control by performing repetitive behaviors or "compulsions" (APA, 2000). The pregnant woman may have persistent thoughts that something is wrong with the baby, or she may become very preoccupied with checking and rechecking to make sure the baby is all right. Although she recognizes that these rituals are excessive, she will still perform them because of the fear that harm will come to her or the baby if she does not. Treatment usually includes antidepressant medication (SSRIs), cognitive-behavioral therapy, and education about how to manage the symptoms of the illness (Fishel, 1998).

PTSD can occur as a result of rape (see Chapter 6). Symptoms include reexperiencing the traumatic event, persistent avoidance of stimuli, and numbing, as well as difficulty sleeping, irritability or angry outbursts, difficulty concentrating, hypervigilance, and exaggerated startle response (APA, 2000). Nurses can support the healing process of persons with PTSD by being alert to what the woman is experiencing during pregnancy and labor.

If the current pregnancy is a result of rape, the woman may be extremely ambivalent about the baby. If the rape occurred some time ago, the whole experience of pregnancy with prenatal examinations can trigger memories of the original trauma. She may avoid prenatal examinations because of the anxiety triggered by bodily touch and vaginal examinations. Some pregnant women with PTSD may feel more comfortable with a female nurse-midwife or a female physician. Giving birth can trigger memories of being out of control, and she may lose contact with reality. The nurse can verbalize understanding of the anxiety and orient to current reality by saying, "You're having an examination to make sure the baby is okay," or, "You're in labor preparing to give birth to your baby. I am your nurse. You're in the hospital. I will check on you frequently. You are safe here." Treatment usually includes psychotherapy and referral to support groups.

Collaborative Care

Benzodiazepines and antidepressants are the most commonly used drugs for the treatment of anxiety disorders (see Table 35-1 and Table 35-2 for FDA categories for these medications). Even though benzodiazepines are the most widely prescribed, antidepressant medications are the treatments of choice. Some pregnant women who have been using benzodiazepines for "anxiety," "nervousness," or insomnia may not realize that these medications may be teratogenic (with consequences including cleft lip and palate), and that their use during pregnancy is not advised—particularly during the first trimester (Kirkwood & Melton, 2005). Note that most of the antianxiety medications are FDA category D (evidence of human fetal risk) or category X (demonstrated fetal abnormalities and use is contraindicated). However, benzodiazepines should not be abruptly discontinued during pregnancy, and they should be tapered sufficiently before the birth to limit neonatal withdrawal syndrome. Nurses should educate women about the dangers of benzodiazepines during pregnancy, assess for use during pregnancy, and help pregnant women find other ways to handle their anxiety and insomnia, or refer them to a psychiatrist who specializes in psychiatric disorders in pregnancy. Nursing strategies to reduce anxiety include empowerment through education; sensory interventions such as music therapy and aromatherapy; behavioral interventions such as breathing exercises, progressive muscle relaxation, guided imagery, and medication (see Table 35-2); and cognitive strategies such as encouraging positive self-talk and questioning negative thinking (Fishel, 1998).

Special Considerations for Medications during Pregnancy. The risks and benefits of drug therapy during pregnancy must always be weighed, and concerns about the risks of untreated depression during pregnancy should be considered (Kando et al., 2005). These concerns include the possibility of low birth weight, suicidality, potential for hospitalization, potential for marital discord, inability to engage in appropriate obstetric care, and difficulty caring for other children (Hendrick & Altshuler, 2002). Even though the basic rule is to avoid administering any medication to a woman who is pregnant, particularly during the first trimester (Kaplan & Sadock, 2005), decisions about the use of medications during pregnancy should be made jointly by the woman, her partner, and the health care providers. If the woman is stable and appears likely to remain well while not taking medication, then discontinuation before pregnancy is a viable option. For those with a history of relapse after medication discontinuation, remaining on the drug during pregnancy is advised (Kando et al.). Even though a pregnant woman should be receiving the lowest therapeutic dose, psychotropic medications may have to be increased over the course of pregnancy to maintain adequate therapeutic serum concentrations and response (Schatzberg & Nemeroff, 2005). Earlier literature indicated that the administration of psychotherapeutic medications at or near birth may cause a baby to be overly sedated at birth and need a respirator, or to be physically dependent on the drug and to require detoxification and treatment of a withdrawal syndrome. More recently, evidence suggests

---

table 35-2 **Antianxiety Medications**

ANTIANXIETY MEDICATIONS	PREGNANCY RISK CATEGORY*	LACTATION RISK CATEGORY*
Alprazolam (Xanax)	D	L3
Buspirone (BuSpar)	B	L3
Chlordiazepoxide (Librium)	D	L3
Clonazepam (Klonopin)	C	L3
Clorazepate (Tranxene)	D	L3
Diazepam (Valium)	D	L3; L4 if used chronically
Flurazepam (Dalmane)	X	L3
Lorazepam (Ativan)	D	L3
Midazolam (Versed)	D	L3
Temazepam (Restoril)	X	L3
Triazolam (Halcion)	X	L3

*Source: Hale, T. (2004). *Medications and mother's milk* (11th ed.). Amarillo, TX: Pharmasoft

B = Animal studies haven't shown fetal risk, but no controlled studies in pregnant women OR animal studies showed adverse effect that was not confirmed in controlled studies in women in first trimester—no risk in later trimesters
C = Animal studies show adverse effects on fetus but no controlled studies in pregnant women OR no studies available
D = Positive evidence of human fetal risk
X = Contraindicated because studies have shown significant and documented risk to infant
L3 = No controlled studies OR studies show minimal nonthreatening effects
L4 = Possibly hazardous

that discontinuation of antidepressants in women near term is unwarranted and may put the mother at unjustified risk; neonatal symptoms occur in a minority of cases and are self-limiting (Koren, Matsiu, Einarson, Knoppert, & Steiner, 2005).

All of the commonly used mood-stabilizing medications such as lithium carbonate, carbamazepine (Tegretol), gabapentin (Neurontin), lamotrigine (Lamictal), and divalproex sodium (Depakote) appear to carry an increased risk of fetal malformations and a potentially deleterious effect on later cognitive development (Stuart & Laraia, 2005) (see Table 35-4 for FDA categories of mood stabilizers). In more recent reviews of epidemiologic data, the risk of Epstein's anomaly is estimated to be quite small—0.05% to 0.1% in infants exposed to lithium during the first trimester. Other side effects in the newborn include muscular hypotonia with impaired breathing and cyanosis ("floppy baby syndrome"), neonatal hypothyroidism, nephrogenic diabetes insipidus, atrial flutter, tricuspid regurgitation, and congestive heart failure (Pigarelli et al., 2005). Mood stabilizers are often taken over the life span by women with bipolar disorder. Women should receive prepregnancy counseling, and those with a single manic episode should have medication tapered gradually and an attempt made to have a lithium-free pregnancy, or, if indicated, reinstitution of lithium after the first trimester. It is recommended that the clinician offer a fetal echocardiogram between weeks 16 and 18 of gestation for women who were treated with lithium during their first trimester of pregnancy.

If the pregnant woman is receiving pharmacologic treatment, the nurse must make sure that the woman is being followed by a psychiatrist or an advanced practice psychiatric nurse. No woman should withdraw abruptly from any psychotropic medication because of the risk of withdrawal symptoms.

▬ SUBSTANCE ABUSE
▬ DURING PREGNANCY

The damaging effects of alcohol and illicit drugs on pregnant women and their unborn babies are well known. Alcohol and other drugs easily pass from a mother to her baby through the placenta. Smoking during pregnancy may have serious health risks, including bleeding complications, miscarriage, stillbirth, prematurity, low birth weight, and sudden infant death syndrome; prenatal exposure to nicotine may lead to dysregulation in the neurodevelopment of the child and higher risk for behavioral problems (Brennan, 2003; Lester, Andreozzi, & Appiah, 2004).

Congenital abnormalities have occurred in infants of mothers who have taken drugs (Stuart & Laraia, 2005). The safest pregnancy is one in which the mother is totally drug- and alcohol-free, with one exception: for pregnant women addicted to heroin, methadone maintenance is safer for the fetus than acute opiate detoxification (Stuart & Laraia). Current use of alcohol is highest among females between

ages of 18 and 24—who are likely to be sexually active with potential for pregnancy (Cook, 2004)

Substance abuse refers to the continued use of substances despite related problems in physical, social, or interpersonal areas (APA, 2000). Recurrent abuse results in failure to fulfill major role obligations, and there may be substance-related legal problems. Any use of alcohol or illicit drugs during pregnancy is considered abuse (APA).

Dual diagnosis is the coexistence of substance abuse and another disorder. Major depression and anxiety disorders are the psychiatric disorders that commonly occur with substance abuse.

Prevalence

Because many pregnant women are reluctant to reveal their use of substances or to reveal the extent of their use, data on prevalence are highly variable. Approximately 12.3% of all mothers report cigarette smoking while pregnant, but this practice is on the decline (Lester et al., 2004). Among pregnant women responding to a national survey, 10% reported alcohol use, 4% reported binge alcohol use, and almost 1% reported heavy alcohol use in the month before the survey (Brady & Ashley, 2005). The Pregnancy Risk Assessment Monitoring System (PRAMS) estimated that the prevalence of alcohol use during pregnancy ranged from 3% to 10% (Brady & Ashley). Women aged 35 or older, non-Hispanic women, women with more than a high school education, and women with higher incomes reported the highest prevalence of alcohol use during pregnancy (Brady & Ashley). The National Pregnancy and Health Survey found that 19% of females used alcohol during pregnancy, and 5% used an illicit drug at least once during pregnancy, including marijuana (3%), and cocaine (1%) (Brady & Ashley). Data from the Maternal Life Study, which oversampled very low-birth-weight infants, found that 35% of pregnant females reported alcohol use and 8% reported marijuana use during pregnancy; meconium toxicology screens were positive for cocaine or opioids in 11% of infants screened (Brady & Ashley). Except for methamphetamine, pregnant women had a lower rate of substance abuse than nonpregnant women (Lester et al., 2004).

Risk Factors

Many factors contribute to substance abuse. Women have a clearer pattern of self-medication and are more likely than men to use a combination of alcohol and prescription drugs. Women begin to use during periods of depression, to relax, to feel more adequate, to lose weight, to decrease stress, or to help them sleep at night. Peer pressure introduces teens to drugs and alcohol; if use begins before age 15, the woman is 4 times more likely to have abuse problems as an adult (Stuart & Laraia, 2005). Lower educational attainment and lower rates of employment are risk factors for turning to substances (Brady & Ashley, 2005). Psychologic factors such as poor self-esteem and a tendency to seek pleasure and avoid pain can play a major role (Stuart

& Laraia). A history of family of origin dysfunction, psychiatric illness, or of physical or sexual abuse greatly increases a woman's risk for developing substance-abuse problems (Brady & Ashley). Both before and during pregnancy, victims of violence are more likely to use multiple substances than nonvictims. Continuation of substance use during pregnancy is more likely among victims of violence than among nonvictims.

Barriers to Treatment

Fewer than 10% of pregnant women who are substance abusers receive treatment for their addictions. Social stigma, labeling, and guilt are significant barriers (Brady & Ashley, 2005). Women often do not seek help because of the fear of losing custody of the child or criminal prosecution. Pregnant women who abuse substances commonly have little understanding of the ways in which these substances affect them, their pregnancies, or their babies. Pregnant women who are substance abusers may not seek prenatal care until labor begins. Often, pregnant women who use psychoactive substances receive negative feedback from society, as well as from health care providers, who not only may condemn them for endangering the life of their fetus, but also may even withhold support as a result. Barriers within the drug treatment system may deter these women as well. Traditionally, substance-abuse treatment programs have not addressed issues that affect pregnant women, such as concurrent need for obstetric care and child care for other children; the long waiting lists and lack of health insurance present further barriers to treatment (Lester et al., 2004). Pregnant women with co-occurring substance abuse and psychiatric disorders face unique barriers because of social stigma attached to both conditions and insufficient knowledge and training to manage coexisting disorders (Brady & Ashley).

Legal Considerations

Because of the risks to the unborn children and financial concerns, pregnant women who abuse substances may now face criminal charges under expanded interpretations of child abuse and drug trafficking statutes (Lester et al., 2004). At least 24 states have attempted to prosecute a pregnant woman on a variety of charges for suspected harm to the fetus (Tillett & Osborne, 2001). Some policymakers have proposed that pregnant women who abuse substances should be jailed, placed under house arrest, or committed to psychiatric hospitals for the remainder of their pregnancies (Stuart & Laraia, 2005). In a survey of obstetricians, pediatricians, and family practice physicians in Michigan, 82% to 83% were in favor of compulsory treatment for illicit drug and alcohol use during pregnancy but opposed to criminal prosecution (Abel & Kruger, 2002). Nurses who screen for substance abuse in pregnancy and encourage prenatal care, counseling, and treatment will be of greater benefit to the mother and child than will prosecution (Foley, 2002).

■ LEGAL TIP Drug Testing During Pregnancy

There is no requirement in the United States for a health care provider to test either the pregnant woman or the newborn for the presence of drugs. However, nurses need to know the practices of the states in which they are working. In some states, a woman whose urine drug screen test is positive at the time of labor and birth must be referred to child protective services. If the mother is not in a drug treatment program or is judged unable to provide care, the infant may be placed in foster care. The U.S. Supreme Court has ruled that in all states it is unlawful to test for drug use without the pregnant woman's permission (Gottlieb, 2001).

Cigarette Smoking and Caffeine Consumption

Cigarettes and caffeine are two examples of legal substances that can be addicting or harmful to the pregnant woman and her fetus and the newborn. Effects of nicotine and caffeine on the fetus and newborn are discussed in Chapter 38.

Cigarette smoking is a major preventable cause of death and illness. Smoking is linked to cardiovascular heart disease, various types of cancers (especially lung and cervical), chronic lung disease, and negative pregnancy outcomes. Tobacco contains nicotine, which is an addictive substance that creates a physical and a psychologic dependence.

The harmful effects of smoking are numerous. Smoking in pregnancy is known to cause a decrease in placental perfusion and is a cause of low birth weight (Bandestra & Accornero, 2006). The oxygen-carrying capacity of hemoglobin is decreased when carbon monoxide passes through the placenta. Furthermore, nicotine causes vasoconstriction, and smokers generally have a nutrient-poor diet. In utero, nicotine targets receptors in the fetal brain to change the pattern of cell proliferation and differentiation, thereby interfering with fetal neuronal development (Lester et al., 2004). Finally, smoking interferes with the body's ability to process essential vitamins and minerals, resulting in calcium loss from the bones, a decreased intestinal synthesis of vitamin B_{12}, and increased use of vitamin C. The woman who smokes during pregnancy is at risk for a variety of complications including ectopic pregnancy, miscarriage, premature rupture of membranes, preterm birth, placenta previa, abruptio placentae, and chorioamnionitis (Lester et al.).

Caffeine is found in society's most popular drinks: coffee, tea, and soft drinks. It is a stimulant that can affect mood and interrupt body functions by producing anxiety and sleep interruptions. Heart arrhythmias may be made worse by caffeine, and there can be interactions with certain medications such as lithium. Birth defects have not been related to caffeine consumption; however, high intake has been related to a slight decrease in birth weight and may also increase the risk of miscarriage (Cnattingius et al., 2000). The FDA recommends that pregnant women eliminate or limit their consumption of caffeine to less than 300 mg per day (3 cups of coffee or cola).

Alcohol

Prenatal alcohol exposure is the single greatest preventable cause of mental retardation (Lester et al., 2004). Alcohol use during pregnancy can cause high blood pressure, miscarriage, premature birth, stillbirth, and anemia (Lester et al., 2004). In addition, women may experience nutritional deficiencies, pancreatitis, alcoholic hepatitis, deficient milk ejection (let-down), and cirrhosis (Cunningham, Leveno, Bloom, Hauth, Gilstrap, & Wenstrom, 2005). A 2010 national health objective is to have 94% of pregnant women abstain from alcohol use (U.S. Department of Health and Human Services [USDHHS], 2000).

Alcohol use during pregnancy can produce "fetal alcohol spectrum disorder" (FASD), which includes fetal alcohol syndrome (FAS), as well as fetal alcohol effects (FAE) and alcohol-related neuro developmental disabilities (ARND). Approximately 40,000 babies per year are born with FASD; however, recent research reveals that antioxidants may lessen the effects of prenatal alcohol exposure in the children of women who are unable or unwilling to curtail their alcohol abuse when pregnant (Lee et al., 2005). Low birth weight, mental retardation, behavioral problems, and learning and physical problems are some of the symptoms of FAS babies (see Chapter 38). Severe facial deformities of FAS occur at day 20 of conception—a time when women may not even suspect they are pregnant. Binge drinking, before a woman recognizes she is pregnant, as well as during the early months of pregnancy, is most likely to cause brain injury in the developing fetus (Maier & West, 2001). Longitudinal studies reported that people affected by FASD have problems such as poor school performance; language difficulties; memory, attention, and judgment problems; poor math, social, and abstract reasoning skills; and impulsivity (Peterson, Nisenholz, & Robinson, 2003).

Accurate data about alcohol abuse are difficult to obtain because alcohol is rapidly absorbed in the small intestine and metabolized in the liver, so it is difficult to test for its presence in blood. The underdiagnosing and underreporting of alcohol use in pregnancy is a major concern of health care providers. Symptoms occurring during alcohol withdrawal can be managed with short-acting barbiturates or benzodiazepines; however, they are potentially teratogenic. Some clinicians recommend avoiding their use if at all possible. Disulfiram (Antabuse), a medication that acts as a deterrent to alcohol ingestion because it produces a dramatic, unpleasant reaction when small amounts of alcohol are consumed, is contraindicated during pregnancy because it is teratogenic (Doering, 2005). Three medications, naltrexone, nalmefene, and acamprosate, have proven efficacious for decreasing alcohol intake; however, they have not been tested in pregnant women and therefore should be avoided (Doering).

Marijuana

Marijuana is a substance derived from the cannabis plant. It is usually rolled into a cigarette and smoked, but it also may be mixed into food and eaten. Marijuana produces an altered state of awareness, relaxation, mild euphoria, and reduced inhibition (Stuart & Laraia, 2005). Prolonged use may lead to apathy, lack of energy, loss of desire to work or be productive, diminished concentration, poor personal hygiene, and preoccupation with marijuana—the amotivational syndrome (Stuart & Laraia). Marijuana readily crosses the placenta and causes increased carbon monoxide levels in the mother's blood, which reduces the oxygen supply to the fetus. Research findings regarding the effects of marijuana on pregnancy are inconsistent; however, it may cause fetal abnormalities (Stuart & Laraia).

Cocaine

Cocaine is a powerful CNS stimulant that blocks the reuptake of norepinephrine and dopamine at the nerve endings. Because more neurotransmitter is present at the synapse, the receptors are continuously activated. It is believed that this causes the euphoria. At the same time, presynaptic supplies of dopamine and norepinephrine are depleted. This causes the "crash" that happens when the effect of the drug wears off (Stuart & Laraia, 2005). The euphoria caused by cocaine is short acting, starting with a 10- to 20-second rush and followed by 15 to 20 minutes of less intense euphoria (Stuart & Laraia). A person who is high on cocaine feels euphoric, energetic, self-confident, and sociable. The relapse rate for clients who try to discontinue cocaine use is very high (Stuart & Laraia).

The smokable form of cocaine is produced by a process called freebasing. Crack is cocaine mixed with baking soda and heated until it reaches its purest form. It is sold in the form of "rocks," which are smoked in pipes. Crack is used by people from all cultures, and the low cost and availability make it the drug of choice among the economically disadvantaged. Because crack is highly addictive, it poses management problems for health care providers who care for pregnant addicts.

Predisposing factors and problems associated with cocaine use in pregnancy are polydrug use, poor nutrition, poverty, sexually transmitted infections, hepatitis B infection, dysfunctional family systems, employment difficulties, stress, anger, poor self-esteem, and previous or present physical, emotional, and sexual abuse. Cocaine use is especially concentrated among poor women of color (Lester et al., 2004). The clinical manifestations of cocaine use include tachycardia, pupillary dilation, and hypertension.

Medical complications of cocaine use in pregnancy range from mild to severe. Some of the less serious medical problems are lack of energy, insomnia, sinusitis, nosebleeds, sore throat, and decreased libido. More serious problems develop as the person's general health deteriorates. These include perforation of the nasal septum, increased cardiovascular stress, tachycardia, systemic hypertension, ventricular arrhythmias, sudden coronary artery spasm, and myocardial infarction (Stuart & Laraia, 2005). Needle-borne diseases such as hepatitis B and acquired immunodeficiency syndrome (AIDS) are common among cocaine users. The tachycardia and subsequent increase in blood pressure are caused by the increasing levels of cat-echolamines produced by the cocaine. During pregnancy, uterine blood vessels are normally maximally dilated, but they vasoconstrict in the presence of catecholamines (Lester et al., 2004). The separation of the placenta (abruption) or the acute onset of preterm labor with long, hard contractions and precipitate birth seen in pregnant women after the intravenous administration of cocaine is probably secondary to acute spasm of uterine blood vessels.

One of the promising treatments for cocaine abuse in pregnancy is acupuncture. A component of traditional Chinese medicine, acupuncture is used to redirect energy flow (*chi*) within the body, reduce cravings, and enhance well-being. The pace and location of the flow of *chi* can be influenced by the insertion of needles at certain points along the meridians to facilitate harmony (Otto, 2003). Evidence from controlled studies of the effectiveness of acupuncture alone or in combination with other therapies has been inconsistent (Vickers, Wilson, & Kleynen, 2002). Further investigation of this therapy is needed.

Opiates

The opiates include opium, heroin, meperidine, morphine, codeine, and methadone. Methadone is used to treat addiction to other opiates. It can be used either to aid withdrawal or to provide maintenance at a stable dose. Women taking methadone may work and live normally, although still addicted to narcotics. Heroin is one of the most commonly abused drugs of this class. It is usually taken by intravenous injection but can be smoked or "snorted." The signs and symptoms of heroin use are euphoria, relaxation, relief from pain, "nodding out" (apathy, detachment from reality, impaired judgment, and drowsiness), constricted pupils, nausea, constipation, slurred speech, and respiratory depression (APA, 2000).

The incidence of heroin use among pregnant women is unknown; however, those women with a dependency on heroin may use multiple drugs. Possible effects on pregnancy include preeclampsia, intrauterine growth restriction, miscarriage, premature rupture of membranes, infections, breech presentation, and preterm labor. Possible effects on the mother include poor nourishment with subsequent vitamin, iron, and folic acid deficiencies; medical complications from frequent use of dirty needles; sexually transmitted infections; and hypertension (Stuart & Laraia, 2005).

The recommended treatment is methadone maintenance combined with psychotherapy. This well-documented approach improves outcomes for both the woman and her fetus (Stuart & Laraia, 2005). The other approach is slow medical withdrawal with methadone, but the safety of this second approach is questionable. In pregnancy, methadone is metabolized more rapidly, leading to withdrawal symptoms in less than 24 hours in many women. Withdrawal symptoms can include fetal hyperactivity and, if severe, preterm labor or fetal death. Women may resort to heroin to alleviate the uncomfortable symptoms. Doses of methadone that increase during the course of pregnancy and are delivered in split doses (morning and evening) are most effective in preventing withdrawal and subsequent heroin use (van der Brink & van Ree, 2003).

Methamphetamine

Described as the No. 1 drug problem in America, approximately 12 million Americans have tried "meth," and 1.5 million are regular users (Jefferson, 2005). Relatively cheap, the highly addictive stimulant is hooking more and more people across the socioeconomic spectrum. Meth makes many users feel hypersexual and uninhibited, thus leads to more sex and less protection from pregnancy. The use among fertile women is creating a new generation of "meth babies" (Jefferson).

The active metabolite of methamphetamine is amphetamine, a CNS stimulant known as both "speed" and meth. Agents used as appetite suppressants or diet pills are closely related substances. The crystalline form of methamphetamine is known as "ice." When smoked, it produces a potent, long-lasting high. Ice enables a person to go without rest or food for 24 hours, only to "crash" for the next 24 hours (Jefferson, 2005). The active ingredient is pseudoephedrine and is easily "cooked," using recipes readily available on the Internet (Jefferson).

Clinical manifestations of methamphetamine use are euphoria, abrupt awakening, increased energy, talkativeness, elation, agitation, hyperactivity, irritability, grandiosity, diaphoresis, weight loss, insomnia, hypertension, increased temperature, ectopic heartbeat, urinary retention, constipation, dry mouth, paranoid delusions, and violent behavior. Seizures, cardiac shock, and death may occur as a result of overdose (Stuart & Laraia, 2005). Most of the effects of amphetamines are similar to those of cocaine.

Although fewer maternal and neonatal complications have been attributed to this class of substances than to cocaine (APA, 2000), the rates of preterm births and of intrauterine growth restriction with smaller head circumference are higher in methamphetamine-exposed pregnant women than in pregnant women who abuse other substances (see Chapter 38).

Phencyclidine

Phencyclidine (PCP) is a synthetic drug known by various names (peace pill, elephant, angel dust, hog). Its use is more prevalent among ethnic minorities and in people between the ages of 18 and 40 years. Its effects are unpredictable and include hostility, aggressiveness, and other bizarre behavior (Stuart & Laraia, 2005). Signs and symptoms of PCP use include confusion, disorientation, euphoria, hallucinations, paranoia, grandiosity, agitation, a tendency toward violence, and antisocial behavior, but the severity of these symptoms depends on the dose. Clinical manifestations include red, dry skin; dilated pupils; nystagmus; ataxia; hypertension; rigidity; and seizures (Stuart & Laraia). Because some effects mimic the signs and symptoms of schizophrenia, a user may be admitted to a psychiatric unit.

The major concerns regarding PCP use in pregnant women are its association with polydrug abuse and the neurobehavioral effects on the neonate. See Table 35-3 for psychologic and physiologic effects of selected illicit drugs.

CARE MANAGEMENT

Assessment and Nursing Diagnoses

The care of the substance-dependent pregnant woman is based on historical data, symptoms, physical findings, and laboratory results. All pregnant women should be asked screening questions for alcohol and drug abuse in the overall assessment at the first prenatal visit. Any judgmental attitude on the part of the health care provider will be evident to the woman and will interfere with the development of trust and with an accurate report of consumption (Morse & Hutchins, 2000). Information about drug use should be obtained by first asking about the woman's intake of over-the-counter and prescribed medications. Next, her use of legal drugs such as caffeine, nicotine, and alcohol should be ascertained. Finally, the woman should be questioned about her use of illicit drugs, such as cocaine, heroin, and marijuana. The approximate frequency and amount should be documented for each drug used (Seidel, Ball, Dains, & Benedict, 2006).

A variety of screening tests are available to screen for alcohol abuse. The CAGE Questionnaire (Ewing, 1984) (Box 35-1) and the Brief Michigan Alcoholism Screening Test (MAST) (Pokorny, Miller, & Kaplan, 1972) are two well-known screens for alcohol use that are often administered by the nurse or included in the written previsit questionnaire. The CAGE is the most popular test used in primary care; however, both the CAGE and MAST focus on alcohol dependency and may not be sensitive to detect the levels of drinking that are considered harmful in pregnancy .

Urine screening for alcohol abuse is unreliable, because alcohol is undetectable within a few hours after ingestion. Abnormal liver function studies can provide diagnostic data about physical effects of alcohol abuse. Urine toxicology testing is often performed to screen for illicit drug use. Drugs may be found in urine days to weeks after ingestion, depending on how quickly they are metabolized and excreted from the body (Gilbert & Harmon, 2003).

In addition to screening for alcohol and drug abuse, the nurse should also screen for physical and sexual abuse and history of psychiatric illness, because these are risk factors in women who abuse substances. Substance-abusing women feel much stigma, shame, and guilt, which leads to

denial of the abuse. If the nurse can help reduce those feelings, the woman will be more apt to confide in the nurse, and that is the first step in receiving help. Asking about how their spouses or partners feel about using substances can reveal whether there are family supports or barriers.

Initial and serial ultrasound studies may be performed to determine the gestational age, because amenorrhea, which is common among drug users, precludes dating on the basis of the history of the last menstrual period. Because of concerns about stillbirth and increased frequency of the birth of small-for-gestational-age infants, as well as the potential for hypoxia, nonstress testing may be performed, at least in the third trimester, in those pregnant women who are known substance abusers.

All states mandate that nurses report suspected child abuse or neglect, and these reports must be made in a timely manner and for each separate incident. Nurses who have filed a report with Children's Protective Services because of a mother's perinatal substance abuse may experience feelings of being torn between the mandated reporting law and trying to maintain some connectedness with the mother. Child custody loss can elicit feelings of grief, anger, or hopelessness in women and can promote or inhibit recovery from their addiction (Lester et al., 2005). Recurrent pregnancies in women who have lost custody of one or more children and who are not in recovery also are common. Information about the women's experiences and the various types of out-of-home placements for children can assist nurses in planning interventions that help mothers process their feelings about custody loss. Nursing diagnoses for the woman who is a substance abuser may include the following:

- *Risk for deficient fluid volume related to*
  −effects of excessive use of psychoactive drugs
- *Risk for imbalanced nutrition: less than body requirements related to*
  −effects of excessive use of psychoactive drugs
- *Risk for injury to self, fetus, or newborn related to*
  −sensory effects of drug
- *Risk for infection related to*
  −lifestyle
  −dehydration and malnutrition
  −method of administration of drug
- *Self-care deficit, bathing or hygiene, related to*
  −effects of substance used
- *Ineffective coping related to*
  −lack of support system
  −low self-esteem
  −lack of anger management techniques
  −denial
- *Risk for impaired parent-infant attachment related to*
  −guilt
  −continuance of substance use
- *Risk for violence (self- and other-directed) related to*
  −maintenance of drug habit
  −effects of substance used
  −lifestyle

box 35-1 CAGE Questionnaire

C Have you ever felt you ought to **CUT DOWN** on your drinking?
A Have people **ANNOYED** you by criticizing your drinking?
G Have you ever felt bad or **GUILTY** about your drinking?
E Have you ever had a drink first thing in the morning to steady your nerves or get rid of a hangover? (**E**YE OPENER)

Text continued on p. 910.

table 35-3 **Psychoactive Substance Effects**

DRUG	PSYCHOLOGIC SIGNS	PHYSIOLOGIC SIGNS
ALCOHOL		
Intoxication	Labile mood	Slurred speech
	Impaired attention	Flushed face
	Irritability	Unsteady gait
	Talkativeness	Nystagmus
Withdrawal	Anxiety	Nausea and vomiting
	Depressed mood	Malaise or weakness
	Maladaptive behavior	Hyperactivity
		Coarse tremor of hands, tongue, eyelids
		Orthostatic hypertension
COCAINE		
Intoxication	Psychomotor agitation	Tachycardia
	Elation	Pupillary dilation
	Grandiosity	Hypertension
	Hypervigilance	Perspiration, chills
	Maladaptive behaviors	Nausea, vomiting
Withdrawal	Depressed mood	Fatigue
	Disturbed sleep	Headache
	Increased dreaming	Convulsions
HEROIN		
Intoxication	Euphoria	Pupillary constriction
	Psychomotor retardation	Drowsiness
	Apathy	Slurred speech
	Maladaptive behavior	
	Impaired attention	
Withdrawal	Insomnia	Lacrimation
		Rhinorrhea
		Pupillary dilation
		Sweating
		Diarrhea
		Yawning
		Mild hypertension
		Tachycardia
		Fever
METHAMPHETAMINE		
Intoxication	Hyperactivity	Tachycardia, palpitations
	Insomnia	Tachypnea
	Restlessness	Nausea, vomiting
	Irritability	Constipation
	Aggressiveness	Impotence
Withdrawal	Depression	Headache
	Increased sleeping	Nausea, vomiting
	Lethargy	Muscle pain
		Weakness
PHENCYCLIDINE (PCP)		
Intoxication	Euphoria	Vertical or horizontal nystagmus
	Psychomotor agitation	Hypertension
	Increased anxiety	Increased heart rate
	Emotional lability	Numbness
	Grandiosity	Decreased response to pain
	Sensation of slowed time	Ataxia, dysarthria
	Synesthesias	
	Maladaptive behaviors	
Withdrawal	No true withdrawal except possible depression.	

- *Hopelessness related to*
  - –inability to stop using substances
- *Powerlessness related to*
  - –lack of resources
  - –relationship with abusive partners
- *Risk for suicide related to*
  - –depression
  - –impulsivity while taking substances

▬ Expected Outcomes of Care

Planning the care for a pregnant woman who is a substance abuser must take into consideration the woman's lifestyle and habits. The ideal long-term outcome would be total abstinence, but the woman may be unable to face that level of commitment at that time. The thought of giving up the substance forever only provokes anxiety. A realistic goal may be to cut down on the use of substances. Short-term outcomes are necessary, and the woman must participate in the formulation of these expected outcomes. The outcomes must be stated as clear behavioral expectations. The expected outcomes may be written as a contract that is then signed by the woman and the nurse, and a copy is given to the woman. Short-term outcomes for the woman and her family may include the following:

- The woman will keep appointments for prenatal and postpartum care for herself and the well-baby care for the infant.
- Fetal effects will be minimized; the baby will be safe.
- The woman's physiologic symptoms will stabilize, and she will be able to care for herself and her infant.
- The woman will develop an attachment to her infant.
- The woman will become involved in a substance abuse treatment program.

▬ Plan of Care and Interventions
▬ *Treatment Programs for Alcohol- and Drug-Dependent Women*

National concern regarding the problem of alcohol and drug use during pregnancy has brought attention to the lack of treatment programs specifically targeted to pregnant women. Any discussion of treatment programs must start with the understanding that substance abuse in women is a complex problem surrounded by multiple individual, familial, and social issues that require many levels of intervention and treatment. The powerlessness of the alcoholic condition and the powerlessness of the female condition act on each other, reinforcing the impotence and hopelessness of both and leaving the woman with few resources to regain a grip on her life.

There is no clear empirical evidence as to what treatment program is best for substance-using mothers (Lester et al., 2005). However, there is general agreement that among major components of programs should be a cognitive-behavioral approach and mostly female staff; programs should address issues of stigmatization, high probability of sexual abuse and physical abuse, lack of social support, need for social services and child care, need for transportation, family support services, medical (particularly women's health) and mental health services, child development services, family planning, respite care, life skills management, pharmacologic services, self-help groups and stress management, and need for support and education in the mothering role (Lester et al.). Drug-free public housing or residential communities may offer an ideal route to stabilization in a safe environment. Treatment must demonstrate cultural sensitivity and responsiveness to recognize ethnicity and culture as an important part of a woman's identity. Other needs of many women include relationship counseling and vocational and legal assistance (Lester et al.).

Women for Sobriety may be a more helpful organization for women than Alcoholics Anonymous (AA) or Narcotics Anonymous, which are based on the 12-step program. The emphasis on powerlessness over addiction and avoidance of codependency found in 12-step programs may further disempower and isolate women, particularly women of color (Saulnier, 1996). The confrontational techniques of the 12-step program, developed to break down denial in men, may be especially threatening to women, who often feel unworthy and full of shame and guilt. In addition, women may be vulnerable to "thirteenth-stepping"—a euphemistic term referring to men who target new, more vulnerable women for dates or sex (Bogart & Pearce, 2003). In one study, 50% of the women experienced thirteenth-stepping behaviors, and two had been raped by men in AA (Bogart & Pearce). Especially vulnerable women, such as those with histories of sexual abuse, should be referred to female-only groups.

Whereas the treatment approach of male substance abusers tends to be oriented toward the individual, substance-abusing women should be viewed within the context of their relationships to others. Women tend to find satisfaction, pleasure, and a sense of worth if they experience their life activities as arising from and leading back to a sense of connection with others. Women who use illicit drugs are likely to be introduced to and supplied with these drugs by men as part of an intimate or sexual relationship. Recognizing the complexities of treating substance-abusing pregnant women may explain why one study reported that pregnant women who received the most treatment in a residential or outpatient treatment program had higher-birth-weight infants than those treated in less intensive programs such as detox only (Daley, Argoriou, McCarty, Callahan, Shepard, & Williams, 2001).

▬ *Nursing Care*

An interdisciplinary, comprehensive model is essential when planning the care for women who abuse substances. Pregnancy presents a window of opportunity for motivating women to stop their abuse of substances; but what, specifically, can the nurse do?

First, nurses must be knowledgeable about how to screen and identify women who abuse substances while pregnant.

They also must maintain a nonjudgmental, nonpunitive attitude. Nurses can advocate for access to woman-centered drug treatment and harm reduction measures to minimize the damage caused by alcohol and drugs (Lester et al., 2005). Collaboration with advanced practice psychiatric nurses will enable nurses to deal with their feelings and provide better care for this challenging group of women. Until the nurse can approach the woman with caring and concern, the therapeutic alliance, which is so important for any change to take place, will not occur. The nurse's role is aimed not only at promoting abstinence, but also at providing a caring, nurturing, and empowering environment in which women can rediscover their values and become authentic, independent decision makers. In a study of nursing students who abused alcohol, Murphy-Parker and Martinez (2005) reported that recovery was possible; however, this optimism may interfere with handling disappointments such as relapse, interpersonal conflict, health deterioration, or other related sequelae.

Second, the nurse should determine the individual's readiness for change. One model for doing this was developed by Prochaska and DiClemente (1992). The five stages of the model illustrate the readiness of women to change. *Precontemplation* is the earliest stage, in which individuals are unaware, unwilling, or discouraged about changing substance use behavior. They will be least responsive to interventions focused on change activities. First they need to take ownership of the problem. *Contemplation* involves an active consideration of the prospects of change. Women engage in information seeking and begin to reevaluate themselves in light of their substance abuse behavior. *Preparation* indicates a readiness to change. They intend to change in the near future and have learned valuable lessons from past change attempts and failures. *Action* involves the overt modification of the problem behavior, and individuals must have the skills to carry out the changes. *Maintenance* is the final stage, and environmental supports are particularly important here, as well as supportive relationships with health care providers.

When working with pregnant adolescents with addictions, the nurse also must consider their developmental stage. A part of normal adolescence often includes experimenting with drugs or alcohol, so how does the nurse know when alcohol or drug use is a problem? Certain patterns, such as drinking to escape reality or drinking to "get wasted," are more dangerous than others. Drinking alone and being secretive about drugs and alcohol also are unhealthy patterns.

Third, the nurse uses supportive nursing interventions such as mutuality and avoidance of confrontation. In mutuality, the nurse conveys to women drug users that their perspective on their life situation is as valid as that of the nurse. Women should be encouraged to describe their views on the role of drug use in their lives, the degree of impairment they are experiencing, and the feasibility of change at this time. Avoidance of confrontation is important because it can be damaging to the nurse-client rela-

tionship. The likely consequences of continued drug use can be presented in a warmly concerned, factual manner rather than as threats.

Fourth, the nurse uses principles of motivational interviewing (Miller & Rollnick, 1991) to effect change. These principles include the following:
- Displaying empathy
- Developing the discrepancy between individuals' perceptions of where they are and where they want to be
- Avoiding argumentation
- Rolling with resistance
- Supporting the woman's sense of self-efficacy

When problematic drug use is suspected, the nurse might ask in a noncritical way, "Are drugs or alcohol any part of this situation you have been describing?" By asking about the role of drugs in self-medication for stressors, the nurse can help the woman reflect on the degree of the problem and avenues for change. The woman can be helped to express the positive aspects of drug use that lead her to continue using and the harmful consequences that she has observed. She can be asked about times she tried to reduce or quit using her drug of choice. What interfered with her success? What times was she successful? What enabled her to succeed at those times? Praise can be given for being able to be successful at some time and optimism expressed that she can be successful again.

An exciting pilot program (The Perinatal Outreach Project) involving public health nurses reported that outreach services provided to 10 pregnant substance-abusing women resulted in a 90% rate of entry into treatment (Corrarino, Williams, Campbell, Amrhein, LoPiano, & Kalachik, 2000). During a home visit, the public health nurse conducted a substance use assessment, and the nurse and the woman jointly agreed to a plan of care with an emphasis on the woman's readiness for change. Key elements of the project were the development of a trusting relationship, a nonjudgmental attitude of staff, and the development of a psychologically healthy and focused interpersonal approach. The other essential elements of the project were the following (Corrarino et al., 2000):
- Assignment of a primary public health nurse with a small caseload
- Flexible home visit plan
- Health education concerning pregnancy-related preventive health care
- Services of substance abuse counselor
- Follow-up at each contact of needs identified
- Referral to community and social services as needed
- Availability of medical social worker for social needs
- Referral to substance abuse treatment when the woman was ready
- Monthly meeting in an interdisciplinary team

▬ Evaluation

Evaluation is difficult in pregnant women with substance abuse problems because the long-range effects cannot be projected. If the goals are realistic and short-term, evaluation is easier. Short-term positive achievements are indicators of some success. Complete abstinence from drugs and assumption of mature adult behaviors within a short time are unrealistic. Long-term care is usually necessary (see Plan of Care).

▬ POSTPARTUM PSYCHOLOGIC ▬ COMPLICATIONS

Mental health disorders in the postpartum period have implications for the mother, the newborn, and the entire family. Such conditions can interfere with attachment to the newborn and family integration, and some may threaten the safety and well-being of the mother, the newborn, and other children. Less than 33% of women with substantial postpartum depression or anxiety symptoms were detected by routine care (Coates, Schaefer, & Alexander, 2004). Because birth is usually thought to be a happy event, a new mother's emotional distress may puzzle and immobilize family and friends. When she most needs the caring attention of loved ones, they may either criticize or withdraw because of their anxiety.

Mood Disorders

Mood disorders are the predominant mental health disorder in the postpartum period (APA, 2000). Up to 70% of women experience a mild depression or "baby blues" after the birth of a child; however, functioning of the woman is usually not impaired. Other women can have more serious depressions that can eventually incapacitate them to the point of being unable to care for themselves or their babies. Postpartum depression occurs in a variety of countries though the manifestations may vary by culture (Goldbort, 2006; Posmontier & Horowitz, 2004). A study among postpartum Hispanic women in three U.S. cities revealed that 42.6% of participants were depressed (Kuo, Wilson, Holman, Fuentes-Afflick, Sullivan, & Minkoff, 2004).

Postpartum depression exerts a moderate to large effect on the interaction of mothers and infants (Beck, 1995a). Although a study in Taiwan showed that postpartum depression had no significant effect on their infants' development (Wang, Chen, Chin, & Lee, 2005), a study in the United Kingdom reported that infants of depressed mothers had significantly poorer weight gain (O'Brien, Heycock, Hanna, Jones, & Cox, 2004). Nurses are strategically positioned to offer anticipatory guidance, to assess the mental

CD: Plan of Care: Substance Abuse During Pregnancy

---

plan of care ▸   Substance Abuse During Pregnancy

NURSING DIAGNOSIS Imbalanced nutrition: less than body requirements related to insufficient intake for prenatal metabolic needs as evidenced by insufficient weight gain for gestational age of fetus

Expected Outcome *Woman will maintain steady weight gain appropriate for trimester of pregnancy.*

Nursing Interventions/Rationales
- Compare current weight to prepregnant weight *to assess if weight is appropriate for trimester of pregnancy.*
- Assess woman's current diet plan and caloric intake *to identify where modifications are necessary.*
- Provide woman with information regarding nutritional requirements during pregnancy *to assist her to provide modifications to diet and promote self-care.*
- Weigh woman frequently *to establish compliance of woman and effectiveness of plan.*

NURSING DIAGNOSIS Ineffective coping related to lack of support system as evidenced by woman's verbalization of concerns

Expected Outcome *Woman will express satisfaction with identified effective coping methods.*

Nursing Interventions/Rationales
- Remain nonjudgmental while listening to woman express feelings and concerns *to promote trust.*
- Assist woman to identify positive coping methods and strengths *to promote involvement in self-care.*
- Encourage woman to take responsibility for activities leading to recovery *to promote self-care, self-esteem, and responsibility for self and fetus's well-being.*
- Refer to appropriate health professionals and support groups *to promote involvement and responsibility in health and well-being of self and fetus.*

NURSING DIAGNOSIS Delayed fetal growth and development related to maternal substance abuse

Expected Outcome *Fetus will exhibit appropriate growth and development during pregnancy.*

Nursing Interventions/Rationales
- Provide information to woman regarding effects of substance abuse on fetus *to reinforce correlation.*
- Monitor fundal height *to determine fetal growth pattern.*
- Assess maternal nutrition and weight gain pattern *to verify potential for fetal growth.*
- Implement fetal assessment testing *to provide data concerning fetal well-being.*

NURSING DIAGNOSIS Situational low self-esteem related to loss of control during pregnancy

Expected Outcome *Woman will identify methods to increase self-esteem.*

Nursing Interventions/Rationales
- Provide reinforcement for positive actions *to encourage woman to accept praise and continue positive actions throughout the pregnancy.*
- Promote the expression of feelings through therapeutic communication *to facilitate ongoing support and trust.*
- Discuss with the woman positive past coping mechanisms and experiences *to promote increase in current self-esteem.*
- Encourage woman to participate in decisions about her care *to promote increased sense of control over care.*
- Refer to support group or individual counseling if needed *to facilitate ongoing support and for expression of feelings.*

health of new mothers, to offer therapeutic interventions, and to make referrals when necessary. Failure to do so may result in tragic consequences. In the rarest of cases, a disturbed mother may kill her infant, other family members, and/or herself (Lehmann, 2004).

The Diagnostic and Statistical Manual (DSM) of Mental Disorders contains the official guidelines for the assessment and diagnosis of psychiatric illness (APA, 2000). However, specific criteria for postpartum depression (PPD) are not listed. Instead, postpartum onset can be specified for any mood disorder either without psychotic features (i.e., PPD) or with psychotic features (i.e., postpartum psychosis) if the onset occurs within 4 weeks of childbirth (APA).

Etiology and Risk Factors

The cause of PPD may be biologic, psychologic, situational, or multifactorial. In a review of literature on nonbiologic interventions (interpersonal and cognitive-behavioral therapy, peer and partner support, nondirective counseling, relaxation/massage therapy, infant sleep interventions, infant-mother relationship therapy, and maternal exercise) to prevent PPD, Dennis (2004c) concluded that effectiveness of most of the approaches could not be measured because of a lack of well-designed studies. Likewise, in a review of biologic interventions to prevent PPD, Dennis (2004b) concluded that methodologic study limitations rendered intervention efficacy equivocal. The studies focused on antidepressants, estrogen and progesterone and thyroid therapy, docosahexanoic acid, and calcium supplementation. Dennis (2004b) did recommend that long-acting progestogen contraceptives should not be given in the postpartum period.

Neurotransmitter deficiencies and psychosocial and marital adjustments in the postpartum period have been related to PPD (APA, 2000; Huang & Mathers, 2001). A personal history or a family history of mood disorder, mood and anxiety symptoms in the antepartal period, as well as postpartum blues increases the risk for PPD (APA, 2000; Linter & Gray, 2006). In a metaanalysis of 84 studies published in the 1990s, Beck (2001) found 13 risk factors for postpartum depression, four of which had not been identified previously as predictors. The effect sizes of the risk factors identified in an updated metaanalysis revealed that 10 predictors have a medium relation with postpartum depression, and three predictors have a small relation (Beck, 2002). A revised version of the Postpartum Depression Predictors Inventory has been published (Beck, 2002). Box 35-2 lists all 13 risk factors for PPD, with those having the greater effect size listed first.

In a population-based sample of 594 mothers around Vancouver, factors predictive of depressive symptomatology at 1 week postpartum included immigration within the last 5 years, history of depression independent of childbirth, diagnosis of preeclampsia, vulnerable personality style, stressful life events, lack of perceived support, lack of readiness for hospital discharge, and dissatisfaction with infant feeding method (Dennis, Janssen, & Singer, 2004).

box 35-2 Risk Factors for Postpartum Depression
• Prenatal depression • Low self-esteem • Stress of child care • Prenatal anxiety • Life stress • Lack of social support • Marital relationship problems • History of depression • "Difficult" infant temperament • Postpartum blues • Single status • Low socioeconomic status • Unplanned/unwanted pregnancy

Source: Beck, C. (2002). Revision of the Postpartum Depression Predictors Inventory. *Journal of Obstetric, Gynecologic, and Neonatal Nursing, 31*(4), 394-402; Beck, C. (2001). Predictors of postpartum depression: An update. *Nursing Research, 50*(5), 275-282.

In a study of low-income women, 51% reported depressive symptoms, stress scores were high, and activity levels were low (Boury, Larkin, & Krummel, 2004). Neither body weight nor steps walked were related to depressive symptoms; however, stress and social support were related to symptoms. Women without symptoms reported significantly less stress than the mild and moderate/severe symptom groups. Mean social support satisfaction was significantly higher for nondepressed women compared to women in the moderate/severe symptom range. Stress and current smoking status explained 46% of the variance in depressive symptoms (Boury et al., 2004).

In addition, multiple births (Davis, Edwards, Mohay, & Wollin, 2003) and fatigue have been found to be important predictors of PPD (Bozoky & Corwin, 2002). As early as 7 days postpartum, fatigue is predictive of depression at postpartum day 28.

Postpartum Depression Without Psychotic Features

PPD is an intense and pervasive sadness with severe and labile mood swings and is more serious and persistent than postpartum blues. Intense fears, anger, anxiety, and despondency that persist past the baby's first few weeks are not a normal part of postpartum blues. Occurring in approximately 10% to 15% of new mothers, these symptoms rarely disappear without outside help. The majority of these mothers do not seek help from any source, and only about 20% consult a health professional. The occurrence of PPD among teenage mothers was more than 2.5 times that for older mothers (Herrick, 2002). African-American mothers were twice as likely as Caucasian mothers to experience PPD. Younger mothers (younger than 20 years) and those with less than a high school education were significantly less likely to seek help and had higher rates of PPD (Herrick). New mothers who had no one to talk to about their problems had a high rate of PPD and a low rate of help seeking.

The symptoms of postpartum major depression do not differ from the symptoms of nonpostpartum mood

CD: Critical Thinking Exercise: Postpartum Depression

EVIDENCE-BASED PRACTICE

Perinatal Depression

BACKGROUND

- Pregnancy and the first 12 months of motherhood can increase the risk of depression for women, which can profoundly affect the children and families of its victims. Symptoms can mimic the discomforts of pregnancy and postpartum fatigue and blues. Perinatal depression may affect from 5% to 25% of new mothers, depending on its definition. Major depression clearly requires intervention, but minor depression is less clear. Many screening tools for depression are modified for use with perinatal women.

OBJECTIVES

- The reviewers set themselves the task to establish the prevalence and incidence of perinatal depression, to examine the validity and reliability of the various screening tools for this population, and to see if screening leads to improved outcomes, such as treatment and improvement. Depression was categorized as major and combined (major and minor).

METHODS

Search Strategy

- After a thorough search of health databases, reference lists, and expert recommendations, the authors identified 59 studies. Studies about incidence and prevalence were retrospective or prospective (stronger design), and included case-controlled studies comparing pregnant and nonpregnant women of similar demographics. For data on screening tools and outcomes, only prospective controlled trials were selected. Publication dates and countries of origin were not noted.

Statistical Analyses

- Similar data were pooled. The reviewers metaanalyzed the data for prevalence and incidence of depression for particular perinatal periods, and for depression screening instruments. Diversity in screening and intervention prevented metaanalysis for outcomes.

FINDINGS

- For major depression, the prevalence was 3%-5% during pregnancy and 1%-5% during the first year. Combined major and minor depression appeared in up to 1 out of 10 pregnant women and 1 out of 8 new mothers.

- The most accurate screening tools for major depression alone appeared to be the Postpartum Depression Screening Scale and the Edinburgh Postnatal Depression Scale, although differences from the Beck Depression Inventory were not significant. The instruments were less sensitive for combined depression.
- Studies of interventions after screening were small and mixed, but showed a beneficial trend with intervention for women at risk for perinatal depression.

LIMITATIONS

- For such a significant public health problem, the research on perinatal depression is sparse. The studies lacked ethnic and socioeconomic diversity. Cost was not addressed.

IMPLICATIONS FOR PRACTICE

- Women undergo psychologic challenges during pregnancy and new motherhood that can bring on new-onset or recurrent depression. Nurses should be alert to risk factors, and sensitive to the differences between normal perinatal fatigue and emotional swings, and onset of depressive symptoms. Women should be taught the symptoms of depression in the same matter-of-fact manner as any other warning signs of physical disease, and screened at each visit. After her 6-week check, the woman is referred back to her generalist, who should be screening all clients routinely for depression, with special sensitivity to the new mother. Women with major depression need intervention, to avoid devastating effects on themselves, their infants, and other family members.

IMPLICATIONS FOR FURTHER RESEARCH

- Future research needs sufficient numbers to provide the power to draw conclusions, and samples that mirror the population's diversity. Comparisons of screening tools would identify accuracy for target populations and perinatal periods, which could influence the best settings for screening. The most promising results were for major depression, so future research should compare established interventions such as medication and psychotherapy. Standardizing screening measures could lead to stronger metaanalyses in the future.

Reference: Gaynes, B., Gavin, N., Meltzer-Brody, S., Lohr, K., Swinson, T., Gartlehner, G., et al. (2005). *Perinatal depression: Prevalence, screening accuracy, and screening outcomes.* AHRQ Publication No. 05-E006-1. Rockville, MD: Agency for Healthcare Research and Quality.

disorders, except that the mother's ruminations of guilt and inadequacy feed her worries about being an incompetent and inadequate parent. In PPD, there may be odd food cravings (often, sweet desserts) and binges with abnormal appetite and weight gain. New mothers report an increased yearning for sleep, sleeping heavily, but awakening instantly with any infant noise, and an inability to go back to sleep after infant feedings. One mother described the onset as related to an inability to breastfeed—no letdown (Reynolds, 2004).

A distinguishing feature of PPD is irritability. These episodes of irritability may flare up with little provocation, and they may sometimes escalate to violent outbursts or dissolve into uncontrollable sobbing. Many of these outbursts are directed against significant others ("He never helps me") or the baby ("She cries all the time, and I feel like hitting her"). Women with postpartum major depressive episodes often have severe anxiety, panic attacks, and spontaneous crying long after the usual duration of baby blues.

Many women feel especially guilty about having depressive feelings at a time when they believe they should be happy. They may be reluctant to discuss their symptoms or their negative feelings toward the child. A prominent feature of PPD is rejection of the infant, often caused by abnormal jealousy (APA, 2000). The mother may be obsessed by the notion that the offspring may take her place in her partner's affections. Attitudes toward the infant may include disinterest, annoyance with care demands, and blaming because of her lack of maternal feeling. When observed, she may appear awkward in her responses to the baby. Obsessive thoughts about harming the child are very frightening to her. Often she does not share these thoughts because of embarrassment, but when she does, other family members become very frightened.

Medical Management

The natural course is one of gradual improvement over the 6 months after birth. However, supportive treatment alone is not efficacious for major postpartum depression. Pharmacologic intervention is needed in most instances. Treatment options include antidepressants, antianxiety agents, and ECT. Alternative therapies such as herbs, dietary supplements, massage, aromatherapy, and acupuncture may be helpful (Weier & Beal, 2004). Psychotherapy focuses on her fears and concerns regarding her new responsibilities and roles, as well as monitoring for suicidal or homicidal thoughts. Support groups may be helpful. For some women, hospitalization is necessary.

Postpartum Depression with Psychotic Features

Postpartum psychosis is a syndrome most often characterized by depression (as described previously), delusions, and thoughts by the mother of harming either the infant or herself (Kaplan & Sadock, 2005). A postpartum mood disorder with psychotic features occurs in 1 to 2 per 1000 births and may occur more often in primiparas (Kaplan & Sadock). Once a woman has had one postpartum episode with psychotic features, there is a 30% to 50% likelihood of recurrence with each subsequent birth (APA, 2000).

Symptoms often begin within days after the birth, although the mean time to onset is 2 to 3 weeks and almost always within 8 weeks of birth (Kaplan & Sadock, 2005). Characteristically, the woman begins to complain of fatigue, insomnia, and restlessness and may have episodes of tearfulness and emotional lability. Complaints regarding the inability to move, stand, or work also are common. Later, suspiciousness, confusion, incoherence, irrational statements, and obsessive concerns about the baby's health and welfare may be present (Kaplan & Sadock). Delusions may be present in 50% of all women, and hallucinations, in about 25%. Auditory hallucinations that command the mother to kill the infant can also occur in severe cases. When delusions are present, they are often related to the infant. The mother may think the infant is possessed by the devil, has special powers, or is destined for a terrible fate (APA, 2000). Grossly disorganized behavior may be manifested as a disinterest in the infant or an inability to provide care. Some will insist that something is wrong with the baby or accuse nurses or family of hurting or poisoning their child. Nurses are advised to be alert for mothers who are agitated, overactive, confused, complaining, or suspicious.

A specific illness included in depression with psychotic features is bipolar disorder (formerly called manic depressive illness). This mood disorder is preceded or accompanied by manic episodes, characterized by elevated, expansive, or irritable moods. Clinical manifestations of a manic episode include at least three of the following symptoms that have been significantly present for at least 1 week: grandiosity, decreased need for sleep, pressured speech, flight of ideas, distractibility, psychomotor agitation, and excessive involvement in pleasurable activities without regard for negative consequences (APA, 2000). Because these women are hyperactive, they may not take the time to eat or sleep, which leads to inadequate nutrition, dehydration, and sleep deprivation. While in a manic state, mothers will need constant supervision when caring for their infant. Mostly they will be too preoccupied to provide child care.

Medical Management

A favorable outcome is associated with a good premorbid adjustment (before the onset of the disorder) and a supportive family network (Kaplan & Sadock, 2005). Because mood disorders are usually episodic, women may experience another episode of symptoms within a year or two of the birth. Postpartum psychosis is a psychiatric emergency, and the mother will probably need psychiatric hospitalization. Antipsychotics and mood stabilizers such as lithium are the treatments of choice (see Table 35-4 and Table 35-5 for FDA categories of risk during pregnancy). If the mother is breastfeeding, some sources recommend that no pharmacologic agents should be prescribed (Kaplan & Sadock), but other sources advise caution while prescribing some agents (Schatzberg & Nemeroff, 2004). It is usually advantageous for the mother to have contact with her baby if she so desires, but visits must be closely supervised. Psychotherapy is indicated after the period of acute psychosis is past.

CRITICAL THINKING EXERCISE

Postpartum Depression

Moiria, 36, gave birth to a 7 lb 4 oz girl 3 weeks ago. She has been diagnosed with postpartum depression, and a tricyclic medication has been prescribed. Moiria is breastfeeding and has concerns about taking the medication.

1. Evidence—Is there sufficient evidence regarding the safety of psychotropic medications and lactation?
2. Assumptions—What assumptions can be made about the following issues?
   a. Lactation risk categories of tricyclic medications
   b. Timing of feeding and medication administration
   c. Risks of discontinuing medications while breastfeeding
3. What is the nursing priority in this situation?
4. Does the evidence objectively support this recommendation?
5. Are there alternative perspectives regarding treatment for postpartum depression for breastfeeding women?

table 35-4 Mood Stabilizers

MOOD STABILIZERS	PREGNANCY RISK CATEGORY*	LACTATION RISK CATEGORY*
Carbamazepine (Tegretol XR)	C	L2
Clonazepam (Klonopin)	C	L3
Gabapentin (Neurontin)	C	L3
Lamotrigene (Lamictal)	C	L3
Lithium carbonate (Eskalith)	D	L4
Topiramate (Topamax)	C	L3
Valproic acid (Depakene, Depakote, & Depakote ER)	D	L2

*Source: Hale, T. (2004). *Medications and mother's milk.* (11th ed.). Amarillo, TX: Pharmasoft.
ER, XR, Extended release.
C = Animal studies show adverse effects on fetus but no controlled studies in pregnant women OR no studies available
D = Positive evidence of human fetal risk
L2 = Drug studied in limited number of breastfeeding women with no adverse effects in infant OR evidence is remote
L3 = No controlled studies OR studies show minimal nonthreatening effects
L4 = Possibly hazardous

▬ CARE MANAGEMENT

Even though the prevalence of PPD is fairly well established, women are unlikely to seek help from a mental health care provider. Primary health care providers can usually recognize severe PPD or postpartum psychosis but may miss milder forms; even if it is recognized, the woman may be treated inappropriately or subtherapeutically (Gold, 2002).

▬ Assessment and Nursing Diagnoses

To recognize symptoms of PPD as early as possible, the nurse should be an active listener and demonstrate a caring attitude (Beck, 1999). Nurses cannot depend on women volunteering unsolicited information about their depression or asking for help. The nurse should observe for signs of depression and ask appropriate questions to determine moods, appetite, sleep, energy and fatigue levels, and ability to concentrate. Examples of ways to initiate conversation include the following: "Now that you have had your baby, how are things going for you? Have you had to change many things in your life since having the baby?" and "How much time do you spend crying?" If the nurse assesses that the new mother is depressed, she or he must ask if the mother has thought about hurting herself or the baby. The woman may be more willing to answer honestly if the nurse says, "Lots of women feel depressed after having a baby, and some feel so badly that they think about hurting themselves or the baby. Have you had these thoughts?"

table 35-5 Antipsychotic Medications

ANTIPSYCHOTIC MEDICATIONS	*PREGNANCY RISK CATEGORY	*LACTATION RISK CATEGORY
TRADITIONAL ANTIPSYCHOTICS		
Chlorpromazine (Thorazine)	C	L3
Fluphenazine (Prolixin)	C	L3
Haloperidol (Haldol)	C	L2
Perphenazine (Trilafon)	C	L3
Thioridazine (Mellaril)	C	L4
Thiothixene (Navane)	C	L4
Trifluoperazine (Stelazine)	unknown	unknown
ATYPICAL ANTIPSYCHOTICS		
Aripiprazole (Abilify)	C	L3
Clozapine (Clozaril)	C	L3
Loxapine (Loxitane)	C	L4
Olanzapine (Zyprexa)	C	L2
Quetiapine (Seroquel)	C	L4
Risperidone (Risperdal)	C	L3
Ziprasidone (Geodon)	C	L4

*Source: Hale, T. (2004). *Medications and mother's milk* (11th ed.). Amarillo, TX: Pharmasoft.
C = Animal studies show adverse effects on fetus but no controlled studies in pregnant women OR no studies available
L2 = Drug studied in limited number of breastfeeding women with no adverse effects in infant OR evidence is remote
L3 = No controlled studies OR studies show minimal nonthreatening effects
L4 = Possibly hazardous

▬ NURSE ALERT

Because mothers with PPD with psychotic features may harm their infants, extra precaution is needed in assessment and intervention. The nurse needs to ask specifically if the mother has had thoughts about harming her baby.

Nurses can use screening tools in assessing whether the depressive symptoms have progressed from postpartum blues to PPD. Examples are the Edinburgh Postnatal Depression Scale (EPDS) (Cox, Holden, & Sagovsky, 1989) (www.wellmother.com) and the Postpartum Depression Predictors Inventory-Revised (PDPI-R) (Beck, 2002).

The EPDS is a self-report assessment designed specifically to identify women experiencing PPD. It has been used and validated in studies in numerous cultures (Dennis, 2004a; Eberhard-Gran, Eskild, & Tambs, 2001) and has even been used to measure depression and anxiety in fathers (partners) (Matthey, Barnett, Howie, & Kavanagh, 2001). The assessment tool asks the woman to respond to 10 statements about the common symptoms of depression. The woman is asked to choose the response that is closest to describing how she has felt for the past week.

Through focused research over at least a decade, Beck (1995a, 1995b, 1998a) continues to refine the postpartum depression assessment tool. The latest revision (PDPI-R) is a list of guided questions for the 13 risk factors found to be related to PPD. The published tool is designed to be used by nurses and other health care providers to elicit information from the woman during an interview during pregnancy and continuing in the postpartum period to assess risk (Beck, 2002). Areas assessed include the predictors of depression as listed in Box 35-2.

If the initial interaction with the woman or analysis of her self-report reveals some question that she might be depressed, a formal screening is helpful in determining the urgency of the referral and the type of provider. Also important is the need to assess the woman's family, because they may be able to offer valuable information, as well as need to express how they have been affected by the woman's emotional disorder (Maley, 2002).

Planning is focused on meeting the individualized needs of the family to ensure safety, especially for the mother and infant and any other children, and to facilitate functional family coping. Nursing diagnoses may include the following:

- *Risk for violence toward self (mother) or children related to*
  −postpartum depression
- *Situational low self-esteem in the mother related to*
  −stresses associated with role changes
- *Compromised family coping related to*
  −increased care needs of mother and infant
- *Risk for impaired parenting related to*
  −inability of depressed mother to attach to infant
- *Risk for injury to newborn related to*
  −mother's depression (inattention to infant's needs for hygiene, nutrition, safety) and psychotropic medications via breast milk

▬ Expected Outcomes of Care

Specific measurable criteria can be developed based on the following general outcomes:
- The mother will no longer be depressed.
- The mother's and infant's physical well-being will be maintained.
- The family will cope effectively.
- Family members will demonstrate continued healthy growth and development.
- The infant will be fully integrated into the family.

▬ Plan of Care and Interventions
▬ On the Postpartum Unit

The postpartum nurse must observe the new mother carefully for any signs of tearfulness and conduct further assessments as necessary. Nurses must discuss PPD to prepare new parents for potential problems in the postpartum period (see Teaching for Self-Care box). The family must be able to recognize the symptoms and know where to go for help. Written materials that explain what the woman can do to prevent depression could be used as part of discharge planning.

Mothers are often discharged from the hospital before the blues or depression occurs. If the postpartum nurse is concerned about the mother, a mental health consult should be requested before the mother leaves the hospital. Routine instructions regarding PPD should be given to whoever comes to take the woman home; for example, "If you notice that your wife (or daughter) is upset or crying a lot, please call the postpartum care provider immediately—don't wait for the routine postpartum appointment."

▬ NURSE ALERT

Because the newborn may be scheduled for a checkup before the mother's 6-week checkup, nurses in well-baby clinics or pediatrician offices should be alert for signs of PPD in new mothers and be knowledgeable about community referral resources.

▬ In the Home and Community

Postpartum home visits can reduce the incidence of or complications from depression. A brief home visit or phone call at least once a week until the new mother returns for her

---

TEACHING FOR SELF-CARE

Activities to Prevent Postpartum Depression
- Educate close family and friends about postpartum emotional problems.
- Take care of yourself: eat a balanced diet, exercise on a regular basis, and get enough sleep. Ask someone to take care of the baby so that you can get a full night's sleep.
- Share your feelings with someone close to you; don't isolate yourself at home.
- Don't overcommit yourself or feel like you need to be a superwoman.
- Don't place unrealistic expectations on yourself.
- Don't be ashamed of having emotional problems after your baby is born—it happens to approximately 15% of women.

postpartum visit may save the life of a mother and her infant; however, home visits may not be feasible or available. Supervision of the mother with emotional complications may become a prime concern. Because depression can greatly interfere with her mothering functions, family and friends may need to participate in the infant's care. This is a time for the extended family and friends to determine what they can do to help, and the nurse can work with them to ensure adequate supervision of and their understanding of the woman's mental illness (Linter & Gray, 2006).

When the woman has PPD, a partner often reacts with confusion, shock, denial, and anger and feels neglected and blamed. The nurse can talk with the woman about how her condition is hard for him too and that he is probably very worried about her. Men oftentimes withdraw or criticize when they are deeply worried about their significant others. The nurse can provide nonjudgmental opportunities for the partner to verbalize feelings and concerns, help the partner identify positive coping strategies, and be a source of encouragement for the partner to continue supporting the woman. Suggestions for partners of women with PPD include helping around the house, setting limits with family and friends, going with her to doctor's appointments, educating yourself, writing down concerns and questions to take to doctor or therapist and be with her—sit quietly, hug her, and tell her you love her (Kleiman, 2000). Both the woman and her partner need an opportunity to express their needs, fears, thoughts, and feelings in a nonjudgmental environment.

Even if the mother is severely depressed, hospitalization can be avoided if adequate resources can be mobilized to ensure safety for both mother and infant. The nurse in home health care will need to make frequent phone calls or home visits to do assessment and counseling. Community resources that may be helpful are temporary child care or foster care, homemaker service, meals on wheels, parenting guidance centers, mother's-day-out programs, and telephone support groups such as Postpartum Support International (www.chss.iup.edu/postpartum) and Depression after Delivery (www.depressionafterdelivery.com).

Referral. Women with moderate to severe PPD should be referred to a mental health therapist, such as an advanced practice psychiatric nurse or psychiatrist, for evaluation and therapy to avoid the effects that PPD can have on the woman and on her relationships with her partner, baby, and other children (Brown, 2001). Inpatient psychiatric hospitalization may be necessary. This decision is made when the safety needs of the mother or children are threatened.

Providing Safety. If delusional thinking about the baby is suspected, the nurse asks, "Have you thought about hurting your baby?" When depression is suspected, the nurse asks, "Have you thought about hurting yourself?" Four criteria measure the seriousness of a suicidal plan: method, availability, specificity, and lethality. Has the woman specified a method? Is the method of choice available? How specific is the plan? If the method is concrete and detailed,

with access to it right at hand, the suicide risk increases. How lethal is the method? The most lethal method is shooting, with hanging a close second. The least lethal is slashing one's wrists. Medication overdose with TCAs does cause death. Avoid TCAs in suicidal women because of their danger in overdose.

■ **NURSE ALERT**

Suicidal thoughts or attempts are among the most serious symptoms of PPD and require immediate assessment and intervention.

■ *Psychiatric Hospitalization*

Women with postpartum psychosis have a psychiatric emergency and must be referred immediately to a psychiatrist who is experienced in working with women with PPD, can prescribe medication and other forms of therapy, and can assess the need for hospitalization.

■ **LEGAL TIP** **Commitment for Psychiatric Care**

If a woman with PPD is experiencing active suicidal ideation or harmful delusions about the baby and is unwilling to seek treatment, legal intervention may be necessary to commit the woman to an inpatient setting for treatment.

Within the hospital setting, the reintroduction of the baby to the mother can occur at the mother's own pace. A schedule is set for increasing the number of hours the mother cares for the baby over several days, culminating in the infant staying overnight in the mother's room. This allows the mother to experience meeting the infant's needs and giving up sleep for the baby, a situation difficult for new mothers even under ideal conditions. The mother's readiness for discharge and caring for the baby is assessed. Her interactions with her baby also are carefully supervised and guided.

Nurses also should observe the mother for signs of bonding with the baby. Attachment behaviors are defined as eye-to-eye contact; physical contact that involves holding, touching, cuddling, and talking to the baby and calling the baby by name; and the initiation of appropriate care. A staff member is assigned to keep the baby in sight at all times. Indirect teaching, praise, and encouragement are designed to bolster the mother's self-esteem and self-confidence.

■ *Psychotropic Medications*

PPD is usually treated with antidepressant medications. If the woman with PPD is not breastfeeding, antidepressants can be prescribed without special precautions. In addition to the TCAs, SSRIs, and SNRIs discussed previously, MAOIs, mood stabilizers, and antipsychotic medications may be prescribed for nonbreastfeeding women.

Hypertensive crisis is the main reason that MAOIs are not prescribed more frequently. The woman should be taught to watch for signs of hypertensive crisis—a throbbing, occipital headache, stiff neck, chills, nausea, flushing, retroorbital pain, apprehension, pallor, sweating, chest pain, and palpitations (Kando et al., 2005). This crisis is brought on by the woman taking any of a large variety of over-the-counter medications or eating foods that contain tyramine, a sympathomimetic pressor amine, which normally is broken down by the enzyme monoamine oxidase. The nurse must do extensive teaching about avoidance of foods and medications that contain tyramine such as pseudoephedrine-containing medications, aged cheese, Chianti wine, avocados, chicken livers, preserved meats, and tap beers (Anaizi, 2006; National Headache Foundation, 2005).

The woman taking mood stabilizers (see Table 35-4) must be taught about the many side effects, and especially, for those taking lithium, the need to have serum lithium levels determined every 6 months. Women with severe psychiatric syndromes such as schizophrenia, bipolar disorder, or psychotic depression will probably require antipsychotic medications (see Table 35-5). Most of these antipsychotic medications can cause sedation and orthostatic hypotension—both of which could interfere with the mother being able to care safely for her baby. They also can cause PNS effects such as constipation, dry mouth, blurred vision, tachycardia, urinary retention, weight gain, and agranulocytosis. CNS effects may include akathisia, dystonias, parkinsonism-like symptoms, tardive dyskinesia (irreversible), and neuroleptic malignant syndrome (potentially fatal). Medication education is especially important when caring for women who are taking antipyschotic medications. The nurse should use discretion in selecting the content to be shared because of the women's altered thought processes and the large number of side/toxic effects. The nurse may choose to do more extensive education with a close family member. The newer, atypical antipsychotic medications such as aripiprazole, olanzapine, quetiapine, risperidone, and ziprasidone are usually safer and have fewer side effects than the older, more traditional antipsychotics; however, their safety in breastfeeding women has not been established.

Psychotropic Medications and Lactation. A major clinical dilemma is the psychopharmacologic treatment of women with PPD who want to breastfeed their infants. In the past, women were told to discontinue lactation. Current beliefs are that although most drugs will diffuse into breast milk, there are very few instances where breastfeeding has to be discontinued (Pigarelli et al., 2005). Several factors influence the amount of drug an infant will receive through breastfeeding: amount of milk produced, the composition of the milk (mature milk versus colostrum), the concentration of the medication, and the extent to which the breast was emptied during a previous feeding (Pigarelli et al.). Infants also vary in their ability to absorb, metabolize, and excrete ingested medication. Premature infants may not have optimal liver function, and kidney function doesn't reach maturity until 2 to 4 months of age.

The FDA has not approved any psychotropic medication for use during lactation. However, most of the medications listed in the position statement from the American Academy of Pediatrics (AAP) are compatible with breastfeeding (AAP, 2001) (see Tables 35-1, 35-2, 35-4, and 35-5 for risk of taking common psychotropic medications during lactation). Almost all of the psychotropic medications are drugs for which the effects on the breastfeeding newborn are "unknown but still may be of concern." The reason for the concern is that although the medications appear to be in low concentrations in breast milk (commonly a milk-to-serum ratio of 0.5 to 1.0), many drugs have a long half-life, and levels may build up in plasma and tissue of nursing infants. Medications that have shorter half-lives tend to accumulate less, and those that are more protein bound do not cross into breast milk as well (Pigarelli et al., 2005). Drugs with lower oral bioavailability and lower lipid solubility are also good choices (Pigarelli et al.). Long-term effects on the newborn are unknown (AAP). Because all psychotropic medications pass through breast milk to the infant, the risks associated with the use of such medication must be weighed against the benefits associated with breastfeeding for both mother and infant.

No controlled trials have examined antidepressant therapy in nursing women; however, numerous case reports and case series have been published (Whitby & Smith, 2005). Most TCAs appear to be safe during breastfeeding, with the exception of doxepin, which is associated with respiratory depression. Although TCAs have been the treatment of choice in the past, SSRIs are gaining popularity because of their superior safety profiles. Of all agents reviewed in the literature, sertraline was the most prescribed, and no adverse effects were reported (Whitby & Smith, 2005). Many of the other SSRIs are well tolerated by breastfed infants. Fluoxetine has resulted in some reports of gastrointestinal problems, irritability, and insomnia (Pigarelli et al., 2005). MAOIs are usually avoided.

The elapsed time between maternal dosing and infant feeding has been shown to affect the amount of antidepressant medication to which the nursling is exposed. Amitriptyline, desipramine, and trazodone appear to reach a peak in breast milk at 4 to 6 hours after an oral dose; peak concentrations of sertraline occurred 7 to 10 hours after the maternal dose (Schatzberg & Nemeroff, 2004). If the mother is using a once-daily medication, administration at bedtime may be advised to increase the interval to the next feeding (Pigarelli et al., 2005). For medications taken multiple times per day, administration of medication immediately after a breastfeeding session will give the longest interval to allow back diffusion of drug from the breast milk as the mother's serum concentration decreases (Spencer, Gonzalez, & Barnhart, 2001). Most of the drugs listed in Tables 35-4 and 35-5 are classified as drugs whose effects on infants are unknown but may be of concern.

Antipsychotic medications are excreted into breast milk. None of these medications has been proven safe during lactation; the AAP does not rate any of the antipsychotic medications as compatible with breastfeeding because the Committee on Drugs found no reports in the literature (AAP, 2001).

With the exception of diazepam, benzodiazepines at relatively low doses present no contraindications to nursing (Schatzberg & Nemeroff, 2004). Diazepam exposure can cause sedation, lethargy, and weight loss in infants (Iqbal, Sobhan, & Ryals, 2002). In contrast to other classes of psychotropic medications, benzodiazepines appear to have lower milk-to-maternal serum ratios.

Mood-stabilizing medications are present in breast milk. With lithium, milk concentrations are 30% to 50% of maternal levels, and serum concentrations in the nursing infant are 10% to 50% of the mother's; thus breastfeeding is usually discouraged (Frankhauser & Freeman, 2005). The AAP considers lithium incompatible with breastfeeding (Viguera, Cohen, Baldessarini, & Nonacs, 2002). Valproic acid appears in low concentrations in human milk and is considered compatible with breastfeeding (Fankhauser & Freeman). There are two case studies of hepatitis and jaundice in nursing infants whose mothers were taking carbamazepine (Fankhauser & Freeman); however, it appears to be compatible with breastfeeding because it is found in breast milk in only a very small quantity (Pigarelli et al., 2005). The benefits of breastfeeding and the potential risks must be carefully considered before using lithium or other mood stabilizers (Fankhauser & Freeman).

In summary, all psychotropic medications studied to date are excreted in breast milk. The known adverse effects of psychotropic agents on infants are limited to case reports. The nursing infant's daily dose of psychotropic agents is less than the maternal daily dose. Psychotropic medications are excreted into breast milk with a specific individual time course, allowing the minimization of infant exposure with continuation of breastfeeding. The long-term neurobehavioral effects of infant exposure to psychotropic medications through breastfeeding are unknown. When selecting psychotropic medications for breastfeeding women, choose those with greatest documentation of prior use, lower FDA risk category, few or no metabolites, and fewer side effects (Schatzberg & Nemeroff, 2004).

Nursing Implications. When breastfeeding women have emotional complications and need psychotropic medications, referral to a mental health care provider who specializes in postpartum disorders is preferred. Depressed women will need the nurse to reinforce the need to take antidepressants as ordered. Because antidepressants do not exert any effect for about 2 weeks and usually do not reach full effect for 4 to 6 weeks, many women discontinue taking the medication on their own. Client and family teaching should reinforce the schedule for taking medications in conjunction with the infant's feeding schedule and to continue taking the medication until therapeutic effects occur.

▬ *Other Treatments for PPD*

Other treatments for PPD include complementary/alternative therapies such as those listed in Box 35-3, ECT, and psychotherapy (group or individual). ECT may be used for women with PPD who have not improved with antidepres-

---

box 35-3 **Possible Alternative/Complementary Therapies for Postpartum Depression**

- Acupuncture
- Acupressure
- Aromatherapy
  - Jasmine
  - Ylang ylang
  - Rose
- Herbal
  - Lavender tea
- Healing touch/therapeutic touch
- Massage
- Relaxation techniques
- Reflexology
- Yoga

Source: Weier, K., & Beal, M. (2004). Complementary therapies and adjuncts in the treatment of postpartum depression. *Journal of Midwifery & Women's Health, 49*(2), 96-104

---

sant therapy. Alternative therapies may be used alone but often are used with other treatments for PPD. Safety and efficacy studies of these alternative therapies are needed to ensure that care and advice is based on evidence (Weier & Beal, 2004).

▬ NURSE ALERT

St. John's wort is often used to treat depression. It has not been proven safe for women who are breastfeeding.

▬ Evaluation

The nurse can be assured that care has been effective if the physical well-being of the mother and infant are maintained, the mother and family are able to cope effectively, and each family member continues to show a healthy adaptation to the presence of the new member of the family (see Plan of Care).

Postpartum Onset of Panic Disorder

Little is known about the risk for and course of panic disorder in the postpartum period. In one study, 147 community women completed an interview and self-report inventories about 8 weeks after childbirth (Wenzel, Haugen, Jackson, & Brendle, 2005). Depending on the particular domain of anxiety being considered, 10% to 50% of women reported anxiety symptoms, and the authors suggested that postpartum anxiety disorders are more common than PPD (Wenzel et al.). In approximately 3% to 5% of women, panic disorder or OCD develops in the postpartum period. Panic attacks are discrete periods in which there is the sudden onset of intense apprehension, fearfulness, or terror (APA, 2000). During these attacks, symptoms such as shortness of breath, palpitations, chest pain, choking, smothering sensations, and fear of losing control are present. Women have reported having intrusive thoughts about terrible injury done to the infant, such as stabbing or burns, sometimes by themselves. Rarely do the women harm the baby. Nurses need only to listen to the mother to hear symptoms of panic

plan of care > Postpartum Depression (PPD)

NURSING DIAGNOSIS Risk for injury to the woman and/or newborn related to woman's emotional state and/or treatment

Expected Outcomes *The mother and newborn will remain free of injury. The woman's family will verbalize understanding of the need for maternal and infant supervision and have a plan to provide that supervision.*

Nursing Interventions/Rationales

- Assess the postpartum woman for risk factors for depression (before discharge) *to determine if she is at risk and in need of prompt interventions or referral.*
- Provide information about signs of PPD to woman and family *to promote prompt recognition of problems.*
- Observe maternal-infant interactions before discharge *to determine appropriateness.*
- Maintain frequent contact with woman by telephone calls and home visits *to determine if further interventions are necessary, because most postpartum mothers are discharged early from the inpatient setting.*
- Counsel woman and family to telephone health care provider if behaviors indicating depression, such as crying, increase *to provide prompt care and referral if necessary and avoid injury to newborn and mother.*
- Provide opportunities for woman and family to verbalize feelings and concerns in a nonjudgmental setting *to promote a trusting relationship.*
- Assess woman for any suicidal thoughts or plans *to provide for safety of woman and infant.*
- Assist family to develop a plan for maternal and infant supervision *to provide for safety of woman and infant.*
- Provide information about community resources for assistance *to ensure care if woman is unable to care for herself or infant.*
- Reinforce teaching or refer breastfeeding mother to lactation consultant *to obtain information regarding effects of antidepressant and antipsychotic medications.*

NURSING DIAGNOSIS Disabled family coping related to postpartum maternal depression as evidenced by family members' denial of woman's illness

Expected Outcomes *Family will identify positive coping mechanisms and initiate a plan to cope with the woman's depression.*

Nursing Interventions/Rationales

- Provide opportunity for family and significant others to verbalize feelings and concerns *to establish a trusting relationship.*
- Give information to the family regarding postpartum depression *to clarify any misconceptions or misinformation.*
- Assist family to identify positive coping mechanisms that have been effective during past crises *to promote active participation in care.*
- Assist family to identify community sources of support *to provide additional resources as needed.*
- Refer family to mental health counselor as needed *to provide further expertise from a mental health professional.*

NURSING DIAGNOSIS Risk for impaired parenting related to inability of mother to attach to infant

Expected Outcomes *Woman demonstrates appropriate attachment behaviors in infant interactions. Woman expresses satisfaction with infant.*

Nursing Interventions/Rationales

- Observe maternal-infant interactions *to assess quality of interactions and to determine need for interventions.*
- Encourage woman to express her anxiety, fears, or other feelings *to allow woman to ventilate her concerns and have them accepted.*
- Encourage the woman to have as much contact with infant as possible *to minimize separation and to promote attachment.*
- Demonstrate infant care and explain infant behaviors *to enhance mother's care abilities and understanding of infant's abilities.*
- Make referrals as needed to community resources *to assist the woman in developing parenting skills or promoting confidence in infant care.*

CD: Plan of Care: Postpartum Depression

---

disorder. Usually these women are so distraught that they will share with whoever will listen. Oftentimes the family has tried to tell them that what they are experiencing is normal, but they know differently. Potential nursing diagnoses for women experiencing postpartum panic disorder include the following:

- *Anxiety related to*
  - −postpartum adaptations and expectations
- *Fear related to*
  - −obsessions
  - −thoughts about harming others
- *Powerlessness related to*
  - −feelings of losing control
- *Deficient knowledge related to*
  - −postpartum mental health problems

Medical Management

Treatment is usually a combination of medications, education, psychotherapy, and cognitive behavioral interven-

tions, along with an attempt to identify any medical or physiologic contributors. Antidepressants such as SSRIs are the treatment of choice, instead of benzodiazepines (Kirkwood & Melton, 2005), and most of the SSRIs are approved in the United States for the treatment of panic disorder and obsessive compulsive disorder. If benzodiazepines are used, avoid diazepam if the mother is nursing because infants can experience sedation, lethargy, and weight loss (Kirkwood & Melton).

Nursing Considerations

The following nursing interventions are suggested:

- Education is a crucial nursing intervention. New mothers should be provided with anticipatory guidance concerning the possibility of panic attacks during the postpartum period. Preparing for the attacks may help offset their unexpected, terrifying nature (Beck, 1998b).
- Empowerment conveys to the woman that she can sort through her fears and expectations and take charge of her life. Women can be reassured that it is common to

feel a sense of impending doom and fear of insanity during panic attacks. These fears are temporary and disappear once the panic attack is over (Beck, 1998b).

- Nurses can help women identify panic triggers that are particular to their own lives. Keeping a diary can help identify the triggers (Beck, 1998b).
- Family and social supports are helpful. The new mother is encouraged to put usual chores on hold and to ask for and accept help.
- Support groups allow these mothers to feel comfort in seeing others like themselves.
- Sensory interventions such as music therapy and aromatherapy are nonintrusive and inexpensive.
- Behavioral interventions such as breathing exercises and progressive muscle relaxation can be helpful (Fishel, 1998).

- Cognitive interventions such as positive self-talk training, reframing and redefining, and reassurance can alter the negative thinking (Fishel, 1998).

community activity

- Identify resources in your community for pregnant women who are substance abusers. What are the services offered, and how accessible are they (i.e., location, time of availability, cost, language other than English)? What services are available after the baby is born, or what type of follow-up is provided? Are the services culturally relevant?
- Alternately, identify resources in the community for women at risk for postpartum depression.

key points

- Because pregnant women may have a history of mental disorder or substance abuse, careful assessment is extremely important at the first and each subsequent prenatal and postnatal visit.
- Values clarification for health care workers may be necessary to assist them in providing nonjudgmental care for substance abusers.
- Alcohol abuse during pregnancy is the leading cause of mental retardation in the United States, and it is entirely preventable.
- Treatment programs must start with an understanding that substance abuse in women is a complex problem surrounded by multiple individual, familial, and social issues that require many levels of intervention and treatment.

- Mood disorders account for most mental health disorders in the postpartum period.
- Identification of women at greatest risk for substance abuse during pregnancy and depression in the postpartum period can be facilitated by use of various screening tools.
- Suicidal thoughts or attempts are among the most serious symptoms of PPD.
- Antidepressant medications are the usual treatment for PPD; however, specific precautions are needed for breastfeeding women.
- Treatment of postpartum onset of panic disorder requires a combination of medication, education, supportive measures, and psychotherapy.

REFERENCES

Abel, E., & Kruger, M. (2002). Physician attitudes concerning legal coercion of pregnant alcohol and drug abusers. *American Journal of Obstetrics and Gynecology, 186*(4), 768-772.

American Academy of Pediatrics (AAP) Committee on Drugs. (2001). The transfer of drugs and other chemicals into human milk. *Pediatrics, 108*(3), 776-789.

American Psychiatric Association. (2000). *Diagnostic and statistical manual of mental disorders* (4th ed., rev.). Washington, DC: American Psychiatric Association Press.

Anaizi, N. (2006). Food-drug interatctions. *The Drug Monitor.* Accessed www.thedrugmonitor.com, August 24, 2006.

Bandestra, E., & Accornero, V. (2006). Infants of substance-abusing mothers. In A. Fanaroff, R. Martin, & M. Walsh, *Fanaroff and Martin's neonatal-perinatal medicine: Diseases of the fetus and infant* (8th ed.). Philadelphia: Mosby.

Beck, C. (1995a). Screening methods for postpartum depression. *Journal of Obstetric, Gynecologic, and Neonatal Nursing, 24*(4), 308-312.

Beck, C. (1995b). Perceptions of nurses' caring by mothers experiencing postpartum depression. *Journal of Obstetric, Gynecologic, and Neonatal Nursing, 24*(9), 819-825.

Beck, C. (1998a). A checklist to identify women at risk for developing postpartum depression. *Journal of Obstetric, Gynecologic, and Neonatal Nursing, 27*(1), 39-46.

Beck, C. (1998b). Postpartum onset of panic disorder. *Image: The Journal of Nursing Scholarship, 30*(2), 131-135.

Beck, C. (1999). *Postpartum depression: Case studies, research, and nursing care.* Washington, DC: AWHONN.

Beck, C. (2001). Predictors of postpartum depression: An update. *Nursing Research, 50*(5), 275-282.

Beck, C. (2002). Revision of the Postpartum Depression Predictors Inventory. *Journal of Obstetric, Gynecologic, and Neonatal Nursing, 31*(4), 394-402.

Bennett, H., Einarson, A., Toddio, A., Koren, G., & Einarson, T. (2004). Prevalence of depression during pregnancy: Systematic review. *Obstetrics and Gynecology, 103*(4), 698-709.

Bogart, C., & Pearce, C. (2003). "13th stepping": Why Alcoholics Anonymous is not always a safe place for women. *Journal of Addictions Nursing, 14*(1), 43-47.

Boury, J., Larkin, T., & Krummel, D. (2004). Factors related to postpartum depressive symptoms in low-income women. *Women's Health, 39*(3), 19-34.

Bozoky, I., & Corwin, E. (2001). Fatigue as a predictor of postpartum depression. *Journal of Obstetric, Gynecologic, and Neonatal Nursing, 31*(4), 436-443.

Brady, T., & Ashley, O. (2005). *Women in substance abuse treatment: Results from alcohol and drug services study* (ADSS). DHHS Publication # SMA 04-3968 analytic series A 26. Rockville MD: Substance and Mental Health Services Administration, Office of Applied Studies.

Brennan, P. (2003). Tobacco consumption during pregnancy and its impact on psychosocial child development. In R. Trembly,

R. Barr, & R. Petros (Eds.) *Encyclopedia of early childhood development* [online]. Montreal, Quebec: Centre of Excellence for early childhood development. Accessed www.excellence-earlychildhood.ca/documents, August 24, 2006.

Brown, C. (2001). Depression and anxiety disorders. *Obstetrics and Gynecology Clinics of North America, 28*(2), 241-268.

Cnattingius, S., Signorello, L., Anneren, G., Clauson, B. Ekbom, A., Ljunger, E., et al. (2000). Caffeine intake and the risk of first-trimester spontaneous abortion. *New England Journal of Medicine, 343*(25), 1839-1845.

Coates, A., Schaefer, C., & Alexander, J. (2004). Detection of postpartum depression and anxiety in a large health plan. *Journal of Behavioral Health Services & Research, 31*(2), 117-133.

Cohen, L., Nonacs, R., Bailey, J., Viguera, A., Reminick, A., Altshuler, L., et al. (2004). Relapse of depression during pregnancy following antidepressant discontinuation: A preliminary prospective study. *Archives of Women's Mental Health, 7*(4), 217-221.

Cook, L. (2004). Educating women about the hidden dangers of alcohol. *Journal of Psychosocial Nursing, 42*(6), 24-31.

Corrarino, J., Williams, C., Campbell, W., Amrhein, E., LoPiano, L., & Kalachik, D. (2000) Linking substance abusing pregnant women to drug treatment services: A pilot program. *Journal of Obstetric, Gynecologic, and Neonatal Nursing, 29*(4), 369-376.

Cox, J., Holden, J., & Sagovsky, R. (1987). Detection of postnatal depression. Development of the 10- item Edinburgh Postnatal Depression Scale. *British Journal of Psychiatry, 150,* 782-786.

Cunningham, G., Leveno, K., Bloom, S., Hauth, J, Gilstrap, L., & Wenstrom, K. (2005). *Williams obstetrics* (22nd ed.). New York; McGraw-Hill.

Daley, M., Argoriou, M., McCarty, D., Callahan, J., Shepard, D., & Williams, C. (2001). The impact of substance abuse treatment modality on birth weight and health care expenditures. *Journal of Psychoactive Drugs, 33*(1), 57-66.

Davis, L., Edwards, H., Mohay, H., & Wollin, J. (2003). The impact of very premature birth on the psychological health of mothers. *Early Human Development, 73*(1-2), 61-70.

Dennis, C. (2004a). Can we identify mothers at risk for postpartum depression in the immediate postpartum period using the Edinburgh Postnatal Depression Scale? *Journal of Affective Disorders, 78*(2), 163-169.

Dennis, C. (2004b). Preventing postpartum depression part 1: A review of biological interventions. *Canadian Journal of Psychiatry, 49*(7), 467-474.

Dennis, C. (2004c). Treatment of postpartum depression. Part 2: A critical review of nonbiological interventions. *Journal of Clinical Psychiatry, 65*(9), 1252-1265.

Dennis, C., Janssen, P., & Singer, J. (2004). Identifying women at-risk for postpartum depression in the immediate postpartum period. *Acta Psychiatrica Scandinavica, 110*(5), 338.

Doering, P. (2005). Substance-related disorders: Alcohol, nicotine, and caffeine. In J. DiPiro, R. Talbert, G. Yee, G. Matzke, B. Wells, & M. Posey (Eds.), *Pharmacotherapy: A pathophysiologic approach* (6th ed). New York: McGraw-Hill.

Eberhard-Gran, M., Eskild, A., & Tambs, K. (2001). Review of validation studies of the Edinburgh Postnatal Depression Scale. *Acta Psychiatrica Scandinavica, 104*(4), 243-249.

Ewing, J. (1984). Detecting alcoholism: The CAGE questionnaire. *Journal of the American Medical Association, 22*(14), 1905-1907.

Fankhauser, M., & Freeman, M. (2005). Bipolar disorder. In J. DiPiro, R. Talbert, G. Yee, G. Matzke, B. Wells, & M. Posey (Eds.), *Pharmacotherapy: A pathophysiologic approach* (6th ed). New York: McGraw-Hill.

Fishel, A. (1998). Nursing management of anxiety and panic. *Nursing Clinics of North America, 33*(1), 135-151.

Fishel, A. (1999). Evidence-based psychosocial therapies. In C. Shea (Ed.), *Advanced practice nursing in psychiatric and mental health care.* St. Louis: Mosby.

Foley, E. (2002). Drug screening and criminal prosecution of pregnant women. *Journal of Obstetric, Gynecologic, and Neonatal Nursing, 31*(2), 133-137.

Gilbert, E., & Harmon, J. (2003). *Manual of high risk pregnancy & delivery* (3rd ed.). St. Louis: Mosby.

Goodman, J. (2005). Women's mental health. *Journal of Obstetric, Gynecologic, and Neonatal Nursing, 34*(2), 245.

Gold, L. (2002). Postpartum disorders in primary care: Diagnosis and treatment. *Primary Care, 29*(1), 27-41.

Goldbort, J. (2006). Transcultural analysis of postpartum depression. *MCN American Journal of Maternal/Child Nursing, 31*(2), 121-126.

Gottlieb, S. (2001). Pregnant women cannot be tested for drugs without consent. *BMJ, 322*(7289), 753.

Hendrick, V., & Altshuler, L. (2002). Management of major depression during pregnancy. *American Journal of Psychiatry, 159*(10), 1667-1673.

Herrick, H. (2002). *Postpartum depression: Who gets help?* Statistical Brief No. 24. Raleigh, NC: Department of Health and Human Services.

Huang, Y., & Mathers, N. (2001). Postnatal depression: Biological or cultural? A comparative study of postnatal women in the UK and Taiwan. *Journal of Advanced Nursing, 33*(3), 279-287.

Iqbal, M., Sobhan, T., & Ryals, T. (2002). Effects of commonly used benzodiazepines on the fetus, the neonate, and the nursing infant. *Psychiatric Services, 53*(1), 39-49.

Jefferson, D. (2005). America's most dangerous drug. *Newsweek,* August 8, 41-48.

Kando, J., Wells, B., & Hayes, P. (2005). Depressive disorders. In J. DiPiro, R. Talbert, G. Yee, G. Matzke, B. Wells, & M. Posey (Eds.), *Pharmacotherapy: A pathophysiologic approach* (6th ed.). New York: McGraw-Hill.

Kaplan, H., & Sadock, B. (2005). *Kaplan & Sadock's comprehensive textbook of psychiatry.* Philadelphia: Lippincott Williams & Wilkins.

Kirkwood, C., & Melton, S. (2005). Anxiety disorders I: Generalized anxiety, panic, and social anxiety disorders. In J. DiPiro, R. Talbert, G. Yee, G. Matzke, B. Wells, & M. Posey (Eds.), *Pharmacotherapy: A pathophysiologic approach* (6th ed). New York: McGraw-Hill.

Kleiman, K. (2000). *The postpartum husband: Practical solutions for living with postpartum depression.* Philadelphia: Xlibris Corp.

Koren, G., Matsiu, D., Einarson, A., Knoppert, D., & Steiner, M. (2005). Is maternal use of SSRI in third trimester of pregnancy harmful to neonates? *Canadian Medical Association Journal, 172*(11), 1457-1459.

Kuo, W, Wilson, T., Holman, S., Fuentes-Afflick, E., Sullivan M., & Minkoff, H. (2004). Depressive symptoms in the immediate postpartum period among Hispanic women in three U.S. cities. *Journal of Immigrant Health, 6*(4), 145-153.

Lee, R., An, S., Kim, S., Rhee, G., Kwack, S., Seok, J., et al. (2005). Neurotoxic effects of alcohol and acetaldehyde during embryonic development. *Journal of Toxicology and Environmental Health Part A, 68*(23-24), 2147-2162.

Lehmann, C. (2004). House committee briefed on postpartum MH issues. *Psychiatric News, 39*(21), 26.

Lester, B., Andreozzi, L., & Appiah, L. (2004). Substance use during pregnancy: Time for policy to catch up with research. *Harm Reduction Journal, 1*(5), 1-44.

Linter, N., & Gray, B. (2006). Childbearing and depression: What nurses need to know. *AWHONN Lifelines, 10*(1), 50-57.

Maier, S., & West, J. (2001). Drinking patterns and alcohol-related-birth defects. *Alcohol Research & Health, 25*(3), 168-174.

Maley, B. (2002). Creating a postpartum depression support group. *AWHONN Lifelines, 6*(1), 62-65.

Matthey, S., Barnett, B., Howie, P., & Kavanagh, D. (2001). Validation of the Edinburgh Postnatal Depression Scale for men, and comparison of item endorsement with their partner. *Journal of Affective Disorders, 64*(2-3), 175-184.

Miller, W., & Rollnick, S. (1991). *Motivational interviewing: Preparing people to change addictive behaviour.* New York: Guilford Press.

Morse, B., & Hutchins, E. (2000). Reducing complications from alcohol use during pregnancy through screening. *Journal of the American Medical Women's Association, 55*(4), 225-227, 240.

Murphy-Parker, D., & Martinez, R. (2005). Nursing students' personal experiences involving alcohol problems. *Archives of Psychiatric Nursing, 19*(3), 150-158.

National Headache Foundation. (2005). *Tyramine.* Accessed www. headaches.org/consumer/topicsheets/tyramine.html, August 24, 2006.

Nulman, I., Rovet, J., Stewart, D., Wolpin, J., Gardner, H., Theis, J., et al. (1997). Neurodevelopment of children exposed in utero to antidepressant drugs. *New England Journal of Medicine, 336*(4), 258-262.

O'Brien, L., Heycock, E., Hanna, M., Jones, P., & Cox, J. (2004.) Postnatal depression and faltering growth: A community study. *Pediatrics, 113*(5), 1242-1247.

Otto, K. (2003). Acupuncture and substance abuse: A synopsis with indications for further research. *American Journal of Addictions, 12*(1), 43-51.

Peterson, J. , Nisenholz, B., & Robinson, G.(2003). *A nation under the influence: America's addiction to alcohol.* Boston: Allyn & Bacon.

Pigarelli, D., Kraus, C., & Potter, B. (2005). Pregnancy and lactation: Therapeutic considerations. In DiPiro, J., Talbert, R., Yee, G., Matzke, G., Wells, B., & Posey. M. (Eds.), *Pharmacotherapy: A pathophysiologic approach* (6th ed.). New York: McGraw-Hill.

Pokorny, A., Miller, B., & Kaplan, H. (1972). The Brief MAST: A shortened version of the Michigan Alcoholism Screening Test. *American Journal of Psychiatry, 129*(3), 342-345.

Posmontier, B., & Horowitz, J. (2004). Postpartum practices and depression prevalences: Technocentric and ethnokinship cultural perspectives. *Journal of Transcultural Nursing, 15*(1), 34-43.

Prochaska, J., & DiClemente, C. (1992). Stages of change in the modification of problem behaviors. In M. Hersen, R. Eisler, & P. Miller (Eds.), *Progress in behavior modification,* Vol. 28. Sycamore, IL: Sycamore.

Reynolds, K. (2004). Living with postpartum depression. *Journal of Psychosocial Nursing, 42*(6), 56-59.

Sanz, E. (2005). SSRI in pregnant women and neonatal withdrawal syndrome. *Lancet, 365*(9458), 482-487.

Saulnier, C. (1996). African-American women in an alcohol intervention group: Addressing personal and political problems. *Substance Use and Misuse, 31*(10),1259-78.

Schatzberg, A., & Nemeroff, C. (Eds.) (2004). *The American Psychiatric Publishing textbook of psychopharmacology.* (3rd ed.). Washington, DC: American Psychiatric Publishing.

Seidel, H., Ball, J., Dains, J., & Benedict, G. (2006). *Mosby's guide to physical examination* (6th ed.). St. Louis: Mosby.

Spencer, J., Gonzalez, L., & Barnhart, D. (2001). Medications in the breast-feeding mother. *American Family Physician, 64*(1), 119-126.

Stowe, J., Strader, J., & Nemeroff, C. (2006). Psychopharmacology during pregnancy andlactation. In A. Schatzberg & C. Nemeroff (Eds.), *Essentials of clinical psychopharmacology* (2nd Ed.). Washington, DC: American Psychiatric Publishing.

Stuart, G., & Laraia, M. (2005). *Principles and practice of psychiatric nursing* (8th ed.). St. Louis: Mosby.

Tillett, J., & Osborne, K. (2001). Substance abuse by pregnant women: Legal and ethical concerns. *Journal of Perinatal and Neonatal Nursing, 14*(4), 1-11.

U.S. Department of Health and Human Services (USDHHS). (2000). *Healthy People 2010.* Washington, DC: Government Printing Office.

van den Brink, W., & van Ree, J. (2003). Pharmacological treatments for heroin and cocaine addiction. *European Neuropsychopharmacology, 13*(6), 476-487.

Vickers, A., Wilson, P., & Kleynen, J. (2002). Effectiveness Bulletin. Acupuncture. *Quality and Safety in Health Care, 11*(1), 92-97.

Viguera, A., Cohen, L., Baldessarini, R., & Nonacs, R. (2002). Managing bipolar disorder during pregnancy: Weighing the risks and benefits. *Canadian Journal of Psychiatry, 47*(5), 426-436.

Wang, S., Chen, C., Chin, C., & Lee, S. (2005). Impact of postpartum depression on the mother-infant couple. *Birth, 32*(1), 39-44.

Weier, K., & Beal, M. (2004). Complementary therapies and adjuncts in the treatment of postpartum depression. *Journal of Midwifery & Women's Health, 49*(2), 96-104.

Wenzel, A., Haugen, E., Jackson, D., & Brendle, J. (2005). Anxiety symptoms and disorders at eight weeks postpartum. *Journal of Anxiety Disorders, 19*(3), 295-311.

Whitby, D., & Smith, K. (2005). The use of tricyclic antidepressants and selective serotonin reuptake inhibitors in women who are breastfeeding. *Pharmacotherapy, 25*(3), 411-425.

Zeskind, P., & Stephens, L. (2004). Maternal selective serotonin reuptake inhibitor use during pregnancy and newborn neurobehavior. *Pediatrics, 113*(2), 368-375.

CHAPTER 36

Karen A. Piotrowski

Labor and Birth Complications

learning objectives

- Differentiate between preterm birth and low birth weight.
- Identify the risk factors for preterm labor.
- Analyze current interventions to prevent preterm birth.
- Discuss the use of tocolytics and antenatal glucocorticoids in preterm labor and birth.
- Evaluate the effects of prescribed bed rest on pregnant women and their families.

- Design a nursing care management plan for women with preterm premature rupture of the membranes (PPROM).
- Summarize the nursing care management for a trial of labor, the induction and augmentation of labor, forceps- and vacuum-assisted birth, cesarean birth, and vaginal birth after a cesarean birth.
- Explain the care of a woman with postterm pregnancy.
- Discuss obstetric emergencies and their appropriate management.

electronic resources

Additional information related to the content in Chapter 36 can be found on

the companion website at *evolve*
http://evolve.elsevier.com/Lowdermilk/MWHC/
- NCLEX Review Questions
- Case Study: Preterm Labor
- Case Study: Postterm Pregnancy
- WebLinks

or on the interactive companion CD
- NCLEX Review Questions
- Case Study: Preterm Labor
- Case Study: Postterm Pregnancy
- Critical Thinking Exercise: Preterm Labor
- Plan of Care: Dysfunctional Labor: Hypotonic Uterine Dysfunction with Protracted Active Phase
- Plan of Care: Preterm Labor

WHEN complications arise during labor and birth, risk of perinatal morbidity and mortality increases. Some complications are anticipated, especially if the woman is identified as at high risk during the antepartum period; others are unexpected or unforeseen. The woman, her family, and the obstetric team can feel devastated when things go wrong. Nurses must recognize these feelings if they are to provide effective support. It is crucial for nurses to understand the normal birth process to prevent and detect deviations from normal labor and birth and to implement nursing measures when complications arise. Optimal care of the laboring woman, the fetus, and the family with complications is possible only when the nurse and other members of the obstetric team use their knowledge and skills in a concerted effort to provide competent and compassionate care. This chapter focuses on the problems of preterm labor and birth, dystocia, postterm pregnancy, and obstetric emergencies.

PRETERM LABOR AND BIRTH

Preterm labor is defined as cervical changes and uterine contractions occurring between 20 and 37 weeks of pregnancy. Preterm birth is any birth that occurs before the completion of 37 weeks of pregnancy (American College of Obstetricians and Gynecologists [ACOG]/American Academy of Pediatrics [AAP], 2002). (A pregnancy ending before 20 weeks gestation is termed a miscarriage.) Preterm labor and birth are the most serious complications of pregnancy because they lead to about 90% of all neonatal deaths, with more than 75% of these deaths occurring in infants born at fewer than 32 weeks of gestation. Preterm birth is second only to congenital anomalies as a cause of infant mortality. In 2003, the preterm birth rate for all races in the United States was 12.3%, an increase of 16% since 1990 when the rate was 10.6% and an increase of 30% since 1981 when the rate was only 9.4%. The very preterm birth rate (birth that occurs before the completion of 32 weeks of pregnancy) was 1.97% in 2003 and representing only a moderate increase from the rate of 1.81% in 1981 (Martin, Hamilton, Sutton, Ventura, Menacker, & Munson, 2005).

Preterm Birth Versus Low Birth Weight

Although they have distinctly different meanings, the terms *preterm birth* or *prematurity* and *low birth weight* are often used interchangeably (Moos, 2004). Preterm birth describes length of gestation (i.e., less than 37 weeks regardless of the weight of the infant), whereas low birth weight describes only weight at the time of birth (i.e., 2500 g or less). Low birth weight is far easier to measure than preterm birth, and thus in many settings and publications, low birth weight has been used as a substitute term for preterm birth. Preterm birth, however, is a more dangerous health condition for an infant because a decreased length of time in the uterus correlates with immaturity of body systems. Low-birth-weight babies can be, but are not necessarily, preterm; low birth weight can be caused by conditions other than preterm birth, such as intrauterine growth restriction (IUGR), a condition of inadequate fetal growth. Pregnant women who have various complications of pregnancy that interfere with uteroplacental perfusion, such as gestational hypertension or poor nutrition, may give birth to a baby at term who is low birth weight because of IUGR.

The incidence of preterm birth in the United States has been increasing for the three largest racial/ethnic groups. The 2003 rate for non-Hispanic black women was 17.8%, whereas the rate for Hispanic women was 11.9%, and the rate for non-Hispanic white women was 11.3%. The preterm birth rate for non-Hispanic black women has been declining slightly since a peak rate of 18.9% in 1991. The very preterm birth rate also has decreased for these women to 3.99% in 2003 (Martin et al., 2005). Despite the decline, the preterm birth rate for non-Hispanic black women still remains substantially higher than for any other racial/ethnic group.

Sociodemographics may play a part in the race-based differences in preterm birth. Preterm birth rates are higher among socially disadvantaged populations, including minorities, women with low levels of education, and women who receive late or no prenatal care (Martin et al., 2005; Maupin et al., 2004). The preterm birth rate is higher among women younger than 15 years of age or older than 45 years (Martin et al.). Multifetal pregnancy from in vitro fertilization also is associated with an increase in preterm births (Moore, 2003).

Predicting Preterm Labor and Birth

The known risk factors for preterm birth are shown in Box 36-1. The risk factors most commonly associated with preterm labor and birth are a history of preterm birth, race, low socioeconomic status, low prepregnancy weight, and multiple gestation (ACOG, 2001; Goldenberg et al., 2003; Martin et al., 2005; Pschirrer & Monga, 2000). Using these risk factors, researchers have tried to determine which women might go into labor prematurely. No risk scoring system has resulted in lowering the preterm birth rate in the United States, however, because at least 50% of all women who ultimately give birth prematurely have no

---

box 36-1 **Risk Factors for Preterm Labor**

DEMOGRAPHIC RISKS
- Nonwhite race
- Age (<17, >35)
- Low socioeconomic status
- Unmarried
- Less than high school education

BIOPHYSICAL RISKS
- Previous preterm labor or birth
- Second-trimester abortion (more than two spontaneous or therapeutic); stillbirths
- Grand multiparity; short interval between pregnancies (<1 year since last birth); family history of preterm labor and birth
- Progesterone deficiency
- Uterine anomalies or fibroids; uterine irritability
- Cervical incompetence, trauma, shortened length
- Exposure to DES (diethylstilbestrol) or other toxic substances
- Medical problems (e.g., diabetes, hypertension, anemia, periodontal disease)
- Small stature (<119 cm in height; <45.5 kg or underweight for height)
- Obesity

- Current pregnancy risks:
  - Multifetal pregnancy
  - Hydramnios
  - Bleeding
  - Placental problems (e.g., placenta previa, abruptio placentae)
  - Infections (e.g., pyelonephritis, recurrent urinary tract infections, asymptomatic bacteriuria, bacterial vaginosis, chorioamnionitis)
  - Gestational hypertension
  - Premature rupture of the membranes
  - Fetal anomalies
  - Inadequate plasma volume expansion; anemia

BEHAVIORAL-PSYCHOSOCIAL RISKS
- Poor nutrition; weight loss or low weight gain
- Smoking (>10 cigarettes a day)
- Substance abuse (e.g., alcohol; illicit drugs, especially cocaine)
- Inadequate prenatal care
- Commutes of more than 1.5 hours each way
- Excessive physical activity (heavy physical work, prolonged standing, heavy lifting, young child care)
- Excessive lifestyle stressors

From Gilbert, E., & Harmon, J. (2003). *Manual of high risk pregnancy and delivery* (3rd ed.). St. Louis: Mosby; Iams, J. (2002). Preterm birth. In S. Gabbe, J. Niebyl, & J. Simpson (Eds.), *Obstetrics: Normal and problem pregnancies* (4th ed.). New York: Churchill Livingstone; Moore, M. (2003). Preterm labor and birth: What have we learned in the past two decades? *Journal of Obstetric, Gynecologic, and Neonatal Nursing, 32*(5), 638-649; Pschirrer, E., & Monga, M. (2000). Risk factors for preterm labor. *Clinics in Obstetrics and Gynecology, 43*(4), 727-734.

identifiable risk factors (Martin et al.). In 2005, the March of Dimes (MOD) began a multi-million dollar research, eduation and awareness campaign to address the problems of prematurity. The Association of Women's Health, Obstetric and Neonatal Nurses (AWHONN), ACOG, and AAP are professional organizations that have partnered with the MOD in this campaign (MOD, 2005). It is important that all women be educated about prematurity not only in early pregnancy but also in the preconception period (Freda & Patterson, 2001; Massett, Greenup, Ryan, Staples, Green, & Maibach, 2003). Unless all women are included in prevention efforts, a widespread reduction of preterm birth rates cannot be expected (Maloni & Damato, 2004; Pschirrer & Monga).

Biochemical Markers

The two most common biochemical markers used in an effort to predict who might experience preterm labor are fetal fibronectin and salivary estriol.

Fetal fibronectins are glycoproteins found in plasma and produced during fetal life. They appear in the cervical canal early in pregnancy, and then again in late pregnancy. Their appearance between 24 and 34 weeks of gestation predicts labor (Bernhardt & Dorman, 2004; Ramsey & Andrews, 2003). The negative predictive value of fetal fibronectins is high (up to 94%). The positive predictive value is lower (46%) (Abrahams & Katz, 2002; Iams & Creasy, 2004). This means that it may be possible to predict who will *not* go into preterm labor but not who will (Bernhardt & Dorman). The test is done during a vaginal examination.

Salivary estriol is a form of estrogen produced by the fetus that is present in plasma at 9 weeks of gestation. Levels of salivary estriol have been shown to increase before preterm birth. Specimens of salivary estriol are collected by the woman in the home. The testing is done every 2 weeks for about 10 weeks. This marker has a high negative predictive value (98%). However, its low positive predictive value (7% to 25%) and high rate of false positive results limits its effectiveness as a screening tool (ACOG, 2001; Bernhardt & Dorman, 2004).

The cost of determining maternal levels of these biochemical markers is high. More research is needed before it will be known if these markers offer valuable assistance that is cost effective in the risk assessment for preterm labor.

Endocervical Length

Another possible predictor of imminent preterm labor is endocervical length. Some studies have suggested that a shortened cervix precedes preterm labor and can be determined by ultrasound measurement (Bernhardt & Dorman, 2004; Colombo & Iams, 2000; Fuchs, Henrich, Osthues, & Dudenhausen, 2004). Women whose cervical length is 35 mm at 24 to 28 weeks of gestation are more likely to have a preterm birth than women whose cervical length exceeds 40 mm (Iams & Creasy, 2004). When a woman has a short cervix combined with a positive fetal fibronectin result, her risk for spontaneous preterm birth is substantially higher than that for women positive for only one marker or none at all (Iams & Creasy).

Causes of Preterm Labor and Birth

The cause of preterm labor is unknown and is assumed to be multifactorial (Iams & Creasy, 2004; Maloni & Damato, 2004) (Box 36-2). Infection is thought to be a major etiologic factor in some preterm labors, but trials of antibiotic therapy for all women at risk have not resulted in statistically significant reductions in preterm births (Iams & Creasy). When cervical, bacterial, or urinary tract infections are present, the risk of preterm birth is increased; thus early, continuous, and comprehensive prenatal care, which can detect and treat infection, is essential in dealing with this aspect of preterm birth prevention. Recent evidence has demonstrated a link between periodontal infection and preterm labor and birth as a result of increased levels of prostaglandins released by the causative pathogens. Although research is ongoing, recommendations for all pregnant women include regular dental care before and during pregnancy, oral assessment as part of prenatal health care, and strict oral hygiene measures (e.g., brushing teeth, using dental floss, rinsing with baking soda and water after vomiting) (Wener & Lavigne, 2004).

Evolve/CD: Case Study: Preterm Labor

box 36-2 Multifactorial Etiology of Preterm Labor and Birth

MATERNAL BEHAVIORS
- Smoking
- Substance use (alcohol or illegal drugs)
- Poor nutrition
- Employment/work involving long hours and periods standing
- Short interpregnancy interval (<1 year)
- Sexual activity

MATERNAL CHARACTERISTICS
- Young or older age
- Previous preterm birth
- Short stature
- Short cervix
- Uterine anomalies
- Diethylstilbestrol exposure
- Prematurely dilated cervix
- Low prepregnancy weight; obesity
- Race (e.g., African-American, Hispanic)
- Unmarried
- Low socioeconomic status
- Intimate partner abuse

OTHER FACTORS
- Inadequate support systems
- Stress
- Uterine irritability
- Multiple gestation
- Late or no prenatal care
- Preterm premature rupture of membranes (PPROM)
- Anemia
- Infection

Not all preterm births can or even should be prevented. About 25% of all preterm births are iatrogenic, that is, babies are intentionally delivered prematurely because of pregnancy complications that put the life or health of the fetus or mother in danger, not because of preterm labor. Another 25% of all preterm births are preceded by spontaneous rupture of the membranes (preterm premature rupture of the membranes) followed by labor. These preterm births are not known to be preventable. About 50% of preterm births, therefore, are possibly amenable to prevention efforts and are considered idiopathic preterm births (Iams & Creasy, 2004).

Sociodemographic factors such as poverty, low educational level, lack of social support, smoking, little or no prenatal care, domestic violence, and stress are thought to contribute to the 50% of preterm births that may be preventable (Gennaro & Hennessy, 2003; Iams & Creasy, 2004). If prenatal care programs are to be effective in reducing the rate of preterm labor and birth, they must address these sociodemographic factors and develop strategies to attract all women to participate, including those at high risk for preterm labor. Addressing the factors that contribute to preterm labor and birth can produce significant results (Maloni & Damato, 2004).

▬ CARE MANAGEMENT

▬ Assessment and Nursing Diagnoses

Because all pregnant women must be considered at risk for preterm labor (as they are for any other pregnancy complication), nursing assessment begins at the time of entry to prenatal care. The onset of preterm labor is often insidious and can be easily mistaken for normal discomforts of pregnancy. It is essential that nurses teach pregnant women how to detect the early symptoms of preterm labor (Box 36-3) (Freda & Patterson, 2001; Witcher, 2002).

The nurse caring for women in a prenatal setting should use modalities that are known to be successful for teaching the pregnant woman about early recognition of preterm symptoms and then reassess the woman at each prenatal visit for the symptoms of preterm labor. Pregnant women also must be taught what to do if the symptoms of preterm labor occur. Some women wait hours or days before contacting a health care provider after preterm labor symptoms have begun. Women may ignore the symptoms because of ignorance regarding their significance or a belief that the symptoms are expected during pregnancy. The symptoms may be attributed to other factors such as the flu, incontinence of urine, or working too hard. Some women will become more vigilant waiting to see if the symptoms subside, go away, or become worse. They may take action by seeking advice about what to do from family or friends, resting more, increasing fluid intake, taking a bath, or rubbing the back or abdomen. Persistence of symptoms and increasing severity finally compel women to seek health care (Weiss, Saks, & Harris, 2002). Waiting too long to see a health care provider could result in inevitable preterm birth without the benefit of the administration of ante-

---

box 36-3 | Signs and Symptoms of Preterm Labor

UTERINE ACTIVITY
- Uterine contractions occurring every 10 minutes or more frequently and persisting for 1 hour or more
- Uterine contractions may be painful or painless

DISCOMFORT
- Lower abdominal cramping similar to gas pains; may be accompanied by diarrhea
- Dull, intermittent low back pain (below the waist)
- Painful, menstrual-like cramps
- Suprapubic pain or pressure
- Pelvic pressure or heaviness; feeling that baby is pushing down
- Urinary frequency

VAGINAL DISCHARGE
- Change in character or increase in amount of usual discharge: thicker (mucoid) or thinner (watery), bloody, brown or colorless, increased amount, odor
- Rupture of amniotic membranes

---

natal corticosteroids (i.e., medication given to accelerate fetal lung maturity). In this event, the neonate is born at higher risk for respiratory distress syndrome and intraventricular hemorrhage.

The nurse must assess the psychosocial and emotional status of women in preterm labor and the impact that treatment (e.g., bed rest, hospitalization) can have on family dynamics. Factors influencing the impact of preterm labor treatment include stability of the support system, financial status, and availability of child support and assistance with household maintenance. Pregnant women who have risk factors for preterm birth are often offered special care with more frequent visits. Although there is no evidence in the literature that this enhanced care results in better outcomes, clinically it makes sense to evaluate at-risk women on a more frequent basis. Freda and Patterson (2001) suggest that the power of nursing care, nursing support, and client education in the care of women at high risk for preterm birth can have an impact on the occurrence and early detection of preterm labor.

Nursing diagnoses relevant for women at risk for preterm birth include the following:

- *Risk for imbalanced fluid volume (maternal) related to*
  - administration of tocolytics to suppress preterm labor
- *Interrupted family processes related to*
  - required limitation on maternal activity associated with preterm labor
- *Impaired physical mobility related to*
  - prescribed bed rest
- *Anticipatory grieving related to*
  - potential for birth of preterm infant
- *Risk for impaired parent-infant attachment related to*
  - care requirements of preterm infant

▪ Expected Outcomes of Care

The nurse develops a plan of care based on each woman's needs. Assessment of each pregnant woman's knowledge of the dangers of preterm birth, the symptoms of preterm labor, and what to do if symptoms should occur is the first step in working toward a positive outcome of pregnancy. Expected outcomes include that the woman will do the following:

- Learn the signs and symptoms of preterm labor and be able to assess herself and her need for intervention.
- Follow teaching suggestions and call her primary health care provider if symptoms occur.
- Not experience preterm symptoms, or if she does, she will take appropriate action.
- Maintain her pregnancy for at least 37 completed weeks.
- Give birth to a healthy, full-term infant.

▪ Plan of Care and Interventions
▪ *Prevention*

Prevention strategies that address risk factors associated with preterm labor and birth are less costly in human and financial terms than the high-tech and often lifelong care required by preterm infants and their families. Programs aimed at health promotion and disease prevention that encourage healthy lifestyles for the population in general and women of childbearing age in particular should be developed to prevent preterm labor and birth (Freda, 2003; Heaman, Sprague, & Stewart, 2001; Tiedje, 2003). One of the most important nursing interventions aimed at preventing preterm birth is the education of pregnant women about the early symptoms of preterm labor, so that if the symptoms occur, the woman can be referred promptly to her primary health care provider for more intensive care (Freda; Moore, 2003) (see Box 36-3). Client education regarding any symptoms of uterine contractions or cramping between 20 and 37 weeks of gestation should be directed toward telling the woman that these symptoms are not normal discomforts of pregnancy, and that contractions or cramping that do not go away should prompt the woman to contact her primary health care provider. Because no one can discriminate between Braxton-Hicks contractions and the contractions of early preterm labor, Freda and Patterson (2001) suggest that the term *Braxton-Hicks contractions* be eliminated from teaching about pregnancy expectations (Fig. 36-1). Preconception and prenatal care should be made available to all women. This care should focus on performing ongoing holistic risk assessment, encouraging women to participate in health-promoting activity (e.g., good nutrition, exercise, stress management), and implementing appropriate medical and psychosocial interventions (Maloni & Damato, 2004).

▪ *Early Recognition and Diagnosis*

Early recognition of preterm labor is essential to implement interventions successfully, such as tocolytic therapy and administration of antenatal glucocorticoids. The diag-

FIG. 36-1 Nurse teaching woman signs and symptoms of preterm labor. (Courtesy Marjorie Pyle, RNC, Lifecircle, Costa Mesa, CA.)

nosis of preterm labor is based on three major diagnostic criteria:

- Gestational age between 20 and 37 weeks
- Uterine activity (e.g., contractions)
- Progressive cervical change (e.g., effacement of 80%, or cervical dilation of 2 cm or greater)

If the presence of fetal fibronectin is used as another diagnostic criterion, a sample of cervical mucus for testing should be obtained before an examination for cervical changes, because the lubricant used to examine the cervix can reduce the accuracy of the test for fetal fibronectin.

The pregnant woman at 30 weeks with an irritable uterus but no documented cervical change is not in preterm labor. Misdiagnosis of preterm labor can lead to inappropriate use of pharmacologic agents that can be dangerous to the health of the woman, the fetus, or both (Abrahams & Katz, 2002; ACOG/AAP, 2002; Iams, 2003).

▪ *Lifestyle Modifications*

Nurses caring for women with symptoms of preterm labor should question the woman about whether she has symptoms when engaged in any of the following activities:

- Sexual activity
- Riding long distances in automobiles, trains, or buses
- Carrying heavy loads such as laundry, groceries, or a small child
- Standing more than 50% of the time
- Heavy housework
- Climbing stairs
- Hard physical work
- Being unable to stop and rest when tired

If symptoms occur when the woman is engaged in any of these activities, the woman should consider what she was doing when the symptoms began, and then consider stopping those activities until 37 weeks of pregnancy when preterm birth is no longer a risk. Counseling about lifestyle modification should be individualized; only women who have symptoms of preterm labor when they are engaged in certain activities need to alter their lifestyles. No specific rules describe which activities are safe for pregnant women

CD: Critical Thinking Exercises: Preterm Labor

and which are not. Each pregnant woman must understand which lifestyle factors might be contributing to her symptoms and be taught to modify only those factors. Sexual activity, for instance, is not contraindicated during pregnancy. If, however, symptoms of preterm labor occur after sexual activity, then that activity may need to be curtailed until 37 weeks of gestation.

▬ Bed Rest

Bed rest is a commonly used intervention for the prevention of preterm birth. Although frequently prescribed, bed rest is not a benign intervention, and there is no evidence in the literature to support the efficacy of this intervention in reducing preterm birth rates. It is a form of care of unknown effectiveness (Enkin et al., 2000; Sosa, Athalbe, Belzian, & Bergel, 2004). The deleterious effects of bed rest on women are well known. After 3 days there is decreased muscle tone, weight loss, calcium loss, and glucose intolerance. Weeks of bed rest lead to bone demineralization, constipation, fatigue, isolation, loneliness, anxiety, and depression. Women often feel that they have lost control over their bodies and pregnancies (Box 36-4). Symptoms often are not resolved by 6 weeks postpartum (Maloni & Park, 2005). The father's constant worry about his partner and baby and increased stress with the assumption of new roles and responsibilities when bed rest is prescribed for his partner also has been documented. Bed rest is costly for society; the estimated economic costs are based on lost wages, household help and child care expenses, and hospital costs (Maloni, Brezinski-Tomasi, & Johnson, 2001;

| box 36-4 | **Adverse Effects of Bed Rest** |

MATERNAL EFFECTS (PHYSICAL)
- Weight loss; indigestion; loss of appetite
- Muscle wasting, weakness; aching muscles
- Bone demineralization and calcium loss
- Decreased plasma volume and cardiac output
- Increased clotting tendency; risk for thrombophlebitis
- Alteration in bowel function
- Sleep disturbance, fatigue
- Prolonged postpartum recovery

MATERNAL EFFECTS (PSYCHOSOCIAL)
- Loss of control associated with role reversals
- Dysphoria—anxiety, depression, hostility, and anger
- Guilt associated with difficulty complying with activity restriction and inability to meet role responsibilities
- Boredom, loneliness
- Emotional lability (mood swings); difficulty concentrating
- Increased stress

EFFECTS ON SUPPORT SYSTEM
- Stress associated with role reversals, increased responsibilities, and disruption of family routines
- Financial strain associated with loss of maternal income and cost of treatment
- Fear and anxiety regarding the well-being of the mother and fetus

---

Youngblut, Madigen, Neff, Deoisres, Siripul, & Brooten, 2000). Prolongation of pregnancy does not necessarily occur despite the increased costs incurred. Women on bed rest need support and encouragement, whether they are at home or are hospitalized. Women who are hospitalized may experience a higher degree of stress when on bed rest than women who remain at home. Nurses can create support groups of hospitalized women on bed rest. Internet resources (e.g., www.pregnancybedrest.com and www.sidelines.com), including chat rooms for women on bed rest at home, as well as family and friends, can be important sources of support for the women and reduce the sense of isolation and loneliness they may feel. Interacting with other women experiencing preterm labor and bed rest has been found to be highly therapeutic (Adler & Zarchin, 2002; Maloni & Kutil, 2000). Women managed at home for preterm labor may use certain strategies when demands from relationships, households, and careers compete with the prescription of bed rest. These strategies included doing more than they are permitted and testing the limits of their activity restriction. Health care providers must recognize the difficulty that women face when placed on bed rest. Exploring with these women the realities of their daily lives helps nurses work with them to set realistic guidelines for activity limitations that the women will follow, thereby avoiding feelings of cheating and its associated guilt. This approach can help to communicate to women that the nurses empathize with the impact that bed rest has on their lives as well as the lives of their families (Sprague, 2004).

▬ Home Care

Women who are at high risk for preterm birth commonly are told that it would be best if they were at home on bed rest for weeks or months. The home care of the woman at risk for preterm birth is a challenge for the nurse, who must assist the woman and her family in dealing with the many difficulties faced by families in which one member is incapacitated. The scope of care given to women in their homes ranges from occasional visits to monitor the maternal and fetal condition, to daily telephone consultation and reading of uterine monitoring strips.

Regardless of the frequency of the visits, nursing care for the woman and family in the home demands organization and a sense of just how this family's life has been disrupted by the loss of activity of this essential family member. Families, who are often anxious regarding the health status of the mother and baby, may need help in learning how to organize time and space or to restructure family routines so that the pregnant woman can remain a part of family activity while still maintaining bed rest. It also is important for the nurse to work toward assisting all the family members to explore their feelings regarding the anxieties of preterm labor and help them to share their feelings with each other (Maloni et al., 2001). The Teaching for Self-Care boxes detail activities for women on bed rest and for their children.

The woman's environment can be modified for convenience by using tables and storage units around her bed

TEACHING FOR SELF-CARE

Suggested Activities for Women on Bed Rest

- Set a routine for daily activities (e.g., getting dressed, moving from the bedroom to a "day bed rest place," having social time, eating meals, self-monitoring fetal and uterine activity).
- Do passive exercises as allowed.
- Review childbirth education information or have a childbirth class at home, if this can be arranged.
- Plan menus and make up grocery shopping lists.
- Shop by phone or Internet
- Read books about high risk pregnancy or other topics.
- Keep a journal of the pregnancy.
- Keep a calendar of your progress.
- Reorganize files, recipes, household budget.
- Update address book.
- Do mending, sewing.
- Listen to iPod/CDs, watch videos/DVDs or television.
- Do crossword puzzles, jigsaw puzzles, etc.
- Do craft projects; make something for the baby.
- Put pictures in photo albums; do scrapbooking.
- Call a friend, family member, or support person each day or use e-mail or online chat room.
- Treat yourself to a facial, manicure, neck massage, or other special treat when you need a lift.

Sources: Gilbert, E., & Harmon, J. (2003). *Manual of high risk pregnancy and delivery* (3rd ed.). St. Louis: Mosby; McCann, M. (2003). *Days in waiting: A guide to surviving bedrest.* St. Paul, MN: deRuyter-Nelson Publications; Moondragon Birthing Services (2005). *Moondragon's pregnancy information: Coping with bedrest during pregnancy.* Accessed www.moondragon.org/pregnancy/bedrestcope.html, September 2, 2006; Tracy, A. (2001). *The pregnancy bedrest book: A survival guide for expectant mothers and their families.* New York: Berkley Publishing Group.

TEACHING FOR SELF-CARE

Activities for Children of Women on Bed Rest

- Schedule brief play periods throughout the day.
- Keep a few favorite toys in a box or basket close to the bed or couch.
- Read to the children.
- Put puzzles together.
- Watch videos, play video games (remote control for television is ideal).
- Play cards or board games.
- Color in coloring books.
- Cut out pictures from magazines and paste on cardboard.
- Play bed basketball with a soft (sponge) ball or rolled up sock and a trash can or empty laundry basket.

Sources: McCann, M. (2003). *Days in waiting: A guide to surviving bedrest.* St. Paul, MN: deRuyter-Nelson Publications; Tracy, A. (2001). *The pregnancy bedrest book: A survival guide for expectant mothers and their families.* New York: Berkley Publishing Group.

to keep essential items within reach (e.g., telephone, television, radio, iPod, CD player, computer with Internet access, snacks, books, magazines, newspapers, and items for hobbies) (Fig. 36-2). Ensuring that the bed or couch is near a window and the bathroom is also helpful. Covering

FIG. 36-2 Woman at home on restricted activity for preterm labor prevention. Note how she has arranged her daytime resting area so that needed items are close at hand. (Courtesy Amy Turner, Cary, NC.)

the bed with an egg crate mattress can relieve discomfort. Women often find that a daily schedule of meals, activities, and hygiene and grooming (e.g., shower, dressing in street clothes, applying make-up) that they create reduces boredom and helps them maintain control and normalcy. Limiting naps, eating smaller but more frequent meals, and performing gentle range of motion exercises can help to reduce some of the detrimental effects of bed rest. It is essential that women and their families recognize that postpartum recovery will be slower as the woman works to regain strength and stamina (Maloni, 2002).

▬ Home Uterine Activity Monitoring (HUAM)

Home uterine monitoring systems were developed to provide uterine monitoring services in the home for women diagnosed with preterm labor. Nurses are usually an integral part of the home uterine monitoring systems to educate and to provide care to the women. The use and effectiveness of HUAM continues to be controversial. Research evidence indicates that HUAM is a form of care unlikely to be beneficial in preventing preterm birth (ACOG, 2001; Enkin et al., 2000). In addition, palpation of the uterus is more effective than a monitor for detecting uterine contractions when a woman is obese (e.g., excessive abdominal adipose tissue) or the gestational age is less than 26 weeks (Abrahams & Katz, 2000). However, a comprehensive evidence-based review of clinical data suggests that if used correctly (e.g., twice daily monitoring of uterine activity and daily nursing care) in clients at risk for preterm birth, HUAM increases the incidence of early diagnosis of preterm labor and prolongation of pregnancy, with fewer preterm births and reduced neonatal morbidity when study groups are compared to control groups of women receiving standard prenatal care in the United States (Morrison & Chauhan, 2003). Research should be continued in this area to determine what place HUAM has, if any, in preterm labor care.

▬ *Suppression of Uterine Activity*

Tocolytics. Should preterm labor occur, women are usually admitted to the hospital for assessment, fetal monitoring, cervical and/or vaginal cultures, and assessment of cervical status, amniotic fluid leakage, and maternal temperature (an early sign of chorioamnionitis). The initiation of tocolytic therapy might be considered at this time. Once the pregnancy has progressed beyond 34 weeks of gestation, the benefits of prolonging the pregnancy do not justify the maternal risk of tocolytic therapy (Witcher, 2002). The use of tocolytics (medications that suppress uterine activity) in an attempt to prevent preterm birth has been the subject of research since the late 1970s. At first, it was thought that use of tocolytic therapy could prolong a threatened pregnancy indefinitely; research has demonstrated that a gain of 48 hours to several days is the best outcome that can be expected if the cervix is less than 6 cm dilated. Once uterine contractions are suppressed, maintenance therapy may be implemented in an attempt to continue the suppression, or tocolytic treatment can be discontinued and resumed only if uterine contractions begin again. Research findings suggest that there appears to be no significant difference when the two tocolytic treatment approaches are compared and that continued maintenance tocolytic ✳ therapy has no more than minimal value (ACOG, 2003a; Berkman et al., 2003; Witcher).

It is now thought that the best reason to use tocolytics is that they afford the opportunity to begin administer- ✳ ing antenatal corticosteroids to accelerate fetal lung maturity and reduce the severity of sequelae in infants born preterm. Time also is provided for maternal transport to a facility with a neonatal intensive care unit (ACOG, 2003a; Anotayanonth, Subhedar, Garner, Neilson, & Harigopal, 2004; Enkin et al., 2000).

The use of tocolysis to suppress preterm labor has increased nearly 50%, from 1.6% in 1990 to 2.1% in 2003 (Martin et al., 2005). The medications used for this purpose include ritodrine (Yutopar), terbutaline (Brethine), magnesium sulfate, indomethacin (Indocin), and nifedipine (Procardia). Ritodrine is the only medication approved by the U.S. Food and Drug Administration (FDA) specifically for the purpose of cessation of uterine contractions; however, magnesium sulfate, terbutaline, and nifedipine are most commonly used in U.S. hospitals though there is no clear first-line tocolytic drug (ACOG, 2003a; Rideout, 2005). These drugs are used on an "unlabeled" basis (i.e., drugs known to be effective for a specific purpose, although not specifically developed and tested for this purpose). Important contraindications exist to the use of all tocolytics (Box 36-5). Because these medications have the potential for serious adverse reactions for mother and fetus, close nursing supervision during treatment is critical (Lehne, 2004) (see Box 36-6 and Medication Guide).

Magnesium sulfate is the most commonly used tocolytic agent, because maternal and fetal/neonatal adverse reactions are less common than with the beta-adrenergic agonists. Although its exact mechanism of action on uterine muscle

---

box 36-5 **Contraindications to Tocolysis**

MATERNAL
- Gestational hypertension (e.g., severe preeclampsia or eclampsia)
- Active vaginal bleeding
- Intrauterine infection (chorioamnionitis)
- Cardiac disease
- Medical or obstetric condition that contraindicates continuation of pregnancy
- Cervical dilation greater than 6 cm

FETAL
- Estimated gestational age more than 34 wk
- Fetal death
- Lethal fetal anomaly
- Acute fetal distress
- Chronic intrauterine growth restriction

---

is unclear, magnesium sulfate does promote relaxation of smooth muscles (Iams, 2002; Witcher, 2002). At the onset of preterm labor, magnesium sulfate is administered via an intravenous infusion (see Medication Guide).

Ritodrine and terbutaline, beta-adrenergic agonist medications for tocolysis, work by relaxing uterine smooth muscle as a result of stimulation of beta$_2$ receptors on uterine smooth muscle. When used, ritodrine is usually administered intravenously as one of the first steps in suppressing preterm labor. Terbutaline is most commonly administered by a subcutaneous injection of 0.25 mg to suppress uterine hyperactivity or by a subcutaneous pump in the home setting. Effectiveness of pump therapy in prolonging gestation is controversial. Terbutaline also may be administered orally. There is no evidence to support the use of terbu- ✳ taline for maintenance therapy (ACOG, 2003a; Witcher, 2002). Beta$_2$-adrenergic agonists have many maternal and fetal cardiopulmonary (e.g., tachycardia) and metabolic

---

box 36-6 **Nursing Care for Women Receiving Tocolytic Therapy**

- Explain the purpose and side effects of tocolytic therapy to woman and her family.
- Position woman on her side to enhance placental perfusion and reduce pressure on the cervix.
- Monitor maternal vital signs including lung sounds and respiratory effort, fetal heart rate (FHR) and pattern, and labor status according to hospital protocol and professional standards.
- Assess mother and fetus for signs of adverse reactions related to the tocolytic being administered.
- Determine maternal fluid balance by measuring daily weight and intake and output (I & O).
- Limit fluid intake to 1500-2500 ml/day, especially if a beta-adrenergic agonist or magnesium sulfate is being administered.
- Provide psychosocial support and opportunities for women and family to express feelings and concerns.
- Offer comfort measures as required.
- Encourage diversional activities and relaxation techniques.

(e.g., hyperglycemia) adverse reactions related to both beta$_1$ and beta$_2$ stimulation and must always be used with extreme caution and careful, conscientious nursing care. Medication administration and nursing care are aimed at maintaining a therapeutic level of medication and avoiding the most serious side effects while maintaining optimal health of the fetus (see Medication Guide).

▬ NURSE ALERT

Caution must be used when administering intravenous fluids to women in preterm labor because this practice can increase the risk for tocolytic-induced pulmonary edema, especially when a beta-adrenergic agonist or magnesium sulfate is used. It is recommended that the total oral and intravenous fluid intake in 24 hours should be restricted to 1500 to 2400 ml. Strict intake and output measurement, daily weight determination, and assessment of pulmonary function (e.g., auscultate lung sounds for crackles; observe for signs of orthopnea) should be instituted (Gilbert & Harmon, 2003; Rideout, 2005; Witcher, 2002).

Nifedipine, a calcium channel blocker, is another tocolytic agent that can suppress contractions. It works by inhibiting calcium from entering smooth muscle cells, thus reducing uterine contractions (Lehne, 2004). The mildness of maternal side effects and the ease of oral administration have increased its use. When the tocolytic effects and maternal tolerance of nifedipine and beta-adrenergic agonists were compared, no significant differences in length of delay

medication guide

Tocolytic Therapy for Preterm Labor

MEDICATION AND ACTION	DOSAGE AND ROUTE	ADVERSE EFFECTS	NURSING CONSIDERATIONS
MAGNESIUM SULFATE CNS depressant; relaxes smooth muscles including uterus	Mix 40 g in 1000 ml intravenous solution, piggyback to primary infusion, and administer using controller pump: Loading dose: 4 to 6 g over 20 min Maintenance dose: 1 to 4 g/hr Use for stabilization only Discontinue within 24 to 48 hours at the maintenance dose or if intolerable adverse reactions occur	*Maternal adverse reactions:* <ul><li>Hot flushes, sweating, nausea and vomiting, dry mouth, drowsiness, blurred vision, diplopia, headache, ileus, generalized muscle weakness, lethargy, dizziness</li><li>Hypocalcemia</li><li>SOB, transient hypotension</li><li>Some reactions may subside when loading dose is completed</li></ul> *Intolerable adverse reactions:* <ul><li>Respiratory rate less than 12</li><li>Pulmonary edema</li><li>Absent DTRs</li><li>Chest pain</li><li>Severe hypotension</li><li>Altered level of consciousness</li><li>Extreme muscle weakness</li><li>Urine output less than 25-30 ml/hr or less than 100 ml/4 hours</li></ul> Serum magnesium level of 10 mEq/L (9 mg/dl) or greater <ul><li>*Fetal/newborn:* (uncommon)</li></ul> *Fetal:* <ul><li>Decreased breathing movement, reduced FHR variability, nonreactive NST</li></ul> *Neonatal:* <ul><li>Hypocalcemia, lethargy, hypotonia, respiratory depression</li></ul>	Assess woman and fetus to obtain baseline before beginning therapy and then before and after each increment; follow frequency of agency protocol Monitor serum magnesium levels with higher doses; therapeutic range is between 4 to 7.5 mEq/L or 5 to 8 mg/dl Discontinue infusion and notify physician if intolerable adverse reactions occur Ensure that calcium gluconate (1 g = 10 ml of 10% solution) is available for emergency administration to reverse magnesium sulfate toxicity Should not be given to women with myasthenia gravis

Continued

Tocolytic Therapy for Preterm Labor

MEDICATION AND ACTION	DOSAGE AND ROUTE	ADVERSE EFFECTS	NURSING CONSIDERATIONS
BETA-ADRENERGIC AGONISTS (BETAMIMETICS): ***Ritodrine (Yutopar)*** **Terbutaline (Brethine)** Relax smooth muscles, inhibiting uterine activity, and causing bronchodilation	*Ritodrine (Yutopar):* Mix 150 mg in 500 ml isotonic intravenous solution Attach to controller pump and piggyback to primary infusion Begin infusion at 0.05 to 0.1 mg/min Increase rate by 0.05 mg every 10 to 20 min until contractions stop, intolerable adverse reactions develop, or a maximum dose of 0.35 mg/min is reached *Terbutaline (Brethine):* Subcutaneous injection of 0.25 mg every 20 min to 3 hours (hold for heart rate greater than 120 beats/min)	*Maternal:* • Shortness of breath, coughing, nasal stuffiness, tachypnea, pulmonary edema • Tachycardia, palpitations, skipped beats • Myocardial ischemia, chest pain • Hypotension • Fluid retention and decreased urine production • Tremors, dizziness, nervousness • Muscle cramps and weakness • Headache • Hyperinsulinemia, hyperglycemia; hypokalemia; hypocalcemia; metabolic acidosis • Nausea and vomiting fever • Altered thyroid function *Fetal/neonatal:* • Tachycardia *Fetal:* • Hyperinsulinemia, hyperglycemia *Neonatal:* • hypoglycemia, hypocalcemia, hyperbilirubinemia, hypotension, ileus	Women should be screened with ECG before therapy begins; maternal heart disease, severe hypertension including preeclampsia, hyperthyroidism, and poorly controlled diabetes mellitus are contraindications Use cautiously if woman has controlled diabetes, migraines Validate that woman is in PTL and is over 20 weeks and less than 35 weeks of gestation Assess woman and fetus to obtain baseline before beginning therapy and then before and after each increment or dose; follow frequency of agency protocol Discontinue infusion and notify physician if the woman exhibits the following: • maternal heart rate greater than 120 to 140 beats/min; arrhythmias, chest pain • BP less than 90/60 • signs of pulmonary edema (e.g., dyspnea, crackles, decreased SaO_2) • fetal heart rate greater than 180 beats/min Ensure that propranolol (Inderal) is available to reverse adverse effects related to cardiovascular function

of birth were found, but significantly fewer maternal side effects occurred with nifedipine. Maternal side effects relate primarily to hypotension and reflex tachycardia that occurs with administration. The decrease in blood pressure that occurs may be helpful for women who are also diagnosed with gestational hypertension. Concerns regarding adverse fetal effects have been reduced. Safety is achieved by following recommended dosages, avoiding concurrent use with magnesium sulfate, and maintaining maternal blood pressure, thereby preserving effective uteroplacental perfusion (ACOG, 2003a; Iams & Creasy, 2004; Rideout, 2005; Witcher, 2002) (see Medication Guide).

Indomethacin, a nonsteroidal antiinflammatory drug (NSAID), has been shown in some trials to suppress preterm labor by blocking the production of prostaglandins.

Two prostaglandins are affected, prostacyclin and thromboxane. The decrease in prostacyclin suppresses uterine contractions, and the decrease in thromboxane suppresses platelet aggregation. However, both of these actions may increase the risk for postpartum hemorrhage. Although NSAIDs pose the lowest risk for maternal adverse reactions, the severity of fetal adverse reactions associated with their use for tocolysis makes them less common than other classes of tocolytic drugs. Risk for premature closure of the ductus arteriosus increases if treatment goes beyond 48 hours or if the gestational age of the fetus is 32 or more weeks. Therefore, limiting the use of indomethacin to a short duration of treatment (e.g., 48 hours) or to women at less than 32 weeks of gestation is recommended (ACOG, 2003a; Iams & Creasy, 2004; Lehne, 2004; Witcher, 2002).

Tocolytic Therapy for Preterm Labor

MEDICATION AND ACTION	DOSAGE AND ROUTE	ADVERSE EFFECTS	NURSING CONSIDERATIONS
CALCIUM CHANNEL BLOCKERS: **Nifedipine (Procardia)** Relax smooth muscles including the uterus by blocking calcium entry	Loading dose: 30 mg, orally Maintenance dose: 10 to 20 mg, orally, every 4 to 6 hr May be used as a first-line tocolytic or to continue treatment after stabilization with magnesium sulfate	*Maternal:* • Transient reflex tachycardia, palpitations • Hypotension • Dizziness, headache, nervousness • Peripheral edema • Fatigue • Nausea • Facial flushing *Fetal/newborn (rare):* • Related to maternal hypotension which would affect uteroplacental perfusion	Avoid concurrent use with magnesium sulfate since severe hypotension can result Assess woman and fetus according to agency protocol, being alert for adverse reactions Do not use sublingual route of administration
PROSTAGLANDIN SYNTHETASE INHIBITORS (NSAIDS): **Indomethacin (Indocin)** Relaxes uterine smooth muscle by inhibiting prostaglandins	Loading dose: 50 mg (rectally) or 50 to 100 mg orally, then 25 to 50 mg orally every 6 hours for 48 hours	*Maternal:* • Nausea and vomiting • Dyspepsia, pyrosis • Dizziness • Oligohydramnios • Reduced platelet aggregation increasing risk for hemorrhage *Fetal:* • Constriction of ductus arteriosus progressing to premature closure • Decrease in renal function with oligohydramnios *Neonate:* • Bronchopulmonary dysplasia, respiratory distress syndrome • Intraventricular hemorrhage • Necrotizing enterocolitis • Hyperbilirubinemia • Pulmonary hypertension	Used when other methods fail only if gestational age is less than 32 weeks Administer for 48 hours or less Do not use for women with bleeding potential (coagulopathy, thrombocytopenia), NSAID-sensitive asthma, peptic ulcer disease, significant renal or hepatic impairment, oligohydramnios Assess woman and fetus according to agency policy, being alert for adverse reactions Determine amniotic fluid volume and function of fetal ductus arteriosus before initiating therapy and within 48 hours of discontinuing therapy; assessment is critical if therapy continues for more than 48 hours Administer with food or use rectal route to decrease GI distress Monitor for signs of postpartum hemorrhage

BP, Blood pressure; *CNS*, central nervous system; *DTRs*, deep tendon reflexes; *ECG*, electrocardiogram; *FHR*, fetal heart rate; *GI*, gastrointestinal; *NSAIDs*, nonsteroidal antiinflammatory drugs; *NST*, nonstress test; *PTL*, preterm labor; *SOB*, shortness of breath.
†NOTE: There are variations in recommended administration protocols; always consult agency protocol, which should be evidence-based.

▬ Promotion of Fetal Lung Maturity

Antenatal Corticosteroids. Antenatal corticosteroids given as intramuscular injections to the mother accelerate fetal lung maturity. In addition, corticosteroid administration has been associated with a decrease in the incidence of neonatal intraventricular hemorrhage and necrotizing enterocolitis (ACOG, 2003a). It is viewed as a form of care likely to be beneficial (Enkin et al., 2000). The National Institutes of Health consensus panel recommended that all women between 24 and 34 weeks of gestation should be given antenatal corticosteroids, most commonly betamethasone and dexamethasone, when preterm birth is threatened, unless there is a medical indication for immediate delivery such as cord prolapse, chorioamnionitis, or abruptio placentae. A corticosteroid should not be given after 34 weeks of gestation unless fetal pulmonary immaturity is confirmed (ACOG, 2002a; National Institutes of Health, 2000). The regimen for administration of antenatal corticosteroids is given in the Medication Guide.

▪ NURSE ALERT

Nurses need to know that a pregnant woman admitted between 24 to 34 weeks of gestation and who is at risk for preterm birth within 7 days should receive antenatal corticosteriods unless she has chorioamnionitis. These drugs require a 24- to 48-hour period to become effective, so timely administration is essential (ACOG, 2002a).

▪ *Management of Inevitable Preterm Birth*

Labor that has progressed to a cervical dilation of 4 cm is likely to lead to inevitable preterm birth. Preterm births in tertiary care centers lead to better neonatal and maternal outcomes. Women considered at risk for inevitable preterm birth should be transferred quickly to such a facility to ensure the best possible outcome. The first dose of antenatal corticosteroids should be given before transfer.

---

medication guide

Antenatal Corticosteroid Therapy with Betamethasone, Dexamethasone

ACTION
- Stimulates fetal lung maturation by promoting release of enzymes that induce production or release of lung surfactant. NOTE: The FDA has not approved these medications for this use (i.e., this is an unlabeled use for obstetrics).

INDICATION
- To prevent or reduce the severity of respiratory distress syndrome in preterm infants between 24 and 34 weeks of gestation

DOSAGE AND ROUTE
- Betamethasone: 12 mg intramuscularly (IM) for 2 doses 24 hr apart
- Dexamethasone: 6 mg IM for 4 doses 12 hr apart

ADVERSE EFFECTS
- Possible maternal infection, pulmonary edema (if given with beta-adrenergic medications), may worsen maternal condition (diabetes, hypertension)

NURSING CONSIDERATIONS
- Give deep IM in gluteal muscle. Teach signs of pulmonary edema. Assess blood glucose levels and lung sounds. Do not give if woman has infection. Use in women with preterm premature rupture of the membranes (PPROM) not universally recommended.

Although maternal transport helps to ensure a better health outcome for the mother and the baby, it may have complications. Women may be transported to tertiary centers far from home, making visits by the family difficult, and increasing the anxiety levels of the woman and her family. Attention to the needs of the woman and her family before, during, and after the transport is essential to comprehensive nursing care for these families.

▪ Evaluation

Evaluation of the nursing care provided for a woman at risk for preterm birth is based on achievement of the expected outcomes of care (Plan of Care).

▪▪ PRETERM PREMATURE RUPTURE OF MEMBRANES

Premature rupture of membranes (PROM) is the rupture of the amniotic sac and leakage of amniotic fluid beginning at least 1 hour before the onset of labor at any gestational age. Preterm premature rupture of the membranes (PPROM) (i.e., membranes rupture before 37 weeks of gestation) occurs in up to 25% of all cases of preterm labor. Infection often precedes PPROM, but the etiology of PPROM remains unknown. PPROM is diagnosed after the woman complains of either a sudden gush of fluid from the vagina, or a slow leak of fluid from the vagina.

Infection is the serious side effect of PPROM that makes it a major complication of pregnancy. Chorioamnionitis is an intraamniotic infection of the chorion and amnion that is potentially life threatening for the fetus and the woman. Most cases of intrauterine infection respond well to antibiotics, yet sepsis can occur and can lead to maternal death. Fetal complications from chorioamnionitis include congenital pneumonia, sepsis, and meningitis (Garite, 2004). Even in the absence of infection, PPROM can precipitate cord prolapse or cause oligohydramnios, leading to cord compression, potentially life-threatening complications for the fetus.

Collaborative Care

Whenever PPROM is suspected, strict sterile technique should be used in any vaginal examination to avoid introduction of infection. A nitrazine or fern test is used to determine if the discharge is amniotic fluid or urine (see the Procedure box in Chapter 21, Tests for Rupture of Membranes). A woman with this diagnosis can be cared for at home, with more frequent visits to her primary health care provider (see Teaching for Self-Care box). Expectant management will continue as long as there are no signs of infection or fetal distress. Nursing support of the woman and her family is critical at this time. She is often anxious about the health of her baby and may fear that she was responsible in some way for the membrane rupture. The nurse should encourage expression of feelings and concerns, provide information, and make referrals as needed (Weitz, 2001).

plan of care ⟩ Preterm Labor

NURSING DIAGNOSIS Deficient knowledge related to recognition of preterm labor

Expected Outcome *Woman and partner delineate the signs and symptoms of preterm labor.*

Nursing Interventions/*Rationales*
- Assess what the woman and partner know about abnormal signs and symptoms during pregnancy *to identify areas of deficit.*
- Discuss signs and symptoms that serve as warning signs of preterm labor *so that the woman or her partner has adequate information to identify problems early.*
- Provide written supplemental materials that include a list of warning signs and instructions regarding what to do if any of the listed signs occur *so that the couple can reinforce and review learning and act swiftly and appropriately should a sign occur.*
- Discuss and demonstrate how to assess and time the contractions *to provide needed skills to assess the signs of labor.*

NURSING DIAGNOSIS Risk for maternal/fetal injury related to recurrence of preterm labor

Expected Outcomes *Woman demonstrates ability to assess self and fetus for signs of recurring labor; maternal-fetal well-being is maintained.*

Nursing Interventions/*Rationales*
- Teach woman/partner how to monitor fetal and uterine contraction activity daily *to provide immediate evidence of a worsening condition.*
- Have woman/partner report rupture of membranes, vaginal bleeding, cramping, pelvic pressure, or low backache to appropriate health care resource immediately *because such symptoms are signs of labor.*
- If home uterine activity monitoring is to be used, teach woman/partner how to use the monitoring device and how to transmit the data to the health care provider via telephone *to enhance correct use of monitoring device and increase the accuracy of detection of early labor.*
- Have woman monitor her weight, diet, fluid intake, and vital signs on a daily basis *to evaluate for potential problems.*
- Have woman limit activities to bed rest with bathroom privileges *to decrease the likelihood of onset of labor.*
- Encourage woman to use a side-lying position *to enhance placental perfusion.*
- Teach woman signs and symptoms of thrombophlebitis and encourage gentle exercise of lower extremities *because pregnancy and limited activity increase risk for clot formation.*
- Counsel woman to abstain from sexual intercourse and nipple stimulation *because such activities may stimulate uterine contractions.*
- Encourage woman to practice relaxation techniques *to decrease uterine tone and decrease anxiety and stress.*

- Teach woman to take tocolytic or other medications per physician's orders *to inhibit uterine contractions.*
- Teach woman/partner about and have them report any medication side effects immediately *to prevent medication-induced complications.*
- Have family arrange for alternative strategies in carrying out the woman's usual roles and functions *to decrease stress and limit temptations to increase activity.*
- If small children are part of the household, encourage family to make alternative arrangements for child care *to enhance woman's adherence to bed rest protocol.*

NURSING DIAGNOSIS Anxiety related to preterm labor and potentially premature neonate

Expected Outcome *Feeling and symptoms of anxiety are reduced.*

Nursing Interventions/*Rationales*
- Provide a calm, soothing atmosphere and teach family to provide emotional support *to facilitate coping.*
- Encourage verbalization of fears *to decrease intensity of emotional response.*
- Involve woman and family in the home management of her condition *to promote a greater sense of control.*
- Help the woman identify and use appropriate coping strategies and support systems *to reduce fear/anxiety.*
- Explore the use of desensitization strategies such as progressive muscle relaxation, visual imagery, or thought stopping *to reduce fear-related emotions and related physical symptoms.*

NURSING DIAGNOSIS Deficient diversional activity related to imposed bed rest

Expected Outcome *Woman will verbalize diminished feelings of boredom.*

Nursing Interventions/*Rationales*
- Assist woman to creatively explore personally meaningful activities that can be pursued from the bed *to ensure activities that have meaning, purpose, and value to the individual.*
- Maintain emphasis on personal choices of the woman *because doing so promotes control and minimizes imposition of routines by others.*
- Evaluate what support and system resources are available in the environment *to assist in providing diversional activities.*
- Explore ways for the woman to remain an active participant in home management and decision making *to promote control.*
- Engage support of family and friends in carrying out chosen activities and making necessary environmental alterations *to ensure success.*
- Encourage woman to use Internet to communicate with other women on bed rest *to obtain support and share feelings.*
- Teach woman about stress management and relaxation techniques *to help manage tension of confinement.*

CD: Plan of Care: Preterm Labor

Frequent biophysical profiles are performed to determine fetal health status and estimate amniotic fluid volume. The woman with PPROM also should be taught how to count fetal movements daily, because a slowing of fetal movement has been shown to be a precursor to severe fetal compromise. Several methods are commonly used to count fetal movements; one method is described in the

Teaching for Self-Care box (see also Chapter 29). Antenatal glucocorticoids may be administered if chorioamnionitis is absent (Weitz, 2001).

Vigilance for signs of infection is a major part of the nursing care and client education after PPROM. The woman must be taught how to keep her genital area clean and that nothing should be introduced into her vagina.

TEACHING FOR SELF-CARE

The Woman with PPROM

- Take your temperature and assess pulse every 4 hours when awake
- Report temperature of more than 38° C
- Remain on modified bed rest
- Insert nothing in the vagina
- Do not engage in sexual activity
- Assess for uterine contractions
- Do fetal movement counts daily
- Do not take tub baths
- Watch for foul-smelling vaginal discharge
- Wipe front to back after urinating or having a bowel movement
- Take antibiotics if prescribed; time frequency for around-the-clock administration; be sure to complete the entire course of treatment
- See primary health care provider as scheduled

PPROM, Preterm premature rupture of membranes.

Signs of infection (e.g., fever, foul-smelling vaginal discharge, maternal and fetal tachycardia) should be reported to the primary health care provider immediately. Prophylactic antibiotic therapy may be ordered in an effort to improve perinatal outcome by preventing infection (Garite, 2004). However, use of prophylactic antibiotics for PROM before labor at term or preterm is a form of care of unknown effectiveness (Enkin et al., 2000).

▬ DYSTOCIA

Dystocia is defined as long, difficult, or abnormal labor; it is caused by various conditions associated with the five factors affecting labor. It is estimated that dystocia occurs in approximately 8% to 11% of all births and is the primary cause for cesarean births (Gregory, 2000). Dystocia can be caused by any of the following:

- Dysfunctional labor, resulting in ineffective uterine contractions or maternal bearing-down efforts (the powers); it is the most common cause of dystocia (Cunningham, Leveno, Bloom, Hauth, Gilstrap, & Wenstrom, 2005)

TEACHING FOR SELF-CARE

Counting Fetal Movements (Kick Counts)

Choose a time of day when you can sit or lie quietly.
Choices for counting strategies:

- Starting at 9 AM, count the baby's movements until you have counted 10. If you have not counted 10 movements in 12 hours, notify your primary health care provider immediately.
- Count 4 movements, 3 times a day after meals. Most people count 4 movements in 1 hour. If you don't, then count for 1 more hour. If at the end of 2 hours, you still have not felt 4 movements, call your primary health care provider immediately.

- Alterations in the pelvic structure (the passage)
- Fetal causes, including abnormal presentation or position, anomalies, excessive size, and number of fetuses (the passenger)
- Maternal position during labor and birth
- Psychologic responses of the mother to labor related to past experiences, preparation, culture and heritage, and support system

These five factors are interdependent. In assessing the woman for an abnormal labor pattern, the nurse must consider the way in which these factors interact and influence labor progress. Dystocia is suspected when there is an alteration in the characteristics of uterine contractions, a lack of progress in the rate of cervical dilation, or a lack of progress in fetal descent and expulsion.

Research also documented a familial occurrence of dystocia. Laboring women whose mothers or sisters experienced dystocia during their labors had an increased risk for experiencing dystocia themselves, possibly related to a genetic factor affecting uterine activity (Berg-Lekas, Hogberg, & Winkvist, 1998).

Dysfunctional Labor

Dysfunctional labor is described as abnormal uterine contractions that prevent the normal progress of cervical dilation, effacement (primary powers), or descent (secondary powers). It is the fourth most common complication of labor and birth and in 2003 occurred at an overall rate of 28.5 per 1000 live births. The highest rate (32.8) occurred among women 40 years of age and older, and the lowest rate (27.3) occurred among women 20 to 24 years of age (Martin et al., 2005).

Gilbert and Harmon (2003) cited several factors that seem to increase a woman's risk for uterine dystocia including the following:

- Body build (e.g., 30 pounds or more overweight, short stature)
- Uterine abnormalities (e.g., congenital malformations; overdistention, as with multiple gestation or hydramnios)
- Malpresentations and positions of the fetus
- Cephalopelvic disproportion (CPD)
- Overstimulation with oxytocin
- Maternal fatigue, dehydration and electrolyte imbalance, and fear
- Inappropriate timing of analgesic or anesthetic administration

Dysfunction of uterine contractions can be further described as being hypertonic or hypotonic.

Hypertonic Uterine Dysfunction

The woman experiencing hypertonic uterine dysfunction, or primary dysfunctional labor, often is an anxious first-time mother who is having painful and frequent contractions that are ineffective in causing cervical dilation or effacement to progress. These contractions usually occur in the latent stage (cervical dilation of less than 4 cm) and are usually uncoordinated (Fig. 36-3). The force of the contractions may be in the midsection of the uterus rather than in the fundus, and the uterus is therefore unable to apply downward pressure to push the presenting part against the cervix. The uterus may not relax completely between contractions (Gilbert & Harmon, 2003).

Women with hypertonic uterine dysfunction may be exhausted and express concern about loss of control because of the intense pain they are experiencing and the lack of progress. Therapeutic rest, which is achieved with a warm bath or shower and the administration of analgesics such as morphine, meperidine (Demerol), hydromorphone (Dilaudid), or nalbuphine (Nubain) to inhibit uterine contractions, reduce pain, and encourage sleep, is usually prescribed for the management of hypertonic uterine dysfunction. After a 4- to 6-hour rest, these women are likely to awaken in active labor with a normal uterine contraction pattern (Gilbert & Harmon, 2003).

Hypotonic Uterine Dysfunction

The second and more common type of uterine dysfunction is hypotonic uterine dysfunction, or secondary uterine inertia. The woman initially makes normal progress into the active stage of labor; then the contractions become weak and inefficient or stop altogether (see Fig. 36-3). The uterus is easily indented, even at the peak of contractions. Intrauterine pressure (IUP) during the contraction (usually less than 25 mm Hg) is insufficient for progress of cervical effacement and dilation (Gilbert & Harmon, 2003). CPD and malpositions are common causes of this type of uterine dysfunction.

A woman with hypotonic uterine dysfunction may become exhausted and be at increased risk for infection.

FIG. 36-3 Uterine contractility patterns in labor. **A,** Typical normal labor. **B,** Subnormal intensity, with frequency greater than needed for optimum performance. **C,** Normal contractions but too infrequent for efficient labor. **D,** Incoordinate activity. **E,** Hypercontractility.

Management usually consists of performing an ultrasound or radiographic examination to rule out CPD and assessing the fetal heart rate (FHR) and pattern, characteristics of amniotic fluid if membranes are ruptured, and maternal well-being. If findings are normal, then measures such as ambulation, hydrotherapy, enema, stripping or rupture of membranes, nipple stimulation, and oxytocin infusion can be used to augment the progress of labor.

Secondary Powers

Secondary powers, or bearing-down efforts, are compromised when large amounts of analgesia are given. Anesthesia may also block the bearing-down reflex and, as a result, alter the effectiveness of voluntary efforts (Mayberry, Wood, Strange, Lee, Heisler, & Nielson-Smith, 2000). Exhaustion resulting from lack of sleep or long labor, and fatigue resulting from inadequate hydration and food intake, reduce the effectiveness of the woman's voluntary efforts. Maternal position can work against the forces of gravity and decrease the strength and efficiency of the contractions. Table 36-1 summarizes the characteristics of dysfunctional labor.

Abnormal Labor Patterns

In 2003, prolonged labor patterns occurred at a rate of 6.8 per 1000 live births. The incidence of prolonged labor patterns was slightly higher (i.e., 7.8 per 1000) among women who were younger than 20 years (Martin et al., 2005).

Six abnormal labor patterns were identified and classified by Friedman (1989) according to the nature of the cervical dilation and fetal descent. The labor patterns seen in normal and abnormal labor are described in Table 36-2.

These patterns may result from a variety of causes, including ineffective uterine contractions, pelvic contractures, CPD, abnormal fetal presentations or position, early use of analgesics, nerve block analgesia/anesthesia, and anxiety and stress. Progress in either the first or second stage of labor can be protracted (prolonged) or arrested (stopped). Abnormal progress can be identified by plotting cervical dilation and fetal descent on a labor graph (partogram) at various intervals after the onset of labor and comparing the resulting curve with the expected labor curve for a nulliparous or multiparous labor. Figure 36-4, *A*, is a labor graph illustrating progress in a normal labor for a primigravida. Figure 36-4, *B*, illustrates major types of deviation from the normal progress of labor. If a woman exhibits an abnormal labor pattern, the primary health care provider should be notified.

However, health care providers must be careful when diagnosing a labor pattern as prolonged and when intervening based on this diagnosis. Cesario (2004) found that although the average length of labor today is similar to that found by Friedman (see Fig. 36-4), a wider range of normal occurs. Parameters to determine if labor is progressing normally may have to be expanded. Criteria defining the differences between false, latent, and active labor should be established. Using hospital admission areas to evaluate a

table 36-1 Dysfunctional Labor: Primary and Secondary Powers

HYPERTONIC UTERINE DYSFUNCTION	HYPOTONIC UTERINE DYSFUNCTION	INADEQUATE VOLUNTARY EXPULSIVE FORCES
DESCRIPTION		
Usually occurs before 4 cm dilation; cause unknown, may be related to fear and tension (primary powers)	Cause may be pelvic contracture and fetal malposition, overdistention of uterus (e.g., twins), or unknown (primary powers)	Involves abdominal and levator ani muscles Occurs in second stage of labor; cause may be related to nerve block anesthetic, analgesia, exhaustion
CHANGE IN PATTERN OF PROGRESS		
Pain out of proportion to intensity of contraction Pain out of proportion to effectiveness of contraction in effacing and dilating the cervix Contractions increase in frequency Contractions uncoordinated Uterus is contracted between contractions, cannot be indented	Contractions decrease in frequency and intensity Uterus easily indentable even at peak of contraction Uterus relaxed between contractions (normal)	No voluntary urge to push or bear down or inadequate or ineffective pushing
POTENTIAL MATERNAL EFFECTS		
Loss of control related to intensity of pain and lack of progress Exhaustion	Infection Exhaustion Psychologic trauma	Spontaneous vaginal birth prevented; assisted birth likely
POTENTIAL FETAL EFFECTS		
Fetal asphyxia with meconium aspiration	Fetal infection Fetal and neonatal death	Fetal asphyxia
CARE MANAGEMENT		
Initiate therapeutic rest measures Administer analgesic (e.g., morphine, nalbuphine, meperidine) if membranes not ruptured or cephalopelvic disproportion not present Relieve pain to permit mother to rest Assist with measures to enhance rest and relaxation (e.g., hydrotherapy)	Rule out cephalopelvic disproportion Stimulate labor with oxytocin (augmentation) Perform amniotomy Assist with measures to enhance the progress of labor (e.g., position changes, ambulation, hydrotherapy)	Coach mother in bearing down with contractions; assist with relaxation between contractions Position mother in favorable position for pushing Reduce epidural infusion rate Assist with low forceps or vacuum-assisted birth Prepare for cesarean birth if nonreassuring fetal status occurs

table 36-2 Labor Patterns in Normal and Abnormal Labor

NORMAL LABOR
1. Dilation: continues
   a. Latent phase: <4 cm and low slope
   b. Active phase: >5 cm or high slope
   c. Deceleration phase: ≥9 cm
2. Descent: active at ≥9 cm dilation

	ABNORMAL LABOR	
PATTERN	**NULLIPARAS**	**MULTIPARAS**
Prolonged latent phase	>20 hr	>14 hr
Protracted active phase dilation	<1.2 cm/hr	<1.5 cm/hr
Secondary arrest: no change	≥2 hr	≥2 hr
Protracted descent	<1 cm/hr	<2 cm/hr
Arrest of descent	≥1 hr	≥ 0.5 hr
Failure of descent	No change during deceleration phase and second stage	
Precipitous labor	>5 cm/hr	10 cm/hr

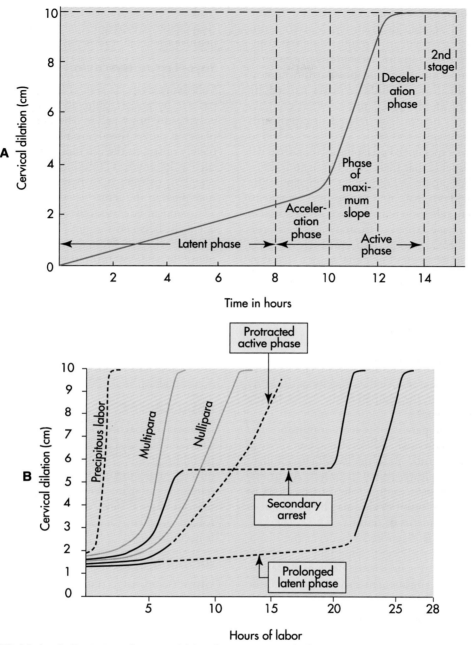

FIG. 36-4 A, Depiction of a normal labor for a primigravida. **B,** Major types of deviation from normal progress of labor may be detected by noting dilation of cervix at various intervals after labor begins. If a woman exhibits an abnormal labor pattern, as depicted by *broken lines*, the primary health care provider should be notified.

woman's labor status is helpful in preventing the premature implementation of labor interventions such as administration of systemic opioid analgesics or induction of epidural analgesia/anesthesia. If a woman is found to be in false or latent (early) labor, she can be sent home if she lives near the hospital or remain in the admissions area until labor becomes active. Women in active labor are admitted to the labor and birth unit.

Maternal morbidity and death may occur as a result of uterine rupture, infection, severe dehydration, and postpartum hemorrhage. The fetus is at increased risk for hypoxia.

A long and difficult labor can have an adverse psychologic effect on the mother, father, and family.

Precipitous Labor

Precipitous labor is defined as labor that lasts less than 3 hours from the onset of contractions to the time of birth. This abnormal labor pattern occurred at a rate of 18.4 per 1000 live births in 2003. Precipitate labor occurred at the highest rate (i.e., 21.5) among women ages 35 to 39 years and at the lowest rate (i.e., 12.8) among women younger than 20 years (Martin et al., 2005).

Precipitous labor may result from hypertonic uterine contractions that are tetanic in intensity. Maternal and fetal complications can occur as a result. Maternal complications include uterine rupture, lacerations of the birth canal, amniotic fluid embolism, and postpartum hemorrhage. Fetal complications include hypoxia caused by decreased periods of uterine relaxation between contractions and intracranial hemorrhage related to rapid birth (Cunningham et al., 2005).

Women who have experienced precipitous labor often describe feelings of disbelief that their labor began so quickly, alarm that their labor progressed so rapidly, panic about the possibility they would not make it to the hospital on time to give birth, and finally, relief when they arrived at the hospital. In addition, women have expressed frustration when nurses would not believe them when they reported their readiness to push. Progress can be so rapid in some women that they may have difficulty remembering the details of their childbirth. They should be provided with an opportunity to discuss their labor and birth with caregivers.

Alterations in Pelvic Structure
Pelvic Dystocia

Pelvic dystocia can occur whenever there are contractures of the pelvic diameters that reduce the capacity of the bony pelvis, including the inlet, the midpelvis, the outlet, or any combination of these planes.

Disproportion of the pelvis is the least common cause of dystocia (Cunningham et al., 2005). Pelvic contractures may be caused by congenital abnormalities, maternal malnutrition, neoplasms, or lower spinal disorders. An immature pelvic size predisposes some adolescent mothers to pelvic dystocia. Pelvic deformities also may be the result of automobile or other accidents or trauma.

An inlet contracture is diagnosed whenever the diagonal conjugate is less than 11.5 cm. The incidence of face and shoulder presentation is increased. Because these presentations interfere with engagement and fetal descent, the risk of prolapse of the umbilical cord is increased. Inlet contracture is associated with maternal rickets and a flat pelvis. Weak uterine contractions may be noted during the first stage of labor in affected women.

Midplane contracture, the most common cause of pelvic dystocia, is diagnosed whenever the sum of the interischial spinous and posterior sagittal diameters of the midpelvis is 13.5 cm or less. Fetal descent is arrested (transverse arrest of the fetal head) in such births because the head cannot rotate internally. These infants are usually born by cesarean, but vacuum-assisted birth has been used safely when the cervix is fully dilated. Midforceps-assisted birth usually is not done because of the increased perinatal morbidity associated with this intervention.

Outlet contracture exists when the interischial diameter is 8 cm or less. It rarely occurs in the absence of midplane contracture. Women with outlet contracture have a long, narrow pubic arch and an android pelvis, and this causes fetal descent to be arrested. Maternal complications include extensive perineal lacerations during vaginal birth because the fetal head is pushed posteriorly.

Soft-Tissue Dystocia

Soft-tissue dystocia results from obstruction of the birth passage by an anatomic abnormality other than that involving the bony pelvis. The obstruction may result from placenta previa (low-lying placenta) that partially or completely obstructs the internal os of the cervix. Other causes, such as leiomyomas (uterine fibroids) in the lower uterine segment, ovarian tumors, and a full bladder or rectum, may prevent the fetus from entering the pelvis. Occasionally, cervical edema occurs during labor when the cervix is caught between the presenting part and the symphysis pubis or when the woman begins bearing-down efforts prematurely, thereby inhibiting complete dilation. Sexually transmitted infections (e.g., human papillomavirus) can alter cervical tissue integrity and thus interfere with adequate effacement and dilation.

Bandl ring, a pathologic retraction ring that forms between the upper and lower uterine segments (see Fig. 18-10), is associated with prolonged rupture of membranes, protracted labor, and increased risk for uterine rupture (Cunningham et al., 2005).

Fetal Causes

Dystocia of fetal origin may be caused by anomalies, excessive fetal size and malpresentation, malposition, or multifetal pregnancy. Complications associated with dystocia of fetal origin include neonatal asphyxia, fetal injuries or fractures, and maternal vaginal lacerations. Although spontaneous vaginal birth is possible in these instances, a low forceps-assisted, vacuum-assisted, or cesarean birth often is necessary.

Anomalies

Gross ascites, large tumors, and open neural tube defects (e.g., myelomeningocele, and hydrocephalus) are fetal anomalies that can cause dystocia. The anomalies affect the relation of the fetal anatomy to the maternal pelvic capacity, with the result that the fetus is unable to descend through the birth canal.

Cephalopelvic Disproportion

Cephalopelvic disproportion (CPD), also called *fetopelvic disproportion* (FPD), is often related to excessive fetal size (i.e., 4000 g or more). It occurred at a rate of 14.6 per 1000 live births in 2003 (Martin et al., 2005).

When CPD is present, the fetus cannot fit through the maternal pelvis to be born vaginally. Excessive fetal size, or *macrosomia*, is associated with maternal diabetes mellitus, obesity, multiparity, or the large size of one or both parents. If the maternal pelvis is too small, abnormally shaped, or deformed, CPD may be of maternal origin. In this case, the fetus may be of average size or even smaller.

Malposition

The most common fetal malposition is persistent occipitoposterior position (i.e., right occipitoposterior [ROP] or left occipitoposterior [LOP]; see Chapter 18), occurring in about 25% of all labors. Labor, especially the second stage, is prolonged; the woman typically complains of severe back pain from the pressure of the fetal head (occiput) pressing against her sacrum. Box 36-7 identifies suggested measures to relieve back pain and facilitate rotation of the fetal occiput to an anterior position, which will facilitate birth (Gilbert & Harmon, 2003; Simkin & Ancheta, 2000; Stremler, Hodnett, Petryshen, Stevens, Weston, & Willan, 2005).

Malpresentation

Malpresentation is the second most commonly reported complication of labor and birth. In 2003, it occurred at a rate of 38.5 per 1000 live births, with the highest rate (i.e., 58.8) among women 40 to 54 years of age (Martin et al., 2005). Breech presentation is the most common form of malpresentation. The four main types of breech presentation are frank breech (thighs flexed, knees extended), complete breech (thighs and knees flexed), and two types of incomplete breech, one in which the knee extends below the buttocks and the other in which the foot extends below the buttocks (Fig. 36-5). Breech presentations are associated with multifetal gestation, preterm birth, fetal and maternal anomalies, hydramnios, and oligohydramnios. Diagnosis is made by abdominal palpation (e.g., Leopold maneuvers) and vaginal examination and usually is confirmed by ultrasound scan (Lanni & Seeds, 2002).

During labor, the descent of the fetus in a breech presentation may be slow because the breech is not as good a dilating wedge as the fetal head; the labor itself usually is not prolonged. There is risk of prolapse of the cord if the membranes rupture in early labor. The presence of meconium in amniotic fluid is not necessarily a sign of

FIG. 36-5 Types of breech presentation. **A,** Frank breech: thighs are flexed on hips; knees are extended. **B,** Complete breech: thighs and knees are flexed. **C,** Incomplete breech: foot extends below the buttocks. **D,** Incomplete breech: knee extends below the buttocks.

fetal distress because it results from pressure on the fetal abdominal wall as it traverses the birth canal. Assessment of FHR and pattern should be used to determine whether the passage of meconium is an expected finding associated with breech presentation or is a nonreassuring sign associated with fetal hypoxia. The fetal heart rate of infants in a breech position is best heard at or above the umbilicus.

Vaginal birth is accomplished by mechanisms of labor that manipulate the buttocks and lower extremities as they emerge from the birth canal (Fig. 36-6). Piper forceps some-

---

box 36-7 **Back Labor—Occiput Posterior Position**

MEASURES TO RELIEVE BACK PAIN AND FACILITATE ROTATION OF FETAL HEAD

Measures to Reduce Back Pain During a Contraction

- *Counterpressure:* apply fist or heel of hand to sacral area
- *Heat or cold applications:* apply to sacral area
- *Double hip squeeze:*
  - Woman assumes a position with hip joints flexed such as knee-chest
  - Partner, nurse, or doula places hands over gluteal muscles and presses with palms of hands up and inward toward the center of the pelvis
- *Knee press:*
  - Woman assumes a sitting position with knees a few inches apart and feet flat on the floor or on a stool
  - Partner, nurse, or doula cups a knee in each hand with heels of hands on top of tibia then presses the knees straight back toward the woman's hips while leaning forward toward the woman

Measures to Facilitate the Rotation of the Fetal Head (May Also Relieve Back Pain)

- *Lateral abdominal stroking:* stroke the abdomen in direction that the fetal head should rotate
- *Hands-and-knees position (all-fours):* can also be accomplished by kneeling while leaning forward over a birth ball, padded chair seat, bed, or over-the-bed table
- *Squatting*
- *Pelvic rocking*
- *Stair climbing*
- *Lateral position:* lie on side toward which the fetus should turn
- *Lunges:* widens pelvis on side toward which woman lunges
  - Woman stands, facing forward, next to/alongside a chair so that she can lunge toward the side the fetal back is on or in the direction of the fetal occiput
  - She places foot on seat of chair with toes pointed toward the back of the chair, then lunges
  - Alternative position for lunge: kneeling

FIG. 36-6 Mechanism of labor in breech presentation. **A,** Breech before onset of labor. **B,** Engagement and internal rotation. **C,** Lateral flexion. **D,** External rotation or restitution. **E,** Internal rotation of shoulders and head. **F,** Face rotates to sacrum when occiput is anterior. **G,** Head is born by gradual flexion during elevation of fetal body.

times are used to deliver the head (see Fig. 36-11). External cephalic version (ECV) may be tried to turn the fetus to a vertex presentation (see Fig. 36-8 and later discussion). Cesarean birth may be necessary (Bowes & Thorp, 2004; Lanni & Seeds, 2002).

Although opinions vary, a cesarean birth is commonly performed when the fetus is estimated to be larger than 3800 g or smaller than 1500 g, if this is a first pregnancy, if labor is ineffective, or if complications occur. Although cesarean birth reduces the risks to the fetus, the maternal risks are increased. ECV also poses risks and is not always successful. Women whose breech presentation occurs late in pregnancy need to be informed of the options for birth, as well as the risks associated with each option.

Face and brow presentations are uncommon and are associated with fetal anomalies, pelvic contractures, and CPD (Fig. 36-7). Vaginal birth is possible if the fetus flexes to a vertex presentation, although forceps often are used.

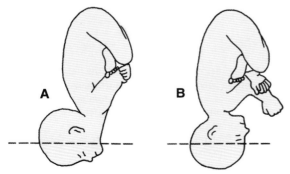

FIG. 36-7 Extension of normally flexed head. Face **(A)** and brow **(B)** presentations.

Cesarean birth is indicated if the presentation persists, if there is fetal distress, or if labor stops progressing.

Cesarean birth is usually necessary for a fetus in a shoulder presentation (i.e., the fetus is in a transverse lie), although ECV may be attempted after 38 weeks of gestation (Bowes & Thorp, 2004).

Multifetal Pregnancy

Multifetal pregnancy is the gestation of twins, triplets, quadruplets, or more infants. Since 1980, the twin birth rate which was 18.9 per 1000 live births has increased by 66%. The twin birth rate was 31.5 per 1000 live births in 2003, a 1% increase over the 2002 rate of 31.1%. The higher-order multiple birth rate was 187.4 per 100,000 live births in 2003 (Martin et al., 2005). The incidence of multiple births increased by more than 500% between 1980 (i.e., 37.0) and 1998 (i.e., 193.5). This increase has been attributed to the use of fertility-enhancing medications and procedures and the older age of childbearing women. When compared with younger women, women age 35 years and older are naturally more likely to have a multifetal pregnancy. Refinements in the treatments used to treat infertility may be responsible for the recent decline in higher-order multiple births (Martin et al.).

Multiple births are associated with more complications (e.g., dysfunctional labor) than single births. The higher incidence of fetal and/or newborn complications and higher risk of perinatal mortality primarily stem from the birth of low-birth-weight infants resulting from preterm birth and/or IUGR in part related to placental dysfunction and twin-to-twin transfusion. Fetuses may experience distress and asphyxia during the birth process as a result of cord prolapse and the onset of placental separation with the birth of the first fetus. As a result, the risk for long-term problems such as cerebral palsy is higher among multiple births.

In addition, fetal complications such as congenital anomalies and abnormal presentations can result in dystocia and an increased incidence of cesarean birth. For example, in only half of all twin pregnancies do both fetuses present in the vertex position, the most favorable for vaginal birth; in one third of the pregnancies, one twin may present in the vertex position and one in the breech (Cunningham et al., 2005).

The health status of the mother may be compromised by an increased risk for hypertension, anemia, and hemorrhage associated with uterine atony, abruptio placentae, and multiple or adherent placentas. Duration of the phases and stages of labor may vary from the duration experienced with singleton births.

Teamwork and planning are essential components of the management of childbirth in multiple pregnancies, especially those of the higher-order multiples. The nurse plays a key role in coordinating the activities of many highly skilled health care professionals. Early detection and care of the maternal, fetal, and newborn complications associated with multiple births are essential to achieve a positive outcome for mother and babies. Maternal positioning and active support are used to enhance labor progress and placental perfusion. Stimulation of labor with oxytocin, epidural anesthesia, forceps and vacuum assistance, and internal or ECV may be used to accomplish the vaginal birth of twins. Cesarean birth is most likely with higher-order multiple births. Each infant may have its own team of health care providers present at the birth. Emotional support that includes expression of feelings and full explanations of events as they occur and of the status of the mother and the fetuses/newborns is important to reduce the anxiety and stress the mother and her family experience. Websites such as www.nomotc.org and www.tripletconnection.org may be helpful for families having a multiple birth.

Position of the Woman

The functional relationship among the uterine contractions, the fetus, and the mother's pelvis are altered by the maternal position. In addition, the position can provide either a mechanical advantage or disadvantage to the mechanisms of labor by altering the effects of gravity and the body-part relations important to the progress of labor. For example, the hands-and-knees position facilitates rotation from a posterior occiput position more effectively than the lateral position. Upright positions such as sitting and squatting facilitate fetal descent during pushing and shorten the second stage of labor (Mayberry et al., 2000; Simkin & Ancheta, 2000). Progress may be compromised by discouraging maternal movement or restricting labor to the recumbent or lithotomy position. The incidence of dystocia in women confined to these positions is increased, resulting in increased need for augmentation of labor or forceps-assisted, vacuum-assisted, or cesarean birth.

Psychologic Responses

Hormones and neurotransmitters released in response to stress (e.g., catecholamines) can cause dystocia. Sources of stress vary for each woman, but pain and the absence of a support person are two recognized factors. Confinement to bed and restriction of maternal movement can be a source of psychologic stress that compounds the physiologic stress caused by immobility in the unmedicated laboring woman. When anxiety is excessive, it can inhibit cervical dilation and result in prolonged labor and increased pain perception. Anxiety also causes increased levels of stress-related hormones (e.g., beta-endorphin, adrenocorticotropic hormone, cortisol, and epinephrine). These hormones act on the smooth muscles of the uterus; increased levels can cause dystocia by reducing uterine contractility.

■ CARE MANAGEMENT

■ Assessment and Nursing Diagnoses

Risk assessment is a continuous process in the laboring woman. Review of the findings obtained during the initial interview conducted at the woman's admission to the labor unit and ongoing observations of her psychologic response to labor may reveal factors that can be a source of dysfunctional labor. These factors may include anxiety or fear, a complication of pregnancy, or previous labor complications. The initial physical assessment and ongoing assessments provide information about maternal well-being; status of labor in terms of the characteristics of uterine contractions and progress of cervical effacement and dilation; fetal well-being in terms of FHR and pattern, presentation, station, and position; and status of the amniotic membranes.

Ultrasound scanning can identify potential dysfunctional labor problems related to the fetus or maternal pelvis. All these assessments contribute to accurate identification of potential and actual nursing diagnoses related to dystocia and maternal-fetal compromise.

Nursing diagnoses that might be identified in women experiencing dystocia include the following:

* *Risk for maternal or fetal injury related to*
  –interventions implemented for dystocia
* *Powerlessness related to*
  –loss of control
* *Risk for infection related to*
  –PPROM
* *Ineffective coping related to*
  –inadequate support system
  –exhaustion secondary to a prolonged labor process
  –pain
* *Risk for impaired parent-infant attachment related to*
  –separation from infant associated with emergency cesarean birth
  –emotional responses to a traumatic childbirth experience

▬ Expected Outcomes of Care

Expected outcomes for the woman with dystocia include that the woman will do the following

- Understand the causes and treatment of dysfunctional labor.
- Use measures recommended by the health care team to enhance the progress of labor and birth.
- Express relief of pain.
- Experience labor and birth with minimal or no complications, such as infection, injury, or hemorrhage.
- Give birth to a healthy infant who has experienced no fetal distress or birth injury.
- Exhibit positive attachment behaviors with newborn.

▬ Plan of Care and Interventions

Nurses assume many caregiving roles when labor is complicated. They also work collaboratively with other health care providers in providing care. Interventions that the nurse may implement or assist with include ECV, trial of labor, cervical ripening with prostaglandins, induction or augmentation with oxytocin, amniotomy, and operative procedures (e.g., forceps- or vacuum-assisted birth) and preoperative and postoperative care for cesarean birth. The nursing role is identified with each of the procedures described.

▬ LEGAL TIP Standard of Care—Labor and Birth Complications

- Document all assessment findings, interventions, and client responses on client record, and monitor strips according to unit protocols, procedures, and policies and professional standards.
- Assess whether the woman (and her family, if appropriate) is fully informed about procedures for which she is consenting.
- Provide full explanations regarding what is happening and what has to be done to help her and her baby.
- Maintain safety in administering medications and treatments correctly.
- Have verbal orders signed as soon as possible.
- Provide care at the acceptable standard (e.g., according to hospital protocols and professional standards).
- If short staffing occurs in the unit and the nurse is assigned additional clients, the nurse should document that rejecting this additional assignment would have placed these clients in danger as a result of abandonment.
- Continue maternal and fetal monitoring until birth according to the policies, procedures, and protocols of the birthing facility, even when a decision to carry out cesarean birth is made.

▬ *Version*

Version is the turning of the fetus from one presentation to another and may be done either externally or internally by the physician.

External Cephalic Version. External cephalic version (ECV) is used to attempt to turn the fetus from a breech or shoulder presentation to a vertex presentation for birth. It may be attempted in a labor and birth setting after 37 weeks of gestation. ECV is accomplished by the exertion of gentle, constant pressure on the abdomen (Fig. 36-8). Before it is attempted, ultrasound scanning is done to determine the fetal position; locate the umbilical cord; rule out placenta previa;

FIG. 36-8 External version of fetus from breech to vertex presentation. This must be achieved without force. **A,** Breech is pushed up out of pelvic inlet while head is pulled toward inlet. **B,** Head is pushed toward inlet while breech is pulled upward.

evaluate the adequacy of the maternal pelvis; and assess the amount of amniotic fluid, the fetal age, and the presence of any anomalies. A nonstress test (NST) is performed to confirm fetal well-being, or the FHR rate and pattern is monitored for a period of time (i.e., 10 to 20 minutes). Informed consent is obtained. A tocolytic agent such as magnesium sulfate or terbutaline often is given to relax the uterus and to facilitate the maneuver (Bowes & Thorp, 2004). Contraindications to ECV include uterine anomalies, previous cesarean birth, CPD, placenta previa, multifetal gestation, and oligohydramnios (Cunningham et al., 2005; Lanni & Seeds, 2002). ECV performed at term to avoid breech birth is a beneficial form of care (Enkin et al., 2000).

Before and during an attempted ECV, the nurse monitors the FHR and pattern, especially for bradycardia and variable decelerations; checks the maternal vital signs; and assesses the woman's level of comfort, because the procedure may cause discomfort. After the procedure is completed, the nurse continues to monitor maternal vital signs, uterine activity, and FHR and pattern, and assess for vaginal bleeding until the woman's condition is stable. Women who are Rh-negative should receive Rh immune globulin, because the manipulation can cause fetomaternal bleeding (Bowes & Thorp, 2004; Lanni & Seeds, 2002).

Internal Version. With internal version, the fetus is turned by the physician who inserts a hand into the uterus and changes the presentation to cephalic (head) or podalic (foot). Internal version may be used in multifetal pregnancies to deliver the second fetus. The safety of this procedure has not been documented; maternal and fetal injury is possible. Cesarean birth is the usual method for managing malpresentation in multifetal pregnancies. The nurse's role is to monitor the status of the fetus and to provide support to the woman.

■ Trial of Labor

A trial of labor (TOL) is the observance of a woman and her fetus for a reasonable period (e.g., 4 to 6 hours) of spontaneous active labor to assess safety of vaginal birth for the mother and infant. It may be initiated if the mother's pelvis is of questionable size or shape, if the fetus is in an abnormal presentation, or if she wishes to have a vaginal birth after a previous cesarean birth. It is a form of care likely to be beneficial when implemented after a previous low-segment cesarean birth (Enkin et al., 2000). Fetal sonography, maternal pelvimetry, or both may be done before a TOL to rule out CPD. The cervix must be ripe (e.g., soft, dilatable). During a TOL, the woman is evaluated for the occurrence of active labor, including adequate contractions, engagement and descent of the presenting part, and effacement and dilation of the cervix.

The nurse assesses maternal vital signs and FHR and pattern and is alert for signs of potential complications. If complications develop, the nurse is responsible for initiating appropriate actions, including notifying the primary health care provider, and for evaluating and documenting the maternal and fetal responses to the interventions. Nurses must recognize that the woman and her partner are often anxious about her health and well-being and that of their baby. Supporting and encouraging the woman and her partner and providing information regarding progress can reduce stress and enhance the labor process and facilitate a successful outcome.

■ Induction of Labor

Induction of labor is the chemical or mechanical initiation of uterine contractions before their spontaneous onset for the purpose of bringing about the birth. In 2003, 20.6% of women who gave birth had their labors induced, which is more than twice the labor induction rate of 9.5% in 1990 (Martin et al., 2005). The induction rate in 2003 for infants born at 37 to 41 weeks of gestation was 21.6% and has been steadily increasing. For infants born after 41 weeks, the rate of induction was 24.2% in 2003. Non-Hispanic white women have the highest induction rate, which in 2003 was 24.7%; the lowest rates were for Asian or Pacific Islanders (i.e.,14%) and Hispanic women (i.e., 13.8%).

Induction may be indicated for a variety of medical and obstetric reasons. These include preeclampsia, diabetes mellitus, chorioamnionitis, and other medical problems; and PROM, postterm gestation, suspected fetal jeopardy (e.g., IUGR), logistic factors such as history of previous rapid birth or distance of the woman's home from the

---

CRITICAL THINKING EXERCISE

Evidence-Based Protocol for Induction

You are a member of a practice committee composed of nurses, midwives, and obstetricians. Your committee has been given the task of developing a new labor induction protocol that is evidence-based. This protocol will be implemented on the labor unit where you work.

1. Evidence—Is there sufficient evidence regarding successful and safe induction of labor to fulfill the task your committee has been assigned?
2. Assumptions—What assumptions can be made about the following issues related to successful and safe labor induction?
   a. Criteria women should meet to be considered as candidates for labor induction
   b. Measures that increase the likelihood of a successful induction
   c. Dosage and administration recommendations
3. Should elective induction be promoted as part of this protocol?
4. Does the evidence objectively support this recommendation?
5. Are there alternative perspectives regarding labor management measures that should be included in the protocol to enhance the success of labor induction?

---

hospital, and fetal death. Under such conditions, the risk to the mother or fetus is less than the risk of continuing the pregnancy (Bowes & Thorp, 2004). Two thirds of the inductions in the United States are elective (i.e., not for medical or obstetric reasons), and it is theorized that elective inductions are in part responsible for the increase in the overall rate of induction. There is evidence that elective induction increases the risk for cesarean birth especially for nulliparous women (Ramsey, Ramin, & Ramin, 2000; Simpson & Atterbury, 2003).

Both chemical and mechanical methods are used to induce labor. Intravenous oxytocin and amniotomy are the most common methods used in the United States. Prostaglandins are increasingly used for inducing labor. The most effective protocol (e.g., dose, frequency) to follow when using prostaglandins continues to be investigated (Simpson, 2002).

Less commonly used methods include stripping of membranes, nipple stimulation (manual or with a breast pump), and acupuncture (Bowes & Thorp, 2004). The ingestion of a laxative (e.g., castor oil), herbal preparations (e.g., green, chamomile, or raspberry tea; blue or black cohosh), or spicy food and administration of a soapsuds enema are other methods (Simpson, 2002). Many folk beliefs exist regarding methods to induce labor. These methods include activity (e.g., walking, exercise, strenuous work, intercourse), fasting, and increasing stress (e.g., frightening the woman). It is important for the nurse to know the practices a woman may believe in and follow, because some of these methods can be harmful (e.g., strenuous activity) (Schaffir, 2002).

table 36-3 **Bishop Score**

	SCORE			
	0	1	2	3
Dilation (cm)	0	1-2	3-4	≥5
Effacement (%)	0-30	40-50	60-70	≥80
Station (cm)	−3	−2	−1	+1, +2
Cervical consistency	Firm	Medium	Soft	
Cervix position	Posterior	Midposition	Anterior	

Success rates for induction of labor are higher when the condition of the cervix is favorable, or inducible. A rating system such as the Bishop score (Table 36-3) can be used to evaluate inducibility. For example, a score of 9 or more on this 13-point scale indicates that the cervix is soft, anterior, 50% or more effaced, and dilated 2 cm or more; and that the presenting part is engaged. Induction of labor is likely to be more successful if the score is 9 or more for nulliparas and 5 or more for multiparas (Gilbert & Harmon, 2003; Simpson, 2002).

■ *Cervical Ripening Methods*

Chemical Agents. Preparations of prostaglandin E_1 and prostaglandin E_2 can be used before induction to "ripen" (soften and thin) the cervix (see Medication Guides). This treatment usually results in a higher success rate for the induction of labor, the need for lower dosages of oxytocin during the induction, and shorter induction times. The use of prostaglandins to increase cervical readiness for induc-

tion of labor is a beneficial form of care (Enkin et al., 2000). In some cases, women will go into labor after the administration of prostaglandin, thereby eliminating the need to administer oxytocin to induce labor (Gilbert & Harmon, 2003; Simpson, 2002). Prostaglandin E_1, although less expensive and more effective than oxytocin or prostaglandin E_2 for inducing labor and birth, is associated with a higher risk for hyperstimulation of the uterus and nonreassuring changes in FHR and pattern. However, when 25 mcg is administered at an interval of every 3 to 6 hours, the rate of hyperstimulation is significantly decreased (Goldberg & Wing, 2003; Simpson & Atterbury, 2003).

Mechanical Methods. Mechanical dilators ripen the cervix by stimulating the release of endogenous prostaglandins. Their use is a form of care with a trade-off between beneficial and adverse effects (Enkin et al., 2000). Balloon catheters (e.g., Foley catheter) can be inserted into the intracervical canal to ripen and dilate the cervix. Hydroscopic dilators (substances that absorb fluid from

medication guide

Cervical Ripening Using Prostaglandin E₁ (PGE₁): Misoprostol (Cytotec)

ACTION ■ PGE₁ ripens the cervix, making it softer and causing it to begin to dilate and efface; stimulates uterine contractions. Note: The FDA has not approved of this medication for cervical ripening (i.e., this is an unlabeled use for obstetrics)

INDICATIONS ■ PGE₁ is used for preinduction cervical ripening (ripen cervix before oxytocin induction of labor when the Bishop score is 4 or less).

DOSAGE AND ADMINISTRATION

- Insert 25 mcg (¼ of a 100-mcg tablet) intravaginally into the posterior vaginal fornix using the tips of index and middle fingers without the use of a lubricant.
- Repeat every 4 to 6 hr as needed until cervix ripens (Bishop score of 8 or greater), or significant adverse reactions occur.
- Tablet, which is not scored, must be cut in the pharmacy to ensure accurate dosage.
- Assist woman to void prior to insertion and to maintain a supine position with a lateral tilt or a side-lying position for 30 to 40 min after insertion.

ADVERSE EFFECTS ■ Higher dosages are more likely to result in adverse reactions such as nausea and vomiting, diarrhea, fever, tachysystole (12 or more uterine contractions in 20 min without alteration of fetal heart rate [FHR] pattern), hyperstimulation of the uterus (tachysystole with nonreassuring FHR patterns), or fetal passage of meconium. Risk for adverse reactions is reduced with lower dosages (i.e., 25 mcg) and longer intervals between doses (i.e., every 6 hours rather than every 4 hours).

NURSING CONSIDERATIONS ■ Explain procedure to woman and her family.

- Ensure that an informed consent has been obtained as per agency policy.
- Assess maternal-fetal unit, before each insertion and during treatment following agency protocol for frequency.
- Assess maternal vital signs and health status, FHR and pattern, and status of pregnancy, including indications for cervical ripening or induction of labor, signs of labor or impending labor, and the Bishop score.
- Recognize that the following contraindicate the use of misoprostol: a nonreassuring FHR pattern; maternal fever, infection, vaginal bleeding, or hypersensitivity; and regular, progressive uterine contractions and history of cesarean birth or uterine scar.
- Use caution if the woman has a history of asthma, glaucoma, or renal, hepatic, or cardiovascular disorders.
- Prepare to swab vagina to remove unabsorbed medication using a saline-soaked gauze wrapped around fingers and to administer terbutaline 0.25 mg subcutaneously or intravenously if significant adverse reactions occur.
- Initiate oxytocin for induction of labor at least 4 hr after last dose of misoprostol was administered, following agency protocol, if ripening has occurred and labor has not begun.
- Document all assessment findings and administration procedures.

medication guide

Cervical Ripening Using Prostaglandin E₂ (PGE₂): Dinoprostone (Cervidil Insert; Prepidil Gel)

ACTION ■ PGE₂ ripens the cervix, making it softer and causing it to begin to dilate and efface; stimulates uterine contractions. Dinoprostone is the only FDA-approved medication for cervical ripening or labor induction.

INDICATIONS ■ PGE₂ is used for preinduction cervical ripening (ripen cervix before oxytocin induction of labor when the Bishop score is 4 or less).

DOSAGE AND ADMINISTRATION

■ **Cervidil**

* Place Cervidil insert (10 mg dinoprostone gradually released over 12 hr) intravaginally into the posterior fornix. Remove after 12 hs or at the onset of labor. Keep insert frozen until ready to use (no rewarming is needed). Uterine contractions usually begin in 5 to 7 hs. Induction may be initiated, if needed, 30 to 60 minutes after the removal of the insert.
* Assist woman to void prior to insertion and to maintain a supine position with a lateral tilt or a side-lying position for 30 to 60 minutes after placement of the insert.

OR

■ **Prepidil**

* Insert Prepidil gel (2.5-ml syringe containing 0.5 mg of dinoprostone) into cervical canal just below internal cervical os or into posterior fornix; a shield can be used to prevent insertion past internal os. Repeat gel insertion in 6 hr as needed to a maximum of 1.5 mg or 3 doses in a 24-hr period. Bring gel to room temperature before administration. Do not force the warming process by using a warm water bath or other source of external heat such as microwave. Continue treatment until maximum dosage is administered or until an effective contraction pattern is established (3 or more uterine contractions in 10 min), cervix ripens (Bishop score of ≥8), or significant adverse reactions occur. Initiate oxytocin for induction of labor, if needed, within 6 to 12 hs after the last instillation of the gel.
* Assist woman to void prior to insertion and to maintain a supine position with a lateral tilt or a side-lying position for 2 hs after insertion of the gel.

ADVERSE EFFECTS ■ Potential adverse reactions include headache, nausea and vomiting, diarrhea, fever, hypotension, tachysystole (12 or more uterine contractions in 20 min without alteration of fetal heart rate [FHR] pattern), hyperstimulation of the uterus (tachysystole with nonreassuring FHR patterns), or fetal passage of meconium. Adverse reactions are more common with intracervical administration.

NURSING CONSIDERATIONS ■ Explain procedure to woman and her family.

* Ensure that an informed consent has been obtained as per agency policy.
* Assess maternal-fetal unit before each insertion and during treatment following agency protocol for frequency.
* Assess maternal vital signs and health status, FHR pattern, and status of pregnancy, including indications for cervical ripening or induction of labor, signs of labor or impending labor, and the Bishop score.
* Recognize that the following contraindicate the use of dinoprostone: a nonreassuring FHR pattern; maternal fever, infection, vaginal bleeding, or hypersensitivity; and regular, progressive uterine contractions and history of cesarean birth or uterine scar.
* Use caution if the woman has a history of asthma, glaucoma, or renal, hepatic, or cardiovascular disorders.
* Allow woman to ambulate after recommended period of bed rest and observation.
* Prepare to swab vagina to remove remaining gel using a saline-soaked gauze wrapped around fingers, or pull string to remove insert and to administer terbutaline 0.25 mg subcutaneously or intravenously if significant adverse reactions occur.
* Follow agency protocol for induction if ripening has occurred and labor has not begun.
* Document all assessment findings and administration procedures.

---

surrounding tissues and then enlarge) also can be used for cervical ripening. Laminaria tents (natural cervical dilators made from desiccated seaweed) and synthetic dilators containing magnesium sulfate (Lamicel) are inserted into the endocervix without rupturing the membranes. As they absorb fluid, they expand and cause cervical dilation. These dilators are left in place for 6 to 12 hours before being removed to assess cervical dilation. Fresh dilators are inserted if further cervical dilation is necessary. Synthetic dilators swell faster than natural dilators and become larger with less discomfort (Simpson, 2002). Amniotomy and membrane stripping also can be used to ripen the cervix (Norwitz, Robinson, & Repke, 2002).

Hydroscopic dilators compare favorably with prostaglandins in terms of their effectiveness in ripening the cervix but are associated with increased discomfort at insertion and during expansion and with a higher incidence of postpartum maternal and newborn infections. They are a reliable alternative when prostaglandins are contraindicated or are unavailable. Nursing responsibilities for women who

have dilators inserted include documenting the number of dilators and sponges inserted during the procedure, as well as the number removed, and assessment for urinary retention, rupture of membranes, uterine tenderness/pain, contractions, vaginal bleeding, and fetal distress (Gilbert & Harmon, 2003; Norwitz et al., 2002; Simpson, 2002).

■ *Amniotomy*

Amniotomy (i.e., artificial rupture of membranes [AROM]) can be used to induce labor when the condition of the cervix is favorable (ripe) or to augment labor if progress begins to slow. Labor usually begins within 12 hours of the rupture; the duration of labor can be decreased by up to 2 hours, especially if combined with oxytocin administration. However, if amniotomy does not stimulate labor, the resulting prolonged rupture may lead to infection. Other potential risks include umbilical cord prolapse and fetal injury. Once an amniotomy is performed, the woman is committed to labor with an unknown outcome for how and when she will give birth. For this reason, amniotomy often is used in combination with oxytocin induction. Evidence from controlled trials clearly demonstrates that amniotomy combined with oxytocin for induction is more effective than either amniotomy or oxytocin alone and is therefore a beneficial form of care (Enkin et al., 2000).

Before the procedure, the woman should be told what to expect; she also should be assured that the actual rupture of the membranes is painless for her and the fetus, although she may experience some discomfort when the Amnihook or other sharp instrument is inserted through the vagina and cervix (see Procedure box).

The presenting part of the fetus should be engaged and well applied to the cervix to prevent cord prolapse. The woman should be free of active infection of the genital tract (e.g., herpes) and human immunodeficiency virus (HIV) infection (Norwitz et al., 2002). The membranes are ruptured with an Amnihook or other sharp instrument and the amniotic fluid allowed to drain slowly. The color, odor, and consistency of the fluid is assessed (i.e., for the presence or absence of meconium or blood). The time of rupture is recorded.

▬ NURSE ALERT

The FHR is assessed before and immediately after the amniotomy to detect any changes (e.g., transient tachycardia is common, but bradycardia and variable decelerations are not) that may indicate cord compression or prolapse.

procedure

Assisting with Amniotomy

PROCEDURE
- Explain to the woman what will be done.
- Assess woman for signs of infection, condition of cervix (e.g., ripeness, dilation), and station of the presenting part.
- Assess fetal heart rate (FHR) before procedure begins to obtain a baseline reading.
- Place several underpads under the woman's buttocks to absorb the fluid.
- Position the woman on a padded bed pan, fracture pan, or rolled up towel to elevate her hips.
- Assist the health care provider who is performing the procedure by providing sterile gloves and lubricant for the vaginal examination.
- Unwrap sterile package containing Amnihook or Allis clamp and pass instrument to the primary health care provider, who inserts it alongside the fingers and then hooks and tears the membranes.
- Reassess the FHR and pattern.
- Assess the color, consistency, and odor of the fluid.
- Assess the woman's temperature every 2 hours or per protocol.
- Evaluate the woman for signs and symptoms of infection.

DOCUMENTATION
- Record the following:
  - Indication for amniotomy
  - Time of rupture
  - Color, odor, consistency and clarity of the fluid
  - FHR and pattern before and after the procedure
  - Maternal status and how well procedure was tolerated

The woman's temperature should be checked at least every 2 hours to rule out infection. If her temperature is 38° C or higher, the primary health care provider should be notified. The nurse assesses for other signs and symptoms of infection, such as maternal chills, uterine tenderness on palpation, foul-smelling vaginal drainage, and fetal tachycardia (Simpson, 2002). Comfort measures, such as frequently changing the woman's underpads and perineal cleansing, are implemented.

▬ Oxytocin

Oxytocin is a hormone normally produced by the posterior pituitary gland; it stimulates uterine contractions. It may be used either to induce labor or to augment a labor that is progressing slowly because of inadequate uterine contractions.

The indications for oxytocin induction or augmentation of labor may include, but are not limited to, the following:
- Suspected fetal jeopardy (e.g., IUGR)
- Inadequate uterine contractions; dystocia
- PROM
- Postterm pregnancy
- Chorioamnionitis
- Maternal medical problems (e.g., woman with severe Rh isoimmunization, inadequately controlled diabetes mellitus, chronic renal disease, or chronic pulmonary disease)
- Gestational hypertension (e.g., preeclampsia, eclampsia)
- Fetal death
- Multiparous women with a history of precipitous labor or who live far from the hospital

The management of stimulation of labor is the same regardless of the indication. Because of the potential dangers associated with the injection of oxytocin in the prenatal and intrapartal periods, the FDA has issued certain restrictions to its use.

Contraindications to oxytocin stimulation of labor include, but are not limited to, the following:
- CPD, prolapsed cord, transverse lie
- Nonreassuring FHR and pattern
- Placenta previa or vasa previa
- Prior classic uterine incision or uterine surgery
- Active genital herpes infection
- Invasive cancer of the cervix

Certain maternal and fetal conditions, although not contraindications to the use of oxytocin to stimulate labor, do require special caution during its administration. These conditions include the following:
- Multifetal presentation
- Breech presentation
- Presenting part above the pelvic inlet
- Abnormal FHR and pattern not requiring emergency birth
- Polyhydramnios
- Grand multiparity
- Maternal cardiac disease; hypertension

Oxytocin use can present hazards to the mother and fetus. These hazards are primarily dose related, with most problems caused by high doses that are given rapidly. Maternal hazards include water intoxication and tumultuous labor with tetanic contractions, which may cause premature separation of the placenta, rupture of the uterus, lacerations of the cervix, or postpartum hemorrhage. These complications can lead to infection, disseminated intravascular coagulation, or amniotic fluid embolism. Women may become anxious or fearful if the induction is not successful because they may then have concerns about the method of birth.

Uterine hyperstimulation reduces the blood flow through the placenta and results in FHR decelerations (bradycardia, diminished variability, late decelerations), fetal asphyxia, and neonatal hypoxia. If the estimated date of birth is inaccurate, physical injury, neonatal hyperbilirubinemia, and prematurity are other hazards.

The primary health care provider writes the order for the induction or augmentation of labor with oxytocin. The nurse implements the order by initiating the primary intravenous infusion and administering the oxytocin solution through a secondary line. The nurse's actions related to assessment and care of a woman whose labor is being induced are guided by hospital protocol and professional standards (Fig. 36-9; Box 36-8).

In the past, the aim of induction was to achieve a contraction pattern that simulates the active phase of labor as quickly as possible. However, research on uterine tolerance to oxytocin has now shown that lower physiologic doses (e.g., initial dose of 0.5 to 1 milliunits/min with increments of 1 to 2 milliunits/min) given over a longer time are as effective as previous protocols. A recommended dosage increment frequency is every 30 to 60 minutes, because 30 to 40 minutes is required for a steady state of oxytocin to be reached and for the full effect of a dosage increment to be reflected in more intense, frequent, and longer contractions (Simpson & Atterbury, 2003). Such an approach reduces the amount of oxytocin required to achieve a spontaneous vaginal birth and decreases the risk for uterine hyperstimula-

tion, dysfunctional labor, operative vaginal birth, cesarean birth, fetal distress, and other adverse reactions such as water intoxication. It is estimated that oxytocin at a rate of 6 milliunits/min will result in successful induction ending in vaginal birth for the majority of pregnant women at term (Norwitz et al., 2002; Simpson, 2002, 2005).

Nursing Considerations. An evidence-based written protocol for the preparation and administration of oxytocin should be established by the obstetric department (physicians, nurses) in each institution. The procedure recommended for a woman who is eligible for induction of labor is discussed in Box 36-8.

■ NURSE ALERT

Oxytocin is discontinued immediately and the primary health care provider notified if uterine hyperstimulation, nonreassuring FHR and pattern, or both occur.

Other nursing interventions, such as administering oxygen by face mask, positioning the woman on her side, and infusing more intravenous fluids are implemented immediately (see Emergency box). Based on the status of the maternal-fetal unit, the primary health care provider may order that the infusion be restarted once the FHR and pattern and uterine activity return to acceptable levels. Depending on the length of time the infusion was discontinued, the induction may be restarted at half the rate that resulted in hyperstimulation (e.g., discontinued for 10 to 20 minutes) or at the same rate as the initial rate (e.g., discontinued for more than 30 to 40 minutes) (Simpson, 2002) (see Plan of Care).

■ *Augmentation of Labor*

Augmentation of labor is the stimulation of uterine contractions after labor has started spontaneously but progress is unsatisfactory. Augmentation is usually implemented

FIG. 36-9 Woman in side-lying position receiving oxytocin. (Courtesy Michael S. Clement, MD, Mesa, AZ.)

EMERGENCY

Uterine Hyperstimulation with Oxytocin

SIGNS

- Uterine contractions lasting >90 sec and occurring more frequently than every 2 min
- Uterine resting tone >20 mm Hg
- Nonreassuring fetal heart rate (FHR) and pattern:
- Abnormal baseline (<110 or >160 beats/min)
- Absent variability
- Repeated late decelerations or prolonged decelerations

INTERVENTIONS

- Maintain woman in side-lying position
- Turn off oxytocin infusion; keep maintenance intravenous (IV) line open; increase rate
- Start administering oxygen by face mask, per protocol or physician's order
- Notify primary health care provider
- Prepare to administer terbutaline (Brethine), 0.25 mg subcutaneously, if ordered to decrease uterine activity
- Continue monitoring FHR and pattern and uterine activity
- Document responses to actions

---

box 36-8 Protocol: Induction of Labor with Oxytocin

CLIENT/FAMILY TEACHING

Explain technique, rationale, and reactions to expect:
- Route and rate for administration of medication
- What "piggyback" is for
- Reasons for use:
  - –Induce labor, improve labor
- Reactions to expect concerning the nature of contractions:
  - –The intensity of contraction increases more rapidly, holds the peak longer, and ends more quickly; contractions will come regularly and more often
- Monitoring to anticipate:
  - –Maternal: blood pressure, pulse, uterine contractions, uterine tone
  - –Fetal: heart rate and pattern, activity/movements
- Success to expect:
  - –A favorable outcome will depend on inducibility of the cervix (e.g., Bishop score of 9)
- Keep woman and support person informed of progress

ADMINISTRATION

Position woman in side-lying or upright position
Assess status of maternal fetal unit
Prepare solution and administer with pump delivery system according to prescribed orders:
- Infusion pump and solution are set up (e.g., 10 units/1000 ml isotonic electrolyte solution)
- Piggyback solution is connected to intravenous (IV) line at proximal port (port nearest point of venous insertion)
- Solution with oxytocin is flagged with a medication label
- Begin induction at 0.5 to 1 milliunits/min (0.5 to 2 milliunits/min is also acceptable)
- Increase dose 1 to 2 milliunits/min at intervals of no less than 30 to 60 min until adequate progress is achieved; reevaluate if dose reaches 20 milliunits/min

MAINTAIN DOSE IF

- Intensity of contractions results in intrauterine pressures of 40 to 90 mm Hg (shown by internal monitor)
- Duration of contractions is 60 to 90 sec
- Frequency of contractions is every 2 to 3 min
- Resting tone of 10 to 15 mm Hg
- Cervical effacement and/or dilation of 1 cm/hr in the active phase

MATERNAL/FETAL ASSESSMENTS

- Monitor blood pressure, pulse, and respirations every 30 to 60 min and with every increment in dose
- Monitor contraction pattern and uterine resting tone every 15 min and with every increment in dose during the first stage and every 5 minutes during the second stage
- Assess intake and output; limit IV intake to 1000 ml/8 hr; output should be 120 ml or more every 4 hr
- Perform vaginal examination as indicated
- Monitor for nausea, vomiting, headache, hypotension
- Assess fetal status using electronic fetal monitoring; evaluate tracing every 15 min and with every increment in dose during the first stage and every 5 minutes during the second stage
- Observe emotional responses of woman and her partner

REPORTABLE CONDITIONS

- Uterine hyperstimulation
- Nonreassuring fetal heart rate (FHR) and pattern
- Suspected uterine rupture
- Inadequate uterine response at 20 milliunits/min

EMERGENCY MEASURES

Discontinue use of oxytocin per hospital protocol:
- Turn woman on her side
- Increase primary IV rate up to 200 ml/hr, unless woman has water intoxication, in which case the rate is decreased to one that keeps the vein open
- Give woman oxygen by face mask at 8 to 10 L/min or per protocol or primary health care provider's order

DOCUMENTATION

- Medication: kind, amount, and times of beginning, increasing dose, maintaining dose, and discontinuing medication
- Reactions of mother and fetus
  - –Pattern of labor
  - –Progress of labor
  - –FHR and pattern
  - –Maternal vital signs
  - –Nursing interventions and woman's response
- Notification of physician or nurse-midwife

From American College of Obstetricians and Gynecologists. (1999). *Induction of labor*. ACOG Practice Bulletin No. 10. Washington, DC: Author; Ruchata, P., Metheby, N., Essenpreis, H., & Borcherding, K. (2002). Current practices in oxytocin dilution and fluid administration for induction of labor. *Journal of Obstetric, Gynecologic, and Neonatal Nursing, 31*(5), 545-550; Simpson, K. (2002). *Cervical ripening and induction and augmentation of labor* (2nd ed.). Washington, DC: AWHONN; Simpson, K., & Atterbury, J. (2003). Trends and issues in labor induction in the United States: Implications for clinical practice. *Journal of Obstetric, Gynecologic, and Neonatal Nursing, 32*(6), 767-779; Simpson, K. (2005). The context and clinical evidence for common nursing practices during labor. *MCN American Journal of Maternal/Child Nursing, 30*(6), 356-363.

---

for the management of hypotonic uterine dysfunction, resulting in a slowing of the labor process (protracted active phase). Common augmentation methods include oxytocin infusion, amniotomy, and nipple stimulation. Noninvasive methods such as emptying the bladder, ambulation and position changes, relaxation measures, nourishment and hydration, and hydrotherapy should be attempted before invasive interventions are initiated. The administration procedure and nursing assessment and care measures for augmentation of labor with oxytocin are similar to those used for induction of labor with oxytocin; protocols for

dosage and frequency of increments may vary (e.g., lower dosages may be needed to achieve spontaneous vaginal birth (Gilbert & Harmon, 2003; Simpson, 2002).

Some physicians advocate active management of labor, that is, the augmentation of labor to establish efficient labor with the aggressive use of oxytocin so that the woman gives birth within 12 hours of admission to the labor unit. Advocates of active management believe that intervening early (as soon as a nulliparous labor is not progressing at least 1 cm/hr) with use of higher pharmacologic oxytocin doses administered at frequent increment intervals (e.g., a

CD: Plan of Care: Dysfunctional Labor

| plan of care | Dysfunctional Labor: Hypotonic Uterine Dysfunction with Protracted Active Phase |

NURSING DIAGNOSIS Risk for injury to mother and/or fetus related to oxytocin augmentation secondary to dysfunctional labor

Expected Outcomes *Maternal-fetal well-being is maintained; labor progresses and birth occurs.*

Nursing Interventions/*Rationales*
- Explain oxytocin protocol to woman and her labor partner *to allay apprehension and enhance participation.*
- Encourage woman to void before beginning protocol *to prevent discomfort and remove a barrier to labor progress.*
- Apply the electronic fetal monitor per hospital protocol and obtain a 15- to 20-min baseline strip *to ensure adequate assessment of fetal heart rate (FHR) and pattern and contractions.*
- Position woman in a side-lying position and administer the oxytocin per physician order using an intravenous (IV) infusion pump *to stimulate uterine activity and provide adequate control of the flow rate.*
- Regulate the oxytocin per protocol (e.g., advancing the dose in increments of 1 to 2 milliunits/min every 30 to 60 min) *to allow adequate evaluation of the woman's response to stimulation and to prevent hyperstimulation and fetal hypoxia.*
- Maintain oxytocin dose and rate when contractions occur every 2 to 3 min with a duration of 40 to 90 sec and intrauterine pressures of 60 to 90 mm Hg (if internal monitoring is used) *to produce effective uterine stimulation without risk of hyperstimulation.*
- Monitor maternal vital signs every 30 to 60 min *to assess for oxytocin-induced hypertension.*
- Monitor contractility pattern and FHR and pattern every 15 min *to assess uterine activity for possible hypertonicity or ineffective uterine response to oxytocin and to detect evidence of fetal distress.*
- Monitor intake, output, and specific gravity (limit intake to 1000 ml/8 hr; output should be at least 120 ml/4 hr) *to assess for urinary retention and prevent water intoxication.*
- Monitor cervical dilation, effacement, and station *to assess progress of labor.*
- If hypertonicity or signs of fetal distress are detected, discontinue oxytocin immediately *to arrest the progress of hypertonicity;* turn woman on her side *to increase placental blood flow;* increase primary IV rate to 200 ml/hr (unless signs of water toxicity are present); administer oxygen per face mask *to enhance placental perfusion;* notify primary health care provider; and continuously monitor maternal vital signs and FHR and pattern *to provide ongoing assessment of maternal/fetal status.*
- Maintain standard precautions and use scrupulous handwashing techniques when providing care *to prevent the spread of infection.*

NURSING DIAGNOSIS Acute pain related to increasing frequency, regularity, intensity, and prolonged peak of contractions as a result of oxytocin augmentation

Expected Outcome *The woman exhibits signs of decreased discomfort.*

Nursing Interventions/*Rationales*
- Prepare woman and labor partner for the change in the nature of the contractions once the oxytocin drip is initiated *to prepare them and allow for more effective coping.*
- Review the use of specific techniques such as conscious relaxation, focused breathing, effleurage, massage, and application of sacral pressure *to increase relaxation, decrease intensity of pain of contractions, and promote use of controlled thought and direction of energy.*
- Provide comfort measures such as frequent mouth care *to prevent dry mouth,* application of damp cloth to forehead and changing of damp gown or bed covers *to relieve discomfort of diaphoresis,* and positioning *to reduce stiffness.*
- Encourage conscious relaxation between contractions *to prevent fatigue, which contributes to increased pain perceptions.*
- Remind woman and labor partner that pharmacologic methods of pain relief including epidural analgesia are available for use during labor *to provide knowledge to help them make decisions about pain control.*
- Monitor level of pain before and after interventions are implemented *to evaluate effectiveness of interventions.*

NURSING DIAGNOSIS Anxiety related to prolonged labor, increased pain, and fatigue

Expected Outcomes *Woman's anxiety is reduced; woman actively participates in the labor process.*

Nursing Interventions/*Rationales*
- Provide ongoing feedback to woman and partner *to allay anxiety and enhance participation.*
- Present care options when possible *to increase feelings of control.*
- Continue to provide comfort measures *to maintain a posture of support and caring and to aid woman in focusing on the labor process.*
- Encourage woman and partner to continue to use those mechanisms that promote effective labor (e.g., breathing, activity, positioning) *to keep woman and partner actively involved in process.*

starting dose of 6 milliunits/min with increases of 6 milliunits/min every 15 minutes to a maximum dose of 40 milliunits/min) shortens labor and is associated with a lower incidence of cesarean birth (Norwitz et al., 2002; Simpson, 2002).

Additional components of the active management of labor include strict criteria to diagnose that the woman is in active labor with 100% effacement, amniotomy within 1 hour of admission of a woman in labor if spontaneous rupture of the membranes has not occurred, and continuous presence of a personal nurse who provides one-on-one care for the woman while she is in labor. When all components are fully implemented, active management of labor is associated with a lower incidence of cesarean birth. Active management of labor continues to be under study in the United States to determine effectiveness and impact on perinatal morbidity and mortality. Thus far results have been disappointing, especially in terms of reducing the rate of cesarean births. The disappointing results have been attributed, in part, to a greater than one-to-one nurse client ratio and the high rate of epidural anesthesia. It is considered to be a form of care of unknown effectiveness (Enkin et al., 2000; Gilbert & Harmon, 2003; Simpson, 2002).

■ Forceps-Assisted Birth

A forceps-assisted birth is one in which an instrument with two curved blades is used to assist in the birth of the fetal head. The cephalic-like curve of the forceps commonly used is similar to the shape of the fetal head, with a pelvic curve to the blades conforming to the curve of the pelvic axis. The blades are joined by a pin, screw, or groove arrangement. These locks prevent the forceps from compressing the fetal skull. Maternal indications for forceps-assisted birth include the need to shorten the second stage of labor in the event of dystocia or to compensate for the woman's deficient expulsive efforts (e.g., if she is tired or has been given spinal or epidural anesthesia), or to prevent worsening of a dangerous condition (e.g., cardiac decompensation).

Fetal indications include birth of a fetus in distress or in certain abnormal presentations; arrest of rotation; or delivery of the head in a breech presentation.

Certain conditions are required for a forceps-assisted birth to be successful. The woman's cervix must be fully dilated to avert lacerations and hemorrhage. The bladder should be empty. The presenting part must be engaged, and a vertex presentation is desired. Membranes must be ruptured so that the position of the fetal head can be determined and the forceps can firmly grasp the head during birth. In addition, CPD should not be present.

Different definitions of forceps applications are found. *Outlet forceps* are used if the fetal scalp is visible on the perineum without manually separating the labia (Fig. 36-10). Outlet forceps are used to shorten the second stage of labor. *Low forceps* refers to the application of forceps to the fetal head that is at least at the +2-cm station. *Midforceps* refers to the application of forceps to the fetal head that is engaged (no higher than station 0) but above the +2 station. In no instances should forceps be applied to an unengaged presenting part.

Nursing Considerations. When a forceps-assisted birth is deemed necessary, the nurse obtains the type of forceps requested by the primary health care provider (Fig. 36-11). The nurse may explain to the mother that the forceps blades fit like two tablespoons around an egg, with the blades in front of the baby's ears. The nurse usually coaches the woman not to push during contractions unless the primary health care provider instructs the women to push as traction is being applied during contractions.

■ NURSE ALERT

Because compression of the cord between the fetal head and the forceps will cause a decrease in FHR, the fetal heart rate and pattern are assessed, reported, and recorded before and after application of the forceps.

If a decrease in FHR occurs, the primary health care provider removes and reapplies the forceps. Ordinarily traction is applied during contractions. After birth, the mother is assessed for vaginal and cervical lacerations (e.g., bleeding that occurs even with a contracted uterus); urine retention, which may result from bladder or urethral injuries; and hematoma formation in the pelvic soft tissues, which may result from blood vessel damage. The infant

FIG. 36-11 Types of forceps. Piper forceps are used to assist delivery of the head in a breech birth.

FIG. 36-10 Outlet forceps-assisted extraction of the head.

should be assessed for bruising or abrasions at the site of the blade applications, facial palsy resulting from pressure of the blades on the facial nerve (cranial nerve VII), and subdural hematoma. Newborn and postpartum caregivers should be told that a forceps-assisted birth was performed.

■ *Vacuum-Assisted Birth*

Vacuum-assisted birth, or vacuum extraction, is a birth method involving the attachment of a vacuum cup to the fetal head and using negative pressure to assist in the birth of the head. Indications for its use are similar to those for outlet forceps. Prerequisites for use include a vertex presentation, ruptured membranes, and absence of CPD (Cunningham et al., 2005). When an operative vaginal birth is required, vacuum assistance is preferred as a beneficial form of care when compared with forceps assistance (Enkin et al., 2002). Forceps- and vacuum-assisted vaginal births have been declining. In 2003, the combined rate was 5.6%, representing a 41% decrease from the 1994 rate of 9.5% (Martin et al., 2005).

When the birth is to be vacuum assisted, the woman is prepared for a vaginal birth in the lithotomy position to allow sufficient traction. The cup is applied to the fetal head, and a caput develops inside the cup as the pressure is initiated (Fig. 36-12). Traction is applied to facilitate descent of the fetal head, and the woman is encouraged to push as suction is applied. As the head crowns, an episiotomy is performed if necessary. The vacuum cup is released and removed after birth of the head. If vacuum extraction is not successful, a forceps-assisted or cesarean birth is then performed.

Risks to the newborn include cephalhematoma, scalp lacerations, and subdural hematoma. Fetal complications can be reduced by strict adherence to the manufacturer's recommendations for method of application, degree of suction, and duration of application. Maternal complications are uncommon but can include perineal, vaginal, or cervical lacerations and soft-tissue hematomas.

Nursing Considerations. The nurse's role for the woman who has a vacuum-assisted birth is one of support person and educator. The nurse can prepare the woman for birth and encourage her to remain active in the birth process by pushing during contractions. The fetal heart rate should

be assessed frequently during the procedure. After birth, the newborn should be observed for signs of trauma and infection at the application site and for cerebral irritation (e.g., poor sucking or listlessness). The newborn may be at risk for hyperbilirubinemia and neonatal jaundice as bruising or a cephalhematoma or subdural hematoma resolves. The parents may need to be reassured that the caput succedaneum will begin to disappear in a few hours. Neonatal caregivers should be told that the birth was vacuum assisted.

■ *Cesarean Birth*

Cesarean birth is the birth of a fetus through a transabdominal incision of the uterus. Whether cesarean birth is planned (scheduled) or unplanned (emergency), the loss of the experience of giving birth to a child in the traditional manner may have a negative effect on a woman's self-concept. An effort is therefore made to maintain the focus on the birth of the baby rather than on the operative procedure.

The purpose of cesarean birth is to preserve the life or health of the mother and her fetus; it may be the best choice for birth when there is evidence of maternal or fetal complications. Since the advent of modern surgical methods and care and the use of antibiotics, maternal and fetal morbidity and mortality have decreased. In addition, incisions are made into the lower uterine segment rather than into the muscular body of the uterus and thus promote more effective healing. However, despite these advances, cesarean birth still poses threats to the health of the mother and infant.

The incidence of cesarean births has increased from less than 5% in 1965 to 29.1% in 2004, the highest rate ever reported in the United States. The primary cesarean birth rate is 20.6% (Hamilton, Martin, Ventura, Sutton, Menaker, & Division of Vital Statistics, 2005), whereas in Canada, the rate was 22.1% in 2001 (Liu et al., 2004). Factors cited in this increase include use of electronic fetal monitoring and epidural anesthesia; an increase in the number of first-time pregnancies, as well as pregnancies at an older age and the decline in the rate of vaginal births after cesarean birth (VBAC). In 2004, the rate of VBACs was 9.2%. Since 1996, the rate of VBACs has declined by 67%. This decline may be due to reports of risks of VBAC, legal pressures, conservative practice guidelines,

FIG. 36-12 Use of vacuum extraction to rotate fetal head and assist with descent. **A,** *Arrow* indicates direction of traction on the vacuum cup. **B,** Caput succedaneum formed by the vacuum cup.

EVIDENCE-BASED PRACTICE

Episiotomy: Does It Really Help?

BACKGROUND

- For decades, research has pointed out that the risks of routine episiotomy generally outweigh their benefits, yet it is still used in one out of three vaginal births in the United States. Its use is heavily influenced by local practice norms, medical training, and practitioner belief that episiotomy will facilitate birth and prevent tearing.

OBJECTIVES

- The reviewers' goal was to report current information about the risks and benefits of episiotomy on obstetric outcomes and long-term impact on urinary or fecal continence, pelvic floor tone, and sexual function. They also sought to compare episiotomy technique and repair.

METHODS

Search Strategy

- After a search of electronic databases, reference lists, and expert consultation, the reviewers identified 45 randomized controlled trials and prospective studies, dated 1980 to 2004. Studies from Canada, Ireland, Malaysia, the United States, and the United Kingdom were mentioned, but other countries of origin were not noted.

Statistical Analyses

- Similar data were pooled. Reviewers calculated relative risk for dichotomous (categoric) data, such as episiotomy type, and weighted mean difference for continuous data, such as number of sutures. Differences between groups outside the 95% confidence interval were accepted as significant.

FINDINGS

- When compared to routine episiotomy, restricted use of episiotomy resulted in less severe perineal trauma, less suturing, higher chance of intact perineum, and earlier resumption of intercourse. When compared to mediolateral episiotomies,

women receiving midline episiotomy groups were able to resume sexual intercourse sooner and had a better cosmetic appearance, but were more prone to anal sphincter injuries. The two-layer repair (leaving the perineal skin unsutured) was beneficial for pain, healing, and cost over the three-layer approach. The evidence favored continuous over interrupted suturing, and absorbable over nonabsorbable sutures. There was little evidence regarding long-term incontinence or pelvic floor defects after episiotomy. Women experienced more dyspareunia with greater perineal trauma.

LIMITATIONS

- Applied definitions of "restricted" and "routine" episiotomies and measures of trauma differed between studies. Blinding the assessor was not possible. Some of the studies did not report randomization adequately.

IMPLICATIONS FOR PRACTICE

- Nurses can educate themselves, their clients, and the health care providers about best perineal practices, and advocate for alternatives to routine episiotomies, which subject women to greater risk of perineal trauma than tears alone. Perineal protective alternatives include maternal positioning (side-lying is most favorable), avoiding fundal pressure, less coached pushing, perineal supports, and lubrication.

IMPLICATIONS FOR FURTHER RESEARCH

- Much more can be learned about long-term urinary and fecal incontinence, and pelvic floor defects and sexual functioning as women are followed into midlife. More infant outcomes and evidence regarding what indications warrant episiotomy would facilitate decision making.

Reference: Viswanathan, M., Hatmann, K., Palmieri, R., Lux, L., Swinson, T., Lohr, K. et al. (2005). *The use of episiotomy in obstetrical care: A systematic review* (AHRQ Publication No. 05-E009-1). Rockville, MD: Agency for Healthcare Research and Quality.

---

and debate regarding the relative benefits and risks of cesarean versus vaginal route for births (Martin et al., 2005). The declining trend in VBACs indicates that once a woman has a cesarean birth it is highly likely (90%) that her subsequent births will also be cesarean (Martin et al., 2005).

As women age, the likelihood of their having a cesarean birth increases. In 2003, women between the ages of 40 and 54 years had a cesarean birth rate of 42.5% more than twice the rate for women younger than 20 years of age, which was 17.2%. The rationale for this difference may be related to a variety of factors including biologic factors, client and physician concerns, and increased rate of multifetal pregnancies (Martin et al., 2005). Women who have private insurance, who are of a higher socioeconomic status, or who give birth in a private hospital are more likely to experience cesarean birth than are women who are poor, who have no insurance, who are receiving public assistance (e.g.,

Medicaid), or who give birth in public hospitals (Gilbert & Harmon, 2003; Moore, 2003).

Approaches for the management of labor and birth to reduce the rate of cesarean births, while increasing the rate of vaginal births after cesarean (VBAC), are presented in Box 36-9. These management approaches involve the combined efforts of health care professionals and pregnant women and their families. The type of nursing care given also may influence the rate of cesarean births. A labor management approach that uses one-to-one support and emphasizes ambulation, maternal position changes, relaxation measures, oral fluids and nutrition, hydrotherapy, and nonpharmacologic pain relief facilitates the progress of labor and reduces the incidence of dystocia (AWHONN, 2000; Hodnett, Gates, Hofmeyr, & Sakala, 2005; Miltner, 2002).

The labor management approach that most consistently reduces the risk for a cesarean birth outcome is continuous, early-onset support of the laboring woman provided by an-

box 36-9 Selected Measures to Reduce Cesarean Birth Rate

EDUCATE WOMEN REGARDING
- Advantages and safety of the home environment for early or latent labor
- Indicators for hospital admission
- Management techniques to use during labor to enhance progress
- Nonpharmacologic measures to reduce pain and discomfort and enhance relaxation
- Safety and effectiveness of TOLAC and VBAC

ESTABLISH ADMISSION CRITERIA FOR WOMEN IN LABOR THAT
- Distinguish clinical manifestations for false labor, latent/early labor, and active labor
- Conduct admission assessments in a separate admissions area
- Send women in false or early/latent labor home or keep them in the admissions area
- Admit women in active labor to the labor and birth unit

USE APPROPRIATE ASSESSMENT TECHNIQUES TO
- Determine status of the maternal-fetal unit
- Establish an individualized rationale for initiating labor interventions such as epidural anesthesia, induction/augmentation, amniotomy, cesarean birth

INITIATE A DOULA PROGRAM THAT
- Provides one-to-one support for women in labor

DEVELOP A PHILOSOPHY OF LABOR MANAGEMENT THAT
- Schedules admission during active labor
- Avoids automatic interventions such as routine induction for spontaneous rupture of membranes at term or postterm pregnancy and cesarean birth for breech presentation, twin gestation, genital herpes, or failure to progress
- Relies on assessment findings reflective of the status of the maternal-fetal unit rather than strict adherence to set ranges for the duration of the stages and phases of labor
- Employs intermittent rather than continuous electronic fetal monitoring of low risk pregnant women
- Focuses on measures that are known to enhance the progress of labor such as upright positions, frequent position changes, ambulation, oral nutrition and hydration, relaxation techniques, hydrotherapy
- Emphasizes nonpharmacologic measures to relieve pain
- Uses nonpharmacologic measures in a manner that reduces their labor-inhibiting effects
- Establishes criteria for repeat elective cesarean birth and TOLAC

TOLAC, Trial of labor after cesarean; *VBAC,* vaginal birth after cesarean.

other woman (e.g., doula, relative, friend, nurse, or nurse-midwife). The greatest reduction in risk for cesarean birth occurs when this woman is not a member of the labor unit staff and is therefore able to spend all of her time providing physical and emotional support (Hodnett et al., 2005).

Indications. Few absolute indications exist for cesarean birth. Today, most are performed primarily for the benefit of the fetus. The most common indications for cesarean birth are related to labor and birth complications. The complications most closely associated with cesarean birth include CPD, malpresentations such as breech and shoulder, placental abnormalities (e.g., previa, abruptio), dysfunctional labor pattern, umbilical cord prolapse, fetal distress, and multiple gestation. Medical risk factors most closely associated with cesarean birth include hypertensive disorders, active genital herpes, positive HIV status, and diabetes (Martin et al., 2005).

Elective Cesarean Birth. Women are requesting cesarean births for reasons other than medical, obstetric, or fetal indications. These reasons include the belief that the surgery will prevent future problems with pelvic support or sexual dysfunction, convenience of planning a date, or having control and choice about when to give birth (Williams, 2005). Some multiparous women may request a cesarean after a previous traumatic vaginal birth or psychologic trauma (Gardner, 2003). In a committee opinion, the American College of Obstetricians and Gynecologists (ACOG) notes that the right of clients to refuse surgery is well known (ACOG, 2003b). It is less clear if they have the right to ask for surgery. The Society of Obstetricians and Gynaecologists of Canada (SOGC)

does not promote elective cesarean and promotes natural childbirth but believes that the final decision as to the safest route for childbirth rests with the woman and her health care provider (SOGC, 2004). It is essential that women are fully informed about the risks and benefits of cesarean birth when they consider requesting elective cesarean (McFarlin, 2004).

Ethical Consideration: Forced Cesarean Birth. A woman's refusal to undergo cesarean birth when indicated for fetal reasons is often described as a maternal-fetal conflict. Health care providers are ethically obliged to protect the well-being of both the mother and the fetus; a decision for one affects the other. If a woman refuses a cesarean birth that is recommended because of fetal jeopardy, health care providers must make every effort to find out why she is refusing and provide information that may persuade her to change her mind. If the woman continues to refuse surgery, then health care providers must decide if it is ethical to get a court order for the surgery; however, every effort should be made to avoid this legal step.

Surgical Techniques. The two main types of cesarean operation are the classic and the lower-segment cesarean incisions. Classic cesarean birth is rarely performed today, although it may be used when rapid birth is necessary and in some cases of shoulder presentation and placenta previa. The incision is made vertically into the upper body of the uterus (Fig. 36-13, *A*). Because the procedure is associated with a higher incidence of blood loss, infection, and uterine rupture in subsequent pregnancies than is lower-segment cesarean birth, vaginal birth after a classic cesarean birth is contraindicated.

SKIN INCISION   UTERINE INCISION

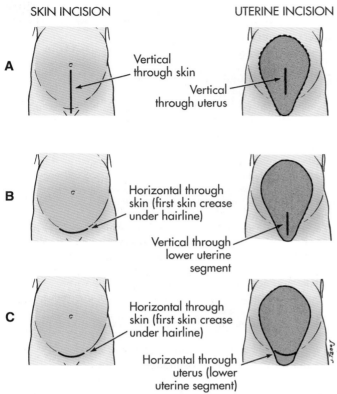

FIG. 36-13 Cesarean birth; skin and uterine incisions. **A,** Classic: vertical incisions of skin and uterus. **B,** Low cervical: horizontal incision of skin; vertical incision of uterus. **C,** Low cervical: horizontal incisions of skin and uterus.

Lower-segment cesarean birth can be achieved through a vertical or transverse incision into the uterus (Fig. 36-13, *B* and *C*). However, the transverse incision is more popular because it is easier to perform, is associated with less blood loss and fewer postoperative infections, and is less likely to rupture in subsequent pregnancies (Bowes & Thorp, 2004; Cunningham et al., 2005).

Complications and Risks. Cesarean births are not without complications for the mother and fetus. Maternal complications include aspiration, pulmonary embolism, wound infection, wound dehiscence, thrombophlebitis, hemorrhage, urinary tract infection, injuries to the bladder or bowel, and complications related to anesthesia. The fetus may be born prematurely if the gestational age has not been accurately determined; fetal injuries can occur during the surgery (Bowes & Thorp, 2004). Besides these risks, the woman is at economic risk because the cost of cesarean birth is higher than that of vaginal birth, and a longer recovery period may require additional expenditures.

Many women who have a cesarean birth speak of having feelings that interfere with their maintaining an adequate self-concept. These feelings include fear, disappointment, frustration at losing control, anger (the "why me" syndrome), and loss of self-esteem related to a change in body image and perceived inability to give birth as they had expected and hoped. Often women experience a delay in their ability to interact with their newborns after birth.

These women are less likely to breastfeed and may even have some difficulty expressing positive feelings about their newborns for some time after birth. They are often less satisfied with their childbirth experience, and report more fatigue and poorer physical functioning during the first few weeks after discharge. Success at mothering and in the recovery process can do much to restore the self-esteem of these women. Some women see the scar as mutilating, and worries concerning sexual attractiveness may surface. Some men are fearful of resuming intercourse because of the fear of hurting their partners. Parents may wonder if a cesarean birth was absolutely necessary, and such feelings may surface even years later. A clear explanation must be given to the woman and her family regarding why the cesarean birth was necessary. Additionally, opportunities should be provided to discuss the childbirth experience in an effort to resolve concerns that may arise after the birth.

Anesthesia. Spinal, epidural, and general anesthetics are used for cesarean births. Epidural blocks are popular because women want to be awake for and aware of the birth experience. However, the choice of anesthetic depends on several factors. The mother's medical history or present condition, such as a spinal injury, hemorrhage, or coagulopathy, may rule out the use of regional anesthesia. Time is another factor, especially if there is an emergency and the life of the mother or infant is at stake. In such a case, general anesthesia will most likely be used unless the woman already has an epidural block in effect. The woman herself is a factor. Either she may not know all the options or may have fears about having "a needle in her back" or about being awake and feeling pain. She needs to be fully informed about the risks and benefits of the different types of anesthesia so that she can participate in the decision whenever there is a choice.

Scheduled Cesarean Birth. Cesarean birth is scheduled or planned if labor and vaginal birth is contraindicated (e.g., complete placenta previa, active genital herpes, positive HIV status), if birth is necessary but labor is not inducible (e.g., hypertensive states that cause a poor intrauterine environment that threatens the fetus), or if this has been decided on by the primary health care provider and the woman (e.g., a repeat cesarean birth).

Women who are scheduled to have a cesarean birth have time to prepare for it psychologically. However, the psychologic responses of these women may differ. Those having a repeat cesarean birth may have disturbing memories of the conditions preceding the initial surgical birth (primary cesarean birth) and of their experiences in the postoperative recovery period. They may be concerned about the added burdens of caring for an infant and perhaps other children while recovering from a surgical operation. Others may feel glad that they have been relieved of the uncertainty about the date and time of the birth and are free of the pain of labor.

Unplanned Cesarean Birth. The psychosocial outcomes of unplanned or emergency cesarean birth are usually more pronounced and negative when compared with the outcomes associated with a scheduled or planned cesarean birth. Women and their families experience abrupt changes in their expectations for birth, postpartum care, and the care of the new baby at home. This may be an extremely traumatic experience for all.

The woman usually approaches the procedure tired and discouraged after an ineffective and difficult labor. Fear predominates as she worries about her own safety and well-being and that of her fetus. She may be dehydrated, with low glycogen reserves. Because preoperative procedures must be done quickly and competently, the time for explanation of the procedures and operation is often short. Because maternal and family anxiety levels are high at this time, much of what is said may be forgotten or misunderstood. The woman may experience feelings of anger or guilt in the postpartum period. Fatigue is often noticeable in these women, and they need much supportive care.

After surgery, counseling strategies that have been implemented by nurses include providing women with opportunities to talk about their birth experience, express feelings about what happened, have their questions answered, address gaps in knowledge or understanding of events, connect the event with emotions and behavior, and talk about future pregnancies. More research is needed to determine how effective these strategies are for these women in influencing their views about the unplanned cesarean birth experience or on future pregnancies (Gamble & Creedy, 2004).

Prenatal Preparation. Concerned professional and lay groups in the community have established councils for cesarean birth to meet the needs of these women and their families. Such groups advocate that a discussion of cesarean birth be included in all parenthood preparation classes. No woman can be guaranteed a vaginal birth, even if she is in good health and there is no indication of danger to the fetus before the onset of labor. For this reason, every woman needs to be aware of and prepared for the possibility of having a cesarean birth.

Childbirth educators stress the importance of emphasizing the similarities and differences between a cesarean and vaginal birth. In support of the philosophy of family-centered birth, many hospitals have instituted policies that permit fathers and other partners and family members to share in these births as they do in vaginal births. Women who have undergone cesarean birth agree that the continued presence and support of their partners helped them respond more positively to the entire experience. In addition to preparing women for the possibility of cesarean birth, childbirth educators should empower women to believe in their ability to give birth vaginally and to seek care measures during labor that will enhance the progress of their labors and reduce their risk for cesarean birth.

Preoperative Care. Family-centered care is the goal for the woman who is to undergo cesarean birth and for her family. The preparation of the woman for cesarean birth is the same as that done for other elective or emergency surgery. The primary health care provider discusses, with the woman and her family, the need for the cesarean

birth and the prognosis for the mother and infant. The anesthesiologist assesses the woman's cardiopulmonary system and describes the options for anesthesia. Informed consent is obtained for the procedure.

Blood and urine tests are usually done a day or two before a planned cesarean birth or on admission to the labor unit. Laboratory tests, most commonly ordered to establish baseline data, include a complete blood cell count and chemistry, blood typing and crossmatching, and urinalysis. Maternal vital signs and blood pressure and FHR and pattern should be assessed according to hospital protocol until the operation begins. Physical preoperative preparation usually includes inserting a retention (Foley) catheter to keep the bladder empty and administering prescribed preoperative medications. Although uncommon, the primary health care provider may order an abdominal-mons shave or a clipping of pubic hair. In the event that general anesthesia will be used, an antacid, administered orally to neutralize gastric secretions in case of aspiration, is a beneficial form of care (Enkin et al., 2000). Intravenous fluids are started to maintain hydration and to provide an open line for the administration of blood or medications if needed.

Removal of dentures, nail polish, and jewelry may be optional, depending on hospital policies and type of anesthesia used. If the woman wears glasses and is going to be awake, the nurse should make sure her glasses accompany her to the operating room so she can see her infant. If the woman wears contact lenses, the nurse can find out whether they can be worn for the birth.

During the preoperative preparation, the support person is encouraged to remain with the woman as much as possible to provide continuing emotional support (if this action is culturally acceptable to the woman and support person). The nurse provides essential information about the preoperative procedures during this time. Although the nursing actions may be carried out quickly if a cesarean birth is unplanned, verbal communication, particularly explanations, is important. Silence can be frightening to the woman and her support person. The nurse's use of touch can communicate feelings of care and concern for the woman. The nurse can assess the woman's and her partner's perceptions about cesarean birth (e.g., the woman feels that she is a failure because she did not have a vaginal birth). As the woman expresses her feelings, the nurse may identify a potential for a disturbance in self-concept during the postpartum period that may need to be addressed. If there is time before the birth, the nurse can teach the woman about postoperative expectations and about pain relief, turning, coughing, and deep-breathing measures.

Intraoperative Care. Cesarean births occur in operating rooms in the hospital's surgical unit or in the labor and birth unit. Once the woman has been taken to the operating room, her care becomes the responsibility of the obstetric team, the surgeon, the anesthesiologist, the pediatrician, and the surgical nursing staff (Fig. 36-14). If possible, the partner, who is dressed appropriately for the operating room, accompanies the mother to the operating room and

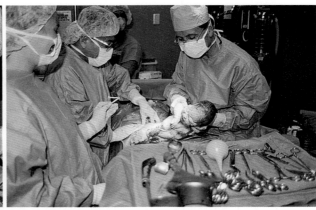

FIG. 36-14 Cesarean birth. **A,** "Bikini" incision has been made, the muscle layer is separated, the abdomen is entered, and the uterus has been exposed and incised; suctioning of amniotic fluid continues as head is brought up through the incision. Note small amount of bleeding. **B,** The neonate's birth through the uterine incision is nearly complete. **C,** A quick assessment is performed; note extreme molding of head resulting from cephalopelvic disproportion. (Courtesy Marjorie Pyle, RNC, Lifecircle, Costa Mesa, CA.)

remains close to her so that continued support and comfort can be provided. In unplanned cesarean birth, the nurse who cared for the woman during labor should be part of the nursing care team in the operating room if possible.

The nurse who is circulating may assist with positioning the woman on the birth (surgical) table. It is important to position her so that the uterus is displaced laterally to prevent compression of the inferior vena cava, which causes decreased placental perfusion. This is usually accomplished by placing a wedge under the hip. A Foley catheter is inserted into the bladder at this time if one is not already in place.

If the partner is not allowed or chooses not to be present, the nurse can stay in communication with him or her and give progress reports whenever possible. If the woman is awake during the birth, the nurse, anesthesiologist, or both can tell her what is happening and provide support. She may be anxious about the sensations she is experiencing, such as the coldness of solutions used to prepare the abdomen and pressure or pulling during the actual birth of the infant. She also may be apprehensive because of the bright lights or the presence of unfamiliar equipment and masked and gowned personnel in the room. Explanations by the nurse can help to decrease the woman's anxiety.

Care of the infant usually is delegated to a pediatrician or a nurse team skilled in neonatal resuscitation, because these infants are considered to be at risk until there is evidence of physiologic stability after the birth.

A crib with resuscitation equipment is readied before surgery. Those responsible for care are expert not only in resuscitative techniques but also in their ability to detect normal and abnormal infant responses. After birth, if the infant's condition permits and the mother is awake, the baby may be placed skin-to-skin on the mother or can be given to the woman's partner to hold (Fig. 36-15). The infant whose condition is compromised is transported after initial stabilization to the nursery for observation and the implementation of appropriate interventions. In some hospitals, the partner may accompany the infant; if not, personnel keep the family informed of the infant's progress, and parent-infant contacts are initiated as soon as possible.

If the family cannot accompany the woman during surgery, the family is directed to the surgical or obstetric waiting room. The physician then reports on the condition of the mother and child to the family members after the birth is completed. Family members may accompany the infant as she or he is transferred to the nursery, giving them an opportunity to see and admire the new baby.

▬ LEGAL TIP   Client Confidentiality

Some mothers/parents want the privilege of informing family and friends of the sex of the infant (if it was not known before birth). Before responding to requests for such information from people waiting outside the birthing area, the nurse should check to see if the mother has given consent for such information to be released and to whom.

Immediate Postoperative Care. Once surgery is completed, the mother is transferred to a recovery room or back to her labor room. After a cesarean birth, women

FIG. 36-15 A, Parents and their newborn. The physician manually removes the placenta, suctions the remaining amniotic fluid and blood from the uterine cavity, and closes the uterine incision, peritoneum, muscle layer, fatty tissue, and finally the skin, while the new family shares some time together. **B,** Parents become better acquainted with their newborn while mother rests after surgery. (Courtesy Marjorie Pyle, RNC, Lifecircle, Costa Mesa, CA.)

have both postoperative and postpartum needs that must be addressed. They are surgical clients as well as new mothers. Nursing assessments in this immediate postbirth period follow agency protocol and include degree of recovery from the effects of anesthesia, postoperative and postbirth status, and degree of pain. If general anesthesia was administered, it is essential that a patent airway be maintained, and the woman positioned to prevent possible aspiration until she is fully alert and responsive. Vital signs are taken every 15 minutes for 1 to 2 hours, or until stable. The condition of the incisional dressing and the fundus and the amount of lochia are assessed, as well as the intravenous intake and the urine output through the retention (Foley) catheter. The woman is helped to turn and do coughing, deep-breathing, and leg exercises. Medications to relieve pain may be administered.

If the baby is present, the mother and her partner are given some time alone with him or her to facilitate bonding and attachment. Breastfeeding can be initiated if the mother feels like trying. If the woman is in a recovery area or in her labor room, she usually is transferred to the postpartum unit after 1 to 2 hours, or once her condition is stable and the effects of anesthesia have worn off (i.e., she is alert, oriented, and able to feel and move extremities) (see Care Path).

Postoperative/Postpartum Care. The attitude of the nurse and other health team members can influence the woman's perception of herself after a cesarean birth. The caregivers should stress that the woman is a new mother first and a surgical client second. This attitude helps the woman perceive herself as having the same problems and needs as other new mothers, while requiring supportive postoperative care.

The woman's physiologic concerns for the first few days may be dominated by pain at the incision site and pain resulting from intestinal gas, and hence the need for pain relief. If epidural anesthesia was used for the surgery, epidural opioids can be given in the immediate postoperative period to provide pain relief for approximately 24 hours. Otherwise, pain medications usually are given parenterally (e.g., intravenously, intramuscularly) every 3 to 4 hours, or patient-controlled analgesia (PCA) may be ordered instead. The most commonly used analgesics include opioids (e.g., hydromorphone, nalbuphine) and NSAIDs (e.g., ketorolac [Toradol]). If opioids are used, an antiemetic (e.g., metoclopramide [Reglan]) is often ordered to be administered either as needed by the woman or around the clock as long as the opioid is used. Other comfort measures such as position changes, splinting of the incision with pillows, and relaxation and breathing techniques (e.g., those learned in childbirth classes) may be implemented.

Women are often the best judges of what their bodies need and can tolerate, including the postoperative ingestion of foods and fluids. If desired by the woman, the early introduction of solid food is safe. Women who eat early have been found to require less analgesia, and gastrointestinal problems do not occur (Abrams, Minassian, & Pickett, 2004). Ambulation and rocking in a rocking chair may relieve gas pains, and avoiding the consumption of gas-forming foods and carbonated beverages may help minimize them (Thomas et al., 1990) (see Teaching for Self-Care box).

Nurses must be alert to a woman's physiologic needs, managing care to ensure adequate rest and pain relief. Mother-baby care (couplet care) for a cesarean birth mother may have to be modified according to her physiologic limitations as a surgical client.

Daily care includes perineal care, breast care, and routine hygienic care, including showering after the dressing has been removed (if showering is acceptable according to the woman's cultural beliefs and practices). The nurse

Text continued on p. 964.

care path ▶ **Cesarean Birth Without Complications: Expected Length of Stay—48 to 72 Hours**

	IMMEDIATE POSTOP CESAREAN	BY FOURTH HOUR AFTER ADMISSION TO PP UNIT	5 TO 24 HOURS	25 TO 48 HOURS	BY DISCHARGE
ASSESSMENTS	Recovery room or PACU admission assessment complete	PP admission assessment and care plan completed			
Vital Signs	q15min × 1 hr; q30min × 4 hr, WNL	q1h × 3, WNL	q4-8h, WNL	q4-8h, WNL	q8h, WNL
Postpartum Assessment	q15min × 1 hr, WNL	q1h × 3, WNL	q4-8h, WNL	q8-12h, WNL	q8-12h, WNL
Abdominal Incision	Dressing dry and intact	Dressing dry and intact	Dressing dry and intact	Dressing off or changed, incision intact	Incision intact; staples may be removed and Steri-Strips in place, incision WNL
Genitourinary	Retention catheter output >30 ml/hr	Retention catheter output >30 ml/hr	Retention catheter output >30 ml/hr; usually discontinued by 24 hours	Catheter discontinued, output >100 ml/void or 240 ml/8 hr	Urine output >240 ml/8 hr
Gastrointestinal		Absent or hypoactive BS	Hypoactive to active BS	Active BS + flatus	Active BS + flatus; may or may not have BM
Musculoskeletal	Alert or easily aroused, can move legs	Alert and oriented, moving all extremities	Ambulating with help	Ambulating unassisted	Ambulating ad lib
Bonding	Evidence of parent-infant bonding; first breastfeeding if desired		Parent-infant bonding continues	Parent-infant bonding progressing	
Laboratory Tests			Intrapartal CBC results on chart or computer; determine Rh status and need for anti-Rh globulin; check for rubella immunity	PP HCT WNL, give anti-Rh globulin if indicated	Give rubella vaccine if indicated
INTERVENTIONS					
IV	IV continues	IV continues	IV continues	IV may be discontinued	
Diet	NPO	Ice chips, sips of clear liquids	Clear liquids	Regular diet or as tolerated	Regular diet
Perineal		Pericare by nurse	Pericare with help	Self-pericare	
Activity	Bed rest	Bed rest	OOB × 3 with help, ADLs assisted, assisted to comfortable position to hold and feed baby	Holds baby comfortably, ambulates without assistance, ADLs unassisted	Activity ad lib

ADLs, Activities of daily living; *BS*, bowel sounds; *BM*, bowel movement; *CBC*, complete blood count; *HCT*, hematocrit; *IM*, intramuscular; *IV*, intravenous; *NPO*, nothing by mouth; *NSAIDs*, nonsteroidal antiinflammatory drugs; *OOB*, out of bed; *PACU*, postanesthesia care unit; *PCA*, patient-controlled analgesia;

	IMMEDIATE POSTOP CESAREAN	BY FOURTH HOUR AFTER ADMISSION TO PP UNIT	5 TO 24 HOURS	25 TO 48 HOURS	BY DISCHARGE
Pulmonary Care	Bed rest Patent airway; O$_2$ discontinued	TCDB q2h with splinting, incentive spirometry q1h if ordered, lungs clear	TCDB q2h, continue incentive spirometry if ordered while awake; lungs clear	TCDB as needed; lungs clear	
Medications	Oxytocin added to IV Pain control: analgesics, IV, or epidural narcotic as ordered	Oxytocin continued Pain control: analgesics—PCA, IV, IM, PO, or epidural narcotic as ordered	Oxytocin may be discontinued Pain control: IV, IM, PO, PCA narcotics or analgesics as needed	Oxytocin discontinued Pain control: PO analgesics, NSAIDs as needed; PCA discontinued; stool softener, PNV as ordered	Rx filled or given to take home
Teaching, Discharge Plan	Breastfeeding, positioning, leg exercises	Verbalize understanding and unit routines, how to achieve rest, TCDB, involution, pain control	*Self:* comfort measures and care; reinforce TCDB and positioning; introduce teaching videos, lactation promotion or suppression *Infant:* handwashing, infant safety, positioning for feeding and burping; if breastfeeding, then positioning baby, latching on, timing, removing from breast	*Self:* diet; activity and rest; bowel and bladder function; perineal care *Infant:* bonding; parent concerns; feeding; infant bath, cord care; need for car seat; newborn characteristics; circumcision care if procedure performed; answer questions	*Self:* home care, signs of complications (infections, bleeding), normal psychologic adjustments, normal ADLs; resumption of sexual activities; contraception; identification of support system at home; self-concept issues related to cesarean birth. Inform whom to call if problems; review need to keep follow-up appointment; provide information about community resources; provide copy of home care instructions *Infant:* parents to demonstrate infant care; reinforce use of booklets for infant care, whom to call if problems; discuss immunization needs; review need to keep follow-up appointments

PNV, prenatal vitamins; *PO,* nothing by mouth; *Postop,* postoperative; *PP,* postpartum; *Rx,* prescription; *TCDB,* turn, cough, deep breathe; *WNL,* within normal limits.

TEACHING FOR SELF-CARE

Postpartum Pain Relief After Cesarean Birth

INCISIONAL
- Splint incision with a pillow when moving or coughing.
- Use relaxation techniques such as music, breathing, and dim lights.

GAS
- Walk as often as you can.
- Do not eat or drink gas-forming foods, carbonated beverages, or whole milk.
- Do not use straws for drinking fluids.
- Take antiflatulence medication if prescribed.
- Lie on your left side to expel gas.
- Rock in a rocking chair.

assesses the woman's vital signs, incision, fundus, and lochia according to hospital policies, procedures, or protocols. Breath sounds, bowel sounds, circulatory status of lower extremities, and urinary and bowel elimination also are assessed. It is important to note maternal emotional status.

During the postpartum period, the nurse also can provide care that meets the psychologic and learning needs of mothers who have had cesarean births. The nurse can explain postpartum procedures to help the woman participate in her recovery from surgery. The nurse can help the woman plan care and visits from family and friends that will allow adequate rest periods. Information on and assistance with infant care can facilitate adjustment to her role as a mother. The woman is supported as she breastfeeds her baby by receiving individualized assistance to comfortably hold and position the baby at her breast. The side-lying position and the use of pillows to support the newborn can enhance comfort and facilitate successful breastfeeding. The partner can be included in infant teaching sessions, and in explanations about the woman's recovery. The couple also should be encouraged to express their feelings about the birth experience. Some parents are angry, frustrated, or disappointed that a vaginal birth was not possible. Some women express feelings of low self-esteem or a negative self-image. Others express relief and gratitude that the baby is healthy and safely born. It may be helpful for them to have the nurse who was present during the birth visit and help fill in "gaps" about the experience. Other psychologic and lifestyle concerns that have been reported include depression, feeling limited in activities, and changes in family interactions (Gamble & Creedy, 2004).

Discharge after cesarean birth is usually by the third postoperative day. The time is often determined by criteria established by the woman's insurance carrier or the federal government (e.g., diagnosis-related groups [DRGs]). The Newborn's and Mother's Health Protection Act of 1996 provides for a length of stay of up to 96 hours for cesarean births. These criteria may not coincide with the woman's physical or psychosocial readiness for discharge. Some states have added home care provisions for mothers who meet appropriate criteria for discharge and choose to leave sooner than the allowed length of stay. This policy recognizes that home care is less costly than hospital care and in most cases is more beneficial for recovery.

In the limited amount of time available before discharge, the nurse needs to provide discharge teaching to prepare women for self-care and newborn care while, at the same time, trying to ensure that the woman is comfortable and able to rest. The nurse must assess the woman's information needs and coordinate the health care team's efforts to meet them.

Discharge teaching and planning should include information about nutrition; measures to relieve pain and discomfort; exercise and specific activity restrictions; time management that includes periods of uninterrupted rest and sleep; hygiene, breast, and incision care; timing for resumption of sexual activity and contraception; signs of complications (see Teaching for Self-Care boxes) and infant care. The nurse assesses the woman's need for continued support or counseling to facilitate her emotional recovery from the birth. The woman's family and friends should be educated regarding her needs during the recovery process, and their assistance should be coordinated before discharge. Referral to support groups (e.g., www.birthrites.org) or to community agencies may be indicated to promote the recovery process further. A postdischarge program of telephone follow-up and home visits can facilitate the woman's full recovery after cesarean birth.

▬ Vaginal Birth After Cesarean

Indications for primary cesarean birth, such as dystocia, breech presentation, or fetal distress, often are nonrecurring. Therefore a woman who has had a cesarean birth may subsequently become pregnant and not have any contraindications to labor and vaginal birth in that pregnancy and may attempt a vaginal birth after cesarean (VBAC).

ACOG (2004a) encourages a trial of labor after cesarean (TOLAC) and VBAC attempt in women who have had one previous cesarean birth by low transverse incision, an adequate pelvis, and no other uterine scars or previous rupture. In addition, a physician must be available throughout active labor and capable of performing an emergency ce-

TEACHING FOR SELF-CARE

Signs of Postoperative Complications After Discharge

Report the following signs to your health care provider:
- Temperature exceeding 38° C
- Painful urination
- Lochia heavier than a normal period
- Wound separation
- Redness or oozing at the incision site
- Severe abdominal pain

sarean birth. TOLAC is relatively safe, but there is a reported risk for uterine rupture of less than 1% compared to a uterine rupture risk of 0.03% to 0.2% with a repeat elective cesarean birth (O'Brien-Abel, 2003) through a lower uterine segment scar. Increased reports of uterine rupture in the United States and Canada in the 1990s have raised concerns about the safety of TOLAC and VBAC. The incidence of uterine rupture appears to be related to the method of the second labor and birth. The rate of uterine rupture is lowest with spontaneous vaginal birth and highest when labor is induced, especially if prostaglandins are used to ripen the cervix. Other factors have been identified that appear to increase the risk of uterine rupture. These risk factors include prior classic uterine incision extending into the fundus, single-layer rather than double-layer uterine closure, 2 or more previous cesarean births, an interdelivery interval of 18 to 24 months or less, maternal age of 30 years or older, postpartum fever, and CPD (Bowes & Thorpe, 2004; Lydon-Rochelle, Hold, Easterling, & Martin, 2001; O'Brien-Abel, 2003; Shipp, 2004).

Women are most often the primary decision makers with regard to choice of birth method. During the antepartal period, the woman should be given information about VBAC and encouraged to choose it as an alternative to repeat cesarean birth, as long as no contraindications exist (Ridley, Davis, Bright, & Sinclair, 2002). VBAC support groups (e.g., www.vbac.com) and prenatal classes can help prepare the woman psychologically for labor and vaginal birth. Women need to believe not only that their efforts during a TOLAC will be successful but also that they are fully capable of doing what is necessary to give birth vaginally (self-efficacy). They must be given the opportunity to discuss their previous labor experience, including feelings of failure and loss of control, and to express concern they may have about how they will manage during their upcoming labor and birth.

This labor should occur in a hospital facility that has the equipment and personnel available to begin the surgery within 30 minutes from the time a decision is made to perform cesarean birth. Therefore, women are strongly advised against attempting VBACs in birth centers (Lieberman, Ernst, Rooks, Stapleton, & Flamm, 2004). Ideally the woman is admitted to the labor unit at the onset of spontaneous labor. In the latent phase of labor, the nurse encourages her to engage in normal activities such as ambulation. In the active phase of labor, FHR and pattern and uterine activity usually are monitored electronically. Nonreassuring FHR patterns (e.g., prolonged decelerations, variable decelerations, and late decelerations) often precede rupture or signal its occurrence. The woman may complain of abdominal, shoulder, or back pain even with an epidural and may exhibit signs of excessive blood loss (Dauphinee, 2004; O'Brien-Abel, 2003). Intravenous access such as a saline lock may be established. The physician or nurse-midwife should be immediately available during active labor.

There is no evidence that administering oxytocin to induce or augment labor or the use of epidural anesthesia is contraindicated, although caution and close monitoring of the laboring woman are urged if these are used (Bowes & Thorp, 2004; Cunningham et al., 2005). However, use of prostaglandins, especially misoprostol (prostaglandin E_1), to ripen the cervix or induce labor is not recommended because they have been associated with an increased risk for uterine rupture (ACOG, 2004a).

Attention should be paid to the woman's psychologic, as well as physical, needs during the TOLAC. Anxiety increases the release of catecholamines and can inhibit the release of oxytocin, thus delaying the progress of labor and possibly leading to a repeat cesarean birth. To alleviate such anxiety, the nurse can encourage the woman to use breathing and relaxation techniques and to change positions to promote labor progress. The woman's partner can be encouraged to provide comfort measures and emotional support. Collaboration among the woman in labor, her partner, the nurse, and other health care providers often results in a successful VBAC. If a TOLAC does not proceed to vaginal birth, the woman will need support and encouragement to express her feelings about having another cesarean birth. It is very important that this outcome not be labeled a failed VBAC. (See Chapter 21 for a full discussion of labor support measures).

CRITICAL THINKING EXERCISE

TOLAC and VBAC

Marie (2-1-0-0-1), a 28-year-old pregnant woman at 32 weeks of gestation, is unsure about how she should give birth. Three years ago she had a cesarean birth with her first pregnancy because of fetal distress. Marie would like to try to have a vaginal birth this time but is afraid that something will go wrong. She asks the nurse at a prenatal visit for help in making the right decision and for advice about what she can do to enhance her chances for a safe vaginal birth. In reviewing Marie's obstetric history the nurse notes that she had a lower segment transverse incision and an uneventful postoperative course with no complications including infection. Her current pregnancy has been progressing well without problems. How should the nurse respond to Marie's request for guidance in making a decision about her upcoming childbirth?

1. Evidence—Is there sufficient evidence to guide Marie in making a decision that will ensure her safety and that of her fetus?
2. Assumptions—What assumptions can be made about the following issues related to TOLAC and VBAC?
   a. Risks Marie faces if she chooses a TOLAC with the goal of a spontaneous vaginal birth
   b. Criteria that Marie should meet to reduce her risk for uterine rupture
   c. Labor management techniques that should be avoided
3. How should the nurse address Marie's request for information about enhancing her chances for a safe vaginal birth?
4. Does the evidence objectively support the nurse's response to Marie's request?
5. Are there alternative perspectives to your conclusion?

TOLAC, Trial of labor after cesarean; *VBAC,* vaginal birth after cesarean.

Evolve/CD: Case Study: Postterm Pregnancy

■ Evaluation

To evaluate the effectiveness of nursing care for a woman experiencing dystocia, the nurse reviews the expected outcomes of care that were met and assesses the woman's and the family's level of satisfaction with the care received.

■ POSTTERM PREGNANCY, LABOR, AND BIRTH

A postterm or postdate pregnancy is one that extends beyond the end of week 42 of gestation, or 294 days from the first day of the last menstrual period. The incidence of postterm pregnancy is estimated to be between 4% and 14%, with an average of 10% (Resnik & Resnik, 2004). In 2003, more than 52% of women gave birth between 27 to 39 weeks of gestation compared to 36% at 40 weeks or later. This represents a trend in recent years away from a watchful waiting approach as women pass their expected date of birth toward use of management techniques such as induction of labor and cesarean birth (Martin et al., 2005).

Many pregnancies are misdiagnosed as prolonged. This can occur because (1) the pregnancy is inaccurately dated because the woman has an irregular menstrual cycle pattern, (2) an accurate date of the last menstrual period is unknown, or (3) entry into prenatal care was delayed or did not occur.

Although the exact cause of true postterm pregnancy is still unknown, a possible cause may be deficiency of placental estrogen and continued secretion of progesterone. Low levels of estrogen may result in a decrease in prostaglandin precursors and reduced formation of oxytocin receptors in the myometrium (Gilbert & Harmon, 2003). A woman who experiences one postterm pregnancy is more likely to experience it again in subsequent pregnancies (Divon, 2002).

Clinical manifestations of postterm pregnancy include maternal weight loss (more than 1.4 kg/wk) and decreased uterine size (related to decreased amniotic fluid), meconium in the amniotic fluid, and advanced bone maturation of the fetal skeleton with an exceptionally hard fetal skull (Gilbert & Harmon, 2003).

Maternal and Fetal Risks

Maternal risks are often related to the birth of an excessively large infant. The woman is at increased risk for dysfunctional labor; birth canal trauma, including perineal lacerations and extension of episiotomy during vaginal birth; postpartum hemorrhage; and infection. Interventions such as induction of labor with prostaglandins or oxytocin, forceps- or vacuum-assisted birth, and cesarean birth (i.e., double the rate) are more likely to be necessary. The woman also may experience fatigue and psychologic reactions such as depression, frustration, and feelings of inadequacy as she passes her estimated date of birth (ACOG, 2004b; Gilbert & Harmon, 2003).

Fetal risks appear to be twofold. The first is the possibility of prolonged labor, shoulder dystocia, birth trauma, and asphyxia from macrosomia. Macrosomia occurs when the placenta continues to provide adequate nutrients to support fetal growth after 40 weeks of gestation. It is estimated to occur in approximately 25% of prolonged pregnancies (Divon, 2002). The second risk is the compromising effects on the fetus of an "aging" placenta. Placental function gradually decreases after 37 weeks of gestation. Amniotic fluid volume (AFV) declines to approximately 800 ml by 40 weeks of gestation and to about 400 ml by 42 weeks of gestation. The resulting oligohydramnios can lead to fetal hypoxia related to cord compression. If placental insufficiency is present, there is a high likelihood of non-reassuring fetal status occurring during labor. Neonatal problems may include asphyxia, meconium aspiration syndrome, dysmaturity syndrome, hypoglycemia, polycythemia, and respiratory distress (Gilbert & Harmon, 2003). Whether an infant born after a postterm pregnancy has neurologic, behavioral, intellectual, or developmental problems must be further investigated (ACOG, 2004b).

Collaborative Care

The management of postterm pregnancy is still controversial. The induction of labor at 41 to 42 weeks is suggested by some authorities as a means of reducing the rate of cesarean birth and stillbirth or neonatal death (Resnik & Resnik, 2004). Others follow a more individualized approach, allowing the pregnancy to proceed to 43 weeks of gestation as long as assessment of fetal well-being with a combination of tests is performed, and the results of the tests are normal. Tests are usually performed on a weekly or twice-weekly basis (Divon, 2002; Myers et al., 2002; Searing, 2001).

Antepartum assessments for postterm pregnancy may include daily fetal movement counts, NSTs, AFV assessments, contraction stress tests (CSTs), biophysical profiles (BPPs), and Doppler flow measurements. The BPP may be the best way of gauging fetal well-being because it combines nonstress testing with real-time ultrasound scanning to assess fetal movements, fetal breathing movements, and the AFV. The woman and her family should be fully informed regarding the tests, including why they are performed and the meaning of the results obtained in terms of the health of the mother and fetus (ACOG, 2004b).

Determining the amniotic fluid index (AFI) is critical in women with postterm pregnancies because a decrease in the amount of amniotic fluid (i.e., oligohydramnios) has been associated with fetal stress as a result of umbilical cord compression. The AFI should be greater than 8, with at least one pocket of amniotic fluid greater than 2 cm, and amniotic fluid should be present throughout the uterine cavity (Gilbert & Harmon, 2003).

Cervical checks usually are performed weekly after 40 weeks of gestation to determine whether the condition of the cervix is favorable for induction (see Table 36-3). Vaginal secretions may be assessed for the amount of fetal fibronectin; a low concentration may predict increased risk for prolonged pregnancy, but results of studies have thus far been inconclusive (Divon, 2002; Gilbert & Harmon, 2003).

During the postterm period, the woman is encouraged to assess fetal activity daily, assess for signs of labor, and keep appointments with her primary health care provider (see Teaching for Self-Care). The woman and her family should be encouraged to express their feelings (e.g., frustration, anger, impatience, fear) about the prolonged pregnancy and should be helped to realize that these feelings are normal. At times the emotional and physical strain of a postterm pregnancy may seem insurmountable. Referral to a support group or another supportive resource may be needed.

If the woman's cervix is favorable, expectant management can be followed but labor is usually induced with oxytocin. If the cervix is not favorable, continued fetal surveillance or a cervical ripening agent (e.g., prostaglandin insert or gel) may be administered, followed by oxytocin induction (ACOG, 2004b; Gilbert & Harmon, 2003; Resnik & Resnik, 2004).

The fetus of a woman with a postterm pregnancy should be monitored electronically for a more accurate assessment of the FHR and pattern. Inadequate fluid volume leads to compression of the cord, which results in fetal hypoxia that is reflected in variable or prolonged deceleration patterns and passage of meconium. If oligohydramnios is present, an amnioinfusion may be performed to restore amniotic fluid volume to maintain a cushioning of the cord. The use of amnioinfusion to treat fetal distress associated with oligohydramnios in labor is a form of care likely to be beneficial. However, it is likely to be ineffective or harmful to perform an amnioinfusion prophylactically (Enkin et al., 2000).

Amnioinfusion may be used to prevent or minimize meconium aspiration syndrome (MAS) by diluting amniotic fluid thickened with meconium passed by a hypoxic fetus. Maternal-fetal risks related to amnioinfusion, although rare, can result from infection and overdistension of the uterine cavity with infused fluid (Gilbert & Harmon, 2003). Accurate assessment of the woman's labor pattern also is important because dysfunctional labor is common.

Emotional support is essential for the woman with a postterm pregnancy and her family. A vaginal birth is anticipated, but the couple should be prepared for a forceps-assisted, vacuum-assisted, or cesarean birth if complications arise. Expected outcomes of care include that the woman and her family use appropriate coping mechanisms to deal with the emotional aspects of her postterm pregnancy and that the woman and her newborn experience no injury during the birth.

▪ OBSTETRIC EMERGENCIES

Shoulder Dystocia

Shoulder dystocia is an uncommon obstetric emergency that increases the risk for fetal/neonatal and maternal morbidity and mortality during the attempt to deliver the fetus vaginally. It is estimated that 0.6% to 1.4% of all vaginal births are complicated by shoulder dystocia (ACOG, 2002b; Bowes & Thorp, 2004; Jevitt, 2005). In this type of dystocia, the head is born, but the anterior shoulder cannot pass under the pubic arch. Fetopelvic disproportion related to excessive fetal size (greater than 4000 g) or maternal pelvic abnormalities may be a cause of shoulder dystocia, although shoulder dystocia can occur in the absence of any known risk factors. There are no accurate methods to predict or to help prevent shoulder dystocia. The nurse should be observant for signs that could indicate the presence of shoulder dystocia, including slowing of the progress of labor and formation of a caput succedaneum that increases in size. When the head emerges, it retracts against the perineum (turtle sign), and external rotation does not occur (ACOG, 2002b; Bowes & Thorp, 2004; Jevitt, 2005).

The fetus and/or newborn is more likely to experience birth injuries related to asphyxia, brachial plexus damage, and fracture, especially of the humerus or clavicle. The mother's primary risk stems from excessive blood loss as a result of uterine atony or rupture, lacerations, extension of the episiotomy, or endometritis.

Collaborative Care

Many maneuvers such as suprapubic pressure and maternal position changes have been suggested and tried to free the anterior shoulder, although no one particular maneuver has been found to be most effective (Bowes & Thorp, 2004). Suprapubic pressure can be applied to the anterior shoulder by using the Mazzanti or Ruben technique (Fig. 36-16) in an attempt to push the shoulder under the symphysis pubis (Baskett, 2002).

In the McRoberts maneuver (Fig. 36-17), the woman's legs are flexed apart, with her knees on her abdomen (Baskett, 2002; Baxley & Gobbo, 2004; Cunningham et al., 2005). This maneuver causes the sacrum to straighten, and the symphysis pubis rotates toward the mother's head; the angle of pelvic inclination is decreased, freeing the shoulder. Suprapubic pressure can be applied at this time. The McRoberts maneuver is the preferred method when a woman is receiving epidural anesthesia.

Having the woman move to a hands-and-knees position (the Gaskin maneuver), a squatting position, or lateral recumbent position also has been used to resolve cases of shoulder dystocia (Baskett, 2002; Bowes & Thorp, 2004; Jevitt, 2005).

TEACHING FOR SELF-CARE

Postterm Pregnancy

- Perform daily fetal movement counts.
- Assess for signs of labor.
- Call your primary health care provider if your membranes rupture, or if you perceive a decrease in or no fetal movement.
- Keep appointments for fetal assessment tests or cervical checks.
- Come to the hospital soon after labor begins.

A   **B**

FIG. 36-16 Application of suprapubic pressure. **A,** Mazzanti technique. Pressure is applied directly posteriorly and laterally above the symphysis pubis. **B,** Rubin technique. Pressure is applied obliquely posteriorly against the anterior shoulder.

FIG. 36-17 McRoberts maneuver. (Modified from Gabbe, S., Niebyl, J., & Simpson, J. [2002]. *Obstetrics: Normal and problem pregnancies* [4ᵗʰ ed.]. New York: Churchill Livingstone.)

Fundal pressure is usually not advised as a method of relieving shoulder dystocia (Nocon, 2000; Simpson & Knox, 2001).

When shoulder dystocia is diagnosed, the nurse helps the woman to assume the position(s) that may facilitate birth of the shoulders, assists the primary health care provider with these maneuvers and techniques during birth, and documents the maneuvers. The nurse also provides encouragement and support to reduce anxiety and fear.

Newborn assessment should include examination for fracture of the clavicle or humerus as well as brachial plexus injuries and asphyxia (Bowes & Thorp, 2004). Maternal as-

sessment should focus on early detection of hemorrhage and trauma to the soft tissue of the birth canal.

Prolapsed Umbilical Cord

Prolapse of the umbilical cord occurs when the cord lies below the presenting part of the fetus. In 2003, prolapse of the umbilical cord occurred in 1.7% of 1000 live births (Martin et al., 2005). Umbilical cord prolapse may be occult (hidden, not visible) at any time during labor whether or not the membranes are ruptured (Fig. 36-18, *A* and *B*). It is most common to see frank (visible) prolapse directly after rupture of membranes, when gravity washes the cord in front of the presenting part (Fig. 36-18, *C* and *D*). Contributing factors include a long cord (longer than 100 cm), malpresentation (breech), transverse lie, or unengaged presenting part.

If the presenting part does not fit snugly into the lower uterine segment (e.g., as in hydramnios), a sudden gush of amniotic fluid that occurs when the membranes rupture may cause the cord to be displaced downward. Similarly the cord may prolapse during amniotomy if the presenting part is high. A small fetus may not fit snugly into the lower uterine segment; as a result, cord prolapse is more likely to occur.

Collaborative Care

Prompt recognition of a prolapsed umbilical cord is important because fetal hypoxia resulting from prolonged cord compression (i.e., occlusion of blood flow to and from the fetus for more than 5 minutes) usually results in central nervous system damage or death of the fetus. Pressure on the cord may be relieved by the examiner putting a sterile gloved hand into the vagina and holding the presenting part off of the umbilical cord (Fig. 36-19, *A* and *B*). The woman is assisted into a position such as a modified Sims (Fig. 36-19, *C*), Trendelenburg, or knee-chest (Fig. 36-19, *D*) position, in which gravity keeps the

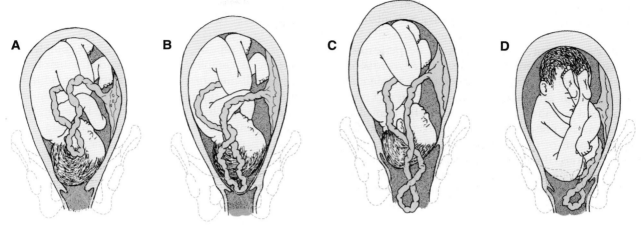

FIG. 36-18 Prolapse of umbilical cord. Note pressure of presenting part on umbilical cord, which endangers fetal circulation. **A,** Occult (hidden) prolapse of cord. **B,** Complete prolapse of cord. Note that membranes are intact. **C,** Cord presenting in front of the fetal head may be seen in vagina. **D,** Frank breech presentation with prolapsed cord.

FIG. 36-19 *Arrows* indicate direction of pressure against presenting part to relieve compression of prolapsed umbilical cord. Pressure exerted by examiner's fingers in **A,** vertex presentation, and **B,** breech presentation. **C,** Gravity relieves pressure when woman is in modified Sims position with hips elevated as high as possible with pillows. **D,** Knee-chest position.

pressure of the presenting part off the cord. If the cervix is fully dilated, a forceps- or vacuum-assisted birth can be performed for the fetus in a cephalic presentation; otherwise, a cesarean birth is likely to be performed. Nonreassuring FHR and pattern (e.g., bradycardia, diminished variability, variable deceleration), inadequate uterine relaxation, and bleeding also can occur as a result of a prolapsed umbilical cord. Indications for immediate interventions are presented in the Emergency box. Ongoing assessment of the woman and her fetus is critical to determine the effectiveness of each action taken. The woman and her family are often aware of the seriousness of the situation; therefore the nurse must provide support by giving explanations for the interventions being implemented and their effect on the status of the fetus.

Rupture of the Uterus

Rupture of the uterus is a rare but very serious obstetric injury that occurs in 1 to 1500 to 2000 births. The most frequent causes of uterine rupture during pregnancy are separation of the scar of a previous classic cesarean birth, uterine trauma (e.g., accidents, surgery), and a congenital uterine anomaly. During labor and birth, uterine rupture may be caused by intense spontaneous uterine contractions, labor stimulation (e.g., oxytocin, prostaglandin), an overdistended uterus (e.g., multifetal gestation), malpresentation, external or internal version, or a difficult forceps-assisted birth. It occurs more commonly in multigravidas than in primigravidas.

A uterine rupture is classified as either complete or incomplete. A complete rupture extends through the entire uterine wall into the peritoneal cavity or broad ligament. An incomplete rupture extends into the peritoneum but not into the peritoneal cavity or broad ligament. Bleeding is usually internal. An incomplete rupture also may be a partial separation at an old cesarean scar and may go unnoticed unless the woman undergoes a subsequent cesarean birth or other uterine surgery.

Signs and symptoms vary with the extent of the rupture and may be silent or dramatic. In an incomplete rupture, pain may not be present. The fetus may or may not have late decelerations, decreased variability, an increased or decreased heart rate, or other nonreassuring signs. The woman may experience vomiting, faintness, increased abdominal tenderness, hypotonic uterine contractions, and lack of progress. Eventually, bleeding and the effects of blood loss will be noted. Fetal heart tones may be lost. In a complete rupture, the woman may complain of sudden, sharp shooting abdominal pain and may state that "something gave way." If she is in labor, her contractions will cease, and pain is relieved. She may exhibit signs of hypovolemic shock caused by hemorrhage (i.e., hypotension, tachypnea, pallor, and cool, clammy skin). If the placenta separates, the FHR will be absent. Fetal parts may be palpable through the abdomen. The nurse should suspect pulmonary embolism if the woman complains of chest pain and difficulty breathing.

Collaborative Care

Prevention is the best treatment. Women who have had a previous classic cesarean birth are advised not to attempt vaginal birth in subsequent pregnancies. Women at risk for uterine rupture are assessed closely during labor. Women whose labor is induced with oxytocin or prostaglandin (especially if their previous birth was cesarean) are monitored for signs of uterine hyperstimulation, because this can precipitate uterine rupture. If hyperstimulation occurs, the oxytocin infusion is discontinued or decreased, and a tocolytic medication may be given to decrease the intensity of the uterine contractions. After giving birth, women are assessed for excessive bleeding, especially if the fundus is firm and signs of hemorrhagic shock are present.

If rupture occurs, the type of medical management depends on the severity. A small rupture may be managed with a laparotomy and birth of the infant, repair of the laceration, and blood transfusions, if needed. For a complete rupture, hysterectomy and blood replacement is the usual treatment.

The nurse's role may include starting intravenous fluids, transfusing blood products, administering oxygen, and assisting with the preparation for immediate surgery. Supporting the woman's family and providing information

---

EMERGENCY

Prolapsed Cord

SIGNS
- Fetal bradycardia with variable deceleration during uterine contraction
- Woman reports feeling the cord after membranes rupture
- Cord is seen or felt in or protruding from the vagina

INTERVENTIONS
- Call for assistance.
- Notify primary health care provider immediately.
- Glove the examining hand quickly and insert two fingers into the vagina to the cervix. With one finger on either side of the cord or both fingers to one side, exert upward pressure against the presenting part to relieve compression of the cord (Fig. 36-19, A and B). Place a rolled towel under the woman's right or left hip.
- Place woman into the extreme Trendelenburg or a modified Sims position (Fig. 36-19, C), or a knee-chest position (Fig. 36-19, D).
- If cord is protruding from vagina, wrap loosely in a sterile towel saturated with warm sterile normal saline solution.
- Administer oxygen to the woman by mask at 8 to 10 L/min until birth is accomplished.
- Start intravenous (IV) fluids or increase existing drip rate.
- Continue to monitor fetal heart rate (FHR) by internal fetal scalp electrode, if possible.
- Explain to woman and support person what is happening and the way it is being managed.
- Prepare for immediate vaginal birth if cervix is fully dilated, or cesarean birth if it is not.

about the treatment is important during this emergency. The associated fetal mortality rate is high (50% to 75%), and the maternal mortality rate may be high if the woman is not treated immediately (Cunningham et al., 2005). Providing information about spiritual support services or suggesting that the family contact their own support system may be warranted.

Amniotic Fluid Embolism

Amniotic fluid embolism (AFE) occurs when amniotic fluid containing particles of debris (e.g., vernix, hair, skin cells, or meconium) enters the maternal circulation and causes the release of endogenous mediators (e.g., histamine, prostaglandins, thromboxane). Pulmonary vessels are obstructed, causing respiratory distress and circulatory collapse. If the woman survives, she is likely to have hemorrhage and disseminated intravascular coagulation. Although AFE is rare, the mortality rate is as high as 80%. About 50% of the neonates who survive have neurologic impairment (Schoening, 2006).

Amniotic fluid is more damaging if it contains meconium and other particulate matter such as mucus, fat globules, lanugo, bacterial products, or debris from a dead fetus because emboli can then form more readily. Maternal death occurs most often when thick meconium is present in the amniotic fluid, because this clogs the pulmonary veins more completely than other debris. Even if death does not occur immediately, serious coagulation problems such as disseminated intravascular coagulopathy usually occur. The substances in the amniotic fluid also can affect pulmonary blood vessels, by causing venospasm or pulmonary hypertension, and cardiac function, by causing left ventricular failure.

Maternal factors (including multiparity, tumultuous labor, abruptio placentae, and oxytocin induction of labor) and fetal problems (including macrosomia, death, and meconium passage) have been associated with an increased risk for the development of AFE (Cunningham et al., 2005). A common first symptom is acute dyspnea, followed by severe hypotension (Schoening, 2006).

Collaborative Care

The immediate interventions for AFE are summarized in the Emergency box. Such medical management must be instituted immediately. Cardiopulmonary resuscitation is often necessary. The woman is usually placed on mechanical ventilation, and blood replacement is initiated; coagulation defects are treated. Although the incidence of possible complications is small, their immediate recognition and the prompt initiation of treatment is important.

■ NURSE ALERT
Automatic blood pressure devices, FHR monitors, and pulse oximeters may be inadequate and inaccurate during extreme clinical conditions. Assessment by a competent nurse is often more accurate than that provided by any one piece of equipment (Curran, 2003).

EMERGENCY

Amniotic Fluid Embolism
SIGNS
Respiratory Distress
- Restlessness
- Dyspnea
- Cyanosis
- Pulmonary edema
- Respiratory arrest

Circulatory Collapse
- Hypotension
- Tachycardia
- Shock
- Cardiac arrest

Hemorrhage
- Coagulation failure: bleeding from incisions, venipuncture sites, trauma (lacerations); petechiae, ecchymoses, purpura
- Uterine atony

INTERVENTIONS
Oxygenate
- Administer oxygen by face mask (8-10 L/min) or resuscitation bag delivering 100% oxygen
- Prepare for intubation and mechanical ventilation
- Initiate or assist with cardiopulmonary resuscitation. Tilt pregnant woman 30 degrees to side to displace uterus

Maintain cardiac output and replace fluid losses
- Position woman on her side
- Administer IV fluids
- Administer blood: packed cells, fresh-frozen plasma
- Insert indwelling catheter, and measure hourly urine output

Correct coagulation failure
Monitor fetal and maternal status
Prepare for emergency birth once woman's condition is stabilized
Provide emotional support to woman, her partner, and family

The nurse's immediate responsibility is to assist with the resuscitation efforts. If the woman survives, she is usually moved to a critical care unit, where hemodynamic monitoring and blood replacement and coagulopathy treatment are implemented. If cardiopulmonary arrest occurs, for optimal fetal survival, a perimortem cesarean delivery should occur within 5 minutes (Curran, 2003).

Support of the woman's partner and family is needed; they will be anxious and distressed. Brief explanations of what is happening are important during the emergency and can be reinforced after the immediate crisis is over. If the woman dies, emotional support and involvement of the perinatal loss support team or other resource for grief counseling is needed. Referral to grief and loss support groups would be appropriate (see Chapter 34). The nursing staff also may need help in coping with feelings and emotions that result from a maternal death.

1. Visit a prenatal clinic in your community. Interview one of the nurses working with women at this clinic and complete the following activities:
   a. Determine the rate of preterm labors and births among the clinic's clients.
   b. Identify risk assessment activities implemented to determine if the clients exhibit factors or characteristics that increase the likelihood that they will experience preterm labor.
   c. Work with the nurses at the clinic to develop an evidence-based preterm labor and birth education program designed to reduce the rate of preterm labors experienced. Outline the components of the program that you and the nurses develop.

2. Interview a childbirth educator to determine what she teaches expectant parents about cesarean birth, including measures to prevent its occurrence. Attend the class when she presents this content to parents. Observe the questions and concerns expressed by parents regarding the possibility of cesarean birth. Discuss this issue with several couples to develop an awareness of accuracy and depth of knowledge they have regarding the potential for this outcome.

- Preterm labor is cervical change (e.g., effacement and dilation) and uterine contractions occurring between 20 weeks and 37 weeks of pregnancy; preterm birth is any birth that occurs before the completion of 37 weeks of pregnancy.
- The cause of preterm labor is unknown and is assumed to be multifactorial; therefore it is not possible to predict with certainty which women will experience preterm labor and birth.
- Because the onset of preterm labor is often insidious and can be mistaken for normal discomforts of pregnancy, nurses should teach all pregnant women how to detect the early symptoms of preterm labor and to call their primary health care provider when symptoms occur.
- Bed rest, a commonly prescribed intervention for preterm labor, has many deleterious side effects and has never been shown to decrease preterm birth rates.
- The best reason to use tocolytic therapy is to achieve sufficient time to administer corticosteroids in an effort to accelerate fetal lung maturity and reduce the severity of respiratory complications in infants born preterm.
- Vigilance for signs of infection is a major part of the care for women with PPROM.
- Dystocia results from differences in the normal relations among any of the five factors affecting labor and is characterized by differences in the pattern of progress in labor.
- Dysfunctional labor occurs as a result of hypertonic uterine dysfunction, hypotonic uterine dysfunction, or inadequate voluntary expulsive forces.
- The functional relations among the uterine contractions, the fetus, and the mother's pelvis are altered by maternal positioning.
- Uterine contractility is increased by the effects of oxytocin and prostaglandin and is decreased by tocolytic agents.
- Cervical ripening using chemical or mechanical measures can increase the success of labor induction.
- Expectant parents benefit from learning about operative obstetrics (e.g., forceps-assisted, vacuum-assisted, or cesarean birth) during the prenatal period.
- The basic purpose of cesarean birth is to preserve the life or health of the mother and her fetus.
- Unless contraindicated, vaginal birth is possible after a previous cesarean birth.
- Labor management that emphasizes one-to-one support of the laboring woman by another woman (e.g., doula, nurse, nurse-midwife) can reduce the rate of cesarean birth and increase the rate of VBACs.
- A postterm pregnancy poses a risk to both the mother and the fetus.
- Obstetric emergencies (e.g., shoulder dystocia, prolapsed cord, rupture of the uterus, and amniotic fluid embolism) occur rarely but require immediate intervention to preserve the health or life of the mother and fetus/newborn.

REFERENCES

Abrahams, C., & Katz, M. (2002). A perspective on the diagnosis of preterm labor. *Journal of Perinatal and Neonatal Nursing, 16*(1), 1-11.

Abrams. B., Minassian, D., & Pickett K. (2004). Maternal nutrition. In R. Creasy, R. Resnik, & J. Iams (Eds): *Maternal-fetal medicine: Principles and practice* (5th ed.). Philadelphia: Saunders.

Adler, C., & Zarchin, Y. (2002). The "Virtual Focus Group": Using the Internet to reach pregnant women on home bed rest. *Journal of Obstetric, Gynecologic, and Neonatal Nursing, 31*(4), 418-427.

American College of Obstetricians and Gynecologists (ACOG). (1999). *Induction of labor.* ACOG Practice Bulletin No. 10. Washington, DC: Author.

American College of Obstetricians and Gynecologists (ACOG). (2001). *Assessment of risk factors for preterm birth.* ACOG Practice Bulletin No. 31. Washington, DC: Author.

American College of Obstetricians and Gynecologists (ACOG). (2002a). *Antenatal corticosteroid therapy for fetal maturation.* ACOG Committee Opinion No. 273. Washington, DC: Author.

American College of Obstetricians and Gynecologists (ACOG). (2002b). *Shoulder dystocia.* ACOG Practice Bulletin No. 40. Washington, DC: Author.

American College of Obstetricians and Gynecologists (ACOG). (2003a). *Management of preterm labor.* ACOG Practice Bulletin No. 43. Washington, DC: Author.

American College of Obstetricians and Gynecologists. (2003b). *New ACOG opinion addresses elective cesarean controversy,* ACOG news release, October, 31, 2003. Washington, DC.: Author.

American College of Obstetricians and Gynecologists (ACOG). (2004a). *Vaginal birth after previous cesarean delivery.* ACOG Practice Bulletin No. 54. Washington, DC: Author.

American College of Obstetricians and Gynecologists (ACOG). (2004b). *Management of postterm pregnancy.* ACOG Practice Bulletin No. 55. Washington, DC: Author.

American College of Obstetricians and Gynecologists & American Academy of Pediatrics (ACOG/AAP). (2002). *Guidelines for perinatal care* (5th ed.). Washington, DC: ACOG.

Anotayanonth, S., Subhedar, N., Garner, P., Neilson, J., & Harigopal, S. (2004), Betamimetics for inhibiting preterm labour. *The Cochrane Database of Systematic Reviews*, 2006, Issue 3. Chichester, UK: John Wiley & Sons.

Association of Women's Health, Obstetric and Gynecologic Nurses (AWHONN). (2000). *Issue: Professional nursing support of laboring women.* Washington, DC: Author.

Baskett, T. (2002). Shoulder dystocia. *Best Practices Research in Clinical Obstetrics and Gynaecology, 16*(10), 57-68.

Baxley, E., & Gobbo, R. (2004). Shoulder dystocia. *American Family Physician, 69*(7), 1610, 1612-1613.

Berg-Lekas, M., Hogberg, U., & Winkvist, A. (1998). Familial occurrence of dystocia. *American Journal of Obstetrics and Gynecology, 179*(1), 117-121.

Berkman, N., Thorp, J., Lohr, K., Carey, T., Hartmann, K., Gavin, N., et al. (2003). Tocolytic treatment for the management of preterm labor: A review of the evidence. *American Journal of Obstetrics and Gynecology, 188*(6), 1648-1659.

Bernhardt, J., & Dorman, K. (2004). Pre-term birth risk assessment tools. Exploring fetal fibronectin and cervical length for validating risk, *AWHONN Lifelines, 8*(1), 38-44.

Bowes, W., & Thorp, J. (2004). Clinical aspects of normal and abnormal labor. In R. Creasy, R. Resnik, & J. Iams (Eds), *Maternal-fetal medicine: Principles and practice* (5th ed.). Philadephia: Saunders.

Cesario, S. (2004). Reevaluation of Friedman's labor curve: A pilot study. *Journal of Obstetric, Gynecologic, and Neonatal Nursing, 33*(6), 713-722.

Colombo, D., & Iams, J. (2000). Cervical length and preterm labor. *Clinical Obstetrics and Gynecology, 43*(4), 735-745.

Cunningham, G., Leveno, K., Bloom, S., Hauth, J, Gilstrap, L., & Wenstrom, K. (2005). *Williams obstetrics* (22nd ed.). New York; McGraw-Hill.

Curran, C. (2003). Intrapartum emergencies. *Journal of Obstetric, Gynecologic, and Neonatal Nursing, 32*(6), 802-813.

Dauphinee, J. (2004). VBAC: Safety for the patient and the nurse. *Journal of Obstetric, Gynecologic, and Neonatal Nursing, 33*(1), 105-115.

Divon, M. (2002). Prolonged pregnancy. In S. Gabbe, J. Niebyl, & J. Simpson (Eds.), *Obstetrics: Normal and problem pregnancies* (4th ed.). New York: Churchill Livingstone.

Enkin, M. Kierse, M., Neilson, J., Crowther, C., Duley, L. Hodnett, E., et al. (2000). *A guide to effective care in pregnancy and childbirth* (3rd ed.). Oxford, NY: Oxford University Press.

Freda, M. (2003). Nursing's contribution to the literature on preterm labor and birth. *Journal of Obstetric, Gynecologic, and Neonatal Nursing, 32*(5), 659-667.

Freda, M., & Patterson, E. (2001). *Preterm birth: Prevention and nursing management* (2nd ed.). March of Dimes nursing module series. White Plains, NY: March of Dimes.

Friedman, E. (1989). Normal and dysfunctional labor. In W. Cohen, D. Acker, & Friedman, E. (Eds.), *Management of labor* (2nd ed.). Rockville, MD: Aspen.

Fuchs, I., Henrich, W., Osthues, K., & Dudenhausen, J. (2004). Sonographic cervical length in singleton pregnancies with intact membranes presenting in threatened preterm labor. *Ultrasound Obstetrics and Gynecology, 24*(5), 554-557.

Gamble, J., & Creedy, D. (2004). Content and processes of postpartum counseling after a distressing birth experience: A review. *Birth, 31*(3), 213-218.

Gardner, P. (2003). Previous traumatic birth: An impetus for requested cesarean birth. *Journal of Perinatal Neonatal Education, 12*(1), 1-5.

Garite, T. (2004). Premature rupture of membranes. In R. Creasy, R. Resnik, & J. Iams (Eds.), *Maternal-fetal medicine: Principles and practice* (5th ed.). Philadephia: Saunders.

Gennaro, S., & Hennessy, M. (2003). Physiological and psychological stress: Impact on preterm birth. *Journal of Obstetric, Gynecologic, and Neonatal Nursing, 32*(5), 669-675.

Gilbert, E., & Harmon, J. (2003). *Manual of high risk pregnancy & delivery* (3rd ed.). St Louis: Mosby.

Goldberg, A., & Wing, D. (2003). Induction of labor: The misoprostol controversy. *Journal of Midwifery & Women's Health, 48*(4), 244-248.

Goldenberg, R., Iams, J., Mercer, B., Meis, P., Moawad, A., Das, A., et al. (2003). What we have learned about the predictors of preterm birth, *Seminars in Perinatology, 27*(3), 636-643.

Gregory, K. (2000). Monitoring risk adjustment and strategies to decrease cesarean rates. *Current Opinion in Obstetrics and Gynecology, 12*(6), 481-486.

Hamilton, B., Martin, J., Ventura, S., Sutton, P., Menaker, F., & Division of Vital Statistics. (2005). Births: Preliminary data from 2004. *National Vital Statistics Report, 54*(8), 1-18.

Heaman, M., Sprague, A., & Stewart, P. (2001). Reducing the preterm birth rate: A population health strategy. *Journal of Obstetric, Gynecologic, and Neonatal Nursing, 30*(1), 20-29.

Hodnett, E., Gates, S. Hofmeyr, G., & Sakala, C. (2005). Continuous support for women during childbirth. *The Cochrane Database of Systematic Reviews*, 2006, Issue 3. Chichester, UK: John Wiley & Sons.

Iams, J. (2002). Preterm birth. In S. Gabbe, J. Niebyl, & J. Simpson (Eds.), *Obstetrics: Normal and problem pregnancies* (4th ed.). New York: Churchill Livingstone.

Iams, J. (2003). Prediction and early detection of pre-term birth. *Obstetrics and Gynecology, 101*(2), 402-412.

Iams, J., & Creasy, R. (2004). Preterm labor and delivery. In R. Creasy, R. Resnik, & J. Iams (Eds.), *Maternal- fetal medicine: Principles and practice* (5th ed.). Philadephia: Saunders.

Jevitt, C. (2005). Shoulder dystocia: Etiology, common risk factors, and management. *Journal of Midwifery & Women's Health, 50*(6), 485-497.

Lanni, S., & Seeds, J. (2002). Malpresentations. In S. Gabbe, J. Niebyl, & J. Simpson (Eds.), *Obstetrics: Normal and problem pregnancies* (4th ed.). New York: Churchill Livingstone.

Lehne, R. (2004). *Pharmacology for nursing care.* Philadelphia: Saunders.

Lieberman, E., Ernst, E., Rooks, J., Stapleton, S., & Flamm, B. (2004). Results of the national study of vaginal birth after cesarean in birth centers. *Obstetrics and Gynecology, 104*(5 Part 1), 933-942.

Liu, S., Rusen, I., Joseph, K., Listen, R., Kramer, M., Wen, S., et al. (2004). Recent trends in caesarean delivery rates and indications for caesarean delivery in Canada. *Journal of Obstetrics and Gynaecology of Canada, 26*(8), 735-742.

Lydon-Rochelle, M., Hold, V., Easterling, T., & Martin, D. (2001). Risk of uterine rupture during labor among women with a prior cesarean delivery. *New England Journal of Medicine, 345*(1), 3-8.

Maloni, J. (2002). Astronauts & pregnancy bed rest: What NASA is teaching us about inactivity. *AWHONN Lifelines, 6*(4), 318-323.

Maloni, J., Brezinski-Tomasi, J., & Johnson, L. (2001). Antepartum bedrest: Effect upon the family. *Journal of Obstetric, Gynecologic, and Neonatal Nursing, 30*(2), 165-173.

Maloni, J., & Damato, E. (2004). Reducing the risk for preterm birth: Evidence and implications for neonatal nurses. *Advances in Neonatal Care, 4*(3), 166-174.

Maloni, J., & Kutil, R. (2000). Antepartum support group for women hospitalized on bedrest. *MCN American Journal of Maternal/Child Nursing, 25*(4), 204-210.

Maloni, J., & Park, S. (2005). Postpartum symptoms after antepartum bedrest. *Journal of Obstetric, Gynecologic, and Neonatal Nursing, 34*(2), 163-171.

March of Dimes. (2005). *March of Dimes prematurity campaign.* Accessed www.marchofdimes.com, September 1, 2006.

Martin, J., Hamilton, B., Sutton, P., Ventura, S., Menacker, F., & Munson, M. (2005). Births: Final data for 2003. *National Vital Statistics Report, 54*(2), 1-115.

Martin, R., & Leaton, M. (2001). Amniotic fluid embolism. *American Journal of Nursing, 101*(3), 43-44.

Massett, H., Greenup, M., Ryan, C., Staples, D., Green, N., & Maibach, E. (2003). Public perceptions about prematurity: A national survey. *American Journal of Preventive Medicine, 24*(2), 120-127.

Maupin, R., Lyman, R., Fatsis, J., Prystowiski, E., Nguyen, A., Wright, C., et al. (2004). Characteristics of women who deliver with no prenatal care. *Journal of Maternal-Fetal & Neonatal Medicine, 16(1)*, 45-50.

Mayberry, L., Wood, S., Strange, L., Lee, L., Heisler, D., & Nielson-Smith, K. (2000). Second stage labor management: Promotion of evidence-based practice and a collaborative approach to patient care. Washington, DC: AWHONN.

McFarlin, B. (2004). Elective cesarean birth: Issues and ethics of informed choice. *Journal of Midwifery & Women's Health, 49*(5), 421-429.

Miltner, R. (2002). More than support: Nursing interventions provided to women in labor. *Journal of Obstetric, Gynecologic, and Neonatal Nursing, 31*(6), 753-761.

Moore, M. (2003). Preterm labor and birth: What have we learned in the past two decades? *Journal of Obstetric, Gynecologic, and Neonatal Nursing, 32*(5), 638-649.

Moos, M. (2004). Understanding prematurity: Sorting fact from fiction. *AWHONN Lifelines, 8*(1), 32-37.

Morrison, J., & Chauhan, S. (2003). Current status of home uterine activity monitoring, *Clinics in Perinatology, 30*(4), 757-801.

Myers, E., Blumrick, R., Christian, A., Santanu Datta, S., Gray, R., Kolimagar, J., et al. (2002). *Management of prolonged pregnancy.* Evidence Report/technology Assessment No. 53 (AHRQ Publication No. 02-E018). Rockville, MD: Agency for Healthcare Research and Quality.

National Institutes of Health. (2000). *Antenatal corticosteroids revisited. Consensus Development Conference Statement.* Maryland: NIH. Accessed http://consensus.nih.gov, September 2, 2006.

Nocon, J. (2000). Shoulder dystocia and macrosomia. In L. Kean, P. Baker, & D. Edlestone (Eds.), *Best practice in labor ward management.* Philadelphia: Saunders.

Norwitz, E., Robinson, J., & Repke, J. (2002). Labor and delivery. In S. Gabbe, J. Niebyl, & J. Simpson (Eds.), *Obstetrics: Normal and problem pregnancies* (4th ed.). New York: Churchill Livingstone.

Pschirrer, E., & Monga, M. (2000). Risk factors for preterm labor. *Clinics in Obstetrics and Gynecology, 43*(4), 727-734.

O'Brien-Abel, N. (2003). Uterine rupture during VBAC trial of labor: Risk factors and fetal response. *Journal of Midwifery & Women's Health, 48*(4), 249-257.

Ramsey, P., & Andrews, W. (2003). Biochemical predictors of preterm labor: Fetal fibronectin and salivary estriol, *Clinics in Perinatology, 30*(4), 701-733.

Ramsey, P., Ramin, K., & Ramin, S. (2000). Labor induction. *Current Opinion in Obstetrics and Gynecology, 12*(6), 463-473.

Resnik, J., & Resnik, R. (2004). Post-term pregnancy. In R. Creasy, R. Resnik, & J. Iams (Eds.), *Maternal-fetal medicine: Principles and practice* (5th ed.). Philadelphia: Saunders.

Rideout, S. (2005). Tocolytics for pre-term labor: What nurses need to know. *AWHONN Lifelines, 9*(1), 56-61.

Ridley, R., Davis, P., Bright, J., & Sinclair, D. (2002). What influences a woman to choose vaginal birth after cesarean? *Journal of Obstetric, Gynecologic, and Neonatal Nursing, 31*(6), 665-672.

Schaffir, J. (2002). Survey of folk beliefs about induction of labor. *Birth, 29*(1), 47-51.

Schoening, A. (2006). Amniotic fluid embolism: Historical perspectives and new possibilities. *MCN American Journal of Maternal/Child Nursing, 31*(2), 78-83.

Searing, K. (2001). Induction vs. post-date pregnancies: Exploring the controversy of who's really at risk. *AWHONN Lifelines, 5*(2), 44-48.

Shipp, T. (2004). Trial of labor after cesarean: So what are the risks? *Clinical Obstetrics and Gynecology, 47*(2), 365-377.

Simkin, P., & Ancheta, R. (2000). *The labor progress handbook.* Malden, MA: Blackwell Science.

Simpson, K. (2002). *Cervical ripening and induction and augmentation of labor* (2nd ed.). Washington, DC: AWHONN.

Simpson, K. (2005). The context and clinical evidence for common nursing practices during labor. *MCN American Journal of Maternal/Child Nursing, 30*(6), 356-363.

Simpson, K., & Atterbury, J. (2003). Trends and issues in labor induction in the United States: implications for clinical practice. *Journal of Obstetric, Gynecologic, and Neonatal Nursing, 32*(6), 767-779.

Simpson, K., & Knox, G. (2001). Fundal pressure during second stage of labor. *MCN American Journal of Maternal/Child Nursing, 26*(6), 64-70.

Society of Obstetricians and Gynaecologists of Canada (SOGC). (2004). News. C-sections on demand—SOGC's position. *Birth, 31*(2), 154.

Sosa C., Athalbe, F., Belzian, J., & Bergel, E. (2004). Bed rest in singleton pregnancies for preventing preterm birth. *The Cochrane Database of Systematic Reviews,* 2006, Issue 3. Chichester, UK: John Wiley & Sons.

Sprague, A. (2004). The evolution of bed rest as a clinical intervention. *Journal of Obstetric, Gynecologic, and Neonatal Nursing, 33*(5), 542-549.

Stremler, R., Hodnett, E., Petryshen, P., Stevens, B., Weston, J., & Willan, A. (2005). Randomized controlled trial of hands-and-knees positioning for occipitoposterior position in labor. *Birth, 32*(4), 243-251.

Thomas, L., Ptak, H., Giddings, L., Moore, L., & Opperman, C. (1990). The effects of rocking, diet modifications, and antiflatulence medication on postcesarean section gas pain. *Journal of Perinatal and Neonatal Nursing, 4*(3), 12-24.

Tiedje, L. (2003). Psychosocial pathways to prematurity: changing our thinking toward a lifecourse and community approach. *Journal of Obstetric, Gynecologic, and Neonatal Nursing, 32*(5), 650-658.

Weiss, M., Saks, N., & Harris, S. (2002). Resolving the uncertainty of preterm symptoms: Women's experiences with the onset of preterm labor. *Journal of Obstetric, Gynecologic, and Neonatal Nursing, 31*(1), 66-76.

Weitz, B. (2001). Premature rupture of the fetal membranes: An update for advanced practice nurses. *MCN American Journal of Maternal/Child Nursing, 26*(2), 86-92.

Wener, M., & Lavigne, S. (2004). Can periodontal disease lead to premature delivery? *AWHONN Lifelines, 8*(5), 422-431.

Williams, D. (2005). The top 10 reasons elective cesarean section should be on the decline. *AWHONN Lifelines, 9*(1), 23-24.

Witcher, P. (2002). Treatment of preterm labor. *Journal of Perinatal and Neonatal Nursing, 16*(1), 25-46.

Youngblut, J., Madigen, E., Neff, D., Deoisres, W., Siripul, P., & Brooten, D. (2000). Employment patterns and timing of birth in women with high-risk pregnancies. *Journal of Obstetric, Gynecologic, and Neonatal Nursing, 29*(2), 137-144.

Postpartum Complications

learning objectives

- Identify causes, signs and symptoms, and medical and nursing management of postpartum hemorrhage.
- Describe hemorrhagic shock as a complication of postpartum hemorrhage including management and hazards of therapy.
- Differentiate the causes of postpartum infection.
- Summarize assessment and care of women with postpartum infection.

- Describe thromboembolic disorders, including incidence, etiology, signs and symptoms, and management.
- Summarize the role of the nurse in the home setting in assessing potential problems and managing care of women with postpartum physiologic complications.

electronic resources

Additional information related to the content in Chapter 37 can be found on

the companion website at **evolve**
http://evolve.elsevier.com/Lowdermilk/MWHC/
- NCLEX Review Questions
- WebLinks

or on the interactive companion CD
- NCLEX Review Questions
- Plan of Care: Postpartum Hemorrhage

COLLABORATIVE efforts of the health care team are needed to provide safe and effective care to the woman and family experiencing postpartum physiologic complications including maternal death. This chapter focuses on hemorrhage and infection.

■ POSTPARTUM HEMORRHAGE

Definition and Incidence

Postpartum hemorrhage (PPH) continues to be a leading cause of maternal morbidity and mortality in the United States (Papp, 2003) and worldwide. It is a life-threatening event that can occur with little warning and is often unrecognized until the mother has profound symptoms. PPH has been traditionally defined as the loss of more than 500 ml of blood after vaginal birth and 1000 ml after cesarean birth (MacMullen, Dulski, & Meagher, 2005). A 10% change in hematocrit between admission for labor and postpartum or the need for erythrocyte transfusion also has been used to define PPH (Cunningham, Leveno, Bloom, Hauth, Gilstrap, & Wenstrom, 2005). However, defining PPH clinically is not a clear-cut undertaking. Diagnosis is often based on subjective observations, with blood loss often being underestimated by as much as 50% (Cunningham et al.).

Traditionally, PPH has been classified as early or late with respect to the birth. Early, acute, or primary PPH occurs within 24 hours of the birth. Late or secondary PPH occurs more than 24 hours but less than 6 weeks postpartum (Cunningham et al., 2005). Today's health care environment encourages shortened stays after birth, thereby increasing the potential for acute episodes of PPH to occur outside the traditional hospital or birth center setting.

Etiology and Risk Factors

It is helpful to consider the problem of excessive bleeding with reference to the stages of labor. From birth of the infant until separation of the placenta, the character and quantity of blood passed may suggest excessive bleeding. For example, dark blood is probably of venous origin, perhaps from varices or superficial lacerations of the birth canal. Bright blood is arterial and may indicate deep lacerations of the cervix. Spurts of blood with clots may indicate partial placental separation. Failure of blood to clot or remain clotted indicates a pathologic condition or coagulopathy such as disseminated intravascular coagulation (see later discussion) (Cunningham et al., 2005).

Excessive bleeding may occur during the period from the separation of the placenta to its expulsion or removal.

975

CRITICAL THINKING EXERCISE

PPH – Prevention and Management

The nursing staff of the labor, delivery, recovery, and postpartum (LDRP) unit are meeting to develop a clinical guideline for orienting new nursing staff on the prevention and management of early postpartum hemorrhage (PPH). The clinical nurse educator has been asked to provide information about what should be included.

1. Evidence—Is there sufficient evidence to draw conclusions about what advice the educator should give?
2. Assumptions—Describe underlying assumptions about each of the following:
   a. Early versus late PPH
   b. Identifying risk factors
   c. Use of oxytocic agents for prevention and management of PPH
3. What implications and priorities for nursing care can be made at this time?
4. Does the evidence objectively support your conclusion?
5. Are there alternative perspectives to your conclusion?

Commonly such excessive bleeding is the result of incomplete placental separation, undue manipulation of the fundus, or excessive traction on the cord. After the placenta has been expelled or removed, persistent or excessive blood loss usually is the result of atony of the uterus or prolapse of the uterus into the vagina. Late PPH may be the result of subinvolution of the uterus, endometritis, or retained placental fragments (Cunningham et al., 2005). Predisposing factors for PPH are listed in Box 37-1.

Uterine Atony

Uterine atony is marked hypotonia of the uterus. Normally, placental separation and expulsion are facilitated by contraction of the uterus, which also prevents hemorrhage from the placental site. The corpus is in essence a basket-weave of strong, interlacing smooth muscle bundles through which many large maternal blood vessels pass (see Fig. 5-3). If the uterus is flaccid after detachment of all or part of the placenta, brisk venous bleeding occurs, and normal coagulation of the open vasculature is impaired and continues until the uterine muscle is contracted.

Uterine atony is the leading cause of PPH. It is associated with high parity, hydramnios, a macrosomic fetus, and multifetal gestation. In such conditions, the uterus is "overstretched" and contracts poorly after the birth. Other causes of atony include traumatic birth, use of halogenated anesthesia (e.g., halothane) or magnesium sulfate, rapid or prolonged labor, chorioamnionitis, use of oxytocin for labor induction or augmentation, and uterine atony in a previous pregnancy (Cunningham et al., 2005; MacMullen et al., 2005; Magann, Evans, Chauhan, Lanneau, Fisk, & Morrison, 2005).

Lacerations of the Genital Tract

Lacerations of the cervix, the vagina, and the perineum also are causes of PPH. Hemorrhage related to lacerations should be suspected if bleeding continues despite a firm, contracted uterine fundus. This bleeding can be a slow trickle, an oozing, or frank hemorrhage. Factors that influence the causes and incidence of obstetric lacerations of the lower genital tract include operative birth, precipitate birth, congenital abnormalities of the maternal soft parts, and contracted pelvis. Other possible causes of lacerations are size, abnormal presentation, and position of the fetus; relative size of the presenting part and the birth canal; previous scarring from infection, injury, or operation; and vulvar, perineal, and vaginal varicosities.

Extreme vascularity in the labial and periclitoral areas often results in profuse bleeding if laceration occurs. Hematomas also may be present.

Lacerations of the perineum are the most common of all injuries in the lower portion of the genital tract. These are classified as first-, second-, third-, and fourth-degree (see Chapter 21). An episiotomy may extend to become either a third- or fourth-degree laceration.

Prolonged pressure of the fetal head on the vaginal mucosa ultimately interferes with the circulation and may produce ischemic or pressure necrosis. The state of the tissues in combination with the type of birth may result in

---

box 37-1 **Risk Factors and Causes of Postpartum Hemorrhage**

Uterine atony	Lacerations of the birth canal
• Overdistended uterus	Retained placental fragments
–Large fetus	Ruptured uterus
–Multiple fetuses	Inversion of the uterus
–Hydramnios	Placenta accreta, increta, percreta
–Distention with clots	Coagulation disorders
• Anesthesia and analgesia	Placental abruption
–Conduction anesthesia	Placenta previa
• Previous history of uterine atony	Manual removal of a retained placenta
• High parity	Magnesium sulfate administration during labor or postpartum
• Prolonged labor, oxytocin-induced labor	period
• Trauma during labor and birth	Chorioamnionitis
–Forceps-assisted birth	Uterine subinvolution
–Vacuum-assisted birth	
–Cesarean birth	

deep vaginal lacerations, with consequent predisposition to vaginal hematomas.

Pelvic hematomas may be vulvar, vaginal, or retroperitoneal in origin. Vulvar hematomas are the most common. Pain is the most common symptom, and most vulvar hematomas are visible. Vaginal hematomas occur more commonly in association with a forceps-assisted birth, an episiotomy, or primigravidity (Benedetti, 2002). During the postpartum period, if the woman reports a persistent perineal or rectal pain or a feeling of pressure in the vagina, a careful examination is made. However, a retroperitoneal hematoma may cause minimal pain, and the initial symptoms may be signs of shock (Benedetti, 2002).

Cervical lacerations usually occur at the lateral angles of the external os. Most are shallow, and bleeding is minimal. More extensive lacerations may extend into the vaginal vault or into the lower uterine segment.

Retained Placenta
Nonadherent Retained Placenta

Nonadherent retained placenta may result from partial separation of a normal placenta, entrapment of the partially or completely separated placenta by an hourglass constriction ring of the uterus, mismanagement of the third stage of labor, or abnormal adherence of the entire placenta or a portion of the placenta to the uterine wall. Placental retention because of poor separation is common in very preterm births (20 to 24 weeks of gestation).

Management of nonadherent retained placenta is by manual separation and removal by the primary health care provider. Supplementary anesthesia is not usually needed for women who have had regional anesthesia for birth. For other women, administration of light nitrous oxide and oxygen inhalation anesthesia or intravenous (IV) thiopental facilitates uterine exploration and placental removal. After this removal, the woman is at continued risk for PPH and for infection.

Adherent Retained Placenta

Abnormal adherence of the placenta occurs for reasons unknown, but it is thought to result from zygotic implantation in an area of defective endometrium so that there is no zone of separation between the placenta and the decidua. Attempts to remove the placenta in the usual manner are unsuccessful, and laceration or perforation of the uterine wall may result, putting the woman at great risk for severe PPH and infection (Cunningham et al., 2005).

Unusual placental adherence may be partial or complete. The following degrees of attachment are recognized:
- *Placenta accreta*—slight penetration of myometrium by placental trophoblast
- *Placenta increta*—deep penetration of myometrium by placenta
- *Placenta percreta*—perforation of uterus by placenta

Bleeding with complete or total placenta accreta may not occur unless separation of the placenta is attempted. With more extensive involvement, bleeding will become profuse when delivery of the placenta is attempted. Treatment includes blood component replacement therapy, and hysterectomy may be indicated (Clark, 2004).

Inversion of the Uterus

Inversion of the uterus after birth is a potentially life-threatening but rare complication. The condition may recur with a subsequent birth. Uterine inversion may be partial or complete. Complete inversion of the uterus is obvious; a large, red, rounded mass (perhaps with the placenta attached) protrudes 20 to 30 cm outside the introitus. Incomplete inversion cannot be seen but must be felt; a smooth mass will be palpated through the dilated cervix. Contributing factors to uterine inversion include fundal implantation of the placenta, vigorous fundal pressure, excessive traction applied to the cord, uterine atony, leiomyomas, and abnormally adherent placental tissue (Bowes & Thorp, 2004). Uterine inversion occurs most often in multiparous women and with placenta accreta or increta. The primary presenting signs of uterine inversion are hemorrhage, shock, and pain.

Prevention—always the easiest, cheapest, and most effective therapy—is especially appropriate for uterine inversion. The umbilical cord should not be pulled on strongly unless the placenta has definitely separated.

Subinvolution of the Uterus

Late postpartum bleeding may occur as a result of subinvolution of the uterus. Recognized causes of subinvolution include retained placental fragments and pelvic infection.

Signs and symptoms include prolonged lochial discharge, irregular or excessive bleeding, and sometimes hemorrhage. A pelvic examination usually reveals a uterus that is larger than normal and that may be boggy.

■ CARE MANAGEMENT
■ Assessment and Nursing Diagnoses

PPH may be sudden and even exsanguinating. The nurse must therefore be alert to the symptoms of hemorrhage and hypovolemic shock and be prepared to act quickly to minimize blood loss (Fig. 37-1 and Box 37-2).

The woman's history should be reviewed for factors that cause predisposition to PPH (see Box 37-1). The fundus is assessed to determine whether it is firmly contracted at or near the level of the umbilicus. Bleeding should be assessed for color and amount. The perineum is inspected for signs of lacerations or hematomas to determine the possible source of bleeding.

Vital signs may not be reliable indicators of shock immediately postpartum because of the physiologic adaptations of this period. However, frequent vital sign measurements during the first 2 hours after birth may identify trends related to blood loss (e.g., tachycardia, tachypnea, decreasing blood pressure).

Assessment for bladder distention is important because a distended bladder can displace the uterus and prevent

FIG. 37-1 Nursing assessments for postpartum bleeding.
CBC, Complete blood count; *IV,* intravenous; *uterotonics,* medications to contract the uterus.

contraction. The skin is assessed for warmth and dryness; nail beds are checked for color and promptness of capillary refill. Laboratory studies include evaluation of hemoglobin and hematocrit levels.

Late PPH develops at least 24 hours after the birth or later in the postpartum period. The woman may be at home when the symptoms occur. Discharge teaching should emphasize the signs of normal involution, as well as potential complications.

Nursing diagnoses for women experiencing PPH include the following:

- *Deficient fluid volume related to*
  −excessive blood loss secondary to uterine atony, lacerations, or uterine inversion
- *Risk for imbalanced fluid volume related to*
  −blood and fluid volume replacement therapy

box 37-2 **Noninvasive Assessments of Cardiac Output in Postpartum Clients Who Are Bleeding**

PALPATION OF PULSES (RATE, QUALITY, EQUALITY)
- Arterial
- Blood pressure

AUSCULTATION
- Heart sounds/murmurs
- Breath sounds

INSPECTION
- Skin color, temperature, turgor
- Level of consciousness
- Capillary refill
- Urinary output
- Neck veins
- Pulse oximetry
- Mucous membranes

OBSERVATION
- Presence or absence of anxiety, apprehension, restlessness, disorientation

---

- *Risk for infection related to*
  - excessive blood loss or exposed placental attachment site
- *Risk for injury related to*
  - attempted manual removal of retained placenta
  - administration of blood products
  - operative procedures
- *Fear or anxiety related to*
  - threat to self
  - deficient knowledge regarding procedures and operative management
- *Risk for impaired parenting related to*
  - separation from infant secondary to treatment regimen
- *Ineffective (peripheral) tissue perfusion related to*
  - excessive blood loss and shunting of blood to central circulation

▬ Expected Outcomes of Care

Expected outcomes of care for the woman experiencing PPH may include that the woman will do the following:
- Maintain normal vital signs and laboratory values.
- Develop no complications related to excessive bleeding.
- Express understanding of her condition, its management, and discharge instructions.
- Identify and use available support systems.

▬ Plan of Care and Interventions
▬ *Medical Management*

Early recognition and acknowledgment of the diagnosis of PPH are critical to care management. The first step is to evaluate the contractility of the uterus. If the uterus is hypotonic, management is directed toward increasing contractility and minimizing blood loss.

The initial management of excessive postpartum bleeding is firm massage of the uterine fundus, expression of any clots in the uterus, elimination of any bladder distention, and continuous IV infusion of 10 to 40 units of oxytocin added to 1000 ml of lactated Ringer's or normal saline solution. If the uterus fails to respond to oxytocin, a 0.2-mg dose of ergonovine (Ergotrate) or methylergonovine (Methergine) may be given intramuscularly to produce sustained uterine contractions. However, it is more common to administer a 0.25-mg dose of a derivative of prostaglandin $F_{2\alpha}$ (carboprost tromethamine) intramuscularly. It also can be given intramyometrially at cesarean birth or intraabdominally after vaginal birth. Oral (400 mcg to 800 mcg) and rectal (1000 mcg) administration of misoprostol has also been used, but there is no consensus ❋ about efficacy for management of postpartum hemorrhage (Gülmezoglu, Forna, Villar, & Hofmeyr, 2004; Magann & Lanneau, 2005). Recombinant Factor VIIa may also be useful in managing PPH but requires testing in clinical trials (McLintock, 2005). See Medication Guide on p. 981 for a comparison of drugs used to manage PPH. In addition to the medications used to contract the uterus, rapid administration of crystalloid solutions and/or blood or blood products will be needed to restore the woman's intravascular volume (Poole & White, 2003).

■ NURSE ALERT

Use of ergonovine or methylergonovine is contraindicated in the presence of hypertension or cardiovascular disease. Prostaglandin $F_{2\alpha}$ should be used cautiously in women with cardiovascular disease or asthma (Bowes & Thorp, 2004).

Hypotonic Uterus. Oxygen can be given to enhance oxygen delivery to the cells. A urinary catheter is usually inserted to monitor urine output as a measure of intravascular volume. Laboratory studies usually include a complete blood count with platelet count, fibrinogen, fibrin split products, prothrombin time, and partial thromboplastin time. Blood type and antibody screen are done if not previously performed (Cunningham et al., 2005).

If bleeding persists, bimanual compression may be considered by the obstetrician or nurse-midwife. This procedure involves inserting a fist into the vagina and pressing the knuckles against the anterior side of the uterus, and then placing the other hand on the abdomen and massaging the posterior uterus with it. If the uterus still does not become firm, manual exploration of the uterine cavity for retained placental fragments is implemented. If the preceding procedures are ineffective, surgical management may be the only alternative. Surgical management options include vessel ligation (uteroovarian, uterine, hypogastric), selective arterial embolization, and hysterectomy (Cunningham et al., 2005).

Bleeding with a Contracted Uterus. If the uterus is firmly contracted and bleeding continues, the source of bleeding still must be identified and treated. Assessment may include visual or manual inspection of the perineum,

EVIDENCE-BASED PRACTICE

Postpartum Hemorrhage and Third-Stage Labor Management

BACKGROUND

- Postpartum hemorrhage is one of the major causes of maternal mortality. After birth, the placenta is forced to separate from the decidua spongiosa of the uterine wall as a result of capillary bleeding and muscular action. The amount of blood loss depends, in part, on the amount of time between separation and clamping of the arterioles by robust uterine contractions. Expectant management of the third stage of labor allows spontaneous delivery of the placenta, aided by gravity or nipple stimulation. This low-intervention style is common in northern Europe, parts of the United States, and home births. Active management, on the other hand, involves combining oxytocin and controlled cord traction in order to decrease total blood loss by decreasing the time of active bleeding. This practice is standard in the United Kingdom and Australia.

OBJECTIVES

- The reviewers sought to compare the effects of active versus expectant management of third-stage labor on maternal blood loss and hemorrhage. Other outcomes included length of third stage, manual removal of placenta, nausea, vomiting, pain, satisfaction, and breastfeeding.

METHODS

Search Strategy

- After searching the Cochrane Pregnancy and Childbirth Group trials register and the Cochrane Controlled Trials register, the authors identified five randomized controlled trials, from Abu Dhabi, Ireland, and the United Kingdom, published 1988 to 1998. The total number of women was not noted.

Statistical Analyses

- Similar data were pooled. Reviewers calculated relative risk for dichotomous (categoric) data, such as nausea and vomiting, and weighted mean difference for continuous data, such as length of third stage. Differences between groups outside the 95% confidence interval were accepted as significant.

FINDINGS

- The active management groups experienced less postpartum hemorrhage, less anemia, and fewer blood transfusions. Prolonged third-stage labor and use of oxytocic drugs were less likely with active management. Breastfeeding rates at discharge and 6 weeks postpartum were higher in the active management group. Adverse effects of active management included nausea, vomiting, headache, and hypertension when ergometrine was used as the oxytocic drug.

LIMITATIONS

- The oxytocic drugs, dose, and route varied. The Dublin study showed more manual placental removal in the active group, in contrast to the other trials. There was inconsistency in pain reports, and suggestion that some of the pain was related to the practice of applying fundal pressure. Blinding subjects and evaluators to the two interventions was not practical.

IMPLICATIONS FOR PRACTICE

- Active management of third-stage labor is recommended to prevent postpartum bleeding and hemorrhage. Ergometrine may cause unpleasant side effects. Active management is beneficial for routine hospital vaginal births, and may offer advantages for low-resource settings, such as home births and birthing centers in developing countries where postpartum hemorrhage complicates so many births.

IMPLICATIONS FOR FURTHER RESEARCH

- Other reviews explore the oxytocic agents used postpartum. The individual risks and benefits of cord traction should be explored, as should the combination of cord traction and nipple stimulation (instead of oxytocic drugs). Much more information is needed to determine the optimum management in low-resource settings, especially the vulnerable populations of developing countries, where even the use of oxytocics may be impractical. The interesting finding about increased breastfeeding in the active management group was unexplained and could be an important benefit.

Reference: Prendiville, W., Elbourne, D., & McDonald, S. (2000). Active versus expectant management in the third stage of labour. *The Cochrane Database of Systematic Reviews,* 2006, Issue 3. Chichester, UK: John Wiley & Sons.

the vagina, the uterus, the cervix, or the rectum and laboratory studies (e.g., hemoglobin, hematocrit, coagulation studies, platelet count). Treatment depends on the source of the bleeding. Lacerations are usually sutured. Hematomas may be managed with observation, cold therapy, ligation of the bleeding vessel, or evacuation. Fluids and or blood replacement may be needed (Benedetti, 2002).

Uterine Inversion. Uterine inversion is an emergency situation requiring immediate recognition, replacement of the uterus within the pelvic cavity, and correction of associated clinical conditions. Tocolytics (e.g., magnesium sulfate, terbutaline) or halogenated anesthetics may be given to relax the uterus before attempting replacement (Cunningham et al., 2005). Medical management of this condition includes repositioning the uterus, giving oxytocin after the uterus is repositioned, treating shock, and initiating broad-spectrum antibiotics (Bowes & Thorp, 2004; Cunningham et al., 2005).

Subinvolution. Treatment of subinvolution depends on the cause. Ergonovine, 0.2 mg every 4 hours for 2 or 3 days, and antibiotic therapy are the most common medications used (Cunningham et al., 2005). Dilation and curettage (D&C) may be needed to remove retained placental fragments or to debride the placental site.

■ Herbal Remedies

Herbal remedies have been used with some success to control PPH after the initial management and control of bleeding, particularly outside the United States. Some herbs have homeostatic actions, whereas others work as oxytocic agents to contract the uterus (Tiran & Mack, 2000). Box 37-3 lists herbs that have been used and their actions.

medication guide

Drugs Used to Manage Postpartum Hemorrhage

DRUG ACTION	SIDE EFFECTS	CONTRAINDICATIONS	DOSAGE AND ROUTE	NURSING CONSIDERATIONS
OXYTOCIN (PITOCIN)				
Contraction of uterus; decreases bleeding	Infrequent: water intoxication; nausea and vomiting	None for PPH	10-40 units/L diluted in lactated Ringer's solution or normal saline at 125 to 200 milliunits/min IV or 10 to 20 units IM	Continue to monitor vaginal bleeding and uterine tone
METHYLERGONOVINE (METHERGINE)*				
Contraction of uterus	Hypertension, nausea, vomiting, headache	Hypertension, cardiac disease	0.2 mg IM every 2-4h up to five doses; 0.2 mg IV only for emergency	Check blood pressure before giving and do not give if >140/90 mm Hg; continue monitoring vaginal bleeding and uterine tone
PROSTAGLANDIN F2α (PROSTIN/15m; HEMABATE)				
Contraction of uterus	Headache, nausea and vomiting, fever, tachycardia, hypertension, diarrhea	Asthma, hypersensitivity	0.25 mg IM or intramyometrially every 15 to 90 min up to eight doses	Continue to monitor vaginal bleeding and uterine tone
MISOPROSTOL (CYTOTEC)†				
Contraction of uterus	Headache, nausea and vomiting, diarrhea	History of allergy to prostaglandins	400 mcg orally (range 200 mcg to 800 mcg) or 1000 mcg rectally	Continue to monitor vaginal bleeding and uterine tone

IM, Intramuscularly; *IV,* intravenously; *PPH,* postpartum hemorrhage.
*Information about methylergonovine may also be used to describe ergonovine (Ergotrate).
†Off-label use; research reports vary in conclusions about dosage and efficacy of use in comparison to other drugs used to manage PPH.

However, published evidence of the safety and efficacy of herbal therapy is lacking. Evidence from well-controlled studies is needed before recommendations for practice are made (Skidmore-Roth, 2004).

■ Nursing Interventions

Immediate nursing care of the woman with PPH includes assessment of vital signs, uterine consistency, bleeding, and administration of oxytocin or other drugs to stimulate uterine contraction according to standing orders or protocols. Venous access is established if not already in place. The primary health care provider, if not present, is notified.

The woman and her family will be anxious about her condition. The nurse can intervene by calmly providing explanations about interventions being performed and the need to act quickly.

After the bleeding has been controlled, the care of the woman with lacerations of the perineum is similar to that of women with episiotomies (analgesia as needed for pain and hot or cold applications as necessary). The need for increased roughage in the diet and increased intake of fluids is emphasized. Stool softeners may be used to assist the

box 37-3 **Herbal Remedies for Postpartum Hemorrhage***

HERB	ACTION
Witch hazel	Homeostatic
Lady's mantle	Homeostatic
Blue cohosh	Oxytocic
Motherwort	Promotes uterine contraction
Shepherd's purse	Promotes uterine contraction
Alfalfa leaf	Promotes uterine contraction; increases availability of vitamin K; increases hemoglobin
Nettle	Increases availability of vitamin K; increases hemoglobin
Raspberry leaf	Homeostatic; promotes uterine contraction
Goldenseal	Promotes uterine contraction

Source: Skidmore-Roth, L. (2004). *Mosby's handbook of herbs and natural supplements* (2nd ed.). St. Louis: Mosby; Tiran, D., & Mack, S. (Eds.). (2000). *Complementary therapies for pregnancy and childbirth* (2nd ed.). Edinburgh: Baillière Tindall.
*Usually used to promote uterine tone after the initial/emergency situation is controlled
NOTE: Readers are advised to check the most current information about each specific herbal therapy to verify dose, methods of administration, side effects, and contraindications.

woman in reestablishing bowel habits without straining and putting stress on the suture lines.

▬ NURSE ALERT

To avoid injury to the suture line, a woman with third- or fourth-degree lacerations is not given rectal suppositories or enemas or digital rectal examinations.

The care of the woman who has experienced an inversion of the uterus focuses on immediate stabilization of hemodynamic status. This requires close observation of her response to treatment to prevent shock or fluid overload. If the uterus has been repositioned manually, care must be taken to avoid aggressive fundal massage.

Discharge instructions for the woman who has had PPH are similar to those for any postpartum woman. In addition, she should be told that she will probably feel fatigue, even exhaustion, and will need to limit her physical activities to conserve her strength. She may need in-

CD: Plan of Care: Postpartum Hemorrhage

---

plan of care ▸ Postpartum Hemorrhage

NURSING DIAGNOSIS Deficient fluid volume related to postpartum hemorrhage

Expected Outcome *Woman will demonstrate fluid balance as evidenced by stable vital signs, prompt capillary refill time, and balanced intake and output.*

Nursing Interventions/Rationales
- Monitor vital signs, oxygen saturation, urine specific gravity, and capillary refill *to provide baseline data.*
- Measure and record amount and type of bleeding by weighing and counting saturated pads. If woman is at home, teach her to count pads and save any clots or tissue. If woman is admitted to hospital, save any clots and tissue for further examination *to estimate type and amount of blood loss for fluid replacement.*
- Provide quiet environment *to promote rest and decrease metabolic demands.*
- Give explanation of all procedures *to reduce anxiety.*
- Begin intravenous (IV) access with 18-gauge or larger needle for infusion of isotonic solution as ordered *to provide fluid or blood replacement.*
- Administer medications as ordered, such as oxytocin, methylergonovine, or prostaglandin $F_2\alpha$, *to increase contractility of the uterus.*
- Insert indwelling urinary catheter *to provide most accurate assessment of renal function and hypovolemia.*
- Prepare for surgical intervention as needed *to stop the source of bleeding.*

NURSING DIAGNOSIS Ineffective tissue perfusion related to hypovolemia

Expected Outcome *Woman will have stable vital signs, oxygen saturation, arterial blood gases, and adequate hematocrit and hemoglobin.*

Nursing Interventions/Rationales
- Monitor vital signs, oxygen saturation, arterial blood gases, and hematocrit and hemoglobin *to assess for hypovolemic shock and decreased tissue perfusion.*
- Assess for any changes in level of consciousness *to assess for evidence of hypoxia.*
- Assess capillary refill, mucous membranes, and skin temperature *to note indicators of vasoconstriction.*
- Give supplementary oxygen as ordered *to provide additional oxygenation to tissues.*
- Suction as needed, and insert oral airway, *to maintain clear, open airway for oxygenation.*
- Monitor arterial blood gases *to provide information about acidosis or hypoxia.*
- Administer sodium bicarbonate if ordered *to reverse metabolic acidosis.*

NURSING DIAGNOSIS Anxiety related to sudden change in health status

Expected Outcome *Woman will verbalize that anxious feelings are diminished.*

Nursing Interventions/Rationales
- Using therapeutic communication, evaluate woman's understanding of events *to provide clarification of any misconceptions.*
- Provide calm, competent attitude and environment *to aid in decreasing anxiety.*
- Explain all procedures *to decrease anxiety about the unknown.*
- Allow woman to verbalize feelings *to permit clarification of information and promote trust.*
- Continue to assess vital signs or other clinical indicators of hypovolemic shock *to evaluate if psychologic response of anxiety intensifies physiologic indicators.*

NURSING DIAGNOSIS Risk for infection related to blood loss and invasive procedures as a result of postpartum hemorrhage

Expected Outcomes *Woman will verbalize understanding of risk factors. Woman will demonstrate no signs of infection.*

Nursing Interventions/Rationales
- Maintain Standard Precautions and use good handwashing technique when providing care *to prevent introduction of or spread of infection.*
- Teach woman to maintain good handwashing technique (particularly before handling her newborn) and to maintain scrupulous perineal care with frequent change and careful disposal of perineal pads *to avoid spread of microorganisms.*
- Monitor vital signs *to detect signs of systemic infection.*
- Monitor level of fatigue and lethargy, evidence of chills, loss of appetite, nausea and vomiting, and abdominal pain, *which are indicative of extent of infection and serve as indicators of status of infection.*
- Monitor lochia for foul smell and profusion *as indicators of infection state.*
- Assist with collection of intrauterine cultures or other specimens for laboratory analysis *to identify specific causative organism.*
- Monitor laboratory values (i.e., white blood cell [WBC] count, cultures) *for indicators of type and status of infection.*
- Ensure adequate fluid and nutritional intake *to promote healthy recovery.*
- Administer and monitor broad-spectrum antibiotics if ordered *to prevent infection.*
- Administer antipyretics as ordered and necessary *to reduce elevated temperature.*

structions in increasing her dietary iron and protein intake and iron supplementation to rebuild lost red blood cell (RBC) volume. She may need assistance with infant care and household activities until she has regained strength. Some women have problems with delayed or insufficient lactation and postpartum depression (PPD). Referrals for home care follow-up or to community resources may be needed, such as Postpartum Support International at www.chss.iup.edu/postpartum.

■ Evaluation

The nurse can be reasonably assured that care was effective to the extent that the expected outcomes were achieved (Plan of Care).

■ HEMORRHAGIC (HYPOVOLEMIC) SHOCK

Hemorrhage may result in hemorrhagic (hypovolemic) shock. Shock is an emergency situation in which the perfusion of body organs may become severely compromised and death may occur. Physiologic compensatory mechanisms are activated in response to hemorrhage. The adrenal glands release catecholamines, causing arterioles and venules in the skin, the lungs, the gastrointestinal tract, the liver, and the kidneys to constrict. The available blood flow is diverted to the brain and the heart and away from other organs, including the uterus. If shock is prolonged, the continued reduction in cellular oxygenation results in an accumulation of lactic acid and acidosis (from anaerobic glucose metabolism). Acidosis (reduced serum pH) causes arteriolar vasodilation; venule vasoconstriction persists. A circular pattern is established; that is, decreased perfusion, increased tissue anoxia and acidosis, edema formation, and pooling of blood further decrease the perfusion. Cellular death occurs. See the Emergency box for assessments and interventions for hemorrhagic shock.

Medical Management

Vigorous treatment is necessary to prevent adverse sequelae. Medical management of hypovolemic shock involves restoring circulating blood volume and treating the cause of the hemorrhage (e.g., lacerations, uterine atony, or inversion). To restore circulating blood volume, a rapid IV infusion of crystalloid solution is given at a rate of 3 ml infused for every 1 ml of estimated blood loss (e.g., 3000 ml infused for 1000 ml of blood loss). Packed RBCs are usually infused if the woman is still actively bleeding and no improvement in her condition is noted after the initial crystalloid infusion. Infusion of fresh-frozen plasma may be needed if clotting factors and platelet counts are below normal values (Cunningham et al., 2005).

Nursing Interventions

Hemorrhagic shock can occur rapidly, but the classic signs of shock may not appear until the postpartum woman has lost 30% to 40% of blood volume. The nurse must con-

---

EMERGENCY

Hemorrhagic Shock

ASSESSMENTS	CHARACTERISTICS
• Respirations	• Rapid and shallow
• Pulse	• Rapid, weak, irregular
• Blood pressure	• Decreasing (late sign)
• Skin	• Cool, pale, clammy
• Urinary output	• Decreasing
• Level of consciousness	• Lethargy → coma
• Mental status	• Anxiety → coma
• Central venous pressure	• Decreased

INTERVENTION
• Summon assistance and equipment.
• Start intravenous infusion per standing orders.
• Ensure patent airway; administer oxygen.
• Continue to monitor status.

---

tinue to reassess the woman's condition, as evidenced by the degree of measurable and anticipated blood loss, and mobilize appropriate resources.

Most interventions are instituted to improve or monitor tissue perfusion. The nurse continues to monitor the woman's pulse and blood pressure. If invasive hemodynamic monitoring is ordered, the nurse may assist with the placement of the central venous pressure (CVP) or pulmonary artery (Swan-Ganz) catheter and monitor CVP, pulmonary artery pressure, or pulmonary artery wedge pressure as ordered (Poole & White, 2003) (see Chapter 34).

Additional assessments to be made include evaluation of skin temperature, color, and turgor, as well as assessment of the woman's mucous membranes. Breath sounds should be auscultated before fluid volume replacement, if possible, to provide a baseline for future assessment. Inspection for oozing at the sites of incisions or injections and assessment of the presence of petechiae or ecchymosis in areas not associated with surgery or trauma are critical in the evaluation for disseminated intravascular coagulation (see later discussion).

Oxygen is administered, preferably by nonrebreathing face mask, at 10 to 12 L/min to maintain oxygen saturation. Oxygen saturation should be monitored with a pulse oximeter, although measurements may not always be accurate in a woman with hypovolemia or decreased perfusion. Level of consciousness is assessed frequently and provides additional indications of blood volume and oxygen saturation. In early stages of decreased blood flow the woman may report "seeing stars" or feeling dizzy or nauseated. She may become restless and orthopneic. As cerebral hypoxia increases, she may become confused and react slowly or not at all to stimuli. Some women complain of headaches (Curran, 2003). An improved sensorium is an indicator of improved perfusion.

Continuous electrocardiographic monitoring may be indicated for the woman who is hypotensive or tachycardic, continues to bleed profusely, or is in shock. A Foley catheter with a urometer is inserted to allow hourly assessment of urinary output. The most objective and least invasive assessment of adequate organ perfusion and oxygenation is urinary output of at least 30 ml/hr (Benedetti, 2002). Blood may be drawn and sent to the laboratory for studies that include hemoglobin and hematocrit levels, platelet count, and coagulation profile.

Fluid or Blood Replacement Therapy

Critical to successful management of the woman with a hemorrhagic complication is establishment of venous access, preferably with a large-bore IV catheter. The establishment of two IV lines facilitates fluid resuscitation. Vigorous fluid resuscitation includes the administration of crystalloids (lactated Ringer's, normal saline solutions), colloids (albumin), blood, and blood components (Benedetti, 2002). Fluid resuscitation must be carefully monitored because fluid overload may occur. Intravascular fluid overload occurs more frequently with colloid therapy. Transfusion reactions may follow administration of blood or blood components, including cryoprecipitates. Even in an emergency, each unit should be checked per hospital protocol. Complications of fluid or blood replacement therapy include hemolytic reactions, febrile reactions, allergic reactions, circulatory overload, and air embolism.

■ LEGAL TIP Standard of Care for Bleeding Emergencies

The standard of care for obstetric emergency situations such as PPH or hypovolemic shock is that provision should be made for the nurse to implement actions independently. Policies, procedures, standing orders or protocols, and clinical guidelines should be established by each health care facility in which births occur and should be agreed on by health care providers involved in the care of obstetric clients.

■ COAGULOPATHIES

When bleeding is continuous and there is no identifiable source, a coagulopathy may be the cause. The woman's coagulation status must be assessed quickly and continuously. The nurse may draw and send blood to the laboratory for studies. Abnormal results depend on the cause and may include increased prothrombin time, increased partial thromboplastin time, decreased platelets, decreased fibrinogen level, increased fibrin degradation products, and prolonged bleeding time. Causes of coagulopathies may be pregnancy complications such as idiopathic thrombocytopenic purpura or von Willebrand disease and disseminated intravascular coagulation.

Idiopathic Thrombocytopenic Purpura

Idiopathic or immune thrombocytopenia purpura (ITP) is an autoimmune disorder in which antiplatelet antibodies decrease the life span of the platelets. Thrombocytopenia, capillary fragility, and increased bleeding time are diagnostic findings. ITP may cause severe hemorrhage after cesarean birth or from cervical or vaginal lacerations. The incidence of postpartum uterine bleeding and vaginal hematomas also is increased. Neonatal thrombocytopenia, a result of the ma-

ternal disease process, occurs in about 50% of cases and is associated with high mortality (Kilpatrick & Laros, 2004).

Medical management focuses on control of platelet stability. If ITP was diagnosed during pregnancy, the woman likely was treated with corticosteroids or IV immunoglobulin. Platelet transfusions are usually given when there is significant bleeding. A splenectomy may be needed if the ITP does not respond to medical management.

von Willebrand Disease

von Willebrand disease (vWD), a type of hemophilia, is probably the most common of all hereditary bleeding disorders. Although vWD is rare, it is among the most common congenital clotting defects in U.S. women of childbearing age (Mannucci, 2004). It results from a factor VIII deficiency and platelet dysfunction that is transmitted as an incomplete autosomal dominant trait to both sexes. Symptoms include a familial bleeding tendency, previous bleeding episodes, prolonged bleeding time (the most important test), factor VIII deficiency (mild to moderate), and bleeding from mucous membranes. Although factor VIII increases during pregnancy, there is still a risk for PPH as levels of von Willebrand (vW) factor begin to decrease (Cunningham et al., 2005).

The woman may be at risk for bleeding for up to 4 weeks postpartum. The treatment of choice is administration of desmopressin, which promotes the release of vW factor and factor VIII. It can be given nasally, intravenously, or orally. Transfusion therapy with plasma products that have been treated for viruses and containing factor VIII and vW factor also may be used (Demers, Derzko, David, Douglas, & Society of Obstetricians and Gynecologists of Canada, 2005; Lee & Abdul-Kadir, 2005). Cryoprecipitate may be used, but products treated for possible donor viruses are considered safer to use (Mannucci, 2001).

Disseminated Intravascular Coagulation

Disseminated intravascular coagulation (DIC) is a pathologic form of clotting that is diffuse and consumes large amounts of clotting factors, including platelets, fibrinogen, prothrombin, and factors V and VII. Widespread external bleeding, internal bleeding, or both can result. DIC also causes vascular occlusion of small vessels resulting from small clots forming in the microcirculation. In the obstetric population, DIC may occur as a result of abruptio placentae, amniotic fluid embolism, dead fetus syndrome (fetus has died but is retained in utero for at least 6 weeks), severe preeclampsia, septicemia, cardiopulmonary arrest, and hemorrhage.

The diagnosis of DIC is made according to clinical findings and laboratory markers. Physical examination reveals unusual bleeding; spontaneous bleeding from the woman's gums or nose may be noted. Petechiae may appear around a blood pressure cuff placed on the woman's arm. Excessive bleeding may occur from the site of a slight trauma (e.g., venipuncture sites, intramuscular or subcutaneous injection sites, nicks from shaving of perineum or abdomen, and injury from insertion of a urinary catheter). Symptoms also may include tachycardia and diaphoresis. Laboratory tests reveal decreased levels of platelets, fibrinogen, proacelerin, antihemophiliac factor, and prothrombin (the factors consumed during coagulation). Fibrinolysis is increased at first but is later severely depressed. Degradation of fibrin leads to the accumulation of fibrin split products in the blood; these have anticoagulant properties and prolong the prothrombin time. Bleeding time is normal, coagulation time shows no clot, clot-retraction time shows no clot, and partial thromboplastin time is increased (Cunningham et al., 2005; Kilpatrick & Laros, 2004; Labelle & Kitchens, 2005) (see Table 37-1). DIC must be distinguished from other clotting disorders before therapy is initiated.

Primary medical management in all cases of DIC involves correction of the underlying cause (e.g., removal of the dead fetus, treatment of existing infection or of preeclampsia or eclampsia, or removal of a placental abruption). Volume replacement, blood component therapy, optimization of oxygenation and perfusion status, and continued reassessment of laboratory parameters are the usual forms of treatment. Plasma levels usually return to normal within 24 hours after birth. Platelet counts usually return to normal within 7 days (Kilpatrick & Laros, 2004).

Nursing interventions include assessment for signs of bleeding and signs of complications from the administration of blood and blood products, administering fluid or blood replacement as ordered, and protecting from injury. Because renal failure is one consequence of DIC, urinary output is monitored, usually by insertion of an indwelling urinary catheter. Urinary output must be maintained at more than 30 ml/hr.

The woman and her family will be anxious or concerned about her condition and prognosis. The nurse offers explanations about care and provides emotional support to the woman and her family through this critical time.

■ THROMBOEMBOLIC DISEASE

A thrombosis results from the formation of a blood clot or clots inside a blood vessel and is caused by inflammation (thrombophlebitis) or partial obstruction of the vessel. Three thromboembolic conditions are of concern in the postpartum period:

- *Superficial venous thrombosis*: Involvement of the superficial saphenous venous system
- *Deep venous thrombosis*: Involvement varies but can extend from the foot to the iliofemoral region
- *Pulmonary embolism*: Complication of deep venous thrombosis occurring when part of a blood clot dislodges and is carried to the pulmonary artery, where it occludes the vessel and obstructs blood flow to the lungs

Incidence and Etiology

The incidence of thromboembolic disease in the postpartum period varies from about 0.5 to 3 per 1000 women (Laros, 2004). The incidence has declined in the last 20 years because early ambulation after childbirth has become the standard practice. The major causes of thromboembolic disease are venous stasis and hypercoagulation, both of which are present in pregnancy and continue into the postpartum period. Other risk factors include cesarean birth, history of venous thrombosis or varicosities, obesity, maternal age older than 35 years, multiparity, and smoking. The risk is also increased in women with associated genetic risk factors (Cunningham et al., 2005; Doyle & Monga, 2004).

Clinical Manifestations

Superficial venous thrombosis is the most frequent form of postpartum thrombophlebitis. It is characterized by pain and tenderness in the lower extremity. Physical examination may reveal warmth, redness, and an enlarged, hardened vein over the site of the thrombosis. Deep vein thrombosis is more common in pregnancy and is characterized by unilateral leg pain, calf tenderness, and swelling (Fig. 37-2). Physical examination may reveal redness and warmth, but women also may have a large amount of clot and have few symptoms (Stenchever, Droegemueller, Herbst, & Mishell, 2001). A positive Homans sign may be present, but further evaluation is needed because the calf pain may be attributed to other causes such as a strained muscle resulting from the birthing position. Other signs and symptoms frequently seen include apprehension, cough, tachycardia, hemoptysis, elevated temperature, and

table 37-1 **Laboratory Abnormalities of Disseminated Intravascular Coagulation (DIC)**

SCREENING TEST	RESULTS
Prothrombin time	Prolonged
Partial thromboplastin time	Normal or shortened
Activated partial thromboplastin time	Prolonged
Thrombin time	Prolonged
Fibrinogen	Decreased
Platelets	Decreased
SPECIAL TESTS	
Fibrin split products (FSP) or Fibrin degradation products (FDP)	Increased
D-Dimers (cross-linked fibrin fragments)	Increased
Factor assays (for Factors V, VII, VIII, X, XIII)	Decreased
Antithrombin	Decreased

Sources: Cunningham, G., Leveno, K., Bloom, S., Hauth, J., Gilstrap, L., & Wenstrom, K. (2005). *Williams obstetrics* (22nd ed.). New York; McGraw-Hill; Kilpatrick, S., & Laros, R. (2004). Maternal hematologic disorders. In R. Creasy, R. Resnick, & J. Iams (Eds.), *Maternal-fetal medicine: Principles and practice* (5th ed.). Philadelphia: Saunders; Labelle, C., & Kitchens, C. (2005). Disseminated intravascular coagulation: Treat the cause, not the lab values. *Cleveland Clinic Journal of Medicine, 72*(5), 377-397; Lewis, H., Heitkemper, M., & Dirksen, S. (2004). *Medical-surgical nursing: Assessment and management of clinical problems* (6th ed). St. Louis: Mosby.

FIG. 37-2 Deep vein thrombophlebitis.

pleuritic chest pain (Laros, 2004). Pulmonary embolism is characterized by dyspnea and tachypnea.

Physical examination is not a sensitive diagnostic indicator for thrombosis. Venography is the most accurate method for diagnosing deep venous thrombosis; however, it is an invasive procedure that exposes the woman and fetus to ionizing radiation and is associated with serious complications. Noninvasive diagnostic methods are more commonly used; these include real-time and color Doppler ultrasound. Cardiac auscultation may reveal murmurs with pulmonary embolism. Electrocardiograms are usually normal. Arterial Po_2 may be lower than normal. A ventilation/perfusion scan, Doppler ultrasound, and pulmonary arteriogram may be used for diagnosis (Laros, 2004).

Medical Management

Superficial venous thrombosis is treated with analgesia (nonsteroidal antiinflammatory agents), rest with elevation of the affected leg, and elastic stockings (Laros, 2004). Local application of heat also may be used. Deep venous thrombosis is initially treated with anticoagulant (usually continuous IV heparin) therapy, bed rest with the affected leg elevated, and analgesia. After the symptoms have decreased, the woman may be fitted with elastic stockings to use when she is allowed to ambulate. IV heparin therapy continues for 3 to 5 days or until symptoms resolve. Oral anticoagulant therapy (warfarin) is started during this time and will be continued for about 3 months. Continuous IV heparin therapy is used for pulmonary embolism until symptoms have resolved. Intermittent subcutaneous heparin or oral anticoagulant therapy is usually continued for 6 months.

Nursing Interventions

In the hospital setting, nursing care of the woman with a thrombosis consists of continued assessments: inspection and palpation of the affected area; palpation of peripheral pulses; checking Homans sign; measurement and comparison of leg circumferences; inspection for signs of bleeding; monitoring for signs of pulmonary embolism including chest pain, coughing, dyspnea, and tachypnea; and respiratory status for presence of crackles. Laboratory reports are monitored for prothrombin or partial thromboplastin times. The woman and her family are assessed for their level of understanding about the diagnosis and their ability to cope during the unexpected extended period of recovery.

Interventions include explanations and education about the diagnosis and the treatment. The woman will need assistance with personal care as long as she is on bed rest; the family should be encouraged to participate in the care if that is what she and they wish. While the woman is on bed rest, she should be encouraged to change positions frequently but not to place the knees in a sharply flexed position that could cause pooling of blood in the lower extremities. She also should be cautioned not to rub the affected area, as this action could cause the clot to dislodge. Once the woman is allowed to ambulate, she is taught how to prevent venous congestion by putting on the elastic stockings before getting out of bed.

Heparin and warfarin are administered as ordered, and the physician is notified if clotting times are outside the therapeutic level. If the woman is breastfeeding, she is assured that neither heparin nor warfarin is excreted in significant quantities in breast milk. If the infant has been discharged, the family is encouraged to bring the infant for feedings as permitted by hospital policy; the mother also can express milk to be sent home.

Pain can be managed with a variety of measures. Position changes, elevating the leg, and application of moist warm heat may decrease discomfort. Administration of analgesics and antiinflammatory medications may be needed.

▬ NURSE ALERT

Medications containing aspirin are not given to women receiving anticoagulant therapy because aspirin inhibits synthesis of clotting factors and can lead to prolonged clotting time and increased risk of bleeding.

The woman is usually discharged home with oral anticoagulants and will need explanations about the treatment schedule and possible side effects. If subcutaneous injections are to be given, the woman and family are taught how to administer the medication and about site rotation. The woman and her family also should be given information about safe care practices to prevent bleeding and injury while she is receiving anticoagulant therapy, such as using a soft toothbrush and an electric razor. She also will need information about follow-up with her health care provider to monitor clotting times and to make sure the correct dose of anticoagulant therapy is maintained. The woman also should use a reliable method of contraception if taking warfarin, because this medication is considered teratogenic (Gilbert & Harmon, 2003).

▬ POSTPARTUM INFECTIONS

Postpartum or puerperal infection is any clinical infection of the genital canal that occurs within 28 days after miscarriage, induced abortion, or childbirth. The definition used in the United States continues to be the presence of a fever of 38° C or more on 2 successive days of the first 10 postpartum days (not counting the first 24 hours after birth) (Cunningham et al., 2005). Puerperal infection is probably the major cause of maternal morbidity and mortality throughout the world; however, it occurs after about 6% of births in the United States (Gibbs, Sweet, & Duff, 2004). Common postpartum infections include endometritis, wound infections, mastitis, urinary tract infections (UTIs), and respiratory tract infections.

The most common infecting organisms are the numerous streptococcal and anaerobic organisms. *Staphylococcus aureus*, gonococci, coliform bacteria, and clostridia are less common but serious pathogenic organisms that also cause puerperal infection. Postpartum infections are more common in women who have concurrent medical or immunosuppressive conditions or who had a cesarean or other operative birth (incidence is 5 to 10 times higher after cesarean births than after vaginal births). Intrapartal factors such as prolonged rupture of membranes, prolonged labor, and internal maternal or fetal monitoring also increase the risk of infection (Gibbs et al., 2004). Factors that predispose the woman to postpartum infection are listed in Box 37-4.

box 37-4 Predisposing Factors for Postpartum Infection

PRECONCEPTION OR ANTEPARTAL FACTORS
- History of previous venous thrombosis, urinary tract infection, mastitis, pneumonia
- Diabetes mellitus
- Alcoholism
- Drug abuse
- Immunosuppression
- Anemia
- Malnutrition

INTRAPARTAL FACTORS
- Cesarean birth
- Prolonged rupture of membranes
- Chorioamnionitis
- Prolonged labor
- Bladder catheterization
- Internal fetal/uterine pressure monitoring
- Multiple vaginal examinations after rupture of membranes
- Epidural analgesia/anesthesia
- Retained placental fragments
- Postpartum hemorrhage
- Episiotomy or lacerations
- Hematomas

Endometritis

Endometritis is the most common postpartum infection. It usually begins as a localized infection at the placental site (Fig. 37-3) but can spread to involve the entire endometrium. Incidence is higher after cesarean birth. Assessment for signs of endometritis may reveal a fever (usually greater than 38° C); increased pulse; chills; anorexia; nausea; fatigue and lethargy; pelvic pain; uterine tenderness; or foul-smelling, profuse lochia (Duff, 2002). Leukocytosis and a markedly increased RBC sedimentation rate are typical laboratory findings of postpartum infections. Anemia also may be present. Blood cultures or intracervical or intrauterine bacterial cultures (aerobic and anaerobic) should reveal the offending pathogens within 36 to 48 hours.

Wound Infections

Wound infections also are common postpartum infections but often develop after the woman is at home. Sites of infection include the cesarean incision and the episiotomy or repaired laceration site. Predisposing factors are similar to those for endometritis (see Box 37-4). Signs of wound infection include erythema, edema, warmth, tenderness, seropurulent drainage, and wound separation. Fever and pain also may be present.

Urinary Tract Infections

Urinary tract infections (UTIs) occur in 2% to 4% of postpartum women. Risk factors include urinary catheterization, frequent pelvic examinations, epidural anesthesia, genital tract injury, history of UTI, and cesarean birth. Signs and symptoms include dysuria, frequency and urgency, low-grade fever, urinary retention, hematuria, and pyuria. Costovertebral angle (CVA) tenderness or flank pain may indicate upper UTI. Urinalysis results may reveal *Escherichia coli*, although other gram-negative aerobic bacilli also may cause UTIs.

FIG. 37-3 Postpartum infection—endometritis.

FIG. 37-4 Mastitis.

Mastitis

Mastitis affects about 1% of women soon after childbirth, most of whom are first-time mothers who are breastfeeding. Mastitis almost always is unilateral and develops well after the flow of milk has been established (Fig. 37-4). The infecting organism generally is the hemolytic *S. aureus*. An infected nipple fissure usually is the initial lesion, but the ductal system is involved next. Inflammatory edema and engorgement of the breast soon obstruct the flow of milk in a lobe; regional, then generalized, mastitis follows. If treatment is not prompt, mastitis may progress to a breast abscess.

Symptoms rarely appear before the end of the first postpartum week and are more common in the second to fourth weeks. Chills, fever, malaise, and local breast tenderness are noted first. Localized breast tenderness, pain, swelling, redness, and axillary adenopathy also may occur. Antibiotics are prescribed. Lactation can be maintained by emptying the breasts every 2 to 4 hours by breastfeeding, manual expression, or breast pump and discarding the milk.

▬ CARE MANAGEMENT

Signs and symptoms associated with postpartum infection were discussed with each infection. Laboratory tests usually performed include a complete blood count, venous blood cultures, and uterine tissue cultures. Nursing diagnoses for women experiencing postpartum infection include the following:

- *Deficient knowledge related to*
  - –cause, management, course of infection
  - –transmission and prevention of infection
- *Impaired tissue integrity related to*
  - –effects of infection process
- *Acute pain related to*
  - –mastitis
  - –puerperal infection
  - –UTI

- *Interrupted family processes related to*
  - –unexpected complication to expected postpartum recovery
  - –possible separation from newborn
  - –interruption in process of realigning relationships after the addition of the new family member
- *Risk for impaired parenting related to*
  - –fear of spread of infection to newborn

The most effective and least expensive treatment of postpartum infection is prevention. Preventive measures include good prenatal nutrition to control anemia and intrapartal hemorrhage. Good maternal perineal hygiene with thorough handwashing is emphasized. Strict adherence by all health care personnel to aseptic techniques during childbirth and the postpartum period is very important.

Management of endometritis consists of IV broad-spectrum antibiotic therapy (cephalosporins, penicillins, or clindamycin and gentamicin) and supportive care, including hydration, rest, and pain relief (French & Smaill, 2004). Antibiotic therapy is usually discontinued 24 hours after the woman is asymptomatic (Gibbs et al. 2004). Assessments of lochia, vital signs, and changes in the woman's condition continue during treatment. Comfort measures depend on the symptoms and may include cool compresses, warm blankets, perineal care, and sitz baths. Teaching should include side effects of therapy, prevention of spread of infection, signs and symptoms of worsening condition, and adherence to the treatment plan and the need for follow-up care. Women may need to be encouraged or assisted to maintain mother-infant interactions and breastfeeding (if allowed during treatment).

Postpartum women are usually discharged to home by 48 hours after birth. This is often before signs of infection are evident. Nurses in birth centers and hospital settings must be able to identify women at risk for postpartum infection and to provide anticipatory teaching and counseling before discharge. After discharge, telephone follow-up, hot lines, support groups, lactation counselors, home visits by nurses, and teaching materials (videos, written materials) are all interventions that can be implemented to decrease the risk of postpartum infections. Home care nurses must be able to recognize signs and symptoms of postpartum infection so that the woman can contact her primary health care provider. These nurses also must be able to provide the appropriate nursing care for women who need follow-up home care.

Treatment of wound infections may combine antibiotic therapy with wound debridement. Wounds may be opened and drained. Nursing care includes frequent wound and vital sign assessments and wound care. Comfort measures include sitz baths, warm compresses, and perineal care. Teaching includes good hygiene techniques (e.g., changing perineal pads front to back handwashing before and after perineal care), self-care measures, and signs of worsening conditions to report to the health care provider. The woman is usually discharged to home for self-care or home nursing care after treatment is initiated in the inpatient setting.

Medical management for UTIs consists of antibiotic therapy, analgesia, and hydration. Postpartum women are usually treated on an outpatient basis; therefore teaching should include instructions on how to monitor temperature, bladder function, and appearance of urine. The woman also should be taught about signs of potential complications and the importance of taking all antibiotics as prescribed. Other suggestions for prevention of UTIs include using proper perineal care, wiping from front to back after urinating or having a bowel movement, and increasing fluid intake.

Because mastitis rarely occurs before the postpartum woman who is breastfeeding is discharged, teaching should include warning signs of mastitis and counseling about prevention of cracked nipples. Management includes intensive antibiotic therapy (e.g., cephalosporins and vancomycin, which are particularly useful in staphylococcal infections), support of breasts, local heat (or cold), adequate hydration, and analgesics.

Almost all instances of acute mastitis can be avoided by using proper breastfeeding technique to prevent cracked nipples. Missed feedings, waiting too long between feedings, and abrupt weaning may lead to clogged nipples and mastitis. Cleanliness practiced by all who have contact with the newborn and new mother also reduces the incidence of mastitis. See Chapter 27 for further information.

community activity

After giving birth, many women are discharged home before an infection can develop. Prepare a "Fact Sheet About Postpartum Infection" that could be distributed to postpartum women upon discharge from the hospitals or birth centers in your community. Include signs and symptoms, and phone numbers and addresses of health care providers who could be contacted. If your community has a large population of clients who do not speak English, consider a fact sheet in Spanish or other language as appropriate.

key points

- Postpartum hemorrhage is the most common and most serious type of excessive obstetric blood loss.
- Hemorrhagic (hypovolemic) shock is an emergency situation in which the perfusion of body organs may become severely compromised, leading to significant risk of morbidity or death for the mother.
- The potential hazards of the therapeutic interventions may further compromise the woman with a hemorrhagic disorder.

- Clotting disorders are associated with many obstetric complications.
- The first symptom of postpartum infection is usually fever greater than 38° C on 2 consecutive days in the first 10 postpartum days (after the first 24 hours).
- Prevention is the most effective and inexpensive treatment of postpartum infection.

REFERENCES

Benedetti, T. (2002). Obstetric hemorrhage. In S. Gabbe, J. Niebyl, & J. Simpson (Eds.), *Obstetrics: Normal and problem pregnancies* (4th ed.). New York: Churchill Livingstone.

Berg, T., & Smith, C. (2002). Pharmacologic therapy for peripartum emergencies. *Clinical Obstetrics and Gynecology, 45*(1), 125-135.

Bowes, W., & Thorp, J. (2004). Clinical aspects of normal and abnormal labor. In R. Creasy, R. Resnick, & J. Iams (Eds.), *Maternal-fetal medicine: Principles and practice* (5th ed.). Philadelphia: Saunders.

Clark, S. (2004). Placenta previa and abruptio placentae. In R. Creasy, R. Resnick, & J. Iams (Eds.), *Maternal-fetal medicine: Principles and practice* (5th ed.). Philadelphia: Saunders.

Cunningham, G., Leveno, K., Bloom, S., Hauth, J., Gilstrap, L., & Wenstrom, K. (2005). *Williams obstetrics* (22nd ed.). New York: McGraw-Hill.

Curran, C. (2003). Intrapartum emergencies. *Journal of Obstetric, Gynecologic, and Neonatal Nursing, 32*(6), 802-813.

Demers, C., Derzko, C., David, M., Douglas, J., & Society of Obstetricians and Gynecologists of Canada. (2005). Gynaecological and obstetric management of women with inherited bleeding disorders. *Journal of Obstetrics and Gynaecology of Canada, 27*(7), 707-732.

Doyle, N., & Monga, M. (2004). Thromboembolic disease in pregnancy. *Obstetrics and Gynecologic Clinics of North America, 31*(2), 319-344.

Duff, P. (2002). Maternal and perinatal infection. In S. Gabbe, J. Niebyl, & J. Simpson (Eds.), *Obstetrics: Normal and problem pregnancies* (4th ed.). New York: Churchill Livingstone.

French, L., & Smaill, F. (2004). Antibiotic regimens for endometritis after delivery. In *The Cochrane Database of Systematic Reviews,* 2006, Issue 3. Chichester UK: John Wiley & Sons.

Gibbs, R., Sweet, R., & Duff, P. (2004). Maternal and fetal infectious disorders. In R. Creasy, R. Resnick, & J. Iams (Eds.), *Maternal-fetal medicine: Principles and practice* (5th ed.). Philadelphia: Saunders.

Gilbert, E., & Harmon, J. (2003). *Manual of high risk pregnancy & delivery* (3rd ed.). St. Louis: Mosby.

Gülmezoglu, A., Forna, F., Villar, J., & Hofmeyr, G. (2004). Prostaglandins for prevention of postpartum haemorrhage. In *The Cochrane Database of Systematic Reviews,* 2006, Issue 3. Chichester, UK: John Wiley & Sons.

Kilpatrick, S., & Laros, R. (2004). Maternal hematologic disorders. In R. Creasy, R. Resnick, & J. Iams (Eds.), *Maternal-fetal medicine: Principles and practice* (5th ed.). Philadelphia: Saunders.

Labelle, C., & Kitchens, C. (2005). Disseminated intravascular coagulation: Treat the cause, not the lab values. *Cleveland Clinic Journal of Medicine, 72*(5), 377-397.

Laros, R. (2004). Thromboembolic disease. In R. Creasy, R. Resnick, & J. Iams (Eds.), *Maternal-fetal medicine: Principles and practice* (5th ed.). Philadelphia: Saunders.

Lee, C., & Abdul-Kadir, R. (2005). von Willibrand disease and women's health. *Seminars in Hematology, 42*(1), 42-48.

Magann, E., Evans, S., Chauhan, S., Lanneau, G., Fisk, A., & Morrison, J. (2005). The length of the third stage of labor and the risk of postpartum hemorrhage. *Obstetrics and Gynecology, 105*(2), 290-293.

Magann, E., & Lanneau, G. (2005). Third stage of labor. *Obstetrics and Gynecologic Clinics of North America, 32*(2), 323-332.

MacMullen, N., Dulski, L., & Meagher, B. (2005). Red alert: Perinatal hemorrhage. *MCN American Journal of Maternal/Child Nursing, 30*(1), 46-51.

Mannucci, P. (2001). How I treat patients with von Willibrand's disease. *Blood, 97*(7), 1915-1919.

Mannucci, P. (2004). Treatment of von Willibrand's disease. *New England Journal of Medicine, 351*(7), 683-694.

McLintock, C. (2005). Postpartum haemorrhage. *Thrombosis Research, 115*(Supp 1), 65-68.

Papp, Z. (2003). Massive obstetric hemorrhage. *Journal of Perinatal Medicine, 31*(5), 408-414.

Poole, J., & White D. (Eds.). (2003). *Obstetrical emergencies for the perinatal nurse.* White Plains, NY: March of Dimes Birth Defects Foundation.

Skidmore-Roth, L. (2004). *Mosby's handbook of herbs and natural supplements* (2nd ed.). St Louis: Mosby

Stenchever, M., Droegemueller, W., Herbst, A., & Mishell, D. (2001). *Comprehensive gynecology* (4th ed.). St Louis: Mosby.

Tiran, D., & Mack, S. (Eds.). (2000). *Complementary therapies for pregnancy and childbirth* (2nd ed.). Edinburgh: Baillière Tindall.

Acquired Problems of the Newborn

learning objectives

- Summarize the care of the newborn with soft tissue, skeletal, and nervous system injuries.
- Describe assessment of infants for birth trauma and for sequelae of a diabetic pregnancy.
- Develop nursing care plans for complications typically seen in infants of mothers with diabetes.
- Describe in detail the assessment of a newborn with a suspected infection.
- Formulate nursing diagnoses for the infant and family for common bacterial and viral infections.

- Interpret the evidence available to guide the care of the infant at risk for group B streptococcus (GBS) sepsis.
- Review implementation and evaluation of care of infants with infections; include their families.
- Distinguish between the effects of maternal use of alcohol, heroin, methadone, marijuana, and cocaine and maternal smoking on the fetus and newborn.
- Describe the assessment and care of a newborn experiencing drug withdrawal; include the infant's family.

electronic resources

Additional information related to the content in Chapter 38 can be found on

the companion website at **evolve**
http://evolve.elsevier.com/Lowdermilk/MWHC/
- NCLEX Review Questions
- WebLinks

or on the interactive companion CD
- NCLEX Review Questions
- Critical Thinking Exercise: Fetal Alcohol Syndrome
- Plan of Care: The Infant of the Mother with Gestational Diabetes
- Plan of Care: The Infant Undergoing Drug Withdrawal

THIS chapter deals with acquired problems of the newborn. *Acquired problems* refer to those conditions resulting from environmental factors rather than genetic circumstances. The focus is on birth trauma, the infant of a mother with diabetes, neonatal infections, and effects of maternal substance abuse.

■ BIRTH TRAUMA

Birth trauma (injury) is physical injury sustained by a neonate during labor and birth. The significance of birth injuries is assessed most accurately by review of recent mortality data. These data show a modest decline in fatal birth injuries. In 1981 birth injuries ranked sixth among major causes of infant mortality in the United States, resulting in 23.8 deaths per 100,000 live births. In 2002, unintentional injuries (which includes birth injuries) ranked sixth and caused 23.5 deaths per 100,000 live births (Martin, Kochanek, Strobino, Guyer, & MacDorman, 2005). Despite improvements in obstetric techniques, increased

use of cesarean surgery for births that would be difficult vaginally, and decreased use of vacuum extraction and version and extraction, birth injuries still are an important source of neonatal morbidity. Therefore the clinician should consider the broad range of birth injuries in the differential diagnosis of neonatal clinical disorders (Mangurten, 2006).

In theory, some birth injuries are avoidable, especially if careful assessment of risk factors and appropriate planning of birth occur. The use of ultrasonography allows antepartum diagnosis of macrosomia, hydrocephalus, and unusual presentations. Elective cesarean birth can be chosen for some pregnancies to prevent significant birth injury (Paige & Moe, 2006). A small percentage of significant birth injuries are unavoidable despite skilled and competent obstetric care, as in especially difficult or prolonged labor or when the infant is in an abnormal presentation (Mangurten, 2006). Some injuries cannot be anticipated until the specific circumstances are encountered during childbirth. Emergency cesarean birth may provide a last-minute salvage, but in these circumstances, the injury may be truly unavoidable. The same injury might be caused in several ways. For example, a cephalhematoma could result from an obstetric technique such as forceps birth or vacuum extraction or from pressure of the fetal skull against the maternal pelvis.

Many injuries are minor and resolve readily in the neonatal period without treatment. Other traumas require some degree of intervention. A few are serious enough to be fatal. The nurse's contribution to the welfare of the newborn begins with early observation and accurate recording. The prompt reporting of signs that indicate deviations from normal permits early initiation of appropriate therapy. Table 38-1 provides an overview of neurologic birth injuries and the sites in which they occur.

▬ CARE MANAGEMENT

▬ Assessment and Nursing Diagnoses

Several factors predispose an infant to birth injuries (Mangurten, 2006; Paige & Moe, 2006). Maternal factors include uterine dysfunction that leads to prolonged or precipitate labor, preterm or postterm labor, and cephalopelvic disproportion. Injury may result from dystocia

table 38-1 Types of Birth Injuries

SITE OF INJURY	TYPE OF INJURY
Scalp	Caput succedaneum
	Subgaleal hemorrhage
	Cephalhematoma
Skull	Linear fracture
	Depressed fracture
	Occipital osteodiastasis
Intracranial	Epidural hematoma
	Subdural hematoma (laceration of falx, tentorium, or superficial veins)
	Subarachnoid hemorrhage
	Cerebral contusion
	Cerebellar contusion
	Intracerebellar hematoma
Spinal cord (cervical)	Vertebral artery injury
	Intraspinal hemorrhage
	Spinal cord transection or injury
Plexus	Erb-Duchenne palsy
	Klumpke paralysis
	Total (mixed) brachial plexus injury
	Horner syndrome
	Diaphragmatic paralysis
	Lumbosacral plexus injury
Cranial and peripheral nerve	Radial nerve palsy
	Medial nerve palsy
	Sciatic nerve palsy
	Laryngeal nerve palsy
	Diaphragmatic paralysis
	Facial nerve palsy

Source: Paige, P., & Moe, P. (2006). *Neurologic disorders.* In G. Merenstein, & S. Gardner, (Eds.). *Handbook of neonatal intensive care* (6th ed.). St. Louis: Mosby.

caused by fetal macrosomia, multifetal gestation, abnormal or difficult presentation (not caused by maternal uterine or pelvic conditions), and congenital anomalies. Intrapartum events that can result in scalp injury include the use of internal monitoring of fetal heart rate (FHR) and collection of fetal scalp blood for acid-base assessment. Obstetric birth techniques can cause injury. Forceps birth, vacuum extraction, version and extraction, and cesarean birth are potential contributory factors. Often more than one factor is present, and multiple predisposing factors may be related to a single maternal condition.

The Apgar score may alert the caregiver to birth injuries and help in identifying infants in need of immediate resuscitation. Flaccid muscle tone, regardless of cause, increases the risk of joint dislocations and separation during the birth process. Flaccid tone in extremities may be traced to nerve plexus injuries or long-bone fractures. A weak or hoarse cry is characteristic of laryngeal nerve palsy as a result of excessive traction on the neck during birth. Pronounced bruising of the skin may preclude accurate assessment for color.

A complete physical assessment of the newborn is performed soon after birth. Because evidence of birth injury may not be apparent at the initial examination, assessment continues during each contact with the neonate. The nursing diagnoses depend on the particular injury incurred; thus the following list represents examples only.

INFANT
* *Impaired physical mobility related to*
  –brachial plexus injury
* *Impaired gas exchange related to*
  –diaphragmatic paralysis (partial or complete)
* *Acute pain related to*
  –injury
* *Injury related to*
  –malpresentation, difficult birth, shoulder dystocia

PARENTS AND FAMILY
* *Anxiety related to deficient knowledge regarding*
  –injury and its cause
  –management and therapy
  –prognosis
* *Anticipatory grieving related to*
  –possible sequelae of the birth injury

▬ Expected Outcomes of Care

Meeting the unique needs of the birth-injured newborn requires constant vigilance. Expected outcomes are established and priorities assigned. Nursing actions are selected in terms of the particular disorder and individual needs of the infant and family. The overall outcomes for care of infants with birth trauma include the following:
* The newborn will have minimal or no sequelae of trauma.
* The infant will receive prompt and appropriate treatment.

- The parents will initiate and maintain a positive parent-child relationship.
- The parents' and family's educational needs regarding the injury and its management will be met.

▪ Plan of Care and Interventions
▪ *Soft-Tissue Injuries*

Caput succedaneum, cephalhematoma, and subgaleal hemorrhage are discussed in Chapter 25.

Subconjunctival (scleral) and retinal hemorrhages result from rupture of capillaries caused by increased *intracranial pressure (ICP)* during birth. They clear within 5 days after birth and usually present no problems; however, parents need reassurance about their presence.

Erythema, ecchymoses, petechiae, abrasions, lacerations, and edema of buttocks and extremities may be present. Localized discoloration may appear over presenting or dependent parts. Ecchymoses and edema may appear anywhere on the body and especially on the presenting body part from the application of forceps. They also may result from manipulation of the infant's body during birth.

Bruises over the face may be the result of face presentation (Fig. 38-1). In a breech presentation, bruising and swelling may be seen over the buttocks or genitalia (Fig. 38-2). The skin over the entire head may be ecchymotic and covered with petechiae caused by a tight nuchal cord. Petechiae, or pinpoint hemorrhagic areas, acquired during birth may extend over the upper portion of the trunk and face. These lesions are benign if they disappear within 2 days of birth and no new lesions appear. Ecchymoses and petechiae may be signs of a more serious disorder, such as thrombocytopenic purpura, if the hemorrhagic areas

FIG. 38-1 Marked bruising on the entire face of an infant born vaginally after face presentation. Less severe ecchymoses were present on the extremities. Phototherapy was required for treatment of jaundice resulting from the breakdown of accumulated blood. (From O'Doherty, N. [1986]. *Neonatology: Micro atlas of the newborn.* Nutley, NJ: Hoffmann-La Roche.)

FIG. 38-2 Swelling of the genitals and bruising of the buttocks after a breech birth. Note the position of the infant's legs. (Courtesy Cheryl Briggs, RN, Annapolis, MD.)

do not disappear spontaneously in 2 days. To differentiate hemorrhagic areas from skin rashes and discolorations such as mongolian spots, the nurse blanches the skin with two fingers. Because extravasated blood remains within the tissues, petechiae and ecchymoses do not blanch.

Forceps injury occurs at the site of application of the instrument. Forceps injury typically has a linear configuration across both sides of the face, outlining the placement of the forceps. The affected areas are kept clean to minimize the risk of secondary infection. These injuries usually resolve spontaneously within several days with no specific therapy.

Accidental lacerations may be inflicted with a scalpel during cesarean birth or with scissors during an episiotomy. These cuts may occur on any part of the body but most often are found on the scalp, buttocks, and thighs. Usually they are superficial, needing only to be kept clean. Butterfly adhesive strips will hold together the edges of more serious lacerations. Rarely are sutures needed.

▪ *Skeletal Injuries*

The newborn's immature, flexible skull can withstand a great degree of deformation (molding) before fracture results. Considerable force is required to fracture the newborn's skull. Two types of skull fractures typically are identified in the newborn: linear fractures and depressed fractures. The location of the fracture and involvement of underlying structures determine its significance.

If an artery lying in a groove on the undersurface of the skull is torn as a result of the fracture, increased ICP will ensue. Unless a blood vessel is involved, linear fractures (which account for 70% of all fractures for this age group) heal without special treatment. Linear fractures are most common in the parietal bones (Uhing, 2004).

The soft skull may become indented without laceration of either the skin or the dural membrane. These depressed fractures, or "ping-pong ball" indentations, may occur during difficult births from pressure of the head on the bony pelvis. They also can occur as a result of injudicious application of forceps. Computed tomography (CT scan) is done to rule out bone fragments or underlying injury of

FIG. 38-3 Fractured clavicle after shoulder dystocia. (From O'Doherty, N. [1986]. *Neonatology: Micro atlas of the newborn.* Nutley, NJ: Hoffmann-La Roche.)

the brain tissue. Management of depressed skull fractures is controversial; many resolve without intervention. Non-surgical elevation of the indentation by using a hand breast pump or vacuum extractor has been reported (Mangurten, 2006). Surgery may be required in the presence of bone fragments or signs of increased ICP (Uhing, 2004).

The clavicle is the bone most often fractured during birth. One study placed the incidence of clavicular fracture at 1.6% of vaginal births (Lam, 2002). Generally the break is in the middle third of the bone (Fig. 38-3). Dystocia, particularly shoulder impaction, is a risk factor in clavicular fracture (Hsu et al., 2002). Other risk factors include vacuum extraction and birth weight greater than 4000 g (Hsu et al.; Lam). Limitation of motion of the arm, crepitus over the bone, and the absence of the Moro reflex on the affected side are diagnostic. Except for use of gentle rather than vigorous handling, no accepted treatment for fractured clavicle exists, and the prognosis is good. A sign posted on the bassinet will alert care providers to the need for careful handling. The figure-eight bandage appropriate for the older child should not be used for the newborn.

The humerus and femur may be fractured during a difficult birth. Fractures in newborns generally heal rapidly. Immobilization is accomplished with slings, splints, swaddling, and other devices.

The parents need support in handling these infants, because they often are fearful of hurting them. Parents are encouraged to practice handling, changing, and feeding the affected neonate under the guidance of nursery personnel. This increases their confidence and knowledge and facilitates attachment. A plan for follow-up therapy is developed with the parents so that the times and arrangements for therapy are acceptable to them.

■ Peripheral Nervous System Injuries

Erb-Duchenne palsy or brachial plexus injury (brachial paralysis of the upper portion of the arm) is the most common type of paralysis associated with a difficult birth, occurring at rates of 0.5 to 2 per 1000 live births (Paige &

Moe, 2006) (Fig. 38-4). An increased risk of brachial plexus injury occurs with birth weights over 4000 g, shoulder dystocia, vaginal breech deliveries, forceps-assisted or vacuum-assisted birth, maternal diabetes, and a prolonged second stage of labor (Mollberg, Hagberg, Bager, Lilja, & Ladfors, 2005). Injury to the upper plexus results from stretching or pulling the head away from the shoulder during the difficult birth. Typical symptoms are a flaccid arm with the elbow extended and the hand rotated inward, absence of the Moro reflex on the affected side, sensory loss over the lateral aspect of the arm, and an intact grasp reflex.

Treatment is by intermittent immobilization across the upper abdomen, proper positioning, and range of motion (ROM) exercises. Gentle manipulation and ROM exercises are delayed until about the tenth day to prevent additional injury to the brachial plexus.

Immobilization may be accomplished with a brace or splint or by pinning the infant's sleeve to his or her shirt.

Damage to the lower plexus, *Klumpke palsy,* is less common. With lower arm paralysis, the wrist and hand are flaccid, the grasp reflex is absent, deep tendon reflexes are present, and dependent edema and cyanosis may be apparent (in the affected hand). Treatment consists of placing the hand in a neutral position, padding the fist, and gently exercising the wrist and fingers.

Parents are taught to position and immobilize the arm or wrist or both. They can gently massage and manipulate the muscles to prevent contractures while the arm is healing. If edema or hemorrhage is responsible for the paralysis, the prognosis is good, and recovery may be expected in a few weeks. If laceration of the nerves has occurred and

FIG. 38-4 Erb-Duchenne paralysis in newborn infant. The Moro reflex was absent in right upper extremity. Recovery was complete. (From O'Doherty, N. [1986]. *Neonatology: Micro atlas of the newborn.* Nutley, NJ: Hoffmann-La Roche.)

healing does not result in return of function within a few months (4 to 6 months or 2 years at the most), surgery may be indicated; however, return of function is variable. Full recovery is expected in 88% to 92% of infants (Paige & Moe, 2006).

Facial paralysis (palsy) (Fig. 38-5) generally is caused by pressure on the facial nerve during birth. Risk factors include a prolonged second stage of labor and forceps-assisted birth. The face on the affected side is flattened and unresponsive to the grimace that accompanies crying or stimulation, and the eye will remain open on the affected side. Moreover, the forehead will not wrinkle. Usually the infant's face appears distorted, especially when crying. Often the condition is transitory, resolving within hours or days of birth. Permanent paralysis is rare.

Treatment involves assistance with feeding, prevention of damage to the cornea of the open eye with the application of artificial tears or taping the eye closed, and supportive care of the parents. Feeding may be prolonged, with the milk flowing out the newborn's mouth around the nipple on the affected side. The mother will need understanding and sympathetic encouragement while learning how to feed and care for the infant, as well as how to hold and cuddle the baby.

Phrenic nerve injury almost always occurs as a component of brachial plexus injury rather than as an isolated problem. Injury is usually the result of traction on the neck and arm during birth. Injury to the phrenic nerve is usually unilateral, but may be bilateral, and results in diaphragmatic paralysis. Cyanosis and irregular thoracic respirations, with no abdominal movement on inspiration, are characteristic of paralysis of the diaphragm. Babies with diaphragmatic paralysis usually require mechanical ventilatory support, at least for the first few days after birth and

FIG. 38-5 Facial paralysis 15 minutes after forceps birth. Absence of movement on affected side is especially noticeable when infant cries. (From O'Doherty, N. [1986]. *Neonatology: Micro atlas of the newborn*. Nutley, NJ: Hoffmann-La Roche.)

are at risk of developing pneumonia. In the presence of persistent respiratory distress, diaphragmatic pacing or surgical correction may be required.

■ Central Nervous System Injuries

All types of intracranial hemorrhage (ICH) occur in newborns. ICH as a result of birth trauma is more likely to occur in the term, large infant. Risk factors for ICH include vacuum extraction or forceps births, precipitous or prolonged second stage of labor, and increased fetal size (Jhawar, Ranger, Steven, & Del Maestro, 2003; Uhing, 2004). In the newborn, more than one type of hemorrhage can and frequently does occur (Hockenberry, 2003).

Subdural hemorrhages (hematomas), a collection of blood in the subdural space, most often are produced by the stretching and tearing of the large veins in the tentorium of the cerebellum, the dural membrane that separates the cerebrum from the cerebellum. When this type of bleeding occurs, the typical history includes a nulliparous mother, with the total labor and birth occurring in less than 2 or 3 hours; a difficult birth involving high forceps or midforceps application; or a large-for-gestational-age (LGA) infant. Subdural hematoma occurs less frequently today because of improvements in obstetric care. However, it is especially serious because of its inaccessibility to aspiration by subdural tap (Hockenberry, 2003).

Subarachnoid hemorrhage, the most common type of ICH, occurs in term infants as a result of trauma and in preterm infants as a result of hypoxia. Small hemorrhages are the most common. Bleeding is of venous origin, and underlying contusion also may occur (Hockenberry, 2003).

The clinical presentation of hemorrhage in the term infant can vary considerably. In many infants, signs are absent, and hemorrhaging is diagnosed only because of abnormal findings on lumbar puncture (e.g., red blood cells in the cerebrospinal fluid [CSF]). The initial clinical manifestations of neonatal subarachnoid hemorrhage may be the early onset of alternating depression and irritability, with refractory seizures or apnea. Occasionally the infant appears normal initially and then has seizures on the second or third day of life, followed by no apparent sequelae.

In general, nursing care of an infant with ICH is supportive and includes monitoring of ventilatory and intravenous therapy, observation and management of seizures, and prevention of increased ICP. Minimal handling to promote rest and reduce stress should guide nursing care (Hockenberry, 2003).

Spinal cord injuries are usually the result of breech births, especially those difficult ones in which version and extraction were used. Brow and face presentations, dystocia, preterm birth, maternal nulliparity, and precipitate birth also have been identified as predisposing factors in these types of injuries. Stretching of the spinal cord, usually by forceful longitudinal traction on the trunk while the head is still firmly engaged in the pelvis, is the most common mechanism of injury. This injury is rarely seen today because cesarean birth is often used for breech presentation (Mangurten, 2006).

Clinical manifestations depend on the severity and location of the injury. High cervical cord injuries are more likely to cause stillbirths or rapid death of the neonate. Lower lesions cause an acute spinal cord syndrome. Common signs of spinal shock include flaccid extremities, diaphragmatic breathing, paralyzed abdominal movements, atonic anal sphincter, and distended bladder. Therapy is supportive and usually unsatisfactory. Infants who survive present a therapeutic challenge that requires combined treatment from many health care providers, including the pediatrician, the neurologist, the neurosurgeon, the urologist, the orthopedist, the nurse, the physical therapist, and the occupational therapist. Parents need to understand fully the implications of severe injury to the spinal cord and the overwhelming implications it presents for the family.

▬ Evaluation

The nurse can be assured that care has been effective if the outcomes for care have been achieved. That is, the injury receives prompt and appropriate therapy, the newborn has no or minimal sequelae of trauma, and the parents understand how to care for the infant.

▬ INFANTS OF DIABETIC MOTHERS

No single physiologic or biochemical event can explain the diverse clinical manifestations seen in the infants of diabetic mothers (IDMs) or infants of gestational diabetic mothers (IGDMs). A better understanding of maternal and fetal metabolism, resulting in stricter control of maternal diabetes and improved obstetric and neonatal intensive care, has led to a decrease in the perinatal mortality rate in diabetic pregnancy. However, maternal diabetes continues to play a significant role in neonatal morbidity and mortality. Compared to nondiabetic pregnancies, mothers with diabetes have twice the risk of stillbirth and two and a half to five times the risk of perinatal mortality (Dunne, Brydon, Smith, & Gee, 2003; Platt et al., 2003). Of infants born to mothers with gestational diabetes, 35% will weigh more than 4000 g (Gillean, Coonrod, Russ, & Bay, 2005). Up to 40% of IDMs may require neonatal intensive care unit (NICU) admission as a result of hypoglycemia or respiratory distress (Watson, Rowan, Neale, & Battin, 2003).

All infants born to mothers with diabetes are at some risk for complications. The degree of risk is affected by the severity and duration of maternal disease. Problems seen in IDMs include congenital anomalies, macrosomia, birth trauma and perinatal asphyxia, respiratory distress syndrome (RDS), hypoglycemia, hypocalcemia and hypomagnesemia, cardiomyopathy, and hyperbilirubinemia and polycythemia.

Pathophysiology

The mechanisms responsible for the problems seen in IDMs are not fully understood. In early pregnancy, fluctuations in blood glucose levels and episodes of ketoaci-dosis are believed to cause congenital anomalies. Later in pregnancy, when the mother's pancreas cannot release sufficient insulin to meet increased demands, maternal hyperglycemia results. Increased amounts of glucose cross the placenta and stimulate the fetal pancreas to release insulin. The combination of the increased supply of maternal glucose and other nutrients and increased fetal insulin results in excessive fetal growth called macrosomia (see later discussion).

Hyperinsulinemia accounts for many of the problems of the fetus or infant. In addition to fluctuating glucose levels, maternal vascular involvement or superimposed maternal infection adversely affects the fetus. Normally, maternal blood has a more alkaline pH than does the carbon dioxide-rich fetal blood. This phenomenon encourages the exchange of oxygen and carbon dioxide across the placental membrane. When the maternal blood is more acidotic than the fetal blood, such as during ketoacidosis, little carbon dioxide or oxygen exchange occurs at the level of the placenta. The mortality rate for unborn babies resulting from an episode of maternal ketoacidosis may be as high as 50% or more (Lindsay, 2006).

Careful control of maternal blood sugars is thought to be important in reducing the rate of diabetic complications. Evidence exists to suggest that the incidence of congenital anomalies can be reduced with preconception glycemic control; however, glycemic control alone may not prevent the development of fetal macrosomia (Walkinshaw, 2005). Neonatal complications such as hypoglycemia and delayed lung maturity may be eliminated, or the incidence decreased, by maintaining control over maternal glucose levels within narrow limits (Piper, 2002; Walkinshaw).

Congenital Anomalies

Congenital anomalies occur in about 2% to 10% of IDMs (Masson et al., 2003; Wyatt et al., 2005). The incidence of congenital heart lesions in these infants is three to five times higher than that in the general population (Knight & Washington, 2006). The incidence is greatest among small-for-gestational-age (SGA) newborns. Intrauterine growth restriction (IUGR) leading to SGA infants is seen in IDMs with severe vascular disease. The most frequently occurring anomalies involve the cardiac, renal, musculoskeletal, and central nervous systems. Elevated fasting blood glucose levels are correlated with an increased risk for anomalies in both type 1 and type 2 diabetics, whereas diabetic women with normal fasting blood glucose levels have a rate of congenital anomalies similar to that seen in nondiabetic pregnancies (Sheffield, Butler-Koster, Casey, McIntire, & Leveno, 2002). The correlation between gestational diabetes and congenital anomalies is controversial, with some studies indicating that the rate of congenital anomalies in infants born to women with gestational diabetes is similar to that of the general populations (Farrell, Neale, & Cundy, 2002; Kelly, Evans, & Messenger, 2005; Langer, 2002) and others identifying a higher rate of anomalies in gestational diabetics (Sheffield et al.). In most defects associated with diabetic pregnancies, the structural abnormality occurs before the eighth week after conception (Kelly et al.). This reinforces the importance of control of blood glucose both before conception and in the early stages of pregnancy.

Coarctation of the aorta, transposition of the great vessels, and atrial or ventricular septal defects are the most common lesions encountered in the IDM. In the genitourinary system, renal agenesis (failure of the kidney to develop) and obstruction of the urinary tract have been associated with maternal diabetes (Nielsen, Norgard, Puho, Rothman, Sorensen, & Czeizel, 2005). CNS anomalies include anencephaly, encephalocele, meningomyelocele, and hydrocephalus. The musculoskeletal system may be affected by *caudal regression syndrome* (*sacral agenesis*, with weakness or deformities of the lower extremities; malformation and fixation of the hip joints; and shortening or deformity of the femurs). Other defects noted in this population include gastrointestinal atresia and urinary tract malformations (see Chapter 39).

Neonatal small left colon syndrome, also called lazy colon syndrome, occurs in up to 50% of IDMs and IGDMs (Thigpen & Kenner, 2003). This syndrome is suspected when failure to pass meconium, abdominal distention, and bile-stained vomitus are noted. Contrast enemas show a greatly diminished caliber of the left colon from the splenic flexure to the anus. The syndrome is transient, with normal bowel function developing early in infancy.

Macrosomia

Despite improvements in the control of maternal blood sugar levels, the incidence of macrosomia is 50% in women with gestational diabetes and 40% in women with type 1 diabetes (Landon, Catalano, & Gabbe, 2002). At birth, the typical LGA infant has a round, cherubic ("tomato" or cushingoid) face, a chubby body, and a plethoric or flushed complexion (Fig. 38-6). The infant has enlarged internal organs (hepatosplenomegaly, splanchnomegaly, cardiomegaly) and increased body fat, especially around the shoulders. The placenta and umbilical cord are larger than average. Because insulin does not cross the blood-brain barrier, the brain is the only organ that is not enlarged. IDMs may be LGA but physiologically immature.

Insulin has been proposed as the primary growth hormone for intrauterine development. Maternal diabetes results in elevated maternal levels of amino acids and free fatty acids, along with hyperglycemia. As the nutrients cross the placenta, the fetal pancreas responds by producing insulin to match the fuel supply. The resulting accelerated protein synthesis, together with a deposition of excessive glycogen and fat stores, is responsible for the typical macrosomic infant. This is the infant most at risk for the neonatal complications of hypoglycemia, hypocalcemia, hyperviscosity, and hyperbilirubinemia. The excessive amounts of metabolic fuels presented to the fetus from the mother and the consequent fetal hyperinsulinism are now understood to represent the basic pathologic mechanism in the diabetic pregnancy (Lindsay, 2006).

The excessive shoulder size in these infants often leads to dystocia, particularly because the head may be smaller

FIG. 38-6 Macrosomia. (From O'Doherty, N. [1986]. *Neonatology: Micro atlas of the newborn.* Nutley, NJ: Hoffmann-La Roche.)

in proportion to the shoulders than in a nonmacrosomic infant. Macrosomic infants, born vaginally or by cesarean birth after a trial of labor, may incur birth trauma such as clavicle fracture or Erb-Duchenne palsy (Gudmundsson, Henningsson, & Lindqvist, 2005). Despite increased vigilance in screening, and improvements in ultrasound techniques, the determination of macrosomia is difficult to make. In one study, the sensitivity of clinical and ultrasonographic prediction of macrosomia was 68% and 58%, respectively (Weiner, Ben-Shlomo, Beck-Fruchter, Goldberg, & Shalev, 2002).

Birth Trauma and Perinatal Hypoxia

Birth injury (resulting from macrosomia or method of birth) and perinatal hypoxia occur in 20% of IGDMs and 35% of IDMs. Examples of birth trauma include cephalhematoma; paralysis of the facial nerve (cranial nerve VII) (see Fig. 38-5); fracture of the clavicle or humerus; brachial plexus paralysis, usually Erb-Duchenne palsy (right upper arm) (see Fig. 38-4); and phrenic nerve paralysis, invariably associated with diaphragmatic paralysis.

Respiratory Distress Syndrome

IDMs and IGDMs are four to six times more likely than normal infants to develop RDS. With improved maternal glucose control, this risk is substantially reduced.

In the fetus exposed to high levels of maternal glucose, synthesis of surfactant may be delayed because of the high fetal serum levels of insulin and/or glucose (Moore, 2002). Fetal lung maturity, as evidenced by a lecithin/sphingomyelin (L/S) ratio of 2:1, is not reassuring if the mother has diabetes mellitus. For the infants of such mothers, an L/S ratio of 3:1 or more or the presence of phosphatidylglycerol (a component of surfactant) in the amniotic fluid is more indicative of adequate lung maturity.

Hypoglycemia

Hypoglycemia (blood glucose levels less than 40 mg/dl in term infants) affects many IDMs, with a reported incidence of 17% to 40% (Evers, de Valk, & Visser, 2004; Watson et al., 2003). LGA and preterm infants have the highest risk. After constant exposure to high circulating levels of glucose, hyperplasia of the fetal pancreas occurs, resulting in hyperinsulinemia. Disruption of the fetal glucose supply occurs with the clamping of the umbilical cord, and the neonate's blood glucose level decreases rapidly in the presence of fetal hyperinsulinism. Hypoglycemia is most common in the macrosomic infant, but blood glucose levels should be monitored in all infants of known or suspected mothers with diabetes.

Asymptomatic or symptomatic hypoglycemia most frequently manifests within the first 1 to 3 hours after birth. Signs of hypoglycemia include jitteriness, apnea, tachypnea, and cyanosis. Significant hypoglycemia may result in seizures. Hypoglycemia is worsened by the presence of hypothermia or respiratory distress.

Hypocalcemia and Hypomagnesemia

Hypocalcemia and hypomagnesemia have been reported to occur in as many as 50% of IDMs (Kalhan & Parimi, 2006). A number of these cases are related to hypoxia or prematurity; however, the overall incidence of hypocalcemia is higher than in nondiabetic pregnancies. Hypomagnesemia is believed to develop because of maternal renal losses that occur in diabetes. Hypocalcemia is associated with preterm birth, birth trauma, and perinatal asphyxia. Signs of hypocalcemia are similar to those of hypoglycemia, but they occur between 24 and 36 hours of age. Hypocalcemia should be considered if therapy for hypoglycemia is ineffective.

Cardiomyopathy

All IDMs need careful observation for **cardiomyopathy** (disease affecting the structure and function of the heart) because an increased heart size is often found in these infants. Two types of cardiomyopathy can occur. Clinicians must be alert to identify the type of lesion correctly so that appropriate therapy is instituted. Both types of lesions are associated with respiratory symptoms and congestive heart failure.

Hypertrophic cardiomyopathy (HCM) is characterized by a hypercontractile and thickened myocardium. The ventricular walls are thickened, as is the septum, which in severe cases results in outflow tract obstructions. The mitral valve is poorly functioning. In *nonhypertrophic cardiomyopathy* (non-HCM), the myocardium is poorly contractile and overstretched. The ventricles are increased in size, and no outflow obstruction is found. Most infants are asymptomatic, but severe outflow obstruction may cause left ventricular heart failure. HCM may be treated with a beta-adrenergic blocker (such as propranolol) to decrease contractility and heart rate. A cardiotonic agent is used to treat non-HCM (such as digoxin, to increase contractility and decrease heart rate). The abnormality usually resolves in 3 to 12 months.

Hyperbilirubinemia and Polycythemia

IDMs are at increased risk of developing hyperbilirubinemia. Many IDMs also are polycythemic. Polycythemia increases blood viscosity, thereby impairing circulation. In addition, this increased number of red blood cells to be hemolyzed increases the potential bilirubin load that the neonate must clear. The excessive red blood cells are produced in extramedullary foci (liver and spleen) in addition to the usual sites in bone marrow; therefore both liver function and bilirubin clearance may be adversely affected. Bruising associated with birth of a macrosomic infant will contribute further to high bilirubin levels.

Nursing Care

Nursing care depends on the neonate's particular problems. General care of the compromised infant is addressed in Chapter 40. If the maternal blood glucose level was well controlled throughout the pregnancy, the infant may require only monitoring. Because euglycemia (normal blood glucose levels) is not always possible, the nurse must promptly recognize and treat any consequences of maternal diabetes that arise. The most common problems of IDMs that require intervention include birth trauma and perinatal asphyxia; RDS; difficult metabolic transition, including hypoglycemia and hypocalcemia; and congenital anomalies (see previous sections and Plan of Care).

■ NEONATAL INFECTIONS

Sepsis

Sepsis (presence of microorganisms or their toxins in blood or other tissues) continues to be one of the most significant causes of neonatal morbidity and mortality. The newborn infant is susceptible to infection. Maternal immunoglobulin (IgM) does not cross the placenta. IgA and IgM require time to reach optimal levels after birth. Phagocytosis is less efficient. Serum complement levels are inadequate; serum complement (C1 through C6) is involved in immunologic reactions, some of which kill or lyse bacteria and enhance phagocytosis. Dysmaturity seen with IUGR and preterm and postdate birth further compromises the neonate's immune system.

Table 38-2 outlines risk factors for neonatal sepsis. Special precautions for preventing infection, as well as prompt recognition when it occurs, are necessary for optimal newborn care. Neonatal infections may be acquired in utero, during birth, during resuscitation, and nosocomially.

Prenatal acquisition of infection occurs by organisms placentally transferred directly into the fetal circulatory system and transmitted from infected amniotic fluid, such as with herpes simplex virus (HSV), cytomegalovirus (CMV), and rubella. Microorganisms also may ascend from the vagina and pass through the cervix. The membranes become infected and may rupture. Infection of the fetal skin and the respiratory or gastrointestinal tract may result.

During birth, contact with an infected birth canal can result in generalized or local infection. The upper airway

EVIDENCE-BASED PRACTICE

Neonatal Hyperbilirubinemia

BACKGROUND

- Neonatal hyperbilirubinemia can lead to kernicterus and serious neurodevelopmental damage. In 1994, the American Academy of Pediatrics published recommendations for the management of healthy newborns with hyperbilirubinemia, using visual inspection of skin for jaundice. Although evidence did not link specific bilirubin levels to adverse outcomes, the recommendations advocated the use of exchange transfusion only when phototherapy failed to decrease total serum bilirubin (TSB) level to below 20 mg/dl. Problems with recommendations included the subjective nature of determining jaundice visually, the lack of precise levels by hours of age, and unknown adverse effects of phototherapy.

OBJECTIVES

- The authors of this review set out to determine what peak bilirubin levels affect neurodevelopmental outcomes of neonates over 34 weeks of gestation and birth weight of 2500 grams, the efficacy of treatments on bilirubin levels and outcomes, and the accuracy of strategies for predicting hyperbilirubinemia.

METHODS

Search Strategy

- After a search of online databases, the reviewers identified 138 articles in this review: 28 on kernicterus, 35 on correlations with risk factors, 21 articles on treatments, and 54 on diagnosis. The studies span 40 years and originate from China, Denmark, India, Israel, Japan, Spain, and the United States. Prospective cohorts, cross-sectional, and longitudinal and retrospective cohort studies were included for neurodevelopmental association with bilirubin levels. Data about treatments came from randomized and nonrandomized controlled trials.

Statistical Analyses

- Similar data were pooled. Reviewers calculated relative risk for dichotomous (categoric) data, such as hearing loss, and weighted mean difference for continuous data, such as TSB level. From that, they calculated the "number needed to treat" (NNT) in order to prevent one baby with rising TSB. Differences between groups outside the 95% confidence interval were accepted as significant.

FINDINGS

- Kernicterus had a mortality rate of at least 10%. It developed in near term/term infants with TSB levels of 22.5 to 54 mg/dl, and at levels as low as 4 mg/dl in infants with sepsis and hemolysis. Levels above 20 mg/dl were associated with a higher risk for central nervous system abnormalities at age 4. Risk for hearing impairment increased at levels above 16 mg/dl. The association of IQ and peak bilirubin level was inconsistent in healthy infants, but lower 4-year IQ was associated with amnionitis and subsequent bilirubinemia.

- The most effective therapy for jaundice in healthy newborns was phototherapy and switching to formula instead of breast milk. Clinicians needed to treat 6 to 10 jaundiced babies at TSB of 15 mg/dl to prevent one case of TSB rising above 20 mg/dl.

- Normative levels of TSB by hours of age could not be standardized.

- Transcutaneous jaundice measurements were best estimated by newer devices, such as Bilicheck and the Colormate III, which accounted for skin pigmentation and were highly predictive of TSB levels.

LIMITATIONS

- The studies span over 45 years of data, across continents, and many definitions of hyperbilirubinemia and neurodevelopmental damage. As with all reviews, the short-term studies are consistent with current quality markers, but may lack tool reliability and validity, while longer-term studies have high attrition rates and variable definitions of normal.

IMPLICATIONS FOR PRACTICE

- New parents need education about jaundice and the need for follow-up, especially in an era where babies are discharged before symptoms are apparent. Nurses can reassure anxious parents that phototherapy is the well-documented treatment to treat rising bilirubin levels. The surprise in this review was the recommendation for a switch to formula during phototherapy. Women will need instruction in pumping and extra support to reestablish breastfeeding.

IMPLICATIONS FOR FURTHER RESEARCH

- A uniform definition of hyperbilirubinemia, kernicterus, and neurodevelopmental markers would help establish a database for metaanalysis. Identification of normative standards by hour, gender, ethnicity, and comorbidity may help predict hyperbilirubinemia. No mention was made of the relationship between the duration of symptoms and outcomes. Cost has not been addressed. Further research is needed to fully explore risks and benefits of switching to formula feeding during phototherapy, since this is interrupting the early, crucial establishment of breastfeeding.

Reference: Ip, S., Glicken, S., Kulig, J., O'Brien, R., & Sege, R. (2003). *Management of neonatal hyperbilirubinemia* (AHRQ Publication No. 03-E011). Rockville, MD: Agency for Healthcare Research and Quality.

and the gastrointestinal tract are the principal pathways for generalized infections. The conjunctiva and the oral cavity are the usual sites of local infection.

Postnatal infection may be acquired during resuscitation or through the introduction of foreign objects such as indwelling catheters or endotracheal tubes. Nursery-acquired infections may be transferred to the infant by the hands of the parents or health care personnel or spread from contaminated equipment. The umbilicus is a receptive site for cutaneous infection leading to sepsis (Edwards, 2006).

Neonatal bacterial infection is classified into two patterns according to the time of presentation. Early-onset or congenital sepsis usually manifests within 24 to 72 hours after birth, progresses more rapidly than later-onset infection, and has a mortality rate between 3% and 50%

plan of care	The Infant of the Mother with Gestational Diabetes

NURSING DIAGNOSIS Risk for injury related to hypoglycemia, hypocalcemia, polycythemia, or hyperbilirubinemia secondary to maternal gestational diabetes

Expected Outcome *Infant will exhibit blood glucose, serum calcium, hematocrit, and serum bilirubin levels that are within normal limits.*

Nursing Interventions/Rationales

- Monitor blood glucose levels (<40 mg/dl indicative of hypoglycemia); and serum calcium levels (<7 mg/dl indicative of hypocalcemia); and serum bilirubin levels (>15 mg/dl indicative of hyperbilirubinemia) *to assess and detect early onset to prevent complications.*
- Observe for signs of hypoglycemia (jitteriness, twitching, lethargy, apathy, convulsions, cyanosis, sweating, eye rolling, refusal to eat); hypocalcemia (jitters, apnea, high-pitched cry, abdominal distention); polycythemia (plethora); and hyperbilirubinemia (jaundice) *to assess and detect signs of onset to prevent complications.*
- Provide early feeding of infant, increased milk feedings/calcium supplements per physician order *to prevent or treat early hypocalcemia;* early and frequent feedings *to reduce hematocrit and enhance excretion of bilirubin in stool.*
- Administer intravenous glucose infusions per physician's order for infants with symptomatic hypoglycemia or those too ill to be fed orally safely *to treat hypoglycemia.*
- Reduce adverse environmental factors (e.g., excessive handling, cold stress, and respiratory distress) *that can predispose infant to hypoglycemia.*

NURSING DIAGNOSIS Impaired gas exchange related to lung immaturity or cardiomyopathy secondary to maternal gestational diabetes

Expected Outcome *Infant will exhibit signs of adequate oxygen supply (respiratory rate, rhythm, and amplitude, and blood gas levels within normal limits).*

Nursing Interventions/Rationales

- Monitor infant's vital signs, oxygen saturation levels, blood gas levels per order, patency of airway *to evaluate pulmonary and circulatory status.*
- Avoid activities that may reduce body temperature and lead to cold stress, *which can induce respiratory distress.*
- Suction as needed *to keep airway patent and prevent aspiration.*
- Have resuscitation equipment and oxygen available *for quick treatment of respiratory distress.*

NURSING DIAGNOSIS Risk for ineffective thermoregulation related to physiologic immaturity; potential for infection related to immature immunologic defenses/environmental exposure

See the Nursing Plan of Care for the normal newborn in Chapter 26.

NURSING DIAGNOSIS Parental anxiety (risk for powerlessness, situational low self-esteem, ineffective coping) related to neonate's condition, management, and prognosis

Expected Outcome *Parents demonstrate understanding of prognosis and therapy for infant.*

Nursing Interventions/Rationales

- Explain potential effects of maternal diabetic condition on newborn *to relieve fear of unknown and support ability to cope.*
- Encourage open communication (e.g., inform parents of ongoing condition, procedures, and treatment; answer questions; correct misperceptions; actively listen to parental concerns) *to provide support and help provide sense of control.*
- Encourage parents to interact with infant and to become involved in care routines *to foster emotional connection.*

(Palazzi, Klein, & Baker, 2006). Early-onset infection is usually caused by microorganisms from the normal flora of the maternal vaginal tract, including group B streptococcus, *Haemophilus influenzae, Listeria monocytogenes, Escherichia coli,* and *Streptococcus pneumoniae* (Venkatesh, Merenstein, Adams, & Weisman, 2006). It is associated with a history of obstetric complications, such as preterm labor, premature rupture of membranes, maternal fever during labor, and chorioamnionitis (Palazzi et al.).

Acquired infection is most frequently seen after 1 to 2 weeks of age and is slower in progression. Bacteria responsible for late-onset sepsis are varied, may be acquired from the birth canal or from the external environment, and include *Staphylococcus aureus, S. epidermidis, Pseudomonas* organisms, and group B streptococcus. The mortality rate for late-onset infection varies between 2% and 40% (Palazzi et al., 2006).

Viral infections may cause miscarriage, stillbirth, intrauterine infection, congenital malformations, and acute dis-

ease. These pathogens also may cause chronic infection, with subtle manifestations that may be recognized only after a prolonged period. It is important to recognize the manifestations of infections in the neonatal period to treat the acute infection and to prevent nosocomial infections in other infants, and to anticipate effects on the infant's subsequent growth and development.

Fungal infections are of greatest concern in the immunocompromised or premature infant. Occasionally, fungal infections such as thrush are found in otherwise healthy term infants.

Septicemia refers to a generalized infection in the bloodstream. Pneumonia, the most common form of neonatal infection, is one of the leading causes of perinatal death and is caused by many of the same organisms that cause sepsis (Edwards, 2006). Bacterial meningitis affects 1 in 2500 live-born infants. Gastroenteritis is sporadic, depending on epidemic outbreaks. Local infections such as conjunctivitis and omphalitis occur frequently, but in-

table 38-2 Risk Factors for Neonatal Sepsis

SOURCE	RISK FACTORS
Maternal	Low socioeconomic status
	Poor prenatal care
	Poor nutrition
	Substance abuse
Intrapartum	Premature rupture of fetal membranes
	Maternal fever
	Chorioamnionitis
	Prolonged labor
	Premature labor
	Maternal urinary tract infection
Neonatal	Twin gestation
	Male
	Birth asphyxia
	Meconium aspiration
	Congenital anomalies of skin or
	mucous membranes
	Galactosemia
	Absence of spleen
	Low birth weight or prematurity
	Malnourishment
	Prolonged hospitalization

From Askin, D. (1995). Bacterial and fungal sepsis in the neonate. *Journal of Obstetric, Gynecologic, and Neonatal Nursing, 24*(7), 635-643.

cidence rates are unavailable. Infection continues to be a significant factor in fetal and neonatal morbidity and mortality.

▬ CARE MANAGEMENT

▬ Assessment and Nursing Diagnoses

The prenatal record is reviewed for risk factors associated with infection and signs and symptoms suggestive of it. Maternal vaginal or perineal infection may be transmitted directly to the infant during passage through the birth canal. Psychosocial history and history of sexually transmitted infections (STIs) may indicate possible human immunodeficiency virus (HIV), hepatitis B virus (HBV), or CMV infection.

Perinatal events also are reviewed. Premature rupture of membranes (PROM) may be caused by maternal or intrauterine infection. Ascending infection may occur after prolonged PROM, prolonged labor, or intrauterine fetal monitoring. A maternal history of fever during labor or the presence of foul-smelling amniotic fluid also may indicate the presence of infection. Antibiotic therapy initiated during labor should be noted. Resuscitation that requires intubation and deep suctioning may result in infection. The neonate's gestational age, maturity, birth weight, and gender all affect the incidence of infection. Sepsis occurs about twice as often and results in a higher mortality rate in male than in female infants. The neonate is assessed for respiratory distress, skin abscesses, rashes, and other indications of infection.

During the postnatal period, the time of onset of suggestive signs is noted. Onset within the first 48 hours of life is more often associated with prenatal or perinatal predisposing factors. Onset after 2 or 3 days more frequently reflects disease acquired at or subsequent to birth.

The earliest clinical signs of neonatal sepsis are characterized by a lack of specificity. The nonspecific signs include lethargy, poor feeding, poor weight gain, and irritability. The nurse or parent may simply note that the infant is just not doing as well as before. Differential diagnosis may be difficult because signs of sepsis are similar to signs of noninfectious neonatal problems such as anemia or hypoglycemia. Additional clinical and laboratory information and appropriate cultures supplement the findings described. Table 38-3 outlines signs of sepsis.

Laboratory studies are performed. Specimens for cultures include blood, nasopharyngeal or oropharyngeal specimens, CSF, stool, and urine. Increased direct (conjugated) bilirubin levels may be found, especially if the infecting microorganism is gram negative. Complete blood cell count with differential is performed to determine the presence of anemia, increased white blood cell count, or decreased white blood cell count (an ominous sign). C-reactive protein may or may not be elevated.

Vigilant assessment continues during and after treatment. The newborn continues to be assessed for sequelae to septicemia. Before the advent of antibiotics, 90% of newborns with sepsis died. Antibiotic therapy decreased mortality rates to between 13% and 45%, depending on the causative organism.

table 38-3 Signs of Sepsis*

SYSTEM	SIGNS
Respiratory	Apnea, bradycardia
	Tachypnea
	Grunting, nasal flaring
	Retractions
	Decreased oxygen saturation
	Acidosis
Cardiovascular	Decreased cardiac output
	Tachycardia
	Hypotension
	Decreased perfusion
Central nervous	Temperature instability
	Lethargy
	Hypotonia
	Irritability, seizures
Gastrointestinal	Feeding intolerance
	Abdominal distention
	Vomiting, diarrhea
Integumentary	Jaundice
	Pallor
	Petechiae

From Askin, D. (1995). Bacterial and fungal sepsis in the neonate. *Journal of Obstetric, Gynecologic, and Neonatal Nursing, 24*(7), 635-643.
*Laboratory findings include neutropenia, increased bands, hypoglycemia or hyperglycemia, metabolic acidosis, and thrombocytopenia.

Sequelae to septicemia include meningitis, disseminated intravascular coagulation (DIC), and septic shock.

Septic shock results from the toxins released into the bloodstream. The most common sign is a decrease in blood pressure, a vital sign often not assessed in the care of the neonate. The infant will often appear gray or mottled and may be noted to have cool extremities. Other signs are rapid, irregular respirations and pulse (similar to septicemia in general).

Any number of nursing diagnoses are possible, depending on the infant's gestational age and birth weight, the organ systems involved, and the nature of the infection. Examples of nursing diagnoses related to neonatal infections include the following:

NEWBORN
- *Risk for infection related to*
  - maternal vaginal (or other) infection
  - resuscitation or ventilation therapy
  - presence of indwelling umbilical catheters, total parenteral nutrition (TPN), parenteral fluids
  - intrauterine electronic fetal monitoring
  - dysmaturity, IUGR, gestational age
- *Ineffective thermoregulation related to*
  - infection
- *Impaired tissue integrity related to*
  - multiple supportive measures (e.g., biometric monitoring, TPN, inhalation therapy)
- *Acute pain related to*
  - multiple supportive measures

PARENTS AND FAMILY
- *Anxiety, fear, or anticipatory grieving related to*
  - uncertainty about infant's prognosis
  - poor prognosis
- *Risk for impaired parenting related to*
  - separation of parent and newborn
  - feelings of inadequacy in caring for infant
- *Powerlessness or spiritual distress related to*
  - perinatal events or newborn's condition
- *Anxiety related to deficient knowledge regarding*
  - newborn's condition, its course, and its management

▪ Expected Outcomes of Care

Planning begins with the development of standards for preventive measures in nurseries and protocols for diagnosis and treatment of infections. Individual assessment findings are used to plan care for each infant. Parents and family are encouraged to participate in planning. Expected outcomes include the following:

Newborn
- The newborn will remain free of sepsis.
- The newborn's early signs of sepsis will be recognized, and appropriate therapy will be instituted.
- If therapy is necessary, the newborn will have no harmful sequelae.

Parents
- Anxiety regarding infant's condition and prognosis will be relieved.
- Parents will interact with newborn and develop caregiving skills.
- Parental anxiety about care of the newborn will be relieved.

▪ Plan of Care and Interventions
▪ *Preventive Measures*

Virtually all controlled clinical trials have demonstrated that effective handwashing is responsible for the prevention of nosocomial infection in nursery units. Nursing is directly or indirectly responsible for minimizing or eliminating environmental sources of infectious agents in the nursery. Measures to be taken include Standard Precautions, careful and thorough cleaning, frequent replacement of used equipment (e.g., changing intravenous tubing per hospital protocol, cleaning resuscitation and ventilation equipment), and disposal of excrement and linens in an appropriate manner. Overcrowding must be avoided in nurseries.

Instillation of antibiotic ointment in newborns' eyes 1 to 2 hours after birth is done to prevent infection, such as from gonorrhea, and chlamydiosis. The skin, its secretions, and its normal flora are natural defenses that protect against invading pathogens. Warm water may be used to remove blood and meconium from the neonate's face, head, and body. A mild nonmedicated soap (in single-use container or in a small bar reserved for a single newborn) can be used with careful water rinsing. The cord can be left to air dry. The stump and base of the cord should be assessed for edema, redness, and purulent drainage.

▪ *Curative Measures*

Breastfeeding or feeding the newborn breast milk from the mother is encouraged. Protective mechanisms exist in breast milk. Colostrum contains immunoglobulin A (IgA), which offers protection against infection in the gastrointestinal tract. Human milk contains iron-binding protein that exerts a bacteriostatic effect on *E. coli*. Human milk also contains macrophages and lymphocytes. The vulnerability of infants to common mucosal pathogens such as respiratory syncytial virus (RSV) may be reduced by passive transfer of maternal immunity in the colostrum and breast milk.

Administering medications, taking precautions when performing treatments, and following isolation procedures also are interventions to be considered when a newborn has an infection.

Monitoring the intravenous infusion rate and administering antibiotics are the nurse's responsibility. If the intravenous fluid the infant is receiving contains electrolytes, vitamins, or other medications, the nurse should check with the hospital pharmacy before adding antibiotics. The antibiotic (or other medication) may be deactivated or may form a precipitate when combined with other substances.

In that case, a piggyback solution of the prescribed fluid is attached with a three-way stopcock at the infusion site.

Care must be taken in suctioning secretions from any newborn's oropharynx or trachea. These secretions may be infected.

Isolation procedures are implemented according to hospital policy as indicated. Isolation protocols are changing rapidly, and the nurse is urged to participate in continuing education and in-service programs to remain up to date.

■ *Rehabilitative Measures*

Rehabilitative measures vary with the individual needs of the neonate. Some neonates will need to be weaned from ventilatory support systems. Those who have sequelae such as mental retardation and epilepsy will require a knowledgeable family and supportive community resources. Some children will require corrective care for problems with dentition, vision, and hearing.

■ Evaluation

The nurse can be reasonably assured that care was effective if the outcomes for care are achieved: The newborn remains free of sepsis or the newborn's early signs of sepsis are recognized and appropriately treated (see Care Path).

TORCH Infections

The occurrence of certain maternal infections during early pregnancy is known to be associated with various congenital malformations and disorders. The most common and best understood infections are traditionally represented by the acronym TORCH (Box 38-1). Additional organisms known to cause congenital infection include enteroviruses and parvovirus, leading some clinicians to suggest the need for a new more comprehensive acronym (Klein, Baker, Remington, & Wilson, 2006). HSV may result in a severe, often fatal systemic illness in neonates. Survivors of herpetic infection may have residual neurologic defects and

---

care path	**Suspected Neonatal Sepsis**
ASSESSMENTS	• Potential maternal risk factors and unstable vital signs, especially temperature instability.
	• Sepsis screen in first hour (complete blood count with differential, platelets, and C-reactive protein [CRP] level) if significant maternal risk factors (prolonged rupture of membranes, maternal temperature) are found or if infant demonstrates physiologic signs of sepsis.
TREATMENT	• Start intravenous (IV) administration of antibiotics by peripheral route.
	• Provide other treatments as needed for additional physiologic problems (ventilator for respiratory distress, incubator or radiant warmer for temperature instability).
POSSIBLE CONSULTATIONS	• Neonatologists and nurse practitioners for care of unstable infants.
	• Medical specialists for care of infants with additional problems (congenital deformities).
	• Lactation consultant, interpreter, social worker, and chaplain as needed or requested.
ADDITIONAL ASSESSMENTS	• Weight and measurements.
	• Blood culture, chest radiograph study, urinalysis, and lumbar puncture, if infant is symptomatic or CRP level is positive.
	• Repeat determination of CRP level in the morning for 2 days. If negative and infant not symptomatic, stop antibiotic treatment.
	• Continuous cardiac and oxygen saturation monitor assessment if infant's condition is unstable.
DIRECT INFANT CARE	• Vital signs every 1 to 2 hours for the first 4 hours, and then every 4 hours.
	• Advance oral feedings as tolerated (infant takes nothing by mouth only if condition is physiologically unstable).
	• Bath done per unit protocol
TEACHING AND DISCHARGE PLANNING	• Initiate on admission. Provide parents with written and oral information on suspected sepsis.
	• Reinforce information and determine parents' understanding of information before discharge. Include information on well-baby care and community follow-up with the family's primary health care provider.

Courtesy Lucile Salter Packard Children's Hospital at Stanford, California.

---

box 38-1 | **TORCH Infections Affecting Newborns**

T Toxoplasmosis
O Other: gonorrhea, syphilis, varicella, hepatitis B virus (HBV), human immunodeficiency virus (HIV)
R Rubella
C Cytomegalovirus (CMV) infections or cytomegalic inclusion disease (CMID)
H Herpes simplex virus (HSV) infection

---

chorioretinitis. The other congenital infections also may result in encephalopathy with various anomalies, including microcephaly, chorioretinitis, intracranial calcifications, microphthalmos, and cataracts. To a certain extent, the varied clinical manifestations of these infections overlap, but a specific diagnosis can be made by the clustering of clinical findings, as well as specific antibody studies.

Toxoplasmosis

Toxoplasmosis is a multisystem disease caused by the protozoan *Toxoplasma gondii* parasite, commonly found in cats, dogs, pigs, sheep, and cattle, with cats being the definitive host. If a woman acquires toxoplasmosis during her pregnancy, there is a 15% risk of fetal transmission for acquisition during the first trimester, 30% for the second trimester, and 60% for the third trimester (Montoya & Rosso, 2005). Fetal infections are estimated to occur at a rate of between 1 and 10 per 10,000 live births (Lopez, Dietz, Wilson, Navin, & Jones, 2000). The diagnosis of toxoplasmosis in the neonate is supported by elevated levels of cord blood serum IgM.

Most neonates (70%) infected with *T. gondii* in utero may be asymptomatic at birth, but in approximately 50%, progressive chorioretinitis develops, and in 40%, central nervous system (CNS) involvement such as hydrocephalus develops in the weeks and months after birth (Martin, 2001). For some infected neonates, hydrocephalus may be the only clinical sign of the disease (Remington, McLeod, Thulliez, & Desmonts, 2006). For others, chorioretinitis may develop during school age or adolescent stages. Up to 30% of infected infants are born with severe manifestations at birth. Clinical features ascribed to *T. gondii* infection include three key findings (classic triad) first described by Sabin (1942): hydrocephalus or microcephaly; chorioretinitis; and cerebral calcifications (Montoya & Liesenfeld, 2004). Transmission of toxoplasmosis from an infected mother to her fetus can be reduced by up to 60% with maternal spiramycin treatment (Montoya & Rosso, 2005).

Severe toxoplasmosis is associated with preterm birth, growth restriction, microcephaly or hydrocephaly, microphthalmos, chorioretinitis, CNS calcification, thrombocytopenia, jaundice, and fever. Petechiae or a maculopapular rash also may be evident (Montoya & Liesenfeld, 2004). The affected infant may be treated with pyrimethamine, as well as oral sulfadiazine; folic acid supplement will be required to prevent anemia (Schmidt, Hogh, Anderson, Hansen, Dalhoff, & Petersen, 2005).

Gonorrhea

With the prophylactic use of silver nitrate or antibiotics, the incidence of gonococcal conjunctivitis is less than 0.5% (Yudin & Gonik, 2006). After rupture of membranes, ascending infection can result in orogastric contamination of the fetus. The organism also may invade mucosal surfaces such as the conjunctiva (ophthalmia neonatorum), the rectal mucosa, and the pharynx. Contamination may occur as the infant passes through the birth canal, or it may occur postnatally from an infected adult. Neonatal gonococcal arthritis, septicemia, meningitis, vaginitis, and scalp abscesses also can develop.

Eye prophylaxis (e.g., with 0.5% erythromycin ointment) is administered at or shortly after birth to prevent ophthalmia neonatorum. The infant with a mild infection often recovers completely with appropriate treatment, such as neonatal ceftriaxone. Rarely infants die of overwhelming infection in the early neonatal period.

Syphilis

Congenital and neonatal syphilis have reemerged in recent years as significant health problems. It is estimated that for every 100 women diagnosed with primary or secondary disease, two to five infants will contract congenital syphilis. If syphilis during pregnancy is untreated, 40% to 50% of neonates born to these women will have symptomatic congenital syphilis. Treatment failure can occur, particularly when treatment is given in the third trimester; therefore infants born to women treated within 4 weeks of birth should be investigated for congenital syphilis. The following factors have been identified as placing the neonate at high risk for exposure to syphilis: crack cocaine use in mother or partner, multiple sexual partners, history of STI, poverty, homelessness, and HIV infection (Woods, 2005).

The mode of transmission in adults is sexual. The infant is usually infected in utero by transplacental infection, but infection of the amniotic fluid also may occur (Woods, 2005). The infant can also contract syphilis during contact with an active genital lesion at birth (Ingall, Sanchez, & Baker, 2006). The risk to the fetus and neonate varies according to the stage of maternal infection, with transmission during primary or secondary syphilis being more common. Untreated maternal disease results in stillbirth in 30% to 40% of cases (Woods). The rate of congenital syphilis is approximately 11.2 cases per 100,000 live births (CDC, 2004). Prompt maternal treatment will eliminate most fetal infections; however, delayed treatment or a failure to obtain treatment may result in fetal effects that range from minor anomalies to preterm birth or fetal death. Damage to the fetus depends on when in gestation the infection occurred and the time that has elapsed before treatment. Congenital syphilis infection may be asymptomatic at birth in up to two thirds of infected infants. A portion of these infants will become symptomatic in the first 2 years of life, whereas others may take up to 20 years before displaying the effects of congenital infection (Woods).

Early congenital syphilis may result in prematurity, hydrops fetalis, and failure to thrive. Hepatosplenomegaly is common, as is jaundice. Hematologic findings include anemia, leukocytosis, and thrombocytopenia. Characteristic bony lesions occur in the long bones, the cranium, and the spine and include osteochondritis, osteomyelitis, and periostitis (Woods, 2005). Other findings include snuffles, mucocutaneous lesions, edema, and a copper-colored maculopapular dermal rash first noticeable on the palms of the hands, the soles of the feet, and in the diaper area and around the mouth and the anus by the end of the first week of life in untreated infants (Woods) (Fig. 38-7). *Condylomata* (elevated wartlike lesions) may be seen on mucous membranes, moist surfaces, or areas of the body affected by friction. Rough, cracked, mucocutaneous lesions of the lips heal to form circumoral radiating scars known as *rhagades*. Other involvement results in exfoliation (separation, flaking) of nails and loss of hair. Iritis and choroiditis are characteristic of infection of the eyes. The following may be noted: nephrotic syndrome secondary to renal infection; hepatitis with jaundice, lymphadenopathy, and inflammation of the pancreas, the testes, and the colon; and a pseudoparalysis of the extremities. In some infants, signs of congenital syphilis do not appear until late in the neonatal period. In these newborns, early signs such as poor feeding, slight hyperthermia, and snuffles may be nonspecific. *Snuffles* refers to the copious clear mucous discharge from the nose.

Medical Management. If the mother was adequately treated before giving birth and serologic testing of the infant does not show syphilis, generally the infant is not treated with antibiotics. The infant is checked for antibody titer (received from the mother through the placenta) every 2 weeks for 3 months, at which time the test result should be negative. Some physicians recommend antibiotic therapy for asymptomatic or inconclusive cases.

Treatment should be carried out in the following situations: when the diagnosis of congenital syphilis is confirmed or suspected, when maternal treatment status is unknown, when the mother is treated within 4 weeks of giving birth or does not respond to treatment, when medi-

cations other than penicillin are used to treat the mother, and when inadequate neonatal follow-up is anticipated (Woods, 2005).

For antibiotic treatment to be effective, an "adequate" blood level must be maintained for an "adequate" period. The suggested medication protocol in the presence of symptomatic systemic disease differs from author to author and from physician to physician. Penicillin G is the usual treatment (Woods, 2005). After 12 hours of antibiotic therapy, the newborn's condition is not considered contagious.

Prognosis. In general, treatment of syphilis is more effective if it is begun early rather than late in the course of the disease. However, a recurrence rate of 5% can be expected. Even adequate treatment of congenital syphilis after birth does not always prevent late (5 to 15 years after initial infection) complications. Potential complications include neurosyphilis, deafness, Hutchinson teeth (notched incisors), saber shins, joint involvement, saddle nose (depressed bridge), gummas (soft, gummy tumors) over the skin and other organs, interstitial keratitis (inflammation of the cornea), rhagades, frontal bossing, and mulberry molars (Woods, 2005).

Varicella-Zoster

The varicella-zoster virus, responsible for chickenpox and shingles, is a member of the herpes family. Approximately 90% of women in the childbearing years are immune; therefore the risk of infection in pregnancy is low, 5 per 10,000 pregnancies (Gershon, 2006).

Varicella transmission to the fetus may occur across the placenta when the disease is contracted in the first half of pregnancy, but this is relatively infrequent. When transmission to the fetus does occur in the early part of pregnancy, the effects on the fetus include limb atrophy, neurologic abnormalities, eye abnormalities, and IUGR.

When maternal infection occurs in the last 3 weeks of pregnancy, 25% of infants born to these mothers will develop clinical varicella (Gershon, 2006). The severity of the infant's illness will increase greatly if maternal infection occurred within 5 days before or 2 days after birth (Tan & Koren, 2006). The mortality rate in severe illness is 30% (Gershon).

Seroimmune pregnant women exposed to active chickenpox can be given varicella-zoster immune globulin (VZIG), which does not reduce the incidence of infection but should decrease the effects of the virus on the fetus. The immunoglobulin must be given within 72 hours of exposure to be effective.

Infants born to mothers in whom chickenpox develops between 5 days before birth and 48 hours after should be given VZIG at birth because of the risk of severe disease (Tan & Koren, 2006). Acyclovir can be used to treat infants with generalized involvement and pneumonia.

Term infants exposed to chickenpox after birth will have a mild or no infection if they are born to immune mothers. In those born to nonimmune mothers, chickenpox may

FIG. 38-7 Neonatal syphilis lesions on hands and feet. (Courtesy Mahesh Kotwal, MD, Phoenix, AZ.)

develop, but the course is not usually severe. Experts are divided as to whether this group of infants should receive VZIG. Infants younger than 28 weeks are at risk regardless of their mother's status and probably benefit from VZIG if exposed to chickenpox.

Hepatitis B Virus

HBV infection during pregnancy is not associated with an increase in malformations, stillbirths, or IUGR; however, approximately 35% of infected fetuses will be born before term (Baley & Toltzis, 2002). The transmission rate of HBV to the newborn is as high as 85% when the mother is seropositive for both hepatitis B surface antigen (HBsAg) and hepatitis B e antigen (HBeAg) (Baley & Toltzis). Transmission occurs transplacentally, serum to serum, and by contact with contaminated urine, feces, saliva, semen, or vaginal secretions during birth. Infants are most frequently infected during birth or in the first few days of life. The rate of transmission is highest when the mother contracts the virus in the third trimester or early in the postpartum period (Bradley, 2006). These mothers will be positive for HBsAg. Transmission may occur through breast milk, but antigens also develop in formula-fed infants at the same or a higher rate, thus breastfeeding is not contraindicated. Diagnosis is made by viral culture of amniotic fluid, as well as the presence of HBsAg and IgM in the cord or baby's serum.

The majority of infants who become HBsAG positive are symptom free at birth, while some show evidence of acute hepatitis with changes in liver function. The mortality rate for full-blown hepatitis is 75%. Infants who become carriers are at high risk for chronic hepatitis, cirrhosis of the liver, or liver cancer even years later.

■ NURSE ALERT

Infants whose mothers have antibodies for HBsAg or in whom hepatitis developed during pregnancy or the postpartum period should be treated with hepatitis B immunoglobulin (HBIG), 0.5 ml intramuscularly, as soon as possible after birth—within the first 12 hours of life. The hepatitis B vaccine also should be given at the same time but in a different site (American Academy of Pediatrics [AAP], 2006; Baley & Toltzis, 2002).

The second dose of vaccine is given at 1 month, and the third dose at 6 months. The vaccine should protect the child for up to 9 years. After the infant has been cleansed thoroughly and has received the vaccine, breastfeeding may be initiated. Vaccination for infants not exposed to HBV is recommended before discharge but may be given by 2 months of age; breastfeeding for these infants may begin before the vaccine is given (Baley & Toltzis, 2002).

Human Immunodeficiency Virus (HIV) and Acquired Immunodeficiency Syndrome (AIDS)

Maternal infection with the retrovirus HIV is discussed in Chapter 8. The focus of this discussion is the neonate at risk for infection with HIV. It is estimated that globally, more than 650,000 children born to HIV-infected women will acquire the virus (Wiysonge, Shey, Shang,

Sterne, Brocklehurst, & Wiysonge, 2005). The majority of cases of pediatric AIDS result from maternal-fetal transmission. Since 1994, when research demonstrated that prenatal treatment of HIV-positive women with zidovudine reduced the vertical transmission of the HIV virus to the fetus, there has been an almost 70% decrease in the risk of transmission, from 25% to 7.6% (Brocklehurst & Volmink, 2002; Connor et al., 1994; Moodley & Moodley, 2004). The risk of perinatal transmission can be further reduced to about 2% when maternal antiretroviral (ARV) prophylaxis is combined with elective cesarean birth (Moodley & Moodley). Universal counseling and screening of pregnant women is recommended in the United States and Canada (AAP & American College of Obstetricians and Gynecologists [ACOG], 2005; CDC, Workowski & Berman, 2006; Chou, Smits, Huffman, Korthuis, & U.S. Preventative Services Task Force, 2005).

Transmission of HIV from the mother to the infant may occur transplacentally at various gestational ages. Transmission close to or at the time of birth is thought to account for 50% to 80% of cases (Baley & Toltzis, 2002). Postnatal transmission through breastfeeding also may occur, with an additional risk of 4% to 22% attributed to breast milk contact (Read & Committee on Pediatric AIDS, 2003). The risk of breast milk transmission is linked to the duration of breastfeeding with an estimated risk of 4% for every 6 months of breastfeeding (Coutsoudis, 2005).

Prevention. A number of factors increase the risk of HIV transmission from mother to fetus. A high viral load correlates strongly with increased transmission, as does a low maternal CD_4 T-lymphocyte count, indicative of severe disease. Asymptomatic women can transmit infection but are less likely than symptomatic women to do so. Chorioamnionitis, rupture of membranes more than 4 hours before birth, and preterm birth also have been shown to increase the risk of HIV transmission to the fetus (Public Health Service Task Force [PHSTF], 2005).

Strategies to prevent HIV acquisition in the fetus and newborn should address these risk factors. Antenatal and postnatal treatment with ARV agents such as zidovudine has been shown to reduce the infant's risk of acquiring HIV (Connor et al., 1994). Combination therapy using highly active antiretroviral therapy (HAART) has almost completely eliminated mother-to-child transmission in developed countries (PHSTF, 2005; Thorne & Newell, 2005). It is unclear what risks these drugs pose to the fetus, particularly in the first trimester (Capparelli, Rakhmanina, & Mirochnick, 2005; Thorne & Newell); however, some data exist that suggest that HAART may increase the risk for preterm birth and that for some ARV drugs, there is an increased risk for congenital anomalies (U.S. Department of Health and Human Services, 2005). It is therefore important that preconception or prenatal counseling include a discussion of the potential risks and benefits of HAART for both the mother and fetus (PHSTF, 2005; Foster & Lyall, 2005). As most mother-to-child transmissions are thought to occur in the last 2 weeks of pregnancy

(Moodley & Moodley, 2004), women who present for prenatal care late in pregnancy would still benefit from antiretroviral therapy. If an infant is born to a mother whose HIV status is unknown, consent should be obtained to test either the mother or the infant so that the infant can receive zidovudine to prevent mother-to-infant transmission (King & Committee on Pediatric AIDS, 2004).

Mode of Birth. For those women with a detectable viral load or those not taking ARV, cesarean births have been shown to reduce contact with maternal virus. For women without a detectable viral load the benefit of a cesarean birth is less clear (Moodley & Moodley, 2004). For vaginal births, transmission risks can be reduced by keeping membranes intact for as long as possible and avoiding invasive testing such as fetal scalp sampling and fetal scalp electrodes, and episiotomies (Moodley & Moodley). HIV-positive women in developed countries should be counseled to avoid breastfeeding.

Diagnosis. Diagnosis of HIV infection in the neonate is complicated by the presence of maternal IgG antibodies, which cross the placenta after 32 weeks of gestation. Three methods to detect HIV virus or its components are available for use in neonates. Viral cultures detect the presence of HIV in the neonate's blood. This sensitive but expensive test requires 4 to 6 weeks for a result. Detection of core protein antigen p24 is less expensive but also less sensitive in neonates. Polymerase chain reaction (PCR) detects HIV DNA or RNA in peripheral blood and is the preferred method of testing for neonates. The accuracy of all HIV tests varies according to the infant's age and is dependent on the viral load in the blood. Newer techniques now make it possible to confirm HIV infection more rapidly than in the past, usually by 1 month of age. Because maternal HIV antibodies cross the placenta, newborns born to infected women should be screened by polymerase chain reaction testing at 48 hours and at 1 to 2 months and 3 to 6 months of age. A positive test should be confirmed immediately by testing a second specimen (National Institutes of Health [NIH] & Health Resources and Services Administration Working Group [HRSA WG] on Antiretroviral Therapy and Medical Management of HIV-Infected Children, 2005). HIV can be excluded with reasonable certainty in nonbreastfed infants who have two or more negative tests after 1 and 4 months of age. Typically the HIV-infected neonate is asymptomatic at birth. In the past, these infants tended to be of lower birth weight than those born to noninfected mothers. No difference is found in the incidence of preterm birth or IUGR between the offspring of zidovudine-treated mothers and those born to HIV-negative women; however, some increased risk of premature birth has been noted when combination therapy is used (European Collaborative Study Group, 2003). Some will have physical effects from concurrent exposure to other STIs or maternal substance abuse of injectable drugs.

Treatment regimens with combination ARV and improved prophylaxis against infections have resulted in major improvements in decreasing the morbidity and mortality of HIV infection in all age groups. Despite this, HIV-infected children continue to have an accelerated disease process relative to adults. In particular, infants who are not diagnosed or treated in infancy continue to have high rates of early and severe disease (Maldonado, 2006).

About one third of infants infected with HIV at birth will become symptomatic within the first 2 years of life, with most of the remaining children expressing symptoms within the first few years of life. Only a few children infected at birth will be asymptomatic by 8 years of age (Maldonado, 2006). Initial presentation for these infants includes nonspecific findings such as failure to thrive, parotitis, oral candidiasis, developmental delay, and recurrent or persistent upper respiratory infections. In these babies, opportunistic infections (caused by an organism that usually does not cause illness) are more common than in HIV-infected adults, but the occurrence of cancer is less common. Common secondary infections include *Pneumocystis carinii* pneumonia, candidiasis, CMV infection, cryptosporidiosis, HSV, herpes zoster, and disseminated varicella.

The age at onset of symptoms predicts the length of survival; the later the onset, the longer the survival.

Care Management. Although it is rare for an infant to be born with symptoms of HIV infection, all infants born to seropositive mothers should be presumed to be HIV positive. Management begins by implementing Standard Precautions. Measures should be undertaken to protect the infant from further exposure to maternal blood and body fluids. The infant's skin should be cleansed with soap and water and alcohol before invasive procedures such as vitamin K administration or heel punctures. Umbilical cord stumps are cleaned meticulously every day until healing is complete. Isolation is not required, and the infant can usually be cared for in the normal nursery. The use of gloves is not required for routine care activities such as dressing or feeding the infant.

Regimens for the prevention of HIV transmission include treatment of the neonate for 6 weeks after birth with zidovudine until the infant's HIV status is determined (PHSTF, 2005).

If a diagnosis of HIV infection in the infant is made, the family should be counseled about conventional and investigational treatment options. It is recommended that therapy be initiated in all HIV-infected infants younger than 12 months of age if they have clinical or immunologic abnormalities, and that therapy also be considered for asymptomatic infants (NIH & HRSA WG, 2005). Aggressive therapy with a combination of antiretroviral drugs is recommended (Capparelli et al., 2005). Monotherapy is no longer recommended for the treatment of known HIV infection, regardless of the age of the client.

Counseling regarding the care of the mothers themselves, the family's care of the infant, and future pregnancies challenges the caregiver. Some parents opt to place the infected infants in foster homes despite the low risk for transmission among members of the same household. Social services are required in these cases. If the parent chooses to keep the infant, home health care may be arranged. For more information and updated information, parents are offered the following resource: the National AIDS hotline, 800-342-AIDS.

The family must be counseled about vaccinations. All HIV-exposed infants should be given routine vaccinations. Vaccination guidelines for infants who have a confirmed HIV infection should be followed (AAP, 2006).

Rubella Infection

Since the rubella vaccination program was begun in 1969, cases of congenital rubella infection have been reduced by 99% (Edlich, Winters, Long, & Gubler, 2005); however, it is still seen occasionally in the newborn. Vaccination failures, lack of compliance, and the migration of nonimmunized persons result in periodic outbreaks of rubella, also known as German measles.

The risk of a congenitally infected infant varies with the gestational age of the fetus when maternal infection occurs. Abnormalities are most severe if the mother contracts the virus during the first trimester and rare if the disease occurs after that time (Cooper & Alford, 2006).

More than two thirds of infected infants show no apparent symptoms at birth, but sequelae may develop years later. Hearing loss, the most common result, appears to be progressive after birth. Congenital rubella syndrome comprises cataracts or glaucoma, hearing loss, and cardiac defects (pulmonary artery stenosis, patent ductus arteriosus, or coarctation of the aorta) (Baley & Toltzis, 2002). Multiple other abnormalities also are present, including IUGR, microphthalmia, hypotonia, hepatosplenomegaly, thrombocytopenic purpura, dermatoglyphic abnormalities, bony radiolucencies, microcephaly, and brain wave abnormalities. Severe infection may result in fetal death. Delayed effects of infection manifest as thyroid dysfunction, diabetes mellitus, growth hormone deficiency, myocarditis, and glaucoma (Baley & Toltzis).

The rubella virus has been cultured in infants for up to 18 months after their birth. These infants are a serious source of infection to susceptible individuals, particularly women in the childbearing years. Extended pediatric isolation is mandatory until the noncontagious stage of rubella has been reached. The infant should be isolated until pharyngeal mucus and urine are free of virus.

Cytomegalovirus Infection

CMV infection during pregnancy may result in miscarriage, stillbirth, or congenital or neonatal cytomegalic inclusion disease (CMID). It is the most common cause of congenital viral infections in humans, occurring in 40,000 newborns in the United States every year (Lombardi & Stronati, 2005). Most (90%) affected infants are asymptomatic at birth; however, hearing loss and learning disabilities have been reported in 10% to 15% of previously asymptomatic infants (Baley & Toltzis, 2002; Lombardi & Stronati, 2005).

The neonate with classic, full-blown CMID displays IUGR and has microcephaly. The neonate also has a rash, jaundice, and hepatosplenomegaly (Fig. 38-8). Anemia, thrombocytopenia, and hyperbilirubinemia are to be expected. Intracranial, periventricular calcification often is noted on x-ray films. Inclusion bodies ("owl's eye" figures) in cells sedimented from freshly voided urine or in liver biopsy specimens are typical.

Elevated levels of cord blood IgM are suggestive of disease. The virus may be isolated from urine or saliva of the newborn. Differential diagnoses include other causes of jaundice, syphilis (positive Venereal Disease Research Laboratories [VDRL] findings), toxoplasmosis (positive Sabin-Feldman dye test result), hemolytic disease of the newborn (positive Coombs' test reaction), or coxsackievirus infection (positive culture).

Despite the extensive, endemic nature of the disease in women and men and its potential for wreaking havoc in perinatal life, critically affected newborns are born only occasionally. Milder forms of the disease often may result when the fetus is affected late in pregnancy. CMV can be transmitted through breast milk while the mother has acute CMV infection. CMV infections acquired after birth are often asymptomatic and have no sequelae. Exceptions to this occur in preterm infants in whom postnatal acquisition of CMV can result in pneumonia, hepatitis, thrombocytopenia, and long-term neurologic sequelae.

Infants infected in utero who are asymptomatic at birth are at risk for late sequelae. Hearing loss may not be apparent until after the first year of life (Pass, 2005). Chorioretinitis, microcephaly, mental retardation, and neuromuscular deficits may occur by 2 years of age. Some children are at risk for a defect in tooth enamel, resulting in severe caries.

Herpes Simplex Virus

HSV infections among newborns are being diagnosed more frequently. The incidence of neonatal herpes simplex infection is estimated to occur in 1 in every 1500 to 2000 live births (Baley & Toltzis, 2002).

FIG. 38-8 Neonatal cytomegalovirus infection. Typical rash seen in a severely affected infant. (Courtesy David A. Clarke, Philadelphia, PA.)

The neonate may acquire the virus by any of four modes of transmission:

- Transplacental infection
- Ascending infection by way of the birth canal
- Direct contamination during passage through an infected birth canal
- Direct transmission from infected personnel or family

Transplacental transmission of HSV infection to the neonate may occur during maternal infection; however, an ascending transcervical infection first involves the intact fetal membranes, causing chorioamnionitis. Transcervical infection can be accelerated by fetal monitoring scalp electrodes. The electrodes break the fetal skin barrier and increase the risk of infection.

Congenital infection is rare and characterized by in utero destruction of normally formed organs. Affected infants are growth restricted. They have severe psychomotor delays, with intracranial calcifications, microcephaly, hypertonicity, and seizures. They have eye involvement, including microphthalmos, cataracts, chorioretinitis, blindness, and retinal dysplasia. Some infants have patent ductus arteriosus, limb anomalies, and recurrent skin vesicles, with a short life expectancy.

Most infants are infected directly during passage through the birth canal. The risk of infection during vaginal birth in the presence of genital herpes has not been clearly delineated. It may be as high as 57% with active primary infection at term (Brown, Wald, Morrow, Selke, Zeh, & Corey, 2003). Primary maternal infections after 32 weeks of gestation have a higher risk for the fetus and newborn than recurrent infections (Baley & Toltzis, 2002). The transmission rate of chronic vaginal herpes from the pregnant woman to her newborn is low, 2% or less (Arvin, Whitley, & Gutierrez, 2006). Passive intrauterine immunity to herpes may be responsible. In 60% to 80% of cases of neonatal HSV infection, the mother has no history or symptoms of infection at the time of birth, but serologic testing reveals evidence of the herpes virus (Kimberlin, 2005).

Postnatal acquisition of the virus and spread within a nursery have been documented by DNA analysis. Both mother and father, as well as maternal breast lesions, have been implicated in neonatal infections. There also is concern regarding symptomatic and asymptomatic shedding among hospital personnel. Nursery personnel with cold sores should practice strict handwashing and wear a mask, but no evidence indicates that they should be removed from the nursery unless they have a herpetic whitlow (primary HSV infection of the terminal segment of a finger) (Baley & Toltzis, 2002).

Clinically, neonatal HSV infections are classified as disseminated infection (25%); CNS disease (30%); or localized infection of the skin, the eye, or the mouth (SEM disease) (45%) (Kimberlin, 2005). Disseminated infections may involve virtually every organ system, but the liver, the adrenal glands, and the lungs are primarily involved. Affected infants exhibit initial symptoms usually in the first week of life but sometimes in the second week, with signs of bacterial sepsis or shock. Clinical manifestations include skin vesicles in about 80% of infants (Kimberlin). Death results from progression of CNS involvement, respiratory distress and pneumonitis, shock, DIC, and bleeding.

In CNS disease, blood-borne seeding of the brain results in multiple lesions of cortical hemorrhagic necrosis. It also can occur alone or in association with oral, eye, or skin lesions. Brain involvement usually manifests in the second to fourth week of life. Skin lesions are apparent in 60% to 70% of the infants, and the CSF of fewer than 50% will reveal the virus. The presenting manifestations include lethargy, poor feeding, irritability, and local or generalized seizures. Almost half of the infants die of neurologic deterioration as late as 6 months after onset, and virtually all survivors have severe sequelae, including microcephaly and blindness (Baley & Toltzis, 2002).

Localized HSV infections most often occur with skin findings or rarely with isolated oral cavity lesions (Fig. 38-9). Without treatment, CNS or disseminated disease develops in 70% of the infants with skin vesicles. Ocular involvement, which can occur alone, may be secondary to either HSV-1 or HSV-2. Ocular disease may not be discovered for months. Microphthalmos, cataracts, optic atrophy, and corneal scarring may result from chorioretinitis, keratitis, and retinal hemorrhage (Baley & Toltzis, 2002).

Care Management. Gloves should be worn when caregivers are in contact with these infants. The neonate's eyes, oral cavity, and skin are inspected carefully for the presence of any lesions. Cultures are obtained from the mouth, the eyes, and any possible lesions. Circumcision, if performed, is delayed until the infant is ready to be discharged. The infant may be discharged with the mother if the infant's cultures are negative for the virus. As long as no suspicious lesions are on the mother's breasts, breastfeeding is allowed. For the infant at risk, prophylactic topical eye ointment (vidarabine) is administered for 5 days for prevention of keratoconjunctivitis. No current recommendations exist for prophylactic systemic therapy; each

FIG. 38-9 Neonatal herpes simplex virus oral lesions. (Courtesy David A. Clarke, Philadelphia, PA.)

case should be considered individually. Blood, urine, and CSF specimens should be cultured when indicated clinically. If herpetic lesions first occur after 6 weeks of life, the risk of dissemination and severe illness is very low (Baley & Toltzis, 2002).

Therapy includes general supportive measures, as well as treatment with vidarabine or acyclovir. Acyclovir is easier to administer and is the most frequently used drug. It is considered safe because only viral replication is inhibited, although long-term sequelae are not yet known. A randomized controlled trial has shown no difference between vidarabine and acyclovir for treatment of HSV. Duration of treatment is 14 days for SEM disease and 21 days for infants with disseminated or CNS disease (Kimberlin, 2005). Continuing therapy may be required in case of recurrence. Ophthalmic ointment should be administered simultaneously (Baley & Toltzis, 2002).

Bacterial Infections
Group B Streptococcus

The most common cause of neonatal sepsis and meningitis in the United States is Group B streptococcus (GBS). From 8% to 28% of pregnant women are colonized at the time of birth. Colonization rates vary with age (increasing with age), race (higher in African-Americans), and gravidity (Yudin & Gonik, 2006).

The incidence of early-onset GBS infection is 1.4 per 1000 live births (Edwards, Nizet, & Baker, 2006). Early-onset GBS infection in the neonate occurs in the first 7 days of life but most commonly manifests in the first 24 hours after birth. Risk factors for the development of early-onset GBS include low birth weight, preterm birth, rupture of membranes of more than 18 hours, maternal fever, previous GBS infant, maternal GBS bacteriuria, and multiple gestation. Usually resulting from vertical transmission from the birth canal, early-onset disease results in a respiratory illness that mimics the symptoms of severe respiratory distress. The infant may rapidly develop septic shock, which has a significant mortality rate. In 2002, guidelines were developed recommending that all pregnant women be screened at 35 to 37 weeks of gestation for GBS colonization, and identified carriers given intravenous penicillin as soon as possible after hospital admission for labor and continue every 4 to 6 hours until the birth of the infant (Schrag, Gorwitz, Fultz-Butts, & Schuchat, 2002). Fig. 38-10 provides an algorithm for the management of pregnancies complicated by GBS.

The practice of giving prophylactic antibiotics to women in labor who are GBS positive has significantly reduced the incidence and severity of early-onset GBS infection in the newborn (Yudin & Gonik, 2006).

Late-onset GBS infections occur between 1 week and 3 months of age, with an average age at onset of 24 days. Of infants with late-onset GBS, 30% develop meningitis, with a mortality rate of 0% to 23%. Of the survivors, 50% develop neurologic damage. The incidence of early onset disease declined significantly after the introduction of

*If no maternal intrapartum prophylaxis for GBS was administered despite an indication being present, data are insufficient on which to recommend a single management strategy.
†Includes complete blood cell count and differential, blood culture, and chest radiograph if respiratory abnormalities are present. When signs of sepsis are present, a lumbar puncture, if feasible, should be performed.
§Duration of therapy varies depending on results of blood culture, cerebrospinal fluid findings, if obtained, and the clinical course of the infant. If laboratory results and clinical course do not indicate bacterial infections, duration may be as short as 48 hours.
¶CBC with differential and blood culture.
**Applies only to penicillin, ampicillin, or cefazolin and assumes recommended dosing regimens (Box 2).
††A healthy-appearing infant who was ≥38 weeks of gestation at delivery and whose mother received ≥4 hours of intrapartum prophylaxis before delivery may be discharged home after 24 hours if other discharge criteria have been met and a person able to comply fully with instructions for home observation will be present. If any one of these conditions is not met, the infant should be observed in the hospital for at least 48 hours and until criteria for discharge are achieved.

FIG. 38-10 Sample algorithm for management of a newborn whose mother received intrapartum antimicrobial agents (IAP) for prevention of early-onset group B streptococcal disease or suspected chorioamnionitis. This algorithm is not an exclusive course of management. Variations that incorporate individual circumstances or institutional preferences may be appropriate. (From Schrag, S., Gorwitz, R., Fultz-Butts, K., & Schuchat, A. [2002]. Prevention of perinatal group B streptococcal disease. Revised guidelines from CDC. *MMWR Morbidity and Mortality Weekly Report, 51*[RR11], 1-22.)

screening and prophylactic treatment protocols; however, the incidence of late-onset disease has remained stable (Edwards et al., 2006).

Escherichia coli

E. coli is the second most common cause of neonatal sepsis and meningitis in the United States. The stated incidence of *E. coli* sepsis is 1 to 2 cases per 1000 births; however, this rate may be declining. *E. coli* is found in the gastrointestinal tract soon after birth and makes up the bulk of human fecal flora. In addition to chorioamnionitis in the mother, *E. coli* also can cause a variety of neonatal infections, including oomphalitis, diarrheal illness, pneumonia, peritonitis, urinary tract infections, and meningitis.

Increasing use of ampicillin in labor as prophylaxis against GBS disease may result in more virulent *E. coli* disease resulting from ampicillin-resistant organisms (Alarcon, Pena, Salas, Sancha, & Omenaca, 2004). Risk factors for the development of *E. coli* infections in the newborn include maternal infection, low birth weight, prolonged rupture of membranes, and septic or traumatic birth. Clinical signs of *E. coli* sepsis are relatively nonspecific and include fever, temperature instability, apnea, cyanosis, jaundice, hepatomegaly, lethargy or irritability, vomiting, abdominal distention, and diarrhea (Askin, 2004).

Staphylococcus aureus

S. aureus is found on the skin, the umbilicus, and the nares in 40% to 90% of neonates in the full-term nursery by 5 days of age (Shinefield & St. Geme, 2001). Despite its presence on the skin, the incidence of *S. aureus* infection is relatively low. This organism does cause periodic epidemic outbreaks within the nursery population in many countries of the world (Shinefield & St. Geme). Conjunctivitis, presenting with purulent eye discharge, is one of the most common manifestations of *S. aureus* infection. Breaks in the skin from intravenous catheters or scalp electrodes present an opportunity for the development of *S. aureus* abscesses. The major sources of colonization by *S. aureus* are the hands of medical and nursing personnel.

Listeriosis

L. monocytogenes is a bacterium capable of producing significant intrapartum illness. Prenatal infection causes chorioamnionitis or endometritis and should be suspected in cases of meconium-stained amniotic fluid in infants younger than 37 weeks of gestation. It also has been implicated as a cause of miscarriage and stillbirth (Bortolussi & Mailman, 2006). With disseminated fetal infection, microabscesses have been reported in the liver, the lungs, and the adrenal glands of stillborn infants. In the United States the incidence of neonatal listeriosis is estimated to be 13 per 100,000 live births (Bortolussi & Mailman). Two forms of neonatal listeriosis are recognized: early-onset and late-onset. Early-onset infections usually present at birth with meconium-stained amniotic fluid, respiratory distress, cyanosis, apnea, and evidence of pneumonia (Bortolussi & Mailman). Listeriosis also can

manifest as meningitis in a late-onset infection (Vergnano, Sharland, Kazembe, Mwansambo, & Heath, 2005).

Chlamydia Infection

Chlamydia trachomatis is an intracellular bacterium that causes neonatal conjunctivitis (20% to 50% of exposed infants) and pneumonia (10% to 20% of exposed infants) (Darville, 2006). Chlamydial infection in pregnancy has also been suggested as a cause of early and late pregnancy loss, stillbirth, premature labor, and postpartum endometritis (Mardh, 2002).

Neonatal chlamydial conjunctivitis (congestion and edema), with minimal discharge, develops 5 days to 2 weeks after birth. Inclusion conjunctivitis is usually self-limiting, but if untreated, chronic follicular conjunctivitis, with conjunctival scarring and corneal microgranulations (Mardh, 2002), has been reported.

Chlamydial pneumonia usually has a gradual onset, between 2 and 12 weeks of age, beginning with rhinorrhea and progressing to tachypnea and coughing. Signs may be quite subtle and often go unrecognized. It is speculated that pneumonia may occur as a result of movement of the organism from the conjunctiva into the lower respiratory tract; however, conjunctivitis is not a prerequisite to pneumonia (Mardh, 2002).

Silver nitrate is not effective against *C. trachomatis,* but erythromycin or tetracycline ointment may prevent ophthalmic infection (Edwards, 2006). Eye prophylaxis is not sufficient to prevent the development of chlamydial pneumonia; therefore infants at risk should be treated with systemic antibiotics such as oral erythromycin syrup.

Fungal Infections
Candidiasis

Candida infections, formerly known as moniliasis, may occur in the newborn. *Candida albicans,* the organism usually responsible, may cause disease in any organ system. It is a yeastlike fungus (producing yeast cells and spores) that can be acquired from a maternal vaginal infection during birth; by person-to-person transmission; or from contaminated hands, bottles, nipples, or other articles. It usually is a benign disorder in the neonate, often confined to the oral and diaper regions (Hockenberry, 2003).

Candidal diaper dermatitis appears on the perianal area, inguinal folds, and lower portion of the abdomen. The affected area is intensely erythematous, with a sharply demarcated, scalloped edge, frequently with numerous satellite lesions that extend beyond the larger lesion. The source of the infection is through the gastrointestinal tract. Treatment is with applications of an antifungal ointment, such as nystatin (Mycostatin) or miconazole 2% (Monistat), with each diaper change. The infant also may be given an oral antifungal preparation to eliminate any gastrointestinal source of infection (Hockenberry, 2003).

Oral candidiasis (thrush, or mycotic stomatitis) is characterized by the appearance of white plaques on the oral mucosa, gums, and tongue. The white patches are easily differentiated from milk curds; the patches cannot be removed and tend to bleed when touched. In most cases, the infant does not seem to be in discomfort from the infection. A few infants seem to have some difficulty swallowing.

Infants who are sick, debilitated, or receiving antibiotic therapy are more susceptible to thrush. Those with conditions such as cleft lip or palate, neoplasms, and hyperparathyroidism seem to be more vulnerable to mycotic infection.

The objectives of management are to eradicate the causative organism, to control exposure to *C. albicans,* and to improve the infant's resistance. Interventions include maintenance of scrupulous cleanliness to prevent reinfection (nursing personnel, parents, others). Good handwashing technique is always essential. Clean surfaces should be provided for neonates. Proper cleanliness of the equipment and environment is ensured. If the infant is breastfeeding, the mother also is treated with topical nystatin.

Medications are administered as ordered. Nystatin is instilled into the newborn's mouth with a medicine dropper after the infant is given sterile water to wash out any residual milk. Nystatin also may be swabbed over mucosa, gums, or tongue. Less frequently, an aqueous solution of gentian violet (1% to 2%) is applied with a swab to oral mucosa, gums, and tongue. The nurse should guard against staining the skin, the clothes, and equipment, and should warn parents about the purple staining of the baby's mouth.

▬ SUBSTANCE ABUSE

Certain maternal behaviors result in perinatal risk. Maternal habits hazardous to the fetus and neonate include drug addiction, smoking, and alcohol abuse. Occasional

withdrawal reactions have been reported in neonates of mothers who use to excess such drugs as barbiturates, alcohol, or amphetamines. Serious reactions are seen in neonates whose mothers abuse psychoactive drugs or are treated with methadone. Almost 50% of pregnancies of women addicted to opioids result in low-birth-weight (LBW) infants who are not necessarily preterm. Alcohol is a teratogen; maternal ethanol abuse during gestation can lead to identifiable fetal alcohol spectrum disorders which include fetal alcohol syndrome (FAS), alcohol-related neurodevelopmental disorders, and alcohol-related birth defects. Maternal substance abuse is discussed in Chapter 35.

The adverse effects of exposure of the fetus to drugs are varied. They include transient behavioral changes such as alterations in fetal breathing movements or irreversible effects such as fetal death, IUGR, structural malformations, or mental retardation. Critical determinants of the effect of the drug on the fetus include the specific drug, the dosage, the route of administration, the genotype of the mother or fetus, and the timing of the drug exposure. Determining the specific effects of individual drugs on the fetus is made difficult by the common practice of polydrug use, errors or omissions in reporting drug use, and variations in the strength, purity, and types of additives found in street drugs. Maternal conditions such as poverty and malnutrition and comorbid conditions such as STIs further compound the difficulty in identifying the presence and consequences of intrauterine drug exposure. Fig. 38-11 shows critical periods in human embryogenesis and the teratogenic effects of drugs. Table 38-4 summarizes the effects of commonly abused substances on the fetus and neonate.

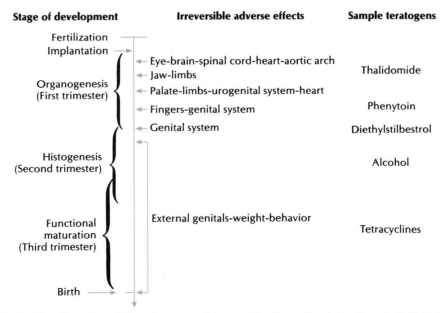

FIG. 38-11 Critical periods in human embryogenesis. (From Reed, M., Aranda, J., & Hales, B. [2006]. Developmental pharmacology. In R. Martin, A. Fanaroff, & M. Walsh (Eds.), *Fanaroff and Martin's neonatal-perinatal medicine: Diseases of the fetus and infant* [8th ed.]. St. Louis: Mosby.

table 38-4 Summary of Neonatal Effects of Commonly Abused Substances

SUBSTANCE	NEONATAL EFFECTS
Alcohol	*Fetal alcohol syndrome* (FAS): craniofacial anomalies, including short eyelid opening, flat midface, flat upper lip groove, thin upper lip; microcephaly; hyperactivity; developmental delays; attention deficits
	Alcohol-related birth defects (ARBD): milder forms of FAS, cardiac anomalies, failure to thrive
Cocaine	Prematurity, small for gestational age, microcephaly, poor feeding, irregular sleep pattern, diarrhea, visual attention problems, hyperactivity, difficult to console, hypersensitivity to noise and external stimuli, irritability, developmental delays, some association with congenital anomalies of the genitourinary tract
Heroin	Low birth weight, small for gestational age, neonatal abstinence syndrome (see Table 38-6)
Amphetamines	Small for gestational age, prematurity, poor weight gain, lethargy
Tobacco	Prematurity, low birth weight, increased risk for sudden infant death syndrome, increased risk for bronchitis, pneumonia, developmental delays

Alcohol

Alcohol ingestion during pregnancy is associated with both acute short-term and long-term effects on the fetus and newborn, which are subsumed under the term *fetal alcohol spectrum disorders (FASDs)*. The quantity of alcohol required to produce fetal effects is unclear, but it is known that infants born to heavy drinkers have twice the risk of congenital abnormalities as those born to moderate drinkers (Stoll & Kliegman, 2004). Alcohol withdrawal can occur in neonates, particularly when maternal ingestion occurs near the time of birth (Greene & Goodman, 2003). Signs and symptoms include jitteriness, increased tone and reflex responses, and irritability. Seizures are also common.

Fetal alcohol syndrome (FAS) is based on minimal criteria of signs in each of three categories: prenatal and postnatal growth restriction; CNS malfunctions, including mental retardation; and craniofacial features such as microcephaly, small eyes or short palpebral fissures, thin upper lip, flat midface, and an indistinct philtrum. Neurologic problems in FAS children include some degree of intelligence quotient (IQ) deficit, attention-deficit disorder, diminished fine motor skills, and poor speech. These children have been shown to lack inhibition, have no stranger anxiety, and lack appropriate judgment skills.

Infants exposed prenatally to alcohol who are affected but do not meet the criteria for FAS may be said to have alcohol-related neurodevelopmental disorders (ARND)

or alcohol-related birth defects (ARBD) (Boyle, 2002). These disorders run the gamut from learning disabilities and behavioral problems to speech or language problems and hyperactivity. Often these problems are not detected until the child goes to school and learning problems become evident. Similar birth defects can be seen with other disorders, such as fetal hydantoin syndrome (from exposure to anti-epileptic drugs); therefore a careful history is needed.

Documentation of FAS has been reported in the literature since the early part of the eighteenth century. The incidence of combined ARND and FAS in the United States is about 9.1 per 1000 population (Bandstra & Accorneo, 2006; Stoll & Kliegman, 2004).

Predictable abnormal patterns of fetal and neonatal morphogenesis are attributed to severe, chronic alcoholism in women who continue to drink heavily during pregnancy. The pattern of growth deficiency begun in prenatal life persists after birth, especially in the linear growth rate, rate of weight gain, and growth of head circumferences.

Ocular structural anomalies are common findings (Fig. 38-12). Limb anomalies and a variety of cardiocirculatory anomalies, especially ventricular septal defects, pose problems for the child. Table 38-5 outlines physical findings in FAS. Mental retardation (IQ of 79 or less at age 7 years), hyperactivity, and fine motor dysfunction (poor hand-to-mouth coordination, weak grasp) add to the handicapping problems that maternal alcoholism can impose. Genital abnormalities are seen in daughters of alcohol-addicted

CRITICAL THINKING EXERCISE

Fetal Alcohol Syndrome

While providing care for Monica during her labor and birth, the nurse learns that Monica admits to smoking marijuana and drinking alcohol early in pregnancy. She claims that she stopped drinking when she found out that she was pregnant. She also said that her friend told her that drinking early in pregnancy will not hurt the baby but wants reassurance from the nurse that that is true. What teaching should the nurse provide for Monica? What features should she look for in Monica's baby that would indicate the presence of fetal alcohol syndrome? What follow-up care should be provided for Monica's baby?

1. Evidence—Is there sufficient evidence to provide Monica with answers to her questions about the effects of alcohol on a fetus?
2. Assumptions—What assumptions can be made about alcohol ingestion during pregnancy?
   a. The risks of drinking alcohol in pregnancy
   b. The effects of alcohol on the fetus
   c. The fit between Monica's beliefs and the implications of a diagnosis of fetal alcohol syndrome
   d. Monica's ability to care for an infant with fetal alcohol syndrome
3. What implications and priorities for nursing can be made at this time?
4. Does the evidence objectively support your conclusion?
5. Are there alternative perspectives to your conclusion?

CD: Critical Thinking Exercise: FAS

FIG. 38-12 Infant with fetal alcohol syndrome. (From Markie-wicz, M., & Abrahamson, E. [1999]. *Diagnosis in color: Neonatology.* St. Louis: Mosby.)

mothers. Two thirds of newborns with FAS are girls; the cause of this altered fetal sex ratio is unknown. Severe and chronic alcoholism (ethanol toxicity), not maternal mal-nutrition, is responsible for the severity and consistency of postnatal performance problems (Bandstra & Accorneo, 2006). High alcohol levels are lethal to the developing em-bryo. Lower levels cause brain and other malformations. Long-term prognosis (no studies are available) is discourag-

table 38-5 Features of Fetal Alcohol Syndrome

AFFECTED PART	CHARACTERISTICS
Eyes	Epicanthal folds, strabismus, ptosis, hypoplastic retinal vessels
Mouth	Poor suck, cleft lip, cleft palate, small teeth
Ears	Deafness
Skeleton	Radioulnar synostosis, fusion of cervical vertebrae, restricted bone growth
Heart	Atrial and ventricular septal defects, tetralogy of Fallot, patent ductus arteriosus
Kidney	Renal hypoplasia, hydronephrosis, urogenital sinus
Liver	Extrahepatic biliary atresia, hepatic fibrosis
Immune system	Increased infections: otitis media, upper respiratory infections, immune deficiencies
Tumors	Nonspecific neoplasms
Skin	Abnormal palmar creases, irregular hair, whorls

From Weiner, L., & Morse, B. (1991). FAS: Clinical perspectives and prevention. In I. Chasnoff (Ed.), *Drugs, alcohol, pregnancy and parenting.* Boston: Kluwer.

ing even in an optimal psychosocial environment, when one considers the combination of growth failure and men-tal retardation.

However, alcohol effects depend not only on the amount of alcohol consumed but also on the interaction of quantity, frequency, type of alcohol, and other drug abuse. Other drugs, such as cigarettes, caffeine, and mari-juana, may potentiate the fetal effects of alcohol consump-tion during gestation.

The infant of a mother who abuses alcohol is faced with many clinical problems. Identification of the prob-lems leads to the medical diagnosis of FAS. The infant may have respiratory distress related to preterm birth, neuro-logic damage, and a "floppy" epiglottis and small trachea. Tracheoepiglottal anomalies may cause cardiopulmonary arrest. Other disorders include recurrent otitis media and hearing loss. Craniofacial features may be important in di-agnosing craniofacial and oral anomalies, dental develop-ment abnormalities, and long-term body growth patterns. Feeding difficulties are related to preterm birth, poor suck-ing ability, and possible cleft palate. The infant may exhibit brain dysfunction, microcephaly, and grand mal seizures.

Long-term effects into childhood may include impaired visuomotor perception and performance, lowered IQ scores, and delayed receptive and expressive language, as well as reduced capacity to process and store factual data. It is now recognized as one of the leading causes of mental retardation in the United States. Although the distinctive facial features of the infant tend to become less evident, the mental capacities never become normal. The lifetime cost of care for one child with FAS in the United States is esti-mated to be $2 million (Lupton, Burd, & Harwood, 2004).

Nursing care involves many of the same strategies used for the care of preterm infants (see Chapter 40). Special ef-forts are made to involve the parents in their child's care and to encourage opportunities for parent-child attachment.

Placing infants in a warm, caring environment with understanding caregivers who can deal with the infant's hyperirritability can lead to improved emotional develop-ment and social functioning (Welch-Carre, 2005). These caregivers provide extensive cuddling and human contact and can deal with the eating problems that typically lead to a diagnosis of failure to thrive. However, these infants may not go home to such an environment. Often the family is dysfunctional.

Heroin

Heroin crosses the placenta and results in IUGR in 50% of exposed infants (Stoll & Kliegman, 2004). Heroin may have a direct growth-inhibiting effect on the fetus, but the exact mechanisms of growth inhibition are not clear. There is an increased rate of stillbirths but not of congenital anomalies.

Many of the medical complications attributed to heroin result from prematurity. Other risks include physical de-pendence in the fetus and the risk of exposure to infections, including hepatitis B and C viruses and HIV. Drug withdrawal in the mother is accompanied by fetal withdrawal, which can lead to fetal death. Maternal detoxification in the first trimester carries an increased risk of miscarriage. Detoxification in pregnancy is not recommended because of possible withdrawal-induced fetal distress (Greene & Goodman, 2003). Methadone is often used in pregnancy to treat maternal drug cravings and prevent withdrawal.

Heroin withdrawal occurs in 75% of infants born to addicted mothers, usually within the first 12 to 48 hours of life (Greene & Goodman, 2003). The signs depend on the length of maternal addiction, the amount of drug taken, and the time of injection before birth. The infant whose mother is taking methadone may not demonstrate signs of withdrawal until a week or so after birth. The symptoms of infants whose mothers used heroin or methadone are similar in nature. Initially the infant may be depressed. The withdrawal syndrome may manifest as a combination of any of the following signs. Most commonly, the infant may be jittery and hyperactive. Usually the infant's cry is shrill and persistent. The infant may yawn or sneeze frequently. The tendon reflexes are increased, but the Moro reflex is decreased. The neonate may exhibit poor feeding and sucking, tachypnea, vomiting, diarrhea, hypothermia or hyperthermia, and sweating. In addition, an abnormal sleep cycle, with absence of quiet sleep and disturbance of active sleep, has been described in these infants (Bandstra & Accorneo, 2006).

If withdrawal is not treated, vomiting, diarrhea, dehydration, apnea, and convulsions may develop. Death may follow. Therapy is individualized. Dehydration and electrolyte imbalance are prevented or treated. Usually one of the following drugs is ordered: phenobarbital, methadone, morphine syrup, or diazepam, singly or in combination.

The use of naloxone (Narcan) is contraindicated in infants born to narcotic addicts because it may cause severe signs and symptoms of narcotic abstinence syndrome and seizures.

The long-term effect on these infants is being studied. The risk of sudden infant death syndrome (SIDS) is 5 to 10 times higher for infants with significant withdrawal problems than for infants in the general population.

Methadone

Methadone, a synthetic opiate, has been the therapy of choice for heroin addiction since 1965. Methadone crosses the placenta. An increasing number of infants have been born to methadone-maintained mothers, who seem to have better prenatal care and a somewhat better lifestyle than those taking heroin (Bandstra & Accorneo, 2006).

Withdrawal, which occurs in 60% of infants born to women on methadone (Greene & Goodman, 2003) resembles heroin withdrawal but tends to be more severe and prolonged. In addition, the incidence of seizures is higher. Seizures usually occur between days 7 and 10. The infants exhibit a disturbed sleep pattern similar to that seen in heroin withdrawal. The infants have a higher birth weight than those in heroin withdrawal, usually appropri-ate for gestational age. No increased incidence of congenital anomalies is seen.

Late-onset withdrawal occurs at 2 to 4 weeks and may continue for weeks or months. A higher incidence of SIDS also has been reported in these infants (Bandstra & Accorneo, 2006). This factor is important for perinatal nurses who coordinate follow-up care for the infant and education for the mother or other caregiver. Community health nurses must know about the potential for withdrawal symptoms to occur.

Therapy for methadone withdrawal is similar to that for heroin withdrawal. The few available follow-up studies of these infants reveal a high incidence of hyperactivity, learning and behavior disorders, and poor social adjustment (Bandstra & Accorneo, 2006).

Marijuana

Marijuana is the most common illicit drug used by pregnant women (Hurd, Wang, Anderson, Beck, Minkoff, & Dow-Edwards, 2005). Marijuana crosses the placenta, and its use during pregnancy may result in a shortened gestation and a higher incidence of IUGR. No specific teratogenic effects have been identified. Some investigators have found a higher incidence of meconium staining of the amniotic fluid (Bandstra & Accorneo, 2006). Symptoms such as jitteriness, tremors, and impaired sleeping have been reported in infants, with persistence into childhood (Dahl, Scher, Williamson, Robles, & Day, 1995). No differences were detected on infant follow-up at 6, 12, and 24 months in general measures of physical growth and development. At 4 years of age, children had poorer scores on memory and verbal tests compared with a control group. Compounding the issue of the effects of marijuana is multidrug use, especially among adolescents, that combines the harmful effects of marijuana, tobacco, alcohol, and cocaine. Long-term follow-up studies on exposed infants are needed.

Cocaine

Cocaine crosses the placenta and is found in breast milk. Considerable controversy exists regarding the effects of cocaine on the fetus and neonate. There is a strong association between maternal cocaine use and both tobacco and marijuana use (Pichini et al., 2005) which makes the determination of cocaine effects difficult. Fetal brain, kidney, and urogenital system malformations have been associated with maternal cocaine ingestion (Langendoerfer, Johnson, & Thureen, 2005). Other reported effects include infarctions to developing organs, resulting in defects such as congenital heart disease, skull defects, ileal atresia, and limb reduction. Infants born to cocaine-abusing mothers show a high rate of perinatal morbidity, IUGR, preterm birth, and placental or cerebral infarction (Bandstra & Accorneo, 2006).

Cocaine-dependent neonates do not experience a process of withdrawal as seen in narcotic-exposed infants but rather show neurotoxic effects of the drug (Greene & Goodman, 2003). Signs of exposure have some of the same characteristics as those of heroin withdrawal but can be highly varied. There may be an increased risk for SIDS. The effects of prenatal exposure to cocaine on neonatal behavior have been studied extensively. Findings indicate that cocaine-exposed infants have limited ability to habituate to stimuli. As these children enter school, they demonstrate a reduced capacity for verbal reasoning and difficulties maintaining attention (Bandstra & Accorneo, 2006). Box 38-2 summarizes neonatal effects of maternal cocaine use.

Miscellaneous Substances

The fetal and neonatal effects of maternal use of methamphetamines in pregnancy are not well known. The effects appear to be dose related. LBW, preterm birth, and perinatal mortality may be consequences of higher doses used throughout pregnancy. A higher incidence of cleft lip and palate and cardiac defects has been reported in infants exposed to amphetamines in utero (Plessinger, 1998). After birth, infants may have bradycardia or tachycardia that resolves as the drug is cleared from the infant's system. Lethargy may continue for several months, along with frequent infections and poor weight gain. Emotional disturbances and delays in gross and fine motor coordination may be seen during early childhood.

Phenobarbital crosses the placenta readily and is subsequently found in high levels in the fetal liver and brain.

box 38-2 Neonatal Effects of Maternal Cocaine Use

PHYSICAL
- Preterm birth
- Decreased length
- Decreased head circumference
- Intrauterine growth restriction (IUGR)
- Cryptorchidism
- Hypospadias
- Hydronephrosis
- Seizures
- Fever
- Congenital heart disease
- Skull defects
- Hypertension
- Cerebral infarction
- Vomiting
- Diarrhea
- Sudden infant death syndrome (SIDS)
- Tachypnea

BEHAVIORAL
- Irritability
- Tremors
- Poor feeding
- Abnormal sleep patterns
- Increased startles
- Disorganized behavior
- Lability
- Poor visual processing
- Difficult to console

Because of its slow metabolic rate, when withdrawal does occur, onset is generally at 2 to 14 days after birth, and duration is about 2 to 4 months. Irritability, crying, hiccups, and sleepiness mark the initial response. During the second stage, the infant is extremely hungry, regurgitates and gags frequently, and demonstrates episodic irritability, sweating, and a disturbed sleep pattern.

Treatment consists of swaddling, frequent feedings, and protection from noxious external stimuli. If no improvement occurs, the neonate should be given phenobarbital and then slowly withdrawn from this drug after control of symptoms (Bandstra & Accorneo, 2006).

Caffeine has not been implicated as a teratogen in humans. Fernandes, Sabharwal, Smiley, Pastuszak, Koren, and Einarson (1998) reported that caffeine consumption of more than 150 mg per day (1.5 to 2 cups per day) was associated with IUGR and LBW. Santos, Victora, Huttly, and Carvalhal (1998) reported no adverse effects in the fetus with consumption of less than 300 mg of caffeine per day.

Tobacco

Cigarette smoking in pregnancy has been found to be associated with birth-weight deficits in the full-term neonate (Reed, Aranda, & Hales, 2006). Specifically, birth weight, head circumference, and length have all been found to be reduced in infants whose mothers smoked during pregnancy (Shankaran et al., 2004). Maternal cigarette smoking is implicated in 21% to 39% of LBW infants. Passive exposure to secondhand smoke by a pregnant woman also may result in the birth of an LBW infant.

The rate of miscarriage and preterm birth is increased in the smoking population. When other variables have been controlled for, no clear association has been found between maternal smoking and congenital anomalies (Reed, Aranda, & Hales, 2006). Nicotine and cotinine, the two pharmacologically active substances in tobacco, are found in higher concentrations in infants whose mothers smoke. These substances can be secreted in breast milk for up to 2 hours after the mother has smoked. Cigarette smoke contains more than 2000 compounds, including carbon monoxide, dioxin, cyanide, and cadmium. Long-term studies show residual effects beyond the neonatal period (Reed et al.). Deficits in growth, in intellectual and emotional development, and in behavior have been documented. These include poor auditory responsiveness, increased fine motor tremors, hypertonicity, and decreased verbal comprehension.

Pregnant women need to be aware of the harmful effects of smoking on their unborn baby's health. These include IUGR, miscarriage, prematurity, and SIDS (Chiriboga, 2003). It is also apparent that the breakdown products from tobacco can be passed to the infant in breast milk. The effects of maternal smoking in breastfed babies includes a reduction in the antiinfective properties of breast milk (Zanardo et al., 2005).

Increasing concern surrounds second-hand smoke and its potential effects on infants and siblings. New evidence suggests that maternal smoking may be linked to an increased incidence of excessive crying and infant colic (Reijneveld, Lanting, Crone, & VanWouwe, 2005; Shenassa & Brown, 2004). Mothers and all others should refrain from smoking near the infant. It is not clear whether the association between smoking and SIDS reflects in utero exposure or passive exposure postnatally, or both.

■ CARE MANAGEMENT

Assessment of the newborn requires a review of the mother's prenatal record. A medical and social history of drug abuse and detoxification is noted. The infant may have IUGR or be preterm with LBW.

The woman who is addicted to narcotics may have infections that compound the risk to the infant, including hepatitis, septicemia, and STIs, including AIDS (Wagner, Katikaneni, Cox, & Ryan, 1998).

The nurse often is the first to observe the signs of drug dependence in the infant. The nurse's observations help the physician differentiate between drug withdrawal and other conditions, such as CNS disorder, sepsis, hypoglycemia, and electrolyte imbalance.

The infant is assessed by means of the guidelines discussed in Chapter 26. The infant's gestational age and maturity are noted. In utero exposure to some drugs results in observable malformations or dysmorphism (abnormality of shape). Neonatal behavior may arouse suspicion. Neonatal abstinence syndrome is the term given to the group of signs and symptoms associated with drug withdrawal in the neonate (Table 38-6). Fig. 38-13 provides an example of a scoring system for assessing withdrawal symptoms. Because many women are multidrug users, the newborn initially may exhibit a confusing complex of signs.

Urine or meconium screening may be used to identify substances abused by the mother. Urine screening is most commonly used, but its sensitivity is limited (Greene & Goodman, 2003). Initially costly and of limited availability, tests of meconium collected on day 1 or 2 of life have been shown to be both sensitive and reliable in detecting the me-

tabolites of several street drugs, including cocaine (Kwong & Shearer, 1998). One study examining urine, hair, and meconium samples for drug use found that although all of these tests were reliable to a greater or lesser degree, the single most reliable method for determining prenatal drug use was a careful history collected by an experienced interviewer (Eyler, Behnke, Wobie, Garvan, & Tebbett, 2005)

■ Nursing Care

Planning for care of the infant born to a substance-abusing mother presents a challenge to the health care team. Parents are included in the planning for the newborn's care and also for the care and support of the mother and her newborn at home. A multidisciplinary approach includes home health or community resource personnel (e.g., regulatory agencies such as child protective services).

Education and social support to prevent the abuse of drugs provide the ideal approach. However, given the scope of the drug abuse problem, total prevention is an unrealistic goal.

Nursing care of the drug-dependent neonate involves supportive therapy for fluid and electrolyte balance, nutrition, infection control, and respiratory care. Swaddling, holding, reducing stimuli, and feeding as necessary may be helpful in easing withdrawal (see Plan of Care). Specific suggestions for providing care to infants experiencing withdrawal are listed in the Teaching for Self-Care box.

Pharmacologic treatment is usually based on the severity of withdrawal symptoms, as determined by an assessment tool (see Fig. 38-13). When indicated, medications are given as ordered. Neonatal tincture of opium (0.4 mg/ml of morphine equivalent), phenobarbital and, less commonly, paregoric may be used to control symptoms (Greene & Goodman, 2003). Treatment may be needed for 2 weeks or more.

Drug dependence in the neonate is physiologic, not psychologic. Thus a predisposition to dependence later in life is not believed to be a factor. However, the psychosocial

Text continued on p. 1020.

table 38-6	Signs of Neonatal Abstinence Syndrome
SYSTEM	**SIGNS**
Gastrointestinal	Poor feeding, vomiting, regurgitation, diarrhea, excessive sucking
Central nervous	Irritability, tremors, shrill cry, incessant crying, hyperactivity, little sleep, excoriations on knees and face, convulsions
Metabolic, vasomotor, respiratory	Nasal congestion; tachypnea; sweating; frequent yawning; increased respiratory rate, >60 breaths/min; fever, >37.2° C

TEACHING FOR SELF-CARE

Care of Infant Experiencing Withdrawal

- Place the infant in a side-lying position with the spine and legs flexed.
- Position the infant's hands in midline with the arms at the side.
- Carry the infant in a flexed position.
- When interacting with the infant, introduce one stimulus at a time when the infant is in a quiet, alert state.
- Watch for time-out or distress signals (gaze aversion, yawning, sneezing, hiccups, arching, mottled color).
- When the infant is distressed, swaddle in a flexed position and rock in a slow, rhythmic fashion.
- Put the infant in a sitting position with chin tucked down for feeding.

NEONATAL ABSTINENCE SCORING SYSTEM

SYSTEM	SIGNS AND SYMPTOMS	SCORE	AM							PM						COMMENTS
CENTRAL NERVOUS SYSTEM DISTURBANCES	Excessive High Pitched (Or other) Cry	2														Daily Weight:
	Continuous High Pitched (Or other) Cry	3														
	Sleeps <1 Hour After Feeding	3														
	Sleeps <2 Hours After Feeding	2														
	Sleeps <3 Hours After Feeding	1														
	Hyperactive Moro Reflex	2														
	Markedly Hyperactive Moro Reflex	3														
	Mild Tremors Disturbed	1														
	Moderate-Severe Tremors Disturbed	2														
	Mild Tremors Undisturbed	3														
	Moderate-Severe Tremors Undisturbed	4														
	Increased Muscle Tone	2														
	Excoriation (Specific Area)	1														
	Myoclonic Jerks	3														
	Generalized Convulsions	5														
METABOLIC/VASOMOTOR/RESPIRATORY DISTURBANCES	Sweating	1														
	Fever <101 (99°-100.8° F./37.2°-38.2° C.)	1														
	Fever >101 (38.4° C. and higher)	2														
	Frequent Yawning (>3-4 Times/Interval)	1														
	Mottling	1														
	Nasal Stuffiness	1														
	Sneezing (>3-4 Times/Interval)	1														
	Nasal Flaring	2														
	Respiratory Rate >60/min	1														
	Respiratory Rate >60/min with Retractions	2														
GASTROINTESTINAL DISTURBANCES	Excessive Sucking	1														
	Poor Feeding	2														
	Regurgitation	2														
	Projectile Vomiting	3														
	Loose Stools	2														
	Watery Stools	3														
	TOTAL SCORE															
	INITIALS OF SCORER															

FIG. 38-13 Neonatal abstinence scoring (NAS) system, developed by L. Finnegan. (From Nelson, N. [1990]. *Current therapy in neonatal-perinatal medicine* [2nd ed.]. St. Louis: Mosby.)

plan of care ▶ The Infant Undergoing Drug Withdrawal

NURSING DIAGNOSIS Risk for injury related to hyperactivity, seizures secondary to passive narcotic addiction resulting from maternal substance abuse during pregnancy

Expected Outcome *Infant exhibits no signs of seizure activity.*

Nursing Interventions/*Rationales*
- Administer phenobarbital, diazepam per physician order *to decrease central nervous system (CNS) irritability and control seizure activity.*
- Decrease environmental stimuli *that may trigger irritability and hyperactive behaviors.*
- Plan care activities carefully *to allow minimal stimulation.*
- Wrap infant snugly and hold infant tightly *to reduce self-stimulation behaviors and protect skin from abrasions.*
- If infant is cocaine addicted, position to avoid eye contact, swaddle infant, use vertical rocking techniques, and use a pacifier *to counter poor organizational response to stimuli and depressed interactive behaviors.*
- Monitor activity level, note the relation between activity level and external stimulation, and stop external stimulation *if it causes activity increase.*

NURSING DIAGNOSIS Imbalanced nutrition: less than body requirements related to CNS irritability, poor suck reflex, vomiting, and diarrhea

Expected Outcome *Infant exhibits ingestion and retention of adequate nutrients and appropriate weight gain.*

Nursing Interventions/*Rationales*
- Feed in frequent, small amounts, elevate head during and after feeding, and burp well *to diminish vomiting and aspiration.*
- Experiment with various nipples *to find one most effective in compensating for poor suck reflex.*
- Monitor weight daily, and maintain strict intake and output *to evaluate success of feeding.*
- If intake is insufficient, feed by oral gavage per physician order *to ensure ingestion of needed nutrients.*
- Have suction available as required *to reduce chances of aspiration.*

NURSING DIAGNOSIS Risk for deficient fluid volume related to diarrhea and vomiting

Expected Outcome *Infant exhibits evidence of fluid homeostasis.*

Nursing Interventions/*Rationales*
- Administer oral and parenteral fluids per physician order and regulate *to maintain fluid balance.*
- Monitor hydration status (skin turgor, weight, mucous membranes, fontanels, urine specific gravity, electrolytes) and intake and output *to evaluate for evidence of dehydration.*

NURSING DIAGNOSIS Ineffective maternal coping, anxiety, powerlessness related to drug use, infant distress during withdrawal

Expected Outcomes *Woman will accept newborn's condition and participate in care activities, showing evidence of maternal-infant bonding process.*

Nursing Interventions/*Rationales*
- Explain effects of maternal drug use on newborn and the withdrawal process *to provide understanding and reality concerning effects of drug use.*
- Encourage open communication (e.g., inform mother of ongoing condition, procedures, and treatment; answer questions; correct misperceptions; actively listen to her concerns) *to provide a sense of respect, provide support, and encourage a sense of control.*
- Encourage mother to interact with infant and to become involved in care routines *to foster emotional connection.*
- Explain how to do care procedures, how to avoid excess stimulation, and how to hold and rock infant *to enhance mother's care abilities and her sense of confidence and control.*
- If the mother is addicted to cocaine, explain infant's inability to interact, gaze aversion, arching back, and lack of response to cuddling *to enhance understanding of infant behaviors.*
- Make appropriate referrals to social agencies for treatment of maternal drug addiction, infant development programs, and other needed support services *to ensure adequate resources for care of self and infant.*

CD: Plan of Care: The Infant Undergoing Drug Withdrawal

---

table 38-7 **Drugs of Abuse Contraindicated During Breastfeeding***

DRUG	REASONS FOR CONCERN
Amphetamine†	Irritability, poor sleeping pattern
Cocaine	Cocaine intoxication
Heroin	Tremors, restlessness, vomiting, poor feeding
Marijuana	Only one report in literature; no effect mentioned; at risk for inhaling smoke, may reduce the protective effects of human milk against infection
Nicotine (smoking)	Shock, vomiting, diarrhea, rapid heart rate, restlessness, decreased milk production
Phencyclidine	Potent hallucinogen

Modified from American Academy of Pediatrics (AAP). (2001). The transfer of drugs and other chemicals into human milk. *Pediatrics, 108*(3), 776-789; Lawrence, R., & Lawrence, R. (2005). *Breastfeeding: A guide for the medical profession* (6th ed.). Philadelphia: Mosby.
*AAP Committee on Drugs strongly believes that breastfeeding mothers should not ingest any substances listed here. Not only are they hazardous to the nursing infant, but they also are detrimental to the physical and emotional health of the mother. This list is obviously not complete; no drug of abuse should be ingested by breastfeeding mothers even though adverse reports are not in the literature.
†Drug is concentrated in human milk.

environment in which the infant is raised may create a tendency to addiction.

The mother requires considerable support. Her need for and her abuse of drugs result in a decreased capacity to cope. The infant's withdrawal signs and decreased consolability stress her coping abilities even further. Home health care, treatment for addiction, and education are important considerations. Sensitive exploration of the woman's options for the care of her infant and herself and for future fertility management may help her see that she has choices. This approach helps communicate respect for the new mother as a person who can make responsible decisions.

The issue of breastfeeding in this population is a difficult one. Although breast milk remains the optimal source of nutrition for these infants, care must be taken to avoid exposing the infant to additional drugs through the breast milk. The American Academy of Pediatrics has compiled a list of drugs contraindicated in breastfeeding (Table 38-7).

---

community activity

Determine what programs are in place in your community to prevent fetal alcohol syndrome (FAS). What community resources exist to support children with FAS and their families? Find two websites that provide information about FAS. Who sponsors these websites, and how does the information on these sites compare to that in your textbook?

---

key points

- A small percentage of significant birth injuries may occur despite skilled and competent obstetric care.
- The same birth injury may be caused in several ways.
- The nurse's primary contribution to the welfare of the neonate begins with early observation, accurate recording, and prompt reporting of abnormal signs.
- Metabolic abnormalities of diabetes mellitus in pregnancy adversely affect embryonic and fetal development.
- Prepregnancy planning and good diabetic control, coupled with strict diabetic control during pregnancy, may prevent the embryonic, fetal, and neonatal conditions associated with pregnancies complicated by diabetes mellitus.
- Infection in the neonate may be acquired in utero, during birth, during resuscitation, and from within the nursery.
- The most common maternal infections during early pregnancy that are associated with various congenital malformations are caused by viruses.

- HIV transmission from mother to infant occurs transplacentally at various gestational ages, perinatally by maternal blood and secretions, and by breast milk.
- The nurse often is the first to observe signs of newborn drug withdrawal.
- Providing high-quality perinatal care to a varied population with multiple conditions is complicated by the special needs of high risk drug-dependent clients.
- Signs and symptoms of infant withdrawal vary in time of onset depending on the type and dose of drug involved.
- Rehabilitative measures must be included in the plan of care for the infant and parents to offer the infant an opportunity for optimal development after discharge.

REFERENCES

Alarcon, A., Pena, P., Salas, S., Sancha, M., & Omenaca, F. (2004). Neonatal early onset *Escherichia coli* sepsis: Trends in incidence and antimicrobial resistance in the era of intrapartum antimicrobial prophylaxis. *Pediatric Infectious Disease Journal, 23*(4), 295-299.

American Academy of Pediatrics Committee on Infectious Diseases. (2006). *Redbook: 2006 Report of the Committee on Infectious Diseases.* (27th ed.). Elk Grove Village, IL: AAP.

American Academy of Pediatrics (AAP) & American College of Obstetricians and Gynecologists (ACOG). (2005). Statement of reaffirmation. Human immunodeficiency virus infection in pregnancy. *Pediatrics, 116*(3), 796. (Original publication: *Pediatrics* [1999], *104*[1], 128).

Arvin, A., Whitley, R., & Gutierrez, K. (2006). Herpes simplex virus infections. In J. Remington, J. Klein, C. Wilson, & C. Baker (Eds.), *Infectious diseases of the fetus and newborn infant.* Philadelphia: Saunders.

Askin, D. (2004). Bacterial infections. In Askin, D. (Ed.), *Infections of the newborn.* Santa Rosa, CA: NICU INK Books.

Baley, J., & Toltzis, P. (2002). Viral infections. In R. Martin, A. Fanaroff, & M. Walsh (Eds.), *Fanaroff and Martin's neonatal-perinatal medicine: Diseases of the fetus and infant* (8th ed.). Philadelphia: Mosby.

Bandstra, E., & Accorneo, V. (2006). Infants of substance-abusing mothers. In R. Martin, A. Fanaroff, & M. Walsh (Eds.), *Fanaroff and Martin's neonatal-perinatal medicine: Diseases of the fetus and infant* (8th ed.). Philadelphia: Mosby.

Bortolussi, R., & Mailman, T. (2006). Listeriosis. In J. Remington, J. Klein, C. Baker, & C. Wilson (Eds.), *Infectious diseases of the fetus and newborn infant* (6th ed.). Philadelphia: Saunders.

Boyle, R. (2002). Effects of certain prenatal drugs on the fetus and newborn. *Pediatrics in Review, 23*(1), 17-24.

Bradley, J. (2006). Hepatitis. In J. Remington, J. Klein, C. Baker, & C. Wilson (Eds.), *Infectious diseases of the fetus and newborn infant.* Philadelphia: Saunders.

Brocklehurst, P., & Volmink, J. (2002). Antiretrovirals for reducing the risk of mother-to-child transmission of HIV infections. *The Cochrane Database of Systematic Reviews,* 2006, Issue 3. Chichester, UK: John Wiley & Sons.

Brown, Z., Wald, A., Morrow, R., Selke, S., Zeh, J., & Corey, L. (2003). Effect of serologic status and cesarean delivery on transmission rates of herpes simplex virus from mother to infant. *Journal of the American Medical Association, 289*(2), 203-209.

Capparelli, E., Rakhmanina, N., & Mirochnick, M. (2005). Pharmacotherapy of perinatal HIV. *Seminars in Fetal and Neonatal Medicine, 10*(2),161-175.

Centers for Disease Control and Prevention (CDC). (2004). Congenital syphilis—United States, 2002. *MMWR Morbidity and Mortality Weekly Report, 53*(31), 716-719.

Centers for Disease Control and Prevention (CDC), Workowski, K., & Berman, S. (2006). Sexually transmitted diseases treatment guidelines, 2006. *MMWR Morbidity and Mortality Weekly Report, Recommendations and Reports, 55*(RR-11), 1-94.

Chiriboga, C. (2003). Fetal alcohol and drug effects. *The Neurologist, 9*(6), 267-279.

Chou, R., Smits, A., Huffman, L., Korthuis, P., & U.S. Preventative Services Task Force. (2005). Prenatal screening for HIV: A review of the evidence for the U.S. Preventative Services Task Force. *Annals of Internal Medicine, 143*(1), 38-54.

Connor, E., Sperling, R., Gelber, R., Kiselev, P., Scott, G., O'Sullivan, M., et al. (1994). Reduction of maternal infant transmission of HIV-1 with zidovudine treatment. Pediatric AIDS Clinical Trials Group Protocol 076 Study Group. *New England Journal of Medicine, 331*(18), 1173-1180.

Cooper, L., & Alford, C. (2006). Rubella. In J. Remington, J. Klein, C. Baker, & C. Wilson (Eds.), *Infectious diseases of the fetus and newborn infant* (6th ed.). Philadelphia: Saunders.

Coutsoudis, A. (2005). Breastfeeding and HIV. *Best Practice and Research. Clinical Obstetrics and Gynaecology, 19*(2), 185-196.

Dahl, R., Scher, M., Williamson, D., Robles, N., & Day. N. (1995). A longitudinal study of prenatal marijuana use: Effects on sleep and arousal at age 3 years. *Archives of Pediatric and Adolescent Medicine, 149*(2), 145-150.

Darville, T. (2006). Chlamydia. In J. Remington, J. Klein, C. Baker, & C. Wilson (Eds.), *Infectious diseases of the fetus and newborn infant* (6th ed.). Philadelphia: Saunders.

Dunne, F., Brydon, P., Smith, K., & Gee, H. (2003). Pregnancy in women with type 2 diabetes: 12 years outcome data 1990-2002. *Diabetic Medicine, 20*(9), 734-738.

Edlich, R., Winters, K., Long, W., & Gubler, K. (2005). Rubella and congenital rubella (German measles). *Long Term Effects of Medical Implants, 15*(3), 319-328.

Edwards, M. (2006). Postnatal bacterial infections. In R. Martin, A. Fanaroff, & M. Walsh (Eds.), *Fanaroff and Martin's neonatal-perinatal medicine: Diseases of the fetus and infant* (8th ed.). Philadelphia: Mosby.

Edwards, M., Nizet, V., & Baker, C. (2006). Group B streptococcal infections. In J. Remington, J. Klein, C. Baker, & C. Wilson (Eds.), *Infectious diseases of the fetus and newborn infant* (6th ed.). Philadelphia: Saunders.

European Collaborative Study Group. (2003). Exposure to antiretroviral therapy in utero or early life: The health of uninfected children born to HIV-Infected women. *Journal of Acquired Immune Deficiency Syndrome, 32*(4), 380-387.

Evers, I., de Valk, H., & Visser, G. (2004). Risk of complications of pregnancy in women with type 1 diabetes: Nationwide prospective study in the Netherlands. *BMJ, 328*(7445), 915-918.

Eyler, F., Behnke, M., Wobie, K., Garvan, C., & Tebbett, I. (2005). Relative ability of biologic specimens and interviews to detect prenatal cocaine use. *Neurotoxicology & Teratology, 27*(4), 677-687.

Farrell, T., Neale, L., & Cundy, T. (2002). Congenital anomalies in the offspring of women with type 1, type 2, and gestational diabetes. *Diabetic Medicine, 19*(9), 322-326.

Fernandes, O., Sabharwal, M., Smiley, T., Pastuszak, A., Koren, G., & Einarson, T. (1998). Moderate to heavy caffeine consumption during pregnancy and relationship to spontaneous abortion and abnormal fetal growth: A meta-analysis. *Reproductive Toxicology, 12*(4), 435-444.

Foster, C., & Lyall, H. (2005). Current guidelines for the management of UK infants born to HIV-1 infected mothers. *Early Human Development, 81*(1), 103-110.

Gershon, A. (2006). Chickenpox, measles and mumps. In J. Remington, J. Klein, C. Baker, & C. Wilson (Eds.), *Infectious diseases of the fetus and newborn infant* (6th ed.). Philadelphia: Saunders.

Gillean, J., Coonrod, D., Russ, R., & Bay, C. (2005). Big infants in the neonatal intensive care unit. *American Journal of Obstetrics and Gynecology, 192*(6), 1948-1955.

Greene, C., & Goodman, M. (2003). Neonatal abstinence syndrome: Strategies for care of the drug-exposed infant. *Neonatal Network, 22*(4), 15-25.

Gudmundsson, S., Henningsson, A., & Lindqvist, P. (2005). Correlation of birth injury with maternal height and birthweight. *British Journal of Obstetrics and Gynaecology, 112*(6), 764-767.

Hockenberry, M. (2003). *Wong's nursing care of infants and children* (7th ed.). St. Louis: Mosby.

Hsu, T., Hung, F., Lu, Y., Ou, C., Roan, C., Kung, F., et al. (2002). Neonatal clavicular fracture: Clinical analysis of incidence, predisposing factors, diagnosis, and outcome. *American Journal of Perinatology, 19*(1), 17-21.

Hurd, Y., Wang, X., Anderson, V., Beck, O., Minkoff, H., & Dow-Edwards, D. (2005). Marijuana impairs growth in mid-gestation fetuses. *Neurotoxicology & Teratology, 27*(2), 221-229.

Ingall, D., Sanchez, P., & Baker, C. (2006). Syphilis. In J. Remington, J. Klein, C. Baker, & C. Wilson (Eds.), *Infectious diseases of the fetus and newborn infant* (6th ed.). Philadelphia: Saunders.

Jhawar, B., Ranger, A., Steven, D., & Del Maestro, R. (2003). Risk factors for intracranial hemorrhage among full-term infants: A case-control study. *Neurosurgery, 52*(3), 581-590.

Kalhan, S., & Parimi, P. (2006). Disorders of carbohydrate metabolism. In R. Martin, A. Fanaroff, & M. Walsh (Eds.), *Fanaroff and Martin's neonatal-perinatal medicine: Diseases of the fetus and infant* (8th ed.). Philadelphia: Mosby.

Kelly, L., Evans, L., & Messenger, D. (2005). Controversies around gestational diabetes. Practical information for family doctors. *Canadian Family Physician, 51*(May), 637-639, 644-646.

Kimberlin, D. (2005). Herpes simplex virus infections in neonates and early childhood. *Seminars in Pediatric Infectious Diseases, 16*(4), 271-281.

King, S., & Committee on Pediatric AIDS. (2004). Evaluation and treatment of the human immunodeficiency virus-1-exposed infant. *Pediatrics, 114*(2), 497-505.

Klein, J., Baker, C., Remington, J., & Wilson, C. (2006). Current concepts of infections of the fetus and newborn infant. In J. Remington, J. Klein, C. Baker, & C. Wilson (Eds.), *Infectious diseases of the fetus and newborn infant* (6th ed.). Philadelphia: Saunders.

Knight, S., & Washington, R. (2006). Cardiovascular disease and surgical interventions. In G. Merenstein, & S. Gardner (Eds.), *Handbook of neonatal intensive care* (6th ed.). St. Louis: Mosby.

Kwong, T., & Shearer, D. (1998). Detection of drug use during pregnancy. *Obstetrics and Gynecology Clinics of North America, 25*(1), 43-64.

Lam, M. (2002). Reappraisal of neonatal clavicular fracture. Relationship between infant size and risk factors. *Journal of Reproductive Medicine, 47*(11), 903-908.

Landon, M., Catalano, P., & Gabbe, S. (2002). In S. Gabbe, J. Niebyl, & J. Simpson (Eds.), *Obstetrics: Normal and problem pregnancies* (4th ed.). New York: Churchill Livingstone.

Langendoerfer, S., Johnson, J., & Thureen, P. (2005). Perinatal drug exposure. In P. Thureen, J. Deacon, J. Hernandez, & D. Hall (Eds.), *Assessment and care of the well newborn* (2nd ed.). St. Louis: Saunders.

Langer, O. (2002). Oral hypoglycemic agents in pregnancy: Their time has come. *Journal of Maternal Fetal, & Neonatal Medicine, 12*(6), 376-383.

Lindsay, C. (2006). Pregnancy complicated by diabetes mellitus. In R. Martin, A. Fanaroff, & M. Walsh (Eds.), *Fanaroff and Martin's neonatal-perinatal medicine: Diseases of the fetus and infant* (8th ed.). Philadelphia: Mosby.

Lombardi, G., & Stronati, M. (2005). Congenital cytomegalovirus infection. *Minerva Pediatrics, 57*(5), 213-27.

Lopez, A., Dietz, V., Wilson, M., Navin, T., & Jones, J. (2000). Preventing congenital toxoplasmosis. *MMWR Morbidity and Mortality Weekly Report, 49*(RR-2), 59-68.

Lupton, C., Burd, L., & Harwood, R. (2004). Cost of fetal alcohol spectrum disorder. *American Journal of Medical Genetics, Part C, Seminars in Medical Genetics, 127*(1), 42-50.

Maldonado, Y. (2006). Acquired immunodeficiency syndrome in the infant. In J. Remington, J. Klein, C. Baker, & C. Wilson (Eds.), *Infectious diseases of the fetus and newborn infant*. Philadelphia: Saunders.

Mangurten, H. (2006). Birth injuries. In R. Martin, A. Fanaroff, & M. Walsh (Eds.), *Fanaroff and Martin's neonatal-perinatal medicine: Diseases of the fetus and infant* (8th ed.). Philadelphia: Mosby.

Mardh, P. (2002). Influence of infection with *Chlamydia trachomatis* on pregnancy outcome, infant health and life-long sequelae in infected offspring. *Best Practice & Research Clinical Obstetrics and Gynaecology, 16*(6), 847-864.

Martin, S. (2001). Congenital toxoplasmosis. *Neonatal Network, 20*(4), 23-30.

Martin, J., Kochanek, K., Strobino, D., Guyer, B., & MacDorman, M. (2005). Annual summary of vital statistics—2003. *Pediatrics, 115*(3), 619-634.

Masson, E., Patmore, J., Brash, P., Baxter, M., Caldwell, G., Gallen, I., et al. (2003). Pregnancy outcome in type 1 diabetes mellitus treated with insulin lispro (Humalog). *Diabetic Medicine, 20*(1), 46-50.

Mollberg, M., Hagberg, H., Bager, B., Lilja, H., & Ladfors, L. (2005). High birthweight and shoulder dystocia: The strongest risk factors for obstetrical brachial plexus palsy in a Swedish population-based study. *Acta Obstetrica Gynecologica Scandinavica, 84*(7), 654-659.

Montoya, J., & Liesenfeld, O. (2004). Toxoplasmosis. *Lancet, 363* (9425), 1965-1976.

Montoya, J., & Rosso, F. (2005). Diagnosis and management of toxoplasmosis. *Clinics in Perinatology, 32*(3), 705-726.

Moodley, J., & Moodley, D. (2004). Management of human immunodeficiency virus infection in pregnancy. *Best Practice & Research Clinical Obstetrics and Gynaecology, 19*(2), 169-183.

Moore, T. (2002). A comparison of amniotic fluid fetal pulmonary phospholipids in normal and diabetic pregnancy. *American Journal of Obstetrics and Gynecology, 186*(4), 641-650.

National Institutes of Health (NIH) & Health Resources and Services Administration Working Group (HRSA WG) on Antiretroviral Therapy and Medical Management of HIV-Infected Children. (March 24, 2005). *Guidelines for the use of antiretroviral agents in pediatric HIV infection*. Accessed http://aidsinfo.nih.gov/guidelines, October 29, 2005.

Nielsen, G., Norgard, B., Puho, E., Rothman, K., Sorensen, H., & Czeizel, A. (2005). Risk of specific congenital abnormalities in offspring of women with diabetes. *Diabetic Medicine, 22*(6), 693-696.

Paige, P., & Moe, P. (2006). Neurologic disorders. In G. Merenstein, & S. Gardner (Eds.), *Handbook of neonatal intensive care* (6th ed.). St. Louis: Mosby.

Palazzi, D., Klein, J., & Baker, C. (2006). Bacterial sepsis and meningitis. In J. Remington, J. Klein, C. Baker, & C. Wilson (Eds.), *Infectious diseases of the fetus and newborn infant*. Philadelphia: Saunders.

Pass, R. (2005). Congenital cytomegalovirus infection and hearing loss. *Herpes, 12*(2), 50-55.

Pichini, S., Puig, C., Zuccaro, P., Marchei, E., Pellegrini, M., Murillo, J., et al. (2005). Assessment of exposure to opiates and cocaine during pregnancy in a Mediterranean city: Preliminary results of the "Meconium Project." *Forensic Science International, 153*(1), 59-65.

Piper, J. (2002). Lung maturation in diabetes in pregnancy: If and when to test. *Seminars in Perinatology, 26*(3), 206-209.

Platt, M., Stanisstreet, M., Casson, I., Howard, C., Walkinshaw, S., Pennycook, S., et al. (2003). St. Vincent's declaration 10 years on: Outcomes of diabetic pregnancies. *Diabetic Medicine, 20*(1), 8, 216-220.

Plessinger, M. (1998). Prenatal exposure to amphetamines. *Obstetrics and Gynecology Clinics of North America, 25*(1), 119-138.

Public Health Service Task Force (PHSTF). (2005). *Recommendations for use of antiretroviral in pregnant HIV-1-infected women for maternal health and interventions to reduce perinatal HIV-1 transmission in the United States*. Accessed www.hivatis.org/guidelines, October 26, 2005.

Read, J., & American Academy of Pediatrics Committee on Pediatric AIDS. (2003). Human milk, breastfeeding, and transmission of human immunodeficiency virus type 1 in the United States. *Pediatrics, 112*(5), 1196-1205.

Reed, M., Aranda, J., & Hales, B. (2006). Developmental pharmacology. In R. Martin, A. Fanaroff, & M. Walsh (Eds.), *Fanaroff and Martin's neonatal-perinatal medicine: Diseases of the fetus and infant* (8th ed.). Philadelphia: Mosby.

Reijneveld, S., Lanting, C., Crone, M., & VanWouwe, J. (2005). Exposure to tobacco smoke and infant crying. *Acta Paediatrica, 94*(2), 217-221.

Remington, J., McLeod, R., Thulliez, P., & Desmonts, G. (2006). Toxoplasmosis. In J. Remington, J. Klein, C. Baker, & C. Wilson (Eds.), *Infectious diseases of the fetus and newborn infant*. Philadelphia: Saunders.

Sabin, A. (1942). Toxoplasmosis: Recently recognized disease of human beings. V. Clinical manifestations of toxoplasmosis in man. *Advances in Pediatrics, 1*(1), 1-56.

Santos, I., Victora, C., Huttly, S., & Carvalhal, J. (1998). Caffeine intake and low birth weight: A population-based case-control study. *American Journal of Epidemiology, 147*(7), 620-627.

Schmidt, D., Hogh, B., Anderson, O., Hansen, S., Dalhoff, K., & Petersen, E. (2005). Treatment of infants with congenital toxoplasmosis: Tolerability and plasma concentrations of sulfadiazine and pyrimethamine. *European Journal of Pediatrics, 165*(1), 19-25.

Schrag, S., Gorwitz, R., Fultz-Butts, K., & Schuchat, A. (2002). Prevention of perinatal group B streptococcal disease. Revised guidelines from CDC. *MMWR Morbidity and Mortality Weekly Report Recommendations and Reports, 51*(RR-11), 1-22.

Shankaran, S., Das, A., Bauer, C., Bada, H., Lester, B., Wright, L., et al. (2004). Association between patterns of maternal substance use and infant birth weight, length, and head circumference. *Pediatrics, 114*(2), e226-e234.

Sheffield, J., Butler-Koster, E., Casey, B., McIntire, D., & Leveno, K. (2002). Maternal diabetes mellitus and infant malformations. *Obstetrics and Gynecology, 100*(5 Pt 1), 925-930.

Shenassa, E., & Brown, M. (2004). Maternal smoking and infantile gastrointestinal dysregulation: The case of colic. *Pediatrics, 114*(4), e497-e505.

Shinefield, H., & St. Geme, J. (2001). Staphylococcal infections. In J. Remington, J. Klein, C. Wilson, & C. Baker (Eds.), *Infectious diseases of the fetus and newborn infant* (6th ed.). Philadelphia: Saunders.

Stoll, B., & Kliegman, R. (2004). Metabolic disturbances. In R. Behrman, *Nelson textbook of pediatrics* (17th ed.). Philadelphia: Saunders.

Tan, M., & Koren, G. (2006). Chickenpox in pregnancy: Revisited. *Reproductive Toxicology, 21*(4), 410-420.

Thigpen, J., & Kenner, K. (2003). Assessment and management of gastrointestinal dysfunction. In C. Kenner, & J. Lott (Eds.), *Comprehensive neonatal nursing* (3rd ed.). Philadelphia: Saunders.

Thorne, C., & Newell, M. (2005). Treatment options for the prevention of mother-to-child transmission of HIV. *Current Opinion Investigative Drugs, 6*(8), 804-811.

Uchil, D., & Arulkumaran, S. (2003). Neonatal subgaleal hemorrhage and its relationship to delivery by vacuum extraction. *Obstetric and Gynecologic Survey, 58*(10), 687-693.

Uhing, M. (2004). Management of birth injuries. *Pediatric Clinics of North America, 51*(4), 1169-1186.

U.S. Department of Health and Human Services. (2005). *Safety and toxicity of individual antiretroviral agents in pregnancy.* Accessed http://aidsinfo.nih.gov/guidelines/default_db2.asp?id=66, October 29, 2005.

Venkatesh, M., Merenstein, G., Adams, K., & Weisman, L. (2006). Infection in the neonate. In G. Merenstein & S. Gardner (Eds.), *Handbook of neonatal intensive care* (6th ed.). St. Louis: Mosby.

Vergnano, S., Sharland, M., Kazembe, P., Mwansambo, C., & Heath, P. (2005). Neonatal sepsis: An international perspective. *Archives of Disease in Childhood Fetal and Neonatal Edition, 90*(3), F220-F224.

Wagner, C., Katikaneni, L., Cox, T., & Ryan, R. (1998). The impact of prenatal drug exposure on the neonate. *Obstetrics and Gynecology Clinics of North America, 25*(1), 169-194.

Walkinshaw, S. (2005). Pregnancy in women with pre-existing diabetes: Management issues. *Seminars in Fetal & Neonatal Medicine, 10*(4), 307-315.

Watson, D., Rowan, J., Neale, L., & Battin, M. (2003). Admissions to neonatal intensive care unit following pregnancies complicated by gestational or type 2 diabetes. *Australia, New Zealand Journal of Obstetrics & Gynaecology, 43*(6), 429-432.

Weiner, Z., Ben-Shlomo, I., Beck-Fruchter, R., Goldberg, Y., & Shalev, E. (2002). Clinical and ultrasonographic weight estimation in large for gestational age fetus. *European Journal of Obstetrics, Gynecology and Reproductive Biology, 105*(1), 20-24.

Welch-Carre, E. (2005). The neurodevelopmental consequences of prenatal alcohol exposure. *Advances in Neonatal Care, 5*(4), 217-229.

Wiysonge, C., Shey, M., Shang, J., Sterne, J., Brocklehurst, P., & Wiysonge, C. (2005). Vaginal disinfection for preventing mother-to-child transmission of HIV infection. *The Cochrane Database of Systematic Reviews,* 2006, Issue 3. Chichester, UK: John Wiley & Sons.

Woods, C. (2005). Syphilis in children: Congenital and acquired. *Seminars in Pediatric Infectious Diseases, 16*(4), 245-257.

Wyatt, J., Frias, J., Hoyme, H., Jovanovic, L., Kaaja, R., Brown, F., et al. (2005). Congenital anomaly rate in offspring of mothers with diabetes treated with insulin lispro during pregnancy. *Diabetic Medicine, 22*(6), 803-807.

Yudin, M., & Gonik, B. (2006). Perinatal infections. In R. Martin, A. Fanaroff, & M. Walsh (Eds.), *Fanaroff and Martin's neonatal-perinatal medicine: Diseases of the fetus and infant* (8th ed.). Philadelphia: Mosby.

Zanardo, V., Nicolussi, S., Cavallin, S., Trevisanuto, D., Barbato, A., Faggian, D., et al. (2005). Effect of maternal smoking on breast milk interleukin-1 alpha, beta-endorphin, and leptin concentrations. *Environmental Health Perspectives, 113*(10), 1410-1413.

Hemolytic Disorders and Congenital Anomalies

learning objectives

- Discuss assessment of the newborn for hyperbilirubinemia.
- Develop a nursing plan of care for the prevention, identification, and management of hyperbilirubinemia in a newborn.
- Compare Rh and ABO incompatibility.
- Explain nursing management to prevent the pathologic consequences of hyperbilirubinemia.
- Review prenatal diagnosis of neonatal disorders.

- Present assessment strategies during the postnatal period to aid in diagnosis of congenital disorders.
- Describe each congenital disorder presented in this chapter and identify the priority of nursing care for each.
- Describe preoperative and postoperative nursing care of the newborn.
- Develop a nursing plan of care for parents of a newborn with a defect or disorder.

electronic resources

Additional information related to the content in Chapter 39 can be found on

the companion website at *evolve*
http://evolve.elsevier.com/Lowdermilk/MWHC/
- NCLEX Review Questions
- WebLinks

or on the interactive companion CD
- NCLEX Review Questions
- Plan of Care: The Infant with Hyperbilirubinemia

THERE are many physiologic alterations that occur in infants during the newborn period. The nurse must be alert to the presence of any deviations from normal, ranging from an obvious congenital anomaly, such as myelomeningocele, to a less obvious deviation such as a congenital heart defect that may not be symptomatic at birth. The nurse must possess the assessment skills necessary to detect any deviation from normal, as well as the knowledge base necessary to participate in the skilled care needed for affected infants. The nurse also must be cognizant of the special needs of the family with a child who is born with or acquires an abnormal condition.

The complications that affect newborns can stem from three basic problems: problems relating to gestational age or intrauterine growth that does not follow normal patterns, such as a preterm birth; acquired problems resulting from maternal or newborn physiologic factors, such as ABO incompatibility or respiratory distress syndrome; and physical problems, such as congenital anomalies or birth defects.

■ HYPERBILIRUBINEMIA

In hyperbilirubinemia, the bilirubin level in the blood is increased. It is characterized by a yellow discoloration of the skin, mucous membranes, sclera, and various organs. This yellow discoloration is referred to as jaundice, or *icterus*. Jaundice is caused primarily by the accumulation in the skin of unconjugated bilirubin, a breakdown product of hemoglobin formed after its release from hemolyzed red blood cells (RBCs). Physiologic jaundice, discussed in Chapters 25 and 26, is the most common abnormal finding in newborns and is usually benign. The challenge in the care of neonates with hyperbilirubinemia is to distinguish physiologic jaundice from a serious clinical pathologic condition.

Physiologic Jaundice

Physiologic jaundice occurs in about half of all healthy term newborns and in 80% of preterm infants (Wong, DeSandre, Sibley, & Stevenson, 2006). It typically arises more than 24 hours after birth. In both Caucasian and African-American infants, it is manifested by a progressive increase in the unconjugated bilirubin level in cord blood from 2 mg/dl to a mean peak of 5 to 6 mg/dl between 60 and 72 hours of age. In Asian and Native-American infants, the level may increase to 10 to 14 mg/dl between 72 and 120 hours of age. Resolution in Caucasian and African-American newborns is evidenced by a rapid decline in the unconjugated bilirubin level to 2 mg/dl by 5 days after birth; in Asian and Native-American infants, this takes 7 to 10 days.

Physiologic jaundice is more common and severe in preterm infants, in whom the serum bilirubin level typically reaches a mean peak of 10 to 12 mg/dl by the fifth day of life. It takes longer for the maximal concentration to be reached in preterm than in full-term infants because the livers of preterm infants are immature, therefore liver function is not fully developed.

Pathologic Jaundice

Pathologic jaundice, or hyperbilirubinemia, is the level of serum bilirubin that, if left untreated, can result in acute bilirubin encephalopathy, which describes the clinical central nervous system findings caused by bilirubin toxicity to the basal ganglia and brainstem nuclei. Bilirubin encephalopathy is used to describe the acute manifestations seen in the first weeks after birth, while the term "kernicterus" is used to describe the chronic and permanent results of bilirubin toxicity (American Academy of Pediatrics [AAP], Subcommittee on Hyperbilirubinemia, 2004). Kernicterus, though rare, still occurs. Adherence to guidelines recently released by the American Academy of Pediatrics (AAP) and followed by a clinical position statement by the Association of Women's Health, Obstetric and Neonatal Nurses (AWHONN, 2005) should result in kernicterus becoming largely preventable. The following findings support a diagnosis of pathologic jaundice and, if encountered in an infant, warrant further investigation (Wong et al., 2006):

* Serum bilirubin concentrations of greater than 4 mg/dl in cord blood
* Clinical jaundice evident within 24 hours of birth
* Total serum bilirubin levels increasing by more than 5 mg/dl in 24 hours or increasing at a rate of 0.5 mg/dl or more over a 4- to 8-hour period
* A serum bilirubin level in a term newborn that exceeds 15 mg/dl at any time or clinical jaundice lasting more than 10 days
* A serum bilirubin level in a preterm newborn that exceeds 10 mg/dl at any time
* Any case of visible jaundice that persists for more than 10 days of life in a term infant or 21 days in a preterm infant, unless the infant is receiving breast milk

AAP guidelines (2004) and the clinical position statement by AWHONN (2005) note the need for universal screening to identify elevated bilirubin level in newborns to facilitate the prevention of acute bilirubin encephalopathy and kernicterus (AWHONN). The use of hour-specific serum bilirubin levels to predict newborns at risk for rapidly

rising levels is an official recommendation by the AAP Subcommittee on Hyperbilirubinemia (2004), for the monitoring of healthy neonates at 35 weeks of gestation or greater before discharge from the hospital. Use of a nomogram helps determine which newborns might need further evaluation after discharge. In many institutions the nomogram is used to determine the infant's risk for development of hyperbilirubinemia requiring medical treatment or closer screening (see Fig. 26-7). Risk factors recognized to place infants in the high risk category include gestational age less than 38 weeks, breastfeeding, previous sibling with significant jaundice, and jaundice appearing before discharge. It is now recommended that healthy infants (35 weeks of gestation or greater) receive follow-up care and assessment of bilirubin within 3 days of discharge if discharged at less than 24 hours and a risk assessment with tools such as the hour-specific nomogram; likewise, newborns discharged at 24 to 47.9 hours should receive follow-up evaluation within 4 days (96 hours), and those discharged between 48 and 72 hours should receive follow-up within 5 days (AAP Subcommittee on Hyperbilirubinemia). Other key elements of the recommendations of the AAP subcommittee include promoting successful breastfeeding; recognizing that visual estimation of the degree of jaundice, particularly in darkly pigmented infants, can lead to errors; and providing parents with written and verbal information about newborn jaundice.

Many potential causes of pathologic hyperbilirubinemia are found in neonates (Box 39-1). The most common are hemolytic disorders of the newborn.

Hemolytic Disease of the Newborn

Hemolytic diseases of the newborn occur most often if the blood groups of the mother and baby are different. The most common are ABO and Rh factor incompatibilities.

box 39-1 Potential Causes of Pathologic Hyperbilirubinemia in Neonates

MATERNAL FACTORS
* Rh and ABO incompatibility
* Maternal infections
* Maternal diabetes
* Oxytocin administration during labor
* Maternal ingestion of sulfonamides, diazepam, or salicylates near time of birth

FETAL/NEWBORN FACTORS
* Prematurity
* Hepatic cell damage by infection or drugs
* Neonatal hyperthyroidism
* Polycythemia
* Intestinal obstruction such as meconium ileus
* Pyloric stenosis
* Biliary atresia
* Sequestered blood (e.g., from cephalhematomas, ecchymosis, or hemangiomas)
* Maternal blood swallowed by neonate

The four major blood groups in the ABO system are A, B, AB, and O. People with type A blood have A antigen; those with type B have B antigen; those with type AB have both A and B antigens; and those with type O have no antigen. In turn, people with type A blood have plasma antibodies to type B blood; those with type B blood have antibodies to type A blood; those with type AB blood have no antibodies; and those with type O blood have antibodies to types A and B blood. If a person is administered or exposed to an incompatible blood type, he or she will form antibodies against the antigen in that blood, with an agglutination, or clumping, occurring as the antibodies in the plasma mix with the antigens of the different blood group.

The Rh factor, a genetically determined factor present on RBCs, can be a major source of incompatibility. Of the several forms of the Rh antigen, the D antigen is the most significant because it causes the most antibody production in a person who is Rh negative. Rh positivity is a dominant trait, so one must inherit the recessive gene from both parents to be Rh negative. A person who has the Rh factor is considered Rh positive; a person without it is considered Rh negative. For example, a mother who has A-negative blood has the A antigen, plasma antibodies to the B antigen, and no Rh factor on her RBCs.

Hemolytic disorders occur when maternal antibodies are present naturally or form in response to an antigen from the fetal blood crossing the placenta and entering the maternal circulation. The maternal antibodies of the immunoglobulin G (IgG) class in turn cross the placenta, causing hemolysis of the fetal RBCs, resulting in hyperbilirubinemia and jaundice.

Rh Incompatibility

Rh incompatibility, or isoimmunization, occurs when an Rh-negative mother has an Rh-positive fetus who inherits the dominant Rh-positive gene from the father. If the mother is Rh negative and the father is Rh positive and homozygous for the Rh factor, all the offspring will be Rh positive. If the father is heterozygous for the factor, there is a 50% chance that each infant born of the union will be Rh positive and a 50% chance that each will be born Rh negative (see Fig. 3-3 on p. 62. An Rh-negative fetus is in no danger because it has the same Rh factor as the mother. An Rh-negative fetus with an Rh-positive mother also is in no danger. Only the Rh-positive fetus of an Rh-negative mother is at risk. From 10% to 15% of all Caucasian couples and about 5% of African-American couples have Rh incompatibility. It is rare in Asian couples.

The incidence of Rh sensitization and resulting hemolytic disease of the newborn has decreased dramatically since the development of $Rh_o(D)$ immune globulin in 1968. New treatment modalities, including early detection and fetal blood transfusions, have improved the outcome of affected fetuses. However, despite continuing research and advances in management modalities, a 1% isoimmunization rate is found among women who are Rh negative, and it continues to be a major factor in fetal and neonatal morbidity and mortality.

The pathogenesis of Rh incompatibility is as follows. Hematopoiesis in the fetus, or the formation of blood cells, begins as early as the eighth week of gestation and, in up to 40% of pregnancies, these cells pass through the placenta into the maternal circulation. If the fetus is Rh positive and the mother Rh negative, the mother forms antibodies against the fetal blood cells—first IgM antibodies that are too large to pass through the placenta, and then later, IgG antibodies that can cross the placenta. The process of antibody formation is called *maternal sensitization.* Sensitization may occur during pregnancy, birth, miscarriage or induced abortion, amniocentesis, external cephalic version, or trauma. Usually women become sensitized in their first pregnancy with an Rh-positive fetus but do not produce enough antibodies to cause lysis (destruction) of fetal blood cells. During subsequent pregnancies, antibodies form in response to repeated contact with the antigen from the fetal blood, and lysis of fetal RBCs results. In approximately 10% to 15% of sensitized mothers, there is no hemolytic reaction in the newborn. In addition, some Rh-negative women, even though exposed to Rh-positive fetal blood, are immunologically unable to produce antibodies to the foreign antigen.

Severe Rh incompatibility results in marked fetal hemolytic anemia, because the fetal erythrocytes are destroyed by maternal Rh-positive antibodies. Although the placenta usually clears the bilirubin resulting from the RBC breakdown, in extreme cases, fetal bilirubin levels increase. This results in fetal jaundice, also known as *icterus gravis.*

The fetus compensates for the anemia by producing large numbers of immature erythrocytes to replace those hemolyzed, thus the name for this condition: erythroblastosis fetalis. In hydrops fetalis, the most severe form of this disease, the fetus has marked anemia, cardiac decompensation, cardiomegaly, and hepatosplenomegaly. Hypoxia results from the severe anemia. In addition, because of the decreased intravascular oncotic pressure involved, fluid leaks out of the intravascular space. This results in generalized edema, as well as effusions into the peritoneal (ascites), pericardial, and pleural (hydrothorax) spaces. The placenta is often edematous, which, along with the edematous fetus, can cause the uterus to rupture.

Intrauterine or early neonatal death may occur as a result of hydrops fetalis, although intrauterine transfusions and early birth of the fetus may avert this. Intrauterine transfusion involves the infusion of Rh-negative, type O blood into the umbilical vein. The frequency of intrauterine transfusions may vary according to institution and fetal hydropic status, but it may be as often as every 2 weeks until the fetus reaches pulmonary maturity at approximately 37 to 38 weeks of gestation. Studies of the use of intrauterine transfusions have demonstrated a high survival rate and low risk of disabilities in the surviving infant (Harkness & Spinnato, 2004).

ABO Incompatibility

ABO incompatibility is more common than Rh incompatibility but causes less severe problems in the affected infant. It occurs if the fetal blood type is A, B, or AB, and the maternal type is O. It occurs rarely in infants with type B blood born to mothers with type A blood. The incompatibility arises because naturally occurring anti-A and anti-B antibodies are transferred across the placenta to the fetus. Unlike the situation that pertains to Rh incompatibility, firstborn infants may be affected because mothers with type O blood already have anti-A and anti-B antibodies in their blood. Such a newborn may have a weakly positive direct Coombs' test (also referred to as a direct antiglobulin test [DAT]). The cord bilirubin level usually is less than 4 mg/dl, and any resulting hyperbilirubinemia usually can be treated with phototherapy. Exchange transfusions are required only occasionally. Although ABO incompatibility is a common cause of hyperbilirubinemia, it rarely precipitates significant anemia resulting from the hemolysis of RBCs.

It is not within the scope of this text to discuss the many potential causes of hemolytic jaundice in childhood. However, in some populations there is a high incidence of glucose-6-phosphate dehydrogenase deficiency (G6PD), which may cause an exaggerated jaundice in a newborn within 24 to 48 hours of birth. G6PD red cells hemolyze at a greater rate than healthy red cells, thus overwhelming the immature neonatal liver's ability to conjugate the indirect bilirubin. Some of the triggers that potentiate hemolysis include vitamin K, acetaminophen, aspirin, sepsis, and exposure to certain chemicals (Reiser, 2004). Treatment is the same as for any newborn with rapidly rising serum bilirubin levels. Other metabolic and inherited conditions that increase hemolysis and may cause jaundice in the infant include galactosemia, Criglar-Najjar disease, and hypothyroidism.

Acute Bilirubin Encephalopathy

The goal of the care given the infant with hyperbilirubinemia is the prevention of acute bilirubin encephalopathy, which is caused by the deposition of bilirubin in the brain, especially within the basal ganglia, the cerebellum, and the hippocampus. This deposition can occur because unconjugated bilirubin is highly lipid soluble, making it capable of crossing the blood-brain barrier if it is not bound to protein. If the concentration of unconjugated bilirubin reaches toxic levels, it results in the yellowish staining of the brain tissue and the necrosis of neurons. Acute bilirubin encephalopathy, which can develop in newborns who show no apparent signs of clinical jaundice, is generally considered to be directly related to the total serum bilirubin level, although these levels alone do not predict the risk of brain injury. In a term infant, a serum bilirubin level of 25 mg/dl is considered the upper limit, beyond which the risk for acute bilirubin encephalopathy increases, although the condition may occur at much lower levels in premature infants or infants with other complications. In some high risk, low-birth-weight infants, a mean peak level of unconjugated bilirubin of even 10 to 12 mg/dl may be associated with the development of acute bilirubin encephalopathy (Juretschke, 2005). Some of the perinatal events that increase the likelihood of acute bilirubin encephalopathy developing, even at these lower bilirubin levels, include hypoxia, asphyxia, acidosis, hypothermia, hypoglycemia, sepsis, treatment with certain medications, and hypoalbuminemia. These conditions interfere with the conjugation of bilirubin or compete for albumin-binding sites. The resulting unconjugated bilirubin can pass through the blood-brain barrier and enter the brain, resulting in acute bilirubin encephalopathy.

Acute bilirubin encephalopathy has been associated with acute and long-term symptoms of neurologic damage; it is never present at birth. The clinical manifestations typically appear between 2 and 6 days after birth and go through several phases as the disease progresses, generally beginning after the bilirubin level has peaked. During the first phase, the newborn is hypotonic and lethargic and shows a poor suck and depressed or absent Moro reflex. These more subtle signs are followed by the appearance of a high-pitched cry, opisthotonos (severe muscle spasm that causes the back to arch acutely), spasticity, hyperreflexia, and often by fever and seizures. All of this occurs over a period of about 24 hours. About half of the affected infants survive, although they often have permanent sequelae including extrapyramidal movement disorders (especially dystonia and athetosis), gaze abnormalities (especially an upward gaze), auditory disturbances (especially sensorineural hearing loss), intellectual deficits (rarely in the mentally retarded range), and enamel dysplasia of the deciduous teeth. Movement abnormalities and auditory disturbances are almost always present.

Kernicterus is used to describe the chronic and permanent results of bilirubin toxicity. The minimal requirement for a diagnosis of kernicteric sequelae is an abnormality in two or more of the five categories described above, with the impairment in at least one area being severe enough to necessitate ongoing specialized therapy and assistance with skills of living (Juretschke, 2005).

■ CARE MANAGEMENT

■ Assessment and Nursing Diagnoses

It is important to determine the blood type and Rh factor of the pregnant woman prenatally. A thorough history must then be obtained in the Rh-negative pregnant woman to assess for the existence of events that could have caused her to develop antibodies to the Rh factor. Such events include (1) previous pregnancy with an Rh-positive fetus; (2) transfusion with Rh-positive blood, which causes immediate sensitization; (3) miscarriage or induced abortion after 8 or more weeks of gestation; (4) amniocentesis performed for any reason; (5) premature separation of the placenta; and (6) trauma.

Because hematopoiesis begins in the fetus during the eighth gestational week, a woman who has had a miscarriage or induced abortion after this time or has previously given birth to a child may have been inoculated with fetal blood at the time of placental separation. During amniocentesis, the needle may cause localized damage to the single layer of cells that separates the maternal and fetal circulation in the placenta, thereby allowing fetal RBCs to enter the maternal circulation.

If any of these events has occurred, the woman's record is checked to determine whether she has received $Rh_o(D)$ immune globulin, such as RhoGAM, which is a commercial preparation of passive antibodies against the Rh factor (see Medication Guide, p. 604). This injection of anti-Rh antibodies destroys any fetal RBCs in the maternal circulation by causing the cells to be phagocytosed before the woman's immune system is activated to produce antibodies.

At the first prenatal visit of an Rh-negative woman with a fetus who may be Rh positive, an indirect Coombs' test should be done to determine whether she has antibodies to the Rh antigen. In this test, the maternal blood serum is mixed with Rh-positive erythrocytes (RBCs). If the Rh-positive RBCs agglutinate or clump, this indicates that maternal antibodies are present or that the mother has been sensitized. The dilution of the specimen of blood at which clumping occurs determines the titer, or level, of maternal antibodies. This titer indicates the degree of maternal sensitization. A level of 1:8 rarely results in fetal jeopardy. If the titer reaches 1:16, amniocentesis is performed to determine optical density (ΔOD) of amniotic fluid to estimate fetal hemolytic process (see Chapter 29). Rising bilirubin levels may indicate the need for an intrauterine transfusion. Genetic testing allows early identification of paternal zygosity at the RhD gene locus, thus allowing earlier detection of the potential for isoimmunization and precluding further maternal or fetal testing (Harkness & Spinnato, 2004).

The indirect Coombs' test is repeated at 28 weeks. If the result remains negative, indicating that sensitization has not occurred, the woman is given an intramuscular injection of $Rh_o(D)$ immune globulin. If the test result is positive, showing that sensitization has occurred, it is then repeated every 4 to 6 weeks to monitor the maternal antibody titer as just described. Examples of nursing diagnoses pertinent to newborns at risk because of hyperbilirubinemia include the following:

- *Risk for injury to neurons and cells in the kidney, pancreas, and intestine related to*
  –hyperbilirubinemia
- *Impaired gas exchange related to*
  –hemolytic anemia
- *Risk for deficient fluid volume related to*
  –phototherapy
- *(Parental) anxiety related to*
  –hyperbilirubinemia, its management, and potential sequelae
- *Risk for impaired skin integrity related to*
  –increased stooling while undergoing phototherapy
- *Ineffective thermoregulation (increased or decreased) related to*
  –phototherapy

▬ Expected Outcomes of Care

Hospital protocols for the care of infants with hyperbilirubinemia are developed as a collaborative effort of the health care team. These protocols are then used to individualize care for the infant and parents. Expected outcomes for care are stated in client-centered terms, as in the following:
- The infant's prenatal and perinatal risk factors will be identified, and intervention will be implemented when appropriate.
- The infant will not develop hyperbilirubinemia or its sequela, kernicterus.
- The infant will have minimal or no sequelae from hyperbilirubinemia and its treatment.
- The infant's serum bilirubin levels will return to normal.
- The infant's parents will demonstrate an understanding of the infant's condition, the therapies, and the possible sequelae of the condition.

▬ Plan of Care and Interventions

Prevention of hyperbilirubinemia is the primary prenatal focus of care. The implementation of interventions focused on the care of the woman whose fetus is considered at risk for hyperbilirubinemia is essential to prevent problems in the newborn. Prenatal control of diabetes mellitus, prevention of maternal infection, avoidance of drugs such as diazepam and salicylates near the time of birth, and prevention of preterm birth reduce the risk.

Early identification of the Rh-negative woman must occur, and care must be taken to prevent sensitization. The Rh-negative woman should be asked about any blood transfusion or any of the other factors already cited that would predispose her to sensitization. $Rh_o(D)$ immune globulin is administered to Rh-negative women whose Coombs' tests are negative (Wong et al., 2006) (Box 39-2).

---

box 39-2 Indications for Amount of $Rh_o(D)$ Immune Globulin to Be Administered

50 mcg
- After chorionic villus sampling, ectopic pregnancy, miscarriage, or abortion before 13 weeks of gestation

300 mcg
- After any of the following events:
  –Miscarriage or elective abortion after 13 weeks of gestation
  –Percutaneous umbilical blood sampling
- Amniocentesis
- Abruptio placentae or placenta previa
- Trauma
- At 28 weeks of gestation
- Within 72 hours of the preterm or term birth of an Rh-positive infant

MORE THAN 300 mcg
- After a large transplacental hemorrhage
- After a mismatched blood transfusion

The fetus and maternal antibody titers are monitored prenatally. Several methods are used to detect fetal anemia; amniocentesis to measure ΔOD 450, percutaneous umbilical blood sampling (PUBS) or cordocentesis, and middle cerebral artery peak systolic velocity (MCA-PSV). Although ultrasound-guided cordocentesis is the gold standard for detecting fetal anemia, MCA-PSV is receiving the most attention as it is a noninvasive means to detect fetal anemia (Harkness & Spinnato, 2004; Shaver, 2004).

If amniocentesis reveals that the ΔOD is high and the fetus is in jeopardy, intrauterine transfusion may be done every 1 to 2 weeks between 26 and 32 weeks. If the endangered fetus is at more than 32 weeks of gestation, a preterm birth may be indicated, usually by cesarean.

Postpartum interventions focus on preventing sensitization in the mother, if it has not occurred already, and treating any complications in the neonate resulting from the hemolysis of RBCs (see Plan of Care). The unsensitized Rh-negative mother whose baby is Rh positive should receive 300 mcg of $Rh_o(D)$ immune globulin within 72 hours of birth. This should prevent her from producing antibodies to the fetal blood cells that entered her bloodstream during the birth.

At birth, the neonate's cord blood is sent to the laboratory to determine the infant's blood type and Rh status. A direct Coombs' test is performed on this cord blood to determine whether there are maternal antibodies in the fetal blood. If antibodies are present, the titer, indicating the degree of maternal sensitization, is measured. If the titer is 1:64, an exchange transfusion is indicated. In addition, the prevention of or prompt therapy for perinatal asphyxia, acidosis, cold stress, sepsis, and hypoglycemia will decrease the newborn's risk for severe hemolytic disease and the susceptibility to kernicterus. Early feeding is initiated to stimulate stooling and thus facilitate the removal of bilirubin.

If pathologic jaundice is present, the cause is determined, and therapeutic management is begun. Phototherapy is used to reduce rapidly increasing serum bilirubin levels. See Chapter 26 for a discussion of phototherapy.

Exchange transfusions are needed infrequently because of the decrease in the incidence of hemolytic disease in newborns resulting from isoimmunization. Other factors must always be considered as well, particularly the clinical condition of the infant, because it is a procedure with potential complications. Guidelines for the initiation of exchange transfusion in relation to serum bilirubin levels in infants of >35 weeks of gestation may be found in the 2004 AAP Clinical Practice Guideline (AAP Subcommittee on Hyperbilirubinemia, 2004). Exchange transfusion is accomplished by alternately removing a small amount of the infant's blood and replacing it with an equal amount of donor blood. Exchange transfusion replaces the RBCs that would otherwise be hemolyzed by circulating maternal antibodies, removes the antibodies responsible for hemolysis, and corrects the anemia caused by hemolysis of the infant's sensitized RBCs. It also reduces the serum bilirubin level in infants who have severe hyperbilirubinemia from any cause. If the infant has Rh incompatibility,

type O Rh-negative blood is used for transfusion, so the maternal antibodies still present in the infant do not hemolyze the transfused blood. Depending on the infant's size, maturity, and condition, amounts of 5 to 20 ml of the infant's blood are removed at one time and replaced with donor blood. The total amount of blood exchanged approximates 170 ml/kg of body weight, or 75% to 85% of the infant's total blood volume. The amount exchanged is limited to 500 ml. During the procedure, the health care team members observe the infection control precautions for invasive procedures.

The infant is monitored closely during and after the procedure, including the heart rate and rhythm, respirations, blood pressure, temperature, pedal pulses, and the presence of edema. Preservatives in donor blood lower the infant's serum calcium level; therefore, calcium gluconate is often given during the exchange transfusion. Symptoms of hypocalcemia include jitteriness, irritability, convulsions, tachycardia, and electrocardiogram changes. The neonate is monitored closely for signs of a blood transfusion reaction as well as hypotension, hypervolemia, temperature instability, and cardiorespiratory compromise.

Planning for rehabilitative measures is necessary if kernicterus occurs. The family will need the services of many community resources to care for the affected child. An interdisciplinary approach that includes social services must be taken (Box 39-3).

■ Evaluation

On a short-term basis, the nurse can consider nursing care to be effective to the degree that the previously described outcomes for care are achieved.

■ CONGENITAL ANOMALIES

The desired and expected outcome of every wanted pregnancy is a normal, functioning infant with a good intellectual potential. Fulfillment of this hope depends on numerous hereditary and environmental factors. Probably all human characteristics have a genetic component, including those that produce symptoms or physical abnormalities that impair the fitness of the person. Some disorders or diseases occur through the influence of a single gene or the combined action of many genes

---

box 39-3 | Monitoring for Jaundice After Early Discharge

If the infant is discharged from the hospital before 48 hours of age, the parents should receive teaching regarding adequate hydration and assessment of the infant for the appearance of jaundice. Appropriate testing and follow-up of the infant should be available. A program of home phototherapy, where available, allows infants to receive treatment of uncomplicated hyperbilirubinemia after discharge from the hospital. For these infants, nurses provide monitoring of treatment and of serum bilirubin levels as outlined by hospital or agency policy.

| plan of care | The Infant with Hyperbilirubinemia |

NURSING DIAGNOSIS Risk for injury related to hemolytic disease and treatment effects

Expected Outcomes *Bilirubin levels decrease with treatment; no evidence exists of harmful effects from phototherapy (e.g., no eye irritation, dehydration, temperature instability, or skin breakdown); and no complications occur from exchange transfusions.*

Nursing Interventions/*Rationales*
- Initiate early feedings *to enhance excretion of bilirubin in stools.*
- Observe skin and mucous membranes for signs of jaundice, indicative of increasing bilirubin levels; monitor serum bilirubin levels *to determine rate of increase and treatment response.*
- Note time of jaundice onset *to help distinguish physiologic from other causes of jaundice.*
- Observe for signs of hypoxia, hypothermia, hypoglycemia, and metabolic acidosis, *which occur as a result of hyperbilirubinemia and increase the risk of brain damage.*
- Initiate phototherapy per physician order *to decrease bilirubin levels.*
- During phototherapy, shield infant's eyes *to prevent damage to corneas and retinas;* keep infant nude and change positions frequently *for maximal body surface exposure;* cleanse skin frequently *to prevent irritation;* maintain adequate fluid intake *to prevent dehydration;* monitor body temperature *to prevent hyperthermia.*
- Before exchange transfusion, keep infant on nothing-by-mouth (NPO) status (2 to 4 hours) *to prevent aspiration;* check donor blood for compatibility *to prevent transfusion reaction;* have resuscitation equipment (oxygen, Ambu bag, endotracheal tubes, laryngoscope) at bedside *in preparation for emergency action.*
- Assist physician with exchange transfusion procedure; track amounts of blood withdrawn and transfused *to maintain balanced blood volume;* maintain body temperature *to avoid hypothermia and cold stress;* monitor vital signs and observe for rash *for indicators of transfusion reaction.*
- After transfusion, continue to monitor vital signs *for transfusion reaction or other complications;* check umbilical cord *for bleeding or signs of infection.*

NURSING DIAGNOSIS Interrupted breastfeeding related to discharge of mother and continued hospitalization of infant

Expected Outcomes *Mother states desire to continue breastfeeding as much as possible and expresses and stores milk when she cannot come to the hospital to nurse the infant.*

Nursing Interventions/*Rationales*
- Encourage the mother to come to hospital to nurse infant as often as feasible for her *to maintain milk supply and encourage bonding.*
- Provide private and comfortable space for nursing that is available 24 hours per day *to support the mother in breastfeeding.*
- Instruct the mother in methods to express and store breast milk *to ensure a safe and adequate milk supply.*
- Provide written educational materials and audiovisual aids *to demonstrate proper techniques for expressing and storing milk and to allow the mother to learn at her own pace.*
- Recommend use of a breast pump and pump according to recommended guidelines (e.g., pump a minimum of 5 times a day; pump a minimum of 100 minutes a day; pump long enough to soften breasts) *to provide maximum stimulation for milk production.*
- Reassure the mother that infant's nutritional needs will be met through expressed milk or other methods *to allay anxiety.*
- Review the daily routine of the mother to advise her on ways *to incorporate pumping into her daily schedule.*
- Provide information about breastfeeding support groups *to help the mother obtain emotional support from other breastfeeding mothers.*

NURSING DIAGNOSIS Parental role conflict related to separation from hospitalized infant and interruptions of family life due to travel to hospital to see infant.

Expected Outcomes *Parents will share responsibilities for child care and home maintenance; parents will visit infant in hospital as often as feasible.*

Nursing Interventions/*Rationales*
- Suggest to parents that they mutually establish a routine for child care for siblings and home maintenance *to enhance communication and provide necessary home activities.*
- Encourage parents to seek assistance and support from friends, relatives, and community groups such as their church *to meet their needs and ensure that a minimal level of appropriate functioning is maintained.*
- Encourage parents to travel to hospital as often as is desirable and feasible *to promote breastfeeding and bonding with infant.*

NURSING DIAGNOSIS Deficient knowledge related to administration of home phototherapy

Expected Outcome *Family demonstrates ability to provide home therapy.*

Nursing Interventions/*Rationales*
- Explore family's willingness to try home phototherapy *to evaluate feasibility of home therapy option.*
- Explore family's understanding of jaundice and proposed therapy *to establish baseline for teaching.*
- Teach family with demonstration–return demonstration, allowing for several practice sessions, and supplement with written materials with pictorial representations *to ensure safe and optimal results.*
- Include the following in your instructions: placement of lamp or fiberoptic unit; proper eye care and patching; proper skin care; proper positioning under lamp; provision of increased fluid intake; monitoring of time under lamp; monitoring of vital signs and skin, eyes, feeding patterns, stooling and voiding patterns; observation for complications *to ensure that the family understands and implements safe and effective use of phototherapy.*
- Stress importance of obtaining the prescribed bilirubin tests on schedule *as a way of tracking success of therapy.*
- Give parents a contact number if they have any questions while carrying out therapy *to offer ongoing support and increase parent comfort.*

inherited from the parents; others result from the action of the intrauterine environment. Many defects appear to occur as the result of multifactorial inheritance, the interaction of multiple genes with environmental factors that affect the embryonic development of the affected system. Examples of these include neural tube defects, congenital heart defects, developmental dysplasia of the hip, and cleft lip or palate.

A congenital disorder is present at birth and can be caused by genetic or environmental factors, or both.

Congenital anomalies are evident in 2% of all live births (Hudgins & Cassidy, 2006), but this number increases to about 6% by age 5 years, by which time anomalies are diagnosed that were previously undetected. In addition, the incidence of congenital malformations in fetuses that are miscarried is higher than that in infants who are born alive, which adds to the overall incidence. Major congenital defects are the leading cause of death in infants younger than 1 year in the United States and account for 20% of neonatal deaths. Although there has been a decrease in the incidence of other causes of neonatal mortality, the death rate associated with most congenital anomalies has essentially remained stable for the last 75 years.

The most common congenital anomalies that cause serious problems in the neonate are congenital heart disease, neural tube defects, cleft lip or palate, clubfoot, and developmental dysplasia of the hip. These are thought to result from the interaction of multiple genetic and environmental factors. Minor anomalies are less apparent but are important to identify because they may be a part of a characteristic pattern of malformations. That is, they may point to the presence of a more serious major anomaly and aid in its diagnosis. When newborns have three or more minor anomalies, there is an approximate 20% risk of a major anomaly or mental retardation (Siegel & Milunsky, 2004). Minor malformations are more common in areas of the body that have variable features, such as the face and distal extremities. Some of the most common malformations include the lack of a helical fold of the pinna, complete or incomplete simian creases, and a capillary hemangioma other than on the face or posterior aspect of the neck.

The seriousness of congenital anomalies in terms of their effect on society is reflected in the more than six million hospital days and $200 billion a year required for the care and treatment of these neonates. Ways of preventing and detecting these anomalies are being improved continuously, as are techniques for the care of the fetus with certain anomalies. Promoting the availability of these services to populations at risk challenges community health care systems. An interdisciplinary team approach is vital for providing holistic care: the surgical treatment, rehabilitation, and education of the child, as well as psychosocial and financial assistance for the parents. Parental disappointment and disillusion add to the complexity of the nursing care needed for these infants.

Cardiovascular System Anomalies

During fetal development, cell division and differentiation of the organs and tissues of a particular body system sometimes occur rapidly. During these various sensitive, or critical, periods, particular body systems are more susceptible to environmental influences than they are later in gestation. For example, the critical period for the cardiovascular system is from week 3 of embryonic development to week 8, when many women may not be aware that they are pregnant.

Congenital heart defects (CHDs) are anatomic abnormalities in the heart that are present at birth, although they may not be diagnosed immediately. Congenital heart disease occurs in 8 in 1000 live births (Green, 2004).

Ventricular septal defect is the most common type of heart defect and acyanotic lesion, and tetralogy of Fallot is the most common type resulting in cyanosis. After prematurity, CHDs, often in association with other congenital anomalies, are the next major cause of death in the first year of life.

The etiology of CHDs is unknown in more than 90% of the cases. This is important for parents to know, because they often feel guilty thinking that they have done something to cause the defect. Maternal factors that are known to be associated with a higher incidence of CHD include the following:

- Viral infections such as rubella
- Ingestion of folic acid antagonists, progesterone, estrogen, lithium, warfarin (Coumadin), or anticonvulsants such as phenytoin
- Use of the acne medication isotretinoin (Accutane)
- Alcohol intake
- Poor nutrition
- Radiation exposure
- Complications of pregnancy such as antepartal bleeding
- Metabolic disorders such as diabetes mellitus and phenylketonuria
- Systemic lupus erythematosus
- Maternal age ≥40 years

There also is an increased likelihood of cardiac disease in low-birth-weight infants, especially those small for gestational age (SGA), as well as in premature infants and those with congenital infections. In addition, CHDs may be associated with other extracardiac defects such as renal agenesis, tracheoesophageal fistula, and diaphragmatic hernias.

Genetic factors are implicated in the pathogenesis of CHDs. As a general rule, these defects are thought to be multifactorial in origin, involving both genetic and environmental influences; however, a familial occurrence of virtually all forms of CHD has been noted. If a family has one affected child, the risk for having a second child with CHD has been thought to be 1% to 3%; the risk for the acquisition of some defects is greater than this. For example, the risk for left-sided lesions such as hypoplastic left heart syndrome and coarctation of the aorta is higher (Hockenberry, 2003). If the father is affected, the risk of having a child with

EVIDENCE-BASED PRACTICE

Maternal Adjustment to Children with Disabilities

BACKGROUND

- As families have grown smaller and prenatal screening more sensitive, there has been an increase in the expectation that every baby will be perfect. The trend toward shorter hospital stays and deinstitutionalization mean that special needs children are more likely to be cared for at home by family. Mothers find themselves stressed with overwhelming responsibilities, and at the same time in need of social support and the chance to grieve and adjust.

OBJECTIVES

- The reviewer sought to metasynthesize the qualitative research, to compare and contrast the experiences of mothers of children with disabilities. Her goal was to provide a multidisciplinary foundation for decision making about clinical practice, government policy, and future research.

METHODS

Search Strategy

- After a thorough search of research databases in nursing, medicine, psychology, and sociology, the author identified 12 qualitative studies, dated 1991 to 1999, representing 179 children of all ages and their mothers from Canada and the United States. Their disabilities included attention deficit disorder with hyperactivity, schizophrenia, asthma, brain injury, birth anomalies, and technologic dependence. The families were Caucasian, Latino, and African-American.

Statistical Analyses

- Qualitative data does not focus on outcomes. It is metasynthesized by comparing the themes and concepts from each study and identifying common thematic patterns. For example, mothers may speak of changing needs, lack of confidence in self or health care provider, fear, and constant vigilance, and the reviewer labels this theme "uncertainty."

FINDINGS

- Themes revealed four developmental milestones for mothers of differently abled children:
  1. Becoming the mother of a disabled child: This included solving the puzzle of what is wrong, diminished maternal role in the hospital, grief for loss of ideal, trusting the health care system, and looking for blame.
  2. Learning a new maternal role: Caregiver burden, family relations, sibling attention, finding support, acceptance of this different child, protecting child's humanity against prejudice and insensitivity by society and medical care providers, and the intensity of mothering a severely dependent child.
  3. Realizing that daily life will never be the same: Adaptation, routine, control, change, restructuring, mastering uncertainty, isolation, grief for lost choices, and identifying realistic and attainable goals.
  4. Acceptance/Denial: Redefining normal, looking for progress, acceptance of chronicity, hope, strength, and life enrichment. The paradox is accepting the child but never giving up hope.

LIMITATIONS

- Such a variety of ages and disabilities might have limited the commonalities found. However, this heterogeneity probably strengthened the generalizability of the themes that emerged. As with all qualitative research, the numbers of subjects are small, but intensively examined. Bias by the examiner is possible, but so is great insight. Financial stressors were not discussed.

IMPLICATIONS FOR PRACTICE

- Nurses need to listen carefully to the mother about her needs and hopes for her child. Nurses need to assess the family's particular circumstances, and engage other family members in caregiving, or arrange for respite care, to lighten the burden on the mother. Acknowledging the humanity and value of each child, and encouraging the mother by helping her gain knowledge and confidence will strengthen the entire family. Most importantly, mothers need hope.

IMPLICATIONS FOR FURTHER RESEARCH

- Metasyntheses specific to each condition might be helpful, and then these could be analyzed together. Much more information is needed about the family dynamics and sibling outcomes of families of children with disabilities. The challenge of such research is the uniqueness of each family makeup, temperament, and resources. Research from other continents besides North America would add culturally diverse insights.

Reference: Nelson, A. (2002). A metasynthesis: Mothering other-than-normal children. *Qualitative Health Research, 12*(4), 515-530.

CHD is 1% to 3%; it is 2% to 10% if the mother is affected. This inherited risk will become more important as children with CHD live longer and reproduce; therefore continuing epidemiologic studies are needed in this area.

In addition, it now appears that a much greater percentage than believed to be true in the past can be attributed to single gene mutations. This recognition is based on animal models, studies of human familial patterns of inheritance, and the finding of cardiovascular defects as a part of syndromes exhibiting mendelian patterns of inheritance. An example of this is the identification of chromosome 22q11 deletions in infants with DiGeorge syndrome. This syndrome affects an estimated 1 in 4000 live births, making this one of the most frequent genetic disorders with congenital heart defects. The gene or genes located in the chromosomal region involved with DiGeorge syndrome appear to play a major role in the development of cardiovascular defects, particularly truncus arteriosus, absent pulmonary valve syndrome, tetralogy of Fallot, pulmonary atresia, and other abnormalities involving the aortic arch.

Chromosomal abnormalities also may be associated with CHDs. For example, 45% of children with trisomy 21, or Down syndrome, have a cardiac defect. Nearly all children who have trisomy 18, the second most common chromosomal abnormality, have cardiac anomalies. About 95% of trisomy 18 fetuses miscarry, and the survivors usually die within the first year of life. Approximately 80% of infants born with trisomy 13 have cardiac defects. In general, cardiovascular surgical intervention has not been offered to infants with trisomies 13 and 18 because of their overall poor prognosis.

Although traditionally CHD has been classified as either cyanotic or acyanotic, a classification that categorizes cardiac defects physiologically is now considered more descriptive. The first of the four categories in this classification includes defects that result in increased pulmonary blood flow, often with congestive heart failure. Examples of the CHDs in this category are atrial and ventricular septal defects and patent ductus arteriosus. The second category includes defects that involve decreased pulmonary blood flow and typically result in cyanosis. The most common example of this type of defect is tetralogy of Fallot; tricuspid atresia is a less common defect in this category. The third category includes those defects that cause obstruction to blood flow out of the heart. Pulmonary stenosis is an example of an obstruction to the flow of blood out of the right side of the heart that causes cyanosis. Coarctation of the aorta and subaortic stenosis are examples of obstructions to the flow of blood out of the left side of the heart that can result in congestive heart failure but not cyanosis. The fourth category comprises those complex cardiac anomalies that involve a flow of mixed saturated and desaturated blood in the heart or great vessels. These include such defects as transposition of the great vessels and total anomalous venous return (Table 39-1; Fig. 39-1).

Severe CHDs often are evident immediately after birth, especially defects that cause cyanosis such as transposition of the great vessels. Infants with these anomalies are transferred directly to special care nurseries or pediatric units. Even though the structural or functional anomalies are always present at birth, some affected newborns may be asymptomatic. Some CHDs, such as a small coarctation of the aorta, become apparent only as the infant or child is exposed to stresses such as growth demands or infection.

If symptoms are present at birth, they may be obvious with the first cry, which may be weak and muffled or loud and breathless. Affected newborns may be cyanotic and unrelieved by oxygen treatment, with the cyanosis increasing whenever the child is in the supine position or cries. The bluish gray, dusky color of cyanotic infants may be mild, moderate, or severe. Other infants may be acyanotic and pale, with or without mottling on exertion, which includes crying, feeding, or stooling.

The affected newborn's activity level varies from restlessness to lethargy, and possibly unresponsiveness, except to pain. Persistent bradycardia (resting heart rate of less than 80 beats/min) or tachycardia (rate exceeding 160 beats/min) may be noted (Askin, 2002). The cardiac rhythm may be abnormal, and murmurs may be heard. Signs of congestive heart failure and decreased tissue perfusion may be evident.

Because the cardiac and respiratory systems function together, cardiac disease may be manifested by respiratory signs and symptoms. The respiratory rate should be determined when the newborn is in a resting state. Abnormal findings may include tachypnea, which is a rate of 60 to 120 breaths/min; retractions with nasal flaring; grunting occurring with or without exertion; and dyspnea, which may worsen when the infant is supine or exerting itself.

A major role of the nurse is to assess infants for abnormal findings, which, if observed, must be reported immediately. Newborns exhibiting these symptoms require prompt diagnosis and appropriate therapy in a neonatal or pediatric intensive care unit. Interventions planned if a nursing diagnosis of decreased cardiac output is made include administering oxygen as ordered, as well as cardiotonic and other medications such as diuretics that rid the body of accumulated fluid, decreasing the workload of the heart by maintaining a thermoneutral environment, feeding with the gavage method if necessary, and preventing crying if this precipitates cyanosis. Various diagnostic tests such as echocardiography and cardiac catheterization are performed to obtain specific information about the defect and the need for surgical intervention. Significant improvements in diagnosis, medical management, and surgical treatment of CHD have caused the death rate to decrease significantly, with the result that more of these children are reaching adulthood.

table 39-1 **Physiologic Classification of Cardiac Defects**

CATEGORIES	EXAMPLES
Defects that result in increased pulmonary blood flow, often with congestive heart failure	Atrial and ventricular septal defects Patent ductus arteriosus
Defects that involve decreased pulmonary blood flow and typically result in cyanosis	Tetralogy of Fallot Tricuspid atresia
Defects that cause obstruction to blood flow out of the heart	Pulmonary stenosis; causes cyanosis Coarctation of the aorta; congestive heart failure, no cyanosis Subaortic stenosis; congestive heart failure, no cyanosis
Complex cardiac anomalies that involve a flow of mixed saturated and desaturated blood in the heart or great vessels	Transposition of the great vessels Total anomalous venous return

Atrial septal defect (ASD)

An ASD is an abnormal opening between the right and left atria. Basically, three types of abnormalities result from incorrect development of the atrial septum. An incompetent foramen ovale is the most common defect. The high ostium secundum defect results from abnormal development of the septum secundum. Improper development of the septum primum produces a basal opening known as an *ostium primum defect*, frequently involving the atrio-ventricular valves. In general, left-to-right shunting of the blood occurs in all atrial septal defects.

Atrial septal defect

Ventricular septal defect (VSD)

A VSD is an abnormal opening between the right and left ventricles. VSDs vary in size and may occur in either the membranous or muscular portion of the ventricular septum. Because of higher pressure in the left ventricle, a shunting of blood from the left to the right ventricle occurs during systole. If pulmonary vascular resistance produces pulmonary hypertension, the shunt of blood is then reversed from the right to the left ventricle, with cyanosis resulting.

Ventricular septal defect

Atrioventricular canal (AVC) defect

An AVC defect is an incomplete fusion of the endocardial cushions. It consists of a low atrial septal defect that is continuous, with a high ventricular septal defect and clefts of the mitral and tricuspid valves, creating a large central atrioventricular valve that allows blood to flow between all four chambers of the heart. Flow is generally from left to right. It is the most common cardiac defect in children with Down syndrome.

Atrio-ventricular canal defect

Patent ductus arteriosus (PDA)

Patent ductus arteriosus

PDA is a vascular connection that, during fetal life, bypasses the pulmonary vascular bed and directs blood from the pulmonary artery to the aorta. Functional closure of the ductus normally occurs soon after birth. If the ductus remains patent after birth, the direction of blood flow in the ductus is reversed by the higher pressure in the aorta.

Coarctation of the aorta (COA)

Coarctation of aorta

COA is characterized by localized narrowing of the aorta near the insertion of the ductus arteriosus, resulting in increased pressure proximal to the defect (head and upper extremities) and decreased pressure distal to the defect (body and lower extremities).

Aortic stenosis (AS)

AS is a narrowing or stricture of the aortic valve, causing resistance to blood flow in the left ventricle, decreased cardiac output, left ventricular hypertrophy, and pulmonary vascular congestion. AS can be valvular, subvalvular, or supravalvular (rare). The most serious sequelae relate to the left ventricular hyper-trophy (increased end-diastolic pressure, pulmonary hypertension, decreased coronary artery perfusion).

Aortic stenosis

Pulmonic stenosis (PS)

PS is a narrowing at the entrance to the pulmonary artery. Resistance to blood flow causes right ventricular hypertrophy and decreased pulmonary blood flow. Pulmonary atresia is the extreme form of PS; no blood flows to the lungs.

Pulmonic stenosis

Tetralogy of Fallot (TOF)

TOF is characterized by the combination of four defects: (1) pulmonary stenosis, (2) ventricular septal defect, (3) overriding aorta, and (4) hypertrophy of the right ventricle. It is the most common defect, causing cyanosis in children surviving beyond 2 years of age. The severity of symptoms depends on the degree of pulmonary stenosis, the size of the ventricular septal defect, and the degree to which the aorta overrides the septal defect.

Pulmonic stenosis Overriding aorta Ventricular septal defect Right ventricular hypertrophy

FIG. 39-1 Congenital heart abnormalities. (Modified from Hockenberry, M. [2003]. *Wong's nursing care of infants and children* [7th ed.]. St. Louis: Mosby.)

Central Nervous System Anomalies

Most congenital anomalies of the central nervous system (CNS) result from defects in the closure of the neural tube during fetal development. Although the cause of neural tube defects (NTDs) is unknown, they are thought to stem from the interaction of many genes that may be influenced by factors in the fetal environment. Environmental influences such as treatment with valproic acid (an anticonvulsant), treatment with methotrexate (a chemotherapeutic medication), and alcohol consumption have been implicated. Excessive maternal body heat exposure during the early first trimester, such as from a significant febrile illness or extensive hot-tub exposure, also may increase the risk of a neural tube defect. Maternal folic acid deficit has a direct bearing on failure of the neural tube to close; therefore folic acid supplementation is recommended for women of childbearing age. Despite an abundance of information about folic acid, many women of childbearing age are unaware of the importance of folic acid intake or choose to ignore it. Neural tube defects also continue to occur because of unplanned pregnancies and the 30% of planned pregnancies that are thought to be folic acid re-

Tricuspid atresia

Tricuspid valvular atresia is characterized by a small right ventricle, a large left ventricle, and usually a diminished pulmonary circulation. Blood from the right atrium passes through an atrial septal defect into the left atrium, mixes with oxygenated blood returning from the lungs, flows into the left ventricle, and is propelled into the systemic circulation. The lungs may receive blood through one of three routes: (1) a small ventricular septal defect, (2) a patent ductus arteriosus, or (3) bronchial vessels.

Transposition of the great vessels (TGV)

TGV is an embryologic defect caused by a straight division of the bulbar trunk without normal spiraling. As a result, the aorta originates from the right ventricle and the pulmonary artery from the left ventricle. An abnormal communication between the two circulations must be present to sustain life.

Total anomalous pulmonary venous connection (TAPVC)

TAPVC is a rare defect characterized by a failure of the pulmonary veins to join the left atrium. Instead, the pulmonary veins are abnormally connected to the systemic venous circuit via the right atrium or various veins draining toward the right atrium (e.g., superior vena cava). The abnormal attachment results in mixed blood being returned to the right atrium and shunted from the right to the left through an atrial septal defect.

Truncus arteriosus (TA)

TA is a retention of the embryologic bulbar trunk. It results from the failure of normal septation and division of this trunk into an aorta and pulmonary artery. This single arterial trunk overrides the ventricles and receives blood from them through a ventricular septal defect. The entire pulmonary and systemic circulation is supplied from this common arterial trunk.

Hypoplastic left heart syndrome (HLHS)

HLHS is characterized by underdevelopment of the left side of the heart, resulting in a hypoplastic left ventricle and aortic atresia. Most blood from the left atrium flows across the patent foramen ovale to the right atrium, to the right ventricle, and out the pulmonary artery. The descending aorta receives blood from the patent ductus arteriosus supplying systemic blood flow.

FIG. 39-1 cont'd

sistant (Rintoul et al., 2002). In the United States, rates of NTDs declined after the introduction of mandatory food fortification with folic acid in 1998 (Mills & Signore, 2004). Increased use of prenatal diagnostic techniques and termination of pregnancies have also made an impact on the overall incidence of birth of infants with NTDs.

Although a neural tube defect is usually an isolated defect, it can occur with some chromosomal abnormalities and syndromes and also with other defects such as cleft palate, ventricular septal defect, tracheoesophageal fistula, diaphragmatic hernia, imperforate anus, and renal anomalies. Some neural tube defects can be diagnosed prenatally with fetal ultrasonography and the finding of elevated levels of alpha-fetoprotein in the amniotic fluid and maternal serum.

Encephalocele and Anencephaly

Encephalocele and anencephaly are abnormalities resulting from failure of the anterior end of the neural tube to close. An encephalocele is a herniation of the brain and meninges through a skull defect. Treatment consists of surgical repair and shunting to relieve hydrocephalus, unless a major brain malformation is present. Most of these infants will have some degree of cognitive deficit. Anencephaly is the absence of both cerebral hemispheres and of the overlying skull. This condition is incompatible with life; many of the infants are stillborn or die within a few days of birth. Comfort measures are provided until the infant eventually dies of respiratory failure.

Spina Bifida

Spina bifida, the most common defect of the CNS, results from failure of the neural tube to close at some point. The two categories of spina bifida are spina bifida occulta and spina bifida cystica. Spina bifida occulta is a malformation in which the posterior portion of the laminas fails to close, but the spinal cord or meninges do not herniate or protrude through the defect. It is usually asymptomatic and may be not diagnosed unless there are associated problems. Spina bifida cystica includes meningocele and myelomeningocele. A meningocele is an external sac that contains meninges and cerebrospinal fluid (CSF) and that protrudes through a defect in the vertebral column. A myelomeningocele is similar, except that it also contains nerves, resulting in motor and sensory deficits below the lesion. A myelomeningocele is visible at birth, most often in the lumbosacral area. It is usually covered with a very fragile, thin membrane (Fig. 39-2). The sac can tear easily, allowing CSF to leak out and providing an entry for infectious agents into the CNS. Myelomeningocele usually is associated with an Arnold-Chiari malformation, which results from the improper development and downward displacement of part of the brain into the cervical spinal canal. This in turn results in the development of hydrocephalus, which affects about 90% of children with myelomeningocele, although it is usually not present at birth. The long-term prognosis in an affected infant can be determined to a large extent at birth, with the degree of neurologic dysfunction related to the level of the lesion, which determines the nerves involved. Many physicians recommend that treatment be instituted regardless of the level of the lesion, unless there is a severe CNS anomaly, advanced hydrocephalus at birth, severe anoxic brain damage, active CNS infection, or a congenital malformation or syndromes incompatible with long-term survival. Prenatal diagnosis makes possible a scheduled cesarean birth, allowing for more careful delivery of the infant's back to try to prevent rupture of the meningeal sac.

A major preoperative nursing intervention for a neonate with a myelomeningocele is to protect the protruding sac from injury, rupture and resultant risk of CNS infection. Such infants should be positioned in a side-lying or prone position to prevent pressure on the sac until surgical repair is done. If the infant is allowed to be held, the nurse or parent must be careful to prevent injury to the sac. The sac should be covered with a sterile, moist, nonadherent dressing, and cared for using sterile techniques. The skin around the defect must be cleansed and dried carefully to prevent breakdown, which would establish a portal of entry for infectious agents. Because a lack of normal innervation may prevent the bladder from emptying completely, the Credé method is used at regular intervals to express urine from the bladder.

Other nursing care involves an assessment of the infant's neurologic function that includes the status of the following: apparent paralysis of lower extremities; the flaccidity and spasticity of muscles below the defect; and sphincter control, as evidenced by the number and character of voidings and stools, as well as the leakage of urine and stool. The infant's head circumference is measured, and other neurologic assessments are performed to determine the presence and degree of hydrocephalus.

A major nursing intervention is providing support and needed information to parents as they begin to learn to cope with an infant who has immediate needs for intensive care and who probably will have long-term needs as well. Surgical repair is often done in the neonatal period, preferably within the first 24 hours. Early closure can prevent CNS infection and trauma to the exposed nerves. It also can prevent stretching of other nerve roots, which can occur as the sac continues to enlarge after birth. Surgical shunt procedures to prevent increasing hydrocephalus may be needed. Other problems, such as infection, are treated as they occur. Additionally, these infants are at increased risk for developing latex sensitivity, so they must not come in direct or secondary contact with any products or equipment containing latex.

Maternal-fetal surgery to repair a fetal myelomeningocele is a significant new development in maternal-fetal intervention. The rationale for this intervention is based on direct and indirect evidence that some of the neural damage resulting from the myelomeningocele is acquired in the later part of gestation, caused by amniotic fluid exposure or trauma to the exposed neural elements. It is believed that closure of the defect will prevent this damage, resulting in less hydrocephalus, lower extremity impairment, and bowel and bladder incontinence (Flake, 2001). Although this seems to be a good treatment option, a number of issues are debated, the most important being that because of the nature and complexity of myelomeningocele, it is difficult to prove benefits that offset the significant mater-

FIG. 39-2 **A,** Myelomeningocele. Note absence of vertebral arches. **B,** Myelomeningocele (spina bifida). (From Zitelli, B., & Davis, H. [1997]. *Atlas of pediatric physical diagnosis.* [3rd ed.]. St. Louis: Mosby.)

nal risk involved. Second, there is a significant likelihood that maternal-fetal surgery will increase the mortality rate and the probability of premature birth with its accompanying problems. The term birth of an infant with myelomeningocele is a viable alternative to fetal repair. Numerous other significant issues have been addressed in the consideration of maternal-fetal surgery for this and other nonlethal anomalies. The National Institutes of Health (NIH) is sponsoring a randomized multiinstitution trial to investigate the open fetal repair of myelomeningocele compared with standard postnatal treatment (Flake).

Hydrocephalus

Hydrocephalus is a condition in which the ventricles of the brain are enlarged as a result of an imbalance between the production and absorption of the CSF. Congenital hydrocephalus usually arises as a result of a malformation in the brain or an intrauterine infection. Approximately one third of all cases of congenital hydrocephalus result from stenosis of the aqueduct of Sylvius in the brain. Hydrocephalus often occurs in conjunction with a myelomeningocele, which blocks the flow of CSF.

An infant with congenital hydrocephalus initially has a bulging anterior fontanel and a head circumference that increases at an abnormal rate, resulting from the increase in CSF pressure (Fig. 39-3). Enlargement of the forehead with depressed eyes that are rotated downward, causing a "setting sun" sign, occurs as the condition worsens. If the surgical shunting of excess CSF from the brain is not done soon after birth, the resulting increasing intracranial pressure will lead to irreversible neurologic damage, as evidenced by palpably widening sutures and fontanels, lethargy, poor feeding, vomiting, irritability, opisthotonic posturing, and a high-pitched, shrill cry.

FIG. 39-3 Mother providing kangaroo care to preterm twins; the one on the right has hydrocephalus. The characteristic appearance is an enlarged head, thinning of the scalp, distended scalp veins, and a full fontanel. (Courtesy Cheryl Briggs, RN, Annapolis, MD.)

Nursing actions appropriate to the needs of a newborn with hydrocephalus include care similar to any high risk newborn. The occipitofrontal circumference of the head is measured daily at its largest point, and neurologic assessments are done frequently. If the infant's head is large, the placement of sheepskin or a special pressure-sensitive air mattress under the infant and frequent position changes are necessary to prevent skin breakdown.

The infant's heavy head should be supported carefully during holding or turning, and positioning in the crib should be done in such a way that a patent airway is maintained. The method, amount, and frequency of feeding are determined by the infant's tolerance and energy level. The nurse should be alert to the possibility of projectile vomiting, which is a frequent occurrence in the presence of increased intracranial pressure, and maintain aspiration precautions. Nonnutritive sucking, touching, and cuddling needs should be met.

Diagnosis is made by computed tomography and magnetic resonance imaging; antenatal diagnosis can be made by fetal ultrasonography. The surgical correction of hydrocephalus involves the placement of a shunt that goes from the ventricles of the brain usually to the peritoneum to allow the drainage of excess CSF. Damaged or destroyed brain tissue cannot be restored. The long-term prognosis in affected infants depends on the presence and extent of such tissue damage, along with the cause of the hydrocephalus; the presence of concurrent neurologic problems; and the long-term success of the shunt procedure.

Microcephaly

Microcephaly refers to a head circumference that measures more than three standard deviations below the mean for age and sex. Brain growth is usually restricted and thus mental retardation is common. Microcephaly can be the result of an autosomal recessive disorder; a chromosomal abnormality; fetal exposure to teratogens such as radiation; alcohol ingestion; and congenital infections such as rubella, toxoplasmosis, or cytomegalovirus. Infants with microcephaly require supportive nursing care and medical observation to determine the extent of the psychomotor retardation that almost always accompanies this abnormality. There is no treatment. Parents need support to learn to care for a child with such cognitive impairment.

Respiratory System Anomalies

Screening for congenital anomalies of the respiratory system is necessary even in infants who are apparently normal at birth. Respiratory distress at birth or shortly thereafter may be the result of lung immaturity or anomalous development. Congenital laryngeal web and bilateral choanal atresia are readily apparent at birth. Respiratory distress caused by diaphragmatic hernia and tracheoesophageal fistula may appear immediately or be delayed, depending on the severity of the defect.

Laryngeal Web and Choanal Atresia

A laryngeal web, which is uncommon, results from the incomplete separation of the two sides of the larynx and is most often between the vocal cords. Choanal atresia (Fig. 39-4) is the most common congenital anomaly of the nose; it is a bony or membranous septum located between the nose and the pharynx. Inability to pass a suction catheter through the nose into the pharynx or cyanosis without obvious respiratory distress usually leads to its detection. Nearly half of the infants with choanal atresia have other anomalies. Infants with either a laryngeal web or choanal atresia require emergency surgery.

Congenital Diaphragmatic Hernia

Congenital diaphragmatic hernia (CDH) results from a defect in the formation of the diaphragm, allowing the abdominal organs to be displaced into the thoracic cavity. It occurs in approximately 1 in 5000 live births (Hartmann, 2004); however, if stillbirths resulting from this defect are included, the incidence increases to 1 in 2000. Herniation of the abdominal viscera into the thoracic cavity may cause severe respiratory distress and represent a neonatal emergency (Fig. 39-5). The defect and herniation may be minimal and easily repaired, or the defect may be so extensive that the viscera present in the thoracic cavity during embryonic life have prevented the normal development of pulmonary and sometimes cardiac tissue. The defect is usually on the left because that is the side of the diaphragm that fuses last.

Most congenital diaphragmatic hernias are discovered prenatally on ultrasound studies. Hernias may be repaired by fetal surgery in some research institutions. Intrauterine surgical correction of CDH has met with poor neonatal

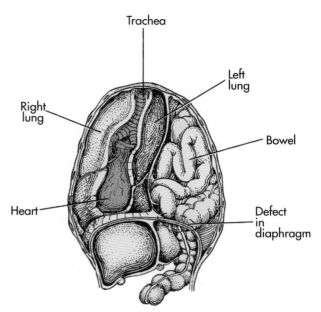

FIG. 39-5 Diaphragmatic hernia. (Used with permission of Ross Products Division, Abbott Laboratories, Inc., Columbus, OH 43216. From Clinical Education Aid #6, Copyright 1963, Ross Products Division, Abbott Laboratories, Inc.)

outcomes in many cases, primarily as a result of tocolysis failure and early birth.

At birth, most affected infants have severe respiratory distress, and respiratory assessment reveals worsening distress as the bowels fill with air. Typically the breath sounds are diminished. Heart sounds may be heard on the right side of the chest because the heart has been displaced there by the abdominal contents. Physical examination reveals a flat or scaphoid abdomen and a prominent ipsilateral chest. Diagnosis can be made on the basis of the x-ray finding of loops of intestine in the thoracic cavity and the absence of intestine in the abdominal cavity.

Surgical repair is performed as soon as the infant is stable. Preoperative nursing interventions include participating in the stabilization of the infant's condition until surgical repair can be done. Inhaled nitrous oxide (NO) has been used in many centers with moderate success to treat the accompanying persistent pulmonary hypertension (Bradshaw, 2004). Gastric contents are aspirated and suction applied to decompress the gastrointestinal tract and prevent further cardiothoracic compromise. Oxygen therapy, mechanical ventilation, and the correction of acidosis are necessary in infants with large defects. As a result of the lung hypoplasia that affected infants sometimes have, pulmonary hypertension occurs. Extracorporeal membrane oxygenation (ECMO) or high-frequency oscillatory ventilation may be used in infants with severe circulatory and respiratory complications (see Chapter 40).

The prognosis depends largely on the degree of fetal pulmonary development and the success of surgical diaphragmatic closure, but the prognosis in severe cases is often poor. The overall survival rate for infants who are symptomatic within the first few hours of life is about

FIG. 39-4 Choanal atresia. Posterior nares are obstructed by membrane or bone either bilaterally or unilaterally. Infant becomes cyanotic at rest. With crying, newborn's color improves. Nasal discharge is present. Snorting respirations often are observed with increased respiratory effort. Newborn may be unable to breathe and eat at the same time. Diagnosis is made by noting inability to pass small feeding tube through one or both nares. (Used with permission of Ross Products Division, Abbott Laboratories, Inc., Columbus, OH 43216. From Clinical Education Aid #6, Copyright 1963, Ross Products Division, Abbott Laboratories, Inc.)

50%, although it has improved recently with the advent of inhaled NO, improved management of high frequency ventilation, and ECMO. Of those who survive, some have chronic lung disease with long-term oxygen dependency, feeding difficulties, and gastroesophageal reflux (GER).

Gastrointestinal System Anomalies

Anomalies in the gastrointestinal (GI) system can occur anywhere along the gastrointestinal tract, from the mouth to the anus. Some anomalies, such as cleft lip, omphalocele, and gastroschisis, are apparent at birth. Others, including cleft palate, esophageal atresia, pyloric stenosis, intestinal obstructions, and imperforate anus, become apparent as the infant is further assessed or becomes symptomatic.

Cleft Lip and Palate

Cleft lip or palate is a commonly occurring congenital midline fissure, or opening, in the lip or palate resulting from failure of the primary palate to fuse (Fig. 39-6). One or both deformities may occur, and nasal deformity may also be present. Multiple genetic and, to a lesser extent, environmental factors (e.g., maternal infection, maternal smoking, radiation exposure, alcohol ingestion, and treatment with medications such as corticosteroids, lithium, retinoids, and phenytoin) appear to be involved in their development.

Cleft lip with or without cleft palate occurs in approximately 1 in 700 live births, while cleft palate alone is less frequent (Mason, Bentz, & Losken, 2002). The defect can

FIG. 39-6 Variations in clefts of lip and palate at birth. **A,** Notch in vermilion border. **B,** Unilateral cleft lip and cleft palate. **C,** Bilateral cleft lip and cleft palate. **D,** Cleft palate. **E,** Infant with complete unilateral cleft lip. Note the feeding tube. (**A-D,** From Hockenberry, M. [2003]. *Wong's nursing care of infants and children* [7th ed.]. St. Louis: Mosby. **E,** From Dickason, E., Silverman, B., & Kaplan J. [1998]. *Maternal-infant nursing care* [3rd ed.]. St. Louis: Mosby.)

range from a simple notch in the lip to complete separation of the lip that extends to the floor of the nose. The treatment for a cleft lip is surgical repair, which usually is done between ages 6 and 12 weeks, if the infant is healthy and free of infection. Advances in surgical techniques have made it possible for some infants, particularly those with unilateral cleft lip, to have a near-normal appearance. The results of the repair depend on the severity of the defect, with more severe bilateral cleft lip requiring surgical repair done in stages.

Anomalies of the palate often occur in association with cleft lip. Cleft palate alone occurs in approximately 1 in 2000 to 2500 live births (Yellon, McBride, & Davis, 2002). It is more common in female infants and occurs more frequently as a constituent of certain syndromes. This defect can range from a cleft in the uvula to a complete cleft of the hard and soft palates that may be unilateral, bilateral, or midline. Feeding is difficult because the cleft lip renders the newborn unable to maintain a seal around a nipple; the cleft palate renders the infant unable to form a vacuum to maintain suction when feeding. In addition, the inability to suck and swallow normally allows milk to pool in the nasopharynx, which increases the likelihood of aspiration. Furthermore, as the infant attempts to suck, milk often comes out through the cleft and out of the nares. Although the degree of difficulty depends on the size of the cleft, feeding problems are greater in infants with a cleft palate than in those with a cleft lip. Breastfeeding can be successful in some infants, particularly if the infant has a cleft lip alone. Bottle feeding also can be successful in some infants. There are special nipples, bottles, and appliances available to aid in feeding (Fig. 39-6, *E*; Fig. 39-7). In general, parents of

FIG. 39-7 *1,* Mead Johnson bottle and nipple for cleft palate. Cleft palate nipple system *(2a)* with valve *(2b)* to regulate flow. Haberman feeder *(3a)* with disc *(3b)* to control flow of milk. *4,* Ross cleft palate assembly. Nipple can be trimmed to accommodate palate size. (Courtesy Shannon Perry, Phoenix, AZ.)

infants with these defects need education and support as they learn to feed their baby, to prevent what should be a normal part of infant care from becoming a very frustrating experience.

The type of surgical repair done to close the cleft palate is based on the degree of the cleft and, as with a cleft lip, if severe, may necessitate repair done in stages. Repair is begun at 6 to 18 months, after some development of the affected area has occurred. Early repair helps avert some of the speech problems that may occur in people with palate defects. Long-term care is often necessary for children with a cleft palate and involves the combined efforts of a health care team comprising acute care and community nurses; social workers; ear, nose, and throat and plastic surgeons; speech therapists; and orthodontists.

Parents of infants with a cleft lip or palate need much support, particularly in the case of a cleft lip, because this is both a cosmetic and functional defect. Recognizing that this may interfere with normal parent-infant bonding in the neonatal period, the nurse must assess for this and intervene appropriately.

Esophageal Atresia and Tracheoesophageal Fistula

Esophageal atresia (EA) and tracheoesophageal fistula (TEF), the most life-threatening anomalies of the esophagus, often occur together, although they can occur singly. Esophageal atresia is a congenital anomaly in which the esophagus ends in a blind pouch or narrows into a thin cord, thus failing to form a continuous passageway to the stomach. TEF is an abnormal connection between the esophagus and the trachea.

Maternal hydramnios is a common finding, particularly if the fetus has an EA without a TEF. Variations of the anomalies are possible, depending on the presence or absence of a TEF, the site of the fistula, and the location and degree of the esophageal obstruction. The most common variant is the combination of a proximal EA, in which the esophagus ends in a blind pouch, with a distal TEF, in which the lower esophagus exits the stomach and is connected to the trachea by a fistula, rather than forming a continuous tube to the upper esophagus (Fig. 39-8). This defect occurs in approximately 1 in 4000 live births (Orenstein, Peters, Khan, Youssef, & Hussain, 2004). The infant with EA or TEF may also show some fetal growth restriction and will thus be SGA. The presence of a midline defect such as EA or TEF is often accompanied by another significant embryonic defect such as a cardiac anomaly, cleft lip and/or palate, or vertebral, genitourinary, or abdominal wall defect (Roaten, Bensard, & Price, 2006).

Infants with the life-threatening anomaly EA with TEF show significant respiratory difficulty immediately after birth. EA with or without TEF results in excessive oral secretions, drooling, and feeding intolerance. When fed, the infant may swallow, but then cough and gag and return the fluid through the nose and mouth. Respiratory distress can result from aspiration or from the acute gastric

FIG. 39-8 Congenital atresia of esophagus and tracheoesophageal fistula. **A,** Upper and lower segments of esophagus end in blind sac, occurring in 5% to 8% of such infants. **B,** Upper segment of esophagus ends in atresia and connects to trachea by fistulous tract, occurring rarely. **C,** Upper segment of esophagus ends in blind pouch; lower segment connects with trachea by small fistulous tract, occurring in 80% to 95% of such infants. **D,** Both segments of esophagus connect by fistulous tracts to trachea, occurring in less than 1% of such infants. Infant may aspirate with first feeding. **E,** Esophagus is continuous but connects by fistulous tract to trachea; known as *H-type*. (From Hockenberry, M. [2003]. *Wong's nursing care of infants and children* [7th ed.]. St. Louis: Mosby.)

distention produced by the TEF. Choking, coughing, and cyanosis occur after even a small amount of fluid is taken by mouth.

Nursing interventions are supportive until surgery is performed.

▪ NURSE ALERT

Any infant with excessive oral secretions and respiratory distress should not be fed orally until a physician is consulted.

The infant with EA and TEF is placed in a semi-Fowler position, which facilitates respiratory efforts and diminishes the reflux of gastric contents into the trachea. A double-lumen catheter is placed in the proximal esophageal pouch and attached to continuous suction to remove secretions and decrease the possibility of aspiration. The infant requires close observation and intervention to maintain a patent airway. Other supportive measures include thermoregulation, maintaining fluid and electrolyte balance intravenously as well as acid-base balance, and prevention of any further complications as a result of an associated defect. Surgical correction, done in one stage if possible, consists of ligating the fistula and anastomosing the two segments of the esophagus. The chances for survival in those infants in a good risk category exceed 95% depending on the presence of associated defects and the infant's birth weight (Konkin, O'Hali, Webber, & Blair, 2003). Many infants with EA and TEF will have postoperative issues related to feeding difficulties such as GER and esophageal strictures requiring periodic dilation.

Omphalocele and Gastroschisis

Omphalocele and gastroschisis are two of the more common congenital defects of the abdominal wall. They are rare, however, with omphalocele occurring in approximately 1 in 3000 to 10,000 live births, whereas the incidence of gastroschisis is about 1 in 6000 live births (Blackburn, 2003).

An omphalocele is a covered defect of the umbilical ring into which varying amounts of the abdominal organs may herniate (Fig. 39-9, *A*). Although it is covered with a peritoneal sac, the sac may rupture during or after birth. Many of the infants born with an omphalocele are preterm and have other serious syndromes or anomalies involving the gastrointestinal, cardiac, genitourinary, musculoskeletal, and nervous systems.

Gastroschisis is the herniation of the bowel through a defect in the abdominal wall to the right of the umbilical cord (Fig. 39-9, *B*). No membrane covers the contents as occurs with an omphalocele. Unlike infants with omphalocele, these infants have less than 10% to 15% likelihood of associated anomalies, most of which are cardiac. Many are of low birth weight and premature.

The preoperative nursing care is similar for infants with either defect. Exposure of the viscera causes problems with thermoregulation and fluid and electrolyte balance. Before closure is performed, the exposed viscera are covered with moistened saline gauze and plastic wrap. In some cases the infant's torso may be placed in an impermeable, clear plastic bowel bag to decrease insensible water losses, maintain thermoregulation, and prevent contamination of the exposed viscera (Roaten et al., 2006). Antibiotics, fluid and electrolyte replacement, gastric decompression, and thermoregulation are needed for physiologic support.

If complete closure is impossible because of the small size of the defect and the large amount of viscera to be replaced, a Silastic silo pouch (Dow Corning, Midland, MI) is created and sewn to the fascia of the abdominal defect. This protects the contents as they are gradually placed back into the abdominal cavity. The defect is closed surgically after the reduction of the contents that have been exposed is completed, which usually takes 7 to 10 days.

Gastric decompression is necessary preoperatively to prevent aspiration pneumonia and to allow as much bowel

FIG. 39-9 A, Omphalocele. **B,** Gastroschisis of bowel and stomach. (**A,** From O'Doherty, N. [1986]. *Neonatology: Micro atlas of the newborn.* Nutley, NJ: Hoffmann-La Roche. **B,** Courtesy Wyeth-Ayerst Laboratories, Philadelphia, PA.)

as possible to be placed into the abdomen during surgery. Surgery is usually performed soon after birth. With improved surgical treatment, nutritional support, and medical management, the prognosis has improved for infants born with an abdominal wall defect (King & Askin, 2003). It is estimated that more than 80% of infants born with an omphalocele survive, as do more than 90% of those born with gastroschisis, although residual feeding difficulties such as GER are not uncommon.

Parental support is essential, because the infant has an obvious disfiguring anomaly that can be shocking and repulsive in appearance. Depending on the size of the defect, the infant may also be critically ill before surgery. The nurse must be aware of the effect this may have on parental bonding and intervene appropriately as the parents cope with this crisis.

Gastrointestinal Obstruction

Congenital intestinal obstruction can occur anywhere in the GI tract and takes one of the following forms: atresia, which is a complete obliteration of the passage; partial obstruction, in which the symptoms may vary in severity and sometimes not be detected in the neonatal period; or malrotation of the intestine, which leads to twisting of the intestine (volvulus) and obstruction. EA, discussed previously, is a type of GI obstruction. Duodenal atresia, midgut malrotation and volvulus, jejunoileal atresia, necrotizing enterocolitis, and meconium ileus are the most common causes of neonatal intestinal obstruction. Meconium ileus is an obstruction caused by impacted meconium and is the earliest sign of cystic fibrosis, a life-threatening chronic illness. Infants with this type of obstruction should be tested for cystic fibrosis, because 95% of infants with meconium ileus have cystic fibrosis.

In addition to polyhydramnios in the pregnant woman, the infant shows the following cardinal signs: bilious vomiting, abdominal distention, and failure to pass normal amounts of meconium in the first 24 hours. High intestinal obstruction is characterized by vomiting, even if the infant is not being fed orally. A low obstruction is characterized primarily by distention, with vomiting occurring later. Abdominal distention can elevate the diaphragm, which causes respiratory difficulties.

Nursing care is aimed at supporting the infant until surgical intervention can be carried out to eliminate the obstruction. Oral feedings are withheld, a nasogastric tube is placed for suction, and intravenous therapy is initiated to provide needed fluid and electrolytes. In infants with an intestinal obstruction, surgery consists of resecting the obstructed area of bowel and anastomosing the nonaffected bowel. In recent years, the survival rate for these infants has risen to 90% to 95% as a result of better treatments, better neonatal intensive care, and a better understanding of the total problem.

Imperforate Anus

Imperforate anus is a term used to describe a wide range of congenital disorders involving the anus and rectum and genitourinary system in many cases (Fig. 39-10). These anomalies are relatively common, with an incidence of approximately 1 in 5000 live births (Roaten et al., 2006). Occurring more in male than in female infants, they result from the failure of anorectal development in weeks 7 and 8 of gestational life. Such infants have no anal opening, and commonly there is also a fistula from the rectum to the perineum or genitourinary system (Fig. 39-11). Types of anorectal malformations include the typical cloaca in females, which involves the vagina, colon, and urethra forming a single common passage in the perineum. Others include the low rectovaginal fistula (female) and rectourethral bulbar fistula (male). Extensive surgical repair is often required in stages for the more complex types of anorectal malformations. In some cases the anomaly may involve stenotic areas, or a thin translucent membrane may cover

FIG. 39-10 Types of imperforate anus. Anal sphincter muscle may be present and intact. **A,** High lesion opening onto perineum through narrow fistulous tract. **B,** High lesion ending in fistulous tract to urinary tract. **C,** Low lesion in bowel passes through puborectal muscle. **D,** High lesion ending in fistulous tract to vagina.

the anal opening. Treatment for such a membrane is excision followed by daily dilation, which parents are taught to do. The preoperative nursing care is similar to that described for other gastrointestinal obstructions. Imperforate anus is often associated with other anomalies, with nearly half having additional genitourinary anomalies, which may complicate long-term care.

FIG. 39-11 Imperforate anus. (From Chessell, G., Jamieson, M., Morton, R., Petrie, J., & Towler, H. [1984]. *Diagnostic picture tests in clinical medicine* [vol. 2]. St. Louis: Mosby.)

Musculoskeletal System Anomalies

The two most common musculoskeletal system anomalies seen in neonates are developmental dysplasia of the hip and congenital clubfoot. Both of these conditions must be detected and treated early for successful correction.

Developmental Dysplasia of the Hip

The broad term developmental dysplasia of the hip (DDH) describes a spectrum of disorders related to abnormal development of one or all of the components of the hip joint that may develop at any time during fetal life, infancy, or childhood. A change in terminology from congenital hip dysplasia (CHD) and congenital dislocation of the hip (CDH) to DDH more properly reflects a variety of hip abnormalities in which there is a shallow acetabulum, subluxation, or dislocation.

The incidence of hip instability of some kind is approximately 10 per 1000 live births. The incidence of frank dislocation or a dislocatable hip is 1.5 per 1000 live births (Brozanski & Bogen, 2002), and approximately 30% to 50% of infants with DDH are born breech (Thompson, 2004).

The cause of DDH is unknown, but certain factors such as sex, birth order, family history, intrauterine position, birth type, joint laxity, and postnatal positioning are believed to affect the risk of DDH. Predisposing factors associated with DDH may be divided into three broad categories: (1) physiologic factors, which includes maternal hormone secretion and intrauterine positioning; (2) mechanical factors, which involves breech presentation, multiple fetus, oligohydramnios, and large infant size; other mechanical factors may include continued maintenance of the hips in adduction and extension that will in time cause a dislocation; and (3) genetic factors, which entail a higher incidence (6%) of DDH in siblings of affected infants, and an even greater incidence (36%) of recurrence if a sibling and one parent were affected.

Three degrees of DDH are illustrated in Fig. 39-12 and are described as follows.
- Acetabular dysplasia (or preluxation)—mildest form of DDH in which there is neither subluxation nor dislocation. There is a delay in acetabular development evidenced by osseous hypoplasia of the acetabular roof that is oblique and shallow, although the cartilaginous roof is comparatively intact. The femoral head remains in the acetabulum.
- Subluxation—The largest percentage of DDH, subluxation, implies incomplete dislocation of the hip and is sometimes regarded as an intermediate state in the development from primary dysplasia to complete dislocation. The femoral head remains in contact with the acetabulum, but a stretched capsule and ligamentum teres cause the head of the femur to be partially displaced. Pressure on the cartilaginous roof inhibits ossification and produces a flattening of the socket.
- Dislocation—The femoral head loses contact with the acetabulum and is displaced posteriorly and superiorly

Normal   Dysplasia   Subluxation   Dislocation

FIG. 39-12 Configuration and relationship of structures in developmental dysplasia of the hip.

over the fibrocartilaginous rim. The ligamentum teres is elongated and taut.

DDH is often not detected at the initial examination after birth; thus, all infants should be carefully monitored for hip dysplasia at follow-up visits throughout the first year of life. In the newborn period dysplasia usually appears as hip joint laxity rather than as outright dislocation. Subluxation and the tendency to dislocate can be demonstrated by the Ortolani or Barlow tests. The Ortolani and Barlow tests are most reliable from birth to 2 or 3 months of age (see Fig. 25-12). Other signs of DDH are shortening of the limb on the affected side (Galeazzi sign, Allis sign), asymmetric thigh and gluteal folds, and broadening of the perineum (in bilateral dislocation).

▬ NURSE ALERT

The Ortolani and Barlow tests must be performed by an experienced clinician to prevent fracture or other damage to the hip. If these tests are performed too vigorously in the first 2 days of life, when the hip subluxates freely, persistent dislocation may occur.

Treatment is begun as soon as the condition is recognized, because early intervention is more favorable to the restoration of normal bony architecture and function. The longer treatment is delayed, the more severe the deformity, the more difficult the treatment, and the less favorable the prognosis. The treatment varies with the age of the child and the extent of the dysplasia. The goal of treatment is to obtain and maintain a safe, congruent position of the hip joint to promote normal hip joint development and ambulation.

The hip joint is maintained by dynamic splinting in a safe position with the proximal femur centered in the acetabulum in an attitude of flexion. Of the numerous devices available, the Pavlik harness is the most widely used, and with time, motion, and gravity, the hip works into a more abducted, reduced position. The harness is worn continuously until the hip is proved stable on clinical and radiographic examination, usually in about 3 to 5 months. If the infant is treated between ages 1 and 8 months, the harness is effective 80% to 90% of the time (Hockenberry, 2003).

If not effective, traction, casting, and even surgery may be necessary to stabilize the hip.

▬ NURSE ALERT

The former practice of double- or triple-diapering for DDH is not recommended because it promotes hip extension, thus worsening proper hip development.

In addition to the major intervention of assessing and helping identify the disorder, another key nursing intervention is teaching the parents about the care of the infant, who will remain in the harness continuously during the treatment. Because this occurs during a time of maximal growth, it will be necessary for them to adjust the infant's care to accommodate the infant's changing needs. Continuing thorough follow-up care is necessary, as is psychosocial support for the family.

Clubfoot

Congenital clubfoot is a congenital deformity of the foot and ankle that includes forefoot adduction, midfoot supination, hindfoot varus, and ankle equinus. Deformities of the foot and ankle are described according to the position of the ankle and foot. The more common positions involve the following variations:

- Talipes varus—An inversion or a bending inward
- Talipes valgus—An eversion or bending outward
- Talipes equinus—Plantar flexion in which the toes are lower than the heel
- Talipes calcaneus—Dorsiflexion, in which the toes are higher than the heel

Most cases of clubfoot are a combination of these positions. The most frequently occurring type (approximately 95%) is the composite deformity *talipes equinovarus* (TEV). In this abnormality, the foot appears C-shaped, pointing downward and inward; the ankle is inverted; and the Achilles tendon is shortened. The foot appears small, wide, and stiff, and the lower leg appears small because of hypoplasia of the calf muscles. Unless treated, further stiffening occurs, and bony changes will result. Unilateral clubfoot is somewhat more common than bilateral clubfoot and may occur as an isolated defect or in association with other dis-

CRITICAL THINKING EXERCISE

Developmental Dysplasia of the Hip (DDH)

Anna, a 4.3 kg Caucasian female, is admitted to the newborn nursery after a breech vaginal birth. She is the first child born to Mr. and Mrs. Robinson. Anna, who appears to be a healthy newborn, is now being examined by the pediatric nurse practitioner (PNP). Anna's vital signs are within normal range and her physical examination is normal except for findings related to her left hip. The assessment findings were followed by an ultrasound, and it was determined that Anna has DDH.

1. Evidence—Are there any predisposing factors presented that would alert the PNP to suspect DDH? Is there evidence to determine her diagnosis and preferred treatment?
2. Assumptions—What assumptions can be made about the following items?
   a. Physical assessment techniques that will be done to assess for DDH
   b. The immediate plan of care for Anna after a diagnosis of DDH
   c. The ability for Mrs. Robinson to breastfeed her daughter
   d. The impact of having an infant with a congenital disorder
   e. The trajectory of Anna's recovery
3. What implications and priorities for nursing care can be made at this time?
4. Does the evidence support your conclusion?
5. Are there alternative perspectives to your conclusion

orders or syndromes, such as chromosomal aberrations, arthrogryposis (a generalized immobility of the joint), cerebral palsy, or spina bifida.

Clubfoot is one of the most common congenital anomalies, occurring in approximately 1.5 per 1000 live births, with two times more male than female infants affected (Trilling & Potts, 2002). The exact cause is unknown, but possibilities include a genetic predisposition, in utero compression, and abnormal embryonic development.

Serial casting is begun shortly after birth, before discharge from the nursery. Successive casts allow for gradual stretching of skin and tight structures on the medial side of the foot. Manipulation and casting are repeated frequently (every week) to accommodate the rapid growth of early infancy. In some cases daily manipulation and stretching of tissues is accomplished with taping and splinting of the affected extremity; a continuous passive motion (CPM) machine may be used several hours daily to stretch and strengthen muscle groups involved (Faulks & Luther, 2005). The extremity or extremities are often casted or splinted until maximum correction is achieved, usually within 8 to 12 weeks. A Denis Browne splint may be used to manage feet that correct with casting and manipulation.

Because these infants are often placed in a cast before discharge, the nurse must teach parents necessary care, including how to protect the cast and assess the toes for neurovascular compromise. This is particularly important because of the potential for the infant to outgrow the cast.

As is true with the birth of any child with an anomaly, the nurse should be supportive of the parents as they learn the ways in which to meet the infant's normal needs, as well as those brought about by the infant's physical problem.

Polydactyly

Occasionally hands or feet are seen with extra digits. In some instances, polydactyly is hereditary. If there is little or no bone involvement, the extra digit is tied with silk suture soon after birth. The finger or toe falls off within a few days, leaving a small scar. When there is bone involvement, surgical repair is indicated.

Genitourinary System Anomalies

Anomalies involving the genitourinary system can be distressing to parents because they may be readily apparent and, in the case of some conditions, because of the concern about sexuality and reproductive functioning. These anomalies range from obvious anomalies of the external genitalia, such as hypospadias, to those involving internal organs that may not be detected but may cause damage to the urinary tract. An example of the latter is an obstruction in the urinary tract that can cause hydronephrosis, which is the abnormal collection of urine in the renal pelvis, which can eventually destroy the kidney.

Hypospadias and Epispadias

Hypospadias constitutes a range of penile anomalies associated with an abnormally located urinary meatus. The meatus can open below the glans penis or anywhere along the ventral surface of the penis, the scrotum, or the perineum. It is the most common anomaly of the penis, affecting approximately 1 in 250 infants (Elder, 2004). The incidence is increasing in the United States (Nelson, Park, Wan, Bloom, Dunn, & Wei, 2005). Hypospadias is classified according to the location of the meatus and the presence or absence of chordee, which is a ventral curvature of the penis (Figs. 39-13, 39-14). The cause is unknown, although it is thought to be of multifactorial inheritance. One large retrospective study found hypospadias to be significantly more prevalent in infants who had uniformly poor intrauterine

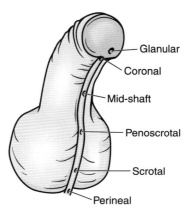

FIG. 39-13 Classification of hypospadias by position of the urethral meatus.

FIG. 39-14 Hypospadias. (Courtesy H. Gil Rushton, MD, Children's National Medical Center, Washington, DC.)

FIG. 39-15 Exstrophy of bladder. (Courtesy H. Gil Rushton, MD, Children's National Medical Center, Washington, DC.)

growth (lower than the 10th percentile) in weight, length, and head circumference (Hussain, Chaghtai, Herndon, Herson, Rosenkrantz, & McKenna, 2002).

Mild cases of hypospadias are often repaired for cosmetic reasons and involve a single surgical procedure. In more severe cases, several operations are required to reconstruct the urethral opening and correct the chordee, thereby straightening the penis. The goals are to improve the appearance of the genitalia, make it possible for the child to urinate in a standing position, and have a sexually adequate organ. These infants are not circumcised because the foreskin may be needed during surgical repair. Repair is done early, often during or soon after the first year of life, so that the child's body image is not impaired. Oral mucosa is sometimes used in reconstruction.

Epispadias, a rare anomaly, results from failure of urethral canalization. About half of the affected infants are males who have a widened pubic symphysis and a broad spadelike penis with the urethral opening on the dorsal surface. In females there is a wide urethra and a bifid clitoris. Severity ranges from mild anomaly to a severe one that is associated with exstrophy of the bladder. Surgical correction is necessary, and affected male infants should not be circumcised.

Exstrophy of the Bladder

The most common bladder anomaly is exstrophy (Fig. 39-15), which often occurs in conjunction with epispadias. It is rare, occurring in approximately 1 in 35,000 to 40,000 live births (Elder, 2004). It results from the abnormal development of the bladder, abdominal wall, and pubic symphysis that causes the bladder, the urethra, and the ureteral orifices to all be exposed. The bladder is visible in the suprapubic area as a red mass with numerous folds, with urine draining from it onto the infant's skin. Immediately after birth the exposed bladder should be covered with a sterile, nonadherent dressing to protect its delicate surface until closure can be performed. It is recommended that reconstructive surgery be started in the neonatal period, preferably with the bladder being closed during the first or second day of

life. Parents will need much support as they deal with caring for an infant who has such an obvious defect. Repair is completed before school age, if possible, although some children never attain normal voiding patterns and later may be considered for surgery for urinary diversion.

Ambiguous Genitalia

Ambiguous genitalia in the newborn (Fig. 39-16) often is discovered by the nurse during a physical assessment. Erroneous or abnormal sexual differentiation may be a genetic aberration, such as congenital adrenal hypoplasia, which can be life threatening because it involves the deficiency of all adrenal cortical hormones. Other possible causes of sexual ambiguity include chromosomal abnormalities, defective sex hormone synthesis in male infants, and the placental transfer of masculinizing agents to female fetuses.

FIG. 39-16 Ambiguous external genitals (i.e., structure can be enlarged clitoral hood and clitoris or malformed penis). (Courtesy Edward S. Tank, MD, Division of Urology, Oregon Health Science University, Portland, OR.)

Gender assignment should be based on data gathered from the following sources: maternal and family history, including the ingestion of steroids during pregnancy, and relatives with ambiguous genitalia or who died during the neonatal period; physical examination; chromosomal analysis (results are available in 2 to 3 days); endoscopy, ultrasonography, and radiographic contrast studies; biochemical tests, such as analysis of urinary steroid excretion, which helps detect several of the adrenal cortical syndromes; and, in some instances, laparotomy or gonad biopsy.

Therapeutic intervention, including any counseling and surgery, should be started as soon as possible. A child born with ambiguous genitalia should not receive a gender assignment until the appropriate gender of rearing may be properly assessed and assigned. An appropriate gender assignment should be based on the following: age at presentation, potential for mature sexual function, potential fertility, and the long-term psychologic and intellectual impact on the child and family. Parents need much support as they learn to deal with this very challenging situation.

Teratoma

A teratoma is an embryonal tumor that may be solid, cystic, or mixed. It is composed of at least two and usually three types of embryonal tissue: ectoderm, mesoderm, and endoderm. This rare tumor in the neonate may occur in the skull, the cervical area, the mediastinum, the abdomen, or the sacral area; more than half are located in the sacrococcygeal area.

The treatment of choice for such neonates is complete surgical resection. Approximately 80% of all teratomas are benign, and no additional therapy is needed after complete resection done in the neonatal period. If the tumor is not surgically resected before the infant is 1 to 2 months old, the likelihood of the teratoma becoming malignant increases rapidly.

■ CARE MANAGEMENT

Prenatal Diagnosis

Refined testing procedures are available to monitor fetal development. Prenatal diagnostic techniques such as amniocentesis, ultrasonography, alpha-fetoprotein measurements, chorionic villus sampling, PUBS, fetal nuchal translucency (FNT) screening, and gene probes contribute information to the database (see Chapter 29). Although they are a valuable adjunct to prenatal care, these tests cannot identify all congenital disorders. Furthermore, ethical issues surround such testing, and the nurse must be prepared to support the family's decision regarding these tests. If a disorder is detected and the family decides to proceed with the pregnancy, the advantage is that appropriate care can be made available for the infant immediately at birth.

In addition to testing, the history and medical information in the prenatal record is reviewed for factors associated with congenital disorders. These factors include various medical, surgical, and social conditions and their

treatments (see Chapter 33); maternal infection (see Chapter 8); maternal endocrine and metabolic disorders (see Chapter 32); and infection and drug dependence in the newborn (see Chapter 38).

Perinatal Diagnosis

Many congenital anomalies require intervention soon after birth. By careful observations in the birth room or nursery, the nurse can identify most of these conditions. An excessive amount of amniotic fluid, hydramnios, is commonly associated with congenital anomalies in the newborn, and such infants should be examined closely at the earliest possible time.

Oligohydramnios, an insufficient amount of amniotic fluid, is associated primarily with anomalies of the urinary tract that prevent normal micturition in utero. It is most often associated with renal agenesis or dysplasia and obstructive lesions in the lower urinary tract. Anomalies of the ears sometimes occur with renal abnormalities. Bilateral renal agenesis, resulting in oligohydramnios, commonly manifests as Potter syndrome, which is characterized by atypical facial appearance consisting of a flat nose, recessed chin, epicanthal folds, and low-set abnormal ears; limb abnormalities; pulmonary hypoplasia; and fetal growth restriction. These conditions may be diagnosed prenatally.

Postnatal Diagnosis

Apgar scoring and a brief assessment are completed for all neonates after birth. Any deviations from normal are reported to the primary health provider immediately. A thorough assessment of all body systems follows, with identification both of visible anomalies and of those that might not be visible.

Some infants have multiple congenital anomalies. A recognized pattern of malformations is referred to as a *syndrome*. The most common, affecting about 1 in every 660 births (Bay & Steele, 2002), is Down syndrome (Fig. 39-17), with the diagnosis confirmed early in the neonatal period.

Genetic Diagnosis

Diagnostic procedures for the detection of genetic disorders are performed after birth at any time from the postnatal period through adulthood. Many tests exist for various disorders; only the most frequently used tests are discussed here.

Newborn Screening

The most widespread use of postnatal testing for genetic disease is the routine screening of newborns for inborn errors of metabolism such as phenylketonuria (PKU), galactosemia, hemoglobinopathy (sickle cell disease and thalassemias) and hypothyroidism; these are the minimum mandatory newborn screening tests in most states in the United States. Newborn screening testing in Canada varies by province.

An inborn error of metabolism (IEM) is the term applied to a large group of disorders caused by a meta-

FIG. 39-17 **A,** Clinical features of Down syndrome. **B,** Simian crease. (From Zitelli, B., & Davis, H. [1997]. *Atlas of pediatric physical diagnosis* [3rd ed.]. St. Louis: Mosby.)

bolic defect that results from the absence of or change in a protein, usually an enzyme, and mediated by the action of a certain gene. These defects can involve any substrate produced from protein, carbohydrate, or fat metabolism. Inborn errors of metabolism are recessive disorders, so a person must receive a defective gene from each parent. The parents usually are unaffected because their normal dominant gene directs the synthesis of sufficient protein to meet their metabolic needs under normal circumstances.

With the advent of new biochemical techniques, it is now possible to detect the abnormal gene responsible for causing an increasing number of these disorders early in the neonatal period so appropriate therapies to prevent further morbidity may be implemented. One screening test, tandem mass spectrometry, has the potential for identifying more than 20 inborn errors of metabolism, in addition to the standard IEMs. With tandem mass spectrometry earlier identification of IEMs may prevent further developmental delays and morbidities in affected children (Fearing & Marsden, 2003).

Phenylketonuria results from a deficiency of the enzyme phenylalanine dehydrogenase (see Chapter 3). The test for PKU is not reliable, however, until the newborn has ingested an ample amount of the amino acid phenylalanine, a constituent of both human and cow's milk.

▬ NURSE ALERT
The nurse must document the initial ingestion of milk and perform the test at least 24 hours after that time.

The current trend toward early infant discharge from the hospital has the potential to cause neonates with a disorder such as PKU to not be screened as frequently as in the past. In response to this, the AAP Committee on Genetics (1996) made the following recommendations:
- Obtain a subsequent sample before age 2 weeks if the initial specimen is collected before the newborn is 24 hours old.
- Designate a primary care provider for all newborns before discharge for adequate newborn screening follow-up.
- Collect the initial specimen as close as possible to discharge or no later than 7 days after birth.

If the infant is found to have PKU, a diet low in phenylalanine is begun soon after birth. Breastfeeding or partial breastfeeding may be possible for some infants if the phenylalanine levels are monitored carefully and remain within acceptable limits (Van Rijn, Bekhof, Dijkstra, Smit, Moddermam, & van Spronsen, 2003). Many affected children have some intellectual impairment. Successful management and outcome is largely dependent on early identification of the condition, modifying the diet, and compliance with the treatment regimen throughout the entire life.

Galactosemia, caused by a deficiency of the enzyme galactose 1-phosphate uridyltransferase, results in the inability to convert galactose to glucose. Galactosemia can be detected by measuring the blood levels of galactose in the urine of newborns suspected of having the disease who have ingested formula containing galactose. Early symptoms are vomiting, weight loss, and CNS symptoms, including poor feeding, drowsiness, and seizures. If the disorder goes untreated, the galactose levels will continue to increase, and the affected infant will show failure to thrive, mental retardation, cataracts, jaundice, hepatomegaly, and cirrhosis of the liver, with death possibly occurring in the first month of life. Therapy consists of eliminating galactose from the diet; this condition precludes breastfeeding since lactose is present in breast milk.

Congenital hypothyroidism results from a deficiency of thyroid hormones; it affects approximately 1 of every 3500 newborns (Kemper & Foster, 2003). All states in the United States routinely screen for hypothyroidism. This can be done by measuring thyroxine (T_4) in a drop of blood obtained from a heel stick at 2 to 5 days of age. At this time the normally expected increase in T_4 is lacking in newborns with hypothyroidism. It is more often included as part of the newborn screen done in the first 24 to 48 hours or before discharge. Neonatal screening consists of an initial filter-paper blood-spot thyroxine (T_4) measurement followed by measurement of thyroid-stimulating hormone (TSH) in specimens with low T_4 values. Early screening may have false-positive results. Treatment is thyroid replacement. In the newborn, thyroid function studies are elevated in comparison with values in older children; therefore it is important to document the timing of the tests. In preterm and sick full-term infants, thyroid function levels are usually lower than in the healthy full-term infant; a repeat T_4 and TSH may be elevated after 30 weeks (corrected age) in newborns born before that time and after resolution of the acute illness in the sick full-term infant.

If the baby is untreated, symptoms usually appear after 6 weeks and include bradycardia; hypothermia; hypotension; hyporeflexia; abdominal distention; umbilical hernia; coarse, dry hair; thick, dry skin that feels cold; anemia; widely patent cranial sutures; and retarded bone age beginning at birth. The most disabling problem, however, is delayed development of the nervous system, leading to severe mental retardation (Hockenberry, 2003).

Cytogenetic Studies

Abnormalities can occur in either the autosomes or the sex chromosomes. Chromosomal disorders often can be diagnosed on the basis of the clinical manifestations alone. However, an infant may have a clinical appearance that is only suggestive of a problem. Cytogenetic studies must be done to confirm or rule out a suspected diagnosis. Newer techniques in molecular cytogenetic analysis make possible a more precise identification of risk for having a fetus affected with a genetic defect such as phenylketonuria.

Disorders in the number or structure of chromosomes can be diagnosed by a *karyotype* (see Fig. 3-1), which is a photographic enlargement of the chromosomes arranged by their numbered pairs.

Abnormalities of the sex chromosomes make up about half of all the chromosomal abnormalities occurring in the newborn. The most common test for sex chromosome abnormalities is the buccal smear, using cells scraped from the mucosa inside the mouth. When prepared and stained, these show the number of inactive X chromosomes, also known as an *X-chromatin mass* or a *Barr body*. Each cell, whether male or female, has one genetically active X chromosome. Therefore a normal female has one active X chromosome and one Barr body, which is on the inactive X chromosome. A normal male has no Barr bodies, because he has only one genetically active X chromosome.

Dermatoglyphics

Dermatoglyphics is the study of the patterns formed by the ridges in the skin on the digits, palms, and soles. These patterns, formed early in development, are strongly correlated with the effects of chromosomes. The addition or deletion of genetic material produces alterations in the loops, swirls, and arches of the finger and toe prints, in the palm lines, and in the flexion creases on the palms of the hands and soles of the feet. Characteristic dermatoglyphic patterns

have been noted for almost all the chromosomal abnormalities, such as Down syndrome.

An infant with Down syndrome may have a single, palmar crease (see simian crease in Fig. 39-17, *B*), a single flexion crease of the fifth digit, and an open-field pattern on the ball of the foot (Matthews & Robin, 2006). The characteristic dermatoglyphic feature in a child with Turner syndrome is the large size of the dermal patterns on the fingers and toes. Certain fingerprint patterns also may be found in those people who have cardiac valvular problems later in life. Asymmetry of palmar ridges has been reported in congenital anomalies such as cleft lip and palate and congenital vertebral anomaly.

Collaborative Care

The nursing diagnoses formulated for an infant born with a congenital anomaly depend on the anomaly the infant has. For example, the diagnoses in an infant born with a CHD causing cyanosis will relate to inadequate oxygenation of body tissues, such as "activity intolerance related to imbalance between oxygen supply and demand." General nursing diagnoses pertaining to the care of neonates with congenital abnormalities include the following:

NEWBORN
- *Risk for injury related to*
  - presence of a congenital disorder
- *Risk for infection related to*
  - anomaly or its treatment
- *Impaired gas exchange, imbalanced nutrition: less than body requirements, or impaired physical mobility related to*
  - congenital anomaly
- *Delayed growth and development related to*
  - inborn error of metabolism

PARENTS AND FAMILY
- *Dysfunctional grieving or spiritual distress related to*
  - birth of a child with a defect
- *Ineffective family coping related to*
  - birth of a child with a defect
- *Deficient knowledge related to*
  - cause of disorder, its management, alternative courses of action, community resources, prognosis, and the care needed by the child after discharge
- *Anxiety related to*
  - uncertainty regarding prognosis or ability to care for child
- *Risk for impaired parenting related to*
  - birth of a child with a disorder or defect

Newborn Care

A collaborative health team approach that includes specialists and community service representatives is needed in the care of infants with some disorders. Surgical intervention in the neonatal period may be necessary for the infant requiring either immediate correction or a palliative procedure to relieve the symptoms of the anomaly until definitive correction can be done. There is also a higher morbidity and mortality rate in neonates than in older children or adults undergoing similar procedures. However, despite these problems unique to neonates, advances in surgical techniques, anesthesia, and the nursing care given in intensive care nurseries have together been responsible for decreasing the risk of surgery in neonates.

The health care team must be highly skilled to meet the needs of these infants. These needs are similar to those of other high risk infants. In addition to stabilization of the infant's condition (oxygenation and perfusion of tissues), other preoperative interventions, such as nasogastric tube placement for abdominal decompression, pain management, and the maintenance of fluid and electrolyte balance, are implemented to manage specific problems.

Postoperatively the infant is returned to the intensive care nursery, where close monitoring is maintained. The infant's respiratory efforts are supported; this often requires mechanical ventilation. Constant surveillance is necessary to detect any respiratory complications resulting from the anesthesia. A pulse oximeter is attached to measure the oxygen saturation in hemoglobin, which closely correlates with arterial oxygen saturation. Oxygen is provided as needed. An indwelling gastric catheter attached to intermittent suction is placed to remove gastric secretions, thereby preventing aspiration and abdominal distention. The infant's fluid, electrolyte, and acid-base balances are monitored and adjusted as needed. Urinary output is monitored and should equal 1 to 2 ml/kg/hr. Other nursing interventions are focused on caring for the surgical site, maintaining thermoregulation, managing pain, and promoting comfort.

Parents and Family Support

While the infant is receiving optimal care, the parents have needs that must be met as they deal with the crisis of having an infant with an abnormal condition. Their reactions are carefully assessed and are likely to be those typical of a grief response. Facilitating their understanding of the information given them about their infant's condition is a vital nursing intervention. A newly diagnosed disorder often implies the need for the implementation of a therapeutic regimen. For example, the disorder may be an inborn error of metabolism, such as PKU, which requires consistent and rigid adherence to a diet. The family may need help with securing the required formula and receiving counseling from the clinical dietitian. The importance of maintaining the diet, keeping an adequate supply of special preparations, and avoiding the use of unauthorized substitutions must be impressed on the family.

Referral to appropriate agencies is another essential component of the follow-up management, and the nurse should make the parents aware of all possible sources of aid, including pertinent literature, parent groups, and national organizations. Many organizations and foundations, such as the Cystic Fibrosis Foundation and the Muscular Dystrophy Association, provide services and counseling

for families of affected children. There are also numerous parent groups the family can join. There they can share experiences and derive mutual support in coping with problems similar to those of other group members. Nurses should be familiar with the services available in their community that provide assistance and education to families with these special problems.

A major nursing function is providing emotional support to the family during all aspects of the care of the child born with a defect or disorder. The feelings stemming from the real or imagined threat posed by a congenital anomaly are as varied as the people being counseled. Responses may include apathy, denial, anger, hostility, fear, embarrassment, grief, and loss of self-esteem (see Chapter 41).

Parents benefit from seeing before-and-after pictures of other babies born with the same defect. Coupled with other verbal and nonverbal supportive care, this visual reassurance may be effective in allaying their concerns.

Families need much information, guidance, and support as they make decisions regarding the care of their infants. Once they have been given the facts and possible consequences and all the assistance they need in problem solving, the final decision regarding a course of action must be their own. It is then incumbent on health care providers to support the decision of the family.

Nurses frequently encounter children with genetic diseases and families in which there is a risk that a disorder may be transmitted to or occur in an offspring. It is a responsibility of nurses to be alert to situations in which persons could benefit from a genetic evaluation and counseling to be aware of the local genetic resources, to aid the family in finding services, and offer support and care for children and families affected by genetic conditions. Local genetic clinics can be located through several sites, such as Gene Tests (www.genetests.org), a publicly funded medical genetics information resource developed for physicians and other health care providers, which is available at no cost to all interested persons. Another resource is the National Society of Genetic Counselors (www.nsgc.org), which lists genetic counselors by states in the United States.

---

community activity

Identify newborn screening procedures in the health care facility in which you provide client care. Describe the current status of newborn screening in your state or province (Canada) including what tests are done. Is tandem mass spectrometry being used? Electronic references include the following:
- U.S. National Screening Status Report (www.genes-r-us.uthscsa.edu)
- Gene Tests—gene Clinics (www.genetests.org)
- Save Babies Through Screening, Inc. (www.savebabies.org)

key points

- Hyperbilirubinemia is caused by a variety of factors, including maternal-fetal Rh and ABO incompatibility.
- Erythroblastosis fetalis leads to anemia, edema, and the cytotoxic effects of unconjugated bilirubin.
- The injection of $Rh_o(D)$ immune globulin in Rh-negative and Coombs' test–negative women bestows passive immunity and also minimizes the possibility of isoimmunization.
- Neonatal exchange transfusion with type O, Rh-negative RBCs serves to treat anemia and acidosis and to remove bilirubin, maternal antibodies, and fetal RBCs that are beginning to hemolyze.
- Major congenital defects are the leading cause of death in term neonates.
- The most common major congenital anomalies that cause serious problems in the neonate are congenital heart disease, neural tube defects, cleft lip or palate, clubfoot, and developmental dysplasia of the hip.

- Minor anomalies may be part of a characteristic pattern of malformations.
- Current technology permits the prenatal diagnosis of many congenital anomalies and disorders.
- The most widespread use of postnatal testing for genetic disease is the routine screening of newborns for inborn errors of metabolism.
- The curative and rehabilitative problems of an infant with a congenital disorder are often complex and require a multidisciplinary approach to care.
- Parents often need special instruction (e.g., meeting nutrition requirements, cast care, or home phototherapy) before they take a high risk infant home.
- The supportive care given to the parents of infants with an abnormal condition must begin at birth or at the time of diagnosis and continue for years.

REFERENCES

American Academy of Pediatrics (AAP) Committee on Genetics. (1996). Newborn screening fact sheets. *Pediatrics, 98*(3), 473-481.

American Academy of Pediatrics (AAP) Subcommittee on Hyperbilirubinemia. (2004). Management of hyperbilirubinemia in the newborn infant 35 or more weeks of gestation. *Pediatrics, 114*(1), 297-316.

Askin, D. (2002). Complications in the transition from fetal to neonatal life. *Journal of Obstetric, Gynecologic, and Neonatal Nursing, 31*(3), 318-327.

Association of Women's Health, Obstetric and Neonatal Nurses (AWHONN). (2005). *Hyperbilirubinemia in the neonate: Risk assessment, screening, and management.* Accessed www.awhonn.org, August 22, 2006.

Bay, C., & Steele, M. (2002). Genetic disorders and dysmorphic conditions. In B. Zitelli, & H. Davis (Eds.), *Atlas of pediatric physical diagnosis* (4th ed.), St. Louis: Mosby.

Blackburn, S. (2003). *Maternal, fetal, and neonatal physiology: A clinical perspective* (2nd ed.). St. Louis: Saunders.

Bradshaw, W. (2004). The use of nitric oxide in neonatal care. *Critical Care Nursing Clinics of North America, 16*(2), 249-255.

Brozanski, B., & Bogen, D. (2002). Neonatology. In B. Zitelli, & H. Davis (Eds.), *Atlas of pediatric physical diagnosis* (4th ed.), St. Louis: Mosby.

Elder, J. (2004). Urologic disorders in infants and children: Anomalies of the bladder. In R. Behrman, R. Kliegman, & H. Jenson (Eds.), *Nelson textbook of pediatrics* (17th ed.). Philadelphia: Saunders.

Faulks, S., & Luther, B. (2005). Changing paradigm for the treatment of clubfeet. *Orthopedics Nursing, 24*(1), 25-30.

Fearing, M., & Marsden, D. (2003). Expanded newborn screening. *Pediatric Annals, 32*(2), 509-515.

Flake, A. (2001). Prenatal intervention: Ethical considerations for life-threatening and non-life-threatening anomalies. *Seminars in Pediatric Surgery, 10*(4), 212-221.

Green, A. (2004). Outcomes of congenital heart disease: A review. *Pediatric Nursing, 30*(4), 280-284.

Harkness, U., & Spinnato, J. (2004). Prevention and management of RhD isoimmunization. *Clinics in Perinatology, 31*(4), 721-742.

Hartman, G. (2004). Diaphragmatic hernia. In R. Behrman, R. Kliegman, & H. Jenson (Eds.), *Nelson textbook of pediatrics* (17th ed.). Philadelphia: Saunders.

Hockenberry, M. (2003). *Wong's nursing care of infants and children* (7th ed.). St. Louis: Mosby.

Hudgins, L., & Cassidy, S. (2006). Congenital anomalies. In R. Martin, A. Fanaroff, & M. Walsh (Eds.), *Fanaroff and Martin's Neonatal-perinatal medicine: Diseases of the fetus and infant* (8th ed.). Philadelphia: Mosby.

Hussain, N., Chaghtai, A., Herndon, C., Herson, V., Rosenkrantz, T., & McKenna, P. (2002). Hypospadias and early gestation growth restriction in infants. *Pediatrics, 109*(3), 473-478.

Juretschke, L. (2005). Kernicterus: Still a concern. *Neonatal Network, 24*(2), 7-19.

Kemper, A., & Foster, C. (2003). Congenital hypothyroidism: A guide for the general pediatrician. *Contemporary Pediatrics, 20*(6), 32-34, 39-40, 42 passim.

King, J., & Askin, D. (2003). Gastroschisis: Etiology, diagnosis, delivery options, and care. *Neonatal Network, 22*(4), 7-12.

Konkin, D., O'Hali, W., Webber, E., & Blair, G. (2003). Outcomes in esophageal atresia and tracheoesophageal fistula. *Journal of Pediatric Surgery, 38*(12), 1726-1729.

Mason, A., Bentz, M., & Losken, W. (2002). Craniofacial syndromes. In B. Zitelli, & H. Davis (Eds.), *Atlas of pediatric physical diagnosis* (4th ed.). St. Louis: Mosby.

Matthews, A., & Robin, N. (2006). Genetic disorders, malformations, and inborn errors of metabolism. In G. Merenstein, & S. Gardner (Eds.), *Handbook of neonatal intensive care* (6th ed.). St. Louis: Mosby.

Mills, J., & Signore, C. (2004). Neural tube defect rates before and after food fortification with folic acid. *Birth Defects Research Part A, Clinical and Molecular Teratology, 70*(11), 844-845.

Nelson, C., Park, J., Wan, J., Bloom, D., Dunn, R., & Wei, J. (2005). The increasing incidence of congenital penile anomalies in the United States. *Journal of Urology, 174*(4 Pt 2), 1573-1576.

Orenstein, S., Peters, J., Khan, S., Youssef, N., & Hussain, S. (2004). The esophagus. In R. Behrman, R. Kliegman, & H. Jenson (Eds.), *Nelson textbook of pediatrics* (17th ed.). Philadelphia: Saunders.

Reiser, D. (2004). Neonatal jaundice: Physiologic variation or patho-logic process. *Critical Care Nursing Clinics of North America, 16*(2), 257-269.

Rintoul, N., Sutton, L., Hubbard, A., Cohen, B., Melchionni, J., Pasquariello, P., et al. (2002). A new look at myelomeningoceles: Functional level, vertebral level, shunting, and the implications for fetal interventions. *Pediatrics, 109*(3), 409-413.

Roaten, J., Bensard, D., & Price, F. (2006). Neonatal surgery. In G. Merenstein & S. Gardner (Eds.), *Handbook of neonatal intensive care* (6th ed.). St. Louis: Mosby.

Shaver, S. (2004). Isoimmunization in pregnancy. *Critical Care Nursing Clinics of North America, 16*(2), 205-209.

Siegel, B., & Milunsky, J. (2004). When should the possibility of a genetic disorder cross your radar screen? *Contemporary Pediatrics, 21*(5), 30-34, 37-38, 40-42 passim.

Thompson, G. (2004). The hip. In R. Behrman, R. Kliegman, & H. Jenson (Eds.), *Nelson textbook of pediatrics* (17th ed.). Philadel-phia: Saunders.

Trilling, J., & Potts, N. (2002). Musculoskeletal alterations. In N. Potts, & B. Mandleco (Eds.), *Pediatric nursing: Caring for children and their families.* Clifton Park, NY: Delmar.

Van Rijn, M., Bekhof, J., Dijkstra, T., Smit, P., Moddermam, P., & van Spronsen, F. (2003). A different approach to breast-feeding of the infant with phenylketonuria. *European Journal of Pediatrics, 162*(5), 323-326.

Wong, R., DeSandre, G., Sibley, E., & Stevenson, D. (2006). Neonatal jaundice and liver disease. In R. Martin, A. Fanaroff, & M. Walsh (Eds.), *Fanaroff and Martin's neonatal-perinatal medicine: Diseases of the fetus and infant* (8th ed.). Philadelphia: Mosby.

Yellon, R., McBride, T., & Davis, H. (2002). Otolaryngology. In B. Zitelli, & H. Davis (Eds.), *Atlas of pediatric physical diagnosis* (4th ed.), St. Louis: Mosby.

Nursing Care of the High Risk Newborn

learning objectives

- Analyze the differences in the characteristics of preterm, near-term, term, postterm, and postmature neonates.
- Discuss respiratory distress syndrome and the approach to treatment.
- Compare methods of oxygen therapy.
- Analyze the appropriate nursing interventions for nutritional care of the preterm infant.
- Discuss the pathophysiology of retinopathy of prematurity and bronchopulmonary dysplasia (BPD) and the risk factors that predispose preterm infants to these problems.

- Discuss pain assessment and management in the preterm infant.
- Describe the signs and symptoms of perinatal asphyxia.
- Analyze the pathophysiology of meconium aspiration syndrome and its clinical signs.
- Plan developmentally appropriate care.
- Discuss the needs of parents of high risk infants.
- Evaluate a neonatal transport plan.
- Explain appropriate responses and interventions the nurse can use in caring for families experiencing anticipatory grief or loss and grief in the neonatal period.

electronic resources

Additional information related to the content in Chapter 40 can be found on

the companion website at **evolve**
http://evolve.elsevier.com/Lowdermilk/MWHC/
- NCLEX Review Questions
- WebLinks

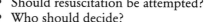

or on the interactive companion CD
- NCLEX Review Questions
- Critical Thinking Exercise: Patent Ductus Arteriosus
- Plan of Care: The High Risk Premature Newborn

MODERN technology and expert nursing care have made important contributions to improving the health and overall survival of high risk infants. However, infants who are born considerably before term and survive are particularly susceptible to the development of sequelae related to their preterm birth. These conditions, which also can occur in term and near-term infants, but not so frequently, include necrotizing enterocolitis, bronchopulmonary dysplasia (BPD), intraventricular and periventricular hemorrhage, and retinopathy of prematurity (ROP). The focus of this chapter is on care of the preterm infant. Care of other high risk infants with gestational age–related problems also is discussed.

■ PRETERM INFANTS

Preterm infants are at risk because their organ systems are immature and they lack adequate reserves of bodily nutrients. The potential problems and care needs of the preterm infant weighing 2000 g differ from those of the term, post-

term, or postmature infant of equal weight. If these infants have physiologic disorders and anomalies as well, these affect the infant's response to treatment. In general, the closer infants are to term from the standpoint of both gestational age and birth weight, the easier their adjustment to the external environment. The cost of the care required by low-birth-weight (LBW) infants is estimated to be in the billions of dollars each year and is increasing as the use of technology increases.

Varying opinions exist about the practical and ethical dimensions of resuscitation of extremely low-birth-weight infants (those infants whose birth weight is 1000 g or less). Ethical issues associated with resuscitation that nurses caring for such infants are confronted with include the following:
- Should resuscitation be attempted?
- Who should decide?
- Is the cost of resuscitation justified?
- Do the benefits of technology outweigh the burdens in relation to the quality of life?

All people involved (health care providers, parents, ethicists, clergy, attorneys) should participate in the discussions in which these controversial issues are addressed.

■ CARE MANAGEMENT

■ Assessment and Nursing Diagnoses

For the high risk infant, an accurate assessment of gestational age (see Chapter 26) is critical in helping the nurse identify the potential problems the newborn is likely to have. The response of the preterm or postterm infant to extrauterine life is different from that of the term infant. By understanding the physiologic basis of these differences, the nurse can assess these infants, determine the response of the preterm or postterm infant, and discern which potential problems are most likely to occur.

■ *Physiologic Functions*

Respiratory Function. The preterm infant is likely to have difficulty making the pulmonary transition from intrauterine to extrauterine life. Numerous problems may affect the respiratory systems of preterm infants and may include the following:
- Decreased number of functional alveoli
- Deficient surfactant levels
- Smaller lumen in the respiratory system
- Greater collapsibility or obstruction of respiratory passages
- Insufficient calcification of the bony thorax
- Weak or absent gag reflex
- Immature and friable capillaries in the lungs
- Greater distance between functional alveoli and the capillary bed

In combination, these deficits severely hinder the infant's respiratory efforts and can produce respiratory distress or apnea.

Respiratory difficulty often follows a progressive pattern. Infants normally breathe between 30 and 60 breaths/min, relying significantly on their abdominal muscles to accomplish this. However, the respiratory rate may increase without a change in rhythm. Early signs of respiratory distress include flaring of the nares and an expiratory grunt. Depending on the cause, retractions may begin as subcostal, suprasternal, or clavicular retractions (Fig. 40-1). If the infant shows increasing respiratory effort—for example, seesaw breathing patterns, retractions, flaring of the nares, expiratory grunts, and/or apneic spells (Fig. 40-2)—this indicates deepening distress. A compromised infant's color progresses from pink to circumoral cyanosis and then to generalized cyanosis. Acrocyanosis deepens. (Acrocyanosis is a normal finding in the neonate, but central cyanosis indicates the existence of an underlying problem.)

Periodic breathing is a respiratory pattern commonly seen in preterm infants. Such infants exhibit 5- to 10-second respiratory pauses followed by 10 to 15 seconds of compensatory rapid respirations. Such periodic breathing should not be confused with apnea, which is a 15- to 20-second ces-

FIG. 40-1 Retractions: Substernal, subcostal, and intercostal retractions are evident. (Courtesy Ross Laboratories, Columbus, OH.)

sation of respiration. The nurse must be prepared to provide oxygen and ventilation as necessary.

Cardiovascular Function. Evaluation of heart rate and rhythm, skin color, blood pressure, perfusion, pulses, oxygen saturation, and acid-base status provides information on the cardiovascular status. The nurse must be prepared to intervene if symptoms of hypovolemia or shock, or both, are found. These symptoms include hypotension, slow capillary refill (longer than 3 seconds), and continued respiratory distress despite the provision of oxygen and ventilation.

An accurate and timely blood pressure reading can assist in making an early diagnosis of cardiorespiratory disease and in monitoring the effects of fluid therapy. Blood pressure readings can be obtained by the Doppler method or by an electronic monitor.

Maintaining Body Temperature. Preterm infants are susceptible to temperature instability as a result of numerous factors. Preterm infants are at high risk for heat loss because of their large body surface area in relation to weight. Other factors that place preterm infants at risk for temperature instability include the following:
- Minimal insulating subcutaneous fat
- Limited stores of brown fat (an internal source for the generation of heat present in normal term infants)
- Fragile capillaries
- Decreased or absent reflex control of skin capillaries (shiver response)
- Inadequate muscle mass activity (rendering the preterm infant unable to produce its own heat)
- Poor muscle tone resulting in more body surface area being exposed to the cooling effects of the environment
- An immature temperature regulation center in the brain

The goal of thermoregulation is to create a **neutral thermal environment (NTE)**, which is the environmental temperature at which oxygen consumption is minimal

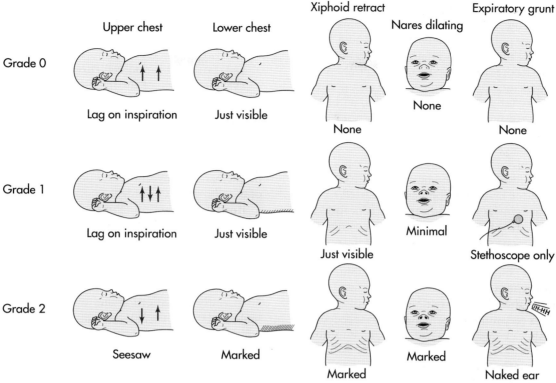

FIG. 40-2   Observation of retractions. Silverman-Anderson index of respiratory distress is determined by grading each of five arbitrary criteria: *grade 0*, no respiratory difficulty; *grade 1*, moderate
difficulty; *grade 2*, maximum difficulty. The retraction score is a sum of these values; a total score of
0 indicates no dyspnea, whereas a total score of 10 indicates maximal respiratory distress. (Modified from Silverman, W., & Anderson, D. [1956]. A controlled clinical trial of effects of water mist on
obstructive respiratory signs, death rate and necropsy findings among premature infants. *Pediatrics,*
17[1], 1-10.)

but adequate to maintain the body temperature (Kenner,
2003). Armed with the knowledge of the four mechanisms
of heat transfer (convection, conduction, radiation, and
evaporation), the nurse can then create an environment
for the preterm infant that prevents temperature instability (see Chapter 25). The infant will be kept in a radiant
warmer or isolette with control settings at a temperature
to maintain the NTE. Because the preterm infant has few
reserves (extra energy calories, minimal or no fat stores),
cold sensitivity is a problem. This infant can easily lose
heat and experience stress from the cold. Physiologically
the infant tries to conserve heat and burns more calories, and the metabolic system goes into overdrive, further stressing the already compromised neonate. There
is mounting evidence to support the need for maintaining a watchful eye on increases in external heat sources
as preterm infants' rectal and nasopharyngeal temperatures change more than might be expected (Simbruner,
Ruttner, Schulze, & Perzlmaier, 2005). The nurse's role
is to prevent or minimize cold stress by recognizing the
risk factors and using intervention strategies to prevent
and treat such stress. Signs of cold stress are listed in Box
40-1. Overheating can also lead to apnea, tachycardia,
and eventually bradycardia, as well as consumption of
calories that the preterm infant cannot afford to expend
(Simbruner et al.).

box 40-1	Signs of Cold Stress
Skin temperature	Decreases before other signs
Respiratory rate	Initially increases, then apneic spells occur
Heart rate	Initially increases, then bradycardia occurs
Skin color	Mottled with acrocyanosis increasing to cyanosis
Physical activity	Increased in term infants without respiratory distress
	Decreased in term infants with respiratory distress
	Decreased in premature infants
Thermoregulatory control	Unstable in premature infants

Central Nervous System Function. The preterm in-
fant's central nervous system (CNS) is susceptible to injury
as a result of the following problems:
- Birth trauma that includes damage to immature
  structures
- Bleeding from fragile capillaries
- An impaired coagulation process, including prolonged
  prothrombin time
- Recurrent anoxic episodes
- Predisposition to hypoglycemia

Research evidence indicates that the developing nervous system has the ability to reorganize neural connection after injury, meaning that some injuries that would be permanent in adults are not so in infants. Certain neurologic signs appear to be predictive of later neurologic abnormalities. These signs include hypotonia, a decreased level of activity, weak cry for more than 24 hours, and an inability to coordinate suck and swallow. Ongoing assessment and documentation of these neurologic signs is needed for the purpose of discharge teaching and making follow-up recommendations, as well as for their predictive value.

A new area of research is "brain nurturing." This refers to examination of brain development as related to postnatal experiences including child care and education (Ito, 2004). Linkages are sought between brain development and long-term conditions such as attention deficit disorder and learning disabilities. The thought is that the brain can be nurtured toward more positive developmental outcomes if these linkages exist.

Maintaining Adequate Nutrition. The goal of neonatal nutrition is to promote normal growth and development. However, the maintenance of adequate nutrition in the preterm infant is complicated by problems with intake and metabolism. The preterm infant has the following disadvantages with regard to intake: weak or absent suck, swallow, and gag reflexes; a small stomach capacity; and weak abdominal muscles. The preterm infant's metabolic functions are compromised by a limited store of nutrients, a decreased ability to digest proteins or absorb nutrients, and immature enzyme systems.

The nurse must continuously assess the infant's ability to take in and digest nutrients. Some preterm infants require gavage or intravenous (IV) feedings instead of oral feedings. An area of research that holds promise for preterm infants is use of minimal enteral nutrition (MEN) that may only be 1 ml/hr (Hawthorne, Griffin, & Abrams, 2004; Tyson & Kennedy, 2002). These feedings stimulate the gastrointestinal system with minute amounts of formula or breast milk, usually given via gavage, so that when enteral feedings can really begin, the gastrointestinal system is primed for nutrient absorption.

Maintaining Renal Function. The preterm infant's immature renal system is unable to (1) adequately excrete metabolites and drugs; (2) concentrate urine; or (3) maintain acid-base, fluid, or electrolyte balance. Therefore intake and output, as well as specific gravity, must be assessed. Laboratory tests must be done to assess acid-base and electrolyte balance. Medication levels also are monitored in preterm infants because certain medications can overwhelm the immature system's ability to excrete them.

Maintaining Hematologic Status. The preterm infant also is particularly predisposed to hematologic problems because of the following problems:

- Increased capillary fragility
- Increased tendency to bleed (prolonged prothrombin time and partial thromboplastin time)

- Slowed production of red blood cells resulting from rapid decrease in erythropoiesis after birth
- Loss of blood due to frequent blood sampling for laboratory tests
- Decreased red blood cell survival related to the relatively larger size of the red blood cell and its increased permeability to sodium and potassium

The nurse assesses such infants for any evidence of bleeding from puncture sites and the gastrointestinal (GI) tract. Infants also are examined for signs of anemia (decreased hemoglobin and hematocrit levels, pale skin, increased apnea, lethargy, tachycardia, and poor weight gain). Amount of blood drawn is recorded.

Resisting Infection. Preterm infants are at increased risk for infection because they have a shortage of stored maternal immunoglobulins, an impaired ability to make antibodies, and a compromised integumentary system (thin skin and fragile capillaries). Preterm infants exhibit various nonspecific signs and symptoms of infection (Box 40-2). Early identification and treatment of sepsis are essential (see Chapter 38). As with all aspects of care, strict attention to handwashing is the single most important measure to prevent iatrogenic infections.

▬ Growth and Development Potential

Although it is impossible to predict with complete accuracy the growth and development potential of each preterm infant, some findings support an anticipated favorable outcome in the absence of ongoing medical sequelae that can affect growth, such as BPD, necrotizing enterocolitis, and CNS problems. The lower the birth weight, the greater the likelihood for negative sequelae. The growth

---

box 40-2 | **Signs and Symptoms of Infection**

Temperature instability
- Hypothermia
- Hyperthermia

Central nervous system changes
- Lethargy
- Irritability

Changes in color
- Cyanosis, pallor
- Jaundice

Cardiovascular instability
- Poor perfusion
- Hypotension
- Bradycardia/tachycardia

Respiratory distress
- Tachypnea
- Apnea
- Retractions, nasal flaring, grunting

Gastrointestinal problems
- Feeding intolerance
- Vomiting
- Diarrhea
- Glucose instability

Metabolic acidosis

and development milestones (e.g., motor milestones, vocalization, growth) are corrected for gestational age until the child is approximately 2½ years old.

The age of a preterm newborn is corrected by adding the gestational age and the postnatal age. For example, an infant born at 32 weeks of gestation 4 weeks ago would now be considered 36 weeks of age. The infant's corrected age at 6 months after the birth date is then 4 months, and the infant's responses are accordingly evaluated against the norm expected for a 4-month-old infant.

Certain measurable factors predict normal growth and development. The preterm infant experiences catch-up body growth during the first 2 years of life; this is most likely to occur when the infant has a normal birth length (Kliegman, 2006). The head is the first to experience catch-up growth, followed by a gain in weight and height. At the infant's discharge from the hospital, which usually occurs between 37 and 40 weeks of postconceptional age, the infant should exhibit the following characteristics:

- An ability to raise the head when prone and to hold the head parallel with the body when tested for the head-lag response
- An ability to cry with vigor when hungry
- An appropriate amount and pattern of weight gain according to a growth grid
- Neurologic responses appropriate for corrected age

At 39 to 40 weeks of corrected age, the infant should be able to focus on the examiner's or parent's face and to follow with his or her eyes.

Of very low-birth-weight (VLBW) (<1500 g) survivors, approximately 15% to 25% will have neurologic and/or cognitive disabilities in varying degrees of severity (Wilson-Costello & Hack, 2006). Research is focused on examining other factors including environmental ones that may cause adverse cognitive and neurodevelopmental outcomes for VLBW and extremely low-birth-weight (ELBW) babies by the time they reach infancy or school age (Vohr et al., 2005).

▬ *Parental Adaptation to Preterm Infant*

The experience of parents whose infant is born prematurely or is otherwise high risk is different from the experience of parents whose infant is born at term and is normal (Davis & Stein, 2004; Holditch-Davis, Cox, Miles, & Belyea, 2003; Swartz, 2005). This may cause parental attachment and the adaptation to the parental role to differ as well.

Parental Tasks. Parents of preterm infants must accomplish numerous psychologic tasks before effective relationships and parenting patterns can evolve. These tasks include the following:

- Experiencing anticipatory grief over the potential loss of an infant. The parent grieves in preparation for the infant's possible death, although the parent clings to the hope that the infant will survive. This process begins during labor and lasts until the infant dies or shows evidence of surviving. Anticipatory grief occurs when families have knowledge of an impending loss, such as when a baby is admitted to a neonatal intensive care unit (NICU) with problems or when a diagnosis of an anencephalic fetus is made with ultrasonography. The baby is still alive, but the prognosis is poor. Being able to anticipate the loss gives families an opportunity to plan, feel more in control of their situation, and say good-bye in a special way. However, some individuals or family members may distance or detach themselves from the experience or from their loved ones as a way of protecting themselves from the pain of loss and grief. How a parent responds to this situation depends on religious, spiritual, and cultural beliefs. These must be considered when planning care. The nurse's role is to advocate for the family so that other health professionals realize that the family is grieving. Being fully present for these families and practicing active listening is important (see Chapter 41).
- The mother's acceptance of her failure to give birth to a healthy, full-term infant. Grief and depression typify this phase, which persists until the infant is out of danger and is expected to survive.
- Resuming the process of relating to the infant. As the baby's condition begins to improve and the baby gains weight, feeds by nipple, and is weaned from the incubator or radiant warmer, the parent can begin the process of developing an attachment to the infant that was interrupted by the infant's critical condition at birth.
- Learning about the ways in which this baby differs in terms of his or her special needs and growth patterns, care giving needs, and growth and development expectations.
- Adjusting the home environment to accommodate the needs of the new infant. Parents are encouraged to limit the number of visitors to minimize exposure of the infant to pathogens. The environmental temperature may have to be altered to optimize conditions for the infant.

Grandparents and siblings also react to the birth of the preterm infant. Parents must deal with the grief of grandparents and the bewilderment and anger of the infant's siblings at the seemingly disproportionate amount of parental time spent on the newborn.

Parental Responses. Parents progress in interactions with their infants from maintaining an *en face* position, stroking, and touching their infant (Fig. 40-3 and Fig. 40-4) to assuming some infant activities, such as feeding, bathing, and changing the infant. Parents go through numerous phases of adjustment as they learn to parent their infant. Nurses assist the transition to parenthood through their teaching and support of parental efforts.

Parenting Disorders. The incidence of physical and emotional abuse has been found to be greater in infants who, because of preterm birth or illness, are separated from their parents for a time after birth. Physical abuse

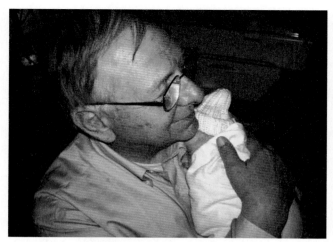

FIG. 40-3 Grandfather with preterm grandchild. (Courtesy Cheryl Briggs, RN, Annapolis, MD.)

includes varying degrees of poor nutrition, poor hygiene, and battering. Emotional abuse ranges from subtle disinterest to outright dislike of the infant to abandonment. Shaken baby syndrome is another possibility with preterm infants. This problem occurs when the child is shaken so violently that brain damage and retinal hemorrhages occur.

■ **NURSE ALERT**

Parents may show preferential treatment toward the brothers and sisters of the infant, discipline the infant harshly for normal behaviors, have extremely high expectations of the infant, or show other types of overt or covert negative parental responses.

Factors surrounding the birth may predispose parents to treat their infant this way because subconsciously they have rejected the infant. These factors might include parental pain and anxiety, a heavy financial burden because of the cost of the infant's care, unresolved anticipatory grief, a threat to self-esteem, or the fact that the infant was the product of an unwanted pregnancy. The goal of health professionals is to identify abuse and neglect early so that further problems can be prevented and, in turn, the incidence of such abuse can be reduced.

Potential nursing diagnoses for high risk infants and their parents include the following:

- *Impaired gas exchange related to*
  –decreased number of functional alveoli
  –deficiency of surfactant
- *Ineffective breathing pattern related to*
  –inadequate chest expansion, secondary to infant position
- *Ineffective thermoregulation related to*
  –immature thermoregulation center
- *Risk for infection related to*
  –invasive procedures
  –decreased immune response

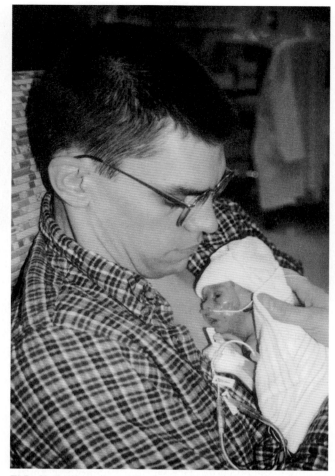

FIG. 40-4 Father providing kangaroo care. (Courtesy Judy Meyr, St. Louis, MO.)

- *Anxiety (parental) related to*
  –lack of knowledge regarding infant condition
  –lack of knowledge regarding infant development
- *Risk for impaired parent/infant attachment*
  –lack of knowledge regarding infant cues

■ **Expected Outcomes of Care**

The plan of nursing care for the preterm infant is directed by the physiologic needs of the infant's immature systems and often involves emergency treatments and procedures. Nursing care is a critical element in determining the infant's chances for survival, as well as normal development. In addition to meeting the infant's physical needs, nursing care is planned in conjunction with parents to promote parent-infant attachment and interaction. Expected outcomes are presented in client-centered terms and include that the infant will do the following:

- Maintain physiologic functioning.
- Maintain adequate nutrition.
- Experience no or minimal hematologic problems.
- Remain free of infection.
- Develop no retinal problems.

- Have no trauma to the immature musculoskeletal system.
- Experience attachment to parents.

Expected outcomes for the parents include that they will do the following:
- Perceive the infant as potentially normal (if this is medically substantiated).
- Provide care competently and comfortably.
- Experience pride and satisfaction in the care of their infant.
- Organize their time and energies to meet the love, attention, and care needs of the other members of the family, as well as their own needs.

▬ Plan of Care and Interventions

The best environment for fetal growth and development is the uterus of a healthy, well-nourished woman. The goal of care for the preterm infant is to provide an extrauterine environment that approximates the healthy intrauterine environment to promote normal growth and development. Physicians, nurses, nurse practitioners, infant developmental specialists, and respiratory therapists work together as a team to provide the intensive care needed.

The admission of a preterm newborn to the intensive care nursery usually represents an emergency situation. Immediately after admission, a rapid initial evaluation is done to determine the infant's need for lifesaving treatment. Resuscitation is started in the birthing unit, and the newborn's need for warmth and oxygen is provided for during transfer to the nursery.

Nursing care is focused on the continuous assessment and analysis of the infant's physiologic status. Nurses fulfill many roles in providing the intensive and extended care that these infants require. In addition, they are the support persons and teachers during the first phase of the parents' adjustment to the birth of their preterm infant.

The nurse uses many technologic support systems to monitor the body responses and maintain the body functions of the infant. Technical skill must be combined with a gentle touch and concern about the traumatic effects of harsh lighting and the volume of machinery noise. The NICU environment may be a major contributing factor to learning and behavioral problems in preterm infants (Symington & Pinelli, 2003). Early interventions within the NICU can have a positive impact on neurobehavioral outcomes (Blauw-Hosper & Hadders-Algra, 2005).

▬ Physical Care

The environmental support measures for the preterm infant typically consist of the following equipment and procedures:
- An incubator or radiant warmer placed over the infant to control body temperature (NTE)
- Oxygen administration, depending on the infant's cardiopulmonary and circulatory status
- Electronic monitors as needed for the observation of respiratory and cardiac functions

- Assistive devices for positioning the infant in neutral flexion and with boundaries
- Clustering of care and minimization of stimulation according to infant cues

Various metabolic support measures that may be instituted consist of the following:
- Parenteral fluids to help support nutrition and maintain normal arterial blood gas (ABG) levels and acid-base balance
- IV access to facilitate the administration of antibiotic therapy if sepsis is a concern
- Blood work to monitor ABG levels, pH, blood glucose levels, electrolytes, and the status of blood cultures

▬ Maintaining Body Temperature

The high risk infant is susceptible to heat loss and its complications. In addition, LBW infants may be unable to increase their metabolic rate because of impaired gas exchange, caloric intake restrictions, or poor thermoregulation. Transepidermal water loss is greater because of skin immaturity in very preterm infants (those at less than 28 weeks of gestation) and can contribute to temperature instability.

High risk infants are cared for in the thermoneutral environment created by use of an external heat source. A probe to an external heat source supplied by a radiant warmer or a servocontrolled incubator is attached to the infant. The infant acts as a thermostat to regulate the amount of heat supplied by the external source. This idealized environment maintains an infant's normal body temperature between 36.5° C and 37.2° C. Maintaining a thermoneutral condition in the youngest, most immature infants decreases the need for them to generate additional heat. As a result, excessive oxygen consumption is prevented in such compromised infants (Blake & Murray, 2002).

▬ Oxygen Therapy

Clinical criteria for identifying the need for oxygen administration include increased respiratory effort, respiratory distress with apnea, tachycardia, bradycardia, and central cyanosis with or without hypotonia. The need for oxygen should be substantiated by biochemical data (arterial oxygen pressure [PaO_2] of less than 60 mm Hg or an oxygen saturation of less than 92%). High risk infants often require saturations of more than 95% to maintain respiratory stability because their hemoglobin levels are frequently low. As the PaO_2 decreases, less oxygen is released from the hemoglobin, which increases the risk for cellular hypoxia.

Oxygen administered to an infant is warmed and humidified to prevent cold stress and drying of the respiratory mucosa. During the administration of oxygen, the concentration, volume, temperature, and humidity of the gas are carefully controlled. Delivery of oxygen for more than a few minutes requires the use of special equipment (hood, nasal cannula, positive-pressure mask, or endotracheal tube) because the concentration of free-flow oxygen cannot be monitored accurately. Free-flow oxygen into an incubator should not be used because the concentration fluctuates dramatically each time the doors or portholes are opened. The indiscriminate use of oxygen may be hazardous. Possible complications of oxygen therapy include retinopathy of prematurity and BPD.

▬ NURSE ALERT
Administration of a therapeutic level of oxygen for a severely depressed infant could cause significant physiologic harm if given to an infant with mild respiratory disease.

Infants who need oxygen should have their respiratory status assessed accurately every 1 to 2 hours; this includes a continuous pulse oximetry reading and at least one ABG measurement (Cifuentes, Segars, & Carlo, 2003). The interventions implemented are then determined on the basis of the findings yielded by the clinical assessment, including telemetry (pulse oximetry or tcPO₂ monitoring) and laboratory tests (Cifuentes et al.). The interventions ordered are those that can directly manage the underlying disease process and range from hood oxygen administration to ventilator therapy.

Hood Therapy. A hood can be used to administer oxygen to infants who do not require mechanical pressure support. The hood is a clear plastic cover that is sized to fit over the head and neck of the infant (Fig. 40-5, *A*). Inside the hood the infant receives the correct amount of oxygen.

The nurse checks the oxygen level every 1 to 2 hours because the concentration must be adjusted in response to the infant's condition.

Nasal Cannula. Infants requiring low-flow amounts of oxygen can benefit from the use of a nasal cannula (Fig. 40-5, *B*). These are of particular value for older infants who are recuperating but still require supplemental oxygen. They are the preferred method for home oxygen administration. They permit the infant to receive an adequate, continuous flow of oxygen while allowing optimal vision, positioning, and parental holding. Infants also can breastfeed while receiving oxygen by this method. However, the nasal prongs must be inspected frequently to make sure they are not partially obstructed by milk or secretions. Nasal cannulas allow easier feedings and psychosocial interactions.

Continuous Positive Airway Pressure Therapy. Infants who are unable to maintain an adequate PaO₂ despite the administration of oxygen by hood or nasal cannula may require the delivery of oxygen by using continuous positive airway pressure (CPAP). CPAP infuses oxygen or air under a preset pressure by means of nasal prongs, a face mask, or an endotracheal tube (Fig. 40-6, *A*). It is often

FIG. 40-6 **A,** Infant receiving ventilatory assistance with nasal continuous positive airway pressure (CPAP). **B,** Infant intubated and on ventilator. (**A,** Courtesy Victoria Langer, RNC, MSN, NNP; from Dickason, E., Silverman, B., & Kaplan, J. [1998]. *Maternal-newborn nursing care* [3rd ed.]. St. Louis: Mosby; **B,** Courtesy Cheryl Briggs, RN, Annapolis, MD.)

FIG. 40-5 **A,** Infant under hood. **B,** Infant with nasal cannula. (**A,** Courtesy Leslie Altimier, MSN, RN, TriHealth, Cincinnati, OH; **B,** Courtesy Cheryl Briggs, RN, Annapolis, MD.)

achieved by sending the oxygen bubbling through water to the infant; this is referred to as bubble CPAP. Research is investigating whether the work of neonatal breathing is improved with bubble CPAP versus variable-flow devices (Liptsen et al., 2005). In either case, an orogastric tube should be used for decompression of the stomach during use of nasal prongs. CPAP increases the functional residual capacity, improves the diffusion time of pulmonary gases, including oxygen, and can decrease pulmonary shunting. If implemented early enough, CPAP may preclude the need for mechanical ventilation (Cifuentes et al., 2003). CPAP can cause vascular shunting in the pulmonary beds, which can lead to persistent pulmonary hypertension and severe respiratory distress.

Mechanical Ventilation. Mechanical ventilation must be implemented if other methods of therapy cannot correct abnormalities in oxygenation (Fig. 40-6, *B*). Its use is indicated whenever blood gas values reveal the existence of severe hypoxemia or severe hypercapnia. The condition of the infant with apnea with bradycardia, ineffective respiratory effort, shock, asphyxia, infection, meconium aspiration syndrome, respiratory distress syndrome, or congenital defects that affect ventilation also may deteriorate and require intubation to reverse the process (Cifuentes et al., 2003). Dexamethasone may be administered to prevent chronic lung disease (Gross, Anbar, & Mettelman, 2005).

The ventilator settings are determined by the infant's particular needs. The ventilator is set to provide a predetermined amount of oxygen to the infant during spontaneous respirations and also to provide mechanical ventilation in the absence of spontaneous respirations. Newer technologies in ventilation allow oxygen to be delivered at lower pressures and in assist modes, thereby preventing the overriding of the infant's spontaneous breathing and providing distending pressures within a physiologic range. Barotrauma and associated complications such as pneumothorax (accumulation of air in the pleural space) and pulmonary interstitial emphysema (PIE) (free air that accumulates in interstitial tissue) are decreased. See Table 40-1 for an explanation of types of mechanical ventilation used in newborns.

Surfactant Administration. Surfactant can be administered as an adjunct to oxygen and ventilation therapy. Before 34 weeks of gestation, most infants do not produce enough surfactant to survive extrauterine life. As a result, lung compliance is decreased, and not enough gas exchange occurs as the lungs become atelectatic and require greater pressures to expand. With administration of artificial surfactant, respiratory compliance is improved until the infant can generate enough surfactant on his or her own. Exogenous surfactant is either artificial or natural and is given in several doses through an endotracheal tube.

table 40-1 Common Methods for Assisted Ventilation in Neonatal Respiratory Distress*

METHOD	DESCRIPTION	HOW PROVIDED
Continuous distending pressure—continuous positive airway pressure (CPAP)	Provides constant distending pressure to airway in spontaneously breathing infant	Nasal prongs Endotracheal tube Face mask Nasal cannula or nasopharyngeal tubes Bubble CPAP uses water resistance
Intermittent mandatory ventilation (IMV)	Allows infant to breathe spontaneously at own rate but provides mechanical cycled respirations and pressure at regular preset intervals; infant may maintain asynchronous ventilation efforts, which diminishes effective gas exchange; uses positive end-expiratory pressure (PEEP)	Endotracheal intubation
Synchronized intermittent mandatory ventilation (SIMV)	Mechanically delivered breaths are synchronized to the onset of spontaneous infant breaths; assist or control (A/C) mode facilitates full inspiratory synchrony; involves signal detection of onset of spontaneous respiration from abdominal movement, thoracic impedance, and airway pressure or flow changes; pressure support ventilation provides an inspiratory pressure assist when spontaneous breathing is detected to decrease infant's work of breathing	Patient-triggered infant ventilator with signal detector and A/C mode; endotracheal tube; SIMV, A/C, and pressure support are also referred to as patient-triggered ventilation
Volume guarantee ventilation	Delivers a predetermined volume of gas using an inspiratory pressure that varies according to the infant's lung compliance (often used in conjunction with SIMV)	Volume guarantee ventilator with flow sensor; endotracheal tube
High-frequency oscillation (HFO)	Application of high-frequency, low-volume, sine-wave flow oscillations to airway at rates between 480 and 1200 breaths/min	Variable-speed piston pump (or loudspeaker, fluidic oscillator); endotracheal tube
High-frequency jet ventilation (HFJV)	Uses a separate, parallel, low-compliant circuit and injector port to deliver small pulses or jets of fresh gas deep into airway at rates between 250 and 900 breaths/min	May be used alone or with low-rate IMV; endotracheal tube

*This is not a comprehensive list of available ventilation modes. For more information, consult specific references on mechanical ventilation such as Donn, S., & Sinha, S. (2003). Invasive and noninvasive neonatal mechanical ventilation. *Respiratory Care, 48*(4), 426-441.

Surfactant has reduced the morbidity and mortality in infants of less than 25 weeks of gestation (Hintz et al., 2005). As with any drug therapy, the infant must be monitored for the occurrence of potential side effects such as a patent ductus arteriosus (PDA) and pulmonary hemorrhage. Use of artificial surfactant has been associated with a significantly reduced length of time on ventilators and oxygen therapy, and an increased survival rate in preterm infants (see Medication Guide).

Extracorporeal Membrane Oxygenation Therapy. Infants with severe pulmonary dysfunction who are older than 34 weeks of gestation may be candidates for extracorporeal membrane oxygenation (ECMO) therapy. ECMO makes use of cardiopulmonary bypass to oxygenate the infant's blood outside the body through a membrane oxygenator. The membrane oxygenator serves as an artificial lung while the infant's lungs heal. Because of the massive systemic anticoagulation therapy required in the pump tubing and the increased risk for hemorrhage, the criteria for its use are very strict, and the use of this therapy is therefore limited (Schwartz, 2003). The risk for intraventricular hemorrhages in preterm infants is particularly high, and for this reason, ECMO therapy cannot be used in them. ECMO has been successful in the treatment of various acute and chronic lung diseases, including meconium aspiration syndrome and persistent pulmonary hypertension of the newborn (Cifuentes et al., 2003).

High-Frequency Ventilation. Other modes of ventilator therapies include high-frequency oscillator ventilation, jet ventilation, flow interruption ventilation, and liquid ventilation (Carlo, Martin, & Fanaroff, 2006; Schwartz, 2003). These methods of high-frequency ventilation work by providing smaller volumes of oxygen at a significantly more rapid rate (more than 300 breaths/min) than do traditional mechanical ventilators. As a result, the intrathoracic pressure is decreased, and along with this, the risk of barotrauma. In liquid ventilation, the surface tension is reduced whereas oxygenation is improved through the re-creation of a fetal lung environment. Instead of air pressure, an experimental oxygenated lipid solution is pumped continuously through the lungs.

Nitric Oxide Therapy. Inhaled nitric oxide (NO), delivered as a gas, causes potent and sustained pulmonary vasodilation in the pulmonary circulation (Schwartz, 2003; Stork, 2006). NO binds with hemoglobin in red blood cells and is inactivated after metabolism. In the few studies conducted with human infants, positive results were seen: oxygen saturation improved, and no toxic effects from methemoglobin or increased levels of nitrogen oxide were documented. NO shows much promise in reducing adverse respiratory sequelae of being born prematurely. Its use has reduced the need for invasive technologies such as ECMO. Neurodevelopmental outcomes are documented as improved at age 2 years following treatment with NO (Mestan, Marks, Hecox, Huo, & Schreiber, 2005).

▄ Weaning from Respiratory Assistance

Respiratory assistance is weaned slowly as the infant's status improves. The infant is ready to be weaned from respiratory assistance once the ABG and oxygen saturation levels are maintained within normal limits. A spontaneous, adequate respiratory effort must be present, and the infant must show improved muscle tone during increased activity. Weaning is done in a stepwise and gradual manner. This may consist of the infant being extubated, placed on CPAP, and then weaned to oxygen by means of a hood or nasal cannula. Throughout the weaning process, the infant's oxygen levels are monitored by pulse oximetry, $tcPO_2$ monitoring, and blood gas levels.

The goal of weaning is the withdrawal of all oxygen support. However, some infants do not achieve this before discharge from the hospital and may require home oxygen therapy for several months. Throughout the weaning period, the infant is assessed for signs and symptoms indicating poor tolerance of the process. These include an increased pulse, respiratory distress, or cyanosis, or a combination of these. If these occur, the amount of oxygen being delivered is increased, and weaning proceeds more slowly while further assessments are done. Underlying causes of intolerance of weaning may be BPD, a PDA, or CNS damage.

▄ Nutritional Care

It is not always possible to provide enteral (by the GI route) nourishment to a high risk infant. Such infants are often too ill or weak to breastfeed or bottle feed because of respiratory distress or sepsis. Early enteral feeding of the asphyxiated neonate with a low Apgar score also is avoided to prevent bowel necrosis. In such cases, nutrition is provided

---

medication guide

Surfactant Replacement: Bovine Lung Extract: Beractant (Survanta) Artificial Surfactant: Colfosceril (Exosurf)

ACTION ▄ These medications provide exogenous surfactant to correct deficiency in lung immaturity.

INDICATIONS ▄ Surfactants are used in the prevention and treatment of respiratory distress syndrome in premature infants. For *prevention,* drug is administered within 15 minutes of birth to infants with clinical manifestations of surfactant deficiency or with a birth weight less than 1250 g. For *treatment,* drug is administered to infants with confirmed diagnosis of respiratory distress syndrome (RDS), preferably within 8 hours of birth.

DOSAGE AND ROUTE ▄ Dosage depends on drug used. Administer via endotracheal tube.

ADVERSE EFFECTS ▄ Adverse reactions include respiratory distress immediately after administration and bradycardia and oxygen desaturation.

NURSING CONSIDERATIONS ▄ Observe infant's condition for changes. Diuresis may occur with improvement. Ventilator settings may need changing as the infant's ability to oxygenate increases.

parenterally. Those infants who require parenteral nutrition may have one or more of the following problems:
- Lack of a coordinated suck-and-swallow reflex
- Inability to suck because of a congenital anomaly
- Respiratory distress requiring aggressive ventilator support
- Asphyxiation with a potential for necrotizing enterocolitis

Type of Nourishment. The types of formulas used, the mode and volume of feeding, and the feeding schedule of the infant are determined on the basis of the findings yielded by assessment of the following variables:
- Initially, the birth weight, and then the current weight of the preterm infant
- Pattern of weight gain or loss (infants weighing less than 1500 g require more energy for growth and thermoregulation and may gain weight poorly with either breast or bottle feedings)
- Presence or absence of suck-and-swallow reflex in all infants at less than 35 weeks of gestation
- Behavioral readiness to take oral feedings
- Physical condition, including presence or absence of bowel sounds, abdominal distention, or bloody stools, as well as presence and degree of respiratory distress or apneic episodes
- Residual from previous feeding, if being gavage-fed
- Malformations (especially GI defects such as gastroschisis, omphalocele or esophageal atresia), including the need for a gastrostomy feeding tube
- Renal function, including urinary output and laboratory values (nitrogen balance, electrolyte balance, glucose level); preterm infants are especially susceptible to altered renal function

Weight and Fluid Loss or Gain. For many reasons, the caloric, nutrient, and fluid requirements of high risk infants are greater than those of the term, normal newborn. One reason is that premature or dysmature (malnourished) newborns often have limited stores of nutrients and fluids. In addition, symptomatic or asymptomatic hypoglycemia, electrolyte imbalances, or other metabolic disturbances can develop in an infant whose nutritional intake is poor. Such hypoglycemia may cause serious damage to carbohydrate-dependent brain cells.

The infant's weight is measured and recorded daily, and the rate of weight loss or gain is calculated. Further depletion of weight and metabolic stores can occur as a result of one or a combination of the following factors:
- Birth asphyxia
- Increased respirations or respiratory effort
- PDA
- Hypothermic environment
- Insensible fluid loss caused by evaporation (with radiant heat or phototherapy)
- Vomiting, diarrhea, and dysfunctional absorption from the GI tract
- Growth demands (a preterm infant's growth rate approximates that of fetal growth during the last trimes-

ter and is at least two times faster than a term infant's growth rate after birth)
- Inability of the renal system to concentrate urine and maintain an adequate rate of urea excretion, as well as infant's inadequate response to antidiuretic hormone

The high risk newborn is predisposed to have weight and fluid losses because of the greater amount of fluid needed to meet the demands of the increased cellular metabolic processes (resulting from stress, repair, or growth). The body weight of preterm infants weighing less than 1500 g consists of 83% to 89% water, compared with the term infant's water content of 71% (Denne, Poindexter, Leitch, Ernst, Lemons, & Lemons, 2002). Most of this water is in the extracellular fluid compartment. Even with the early institution of fluid and nutrition intake, the preterm infant's weight and fluid losses seem exaggerated. Inadequate fluid intake, resulting from either delayed administration or insufficient volume, can further cause weight and fluid losses in the preterm infant.

Insensible water loss (IWL) is an evaporative loss that occurs largely through the skin. Approximately 30% of this IWL comes from the respiratory tract. The total IWL in a normal infant ranges anywhere from 30 to 60 ml/kg/24 hr. The effects of radiant warmers, incubators, phototherapy, and other factors can augment the IWL. Humidifying the respiratory gases administered can prevent some of this loss.

During the first week of extrauterine life, the preterm infant can lose up to 15% of his or her birth weight. In contrast, a weight loss of up to only 10% is acceptable in a term, appropriate-for-gestational-age (AGA) infant. After the initial week, a preterm infant's loss or gain during each 24-hour period should not exceed 2% of the previous day's weight. (To calculate a weight loss or gain, see Box 40-3.)

Increased stooling or voiding, increased evaporative losses, inadequate volume or incorrect fluid administration, and problems with malabsorption may cause weight loss. Implementation of interventions and frequent reassessment of the infant and its environment are necessary to correct the problems. Such interventions include adjusting the incubator temperature; "swamping" or providing high

---

box 40-3 | **Calculation of a Weight Loss or Gain**

EXAMPLE 1

Day 1	1750 g (birth weight)
Day 3	1680 g
	70 g loss

$$\frac{70}{1750} = \frac{X\%}{100\%}$$

$$1750X = 7000$$

$$1750\overline{)7000.0} = 4.0$$

X = 4.0% weight loss

EXAMPLE 2

Day 3	1680 g
Day 4	1720 g
	40 g gain

$$\frac{40}{1680} = \frac{X\%}{100\%}$$

$$1680X = 4000$$

$$1680\overline{)4,000.00} = 2.38$$

X = 2.4% weight gain

levels of humidity under a cover over the radiant warmer; monitoring and adjusting the volume and type of fluids being administered; assessing the urinary output, including the specific gravity; and assessing the blood glucose levels. The glucose determinations are used to assess urine osmolarity and hence renal function. High glucose levels (greater than 125 mg/dl) can stimulate an excessive osmotic diuresis (Hockenberry, 2003).

Weight gain may be due to overfeeding or fluid retention. The nurse reports and records the findings and continues to assess the infant's fluid status, urinary output, and blood glucose levels. The interventions implemented are determined by the infant's specific disorder and nutritional needs.

Elimination Patterns. The infant's elimination patterns also are assessed. This includes the frequency of urination, as well as the amount, color, pH, and specific gravity of the urine. The assessment of the infant's bowel movements includes the frequency of stooling and the character of the stool, as well as whether there is constipation, diarrhea, or loss of fats (steatorrhea). All of these findings are documented. The nurse may request guaiac tests to assess for blood in the stool, tests to detect stool-reducing substances, and a pH determination to assess for malabsorption. Infants with unexplained abdominal dis-

tention are assessed carefully to rule out the presence of hypomotility or obstructions of the GI tract.

Oral Feeding. Nourishment by the oral route is preferred for the infant who has adequate strength and GI function. The best milk for an infant is that of its mother. Breast milk may be fed by breast, bottle, or cup. Formula may be fed by bottle or a supplementer (see Fig. 27-2). Throughout the feeding, the nurse assesses the newborn's tolerance of the procedure. The nurse assists the mother by providing support and help as necessary when the infant breastfeeds. Referral to a lactation consultant is important.

The needs of the high risk infant must be considered when determining the type and frequency of the feedings. Many high risk infants cannot suck well enough to breast-feed or bottle feed until they have recovered from their initial illness or matured physically (corrected age more than 32 weeks of gestation). Mothers of high risk infants are encouraged to continue pumping breast milk, especially if theirs is a very premature infant who may not breastfeed for many weeks. Because of the significant breastfeeding attrition rates among these mothers, they need support and encouragement every few days to continue pumping while their infant is not yet able to nurse. If no breast milk is available (from the mother or a milk bank), commercial formula is used. The calories, protein, and mineral content of commercial formulas vary (see Chapter 27). The type of nipple selected ("preemie," regular, orthodontic) depends on the infant's ability to suck from the specific type of nipple. The nurse also considers the energy the infant needs to expend in the process. However, the current practice of delaying breastfeeding until the baby is able to effectively bottle-feed is not evidence-based since studies continue to confirm that breastfeeding is less stressful than bottle-feeding (Callen & Pinelli, 2005).

Overfeeding of the preterm infant should be avoided because this can lead to abdominal distention, with apnea, vomiting, and possibly aspiration of the feeding. The nurse monitors the infant's abdominal girth when distention is obvious.

Gavage Feeding. Gavage feeding is a method of providing nourishment to the infant who is compromised by respiratory distress, the infant who is too immature to have a coordinated suck-and-swallow reflex, or the infant who is easily fatigued by sucking. In gavage feeding, breast milk or formula is given to the infant through a nasogastric or orogastric tube (Fig. 40-7). This spares the infant the work of sucking.

Gavage feeding can be done either with an intermittently placed tube providing a bolus feeding or continuously through an indwelling catheter. Infants who cannot tolerate large bolus feedings (those on ventilators for more than a week) are given continuous feedings. Minimal enteral nutrition (MEN) may be used to stimulate or prime the GI tract to achieve better absorption of nutrients when bolus or regular intermittent gavage feedings can be given (Hawthorne et al., 2004; Tyson & Kennedy, 2002). Breast milk or formula can be supplied intermittently by using

---

CRITICAL THINKING EXERCISE

Preterm Infant

After having two full-term pregnancies, Charlotte gave birth to her third baby at 28 weeks of gestation. She was transported to a tertiary center prior to the birth so that the infant would receive the care needed. Charlotte lives 60 miles from the city in which the tertiary center is located, and she is to be discharged tomorrow. It is anticipated that the infant will require a stay in the NICU for at least 8 more weeks. You have been caring for Charlotte and are preparing her for discharge. You have spoken to the nurse caring for the baby. The infant is stable at present, receiving a small amount of oxygen, and has started gavage feeding. The intravenous (IV) line is to be discontinued when the infant can tolerate adequate amounts of milk. The nursery has asked for breast milk from Charlotte to feed the baby.

1. Evidence—Is there sufficient evidence to draw conclusions about what to tell Charlotte about her own recovery and the expected progress of the baby?
2. Assumption—What assumptions can be made about the following?
   a. Charlotte's postpartum recovery
   b. The infant's expected progress
   c. The possibility of Charlotte furnishing breast milk for the baby
   d. The long-term outcome for the baby
3. What implications and priorities for nursing care can be drawn at this time?
4. Does the evidence objectively support your conclusion?
5. Are there alternative perspectives to your conclusion?

to prevent the loss of gastric electrolytes. Feeding is usually stopped if the residual is greater than a quarter of the feeding and is not resumed until the infant can be assessed for a possible feeding intolerance.

The orogastric route for gavage feedings is preferred because most infants are preferential nose breathers. Also when indwelling nasogastric tubes are used, there is a tendency toward nares necrosis; however, some infants do not tolerate oral tube placement. A small nasogastric feeding tube can be placed in older infants who would otherwise gag or vomit or in ones who are learning to suck. To insert the tube and give the feeding, the nurse should follow the sequence given in the Procedure boxes.

Gastrostomy Feedings. Infants with certain congenital malformations require gastrostomy feedings. This involves the surgical placement of a tube through the skin of the abdomen into the stomach. The tube is then taped in an upright position to prevent trauma to the incision site. After the site heals, the nurse initiates small bolus feedings per the physician's orders. Feedings by gravity are done slowly over 20- to 30-minute periods. Special care must

FIG. 40-7 Gavage feeding. **A,** Measurement of gavage feeding tube from tip of nose to earlobe and to midpoint between end of xyphoid process and umbilicus. Tape may be used to mark correct length on tube. **B,** Insertion of gavage tube by using orogastric route. **C,** Indwelling gavage tube, nasogastric route. After feeding by orogastric or nasogastric tube, infant is propped on right side for 1 hour to facilitate emptying of stomach into small intestine. Note rolled towel for support. (**A** and **B,** Courtesy Marjorie Pyle, RNC, Lifecircle, Costa Mesa, CA.)

a syringe with gravity-controlled flow, or it can be given continuously by using an infusion pump. The type of fluid instilled is recorded with every syringe change. The volume of the continuous feedings is recorded hourly, and the residual gastric aspirate is measured every 4 hours. Residuals of less than a fourth of a feeding can be refed to the infant

procedure

Inserting a Gavage Feeding Tube

1. Measure the length of the gavage tube from the tip of the nose to the lobe of the ear to the midpoint between the xiphoid process and the umbilicus (see Fig. 40-7, *A*). Mark the tube with a piece of tape.
2. Lubricate the tip of the tube with sterile water and insert gently through the nose or mouth (see Fig. 40-7, *B*) until the predetermined mark is reached. Placement of the tube in the trachea will cause the infant to gag, cough, or become cyanotic.
3. Check correct placement of the tube by
   a. Pulling back on the plunger to aspirate stomach contents. Lack of fluid is not necessarily evidence of improper placement. Respiratory secretions may be mistaken for stomach contents; however, the pH of the stomach contents is much lower (more acidic) than the pH of respiratory secretions.
   b. Injecting a small amount of air (1 to 3 ml) into the tube while listening for gurgling or by using a stethoscope placed over the stomach. Ensure that the tube is inserted to the mark; it is possible to hear air entering the stomach even if the tube is positioned above the gastroesophageal (cardiac) sphincter.
4. Tape the tube in place and also tape it to the cheek to prevent accidental dislodgment and incorrect positioning (see Fig. 40-7, *C*).
   a. Assess the infant's skin integrity before taping the tube.
   b. Edematous or very premature infants should have a pectin barrier placed under the tape to prevent abrasions.*
5. Tube placement must be assessed before each feeding.

* Houska-Lund, C., & Durand, D. (2006). Skin and skin care. In G. Merenstein & S. Gardner (Eds.), *Handbook of neonatal intensive care* (6th ed.). St. Louis: Mosby.

procedure

Gavage Feeding

- To begin the feeding, connect the barrel of a syringe to the gavage tube. While crimping the feeding tube, pour the specified amount of breast milk or formula into the syringe.
- Release the crimp in the tube and allow the feeding to flow down by gravity. The infant usually tolerates the feeding better if the rate approximates that of an oral feeding (about 1 ml/min).
- The parent or nurse can swaddle or hold the infant to help the infant associate the feeding with positive interactions. Some parents like to do kangaroo care while gavage feeding their infant. The parents are encouraged to talk to their infant during the feedings.
- Once the prescribed volume has been delivered, the nurse crimps or pinches the tube and removes the syringe.
- The gavage tube is capped (or the nurse continues to pinch it) while removing it in one steady motion. Capping the tube (or pinching it off) prevents breast milk or formula from leaking from the tube and being aspirated during removal of the tube.
- After the feeding, position the infant on the right side to prevent aspiration (see Fig. 40-7, C).
- Document the procedure: the size of the feeding tube, the amount and quality of the residual from the previous feeding, the type and quantity of fluid instilled (sterile water, breast milk, or formula), and the infant's response to the procedure.

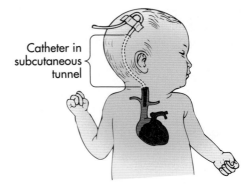

FIG. 40-8 Total parenteral nutrition (TPN). Close-up showing infusion site and internal placement of catheter into descending vena cava.

Catheter in subcutaneous tunnel

be taken to prevent rapid bolusing of the fluid because this may lead to abdominal distention, GI reflux into the esophagus, or respiratory compromise. Meticulous skin care at the tube insertion site is necessary to prevent skin breakdown or infections. In addition, intake and output are monitored scrupulously because these infants are prone to diarrhea until regular feedings are established.

Parenteral Fluids. Feeding supplemental parenteral fluids is indicated for infants who are unable to obtain sufficient fluids or calories by enteral feeding (Fig. 40-8). Some of these infants are dependent on total parenteral nutrition (TPN) for extensive periods. The nurse assesses and documents the following in infants receiving parenteral fluids or TPN:

- Type and infusion rate of the solution
- Functional status of the infusion equipment, including the tubing and infusion pump
- Infusion site for possible complications (phlebitis, infiltration, dislodgment)
- Caloric intake
- Infant's responses to therapy

The physician or nurse practitioner orders TPN per the hospital protocol. These orders must specify the electrolytes and nutrients desired, as well as the volume and rate of infusion. The amounts of calories, protein, and fat are determined on the basis of the individual infant's energy needs (Wyckoff, McGrath, Griffin, Malan, & White-Traut, 2003).

While caring for the infant receiving parenteral fluids or TPN, the nurse secures and protects the insertion site. In addition to observing the principles of asepsis, the nurse must observe the principles of neonatal skin care (Lund & Kuller, 2003). The nurse also should inspect the infusion site for signs of infiltration and reposition the infant frequently to maintain body alignment and protect the site. Parents of infants need to be given explanations about TPN and the way in which the IV equipment and solutions affect their infant.

Advancing Infant Feedings. Feedings are advanced as assessment data and the infant's ability to tolerate the feedings warrant. Documentation of a preterm infant's sucking patterns also can be used to determine its readiness to nipple feed. Feedings are advanced from passive (parenteral and gavage) to active (nipple and breastfeeding). At each step, the nurse must carefully assess the infant's response to prevent overstressing the infant.

The infant receiving nutrition parenterally is gradually weaned off of this type of nutrition. To do this, the nourishment given by continuous or intermittent gavage feedings is increased while the parenteral fluids are decreased. Even the smallest infant is sometimes given MEN to stimulate the GI system to mature and to enhance caloric intake (Wyckoff et al., 2003).

Feedings are advanced slowly and cautiously because, if feedings are advanced too rapidly, the infant may vomit (with an attendant risk of aspiration), with diarrhea, abdominal distention, and apneic episodes. Rapid advancement of feedings also may cause fluid retention with cardiac compromise or a pronounced diuresis with hyponatremia.

If the infant needs additional calories, a commercial human milk fortifier can be added to the gavaged breast milk, or the number of calories per 30 ml of commercial formula can be increased. Soy and elemental formulas are used only for infants with very special dietary needs, such as allergies to cow's milk or chronic malabsorption. Calories in breast milk can be lost if the cream separates and adheres to the tubing during continuous infusion. This problem is decreased if microbore tubing is used for both continuous and intermittent gavage feedings.

The infant receiving gavage feedings progresses to bottle feeding or breast milk feedings. To do this, the gavage feedings are decreased as the infant's ability to suckle breast milk or formula improves. Often during this transition, the infant is fed by both nipple and gavage feeding to ensure the intake of both the prescribed volume of food and nutrients. However, when there is an indwelling tube, during nipple feedings, some infants experience an increased respiratory effort, so nurses must watch for this. The parents need support during this transition because many families measure their parenting competence by how well they can feed their infant. For breastfed infants, weighing before and after a feeding provides documentation of intake (1 gram gain = 1 ml intake), but should be used judiciously (Hall, Shearer, Mogan, & Berkowitz, 2002).

As the time of discharge nears, the appropriate method of feeding, as well as the assessments pertaining to the method (e.g., tolerance of feedings, status of gavage tube placement), are reviewed with the parents. The parents should be encouraged to interact with the infant by talking and making eye contact with the infant during the feeding. This interaction is encouraged to stimulate the psychosocial development of the infant and to facilitate bonding and attachment.

Nonnutritive Sucking. If the gavage or the parenteral route nourishes the infant, nonnutritive sucking is encouraged (Fig. 40-9) for several reasons. Allowing the infant to suck on a pacifier during gavage or between oral feedings may improve oxygenation. In addition, such nonnutritive sucking may lead to a decreased energy expenditure with less restlessness and to positive weight gain, and promote faster attachment to the nipple when oral feedings are initiated (Wyckoff et al., 2003).

Mothers of preterm infants should be encouraged to let their preterm infants start sucking at the breast during kangaroo care (skin-to-skin) because some infant's suck-and-swallow reflexes may be coordinated as early as 32 weeks of gestation.

Infants with intrauterine growth restriction (IUGR) may have an age-appropriate sucking reflex but require thermoregulatory support, making it difficult to breastfeed. These infants also may benefit from nonnutritive sucking at the breast for short periods.

▰ Environmental Concerns

Infants in NICUs also are exposed to high levels of auditory input from the various machine alarms, and this can have adverse effects (Fig. 40-10). In addition, continuous noise levels of 45 to 85 decibels (db) are common in NICUs. An incubator alone produces a constant noise level of 60 to 80 db, and each new piece of life-support equipment used adds another 20 db to the background noise. The infant's hearing may be damaged if it is exposed to a constant decibel level of 90 db or frequent decibel swings higher than 110 db. Cochlear damage has been recognized as a side effect of the NICU environment. Thus both conductive and sensorineural hearing losses have been identified in NICU graduates; these losses lead to long-term speech and language deficits (Haubrich, 2003; Krueger, Wall, Parker, & Nealis, 2005). Based on research findings, Johnson (2003) developed and tested a protocol aimed at noise reduction in the NICU (Box 40-4). It needs to be tested for developmental long-term outcomes.

Respiratory equipment or a phototherapy mask may alter the infant's vision, making it difficult for the infant to interact with caregivers and family members. The infant also may be unable to establish diurnal and nocturnal rhythms because of the continuous exposure to overhead lighting. In addition, sedation or pain medications affect the way in which the infant perceives the environment.

An additional concern in the care of infants is that some drugs used for infant therapy can potentiate environmental hazards. Diuretics (especially furosemide [Lasix]), antibiotics (gentamicin), and antimalarial agents can potentiate noise-induced hearing loss (Haubrich, 2003).

FIG. 40-9 Nonnutritive sucking. (Courtesy Cheryl Briggs, RN, Annapolis, MD.)

FIG. 40-10 Significant environmental stimulation. Note bed, wall oxygen attachments, monitor, ventilator, incubator, and pumps, all of which have alarm systems. (Courtesy Marjorie Pyle, RNC, Lifecircle, Costa Mesa, CA.)

box 40-4 5-Step Process to Develop Noise Reduction Protocol

1. *Assess the NICU environment.* Determine the current noise levels in the NICU.
2. *Develop the protocol.* Findings of the assessment are used to develop the protocol to reduce noise. Sources of noise are analyzed to examine feasibility of change, barriers to change, cost of change, and implications for practice.
3. *Provide educational preparation for the staff.* Provide in-service education and informational posters as well as clear guidelines to guide staff in noise reduction.
4. *Implement the protocol.* Implementation occurs after staff become familiar with the protocol and aware of caregiving activities that contribute to noise.
5. *Evaluate the progress.* Taking intermittent sound level measurements is the most effective way to evaluate progress.

Source: Johnson, A. (2003). Adapting the neonatal intensive care environment to decrease noise. *Journal of Perinatal and Neonatal Nursing, 17*(4), 280-288.

Research is ongoing to determine effects of light and noise on the preterm infant. Long-term problems are the focus of much research (Symington & Pinelli, 2003). Cycling of light and covering of isolettes to reduce direct light hitting the retina are two areas of research. The retina of the immature infant has little protection from the nearly translucent eyelid, thus allowing light to almost continuously penetrate the retina unless it is artificially protected by dimming the lights or using isolette covers. Brandon, Holditch-Davis, and Belyea (2003) have found that cycled lighting on the preterm infant has resulted in more positive growth patterns than if they are kept in very dim light. Light and sound are known adverse stimuli that add to an already stressed preterm infant. The result is stress cues, increased metabolic rates, increased oxygen and caloric use, and depression of the immune system. The nurse must monitor the macroenvironment and the microenvironment (unit and immediate environments) for sources of overstimulation. Providing a developmentally supportive environment can lead to decreased complications and lengths of stay. There are national recommendations for sound and light levels in the NICU.

▬ NURSE ALERT

Routine hearing screening should be performed in all infants before discharge, with universal screening completed by no later than the third month of life.

Nurses can modify the environment to provide a developmentally supportive milieu. In that way, the infant's neurobehavioral and physiologic needs can be met better, the infant's developing organization can be supported, and growth and development fostered (Symington & Pinelli, 2003).

▬ *Developmental Care*

The goal of developmental care is to support each infant's efforts to become as well organized, competent, and stable as possible (Kenner & McGrath, 2004). Developmental care includes all care procedures and the physical and social aspects of care in the NICU (Als et al., 2004). The caregiver uses the infant's own behavior and physiologic functioning as the basis for planning care and providing interventions. Through caregiver observation, the infant's strengths, thresholds for disorganization, and areas in which the infant is vulnerable can be identified (Als et al.). The family is included in developmental care as the primary coregulators (Als et al.). Working together, the family and other caregivers provide opportunities to enhance the strengths of the family and the infant and to reduce the stress that is associated with the birth and care of high risk infants. In some settings, a "cuddler" participates in the care (a specially trained adult volunteer who holds, reads to, talks to, and consoles infant when the parents are unable to visit) (Steuber, Carroll, McCoy, & Nurney, 2002). Mothers of preterm infants need to be taught the importance of interactions with their infant since they tend to do this less than mothers of term infants (Holditch-Davis, Cox et al. 2003).

Reducing light and noise levels by instituting "quiet hours" during each 8 hour shift and positioning are just two of the ways in which nurses can support infants in their development. Sleep interruptions are minimized, and positioning and bundling the infant help promote self-regulation and prevent disorganization (Symington & Pinelli, 2003).

Positioning. The motor development of preterm infants permits less flexion than that in their term counterparts. Caregivers can provide a variety of positions for infants; side-lying and prone are preferred to supine (but only in the nursery) (Fig. 40-11). Body containment with use of blanket rolls, swaddling, holding the infant's arms in a crossed position, and secure holding provide boundaries and promote self-regulation during feeding, procedures, and other stressful interventions (Hendricks-Muñoz, Prendergast, Caprio, & Wasserman, 2002). The prone position encourages flexion of the extremities; a sling or hip roll assists in maintenance of flexion. Use of a sheepskin prevents abrasion of the knees. However, there is some concern that fibers from sheepskin can be breathed in if the infant's face is positioned near the sheepskin itself, so it should be used with caution. Hold-

FIG. 40-11 Positioning of infant while receiving neonatal care. (Courtesy Leslie Altimier, MSN, RN, TriHealth, Cincinnati, OH.)

ing the limbs close to the body when the infant is moved decreases stimulation that produces jerky, uncoordinated movements (Hockenberry, 2003). Proper body alignment is necessary to prevent developmental problems that may affect the ability to walk as the child matures.

Reducing Inappropriate Stimuli. Staff can reduce unnecessary noise by closing doors or portholes on incubators quietly, placing only necessary objects gently on top of incubators, keeping radios at low volume, speaking quietly, and handling equipment noiselessly. Earmuffs for the infant may be used to reduce auditory input (Hockenberry, 2003).

Infants can be protected from light by dimming the lights during the night, placing a blanket over the incubator (Fig. 40-12), or covering the infant's eyes with a mask. Sleep-wake cycles can be induced with such measures. Infants need periods when they are completely undisturbed (Hockenberry, 2003).

Infant Communication. Infants communicate their needs and ability to tolerate sensory stimulation through physiologic responses. The nurses and parents of high risk infants must therefore be alert to such cues. Although term infants may thrive on stimulation, this same stimulation in high risk infants can instead provoke physical symptoms of stress and anxiety (Symington & Pinelli, 2003).

Problems with noxious stimuli and barriers to normal contact may cause anxiety and tension. Clues to overstimulation include averting the gaze, hiccuping, gagging, or regurgitating food. Term infants exhibit a startle reflex, and preterm infants move all of their limbs in an uncoordinated fashion in response to noxious stimuli. An irregular respiratory rate or an increased heart rate may develop in severely distressed infants, and they may then be unable to regain a calm state.

A relaxed infant state is indicated by stabilization of vital signs, closed eyes, and a relaxed posture. Nonintubated infants may make soothing verbal sounds when they are relaxed. Infants requiring artificial ventilation cannot cry audibly and often show their distress through posturing; they relax once their needs are met. As high risk infants

heal and mature, they increasingly respond to stimuli in a self-regulated manner rather than with a dissociated response. Infants who do not show increased self-regulation should be evaluated for a neurologic problem.

Infant Stimulation. A neonatal individualized developmental care and assessment program (NIDCAP) routinely integrates aspects of neurodevelopmental theory with caregivers' observations, environmental interventions, and parental support (Hendricks-Muñoz et al., 2002). Routine reassessment is built into the program's design. Developmental stimuli may consist of such simple measures as placing a waterbed mattress on the top of the infant's mattress or kangaroo (skin-to-skin) holding. The simplest calming technique is to contain the infant's extremities close to the body with both hands. The care of the infant is organized to allow extended periods of undisturbed rest and sleep. Pain medications or sedatives should be administered consistently, per the unit's protocol.

Infants acquire a sense of trust as they learn the feel, sound, and smell of their parents. High risk infants also must learn to trust their caregivers to obtain comfort (Fig. 40-13 and Fig. 40-14). However, caregivers in the nursery

FIG. 40-13 Mother interacts with her preterm infant by touch. (Courtesy Michael S. Clement, MD, Mesa, AZ.)

FIG. 40-12 Infant in double-walled incubator with a blanket for a light shield. (Courtesy Marjorie Pyle, RNC, Lifecircle, Costa Mesa, CA.)

FIG. 40-14 Father interacts with his newborn by stroking and touching infant with fingertips. (Courtesy Michael S. Clement, MD, Mesa, AZ.)

also may inflict pain as part of the care they must give. For this reason, it is important for both the parents and the caregivers of infants to use comforting interventions such as removing painful stimuli, stopping hunger, and changing wet or soiled clothing to foster trust. They can offer nonnutritive sucking opportunities or use oral sucrose for pain relief and topical creams before procedures to avoid the sensation of pain. All of these techniques are part of developmental, supportive care.

When the infant is ready for stimulation, the nurse has many options. All infants can tolerate being held, even if only for short periods. Additional ways for the nurse or parents to stimulate infants include cuddling, rocking, singing, use of music therapy, and talking to the infant. These activities are beneficial, increase weight gain, and decrease time to discharge (Standley, 2002). Stroking the infant's skin during medical therapy can provide tactile stimulation. The caregiver responds to the infant's cues by offering reassurance, providing nonnutritive sucking, stroking the infant's back, and talking to the infant. Infant massage is gaining evidence as a way to promote weight gain (Diego, Field, & Hernandez-Reif, 2005).

Mobiles and decals that can be changed frequently also may be placed within the infant's visual range to stimulate the infant visually. Wind-up musical toys provide rhythmic distractions as long as they are not too loud. If the infant is receiving phototherapy, the protective eye patches are removed periodically (e.g., during feeding) so that the infant can see the caregiver's face for short, comforting sessions.

Kangaroo Care. Kangaroo care (skin-to-skin holding) (see Fig. 40-4) helps infants to interact directly with their parents. In this technique, the infant, dressed only in a diaper, is placed directly on the parent's bare chest and then covered with the parent's clothing or a warmed blanket. In this way, the parent's body temperature also functions as an external heat source that enhances the infant's temperature regulation. Even ventilator-dependent infants weighing less than 1000 g have been found to benefit from this measure, although they usually tolerate it for only 30 minutes or less at a time.

Kangaroo holding was originally developed in Bogotá, Colombia, where radiant warmers and incubators were in severely short supply. Although such care has its roots in severe economic hardships, it stems from a deep respect for natural processes. Infants and parents who participate in kangaroo care have been observed to have dramatically better outcomes (Beal & Wood, 2005; Kledzik, 2005). The mothers report increased breast milk output and fewer feelings of helplessness related to their experiences in the NICU. The infants have been found to maintain their temperatures and oxygenation levels better and to experience fewer episodes of crying, apnea, and periodic respirations. They also have been observed to be alert and quiet longer and to have slightly higher heart rates. Kangaroo care also meets developmental needs by fostering neurobehavioral development.

▬ *Parental Support*

The nurse as the support person and teacher is responsible for shaping the environment and making the care giving responsive to the needs of the parents and infant. Nurses are instrumental in helping parents learn who their infant is and to recognize behavioral cues in his or her development and using these cues in the care they provide (Liaw, Yuh, & Chang, 2005).

If a high risk birth has been anticipated, the family can be given a tour of the NICU or shown a video to prepare them for the sights and activities of the unit. After the birth, the parents can be given a booklet, be shown a video, or have someone describe what they will see when they go to the unit to see their infant. As soon as possible, the parents should see and touch their infant so that they can begin to acknowledge the reality of the birth and the infant's true appearance and condition. They will need encouragement as they begin to accomplish the psychologic tasks imposed by the high risk birth. For the following reasons, a nurse or physician should be present during the parents' first visit to see the infant:

- To help them "see" the infant rather than focus on the equipment. The importance and purpose of the apparatus that surrounds their infant also should be explained to them.
- To explain the characteristics normal for an infant of their baby's gestational age; in this way parents do not compare their child with a term, healthy infant.
- To encourage the parents to express their feelings about the pregnancy, labor, and birth and the experience of having a high risk infant.
- To assess the parents' perceptions of the infant to determine the appropriate time for them to become actively involved in care.

As soon as possible after the birth, the parents are given the opportunity to meet the infant in the *en face* position, to touch the infant, and to see his or her favorable characteristics. Mothers often state that their greatest source of stress is the appearance of their baby (Miles, Burchinal, Holditch-Davis, Brunssen, & Wilson, 2002). As soon as possible, depending primarily on her physical condition, the mother is encouraged to visit the nursery as desired and help with the infant's care. When the family cannot be present physically, staff members devise appropriate methods to keep them in almost constant touch with the newborn, such as with daily phone calls, notes written as if by the infant, or photographs of the infant.

Some hospitals have support groups for the parents of infants in NICUs. These groups help parents experiencing anxiety and grief by encouraging them to share their feelings. Hospitals also often arrange to have an experienced NICU parent make contact with a new group member to provide additional support. The volunteer parents provide support by making hospital visits, phone calls, and home visits. Mothers in particular are prone to posttraumatic stress that may hinder their ability to interact or care for their infant (Holditch-Davis, Bartlett, Blickman, & Miles, 2003).

They need help in expressing their feelings and, when appropriate, referral for psychologic or family counseling.

Many NICUs use volunteers in varying capacities. After they have gone through the orientation program, volunteers can perform tasks such as holding the infants, stocking bedside cabinets, assembling parent packets, and, in some nurseries, feeding the infants.

Some high risk infants can be discharged earlier than the expected time. The criteria showing an infant's readiness for early discharge are that the infant's physiologic condition is stable, the infant is receiving adequate nutrition, and the infant's body temperature is stable. The parents, or other caregivers, also need to exhibit a physical, emotional, and educational readiness to assume responsibility for the care of the infant. Ideally, the home environment is adequate for meeting the needs of the infant. The parents also need to show that they know the way to take the infant's temperature, know the signs and symptoms to report, and understand the dietary needs of the infant. Resources for parents and health care providers include http://premature-infant.com, www.vort.com/age/premature.html, www.neonatology.org, and www.familyvillage.wisc.edu.

■ Parent Education

Cardiopulmonary Resuscitation. Sudden infant death syndrome (SIDS) is 8 to 10 times more likely to develop in preterm infants than in term infants. Furthermore, it has been found that infants discharged from an NICU are about twice as likely to die unexpectedly during the first year of life as are infants in the general population. Instruction in cardiopulmonary resuscitation (CPR) is essential for parents of all infants but especially for those of infants at risk for life-threatening events (see Chapter 28). Infants considered at risk include those who are preterm, have apnea or bradycardia spells, or have a tendency to choke. Before taking their infant home, parents must be able to administer CPR. All parents should be encouraged to obtain instruction in CPR at their local Red Cross or other community agency, if it is not provided by the NICU.

■ Evaluation

The nurse uses the previously stated expected outcomes of care to evaluate the effectiveness of the physical and psychosocial aspects of care (see Plan of Care).

■ COMPLICATIONS IN HIGH ■ RISK INFANTS

Respiratory Distress Syndrome

Respiratory distress syndrome (RDS) refers to a lung disorder usually affecting preterm infants. Maternal and fetal conditions associated with a decreased incidence and severity of RDS include female infant, African-American race, maternal gestational hypertension, maternal drug abuse, maternal steroid therapy (betamethasone), chronic retroplacental abruption, prolonged rupture of membranes, and IUGR. The incidence and severity of RDS increase with a decrease in the gestational age. Perinatal asphyxia, hypovolemia, male infant, Caucasian race, maternal diabetes (types 1 and 2), second-born twin, familial predisposition, maternal hypotension, cesarean birth without labor, hydrops fetalis, and third-trimester bleeding are all factors that place an infant at increased risk for RDS. The incidence of RDS in infants weighing less than 1500 g is between 40% and 60% (Cifuentes et al., 2003; Schwartz, 2003).

RDS is caused by a lack of pulmonary surfactant, which leads to progressive atelectasis, loss of functional residual capacity, and a ventilation/perfusion imbalance with an uneven distribution of ventilation. This surfactant deficiency may be caused by insufficient surfactant production, abnormal composition and function, disruption of surfactant production, or a combination of these factors. The weak respiratory muscles and an overly compliant chest wall, common among preterm infants, further compromise the sequence of events that occurs. Lung capacity is further compromised by the presence of proteinaceous material and epithelial debris in the airways. The resulting decreased oxygenation, cyanosis, and metabolic or respiratory acidosis can cause the pulmonary vascular resistance (PVR) to be increased. This increased PVR can lead to right-to-left shunting and a reopening of the ductus arteriosus and foramen ovale (Fig. 40-15).

Clinical symptoms of RDS are listed in Box 40-5. These respiratory signs usually appear immediately after birth or within 6 hours of birth. Physical examination reveals crackles, poor air exchange, pallor, the use of accessory muscles (retractions) and, occasionally, apnea. Radiographic findings include a uniform reticulogranular appearance and air bronchograms (Rodriguez, Martin, & Fanaroff, 2006). The infant's clinical course typically is variable, with usually an increased oxygen requirement and increased respiratory effort as atelectasis, a loss of functional residual capacity, and ventilation/perfusion imbalance worsen.

However, RDS is a self-limiting disease, with the respiratory symptoms abating after 72 hours. This disappearance of respiratory signs coincides with the production of surfactant in the type 2 cells of the alveoli.

The treatment for RDS is supportive. Adequate ventilation and oxygenation must be established and maintained in an attempt to prevent ventilation/perfusion mismatch and atelectasis. Exogenous surfactant may be administered

---

box 40-5 Clinical Signs of Respiratory Distress Syndrome

- Tachypnea
- Grunting
- Flaring
- Retractions
- Cyanosis
- Increased work of breathing
- Hypercapnia
- Respiratory or mixed acidosis
- Hypotension and shock

CD: Plan of Care: The High Risk Premature Newborn

NURSING DIAGNOSIS Ineffective breathing pattern related to pulmonary and neuromuscular immaturity, decreased energy, fatigue

Expected Outcomes *Infant exhibits adequate oxygenation (i.e., arterial blood gases [ABGs] and acid-base within normal limits [WNL]; oxygen saturations 92% or greater; respiratory rate and pattern WNL; breath sounds clear; and absence of grunting, nasal flaring, minimal retractions, skin color WNL).*

Nursing Interventions/*Rationales*
- Position neonate prone or supine, avoiding neck hyperextension *to promote optimum air exchange.* Use a side-lying position after feeding or in cases of excessive mucus production *to avoid aspiration.* Avoid Trendelenburg position *because it can cause increased intracranial pressure and reduce lung capacity.*
- Suction nasopharynx, trachea, and endotracheal tube as indicated *to remove mucus.* Avoid oversuctioning *because it can cause bronchospasm, bradycardia, and hypoxia and predispose neonate to intraventricular hemorrhage.*
- Administer percussion, vibration, and postural drainage as prescribed *to facilitate drainage of secretions.*
- Administer oxygen and monitor neonatal response *to maintain oxygen saturation.*
- Maintain a neutral thermal environment *to conserve oxygen use.*
- Monitor arterial blood gases, acid-base balance, oxygen saturation, respiratory rate and pattern, breath sounds, and airway patency; observe for grunting, nasal flaring, retractions, and cyanosis *to detect signs of respiratory distress.*

NURSING DIAGNOSIS Ineffective thermoregulation related to immature temperature regulation and minimal subcutaneous fat stores

Expected Outcome *Infant exhibits maintenance of stable body temperature within normal range for postconceptional age (36.5° C to 37.2° C).*

Nursing Interventions/*Rationales*
- Place neonate in a prewarmed radiant warmer *to maintain stable temperature.*
- Place temperature probe on neonatal abdomen *to control heat levels in radiant warmer.*
- Take axillary temperature periodically *to monitor temperature and cross-check functioning of warmer unit.*
- Avoid infant exposure to cool air and drafts, cold scales, cold stethoscopes, cold examination tables, and prolonged bathing *that predispose the infant to heat loss.*
- Monitor probe frequently *since detachment can cause overheating or warmer-induced hyperthermia.*
- Transfer infant to a servocontrolled open warmer bed or incubator *when temperature has stabilized.*

NURSING DIAGNOSIS Risk for infection related to immature immune system

Expected Outcome *Infant exhibits no evidence of nosocomial infection.*

Nursing Interventions/*Rationales*
- Institute scrupulous handwashing techniques before and after handling neonate, ensure all supplies and/or equipment are clean before use, and ensure strict aseptic technique with invasive procedures *to minimize exposure to infective organisms.*
- Prevent contact with persons who have communicable infections, and instruct parents in infection-control procedures *to minimize infection risk.*

- Administer prescribed antibiotics *to provide coverage for infection during sepsis workup.*
- Continuously monitor vital signs for stability *since instability, hypothermia, or prolonged temperature elevations serve as indicators for infection.*

NURSING DIAGNOSIS Risk for imbalanced nutrition: less than body requirements related to inability to ingest nutrients secondary to immaturity

Expected Outcomes *Infant receives adequate amount of nutrients with sufficient caloric intake to maintain positive nitrogen balance; demonstrates steady weight gain.*

Nursing Interventions/*Rationales*
- Administer parenteral fluid/total parenteral nutrition (TPN) as prescribed *to provide adequate nutrition and fluid intake.*
- Monitor for signs of intolerance to TPN, *which can interfere with effective replenishment of nutrients.*
- Periodically assess readiness to orally feed (i.e., strong suck, swallow, and gag reflexes) *to provide appropriate transition from TPN to oral feeding as soon as neonate is ready.*
- Advance volume and concentration of formula when orally feeding per unit protocol *to avoid overfeeding and feeding intolerance.*
- If mother desires to breastfeed when neonate is stable, demonstrate how to express milk *to establish and maintain lactation until infant can breastfeed.*

NURSING DIAGNOSIS Risk for deficient fluid volume/excess fluid volume related to immature physiology

Expected Outcome *Infant exhibits evidence of fluid homeostasis.*

Nursing Interventions/*Rationales*
- Administer parenteral fluids as prescribed and regulate carefully *to maintain fluid balance.* Avoid hypertonic fluids such as undiluted medications, and concentrated glucose *because they can cause excess solute load on immature kidneys.*
- Implement strategies (e.g., use of plastic covers and increase of ambient humidity) *that minimize insensible water loss.*
- Monitor hydration status (i.e., skin turgor, blood pressure, edema, weight, mucous membranes, fontanels, urine specific gravity, electrolytes) and intake and output *to evaluate for evidence of dehydration or overhydration.*

NURSING DIAGNOSIS Risk for impaired skin integrity related to immature skin structure, immobility, or invasive procedures

Expected Outcome *Infant's skin remains intact, with no evidence of irritation or injury.*

Nursing Interventions/*Rationales*
- Cleanse skin as needed with plain warm water and apply moisturizing agents to skin *to prevent dryness and reduce friction across skin surface.*
- When performing procedures: minimize use of tape and apply a skin barrier between tape and skin; use transparent elastic film for securing central and peripheral lines; use limb electrodes for monitoring or attach with hydrogel and rotate electrodes frequently; remove adhesives with soap and water rather than alcohol or acetone-based adhesive removers *to minimize skin damage.*
- Monitor use of thermal devices such as warmers or heating pads carefully *to prevent burns.*

plan of care	The High Risk Premature Newborn—cont'd

Nursing Interventions/*Rationales*

- Monitor skin closely for evidence of redness, rash, irritation, bruising, breakdown, ischemia, and infiltration *to detect and treat potential complications early.*

NURSING DIAGNOSIS Risk for injury related to increased intracranial pressure (ICP) and intraventricular hemorrhage secondary to immature central nervous system

Expected Outcome *Infant will exhibit normal ICP with no evidence of intraventricular hemorrhage.*

Nursing Interventions/*Rationales*

- Institute minimum stimulation protocol (i.e., minimal handling, clustering care techniques, avoidance of sudden head movements to one side, undisturbed sleep periods, light variations to simulate day and night, limiting personnel and equipment noise in environment) *to decrease stress responses, which can increase ICP.*
- Institute ordered pharmacologic and nonpharmacologic pain control methods *to manage pain and reduce physical stress.*
- Avoid hypertonic solutions and medications *since they increase cerebral blood flow.*
- Elevate head of bed 15 to 20 degrees *to decrease ICP.*
- Monitor vital signs *for evidence of ICP.*
- Recognize signs of overstimulation (i.e., flaccidity, yawning, irritability, crying, staring, active averting) *so stimulation can be stopped to allow rest.*

NURSING DIAGNOSIS Impaired parenting related to separation and interruption of parent/infant attachment secondary to premature birth

Expected Outcomes *Parents establish contact with neonate; demonstrate competent parenting skills and willingness to care for neonate.*

Nursing Interventions/*Rationales*

- Before parents' first visit to the NICU, prepare them by explaining what the neonate will look like, and what the equipment will look like and its function *to diminish fear and decrease sense of shock.*

- Keep parents informed about infant's condition (improvements and setbacks) and important aspects of infant's care; encourage and answer parental questions; actively listen to parents' concerns *to establish trust, open communication, and caring atmosphere to aid in coping.*
- Encourage parents to visit the NICU often; to name infant (if that is culturally appropriate); to touch, hold, or caress infant as physical condition permits; to be actively involved in infant's care; to bring personal items (i.e., clothing, stuffed animals, or pictures of family) *to allow for formation of emotional bond.*
- Reinforce parents' involvement and praise care endeavors *to increase self-confidence in their contribution.*
- Encourage parents to bring other siblings to visit; explain to siblings what they are seeing; encourage siblings to draw pictures or write letters for infant and place in or near infant's crib *to promote family involvement, help ease sibling fears, and let them contribute to infant's care.*
- Refer parents to social services as needed *to ensure comprehensive care.*

NURSING DIAGNOSIS Anticipatory grieving related to perceived loss of premature infant

Expected Outcomes *Parents express feelings about the potential loss and seek support from staff, family, clergy, and other support systems.*

Nursing Interventions/*Rationales*

- Encourage parents to express feelings about perceived loss of infant *to reinforce reality and help alleviate guilt.*
- Encourage parents to use family, friends, clergy, and other support persons *to enhance coping ability.*
- Plan time on each shift to sit and listen to parents *to demonstrate concern, empathy, and support.*
- Inform parents about support groups in the facility and the community *to encourage parents to use available resources.*

---

at birth or shortly after birth, and this has the effect of altering the typical course of RDS. Positive-pressure ventilation, bubble CPAP, and oxygen therapy may be needed during the respiratory illness. However, the prevention of complications associated with mechanical ventilation also is critical. These complications include pulmonary interstitial emphysema, pneumothorax, pneumomediastinum, and pneumopericardium. The mortality and morbidity rates associated with RDS are attributed to the immature organ systems of the infant and the complications associated with the treatment of the disease (Rodriguez et al., 2006).

Acid-base balance is evaluated by monitoring the ABG values (Table 40-2). Frequent blood sampling requires arterial access either by umbilical artery catheterization or by a peripheral arterial line. Pulse oximetry and transcutaneous carbon dioxide and oxygen monitors document trends in ventilation and oxygenation. Capillary blood gas values indicate the pH and Pco_2 status in infants who are in more stable condition.

The maintenance of an NTE continues to be of critical importance in infants with RDS because infants with hypoxemia are unable to increase their metabolic rate when cold stressed (Rodriguez et al., 2006).

The clinical and radiographic presentation (radiodense lung fields and air bronchograms) of neonatal pneumonia may be similar to that of RDS. Fluid in the minor tissue also may be noted in infants with neonatal pneumonia. Therefore sepsis evaluation, including blood culture and complete blood count (CBC) with differential, is done in infants with RDS to rule out neonatal pneumonia. Occasionally a lumbar puncture is done as part of the sepsis evaluation. Broad-spectrum antibiotics are begun while the results of cultures are awaited.

Fluid and nutrition must be maintained in the critically ill infant with RDS. Parenteral nutrition can be implemented to provide protein and fats to promote a positive nitrogen balance. Daily monitoring of the electrolyte values, urinary output, specific gravity, and weight help evaluate the infant's hydration status.

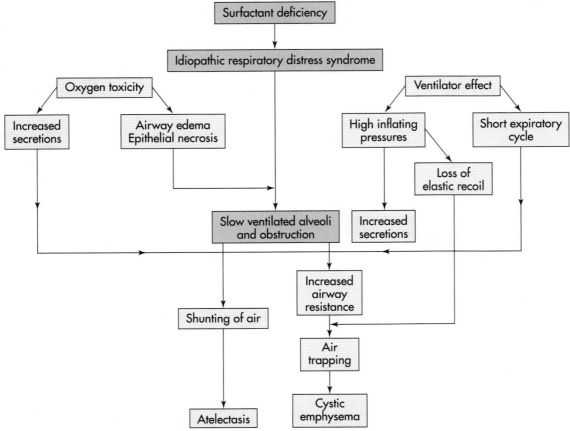

FIG. 40-15 Pathogenesis of respiratory distress syndrome (RDS). (From Hagedorn, M., Gardner, S., Dickey, L., & Abman, S. [2006]. Respiratory diseases. In G. Merenstein, & S. Gardner. [Eds.], *Handbook of neonatal intensive care* [6th ed.]. St. Louis: Mosby.)

table 40-2 Normal Arterial Blood Gas Values for Neonates

VALUE	RANGE
pH	7.32-7.49
Arterial oxygen pressure (PaO_2)	60-70 mm Hg
Carbon dioxide pressure ($PaCO_2$)	26-41 mm Hg
Bicarbonate (HCO_3)	16-24 mEq/L
Oxygen saturation	40%-90%

From Pagana, K., & Pagana, T. (2005). *Mosby's diagnostic and laboratory test reference* (7th ed.). St. Louis: Mosby.

Frequent blood sampling may make blood transfusions necessary. The critically ill infant usually needs to have a venous hematocrit level of more than 40% to maintain adequate oxygen-carrying capacity.

▬ NURSE ALERT

Directed-donor blood may be requested. This donor blood usually is obtained from a family member or close friend of the family who has the same blood type as the infant or a compatible blood type. It may be necessary to notify the infant's family of the potential need for blood transfusion on admission to allow for the processing of directed-donor blood.

Reassuring the family that stringent testing of all blood products is done may alleviate some of their anxiety about the transmission of blood-borne pathogens such as human immunodeficiency virus (HIV) and hepatitis B. Because some religions prohibit the use of blood transfusions, it is critical to obtain a complete history from the family, including their religious preference. Alternative strategies for maintaining the hematocrit may be used in these instances.

Complications Associated with Oxygen Therapy
Retinopathy of Prematurity

Retinopathy of prematurity (ROP) is a complex multi-cause disorder that affects the developing retinal vessels of preterm infants. The normal retinal vessels begin to form in utero at approximately 16 weeks in response to an unknown stimulus. These vessels continue to develop until they reach maturity at approximately 42 to 43 weeks after conception. Once the retina is completely vascularized, the retinal vessels are not susceptible to ROP. The mechanism of injury in ROP is unclear. Oxygen tensions that are too high for the level of retinal maturity initially result in vasoconstriction. After oxygen therapy is discontinued, neovascularization occurs in the retina and vitreous, with capillary hemorrhages, fibrotic resolution, and possible retinal detachment. Cicatricial (scar) tissue formation and consequent visual impairment may be mild or severe. The entire disease process in severe cases may take as long as 5 months to evolve. Examination by an ophthalmologist before discharge and a schedule for repeated examinations thereafter are recommended for the parents' guidance.

The key to the management of ROP is prevention of preterm birth and early detection. Circumferential cryopexy, laser photocoagulation, vitamin E therapy, and decreasing the intensity of ambient light are used in the prevention and treatment of ROP, with varying results (Phelps, 2006). Research is being done to examine the impact of the NICU environment on the development of ROP in relation to light that shines directly through the very thin eyelid of very immature infants. Ambient lighting in the NICU is known to have an effect on the developing eye; although it may not directly cause ROP, it does contribute to other visual problems for the preterm infant. Another potential contributor to ROP is hyperglycemia, which apparently fosters vasoproliferation (Ertl, Gyarmati, Gaal, & Szabo, 2006). This factor needs much more study.

Bronchopulmonary Dysplasia

Bronchopulmonary dysplasia (BPD) is a chronic pulmonary iatrogenic condition caused by barotrauma from pressure ventilation and oxygen toxicity. The etiology of BPD is multifactorial and includes pulmonary immaturity, surfactant deficiency, lung injury and stretch, barotrauma, inflammation caused by oxygen exposure, fluid overload, ligation of a PDA, and a familial predisposition. With the advent of prenatal use of maternal steroids when preterm birth is expected coupled with use of exogenous surfactant in the neonate, most BPD or chronic lung disease (CLD) has been eliminated.

Clinical signs of BPD include tachypnea, retractions, nasal flaring, increased work of breathing, exercise intolerance (to handling and feeding), and tachycardia. Auscultation of the lung fields in affected infants typically reveals crackles, decreased air movement, and occasionally expiratory wheezing. The treatment for BPD includes oxygen therapy, nutrition, fluid restriction, and medications (diuretics, corticosteroids, bronchodilators). However, the key to the management of BPD is prevention by preventing prematurity and RDS and by using surfactant and other less toxic therapies. Use of high-frequency ventilation and nitric oxide has contributed to the decline of this condition.

The prognosis for infants with BPD depends on the degree of pulmonary dysfunction. Most deaths occur within the first year of life as a result of cardiorespiratory failure, sepsis, or respiratory infection; in some infants, the deaths are sudden and unexplained (Cifuentes et al., 2003; Schwartz, 2003).

Patent Ductus Arteriosus

The ductus arteriosus is a normal muscular contractile structure in the fetus connecting the left pulmonary artery and the dorsal aorta. The duct constricts after birth as oxygenation, the levels of circulating prostaglandins, and the muscle mass increase. Other factors that promote ductal closure include catecholamines, low pH, bradykinin, and acetylcholine. When the fetal ductus arteriosus fails to close after birth, patent ductus arteriosus (PDA) occurs. During the first few days of life when a preterm or sick infant is under stress, this ductus arteriosus can reopen, leading to mottling and cyanosis. It may last only a few minutes until the stress is past, or it may remain open if the infant is quite unstable. The incidence of PDA in preterm infants is 20%, with an increasing incidence in VLBW infants and those with pulmonary disease (Carlo et al., 2006).

The clinical presentation in an infant with a PDA includes systolic murmur, active precordium, bounding peripheral pulses, tachycardia, tachypnea, crackles, and hepatomegaly. The systolic murmur is heard best at the second or third intercostal space at the upper left sternal border. An increased left ventricular stroke volume causes an active precordium. In addition, a widened pulse pressure may result in an increase in peripheral pulses.

Radiographic studies in infants with PDA typically show cardiac enlargement and pulmonary edema. ABG findings reveal hypercapnia and metabolic acidosis. Echocardiography can demonstrate a PDA and can measure the amount of blood shunting across the PDA.

The PDA can be managed medically or surgically. Medical management consists of ventilatory support, fluid restriction, and the administration of diuretics and indomethacin. Indomethacin is a prostaglandin synthetase inhibitor that blocks the effect of the arachidonic acid products on the ductus and causes the PDA to constrict (Rodriguez et al., 2006). Some evidence indicates that use of indomethacin may contribute to the incidence of ROP, but further research must be done. Ventilatory support is adjusted based on the ABG values. Fluid restriction is implemented to decrease cardiovascular volume overload in association with the diuretic therapy. Surgical ligation is done when a PDA is clinically significant and medical management has failed (Rodriguez et al.).

The nursing care of the infant with PDA focuses on supportive care. The infant needs an NTE, adequate oxygenation, meticulous fluid balance, and parental support.

Germinal Matrix Hemorrhage-Intraventricular Hemorrhage

Germinal matrix hemorrhage-intraventricular hemorrhage (GMH-IVH) is one of the most common types of brain injury that occurs in neonates and is among the most severe from the standpoint of both short-term and long-term outcomes. The true incidence of GMH-IVH is unknown, but the incidence is decreasing. The average incidence ranges from 5% to 11% (de Vries, 2006). The decline in

CD: Critical Thinking Exercise: Patent Ductus Arteriosus

incidence is attributed to the prenatal use of corticosteroids and postnatal use of surfactant.

The pathogenesis of GMH-IVH includes intravascular factors (fluctuating or increasing cerebral blood flow, increases in cerebral venous pressures, and coagulopathy), vascular factors, extravascular factors, and nursery care. GMH-IVH events typically occur within the first hours or days of life. The exact location of this hemorrhage varies with gestational age. In the very immature infant (younger than 28 weeks), it usually occurs in or adjacent to the germinal matrix.

GMH-IVH is classified according to a grading system of I to III, with grade I being the least severe, and grade III, the most severe (de Vries, 2006) (Table 40-3).

The long-term neurodevelopmental outcome is determined by the severity of the GMH-IVH. Infants with small hemorrhages usually have good outcomes; infants with posthemorrhagic ventricular dilation and those that require shunt diversion often have long-term morbidity (de Vries, 2006). Hemorrhage associated with a lesion in the area of the periventricular white matter results in necrosis that alters cerebral brain flow in the affected area. This condition is referred to as periventricular leukomalacia (PVL).

Nursing care focuses on recognition of factors that increase the risk of GMH-IVH and PVL, interventions to decrease the risk of bleeding, and supportive care to infants who have bleeding episodes. The infant is positioned with the head in midline and the head of the bed elevated slightly to prevent or minimize fluctuations in intracranial blood pressure. NTE is maintained, as well as oxygenation. Rapid infusions of fluids should be avoided. Blood pressure is monitored closely for fluctuations. The infant is monitored for signs of pneumothorax because it often precedes GMH-IVH.

table 40-3 Grading System for Neonatal Intraventricular Hemorrhage

DESCRIPTION	GENERIC TERM
Grade I: Germinal matrix hemorrhage	GMH-IVH
Grade II: Intraventricular hemorrhage without ventricular dilation	GMH-IVH
Grade III: Intraventricular hemorrhage with acute ventricular dilation (clot fills >50% of the ventricle)	GMH-IVH and ventriculomegaly
Intraparenchymal lesion— describe size, location	Intraparenchymal hemorrhage

GMH, Germinal matrix hemorrhage; *IVH,* intraventricular hemorrhage. From de Vries, L. (2006). Intracranial hemorrhage and vascular legions. In R. Martin, A. Fanaroff, & M.Walsh (Eds.). *Fanaroff and Martin's neonatal-perinatal medicine: Diseases of the fetus and infant* (8th ed.). Philadelphia: Mosby.

Necrotizing Enterocolitis

Necrotizing enterocolitis (NEC) is an acute inflammatory disease of the GI mucosa, commonly complicated by perforation. This often fatal disease occurs in about 2% to 5% of newborns in NICUs. Although the cause is unknown, the factors listed in Box 40-6 are known to contribute to its development. Breastfeeding seems to lower the incidence of NEC, as does use of minimal enteral nutrition.

Reversal of perinatal asphyxia within 30 minutes may prevent GI tract insult and thus prevent the pathophysiologic events that trigger NEC. After 30 minutes, the distribution of cardiac output tends to be directed more toward the heart and brain and away from the abdominal organs. Therefore prompt birth of the intrauterine-asphyxiated fetus or ventilation of the asphyxiated newborn may be beneficial to the GI tract, as well as to other organs.

The onset of NEC in the term infant usually occurs between 4 and 10 days after birth. In the preterm infant, the onset may be delayed for up to 30 days. The signs of developing NEC are nonspecific, which is characteristic of many neonatal diseases. Some generalized signs include decreased activity, hypotonia, pallor, recurrent apnea and bradycardia, decreased oxygen saturation values, respiratory distress, metabolic acidosis, oliguria, hypotension, decreased perfusion, temperature instability, and cyanosis. GI symptoms include abdominal distention, increasing or bile-stained residual gastric aspirates, vomiting (bile or blood), grossly bloody stools, abdominal tenderness, and erythema of the abdominal wall.

A diagnosis of NEC is confirmed by a radiographic examination that reveals bowel loop distention, pneumatosis intestinalis (air in the wall of the bowel), pneumoperitoneum, portal air, or a combination of these findings. The abnormal radiographic findings are caused by the bacterial colonization of the GI tract associated with NEC, resulting in ileus. Pneumatosis intestinalis, pneumoperitoneum, and portal air are caused by gas produced by the bacteria that invade the wall of the intestines and escape into the peritoneum and portal system when perforation occurs. The laboratory evaluation in such infants consists of a CBC with differential, coagulation studies, ABG analysis, measurement of serum electrolyte levels, and blood culture. The white blood cell count on the CBC may be either

box 40-6 Proposed Risk Factors for Necrotizing Enterocolitis

- Asphyxia
- Respiratory distress syndrome
- Umbilical artery catheter
- Exchange transfusion
- Early enteral feedings/hyperosmolar feedings
- Patent ductus arteriosus
- Congenital heart disease
- Polycythemia
- Anemia
- Shock
- Gastrointestinal infection

increased or decreased. The platelet count and coagulation study findings may be abnormal, showing thrombocytopenia and disseminated intravascular coagulation (DIC). Electrolyte levels may be abnormal, with leaking capillary beds and fluid shifts with the infection.

Treatment in such infants is supportive. Oral or tube feedings are discontinued to rest the GI tract. An orogastric tube is placed and attached to low wall suction to provide gastric decompression. Parenteral therapy (often TPN) is begun. Because NEC is an infectious disease, control of the infection is imperative, with an emphasis on careful handwashing before and after infant contact. Antibiotic therapy may be instituted, and surgical resection is performed if perforation or clinical deterioration occurs. Therapy is usually prolonged, and recovery may be delayed by the formation of adhesions, the development of the complications associated with bowel resection, the occurrence of short-bowel syndrome (especially if the ileocecal valve is removed), or the development of intolerance to oral feedings. Some of these infants are candidates for intestinal transplants if they truly have short-bowel syndrome.

A decrease in the incidence of NEC correlates with feedings of breast milk (Caplan, 2006). Use of natural prophylactic probiotics such as *Bifidobacteria infantis, Streptococcus thermophilus,* and *Bifidobacteria bifuus* to enhance bowel flora appears to decrease the incidence of NEC. Bin-Nun and colleagues (2005) found a decreased incidence and severity of NEC when it did occur among those infants given probiotics as compared to those who did not receive the supplement.

■ INFANT PAIN RESPONSES

The physiology of pain and pain assessment in the newborn were discussed in Chapter 26. This discussion focuses on pain assessment and management in the preterm infant.

Pain Assessment

Assessment of pain in the neonate is difficult because evaluation must be based on physiologic changes and behavioral observations. Pain is now considered the fifth vital sign, and its assessment is a requirement of the Joint Commission on Accreditation of Healthcare Organizations (JCAHO). A scale that examines multiple dimensions is more accurate (Spence, Gillies, Harrison, Johnston, & Nagy, 2005). Although behaviors such as vocalizations, facial expressions, body movements, and general state are common to all infants, they vary with different situations. Crying associated with pain is more intense and sustained. Facial expression is the most consistent and specific characteristic; scales are available for systematic evaluation of facial features, such as eye squeeze, brow bulge, and open mouth and taut tongue (Walden & Franck, 2003) (see Fig. 26-20). Most infants respond with increased body movements, but the infant may be experiencing pain even when lying quietly with eyes closed. The preterm infant's response to pain may be behaviorally blunted or absent.

An infant who receives a muscle-paralyzing agent such as vecuronium will be incapable of mounting a behavioral or visible pain response (Box 40-7), yet the infant still feels the pain.

■ NURSE ALERT

When in doubt about the presence of pain in infants, base your decision for the need for intervention on the following rule: Whatever is painful to an adult or child is painful to an infant unless proved otherwise. Anticipate pain; do not wait for pain symptoms to appear before intervening.

Several tools have been developed for the assessment of pain in the neonate. The CRIES assessment tool is discussed in Chapter 26 (see Table 26-3). Other instruments that are used are the Pain Assessment Tool (PAT) (Hodgkinson, Bear, Thorn, & Van Blaricum, 1994); Scale for Use in Newborns (SUN) (Blauer & Gerstmann, 1998); Behavioral Pain Score (BPS) (Pokela, 1994); Distress Scale for Ventilated Newborn Infants (DSVNI) (Sparshott, 1995); Neonatal Infant Pain Scale (NIPS) (Lawrence, Alcock, McGrath, Kay, MacMurray, & Dulberg, 1993); and the Premature Infant Pain Profile (PIPP) (Stevens, Johnston, Petryshen, & Taddio, 1996). The PIPP is one of the most widely used scales for preterm infants since it considers behavioral, physiologic, and contextual indicators (Stevens, Johnston, Franck, Petryshen, Jack, & Foster, 1999; Walden & Franck, 2003).

Memory of Pain

Preterm infants are subjected to a variety of repeated noxious stimuli, including multiple heel sticks, venipuncture, endotracheal intubation and suctioning, arterial sticks, chest tube placement, and lumbar puncture. The effects of pain caused by such procedures are not fully known, but researchers have begun to investigate potential consequences. From preliminary reports, it appears that a rewiring of the pain responses occurs in preterm infants who have been subjected to multiple painful treatments early in their lives. The nervous system networks of the preterm infant appear more dense and have more branches than those in the average infant, leading to the conclusion that the pain threshold and sensitivity in once preterm infants is heightened for life. There are also changes when the infant has undergone anesthesia (Anand, Johnston, Oberlander, Taddio, Lehr, & Walco, 2005; Aranda, Carlo, Hummel, Thomas, Lehr, & Anand, 2005).

Nurses' anecdotal reports suggest that infants show memory by exhibiting defensive behaviors when painful procedures are repeated. Nurses often describe infants who stiffen and withdraw when touched because human touch has repeatedly been associated with pain. Such infants often become hypervigilant and gaze intently at the hands rather than at the eyes of people who approach them.

These reports not only indicate that infants remember painful events but also show that continual exposure to pain affects development, especially in response to human contact.

---

box 40-7 **Manifestations of Acute Pain in the Neonate**

PHYSIOLOGIC RESPONSES
Vital Signs: Observe for Variations
- Increased heart rate
- Increased blood pressure
- Rapid, shallow respirations

Oxygenation
- Decreased transcutaneous O_2 saturation ($tcPO_2$)
- Decreased arterial O_2 saturation (SaO_2)

Skin: Observe Color and Character
- Pallor or flushing
- Diaphoresis
- Palmar sweating

Other Observations
- Increased muscle tone
- Dilated pupils
- Decreased vagal nerve tone
- Increased intracranial pressure
- Laboratory evidence of metabolic or endocrine changes
  - Hyperglycemia
  - Lowered pH
  - Elevated corticosteroids

BEHAVIORAL RESPONSES
Vocalizations: Observe Quality, Timing, and Duration
- Crying
- Whimpering
- Groaning

Facial Expression: Observe Characteristics, Timing, and Orientation of Eyes and Mouth (see Chapter 26, Fig. 26-20)
- Grimaces
- Brow furrowed
- Chin quivering
- Eyes tightly closed
- Mouth open and squarish

Body Movements and Posture: Observe Type, Quality, and Amount of Movement or Lack of Movement; Relationship to Other Factors
- Limb withdrawal
- Thrashing
- Rigidity
- Flaccidity
- Fist clenching

Change in State: Observe Sleep, Appetite, Activity Level
- Changes in sleep/wake cycles
- Changes in feeding behavior
- Changes in activity level
- Fussiness, irritability
- Listlessness

From Hockenberry, M. (2003). *Wong's nursing care of infants and children* (7th ed.). St. Louis: Mosby.

Consequences of Untreated Pain in Infants

Despite current research on the neonate's experience of pain, infant pain remains inadequately managed. The mismanagement of infant pain is partially due to misconceptions regarding the effects of pain on the neonate, as well as a lack of knowledge of immediate and long-term consequences of untreated pain. Infants respond to noxious stimuli through physiologic indicators (increased heart rate and blood pressure, variability in heart rate and intracranial pressure, and decreases in arterial oxygen saturations and skin blood flow) and behavioral indicators (muscle rigidity, facial expression, crying, withdrawal, and sleeplessness). The physiologic and behavioral indicators, as well as a variety of neurophysiologic responses to noxious stimulation, are responsible for short-term and long-term consequences of pain.

Pain Management

The International Evidence-Based Group for Neonatal Pain developed a Consensus Statement for the Prevention and Management of Pain in the Newborn (Anand, 2001). This statement states that pain must be anticipated and prevented to avoid long-term consequences. Nonpharmacologic measures to alleviate pain include repositioning, swaddling, containment, cuddling, rocking, music, reduc-

ing environmental stimulation, tactile comfort measures, nonnutritive sucking, and use of oral sucrose (Walden & Franck, 2003). However, nonpharmacologic measures may not be sufficient to decrease physiologic distress, even if behavioral responses such as crying are lessened (Walden & Franck). In preterm infants, additional stimulation such as stroking or environmental light or noise may *increase* physiologic distress (Walden & Franck). The impact of the NICU environment must be considered along with other forms of stimuli that may produce stress and pain.

Morphine is the most widely used opioid analgesic for pharmacologic management of neonatal pain, with fentanyl as an effective alternative. Continuous or bolus epidural or IV infusion of opioids provides effective and safe pain control (Stork, 2006; Walden & Franck, 2003). Other methods of relieving pain are epidural/intrathecal infusion, local and regional nerve blocks, and topical anesthetics, as well as general anesthesia for surgery (Stork; Walden & Franck).

Parents are universally concerned that their infants are feeling pain during procedures. Nurses need to address these concerns and encourage the parents to speak with the health care professionals involved. Parents have the right to withhold consent for invasive procedures and are entitled to honest answers from those responsible for the infant's care. When appropriate, they also can help provide comfort measures for the infant. Kangaroo care is one method of parental intervention that comforts and calms the infant.

Parents want to know that nurses recognize pain in their infants and that the infants will be comfortable when they, the parents, are not present. They want to know that the nurse will advocate for comfort care for their baby. Although pain is considered a fifth vital sign, it cannot be assessed only at the time of vital signs. It must receive an ongoing evaluation of the pain level and the effectiveness of comfort measures used. This assessment is not lengthy but can be as simple as walking to the bedside and really looking at the infant's color, posture, movements, and breathing. Pain is a real phenomenon that is preventable in many instances. Pain management is a standard of care, and it is considered unethical not to prevent and effectively treat pain. Another growing area of neonatal nursing is end-of-life and palliative care. Most of this care centers on pain management. Palliative care is really comfort care that supports the needs of the preterm, sick neonate.

▬ NEAR-TERM INFANTS

Near-term infants are those born between 34 and 37 weeks of gestation (Wang, Dorer, Fleming, & Catlin, 2004). Some literature defines near term as 35 to 37 weeks (Medoff-Cooper, Bakewell-Sachs, Buus-Frank, & Santa-Donato, 2005). In practice these infants are often thought of as functionally at term and are treated as such. They usually have normal Apgar scores. However, these infants are at increased risk for problems when compared to term infants. In a study comparing near-term and full-term infants on length of stay and medical problems encountered, Wang and associates found important differences in hospital courses and clinical outcomes. Almost one third of the near-term infants had respiratory distress, and discharge was delayed for many of those. The near-term infants experienced temperature instability; hypoglycemia and poor feeding necessitating intravenous therapy; jaundice; evaluation for sepsis three times as often as term infants, and treatment with antibiotics.

The Association of Women's Health, Obstetric and Neonatal Nurses (AWHONN) announced an initiative in 2005 to build awareness of near-term infants and to improve their care (Medoff-Cooper et al., 2005). The Association listed five things that parents of near-term infants should know and observe for (What the parents of near-term infants need to know, 2005):

1. *Feeding.* Near-term infants need to be fed more often, since they eat less. They may also have difficulty coordinating sucking and swallowing. Breastfeeding may be more problematic and necessitate the assistance of a professional.
2. *Sleeping.* Near-term infants may be sleepier than term infants and may need to be awakened for feedings.
3. *Breathing.* Near-term infants may have had respiratory distress after birth and may be prone to respiratory problems.
4. *Temperature.* Since they have less body fat than term infants, near-term infants may have more difficulty regulating their temperatures.
5. *Infections and jaundice.* The immune systems of near-term infants are immature; thus they are more likely to experience infections. They are also more likely to have jaundice.

The goal of these efforts is to raise the awareness of health care providers to the risks associated with near-term birth and to match the care environment with the needs of the near-term infant (Medoff-Cooper et al., 2005).

▬ POSTMATURE INFANTS

A pregnancy that is prolonged beyond 42 weeks is a post-term pregnancy, and the infant who is born is called *postmature.* Postmaturity can be associated with placental insufficiency, resulting in a fetus that has a wasted appearance (dysmaturity) at birth because of loss of subcutaneous fat and muscle mass. Meconium staining of the fingernails may be noted, and the hair and nails may be long. The skin may peel off. Not all postmature infants will show signs of dysmaturity; some will continue to grow in utero and be large at birth.

The perinatal mortality rate is significantly higher in the postmature fetus and neonate. One reason for this is that during labor and birth, the increased oxygen demands of the postmature fetus may not be met. Insufficient gas exchange in the postmature placenta also increases the likelihood of intrauterine hypoxia, which may result in the passage of meconium in utero, thereby increasing the risk for meconium aspiration syndrome (MAS). Of all the deaths that occur in postmature newborns, half occur during labor and birth, about one third occur before the onset of labor, and one sixth occur during the postpartum period.

Meconium Aspiration Syndrome

Meconium staining of the amniotic fluid can be indicative of nonreassuring fetal status, especially in a vertex presentation. It appears in 8% to 20% of all births. Many infants with meconium staining exhibit no signs of depression at birth; however, the presence of meconium in the amniotic fluid necessitates careful supervision of labor and close monitoring of fetal well-being. Use of amnioinfusion has decreased some of the incidence of MAS (Yoder, Kirsch, Barth, & Gordon, 2002). This procedure thins any meconium particles that may be present in the amniotic fluid, thus decreasing the chance of thick meconium being aspirated at the time of birth. Because these infants are surfactant deficient, one method of prevention of MAS is to use surfactant lavages immediately after birth. The findings indicate that outcomes for these infants are better than those of their counterparts who received no surfactant lavages (i.e., they were weaned from mechanical ventilation quicker, had less full-blown MAS, and had better oxygenation patterns) (Wiswell et al., 2002). Although this was a randomized multicenter trial, more research is needed.

The presence of a team skilled at neonatal resuscitation is required at the birth of any infant with meconium-stained amniotic fluid (Bloom, (2006). The hypopharynx of the infant of a baby born through meconium should be suctioned after birth of the head and before birth of the shoulders. *Vigorous infants* need no special handling (American Heart Associaton, 2006; Vain, Szyld, Prudent, Wiswell, Aguilar, & Vivas, 2004).

If the infant is very depressed and the meconium is not removed from the airway at birth, it can migrate down to the terminal airways, causing mechanical obstruction leading to MAS. It also is possible that the fetus aspirated meconium in utero. Such meconium aspiration can cause a chemical pneumonitis. These infants may develop persistent pulmonary hypertension of the newborn, further complicating their management.

Persistent Pulmonary Hypertension of the Newborn

The term *persistent pulmonary hypertension of the newborn (PPHN)* is applied to the combined findings of pulmonary hypertension, right-to-left shunting, and a structurally normal heart. PPHN may be either a single entity or the main component of MAS, congenital diaphragmatic hernia, RDS, hyperviscosity syndrome, or neonatal pneumonia or sepsis. PPHN also is called *persistent fetal circulation (PFC)* because the syndrome includes a reversion to fetal pathways for blood flow.

A brief review of the characteristics of fetal blood flow can help in the visualization of the problems with PPHN (see p. 321-322, Fig. 13-9). In utero, oxygen-rich blood leaves the placenta via the umbilical vein, goes through the ductus venosus, and enters the inferior vena cava. From there it empties into the right atrium and is mostly shunted across the foramen ovale to the left atrium, effectively bypassing the lungs. This blood enters the left ventricle, leaves via the aorta, and preferentially perfuses the carotid and coronary arteries. Thus the heart and brain receive the most oxygenated blood. Blood drains from the brain into the superior vena cava, reenters the right atrium, proceeds to the right ventricle, and exits via the main pulmonary artery. The lungs are a high-pressure circuit, needing only enough perfusion for growth and nutrition. The ductus arteriosus (connecting the main pulmonary artery and the aorta) is the path of least resistance for the blood leaving the right side of the fetal heart, shunting most of the cardiac output away from the lungs and toward the systemic system. This *right-to-left shunting* is the key to fetal circulation.

After birth, both the foramen ovale and the ductus arteriosus close in response to various biochemical processes, pressure changes within the heart, and dilation of the pulmonary vessels. This dilation allows virtually all of the cardiac output to enter the lungs, become oxygenated, and provide oxygen-rich blood to the tissues for normal metabolism. Any process that interferes with this transition from fetal to neonatal circulation may precipitate PPHN. PPHN characteristically proceeds into a downward spiral of exacerbating hypoxia and pulmonary vasoconstriction. Prompt recognition and aggressive intervention are required to reverse this process.

The infant with PPHN is typically born at term or after term and has tachycardia and cyanosis. Management depends on the underlying cause of the persistent pulmonary hypertension. The use of ECMO has improved the chances of survival in these infants (see earlier discussion); however, it is considered a very invasive procedure. Use of nitric oxide (NO) as a pharmacologic intervention has increased in the last few years with great success. NO acts as a vasodilator to decrease the pulmonary hypertension while increasing oxygenation (Zahka & Bengur, 2006). This therapy is proving to work well either alone or with high-frequency ventilation. Another pharmacologic treatment is use of exogenous surfactant, since some of these infants appear to be surfactant deficient. Use of environmental strategies such as decreasing adverse stimuli (excessive light and noise) to decrease stress is another area of ongoing research. This intervention is used in conjunction with other therapies.

Another mode of treatment for PPHN and other respiratory disorders of the newborn is high-frequency ventilation, a group of assisted ventilation methods that deliver small volumes of gas at high frequencies and limit the development of high airway pressure, thus reducing barotrauma. High-frequency ventilation decreases carbon dioxide while increasing oxygenation. It can be effectively used in conjunction with NO (Zahka & Bengur, 2006). It is important to understand that PPHN is considered a cardiovascular and a respiratory problem. The lungs of these infants are healthy, but the hypertension of the cardiovascular system leads to their oxygenation problems.

▬ COLLABORATIVE CARE

To ensure the safe birth of the fetus, it becomes important to determine whether the pregnancy is actually prolonged and also whether there is any evidence of fetal jeopardy as a result.

Most postmature infants are oversized but otherwise normal, with advanced development and bone age. A postmature infant will have some, but not necessarily all, of the following physical characteristics:

- Generally a normal skull, but the reduced dimensions of the rest of the body in the presence of dysmaturity make the skull look inordinately large
- Dry, cracked (desquamating), parchment-like skin at birth
- Hard nails extending beyond the fingertips
- Profuse scalp hair
- Depleted subcutaneous fat layers, leaving the skin loose and giving the infant an "old person" appearance
- Long and thin body

- Absent vernix
- Often meconium staining (golden yellow to green) of skin, nails, and cord, indicative of a hypoxic episode in utero or a perinatal infection such as listeriosis
- May have an alert, wide-eyed appearance symptomatic of chronic intrauterine hypoxia

Possible nursing diagnoses for the postmature infant include the following:

- *Impaired gas exchange related to*
  - –decreased number of functional alveoli
  - –deficiency of surfactant
  - –cardiovascular hypertension in the pulmonary tree
- *Ineffective breathing pattern related to*
  - –inadequate chest expansion, secondary to infant position
  - –environmental stimuli
  - –pain
  - –pulmonary hypertension
- *Ineffective thermoregulation related to*
  - –immature thermoregulation center
  - –exposure to cold air or increased factors promoting thermal loss
  - –lack of subcutaneous tissue and fat stores
- *Risk for infection related to*
  - –invasive procedures
  - –decreased immune response
  - –immature skin or very thin, friable skin
- *Anxiety (parental) related to*
  - –lack of knowledge regarding infant condition
  - –lack of knowledge regarding infant cues
  - –fear of death of infant
  - –feeling powerless in the situation/inability to protect infant from harm
- *Anticipatory grieving (parental) related to*
  - –fear of infant's death
  - –lack of knowledge about what to expect
  - –lack of clear communication on part of health care team

Immediate outcomes of care are that the postmature newborn will do the following:
- Initiate and maintain respirations.
- Experience no CNS trauma or infection.
- Have any birth trauma identified and treated promptly without sequelae.

The long-term expected outcome is that the infant will not experience adverse effects of postmaturity.

The immediate care rendered to postmature infants is similar to that given to preterm infants. Potential complications experienced by postmature infants include polycythemia, hypothermia, hypoglycemia, and meconium aspiration. See other sections for the management and care of infants with these complications.

The nurse can be assured that care was effective when the short-term outcomes for care have been achieved. Long-term follow-up will be needed to evaluate whether any adverse effects are a result of postmaturity.

▬ OTHER PROBLEMS RELATED TO GESTATION

Small for Gestational Age and Intrauterine Growth Restriction

Infants who are small for gestational age (SGA; e.g., weight is below the 10th percentile expected at term) and infants who have IUGR (rate of growth does not meet expected growth pattern) are considered high risk, with the perinatal mortality rate 5 to 20 times greater than that for the normal term infant (Kliegman, 2006). In some cases, a genetic linkage is possible, since maternal genes have been implicated when the incidence of infants who are SGA runs in families. The maternal genes must regulate the fetal growth potential through uteroplacental circulation effects (Kliegman). Women with chronic illness or suboptimal nutrition also are at risk for producing an SGA infant, since the nutrients to the fetus are diminished. Thus, although the underlying cause of the SGA circumstance can affect the condition of the infant, common problems that affect SGA and IUGR infants are predictable: perinatal asphyxia, meconium aspiration, hypoglycemia, polycythemia, and heat loss.

Perinatal Asphyxia

Commonly, IUGR infants have been exposed to chronic hypoxia for varying periods before labor and birth. Labor is a stressor to the normal fetus, but it is an even greater stressor for the growth-restricted fetus. The chronically hypoxic infant is severely compromised even by a normal labor and has difficulty compensating after birth. Appropriate management and resuscitation are essential for these depressed infants.

The birth of SGA babies with perinatal asphyxia may be associated with a maternal history of heavy cigarette smoking; preeclampsia; low socioeconomic status; multifetal gestation; gestational infections such as rubella, cytomegalovirus, and toxoplasmosis; advanced diabetes mellitus; and cardiac problems. The nursing staff must be alert to and prepared for possible perinatal asphyxia during the birth of an infant to a woman with such a history. Sequelae to perinatal asphyxia include MAS and hypoglycemia.

Hypoglycemia

All stressed infants are at risk for the development of hypoglycemia. Such stress may include perinatal asphyxia and IUGR. The definition of hypoglycemia differs for the term and the preterm infant. Hypoglycemia occurring within the first 3 days of life in the term infant is defined as a blood glucose level of less than 40 mg/dl; that occurring in the preterm infant within the same time frame is defined as a blood glucose level of less than 25 mg/dl. Symptoms of hypoglycemia include poor feeding, hypothermia, and diaphoresis. CNS symptoms can include tremors and jitteriness, weak cry, lethargy, floppy posture, convulsions, or coma. Diagnosis is confirmed by blood glucose determinations performed by the laboratory, when suspected, or by unit visual methods with reagent strips such as Chemstrip-BG or Dextrostix (Kliegman, 2006).

Polycythemia

Polycythemia or hyperviscosity of the blood is another common problem of the SGA infant. The plasma volume may be on average 52 ml/kg (normal, 43 ml/kg) (Kliegman, 2006). This condition is a result of fetal hypoxia and intrauterine stress that forces the body to produce more red blood cells in an attempt to provide oxygen to the developing fetus. This condition can compromise blood circulation and oxygenation, and lead to further hypoglycemia and hypoxia in extrauterine life. A partial exchange transfusion to reduce the viscosity of the blood may be necessary.

Heat Loss

For numerous reasons, SGA infants are particularly susceptible to temperature instability, and close attention must be paid to maintain thermoneutrality for them. They have less muscle mass, less brown fat, less heat-preserving subcutaneous fat, and little ability to control skin capillaries. Nursing considerations in these infants focus on the maintenance of thermoneutrality to promote recovery from perinatal asphyxia, because cold stress jeopardizes such recovery (Kliegman, 2006).

▬ COLLABORATIVE CARE

Several physical findings are characteristic of the SGA neonate:

- Generally a normal skull, but the reduced dimensions of the rest of the body make the skull look inordinately large
- Reduced subcutaneous fat stores
- Loose and dry skin
- Diminished muscle mass, especially over buttocks and cheeks
- Sunken abdomen (scaphoid) as opposed to the well-rounded abdomen seen in normal infants
- Thin, yellowish, dry, and dull umbilical cord (normal cord is gray, glistening, round, and moist)
- Sparse scalp hair
- Wide skull sutures (inadequate bone growth)

The nursing care given to the SGA infant is determined by the nature of the clinical problems and is the same as that given to the preterm infant with the same problems. Maintaining a clear airway and preventing cold stress support gas exchange. Hypoglycemia is treated with oral feedings (e.g., breast milk, formula, dextrose solution) per the hospital protocol. Parenteral infusions may be necessary. If polycythemia is present, assessment of the cardiovascular circulation is important, and assistance with a partial exchange transfusion may be necessary. To assist with thermoregulation, an external heat source (radiant warmer or incubator) is used until the infant's temperature is stabilized. The nursing support given to parents is similar to that given to parents of preterm infants.

Large for Gestational Age

The large for gestational age (LGA), or oversized, infant traditionally has been regarded as one weighing 4000 g or more at birth. An infant is considered LGA at any gesta-

tion when the weight is above the 90th percentile on growth charts or two standard deviations above the mean weight for gestational age. Certain fetal disorders also can result in LGA infants. These include transposition of the great vessels and Beckwith-Wiedemann syndrome.

Birth trauma, especially in infants with a breech or shoulder presentation, is a serious hazard for the oversized neonate. Asphyxia or CNS injury, or both, may occur. All pregnancies of more than 42 weeks of gestation must be carefully evaluated. All large fetuses are monitored during a trial of labor, and preparation is made for cesarean birth if a nonreassuring fetal status or poor progress of labor occurs. LGA newborns may be preterm, term, or postterm; they may be the infants of mothers who are diabetic (or prediabetic); and they may be postmature. Each of these problems has special concerns. Regardless of any coexisting potential problems, the oversized infant is at risk just by virtue of its size.

▬ COLLABORATIVE CARE

The nurse assesses the LGA infant for gestational age, hypoglycemia, and trauma resulting from vaginal or cesarean birth. The blood glucose levels of LGA infants are monitored, and any hypoglycemia is corrected. Any specific birth injuries are identified and treated appropriately. Care depends on the LGA infant's condition.

▬ DISCHARGE PLANNING

Discharge planning for the high risk infant begins at the time of admission. Throughout the infant's hospitalization, the discharge planning coordinator gathers information from all of the health care team members. This information is used to determine the infant's and family's readiness for discharge. Nurses are very influential members of the planning team because as the direct caregivers throughout the infant's hospitalization, they have a firsthand knowledge of the infant and the family.

As the home care needs of the infant's parents are assessed, steps are taken to eliminate any knowledge deficits. Information is provided about infant care, especially as it pertains to the particular infant's home needs (e.g., the administration of oxygen, gastrostomy feedings). Parent education includes having them give return demonstrations of their infant care skills to show whether they are becoming increasingly independent in the provision of this care. Parents also should obtain an age-appropriate car seat before the discharge of their infant. Instruction in infant CPR should be offered to all parents before discharge. With the emphasis on the American Academy of Pediatrics (AAP) Back-to-Sleep program to reduce the incidence of SIDS, it may be necessary to place the infant in the supine position before discharge to challenge the infant's ability to tolerate this position. Because the parents saw their infant in a prone or side-lying position while sick; they need to understand the importance of use of the new positioning on the back once the infant is stable and at home.

EVIDENCE-BASED PRACTICE

Enriched Formula for Low-Birth-Weight Infants

BACKGROUND

- Preterm and low-birth-weight (LBW) (less than 2.5 kg) infants have fewer nutrient reserves than term babies, yet are more vulnerable to physiologic stresses that increase nutritional demands, such as respiratory distress, cold stress, or infection. Smaller infants may not be able to take in and process enough calories and protein to compensate for the deficit. Consequently, preterm and LBW infants remain growth restricted (below the 10th percentile for equivalent gestational age), sometimes for years. Nutritional deficiency has been linked with poor bone density, cardiovascular disease, insulin resistance, high blood pressure, and obesity in later life. Many hospitals start calorie- and protein-enriched formula for their smallest clients. Compared to breast milk, 100 ml of standard formula has 68 kcal and 1.4 to 1.5 g of protein, while preterm formula started in hospital may have 80 kcal and 2 to 2.4 g of protein. Infants are then sent home with formula that has 72 to 74 kcal and 1.8 g of protein per 100 ml. Some calorie-enriched formula is poorly tolerated as a result of decreased gastric motility.

OBJECTIVES

- The reviewers' goal was to compare the growth and development of preterm and LBW infants fed standard versus enriched (at least 72 kcal and 1.6 g of protein per 100 ml) formula. They included exclusively formula-fed babies, as well as breastfed babies who were supplemented with enriched formula. Outcomes included weight, height, head circumference, neurodevelopmental outcomes on a validated scale, IQ, educational achievement, bone mineralization and growth, feed tolerance, and blood pressure.

METHODS

Search Strategy

- After a thorough search of the Cochrane Central Register of Controlled Trials and databases, conferences, and references, the authors identified six randomized or quasi-randomized controlled trials that were double-blinded. They were dated 1992 to 2004, representing 424 infants from Europe, Israel, and North America.

Statistical Analyses

- Similar data were pooled. Reviewers calculated relative risk for dichotomous (categoric) data, such as feeding intolerance, and weighted mean difference for continuous data, such as head circumference. Differences between groups outside the 95% confidence interval were accepted as significant.

FINDINGS

- At 18 months, there were no differences found between standard and enriched formula groups in weight or head circumference. There was a significant difference in height of 1 cm at 18 months, favoring the enriched formula. No differences were found in neurodevelopmental scores (Bayley Scales Mental Development Index and Psychomotor Development Index). Bone mineralization was similar. There were no differences in feed tolerance. Two studies reported that infants fed enriched formula drank less milk than the standard formula group. This caused their calorie intake to equalize, although the enriched group still received more protein.

LIMITATIONS

- There is still limited evidence as to the longer-term outcomes of linear growth and neurodevelopmental milestones. The studies are fairly small. There were some differences in the formulas and the other additives, such as minerals, that might also potentiate growth.

IMPLICATIONS FOR PRACTICE

- It does not appear that enriched formula is harmful, but there is limited evidence to recommend it for catch-up growth of the preterm or the LBW infant.

IMPLICATIONS FOR FURTHER RESEARCH

- Future research may establish whether outcomes at 18 months can predict longer-term outcomes. There were no trials measuring cognitive or educational levels, evidence of rickets, or blood pressure, or the longer-term metabolic or cardiovascular outcomes. Future research should address the possible combinations of minerals and vitamins with protein that can foster absorption and growth. Breastfeeding, alone or supplemented with some enrichment, should be included in any future discussion of infant feeding, since its advantages for vulnerable infants are well documented.

Reference: Henderson, G., Fahey, T., & McQuire, W. (2005). Calorie and protein-enriched formula versus standard term formula for improving growth and development in preterm or low birth weight infants following hospital discharge. *The Cochrane Database of Systematic Reviews*, 2006, Issue 3. Chichester, UK: John Wiley & Sons.

As the home care of medically fragile clients is expanded to the pediatric population, early teaching and planning become a necessity. With the advent of managed care and cost-effective care strategies, more facilities using vertical integration of services thus provide home care as part of their inpatient continuum of care. These institutions are investigating such home care options as one way to provide long-term care for the compromised infant. If the infant requires palliative care or is considered to be dying, hospice and palliative care are available in some areas of the country. Problems still exist with insurance coverage for these services in some states, but many discharge coordinators are able to obtain payment when the services are coupled with home care (Association of Pediatric Oncology Nurses (APON), National Association of Neonatal Nurses (NANN), & Society of Pediatric Nurses (SPN), 2002).

Referrals for appropriate resources should be made whether the infant just needs follow-up or is going home to die. Social service involvement is especially important for young or psychosocially high risk parents (e.g., substance abusers or those with a mental illness). Social services also can provide parents with information about financial assistance (e.g., Temproary Asistance for Needy Families (TANF) (http://aspe.hhs.gov/hsp/abbrev/afdc-tanf.htm), Medicaid, Crippled Children's Program, Social Security Disability). Appropriate genetic counseling, referral, and follow-up should be provided.

Infants with developmental disabilities, or those infants who may be at risk for further problems (preterm, infants), are referred to appropriate community programs. Federal Public Law 102-119 mandates that community resources be available to those children and families with special educational and medical needs (Robinson & Driscoll, 2003). Such services range from family counseling to physical therapy. Some hospitals also offer infant stimulation and development programs for the parents of at-risk infants. This law recognizes nursing as one of the 10 qualified disciplines that can provide these services. Federal Public Law 106-402 contains four grant programs to assist those with developmental disabilities to reach their maximum potential (www.acf.hhs.gov/programs/add/Factsheet.html).

Referrals are made for home health assistance, as appropriate (some medical plans cover these services). These health care providers can perform actual nursing functions, as well as provide some relief from the emotional burden of caring for an infant with medical problems. Special attention should be given to parents' feelings of uncertainty, anxiety, and overwhelming frustration. Parents often have these emotions during the planning for an infant's home care, especially if the infant has had a severe or prolonged illness (Holditch-Davis, Bartlett et al., 2003; Miles et al., 2002).

▬ TRANSPORT TO A REGIONAL CENTER

If a hospital is not equipped to care for a high risk mother and fetus or a high risk infant, transfer to a specialized perinatal or tertiary care center is arranged. Maternal transport ideally occurs with the fetus in utero because this has two distinct advantages: (1) The associated neonatal morbidity and mortality are decreased; and (2) infant-parent attachment is supported, thereby avoiding separation of the parents and infant.

For a variety of reasons, however, it is not always possible to transport the mother before the birth. These reasons include imminent birth and unanticipated problems; therefore, physicians and nurses in level 1 and 2 facilities must have the skills and equipment necessary for making an accurate diagnosis and implementing emergency interventions to stabilize the infant's condition until transport can occur (Box 40-8) (Pettett, Pallotto, & Merenstein, 2006). The goal of these interventions is to maintain the infant's

condition within the normal physiologic range. Specific attention is given to the following areas:
- Vital signs
- Oxygen and ventilation
- Thermoregulation
- Acid-base balance
- Fluid and electrolyte levels
- Glucose level
- Developmental interventions

The transport team may consist of physicians, nurse practitioners, nurses, and respiratory therapists. Commonly the team consists of a nurse trained in neonatal intensive care and a respiratory therapist. The team must have expertise in resuscitation, stabilization, and provision of critical care during the transport which can occur on the ground or in the air (Fig. 40-16, *B*). In a neonatal transport, the team should provide information for the parents about the tertiary center (Box 40-9). Transport teams can integrate an individual developmental plan of care into their caregiving efforts, thereby initiating multidisciplinary interventions early in the infant's life.

The birth of any high risk infant can cause profound parental stress. Parents can grieve the loss of the ideal infant. They are fearful of the possible eventual outcomes for the infant. They also must deal with the technologic world surrounding their infant, and amid all the equipment, it is sometimes difficult for them to perceive the infant and respond to its needs. Parents of high risk infants who have been transported to regional centers therefore need special support. As one way to deal with this problem, many intensive care units provide the family with a handbook or pictures of the tertiary care unit to help them understand what is going on around them. Parents should have the name and telephone number of a contact person at the regional center.

▬ TRANSPORT FROM A REGIONAL CENTER

Infants may need to be transferred back to the referring facility. Often preterm infants who require thermoregulation and gavage feedings can be cared for in community hospitals closer to the parents' home. This back transfer allows parents to visit their infant more easily and to work with their personal health care provider on the long-range expected outcomes for the infant. Specialized incubators make these trips possible (see Fig. 40-16, *A*). However, parents may express mixed feelings about such return transports and may be reluctant to adapt to a different facility and group of caregivers. To minimize some of these concerns, it is important to give the parents very clear information about return transports during the initial discharge planning.

Although at the time of discharge, parents may not recognize the need for information on the various resources available to help them in the care of their infant, they can be given such lists of agencies and telephone numbers for later use. Providing them with a client-specific directory box 40-8 **Neonatal Resuscitation Supplies and Equipment**

SUCTION EQUIPMENT

Bulb syringe
Mechanical suction and tubing
Suction catheters, 5F or 6F, 8F, 10F, 12F or 14F
8F feeding tube and 20 ml syringe
Meconium aspirator

BAG-AND-MASK EQUIPMENT

Device for delivering positive-pressure ventilation, capable of
    delivering 90% to 100%
Face masks, newborn and premature sizes (cushioned-rim masks
    preferred)
Oxygen source with flowmeter (flow rate up to 10 L/min) and
    tubing

INTUBATION EQUIPMENT

Laryngoscope with straight blades, No. 0 (preterm) and No. 1
    (term)
Extra bulbs and batteries for laryngoscope
Endotracheal tubes, 2.5-, 3, 3.5-, 4-mm internal diameter (ID)
Stylet (optional)
Scissors
Tape or securing device for endotracheal tube
Alcohol sponges
CO_2 detector or capnograph
Laryngeal mask airway (optional)

MEDICATIONS

Epinephrine, 1:10,000 (0.1 mg/ml): 3 ml or 10 ml ampules
Isotonic crystalloid (normal saline or Ringer's lactate) for vol-
    ume expansion: 100 or 250 ml
Sodium bicarbonate, 4.2% (5 mEq/10 ml): 10 ml ampules
Naloxone hydrochloride, 0.4 mg/ml: 1-ml ampules; or 1.0 mg/ml:
    2-ml ampules
Dextrose, 10%: 250 ml
Normal saline for flushes
Umbilical vessel catheterization supplies
    Sterile gloves
    Scalpel or scissors
    Antiseptic prep solution
    Umbilical tape
    Umbilical catheters, 3.5F, 5F
    Three-way stopcock
Syringes: 1, 3, 5, 10, 20, 50 ml
Needles: 25-, 21-, 18-gauge, or puncture device for needleless
    system

MISCELLANEOUS

Gloves and appropriate personal protection
Radiant warmer or other heat source
Firm, padded resuscitation surface
Clock with second hand (timer optional)
Warmed linens
Stethoscope (neonatal head preferred)
Tape, ½- or ¾- inch
Cardiac monitor and electrodes or pulse oximeter and probe
    (optional for delivery room)
Oropharyngeal airways (0, 00, and 000 sizes or 30, 40, and
    50-mm lengths)

Used with permission of the American Academy of Pediatrics. (2006). *Textbook of neonatal resuscitation* (5th ed.). Elk Grove Village, IL: Author.

A B

FIG. 40-16   A, Total life support system for transport of high risk newborns. **B,** Life Flight helicopter to transport infant. (**A,** Courtesy UNC Hospitals, Carolina Air Care, Chapel Hill, NC. **B,** Courtesy OSF St. Francis Medical Center, Peoria, IL.)

box 40-9 **Information for Parents About the Tertiary Center**

- Exact location of the unit—address, map
- Visiting hours and hospital rules
- Telephone numbers
- Names of individuals likely to be involved with the baby's care
- Information of the special care unit—what it is, what it does
- Location of parking facilities, nearby lodging, and rules regarding young children (siblings)
- Any particular rules or regulations regarding the special care unit

From Pettett, G., Pallotto, E., & Merenstein. (2006). Perinatal transport. In G. Merenstein, & S. Gardner, (Eds.). *Handbook of neonatal intensive care* (6th ed.). St. Louis: Mosby.

covering special programs, social support, community, and funding resources can help them make the transition to the home care of their infants. As the nurse continually reinforces the idea that the infant will go home, this will prompt the parents to plan for the days ahead and therefore be ready to take their infant home when the time comes.

▬ ANTICIPATORY GRIEF

Families experience anticipatory grief when they are told of the impending death of their infant. Anticipatory grief prepares and protects parents who are facing a loss. Parents who have an infant with a debilitating disease (with or without a congenital deformity), but one that may not necessarily threaten the life of the child, also may experience anticipatory grief. An alteration in relationships, a change in lifestyle, and a very real threat to their hopes and dreams for the future may affect the day-to-day interaction of the family with their infant and the staff. Nurses can help facilitate the family's grieving process. If the nurse observes that a family member's day-to-day interactions with the infant change, the nurse should assess the situation and request psychosocial support or intervention by a chaplain or social worker, if necessary.

Loss of an Infant

Parents who know their infant is going to die have a very difficult time. Before the infant's death, the parents need to direct their attention, energy, and caregiving activities toward the dying infant. However, some parents find it difficult to visit their infant even for short periods once a terminal diagnosis has been made. Grandparents also grieve but often are unsure how to comfort their own child (the infant's parent) during the period of impending death. Health care professionals can help by involving the family in the infant's care, providing privacy, answering questions, and preparing them for the inevitability of the death (see Chapter 41). Today there is a growing emphasis on hospice

and palliative care for infants and their families (End-of-Life Nursing Education Consortium (ELNEC), 2005).

The nursing staff also experiences grief. Many primary staff nurses find themselves grieving as if the infant were their own because they often have been the health professional that has worked closely with the infant and family for weeks, or even months. Managers and other staff members must acknowledge this grief. Talking about the infant or attending the funeral may help the affected staff members resolve their feelings about the infant's death (ELNEC, 2005).

community activity

Access the website of your local and state health department. What services are available for parents of high risk infants? Are follow-up clinics available? Are there groups for parents of high risk infants? What parent education materials are available? Are there multilingual services and materials available? Is there an active local chapter of AWHONN?

key points

- Preterm infants are at risk for problems stemming from the immaturity of their organ systems.
- Nurses who work with preterm and other high risk infants observe them for respiratory distress and other early symptoms of physiologic disorders.
- The adaptation of parents to preterm or high risk infants differs from that of parents to normal term infants.
- Nurses can facilitate the development of a positive parent-child relationship.
- Nurses' skills in interpreting data, making decisions, and initiating therapy in newborn intensive care units are crucial to ensuring infants' survival.
- Pain management requires vigilant ongoing assessment, anticipation of painful events, and early interventions to prevent and diminish such a response.
- Nurses need to assess the macroenvironments and microenvironments of the infant and family to create a developmentally positive atmosphere.
- Developmental care is a philosophy that embraces family-centered care and awareness of the impact of environmental stimuli on the physical and psychologic well-being of the infant and family.
- Parents need special instruction (e.g., CPR, oxygen therapy, suctioning, developmental care) before they take home a high risk infant.
- SGA infants are considered at risk because of fetal growth restriction.
- The high incidence of nonreassuring fetal status among postmature infants is related to the progressive placental insufficiency that can occur in a postterm pregnancy.
- Specially trained nurses may transport high risk infants to and from special care units.
- Parents need assistance with coping with anticipatory grief or loss and grief.

REFERENCES

Als, H., Duffy, F., McAnulty, G., Rivkin, M., Vajapeyam, S., Mulkern, R., et al. (2004). Early experience alters brain function and structure. *Pediatrics, 113*(4), 846-857.

American Heart Association. (2006). 2005 American Heart Association (AHA) guidelines for cardiopulmonary resuscitation (CPR) and Emergency Cardiovascular Care (ECC) of pediatric and neonatal patients: Pediatric basic life support. *Pediatrics, 117*(5), e989-e1004.

Anand, K. (2001). Consensus statement for the prevention and management of pain in the newborn: International Evidence-Based Group for Neonatal Pain. *Archives of Pediatric and Adolescent Medicine, 155*(2), 173-180.

Anand, K., Johnston, C., Oberlander, T., Taddio, A., Lehr, V., & Walco, G. (2005). Analgesia and local anesthesia during invasive procedures in the neonate. *Clinical Therapies, 27*(6), 844-876.

Aranda, J., Carlo, W., Hummel, P., Thomas, R., Lehr, V., & Anand, K. (2005). Analgesia and sedation during mechanical ventilation in neonates. *Clinical Therapies, 27*(6), 877-899.

Association of Pediatric Oncology Nurses (APON), National Association of Neonatal Nurses (NANN), & Society of Pediatric Nurses (SPN). (2002). *Precepts of palliative care for children/adolescents and their families.* Chicago, IL: Last Acts.

Association of Women's Health, Obstetric, and Neonatal Nurses (AWHONN). (2005). What the parents of near-term infants need to know. (June 12, 2005). News release. Accessed www.awhonn.org, May 11, 2006.

Beal, J., & Wood, S. (2005). Implications of kangaroo care for growth and development in preterm infants. *MCN American Journal of Maternal/Child Nursing, 30*(5), 338.

Bin-Nun, A., Bromiker, R., Wilschanski, M., Kaplan, M., Rudensky, B., Caplan, M., et al. (2005). Oral probiotics prevent necrotizing enterocolitis in very low birth weight neonates. *Journal of Pediatrics, 147*(2), 192-196.

Blake, W., & Murray, J. (2006). Heat balance. In G. Merenstein & S. Gardner. (Eds.), *Handbook of neonatal intensive care* (6th ed.). St. Louis: Mosby.

Blauer, T., & Gerstmann, D. (1998). A simultaneous comparison of three neonatal pain scales during common NICU procedures. *Clinical Journal of Pain, 14*(1), 39-47.

Blauw-Hosper, C., & Hadders-Algra, M. (2005). A systematic review of the effects of early intervention on motor development. *Developmental Medicine & Child Neurology, 47*(6), 421-432.

Bloom, R. (2006). Delivery room resuscitation of the newborn. Part 4. Chest compression, medications, and special problems. In R. Martin, A. Fanaroff, & M. Walsh (Eds.), *Fanaroff and Martin's neonatal-perinatal medicine: Diseases of the fetus and infant* (8th ed.). Philadelphia: Mosby.

Brandon, D., Holditch-Davis, D., & Belyea, M. (2003). Preterm infants born at less than 31 weeks' gestation have improved growth in cycled light compared with continuous near darkness. *Journal of Pediatrics, 142*(4), 451-452.

Callen, J., & Pinelli, J. (2005). A review of the literature examining the benefits and challenges, incidence and duration, and barriers to breastfeeding in preterm infants. *Advances in Neonatal Care, 5*(2), 72-88.

Caplan, M. (2006). Neonatal necrotizing enterocolitis. In R. Martin, A. Fanaroff, & M. Walsh (Eds.), *Fanaroff and Martin's neonatal-perinatal medicine: Diseases of the fetus and infant* (8th ed.). Philadelphia: Mosby.

Carlo, W., Martin, R., & Fanaroff, A. (2006). Assisted ventilation and complications of respiratory distress. In R. Martin, A. Fanaroff, & M. Walsh (Eds.), *Fanaroff and Martin's neonatal-perinatal medicine: Diseases of the fetus and infant* (8th ed.). Philadelphia: Mosby.

Cifuentes, J., Segars, A., & Carlo, W. (2003). Assessment and management of neonatal respiratory system disorders. In C. Kenner, & J. Lott (Eds.), *Comprehensive neonatal nursing care: A physiologic perspective.* St. Louis: Saunders.

Davis, D., & Stein, M. (2004). *Parenting your premature baby and child: The emotional journey.* Golden, CO: Fulcrum.

Denne, S., Poindexter, B., Leitch, C., Ernst, J., Lemons, P., & Lemons, J. (2006). Nutrition and metabolism in the high-risk neonate. In R. Martin, A. Fanaroff, & M. Walsh (Eds.), *Fanaroff and Martin's neonatal-perinatal medicine: Diseases of the fetus and infant* (8th ed.). Philadelphia: Mosby.

de Vries, L. (2006). Intracranial hemorrhage and vascular lesions. In R. Martin, A. Fanaroff, & M. Walsh (Eds.), *Fanaroff and Martin's neonatal-perinatal medicine: Diseases of the fetus and infant* (8th ed.). Philadelphia: Mosby.

Diego, M., Field, T., & Hernandez-Reif, M. (2005). Vagal activity, gastric motility, and weight gain in massaged preterm neonates. *Journal of Pediatrics, 147*(1), 50-55.

End-of-Life Nursing Education Consortium (ELNEC) (Pediatric). (2005). *End-of-Life Nursing Education Consortium Training (Pediatric).* Washington, DC: American Association of Colleges of Nursing and City of Hope.

Ertl, T., Gyarmati, J., Gaal, V., & Szabo, I. (2006). Relationship between hyperglycemia and retinopathy of prematurity in very low birth weight infants. *Biology of the Neonate, 89*(1), 56-59.

Gross, S., Anbar, R., & Mettelman, B. (2005). Follow-up at 15 years of preterm infants from a controlled trial of moderately early dexamethasone for the prevention of chronic lung disease. *Pediatrics, 115*(3), 681-687.

Hall, W., Shearer, K., Mogan, J., & Berkowitz, J. (2002). Weighing preterm infants before & after breastfeeding: Does it increase maternal confidence and competence? *MCN American Journal of Maternal/Child Nursing, 27*(6), 318-327.

Haubrich, K. (2003). Assessment and management of auditory dysfunction. In C. Kenner, & J. Lott (Eds.), *Comprehensive neonatal nursing: A physiologic perspective* (3rd ed.). St. Louis: Saunders.

Hawthorne, K., Griffin, I., & Abrams, S. (2004). Current issues in nutritional management of very low birth weight infants. *Minerva Pediatrica, 56*(4), 359-372.

Hendricks-Muñoz, K., Prendergast, C., Caprio., M., & Wasserman, R. (2002). Developmental care: The impact of Wee Care developmental care training on short-term infant outcome and hospital costs. *Newborn and Infant Nursing Reviews, 2*(1), 39-45.

Hintz, S., Poole, W., Wright, L., Fanaroff, A., Kendrick, D., Laptook, A., et al. (2005). Changes in mortality and morbidities among infants born at less than 25 weeks during the post-surfactant era. *Archives of Disease in Childhood. Fetal & Neonatal Edition, 90*(2), F128-F133.

Hockenberry, M. (2003). *Wong's nursing care of infants and children* (7th ed.). St. Louis: Mosby.

Hodgkinson, K., Bear, M., Thorn, J., & Van Blaricum, S. (1994). Measuring pain in neonates: Evaluating an instrument and developing a common language. *Australian Journal of Advanced Nursing, 12*(1), 17-22.

Holditch-Davis, D., Bartlett, T., Blickman, A., & Miles, M. (2003). Posttraumatic stress symptoms in mothers of premature infants. *Journal of Obstetric, Gynecologic, and Neonatal Nursing, 32*(2), 161-171.

Holditch-Davis, D., Cox, M., Miles, M., & Belyea, M. (2003). Mother-infant interactions of medically fragile infants and non-chronically ill premature infants. *Research in Nursing & Health, 26*(4), 300-311.

Ito, M. (2004). 'Nurturing the brain' as an emerging research field involving child neurology. *Brain Development, 26*(7), 429-433.

Johnson, A. (2003). Adapting the neonatal intensive care environment to decrease noise. *Journal of Perinatal and Neonatal Nursing, 17*(4), 280-288.

Kenner, C. (2003). Resuscitation and stabilization of the newborn. In C. Kenner, & J. Lott (Eds.), *Comprehensive neonatal nursing care: A physiologic perspective* (3rd ed.). St. Louis: Saunders.

Kenner, C., & McGrath, J. (2004). *Developmental care of newborns & infants: A guide for health professionals.* St. Louis: Mosby.

Kledzik, T. (2005). Holding the very low birth weight infant: Skin-to-skin techniques. *Neonatal Network, 24*(1), 7-14.

Kliegman, R. (2006). Intrauterine growth restriction. In R. Martin, A. Fanaroff, & M. Walsh (Eds.), *Fanaroff and Martin's neonatal-perinatal medicine: Diseases of the fetus and infant* (8th ed.). Philadelphia: Mosby.

Krueger, C., Wall, S., Parker, L., & Nealis, R. (2005). Elevated sound levels within a busy NICU. *Neonatal Network, 24*(6), 33-37.

Lawrence, J., Alcock, D., McGrath, P., Kay, J., MacMurray, S., & Dulberg, C. (1993). The development of a tool to assess neonatal pain. *Neonatal Network, 12*(6), 59-66.

Liaw, J., Yuh, Y., & Chang, L. (2005). A preliminary study of the associations among preterm infant behaviors. *Journal of Nursing Research, 13*(1), 1-10.

Liptsen, E., Aghai, Z., Pyon, K., Saslow, J., Nakhla, T., Long, J., et al. (2005). Work of breathing during nasal continuous positive airway pressure in preterm infants: A comparison of bubble vs variable-flow devices. *Journal of Perinatology, 25*(7), 453-458.

Lund, C., & Kuller, J. (2003). Assessment and management of the integumentary system. In C. Kenner, & J. Lott (Eds.), *Comprehensive neonatal nursing care: A physiologic perspective* (3rd ed.). St. Louis: Saunders.

Medoff-Cooper, B., Bakewell-Sachs, S., Buus-Frank, M., & Santa-Donato, A. (2005). The AWHONN near-term infant initiative: A conceptual framework for optimizing health for near-term infants. *Journal of Obstetric, Gynecologic, and Neonatal Nursing, 34*(6), 666-671.

Mestan, K., Marks, J., Hecox, K., Huo, D., & Schreiber, M. (2005). Neurodevelopmental outcomes of premature infants treated with inhaled nitric oxide. *New England Journal of Medicine, 353*(1), 23-32.

Miles, M., Burchinal, P., Holditch-Davis, D., Brunssen, S., & Wilson, S. (2002). Perceptions of stress, worry, and support in Black and White mothers of hospitalized, medically fragile infants. *Journal of Pediatric Nursing, 17*(2), 82-88.

Pettett, G., Pallotto, E., & Merenstein, G. (2006). Perinatal transport. In G. Merenstein & S. Gardner (Eds.), *Handbook of neonatal intensive care* (6th ed.). St. Louis: Mosby.

Phelps, D. (2006). Retinopathy of prematurity. In R. Martin, A. Fanaroff, & M. Walsh (Eds.), *Fanaroff and Martin's neonatal-perinatal medicine: Diseases of the fetus and infant* (8th ed.). Philadelphia: Mosby.

Pokela, M. (1994). Pain relief can reduce hypoxemia in distressed neonates during routine treatment procedures. *Pediatrics, 93*(3), 379-383.

Robinson, T., & Driscoll, K. (2003). Legal and ethical issues of neonatal care. In C. Kenner, & J. Lott (Eds.), *Comprehensive neo-natal nursing care: A physiologic perspective* (3rd ed.). St. Louis: Saunders.

Rodriguez, R., Martin, R., & Fanaroff, A. (2006). Respiratory distress syndrome and its management. In R. Martin, A. Fanaroff, & M. Walsh (Eds.), *Fanaroff and Martin's neonatal-perinatal medicine: Diseases of the fetus and infant* (8th ed.). Philadelphia: Mosby.

Schwartz, J. (2003). New technologies applied to the management of the respiratory system. In C. Kenner, & J. Lott (Eds.), *Comprehen-*

sive neonatal nursing care: A physiologic perspective (3rd ed.). St. Louis: Saunders.

Simbruner, G., Ruttner, E., Schulze, A., & Perzlmaier, K. (2005). Premature infants are less capable of maintaining thermal balance of head and body with increases of thermal environment than with decreases. *American Journal of Perinatology, 22*(1), 25-33.

Sparshott, M. (1995). Assessing the behaviour of the newborn infant. *Paediatric Nursing, 7*(7), 14-16, 36.

Spence, K., Gillies, D., Harrison, D., Johnston, L., & Nagy, S. (2005). A reliable pain assessment tool for clinical assessment in the neonatal intensive care unit. *Journal of Obstetric, Gynecologic, and Neonatal Nursing, 34*(10), 80-86.

Standley, J. (2002). A meta-analysis of the efficacy of music therapy for premature infants. *Journal of Pediatric Nursing, 17*(20), 107-114.

Steuber, K., Carroll, D., McCoy, S., & Nurney, E. (2002). Cuddler volunteers: A very special part of the NICU team. *Central Lines, 18*(4), 4-6.

Stevens, B., Johnston, C., Petryshen, P., & Taddio, A. (1996). Premature Infant Pain Profile: Development and initial validation. *Clinical Journal of Pain, 12*(1), 13-22.

Stevens, B., Johnston, C., Franck, L., Petryshen, P., Jack, A., & Foster, G. (1999). The efficacy of developmentally sensitive interventions and sucrose for relieving procedural pain in very low birth weight neonates. *Nursing Research, 48*(1), 35-43.

Stork, E. (2006). Therapy for cardiorespiratory failure. In R. Martin, A. Fanaroff, & M. Walsh (Eds.), *Fanaroff and Martin's neonatal-perinatal medicine: Diseases of the fetus and infant* (8th ed.). Philadelphia: Mosby.

Swartz, M. (2005). Parenting preterm infants: A meta-synthesis. *MCN American Journal of Maternal/Child Nursing, 30*(2), 115-120.

Symington, A., & Pinelli, J. (2003). Developmental care for promoting development and preventing morbidity in preterm infants (review). *The Cochrane Database of Systematic Reviews,* 2006, Issue 3. Chichester, UK: John Wiley & Sons.

Tyson, J., & Kennedy, K. (2002). Trophic feedings for parenterally fed infants (review). *The Cochrane Database of Systematic Reviews,* 2006, Issue 3. Chichester, UK: John Wiley & Sons.

Vain, N., Szyld, E., Prudent, L., Wiswell, T. Aguilar, A., & Vivas, N. (2004). Oropharyngeal and nasopharyngeal suctioning of meconium-stained neonates before delivery of their shoulders: Multicentre, randomized controlled trial. *Lancet, 14*(364), 597-602.

Vohr, B., Wright, L., Dusick, A., Mele, L., Verter, J., Steichen, J., et al. (2005). Infants in the National Institute of Child Health and Human Development Neonatal Research Network, 1993-1994. *Pediatrics, 105*(6), 1216-1226.

Walden, M., & Franck, L. (2003). Identification, management, and prevention of newborn/infant pain. In C. Kenner, & J. Lott (Eds.), *Comprehensive neonatal nursing care: A physiologic perspective* (3rd ed.). St. Louis: Saunders.

Wang, M., Dorer, D., Fleming, M., & Catlin, E. (2004). Clinical outcomes of near-term infants. *Pediatrics, 114*(2), 372-376.

Wilson-Costello, D., & Hack, M. (2006). Follow-up for high-risk neonates. In R. Martin, A. Fanaroff, & M. Walsh (Eds.), *Fanaroff and Martin's neonatal-perinatal medicine: Diseases of the fetus and infant* (8th ed.). Philadelphia: Mosby.

Wiswell, T., Knight, G., Finer, N., Donn, S., Desai, H., Walsh, W., et al. (2002). A multicenter, randomized, controlled trial comparing Surfaxin (Lucinactant) lavage with standard care for treatment of meconium aspiration syndrome. *Pediatrics, 109*(6), 1081-1087.

Wyckoff, M., McGrath, J., Griffin, T., Malan, J., & White-Traut, R. (2003). Nutrition: Physiologic basis of metabolism and management of enteral and parenteral nutrition. In C. Kenner, & J.

Lott (Eds.), *Comprehensive neonatal nursing: A physiologic perspective* (3rd ed.). St. Louis: Saunders.

Yoder, B., Kirsch, E., Barth, W., & Gordon, M. (2002). Changing obstetric practices associated with decreasing incidence of meconium aspiration syndrome. *Obstetrics and Gynecology, 99*(5 Pt 1), 731-739.

Zahka, K., & Bengur, A. (2006). Cardiovascular problems of the neonate. In R. Martin, A. Fanaroff, & M. Walsh (Eds.), *Fanaroff and Martin's neonatal-perinatal medicine: Diseases of the fetus and infant* (8th ed.). Philadelphia: Mosby.

Grieving the Loss of a Newborn

learning objectives

- Describe emotional, behavioral, cognitive, and physical responses commonly experienced during the grieving process associated with perinatal loss.
- Understand the personal and societal issues that may complicate responses to perinatal loss.
- Formulate appropriate nursing diagnoses for parents experiencing perinatal loss.

- Identify specific nursing interventions to meet the special needs of parents and their families related to perinatal loss and grief.
- Differentiate among helpful and nonhelpful responses in caring for parents experiencing loss and grief.

electronic resources

Additional information related to the content in Chapter 41 can be found on

the companion website at *evolve*
http://evolve.elsevier.com/Lowdermilk/MWHC/
- NCLEX Review Questions
- WebLinks

or on the interactive companion CD
- NCLEX Review Questions
- Plan of Care: Fetal Death: 24 Weeks of Gestation

BECOMING a parent is an important developmental milestone that is anticipated by most men and women in our society. Becoming a parent gives one social status, expands one's capacity for caring and loving for another, and adds immense responsibility to one's life. However, pregnancy and birth can also be associated with loss. During pregnancy, parents plan for the birth, imagine what the birth will be like, and develop an image of the appearance of the baby. The reality of childbirth may not be what the parents have dreamed of or hoped for. In particular, the experience of preterm labor and birth or cesarean birth involves loss of the expected pregnancy and birth plans. Parents also may grieve over the sex or appearance of their child. For some parents, loss is associated with the birth of an infant who has a birth defect or chronic illness.

Although having children can be a strong desire and goal for women and men, not everyone is successful in achieving parenthood. For some couples, infertility may thwart their plans and desires for parenthood and cause intense feelings of grief (Johansson & Berg, 2005). When couples undergo infertility treatments, feelings of loss may intensify, especially when treatments fail and/or a pregnancy ends in an ectopic pregnancy loss or miscar-

riage (Freda, Devine, & Semelsberger, 2003; Johansson & Berg).

Many women and their partners, whether infertile or not, can experience perinatal loss. This includes ectopic pregnancy or fetal death, miscarriage, and induced abortion, all of which occur in the early months of pregnancy. These losses are often called "hidden" or "silent" because others in the women's network may not even know about the pregnancy and subsequent loss, or because family and friends may not feel comfortable bringing up the loss with the woman and her partner (Bennett, Litz, Lee, & Shira, 2005; Bowles et al., 2000). Women and their partners may suddenly be confronted with *stillbirth*, the birth of an infant who is not alive (Hughes, Turton, Hopper, & Evans, 2002). Stillbirth is particularly devastating because it occurs suddenly and late in the pregnancy when expectant parents are preparing for the birth of a healthy infant. Couples also experience intense grief after infant death. This includes birth of a preterm infant or an infant with severe congenital anomalies or other serious health problems who survives only a few hours or who dies after days, weeks, or months in an intensive care unit. Many of these parents are confronted with making difficult end-of-life decisions about their baby (Kavanaugh, Savage, Kilpatrick,

Kimura, & Hershberger, 2005; Moseley, Church, Hempel, Yuan, Goold, & Freed, 2004).

There has been a considerable decline in infant mortality during the 1990s; in 1991 the rate was 8.9 per 1000 live births, in 2001 it was 6.9, and in 2003 it was 7.0 (Hoyert, Mathews, Menacker, Strobino, & Guyer, 2006). Approximately 20 of each 1000 pregnancies are ectopic pregnancies, taking place outside the uterus, usually in a uterine tube (Sepilian & Wood, 2005). It is estimated that miscarriage occurs in approximately 15% of all pregnancies (American College of Obstetricians and Gynecologists, 2001). In addition, each year approximately 5 of every 1000 births end in stillbirth or fetal deaths (those occurring after 20 weeks of gestation) (Ananth, Liu, Kinzler, & Kramer, 2005). Newborn death, death of a baby born showing signs of life such as respiratory effort, heart rate, pulsating cord at birth, and/or muscle irritability, regardless of gestational age, accounts for numerous deaths each year in the United States. The primary cause of infant death is birth defects (137.6 per 100,000 live births) (March of Dimes, 2005). Prematurity accounted for approximately 70% of all neonatal deaths, and extremely preterm infants accounted for 58% of deaths in 2001 (Centers for Disease Control and Prevention [CDC], 2004). Other causes of infant mortality are sudden infant death syndrome, maternal complications of pregnancy, and respiratory distress syndrome. African-American women experience pregnancy and infant losses at rates twice those of Caucasian women and women of other ethnic minority groups (Ananth et al.; Van, 2001).

The infant mortality rates in many countries across the world are staggeringly high, mostly due to infections, birth asphyxia and trauma, and preterm birth (which is also associated with maternal infection) (World Health Organization [WHO], 2005).

Thus parents can experience grief before or during the childbearing experience. Grief involves the painful emotions and related behavioral and physical responses to a major loss (Capitulo, 2004; Miles, 2005). Grief can be particularly difficult with perinatal losses for a number of reasons. One is the societal belief that there are no barriers to getting pregnant. Another is the expectation that once a woman is pregnant, the outcome will be a healthy live infant. As a result, our society tends to minimize perinatal loss and to lack understanding of the associated pain (Bennett et al., 2005; Malacrida, 1999). Women and men who undergo perinatal losses often struggle with these issues alone and may not receive the support they need because many perinatal losses are hidden or private.

Perinatal losses may be intensified for couples who delay pregnancy until the woman's career and the family's financial status is at the right point to take on the responsibilities of a child. Feelings of helplessness and loss of control can be very difficult when the couple experiences infertility or miscarriage. In many instances of perinatal loss, the lack of an identified cause for the loss can complicate grief. This is particularly difficult for women, who often

feel personally responsible for infertility, miscarriage, and infant death. Some couples endure repeated losses, which can be devastating. Further, society allows too little time for mothers grieving a perinatal loss and even less for men. All of these issues can reduce the support to bereaved parents. Parents in a Canadian study reported that social support from families and friends fell short of expectations, and they interpreted this inattention as an indication that the death of their baby was not an important life event (Malacrida, 1999).

Nurses have a powerful influence on how parents experience and cope with perinatal loss (Capitulo, 2005; Corbet-Owen & Kruger, 2001; Lundqvist, Nilstun, & Dykes, 2002b; Saflund, Sjogren, & Wredling, 2004). Nurses encounter these parents in a variety of settings, including the antepartum, labor and birth, neonatal, postpartum, and gynecologic units of hospitals, and obstetric, gynecologic, and infertility outpatient clinics and general medical offices. In these settings, nurses have opportunities to provide sensitive and caring interventions to parents. Parents have reported that their nurses were an important resource in helping them cope with their grief.

Nurses in many inpatient settings have developed protocols that provide clear direction to all staff in how to help parents through this difficult process. In some units, experienced nurses or social workers who are particularly comfortable in helping bereaved parents are designated as perinatal grief consultants. They are available to help parents but also to help prepare the staff for their role with parents. In addition, many institutions now have follow-up programs involving telephone calls, home visits, and support groups that are effective in helping parents after discharge. It is important, then, that dealing with perinatal loss be included in nursing curricula and in-service training for staff nurses.

The focus of this chapter is to prepare the nurse to provide sensitive, supportive, and therapeutic interventions to parents experiencing perinatal loss in a variety of settings. An overview of the grief process is presented as a guide for assessing and understanding the responses of bereaved women, men, and their families. Guidelines for intervention are given, and specific intervention approaches are discussed.

▰ GRIEF RESPONSES

Grief or bereavement has been described as a cluster of painful responses experienced by individuals coping with the death of someone with whom they had a close relationship, generally a relative or close friend (Lindemann, 1944). Many authors believe there are overlapping phases in the grief process, but most do not believe that grief is experienced in "stages." Based on years of clinical work with bereaved parents and building on the conceptualization of others regarding grief following the death of a spouse, Miles developed a model of parental grief (Miles, 1984; 2005).

Parental grief responses occur in three overlapping phases (Box 41-1). There is an early period of acute distress and shock followed by a period of intense grief that includes emotional, cognitive, behavioral, and physical responses. The phase of reorganization is reached when parents return to their usual level of functioning in society, although the pain associated with the death remains. The duration of grief varies with the individual, but there is general agreement that grief is a long-term process that can extend for months and years. With a very close relationship such as with one's baby, some aspects of grief never truly end.

Acute Distress

The loss of a pregnancy or the death of an infant is an acute and distressing experience for mothers and fathers. The loss encompasses a loss of their identity as a mother or father and the loss of their many dreams related to parenthood. Lundqvist, Nilstun, and Dykes (2002a) have labeled this experience for mothers as an "ambivalent transition into motherhood." The immediate reaction to news of a perinatal loss or infant death encompasses a period of acute distress. Parents generally are in a state of shock and numbness. They may feel a sense of unreality, loss of innocence, and powerlessness as though they were in a bad dream or in a fog or trancelike state. Disbelief and denial can occur (Lundqvist et al., Rillstone & Hutchinson, 2001). Sadness, devastation, and depression as well as intense outbursts of emotion and crying are common. However, lack of affect, euphoria, and calmness may occur and may reflect numbness, denial, or a personal way of coping with stress.

---

box 41-1 **Conceptual Model of Parental Grief**

PHASE OF ACUTE DISTRESS
- Shock
- Numbness
- Intense crying
- Depression

PHASE OF INTENSE GRIEF
- Loneliness, emptiness, and yearning
- Guilt
- Anger, resentment, bitterness, irritability
- Fear and anxiety (especially about getting pregnant again)
- Disorganization
- Difficulties with cognitive processing
- Sadness and depression
- Physical symptoms

REORGANIZATION
- Search for meaning
- Reduction of distress
- Reentering normal life activities with more enthusiasm
- Can make future plans, including decision about another pregnancy

Adapted from Miles, M. (1980). *The grief of parents...when a child dies.* Oak Brook, IL: Compassionate Friends; Miles, M. (1984). Helping adults mourn the death of a child. In H. Wass, & C. Corr (Eds.), *Childhood and death.* New York: Hemisphere.

Much of the literature and research on grief after perinatal loss and infant death has focused on the mother. Likewise, much of the attention during the time of a loss is on the mother; the father is expected to be her main support but is often not acknowledged as grieving, too. The response of fathers may be more variable than that of mothers and depends on the level of identification with the pregnancy. With early miscarriage or ectopic pregnancy, some fathers may not yet have developed a strong investment in the wished-for child. However, many fathers are profoundly affected and do grieve deeply for a perinatal loss, yet their feelings are often ignored (McCreight, 2004; Samuelsson, Radestad, & Segesten, 2001).

Fathers are distressed by the grief of the mother and often feel helpless as to how to help her with the intense pain. Some fathers appear stoic and unemotional to maintain the societal expectation that they be "strong" for the mother and other family members. It is important to realize that fathers may be experiencing deep pain beneath their calm and quiet appearance and need help in acknowledging these feelings. Because many fathers do not easily share feelings or ask for help, special efforts are needed to help them realize that they too have a right to support from others in their pain.

During this time of acute distress, parents face the first task of grief, accepting the reality of the loss. The pregnancy has ended or the baby has died, and their life has changed. Although parents are often required to make many decisions, such as having an autopsy, naming the infant, and funeral arrangements, normal functioning is impeded, and decisions are difficult to make. These decisions are especially painful and difficult for young couples who have limited or no previous experience with death. Grandparents are often called on to help make difficult decisions regarding funeral arrangements and/or disposition of the body because they have more life experience with taking care of these painful, yet required arrangements. However, some well-meaning grandparents and other family members may try to take over all the decisions that must be made. It is critical that the nurse remember that a very important role is always to be a client advocate and that the parents themselves should approve the final decisions.

Intense Grief

The phase of intense grief encompasses many difficult emotions as the parents work through their pain and adjust to life without the wished-for child. In the early months after the loss, parents often experience feelings of loneliness, emptiness, and yearning. The mother may report that her arms ache to hold or nurse her baby and that she wakes to the sound of a baby crying. When her milk comes in, it is particularly poignant when there is no baby to take to breast. Both mothers and fathers may be preoccupied with thoughts about the wished-for child. Some women cope with these feelings by avoiding memories and by not talking about the baby, whereas others want to reminisce and discuss their loss over and over. Deciding what to do about the nursery and baby clothes is particularly difficult during this period. Some women want the room taken down before they go home, whereas others want the room left intact until they have had time to grieve their loss. It is not unusual for a grandparent or other family member to want to rush home to take down the nursery with the thought that they would be sparing additional painful grief. In fact, their actions might only complicate the grief if parents were not involved in the decision. The bereaved parents, in their own time frame, must go through these types of experiences so that healing can take place.

During this phase of intense grief, guilt may emerge from the deep feelings of helplessness in not somehow preventing the pregnancy loss or the death of the infant. Mothers are particularly vulnerable to feel guilt because of their sense of responsibility for the well-being of the fetus and baby. With many perinatal losses, there is no clear cause of the event, leaving the woman to speculate about what she might have done or not done to cause the loss. Guilt also may be intense if a mother thinks she is being punished for some unrelated event such as having had a prior induced abortion. Such self-blame is torture for mothers, and they need repeated emotional reassurance that they were not at fault. Guilt can occur when one is enjoying life again and experiencing happiness despite the loss of the infant.

Other common responses during this phase of grief are anger, resentment, bitterness, or irritability. Anger is particularly poignant if the loss is perceived as senseless, and there is a need to blame others. Anger may be focused on the health care team who failed to save the pregnancy or infant. For some parents, anger is vented toward a God who allowed the loss to occur. This can lead to a spiritual crisis. Anger also occurs toward family, friends, and peers when they do not provide the support bereaved parents need and want. Some parents focus their resentment on parents who do not appreciate their children or who neglect and abuse them. A sense of bitterness or generalized irritability, rather than frank anger, may be another response.

Fear and anxiety can occur during the grief process as a profound worry that something else bad might happen to another. Fear and anxiety are particularly poignant when the couple thinks about another pregnancy (Cote-Arsenault & Marshall, 2000; Rillstone & Hutchinson, 2001). Some parents, especially mothers, are almost obsessed with the desire to become pregnant again; others struggle with whether they can cope with another potential loss.

Deep sadness and depression occur when the parent is faced with the full awareness of the reality of the loss. This often occurs several months after a perinatal loss and can continue for some time. Sadness and depression are often accompanied by disorganization and problems with cognitive processing. This leads to behavioral changes such as difficulty in getting things done, an inability to concentrate, restlessness, confused thought processes, difficulty in solving problems, and poor decision making. Disorganization and depression often cause difficulties in keeping up with work and family expectations. Additionally, parents return-

ing to work face issues such as handling well-meaning but painful comments or the silence of co-workers.

Physical symptoms of grief include fatigue, headaches, dizziness, or backaches. Parents are at risk for developing health problems, such as colds or hypertension. The grieving process makes it difficult for bereaved parents to sleep. Their appetites may be depressed or voracious. Lack of sleep and inadequate nutrition and fluids can complicate other grief responses.

Grief responses are very personal, ongoing, and difficult to cope with. Some parents may suppress or deny their feelings because of societal indifference toward pregnancy loss and infant death. Suppression of feelings may, on the surface, be more socially acceptable. However, denying the pain of grief may lead to eventual physical and emotional distress or illness. Many parents, especially mothers, want to tell their story over and over. This helps them actualize the loss and face their feelings. Sometimes parents begin to think they are the only individuals who have ever had such a rough time and that they may be going crazy. Although bereaved parents have many ups and downs for many months and even years after a child's death, few parents actually become mentally ill or commit suicide. Knowing that these feelings are normal and that others have felt the same is helpful. The grief process during this phase is often difficult for fathers (Samuelsson et al., 2001). Some may continue to have difficulty sharing their feelings. A rift can occur if one parent, usually the mother, wants to talk about the loss and pain, and the other parent, often but not always the father, withdraws. Other signs of problems include reliance on alcohol and drugs, extramarital affairs, prolonged hours at work, and overinvolvement in activities outside the home as an escape.

Reorganization

From the time of the pregnancy loss or infant death, parents attempt to understand "why?" This leads to a long and intense search for meaning. At first the "why" is focused on the cause of death. Finding few good answers, parents focus next on "why me, why mine?" These questions lead some parents into an existential search about the meaning of life and death. "What does my loss mean to my life?" "What is life all about?" "What do I do with the rest of my life?" This search continues into the phase of reorganization and may lead to profound changes in the parents' views about the fragility of life.

Time helps to ease slowly the painful feelings of grief. Over time, the feelings become less painful. Reorganization occurs when the parent is better able to function at home and work, experiences a return of self-esteem and confidence, can cope with new challenges, and has placed the loss in perspective. Reorganization begins to peak sometime after the first year as parents begin to achieve the task of moving on with their lives. Enjoying the simple pleasures of life without feeling guilty, nurturing self and others, developing new interests, and reestablishing relationships are all signs of moving on. For some women and

EVIDENCE-BASED PRACTICE

Measuring the Unmeasurable: Perinatal Grief Scale

BACKGROUND

- Throughout the last century, perinatal loss became the exception and not the rule. Cultural changes in the 1970s created increased client expectations of control during childbirth, self-help movements, and open discussion of the stages of dying and grieving. To understand the grief of perinatal loss, social scientists faced the challenge of measuring this powerful, profound emotion. Since the Perinatal Grief Scale (PGS) was presented in 1988, it has been used in many studies as a tool to quantify and predict the impact of perinatal loss. The PGS is a 33-item test, using Likert-type responses (strongly agree to strongly disagree) to various statements of grief.

OBJECTIVES

- The original PGS authors sought further validation of the tool. Their goals were to compare the internal consistency reliability of the PGS, establish normative ranges for screening, and compare groups across cultures and times.

METHODS

Search Strategy

- Every article that referenced the original publications about the PGS or requested to use the tool was evaluated. The reviewers also thoroughly searched research databases. The authors identified 22 empirical studies, presented from 1988 to 1999, representing 1803 women and 654 men (total 2457) from the United States, the United Kingdom, the Netherlands, and Germany. The types of losses included miscarriage, stillbirth, newborn loss, ectopic pregnancy, adoption, and elective abortion.

Statistical Analyses

- Metaanalysis indicated strong internal consistency reliability (all items seem to measure the same phenomenon similarly) and external validity (generalizability) of the PGS tool. The number of subjects enabled the establishment of a normal range of grief by determining that 97.5% of newly bereaved parents' scores fall below 91. Therefore, a score above 91 was accepted as reflecting severe distress. No normal low range was established. It was speculated that grief scores would decline across time. Group scores were compared, as were stages of pregnancy and birth at time of loss.
- High benchmarks were also set for the three subscale groups which showed progressive psychologic decline: active grief, difficulty coping (more severe), and despair (most severe).

FINDINGS

- Women's scores exceeded men's scores, but not to the level of significance. Grief scores decreased across 2 years. There were significantly higher grief scores in groups recruited from grief groups or advertisements than from parents referred by health care workers. This may account for the significantly higher scores in the U.S. samples, who were mostly recruited through advertisements and groups, as compared to the European cohorts, who were mostly referrals from hospitals. Strong marriages and the perception of social support were consistently related to lower grief scores. Pre-loss poor mental health, such as neuroticism, led to significantly higher grief. Grief scores showed a pattern of increasing with increasing gestation, but not to the level of significance. In the United States, low socioeconomic status was significantly associated with higher grief scores; this disparity was less marked in Europe.

LIMITATIONS

- Diversity was lacking in the U.S. samples, which were largely white and middle class. Groups and advertisements may attract people seeking relief from more severe grief; this sample bias may confound the comparison of scores between the United States and Europe. Cultural bias and wording may also have influenced results.

IMPLICATIONS FOR PRACTICE

- Nurses can identify those at risk for poor adaptation, and counsel the bereaved parents that healing will take years, social support, and a strong marriage. Clients with high PGS scores that do not improve across time, or who seem to be slipping into measurable despair on the subscale, can be referred to grief specialists.

IMPLICATIONS FOR FURTHER RESEARCH

- Research is needed with more diverse cohorts. The PGS can be used to explore the grief patterns of men and other family/support members. Researchers can examine the lower end of the grief scale, to distinguish functional results from denial, which may prove to be a bigger problem later on. Research can determine whether those seeking groups have higher baseline scores, or whether self-help groups are not as effective for alleviating grief as some hospital interventions. In-depth research is still needed on ectopic pregnancy, second trimester abortions for genetic abnormalities, and elective abortion.

Reference: Toedter, L., Lasker, L., & Janssen, H. (2001). International comparison of studies using the Perinatal Grief Scale: A decade of research on pregnancy loss. *Death Studies, 25*(3), 205-228.

families, another pregnancy and the birth of a subsequent child is an important step in moving on with their lives; however, the term "recovery" is used because the grief related to perinatal loss can continue in varying degrees for life.

Parents have shared that they will never forget the baby who has died, and they are not the same persons as before the loss. The term "bittersweet grief," refers to the grief response that occurs with reminders of the loss. This typically happens at special anniversary dates related to the

loss. Grief feelings also can be triggered during subsequent pregnancies and after birth (Cote-Arsenault & Marshall, 2000; Rillstone & Hutchinson, 2001) (Box 41-2).

Resuming the sexual relationship is an important aspect of recovery but can be very complicated. Many parents are comforted with the belief that their babies were conceived in love, lived in love, and died in love. Their love and intimacy created this child, and parents may believe that they may never experience joy and closeness again. Once the doctor has given permission for resumption of sexual

Presents Thoughts and Feelings About Your Loss

Each of the items is a statement of thoughts and feelings that some people have concerning a loss such as yours. There are no right or wrong responses to these statements. For each item, circle the number that best indicated the extent to which you agree or disagree with it at the present time. If you are not certain, use the "neither" category. Please try to use this category only when you truly have no opinion.

	Strongly Agree	Agree	Neither Agree nor Disagree	Disagree	Strongly Disagree
1. I feel depressed.	1	2	3	4	5
2. I find it hard to get along with certain people.	1	2	3	4	5
3. I feel empty inside.	1	2	3	4	5
4. I can't keep up with my normal activities.	1	2	3	4	5
5. I feel a need to talk about the baby.	1	2	3	4	5
6. I am grieving for the baby.	1	2	3	4	5
7. I am frightened.	1	2	3	4	5
8. I have considered suicide since the loss.	1	2	3	4	5
9. I take medicine for my nerves.	1	2	3	4	5
10. I very much miss the baby.	1	2	3	4	5
11. I feel I have adjusted well to the loss.	1	2	3	4	5
12. It is painful to recall memories of the loss.	1	2	3	4	5
13. I get upset when I think about the baby.	1	2	3	4	5
14. I cry when I think about him/her.	1	2	3	4	5
15. I feel guilty when I think about the baby.	1	2	3	4	5
16. I feel physically ill when I think about the baby.	1	2	3	4	5
17. I feel unprotected in a dangerous world since he/she died.	1	2	3	4	5
18. I try to laugh, but nothing seems funny anymore.	1	2	3	4	5
19. Time passes so slowly since the baby died.	1	2	3	4	5
20. The best part of me died with the baby.	1	2	3	4	5
21. I have let people down since the baby died.	1	2	3	4	5
22. I feel worthless since he/she died.	1	2	3	4	5
23. I blame myself for the baby's death.	1	2	3	4	5
24. I get cross at my friends and relatives more than I should.	1	2	3	4	5
25. Sometimes I feel like I need a professional counselor to help me get my life back together again.	1	2	3	4	5
26. I feel as though I'm just existing and not really living since he/she died.	1	2	3	4	5
27. I feel so lonely since he/she died.	1	2	3	4	5
28. I feel somewhat apart and remote, even among friends.	1	2	3	4	5
29. It's safer not to love.	1	2	3	4	5
30. I find it difficult to make decisions since the baby died.	1	2	3	4	5
31. I worry about what my future will be like.	1	2	3	4	5
32. Being a bereaved parent means being a "Second-Class Citizen."	1	2	3	4	5
33. It feels great to be alive.	1	2	3	4	5

Scoring Instructions

The total PGS score is arrived at by first reversing all of the items except 11 and 33. By reversing the items, higher scores now reflect more intense grief. Then add the scores together. The result is a total scale consisting of 33 items with a possible range of 33-165.

The three subscales consist of the sum of the scores of 11 items each, with a possible range of 11-55.

Subscale 1 Active Grief	Subscale 2 Difficulty Coping	Subscale 3 Despair
1	2	9
3	4	15
5	8	16
6	*11	17
7	21	18
10	24	20
12	25	22
13	26	23
14	28	29
19	30	31
27	*33	32

*Do not reverse.

FIG. 41-1 The Perinatal Grief Scale (33-item short version). (From Toedter, L., Lasker, J., & Janssen, H. [2001]. International comparison of studies using the Perinatal Grief Scale: A decade of research on pregnancy loss. *Death Studies, 25*[3], 205-228.)

box 41-2 **Bittersweet Grief**

To Jessica Mayo—on her eleventh birthday
Sunday, November 18, 1990
"The child who is born on the Sabbath day,
    is bonny and blithe and good and gay."
Sundays are special days.
. . . a day of rest, a day to play.
A day to reflect on days past.
. . . a day to thank God for all that we bless.
I bless your memory.
I wish you were here.
On your eleventh birthday I still want to share.
. . . Your dreams of the future.
. . . Our memories past.
My baby's first cry.
My daughter's first laugh.
I was told you were an angel in heaven above.
Eleven years later, I'm an expert . . .
At long-distance love.
On your third birthday I wrote my first poem
to you.
Eight years later, it's still true
". . . no birthday cake,
no presents unwrapped . . .
no pictures of you in your party hat.
But the candles are lit,
Never to go out
For they burn forever in my heart.
Love, Mom"
    Kathie Rataj Mayo
    1990

Used with permission of Bereavement Services. Copyright Lutheran Hospital—La Crosse, Inc., a Gundersen Lutheran Affiliate, La Crosse, WI.

activities, parents may find it emotionally very difficult. Some couples may have an increased need for sexual activity in an attempt for closeness and healing, whereas others have a decreased desire for sexual intimacy. It is important that clients be aware of some possible deep need from inside themselves to stop the emotional pain. Difficulties arise when the needs of the couple differ.

Sexuality also brings with it decisions about a future pregnancy. Some are eager to have another child, although one child cannot replace the one who died, and the grief will continue despite being pregnant. Other parents have a deep fear of experiencing the pain of loss again, which can make the resumption of sexual activity difficult. These ambivalent feelings are normal, and couples will find themselves moving back and forth between the emotions of exhilaration and fear. The subsequent pregnancy after a loss is often filled with guarded emotions and great anxiety (Cote-Arsenault & Marshall, 2000; Rillstone & Hutchinson, 2001). The excitement that many others experience with a pregnancy is very different for previously bereaved parents. For some, this emotional distress can affect maternal attachment to the new baby (Armstrong, 2002). Fathers also reported anxiety about the outcome of the next pregnancy and increased their vigilance (Armstrong, 2001). Couples often mark the progress of the pregnancy in terms of fetal development, waiting anxiously until the number of weeks of the previous loss are passed. In some cases, the fear of repeated loss, especially after a stillbirth, is so great that induction of labor is considered if lung maturity studies can confirm that the baby is mature. Support groups have been found important in helping women through pregnancies after loss (Cote-Arsenault & Freije, 2004).

▬ FAMILY ASPECTS OF GRIEF

Grandparents and Siblings

It is extremely important for the nurse taking care of these clients to keep in mind that they have an entire family to minister to, including especially grandparents and siblings. Grandparents have hopes and dreams for a grandchild; these have been shattered. The grief of grandparents is often complicated by the fact that they are experiencing intense emotional pain by witnessing and feeling the immense grief of their own child. It is extremely difficult to watch their son or daughter experience unimaginable emotional trauma with very few ways to comfort and end their pain. As a result, the grief response may be complicated or delayed for grandparents. On occasions, some grandparents experience immense "survivor guilt" because they feel the death is out of order as they are alive and their grandchild has died.

The siblings of the expected infant also experience a profound loss. Most children have been prepared for having another child in the family once the pregnancy is confirmed. These children come in all ages and stages of development, and this must be considered in understanding how they view the event and their loss experience. A young child will respond more to the response of his or her parents, picking up on the fact that they are behaving differently and are extremely sad. This can cause clinging, altered eating and sleeping patterns, or acting out behaviors, yet it is a time when parents have limited patience for responding to and meeting the needs of the child. Older children have a more complete understanding of the loss. School-aged children may be frightened by the entire event, whereas teens may understand fully but feel awkward in responding.

Older siblings need to be included in grieving rituals to the extent the parents and the child feel comfortable. They may need to see the baby to actualize the loss. Nurses need to have a basic understanding about how children view death and grieve to reach out to siblings in an appropriate and sensitive manner. Nurses also need to help parents recognize and be sensitive to the grief of siblings, include them in family rituals, and keep the baby alive in the family memory (Wilson, 2001).

▬ CARE MANAGEMENT

Nursing care of mothers and fathers experiencing a perinatal loss begins the first time the parents are faced with the potential loss of their pregnancy or death of their infant. Supportive interventions are important both at the time of the loss and after the parents have returned home.

▬ Assessment and Nursing Diagnoses

An important step in the nursing process involves assessment. Several key areas to address include the following:

- The nature of the parental attachment with the pregnancy or infant, the meaning of the pregnancy and infant to the parent, and the related losses they are experiencing. Each pregnancy and birth has a special meaning to parents. Whether a woman has experienced a miscarriage or ectopic pregnancy, stillbirth, or death of an infant, it is important to gain some understanding of parents' perceptions of their unique loss. The meaning of the loss is determined by familial and cultural systems of the parents. In one study, feelings about perinatal loss ranged from feeling devastated to feeling relieved (Corbet-Owen & Kruger, 2001). Listening to parents tell their story and being sensitive to the language used to describe their experience can help one gain an understanding of the meaning of the loss. Open-ended questions are helpful: "Tell me about your labor and birth with Mia." Or "When did you know you were miscarrying?" Mothers who have had a previous pregnancy loss may feel less attached, which can increase their feelings of guilt when a loss occurs.
- The circumstances surrounding the loss, including the level of preparation for the loss and the parents' level of understanding about the cause of the loss or death, and any related unresolved issues are important. While listening to the parents' stories, it is important to uncover any special experiences that may make their losses even more poignant. A history of infertility, repeated pregnancy losses, a previous stillbirth, or infant death can make this loss even more painful. In addition, other life circumstances such as illness of another family member, loss of a job, or other family stresses can increase the distress of parents. It also is helpful to know whether the mother and father perceived the loss to be totally unexpected, or whether they had some forewarning or preparation.
- The immediate response of the mother and father to the loss, whether their responses are complementary or problematic, and how their responses match with their past experiences, personalities, and behavioral and cultural backgrounds. An understanding of the usual responses to grief described earlier can be helpful in attempting to understand the unique grief responses of the mother and the father and other family members. As nurses work with families, they may uncover information about how the individual or family responded to a previous loss, or a personality or behavioral trait that may be involved in their responses to this grief. In particular, it is important to know about any history of infertility, previous pregnancy losses, or infant deaths and evaluate how that might affect parental responses. It also is important to be sensitive to different expectations during grief for men and women from different cultural groups (see section on cultural and spiritual needs of parents later in this chapter).

- The social support network of the parent (e.g., extended family, friends, co-workers, church) and the extent to which it has been activated. Support during a perinatal loss is important to most couples. However, it is important to assess the amount of support and the type of support from others that a couple wants. Some prefer to handle the tragedy alone for a time. Others want assistance in calling other family members, friends, and clergy to be with them and to help them with decisions.

Nursing diagnoses may include physiologic and psychosocial problems experienced by the individual mother or father, or problems occurring within the couple or family because of the loss and subsequent grief. Examples of nursing diagnoses include the following:

- *Anxiety related to*
  - lack of experience regarding how to manage the loss
  - worry about the partner
  - intense concern over not achieving a pregnancy
  - becoming pregnant again with risk of another loss
- *Ineffective family coping related to*
  - inability to make decisions as a family
  - difficulties in communication within the family
  - conflicting coping patterns between mother and father
- *Powerlessness related to*
  - high risk pregnancy and birth
  - unexpected cesarean birth
  - inability to prevent the infant's death
- *Interrupted family processes related to*
  - maternal depression leading to changes in role function
  - inadequate communication of feelings between the grieving mother and father
  - lack of expected support from family
  - behavioral and emotional reactions of siblings
  - grief within the family system including grandparents and other relatives
- *Ineffective sexuality patterns between the mother and father related to*
  - guilt and fear associated with sexuality
  - loss of pleasure in sexual intercourse
  - differences in desires of each partner
  - fear of getting pregnant again
- *Fatigue and disturbed sleep pattern related to*
  - inability to fall asleep because of grief
  - waking in the night and thinking about the loss
  - loss of sleep
- *Dysfunctional grieving related to*
  - prolonged denial or avoidance of the loss
  - intense guilt related to the loss
  - continued anger about the loss
  - serious depressive symptoms and despair
  - loss of self-esteem
  - intense grieving patterns that continue for more than a year
  - social isolation due to grief

- *Situational low self-esteem related to*
  - prolonged feelings of poor self-worth because of the loss
  - feeling unworthy of having a child
- *Spiritual distress related to*
  - anger with God
  - confusion about why prayers were not answered
- *Disturbed thought processes related to*
  - difficulty making decisions
  - inability to get organized
  - poor work performance
  - confused thinking

■ Expected Outcomes of Care

Expected outcomes are set and priorities assigned in client-centered terms according to the mutual goals chosen by the client and the nurse. Nursing actions are then selected to meet the expected outcomes, which may include that the woman/family will do the following:

- Actualize the loss.
- Feel supported by the nursing staff throughout their hospital stay and when visiting the clinic.
- Share experiences and verbalize feelings of grief as much as is culturally and personally appropriate.
- Understand the normal grief responses they and others in the family may experience at the time of and after the loss.
- Demonstrate increasing independence in participating in and making decisions that meet their needs and reflect their religious and cultural beliefs.
- Identify family, spiritual, health care, and community resources for support.
- Discuss problems or issues involving relationships with each other and family.
- Verbalize satisfaction with the care and support provided by their health care professionals.

■ Plan of Care and Interventions

Interventions and support for parents from the nursing and medical staff after a perinatal loss or infant death are extremely important in their healing. Although parents often cannot recall details of their experiences at the time of death, they may recall vividly minor events that were perceived as particularly painful or particularly helpful. However, care must be individualized for each parent and family. Parents whose infants were stillborn noted that nurses were important in supporting them during periods of chaos, helping them meet and separate from the baby, and providing bereavement support (Saflund et al., 2004). In another study, mothers recalled two years after the death of their newborns the importance of nursing support that encouraged, enhanced self-esteem, and was empathetic and comforting as helping them overcome feelings of powerlessness by feeling empowered (Lundqvist et al., 2002b). In a large longitudinal study of parents after a perinatal death, Rand, Kellner, Revak-Lutz, and Massey (1998) found that

---

CRITICAL THINKING EXERCISE

The Bereaved Couple

Marsha gave birth to a stillborn 17-week fetus. This is her second miscarriage. She has been diagnosed with premature dilation of the cervix. She and her husband, Andrew, are in the labor, delivery, recovery room (LDRP) room 1 hour after the birth. Both are crying softly. Andrew has his arm around Marsha and is trying to comfort her. You have just come on duty and are assigned to care for the couple. When you enter the room, Marsha says, "Why did this happen? I want a baby so badly. I did everything right; I did exactly what the doctor told me to do. My sister has five children and she didn't even want the last one. What is the matter with me? Why is God doing this to us?" How should you respond to Marsha's questions? What can you do to comfort the couple? Should they see the baby?

1. Evidence—Is there sufficient evidence to draw conclusions about factors interfering with healthy bereavement? About appropriate support related to accepting the death of the baby? Is the fact that this is Marsha's second miscarriage a factor in her grief?
2. Assumptions—What assumptions can be made about the following factors?
   a. A diagnosis of premature dilation of the cervix
   b. A second miscarriage
   c. The importance of the father's support
   d. Andrew's need for an outlet for his grief
3. What implications and priorities for nursing care can be drawn at this time?
4. Does the evidence objectively support your conclusion?
5. Are there alternative perspectives to your conclusion?

---

parents appreciated the opportunity to make choices about their needs. The authors suggested that providers should not bias parents or make presumptions that would limit their choices or force them to make choices they do not want.

Furthermore, the cultural and spiritual beliefs and practices of individual parents and families must be considered. The interventions discussed later are general ideas about what may be helpful to parents.

■ *Help the Mother, the Father, and Other Family Members Actualize the Loss*

When a loss or death occurs, the nurse should be sure that parents have been honestly told about the situation by their physician or others on the health care team. It is important for their nurse to be with them during this time. With early pregnancy loss, it is recommended that the terminology "miscarriage" be used consistently (Cameron & Penney, 2005). With infant death, caregivers should use the words "dead" and "died," rather than "lost" or "gone," to assist the bereaved in accepting this reality. Parents need opportunities to tell their story about the events, experiences, and feelings surrounding the loss. This can help them come to terms with the reality of their loss. Listening to their pain and allowing time for them to absorb the information is important.

One way of actualizing the loss is to tell the parents the sex of the baby and give them the option of naming the fetus or to help them to name an infant who has died. Choosing a name helps make the baby a member of their family so that the baby can be remembered in a special way. Once the baby is named, the nurse should use the name when referring to the baby. Although naming can be helpful, it is important not to create the sense that the parents must name the "baby," especially in the case of a early pregnancy loss.

▬ NURSE ALERT

A caution about naming is important. It is very important to be sensitive about naming. This is an individual decision that should never be imposed on parents. Beliefs and needs vary widely across individuals, cultures, and religions. Cultural taboos and rules in some religious faiths prohibit the naming of an infant who has died.

It may be helpful for mothers and fathers to see the fetus or baby as a way of becoming acquainted and of separating. Many professionals, based on vast clinical experiences with parents, believe that seeing the fetus/baby helps parents face the reality of the loss, reduces painful fantasies, and offers an opportunity for closure. This intervention has recently been questioned as the result of a longitudinal study of a small group of mothers in England (Hughes et al., 2002). These authors strongly urge that parents never be made to feel they "should" see or hold their baby when this is something that they do not really want. Encouraging reluctant parents to hold or see their dead child by telling them that not seeing the child could make mourning more difficult is inappropriate. Obviously, this subject must be approached very carefully. A question such as, "Some parents have found it helpful to see their baby. Would you like time to consider this?" Because the need or willingness to see also may vary between the mother and father, it is extremely important to determine what each parent really wants. This should not be a joint decision made by one person or a decision made for the parents by grandparents or others. It is a good policy for the nurse to first tell them about this option and then give them time to think about it. Later the nurse can return and ask each parent individually what they decided.

In preparation for the visit with the baby, parents appreciate explanations about what to expect. Descriptions of how their baby looks is important. For example, babies may have red, peeling skin like a bad sunburn, dark discoloration similar to bruises, molding of the head that makes the head look soft and swollen, or birth defects. The nurse should make the baby look as normal as possible, and remember that parents see their baby with different eyes from health care professionals. Bathing the baby, applying lotion to the baby's skin, combing hair, placing identification bracelets on the arm and leg, dressing the baby in a diaper and special outfit, sprinkling powder in the baby's blanket, and wrapping the baby in a pretty blanket conveys to the parents that their baby has been cared for in a special way (Fig. 41-2). If the baby has been in the morgue, he or she can be placed underneath a warmer for 20 to 30 minutes and wrapped in a warm blanket before being brought to the parents. Cold cream rubbed over stiffened joints can help in positioning the baby. The use of powder and lotion stimulates the parent's senses and provides pleasant memories of their baby.

When bringing the baby to the parents, it is important to treat the baby as one would a live baby. Holding the baby close, touching a hand or cheek, using the baby's name, and talking with the parents about the special features of their child conveys that it is all right for them to do likewise. If a baby has a congenital anomaly, the nurse can desensitize the family by pointing out aspects of the baby that are normal. Nurses can help parents explore the baby's body as they desire. Parents often seek to identify family resemblance. A good question might be: "Who in your family does Michael resemble?"

Some families may like to have the opportunity to bathe and dress their baby. Although the skin may be fragile, parents can still apply lotion with cotton balls, sprinkle powder, tie ribbons, fasten the diaper, and place amulets, medallions, rosaries, or special toys or mementos in their baby's hands or alongside their baby. Volunteer women in communities across the country make special burial clothes to give parents at this difficult time. Parents may want to perform other parenting activities, such as combing the hair, dressing the baby in a special outfit, wrapping the baby in a blanket, or placing the baby in a crib.

Parents need to be offered time alone with their baby if they wish. They also need to know when the nurse will return and how to call if they should need anything. If at all possible, the family should be placed in a private room and, when possible, the room should have a rocking chair for the parents to sit in when holding their baby. This offers the mother and father special time together with their baby and with other family members (Fig. 41-3). Marking the door to the room with a special card can be helpful in

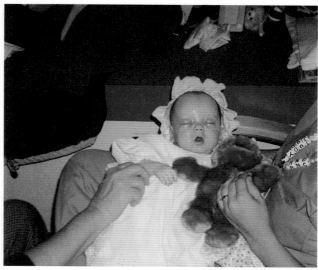

FIG. 41-2 Laura. (Courtesy Amy and Ken Turner, Cary, NC.)

FIG. 41-3 Laura's family members say a special good-bye. (Courtesy Amy and Ken Turner, Cary, NC.)

reminding the staff that this family has experienced a loss (Fig. 41-4).

It is difficult to predict how long and how often parents will need to spend time with their baby. These moments are the only ones they will have to parent their child while their child's physical presence is still with them. Some parents need only a few minutes; others need hours. It is extremely painful for some parents to say good-bye to their baby. They will tell the nurse when they are ready verbally and nonverbally. The nurse should watch for cues that the parents have had enough time with their baby, such as when parents are no longer holding their child close to them or have placed the baby back in the crib. Asking parents whether they have had enough time may make parents feel that the nurse thinks they have had enough time, which may not be the case. Heiman, Yankowitz, and Wilkins (1997) found that 85% of parents in their study would have appreciated additional opportunities to see their baby, and 44% felt they did not have adequate time with the baby. Thus sensitivity to parental needs in actualizing the loss and coping with the

FIG. 41-4 Door card for room of mother who has had a perinatal loss. (Used with permission of Bereavement Services. Copyright Lutheran Hospital—La Crosse, Inc., A Gundersen Lutheran Affiliate, La Crosse, WI.)

reality of the death is essential for their healing. Grandparents should be offered the same opportunities to hold, rock, swaddle, and love their grandchildren so that their grief is started in a healthy way.

▬ Help the Parents with Decision Making

At a time when they are experiencing the great distress of a perinatal loss, and especially if the loss was of an infant, parents have many decisions to make. Mothers, fathers, and extended families look to the medical and nursing staff for guidance in knowing what decisions they must and can make, and in understanding the options related to those decisions. Thus it is a primary responsibility of the nurse to help them and to advocate for them, because decisions made during the time of their loss will provide their memories for a lifetime.

One decision might be related to conducting an autopsy. An autopsy can be very important in answering the question "why" if there is a chance that the cause of death can be determined. This information can be helpful in processing grief and perhaps preventing another loss. However, the cost of an autopsy must be considered. Autopsies are not covered by insurance and are expensive. Some parents may feel that their baby has been through enough and prefer not to have further information about the cause of death. Some religions prohibit autopsy or limit the choice to times when it may help prevent another loss. Options for the type of autopsy, such as excluding the head, are available to parents. Parents may need time to make this decision. There is no need to rush them, unless there was evidence of contagious disease or maternal infection at the time of death.

Organ donation can be an aid to grieving and an opportunity for the family to see something positive associated with their experience. The federal "Gift of Life Act" and HCFA-3005-F, enacted in 1998, shifted the responsibility for determining organ donation potential from the hospital staff to the state's organ procurement organization

(OPO). States and hospitals have clear procedures for how and when to call the OPO. Generally, if a death certificate is issued, a call must be made to the OPO. Once contacted, they will decide whether to talk to the family, and either an OPO representative or a designated requester will contact them. This allows requests to be made by trained personnel in a consistent and compassionate manner. The most common donation is of cornea; donation of cornea from a baby can occur if the baby was born alive at 36 weeks of gestation or later.

Another important decision relates to spiritual rituals that may be helpful and important to parents. Support from the clergy is an option that should be offered to all parents. Parents may wish to have their own pastor, priest, rabbi, or spiritual leader contacted, or they may wish to see the hospital's chaplain. They may choose to do neither. Members from the clergy may offer the parents the opportunity for baptism when appropriate. Other rituals that may be important include a blessing, a naming ceremony, anointing, ritual of the sick, memorial service, or prayer.

One of the major decisions parents must make has to do with disposition of the body. Parents should be given information about the choices for the final disposition of their baby, regardless of gestational age. The nurses must be aware, however, of cultural and spiritual beliefs that may dictate the choices of parents, issues related to the cost of burial, alternatives to burial, and state laws related to burial. A baby younger than 20 weeks of gestation is considered a product of conception, whereas embryos, uterine tubes removed with an ectopic pregnancy, and tissue from a pregnancy obtained during a dilation and curettage are all considered tissue. Many hospitals will make arrangements for the cremation of these infants or tissue. The nurse should know the hospital's policies and procedures and answer the parents' questions honestly. In most states, if a fetus is at least 20 weeks and 1 day of gestational age or is born alive, it is the parents' responsibility to make the final arrangements for their baby, although some hospitals will offer free cremation. In this case, the family would not get the ashes.

■ LEGAL TIP Laws Regarding Live Birth

Laws in all states govern what constitutes a live birth. In most states a live birth is considered to be any products of conception expelled from a woman that show any signs of life. Signs of life are considered to be any muscle irritability, respiratory effort, or heart rate, regardless of gestational age. All nurses should be knowledgeable about their state laws regarding what constitutes a live birth and what forms must be completed and filed in the case of fetal death, stillbirth, or newborn death.

Final disposition of all identifiable babies, regardless of gestational age, includes burial or cremation. Depending on the cemetery's policies, babies in caskets or the ashes from cremated babies can be buried in a special place designated for babies, at the foot of a deceased relative, in a separate plot, or in a mausoleum. Ashes also may be scattered in a designated area; many states have regulations regarding where ashes can be scattered. A local funeral director or a state's Vital Statistics Bureau should have information about the state's rules, codes, and regulations regarding live births, burial requirements, transportation of the deceased by parents, and cremation.

In making final arrangements for their baby, parents may want a special service. They may choose to have a service in the hospital chapel, visitation at a funeral home or their own home, a funeral service, or a graveside service. Parents can make any of these services as special, personal, and memorable as they like. They can choose special music, poetry, or prose written by themselves or others.

If the family has decided on a funeral and burial, they still have decisions about what funeral home to call and where to bury the baby. Many couples may be living in an area distant from their family homes, and they may want to bury their child in their hometown or family cemetery. If the family desires cremation, they may want to have the option of obtaining the ashes. It is important to determine whether this will be done by the facility conducting the cremation.

Parents' hopes, dreams, self-esteem, and role expectations have been shattered with a perinatal loss; thus they may have many needs. Unmet needs can form the basis of "if only" that may plague a mother or family for a lifetime and can be the foundation for the development of complicated bereavement. However, it is difficult for parents to know exactly what they can expect or what they need; thus the nurse as an advocate should lead by offering various options that might meet specific needs. When a mother or family is able to verbalize needs, it is extremely important for the nurse to respond positively and do everything to see that the request is met.

Families become unaware of time frames and do not care about the change of shifts or any needs the hospital system might have in "moving things along." When families are pushed or rushed into making decisions, in most cases, they make a decision in response to the health care system's needs, not their own. The timing for actions such as naming the baby, seeing and holding the baby, disposition of the body, and funeral arrangements should never be rushed. In some cases, the mother may be discharged home before these decisions are made. Then the family can think about them in the comfort of their home and contact the hospital in the following days to give their answers.

■ *Help the Bereaved to Acknowledge and Express Their Feelings*

One of the most important goals of the nurse is to validate the experience and feelings of the parents by encouraging them to tell their stories and listening with care (Corbet-Owen & Kruger, 2001). At the very least, the nurse should acknowledge the loss with a simple but sincere comment such as "I'm sorry about the baby." Helping the parents to talk about their loss and the meaning it has for their lives and to share their emotional pain is the next step. "Tell me about what happened." Because nurses tend to be very focused on the physical and emotional needs of the mother, it is especially important to ask the father directly about his views of what happened and his feelings of loss.

The nurse should listen patiently during the story of loss or grief, but listening is hard work and can be painful for the helper. The feelings and emotions of expressed grief can overwhelm health care professionals. Being with someone who is terribly sad and crying or sobbing can be extremely difficult. The initial impulse to reduce one's sense of helplessness is to say or do something that you think will reduce their pain. Although such a response may seem supportive at the time, it can stifle the further expression of emotion. Bereaved parents have identified many unhelpful responses made to them by well-meaning health care professionals, family, and friends. The nurse should resist the temptation to give advice or to use clichés in offering support to the bereaved (Box 41-3). Nurses need to be comfortable with their own feelings of grief and loss to support and care for bereaved persons effectively. The nurse should have a presence of self, the willingness to be alongside, quietly supporting the bereaved in whatever expressions of feelings or emotions are appropriate for them. This presence leaves parents feeling that they were cared for. Leaning forward, nodding the head, and saying "Uh-huh" or "Tell me more" is often encouragement enough for the bereaved person to tell his or her story. Sitting through the silence can be therapeutic; silence gives the bereaved person an opportunity to collect thoughts and to process what he or she is sharing. Furthermore, careful assessment is important before using touch as a therapeutic technique.

| box 41-3 | **What to Say and What Not to Say to Bereaved Parents** |

WHAT TO SAY
- "I'm sad for you."
- "How are you doing with all of this?"
- "This must be hard for you."
- "What can I do for you?"
- "I'm sorry."
- "I'm here, and I want to listen."

WHAT NOT TO SAY
- "God had a purpose for her."
- "Be thankful you have another child."
- "The living must go on."
- "I know how you feel."
- "It's God's will."
- "You have to keep on going for her sake."
- "You're young; you can have others."
- "We'll see you back here next year, and you'll be happier."
- "Now you have an angel in heaven."
- "This happened for the best."
- "Better for this to happen now, before you knew the baby."
- "There was something wrong with the baby anyway."

Used with permission of Bereavement Services. Copyright Lutheran Hospital—La Crosse, Inc., a Gundersen Lutheran Affiliate, La Crosse, WI.

For some, touch is a meaningful expression of concern, but for others it is an invasion of privacy.

Bereaved parents have many questions surrounding the event of their loss that can leave them feeling guilty. This is particularly true for mothers. Such questions include "What did I do?" "What caused this to happen?" "What do you think I should have, could have done?" Part of the grief process for bereaved parents is figuring out what happened, their role in the loss, why it happened to them, and why it happened to their baby. The nurse should recognize that the answers to these questions must be answered by the bereaved themselves; it is part of their healing. For example, a bereaved mother might ask, "Do you think that this was caused by painting the baby's room?" An appropriate response might be, "I understand you need to find an answer for why your baby died, but we really don't know why she died. What are some of the other things you have been thinking about?" Trying to give bereaved parents answers when there are no clear answers or trying to squelch their guilt feelings by telling them they should not feel guilty does not help them process their grief. In reality, many times there are no definite answers to the question of why this terrible thing has happened to them. However, factual information, such as data about the frequency of miscarriages in pregnant women or the fact that there usually is no clear cause of a stillbirth, can be helpful.

Feelings of anger, guilt, and sadness can occur immediately but often become more problematic in the early days and months after a loss. When a bereaved person expresses feelings of anger, it can be helpful to identify the feeling by simply saying, "You sound angry," or "You look angry." The nurse's willingness to sit down and listen to these feelings of anger can help the bereaved move past those surface feelings into the underlying feelings of powerlessness and helplessness in not being able to control the many aspects of the situation.

■ Normalize the Grief Process and Facilitate Positive Coping

While helping parents share their feelings of pain, it is critical to help them understand their grief responses and feel they are not alone in these painful responses. Most parents are not prepared for the raw feelings that they experience or the fact that these painful, complex feelings and related behavioral reactions continue for many weeks or months. Thus reassuring them of the normality of their responses and preparing them for the length of their grief is important.

The nurse can help the parent be prepared for the emptiness, loneliness, and yearning; for the feelings of helplessness that can lead to anger, guilt, and fear; and for the cognitive processing problems, disorganization, difficulty making decisions; and sadness and depression that are part of the grief process. Books and pamphlets about grief, if short and sensitive, can be given to parents to take home. Many parents have reported feelings of fear that they were going crazy because of the many emotions and behavioral responses that leave them feeling totally out of control in the months after the loss.

It is essential for the nurse to reassure and educate bereaved parents about the grief process, including the physical, social, and emotional responses of individuals and families. Offering health teaching on the bereavement process alone is not enough, however. In the initial days after a loss, other strategies might include follow-up phone calls, referrals to a perinatal grief support group, or providing a list of publications or websites intended for helping parents who have experienced a perinatal loss (e.g., www.compassionatefriends.org, www.griefnet.org, www.growthhouse.org, www.natonalshareoffice.com). As with any referral, however, the nurse should first read the materials or check out the websites.

To reduce relationship problems that can occur in grieving couples, it is particularly important to help them understand that they may respond and grieve in very different ways (Abboud & Liamputtong, 2005). Discongruent grieving can lead to serious marital problems and be a risk factor for complicated bereavement. Remind the couple of the importance of being understanding and patient with each other. A father may need encouragement to be able to share his grief with his wife, because of the desire to protect the woman from his pain or the need to appear strong (McCreight, 2004; Samuelsson et al., 2001).

Nurses can reinforce positive coping efforts and attempt to prevent negative coping (Abboud & Liamputtong, 2005). They can remind the parents of the importance of being patient and being good to themselves during the grief process. Additional suggestions are to encourage attempts to resume normal activities; reinforce and encourage positive ways to hold onto memories of the pregnancy or baby, while letting go; and help the parent to organize a plan for daily activities, if needed. In particular, nurses should discourage overdependence on drugs and alcohol.

■ Meet the Physical Needs of the Postpartum Bereaved Mother

Coping with loss and grief after childbirth can be an overwhelming experience for the woman and her family. One particularly difficult aspect of the loss is the sound of crying babies and the happiness of other families on the unit who have given birth to healthy infants. The mother should be given the opportunity to decide if she wants to remain on the maternity unit or be moved to another hospital unit. She also should be helped to understand the pluses and minuses of each choice. Postpartum care as well as grief support may not be as good on another hospital unit where the staff are not experienced in postpartum and bereavement care.

The physical needs of a bereaved mother are the same as those of any woman who has given birth. The cruel reality for many bereaved mothers is that their milk may come in with no baby to nurse, their afterpains remind them of their emptiness, and gas pains feel as though a baby is still moving inside. The nurse should assure that the mother receives appropriate medications to reduce these physical symptoms. Adequate rest, diet, and fluids must be offered to replenish her physical strength.

Mothers need postpartum care instructions on discharge. They also need ideas about how to cope with problems with sleep such as decreasing food or fluids that contain caffeine, limiting alcohol and nicotine consumption, exercising regularly, using strategies for rest, taking a warm bath or drinking warm milk before bedtime, relaxation exercises, restful music, or a massage. Furthermore, the couple needs to be encouraged and supported in maintaining their relationship and keeping open channels of communication. They also need to be prepared for some of the issues related to resuming sexual relations after perinatal loss.

■ Assist the Bereaved in Communicating with, Supporting, and Getting Support from Family

Providing sensitive care to bereaved parents means including their families in the grief process. Grandparents and siblings are particularly important when a perinatal loss has occurred. However, it is up to the parents to decide to what extent they want family involved in their grief process. If it is the parents' desire, children, grandparents, extended family members, and friends should be allowed to be involved in the rituals surrounding the death, such as seeing and holding the baby. Such visits afford others the opportunity to become acquainted with the baby, to understand the parents' loss, to offer their support, and to say goodbye (see Fig. 41-3). This experience helps parents explain to their surviving children who their brother or sister was and what death means, offers the children answers to their questions in a concrete manner, and helps the children in expressing their grief (Wilson, 2001). Involving extended family and friends enables the parents to mobilize their social support system of people who will support the family not only at the time of loss but also in the future.

Parents also need information about how grief affects a family. They may need help in understanding and coping with the potential differing responses of various family members. Frustrations may arise because of the insensitive or inadequate responses of other family members. Parents may need help in determining ways to let family members know how they feel and what they need.

■ Create Memories for Parents to Take Home

Parents may want tangible mementos of their baby to allow them to actualize the loss. Some may want to bring in a previously purchased baby book. Special memory books, cards, and information on grief and mourning are available for purchase by parents or hospitals or clinics through national perinatal bereavement organizations (Fig. 41-5).

The nurse can provide information about the baby's weight, length, and head circumference to the family. Footprints and handprints can be taken and placed with the other information on a special card or in a memory or

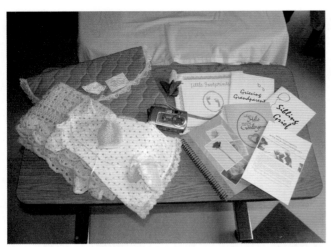

FIG. 41-5 A memory kit assembled at John C. Lincoln Hospital, Phoenix, AZ. Memory kits may include pictures of the infant, clothing, death certificate, footprints, identification bands, fetal monitor printout, and ultrasound picture. (Courtesy Julie Perry Nelson, Gilbert, AZ.)

baby book. Sometimes it is difficult to obtain good handprints or footprints. Application of alcohol or acetone on the palms or soles can help the ink adhere to make the prints clearer, especially for small babies. When making prints, have a hard surface underneath the paper to be printed. The baby's heel or palm is placed down first, and the foot or hand is rolled forward, keeping the toes or fingers extended. It may be helpful to have assistance in this procedure. If the print does not turn out, tracing around the baby's hands and feet can be done, although this distorts the actual size. A form of plaster of paris can also be used to make an imprint of the baby's hand or foot.

Parents often appreciate articles that were in contact with or used in caring for the baby. This might include the tape measure used to measure the baby, baby lotions, combs, clothing, hats, blankets, crib cards, and identification bands. The identification band helps the parents remember the size of the baby and personalizes the mementos. The nurse should ask parents if they wish to have these articles before giving them to the parents. A lock of hair may be another important keepsake. Parents must be asked for permission before cutting a lock of hair, which can be removed from the nape of the neck where it is not noticeable.

For some, pictures are the most important memento. Photographs are generally taken whenever there is an identifiable baby and when it is culturally acceptable to the family. It does not matter how tiny the baby is, what the baby looks like, or how long the baby has been dead. Pictures should include close-ups of the baby's face, hands, and feet and photos of the baby clothed and wrapped in a blanket as well as unclothed. If there are any congenital anomalies, close-ups of the anomalies also should be taken. Flowers, blocks, stuffed animals, or toys can be placed in the background to make the picture more special. Parents may want their pictures taken holding the baby. Keeping a

camera nearby and taking pictures when parents are spending special time with their baby can provide special memories. Some parents may have their own camera or video camera and would like the nurse to record them as they bathe, dress, hold, or diaper their baby.

■ *Communicate Using a Caring Framework*

Mothers, fathers, and extended families look to the nursing staff for support and understanding during the time of loss. Nurses have an important role in providing sensitive care to parents at the time of a perinatal loss. One model for conceptualizing intervention is that developed by Swanson-Kauffman based on her research with women experiencing perinatal loss (Swanson, 2001). The framework identifies five components in a caring concept:

1. Knowing
2. Being with
3. Doing for
4. Enabling
5. Maintaining belief

Knowing implies that the nurse has taken the time to understand the perception of the loss and its meaning to the woman and her family. *Being with* involves how the nurse conveys acceptance of the various feelings and perceptions of each family member. *Doing for* refers to the activities performed by the nurse that provide physical care, comfort, and safety for the woman and her family. This may include offering pain medication or sitz baths, maintaining the patency of the intravenous line, performing postpartum checks, and giving back rubs. *Enabling* occurs when the nurse offers the woman and her family options for care. Offers of information, anticipatory guidance, choices for decision making, and support during hospitalization and after discharge help the family feel more in control of a situation in which they feel very much out of control. Enabling raises their self-esteem and allows them to feel more comfortable in asking for options according to their needs for memories and closure, rather than to the nurse's perception of their needs. *Maintaining belief* involves encouraging the woman and her family to believe in their own ability to pick up the pieces and begin to heal. The nurse spends time with the family, learns their inner strengths and coping abilities, and points out these inner resources to the family by saying, "I know this is a difficult time for you, but I have seen some of your inner strength and know that you will be able to make it through all of this."

■ *Be Concerned About Cultural and Spiritual Needs of Parents*

Given the growing diversity of the American culture, parents who experience perinatal loss can be from widely diverse cultural, ethnic, and spiritual groups. Many of the emotional responses and suggested interventions in this chapter are based on middle-class European-American views. Although there are likely no particular differences in the individual, intrapersonal experiences of grief based on culture, ethnicity, or religion, there are complex differences in the meaning of children and parenthood, the role of women and men, the beliefs and knowledge about modern medicine, views about death, mourning rituals and traditions, and behavioral expressions of grief (Bennett et al., 2005; Hughes et al., 2002). Thus the nurse must be sensitive to the responses and needs of parents from various cultural backgrounds and religious groups. To do this, the nurse needs to be aware of her own values and beliefs and acknowledge the importance of understanding and accepting the values and beliefs of others who are different or even in conflict (Chichester, 2005). Furthermore, it is critical to understand that the individual and unique responses of a parent to a perinatal loss cannot be entirely predicted by their cultural or spiritual backgrounds. Each mother and father must be approached first as an individual needing support during a profoundly difficult and distressing life experience.

It would be impossible to address all of the specific differences and needs of parents from diverse cultural and religious groups because of the complexity of this task and the lack of adequate research in this area of practice. Instead, we present some key concepts and give a few examples of areas of particular concern. For more detailed discussion of this topic, the reader is referred to an article by Melanie Chichester (2005).

The cultural meaning of children has a strong impact on the response of parents, extended family, and the community when an infant dies or is stillborn. For example, death of an infant or having a stillborn child shakes the foundation of a Jewish family and is surrounded by many cultural traditions, such as naming of the baby, burial, and mourning rituals (Shuzman, 2003). Likewise, in Hispanic families, children are deeply valued. Culture and religious beliefs often affect decision making surrounding stillbirth or death of an infant. Autopsies and/or cremation are not allowed by some religious groups, except under unusual circumstances. Making a decision to end life-sustaining measures may be more difficult for some groups. African-American parents were less likely than Caucasians to make a decision to stop life-sustaining treatments in a mortally ill infant (Moseley et al., 2004). Picture taking may conflict with beliefs of some cultures, such as among some Native Americans, Eskimos, Amish, Hindus, and Muslims. Families from these cultures should be sensitively offered this opportunity but not pushed into having a picture taken. In many cultures, decisions do not reside solely in the individual woman or couple but in the extended family. In Hispanic families, the concept of "La Familia" is critical. Family decisions are usually made together and may be communicated through someone appointed by the family rather than the parents (Chichester, 2005). In Muslim families, decisions are made by the father.

Culture and religious beliefs also influence the customs following death. Many religious groups have rituals such as prayers, ritualistic washing and shrouding, or anointing with oil that are performed at the time of death. It is critical to ask parents about their needs as they relate to

rituals at the time of and following death. For example, baptism is extremely important for Roman Catholics and some, but not all, Protestant groups. Baptism can be performed by a lay person, such as a nurse, in an emergency situation when a priest cannot be there in a timely fashion (Box 41-4).

Expressions of grief may also vary across cultures from quiet and stoic to dramatic and hysterical responses. Muslims view death as a part of life and believe a baby's death is God's will. The Muslim mother may cry but loud wailing is not acceptable. The tearing of a garment, *keria*, may be done at the time of a death by Jewish parents. Hispanic parents and family members may be very demonstrative in their grief with loud wailing and weeping (Purnell & Paulanka, 2003). African-American women were found to use self-healing strategies that reflect inner processes, resources, and remedies (Van, 2001).

■ Provide Sensitive Care at and After Discharge

When leaving the hospital, mothers are often taken out in a wheelchair. This can be a devastating experience for the mother who has experienced a pregnancy loss. Leaving the hospital without a baby in her arms is a very empty and painful experience. It is especially difficult if others are seen leaving with babies; thus the discharge of mothers and fathers who have experienced a perinatal loss should be done with great sensitivity to their feelings. They should not be discharged at a time when other mothers with live babies are leaving. Giving the mother a special flower to carry in her arms can be a thoughtful gesture.

The grief of the mother and her family does not end with discharge; rather it really begins once they return home, attend the funeral, and start to live their lives without their baby. There are numerous models for providing follow-up care to parents after discharge and, although there is no solid evidence from sound clinical trials regarding the benefit of these programs (Chambers & Chan, 2000), nonexperimental studies and clinical evaluations suggest these programs are helpful (Cote-Arsenault & Freije, 2004; Heiman et al., 1997; Reilly-Smorawski, Armstrong, &

---

box 41-4 | Infant Baptism

In an emergency, baptism may be performed by anyone by pouring water over the forehead (or products of conception) and saying "I baptize you in the name of the Father and of the Son and of the Holy Spirit." The person performing the baptism needs only to have the intention of baptizing and does not necessarily have to believe in infant baptism for the baptism to be valid. If the infant has no signs of life, the person performing the baptism can add "If you are alive, I baptize you..." In the Greek Orthodox tradition, baptism is only for the living; thus a miscarried or stillborn infant would not be baptized. If the infant is born alive and in serious danger of death, the infant can be lifted up while saying "The servant of God is baptized in the name of the Father and the Son and the Holy Spirit."

Catlin, 2002; Rich, 2000). Programs include hospital-based bereavement teams who provide support during hospitalization and follow-up contacts.

Phone calls after a loss may be helpful to some parents; however, it must be determined which parents do not want a follow-up call. Follow-up calls let the parents know they are still thought of and cared about. The calls are made at predictably difficult times such as the first week at home, 1 month to 6 weeks later, 4 to 6 months after the loss, and at the anniversary of the death. Families who experienced a miscarriage, ectopic pregnancy, or death of a preterm baby may appreciate a phone call on the estimated date of birth. The calls provide an opportunity for parents to ask questions, share their feelings, seek advice, and receive information to help them in processing their grief.

A grief conference can be planned when parents return for an appointment with their doctor, nurses, and other health care providers. At the conference, the loss or death of the infant is discussed in detail, parents are given information about the baby's autopsy report and genetic studies, and they have opportunities to ask the questions that have arisen since their baby's death. Parents appreciate the opportunity to review the events of hospitalization, go over the baby's and/or mother's chart with their primary health care provider, and talk with those who cared for them and their baby during hospitalization. This is an important time to help parents understand the cause of the loss, or to accept the fact that the cause will forever be unknown. This gives health care professionals the opportunity to assess how the family is coping with their loss and provide additional information and education on grief.

Some parents are very interested in finding a perinatal or parent grief support group. The opportunity to talk with others who have been through similar experiences, share memories of the pregnancy and the baby, and gain an understanding of the normality of the grief process have been generally found to be supportive (Cote-Arsenault & Freije, 2004; Reilly-Smorawski et al., 2002). Over time, it may be the only place where bereaved parents can talk about the wished-for child and their grief. However, not all parents find such groups helpful (DiMarco, Menke, & McNamara, 2001).

When referring to a group, it is important to know something about the group and how it operates. For example, if a group has a religious base for their interventions, a nonreligious parent would not likely find the group to be helpful. If parents experiencing a perinatal loss are referred to a general parental grief group, they might feel overwhelmed with the grief of parents whose older children have died of cancer, suicide, or homicide. In addition, the grief of parents following a perinatal loss might be minimized by other parents. Thus the needs of the parents must be matched with the focus of the group.

▬ *Provide Postmortem Care*

Preparation of the baby's body and transport to the morgue depends on the procedures and protocols developed by individual hospitals. The Joint Committee on Accreditation of Healthcare Organizations (www.jcaho.org) requires that appropriate care is offered to the body after death. A sensitive and respectful approach for taking the fetus or infant to the morgue is the use of a "burial cradle" which makes the process more dignified for parents and the nursing staff. These Styrofoam miniature coffins have a quilted lining and can be obtained from Zerbell's Bay Memorials (321 South 15th Street, Escanaba, MI, 906-786-2609) (Fig. 41-6). Postmortem care can be an emotional and sometimes difficult task for the nurse. However, nurses may find that providing postmortem care helps them find closure in their own grief related to a perinatal loss. This is particularly true for neonatal intensive care nurses who have cared for an infant for several hours, days, or weeks.

▬ Evaluation

The evaluation of nursing care is made more difficult by the shock and numbness of the bereavement process and the varied grief responses of the parents and other family members during hospitalization. The achievement of expected outcomes is assured when positive integration of the perinatal loss is expressed by the family (see Plan of Care).

One approach to evaluation is the use of checklists. Many hospitals have checklists used in providing care, mobilizing members of the multidisciplinary health care team, communicating options the family has chosen, and keeping track of all the details in meeting the needs of bereaved parents (Figs. 41-7 and 41-8). Such checklists may be a permanent part of the chart. Documentation in the nursing notes of primary concerns, grief responses, health teaching, health care advice, and any referrals of the mother or other family members is essential to ensure continuity and consistency of care.

FIG. 41-6 Burial cradle. (Courtesy Shannon Perry, Phoenix, AZ.)

plan of care **Fetal Death: 24 Weeks of Gestation**

NURSING DIAGNOSIS Dysfunctional grieving related to fetal death, as evidenced by intense expressions of grief for prolonged period of time

Expected Outcome *Parents will identify appropriate ways to deal with grief.*

Nursing Interventions/*Rationales*
- Prepare family for viewing fetus by cleaning body and wrapping in clean blanket *to initiate and support the grieving process in a supportive setting.*
- Allow family quiet time to hold and view fetus. Take pictures for family to keep *to provide reality to death and support the grieving process.*
- Provide a certificate for the family with vital statistics, along with identification bands, lock of hair (with parental permission), and footprints *to provide reality of situation and support the grieving process.*
- Provide spiritual support as needed to assist with religious services, such as baptism and memorial services, *to assist with religious practices.*
- Refer to appropriate community support groups *to facilitate grieving with group input and to share experiences.*

NURSING DIAGNOSIS Situational low self-esteem related to fetal death as evidenced by mother's/family's intense feelings of guilt

Expected Outcomes *Mother/family will exhibit positive self-comments and adapt to death of fetus in a timely manner.*

Nursing Interventions/*Rationales*
- Provide private time for expressions of feelings through therapeutic communication and active listening *to validate feelings.*
- Identify mother's/family's perception and feelings about fetal death *to correct any misconceptions and alleviate guilt.*
- Assist mother/family to identify positive coping mechanisms and support systems *to promote feelings of self-worth.*
- Refer to appropriate health professionals for further evaluation and counseling, such as social services, *to provide ongoing assistance as needed.*

NURSING DIAGNOSIS Spiritual distress related to perinatal loss

Expected Outcome *Parents will verbalize a decrease in spiritual distress.*

Nursing Interventions/*Rationales*
- Assess parent's spiritual preference *to reinforce parent's own beliefs.*
- Assist with spiritual rituals for parents and infant *to promote comfort for parents.*
- Provide opportunity for parents to express feelings about perinatal loss *to facilitate the grief process.*
- Assist parents in contacting the facility's chaplain or personal spiritual advisor *to provide spiritual support.*
- Attend memorial service/funeral if feasible *to provide support to parents and to help process grief of health care provider.*

NURSING DIAGNOSIS Interrupted family processes related to inadequate communication of feelings between mother and father and other family members

Expected Outcome *Mother and father will discuss feelings involving relationship with each other and family members*

Nursing Interventions/*Rationales*
- Provide information to parents about how grief affects a family *to faciliate expression of grieving among family members.*
- Encourage mother and father to talk about their loss and its meaning to the family *to help the bereaved to acknowledge and express their feelings.*
- Offer follow-up contact (e.g., phone calls, grief conference) *to provide opportunity for parents to ask questions, share feelings, and to receive information to help them in processing their grief.*
- Refer family to perinatal or family support group if appropriate *to facilitate communication and sharing of the experience of loss with other who have ad similar experiences.*

CD: Plan of Care: Fetal Death

SPECIAL LOSSES

Prenatal Diagnoses with Negative Outcome

Early prenatal diagnostic tests such as ultrasonography, chorionic villus sampling, and amniocentesis can determine the well-being of the embryo or fetus. Reasons for prenatal testing include history of chromosomal abnormality in the family; three or more miscarriages; maternal age over 35 years; lack of fetal growth, movement, or heartbeat; and diabetes mellitus or other chronic illnesses. If the health care provider is certain that the baby has a serious genetic defect that would lead to death in utero or after birth (congenital anomalies incompatible with life or genetic disorders with severe mental retardation), the choice of interruption of a pregnancy via dilation and evacuation or induction of labor may be offered (Burgoine, Van Kirk, Romm, Edelman, Jacobson, & Jensen, 2005).

Foreknowledge of a prenatal diagnosis along with perception of the future low health status of the baby as well as multiple congenital problems intensify the grief response (Hunfeld, Tempels, Passchier, Hazebroek, & Tibboel, 1999). The decision to terminate a pregnancy is a difficult decision and can pave the way for feelings such as guilt, despair, sadness, depression, and anger. The parent who decides to continue the pregnancy needs intensive support from the nursing staff. The time of labor and birth can be particularly difficult. The nurse should remember that parents may be grieving not only the loss of the perfect child but the loss of expectations for their child's future. Thus, nurses should assess how these parents feel about the experience, offer options for their memories as appropriate, and be a support person and good listener. Healing can take place when words can be given to feelings. A new model, perinatal hospice programs for parents

Text continued on p. 1110.

SAMPLE

RTS Bereavement Services
CHECKLIST FOR ASSISTING PARENT(S) EXPERIENCING
MISCARRIAGE/ECTOPIC PREGNANCY

RTS Counselor _____   Date _____
Mother's name _____   Age _____ Due date _____
Date of beginning of miscarriage _____   Date of surgery _____
# of Miscarriages _____ # of Children _____   Religion _____
Address _____   Occupation _____
Phone number (   ) _____   Marital status _____
Father's name _____   Age _____ Occupation _____
Address _____   Phone number (   ) _____
Baby's name _____   Sex _____
Support people available _____   Children's names: _____
Problem areas _____   Physician _____
OK to send written material to home address ☐ Yes ☐ No

Date	Time	See Miscarriage Protocol RTS Manual	Comments	Initials
		Notify/Assign RTS counselor ☐ Yes ☐ No		
		Pastoral Care ☐ Yes ☐ No		
		Offered: ☐ Blessing ☐ Memorial Service ☐ Naming Ceremony ☐ Burial		
		Asked: "Would you like someone with you now?" ☐ Yes ☐ No		
		D&C/Surgical procedure discussed ☐ Yes ☐ No		
		Saw baby or tissue ☐ Mother ☐ Father		
		Touched and/or held baby ☐ Mother ☐ Father		
		If RH negative, RhoGAM given within 72 hrs ☐ Yes ☐ No		
		Patient's room flagged with door card ☐ Yes ☐ No		
		Photos taken: ☐ 35 mm ☐ Polaroid ☐ Given to parents ☐ On file		
		Footprints & handprints/weight & length: ☐ Given to parents ☐ On file		
		Grief process discussed ☐ Yes ☐ No		
		Incongruent grief discussed ☐ Yes ☐ No		
		Grief packet given ☐ Yes ☐ No		
		Info Brochure given to parents re: RTS PSG ☐ Yes ☐ No		
		Name/business card given ☐ Yes ☐ No		
		Regular OB/Midwife notified _____ ☐ Memo ☐ Verbally		
		Childbirth Educator notified _____ ☐ Yes ☐ No		
		Telephone number verified ☐ Yes ☐ No Optimal call time _____		
		Preg & Inf Loss Card sent to RTS Secretary ☐ Yes ☐ No		
		Given option to transfer from Maternity Unit ☐ Yes ☐ No		
		Genetic Studies ordered ☐ Yes ☐ No		
		Sex determination desired (tissue in NS only) ☐ Yes ☐ No		
		Would like another parent to call: ☐ Yes ☐ No ☐ Ask later		
		Parent contact: _____ Follow-up calls: eg. ☐ 1 wk, ☐ 3 wk, ☐ 4 mo, ☐ due date/anniv. date		

Forms for burial or cremation of:
  a) Products of conception - 2 copies of "Request for Return of Products of Conception to Patients" (1 copy-chart, 1 copy-lab). Obtain forms from histology.
  b) Identifiable baby less than 20 wk or less than 350 gm - 2 copies of "Request for Return of Products of Conception to Patients" (1-chart, 1-lab). "Notice of Removal" #DOH 5043 - Responsible party for burial signs this form (either parent or a funeral director). Pink copy goes to responsible party. "Final Disposition of a Human Corpse" #DOH 5045 is required for any age identifiable baby that goes across state lines.
Note: Some cemeteries may require a "Final Disposition of a Human Corpse" report for their own recordkeeping.

FIG. 41-7 Sample checklist for assisting parents experiencing miscarriage/ectopic pregnancy. (Used with permission of Bereavement Services. Copyright Lutheran Hospital—La Crosse, Inc., A Gundersen Lutheran Affiliate, La Crosse, WI.)

RTS Bereavement Services
CHECKLIST FOR ASSISTING PARENT(S) EXPERIENCING STILLBIRTH OR NEWBORN DEATH

SAMPLE

Mother's discharge date: _____

Mother's name: _____

Address: _____

Phone number: ( )_____

Father's name: _____

Address: _____

Phone number: ( )_____

Optimal call time: _____

RTS Counselor: _____

Unit: _____ Ext _____

Regular OB MD/Midwife: _____

Religion: _____

Age _____ Gr ___ Para ___ L.C. ___ Due date _____

Previous loss: _____

Date/Time delivered: _____

Date/Time death: _____

Baby's name: _____ Sex: _____

Children's name(s): _____ Age: _____

_____ Age: _____

_____ Age: _____

Support people

Attending MD &/or Pediatrician _____

Notify Peds Nurse Practitioner _____

Date	Time			Comments	Initials
		Notify/Assign RTS counselor	☐ Yes ☐ No		
		Pastoral Care notified	☐ Yes ☐ No		
		Funeral Home notified: ☐ Yes ☐ No Family Burial:	☐ Yes ☐ No		
		Saw baby when born and/or after delivery:	☐ Mother ☐ Father		
		Touched and/or held baby:	☐ Mother ☐ Father		
			☐ Siblings ☐ Grandparents ☐ Friends		
		Offered private time with their baby:	☐ Yes ☐ No		
		Baptism offered: (use seashell as vessel, give to parents)	☐ Yes ☐ No		
		Remembrance of Blessing offered:	☐ Yes ☐ No		
		(can offer for any perinatal loss)	☐ Given to parents		
		Given option to transfer off Maternity Unit:	☐ Yes ☐ No		
		Patient's room flagged with door card	☐ Yes ☐ No		
		Autopsy: ☐ Yes ☐ No Genetic studies: ☐ Yes ☐ No			
		Genetic Associate notified:	☐ Yes ☐ No		
		Regular Physician/Midwife notified of death:	☐ Yes ☐ No		
		Memo sent to Physician/Midwife:	☐ Yes ☐ No		
		Section of Fetal monitor strip:	☐ Given to parents ☐ On file		
		ID Bands/Crib cards/Tape measure:	☐ Given to parents ☐ On file		
		Footprints/Handprints/Weight/Length recorded on "In Memory Of" sheet:	☐ Given to parents ☐ On file		
		Lock of hair offered: (ask permission)	☐ Yes ☐ No		
			☐ Given to parents ☐ On file		
		Mementos (clothing, hat, blanket, pacifier, crib cards, basin, baby ring, bear, thermometer, silk flower)	☐ Given to parents ☐ On file		
		Complimentary birth keepsake	☐ Given to parents ☐ On file		
		RTS Photos taken: (clothed, unclothed, w. props, family photo)			
		1) Polaroid - 3 or more	☐ Given to parents ☐ On file		
		2) 35 mm (6-12 pictures)	☐ Given to parents ☐ On file		
		3) Medical photos:	☐ Yes ☐ No		

FIG. 41-8 Sample checklist for assisting parents experiencing stillbirth or newborn death. (Used with permission of Bereavement Services. Copyright Lutheran Hospital—La Crosse, Inc., A Gundersen Lutheran Affiliate, La Crosse, WI.)

Continued

Date	Time		Comments	Initials
		Informed about postponing funeral until mother is able to attend: ☐ Yes ☐ No		
		Services/Funeral arrangements, options discussed: ☐ Self-transport ☐ Gravesite service ☐ Visitation ☐ Hospital chapel ☐ Cremation ☐ Funeral home ☐ Burial at foot or head of relative's grave ☐ Specific area for babies in cemetery ☐ Plan own service		
		Funeral arrangements made by: ☐ Mother ☐ Father Discussed: ☐ Seeing baby at funeral home ☐ Taking pictures there ☐ Providing outfit/toy for baby ☐ Dressing baby at funeral home		
		Grief information packet given to: ☐ Mother ☐ Father		
		Discussed grief process/incongruent grief with: ☐ Mother ☐ Father		
		Discussed grief conference: ☐ Yes ☐ No		
		RTS Parents Support Group brochure given to: ☐ Mother ☐ Father		
		RTS business card given to: ☐ Mother ☐ Father		
		Pregnancy & Infant Loss Card sent to RTS secretary: ☐ Yes ☐ No		
		Follow-up calls: 1 week: . . . . 3 weeks: . . . . Due date: . . . . 6-10 months: . . . . Anniversary date:		
		Grief conference planned with parents: Date _____ Time _____ Place _____ Letter of confirmation sent: ☐ Yes ☐ No		
		Parent Support Group, first meeting attended: Date: _____ Follow-up meetings attended: Dates _____		
		Would like another parent to call: ☐ Yes ☐ No ☐ Ask later Parent contact: _____		

Forms Needed: Report of fetal death (Photocopy and save for mother.)
                 Autopsy if ordered
                 Record of death
                 Genetics protocol (folder) if ordered
                 Notice of removal of a human corpse from an institution
                 Final disposition form
                 If funeral home involved - Final disposition will be completed by them.
                 Original certificate of death (for NB death only)

Note: <u>Family Burial</u> - Check with your funeral home.

** You may wish to list your hospital and state forms that are necessary, as required by your state laws and your institution.

FIG. 41-8 cont'd

experiencing prenatal diagnoses of lethal birth defects, has been effective in helping families before and after their loss is actualized (Calhoun, Napolitano, Terry, Bussey, & Hoeldtke, 2003).

Loss of One in a Multiple Birth

The death of a twin or baby in a multifetal gestation during pregnancy, labor, birth, or after birth requires parents to parent and grieve at the same time. Such a death imposes a confusing and ambivalent induction into parenthood (Bryan, 2005; Swanson-Kauffman, 1988). Parents may feel torn regarding how they should feel. They may have difficulty parenting their surviving child with all the joy and enthusiasm of new parents because their surviving child re-

minds them of what they have lost. Yet, they may also have difficulty fully grieving their loss because their surviving child demands their attention. These parents could be at risk for altered parenting and complicated bereavement.

It is important to help the parents acknowledge the birth of all their babies. Parents should be treated as bereaved families, and all the options previously discussed should be offered. Pictures should be taken of the babies and parents should be offered the opportunity to hold their babies in their arms and have time to say good-bye to the baby who has died.

Bereaved parents should be warned that well-meaning family members or friends may say, "Well, at least you have the other baby," implying that there should be no grief because they are lucky to have one at all. Parents need to be able to anticipate insensitivity to their loss and be empowered to say to those people, "That is not how I feel." By simply setting a boundary on what their feelings are, they are able to acknowledge the baby who died and then have an opportunity to share more about their feelings if they so choose.

Bereaved parents of multiples have special problems in coping with life without their anticipated "extra special" family, telling their surviving child about his or her twin, dealing with the possibility of that child's feelings of survivor guilt, and deciding on how to celebrate birthdays, death days, or special holidays.

Adolescent Grief

Adolescent pregnancy accounts for many births in the United States. Each year, many adolescents experience perinatal loss, particularly as elective abortion or miscarriage. Adolescents grieve the loss of their babies through miscarriage, stillbirth, or newborn death and have significant emotional, social, and cognitive responses (Wheeler & Austin, 2001). These teens need emotional support from the nurses who care for them.

Often nurses and other health care professionals, as well as family members, believe that the adolescent's loss of her baby was for the best, so that the adolescent can move on with her life. Adolescent girls, then, may not receive the support they need from staff and family. In addition, adolescent girls usually may not have the support from the father of the baby as compared with older women who have a perinatal loss; thus there is a great need to provide sensitive care to all adolescents who experience any type of perinatal loss.

The first step for the nurse in caring for a bereaved adolescent is to acknowledge the significance of giving birth, no matter what age the mother might be. Second, the nurse should make additional efforts to develop a trusting relationship in working with the adolescent. Third, the nurse should offer options for saying good-bye, anticipatory guidance, support, and information to meet the adolescent at the point of her need. It may take longer for adolescents to process their grief because of their level of cognitive and emotional maturation. Being patient, saving mementos, and giving the adolescent information on how to contact the nurse are interventions that can help the adolescent accept the reality of the loss and process her grief.

■ COMPLICATED BEREAVEMENT

Although most parents cope adequately with the pain of their grief and return to some level of normal functioning, some parents have extremely intense grief reactions that last for a very long time; this response is complicated bereavement. A long pre-loss pregnancy (i.e., the fetus/infant died in late gestation), a more neurotic personality, more preexisting psychiatric symptoms, and not having other living children are important risk factors for stronger grief reactions (Janssen, Cuisinier, de Graauw, & Hoogduin, 1997; Malacrida, 1999). A study by Swanson (2000) found that women most at risk for depressive symptoms after a miscarriage attributed higher personal significance to the loss, lacked social support, showed lower emotional strength, used passive coping, were low-income, and did not conceive another pregnancy by a year later.

Evidence of complicated grief includes continued yearning and loneliness, intense and continued guilt or anger, relentless depression or anxiety that interferes with role functioning, abuse of drugs (including prescription medications) or alcohol, severe relationship difficulties, high depressive symptomatology, low self-esteem, feelings of inadequacy, and suicidal thoughts or threats years after the loss has occurred (Swanson, 2000). Symptoms of posttraumatic stress include reliving the trauma, avoiding things and places that are reminders, and disassociation (Bowles et al., 2000). Parents showing signs of complicated grief or posttraumatic stress should be referred for counseling. It is the responsibility of a qualified mental health professional to determine whether the parents are experiencing a normal, albeit intense grief response or whether they are also having a serious mental health problem such as depression. However, it is important when referring to a therapist or counselor that the referral be to one who is experienced in grief counseling and knows how to help the bereaved, because some therapists and counselors do not have an understanding of the special needs related to grief.

Making an appointment for counseling or therapy is a big step. The highest number of cancellations and "no shows" in a therapist's practice are intakes, or first visits; therefore, anything the nurse can do for a family or individual to help with that major hurdle would be helpful. However, it also is important to remember that people may have symptoms but may not, for whatever reason, be ready to deal directly with these symptoms or may not have the energy to make the call. Enlisting a family member to encourage parents to seek such assistance may be helpful.

---

community activity

Visit or call a mortuary. Interview one of the personnel regarding services following an infant death and infant burial. What supports are available to parents? Are infant caskets or burial urns available? What choices do parents have? What is the cost of such services? Discuss your findings in a conference with your classmates.

---

key points

- Parental and infant attachment can begin before pregnancy with many hopes and dreams for the future.
- The gestational age of the baby influences neither the severity of the grief response nor the bereavement process.
- When a baby dies, all members of a family are affected, but no two family members grieve in the same way.

Continued

---

key points—cont'd

• When birth represents death, the role of the nurse is critical in caring for the woman and her family, regardless of the age of the woman or stage of gestation.

• An understanding of the grief process is fundamental in the implementation of the nursing process.

• Assessment of each family member's perception and experience of the loss is important.

• Therapeutic communication and counseling techniques can help families identify their feelings, feel comfortable in expressing their grief, and understand their bereavement process.

• Follow-up after discharge can be an important component in providing care to families who have experienced a loss.

• Nurses need to be aware of their own feelings of grief and loss to provide a nonjudgmental environment of care and support for bereaved families.

REFERENCES

Abboud, L., & Liamputtong, P. (2005). When pregnancy fails: Coping strategies, support networks and experiences with health care of ethnic women and their partners. *Journal of Reproductive and Infant Psychology, 23*(1), 3-18.

American College of Obstetricians and Gynecologists. (2001). Management of recurrent early pregnancy loss: *ACOG Practice Bulletin*, No. 24. Washington, DC: Author.

Ananth, C., Liu, S., Kinzler, W., & Kramer, M. (2005). Stillbirths in the United States, 1981-2000: An age, period, and cohort analysis. *American Journal of Public Health, 95*(12), 2213-2217.

Armstrong, D. (2001). Exploring fathers' experiences of pregnancy after a prior perinatal loss. *MCN American Journal of Maternal/Child Nursing, 26*(3), 147-153.

Armstrong, D. (2002). Emotional distress and prenatal attachment in pregnancy after perinatal loss. *Journal of Nursing Scholarship, 34*(4), 339-345.

Bennett, S., Litz, B., Lee, B., & Shira, M. (2005). The scope and impact of perinatal loss: Current status and future directions. *Professional Psychology, Research and Practice, 36*(2), 180-187.

Bowles, S., James, L., Solursch, D., Yancey, M., Epperly, T., Folen, R., et al. (2000). Acute and post-traumatic stress disorder after spontaneous abortion. *American Family Physician, 61*(6), 1689-1696.

Bryan, E. (2005). Psychological aspects of prenatal diagnosis and its implications in multiple pregnancies. *Prenatal Diagnosis, 25*(9), 827-834.

Burgoine, G., Van Kirk, S., Romm, J., Edelman, A., Jacobson, S., & Jensen, J. (2005). Comparison of perinatal grief after dilation and evacuation or labor induction in second trimester terminations for fetal anomalies. *American Journal of Obstetrics and Gynecology, 192*(6), 1928-1932.

Calhoun, B., Napolitano, P., Terry, M., Bussey, C., & Hoeldtke, N. (2003). Perinatal hospice: Comprehensive care for the family of the fetus with a lethal condition. *Journal of Reproductive Medicine, 48*(5), 343-348.

Cameron, M., & Penney, G. (2005). Terminology in early pregnancy loss: What women hear and what clinicians write. *Journal of Family Planning and Reproductive Health Care, 31*(4), 313-314.

Capitulo, K. (2004). Perinatal grief online. *MCN American Journal of Maternal/Child Nursing, 29*(5), 305-311.

Capitulo, K. (2005). Evidence for healing interventions with perinatal bereavement. *MCN American Journal of Maternal/Child Nursing, 30*(6), 389-396.

Centers for Disease Control and Prevention (CDC). (2004). Racial/ethnic disparities in neonatal mortality–United States, 1989-2001. *MMWR Morbidity and Mortality Weekly Report, 53*(29), 655-658.

Chambers, H., & Chan, F. (2000). Support for women/families after perinatal death. *The Cochrane Database of Systematic Reviews,* 2006, Issue 3. Chichester, UK: John Wiley & Sons.

Chichester, M. (2005). Multicultural issues in perinatal loss. *AWHONN Lifelines, 9*(4), 312-320.

Corbet-Owen, C., & Kruger, L. (2001). The health system and emotional care: Validating the many meanings of spontaneous pregnancy loss. *Family Systems of Health, 19*(4), 411-417.

Cote-Arsenault, D., & Freije, M. (2004). Support groups helping women through pregnancies after loss. *Western Journal of Nursing Research, 26*(6), 650-670.

Cote-Arsenault, D., & Marshall, R. (2000). One foot in-one foot out: Weathering the storm of pregnancy after perinatal loss. *Research in Nursing & Health, 23*(6), 473-485.

DiMarco, M., Menke, E., & McNamara, T. (2001). Evaluating a support group for perinatal loss. *MCN American Journal of Maternal/Child Nursing, 26*(3), 135-140.

Freda, M., Devine, K., & Semelsberger, C. (2003). The lived experience of miscarriage after infertility. *MCN American Journal of Maternal/Child Nursing, 28*(1), 16-23.

Heiman, J., Yankowitz, J., & Wilkins, J. (1997). Grief support programs: Patients' use of services following the loss of a desired pregnancy and degree of implementation in academic centers. *American Journal of Perinatology, 14*(10), 587-591.

Hoyert, D., Mathews, T., Menacker, F., Strobino, D., & Guyer, B. (2006). Annual summary of vital statistics: 2004. *Pediatrics, 117*(1), 168-183.

Hughes, P., Turton, P., Hopper, E., & Evans, C. (2002). Assessment of guidelines for good practice in psychosocial care of mothers after stillbirth: A cohort study. *Lancet, 360*(9327), 114-118.

Hunfeld, J., Tempels, A., Passchier, J., Hazebroek, F., & Tibboel, D. (1999). Brief report: Parental burden and grief one year after the birth of a child with congenital anomaly. *Journal of Pediatric Psychology, 24*(6), 515-520.

Janssen, H., Cuisinier, M., de Graauw, K., & Hoogduin, K. (1997). A prospective study of risk factors predicting grief intensity following pregnancy loss. *Archives of General Psychiatry, 54*(1), 56-61.

Johansson, M., & Berg, M. (2005). Women's experiences of childlessness 2 years after the end of in vitro fertilization treatment. *Scandinavian Journal of Caring Sciences, 19*(1), 58-63.

Kavanaugh, K., Savage, T., Kilpatrick, S., Kimura, R., & Hershberger, P. (2005). Life support decisions for extremely premature infants: Report of a pilot study. *Journal of Pediatric Nursing, 20*(5), 347-359.

Lindemann, E. (1944). Symptomatology and management of acute grief. *American Journal of Psychiatry, 151*(6 Suppl), 155-160.

Lundqvist, A., Nilstun, T., & Dykes, A. (2002a). Experiencing neonatal death: An ambivalent transition into motherhood. *Pediatric Nursing, 28*(6), 621-625.

Lundqvist, A., Nilstun, T., & Dykes, A. (2002b). Both empowered and powerless: Mother's experiences of professional care when their newborn dies. *Birth, 29*(3), 192-199.

Malacrida, C. (1999). Complicating mourning: The social economy of perinatal death. *Qualitative Health Research, 9*(4), 504-519.

March of Dimes. (2005). *Perinatal statistics.* Accessed www.marchofdimes.com/peristats, May 8, 2006.

McCreight, B. (2004). A grief ignored: Narratives of pregnancy loss from a male perspective. *Sociology of Health & Illness, 26*(3), 326-350.

Miles, M. (1984). Helping adults mourn the death of a child. In H. Wass, & C. Corr (Eds.), *Childhood and death.* New York: Hemisphere.

Miles, M. (2005). A conceptual model of parental grief: Guidelines for assessing and understanding their pain. Unpublished paper submitted for publication.

Moseley, K., Church, A., Hempel, B., Yuan, H., Goold, S., & Freed, G. (2004). End-of-life choices for African-American and white infants in a neonatal intensive-care unit: A pilot study. *Journal of the National Medical Association, 96*(7), 933-937.

Purnell, L., & Paulanka, B. (Eds.). (2003). *Transcultural health care: A culturally competent approach.* Philadelphia: F.A. Davis.

Rand, C., Kellner, K., Revak-Lutz, R., & Massey, J. (1998). Parental behavior after perinatal death: Twelve years of observations. *Journal of Psychosomatic Obstetrics and Gynaecology, 19*(1), 44-48.

Reilly-Smorawski, B., Armstrong, V., & Catlin, E. (2002). Bereavement support for couples following death of a baby: Program development and 14-year exit analysis. *Death Studies, 26*(1), 21-37.

Rich, D. (2000). The impact of postpregnancy loss services on grief outcome: Integrating research and practice in the design of perinatal bereavement programs. *Illness, Crisis, & Loss, 8*(3), 244-264.

Rillstone, P., & Hutchinson, S. (2001). Managing the reemergence of anguish: Pregnancy after a loss due to anomalies. *Journal of Obstetric, Gynecologic, and Neonatal Nursing, 30*(3), 291-298.

Saflund, K., Sjogren, B., & Wredling, R. (2004). The role of caregivers after a stillbirth: Views and experiences of parents. *Birth, 31*(2), 132-137.

Samuelsson, M., Radestad, I., & Segesten, K. (2001). A waste of life: Fathers' experience of losing a child before birth. *Birth, 28*(2), 124-130.

Sepilian, V., & Wood, E. (2005). *Ectopic pregnancy.* Accessed www.emedicine.com/med/topic3212.htm, May 8, 2006.

Shuzman, E. (2003). Facing stillbirth or neonatal death: Providing culturally appropriate care for Jewish families. *AWHONN Lifelines, 7*(6), 537-543.

Swanson, K. (2000). Predicting depressive symptoms after miscarriage: A path analysis based on the Lazarus paradigm. *Journal of Women's Health & Gender-Based Medicine, 9*(2), 191-206.

Swanson, K. (2001). A program of research on caring. In M. Parker (Ed.), *Nursing theories and nursing practice.* Philadelphia: F.A. Davis.

Swanson-Kauffman, K. (1988). There should have been two: Nursing care of parents experiencing perinatal death of a twin. *Journal of Perinatal and Neonatal Nursing, 2*(2), 78-86.

Van, P. (2001). Breaking the silence of African American women: Healing after pregnancy loss. *Health Care for Women International, 22*(3), 229-243.

Wheeler, S., & Austin, J. (2001). The impact of early pregnancy loss on adolescents. *MCN American Journal of Maternal/Child Nursing, 26*(3), 154-159.

Wilson, R. (2001). Parents' support of their other children after a miscarriage or perinatal death. *Early Human Development, 61*(2), 55-65.

World Health Organization (WHO). (2005). Making pregnancy safer. Accessed www.who.int/making_pregnancy_safer/en/, May 8, 2006.

Glossary

abdominal Belonging or relating to the abdomen and its functions and disorders.

  a. birth Birth of a child through a surgical incision made into the abdominal wall and uterus; cesarean birth.

  a. pregnancy Implantation of a fertilized ovum outside the uterus but inside the peritoneal cavity.

ABO incompatibility Hemolytic disease that occurs when the mother's blood type is O and the newborn's is A, B, or AB.

abortion Termination of pregnancy before the fetus is viable and capable of extrauterine existence, usually less than 20 weeks of gestation (or when the fetus weighs less than 500 g); miscarriage.

  complete a. Abortion in which fetus and all related tissue have been expelled from the uterus.

  elective a. Termination of pregnancy chosen by the woman that is not required for her physical safety.

  habitual (recurrent) a. Loss of three or more successive pregnancies for no known cause.

  incomplete a. Loss of pregnancy in which some but not all the products of conception have been expelled from the uterus.

  induced a. Loss of pregnancy, intentionally produced by woman or others.

  inevitable a. Threatened loss of pregnancy that cannot be prevented or stopped and is imminent.

  missed a. Loss of pregnancy in which the products of conception remain in the uterus after the fetus dies.

  septic a. Loss of pregnancy in which there is an infection of the products of conception and the uterine endometrial lining, usually resulting from attempted termination of early pregnancy.

  spontaneous a. Loss of pregnancy that occurs naturally without interference or known cause; preferred term is *miscarriage.*

  therapeutic a. Pregnancy that has been intentionally terminated for medical reasons.

  threatened a. Possible loss of a pregnancy; early symptoms are present (e.g., the cervix begins to dilate).

abruptio placentae Partial or complete premature separation of a normally implanted placenta.

abstinence Refraining from sexual intercourse periodically or permanently.

acceleration Increase in fetal heart rate, usually seen as a reassuring sign.

accreta, placenta See *placenta accreta.*

acculturation Changes that occur within one group or among several groups when people from different cultures come in contact with one another.

acidosis Increase in hydrogen ion concentration resulting in a lowering of blood pH below 7.35.

acoustic stimulation test Antepartum test to elicit fetal heart rate response to sound; performed by applying sound source (laryngeal stimulator) to maternal abdomen over the fetal head.

acquaintance Process used by parents to get to know or become familiar with their new infant; an important step in *attachment.*

acrocyanosis Peripheral cyanosis; blue color of hands and feet in most infants at birth that may persist for 7 to 10 days.

active phase Phase in first stage of labor from 4 to 7 cm dilation.

acupressure Massage technique applied to specific points along certain energy pathways of the body called meridians. A form of treatment based in the theories of traditional Chinese medicine.

acupuncture A form of treatment using slender needles to stimulate points along energy pathways to correct, enhance, and rebalance the flow of body energy.

adequate intakes (AIs) Recommended nutrient intakes estimated to meet the needs of almost all healthy people in the population. They are provided for nutrients or age-group categories when the available information is not sufficient to warrant establishing recommended dietary allowances.

adnexa Adjacent or accessory parts of a structure.

  uterine a. Ovaries and uterine (fallopian) tubes.

adult respiratory distress syndrome (ARDS) Set of symptoms including decreased compliance of lung tissue, pulmonary edema, and acute hypoxemia. The condition is similar to respiratory distress syndrome of the newborn.

afterbirth pains (afterpains) Painful uterine cramps that occur intermittently for approximately 2 or 3 days after birth and that result from contractile efforts of the uterus to return to its normal involuted condition.

afterload Ventricular wall tension during systole, or the resistance the blood meets as it is ejected from the ventricles.

AGA Appropriate (growth) for gestational age.

alkalosis Abnormal condition of body fluids characterized by a tendency toward an increased pH, such as from an excess of alkaline bicarbonate or a deficiency of acid.

allopathic, standard, or Western medicine Interchangeable terms used to describe the current U.S. health care system. With foundations in germ theory and reductionism, standard medical practice often focuses on one body system or disease complex. Treatments are often pharmaceutical or surgical and produce effects that are different from those of the disease complex.

alpha-fetoprotein (AFP) Fetal antigen; elevated levels in amniotic fluid are associated with neural tube defects.

alternative and complementary therapies Nontraditional approaches to health care and healing, often philosophically different from Western medicine. Often involve interventions that are said to induce healing from within the client or improve the internal environment so that the body, mind, or spirit can heal. Often referred to as "natural healing." Might be used in place of or in conjunction with standard health care practices. Also defined as therapeutic modalities not commonly taught by U.S. medical schools or available in U.S. hospitals. *Alternative therapy* often refers to those modalities used in place of conventional (or other) health care. *Complementary therapy* refers to those modalities used in conjunction with conventional (or other) health care. Many therapies can be either alternative or complementary.

amenorrhea Absence or suppression of menstruation.

amniocentesis Procedure in which a needle is inserted through the abdominal and uterine walls into the amniotic fluid; some fluid is withdrawn; used for assessment of fetal health and maturity.

amnioinfusion Infusion of normal saline warmed to body temperature through an intrauterine catheter into the uterine cavity in an attempt to increase the fluid around the umbilical cord and prevent compression during uterine contractions.

amnion Inner membrane of two fetal membranes that form the sac and contain the fetus and the fluid that surrounds it in utero.

amnionitis Inflammation of the amnion, occurring most frequently after early rupture of membranes.

amniotic Pertaining or relating to the amnion.

  a. fluid Fluid surrounding fetus derived primarily from maternal serum and fetal urine.

  a. fluid embolism Embolism resulting from amniotic fluid entering the maternal bloodstream during labor and birth after rupture of membranes; this is often fatal to the woman if it is a pulmonary embolism.

  a. fluid index (AFI) Estimation of amount of amniotic fluid by means of ultrasound to determine excess or decrease.

  a. sac Membrane "bag" that contains the fetus and fluid before birth.

amniotomy Artificial rupture of the fetal membranes (AROM), using a plastic Amnihook or surgical clamp.

analgesia Absence of pain without loss of consciousness.

analgesic Any medication or agent that relieves pain.

android pelvis Male type of pelvis; heart-shaped inlet.

anencephaly Congenital deformity characterized by the absence of cerebrum, cerebellum, and flat bones of the skull.

anesthesia Partial or complete absence of sensation with or without loss of consciousness.

aneuploidy Having an abnormal number of chromosomes.

anovulatory Failure of the ovaries to produce, mature, or release eggs.

antenatal Occurring before or formed before birth (newborn).

  a. glucocorticoids Medications given 24 hours before a preterm birth between 24 and 34 weeks of gestation to accelerate fetal lung maturation.

antepartal Before labor (maternal).

anthropoid pelvis Pelvis in which the anteroposterior diameter is equal to or greater than the transverse diameter; oval inlet.

anthropometric measurements Body measurements, such as height and weight.

antibody Specific protein substance made by the body that exerts restrictive or destructive action on specific antigens, such as bacteria, toxins, or Rh factor.

anticipatory grief Feelings of grief that develop before, rather than after, a loss.

antigen Protein foreign to the body that causes the body to develop antibodies (e.g., bacteria, dust, Rh factor).

Apgar score Numeric expression of the condition of a newborn obtained by rapid assessment at 1 and 5 minutes of age; developed by Dr. Virginia Apgar.

apnea Cessation of respirations for more than 15 seconds associated with generalized cyanosis.

areola Pigmented ring of tissue surrounding the nipple.

arterial pressure catheter A Teflon intravenous catheter, usually 20 gauge, that is placed in an artery and connected to a hemodynamic monitor by means of a pressure line to provide continuous measurements of the systolic, diastolic, and mean arterial blood pressures.

arteriolar vasospasm Diameter of arteriolar vessels diminishes, impeding blood flow to all organs and raising blood pressure.

Asherman syndrome Intrauterine adhesions after inflammation and infection; one cause of impaired fertility.

asphyxia Decreased oxygen with or without excess of carbon dioxide in the body.

perinatal a. Condition occurring in utero with the following biochemical changes: hypoxemia (lowering of PO_2), hypercapnia (increase in PCO_2), and respiratory and metabolic acidosis (reduction of blood pH).

aspiration pneumonia Inflammatory condition of the lungs and bronchi caused by the inhalation of vomitus containing acid gastric contents.

assimilation Occurs when a cultural group loses its identity and becomes part of the dominant culture.

assisted reproductive therapies (ARTs) Treatments for infertility, including in vitro fertilization procedures, embryo adoption, embryo hosting, and therapeutic insemination.

asynclitism Oblique presentation of the fetal head at the superior strait of the pelvis; the pelvic planes and those of the fetal head are not parallel.

atony Absence of muscle tone.

atresia Absence of a normally present passageway.
  biliary a. Absence of the bile duct.
  choanal a. Complete obstruction of the posterior nares, which open into the nasopharynx, with membranous or bony tissue.
  esophageal a. Congenital anomaly in which the esophagus ends in a blind pouch or narrows into a thin cord, thus failing to form a continuous passageway to the stomach.

attachment A specific and enduring affective tie to another person.

attitude Body posture or position.
  fetal a. Relation of fetal parts to each other in the uterus (e.g., all parts flexed; all parts flexed except neck, which is extended).

augmentation of labor Stimulation of ineffective uterine contractions after labor has started spontaneously but is not progressing satisfactorily.

autoimmune disorders Body produces antibodies against itself, causing tissue damage.

autoimmunization Development of antibodies against constituents of one's own tissues (e.g., a man may develop antibodies against his own sperm).

autolysis "Self-digestive" process by which the uterus returns to a nonpregnant state after childbirth. The decrease in estrogen and progesterone levels after childbirth results in this destruction of excess hypertrophied uterine tissue.

autosomal inheritance Characteristics transmitted by genes on the autosomes, not the sex chromosomes.

autosomes Any of the paired chromosomes other than the sex (X and Y) chromosomes.

azoospermia Absence of sperm in the semen.

bag of waters Lay term for the sac containing amniotic fluid and fetus.

ballottement (1) Movability of a floating object, such as a fetus. (2) Diagnostic technique using palpation: a floating object, when tapped or pushed, moves away and then returns to touch the examiner's hand.

Bandl ring Abnormally thickened ridge of uterine musculature between the upper and lower segments that occurs after a mechanically obstructed labor, with the lower segment thinning abnormally.

Bartholin glands Two small glands situated on either side of the vaginal orifice that secrete small amounts of mucus during coitus and that are homologous to the bulbourethral glands in the male.

basal body temperature Lowest body temperature of a healthy person taken immediately after awakening and before getting out of bed.

basalis, decidua See *decidua basalis*.

baseline fetal heart rate Average fetal heart rate between uterine contractions.

bearing-down effort "Secondary powers"; energy exerted by the woman during contractions to push out the baby.

Bell's palsy Peripheral facial paralysis of the facial nerve (cranial nerve VII), causing the muscles of the unaffected side of the face to pull the face into a distorted position.

bereavement The feelings of loss, pain, desolation, and sadness that occur after the death of a loved one.

best practice A program or service that has been recognized for excellence.

bicornuate uterus Anomalous uterus that may be either a double or single organ with two horns.

bilateral tubal ligation Female sterilization, in which both uterine tubes are blocked to prevent conception.

biliary atresia See *atresia, biliary*.

bilirubin Yellow or orange pigment that is a breakdown product of hemoglobin. It is carried by the blood to the liver, where it is chemically changed and excreted into the bile or is conjugated and excreted by the kidneys.

Billings method See *ovulation method*.

bimanual Performed with both hands.
  b. palpation Examination of a woman's pelvic organs done by placement of one hand on the abdomen and one or two fingers of the other hand in the vagina.

biofeedback Technique that teaches the client to consciously control certain body functions usually thought of as unconscious (e.g., breathing, heart rate). Often involves electronic instrumentation that provides immediate visual and auditory feedback to assist the learning process.

biophysical profile (BPP) Noninvasive assessment of the fetus and its environment using ultrasonography and uterine fetal monitoring; includes fetal breathing movements, gross body movements, fetal tone, reactive fetal heart rate, and qualitative amniotic fluid volume.

biopsy Removal of a small piece of tissue for microscopic examination and diagnosis.

biorhythmicity Cyclic changes that occur with established regularity, such as sleeping and eating patterns.

biparietal diameter Largest transverse diameter of the fetal head; extends from one parietal bone to the other.

birth plan A tool by which parents can explore their childbirth options and choose those that are most important to them.

birth rate Number of live births per 1000 population per year. See also *fertility.*

Bishop score Rating system to evaluate inducibility of the cervix; a higher score increases the rate of successful induction of labor.

bittersweet grief The resurgence of feelings and emotions that occur on remembering a loved one after the bereavement process has lessened.

blastocyst Stage in the development of a mammalian embryo, occurring after the morula stage, that consists of an outer layer, or trophoblast, and a hollow sphere of cells enclosing a cavity.

bloody show Vaginal discharge that originates in the cervix and consists of blood and mucus; increases as cervix dilates during labor.

body mass index (BMI) Method of calculating appropriateness of weight for height (BMI = Weight [kilograms]/Height^2 [meters]).

Bradley method Husband-coached childbirth using breathing techniques.

bradycardia Baseline fetal heart rate below 110 beats per minute.

Braxton Hicks sign Mild, intermittent, painless uterine contractions that occur during pregnancy. These contractions occur more frequently as pregnancy advances but do not represent true labor.

Brazelton assessment Method for assessing the interactional behavior of a newborn.

breakthrough bleeding Escape of blood occurring between menstrual periods; may be noted by women using chemical contraception (birth control pills).

breast self-examination (BSE) Self-examination of the breasts.

breech presentation Presentation in which buttocks or feet are nearest the cervical opening and are born first; occurs in approximately 3% of all births.
> **complete b.p.** Simultaneous presentation of buttocks, legs, and feet.
> **footling (incomplete) b.p.** Presentation of one or both feet.
> **frank b.p.** Presentation of buttocks, with hips flexed so that thighs are against abdomen.

bronchopulmonary dysplasia (BPD) Pulmonary condition affecting preterm infants who have experienced respiratory failure and have been oxygen dependent for more than 28 days.

brown fat Source of heat unique to neonates that is capable of greater thermogenic activity than ordinary fat. Deposits are found around the adrenals, the kidneys, and the neck, between the scapulas, and behind the sternum for several weeks after birth.

bruit, uterine See *uterine bruit.*

calendar method See *rhythm method.*

candidiasis Infection of the skin or mucous membrane by a yeastlike fungus, formerly called *moniliasis; Candida albicans;* see *thrush.*

capillary hydrostatic pressure Pressure in the arterial capillary system to promote the movement of fluid across the semipermeable membrane of the capillary wall from the vessel into the interstitial space. Measured as the pulmonary capillary wedge pressure (PCWP).

capsularis, decidua See *decidua capsularis.*

caput Occiput of fetal head appearing at the vaginal introitus preceding birth of the head.
> **c. succedaneum** Swelling of the tissue over the presenting part of the fetal head caused by pressure during labor.

carcinoma Malignant, often metastatic epithelial neoplasm; cancer.

cardiac decompensation A condition of heart failure in which the heart is unable to maintain a sufficient cardiac output.

cardiac output (CO) Volume of blood ejected from the left ventricle in 1 minute, measured in liters per minute. Cardiac output is the product of stroke volume and heart rate (CO = HR × SV).

cardinal movements of labor The mechanism of labor in a vertex presentation; includes engagement, descent, flexion, internal rotation, extension, external rotation (restitution), and expulsion.

carpal tunnel syndrome Pressure on the median nerve at the point at which it goes through the carpal tunnel of the wrist. It causes soreness, tenderness, and weakness of the muscles of the thumb.

carrier Individual who carries a gene that does not exhibit itself in physical or chemical characteristics but that can be transmitted to children (e.g., a female carrying the trait for hemophilia, which is expressed in male offspring).

cephalhematoma NOTE: This is spelled *cephalohematoma* in some sources. Extravasation of blood from ruptured vessels between a skull bone and its external covering, the periosteum. Swelling is limited by the margins of the cranial bone affected (usually parietals).

cephalic Pertaining to the head.
> **c. presentation** Presentation of the fetal head.

cephalopelvic disproportion (CPD) Condition in which the infant's head is of such a shape, size, or position that it cannot pass through the mother's pelvis; can also be caused by maternal pelvic problems.

cerclage Use of nonabsorbable suture to keep a prematurely dilating cervix closed; released when pregnancy is at term to allow labor to begin, or left in place and birth by cesarean.

cervical cap Individually fitted contraceptive barrier for the cervix.

cervical conization Excision of a cone-shaped section of tissue from the endocervix.

cervical funneling Effacement of the internal cervical os.

cervical intraepithelial neoplasm (CIN) Uncontrolled and progressive abnormal growth of cervical epithelial cells.

cervical mucus method See *ovulation method.*

cervical os "Mouth" or opening to the cervix.

cervical ripening Process of effecting physical softening and distensibility of the cervix in preparation for labor and birth.

cervix Lowest and narrow end of the uterus; the "neck." The cervix is situated between the external os and the body, or corpus, of the uterus, and its lower end extends into the vagina.

cesarean birth Birth of a fetus by an incision through the abdominal wall and uterus.

Chadwick sign Violet color of vaginal mucous membrane that is visible from about the fourth week of pregnancy; caused by increased vascularity.

chloasma Increased pigmentation over bridge of nose and cheeks of pregnant women and some women taking oral contraceptives; also known as mask of pregnancy.

choanal atresia See *atresia, choanal.*

cholecystitis Acute or chronic inflammation of the gallbladder.

cholelithiasis Presence of gallstones in the gallbladder.

choreoathetoid cerebral palsy Condition characterized by both choreiform (jerky, ticlike, twitching) and athetoid (slow, writhing) movements.

chorioamnionitis Inflammatory reaction in fetal membranes to bacteria or viruses in the amniotic fluid, which then become infiltrated with polymorphonuclear leukocytes.

chorion Fetal membrane closest to the intrauterine wall that gives rise to the placenta and continues as the outer membrane surrounding the amnion.

chorionic villus Tiny vascular protrusions on the chorionic surface that project into the maternal blood sinuses of the uterus and that help form the placenta and secrete human chorionic gonadotropin.

chorionic villus sampling (CVS) Removal of fetal tissue from placenta for genetic diagnostic studies.

chromosome Element within the cell nucleus carrying genes and composed of DNA and proteins.

circumcision

female c. Religious or cultural removal of a portion of the clitoris and labia; practiced in some Third World countries but illegal in the United States. Mutilating procedure that can cause problems in childbirth.

male c. Excision of the prepuce (foreskin) of the penis, exposing the glans; may be done for religious or cultural reasons.

claiming process Process by which the parents identify their new baby in terms of likeness to other family members, differences, and uniqueness.

cleft lip Incomplete closure of the lip. Lay term used is harelip.

cleft palate Incomplete closure of the palate or roof of mouth; a congenital fissure.

climacteric The period of a woman's life when she is passing from a reproductive to a nonreproductive state, with regression of ovarian function. The cycle of endocrine, physical, and psychosocial changes that occurs during the termination of the reproductive years. Also called *climacterium.*

clinical benchmark Process used to compare one's own performance against the performance of the best in an area of service.

clitoris Female organ analogous to male penis; a small, ovid body of erectile tissue situated at the anterior junction of the vulva.

clubfoot Congenital deformity in which portions of the foot and ankle are twisted out of a normal position.

Cochrane Pregnancy and Childbirth Database Database of up-to-date systematic reviews and dissemination of results of randomized controlled trials of health care.

cohabitating-parent family Family form in which children live with two unmarried biologic parents or two adoptive parents.

coitus Penile-vaginal intercourse.

c. interruptus Intercourse during which the penis is withdrawn from the vagina before ejaculation.

cold stress Excessive loss of heat that results in increased respirations and nonshivering thermogenesis to maintain core body temperature.

colloid osmotic pressure (COP) Pressure in the arterial capillary system to prevent the movement of fluid across the semipermeable membrane of the capillary wall from the vessel into the interstitial space. The COP measures the "pulling" pressure of proteins in the plasma to retain fluid inside the vessel.

colostrum The fluid in the breast from pregnancy into the early postpartal period. It is rich in antibodies, which provide protection from many diseases; high in protein, which binds bilirubin; and laxative-acting, which speeds the elimination of meconium and helps loosen mucus.

colposcopy Examination of vagina and cervix with a colposcope to identify neoplastic or other changes.

complete abortion See *abortion, complete.*

complete breech presentation See *breech presentation, complete.*

complicated bereavement The persistent feelings of anger, guilt, loss, pain, and sadness over time that lead to feelings of hopelessness, helplessness, and diminishing self-worth. Signs and symptoms are those of clinical depression, which is different from the normal expression of bereavement.

conception Union of the sperm and ovum resulting in fertilization; formation of the one-celled zygote.

conceptional age In fetal development the number of completed weeks since the moment of conception. Because the moment of conception is almost impossible to determine, conceptional age is estimated at 2 weeks less than gestational age.

conceptus Embryo or fetus, fetal membranes, amniotic fluid, and the fetal portion of the placenta.

condom Mechanical barrier worn on the penis for contraception or to protect against sexually transmitted infections (STIs); a "rubber."

condyloma acuminatum (plural condylomata acuminata) Wartlike growth(s) on the skin usually seen near the anus or external genitals caused by human papillomavirus (HPV); genital warts. (Must be differentiated from condyloma latum seen in secondary syphilis.)

congenital Present or existing before birth as a result of either hereditary or prenatal environmental factors.

congenital rubella syndrome Complex of problems, including hearing defects, cardiovascular abnormalities, and cataracts, caused by maternal rubella in the first trimester of pregnancy.

conjoined twins See *twins, conjoined.*

conjugate
  diagonal c. Radiographic measurement of distance from inferior border of symphysis pubis to sacral promontory; may be obtained by vaginal examination; normal is 12.5 to 13 cm.
  true c. (conjugata vera) Radiographic measurement of distance from upper margin of symphysis pubis to sacral promontory; 1.5 to 2 cm less than diagonal conjugate.

conjunctivitis Inflammation of the mucous membrane that lines the eyelids and is reflected onto the eyeball.

conscious relaxation Technique used to release the mind and body from tension through conscious effort and practice.

contraception Prevention of impregnation or conception.

contractility Force and velocity of ventricular contractions when preload and afterload are held constant.

contraction ring See *Bandl ring.*

contractions In labor, involuntary rhythmic tightenings of uterine muscle that act to expel the fetus and placenta from uterus.
  duration Period from the beginning of the contraction to the end.
  frequency How often the contractions occur—the period from the beginning of one contraction to the beginning of the next.

intensity Strength of the contraction at its peak.

interval Period between uterine contractions, timed from the end of one contraction to the beginning of the next.

resting tone The tension in the uterine muscle between contractions.

contraction stress test (CST) Test to stimulate uterine contractions for the purpose of assessing fetal response; a healthy fetus does not react to contractions, whereas a compromised fetus demonstrates late decelerations in the fetal heart rate that are indicative of uteroplacental insufficiency.

Coombs' test Indirect: determination of Rh-positive antibodies in maternal blood; direct: determination of maternal Rh-positive antibodies in fetal cord blood. A positive test result indicates the presence of antibodies or titer.

corpus luteum Yellow body. After rupture of the graafian follicle at ovulation, the follicle develops into a yellow structure that secretes progesterone and some estrogen in the second half of the menstrual cycle, atrophying about 3 days before sloughing of the endometrium in menstrual flow. If impregnation occurs, it continues to produce the hormones until the placenta can take over this function.

corrected age Taking into account the gestational age and the postnatal age of a preterm infant when determining expectations for development.

cotyledon One of the 15 to 28 visible segments of the placenta on the maternal surface, each made up of fetal vessels, chorionic villus, and an intervillous space.

counterpressure Pressure to sacral area of back during uterine contractions.

couplet care One nurse, educated in both mother and infant care, functions as the primary nurse for both mother and infant (also known as mother-baby care or single-room maternity care).

Couvade syndrome The phenomenon of expectant fathers' experiencing pregnancy-like symptoms.

Couvelaire uterus See *uterus, Couvelaire.*

CPAP Continuous positive airway pressure.

cradle cap Common seborrheic dermatitis of infants consisting of thick, yellow, greasy scales on the scalp.

creatinine Substance found in blood and muscle; measurement of levels in maternal urine correlates with amount of fetal muscle mass and therefore fetal size.

crib death Unexpected and sudden death of an apparently normal and healthy infant that occurs during sleep and with no physical or autopsy-derived evidence of disease. Also referred to as *sudden infant death syndrome (SIDS).*

cri-du-chat syndrome Rare congenital disorder recognized at birth by a kitten-like cry, which may prevail for weeks and then disappear. Other characteristics include low birth weight, microcephaly, "moon face," wide-set eyes, strabismus, and low-set misshapen ears. Infants are hypotonic; heart defects and mental and physical retardation are common. Also called *cat-cry syndrome.*

crowning Stage of birth when the top of the fetal head can be seen at the vaginal orifice as the widest part of the head distends the vulva.

cryosurgery Local freezing and removal of tissue without injury to adjacent tissue and with minimal blood loss, done with special equipment.

cul-de-sac of Douglas Pouch formed by a fold of the peritoneum dipping down between the anterior wall of the rectum and the posterior wall of the uterus; also called *Douglas's cul-de-sac, pouch of Douglas,* and *rectouterine pouch.*

culdocentesis Puncture of cul-de-sac of Douglas through the vagina for aspiration of fluid.

Cullen's sign Faint, irregularly formed, hemorrhagic patches on the skin around the umbilicus. The discolored skin is blue-black and becomes greenish brown or yellow. Cullen's sign may develop in undiagnosed ruptured intraabdominal ectopic pregnancy.

cultural competence Awareness, acceptance, and knowledge of cultural differences and adaptation of services to acknowledge and support the culture of the client.

cultural context Setting in which one considers the individual's and the family's beliefs and practices (culture).

cultural prescriptions Practices that are expected or acceptable.

cultural proscriptions Forbidden or taboo practices.

curettage (curet or curette) Scraping of the endometrium lining the uterus with a curette to remove the contents of the uterus (as is done after an incomplete miscarriage or induced abortion) or to obtain specimens for diagnostic purposes.

cycle of violence Pattern of three phases: period of increasing tension, the abusive episode, and a period of contrition and kindness.

cystocele Bladder hernia: injury to the vesicovaginal fascia during labor and birth may allow herniation of the bladder into the vagina.

daily fetal movement counts (DFMCs) Maternal assessment of fetal activity; the number of fetal movements within a specific time are counted.

death Cessation of life.
> **fetal d.** Death of the fetus after 20 weeks of gestation and before birth, with absence of any signs of life after birth.
> **infant d.** Death during the first year of life.
> **maternal d.** Death of a woman as a result of a pregnancy or birth-related problem.
> **neonatal d.** Death of a newborn within the first 28 days after birth.
> **perinatal d.** Death of a fetus of 20 weeks of gestation or older, or death of a neonate 28 days old or younger.

deceleration Slowing of fetal heart rate attributed to a parasympathetic response and described in relation to uterine contractions.
> **early d.** Onset corresponding to onset of uterine contraction, related to fetal head compression.
> **late d.** Onset after peak of contraction, continuing into interval after contraction; caused by uteroplacental insufficiency.
> **prolonged d.** Episode of slowing of fetal heart rate lasting longer than 2 minutes.
> **variable d.** Onset at any time unrelated to contraction; caused by cord compression.

decidua Mucous membrane, lining of uterus, or endometrium of pregnancy that is shed after giving birth.
> **d. basalis** Maternal aspect of the placenta made up of uterine blood vessels, endometrial stroma, and glands. It is shed in lochial discharge after the birth.
> **d. capsularis** That part of the decidual membranes surrounding the chorionic sac.
> **d. vera** Nonplacental decidual lining of the uterus.

decrement Decrease or stage of decline, as of a contraction.

deep tendon reflexes (DTRs) Reflex caused by stimulation of tendons, such as elbow, wrist, knee, triceps, and ankle jerk reflexes.

delivery (birth) Expulsion of the child with placenta and membranes by the mother or their extraction by the obstetric practitioner.
> **abdominal d.** See *abdominal birth.*

ΔOD_{450} (delta OD_{450}) Delta optical density (or absorbance) at 450 nm, obtained by spectral analysis of amniotic fluid. This prenatal test is used to measure the degree of hemolytic activity in the fetus and to evaluate fetal status in women sensitized to the Rh factor.

demand feeding Feeding a newborn every third hour or when the baby cries to be fed, whichever comes first.

deoxyribonucleic acid (DNA) Intracellular complex protein that carries genetic information, consisting of two purines (adenine and guanine) and two pyrimidines (thymine and cytosine).

DES Diethylstilbestrol; female fetus is predisposed to reproductive tract malformations and (later) dysplasia if her mother ingested this medication during pregnancy.

desquamation Shedding of epithelial cells of the skin and mucous membranes.

developmental dysplasia of the hip Abnormal development of the hip joint, resulting in instability of the hip causing one or both of the femoral heads to be displaced from the acetabulum (hip socket).

diabetes mellitus Systemic disorder of carbohydrate, protein, and fat metabolism; caused by deficient insulin production or ineffective use of insulin at the cellular level.

diaphragmatic hernia Congenital malformation of diaphragm that allows displacement of the abdominal organs into the thoracic cavity.

diastasis recti abdominis Separation of the two rectus muscles along the median line of the abdominal wall. This is often seen in women with repeated childbirths or with a multiple gestation (e.g., triplets). In the newborn it is usually attributable to incomplete development.

Dick-Read method An approach to childbirth based on the premise that fear of pain produces muscular tension, producing pain and greater fear. The method includes teaching physiologic processes of labor, exercise to improve muscle tone, and techniques to assist in relaxation and prevent or interrupt the fear-tension-pain mechanism.

dietary reference intakes (DRIs) New nutritional recommendations being prepared for the United States, consisting of the recommended dietary allowances, adequate intakes, and tolerable upper intake levels; the upper limit of intake associated with low risk in almost all members of a population.

dilation and curettage (D&C) Vaginal procedure in which the cervical canal is stretched enough to admit passage of an instrument called a curette (or curet). The endometrium of the uterus is scraped with the curette to empty the uterine contents or to obtain tissue for examination.

dilation of cervix Stretching of the external os from an opening a few millimeters in size to an opening large enough to allow the passage of the infant.

disorganization A dimension of bereavement characterized by depression, anorexia, difficulty in concentration, and a generalized feeling of not feeling good about oneself physically and emotionally.

disparate twins See *twins, disparate.*

disseminated intravascular coagulation (DIC) Pathologic form of coagulation in which clotting factors are consumed to such an extent that generalized bleeding can occur; associated with abruptio placentae, eclampsia, intrauterine fetal demise, amniotic fluid embolism, and hemorrhage.

dizygotic Related to or proceeding from two zygotes (fertilized ova).

dizygotic twins See *twins, dizygotic.*

dominant trait Gene that is expressed whenever it is present in the heterozygous gene state (e.g., brown eyes are dominant over blue).

Doppler blood flow analysis Device for measuring blood flow noninvasively in the fetus and placenta to detect intrauterine growth restriction.

Douglas's cul-de-sac See *cul-de-sac of Douglas.*

doula Experienced assistant hired to give the woman support during labor and birth.

Down syndrome Abnormality involving the occurrence of a third chromosome, rather than the normal pair (trisomy 21), that characteristically results in a typical picture of mental retardation and altered physical appearance. This condition was formerly called *mongolism.*

dry labor Lay term referring to labor in which amniotic fluid has already escaped. A "dry birth" does not exist.

ductus arteriosus In fetal circulation an anatomic shunt between the pulmonary artery and arch of the aorta. It is obliterated after birth by a rising PO_2 and a change in intravascular pressures in the presence of normal pulmonary function. It normally becomes a ligament after birth but in some instances remains patent.

ductus venosus In fetal circulation, a blood vessel carrying oxygenated blood between the umbilical vein and the inferior vena cava, bypassing the liver. It is obliterated and becomes a ligament after birth.

Duncan's mechanism Delivery of placenta with the maternal surface presenting, rather than the shiny fetal surface.

dysfunctional labor Abnormal uterine contractions that prevent normal progress of cervical dilation and effacement.

dysfunctional uterine bleeding (DUB) Abnormal bleeding from the uterus for reasons that are not readily established.

dysmaturity See *intrauterine growth restriction (IUGR).*

dysmenorrhea
   primary d. Painful menstruation beginning 2 to 6 months after menarche, related to ovulation.
   secondary d. Painful menstruation related to organic disease such as endometriosis, pelvic inflammatory disease, or uterine neoplasm.

dyspareunia Painful sexual intercourse, for either sex.

dysplasia Any abnormal development of tissues or organs.

dystocia Prolonged, painful, or otherwise difficult birth because of mechanical factors produced by the passenger (the fetus), the passage (the pelvis and soft tissues of the birth canal of the mother), inadequate powers (uterine and other muscular activity), or maternal position.

ecchymosis Bruise; bleeding into tissue caused by direct trauma, serious infection, or bleeding diathesis.

eclampsia Severe complication of pregnancy of unknown cause and occurring more often in the primigravida; characterized by tonic and clonic convulsions, coma, high blood pressure, albuminuria, and oliguria occurring during pregnancy or shortly after birth.

ectoderm Outer layer of embryonic tissue giving rise to skin, nails, and hair.

ectopic Out of normal place.
   e. pregnancy Implantation of the fertilized ovum outside of its normal place in the uterine cavity. Locations include the abdomen, the uterine tubes, and the ovaries.

edema Generalized accumulation of interstitial fluid.
   dependent e. Edema of lower or most dependent parts of body where hydrostatic pressure is greater.
   pitting e. Edema that leaves a small depression or pit when pressure is applied to a swollen area.

effacement Thinning and shortening or obliteration of the cervix that occurs during late pregnancy or labor or both.

effleurage Gentle stroking used in massage.

Eisenmenger syndrome Pulmonary hypertension characterized by elevated pulmonary vascular resistance and right-to-left (or bidirectional) shunting in either atria or ventricles.

ejaculation Sudden expulsion of semen from the male urethra.

elective abortion See *abortion, elective.*

electronic fetal monitoring (EFM) Electronic surveillance of fetal heart rate by external and internal methods.

embolus Any undissolved matter (solid, liquid, or gaseous) that is carried by the blood to another part of the body and obstructs a blood vessel.

embryo Conceptus from the second or third week of development until about the eighth week after conception, when mineralization (ossification) of the skeleton begins. This period is characterized by cellular differentiation and predominantly hyperplastic growth.

emergency contraception Contraception that should be taken by a woman as soon as possible but within 120 hours of unprotected intercourse or birth control mishap to prevent unintended pregnancy.

emotional lability Rapid mood changes from irritability to anger or sadness to joy and cheerfulness; often seen in the first trimester of pregnancy.

endocarditis Inflammation of the inner layer of the heart muscle (endocardium).

endocervical Pertaining to the interior of the canal of the cervix of the uterus.

endocrine glands Ductless glands that secrete hormones into the blood or lymph.

endometriosis Tissue closely resembling endometrial tissue but located outside the uterus in the pelvic cavity. Symptoms may include pelvic pain or pressure, dysmenorrhea, dyspareunia, abnormal bleeding from the uterus or rectum, and sterility.

endometritis Postpartum uterine infection, often beginning at the site of the placental implantation.

endometrium Inner lining of the uterus that undergoes changes caused by hormones during the menstrual cycle and pregnancy; decidua.

endorphins Endogenous opioids secreted by the pituitary gland that act on the central and peripheral nervous systems to reduce pain.

energy healing A variety of techniques and disciplines that are said to augment, modulate, stimulate, or remedy certain deficiencies or blocks in the human energy system.

en face Face-to-face position in which the parent's and infant's faces are approximately 20 cm apart and on the same plane.

engagement In obstetrics, the entrance of the fetal presenting part into the superior pelvic strait and the beginning of the descent through the pelvic canal.

engorgement Distention or vascular congestion. In obstetrics, the process of swelling of the breast tissue brought about by an increase in blood and lymph supply to the breast, which precedes true lactation. It lasts about 48 hours and usually reaches a peak between the third and fifth postbirth days.

engrossment A parent's absorption, preoccupation, and interest in his or her infant; term typically used to describe the father's intense involvement with his newborn.

entrainment Phenomenon observed in the microanalysis of sound films in which the speaker moves several parts of the body and the listener responds to the sounds by moving in ways that are coordinated with the rhythm of the sounds. Infants have been observed to move in time to the rhythms of adult speech but not to random noises or disconnected words or vowels.

epicanthus Fold of skin covering the inner canthus and caruncle that extends from the root of the nose to the median end of the eyebrow; characteristically found in certain races but may occur as a congenital anomaly.

epidural block Type of regional anesthesia produced by injection of a local anesthetic into the epidural (peridural) space.

epidural blood patch A patch formed by a few millimeters of the mother's blood occluding a tear or hole in the dura mater around the spinal cord.

episiotomy Surgical incision of the perineum at the end of the second stage of labor to facilitate birth and to avoid laceration of the perineum.

episodic changes Changes from baseline patterns in the fetal heart rate that are not associated with uterine contractions.

epispadias Defect in which the urethral canal terminates on the dorsum of the penis or above the clitoris (rare).

Epstein's pearls Small, white blebs found along the gum margins and at the junction of the soft and hard palates. They are a normal manifestation and are typically seen in the newborn. Similar to *Bohn's nodules.*

epulis Tumorlike benign lesion of the gingiva seen in pregnant women.

Erb-Duchenne paralysis Paralysis caused by physical injury to the upper brachial plexus, occurring most often in childbirth from forcible traction during birth. The signs of Erb's paralysis include loss of sensation in the arm and paralysis and atrophy of the deltoid, the biceps, and the brachialis muscles. Also called *Erb's palsy.*

erythema toxicum Innocuous pink papular neonatal rash of unknown cause, with superimposed vesicles appearing within 24 to 48 hours after birth and resolving spontaneously within a few days.

erythroblastosis fetalis Hemolytic disease of the newborn, usually caused by isoimmunization resulting from Rh incompatibility or ABO incompatibility.

esophageal atresia See *atresia, esophageal.*

estimated date of birth (EDB) Approximate date of birth. Usually determined by calculation using Nägele's rule; "due date"; also called expected date of delivery (EDD).

estradiol An estrogen.

estriol Major metabolite of estrogen that increases during the second half of pregnancy with an intact fetoplacental unit (normal placenta, normal fetal liver and adrenals) and normal maternal renal function.

estrogen Female sex hormone produced by the ovaries and the placenta.

estrogen replacement therapy (ERT) Exogenous estrogen given to women during and after menopause to prevent hot flashes, mood changes, osteoporosis, and genitourinary symptoms.

ethics Systematic inquiry into the principles of right and wrong conduct, of virtue and vice, and of good and evil as they relate to conduct.

ethnocentrism Belief in the rightness of one's culture's way of doing things.

eutocia Normal or natural labor or birth.

evidence-based practice Practice based on analysis of research findings.

exchange transfusion Replacement of 75% to 85% of circulating blood by withdrawal of the recipient's blood and injection of a donor's blood in equal amounts, the purposes of which are to prevent an accumulation of bilirubin in the blood above a dangerous level, to prevent the accumulation of other by-products of hemolysis in hemolytic disease, and to correct anemia and acidosis.

expulsive Having the tendency to drive out or expel.

   e. contractions Labor contractions that are characteristic of the second stage of labor.

extended family Family form that includes the nuclear family and other blood-related persons.

external cephalic version (ECV) Turning the fetus to a vertex position by exertion of pressure on the fetus externally through the maternal abdomen.

extracorporeal membrane oxygenation (ECMO) Oxygenation of blood external to body using cardiopulmonary bypass and a membrane oxygenator. Used primarily for newborns with refractory respiratory failure or meconium aspiration syndrome.

extrauterine Occurring outside the uterus.

   e. pregnancy Pregnancy in which the fertilized ovum implants itself outside the uterus.

extrusion reflex Infant automatically extends tongue when it is stimulated.

facies Pertaining to the appearance or expression of the face; certain congenital syndromes typically cause a specific facial appearance.

FAD Fetal activity determination; also called *fetal activity test (FAT).*

failure to thrive Condition in which neonate's or infant's growth and development patterns are below the norms for age.

fallopian tubes Two canals or oviducts extending laterally from each side of the uterus through which the ovum travels, after ovulation, to the uterus; also called uterine tubes.

false labor Uterine contractions that do not result in cervical dilation, are irregular, are felt more in front, often do not last more than 20 seconds, and do not become longer or stronger.

false pelvis Part of the pelvis superior to a plane passing through the linea terminalis (brim or outlet).

family dynamics Process by which family members assume varying social roles.

family functions Activities carried out within families for the well-being of family members, including biologic, economic, educational, psychologic, and sociocultural aspects.

family stress theory Theory that explains how families react and adapt to stressors that they experience.

family systems theory Theory that conceptualizes the family as a unit and focuses on observing interactions among family members.

feeding readiness cues Infant responses that indicate optimal times to begin a feeding. The baby may make mouthing motions, suck a fist, or awaken and cry.

Ferguson reflex Reflex contractions of the uterus after stimulation of the cervix.

ferning (arborization) test The appearance of a fernlike pattern found on slides of certain fluids.

   ovulation f.t. Test in which cervical mucus, placed on a slide, dries in a branching pattern in the presence of high estrogen levels at the time of ovulation.

fertile period Period before and after ovulation during which the human ovum can be fertilized; usually between 3 days before and 4 days after ovulation.

fertility Quality of being able to reproduce; also number of births per 1000 women ages 15 through 44 years. See also *birth rate.*

fertility awareness methods (FAMs) Methods of family planning that identify the beginning and end of the fertile period of the menstrual cycle.

fertilization Union of an ovum and a sperm.

fetal Pertaining or relating to the fetus.

   f. alcohol effect (FAE) Lesser set of the same symptoms that make up fetal alcohol syndrome.

   f. alcohol syndrome (FAS) Congenital abnormality or anomaly resulting from excessive maternal alcohol intake during pregnancy. It is characterized by typical craniofacial and limb defects, cardiovascular defects, intrauterine growth restriction, and developmental delay.

   f. asphyxia See *asphyxia, fetal.*

   f. attitude See *attitude, fetal.*

f. compromise Evidence such as a nonreassuring fetal heart rate pattern that indicates the fetus may be in jeopardy.

f. death See *death, fetal*.

f. heart rate (FHR) Beats per minute of the fetal heart. Normal range is 110 to 160 beats per minute.

f. lie Relation of the fetal spine to the maternal spine; that is, in vertical lie, maternal and fetal spines are parallel and the fetal head or breech presents; in transverse lie, fetal spine is perpendicular to the maternal spine and the fetal shoulder presents.

f. membrane See *membrane*.

f. presentation The part of the fetus that enters the pelvic inlet first.

f. scalp spiral electrode Internal signal source for electronically monitoring the fetal heart rate.

f. tobacco syndrome Diagnostic term applicable to infants who fit the following criteria: mother who smoked more than 5 cigarettes a day during pregnancy and had no prenatal evidence of hypertension; infant has symmetric growth restriction, weighs less than 2500 g, and has no other cause of intrauterine growth restriction.

fetotoxic Poisonous or destructive to the fetus.

fetus Child in utero from approximately the eighth week after conception until birth.

fibroid Fibrous, encapsulated connective tissue tumor, especially of the uterus; leiomyoma.

fimbria Structure resembling a fringe, particularly the fringelike end of the uterine tube.

first stage of labor Stage of labor from the onset of regular uterine contractions to full dilation of the cervix.

fissure Groove or open crack in tissue.

fistula Abnormal tubelike passage that forms between two normal cavities, possibly congenital or caused by trauma, abscesses, or inflammatory processes.

flaccid Having relaxed, limp, or absent muscle tone.

flaring of nostrils Widening of nostrils (alae nasi) during inspiration in the presence of air hunger; sign of respiratory distress.

flexion Opposite of extension. In obstetrics, resistance to the descent of the baby down the birth canal causes the head to flex, or bend, so that the chin approaches the chest. Thus the smallest diameter (suboccipitobregmatic) of the vertex presents.

follicle Small secretory cavity or sac.

graafian f. Mature, fully developed ovarian cyst containing the ripe ovum. The follicle secretes estrogens, and after ovulation the corpus luteum develops within the ruptured graafian follicle and secretes estrogen and progesterone.

follicle-stimulating hormone (FSH) Hormone produced by the anterior pituitary during the first half of the menstrual cycle. Stimulates development of the graafian follicle.

fontanel Broad area, or soft spot, consisting of a strong band of connective tissue contiguous with cranial bones and located at the junctions of the bones.

anterior f. Diamond-shaped area between the frontal and two parietal bones just above the baby's forehead at the junction of the coronal and sagittal sutures.

mastoid f. Posterolateral fontanel, usually not palpable.

posterior f. Small, triangular area between the occipital and parietal bones at the junction of the lambdoidal and sagittal sutures.

sagittal f. Soft area located in the sagittal suture, halfway between the anterior and posterior fontanels; may be palpated in normal newborns and in some neonates with Down syndrome.

sphenoid f. Anterolateral fontanel usually not palpable.

footling (incomplete) breech presentation See *breech presentation, footling*.

foramen ovale Septal opening between the atria of the fetal heart. The opening normally closes shortly after birth, but if it remains patent, surgical repair usually is necessary.

forceps Curved-bladed instruments used to protect head of fetus during birth and to apply traction to assist birth.

forceps-assisted birth Birth in which forceps are used to assist in delivery of the fetal head.

foreskin Prepuce, or loose fold of skin covering the glans penis.

fornix Any structure with an arched or vaultlike shape.

f. of the vagina Anterior and posterior spaces, formed by the protrusion of the cervix into the vagina, into which the upper vagina is divided.

fourth stage of labor Initial period of recovery from childbirth. It is usually considered to last for the first 1 to 2 hours after the expulsion of the placenta.

fourth trimester Another term for the puerperium; the 3-month interval after the birth of the newborn that includes return of the reproductive organs to their nonpregnant state and psychologic adaptation to parenthood.

frank breech presentation See *breech presentation, frank*.

fraternal twins Nonidentical twins who come from two separate fertilized ova.

free-standing birth center A center that provides prenatal care, labor and birth, and postbirth care outside of a hospital setting.

frenulum Thin ridge of tissue in midline of undersurface of tongue extending from its base to varying distances from the tip of the tongue.

friability Easily broken. May refer to a fragile condition of the cervix, especially during pregnancy, that causes the cervix to bleed easily when touched.

Friedman's curve Labor curve; pattern of descent of presenting part and of dilation of cervix; partogram.

FSH See *follicle-stimulating hormone.*

fundus Dome-shaped upper portion of the uterus between the points of insertion of the uterine tubes.

funic souffle See *souffle, funic.*

funis Cordlike structure, especially the umbilical cord.

galactorrhea Lactation not associated with childbirth or breastfeeding; a symptom of a pituitary gland tumor.

galactosemia Inherited, autosomal recessive disorder of galactose metabolism, characterized by a deficiency of the enzyme galactose-1-phosphate uridyltransferase.

gamete Mature male or female germ cell; the mature sperm or ovum.

gastroschisis Abdominal wall defect at base of umbilical stalk.

gastrostomy Surgical creation of an artificial opening into the stomach through the abdominal wall, performed to feed a client when oral feeding is not possible.

gate control theory Proposed in 1965 by Melzack and Wall, this theory explains the neurophysical mechanism underlying the perception of pain: The capacity of nerve pathways to transmit pain is reduced or completely blocked by using distraction techniques.

gavage Feeding by means of a tube passed through the nose or mouth to the stomach.

gene Factor on a chromosome responsible for hereditary characteristics of offspring.

genetic Dependent on the genes. A genetic disorder may or may not be apparent at birth.

genetic counseling Process of determining the occurrence or risk of occurrence of a genetic disorder within a family and of providing appropriate information and advice about the courses of action that are available, whether care of a child already affected, prenatal diagnosis, termination of a pregnancy, sterilization, or artificial insemination is involved.

genitalia Organs of reproduction.

genogram Pictorial representation of family relationships and health history.

genome Complete copy of genetic material in an organism.

genotype Hereditary combinations in an individual determining physical and chemical characteristics. Some genotypes are not expressed until later in life (e.g., Huntington's chorea); some hide recessive genes, which can be expressed in offspring; and others are expressed only under the proper environmental conditions (e.g., diabetes mellitus appearing under the stress of obesity or pregnancy).

gestation Period of intrauterine fetal development from conception through birth; the period of pregnancy.

gestational age In fetal development, the number of completed weeks counting from the first day of the last normal menstrual cycle.

gestational diabetes Glucose intolerance first recognized during pregnancy.

gestational trophoblastic neoplasia (GTN) Persistent trophoblastic tissue that is presumed to be malignant.

GIFT Gamete intrafallopian transfer of ova and washed sperm into uterine tubes.

gingivitis Inflammation of the gums characterized by redness, swelling, and tendency to bleed.

glans penis Smooth, round head of the penis, analogous to the female glans clitoris.

glomerulonephritis Noninfectious disease of the glomerulus of the kidney, characterized by proteinuria, hematuria, decreased urine production, and edema.

glucose tolerance test A test of the body's ability to use carbohydrates; used as a screening measure for gestational diabetes.

glycosuria Presence of glucose (a sugar) in the urine.

glycosylated hemoglobin (GHb) Glycohemoglobin, a minor hemoglobin with glucose attached. GHb/Hb A_{1c} concentration represents the average blood glucose level over the previous several weeks and is a measurement for glycemic control in diabetic therapy.

gonad Gamete-producing, or sex, gland; the ovary or testis.

gonadotropic hormone Hormone that stimulates the gonads.

gonadotropin-releasing hormone (GnRH) Hormone released from the hypothalamus that stimulates pituitary gland to produce follicle-stimulating hormone (FSH) and luteinizing hormone (LH).

Goodell sign Softening of the cervix, a probable sign of pregnancy, occurring during the second month.

graafian follicle (vesicle) See *follicle, graafian.*

gravida Pregnant woman.

gravidity Number of times a woman has been pregnant.

grief responses The physical, emotional, social, and cognitive responses to the death of a loved one.

grieving process A complex of somatic and psychologic symptoms associated with some extreme sorrow or loss, specifically the death of a loved one.

growth spurts Times of increased neonatal growth that usually occur at approximately 6 to 10 days, 6 weeks, 3 months, and 4 to 5 months. The increased caloric needs necessitate more frequent feedings to increase the amount of milk produced.

grunt, expiratory Sign of respiratory distress (hyaline membrane disease [respiratory distress syndrome, or RDS] or advanced pneumonia) indicative of the body's attempt to hold air in the alveoli for better gaseous exchange.

guided imagery The use of imagination and thought processes in a purposeful way to change certain physiologic and emotional conditions.

gynecoid pelvis Pelvis in which the inlet is round instead of oval or blunt; typical female pelvis.

gynecology Study of the diseases of the female, especially of the genital, urinary, and rectal organs.

habitual (recurrent) abortion See *abortion, habitual.*

habituation An acquired tolerance from repeated exposure to a particular stimulus. Also called *negative adaptation;* a decline and eventual elimination of a conditioned response by repetition of the conditioned stimulus.

harlequin sign Rare color change of no pathologic significance occurring between the longitudinal halves of the neonate's body. When infant is placed on one side, the dependent half is noticeably pinker than the superior half.

healing touch A combination of energetic healing techniques used by nurses and other health care professionals.

health promotion Motivation to increase well-being and actualize health potential.

Hegar sign Softening of the lower uterine segment that is classified as a probable sign of pregnancy and that may be present during the second and third months of pregnancy and is palpated during bimanual examination.

HELLP syndrome Condition characterized by *h*emolysis, *e*levated *l*iver enzymes, and *low p*latelet count; a form of severe preeclampsia.

hematocrit Volume of red blood cells per deciliter (dl) of circulating blood; packed cell volume (PCV).

hematoma Collection of blood in a tissue; a bruise or blood tumor.

hematopoiesis Production of blood cells.

hemoconcentration Increase in the number of red blood cells in proportion to the volume, resulting from either a decrease in plasma volume or increased erythropoiesis.

hemodilution An increase in fluid content of blood, resulting in diminution of the proportion of formed elements.

hemoglobin Component of red blood cells consisting of globin, a protein, and hematin, an organic iron compound.

    h. electrophoresis Test to diagnose sickle cell disease in newborns. Cord blood is used.

hemolytic disease of the newborn Breakdown of fetal red blood cells by maternal antibodies, usually from an Rh-negative mother.

hemorrhagic disease of newborn Bleeding disorder during first few days of life based on a deficiency of vitamin K.

hemorrhagic shock Clinical condition in which the peripheral blood flow is inadequate to return sufficient blood to the heart for normal function, particularly oxygen transport to the organs or tissue.

hereditary Pertaining to a trait or characteristic transmitted from parent to offspring by way of the genes; used synonymously with the term *genetic.*

hermaphrodite Person having genital and sexual characteristics of both sexes.

heterozygous Having two dissimilar genes at the same site, or locus, on paired chromosomes (e.g., at the site for eye color, one chromosome carrying the gene for brown, the other for blue).

high risk Increased possibility of suffering harm, damage, loss, or death. See also *risk factor.*

hirsutism Condition characterized by the excessive growth of hair.

holism Philosophy that states that the whole is greater than the sum of its parts. In healing, refers to consideration and treatment of the whole client as a unified being. May include alternative and complementary modalities, but it is more a philosophic base than a modality in and of itself.

holistic medicine Health care treatment with techniques not commonly taught in U.S. medical schools or widely available in U.S. hospitals. May include a variety of disciplines involving diet, exercise, vitamin and nutritional supplements, bodywork, or alternative pharmacologic agents. Philosophy of medicine that encompasses holism.

holistic nursing Nursing practice that stems from the philosophy of holism, one that views the client as an integrated whole, and influenced by a variety of internal and external factors, including the biopsychosocial and spiritual dimensions of the person.

Homans sign Early sign of phlebothrombosis of the deep veins of the calf, in which there are complaints of pain when the leg is in extension and the foot is dorsiflexed.

home birth Planned birth of the child at home, usually done under the supervision of a midwife.

homologous Similar in structure or origin but not necessarily in function.

homologous insemination Insemination in which the semen specimen is provided by the husband. The procedure is used primarily in cases of impotence or when the husband is incapable of sexual intercourse because of some physical disability.

homosexual family Family in which parents form a homosexual union. Children may be the offspring of a previous heterosexual union, adopted, or conceived by one or both members of a homosexual couple through artificial insemination.

homozygous Having two similar genes at the same locus, or site, on paired chromosomes.

hormone Chemical substance produced in an organ or gland that is conveyed through the blood to another organ or part of the body, stimulating it to increased functional activity or secretion. See also specific hormones.

hormone replacement therapy (HRT) Progestin and estrogen given for menopausal symptoms. See *estrogen replacement therapy.*

hot flash (flush) Transient sensation of warmth experienced by some women during or after menopause, resulting from autonomic vasomotor disturbances that accompany changes in the neurohormonal activity of the ovaries, the hypothalamus, and the pituitary gland.

human chorionic gonadotropin (hCG) Hormone that is produced by chorionic villus; the biologic marker in pregnancy tests.

hyaline membrane disease (HMD) See *respiratory distress syndrome (RDS)*.

hydatidiform mole (molar pregnancy) Gestational trophoblastic neoplasm usually resulting from fertilization of egg that has no nucleus or an inactivated nucleus.

hydramnios (polyhydramnios) Amniotic fluid in excess of 1.5 liters; often indicative of fetal anomaly and frequently seen in poorly controlled, insulin-dependent, diabetic pregnant women even if there is no coexisting fetal anomaly.

hydrocele Collection of fluid in a saclike cavity, especially in the sac that surrounds the testis, causing the scrotum to swell.

hydrocephalus Accumulation of fluid in the subdural or subarachnoid spaces.

hydrops fetalis Most severe expression of fetal hemolytic disorder, a possible sequela to maternal Rh isoimmunization; infants exhibit gross edema (anasarca), cardiac decompensation, and profound pallor from anemia, and seldom survive.

hymen Membranous fold that normally partially covers the entrance to the vagina.

hyperbilirubinemia Elevation of unconjugated serum bilirubin concentrations.

hyperemesis gravidarum Abnormal condition of pregnancy characterized by protracted vomiting, weight loss, and fluid and electrolyte imbalance.

hyperesthesia Unusual sensitivity to sensory stimuli, such as pain or touch.

hyperglycemia Excess glucose in the blood.

hyperplasia Increase in number of cells; formation of new tissue.

hyperreflexia Increased action of the reflexes.

hyperthyroidism Excessive functional activity of the thyroid gland.

hypertonic uterine dysfunction Uncoordinated, painful, frequent uterine contractions that do not cause dilation and effacement; primary dysfunctional labor.

hypertrophic cardiomyopathy Enlargement and loss of elasticity of the heart muscle, that is, the septum and the left ventricle, causing impaired filling during diastole and resulting in decreased cardiac output.

hypertrophy Enlargement, or increase in size, of existing cells.

hyperventilation Rapid, shallow (or prolonged, deep) respirations resulting in respiratory alkalosis: a decrease in H^+ concentration and PCO_2 and an increase in the blood pH and the ratio of $NaHCO_3$ to H_2CO_3.

Symptoms may include faintness, palpitations, and carpopedal (hands and feet) muscular spasms.

hypocalcemia Deficiency in calcium often seen in preterm infants, in infants of diabetic mothers, or after long, stressful labor in full-term infants.

hypofibrinogenemia Deficient level of a blood-clotting factor, fibrinogen, in the blood; in obstetrics, it occurs after complications of abruptio placentae or retention of a dead fetus.

hypogastric arteries Branches of the right and left iliac arteries carrying deoxygenated blood from the fetus through the umbilical cord, where they are known as umbilical arteries, to the placenta.

hypoglycemia Less than normal amount of glucose in the blood, usually caused by administration of too much insulin, excessive secretion of insulin by the islet cells of the pancreas, or dietary deficiency.

hypospadias Anomalous positioning of urinary meatus on undersurface of penis or close to or just inside the vagina.

hypothalamus Portion of the diencephalon of the brain forming the floor and part of the lateral wall of the third ventricle. It activates, controls, and integrates the peripheral autonomic nervous system, endocrine processes, and many somatic functions, such as body temperature, sleep, and appetite.

hypothermia Temperature that falls below normal range, that is, below 35° C, usually caused by exposure to cold.

hypothyroidism Deficiency of thyroid gland activity with underproduction of thyroxine.

hypotonic uterine dysfunction Weak, ineffective uterine contractions usually occurring in the active phase of labor; often related to cephalopelvic disproportion (CPD) or malposition of the fetus.

hypoxemia Reduction in arterial PO_2 resulting in metabolic acidosis by forcing anaerobic glycolysis, pulmonary vasoconstriction, and direct cellular damage.

hypoxia Insufficient availability of oxygen to meet the metabolic needs of body tissue.

hysterectomy Surgical removal of the uterus.
   TAH-BSO Total abdominal hysterectomy and bilateral salpingo-oophorectomy; removal of uterus, both tubes, and both ovaries.
   TVH Total vaginal hysterectomy.

hysterosalpingography Recording by x-rays of the uterus and uterine tubes after they are injected with radiopaque material.

hysterotomy Surgical incision into the uterus.

iatrogenic Caused by a health care provider's words, actions, or treatment.

icterus neonatorum Jaundice in the newborn.

idiopathic peripartum cardiomyopathy A primary disease of the heart muscle with no apparent cause, occurring during the peripartum period.

IDM Infant of a diabetic mother.

immunity

acquired i. Protection against microorganisms that develops in response to actual infection or transfer of antibody from an immune donor.

active i. Protection against specific microorganisms that develops in response to actual infection or vaccination.

natural i. Nonspecific protection against microorganisms. Natural immunity is the first line of defense and includes skin and phagocytic cells.

passive i. Protection against specific microorganisms that develops in response to the transfer of antibody or lymphocytes from an immune donor.

immunocompetent Ability of the immune system to respond appropriately to foreign antigens and to develop antigen-specific antibodies.

immunoglobulin Antibody present in serum and external secretions of the body.

IgA Primary immunoglobulin in colostrum.

IgG Transplacentally acquired immunoglobulin that confers passive immunity to the fetus against the infections to which the mother is immune.

IgM Immunoglobulin that neonate can manufacture soon after birth. Fetus produces it in the presence of amnionitis.

immunology The study of the components essential to the recognition and disposal of foreign (nonself or antigenic) material and maintenance of body defenses.

impaired fertility Inability to conceive or to carry fetus to live birth at a time a couple chooses to do so.

implantation Embedding of the fertilized ovum in the uterine mucosa; nidation.

impotence Term designating a man's inability, partial or complete, to perform sexual intercourse or to achieve orgasm; erectile dysfunction.

inborn error of metabolism Hereditary deficiency of a specific enzyme needed for normal metabolism of specific chemicals (e.g., deficiency of phenylalanine hydroxylase results in phenylketonuria [PKU]; a deficiency of hexosaminidase results in Tay-Sachs disease).

incompetent cervix Cervix that is unable to remain closed until a pregnancy reaches term because of a mechanical defect in the cervix resulting in dilation and effacement usually during the second or early third trimester of pregnancy. *Premature dilation of the cervix* is the preferred term.

incomplete abortion See *abortion, incomplete.*

increment Increase, or buildup, as of a contraction.

induced abortion See *abortion, induced.*

induction Stimulation of uterine contractions before the spontaneous onset of labor.

inertia Sluggishness or inactivity; in obstetrics, refers to the absence or weakness of uterine contractions during labor.

inevitable abortion See *abortion, inevitable.*

infant Child who is under 1 year of age.

infective endocarditis Inflammation of the inner layer of the heart muscle (endocardium), caused by a bacterial infection.

infertility Decreased capacity to conceive.

informed consent Choice based on full comprehension of relevant information.

inhalation analgesia Reduction of pain by administration of anesthetic gas. Occasionally given during the second stage of labor. Consciousness is retained to allow the woman to follow instructions and to avoid the adverse effects of general anesthesia.

inlet Passage leading into a cavity.

pelvic i. Upper brim of the pelvic cavity.

insemination Introduction of semen into the vagina or uterus for impregnation.

therapeutic donor i. Introduction of donor semen by instrument injection into the vagina or uterus for impregnation.

insensible water loss Evaporative water loss that occurs mainly through the skin and respiratory tract.

insulin Hormone produced by the beta cells of the pancreatic islets of Langerhans; promotes glucose transport into the cells; aids in protein and lipid synthesis.

integrative health care Encompasses complementary and alternative therapies in combination with conventional Western modalities of treatment.

internal os Inside mouth or opening (cervix).

intertuberous diameter Distance between ischial tuberosities. Measured to determine dimension of pelvic outlet.

intervillous space Irregular space in the maternal portion of the placenta, filled with maternal blood and serving as the site of maternal-fetal gas, nutrient, and waste exchange.

intoxication Development of a reversible substance-specific syndrome caused by the recent ingestion of or exposure to a substance. The symptoms of intoxication are attributable to the direct physiologic effects of the substance on the central nervous system.

intrapartum During labor and birth.

intrathecal Within the subarachnoid space.

intrauterine device (IUD) Small plastic or metal form placed in the uterus to prevent implantation of a fertilized ovum.

intrauterine growth restriction (IUGR) Fetal undergrowth of any cause, such as deficient nutrient supply or intrauterine infection, or associated with congenital malformation; birth weight below population 10th percentile corrected for gestational age.

intrauterine pressure catheter (IUPC) Catheter inserted into uterine cavity to assess uterine activity and pressure by electronic means.

intrauterine resuscitation Interventions initiated when nonreassuring fetal heart rate patterns are noted and are directed at improving intrauterine blood flow.

introitus Entrance into a canal or cavity such as the vagina.

intussusception Prolapse of one segment of bowel into the lumen of the adjacent segment.

in utero Within or inside the uterus.

inversion Turning end for end, upside down, or inside out.

   i. of uterus Condition in which the uterus is turned inside out so that the fundus intrudes into the cervix or vagina, caused by a too vigorous removal of the placenta before it is detached by the natural process of labor.

in vitro fertilization Fertilization in a culture dish or test tube.

involution (1) Rolling or turning inward. (2) Reduction in size of the uterus after birth and its return to its nonpregnant condition.

isoimmune hemolytic disease Breakdown (hemolysis) of fetal or neonatal Rh-positive red blood cells because of Rh antibodies formed by an Rh-negative mother who had been previously exposed to Rh-positive red blood cells.

isoimmunization Development of antibodies in a species of animal with antigens from the same species (e.g., development of anti-Rh antibodies in an Rh-negative person).

ITP Idiopathic thrombocytopenic purpura.

IVF-ET In vitro fertilization and embryo transfer.

jaundice Yellow discoloration of the body tissues caused by the deposit of bile pigments (unconjugated bilirubin); icterus.

   breast milk j. Term used by some clinicians to describe late-onset (after day 5) jaundice in the breastfed infant. A cause for this phenomenon has not been conclusively identified. See *physiologic j.*

   pathologic j. Jaundice usually first noticeable within 24 hours after birth; caused by some abnormal condition such as an Rh or ABO incompatibility and resulting in bilirubin toxicity (e.g., kernicterus).

   physiologic j. Yellow tinge to skin and mucous membranes in response to increased serum levels of unconjugated bilirubin; not usually apparent until after 24 hours; also called *neonatal jaundice, physiologic hyperbilirubinemia.*

kangaroo care Skin-to-skin infant care, used especially for preterm infants, which provides warmth to infant. Infant is placed naked or diapered against mother's or father's bare chest and is covered with parent's shirt or a warm blanket.

karyotype Schematic arrangement of the chromosomes within a cell to demonstrate their numbers and morphology.

Kegel exercises Pelvic muscle exercises to strengthen the pubococcygeal muscles.

kernicterus Bilirubin encephalopathy involving the deposit of unconjugated bilirubin in brain cells, resulting in death or impaired intellectual, perceptive, or motor function and adaptive behavior.

ketoacidosis The accumulation of ketone bodies in the blood as a consequence of hyperglycemia; leads to metabolic acidosis.

key informants Individuals in positions of leadership who can provide information about a situation.

Kleihauer-Betke test Laboratory test that detects the presence of fetal blood cells in the maternal circulation.

labia majora Two folds of skin containing fat and covered with hair that lie on either side of the vaginal opening and form each side of the vulva. (Singular, *labium majus.*)

labia minora Two thin folds of delicate, hairless skin inside the labia majora. (Singular, *labium minus.*)

labor Series of processes by which the fetus is expelled from the uterus; parturition; childbirth.

   active phase Phase in first stage of labor from 4 to 7 cm of cervical dilation.

   first stage Stage of labor from the onset of regular uterine contractions to full dilation of the cervix.

   latent phase Phase in first stage of labor from 0 to 3 cm of cervical dilation.

   second stage Stage of labor from full dilation of the cervix to the birth of the baby.

   third stage Stage of labor from the birth of the baby to the expulsion of the placenta.

   transition phase Phase in first stage of labor from 8 to 10 cm of cervical dilation.

labor, delivery, recovery (LDR) A single room where all steps of the birth process occur. Avoids having to move the woman to different rooms for each phase of the birth process. The woman is moved to a postpartum room after recovery.

labor, delivery, recovery, postpartum (LDRP) A single room where all steps of the birth process and hospitalization occur. The woman stays in the same room throughout her hospitalization.

laceration Irregular tear of wound tissue; in obstetrics, it usually refers to a tear in the perineum, the vagina, or the cervix caused by childbirth.

lactase Enzyme necessary for the digestion of lactose.

lactation Function of secreting milk or period during which milk is secreted.

   l. consultant A health care professional who has specialized training in breastfeeding.

   l. suppression Stopping the production of breast milk through the use of medication (rare) or nonpharmacologic interventions.

lactogen Medication or other substance that enhances the production and secretion of milk.

lactogenesis stage I Initial synthesis of milk components (colostrum) that begins during pregnancy.

lactogenesis stage II Beginning of milk production 2 to 5 days postpartum.

lactose intolerance Inherited absence of the enzyme lactose.

lactosuria Presence of lactose in the urine during late pregnancy and during lactation. Must be differentiated from glycosuria.

Lamaze (psychoprophylaxis) method Method of preparation for childbirth developed in the 1950s by a French obstetrician, Fernand Lamaze, that gained popularity in the United States in the 1960s. It requires practice at home and coaching during labor and birth. The goals are to minimize fear and the perception of pain and to promote positive family relationships by using both mental and physical preparation.

Laminaria tent Cone of dried seaweed that swells as it absorbs moisture. Used to dilate the cervix nontraumatically in preparation for an induced abortion or in preparation for induction of labor.

lanugo Downy, fine hair characteristic of the fetus between 20 weeks of gestation and birth that is most noticeable over the shoulders, the forehead, and the cheeks but is found on nearly all parts of the body except the palms of the hands, the soles of the feet, and the scalp.

laparoscopy Examination of the interior of the abdomen by insertion of a small telescope through the anterior abdominal wall.

large for gestational age (LGA) Exhibiting excessive growth for gestational age.

last menstrual period (LMP) Date of the first day of the last menstrual bleeding.

latch-on Attachment of the infant to the breast for feeding.

lecithin A phospholipid that decreases surface tension; surfactant.

lecithin/sphingomyelin ratio Ratio of lecithin to sphingomyelin in the amniotic fluid. It is used to assess maturity of the fetal lung.

leiomyoma Benign smooth muscle tumor.

Leopold maneuvers Four maneuvers for diagnosing the fetal position by external palpation of the mother's abdomen.

letdown or letdown reflex See *milk ejection reflex.*

letting-go phase Interdependent phase after birth in which the mother and family move forward as a system with interacting members.

leukorrhea White or yellowish mucous discharge from the cervical canal or the vagina that may be normal physiologically or caused by pathologic states of the vagina and endocervix (e.g., *Trichomonas vaginalis* infections).

LH See *luteinizing hormone (LH).*

libido Sexual drive.

lie Relationship existing between the long axis of the fetus and the long axis of the mother. In a longitudinal lie, the fetus is lying lengthwise or vertically, whereas in a transverse lie, the fetus is lying crosswise or horizontally in the uterus.

lightening Sensation of decreased abdominal distention produced by uterine descent into the pelvic cavity as the fetal presenting part settles into the pelvis. It usually occurs 2 weeks before the onset of labor in nulliparas.

linea nigra Line of darker pigmentation seen in some women during the latter part of pregnancy that appears on the middle of the abdomen and extends from the symphysis pubis toward the umbilicus.

linea terminalis Line dividing the upper (false) pelvis from the lower (true) pelvis.

lithotomy position Position in which the woman lies on her back with her knees flexed and with thighs abducted and rotated externally.

live birth Birth in which the neonate, regardless of gestational age, manifests any heartbeat, breathes, or displays voluntary movement.

local infiltration anesthesia Process by which a substance such as a local anesthetic drug is deposited within the tissue to anesthetize a limited region.

lochia Vaginal discharge during the puerperium consisting of blood, tissue, and mucus.

   l. alba Thin, yellowish to white, vaginal discharge that follows lochia serosa on about the tenth day after birth and that may last from 2 to 6 weeks postpartum.

   l. rubra Red, distinctly blood-tinged vaginal flow that follows birth and lasts 2 to 4 days.

   l. serosa Serous, pinkish brown, watery vaginal discharge that follows lochia rubra until about the tenth day after birth.

low birth weight (LBW) An infant birth weight of less than 2500 g.

low spinal (saddle) block anesthesia Type of regional anesthesia produced by injection of a local anesthetic solution into the cerebrospinal fluid intrathecal (subarachnoid) space in the spinal canal.

L/S ratio See *lecithin/sphingomyelin ratio.*

lunar month Four weeks (28 days).

luteinizing hormone (LH) Hormone produced by the anterior pituitary that stimulates ovulation and the development of the corpus luteum.

luteotropin hormone (LTH) Lactogenic hormone; prolactin; an adenohypophyseal hormone.

lysozyme Enzyme with antiseptic qualities that destroys foreign organisms and that is found in blood cells of the granulocytic and monocytic series and is also normally present in saliva, sweat, tears, and breast milk.

maceration (1) Process of softening a solid by soaking it in a fluid. (2) Softening and breaking down of fetal skin from prolonged exposure to amniotic fluid as seen in a postterm infant. Also seen in a dead fetus.

macroglossia Hypertrophy of tongue or tongue large for oral cavity; seen in some preterm neonates and in neonates with Down syndrome.

macrophage Any phagocytic cell of the reticuloendothelial system, including Kupffer cells in the liver, splenocytes in the spleen, and histocytes in the loose connective tissue.

macrosomia Large body size as seen in neonates of diabetic or prediabetic mothers.

magnetic resonance imaging (MRI) Noninvasive nuclear procedure for imaging tissues with high fat and water content; in obstetrics, uses include evaluation of fetal structures, placenta, and amniotic fluid volume.

malpractice Professional negligence that is the proximate cause of injury or harm to a client, resulting from a lack of professional knowledge, experience, or skill that can be expected in others in the profession or from a failure to exercise reasonable care or judgment in the application of professional knowledge, experience, or skill.

mammary gland Compound gland of the female breast that is made up of lobes and lobules that secrete milk for nourishment of the young. Rudimentary mammary glands exist in the male.

mammography X-ray examination technique used to screen for and evaluate breast lesions.

managed care System of guiding care to promote efficiency and cost-effectiveness.

Marfan syndrome An inherited disorder that is an autosomal dominant trait resulting in an abnormal condition characterized by elongation of the bones, causing significant musculoskeletal disturbances. Also usually associated with cardiovascular and eye abnormalities.

married-blended family Family formed as a result of divorce and remarriage, consisting of unrelated family members (stepparents, stepchildren, stepsiblings).

married-parent family Family form in which male and female partners are married and live with their children as an independent unit; parents can be biologic or adoptive.

mask of pregnancy See *chloasma.*

mastectomy Excision, or removal, of the breast.
   modified radical m. Removal of breast tissue, skin, and axillary nodes.

mastitis Infection in a breast, usually confined to a milk duct, characterized by influenza-like symptoms and redness and tenderness in the affected breast.

maternal adaptation Process that a woman goes through in adjusting to her version of the maternal role; includes three phases: taking in, taking hold, and letting go.

maternal mortality Death of a woman that is related to childbearing.

maturation (1) Process of attaining maximum development. (2) In biology, a process of cell division during which the number of chromosomes in the germ cells (sperm or ova) is reduced to one half the number (haploid) characteristic of the species.

maturational crisis Crisis that arises during normal growth and development, such as puberty.

McDonald sign Easy flexion of the fundus on the cervix.

mean arterial pressure (MAP) Average of systolic and diastolic blood pressures. A MAP of greater than 90 mm Hg in the second trimester is associated with an increase in the incidence of preeclampsia in the third trimester.

meatus Opening from an internal structure to the outside (e.g., urethral meatus).

mechanical ventilation Technique used to provide predetermined amount of oxygen; requires intubation.

meconium First stools of infant: viscid, sticky; dark greenish brown, almost black; sterile; odorless.
   m. aspiration syndrome (MAS) Function of fetal hypoxia: With hypoxia, the anal sphincter relaxes and meconium is released; reflex gasping movements draw meconium and other particulate matter in the amniotic fluid into the infant's bronchial tree, obstructing the airflow after birth.
   m. ileus Lower intestinal obstruction by thick, putty-like, inspissated (dried) meconium that may be the result of deficiency of trypsin production in the newborn with cystic fibrosis.
   m.-stained fluid In response to hypoxia, fetal intestinal activity increases and the anal sphincter relaxes, resulting in the passage of meconium, which imparts a greenish coloration; normally seen in breech presentations.

meditation Any activity that focuses the attention in the present moment and quiets and relaxes the mind and body in the process.

meiosis Process by which germ cells divide and decrease their chromosomal number by one half.

membrane(s) Thin, pliable layer of tissue that lines a cavity or tube, separates structures, or covers an organ or structure; in obstetrics, the amnion and chorion surrounding the fetus.
   artificial rupture of m. (AROM) Rupture of membranes using a plastic Amnihook or surgical clamp.
   premature rupture of m. (PROM) Rupture of amniotic sac and leakage of amniotic fluid beginning at least 1 hour before onset of labor at any gestational age.
   preterm premature rupture of m. (PPROM) PROM that occurs before 37 weeks of gestation.
   spontaneous rupture of m. (SROM) Rupture of membranes by natural means.

menarche Onset, or beginning, of menstrual function.

meningomyelocele Saclike protrusion of the spinal cord through a congenital defect in the vertebral column.

menopausal hormone therapy (MHT) Hormonal therapy for menopausal symptoms, usually estrogen and progestin.

menopause From the Greek words *mensis* (month) and *pausis* (cessation), the actual permanent cessation of menstrual cycles; so diagnosed after 1 year without menses.

menorrhagia Abnormally profuse or excessive menstrual flow.

menses (menstruation) (Latin plural of *mensis* "month.") Periodic vaginal discharge of bloody fluid from the nonpregnant uterus that occurs from the age of puberty to menopause.

mentum Chin, a fetal reference point in designating position (e.g., "left mentoanterior" [LMA], meaning that the fetal chin is presenting in the left anterior quadrant of the maternal pelvis).

mesoderm Embryonic middle layer of germ cells giving rise to all types of muscles, connective tissue, bone marrow, blood, lymphoid tissue, and urogenital system.

metastasis Process by which tumor cells spread from site of origin to distant parts of the body.

metrorrhagia Abnormal bleeding from the uterus, particularly when it occurs at any time other than the menstrual period.

microcephaly Congenital anomaly characterized by abnormal smallness of the head in relation to the rest of the body and by underdevelopment of the brain, resulting in some degree of mental retardation.

midwife One who practices the art of helping a woman to give birth.

> **certified nurse m.** Registered nurse with advanced education in midwifery.

> **direct entry m.** Certified midwife educated only in the discipline of midwifery.

> **lay m.** Midwife who learned skills through practice; has no formal education in midwifery.

milia Unopened sebaceous glands appearing as tiny, white, pinpoint papules on forehead, nose, cheeks, and chin of a neonate that disappear spontaneously in a few days or weeks.

milk ejection reflex (MER) Release of milk caused by the contraction of the myoepithelial cells within the milk glands in response to oxytocin; also called *letdown*.

milk-leg Thrombophlebitis of femoral vein resulting in edema of leg and pain; may occur after difficult vaginal birth.

milk transfer Infant's removal of milk from the breast, which is dependent on correct latch-on and the efficiency of the baby's suck, as well as the mother's milk ejection reflex.

miscarriage Spontaneous abortion; lay term usually referring to the loss of the fetus.

missed abortion See *abortion, missed*.

mitosis Process of somatic cell division in which a single cell divides, but both of the new cells have the same number of chromosomes as the first.

mitral valve prolapse (MVP) A disorder in which one or both of the cusp(s) of the mitral valve protrude backward into the left atrium during ventricular systole, resulting in incomplete closure of the valve. A midsystolic click or a late systolic murmur may be heard.

mitral valve stenosis Narrowing of the opening of the mitral valve caused by stiffening of valve leaflets, obstructing the blood flow from the atrium to the ventricle.

mittelschmerz Abdominal pain in the region of an ovary during ovulation that usually occurs midway through the menstrual cycle. Present in many women, mittelschmerz is useful for identifying ovulation, thus pinpointing the fertile period of the cycle.

molding Overlapping of cranial bones or shaping of the fetal head to accommodate and conform to the bony and soft parts of the mother's birth canal during labor.

mongolian spot Bluish gray or dark nonelevated pigmented area usually found over the lower back and buttocks present at birth in some infants, primarily nonwhite. The spot usually fades by school age.

mongolism See *Down syndrome*.

moniliasis See *candidiasis*.

monosomy Chromosomal aberration characterized by the absence of one chromosome from the normal diploid complement.

monozygotic Originating or coming from a single fertilized ovum, such as identical twins.

monozygotic twins See *twins, monozygotic*.

mons veneris Pad of fatty tissue and coarse skin that overlies the symphysis pubis in the woman and that, after puberty, is covered with hair.

Montgomery glands (tubercles) Small, nodular prominences (sebaceous glands) on the areolas around the nipples of the breasts that enlarge during pregnancy and lactation.

mood disorders Disorders that have a disturbance in the prevailing emotional state as the dominant feature. Cause is unknown.

moratorium phase The second developmental task experienced by expectant fathers as identified by May. During this phase the expectant father adjusts to the reality of pregnancy.

morbidity (1) Condition of being diseased. (2) Number of cases of disease or of sick persons in relation to a specific population; incidence.

morning sickness Nausea and vomiting that affect some women during the first few months of their pregnancy; may occur at any time of day.

Moro reflex Normal, generalized reflex in a young infant elicited by a sudden loud noise or by striking the table next to the child, resulting in flexion of the legs, an embracing posture of the arms, and usually a brief cry. Also called *startle reflex*.

mortality (1) Quality or state of being subject to death. (2) Number of deaths in relation to a specific population; incidence.

fetal m. Number of fetal deaths per 1000 births (or per live births). See also *death, fetal*.

infant m. Number of deaths per 1000 children 1 year of age or younger.

maternal m. Number of maternal deaths per 100,000 births.

neonatal m. Number of neonatal deaths per 1000 births (or per live births). See also *neonatal mortality*.

perinatal m. Combined fetal and neonatal mortality. See also *death, perinatal*.

morula Developmental stage of the fertilized ovum in which there is a solid mass of cells resembling a mulberry.

mosaicism Condition in which some somatic cells are normal, whereas others show chromosomal aberrations.

mourning The process of finding the answers to the questions surrounding the loss, coping with grief responses, and determining how to live again.

multifetal pregnancy Pregnancy in which there is more than one fetus in the uterus at the same time; multiple pregnancy.

multigravida Woman who has been pregnant 2 or more times.

multipara Woman who has carried two or more pregnancies to viability, whether they ended in live infants or stillbirths.

mutation Change in a gene or chromosome in gametes that may be transmitted to offspring.

mutuality Component of parent-infant attachment; infant behaviors and characteristics call forth corresponding parent behaviors and characteristics.

myelomeningocele External sac containing meninges, spinal fluid, and nerves that protrudes through defect in vertebral column.

Nägele's (or Naegele's) rule Method for calculating the estimated date of birth (EDB) or "due date."

narcotic antagonist A compound such as naloxone (Narcan) that promptly reverses the effects of narcotics such as meperidine (Demerol).

natal Relating or pertaining to birth.

navel Depression in the center of the abdomen, where the umbilical cord was attached to the fetus; umbilicus.

necrotizing enterocolitis (NEC) Acute inflammatory bowel disorder that occurs primarily in preterm or low-birth-weight neonates. It is characterized by ischemic necrosis (death) of the gastrointestinal mucosa, which may lead to perforation and peritonitis; formula-fed infants are at higher risk for this disease.

negligence Commission of an act that a prudent person would not have done or the omission of a duty that a prudent person would have fulfilled, resulting in injury or harm to another person. In particular, in a malpractice suit a professional person is negligent if harm to a client results from such an act or such a failure to act, but it must be proved that other prudent persons of the same profession would ordinarily have acted differently under the same circumstances.

neonatal abstinence syndrome Signs and symptoms associated with drug withdrawal in the neonate.

neonatal mortality Statistical rate of infant death during the first 28 days after live birth, expressed as the number of such deaths per 1000 live births in a specific geographic area or institution in a given period of time.

neonatal narcosis Central nervous system depression in the newborn caused by a narcotic; may be exhibited by respiratory depression, hypertonia, lethargy, and delay in temperature regulation.

neonatology Branch of medicine that studies care of the neonate.

neoplasia Growth of new tissue; tumor that serves no physiologic function; may be benign or malignant.

neural tube Tube formed from fusion of the neural folds from which develop the brain and spinal cord.

n. t. defect Improper development of tube, resulting in malformation of brain or spinal cord; see alpha-fetoprotein.

neutral thermal environment (NTE) Environment that enables the neonate to maintain a body temperature of at least 36.5° C with minimum use of oxygen and energy.

nevus Natural blemish or mark; a congenital circumscribed deposit of pigmentation in the skin; mole.

n. flammeus Port-wine stain; reddish, usually flat, discoloration of the face or neck. Because of its large size and color, it is considered a serious deformity.

n. vasculosus (strawberry hemangioma) Elevated lesion of immature capillaries and endothelial cells that regresses over a period of years.

nidation Implantation of the fertilized ovum in the endometrium, or lining, of the uterus.

nipple confusion Difficulty experienced by some infants in mastering breastfeeding after having been given a pacifier or bottle. This problem appears to be more related to tactile sensation than flow of liquid.

nonmaleficence The principle in bioethics directing us to act so as to avoid causing harm.

nonnutritive sucking Use of a pacifier by infants.

nonreassuring fetal heart rate pattern Fetal heart rate pattern that indicates the fetus is not well oxygenated and requires intervention.

nonshivering thermogenesis Infant's method of producing heat from brown fat by increasing metabolic rate.

nonstress test (NST) Evaluation of fetal response (fetal heart rate) to natural contractile uterine activity or to an increase in fetal activity.

no-parent family Family form in which children live independently in foster or kinship care, such as living with a grandparent.

normoglycemia Blood glucose level within normal limits; glycemic control.

nosocomial Pertaining to a hospital.

nuchal cord Encircling of fetal neck by one or more loops of umbilical cord.

nuclear family Family form consisting of parents and their dependent children.

nulligravida Woman who has never been pregnant.

nullipara Woman who has not yet carried a pregnancy to viability.

nurse practitioner Registered nurse who has additional education to practice nursing in an expanded role.

observer style Characteristic style described by May that is displayed by expectant fathers who show a detached approach to involvement in their partner's pregnancy.

occipitobregmatic Pertaining to the occiput (the back part of the skull) and the bregma (junction of the coronal and sagittal sutures) or anterior fontanel.

occiput Back part of the head or skull.

oligohydramnios Abnormally small amount or absence of amniotic fluid; often indicative of fetal urinary tract defect.

oligomenorrhea Abnormally light or infrequent menstruation.

oliguria Urine output below 25 to 30 ml by the kidneys for 2 consecutive hours (in adults).

omphalitis Inflammation of the umbilical stump characterized by redness, edema, and purulent exudate in severe infections.

omphalocele Congenital defect resulting from failure of closure of the abdominal wall or muscles and leading to hernia of abdominal contents through the navel.

oocyte Primordial or incompletely developed ovum.

oogenesis Formation and development of the ovum.

operculum Plug of mucus that fills the cervical canal during pregnancy.

ophthalmia neonatorum Infection in the neonate's eyes usually resulting from gonorrheal or other infection contracted when the fetus passes through the birth canal (vagina).

opisthotonos Tetanic spasm resulting in an arched, hyperextended position of the body.

oral glucose tolerance test Test for blood glucose after oral ingestion of a concentrated sugar solution.

orchitis Inflammation of one or both of the testes, characterized by swelling and pain, often caused by mumps, syphilis, or tuberculosis.

orifice Normal mouth, entrance, or opening to any aperture.

os Mouth, or opening.
  external o. (o. externum) External opening of the cervical canal.
  internal o. (o. internum) Internal opening of the cervical canal.
  o. uteri Mouth, or opening, of the uterus.

ossification Mineralization of fetal bones.

osteoporosis Deossification of bone tissue resulting in structural weakness; decreased bone mass increasing risk of fractures, especially after menopause.

outcomes-oriented care Measures effectiveness of care against benchmarks or standards.

outlet Opening by which something can leave.
  pelvic o. Lower aperture, or opening, of the true pelvis.

ovary One of two glands in the female situated on either side of the pelvic cavity that produces the female reproductive cell, the ovum, and two known hormones, estrogen and progesterone.

ovulation Periodic ripening and discharge of the ovum from the ovary, usually 14 days before the onset of menstrual flow.
  o. method Control of fertility using evaluation of cervical mucus throughout the menstrual cycle; ovulation occurs just after the appearance of the peak mucus sign; Billings method.

ovum Female germ, or reproductive cell, produced by the ovary; egg.

oxygen toxicity Oxygen overdosage that results in pathologic tissue changes (e.g., retinopathy of prematurity, bronchopulmonary dysplasia).

oxytocics Drugs that stimulate uterine contractions, thus accelerating childbirth and preventing postbirth hemorrhage. They may be used to increase the letdown reflex during lactation.

oxytocin Hormone produced by the posterior pituitary that stimulates uterine contractions and the release of milk in the mammary gland (letdown reflex).
  o. challenge test (OCT) Evaluation of fetal response (fetal heart rate) to contractile activity of the uterus stimulated by exogenous oxytocin (Pitocin).

Paco$_2$ Partial pressure of carbon dioxide in arterial blood.

palmar erythema Rash on the surface of the palms sometimes seen in pregnancy.

panic disorder Repeated, unprovoked episodes of intense fear, which develop without warning and are not related to any specific event.

Pao$_2$ Partial pressure of oxygen in arterial blood.

Papanicolaou (Pap) test Microscopic examination using scrapings from the cervix, endocervix, or other mucous membranes that will reveal, with a high degree of accuracy, the presence of premalignant or malignant cells.

para Usually expressed as a number that refers to parity. See *parity*.

paracervical block Type of regional anesthesia produced by injection of a local anesthetic into the lower uterine segment just beneath the mucosa adjacent to the outer rim of the cervix (3 and 9 o'clock positions).

parental adjustment Process that a person goes through in adapting to the parental role; includes three stages: expectations, reality, and transition to mastery.

parity Number of past pregnancies that have reached viability, regardless of whether the infant or infants were alive or stillborn. See *para.*

parturient Woman giving birth.

parturition Process or act of giving birth.

patent Open.

pathogen Substance or organism capable of producing disease.

pathologic jaundice See *jaundice, pathologic.*

pelvic Pertaining or relating to the pelvis.

    p. exenteration Surgical removal of all female reproductive organs and adjacent tissues.

    p. inflammatory disease (PID) Infection of internal reproductive structures and adjacent tissues usually secondary to sexually transmitted infections.

    p. inlet See *inlet, pelvic.*

    p. outlet See *outlet, pelvic.*

    p. relaxation Refers to the lengthening and weakening of the fascial supports of pelvic structures.

    p. tilt (rock) Exercise used to help relieve low back discomfort during menstruation and pregnancy.

pelvimetry Measurement of dimensions and proportions of the pelvis to determine its capacity and ability to allow the passage of the fetus through the birth canal.

pelvis Bony structure formed by the sacrum, the coccyx, the innominate bones, and the symphysis pubis and the ligaments that unite them.

    android p. See *android pelvis.*

    anthropoid p. See *anthropoid pelvis.*

    gynecoid p. See *gynecoid pelvis.*

    platypelloid p. See *platypelloid pelvis.*

    true p. Pelvis below the linea terminalis.

penis Male organ used for urination and copulation.

percutaneous umbilical blood sampling (PUBS) Procedure during which the fetal umbilical vessel is accessed for blood sampling or for transfusions.

perimenopause Period of transition of changing ovarian activity before menopause and through first few years of amenorrhea.

perinatal Of or pertaining to the time and process of giving birth or being born.

perinatal loss Death of a fetus or infant through the twenty-eighth day after birth.

perinatal period Period extending from the twentieth or twenty-eighth week of gestation through the end of the twenty-eighth day after birth.

perinatologist Physician who specializes in fetal and neonatal care.

perineum Area between the vagina and the rectum in the female and between the scrotum and the rectum in the male.

periodic abstinence Contraceptive method in which a woman abstains from sexual intercourse during the fertile period of her menstrual cycle; also referred to as natural family planning (NFP) because no other form of birth control is used during this period; see *rhythm method.*

periodic breathing Sporadic episodes of cessation of respirations for periods of 10 seconds or less not associated with cyanosis, typically noted in preterm infants.

periodic changes Changes from baseline of the fetal heart rate that occur with uterine contractions.

periods of reactivity (newborn infant) First period (within 30 minutes after birth): brief cyanosis, flushing with crying; crackles, nasal flaring, grunting, retractions; heart sounds loud, forceful, irregular; alert; mucus; no bowel sounds; followed by period of sleep. Second period (4 to 8 hours after birth): swift color changes; irregular respiratory and heart rates; mucus with gagging; meconium passage; temperature stabilizing.

peripartum heart failure Inability of the heart to maintain an adequate cardiac output. Heart failure occurring during pregnancy.

periventricular hemorrhage Intraventricular hemorrhage, a common type of brain injury in preterm infants; prognosis depends on severity of hemorrhage.

pessary Device placed inside the vagina to function as a supportive structure for the uterus.

petechiae Pinpoint hemorrhagic areas caused by numerous disease states involving infection and thrombocytopenia and occasionally found over the face and trunk of the newborn because of increased intravascular pressure in the capillaries during birth.

pH Hydrogen ion concentration.

phenotype Expression of certain physical or chemical characteristics in an individual resulting from interaction between genotype and environmental factors.

phenylketonuria (PKU) Recessive hereditary disease that results in a defect in the metabolism of the amino acid phenylalanine caused by the lack of an enzyme, phenylalanine hydroxylase, that is necessary for the conversion of the amino acid phenylalanine into tyrosine. If PKU is not treated, brain damage may occur, causing severe mental retardation.

phimosis Tightness of the prepuce, or foreskin, of the penis.

phlebitis Inflammation of a vein with symptoms of pain and tenderness along the course of the vein, inflammatory swelling and acute edema below the obstruction, and discoloration of the skin because of injury or bruise to the vein, possibly occurring in acute or chronic infections or after procedures or childbirth.

phlebothrombosis Formation of a clot or thrombus in the vein; inflammation of the vein with secondary clotting.

phosphatidylglycerol A phospholipid, a component of pulmonary surfactant; its presence in amniotic fluid is considered a sign of fetal lung maturity when the pregnancy is complicated by maternal diabetes.

phototherapy Utilization of lights to reduce serum bilirubin levels by oxidation of bilirubin into water-soluble compounds that are then processed in the liver and excreted into bile and urine.

physiologic jaundice See *jaundice, physiologic.*

phytoestrogens Plant compounds that have a weak estrogenic effect in the human body; used in the management of menopause as an alternative or complement to conventional hormone replacement therapy.

pica Unusual craving during pregnancy (e.g., of laundry starch, dirt, red clay).

pinch test Determines if nipples are everted or inverted by placing thumb and forefinger on areola and pressing inward. The nipple will stand erect or invert.

placenta Latin, flat cake; afterbirth, specialized vascular disk-shaped organ for maternal-fetal gas and nutrient exchange. Normally it implants in the thick muscular wall of the upper uterine segment.

   abruptio p. See *abruptio placentae.*

   battledore p. Umbilical cord insertion into the margin of the placenta.

   circumvallate p. Placenta having a raised white ring at its edge.

   p. accreta Invasion of the uterine muscle by the placenta, thus making separation from the muscle difficult if not impossible.

   p. increta Deep penetration in myometrium by placenta.

   p. percreta Perforation of uterus by placenta.

   p. previa Placenta that is abnormally implanted in the thin, lower uterine segment and that is typed according to proximity to cervical os: total—completely occludes os; partial—does not occlude os completely; and marginal—edge of placenta encroaches on margin of internal cervical os.

   p. succenturiata Accessory placenta.

placental Pertaining or relating to the placenta.

   p. infarct Localized, ischemic, hard area on the fetal or maternal side of the placenta.

   p. souffle See *souffle, placental.*

platypelloid pelvis Broad pelvis with a shortened anteroposterior diameter and a flattened, oval, transverse shape.

plethora Deep, beefy-red coloration of a newborn caused by an increased number of blood cells (polycythemia) per volume of blood.

plugged ducts Milk ducts blocked by small curds of dried milk.

podalic Concerning or pertaining to the feet.

   p. version Shifting of the position of the fetus so as to bring the feet to the outlet during labor.

polycythemia Increased number of erythrocytes per volume of blood, which may be caused by large placental transfusion, fetus transfusion, or maternal-fetal transfusion; or it may be attributable to hypovolemia resulting from movement of fluid out of vascular into interstitial compartment.

polydactyly Excessive number of digits (fingers or toes).

polyhydramnios See *hydramnios.*

polyp Small tumorlike growth that projects from a mucous membrane surface.

polyuria Excessive secretion and discharge of urine by the kidneys.

position Relationship of an arbitrarily chosen fetal reference point, such as the occiput, the sacrum, the chin, or the scapula on the presenting part of the fetus to its location in the front, the back, or the sides of the maternal pelvis.

positive signs of pregnancy Definite indication of pregnancy (e.g., hearing the fetal heartbeat, visualization and palpation of fetal movement by the examiner, sonographic examination).

posterior Pertaining to the back.

   p. fontanel See *fontanel, posterior.*

postmature infant Infant born at or after the beginning of week 43 of gestation or later and exhibiting signs of dysmaturity.

postnatal Happening or occurring after birth (newborn).

postpartum Happening or occurring after birth (mother).

   p. blues A letdown feeling, accompanied by irritability and anxiety, which usually begins 2 to 3 days after giving birth and disappears within a week or two. Sometimes called the "baby blues."

   p. depression Depression occurring within 6 months of childbirth, lasting longer than postpartum blues and characterized by a variety of symptoms that interfere with activities of daily living and care of the baby.

   p. hemorrhage Excessive bleeding after childbirth; traditionally defined as a loss of 500 ml or more after a vaginal birth.

   p. psychosis Symptoms begin as postpartum blues or depression but are characterized by a break with reality. Delusions, hallucinations, confusion, delirium, and panic can occur.

postterm pregnancy Pregnancy prolonged past 42 weeks of gestation (also called *postdate pregnancy*).

posttraumatic stress disorder An anxiety disorder characterized by an acute emotional response to a traumatic event or situation such as sexual abuse.

precipitous labor Rapid or sudden labor of less than 3 hours beginning from onset of cervical changes to completed birth of neonate.

preconception care Care designed for health maintenance before pregnancy.

preeclampsia Disease encountered after 20 weeks of gestation or early in the puerperium; a vasospastic disease process characterized by increasing hypertension, proteinuria, and hemoconcentration.

pregestational diabetes Diabetes mellitus type 1 or type 2 that exists before pregnancy.

pregnancy Period between conception through complete birth of the products of conception. The usual duration of pregnancy in the human is 280 days, 9 calendar months, or 10 lunar months.

abdominal p. See *abdominal gestation.*

ectopic p. See *ectopic pregnancy.*

extrauterine p. See *extrauterine pregnancy.*

preload The stretch of myocardial fiber at end-diastole. The ventricular end-diastole pressure and volume reflect this parameter.

premature dilation of the cervix See *incompetent cervix.*

premature infant Infant born before completing week 37 of gestation, irrespective of birth weight; preterm infant.

premature rupture of membranes (PROM) See *membrane(s).*

premenstrual syndrome Syndrome of nervous tension, irritability, weight gain, edema, headache, mastalgia, dysphoria, and lack of coordination occurring during the last few days of the menstrual cycle preceding the onset of menstruation.

premonitory Serving as an early symptom or warning.

prenatal Occurring or happening before birth.

prepartum Before birth; before giving birth.

prepuce Fold of skin, or foreskin, covering the glans penis of the male.

p. of the clitoris Fold of the labia minora that covers the glans clitoris.

presentation That part of the fetus that first enters the pelvis and lies over the inlet: may be head, face, breech, or shoulder.

breech p. See *breech presentation.*

cephalic p. See *cephalic presentation.*

presenting part That part of the fetus that lies closest to the internal os of the cervix.

pressure edema Edema of the lower extremities caused by pressure of the heavy pregnant uterus against the large veins; edema of the fetal scalp after cephalic presentation (caput succedaneum).

presumptive signs of pregnancy Manifestations that are suggestive of pregnancy but are not absolutely positive. These include the cessation of menses, Chadwick sign, morning sickness, and quickening.

preterm birth Birth occurring before 37 weeks of gestation.

preterm premature rupture of membranes (PPROM) See *membrane(s).*

prevention Actions taken out of the desire to avoid illness, detect it early, or maintain optimal functioning when illness is present.

previa, placenta See *placenta previa.*

primary survey The immediate response after trauma: the ABCs of resuscitation: establishment and maintenance of an airway, ensuring adequate breathing, and maintenance of an adequate circulatory volume.

primigravida Woman who is pregnant for the first time.

primipara Woman who has carried a pregnancy to viability whether the child is dead or alive at the time of birth.

probable signs of pregnancy Manifestations or evidence that indicates that there is a definite likelihood of pregnancy. Among the probable signs are enlargement of abdomen, Goodell sign, Hegar sign, Braxton Hicks sign, and positive hormonal tests for pregnancy.

prodromal Serving as an early symptom or warning of the approach of a disease or condition (e.g., prodromal labor).

progesterone Hormone produced by the corpus luteum and placenta whose function is to prepare the endometrium of the uterus for implantation of the fertilized ovum, develop the mammary glands, and maintain the pregnancy.

prolactin A pituitary hormone that triggers milk production.

prolapsed cord Protrusion of the umbilical cord in advance of the presenting part.

proliferative phase of menstrual cycle Preovulatory, follicular, or estrogen phase of the menstrual cycle.

promontory of the sacrum Superior projecting portion of the sacrum at the junction of the sacrum and L5.

prophylactic (1) Pertaining to prevention or warding off of disease or certain conditions. (2) Condom, or "rubber."

proscription The understanding that something is forbidden; taboo.

prostaglandin (PG) Substance present in many body tissues; has a role in many reproductive tract functions; used to induce abortions, cervical ripening for labor induction.

proteinuria Presence of protein in urine.

pruritus Itching.

pseudocyesis Condition in which the woman has all the usual signs of pregnancy, such as enlargement of the abdomen, cessation of menses, weight gain, and morning sickness, but is not pregnant; phantom or false pregnancy.

pseudopregnancy See *pseudocyesis.*

psychoprophylaxis Mental and physical education of the parents in preparation for childbirth, with the goal of minimizing fear and pain and promoting positive family relationships (Lamaze).

ptyalism Excessive salivation.

puberty Period in life in which the reproductive organs mature and one becomes functionally capable of reproduction.

pubic Pertaining to the pubis.

pubis Pubic bone forming the front of the pelvis.

pudendal block Injection of a local anesthetizing drug at the pudendal nerve root to produce numbness of the genital and perianal region.

puerperal infection Infection of the pelvic organs during the postbirth period; childbed fever.

puerperium Period after the third stage of labor and lasting until involution of the uterus takes place, usually about 3 to 6 weeks.

pulmonary artery catheter (PAC) A flow-directed, balloon-tipped multilumen catheter made of polyvinyl chloride that is inserted into the pulmonary artery to provide continuous measurements of pulmonary artery pressure when the balloon is deflated and pulmonary capillary wedge pressures when the balloon is inflated. Sometimes called a Swan-Ganz catheter.

pulmonary artery pressure (PAP) Systolic and diastolic pressures of blood in the pulmonary artery; reflects right afterload.

pulmonary capillary wedge pressure (PCWP) Pressure when the balloon of the pulmonary artery catheter (PAC) is inflated to obstruct right-sided pressures and to reflect left-sided pressures. Value is obtained during diastole, with the mitral valve open; it reflects left preload.

pulmonary vascular resistance A measure for the tension required for the ejection of blood from the right ventricle into the circulation (afterload).

pulse oximetry Noninvasive method of monitoring oxygen levels by detecting the amount of light absorbed by oxygen-carrying hemoglobin.

pyrosis A burning sensation in the epigastric and sternal region from stomach acid (heartburn).

quickening Maternal perception of fetal movement; usually occurs between weeks 16 and 20 of gestation.

radioimmunoassay Pregnancy test that tests for the beta subunit of human chorionic gonadotropin using radioactively labeled markers.

rape-trauma syndrome Characteristic symptoms seen in victims of rape and consisting of several phases; similar to posttraumatic stress syndrome.

recessive trait Genetically determined characteristic that is expressed only when present in the homozygotic state.

reciprocity Type of body movement or behavior that provides the observer with cues, such as the behavioral cues infants provide to parents and parents' responses to cues.

recommended dietary allowances (RDAs) Recommended nutrient intakes estimated to meet the needs of almost all (97% to 98%) of the healthy people in the population.

rectocele Herniation or protrusion of the rectum into the posterior vaginal wall.

referred pain Discomfort originating in a local area such as the cervix, the vagina, or the perineal tissues but felt in the back, the flanks, or the thighs.

reflection Looking within for solutions and answers to certain dilemmas; using intuition and inner wisdom as guides for attainment of healing.

reflex Automatic response built into the nervous system that does not need the intervention of conscious thought (e.g., in the newborn, rooting, gagging, grasp).

reflex bradycardia Slowing of the heart in response to a particular stimulus.

refractory oliguria Oliguria not corrected with fluid challenge.

regional anesthesia Anesthesia of an area of the body by injection of a local anesthetic to block a group of sensory nerve fibers.

regurgitate Vomiting or spitting up of solids or fluids.

relaxation The absence or alleviation of mental, physical, and emotional tension through purposeful activities that quiet the mind and body.

residual urine Urine that remains in the bladder after urination.

respiratory distress syndrome (RDS) Condition resulting from decreased pulmonary gas exchange, leading to retention of carbon dioxide (increase in arterial PCO_2). Most common neonatal causes are prematurity, perinatal asphyxia, and maternal diabetes mellitus; hyaline membrane disease (HMD).

restitution In obstetrics, the turning of the fetal head to the left or right after it has completely emerged from the introitus as it assumes a normal alignment with the infant's shoulders.

resuscitation Restoration of consciousness or life in one who is apparently dead or whose respirations or cardiac function or both have ceased.

retained placenta Retention of all or part of the placenta in the uterus after birth.

retinopathy of prematurity (ROP) Associated with hyperoxemia, resulting in eye injury and blindness in premature infants.

retraction (1) Drawing in or sucking in of soft tissues of chest, indicative of an obstruction at any level of the respiratory tract from the oropharynx to the alveoli. (2) Retraction of uterine muscle fiber. After contracting, the muscle fiber does not return to its original length but remains slightly shortened, a unique attribute of uterine muscle that aids in preventing postdelivery hemorrhage and results in involution.

retroflexion Bending backward.
    r. of uterus Condition in which the body of the uterus is bent backward at an angle with the cervix, the position of which usually remains unchanged.

retrolental fibroplasia (RLF) See *retinopathy of prematurity.*

retroversion Turning or a state of being turned back.
    r. of uterus Displacement of the uterus; the body of the uterus is tipped backward with the cervix pointing forward toward the symphysis pubis.

rheumatic heart disease Permanent damage of the heart muscle and valves secondary to an autoimmune reaction in the heart tissue precipitated by rheumatic fever.

Rh factor Inherited antigen present on erythrocytes. The individual with the factor is known as positive for the factor.

Rh immune globulin (RhIg) Solution of gamma globulin that contains Rh antibodies. Intramuscular administration of Rh immune globulin prevents sensitization in Rh-negative women who have been exposed to Rh-positive red blood cells.

rhythm method Contraceptive method in which a woman abstains from sexual intercourse during the ovulatory phase of her menstrual cycle; calendar method; see *periodic abstinence.*

ribonucleic acid (RNA) Element responsible for transferring genetic information within a cell; a template, or pattern.

ring of fire Burning sensation as vagina stretches and fetal head crowns.

risk factors Factors that cause a person or a group of people to be particularly vulnerable to an unwanted, unpleasant, or unhealthful event.

Ritgen maneuver Procedure used to control the birth of the head.

rooming-in unit Maternity unit designed so that the newborn's crib is at the mother's bedside or in a nursery adjacent to the mother's room.

rooting reflex Normal response of the newborn to move toward whatever touches the area around the mouth and to attempt to suck. This reflex usually disappears by 3 to 4 months of age.

rotation In obstetrics, the turning of the fetal head as it follows the curves of the birth canal downward.

rubella vaccine Live attenuated rubella virus given to clients who have not had rubella or who are serologically negative. Exposure to the rubella virus through vaccination causes the client to form antibodies, producing active immunity.

rugae Folds in the vaginal mucosa and the scrotum.

sac, amniotic See *amniotic sac.*

sacroiliac Of or pertaining to the sacrum and ilium.

sacrum Triangular bone composed of five united vertebrae and situated between L5 and the coccyx; forms the posterior boundary of the true pelvis.

safe passage Normal uneventful birth process for mother and child.

safe period The days in the menstrual cycle that are not designated as fertile days, that is, before and after ovulation.

safer sex Use of protection whenever body fluids (semen, blood, vaginal secretions) are exchanged.

sagittal suture Band of connective tissue separating the parietal bones, extending from the anterior to the posterior fontanel.

salpingo-oophorectomy Removal of a uterine tube and an ovary.

Schultze mechanism Delivery of the placenta with the fetal surfaces (shiny in appearance) presenting.

scrotum Pouch of skin containing the testes and parts of the spermatic cords.

secondary survey A complete physical assessment of all body systems after immediate resuscitation and stabilization after trauma to mother and fetus.

second stage of labor Stage of labor from full dilation of the cervix to the birth of the baby.

secretory phase of menstrual cycle Postovulatory, luteal, progestational, premenstrual phase of menstrual cycle; 14 days in length.

secundines Fetal membranes and placenta expelled after childbirth; afterbirth.

self-care Client provides care for self as part of plan of care.

semen Thick, white, viscid secretion discharged from the urethra of the male at orgasm; the transporting medium of the sperm.

semen analysis Examination of semen specimen to determine liquefaction, volume, pH, sperm density, and normal morphology.

sensitization Development of antibodies to a specific antigen.

sensory behavior Responses of the five senses; indicate a readiness for social interaction.

sepsis Bacterial infections of the bloodstream.

septic abortion See *abortion, septic.*

sex chromosome Chromosome associated with determination of sex: the X (female) and Y (male) chromosomes. The normal female has two X chromosomes, and the normal male has one X and one Y chromosome.

sexual decision making Selection of choices concerned with intimate and sexual behavior.

sexual history Past and present health conditions, lifestyle behaviors, knowledge, and attitudes related to sex and sexuality.

sexuality The part of life that has to do with being male or female.

sexually transmitted infections (STIs) Infections transmitted as a result of sexual activity with an infected individual; also called sexually transmitted diseases (STDs).

sexual response cycle The phases of physical changes that occur in response to sexual stimulation and sexual tension release.

shake test "Foam" test for lung maturity of fetus; more rapid than determination of lecithin/sphingomyelin ratio.

sibling rivalry Negative behaviors exhibited by siblings in response to the addition of a new baby in the family.

sickle cell hemoglobinopathy Abnormal crescent-shaped red blood corpuscles in the blood.

Sims' position Position in which the client lies on the left side with the right knee and thigh drawn upward toward the chest.

single-parent family Family form characterized by one parent (male or female) in the household. This may result from loss of spouse by death, divorce, separation, desertion, or birth of a child to a single woman.

single-room maternity care (SRMC) Variation of care sites where one nurse provides care to a mother and infant, that is, mother-baby units, LDRPs.

singleton A single fetus.

situational crisis Crisis that arises suddenly in response to an external event or a conflict concerning a specific circumstance. The symptoms are transient, and the episode is usually brief.

sitz bath Application of moist heat to the perineum by sitting in a tub or basin filled with warm water.

sleep-wake cycles Variations in states of newborn consciousness.

small for gestational age (SGA) Inadequate growth for gestational age.

smegma Whitish secretion around labia minora and under foreskin of penis.

somatic pain Perineal discomfort resulting from stretching of perineal tissues.

sonogram See *ultrasonography.*

souffle Soft, blowing sound or murmur heard by auscultation.

  funic s. Soft, muffled, blowing sound produced by blood rushing through the umbilical vessels and synchronous with the fetal heart sounds.

  placental s. Soft, blowing murmur caused by the blood current in the placenta and synchronous with the maternal pulse.

  uterine s. Soft, blowing sound made by the blood in the arteries of the pregnant uterus and synchronous with the maternal pulse.

sperm Male sex cell. Also called *spermatozoon, spermatozoa.*

spermatogenesis Process by which mature spermatozoa are formed, during which the diploid chromosome number (46) is reduced by half (haploid, 23).

spermicide Chemical substance that kills sperm by reducing their surface tension, causing the cell wall to break down by a bactericidal effect or by creating a highly acidic environment. Also called *spermatocide.*

spina bifida occulta Congenital malformation of the spine in which the posterior portion of the lamina of the vertebrae fails to close but there is no herniation or protrusion of the spinal cord or meninges through the defect. The newborn may have a dimple in the skin or growth of hair over the malformed vertebrae.

spinnbarkeit Formation of a stretchable thread of cervical mucus under estrogen influence at time of ovulation.

spirituality The individual's connection to his or her own values, purpose, and meaning of life. May encompass organized religion or belief in higher power or authority. Recognition of wisdom, imagination, spirit, intuition. A perception of the unity of nature and the interconnectedness of all beings. Inner strength.

splanchnic engorgement Excessive filling or pooling of blood within the visceral vasculature that occurs after the removal of pressure from the abdomen, such as birth of an infant, removal of an excess of urine from bladder, or removal of large tumor.

spontaneous abortion See *abortion, spontaneous.*

spontaneous rupture of membranes (SROM) Rupture of membranes by natural means.

squamocolumnar junction Site in the endocervical canal where columnar epithelium and squamous epithelium meet; also called *transformation zone.*

squamous intraepithelial lesion (SIL) Term used to describe neoplastic changes of the cervix.

square window Angle of wrist between hypothenar prominence and forearm; one criterion for estimating gestational age of neonate.

standard body weight An appropriate weight for height; a body mass index (BMI) within the normal range.

standard of care Level of practice that a reasonable, prudent nurse would provide.

state-related behavior Behavioral responses dependent on current state of infant.

station Relationship of the presenting fetal part to an imaginary line drawn between the ischial spines of the pelvis.

sterility (1) State of being free from living microorganisms. (2) Complete inability to reproduce offspring.

sterilization Process or act that renders a person unable to produce children.

stillbirth The birth of a baby after 20 weeks of gestation and 1 day or weighing 350 g (depending on the state code) that does not show any signs of life.

stress urinary incontinence (SUI) Loss of urine occurring with increased abdominal pressure (e.g., with coughing or sneezing).

striae gravidarum ("stretch marks") Shining reddish lines caused by stretching of the skin, often found on the abdomen, thighs, and breasts during pregnancy. These streaks turn to a fine pinkish white or silver tone in time in fair-skinned women and brownish in darker-skinned women.

stroke volume Volume of blood ejected from the left ventricle during one cardiac cycle.

subculture Group existing within a larger cultural system that retains its own characteristics.

subinvolution Failure of a part (e.g., the uterus) to reduce to its normal size and condition after enlargement from functional activity (e.g., pregnancy).

suboccipitobregmatic diameter Smallest diameter of the fetal head—follows a line drawn from the middle of the anterior fontanel to the undersurface of the occipital bone.

supine hypotension Shock; fall in blood pressure caused by impaired venous return when gravid uterus presses on ascending vena cava, when woman is lying flat on her back; vena cava syndrome.

supply meets demand Physiologic basis for determining milk production. The volume of milk produced equals the amount of milk removed from the breast.

support systems Network from which people receive help in times of crisis.

surfactant Phosphoprotein necessary for normal respiratory function that prevents the alveolar collapse (atelectasis). See also *lecithin* and *L/S ratio.*

suture (1) Junction of the adjoining bones of the skull. (2) Procedure uniting parts by sewing them together.

Svo₂ monitoring Percentage of saturation of hemoglobin with oxygen in mixed venous and arterial blood monitored with a fiberoptic pulmonary artery catheter that is connected to a bedside microprocessor. The Svo₂ reflects the balance between oxygen delivery and oxygen use.

symphysis pubis Fibrocartilaginous union of the bodies of the pubic bones in the midline.

synchrony Fit between an infant's cues and the parent's response.

syndactyly Malformation of digits, often seen as a fusion of two or more toes to form one structure.

systemic analgesia Analgesics administered either intramuscularly or intravenously that cross the blood-brain barrier and provide central analgesic effects.

systemic lupus erythematosus (SLE) A chronic inflammatory connective tissue disease affecting many systems, that is, the integumentary, renal, and nervous systems.

systemic vascular resistance (SVR) A measure of the tension required for the ejection of blood from the left ventricle into the circulation (afterload) and is derived by calculation as follows: SVR = [(MAP − CVP)/CO] × 80.

tachycardia Baseline fetal heart rate above 160 beats per minute.

tachypnea Excessively rapid respiratory rate (e.g., in neonates, respiratory rate of 60 breaths/min or more).

taking-hold phase Period after birth characterized by a woman becoming more independent and more interested in learning infant care skills; learning to be a competent mother is an important task.

taking-in phase Period after birth characterized by the woman's dependency; maternal needs are dominant, and talking about the birth is an important task.

talipes equinovarus Deformity in which the foot is extended and the person walks on the toes.

telangiectasia Permanent dilation of groups of superficial capillaries and venules.

telangiectatic nevi ("stork bites") Clusters of small, red, localized areas of capillary dilation frequently seen in neonates at the nape of the neck or lower occiput, upper eyelids, and nasal bridge that can be blanched with pressure of a finger.

telemedicine Use of communication technologies and electronic information to provide or support health care when participants are separated by distance.

telephonic nursing Services such as warm lines, nurse advice lines, and telephonic nursing assessments.

teratogenic agent Any drug, virus, or irradiation, the exposure to which can cause malformation of the fetus.

teratogens Nongenetic factors that cause malformations and disorders in utero.

teratoma Tumor composed of different kinds of tissue, none of which normally occurs together or at the site of the tumor.

term infant Live infant born between weeks 38 and 42 of completed gestation.

term pregnancy Gestation that continues until at least 38 weeks.

testis One of the glands contained in the male scrotum that produces the male reproductive cell, or sperm, and the male hormone, testosterone; testicle.

tetany, uterine Extremely prolonged uterine contractions.

thalassemia An anemia affecting Mediterranean and Southeast Asian populations in which there is an insufficient amount of hemoglobin produced to fill the red blood cells.

therapeutic abortion See *abortion, therapeutic.*

therapeutic donor insemination See *insemination, therapeutic donor.*

therapeutic rest Administration of analgesics to decrease pain and induce rest for management of hypertonic uterine dysfunction.

therapeutic touch A modern interpretation of the laying-on-of-hands for healing, as interpreted by Dolores Krieger, PhD, RN, and Dora Kunz, a noted healer. Originally taught within nursing programs.

thermal shift Drop and subsequent rise in basal body temperature around the time of ovulation.

thermistor probe Automatic sensor used to monitor skin temperature of infant under radiant warmer.

thermogenesis Creation or production of heat, especially in the body.

thermoregulation Control of temperature.

third stage Stage of labor from the birth of the baby to the expulsion of the placenta.

threatened abortion See *abortion, threatened.*

thrombocytopenia Abnormal hematologic condition in which the number of platelets is reduced, usually by destruction of erythroid tissue in bone marrow because of certain neoplastic diseases or an immune response to a drug.

thrombocytopenic purpura Hematologic disorder characterized by prolonged bleeding time, decreased number of platelets, increased cell fragility, and purpura, which result in hemorrhages into the skin, the mucous membranes, the organs, and other tissue.

thromboembolism Obstruction of a blood vessel by a clot that has become detached from its site of formation.

thrombophlebitis Inflammation of a vein with secondary clot formation.

thrombus Blood clot obstructing a blood vessel that remains at the place it was formed.

thrush Fungal infection of the mouth or throat that is characterized by the formation of white patches on a red, moist, inflamed mucous membrane and is caused by *Candida albicans*.

toco- (toko-) Combining form that means childbirth or labor.

tocolysis See *tocolytic therapy*.

tocolytic therapy Medications used to relax the uterus, to suppress preterm labor, or for version.

tocotransducer Electronic device for measuring uterine activity transabdominally.

TORCH infections Infections caused by organisms that damage the embryo or fetus; acronym for *t*oxoplasmosis, *o*ther (e.g., syphilis), *r*ubella, *c*ytomegalovirus, and *h*erpes simplex.

toxicology screen Laboratory analysis of blood or urine to test for alcohol or drug content. Urine drug screening is the most common because it is noninvasive.

toxic shock syndrome A severe acute disease usually caused by *Staphylococcus aureus;* associated with high-absorbency tampon use during menstruation.

tracheoesophageal fistula Congenital malformation in which there is an abnormal tubelike passage between the trachea and esophagus.

traditional Chinese medicine Ancient methods of healing that combine herbs, energy healing, and movement as a pathway to health. Seeks to heal on deeper levels, rather than just treat symptoms.

transformation zone See *squamocolumnar junction*.

transition—labor See *transition phase*.

transition period—newborn Period from birth to 4 to 6 hours later; infant passes through period of reactivity, sleep, and second period of reactivity.

transition phase Phase in first stage of labor from a cervical dilation of 8 to 10 cm.

transition to parenthood Period of time from the preconception parenthood decision through the first months after birth of the baby, during which parents define their parental roles and adjust to parenthood.

translocation Condition in which a chromosome breaks and all or part of that chromosome is transferred to a different part of the same chromosome or to another chromosome.

trial of labor (TOL) Period of observation to determine if a laboring woman is likely to be successful in progressing to a vaginal birth.

Trichomonas vaginitis Inflammation of the vagina caused by *Trichomonas vaginalis,* a parasitic protozoon, and characterized by persistent burning and itching of the vulvar tissue and a profuse, frothy, white discharge.

trimester One of three periods of about 3 months each into which pregnancy is divided.

trisomy Condition whereby any given chromosome exists in triplicate instead of the normal duplicate pattern.

trophoblast Outer layer of cells of the developing blastodermic vesicle that develops the trophoderm or feeding layer, which will establish the nutrient relationships with the uterine endometrium.

trophoblastic disease A condition in which trophoblastic cells covering the chorionic villus proliferate and undergo cystic changes, which may be malignant.

tubal ligation Abdominal procedure in which the uterine tubes are tied off and a section is removed to interrupt tubal continuity and thus sterilize the woman.

tubercles of Montgomery Small papillae on surface of nipples and areolae that secrete a fatty substance that lubricates the nipples.

twins Two neonates from the same impregnation developed within the same uterus at the same time.
  conjoined t. Twins who are physically united; Siamese twins.
  disparate t. Twins who are different (e.g., in weight) and distinct from one another.
  dizygotic t. Twins developed from two separate ova fertilized by two separate sperm at the same time; fraternal twins.
  monozygotic t. Twins developed from a single fertilized ovum; identical twins.

ultrasonography Use of high-frequency sound waves for a variety of obstetric diagnoses and for fetal surveillance.

ultrasound transducer External signal source for monitoring fetal heart rate electronically.

umbilical cord (funis) Structure connecting the placenta and the fetus and containing two arteries and one vein encased in a tissue called Wharton's jelly. The cord is ligated at birth and severed; the stump falls off in 4 to 10 days.

umbilicus Navel, or depressed point in the middle of the abdomen that marks the attachment of the umbilical cord during fetal life.

urethra Small tubular structure that drains urine from the bladder.

urinary frequency Need to void often or at close intervals.

urinary meatus Opening, or mouth, of the urethra.

uterine Referring or pertaining to the uterus.
  u. adnexa See *adnexa, uterine*.
  u. atony Relaxation of uterus; leads to postpartum hemorrhage.
  u. bruit Abnormal sound or murmur heard while auscultating the uterus.
  u. ischemia Decreased blood supply to the uterus.
  u. prolapse Falling, sinking, or sliding of the uterus from its normal location in the body.
  u. souffle See *souffle, uterine*.

uteroplacental insufficiency (UPI) Decline in placental function—exchange of gases, nutrients, and wastes—leading to fetal hypoxia and acidosis; evidenced by late fetal heart rate decelerations in response to uterine contractions.

uterus Hollow muscular organ in the female designed for the implantation, containment, and nourishment of the fetus during its development and expulsion of fetus during labor and birth; also organ of menstruation.

   Couvelaire u. Interstitial myometrial hemorrhage after premature separation (abruption) of placenta. A purplish-bluish discoloration of the uterus and boardlike rigidity of the uterus are noted.

   inversion of u. See *inversion of uterus.*

   retroflexion of u. See *retroflexion of uterus.*

   retroversion of u. See *retroversion of uterus.*

vaccination Intentional injection of antigenic material given to stimulate antibody production in the recipient.

vacuum-assisted birth Birth involving attachment of vacuum cup to fetal head and using negative pressure to assist in birth of the fetus.

vacuum curettage Uterine aspiration method of early abortion.

vagina Normally collapsed musculomembranous tube that forms the passageway between the uterus and the entrance to the vagina (introitus).

vaginal birth after cesarean (VBAC) Giving birth vaginally after having had a previous cesarean birth.

vaginismus Intense, painful spasm of the muscles surrounding the vagina.

Valsalva maneuver Any forced expiratory effort against a closed airway such as holding one's breath and tightening the abdominal muscles (e.g., pushing during the second stage of labor).

variability Normal irregularity of fetal cardiac rhythm; fluctuations in the baseline FHR.

varicocele Enlargement of veins of the spermatic cord.

varicosity (varicose veins) Swollen, distended, and twisted veins that may develop in almost any part of the body but are most commonly seen in the legs, caused by pregnancy, obesity, congenital defective venous valves, and occupations requiring much standing.

vasectomy Ligation or removal of a segment of the vas deferens, usually done bilaterally to produce sterility in the male.

VDRL test Abbreviation for Venereal Disease Research Laboratories test, a serologic flocculation test for syphilis.

vernix caseosa Protective gray-white fatty substance of cheesy consistency covering the fetal skin.

version Act of turning the fetus in the uterus to change the presenting part and facilitate birth.

   external cephalic v. See *external cephalic version.*

   podalic v. Shifting of the fetus's position so as to bring the feet to the outlet during birth.

vertex Crown or top of the head.

   v. presentation Presentation in which the fetal head is nearest the cervical opening and is born first.

very low birth weight (VLBW) Refers to infant weighing 1500 g or less at birth.

viable, viability Capable, capability of living, as in a fetus that has reached a stage of development, usually 22 menstrual weeks (20 weeks of gestation), which will permit it to live outside the uterus.

visceral pain Discomfort from cervical changes and uterine ischemia located over the lower portion of the abdomen and radiating to the lumbar area of the back and down the thighs.

vulva External genitalia of the female that consist of the labia majora, the labia minora, the clitoris, the urinary meatus, and the vaginal introitus.

vulvar self-examination (VSE) Systematic examination of the vulva by the woman.

vulvectomy Surgical removal of all or parts of the vulva.

walking survey Using one's senses while traveling through a community to obtain information about sociocultural characteristics and the environment, housing, transportation, and local community agencies.

warm line A help line, or consultation service, for families; most often accessed for support of newborn care and postpartum care after hospital discharge.

weaning Process of changing from breastfeeding or bottle feeding to drinking from a cup.

Wharton's jelly White, gelatinous material surrounding the umbilical vessels within the cord.

witch's milk Secretion of a whitish fluid for about a week after birth from enlarged mammary tissue in the neonate, presumably resulting from maternal hormonal influences.

withdrawal (1) Physiologic or cognitive changes that occur after removal of the substance in the substance-dependent person; (2) removing the penis from the vagina before ejaculation (coitus interruptus).

womb See *uterus.*

X chromosome Sex chromosome in humans existing in duplicate in the normal female and singly in the normal male.

X linkage Genes located on the X chromosome.

Y chromosome Sex chromosome in the human male necessary for the development of the male gonads.

ZIFT Zygote intrafallopian transfer.

zona pellucida Inner, thick membranous envelope of the ovum.

zygote Cell formed by the union of two reproductive cells or gametes; the fertilized ovum resulting from the union of a sperm and an ovum.

Index

Page numbers followed by f indicate figure(s); t, table(s); b, box(es) and boxed material.

1145